Register Now for Online Access to Your Book!

AF208083

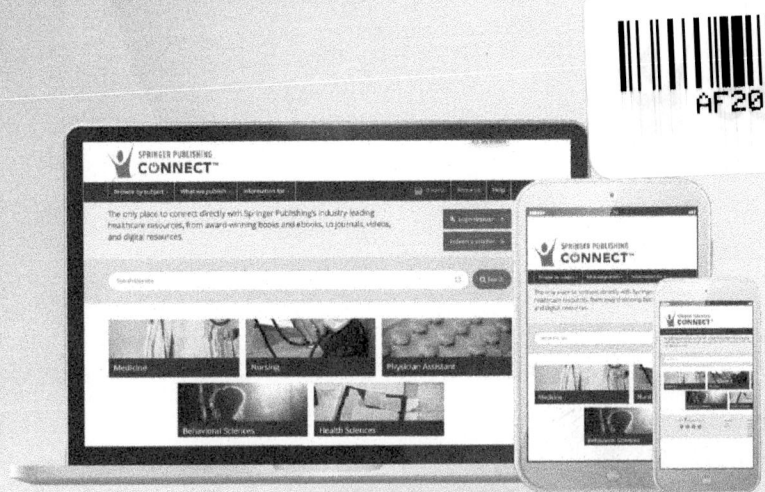

Your print purchase of *The APRN and PA's Complete Guide to Prescribing Drug Therapy 2024,* **includes online access to the contents of your book**—increasing accessibility, portability, and searchability!

Access today at:

http://connect.springerpub.com/content/reference-book/978-0-8261-7935-7
or scan the QR code at the right with your smartphone. Log in or register, then click "Redeem a voucher" and use the code below.

> **MBS3CLJV**

Having trouble redeeming a voucher code?
Go to https://connect.springerpub.com/redeeming-voucher-code

If you are experiencing problems accessing the digital component of this product, please contact our customer service department at cs@springerpub.com

The online access with your print purchase is available at the publisher's discretion and may be removed at any time without notice.

Publisher's Note: New and used products purchased from third-party sellers are not guaranteed for quality, authenticity, or access to any included digital components.

Scan here for quick access.

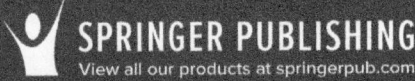

SPRINGER PUBLISHING
View all our products at springerpub.com

The APRN and PA's Complete Guide to
Prescribing Drug Therapy

2024

Mari J. Wirfs, PhD, MN, RN, APRN, ANP-BC, FNP-BC, CNE, NRCME, began her career with an ASN (1968, Dekalb College), and subsequently completed a BSN (1970, Georgia State University), MS (1975, Emory University), Post-Master's Certificates in Primary Care of the Adult (1997) and Family (1997, LSU Health Sciences Center), and PhD in Higher Education Administration and Leadership (1991, University of New Orleans). She is a nationally certified Adult Nurse Practitioner (1997, American Nurses Credentialing Center), Family Nurse Practitioner (1998, American Academy of Nurse Practitioners), and Certified Nurse Educator (2008, National League for Nursing). Her career spans 50+ years inclusive of collegiate undergraduate and graduate nursing education and clinical practice in critical care, pediatrics, psychiatric–mental health nursing, and advanced practice primary care nursing. During her academic career, she has achieved the rank of professor with tenure in two university systems.

Dr. Wirfs was a founding member of the medical staff in the establishment of Baptist Community Health Services, a community-based non-profit primary care clinic founded post-Hurricane Katrina in the New Orleans Lower Ninth Ward. From 2002 to 2022, Dr. Wirfs served as clinical director and primary care provider at the Family Health Care Clinic, serving faculty, staff, students, and their families at New Orleans Baptist Theological Seminary (NOBTS). During that time, she also served as adjunct graduate faculty, teaching neuropsychology and psychopharmacology, in the NOBTS Guidance and Counseling program. She is a long-time member of the National Organization of Nurse Practitioner Faculties (NONPF), Sigma Theta Tau International Honor Society of Nursing, and several other academic honor societies.

During her career, Dr. Wirfs has completed, published, and presented six quantitative research studies focusing on academic leadership, nursing education, and clinical practice issues, including one for the Army Medical Department conducted during her 8-year reserve service in the U.S. Army Nurse Corps. Her publications include co-authored family primary care certification review books and study materials. Her first prescribing guide, *Clinical Guide to Pharmacotherapeutics for the Primary Care Provider,* was published by Advanced Practice Education Associates (APEA) from 1999 to 2014. Other reference books published by Dr. Wirfs have included *The APRN's Complete Guide to Prescribing Drug Therapy* (2016–2021), *The APRN's Complete Guide to Prescribing Pediatric Drug Therapy* (2017), and *The PA's Complete Guide to Prescribing Drug Therapy* (2017), published by Springer Publishing Company. *The APRN's Complete Guide to Prescribing Pediatric Drug Therapy 2018* was awarded second place, **Book of the Year 2017** in the Child Health Category, by the *American Journal of Nursing (AJN),* the official publication of the **American Nurses Association (ANA).** The panel of judges included the co-founder of the nurse practitioner role and first nurse practitioner program, Dr. Loretta C. Ford, Professor Emerita.

Dr. Wirfs entered semi-retirement in 2022, working as a floating PRN Family Nurse Practitioner for Concentra Occupational Health and Urgent Care sites in the metropolitan New Orleans area. She retired from clinical APRN practice in July, 2023. In her retirement, she continues to update and expand *The APRN and PA's Complete Guide to Prescribing Drug Therapy* (launched in 2022 by Springer Publishing Company).

The APRN and PA's Complete Guide to Prescribing Drug Therapy

2024

Mari J. Wirfs, PhD, MN, RN, APRN, ANP-BC, FNP-BC, CNE, NRCME

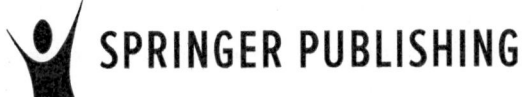 SPRINGER PUBLISHING

Springer Publishing Company, LLC
www.springerpub.com

Acquisitions Editor: John Zaphyr
Composition: Exeter Premedia Services Private Ltd.

ISBN: 978-0-8261-4206-1
e-book ISBN: 978-0-8261-4207-8
DOI: 10.1891/9780826142078

23 24 25 26 / 5 4 3 2 1

This book is a reference guide for healthcare providers. The information has been extrapolated from a variety of professional sources and is presented in condensed and summary form. It is not intended to replace or substitute for complete and current manufacturer prescribing information, current research, or knowledge and experience of the user. For complete prescribing information, including toxicities, drug interactions, contraindications, warnings, and precautions, the reader is referred to the manufacturer's package insert and the published literature. The inclusion of a particular brand name neither implies nor suggests that the author or publisher advises or recommends the use of that particular product or considers it superior to similar products available by other brand names. Neither the author nor the publisher makes any warranty, expressed or implied, with respect to the information, including any errors or omissions, herein.

Library of Congress Cataloging-in-Publication Data
Names: Wirfs, Mari J., author.
Title: The APRN and PA's complete guide to prescribing drug therapy 2024 / Mari J.
  Wirfs.
Description: New York, NY: Springer Publishing Company, LLC, [2024] |
  Includes bibliographical references and index.
Identifiers: LCCN 2017008900| ISBN 9780826142061 | ISBN 9780826142078 (ebook)
Subjects: | MESH: Drug Therapy—nursing | Advanced Practice Nursing—methods
  | Handbooks
Classification: LCC RM301 | NLM WY 49 | DDC 615.1—dc23
LC record available at https://lccn.loc.gov/2017008900

Contact us to receive discount rates on bulk purchases.
For more information please contact: sales@springerpub.com

Publisher's Note: New and used products purchased from third-party sellers are not guaranteed for quality, authenticity, or access to any included digital components.

Printed in the United States of America.

CONTENTS

Reviewers   *xv*
Preface and Acknowledgments   *xvii*
Quick Check Prescribing Reminders   *xviii*

SECTION I: DRUG THERAPY BY CLINICAL DIAGNOSIS

3-Day Fever (Roseola Infantum)   *557*
Acetaminophen Overdose   *1*
Achondroplasia   *1*
Acne Rosacea   *2*
Acne Vulgaris   *3*
Acromegaly   *7*
Actinic Keratosis (AK)   *8*
Acute Bacterial Skin and Skin Structure Infection (ABSSSI)   *142*
Acute Exacerbation of Chronic Bronchitis (AECB)   *68*
Acute Urinary Tract Infection (UTI)   *641*
Adrenocortical Insufficiency   *9*
African Sleeping Sickness (*Human African Trypanosomiasis* [HAT])   *10*
Agammaglobulinemia, Congenital or X-linked (see Immunodeficiency: Primary, Humoral, PHI)   *348*
Alcohol Dependence   *11*
Alcohol Withdrawal Syndrome   *11*
Allergic Reaction: General   *12*
Allergic Rhinitis   *549*
Allergic Sinusitis   *549*
Allergies: Multi-Food   *12*
Allergy: Peanut (*Arachis hypogaea*)   *474*
Alopecia Areata   *12*
Alpha-1 Antitrypsin (AAT) Deficiency   *13*
Alzheimer's Disease (AD)   *13*
Amebiasis   *17*
Amebic Dysentery (*see* Amebiasis)   *17*
Amebic Liver Abscess   *17*
Amenorrhea: Secondary   *17*
American Trypanosomiasis (*see* Chagas Disease)   *146*
Amyotrophic Lateral Sclerosis (ALS, Lou Gehrig's Disease)   *18*
Anaphylaxis   *21*
Anemia: Beta Thalassemia-Associated   *21*
Anemia of Chronic Kidney Disease (CKD)   *22*
Anemia of Chronic Renal Failure (CRF)   *22*
Anemia: Folic Acid Deficiency   *24*
Anemia: Hemolytic   *24*
Anemia: Iron Deficiency   *25*
Anemia: Megaloblastic/Pernicious   *26*
Anemia: Pernicious   *26*
Anesthesia: Procedural Sedation   *26*

Angina Pectoris: Stable   *28*
Angioedema, Hereditary (HAE)   *296*
Angiofibroma, Facial, Associated with Tuberous Sclerosis   *27*
Ankylosing Spondylitis (*see* Osteoarthritis)   *434*
Anorexia/Cachexia   *30*
Anthrax (*Bacillus anthracis*)   *31*
Anxiety Disorder: Generalized (GAD)   *32*
Anxiety Disorder: Social (SAD)   *32*
Aphasia, Expressive: Stroke-induced   *36*
Aphthous Stomatitis (Mouth Ulcer, Canker Sore)   *37*
Arterial Insufficiency   *482*
Arthritis: Gouty   *261*
Ascariasis   *557*
Aphthous Stomatitis (Mouth Ulcer, Canker Sore)   *37*
Aspergillosis (*Scedosporium apiospermum, Fusarium* spp.)   *38*
Asthma   *38*
Asthma-COPD Overlap Syndrome (ACOS)   *46*
Asthma: Severe, Eosinophilia   *47*
Athlete's Foot   *599*
Atonic Bladder   *353*
Atrophic Vaginitis   *49*
Attention Deficit Hyperactivity Disorder (ADHD)   *50*
Atypical Hemolytic Uremic Syndrome (aHUS)   *284*
Bacterial Endocarditis: Prophylaxis   *55*
Bacterial Vaginosis (BV, *Gardnerella Vaginalis*)   *56*
Baldness: Male Pattern   *57*
Bartonella Infection (Cat Scratch Fever)   *141*
Basal Cell Carcinoma (BCC)   *76*
Bell's Palsy   *57*
Benign Essential Tremor   *58*
Benign Prostatic Hyperplasia (BPH)   *58*
Beta Thalassemia   *59*
Bile Acid Deficiency   *60*
Binge Eating Disorder   *60*
Bipolar Disorder   *60*
Bite: Cat   *65*
Bite: Dog   *65*
Bite: Human   *66*
Bladder Cancer   *77*
Blastomycosis   *38*
Blepharitis   *67*
Blepharoconjunctivitis: Bacterial   *161*
Blepharoptosis, Acquired (Droopy Eyelid)   *67*
Bloating (*see* Flatulence)   *245*
Boil (*see* Skin Infection: Bacterial)   *573*
Bordetella (Pertussis)   *482*

Bowel Resection With Primary Anastomosis   68
Breast Abscess (see Mastitis)   387
Breast Cancer   78
Bronchiolitis   68
Bronchitis: Acute (AECB, Acute Exacerbation of Chronic Bronchitis)   68
Bronchitis: Chronic (COPD, Chronic Obstructive Pulmonary Disease)   71
Bulimia Nervosa   75
Burn: Major   75
Burn: Minor   76
Bursitis   76
C1 Esterase Inhibitor Deficiency   296
Cachexia   30
Calcium Deficiency   339
Callused Skin   572
Cancer: Basal Cell Carcinoma (BCC)   76
Cancer: Bladder, Urothelial   77
Cancer: Breast   78
Cancer: Cervical   86
Cancer: Colorectal   86
Cancer: Endometrial   87
Cancer: Epithelial, Epithelioid Sarcoma   88
Cancer: Esophageal   90
Cancer: Fallopian Tube   88
Cancer: Gastric   90
Cancer: Gastroesophageal   90
Cancer: Gastrointestinal Stromal Tumor   91
Cancer: Glioblastoma Multiforme   92
Cancer: Hepatocellular Carcinoma (HCC) (see Cancer: Liver)   99
Cancer: Kidney   93
Cancer: Leukemia   96
Cancer: Liver   99
Cancer: Lung   102
Cancer: Lymphoma   108
Cancer: Melanoma   116
Cancer: Merkel Cell Carcinoma (MCC)   119
Cancer: Multiple Myeloma   120
Cancer: Ovarian   122
Cancer: Pancreatic   124
Cancer: Peritoneal   125
Cancer: Prostate   127
Cancer: Renal Cell Carcinoma (RCC)   93
Cancer: Squamous Cell Carcinoma (SCC)   130
Cancer: Thyroid   131
Cancer: Tumor, Solid   132
Cancer: Urothelial Carcinoma (UC)   133
Candidiasis: Abdomen, Bladder, Esophagus, Kidney   134
Candidiasis: Oral (Thrush)   134
Candidiasis: Skin   135
Candidiasis: Vulvovaginal (Moniliasis)   136
Canker Sore (see Aphthous Stomatitis)   37
Cannabinoid Hyperemesis Syndrome (CHS)   138
Carbuncle (see Skin Infection: Bacterial)   573
Carcinoid Syndrome Diarrhea (CSD)   140
Cardiomyopathy of Transthyretin-Mediated Amyloidosis   140
Carpal Tunnel Syndrome (CTS)   140
Cataplexy   409

Cat Bite   65
Cat Scratch Fever (Bartonella Infection)   141
Cellulite   141
Cellulitis   142
Cerumen Impaction   145
Cervical Cancer   86
Chagas Disease (American Trypanosomiasis)   146
Chalazion: Inflamed Meibomian Cyst, (see Stye)   580
Chancroid   146
Chemotherapy-Induced Nausea/Vomiting (CINV)   147
Chest Wall Syndrome (Costochondritis)   171
Chickenpox (Varicella)   149
Chikungunya Virus   150
Chikungunya-Related Arthritis   150
Chlamydia trachomatis   150
Chloasma   387
Cholangitis, Primary Biliary (PBC)   152
Cholelithiasis   153
Cholera (Vibrio cholerae)   154
Cholestasis   154
Christmas Disease   285
Chronic Idiopathic Constipation (CIC)   168
Chronic Obstructive Pulmonary Disease (COPD)   71
Chronic Renal Failure (CRF)   22
Churg-Strauss Syndrome (see Eosinophilic Granulomatosis With Polyangiitis [EGWPA])   235
Clostridioides difficile Infection (CDI)   156
Clostridium tetani (Tetanus)   591
Cluster Headache   270
Cluster Seizures   566
Cold Agglutinin Disease (CAD)   159
Cold Sore   300
Colic: Infantile   159
Colitis   519
Colon Cleanse   160
Colonoscopy Prep   160
Common Cold (URI, Viral Upper Respiratory Infection)   160
Community-Acquired Pneumonia (CAP)   492
Complicated Intra-Abdominal Infection (cIAI)   363
Complicated Urinary Tract Infection (cUTI)   640
Condyloma Acuminata (Venereal Wart)   655
Conjunctivitis: Allergic (Vernal)   165
Conjunctivitis/Blepharoconjunctivitis: Bacterial   161
Conjunctivitis: Chlamydial   164
Conjunctivitis: Fungal   165
Conjunctivitis: Gonococcal   165
Conjunctivitis: Viral   168
Constipation: Chronic Idiopathic (CIC)   168
Constipation: Occasional, Intermittent   169
Constipation: Opioid-Induced (OIC)   428
COPD (see Bronchitis: Chronic or Emphysema)   71
Corneal Edema   171
Corneal Ulceration   171
Coronavirus (COVID-19)   171
Costochondritis (Chest Wall Syndrome)   171

COVID-19 (*Coronavirus*)   *171*
Coxsackievirus (Hand, Foot, and Mouth
  Disease)   *268*
Cradle Cap (*see* Dermatitis: Seborrheic)   *204*
Cramps: Abdominal, Intestinal   *174*
Crohn's Disease   *175*
Cryptosporidiosis (*Cryptosporidium parvum*)   *179*
Cryptosporidium parvum (Cryptosporidiosis)   *179*
Cushing's Syndrome   *179*
Cutaneous Larvae Migrans (Hookworm)   *304*
Cutaneous T-Cell Lymphoma (*see* Cancer:
  Lymphoma)   *108*
Cyclospora cayetanensis (Cyclosporiasis)   *182*
Cyclosporiasis (*Cyclospora cayetanensis*)   *179*
Cystic Fibrosis (CF)   *182*
Cystinuria   *184*
Cystitis (UTI, Urinary Tract Infection)   *640*
Cytomegalovirus (CMV), CMV Retinitis   *186*
Cytomegalovirus (CMV): Posttransplant   *185*
Dandruff (*see* Dermatitis: Seborrheic)   *204*
Decubitus Ulcer   *633*
Deep Vein Thrombosis (DVT) Prophylaxis   *187*
Dehydration   *187*
Delirium: End-of-Life   *187*
Delirium Tremens   *187*
Dementia   *188*
Dengue Fever (Dengue Virus)   *189*
Dental Abscess   *190*
Dental Procedure Prophylaxis (*see* Bacterial
  Endocarditis: Prophylaxis)   *55*
Denture Irritation   *191*
Depression, Major Depressive Disorder (MDD)   *191*
Depression: Postpartum   *196*
Depression: Treatment-Resistant (TRD)   *196*
Dermatitis: Atopic (Eczema)   *197*
Dermatitis: Contact   *201*
Dermatitis: Diaper (*see* Diaper Rash)   *208*
Dermatitis: Genus *Rhus* (Poison Oak, Poison Ivy, Poison
  Sumac)   *203*
Dermatitis: Seborrheic   *204*
Dermatomyositis   *502*
Diabetes Mellitus, Type 1 (T1DM)   *613*
Diabetes Mellitus, Type 2 (T2DM)   *619*
Diabetic Macular Edema   *206*
Diabetic Neuropathic Pain   *480*
Diabetic Peripheral Neuropathy (DPN)   *208*
Diabetic Retinopathy   *206*
Diaper Rash   *210*
Diarrhea: Acute   *211*
Diarrhea: Carcinoid Syndrome (CSD)   *212*
Diarrhea: Chronic   *213*
Diarrhea: Traveler's   *213*
Digitalis Toxicity   *214*
Diphtheria (*Corynebacterium diphtheriae*)   *214*
Distributive Shock   *568*
Diverticulitis   *215*
Diverticulosis   *216*
Dog Bite   *65*
Donovanosis (Granuloma Inguinale)   *265*
Dravet Syndrome   *377*
Drooling   *216*

Droopy Eyelid (Blepharoptosis, Acquired)   *67*
Dry Eye Disease/Syndrome (Keratoconjunctivitis
  [Sicca])   *216*
Dry Mouth Syndrome   *572*
Duchenne Muscular Dystrophy (DMD)   *218*
Dust Mite Allergy   *219*
Dysentery (*see* Amebiasis)   *17*
Dysfunctional Uterine Bleeding (DUB)   *220*
Dyshidrosis   *220*
Dyshidrotic Eczema (Dyshidrosis, Pompholyx)   *220*
Dyslipidemia (Hypercholesterolemia, Hyperlipidemia,
  Mixed Dyslipidemia)   *220*
Dysmenorrhea: Primary   *225*
Dyspareunia (Postmenopausal Painful
  Intercourse)   *226*
Dyspepsia/Gastritis   *247*
Eating Disorder: Anorexia Nervosa   *60*
Eating Disorder: Binge   *60*
Eating Disorder: Bulimia Nervosa   *75*
Ebola Zaire Disease (*Zaire ebolavirus*)   *226*
Eczema (Atopic Dermatitis)   *197*
Edema   *228*
Emphysema   *230*
Encopresis   *232*
End-of-Life Delirium   *187*
Endometrial Cancer   *87*
Endometriosis   *232*
Enteritis   *516*
Enterobius vermicularis (*see* Pinworm)   *488*
Enuresis: Primary, Nocturnal   *235*
Eosinophilic Granulomatosis With Polyangiitis (EGPA,
  formerly Churg-Strauss Syndrome)   *235*
Epicondylitis   *236*
Epididymitis   *236*
Epithelioid Sarcoma   *88*
Epstein-Barr Virus (EBV; *see* Mononucleosis)   *396*
Erectile Dysfunction (ED)   *237*
Erosive Esophagitis   *238*
Erysipelas   *238*
Erythema Chronicum Migrans (Lyme Disease)   *382*
Erythema Infectiosum (Fifth Disease)   *245*
Erythropoietic Protoporphyria (EPP)   *238*
Esophageal Cancer   *90*
Esophagitis, Erosive   *238*
Exanthem Subitum (Roseola Infantum)   *557*
Excessive Daytime Sleepiness   *409*
Exocrine Pancreas Insufficiency (EPI)   *238*
Extrapyramidal Side Effects (EPS)   *238*
Eyelashes, Thin/Sparse (Hypotrichosis)   *347*
Eye Pain   *241*
Facial Hair: Excessive/Unwanted   *241*
Fascioliasis (Fasciola gigantica, Fasciola
  hepatica)   *379*
Fecal Odor   *241*
Fever (Pyrexia)   *241*
Fever Blister   *300*
Fibrocystic Breast Disease   *243*
Fibroid Tumor (Uterine Leiomyomata)   *650*
Fibromyalgia   *244*
Fifth Disease (Erythema Infectiosum)   *245*
Flatulence   *245*

Flu   356
Fluoridation, Water, <0.6 PPM   246
Folic Acid Deficiency (Anemia)   24
Folliculitis   246
Folliculitis Barbae   246
Foreign Body: Esophagus   247
Foreign Body: Eye   247
Furuncle   573
Gardnerella vaginalis (BV, Bacterial Vaginosis)   56
Gastritis/Dyspepsia   247
Gastritis-Related Nausea/Vomiting   247
Gastroesophageal Reflux (GER)   248
Gastroesophageal Reflux Disease (GERD)   248
Gastrointestinal Stromal Tumor (GIST)   91
Gaucher Disease, Type 1   251
Generalized Anxiety Disorder (GAD)   32
Genital Herpes (see Herpes Genitalis, HSV Type II)   299
Genital Warts   655
German Measles (Rubella)   558
Giant Cell Arteritis (GCA)/Temporal Arteritis   253
Giardiasis (Giardia lamblia)   254
Gingivitis/Periodontitis   254
Glaucoma: Open-Angle   255
Glioblastoma Multiforme   92
Golfer's Elbow (see Epicondylitis)   236
Gonococcal Pharyngitis   483
Gonorrhea (Neisseria gonorrhoeae)   258
Gout   259
Gouty Arthritis   261
Graft Versus Host Disease (GVHD)   263
Granuloma Inguinale (Donovanosis)   265
Granulomatosis, Wegener's Granulomatosis   265
Grave's Eye Disease   596
Growth Failure   266
Growth Hormone Deficiency (GHD)   267
Haemophilus influenzae b (Hib)   268
Hair Loss (see Baldness: Male Pattern)   57
Hand, Foot, and Mouth Disease (Coxsackievirus)   268
Hansen's Disease   269
Headache: Cluster   270
Headache: Migraine   270
Headache: Tension (Muscle Contraction Headache)   277
Headache: Vascular   270
Heartburn (see GER/GERD)   248
Heart Failure (HF)   278
Helicobacter pylori (H. pylori) Infection   283
Hemolytic Anemia   24
Hemolytic Uremia Syndrome: Atypical (aHUS)   284
Hemophagocytic Lymphohistiocytosis (HLH)   285
Hemophilia A (Congenital Factor VIII Deficiency)   285
Hemophilia B   285
Hemorrhoids   289
Hepatic Porphyria, Acute (AHP)   291
Hepatitis A (HAV)   291
Hepatitis B (HBV)   292
Hepatitis C (HCV)   294
Hepatocellular Carcinoma (HCC) (see Cancer: Liver)   99
Hereditary Angioedema (HAE)   296
Herpangina   298
Herpes Facialis (HSV Type I)   300
Herpes Genitalis (HSV Type II)   299
Herpes Labialis (HSV Type I)   300
Herpes Simplex Virus Type I (HSV I, Herpes Facialis/Labialis)   300
Herpes Simplex Virus Type II (HSV II, Genital Herpes)   299
Herpes Zoster (HZ, Shingles)   301
Herpes Zoster Ophthalmicus (HZO)   302
Herpetic Dendritic   302
Hib (see Haemophilus influenzae b)   268
Hiccups: Intractable   303
Hidradenitis Suppurativa   303
Histoplasmosis   38
Hives (Urticaria)   648
Homocystinuria   304
Hookworm (Uncinariasis, Cutaneous Larvae Migrans)   304
Hordeolum (see Stye)   580
Hospital-Acquired Bacterial Pneumonia (HABP)   489
Human Bite   66
Human Immunodeficiency Virus (HIV) Infection   305
Human Immunodeficiency Virus (HIV): Non-Occupational Post-Exposure Prophylaxis (nPEP)   305
Human Immunodeficiency Virus (HIV): Occupational Post-Exposure Prophylaxis (oPEP)   305
Human Immunodeficiency Virus (HIV): Pre-Exposure Prophylaxis (PrEP)   305
Human Papillomavirus (HPV, Venereal Wart)   317
Huntington Disease-Associated Chorea   318
Hyperammonemia   318
Hypercalcemia   319
Hypercholesterolemia   220
Hyperemesis Gravidarum   319
Hypereosinophilia Syndrome (HES)   47
Hyperhidrosis (Perspiration, Excessive)   320
Hyperhomocysteinemia   321
Hyperkalemia   322
Hyperlipidemia   220
Hyperparathyroidism (HPT)   323
Hyperphosphatemia   324
Hyperpigmentation   325
Hyperprolactinemia   326
Hypertension: Primary, Essential   326
Hyperthyroidism   337
Hypertriglyceridemia   338
Hyperuricemia   259
Hypoactive Sexual Desire Disorder (HSDD, Low Libido)   380
Hypocalcemia   339
Hypoglycemia: Acute   341
Hypogonadism   588
Hypokalemia   343
Hypomagnesemia   344

Hypoparathyroidism   344
Hypophosphatasia (Osteomalacia, Rickets)   345
Hypophosphatemia, X-Linked (XLH)   345
Hypopnea Syndrome   575
Hypotension: Neurogenic, Orthostatic   345
Hypotestosteronemia   588
Hypothyroidism   346
Hypotrichosis (Thin/Sparse Eyelashes)   347
Idiopathic Gastric Acid Hypersecretion
    (IGAH)   248
Idiopathic (Immune) Thrombocytopenia Purpura
    (ITP)   347
Idiopathic Peripheral Neuritis   368
Idiopathic Pulmonary Fibrosis (IPF)   534
Immunodeficiencies, Severe, Combined (see
    Immunodeficiency: Primary Humoral,
    PHI)   348
Immunodeficiency, Common Variable (see
    Immunodeficiency: Primary Humoral,
    PHI)   348
Immunodeficiency: Primary Humoral (PHI)   348
Immunoglobulin A Nephropathy, Primary
    (IGAN)   414
Impetigo Contagiosa (Indian Fire)   351
Impotence (see ED, Erectile Dysfunction)   237
Incontinence: Fecal   353
Incontinence: Urinary Overactive Bladder   353
Incontinence: Urinary Overflow, Atonic
    Bladder   353
Incontinence: Urinary Stress   353
Incontinence: Urinary Urge   353
Indian Fire (Impetigo Contagiosa)   351
Infectious Mononucleosis   396
Influenza, Seasonal (Flu)   356
Insect Bite/Sting   358
Insomnia   359
Intermittent Claudication (PAD, Peripheral Artery
    Disease)   482
Interstitial Cystitis   361
Intertrigo   362
Intra-Abdominal Infection: Complicated (cIAI)   363
Iritis: Acute   364
Iron Deficiency (Anemia)   25
Iron Overload   364
Irritable Bowel Syndrome With Constipation
    (IBS-C)   365
Irritable Bowel Syndrome With Diarrhea
    (IBS-D)   366
Japanese Encephalitis Virus (JEV)   368
Jock Itch (Tinea Cruris)   598
Juvenile Idiopathic Arthritis (JIA)   368
Juvenile Rheumatoid Arthritis (JRA)   371
Keratitis   371
Keratitis: Allergic (Vernal)   374
Keratitis: Neurotrophic   374
Keratitis/Keratoconjunctivitis: Herpes Simplex   374
Keratitis/Keratoconjunctivitis: Vernal   375
Keratoconjunctivitis: Allergic (Vernal)   165
Keratoconjunctivitis (Sicca)   216
Kidney Cancer   93

Kidney Stones   646
Labyrinthitis   375
Lactose Intolerance   375
Lambert-Eaton Myasthenic Syndrome (LEMS)   375
Larva Migrans: Cutaneous   376
Larva Migrans: Visceral   376
Lead Encephalopathy   376
Lead Poisoning   376
Lead Toxicity   376
Leg Cramps: Nocturnal, Recumbency   376
Leishmaniasis: Cutaneous   376
Leishmaniasis: Mucosal   376
Leishmaniasis: Visceral   376
Lennox-Gastaut Syndrome (LGS)   377
Lentigines: Benign, Senile   379
Leprosy   269
Leukemia   96
Lice (see Pediculosis)   475
Listeria monocytogenes (Listeriosis)   379
Listeriosis (Listeria monocytogenes)   379
Liver Cancer   99
Liver Flukes   379
Lou Gehrig's Disease (ALS, Amyotrophic Lateral
    Sclerosis)   18
Low Back Strain (LBS)   380
Low Libido (see HSDD, Hypoactive Sexual Desire
    Disorder)   380
Lung Cancer   102
Lupus Nephritis   382
Lyme Disease (Erythema Chronicum Migrans)   382
Lymphadenitis   383
Lymphogranuloma Venereum   383
Macular Degeneration   206
Macular Edema   206
Macular Edema: Diabetic   206
Magnesium Deficiency   344
Major Depressive Disorder (MDD)   191
Malaria (Plasmodium falciparum, Plasmodium
    vivax)   384
Mastitis (Breast Abscess)   387
Megaloblastic Anemia (Vitamin B$_{12}$ Deficiency)   26
Melanoma   116
Melasma/Chloasma   387
Ménière's Disease   388
Meningitis (Neisseria meningitidis)   388
Menometrorrhagia: Irregular Heavy Menstrual
    Bleeding   389
Menopause   390
Menorrhagia: Heavy Cyclical Menstrual
    Bleeding   389
Merkel Cell Carcinoma   119
Mesothelioma   393
Metastatic High-Risk Castration-Sensitive Prostate
    Cancer (CSPC)   516
Methamphetamine-Induced Psychosis   394
Migraine Headache   270
Mitral Valve Prolapse (MVP)   396
Moniliasis (Vulvovaginal Candidiasis)   136
Mononucleosis (Mono)   396
Motion Sickness   396

Mouth Ulcer (Aphthous Stomatitis)   *37*
Multi-Food Allergies   *12*
Multiple Myeloma   *120*
Multiple Sclerosis (MS)   *397*
Mumps (Infectious Parotitis, *Paramyxovirus*)   *403*
Muscle Contraction Headache (Tension
    Headache)   *277*
Muscle Strain   *403*
Myasthenia Gravis (MG)   *406*
Mycobacterium leprae   *269*
Mycobacterium tuberculosis (TB)   *609*
Mycoplasma Pneumonia   *496*
Myelodysplastic Syndromes (MDS)   *407*
Myelofibrosis   *408*
Myositis (*see* Polymyositis)   *502*
Narcolepsy   *409*
Narcotic Dependence (*see* Opioid Dependence)   *423*
Nausea/Vomiting: Chemotherapy-Induced
    (CINV)   *413*
Nausea/Vomiting of Pregnancy   *319*
Nausea/Vomiting: Opioid-Induced   *429*
Nausea/Vomiting: Post-Anesthesia (PONV)   *414*
Neisseria meningitidis (Meningitis)   *388*
Nephropathy: Primary, Immunoglobulin A   *414*
Nerve Agent Poisoning   *415*
Neurogenic Detrusor Overactivity (NDO)   *415*
Neurogenic, Hypotension   *345*
Neuromyelitis Optica Spectrum Disorder
    (NMOSD)   *416*
Neuropathic Pain: Generalized   *480*
Neuropathic Pain: Peripheral   *480*
Neurotrophic Keratitis   *374*
Neutropenia   *416*
Neutropenia: Chemotherapy-Associated   *416*
Neutropenia: Febrile   *416*
Neutropenia: Myelosuppression-Associated   *416*
Nicotine Withdrawal Syndrome   *602*
Nocturnal Enuresis (Primary Enuresis)   *235*
Nocturnal Polyuria   *506*
Non-24 Sleep-Wake Disorder   *418*
Non-Hodgkin's Lymphoma (see Cancer:
    Lymphoma)   *108*
nPrEP (Non-Occupational HIV Pre-Exposure
    Prophylaxis)   *305*
Obesity   *418*
Obsessive-Compulsive Disorder (OCD)   *421*
Obstructive Sleep Apnea (OSA)   *575*
Ocular Hypertension   *255*
Odor: Fecal   *241*
Onychomycosis (Fungal Nail)   *422*
Ophthalmia Neonatorum: Chlamydial   *423*
Ophthalmia Neonatorum: Gonococcal   *423*
Opioid Dependence   *423*
Opioid-Induced Constipation (OIC)   *428*
Opioid-Induced Nausea/Vomiting (OINV)   *429*
Opioid Overdose/Opioid Reversal   *430*
Opioid Use Disorder (OUD)   *423*
Opioid Withdrawal Syndrome   *423*
Organ Transplant Rejection Prophylaxis
    (OTRP)   *431*
Orthostatic Hypotension   *345*

Osgood-Schlatter Disease   *433*
Osteoarthritis   *434*
Osteomalacia (Hypophosphatasia, Rickets)   *345*
Osteoporosis   *439*
Osteoporosis Prophylaxis (*see* Osteoporosis)   *439*
Otitis Externa   *444*
Otitis Media: Acute   *445*
Otitis Media: Serous (SOM)   *448*
Otitis Media With Effusion (OME)   *448*
Overactive Bladder   *353*
Overdose: Opioid   *430*
Overflow Urinary Incontinence   *353*
Ovulation Induction   *448*
Paget's Disease: Bone   *449*
Pain   *450*
Painful Intercourse (Postmenopausal
    Dyspareunia)   *226*
Pancreatic Enzyme Deficiency   *238*
Pancreatic Enzyme Insufficiency   *462*
Panic Disorder   *464*
Parathyroid Hormone Deficiency   *344*
Parkinsonism (*see also* Parkinson's Disease)   *466*
Parkinsonism: Carbonmonoxide Intoxication   *472*
Parkinsonism: Manganese Intoxication   *472*
Parkinsonism: Postencephalitic   *472*
Parkinson's Disease (PD)   *466*
Paronychia (Periungual Abscess)   *472*
Parotitis: Infectious (Mumps)   *403*
Paroxysmal Nocturnal Hemoglobinuria (PNH)   *472*
Peanut Allergy (*Arachis hypogaea*)   *474*
Pediculosis Humanus Capitis (Head Lice)   *475*
Pediculosis Phthirus (Pubic Lice)   *475*
Pelvic Inflammatory Disease (PID)   *476*
Pemphigus Foliaceus (PF)   *476*
Pemphigus Vulgaris (PV)   *476*
Peptic Ulcer Disease (PUD)   *477*
Periodontitis   *254*
Peripheral Artery Disease (PAD)   *462*
Peripheral Neuritis: Diabetic   *480*
Peripheral Neuritis: Idiopathic   *480*
Peripheral Neuropathic Pain   *480*
Peripheral Vascular Disease (PVD)   *482*
Peritoneal Cancer   *125*
Periungual Abscess (Paronychia)   *472*
Perleche (Angular Stomatitis)   *482*
Pernicious Anemia (Vitamin B_{12} Deficiency)   *26*
Perspiration: Excessive (Hyperhidrosis)   *320*
Pertussis (Whooping Cough)   *482*
Pharyngitis: Gonococcal   *483*
Pharyngitis: Streptococcal (Strep Throat)   *484*
Phenylketonuria (PKU)   *485*
Pheochromocytoma   *486*
Pheochromocytoma: Unresectable, Locally Advanced,
    or Metastatic   *487*
Phthirus (Pubic Lice)   *475*
Pinworm (*Enterobius vermicularis*)   *488*
Pityriasis Alba   *488*
Pityriasis Rosea   *488*
Plague (*Yersinia pestis*)   *489*
Plantar Wart (Verruca Plantaris)   *655*
Plaque Psoriasis   *519*

Pneumococcal Pneumonia   *497*

Pneumocystis jirovecii (Pneumonia)   *498*

Pneumonia: Bacterial, Hospital-Acquired (HABP)   *489*

Pneumonia: Bacterial, Ventilator-Associated (VABP)   *490*

Pneumonia: Chlamydial   *492*

Pneumonia: Community-Acquired (CAP)   *492*

Pneumonia: Community-Acquired Bacterial (CABP)   *492*

Pneumonia: Legionella   *496*

Pneumonia: Mycoplasma   *496*

Pneumonia: Pneumococcal   *497*

Pneumonia: *Pneumocystis jirovecii*   *498*

Poliomyelitis (*Poliovirus*)   *498*

Poliovirus (Poliomyelitis)   *498*

Polyangiitis   *499*

Polyarticular Juvenile Idiopathic Arthritis (PJIA)   *368*

Polycystic Kidney Disease, Autosomal Dominant (ADPKD)   *500*

Polycystic Ovarian Syndrome (PCOS, Stein-Leventhal Disease)   *500*

Polycythemia Vera   *500*

Polymyalgia Rheumatica   *501*

Polymyositis   *502*

Polyneuropathy, Chronic Inflammatory Demyelinating Polymyositis (CIDP)   *503*

Polyps: Nasal   *505*

Polyuria: Nocturnal   *506*

Pompholyx (Dyshidrosis, Dyshidrotic Eczema)   *220*

Postanesthesia Nausea/Vomiting   *414*

Postherpetic Neuralgia (PHN)   *507*

Postmenopausal Dyspareunia   *226*

Postpartum Depression   *196*

Posttramatic Stress Disorder (PTSD)   *510*

Posttransplant Cytomegalovirus (CMV)   *185*

Potassium Deficiency   *343*

Potassium Excess   *322*

Precedes Merkel Cell Carcinoma (MCC)   *119*

Precocious Puberty, Central (CPP)   *512*

Pregnancy   *514*

Premenstrual Dysphoric Disorder (PMDD)   *514*

PrEP (HIV Pre-Exposure Prophylaxis)   *305*

Presbyopia   *515*

Pressure Sore (Decubitus Ulcer)   *633*

Primary Biliary Cholangitis (PBC)   *152*

Primary Humoral Immunodeficiency (PHI)   *348*

Primary Immunoglobulin A Nephropathy (IGAN)   *414*

Proctitis: Acute   *516*

Proctocolitis, Enteritis   *516*

Prostate Cancer   *127*

Prostatitis: Acute   *516*

Prostatitis: Chronic   *516*

Pruritus   *517*

Pruritus Ani (*see* Pruritis, *see* Hemorrhoids)   *517*

Pseudobulbar Affect (PBA) Disorder   *518*

Pseudogout   *518*

Pseudomembranous Colitis   *519*

Pseudorubella (Roseola Infantum)   *557*

Psittacosis   *519*

Psoriasis   *519*

Psoriatic Arthritis   *526*

Puberty: Central Precocious (CPP)   *512*

Pulmonary Arterial Hypertension (PAH, WHO Group I)   *532*

Pulmonary Fibrosis, Idiopathic (IPF)   *534*

Pupillary Dilation: Short-Term   *536*

Pyelonephritis: Acute   *536*

Pyelonephritis: Acute, Complicated (aCP)   *536*

Pyrexia (Fever)   *241*

Pyruvate Kinase (PK) Deficiency   *24*

Rabies (*Lyssavirus*)   *538*

Red Measles (Rubeola, 3-Day Measles)   *558*

Renal Calculi   *646*

Renal Cell Carcinoma   *93*

Respiratory Syncytial Virus (RSV)   *539*

Restless Legs Syndrome (RLS)   *540*

Retinitis: *Cytomegalovirus* (CMV)   *185*

Rett Syndrome   *541*

Rheumatoid Arthritis (RA)   *541*

Rhinitis Medicamentosa   *554*

Rhinitis: Vasomotor   *556*

Rhinitis/Sinusitis: Allergic   *549*

Rhinosinusitis: Acute Bacterial (ABRS)   *571*

Rhinosinusitis: Chronic, With Nasal Polyps (CRSwNP)   *553*

Rickets (Hypophosphatasia, Osteomalacia)   *345*

Rickettsia rickettsii (Rocky Mountain Spotted Fever)   *556*

Ringworm   *597*

River Blindness (Onchocerciasis)   *556*

Rocky Mountain Spotted Fever (RMSF, *Rickettsia rickettsii*)   *556*

Rosacea (Acne Rosacea)   *2*

Roseola Infantum (Exanthem Subitum, Sixth Disease)   *557*

Rotavirus Gastroenteritis   *557*

Roundworm (Ascariasis)   *557*

Rubella (German Measles)   *558*

Rubeola (Red Measles)   *558*

Salmonella typhi (Typhoid Fever)   *632*

Salmonellosis   *559*

Sarcoptes scabiei (Scabies)   *559*

Scabies (*Sarcoptes scabiei*)   *559*

Scarlatina (Scarlet Fever)   *560*

Scarlet Fever (Scarlatina)   *560*

Schistosomiasis   *560*

Schizoaffective Disorder   *561*

Schizophrenia   *561*

Schizophrenia With Comorbid Personality Disorder   *561*

Sebaceous Cyst: Infected (*see* Skin Infection)   *573*

Seborrhea (*see* Seborrheic Dermatitis)   *204*

Seizure, Cluster   *566*

Seizure Disorder   *566*

Septic Shock   *568*

Serous Otitis Media (SOM)   *448*

Sexual Assault (STD/STI/VD Exposure)   *566*

Shift Work Sleep Disorder (SWSD)   *576*

Shigellosis (Genus *Shigella*)   *567*

Shingles (Herpes Zoster)   *301*

Shock: Septic, Distributive   568
Sickle Cell Disease (SCD)   568
Sinusitis: Allergic   549
Sinusitis/Rhinosinusitis: Acute Bacterial
    (ABRS)   571
Sixth Disease (*see* Roseola Infantum)   557
Sjögren-Larsson Syndrome (SLS)   572
Skin: Callused   572
Skin Infection: Bacterial (Carbuncle, Folliculitis,
    Furuncle)   573
Sleep Apnea: Obstructive (Hypopnea
    Syndrome)   575
Sleepiness: Excessive Shift-Work Sleep Disorder
    (SWSD)   576
Sleep-Wake Disorder: Non-24   418
Smallpox (Variola Major)   576
Solar Keratosis (Actinic Keratosis)   8
Spasticity of Cerebral or Spinal Origin   577
Spinal Muscular Atrophy (SMA)   577
Spondylitis, Ankylosing   434
Sprain   578
Squamous Cell Carcinoma (SCC)   130
Status Asthmaticus   578
Status Epilepticus   579
STD/STI/VD Exposure, Sexual Assault   566
Stein-Leventhal Disease (PCOS, Polycystic Ovarian
    Syndrome)   500
Stomatitis: Angular (Perleche)   482
Stomatitis (Aphthous Stomatitis)   37
Stress Urinary Incontinence   353
Stroke-Induced Expressive Aphasia   36
Strongyloides stercoralis (Threadworm)   593
Stye (Hordeolum)   580
Sunburn   580
Swimmer's Ear (Otitis Externa)   444
Syphilis (*Treponema pallidum*)   581
Systemic Juvenile Idiopathic Arthritis (SJIA)   368
Systemic Lupus Erythematosus (SLE)   582
Takayasu Arteritis   585
Tapeworm (Cestode)   585
Tardive Dyskinesia   586
Temporal Arteritis   253
Temporomandibular Joint (TMJ) Disorder   586
Tennis Elbow (*see* Epicondylitis)   236
Tenosynovial Giant Cell Tumor (TGCT)   587
Tension Headache   277
Testosterone Deficiency   588
Tetanus (*Clostridium tetani*)   591
Threadworm (*Strongyloides stercoralis*)   593
Thrombocytopenia Purpura, Idiopathic (Immune)
    (ITP)   593
Thrombocytopenia Purpura, Thrombotic, Acquired
    Autoimmune (aTTP)   594
Thrush (Oral Candidiasis)   134
Thyroid Cancer   595
Thyroid Eye Disease   596
Thyroid Hormone Deficiency   346
Thyroid Hormone Excess   338
Tic Douloureux (Trigeminal Neuralgia)   608
Tickborne Encephalitis Prophylaxis   596
Tinea Capitis   597

Tinea Corporis   597
Tinea Cruris (Jock Itch)   598
Tinea Pedis (Athlete's Foot)   599
Tinea Versicolor   601
Tobacco Cessation Syndrome   602
Tobacco Dependence   602
Tonsillitis: Acute   603
Toxoplasmosis   605
Traveler's Diarrhea   213
Treatment-Resistant Depression (TRD)   196
Tremor: Benign Essential   58
Trichinosis (*Trichinella spiralis*)   605
Trichomoniasis (*Trichomonas vaginalis*)   606
Trichotillomania   607
Trichuriasis (Whipworm)   656
Trigeminal Neuralgia (Tic Douloureux)   608
Tuberculosis (TB): Pulmonary (*Mycobacterium
    tuberculosis*)   609
Tuberculosis (TB): Treatment-Resistant   609
Type 1 Diabetes Mellitus (T1DM)   613
Type 2 Diabetes Mellitus (T2DM)   619
Typhoid Fever (*Salmonella typhi*)   632
Ulcer: Diabetic, Lower Extremity   633
Ulcer: Decubitus/Pressure   633
Ulcer: Neuropathic (Lower Extremity)   633
Ulcer: Pressure/Decubitus   633
Ulcer: Venous Insufficiency (Lower Extremity)   633
Ulcerative Colitis (UC)   634
Uncinariasis (Hookworm, Cutaneous Larvae
    Migrans)   304
Upper Respiratory Infection (URI)   160
Upper Respiratory Infection (URI, Common
    Cold)   160
Urethritis: Non-Gonococcal (NGU)   638
Urge Urinary Incontinence   353
Urinary Overflow Incontinence   353
Urinary Retention: Unobstructive   639
Urinary Stress Incontinence   353
Urinary Tract Infection, Complicated (cUTI)   640
Urinary Tract Infection (UTI, Acute Cystitis)   641
Urinary Urge Incontinence   353
Urolithiasis (Renal Calculi, Kidney Stones)   646
Urothelial Carcinoma   77
Urticaria: Acute (Hives)   648
Urticaria: Mild, Chronic Idiopathic (CIU)   648
Uterine Fibroid Tumors (Uterine Leiomyomas)   650
Uterine Leiomas (Uterine Fibroid Tumors)   650
Uveitis: Posterior, Chronic, Non-Infectious   652
Vaginal Irritation: External   652
Varicella (Chickenpox)   149
Varicose Veins   652
Variola Major (Smallpox)   576
Vascular Headache (Migraine Headache)   270
Vasomotor Rhinitis   556
Venereal Wart   655
Venous Insufficiency Ulcer: Lower Extremity   633
Ventilator-Associated Bacterial (VABP)
    Pneumonia   490
Verruca Plantaris (Plantar Wart)   655
Verruca Vulgaris (Common Wart)   655
Vertigo   653

Vibrio cholerae (Cholera)   *154*
Vitamin B12 Deficiency   *26*
Vitiligo   *653*
Vomiting   *147*
von Willebrand Disease   *285*
Wagener's Granulomatosis   *265*
Waldenström's Macroglobulinemia   *654*
Wart: Common (Verruca Vulgaris)   *654*
Wart: Plantar (Verruca Plantaris)   *655*
Wart: Venereal, Human Papillomavirus (HPV),
   Condyloma Acuminata   *655*
West Nile Virus (WNV)   *656*
Whipworm (Trichuriasis)   *656*
Whooping Cough (Pertussis)   *482*
Wilson's Disease   *657*
Wiskott-Aldrich Syndrome (*see* Immunodeficiency:
   Primary, Humoral [PHI])   *348*
Wound: Infected, Non-Surgical, Minor   *658*
Wrinkles: Facial   *660*
Xerosis   *661*
Yellow Fever   *661*
Yersinia pestis (Plague)   *489*
Zaire ebolavirus (Ebola Zaire Disease)   *226*
Zika Syndrome, Congenital (CZS)   *661*
Zika Virus/Congenital Zika Syndrome (CZS)   *661*
Zollinger-Ellison Syndrome   *662*

SECTION II: APPENDICES

Appendix A. U.S. Schedule of Controlled
   Substances   *665*
*Appendix B. Blood Pressure Guidelines
   *Appendix B.1. Blood Pressure Classifications (≥18
   Years)
   *Appendix B.2. Blood Pressure Classifications (<18
   Years)
   *Appendix B.3. Identifiable Causes of Hypertension
   (JNC-9)
   *Appendix B.4. Cardiovascular Disease (CVD) Risk
   Factors (JNC-9)
   *Appendix B.5. Diagnostic Workup of Hypertension
   (JNC-9)
   *Appendix B.6. Recommendations for Measuring
   Blood Pressure (JNC-9)
   *Appendix B.7. Patient-Specific Factors to
   Consider When Selecting Drug Treatment for
   Hypertension (JNC-9 and ASH)
   *Appendix B.8. Blood Pressure Treatment
   Recommendations (JNC-9)
*Appendix C. Target Lipid Recommendations (ATP-IV)
   *Appendix C.1. Target TC, TRG, HDL-C, Non-HDL-C
   *Appendix C.2. Target LDL-C (ATP-IV)
   *Appendix C.3. Non-HDL-C Classifications
   (ATP-IV)
*Appendix D. Effects of Selected Drugs on Insulin
   Activity
*Appendix E. Glycosylated Hemoglobin (HbA1c) and
   90-Day Average Blood Glucose Equivalent
*Appendix F. Routine Immunization Recommendations

*Appendix F.1. Administration of Vaccines
*Appendix F.2. Contraindications to Vaccines
*Appendix F.3. Route of Administration and Dose of
   Vaccines
*Appendix F.4. Adverse Reactions to Vaccines
*Appendix F.5. Minimum Interval Between Vaccine
   Doses
Appendix F.6. Childhood (Birth-12 Years)
   Immunization Schedule   *665*
Appendix F.7. Childhood (Birth-12 Years)
   Immunization Catch-Up Schedule   *666*
Appendix F.8. Recommended Adult Immunization
   Schedule   *666*
Appendix G. Contraceptives   *666*
   Appendix G.1. Non-Hormonal Vaginal
   Contraceptives   *666*
   Appendix G.2. Hormonal Contraceptive
   Contraindications and
   Recommendations   *666*
   Appendix G.3. 28-Day Oral Contraceptives With
   Estrogen and Progesterone Content   *667*
   Appendix G.4. Extended-Cycle Oral
   Contraceptives   *673*
   Appendix G.5. Progesterone-Only Oral
   Contraceptives ("Mini-Pill")   *674*
   *Appendix G.6. Injectable Contraceptives
   *Appendix G.6.1. Injectable Progesterone
   Appendix G.7. Transdermal Contraceptives   *674*
   Appendix G.8. Contraceptive Vaginal Rings   *674*
   Appendix G.9. Subdermal Contraceptives   *675*
   Appendix G.10. Intrauterine Contraceptives   *675*
   Appendix G.11. Emergency Contraception   *675*
*Appendix H. Anesthetic Agents for Local Infiltration
   and Dermal/Mucosal Membrane Application
*Appendix I. NSAIDs
Appendix J. Topical Corticosteroids by Potency   *676*
Appendix K. Oral Corticosteroids   *678*
Appendix L. Parenteral Corticosteroids   *679*
Appendix M. Inhalational Corticosteroids   *680*
Appendix N. Antiarrhythmia Drugs   *681*
Appendix O. Antineoplasia Drugs   *682*
Appendix P. Antipsychosis Drugs   *692*
Appendix Q. Anticonvulsant Drugs   *694*
Appendix R. Anti-HIV Drugs   *696*
Appendix S. Anticoagulants   *698*
   Appendix S.1. Coumadin Titration and Dose
   Forms   *698*
   Appendix S.2. Coumadin Over-Anticoagulation
   Reversal   *699*
   Appendix S.3. Agents That Inhibit Coumadin's
   Anticoagulation Effects   *699*
Appendix T. Low Molecular Weight Heparins   *699*
Appendix U. Factor Xa Inhibitors   *699*
Appendix V. Direct Thrombin Inhibitors   *701*
Appendix W. Platelet Aggregation Inhibitors   *702*
Appendix X. Protease-Activated Receptor-1 (PAR-1)
   Inhibitors   *703*
*Appendix Y. Prescription Prenatal Vitamins

---

*Online only; available at connect.springerpub.com/content/reference-book/978-0-8261-7935-7/section/sectionII/appendix.

*Appendix Z. Drugs for the Management of Allergy, Cough, and Cold Symptoms
Appendix AA. Systemic Anti-Infectives *703*
Appendix BB. Antibiotic Dosing by Weight for Liquid Forms *710*
  Appendix BB.1. *acyclovir* (G) (Zovirax Suspension) *710*
  Appendix BB.2. *amantadine* (G) (Symmetrel Syrup) *711*
  Appendix BB.3. *amoxicillin* (G) (Amoxil Suspension, Trimox Suspension) *711*
  Appendix BB.4. *amoxicillin+clavulanate* (G) (Augmentin Suspension) *712*
  Appendix BB.5. *amoxicillin+clavulanate* (G) (Augmentin ES 600 Suspension) *712*
  Appendix BB.6. *ampicillin* (G) (Omnipen Suspension, Principen Suspension) *712*
  Appendix BB.7. *azithromycin* (G) (Zithromax Suspension, Zmax Suspension) *713*
  Appendix BB.8. *cefaclor* (G) (Ceclor Suspension) *713*
  Appendix BB.9. *cefadroxil* (G) (Duricef Suspension) *714*
  Appendix BB.10. *cefdinir* (G) (Omnicef Suspension) *714*
  Appendix BB.11. *cefixime* (G) (Suprax Oral Suspension) *714*
  Appendix BB.12. *cefpodoxime proxetil* (G) (Vantin Suspension) *715*
  Appendix BB.13. *cefprozil* (G) (Cefzil Suspension) *715*
  Appendix BB.14. *ceftibuten* (G) (Cedax Suspension) *715*
  Appendix BB.15. *cephalexin* (G) (Keflex Suspension) *716*
  Appendix BB.16. *clarithromycin* (G) (Biaxin Suspension) *716*
  Appendix BB.17. *clindamycin* (G) (Cleocin Pediatric Granules) *716*
  Appendix BB.18. *dicloxacillin* (G) (Dynapen Suspension) *717*
  Appendix BB.19. *doxycycline* (G) (Vibramycin Syrup/ Suspension) *717*
  Appendix BB.20. *erythromycin estolate* (G) (Ilosone Suspension) *717*
  Appendix BB.21. *erythromycin ethylsuccinate* (G) (E.E.S. Suspension, EryPed Drops/ Suspension) *718*
  Appendix BB.22. *erythromycin+sulfamethoxazole* (G) (Eryzole, Pediazole) *719*
  Appendix BB.23. *fluconazole* (G) (Diflucan Suspension) *719*
  Appendix BB.24. *furazolidone* (G) (Furoxone Liquid) *719*
  Appendix BB.25. *griseofulvin, microsize* (G) (Grifulvin V Suspension) *719*
  Appendix BB.26. *itraconazole* (G) (Sporanox Solution) *720*
  Appendix BB.27. *Loracarbef* (G) (Lorabid Suspension) *720*
  Appendix BB.28. *nitrofurantoin* (G) (Furadantin Suspension) *720*
  Appendix BB.29. *penicillin v potassium* (G) (Pen-Vee K Solution, Veetids Solution) *720*
  Appendix BB.30. *rimantadine* (G) (Flumadine Syrup) *721*
  Appendix BB.31. *tetracycline* (G) (Sumycin Suspension) *721*
  Appendix BB.32. *trimethoprim* (G) (Primsol Suspension) *721*
  Appendix BB.33. *trimethoprim+sulfamethoxazole* (G) (Bactrim Suspension, Septra Suspension) *722*
  Appendix BB.34. *vancomycin* (G) (Vancocin Suspension) *722*

Resources *723*
Index: Brand/Generic Drug Name Cross-Reference With FDA Pregnancy Category and Controlled Drug Category *731*
Key *Inside Back Cover*

---

*Online only; available at connect.springerpub.com/content/reference-book/978-0-8261-7935-7/section/sectionII/appendix.

Kelley M. Anderson, PhD, FNP, Assistant Professor of Nursing, Georgetown University School of Nursing and Health Studies, Washington, DC

Kathleen Bradbury-Golas, DNP, RN, FNP-C, ACNS-BC, Associate Clinical Professor, Drexel University, Philadelphia, Pennsylvania; Family Nurse Practitioner, Virtua Medical Group, Hammonton and Linwood, New Jersey

Lori Brien, MS, ACNP-BC, Instructor, Advanced Practice Nursing Department, Georgetown University School of Nursing and Health Studies, Washington, DC

Jill Cash, MSN, APN, CNP, Nurse Practitioner, Logan Primary Care, West Frankfort, Illinois

Catherine M. Concert, DNP, RN, FNP-BC, AOCNP, NE-BC, CNL, CGRN, Nurse Practitioner-Radiation Oncology, Laura and Isaac Perlmutter Cancer Center, New York University Langone Medical Center; Clinical Assistant Professor, Pace University Lienhard School of Nursing, New York, New York

Kate DeMutis, MSN, CRNP, Senior Lecturer, Adult-Gerontology Primary Care Nurse Practitioner Program, Centralized Clinical Site Coordinator-Primary Care, University of Pennsylvania School of Nursing, Philadelphia, Pennsylvania

Gaye M. Douglas, DNP, MEd, APRN-BC, Assistant Professor of Nursing, Francis Marion University, Florence, South Carolina

Brenda Douglass, DNP, APRN, FNP-C, CDE, CTTS, Coordinator of Clinical Faculty, Assistant Clinical Professor, Drexel University College of Nursing and Health Professions, Philadelphia, Pennsylvania

Aileen Fitzpatrick, DNP, RN, FNP-BC, Clinical Assistant Professor, Pace University Lienhard School of Nursing, New York, New York

Nancy M. George, PhD, RN, FNP-BC, FAANP, Director of DNP Program, Associate Clinical Professor, Wayne State University College of Nursing, Detroit, Michigan

Tracy P. George, DNP, APRN-BC, CNE, Assistant Professor of Nursing, Amy V. Cockcroft Fellow 2016-2017, Francis Marion University, Florence, South Carolina

Cheryl Glass, MSN, WHNP, RN-BC, Clinical Research Specialist, KePRO, TennCare's Medical Solutions Unit, Nashville, Tennessee

Kathleen Gray, DNP, FNP-C, Assistant Professor, Georgetown School of Nursing and Health Studies, Washington, DC

Norma Stephens Hannigan, DNP, MPH, FNP-BC, DCC, FAANP, Clinical Professor of Nursing, Coordinator, Accelerated Second Degree (A2D) Program/Sophomore Honors Program, Hunter College, CUNY Hunter-Bellevue School of Nursing, New York, New York

Ella T. Heitzler, PhD, WHNP, FNP, RNC-OB, Assistant Professor, Georgetown University School of Nursing and Health Studies, Washington, DC

Mary T. Hickey, EdD, RN, Clinical Professor of Nursing, Hunter College, CUNY Hunter-Bellevue School of Nursing, New York, New York

Deborah L. Hopla, DNP, APRN-BC, Assistant Professor of Nursing, Director MSN/FNP Track, Amy V. Cockcroft Fellow, Francis Marion University, Florence, South Carolina

Julia M. Hucks, MN, APRN-BC, Assistant Professor of Nursing, Family Nurse Practitioner, Francis Marion University, Florence, South Carolina

Honey M. Jones, DNP, ACNP-BC, Acute Care Nurse Practitioner, Duke University Medical Center; Clinical Associate Faculty, MSN Program, Duke University School of Nursing, Durham, North Carolina

Melissa H. King, DNP, FNP-BC, ENP-BC, Director of Advanced Practice Providers, Director of TelEmergency, Department of Emergency Medicine, University of Mississippi Medical Center, Jackson, Mississippi

Brittany M. Newberry, PhD, MSN, MPH, APRN, ENP, FNP, Board Certified Emergency and Family Nurse Practitioner; Vice President Education and Professional Development of Hospital MD; Chair, Practice Committee of American Academy of Emergency Nurse Practitioners; Adjunct Faculty, Emory University School of Nursing, Atlanta, Georgia

Andrea Rutherfurd, MS, MPH, FNP-BC, Clinical Faculty Advisor, Adjunct Instructor, FNP Program, Georgetown University School of Nursing and Health Studies, Washington, DC

Samantha Venable, MSN, RN, FNP, Family Nurse Practitioner, Correctional Nursing, Trabuco Canyon, California

Michael Watson, DNP, APRN, FNP-BC, Lead Family Nurse Practitioner, Emergency Department, Wadley Regional Medical Center, Texarkana, Texas

PREFACE

The APRN and PA's Complete Guide to Prescribing Drug Therapy 2024 is a prescribing reference intended for healthcare providers in all clinical practice settings who are involved in management of patients with acute, episodic, and chronic health problems and needs for health promotion and disease prevention. It is organized in a concise, easy-to-read format. Comments are interspersed throughout, including such clinically useful information as laboratory values to be monitored, patient teaching points, and safety information. If pediatric indications for a drug have not been established or a drug is not recommended for a pediatric subgroup, this information is noted accordingly.

This reference is divided into two major sections. **Section I** presents drug treatment regimens for over 600 clinical diagnoses. Drugs are listed alphabetically by generic name, followed by OTC availability; DEA schedule (I, II, III, IV, V); generic availability (G); dosing regimens; brand/trade name(s); dose forms; whether tablets, caplets, or chew tabs are single- (*), cross- (**), or tri-scored (***); flavors of chewable, sublingual, buccal, and liquid forms; and information regarding additives (dye-free, sugar-free, preservative-free or preservative type, alcohol-free or alcohol content). Non-pharmaceutical products and drugs that received initial FDA approval on or after June 30, 2015, do not have an FDA pregnancy letter designation. US FDA pregnancy category Not Assigned: The FDA amended the pregnancy labeling rule for prescription drug products to require labeling that includes a summary of risk, a discussion of the data supporting that summary, and relevant information to help healthcare providers make prescribing decisions and counsel women about the use of drugs during pregnancy. Accordingly, the former A, B, C, D, F designations have been removed and replaced with the drug's FDA-approved risk summary. Use of a specific drug in pregnancy and breastfeeding is addressed in narrative form in the drug's "Comment" section. *Healthcare providers may access the full product label (i.e., mfr pkg insert) by visiting https://www.accessdata.fda.gov/scripts/cder/daf/. Visit https://www.drugs. com/pregnancy-categories.html to view the FDA Pregnancy and Lactation Labeling Final Rule (PLLR).*

Section II presents clinically useful information in table format, including JNC-8 and ASH recommendations for hypertension management, childhood immunization recommendations, brand/trade name drugs (with contents) for management of common respiratory symptoms, anti-infectives by classification, pediatric dosing by weight for liquid forms, glucocorticosteroids by potency and route of administration, and contraceptives by route of administration and estrogen and/or progesterone content. An alphabetical cross-reference index of drugs by generic and brand/trade name, with FDA pregnancy category and controlled drug schedule, facilitates quick identification of drugs by alternate names and page location(s).

Selected diseases and diagnoses (e.g., angina, attention deficit hyperactivity disorder [ADHD], growth failure, glaucoma, Parkinson's disease, multiple sclerosis, cystic fibrosis) and selected drugs (e.g., antineoplastics, antipsychotics, antiarrhythmics, anti-HIV drugs, anticoagulants) are included because patients are frequently referred to primary care providers by specialists for follow-up monitoring and ongoing management. Further, the shifting healthcare paradigm is such that with expanding roles and patient empowerment through education, initial diagnosis and initiation of treatment is increasing in primary care with measurable increases in access to quality healthcare and improved patient self-care. *The user is referred to the manufacturer's package insert for available animal studies and human clinical summaries.* Several diseases are included that may not be prevalent in North America but have been identified in other parts of the world. Endemic diseases for which there is no FDA-approved drug treatment are also included with known transmission and treatment interventions. Accordingly, this guide serves primary care providers internationally. Today's healthcare providers are in an era of rapidly expanding knowledge in the field of genomics, and thus each new edition of this prescribing guide contains new drug classes and new FDA-approved drugs.

For quick reference to pediatric weight-based dosing of a drug, the user is directed to the dose-by-weight table for that drug in the appendices. Potential safe, efficacious prescribing and monitoring of drug therapy regimens require adequate knowledge about (a) pharmacodynamics and pharmacokinetics of drugs, (b) concomitant therapies, and (c) individual patient characteristics (e.g., age, weight, current/past medical history, physical examination findings, hepatic and renal function, comorbidities and risk factors). Users of this guide are encouraged to utilize the manufacturer's package insert, recommendations and guidance of specialists, standard-of-practice protocols, and current research literature for more comprehensive information about specific drugs (e.g., special precautions, drug-drug and drug-food interactions, risk versus benefit, age-related considerations, potential adverse reactions, and appropriate patient-centered care).

ACKNOWLEDGMENTS

This publication, which we consider to be a "must have" for students, academicians, and practicing clinicians, represents the culmination of Springer Publishing Company's and Exeter Premedia's collaborative team effort. The work of reviewers from academia and clinical practice was essential to the process, and their contributions are greatly appreciated. I am proud of my association with these dedicated professionals, and I thank them on behalf of the healthcare community worldwide for supporting the end goal of quality healthcare for all people.

Sincerely, Dr. Mari J. Wirfs

Angiotensin-converting enzyme inhibitors (ACEIs) and **angiotensin II receptor blockers (ARBs)** are contraindicated in the 2nd and 3rd trimesters of pregnancy. Addition of a daily ACEI or ARB is strongly recommended for renal protection in patients with hypertension and/or diabetes. The "ACE inhibitor cough," a dry cough, is an adverse side effect produced by an accumulation of bradykinins that occurs in 5%-10% of the population and typically resolves within a few days of discontinuing the drug.

Alcohol is contraindicated with concomitant **narcotic analgesics, benzodiazepines, selective serotonin reuptake inhibitors (SSRIs), antihistamines, tricyclic antidepressants (TCAs),** and other sedating agents due to risk of oversedation.

Alpha-1 blockers have a potential adverse side effect of sudden hypotension, especially with first dose. Alert the patient regarding this "first-dose effect" and recommend the patient sit or lie down to take the first dose. Usually start at lowest dose and titrate upward.

Antidepressant monotherapy should be avoided until any presence of (hypo) mania or positive family history for bipolar spectrum disorder has been ruled out as antidepressant monotherapy can induce mania in the bipolar patient.

For patients 65 years of age and older, consult the **May 2017 Beers Criteria** for Potentially Inappropriate Medication (PIM) Use in Older Adults, to help improve the safety of prescribing medications for older adults, presented in table format at:
https://www.priorityhealth.com/provider/clinical-resources/medication-resources/~/media/documents/pharmacy/cms-high-risk-medications.pdf

Aspirin is contraindicated in children and adolescents with *varicella* or other viral illness, and 3rd trimester of pregnancy.

Beta-blockers, by all routes of administration, are generally contraindicated in severe chronic obstructive pulmonary disease (COPD), history of or current bronchial asthma, sinus bradycardia, and second- or third-degree atrioventricular (AV) block. Use a cardiospecific beta-blocker where appropriate in these cases.

A **biosimilar** product is one that has been FDA-approved based on data demonstrating that it is highly similar to a previously FDA-approved biological product, known as the reference product. Accordingly, the FDA has determined that there are no clinically meaningful differences between the biosimilar product and the reference product (e.g., **Cyltezo** [*adalimumab-adbm*] is biosimilar to **Humira** [*adalimumab*]). A biosimilar product has been demonstrated for the condition(s) of use (e.g., indication(s), dosing regimen(s)), strength(s), dosage form(s), and route(s) of administration described in its full prescribing information in the manufacturer's package insert.

An **interchangeable product (IP)** is a biological product that is approved based on data demonstrating that it is highly similar to an FDA-approved reference product (RP) and that there are no clinically meaningful differences between the products; it can be expected to produce the same clinical result as the RP in any given patient; and if administered more than once to a patient, the risk in terms of safety or diminished efficacy from alternating or switching between use of the RP and IP is not greater than that from the RP without such alternation or switch. For example, Interchangeability of **Semglee** has been demonstrated for the condition(s) of use, strength(s), dosage form(s), and route(s) of administration as described in the mfr pkg insert. **Semglee** *(IP; insulin glargine-yfgn)* is interchangeable with **Lantus** *(RP; insulin glargine).*

The FDA **Breakthrough Therapy Designation (BTD)** is intended to expedite the development and review of a drug candidate that is planned for use, alone or in combination with one or more other drugs, to treat a serious or life-threatening disease or condition when preliminary clinical evidence indicates that the drug may demonstrate substantial improvement over existing therapies on one or more clinically significant endpoints. The benefits of Breakthrough Therapy Designation include the same benefits as Fast Track Designation (FTD), plus an organizational commitment involving the FDA's senior managers with more intensive guidance from the FDA (e.g., *Zulresso [brexanolone]* received the FDA Breakthrough Therapy Designation for treatment of postpartum depression).

Calcium channel blockers may cause the adverse side effect of pedal edema (feet, ankles, lower legs) that resolves with discontinuation of the drug.

Codeine is known to be excreted in breast milk: <12 years, not recommended; 12-<18 years, use extreme caution; not recommended for children and adolescents with asthma or other chronic breathing problem. The FDA and the European Medicines Agency (EMA) are investigating the safety of using *codeine*-containing medications to treat pain, cough, and colds in children 12-<18 years because of the potential for serious side effects, including slowed or difficult breathing.

Check **drug interactions** at https://www.drugs.com/drug_interactions.php.

Check FDA **drug recalls, market withdrawals, and safety alerts** at http://www.fda.gov/Safety/Recalls/default.htm.

Contraceptives that are estrogen-progesterone combinations and **progesterone-only** are contraindicated in pregnancy (pregnancy category X).

Corticosteroids increase blood sugar in patients with diabetes and decrease immunity; therefore, consider risk versus benefit in susceptible patients, use lowest effective dose, and taper gradually to discontinue.

Diclofenac is contraindicated with *aspirin* allergy and, as with all other non-steroidal anti-inflammatory drugs (NSAIDs), should be avoided in late pregnancy (≥30 weeks) because it may cause premature closure of the ductus arteriosus.

Erythromycin may increase INR with concomitant warfarin, as well as increase serum level of digoxin, benzodiazepines, and statins.

Finasteride, a 5-alpha reductase inhibitor, is associated with low but increased risk of high-grade prostate cancer. Pregnant females should not touch broken tablets.

Fluoroquinolones and **quinolones** are contraindicated <18 years of age, pregnancy, and breastfeeding. *Exception:* In the case of anthrax, *ciprofloxacin* is indicated for patients <18 years of age and dose is based on mg/kg body weight. There is risk of tendonitis or tendon rupture (e.g., *ciprofloxacin, gemifloxacin, levofloxacin, moxifloxacin, norfloxacin, ofloxacin*).

Fluoroquinolones can increase the risk of aortic dissection or aortic aneurysm rupture and should not be used in patients at increased risk (including patients with peripheral artery disease, hypertension, Marfan syndrome, Ehlers-Danlos syndrome, and older adults) unless there is no other available treatment option.

The U.S. Preventive Services Task Force (USPSTF) recommends against using **hormone replacement therapy** (HRT) for primary prevention of chronic conditions among postmenopausal women. The harms associated with combined use of estrogen and a progestin, such as increased risks of invasive breast cancer, venous thromboembolism, and coronary heart disease, far outweigh the benefits.

Ibuprofen is contraindicated in children <6 months of age and in the 3rd trimester of pregnancy.

Live vaccines are contraindicated in patients who are immunosuppressed or receiving immunosuppressive therapy, including immunosuppressive levels of corticosteroid therapy.

Metronidazole and *tinidazole* are contraindicated in the 1st trimester of pregnancy. Alcohol is contraindicated during treatment with oral forms and for 72 hours after therapy due to a possible *disulfiram*-like reaction (nausea, vomiting, flushing, headache).

When prescribing **opioid analgesics**, presumptive urine **drug testing** (UDT) should be performed when opioid therapy for chronic pain is initiated, along with subsequent use as adherence monitoring, using in-office point of service testing to identify patients who are non-compliant or abusing prescription drugs or illicit drugs. American Society of Interventional Pain Physicians (ASIPP)

Orphan Drug designation means the drug is a first-in-class and/or the drug is for treatment of a rare disease and/or the drug is a first and only treatment for a disease and the application for FDA approval has received priority review as incentive to assist and encourage the development of drugs for rare diseases.

Oral **phosphodiesterase type 5 (PDE5) inhibitors** are contraindicated in patients taking nitrates due to risk of hypotension or syncope (e.g., *avanafil, sildenafil, tadalafil, vardenafil*).

Chronic long-term **proton pump inhibitor (PPI)** use carries a risk to renal function (consider risk-benefit and alternative treatment). PPIs should be discontinued, and should not be initiated, in patients with acute kidney injury (AKI) and chronic kidney disease (CKD).

Statins are strongly recommended as adjunctive therapy for patients with diabetes, with <u>or</u> without abnormal lipids.

Sulfonamides (e.g., *sulfamethoxazole, trimethoprim*) are not recommended in pregnancy <u>or</u> lactation. CrCl 15-30 mL/min: reduce dose by ½; CrCl <15 mL/min: not recommended. Contraindicated with glucose-6-phosphate dehydrogenase deficiency (G6PD). A high fluid intake is indicated during sulfonamide therapy to avoid crystallization in the kidneys.

Tetracyclines are contraindicated in children <8 years of age, pregnancy, and breastfeeding (discolors developing tooth enamel). A side effect may be photosensitivity (photophobia). Do not take with antacids, calcium supplements, milk <u>or</u> other dairy, <u>or</u> within 2 hours of taking another drug (e.g., *doxycycline, minocycline*).

Tramadol is known to be excreted in breast milk. The FDA and the European Medicines Agency (EMA) are investigating the safety of using *tramadol*-containing medications to treat pain in children 12-18 years because of the potential for serious side effects, including slowed <u>or</u> difficult breathing.

The **Transmucosal Immediate Release Fentanyl (TIRF) Risk Evaluation and Mitigation Strategy (REMS)** program is an FDA-required program designed to ensure informed risk-benefit decisions before initiating treatment, and while patients are being treated to ensure appropriate use of TIRF medicines. The purpose of the TIRF REMS Access program is to mitigate the risk of misuse, abuse, addiction, overdose, and serious complications due to medication errors with the use of TIRF medicines. You must enroll in the TIRF REMS Access program to prescribe, dispense, **or** distribute TIRF medicines. To register, call the TIRF REMS Access program at 1-866-822-1483 **or** register online at https://www.tirfremsaccess.com/TirfUI/rems/home.action.

SECTION I

DRUG THERAPY BY CLINICAL DIAGNOSIS

ACETAMINOPHEN OVERDOSE

ANTIDOTE/CHELATING AGENT

▷ *acetylcysteine* (G) *Loading dose:* 150 mg/kg administered over 15 minutes; *Maintenance:* 50 mg/kg administered over 4 hours; then 100 mg/kg administered over 16 hours
Pediatric: same as adult

Acetadote *Vial: soln for IV infusion after dilution:* 200 mg/ml (30 ml; dilute in D5W) (preservative-free)
Comment: *Acetaminophen* overdose is a medical emergency due to the risk of irreversible hepatic injury. An IV infusion of *acetylcysteine* should be started as soon as possible and within 24 hours if the exact time of ingestion is unknown. Use a serum *acetaminophen* nomogram to determine need for treatment. Extreme caution is needed if used with concomitant hepatotoxic drugs.

ACHONDROPLASIA

C-TYPE NATRIURETIC PEPTIDE (CNP) ANALOG

▷ *vosoritide* not indicated in adults due to epiphyseal closure
Pediatric: <5 years: safety and efficacy not established; ≥5 years, prior to epiphyseal closure: Ensure adequate food and fluid intake prior to administration, including approximately 240-300 ml of fluid in the hour prior to dose administration; Recommended dose is weight-based; Administer SC at approximately the same time once daily; Recommended sites: front middle of the thigh, lower part of the abdomen at least 2 inches (5 centimeters) away from the navel, top of the buttocks, or back of the upper arm. Rotate sites. The same injection area should not be used for 2 consecutive days; do not inject **Voxzogo** administer into sites that are red, swollen, or tender; reconstitute dose prior to use and administer injection within 3 hours; injection volume is based on both the patient's weight and the concentration of reconstituted **Voxzogo**; monitor growth and adjust dose according to changes in body weight; permanently discontinue upon closure of the epiphyses; see mfr pkg insert for full prescribing information, preparation, and administration instructions; see dosing table below

Recommended Daily Dose and Injection Volume by Actual Weight and Vial Strength			
Actual Body Weight	Vial Strength*	Dose	Injection Volume
10-11 kg	0.4 mg	0.24 mg	0.3 ml
12-16 kg	0.56 mg	0.28 mg	0.35 ml
17-21 kg	0.56 mg	0.32 mg	0.4 ml
22-32 kg	0.56 mg	0.4 mg	0.5 ml
33-43 kg	1.2 mg	0.5 mg	0.25 ml
44-59 kg	1.2 mg	0.6 mg	0.3 ml
60-89 kg	1.2 mg	0.7 mg	0.35 ml
≥90 kg	1.2 mg	0.8 mg	0.4 ml

*The concentration of *vosoritide* in reconstituted 0.4 mg vial and 0.56 mg vial is 0.8 mg/ml. The concentration of *vosoritide* in reconstituted 1.2 mg vial is 2 mg/ml.

Voxzogo *Vial:* 0.4, 0.56, 1.2 mg, single-dose, pwdr, w. co-packaged diluent syringe, diluent transfer needle (23 gauge), and single-dose administration syringe (30 gauge), both with needle retraction safety devices
Comment: **Voxzogo** is a C-type natriuretic peptide (CNP) analog indicated to increase linear growth in pediatric patients with achondroplasia who are ≥5 years of age with open epiphyses. This indication is approved under accelerated approval based on an improvement in annualized growth velocity. Continued approval for this indication may be contingent upon verification and description of clinical

(*continued*)

benefit in confirmatory trial(s). Transient decreases in BP have been reported; assure adequate food and fluids and monitor BP. *eGFR <60 ml/min/1.73 m²*: Not recommended. The most common adverse reactions (incidence >10%) have been injection site erythema, injection site swelling, vomiting, injection site urticaria, arthralgia, decreased BP, and gastroenteritis. Monitor and assess the patient's body weight, growth, and physical development regularly every 3-6 months. Permanently discontinue **Voxzogo** upon confirmation of no further growth potential, indicated by closure of epiphyses. Caregivers may administer **Voxzogo** after proper training by a healthcare professional on preparation and administration. In a fertility and reproductive animal study, including males and females at doses up to 540 mcg/kg/day (15 times the exposure at the maximum recommended human dose [MRHD]), *vosoritide* had no effect on mating performance, fertility, or litter characteristics. There are no available data on *vosoritide* use in pregnant females to evaluate for a drug-associated risk of major birth defects, miscarriage, or adverse maternal or fetal outcomes. In animal reproduction studies, there was no evidence of embryo-fetal toxicity or congenital malformations. There is no information regarding the presence of *vosoritide* in human milk or effects on the breastfed infant. *Vosoritide* is present in animal milk. Developmental and health benefits of breastfeeding should be considered along with the mother's clinical need for **Voxzogo** and any potential adverse effects on the breastfed infant from **Voxzogo** or from the underlying maternal condition.

ACNE ROSACEA

Comment: All acne rosacea products should be applied sparingly to clean, dry skin as directed. Avoid use of topical corticosteroids.
▷ *ivermectin* (G) apply bid
    Soolantra *Crm:* 1% (30 gm)
    Comment: Soolantra is a macrocyclic lactone. Exactly how it works to treat rosacea is unknown.

TOPICAL ALPHA-1A ADRENOCEPTOR AGONIST
▷ *oxymetazoline hcl* (G) apply a pea-sized amount once daily in a thin layer covering the entire face (forehead, nose, cheeks, and chin), avoiding the eyes and lips; wash hands immediately
  Pediatric: <18 years: not recommended; ≥18 years: same as adult
    Rhofade *Crm:* 1% (30 gm tube)
    Comment: Rhofade acts as a vasoconstrictor. Use with caution in patients with cerebral or coronary insufficiency, Raynaud's phenomenon, thromboangiitis obliterans, scleroderma, or Sjögren's syndrome. Rhofade may increase the risk of angle closure glaucoma in patients with narrow-angle glaucoma. Advise patients to seek immediate medical care if signs and symptoms of potentiation of vascular insufficiency or acute angle closure glaucoma develop.

TOPICAL ALPHA-2 AGONIST
▷ *brimonidine* (G) apply to affected area once daily
  Pediatric: <18 years: not recommended; ≥18 years: same as adult
    Mirvaso *Gel:* 0.33% (30, 45 gm tube; 30 gm pump)
    Comment: Mirvaso is indicated for persistent erythema; *brimonidine* constricts dilated facial blood vessels to reduce redness.

TOPICAL ANTIMICROBIALS
▷ *azelaic acid* (G) apply to affected area bid
    Azelex *Crm:* 20% (30, 50 gm)
    Finacea *Gel:* 15% (30 gm); *Foam:* 15% (50 gm)
▷ *metronidazole* apply to clean dry skin
    MetroCream apply bid
      Emol crm: 0.75% (45 gm)
    MetroGel apply once daily
      Gel: 1% (60 gm tube; 55 gm pump)
    MetroLotion apply bid
      Lotn: 0.75% (2 oz)
▷ *minocycline* topical foam apply to affected areas once daily; gently rub into the skin
  Pediatric: <9 years: not recommended; ≥9 years: same as adult
    Amzeeq *Aerosol can:* 4% (30 gm)
    Comment: Amzeeq *(minocycline)* is a tetracycline-class drug indicated for the treatment of inflammatory lesions of non-nodular moderate-to-severe acne vulgaris in patients >9 years of age. The propellant in **Amzeeq** is flammable. Instruct the patient to avoid fire, flame, and smoking during and immediately following application. Use of tetracycline class of drugs orally during the 2nd and 3rd trimesters of pregnancy and during infancy and childhood up to the age of 8 years may cause permanent discoloration of the teeth (yellow-gray-brown) and reversible inhibition of bone growth. If *Clostridium difficile*-associated diarrhea occurs, discontinue **Amzeeq**. If liver injury is suspected, discontinue **Amzeeq**. Patients who are on anticoagulant therapy may require downward adjustment of their

anticoagulant dosage. Avoid co-administration with penicillins. **Amzeeq** may cause fetal harm when used during pregnancy. Breastfeeding is not recommended while using **Amzeeq**.

▷ *sodium sulfacetamide* (G) apply 1-3 x daily

    Klaron *Lotn:* 10% (2 oz)

▷ *sodium sulfacetamide+sulfur*

    Clenia Emollient Cream apply 1-3 x daily

        Wash: sod sulfa 10%+sulfur 5% (10 oz)

    Clenia Foaming Wash wash affected area once or twice daily

        Wash: sod sulfa 10%+sulfur 5% (6, 12 oz)

    Rosula Gel apply 1-3 x daily

        Gel: sod sulfa 10%+sulfur 5% (45 ml)

    Rosula Lotion apply tid

        Lotn: sod sulfa 10%+sulfur 5% (45 ml) (alcohol-free)

    Rosula Wash wash bid

        Clnsr: sod sulfa 10%+sulfur 5% (335 ml)

ORAL ANTIMICROBIALS

▷ *doxycycline* (G) 40-100 mg bid

    Pediatric: <8 years: not recommended; ≥8 years, <100 lb: 2 mg/lb on the first day in 2 divided doses, followed by 1 mg/lb/day in 1 or 2 divided doses; ≥8 years, ≥100 lb: same as adult; *see* Appendix BB.19.

    doxycycline (G) (Vibramycin Syrup/Suspension) *for dose by weight*

    Acticlate *Tab:* 75, 150**mg

    Adoxa *Tab:* 50, 75, 100, 150 mg ent-coat

    Doryx *Tab:* 50, 75, 100, 150, 200 mg del-rel

    Doxteric *Tab:* 50 mg del-rel

    Monodox *Cap:* 50, 75, 100 mg

    Oracea *Cap:* 40 mg del-rel

    Vibramycin *Tab:* 100 mg; *Cap:* 50, 100 mg; *Syr:* 50 mg/5 ml (raspberry-apple) (sulfites); *Oral susp:* 25 mg/5 ml (raspberry)

    Vibra-Tab *Tab:* 100 mg film-coat

▷ *minocycline* (G) 200 mg on the first day; then 100 mg q 12 hours x 9 more days

    Pediatric: <8 years: not recommended; ≥8 years, <100 lb: 2 mg/lb on the first day in 2 divided doses, followed by 1 mg/lb q 12 hours x 9 more days; ≥8 years, ≥100 lb: same as adult

    Dynacin *Cap:* 50, 100 mg

    Minocin *Cap:* 50, 75, 100 mg; *Oral susp:* 50 mg/5 ml (60 ml) (custard) (sulfites, alcohol 5%)

ACNE VULGARIS

ORAL CONTRACEPTIVES

see Appendix G. Contraceptives
see Appendix G.5. Progesterone-Only Oral Contraceptives ("Mini-Pill")

Comment: In their 2016 published report, researchers concluded different hormonal contraceptives have significantly varied effects on acne. Women (n = 2,147) who were using a hormonal contraceptive at the time of their first consultation for acne comprised the study sample. Participants completed an assessment at baseline to report how the contraceptive affected their acne. Then the researchers used the Kruskal-Wallis test and logistic regression analysis to compare the outcomes by contraceptive type. On average, the vaginal ring and combined oral contraceptives (COCs) improved acne, whereas depot injections, subdermal implants, and hormonal intrauterine devices worsened acne. In the COC categories, *drospirenone* was the most helpful in improving acne, followed by *norgestimate* and *desogestrel*, and then *levonorgestrel* and *norethindrone*. Although triphasic progestin dosage had a positive effect on acne, estrogen dosage did not.

Comment: Off-label use of spironolactone in the treatment of acne vulgaris—In the clinical experience of Julie C. Harper, MD, an increasing number of women with acne are turning to off-label, long-term treatment with spironolactone. "Spironolactone is fairly accessible, inexpensive, and effective for our patients," Dr. Harper, a dermatologist who practices in Birmingham, Alabama, said at the Hawaii Dermatology Seminar provided by MedscapeLIVE! An aldosterone receptor antagonist commonly used to treat high blood pressure and heart failure also has antiandrogenic properties with a proven track record of treating acne and hirsutism. It reduces androgen production, inhibits 5-alpha reductase, and increases sex hormone binding globulin. The dosing range for treating acne is 25 mg to 200 mg per day, but Dr. Harper prefers a maximum dose of 100 mg per day. According to a systematic review of its use for acne in adult women, the most common side effect is menstrual irregularity, while other common side effects include breast tenderness/swelling, fatigue, and headaches.

TOPICAL ANDROGEN RECEPTOR INHIBITOR

▷ *clascoterone* apply a thin layer to affected area bid (morning and evening)
Pediatric: <12 years: <u>not</u> recommended; ≥12 years: same as adult
    Winlevi *Crm:* 1%
    Comment: **Winlevi** is a first-in-class topical androgen receptor inhibitor for the treatment of acne vulgaris. Hypothalamic-pituitary-adrenal (HPA) axis suppression may occur during <u>or</u> after treatment with *clascoterone.* Attempt to withdraw use if HPA suppression occurs. Pediatric patients may be more susceptible to systemic toxicity. Elevated potassium level has been observed in some subjects during clinical trials. The most common adverse reactions (incidence 7%-12%) have been erythema, reddening, pruritis, and scaling/dryness. Additionally, edema, stinging, and burning have occurred in >3% of patients and were reported in a similar percentage of patients treated with the vehicle. There are <u>no</u> available data on **Winlevi** cream use in pregnant females to evaluate for an associated risk of major birth defects, miscarriage, <u>or</u> adverse maternal <u>or</u> fetal outcomes. There are <u>no</u> data regarding the presence of *clascoterone* <u>or</u> its metabolite in human milk <u>or</u> effects on the breastfed infant.

TOPICAL ANTIMICROBIALS

Comment: All topical antimicrobials should be applied sparingly to clean, dry skin.
▷ *azelaic acid* **(G)** apply to affected area bid
    Azelex *Crm:* 20% (30, 50 gm)
    Finacea *Gel:* 15% (30 gm); *Foam:* 15% (50 gm)
▷ *benzoyl peroxide* **(G)**
    Comment: *Benzoyl peroxide* may discolor clothing and linens.
    Benzac W initially apply to affected area once daily; increase to bid-tid as tolerated
      Gel: 2.5, 5, 10% (60 gm)
    Benzac W Wash wash affected area bid
      Wash: 5% (4, 8 oz), 10% (8 oz)
    Benzagel apply to affected area one <u>or</u> more times a day
      Gel: 5, 10% (1.5, 3 oz) (alcohol 14%)
    Benzagel Wash wash affected area bid
      Gel: 10% (6 oz)
    Desquam-X 5 wash affected area bid
      Wash: 5% (5 oz)
    Desquam-X 10 wash affected area bid
      Wash: 10% (5 oz)
    Triaz apply to affected area daily bid
      Lotn: 3, 6, 9% (bottle), 3% (tube); *Pads:* 3, 6, 9% (jar)
    ZoDerm apply once <u>or</u> twice daily
      Gel: 4.5, 6.5, 8.5% (125 ml); *Crm:* 4.5, 6.5, 8.5% (125 ml); *Clnsr:* 4.5, 6.5, 8.5% (400 ml)
▷ *clindamycin* topical apply to affected area bid
    Pediatric: <12 years: <u>not</u> recommended; ≥12 years: same as adult
    Cleocin T *Pad:* 1% (60/pck; alcohol 50%); *Lotn:* 1% (60 ml); *Gel:* 1% (30, 60 gm); *Soln w. applicator:* 1% (30, 60 ml) (alcohol 50%)
    Clindagel *Gel:* 1% (42, 77 gm)
    Evoclin Foam: 1% (50, 100 gm) (alcohol)
▷ *clindamycin+benzoyl peroxide* topical apply to affected area once daily
    Pediatric: <12 years: <u>not</u> recommended; ≥12 years: same as adult
    Acanya (G) apply to affected area once daily-bid
      Gel: clin 1.2%+benz 2.5% (50 gm)
    BenzaClin (G) apply to affected area bid
      Gel: clin 1%+benz 5% (25, 50 gm)
    Duac apply daily in the evening
      Gel: clin 1%+benz 5% (45 gm)
    Onexton Gel (G) apply to affected area once daily
      Gel: clin 1.2%+benz 3.75% (50 gm pump) (alcohol-free) (preservative-free)
▷ *dapsone* topical **(G)** apply to affected area bid
    Pediatric: <12 years: <u>not</u> recommended; ≥12 years: same as adult
    Aczone *Gel:* 5, 7.5% (30, 60, 90 gm pump)
▷ *erythromycin+benzoyl peroxide* initially apply to affected area once daily; increase to bid as tolerated
    Benzamycin Topical Gel *Gel:* eryth 3%+benz 5% (46.6 gm/jar)
▷ *minocycline* topical foam apply to affected areas once daily; gently rub into the skin
    Pediatric: <9 years: <u>not</u> recommended; ≥9 years: same as adult
    Amzeeq *Aerosol can:* 4% (30 gm)

Comment: Amzeeq *(minocycline)* is a tetracycline-class drug indicated for treatment of inflammatory lesions of non-nodular moderate-to-severe acne vulgaris in patients >9 years of age. The propellant in **Amzeeq** is flammable. Instruct the patient to avoid fire, flame, and smoking during and immediately following application. Use of tetracycline class of drugs orally during the 2nd and 3rd trimesters of pregnancy and during infancy and childhood up to the age of 8 years may cause permanent discoloration of the teeth (yellow-gray-brown) and reversible inhibition of bone growth. If *Clostridioides difficile*-associated diarrhea occurs, discontinue **Amzeeq**. If liver injury is suspected, discontinue **Amzeeq**. Patients who are on anticoagulant therapy may require downward adjustment of their anticoagulant dosage. Avoid co-administration with penicillins. **Amzeeq** may cause fetal harm when used during pregnancy. Breastfeeding is <u>not</u> recommended while using **Amzeeq**.

▷ *sodium sulfacetamide* **(G)** apply tid
   Klaron *Lotn:* 10% (2 oz)

ORAL ANTIMICROBIALS
▷ *doxycycline* **(G)** 100 mg bid
   Pediatric: <8 years: <u>not</u> recommended; ≥8 years, <100 lb: 2 mg/lb on first day in 2 divided doses, followed by 1 mg/lb/day in 1-2 divided doses; ≥8 years, ≥100 lb: same as adult; *see* Appendix BB.19. *doxycycline* **(G)** (Vibramycin Syrup/Suspension) *for dose by weight*
   Acticlate *Tab:* 75, 150**mg
   Adoxa *Tab:* 50, 75, 100, 150 mg ent-coat
   Doryx *Tab:* 50, 75, 100, 150, 200 mg del-rel
   Doxteric *Tab:* 50 mg del-rel
   Monodox *Cap:* 50, 75, 100 mg
   Oracea *Cap:* 40 mg del-rel
   Vibramycin *Tab:* 100 mg; *Cap:* 50, 100 mg; *Syr:* 50 mg/5 ml (raspberry-apple) (sulfites); *Oral susp:* 25 mg/5 ml (raspberry)
   Vibra-Tab *Tab:* 100 mg film coat
▷ *erythromycin base* **(G)** 250 mg qid, 333 mg tid <u>or</u> 500 mg bid x 7-10 days; then taper to lowest effective dose
   Pediatric: <45 kg: 30-50 mg in 2-4 divided doses x 7-10 days; ≥45 kg: same as adult
   Ery-Tab *Tab:* 250, 333, 500 mg ent-coat
   PCE *Tab:* 333, 500 mg
▷ *erythromycin ethylsuccinate* **(G)** 400 mg qid x 7-10 days
   Pediatric: 30-50 mg/kg/day in 4 divided doses x 7-10 days; may double dose with severe infection; max 100 mg/kg/day; *see* Appendix BB.21. *erythromycin ethylsuccinate* **(G)** (E.E.S. Suspension, Ery-Ped Drops/ Suspension) *for dose by weight*
   EryPed *Oral susp:* 200 mg/5 ml (100, 200 ml) (fruit), 400 mg/5 ml (60, 100, 200 ml) (banana); *Oral drops:* 200, 400 mg/5 ml (50 ml) (fruit); *Chew tab:* 200 mg wafer (fruit)
   E.E.S. *Oral susp:* 200, 400 mg/5 ml (100 ml) (fruit)
   E.E.S. Granules *Oral susp:* 200 mg/5 ml (100, 200 ml) (cherry)
   E.E.S. 400 Tablets *Tab:* 400 mg
▷ *minocycline* **(G)** initially 50-200 mg/day in 2 divided doses; reduce dose to once daily after improvement
   Pediatric: <8 years: <u>not</u> recommended; ≥8 years: same as adult
   Dynacin *Cap:* 50, 100 mg
   Minocin *Cap:* 50, 75, 100 mg; *Oral susp:* 50 mg/5 ml (60 ml) (custard) (sulfites, alcohol 5%)
   Minolira *Tab:* 105, 135 mg ext-rel
   Solodyn *Tab:* 55, 65, 80, 105, 115 mg ext-rel
   Comment: Once-daily dosing of **Minolira** <u>or</u> **Solodyn**, extended-release *minocyclines*, is approved for inflammatory lesions of non-nodular moderate-to-severe acne vulgaris in patients ≥12 years of age. The recommended dose of **Solodyn** is 1 mg/kg once daily × 12 weeks.
▷ *sarecycline* 1 tab daily with <u>or</u> without food; <9 years: <u>not</u> recommended; ≥9 years: 33-54 kg: 60 mg; 55-84 kg: 100 mg; *85-136 kg:* 150 mg
   Seysara *Tab:* 60, 100, 150 mg
   Comment: Seysara is a first-in-class, *tetracycline*-derived, once daily treatment for inflammatory lesions of non-nodular moderate-to-severe acne. Efficacy of **Seysara** beyond 12 weeks and safety beyond 12 months have <u>not</u> been established. **Seysara** has <u>not</u> been evaluated in the treatment of infections. To reduce the development of drug-resistant bacteria as well as to maintain the effectiveness of other antibacterial drugs, **Seysara** should be used <u>only</u> as indicated. If *Clostridioides difficile*-associated diarrhea (antibiotic-associated colitis) occurs, discontinue **Seysara**. Central nervous system side effects, including light headedness, dizziness, <u>or</u> vertigo, have been reported with *tetracycline* use. Patients who experience these symptoms should be cautioned about driving vehicles <u>or</u> using hazardous machinery. These symptoms may disappear during therapy and when the drug is discontinued. **Seysara** may cause intracranial hypertension; discontinue **Seysara** if symptoms occur. Photosensitivity can occur with

(continued)

Seysara; minimize or avoid exposure to natural or artificial sunlight. *Tetracycline* is contraindicated in patients <8 years of age and during pregnancy and lactation (discolors developing tooth enamel). A side effect may be photosensitivity (photophobia). Avoid co-administration with retinoids and penicillin. Decrease anticoagulant dosage as appropriate. Monitor for toxicities of drugs that may require dosage reduction (e.g., P-glycoprotein substrates) and monitor for toxicities. Do not take with antacids, calcium supplements, iron preparations, milk or other dairy, or within 2 hours of taking another drug.

▶ tetracycline (G) initially 1 gm/day in 2-4 divided doses; after improvement, 125-500 mg daily
 Pediatric: <8 years: not recommended; ≥8 years, <100 lb: 25-50 mg/kg/day in 2-4 divided doses; ≥8 years, ≥100 lb: same as adult; *see Appendix BB.31.* tetracycline (G) (Sumycin Suspension) *for dose by weight*
 Achromycin V *Cap:* 250, 500 mg
 Sumycin *Tab:* 250, 500 mg; *Cap:* 250, 500 mg; *Oral susp:* 125 mg/5 ml (100, 200 ml) (fruit) (sulfites)

TOPICAL RETINOIDS

Comment: Wash affected area with a soap-free cleanser; pat dry and wait 20 to 30 minutes; then apply sparingly to affected area; use only once daily in the evening. Avoid applying to eyes, ears, nostrils, and mouth.

▶ adapalene apply once daily at HS
 Pediatric: <12 years: not recommended; ≥12 years: same as adult
 Differin *Crm:* 0.1% (45 gm); *Gel:* 0.1, 0.3% (45 gm) (alcohol-free); *Pad:* 0.1% (30/pck) (alcohol 30%); *Lotn:* 0.1% (2, 4 oz)

▶ tazarotene (G) apply to affected area once daily at HS
 Pediatric: <12 years: not recommended; ≥12 years: same as adult
 Arazlo *Tube:* 0.045% (45 gm)
 Comment: Arazlo *(tazarotene)* is a lotion formulation of retinoid *tazarotene* approved for the topical treatment of acne vulgaris in patients ≥9 years of age.
 Avage Cream *Crm:* 0.1% (30 gm)
 Tazorac Cream *Crm:* 0.05, 0.1% (15, 30, 60 gm)
 Tazorac Gel *Gel:* 0.05, 0.1% (30, 100 gm)

▶ tretinoin (G) apply sparingly to affected area once or twice daily
 Comment: Dryness, pain, erythema, irritation, and exfoliation may occur during treatment. Avoid paranasal creases and mucous membranes. Minimize exposure to sunlight and sunlamps. Use sunscreen and protective clothing when sun exposure cannot be avoided. Use with caution if allergic to fish due to potential for allergenicity to fish protein.
 Pediatric: <12 years: not recommended; ≥12 years: same as adult
 Altreno *Lotn:* 0.05% (45 gm tube)
 Comment: Altreno is indicated for children >9 years of age. Apply a thin film to affected area bid.
 Atralin Gel *Gel:* 0.05% (45 gm)
 Avita *Crm:* 0.025% (20, 45 gm); *Gel:* 0.025% (20, 45 gm)
 Retin-A Cream *Crm:* 0.025, 0.05, 0.1% (20, 45 gm)
 Retin-A Gel *Gel:* 0.01, 0.025% (15, 45 gm) (alcohol 90%)
 Retin-A Liquid *Soln:* 0.05% (alcohol 55%)
 Retin-A Micro Gel *Gel:* 0.04, 0.08, 0.1% (20, 45 gm)
 Tretin-X Cream *Crm:* 0.075% (35 gm) (parabens-free, alcohol-free, propylene glycol-free)

▶ trifarotene 0.005% cream apply a thin layer to the affected areas of the face, chest, shoulders, and/or back once daily, in the evening, to clean and dry skin; avoid contact with the eyes, lips, paranasal creases, and mucous membranes
 Pediatric: <9 years: not recommended; ≥9 years: same as adult
 Aklief *Pump:* 30, 45, 75 gm

TOPICAL RETINOID+ANTIMICROBIAL COMBINATIONS

Comment: Wash affected area with a soap-free cleanser; pat dry and wait 20-30 minutes; then apply sparingly to affected area; use only once daily in the evening. Avoid the eyes, ears, nostrils, and mouth.

▶ adapalene+benzoyl peroxide (G) apply a thin film once daily
 Pediatric: <18 years: not recommended
 Epiduo Gel *Gel:* adap 0.1%+benz 2.5% (45 gm)
 Epiduo Forte Gel *Pump gel:* adap 0.3%+benz 2.5% (15, 30, 45, 60 gm)

▶ tretinoin 0.1% cream+benzoyl peroxide 3%
 Pediatric: <9 years: not recommended; ≥9 years: same as adult
 Twyneo *Crm:* 0.1%/3% (50 gm bottle w. pump)
 Comment: Twyneo is a once-daily, fixed-dose, combination of *benzoyl peroxide+tretinoin* indicated for the treatment of acne vulgaris in patients ≥9 years of age. Core shell structures separate micro-encapsulated *tretinoin* crystals and *benzoyl peroxide* crystals, enabling inclusion of the two active ingredients in the cream. Severe hypersensitivity reactions, including anaphylaxis and angioedema, have been reported with use of *benzoyl peroxide* products. Pain, dryness, exfoliation, erythema, and irritation may occur with use of Twyneo. Avoid application of Twyneo to cuts, abrasions, and eczematous or sunburned skin. Minimize unprotected exposure to sunlight and sunlamps. Use sunscreen and

protective clothing when sun exposure cannot be avoided. While available studies cannot definitively establish the absence of risk, published data from multiple, prospective, controlled, observational studies on the use of topical *tretinoin* products during pregnancy have not identified an association with topical tretinoin and major birth defects or miscarriage. There are no data on the presence of **benzoyl peroxide** and *tretinoin* or its metabolites in human milk or effects on the breastfed infant. Developmental and health benefits of breastfeeding should be considered along with the mother's clinical need for **Twyneo** and any potential adverse effects on the breastfed infant from **Twyneo** or from the underlying maternal condition.

➤ *tretinoin+clindamycin* (G) apply a thin film once daily
  Pediatric: <18 years: not recommended
    Ziana *Gel:* tret 0.025%+clin 1.2% (30, 60 gm)

ORAL RETINOID

Comment: Oral retinoids are indicated only for severe recalcitrant nodular acne unresponsive to conventional therapy, including systemic antibiotics.

➤ *isotretinoin* initially 0.5-1 mg/kg/day in 2 divided doses; maintenance 0.5-2 mg/kg/day in 2 divided doses x 4-5 months; may repeat only if necessary 2 months following cessation of first treatment course
  Pediatric: <12 years: not recommended; ≥12 years: same as adult
    Absorica *Cap:* 10, 20, 25, 30, 35, 40 mg
    Absorica LD *Cap:* 8, 16, 20, 24, 28, 32 mg
    Comment: Absorica/Absorica LD strengths have different bioavailability and are not substitutable. **Absorica** dosing is 0.5 to 1 mg/kg/day administered in two divided doses without regard to meals for 15 to 20 weeks. **Absorica LD** dosing is 0.4 to 0.8 mg/kg/day administered in two divided doses without regard to meals for 15 to 20 weeks.
    Accutane *Cap:* 10, 20, 40 mg (parabens)
    Amnesteem *Cap:* 10, 20, 40 mg (soy)
  Comment: *Isotretinoin* is highly teratogenic and therefore female patients should be counseled prior to initiation of treatment as follows: Two negative pregnancy tests are required prior to initiation of treatment and monthly thereafter. Not for use in females who are or who may become pregnant or who are breastfeeding. Two effective methods of contraception should be used for 1 month prior to, during, and continuing for 1 month following completion of treatment. Low-dose *progestin* (mini-pill) may be an *inadequate* form of contraception. No refills; a new prescription is required every 30 days and prescriptions must be filled within 7 days. Serum lipids should be monitored until response is established (usually initially and again after 4 weeks). Bone growth, serum glucose, ESR, RBCs, WBCs, and liver enzymes should be monitored. Blood should not be donated during, or for 1 month after, completion of treatment. Avoid the sun and artificial UV light. *Isotretinoin* should be discontinued if any of the following occurs: visual disturbances, tinnitus, hearing impairment, rectal bleeding, pancreatitis, hepatitis, significant decrease in CBC, hyperlipidemia (particularly hypertriglyceridemia). Advise patients and/or their caregivers/families that oral *isotretinoin* may cause depression, psychosis, suicidal ideation, suicide attempts, and aggressive or violent behavior and to inform their healthcare provider immediately if any of these signs/symptoms occur. **Absorica/Absorica LD, Accutane,** and **Amnesteem** are available only through a restricted program called the iPLEDGE REMS and are available only from certified pharmacies participating in the program. Inform patients of reproductive potential that they must (1) sign an informed consent form to be enrolled in the program, (2) comply with the pregnancy testing and contraception requirements, (3) demonstrate comprehension of the safe-use conditions of the program every month, and (4) obtain the prescription within 7 days of the pregnancy test collection. Because of the potential for serious adverse reactions in nursing infants from *isotretinoin*, advise patients that breastfeeding is not recommended during treatment with oral *isotretinoin* and for at least 8 days after the last dose.

ACROMEGALY

GROWTH HORMONE RECEPTOR ANTAGONIST

➤ *pegvisomant* *Loading dose:* 40 mg SC; *Maintenance:* 10 mg SC daily; titrate by 5 mg (increments or decrements, based on insulin-like growth factor 1 [IGF-1] levels) every 4 to 6 weeks; max 30 mg/day
  Pediatric: <12 years: not recommended; ≥12 years: same as adult
    Somavert *Inj:* 10, 15, 20 mg
  Comment: Prior to initiation of *pegvisomant*, patients should have baseline fasting serum glucose, HgbA1c, serum K+ and Mg++, liver function tests (LFTs), EKG, and gall bladder ultrasound.

CYCLOHEXAPEPTIDE SOMATOSTATIN

➤ *pasireotide* administer SC in the thigh or abdomen; initial dose is 0.6 mg or 0.9 mg bid; titrate dose based on response and tolerability; for patients with moderate hepatic impairment *(Child-Pugh Class B),* the recommended initial dosage is 0.3 mg bid and max dose is 0.6 mg bid; avoid use in patients with severe hepatic impairment *(Child-Pugh Class C)*
  Pediatric: <12 years: not recommended; ≥12 years: same as adult
    Signifor LAR *Amp:* 0.3, 0.6, 0.9 mg/ml, single-dose, long-act rel (LAR), susp for inj

SOMATOSTATIN ANALOG
▷ *octreotide acetate*

Comment: *Octreotide acetate* is indicated for reduction of growth hormone (GH) and insulin-like growth factor 1 (IGF-1) (somatomedin C) in adult patients with acromegaly who have had inadequate response to or cannot be treated with surgical resection, pituitary irradiation, and bromocriptine mesylate at maximally tolerated doses. Monitor patients treated with *octreotide acetate* for cholelithiasis. Glucose monitoring is recommended and antidiabetic treatment may need adjustment. Hypothyroidism may occur; monitor thyroid levels periodically. Bradycardia, arrhythmia, or conduction abnormalities may occur; use with caution in at-risk patients. Common adverse side effects may include diarrhea, cholelithiasis, abdominal pain, and flatulence. Advise premenopausal females of the potential for an unintended pregnancy. Although acromegaly may lead to infertility, there are reports of pregnancy in acromegalic women. In women with active acromegaly who have been unable to become pregnant, normalization of GH and IGF-1 (somatomedin C) may restore fertility. Female patients of child-bearing potential should be advised to use adequate contraception during treatment with *octreotide*.

PARENTERAL FORMS
▷ *octreotide acetate*

Bynfezia Pen initiate at 50 mcg SC tid; typical dose is 100 mcg SC tid
  Prefilled Pen: 2.5 mg/ml (2,500 mcg/ml 2.8 ml), single-patient-use
Sandostatin initiate at 50 mcg SC tid; IGF-I (somatomedin C) levels every 2 weeks can be used to guide titration; goal is to achieve growth hormone (GH) levels <5 ng/ml or IGF-I (somatomedin C) levels <1.9 unit/ml (males) and <2.2 unit/ml (females); the most common effective dose is 100 mcg SC tid; some patients require up to 500 mcg SC tid for maximum effectiveness; >300 mcg/day seldom results in additional biochemical benefit; if dose increase fails to provide additional benefit, the dose should be reduced; IGF-I (somatomedin C) or GH levels should be re-evaluated at 6-month intervals
  Vial: 200, 1000 mcg/5 ml, multidose; *Amp:* 50, 100, 500 mcg/ml
Comment: **Sandostatin** should be withdrawn yearly for approximately 4 weeks from patients who have received irradiation to assess disease activity. If GH or IGF-I (somatomedin C) levels increase and signs and symptoms recur, **Sandostatin** therapy may be resumed.
Sandostatin LAR Depot after administering **Sandostatin** 50 mcg SC tid for 2 weeks, initiate **Sandostatin LAR Depot** suspension 20 mg IM intragluteally once every 4 weeks for 3 months
  Vial: 10, 20, 30 mg/6 ml, single-use
Comment: **Sandostatin LAR Depot** is indicated for the treatment of patients with acromegaly who have first responded to **Sandostatin** with achievement of GH levels <5 ng/ml or IGF-I (somatomedin C) levels <1.9 units/ml (males) and <2.2 units/ml (females).

ORAL FORM
▷ **Mycapssa** initiate at 40 mg daily, as 20 mg bid; titrate in increments of 20 mg; max 80 mg/day; monitor insulin-like growth factor 1 (IGF-1) levels and the patient's signs and symptoms every 2 weeks during the dose titration or as indicated once the maintenance dose is achieved; monitor IGF-1 levels and the patient's signs and symptoms monthly or as indicated; *end-stage renal disease (ESRD):* initiate at 20 mg once daily; titrate and adjust maintenance dose based on IGF-1 levels, signs and symptoms, and tolerability; take with a glass of water on an empty stomach, at least 1 hour before a meal or at least 2 hours after a meal
  Cap: 20 mg del-rel
Comment: **Mycapssa** is an oral form of *octreotide* indicated for long-term maintenance treatment of patients with acromegaly who have responded to and tolerated treatment with parenteral *octreotide* or *lanreotide*. The most common adverse reactions (incidence >10%) are nausea, diarrhea, headache, arthralgia, asthenia, hyperhidrosis, peripheral swelling, increased blood glucose, vomiting, abdominal discomfort, dyspepsia, sinusitis, and osteoarthritis. Concomitant use of **Mycapssa** with other drugs mainly metabolized by CYP3A4 that have a narrow therapeutic index (e.g., *quinidine*) should be used with caution.

ACTINIC KERATOSIS (AK)

▷ *aminolevulinic acid 10%* clean and prepare all lesions prior to applying gel 1 mm thick and include 5 mm of the surrounding skin; max application area is 20 cm² and max 2 gm per treatment; apply an occlusive dressing x 3 hours; photodynamic therapy involves preparation of lesions, application of **Ameluz**, occlusion, and illumination with BF-RhodoLED only by a qualified healthcare provider; remove the remaining gel at the end of the treatment; may re-treat in 3 months after the initial treatment; see BF-RhodoLED user manual for detailed lamp safety and operating instructions
  Pediatric: <18 years: not recommended; ≥18 years: same as adult
  Ameluz *Gel:* 10% (2 gm tube) 100 mg/gm of *aminolevulinic acid hcl* (equivalent to 78 mg/gm *aminolevulinic acid*) (xanthan gum, soybean phosphatidylcholine, polysorbate 80, medium-chain triglycerides, dibasic sodium phosphate, monobasic sodium phosphate, propylene glycol, sodium benzoate, isopropyl alcohol)
  Comment: Ameluz (*aminolevulinic acid*) 10% gel, a porphyrin precursor, in combination with photodynamic therapy using BF-RhodoLED lamp, is indicated for the lesion- and field-directed treatment

of actinic keratoses of mild-to-moderate severity on the face and scalp. The most common adverse reactions (incidence ≥10%) have been application site erythema, pain/burning, irritation, edema, pruritus, exfoliation, scab formation, induration, and vesicles. Concomitant use of other photosensitizing agents may increase the risk of phototoxic reaction to photodynamic therapy (e.g., St. John's wort, *griseofulvin*, thiazide diuretics, sulfonylureas, phenothiazines, sulfonamides, quinolones, and tetracyclines). The patient and the healthcare provider must wear protective eyewear before and during operation of the BF-RhodoLED lamp. Treated lesions should be protected from sunlight exposure for 48 hours posttreatment. Special care should be taken to avoid bleeding during lesion preparation in patients with inherited or acquired a coagulation disorder. Avoid direct contact of **Ameluz** with the eyes and mucous membranes. There are no human or animal reproductive studies of **Ameluz** use in pregnancy to inform a drug-associated risk. Systemic absorption of *aminolevulinic acid* is negligible. No data are available regarding the presence of *aminolevulinic acid* in human milk or effects on the breastfed infant; however, breastfeeding is not expected to result in infant exposure to the drug due to negligible systemic absorption.

➤ *diclofenac sodium* 3% (G) apply to lesions bid x 60-90 days; pregnancy: not recommended ≥30 weeks
Pediatric: <12 years: not established; ≥12 years: same as adult
    Solaraze Gel *Gel:* 3% (50 gm) (benzyl alcohol)
    Comment: *Diclofenac* is contraindicated with **aspirin** allergy. As with other NSAIDs, **Solaraze Gel** should be avoided in late pregnancy (≥30 weeks) because it may cause premature closure of the ductus arteriosus.
    Voltaren Gel apply qid; avoid non-intact skin
        Gel: 1% (100 gm)

➤ *fluorouracil* (G) apply to lesion(s) daily-bid until erosion occurs, usually 2-4 weeks
Pediatric: <12 years: not recommended; ≥12 years: same as adult
    Carac *Crm:* 0.5% (30 gm)
    Efudex (G) *Crm:* 5% (25 gm); *Soln:* 2, 5% (10 ml w. dropper)
    Fluoroplex *Crm:* 1% (30 gm); *Soln:* 1% (30 ml w. dropper)

➤ *imiquimod* (G)
Pediatric: <18 years: not recommended; ≥18 years: same as adult
    Aldara (G) rub into lesions before bedtime and remove with soap and water 8 hours later; treat 2 times per week; max 16 weeks
        Crm: 5% (single-use pkts/carton)
    Zyclara rub into lesions before bedtime and remove with soap and water 8 hours later; treat for 2-week cycles separated by a 2-week no-treatment cycle; max 2 packs per application; max 1 treatment course per area
        Crm: 3.75% (single-use pkts; 28/carton) (parabens)

➤ *ingenol mebutate* (G) limit application to one contiguous skin area of about 25 cm² using one unit-dose tube; allow treated area to dry for 15 minutes; wash hands immediately after application; may remove with soapy water after 6 hours; *Face and scalp:* apply 0.015% gel to lesions once daily x 3 days; *Trunk and extremities:* apply 0.05% gel to lesions once daily x 2 days
Pediatric: <18 years: not recommended; ≥18 years: same as adult
    Picato *Gel:* 0.015% (3 single-use tubes), 0.05% (2 single-use tubes)

Src KINASE AND TUBULIN POLYMERIZATION INHIBITOR

➤ *tirbanibulin* apply to the treatment field on the face or scalp once daily for 5 consecutive days using 1 single-dose packet per application
Pediatric: <18 years: not established; ≥18 years: same as adult
    Klisyri *Oint:* 1%, single-dose pkts (25 mg/pkt)
    Comment: **Klisyri** *(tirbanibulin)* is a first-in-class dual Src kinase and tubulin polymerization inhibitor for the topical treatment of actinic keratosis on the face or scalp. The most common adverse reactions (incidence ≥2%) have been local skin reactions, application site pruritus, and application site pain.

ADRENOCORTICAL INSUFFICIENCY

CORTICOSTEROID

➤ *hydrocortisone granules* individualize the dose, using the lowest possible dosage; *Recommended starting replacement dose:* 8 to 10 mg/m² daily (higher doses may be needed based on the patient's age and symptoms of the disease; lower starting doses may be sufficient in patients with residual but decreased endogenous cortisol production; round the dose to the nearest 0.5 mg or 1 mg); more than one capsule may be needed to supply the required dose; divide the total daily dose into 3 doses and administer tid; older patients may have their daily dose divided by 2 and administered bid; do not swallow the capsule, do not chew or crush the granules; see the mfr pkg insert for full prescribing information and for detailed administration instructions
    Alkindi Sprinkle *Cap:* 0.5, 1, 2, 5 mg oral granules
    Comment: **Alkindi Sprinkle** is indicated as replacement therapy in pediatric patients with adrenocortical insufficiency. Use the minimum dosage to achieve desired clinical response. Common adverse reactions for corticosteroids include fluid retention, alteration in glucose tolerance, elevation in blood pressure, behavioral and mood changes, increased appetite, and weight gain. Corticosteroids decrease bone

(continued)

formation and increase bone resorption, which may lead to inhibition of bone growth and development of osteoporosis. Use may be associated with severe psychiatric adverse reactions, such as euphoria, mania, psychosis with hallucinations, and delirium or depression. Symptoms typically emerge within a few days or weeks of starting the treatment. Most reactions resolve after either dose reduction or withdrawal. Cataracts, glaucoma, and central serous chorioretinopathy have been reported with prolonged use of high doses. Monitor patients for blurred vision or other visual disturbances. Prolonged use with supraphysiologic doses may cause Cushing's syndrome. Monitor patients for signs and symptoms of Cushing's syndrome every 6 months; pediatric patients under 1 year of age may require more frequent monitoring. Long-term use in excessive doses may cause growth retardation; monitor the patient's growth. Excessive doses may increase the risks of new infections or exacerbation of latent infections with any pathogen, including any viral, bacterial, fungal, protozoan, or helminthic infections. Monitor patients for signs and symptoms of infections. Treat all infections seriously and initiate stress dosing of corticosteroids early. Undertreatment or sudden discontinuation of therapy may lead to adrenocortical insufficiency, adrenal crisis, and death. Increase the dose during periods of stress. Switch patients who are vomiting, severely ill, or unable to take oral medications to parenteral corticosteroid formulations.

AFRICAN SLEEPING SICKNESS (*HUMAN AFRICAN TRYPANOSOMIASIS* [HAT])

NITROIMIDAZOLE ANTIBACTERIAL

▷ *fexinidazole* (*African trypanosomiasis* [African sleeping sickness]); administer once daily with food, at about the same time each day; do not break or crush tablets; see dosing table below

Recommended Dosage of Fexinidazole Tablets for Patients >6 Years, >20 kg				
Age/Wt	Dose Type	Dose/Day	# Tablets	# Days
>6 years >35 kg	Loading	1,800 mg	3	4
	Maintenance	1,200 mg	2	6
>6 years 20-35kg	Loading	1,200 mg	2	4
	Maintenance	600 mg	1	6

Pediatric: <6 years: safety and efficacy not established; ≥6 years, ≥20 kg: administer once daily with food each, at about the same time each day; do not break or crush tablets; see dosing table above
Fexinidazole Tablets *Tab:* 600 mg
Comment: Fexinidazole Tablets is a nitroimidazole antimicrobial indicated for the treatment of both first-stage (hemolymphatic) and second-stage (meningoencephalitic) human African trypanosomiasis (HAT) due to *Trypanosoma brucei gambiense* in patients ≥6 years of age and weighing ≥20 kg. *Limitations of use:* Due to the decreased efficacy observed in patients with severe second-stage HAT (cerebrospinal fluid white blood cell count [CSF-WBC] >100 cells/μL) due to *T. brucei gambiense disease*, **Fexinidazole Tablets** should only be used in these patients if there are no other available treatment options. *Contraindications to use:* known hypersensitivity to *fexinidazole* and/or *nitroimidazole* drugs, hepatic impairment, and Cockayne syndrome. Avoid use in patients with severe renal impairment. Avoid use of herbal medicines and supplements (see mfr pkg insert for complete list of clinically significant drug interactions). The most common adverse reactions (incidence >10%) have been headache, vomiting, insomnia, nausea, asthenia, tremor, decreased appetite, dizziness, hypocalcemia, dyspepsia, back pain, upper abdominal pain, and hyperkalemia. *Fexinidazole* has decreased efficacy in severe HAT caused by *T. brucei gambiense*. Prolongation of the QT interval due to **Fexinidazole Tablets** occurs in a concentration-dependent manner. Avoid use of *fexinidazole* in patients with known prolongation, proarrhythmic conditions, and concomitant use with drugs that prolong the QT interval, those that block cardiac potassium channels, and/or those that induce bradycardia or are inducers of hepatic CYP450. Neuropsychiatric adverse reactions such as agitation, anxiety, abnormal behavior, depression, suicidal ideation, nightmares, hallucination, and personality change have been observed during treatment with *fexinidazole*; inform patients and their caregivers of the risk. If any of these adverse reactions occur or if the patient has a known psychiatric disorder, consider alternative therapy or increased monitoring of the patient and/or hospitalization. Avoid concomitant use of drugs which may cause neutropenia and monitor leukocyte count periodically. Monitor patients with neutropenia for symptoms or signs of infection. Evaluate liver-related laboratory tests at the start and during treatment. Alcohol use when the patient is receiving treatment with a *nitroimidazole*-class drug can cause a disulfiram-like reaction, which may include a psychotic reaction. Advise patients to avoid consumption of alcohol during treatment and for at least 48 hours after completing treatment. There are adverse effects on maternal and fetal outcomes associated with untreated HAT due to *T. brucei gambiense* in pregnancy and disease progression may occur. Pregnant females should be treated for HAT due to *T. brucei gambiense* during pregnancy to prevent vertical transmission. For timing of treatment

during pregnancy, consider the benefits to the mother and the potential risks to the fetus. Available data from clinical trials of *fexinidazole* use in pregnant females have been insufficient to evaluate for a drug-associated risk of major birth defects or miscarriage. In embryo/fetal animal studies, there were no effects on prenatal development when *fexinidazole* was administered during organogenesis at a dose similar to the human clinical dose based on area under the curve (AUC) comparisons. There are no data on the presence of *fexinidazole* in human milk and there are no reports of adverse effects to the breastfed infant associated with *fexinidazole* exposure through breast milk. Developmental and health benefits of breastfeeding should be considered along with the mother's clinical need for **Fexinidazole Tablets** and any potential adverse effects on the breastfed infant from *fexinidazole* or from the underlying maternal condition.

ALCOHOL DEPENDENCE, DETOXIFICATION/ALCOHOL WITHDRAWAL SYNDROME

ALCOHOL WITHDRAWAL SYNDROME
Comment: Total length of time of a given detoxification regimen and/or length of time of treatment at any dose reduction level may be extended based on patient-specific factors, including potential or actual seizure, hallucinosis, and increased sympathetic nervous system activity (severe anxiety, unwanted elevation in vital signs). If any of these symptoms are anticipated or occur, revert to an earlier step in the dosing regimen to stabilize the patient, extend the detoxification timeline, and consider appropriate adjunctive drug treatments (e.g., anticonvulsants, antipsychotic agents, antihypertensive agents, sedative hypnotics agents).

▷ *chlordiazepoxide* (IV)(G)
  Pediatric: <18 years: not recommended; ≥18 years: same as adult
    Librium 50-100 mg q 6 hours x 24-72 hours; then q 8 hours x 24-72 hours; then q 12 hours x 24-72 hours; then daily x 24-72 hours
      Cap: 5, 10, 25 mg
    Librium Injectable 50-100 mg IM or IV; then 25-50 mg IM tid-qid prn; max 300 mg/day
      Inj: 100 mg
▷ *clorazepate* (IV)(G) in the following dosage regimen: *Day 1:* 30 mg initially, followed by 30-60 mg in divided doses; *Day 2:* 45-90 mg in divided doses; *Day 3:* 22.5-45 mg in divided doses; *Day 4:* 15-30 mg in divided doses; thereafter, gradually reduce the daily dose to 7.5-15 mg; then discontinue when the patient's condition is stable; max dose 90 mg/day
  Pediatric: <18 years: not recommended; ≥18 years: same as adult
    Tranxene *Tab:* 3.75, 7.5, 15 mg
    Tranxene T-Tab *Tab:* 3.75*, 7.5*, 15*mg
▷ *diazepam* (IV)(G) 2-10 mg q 6 hours x 24-72 hours; then q 8 hours x 24-72 hours; then q 12 hours x 24-72 hours; then daily x 24-72 hours
  Pediatric: <18 years: not recommended; ≥18 years: same as adult
    Diastat *Rectal gel delivery system:* 2.5 mg
    Diastat AcuDial *Rectal gel delivery system:* 10, 20 mg
    Valium *Tab:* 2*, 5*, 10*mg
    Valium Injectable *Vial:* 5 mg/ml (10 ml); *Amp:* 5 mg/ml (2 ml); *Prefilled syringe:* 5 mg/ml (5 ml)
    Valium Intensol Oral Solution *Conc oral soln:* 5 mg/ml (30 ml w. dropper) (alcohol 19%)
    Valium Oral Solution *Oral soln:* 5 mg/5 ml (500 ml) (wintergreen-spice)
▷ *oxazepam* 10-15 mg tid-qid x 24-72 hours; decrease dose and/or frequency every 24-72 hours; total length of therapy 5-14 days; max 120 mg/day
  Pediatric: <18 years: not recommended; ≥18 years: same as adult
    Cap: 10, 15, 30 mg

ABSTINENCE THERAPY
Gamma-Aminobutyric Acid (GABA) Taurine Analog
▷ *acamprosate* (G) 666 mg tid; begin therapy during abstinence; continue during relapse; *CrCl 30-50-ml/min:* max 333 mg tid; *CrCl <30 ml/min:* contraindicated
  Pediatric: <18 years: not recommended; ≥18 years: same as adult
    Campral *Tab:* 333 mg ext-rel
    Comment: Campral does not eliminate or diminish alcohol withdrawal symptoms.

AVERSION THERAPY
▷ *disulfiram* (G)
  Pediatric: <18 years: not recommended; ≥18 years: same as adult
    Antabuse 500 mg once daily x 1 to 2 weeks; then 250 mg once daily
      Tab: 250, 500 mg; *Chew tab:* 200, 500 mg
    Comment: *Disulfiram* use requires informed consent. Contraindications include severe cardiac disease, psychosis, and concomitant use of *isoniazid, phenytoin, paraldehyde*, and topical and systemic alcohol-containing products. Approximately 20% remains in the system for 1 week after discontinuation.

ALLERGIC REACTION: GENERAL

Oral Second-Generation Antihistamines *see* Appendix BB. Drugs for the Management of Allergy, Cough, and Cold Symptoms online at https://connect.springerpub.com/content/reference-book/978-0-8261-7935-7/back-matter/part02/back-matter/bmatter27
Topical Corticosteroids *see* Appendix J. Topical Corticosteroids by Potency
Parenteral Corticosteroids *see* Appendix L. Parenteral Corticosteroids
Oral Corticosteroids *see* Appendix M. Oral Corticosteroids

FIRST-GENERATION PARENTERAL ANTIHISTAMINE
➤ *diphenhydramine* (G) 25-50 mg IM immediately; then q 6 hours prn
  Pediatric: <12 years: see mfr pkg insert: 1.25 mg/kg up to 25 mg IM x 1 dose; then every 6 hours prn
    Benadryl Injectable *Vial:* 50 mg/ml (1 ml single-use); 50 mg/ml (10 ml multidose); *Amp:* 10 mg/ml (1 ml); *Prefilled syringe:* 50 mg/ml (1 ml)

FIRST-GENERATION ORAL ANTIHISTAMINES
➤ *diphenhydramine* (G) 25-50 mg q 6-8 hours; max 100 mg/day
  Pediatric: <2 years: <u>not</u> recommended; 2-6 years: 6.25 mg every 4-6 hours; max 37.5 mg/day; >6-12 years: 12.5-25 mg every 4-6 hours, max 150 mg/day; >12 years: same as adult
    Benadryl (OTC) *Chew tab:* 12.5 mg (grape) (phenylalanine); *Liq:* 12.5 mg/5 ml (4, 8 oz); *Cap:* 25 mg; *Tab:* 25 mg; *Dye-free soft gel:* 25 mg; *Dye-free liq:* 12.5 mg/5 ml (4, 8 oz)
➤ *hydroxyzine* (G) 50-100 mg qid; max 600 mg/day
  Pediatric: <6 years: 50 mg/day divided qid; ≥6 years: 50-100 mg/day divided qid
    Atarax *Tab:* 10, 25, 50, 100 mg; *Syr:* 10 mg/5 ml (alcohol 0.5%)
    Vistaril *Cap:* 25, 50, 100 mg; *Oral susp:* 25 mg/5 ml (4 oz) (lemon)

ALLERGIES: MULTI-FOOD

Comment: Eight food types cause about 90% of food allergy reactions—*milk* (mostly in children), *eggs, peanuts, tree nuts* (e.g., walnuts, almonds, pine nuts, Brazil nuts, and pecans), *soy, wheat* (and other grains with gluten, including barley, rye, and oats), *fish* (mostly in adults), and *shellfish* (mostly in adults). Combining *omalizumab* with oral immunotherapy (OIT) significantly improves the effectiveness of OIT in children with multiple food allergies, according to the results of a recent study. Researchers conducted a blinded, phase 2 clinical trial including children aged 4 to 15 years who had multi-food allergies validated by double-blind, placebo-controlled food challenges. Participants were randomly assigned (3:1) to either receive *omalizumab* with multi-food oral immunotherapy <u>or</u> placebo. *Omalizumab* and placebo were administered for 16 weeks, with OIT beginning at 8 weeks. Overall, at week 36, a significantly greater proportion of the *omalizumab*-treated participants passed the double-blind, placebo-controlled food challenges compared with placebo (83% vs 33%). No serious <u>or</u> severe adverse events were reported. In multi-food allergic patients, *omalizumab* improves the efficacy of multi-food oral immunotherapy and enables safe and rapid desensitization.

IMMUNOGLOBULIN E (IGE) BLOCKER (IMMUNOGLOBULIN G1K [IGG1K] MONOCLONAL ANTIBODY)
➤ *omalizumab* 150-375 mg SC every 2-4 weeks based on body weight and pretreatment serum total IgE level; max 150 mg/injection site; approved for patient self-administration after education by a qualified healthcare provider
  Pediatric: <12 years: <u>not</u> recommended; 30-90 kg + IgE >30-100 IU/ml: 150 mg every 4 weeks; 90-150 kg + IgE >30-100 IU/ml <u>or</u> 30-90 kg + IgE >100-200 IU/ml <u>or</u> 30-60 kg + IgE >200-300 IU/ml: 300 mg q4h; >90-150 kg + IgE >100-200 IU/ml <u>or</u> >60-90 kg + IgE >200-300 IU/ml: <u>or</u> 30-70 kg + IgE >300-400 IU/ml: 225 mg every 2 weeks; >90-150 kg + IgE >200-300 IU/ml <u>or</u> >70-90 kg + IgE >300-400 IU/ml <u>or</u> 30-70 kg + IgE >400-500 IU/ml <u>or</u> 30-60 kg + IgE >500-600 IU/ml <u>or</u> 30-60 kg + IgE >600-700 IU/ml 375 mg every 2 weeks; ≥12 years: same as adult
    Xolair *Vial:* 150 mg, single-dose, pwdr for SC injection after reconstitution; *Prefilled syringe:* 75 mg/0.5 ml, 150 mg/1 ml, single-dose (preservative-free)

ALOPECIA AREATA

JANUS KINASE (JAK) INHIBITOR
➤ *baricitinib* *Recommended dose:* 2 mg once daily; take with <u>or</u> without food; increase dose to 4 mg once daily if the response to treatment is <u>not</u> adequate; for patients with nearly complete <u>or</u> complete scalp hair loss, with <u>or</u> without substantial eyelash <u>or</u> eyebrow hair loss, consider treating with 4 mg once daily; once patients achieve an adequate response to treatment with 4 mg, decrease the dosage to 2 mg once daily
  Pediatric: safety and efficacy <u>not</u> established
    Olumiant *Tab:* 1, 2, 4 mg
    Comment: Olumiant is indicated for the treatment of adult patients with severe alopecia areata. See the mfr pkg insert for full prescribing information including a boxed warning regarding serious infections, mortality, malignancy, major adverse cardiovascular events (MACE), and thrombosis. Advise patients

(continued)

of the potential benefits and risks of treatment with **Olumiant** and advise patients to read the FDA-approved patient labeling (Medication Guide). Limited data on **Olumiant** use in human pregnancy are not sufficient to inform a drug-associated risk of major birth defects or miscarriage. Exclude pregnancy prior to initiating treatment with **Olumiant**. Females of reproductive potential should be informed of the risks to the fetus and advised to use effective contraception during treatment. Because of the potential for serious adverse reactions in breastfed infants, advise **Olumiant**-treated mothers not to breastfeed. Report pregnancies to Eli Lilly at 1-800-LillyRx (1-800-545-5979). To report suspected adverse reactions, contact Eli Lilly at 1-800-LillyRx (1-800-545-5979) or FDA at 1-800-FDA-1088 or www.fda.gov/medwatch.

ALPHA-1 ANTITRYPSIN (AAT) DEFICIENCY

Comment: Alpha-1 antitrypsin (AAT, a major circulating serine protease inhibitor) deficiency is a common genetic (autosomal co-dominant) condition characterized by low serum levels of AAT. Absence of deficiency of AAT accelerates lung tissue degradation and increases the risk of development of chronic obstructive pulmonary disease (COPD) and early-onset emphysema, particularly in smokers. Extrapulmonary complications of ATT deficiency include liver disease (onset as early as childhood), granulomatosis with polyangiitis (GPA, previously known as Wegener's granulomatosis), vasculitis, and necrotizing panniculitis. Management of symptomatic AAT and exacerbations includes bronchodilators (LABA/LAMA) and inhaled corticosteroids in line with the management of COPD symptoms and exacerbations (Global Initiative for Chronic Obstructive Lung Disease [GOLD]). Management of ATT includes smoking cessation; avoidance of environmental pollutants; immunizations against influenza, pneumonia, and hepatitis; antibiotic therapy as needed (with *amoxicillin* or a macrolide); and management in a critical care setting for acute respiratory distress/failure. Pharmacologic management of AAT deficiency may also include AAT infusion therapy (with alpha-1 proteinase inhibitor, the only treatment to slow disease progression). *Brand names:* **Aralast, Glassia, Prolastin, Prolastin-C,** and **Zemaira.**

▷ *alpha-1 proteinase inhibitor (human)* (G) recommended dosage of **Aralast** is 60 mg/kg administered once weekly via IV infusion, by a qualified healthcare provider, at a rate not exceeding 0.08 ml/kg; if any adverse event occurs, the rate should be reduced or the infusion interrupted until the symptoms subside; the infusion may then be resumed at a rate tolerated; refer to mfr pkg insert for detailed preparation directions and administration protocol
Pediatric: safety and effectiveness in pediatric patients not established
    Aralast *Vial:* 25 ml/0.5 gm, 50 ml/1 gm (1 single-use vial of product + 1 single-use vial of diluent + 1 double-ended transfer needle and 1-20 micron filter; sterile, stable, lyophilized preparation of preservative-free purified human alpha-1-proteinase inhibitor (a1-PI), also known as alpha-1-antitrypsin, for reconstitution with diluent provided; do not administer or mix with other agents or diluting solutions; when reconstituted, concentration of a1-PI is not less than 16 mg/ml and the specific activity is not less than 0.55 mg active a1-PI/mg total protein; refrigerate; do not freeze; administer within 3 hours after the reconstituted product is warmed to room temperature; discard partially used vials
    Comment: Aralast is an a1-PI (human) indicated for chronic augmentation therapy in patients with congenital deficiency of a1-PI with clinically evident emphysema. Clinical and biochemical studies have demonstrated that with such therapy, **Aralast** is effective in maintaining target serum a1-PI trough levels and increasing a1-PI levels in epithelial lining fluid (ELF). Clinical data demonstrating the long-term effects of chronic augmentation or replacement therapy of individuals with **Aralast** are not available. **Aralast** is not indicated as therapy for lung disease patients in whom congenital a1-PI deficiency has not been established. **Aralast** is contraindicated in individuals with selective immunoglobulin A (IgA) deficiencies (IgA level <15 mg/dl) who have known antibody against IgA since they may experience a severe reaction, including anaphylaxis, to IgA which may be present. **Aralast** is prepared from large pools of human plasma by using the Cohn-Oncley cold alcohol fractionation process, followed by purification steps including polyethylene glycol and zinc chloride precipitations and ion exchange chromatography. To reduce the risk of viral transmission, the manufacturing process includes treatment with a solvent detergent (SD) mixture (tri-n-butyl phosphate and polysorbate 80) to inactivate enveloped viral agents, such as HIV and hepatitis B and C. In addition, a nanofiltration step is incorporated prior to final sterile filtration to reduce the risk of transmission of non-enveloped viral agents. It is not known whether **Aralast** can cause fetal harm when administered to pregnant females or can affect reproductive capacity. It is not known whether a1-PI is excreted in human milk.

ALZHEIMER'S DISEASE

NUTRITIONAL SUPPLEMENT

▷ *l-methylfolate calcium (as Metafolin)+methylcobalamin+n-acetyl cysteine* take 1 cap once daily
    Cerefolin *Cap:* metafo 5.6 mg+methyl 2 mg+n-ace cys 600 mg (gluten-free, yeast-free, lactose-free)
    Comment: Cerefolin is indicated in the dietary management of patients treated for early memory loss, with emphasis on those at risk for neurovascular oxidative stress, hyperhomocysteinemia, mild-to-moderate cognitive impairment with or without vitamin B12 deficiency, vascular dementia, or Alzheimer's disease.

AMYLOID BETA-DIRECTED ANTIBODY

▷ *aducanumab-avwa Dilute dose* in 100 ml of 0.9% NaCl inj; *administer* via IV infusion over approximately 1 hour, with a 0.2 or 0.22 micron in-line filter; *Dose titration* is required for treatment initiation; *Recommended maintenance dose:* 10 mg/kg via IV infusion once every four weeks; confirm the presence of amyloid beta pathology prior to initiating treatment; obtain a recent (within 1 year) brain MRI prior to initiating treatment and prior to the 5th, 7th, 9th, and 12th infusions; if radiographically observed amyloid-related imaging abnormalities (ARIA) occurs, treatment recommendations are based on type, severity, and presence of symptoms.

> Aduhelm *Vial:* 170 mg/1.7 ml (100 mg/ml), 300 mg/3 ml (100 mg/ml), single-dose, soln for dilution in 100 ml of 0.9% NaCl inj and IV infusion with a 0.2 or 0.22 micron in-line filter (not included)
> **Comment:** Treatment with **Aduhelm** should be initiated in patients with mild cognitive impairment or mild dementia stage of disease, the population in which treatment was initiated in clinical trials. There are no safety or effectiveness data on initiating treatment at earlier or later stages of the disease than were studied. This indication is approved under accelerated approval based on reduction in amyloid beta plaques observed in patients treated with **Aduhelm**. Continued approval for this indication may be contingent upon verification of clinical benefit in confirmatory trial(s). Enhanced clinical vigilance for ARIA is recommended during the first 8 doses of treatment with **Aduhelm**, particularly during titration. If the patient experiences symptoms which could be suggestive of ARIA, clinical evaluation should be performed, including MRI testing if indicated. Angioedema and urticaria have occurred; if a hypersensitivity reaction occurs, promptly discontinue the infusion of **Aduhelm** and initiate appropriate therapy. The common reported adverse reactions (incidence ≥10% compared to placebo) have been (ARIA-E) [brain], headache, (ARIA-H) [brain] microhemorrhage, (ARIA-H) [brain] superficial siderosis, and fall. If radiographically observed ARIA occurs, treatment recommendations are based on type, severity, and presence of symptoms.

▷ *lecanemab-irmb Recommended dose:* 10 mg/kg (e.g., 10 mg x 70 kg = 700 mg); dilute dose in 0.9% NaCl; administer via IV infusion over approximately 1 hour via a terminal low-protein binding 0.2 micron in-line filter once every 2 weeks; *Infusion-related reaction:* infusion rate may be reduced or the infusion may be discontinued, and appropriate treatment administered as clinically indicated; consider premedication at subsequent dosing with antihistamines, non-steroidal anti-inflammatory drugs, or corticosteroids

> Leqembi *Vial:* 200 mg/2 ml, 500 mg/5 ml (100 mg/ml), single-dose, soln for dilution and IV infusion
> **Comment:** **Leqembi** is an amyloid beta-directed antibody indicated for the treatment of Alzheimer's disease. **Leqembi** was approved under the Accelerated Approval Pathway (AAP). Continued approval for this indication may be contingent upon verification of clinical benefit in a confirmatory trial. Treatment with **Leqembi** should be initiated in patients with mild cognitive impairment or mild dementia stage of disease, the population in which treatment was initiated in clinical trials. There are no safety or efficacy data on initiating treatment at earlier or later stages of the disease than were studied. Confirm the presence of amyloid beta pathology prior to initiating treatment. Obtain a recent (within 1 year) brain MRI prior to initiating treatment to evaluate for preexisting amyloid-related imaging abnormalities (ARIA), and repeat the MRI prior to the 5th, 7th, and 14th infusion. If radiographically observed ARIA occurs, treatment recommendations are based on type, severity, and presence of symptoms. There are no contraindications to Alzheimer's disease treatment with **Leqembi**. The most common adverse reactions (10% and higher incidence compared to placebo) reported have been infusion-related reactions, headache, and ARIA-edema.

REVERSIBLE ANTICHOLINESTERASE INHIBITORS (RAIs)

Comment: Reversible anticholinesterase inhibitor (RAI) drugs do not halt disease progression. They are indicated for early-stage disease; not effective in severe dementia. If treatment is stopped for more than several days, retitrate from lowest dose. Side effects include nausea, anorexia, dyspepsia, diarrhea, headache, and dizziness. Side effects tend to resolve with continued treatment. Peak cognitive improvements are seen 12 weeks into therapy (increased spontaneity, reduced apathy, lessened confusion, and improved attention, conversational language, and performance of daily routines).

▷ *donepezil* (G) initially 5 mg q HS, increase to 10 mg after 4-6 weeks as needed; max 23 mg/day

> Aricept *Tab:* 5, 10, 23 mg
> Aricept ODT *ODT tab:* 5, 10 mg orally-disint

▷ *donepezil transdermal system Recommended starting dose:* 5 mg/day; after 4 to 6 weeks, may increase dose to the max recommended 10 mg/day; if the patient has been on 5 mg/day oral *donepezil* for at least 4-6 weeks, or on 10 mg/day of oral *donepezil*, the recommended starting **Adlarity** dose is 10 mg/day; store in the refrigerator between 2°C to 8°C (36°F to 46°F); do not freeze; allow the pouch to reach room temperature before opening and removing the new transdermal system for application; remove and replace once weekly on the same day each week
Pediatric: not indicated

> Adlarity *Transdermal system:* 5, 10 mg/day (4 pouches/carton)
> **Comment:** **Adlarity** is a once-weekly transdermal formulation of the approved acetylcholinesterase inhibitor *donepezil* indicated for the treatment of patients with mild, moderate, and severe dementia of the Alzheimer's type. Contraindications to **Adlarity** are known hypersensitivity to *donepezil* or to *piperidine derivatives* or history of allergic contact dermatitis with use of **Adlarity**. Because of the

mechanism of action, cholinesterase inhibitors, including **Adlarity**, have the potential to interfere with the activity of anticholinergic medications. Cholinomimetics and other cholinesterase inhibitors have a synergistic effect which may be expected when **Adlarity** is administered concurrently with *succinylcholine* (e.g., exaggerated succinylcholine-type muscle relaxation during anesthesia) or similar neuromuscular blocking agents (e.g., vagotonic effects on the sinoatrial [SA] and atrioventricular [AV] nodes manifesting as bradycardia <u>or</u> heart block), and should be prescribed with caution to patients with a history of asthma <u>or</u> obstructive pulmonary disease (e.g., COPD), <u>or</u> bladder outflow obstruction. **Adlarity** can cause vomiting; patients should be observed closely at initiation of treatment and after dose increase. Patients should be monitored closely for symptoms of active <u>or</u> occult gastrointestinal (GI) bleeding, especially those at increased risk of developing ulcers. Cholinomimetics, including **Adlarity**, are believed to have some potential to cause generalized convulsions. The most common adverse reactions (>5% with *donepezil* tablets and twice the placebo rate) have been nausea, diarrhea, insomnia, vomiting, muscle cramps, fatigue, and anorexia. To report suspected adverse reactions, contact Corium 1-800-910-8432 <u>or</u> FDA at 1-800-FDA-1088 <u>or</u> www.fda.gov/medwatch.

▷ *galantamine* initially 4 mg bid x at least 4 weeks; usual maintenance 8 mg bid; max 16 mg bid
    Razadyne *Tab:* 4, 8, 12 mg
    Razadyne ER *Tab:* 8, 16, 24 mg ext-rel
    Razadyne Oral Solution *Oral soln:* 4 mg/ml (100 ml w. calib pipette)

▷ *rivastigmine* (G)
    Exelon initially 1.5 mg bid, increase every 2 weeks as needed; max 12 mg/day; take with food
        Cap: 1.5, 3, 4.5, 6 mg
    Exelon Oral Solution initially 1.5 mg bid; may increase by 1.5 mg bid at intervals of at least 2 weeks; usual range 6-12 mg/day; max 12 mg/day; if stopped, restart at the lowest dose and retitrate; may take directly from syringe <u>or</u> mix with water, fruit juice, <u>or</u> cola
        Oral soln: 2 mg/ml (120 ml w. dose syringe)
    Exelon Patch initially apply 4.6 mg/24 hr patch; if tolerated, may increase to 9.5 mg/24 hr patch after 4 weeks; max 13.3 mg/24 hr; change patch daily; apply to clean, dry, hairless, intact skin; rotate application site; allow 14 days before applying new patch to the same site
        Patch: 4.6, 9.5, 13.3 mg/24 hr trans-sys (30/carton)

▷ *tacrine* initially 10 mg qid, increase 40 mg/day q 4 weeks as needed; max 160 mg/day
    Cognex *Cap:* 10, 20, 30, 40 mg
    Comment: Transaminase levels should be checked every 3 months while taking **Cognex**.

N-METHYL-D-ASPARTATE (NMDA) RECEPTOR ANTAGONIST

▷ *memantine* (G)
    Namenda initially 5 mg once daily; titrate weekly in 5 mg/day increments; *Week 2:* 5 mg bid; *Week 3:* 5 mg AM and 10 mg PM; *Week 4:* 10 mg bid; *CrCl 5-29 ml/min:* max 5 mg bid
        Tab: 5, 10 mg
    Namenda Oral Solution initially 5 mg once daily; titrate weekly in 5 mg increments administered bid
        Oral soln: 2 mg/ml (360 ml) (peppermint) (sugar-free, alcohol-free)
    Namenda Titration Pak
        Cap: 7 x 7 mg, 7 x 14 mg, 7 x 21 mg, 7 x 28 mg/pck
    Namenda XR initially 7 mg once daily; titrate in 7 mg increments weekly; max 28 mg once daily; do <u>not</u> divide doses
        Cap: 7, 14, 21, 28 mg ext-rel
    Comment: *Memantine* does <u>not</u> halt disease progression. It is indicated for moderate-to-severe dementia.

NMDA RECEPTOR ANTAGONIST+ ACETYLCHOLINE-ESTERASE INHIBITOR COMBINATION

▷ *memantine+donepezil* (G) initiate one 28/10 dose daily in the evening after stabilized on *memantine* and *donepezil* separately; start the day after the last dose of *memantine* and *donepezil* taken separately; swallow whole <u>or</u> open cap and sprinkle on applesauce; *CrCl 5-29 ml/min:* take one 14/10 dose once daily in the evening
    Namzaric
        Cap: **Namzaric 7/10** mem 7 mg+done 10 mg
            Namzaric 14/10 mem 14 mg+done 10 mg
            Namzaric 21/10 mem 21 mg+done 10 mg
            Namzaric 28/10 mem 28 mg+done 10 mg

ERGOT ALKALOID (DOPAMINE AGONIST)

▷ *ergoloid mesylate* 1 mg tid
    Hydergine *Tab:* 1 mg
    Hydergine LC *Cap:* 1 mg
    Hydergine Liquid *Liq:* 1 mg/ml (100 ml w. calib dropper) (alcohol 28.5%)

AGITATION ASSOCIATED WITH DEMENTIA DUE TO ALZHEIMER'S DISEASE

▷ *brexpiprazole* administer once daily with <u>or</u> without food; dose increases should occur at weekly intervals based on the patient's clinical response and tolerability; *Recommended starting dose:* 0.5 mg once daily on

(continued)

days 1 through 7; *then,* increase the dose on days 8 through 14 to 1 mg once daily; *then* on day 15 increase the dose to 2 mg once daily; *Recommended target dose:* 2 mg once daily; the dose can be increased to the max recommended daily dose of 3 mg once daily after at least 14 days based on clinical response and tolerability
Pediatric: not indicated

Rexulti *Tab:* 0.25, 0.5, 1, 2, 3, 4 mg

Comment: Rexulti is an atypical antipsychotic indicated for the treatment of major depressive disorder (MDD), schizophrenia, and agitation associated with dementia due to Alzheimer's disease. This new approval makes **Rexulti** the first and only pharmacologic treatment approved in the United States for agitation associated with dementia due to Alzheimer's disease. **Rexulti** is not approved for use in older adults with dementia-related psychosis. **Rexulti** is not indicated as an "as needed" (prn) treatment for agitation associated with dementia due to Alzheimer's disease. **Rexulti is not approved for the treatment of people with dementia-related psychosis without agitation that may happen with dementia due to Alzheimer's disease.** If co-administered with strong CYP2D6 or CYP3A4 inhibitors, administer half of the usual dose of **Rexulti**. If co-administered with strong/moderate CYP2D6 inhibitors and strong/moderate CYP3A4 inhibitors, administer 1/4 of the usual **Rexulti** dose. If the patient is a known CYP2D6 poor metabolizer and is taking a strong/moderate CYP3A4 inhibitor, administer 1/4 of the usual **Rexulti** dose. If co-administered with strong CYP3A4 inducers, double the usual dose of **Rexulti** and further adjust the **Rexulti** dose based on clinical response. The most common side effects among patients with agitation associated with dementia due to Alzheimer's disease include headache, dizziness, urinary tract infection, nasopharyngitis, and sleep disturbances (both somnolence and insomnia). The **Rexulti** drug label (mfr pkg insert) contains a boxed warning that elderly patients with dementia-related psychosis treated with antipsychotic drugs are at an increased risk of death. Therefore, use of **Rexulti** in these patients is contraindicated. Closely monitor patients for signs and symptoms of neuroleptic malignant syndrome (NMS); if this occurs, immediately discontinue **Rexulti,** evaluate, and treat as appropriate. Closely monitor patients for signs and symptoms of tardive dyskinesia (TD); if this occurs, discontinue **Rexulti** if clinically appropriate. Monitor patients for metabolic changes, such as hyperglycemia/diabetes mellitus, dyslipidemia, and weight gain. Leukopenia, neutropenia, and agranulocytosis may develop. Obtain complete blood counts (CBCs) in patients with preexisting low white blood cell count (WBC) or history of leukopenia or neutropenia. Consider discontinuing **Rexulti** if a clinically significant decline in WBC occurs in the absence of other causative factor. Advise patients and caregivers that orthostatic hypotension and/or syncope may occur. Monitor heart rate (HR) and blood pressure (BP), especially patients with known cardiovascular or cerebrovascular disease, and avoid dehydration. Use **Rexulti** cautiously in patients with a history of seizures or with conditions that lower the seizure threshold. Adequate and well-controlled studies have not been conducted with **Rexulti** in human pregnancy to inform drug-associated risks. In animal reproduction studies, no teratogenicity was observed with oral administration of *brexpiprazole* during organogenesis at doses up to 73 and 146 times, respectively, of the maximum recommended human dose (MRHD) of 4 mg/day on a mg/m^2 basis. However, when administered *brexpiprazole* during the period of organogenesis through lactation, the number of perinatal deaths of pups increased at 73 times the MRHD. Extrapyramidal and/or withdrawal symptoms, including agitation, hypertonia, hypotonia, tremor, somnolence, respiratory distress, and feeding disorder have been reported in neonates whose mothers were exposed to antipsychotic drugs during the 3rd trimester of pregnancy. These symptoms have varied in severity. Some neonates recovered within hours or days without specific treatment; others required prolonged hospitalization. Monitor neonates for extrapyramidal and/or withdrawal symptoms and manage symptoms appropriately. There is a pregnancy exposure registry that monitors pregnancy outcomes in women exposed to **Rexulti** during pregnancy. For more information contact the National Pregnancy Registry for Atypical Antipsychotics at 866-961-2388 or http://womensmentalhealth.org/clinical-and-research-programs/pregnancyregistry/. Lactation studies have not been conducted to assess the presence of *brexpiprazole* in human milk or effects of *brexpiprazole* on the breastfed infant. However, *brexpiprazole* is present in animal milk. Developmental and health benefits of breastfeeding should be considered along with the mother's clinical need for **Rexulti** and any potential adverse effects on the breastfed infant from **Rexulti** or from the underlying maternal condition. To report suspected adverse reactions, contact Otsuka America Pharmaceutical at 800-438-9927 or FDA at 800-FDA-1088 or www.fda.gov/medwatch.

May, 2023—Agitation is a neuropsychiatric symptom in Alzheimer's dementia and one of the most complex and stressful aspects of caring for people living with the condition. "Agitation is one of the most common and challenging aspects of care among patients with dementia due to Alzheimer's disease. 'Agitation' can include symptoms ranging from pacing or restlessness to verbal and physical aggression," said Tiffany Farchione, MD, director of the Division of Psychiatry in the FDA's Center for Drug Evaluation and Research. "These symptoms are leading causes of assisted living or nursing home placement and have been associated with accelerated disease progression." It is reported in approximately half of people with Alzheimer's dementia and is associated with earlier nursing home placement. The FDA had previously granted priority review of **Rexulti** for the new indication. Priority review is a designation for a drug application that represents a significant improvement in the safety and/or effectiveness of the treatment, diagnosis, or prevention of a serious medical condition. The priority review and approval was based on two Phase 3, 12-week, randomized, double-blind, placebo-controlled fixed-dose studies that evaluated the frequency of agitation symptoms in patients with dementia due to Alzheimer's disease based on the Cohen-Mansfield Agitation Inventory (CMAI) total score. The primary endpoint was a change in agitation symptom frequency (CMAI total score) from baseline at week 12 in both studies. *Brexpiprazole* patients with agitation associated with dementia due to Alzheimer's disease achieved a 31% greater reduction in frequency of agitation symptoms from baseline versus placebo. Overall, the data showed *brexpiprazole* as being well-tolerated with a low incidence of discontinuations and with a safety profile consistent with the known safety profile of *brexpiprazole* for other indications. —From www.Drugs.com

AMEBIASIS

AMEBIASIS (INTESTINAL)
➤ *diiodohydroxyquin (iodoquinol)* (G) 650 mg tid pc x 20 days
Pediatric: <6 years: 40 mg/kg/day in 3 divided doses pc x 20 days; max 1.95 gm; 6-12 years: 420 mg tid pc x 20 days
Tab: 210, 650 mg
➤ *metronidazole* (G) 750 mg tid x 5-10 days use in pregnancy is <u>not</u> recommended in the 1st trimester
Pediatric: 35-50 mg/kg/day in 3 divided doses x 10 days
Flagyl *Tab:* 250*, 500*mg
Flagyl 375 *Cap:* 375 mg
Flagyl ER *Tab:* 750 mg ext-rel
➤ *paromomycin* 25-35 mg/kg/day in 3 divided doses x 5-10 days
Pediatric: same as adult
Humatin *Cap:* 250 mg
➤ *tinidazole* 2 gm daily x 3 days; take with food
Pediatric: <3 years: <u>not</u> recommended; ≥3 years: 50 mg/kg daily x 3 days; take with food; max 2 gm/day
Tindamax *Tab:* 250*, 500*mg
Comment: Other than for use in the treatment of *giardiasis* and *amebiasis* in pediatric patients older than 3 years of age, the safety and effectiveness of *tinidazole* in pediatric patients have <u>not</u> been established. *Tinidazole* is excreted in breast milk in concentrations similar to those seen in serum and can be detected in breast milk for up to 72 hours following administration. Interruption of breastfeeding is recommended during *tinidazole* therapy and for 3 days following the last dose.

AMEBIASIS (EXTRAINTESTINAL)
➤ *chloroquine phosphate* (G) 1 gm PO daily x 2 days; then 500 mg daily x 2 to 3 weeks <u>or</u> 200-250 mg IM daily x 10-12 days (when oral therapy is impossible); use with intestinal amebicide
Pediatric: see mfr pkg insert
Aralen *Tab:* 500 mg; *Amp:* 50 mg/ml (5 ml)

AMEBIC LIVER ABSCESS

ANTI-INFECTIVES
➤ *metronidazole* (G) 250 mg tid <u>or</u> 500 mg bid <u>or</u> 750 mg daily x 7 days
Pediatric: <12 years: <u>not</u> recommended; ≥12 years: same as adult
Flagyl *Tab:* 250*, 500*mg
Flagyl 375 *Cap:* 375 mg
Flagyl ER *Tab:* 750 mg ext-rel
➤ *tinidazole* 2 gm once daily x 3-5 days; take with food
Pediatric: <3 years: <u>not</u> recommended; ≥3 years: 50 mg/kg once daily x 3-5 days; take with food; max 2 gm/day
Tindamax *Tab:* 250*, 500*mg
Comment: Other than for use in the treatment of *giardiasis* and *amebiasis* in pediatric patients older than 3 years of age, safety and effectiveness of *tinidazole* in pediatric patients have <u>not</u> been established. *Tinidazole* is excreted in breast milk in concentrations similar to those seen in serum and can be detected in breast milk for up to 72 hours following administration. Interruption of breastfeeding is recommended during *tinidazole* therapy and for 3 days following the last dose.

AMENORRHEA: SECONDARY

➤ *estrogen+progesterone*
Premarin (*estrogen*) 0.625 mg daily x 25 days; then 5 days off; repeat monthly
Provera (*progesterone*) 5-10 mg last 10 days of cycle; repeat monthly
➤ *estrogen replacement*
see Menopause

(continued)

▷ *human chorionic gonadotropin* 5,000-10,000 units IM x 1 dose following last dose of menotropins
    Pregnyl *Vial:* 10,000 units (10 ml) w. diluent (10 ml)
▷ *medroxyprogesterone Monthly:* 5-10 mg last 5-10 days of cycle; begin on the 16th or 21st day of cycle; repeat monthly; *One-time only:* 10 mg once daily x 10 days
    Amen *Tab:* 10 mg
    Provera *Tab:* 2.5, 5, 10 mg
▷ *norethindrone* 2.5-10 mg daily x 5-10 days
    Aygestin *Tab:* 5 mg
▷ *progesterone, micronized* (G) 400 mg q HS x 10 days
    Prometrium *Cap:* 100, 200 mg
Comment: Administration of *progesterone* induces optimum secretory transformation of the *estrogen*-primed endometrium. Administration of *progesterone* is contraindicated in breast cancer, undiagnosed vaginal bleeding, genital cancer, severe liver dysfunction or disease, missed abortion, thrombophlebitis, thromboembolic disorders, cerebral apoplexy, and pregnancy.

AMYOTROPHIC LATERAL SCLEROSIS (ALS, LOU GEHRIG'S DISEASE)

▷ *sodium phenylbutyrate+taurursodiol Recommended dose:* 1 packet (3 gm *sodium phenylbutyrate*+1 gm *taurursodiol*) administered orally or via feeding tube as follows: *Initial dose:* 1 packet daily for the first 3 weeks; *Maintenance dose:* 1 packet bid; empty contents of 1 packet into a cup containing 8 oz of room-temperature water and stir vigorously prior to administration; take within 1 hour of preparation; administer before a snack or meal; reconstituted suspension may be stored for up to 1 hour at room temperature; discard any unused reconstituted suspension after 1 hour
Pediatric: safety and efficacy not established
    Relyvrio *Pkt:* 3 gm *sodium phenylbutyrate* and 1 gm *taurursodiol*, single-dose, for oral suspension (7, 56 dose pkts/carton) (mixed berry) (sorbitol, sucralose)
    Comment: Relyvrio is a neuroprotective therapy for the treatment of amyotrophic lateral sclerosis (ALS) in adults. The most common adverse reactions (incidence at least 15% and at least 5% greater than placebo) have been diarrhea, abdominal pain, nausea, and upper respiratory tract infection. **Relyvrio** contains *taurursodiol*, which is a bile acid. In patients with disorders that interfere with bile acid circulation, there may be an increased risk of worsening diarrhea and patients should be monitored appropriately for this adverse reaction. Pancreatic insufficiency, intestinal malabsorption, or intestinal diseases that may alter the concentration of bile acids may also lead to decreased absorption of either of the components of **Relyvrio**. Because different enterohepatic circulation, pancreatic, and intestinal disorders have varying degrees of severity, consider consulting with a specialist. Patients with disorders of enterohepatic circulation (e.g., biliary infection, active cholecystitis), severe pancreatic disorders (e.g., pancreatitis), and intestinal disorders that may alter concentrations of bile acids (e.g., ileal resection, regional ileitis) were excluded from the study; therefore, there is no clinical experience in patients with these conditions. **Relyvrio** has a high sodium content. Each initial daily dose of one packet contains 464 mg of sodium. Each maintenance dose of two packets daily contains 928 mg of sodium. In patients sensitive to salt intake (e.g., those with heart failure, hypertension, or renal impairment), consider the amount of daily sodium intake in each dose of **Relyvrio** and monitor appropriately. No dose adjustment is needed for patients with mild renal impairment. Avoid use in patients with moderate or severe renal impairment. No dose adjustment is needed for patients with mild hepatic impairment. Avoid use in patients with moderate or severe hepatic impairment. See the mfr pkg insert for full prescribing information, including a complete list of clinically significant drug interactions. There are no available data on **Relyvrio** use in pregnant women to evaluate for a drug-associated risk of major birth defects, miscarriage, or other adverse maternal or fetal outcomes. However, in animal studies, administration of *sodium phenylbutyrate* and *taurursodiol* throughout pregnancy and lactation resulted in increased offspring mortality at all doses tested, which were less than or similar to the clinical doses. There are no data on the presence of *sodium phenylbutyrate* or *taurursodiol* in human milk or effects on the breastfed infant. Developmental and health benefits of breastfeeding should be considered along with the mother's clinical need for **Relyvrio** and any potential adverse effects on the breastfed infant from **Relyvrio** or from the underlying maternal condition. To report suspected adverse reactions, contact Amylyx Pharmaceuticals at 877-374-1208 or FDA at 800-FDA-1088 or www.fda.gov/medwatch.

PYRAZOLONE FREE RADICAL SCAVENGER

▷ *edaravone* the dosing regimens are the same for IV and oral forms; *Initial treatment cycle:* once daily dosing x 14 days followed by a 14-day drug-free period; *Subsequent treatment cycles:* once daily dosing x 10 days out of 14-day periods, followed by 14-day drug-free periods; **Radicava:** recommended dose is 60 mg administered as an IV infusion over 60 minutes; **Radicava ORS:** recommended dose is 105 mg (5 ml) administered orally or via feeding tube in the morning after overnight fasting; food should not be consumed for 1 hour after administration, except water
Pediatric: not indicated

Radicava *IV bag:* 30 mg/100 ml (0.3 mg/ml, 100 ml), single-dose, soln for IV infusion (2 bags/carton)
Radicava ORS *Oral susp:* 105 mg/5 ml, multidose amber glass bottle; *Radicava ORS Starter Kit (14-day treatment cycle):* includes 2 inner cartons, each containing 1 bottle of 735 mg/35 ml (105 mg/5 ml dose), 2 oral dosing syringes, and 1 bottle adapter; *Radicava ORS Kit (10-day treatment cycle):* includes 1 bottle of 1,050 mg/50 ml (105 mg/5 ml dose) with 2 oral dosing syringes and one bottle adapter
Comment: The most common adverse reactions (at least 10% of patients treated with **Radicava** and greater than placebo) have been contusion, gait disturbance, and headache. **Radicava** and/or **Radicava ORS** are contraindicated in patients with a history of hypersensitivity to *edaravone* or any of the inactive ingredients in **Radicava** and/or **Radicava ORS**. *Hypersensitivity Reactions:* Advise patients to seek immediate medical care. *Sulfite Allergic Reactions:* **Radicava** and **Radicava ORS** contain sodium bisulfite, which may cause allergic type reactions, including anaphylaxis and asthmatic episodes in susceptible people. In the event a hypersensitivity reaction occurs, appropriate medical interventions should be provided as indicated. Based on animal reproductive and developmental studies, **Radicava** can cause fetal harm (such as stillbirths, offspring mortality, and delayed physical development). Advise pregnant females and females of reproductive potential of the risk. Advise females of reproductive potential to use effective contraception. Reproductive and developmental toxicology studies of *edaravone* using the oral route have not been conducted. There are no data on the presence of *edaravone* in human milk. *Edaravone* and its metabolites are excreted in the milk of lactating animals. Developmental and health benefits of breastfeeding should be considered along with the mother's clinical need for **Radicava** and/or **Radicava ORS** and any potential adverse effects on the breastfed infant from the drug or from the underlying maternal condition. To report suspected adverse reactions, contact Mitsubishi Tanabe Pharma America at 888-292-0058 or FDA at 1-800-FDA-1088 or www.fda.gov/medwatch.

GLUTAMATE INHIBITOR

▷ **riluzole** 50 mg bid; take at least 1 hour before or 2 hours after a meal; measure serum aminotransferases before and during treatment
Exservan *Oral film:* 50 mg
Comment: **Exservan** is an oral film formulation of the approved glutamate inhibitor *riluzole* for the treatment of patients with ALS who have difficulty swallowing. Use of **Exservan** is not recommended in patients with baseline elevations of serum aminotransferase >5 times the upper limit of normal (ULN); discontinue **Exservan** if there is evidence of liver dysfunction. Monitor the patient for signs and symptoms of neutropenia and advise them to report any febrile illness. Discontinue **Exservan** if interstitial lung disease develops. Co-administration of strong-to-moderate CYP1A2 inhibitors may increase **Exservan**-associated adverse reactions. Co-administration of strong-to-moderate CYP1A2 inducers may result in decreased **Exservan** efficacy. **Exservan**-treated patients who take other hepatotoxic drugs may be at increased risk for hepatotoxicity. The most common adverse reactions (incidence ≥5% and greater than placebo) have been oral hypoesthesia, asthenia, nausea, decreased lung function, hypertension, and abdominal pain. Based on animal data, **Exservan** may cause fetal harm. Decreased embryo/fetal viability, growth, and functional development was observed at clinically relevant doses. Women should be advised of a possible risk to the fetus associated with use of **Exservan** during pregnancy. There are no data on the presence of *riluzole* in human milk or effects on the breastfed infant. *Riluzole* or its metabolites have been detected in milk of lactating animals. Developmental and health benefits of breastfeeding should be considered along with the mother's clinical need for **Exservan** and any potential adverse effects on the breastfed infant from **Exservan** or from the underlying maternal condition.

ANTISENSE OLIGONUCLEOTIDE

▷ **tofersen** *Recommended dose:* 100 mg (15 ml) per intrathecal IVP over 1 to 3 minutes; initiate treatment with 3 loading doses administered at 14-day intervals; *Maintenance dose:* administer once every 28 days; allow vial to warm to room temperature prior to administration; administer within 4 hours of removal from the vial; prior to administration, remove approximately 10 ml of cerebrospinal fluid (CSF); store refrigerated between 2°C to 8°C (36°F to 46°F) in the original carton to protect from light; do not freeze; if no refrigeration is available, **Qalsody** may be stored in its original carton, protected from light at or below 30°C (86°F) for up to 14 days; if removed from the original carton, unopened vials may be removed from and returned to the refrigerator, if necessary, for not more than 6 hours per day at or below 30°C (86°F) for a maximum of 6 days (36 cumulative hours)
Pediatric: safety and efficacy not established
Qalsody *Vial:* 100 mg/15 ml (6.7 mg/ml), single-dose, soln for intrathecal administration (preservative-free)
Comment: **Qalsody** is an antisense oligonucleotide indicated for the treatment of amyotrophic lateral sclerosis (ALS) in adults who have a mutation in the superoxide dismutase 1 (SOD1) gene. This indication is approved under accelerated approval based on reduction in plasma neurofilament light chain (NfL) observed in patients treated with **Qalsody**. Neurofilaments are proteins that are released from neurons when they are damaged, making them a marker of neurodegeneration. The most common adverse reactions (incidence ≥10% of patients treated with **Qalsody** and greater than placebo)

(continued)

were pain, fatigue, arthralgia, cerebrospinal fluid white blood cell (CSF-WBC) increase, and myalgia. Serious neurologic events have been reported. These include myelitis, radiculitis, papilledema, elevated intracranial pressure (ICP), and aseptic meningitis. Monitor for signs and symptoms. Diagnostic workup and treatment should be initiated according to standard of care. Continued FDA approval for this indication may be contingent upon verification of clinical benefit in confirmatory trial(s). The ongoing Phase 3 ATLAS study of *tofersen* in people with presymptomatic *SOD1*-ALS serves as the confirmatory trial. **Qalsody** is a first-of-its-kind treatment, the first approved treatment to target a genetic cause of ALS. Efficacy of **Qalsody** was assessed in a 28-week randomized, double-blind, placebo-controlled clinical study in patients 23-78 years of age with weakness attributable to ALS and a *SOD1* mutation confirmed by a central laboratory. One hundred eight patients were randomized 2:1 to receive treatment with either **Qalsody** 100 mg (n=72) or placebo (n=36) for 24 weeks (3 loading doses followed by 5 maintenance doses). Concomitant *riluzole* and/or *edaravone* use was allowed in patients, and at baseline 62% of patients were taking *riluzole*, and 8% were taking *edaravone*. Over 28 weeks in VALOR, participants in the primary analysis population (n=60) treated with **Qalsody** experienced less decline from baseline as measured by the Revised Amyotrophic Lateral Sclerosis Functional Rating Scale (ALSFRS-R) compared to placebo, though the results were not statistically significant (**Qalsody**-placebo adjusted mean difference [95% CI]: 1.2 [-3.2, 5.5]). In the overall intent-to-treat population (n=108), **Qalsody**-treated participants experienced a 55% reduction in plasma NfL compared to a 12% increase in placebo-treated participants (difference in geometric mean ratios for **Qalsody** to placebo: 60%; nominal $p<.0001$). Additionally, levels of CSF SOD1 protein, an indirect measure of target engagement, were reduced by 35% in the **Qalsody**-treated group compared to 2% in the corresponding placebo group (difference in geometric mean ratios for **Qalsody** to placebo: 34%; nominal $p<.0001$). At an interim analysis at 52 weeks of participants who had completed VALOR and enrolled in an open-label extension (OLE) study, reductions in NfL were seen in participants previously receiving placebo and who initiated **Qalsody** in the OLE, similar to the reductions seen in participants treated with **Qalsody** in VALOR. Earlier initiation of **Qalsody** compared to placebo/delayed start of **Qalsody** was associated with a declining trend in measures of clinical function (ALSFRS-R), respiratory strength (slow vital capacity percent predicted), and muscle strength (handheld dynamometry megascore), although they were not statistically significant. **Qalsody** was also associated with a non-statistically significant trend toward reduction in risk of death or permanent ventilation. These exploratory analyses should be interpreted with caution given the limitations of data collected outside of controlled study, which may be subject to confounding. Approval of **Qalsody** was supported by 12-month integrated results from VALOR and its OLE comparing earlier initiation of *tofersen* (at the start of VALOR) to delayed initiation of *tofersen* (6 months later, in the OLE). In addition to the ongoing OLE of VALOR, **Qalsody** is being studied in the Phase 3, randomized, placebo-controlled ATLAS study to evaluate whether **Qalsody** can delay clinical onset when initiated in presymptomatic individuals with a *SOD1* genetic mutation and biomarker evidence of disease activity (elevated plasma NfL). The primary efficacy endpoint is the proportion of participants with emergence of clinically manifest ALS. ATLAS currently has an enrollment rate of more than 50% with clinical trial sites in 14 countries worldwide and an estimated primary completion date in 2026. More details about ATLAS (NCT04856982) can be found at clinicaltrials.gov. Up to 15% of people living with ALS are thought to have a genetic form of the disease, whether or not they have a known family history. As genetic testing is not broadly available, Biogen sponsors a genetic testing program, *ALS Identified*, for people living with ALS and their families in the United States. Sponsored by Biogen and offered through Invitae, the *ALS Identified* program facilitates access to genetic counseling and testing for all individuals ≥18 years of age within the United States and Puerto Rico with a clinical diagnosis of ALS or a family history of ALS at no charge. More information about *ALS Identified* is available at insideALS.com, a website designed in collaboration with outside medical experts and the ALS community that offers continuous updates on the emerging science that provides insights and information to the ALS community. There are no adequate data on developmental risks associated with the use of **Qalsody** in human pregnancy to evaluate for a drug-associated risk of major birth defects, miscarriage, or other adverse maternal or fetal outcomes. Animal studies have not demonstrated any adverse fetal outcomes. There are no data on the presence of *tofersen* or its metabolites in human milk or effects on the breastfed infant. Animal studies have detected *tofersen* in the milk of lactating animals following subcutaneous administration. Developmental and health benefits of breastfeeding should be considered along with the mother's clinical need for **Qalsody** and any potential adverse effects on the breastfed infant from **Qalsody** or from the underlying maternal condition. To report suspected adverse reactions, contact Biogen at 877-725-7639 or FDA at 800-FDA-1088 or www.fda.gov/medwatch.

April 26, 2023—"The FDA has approved the first treatment that takes a genetics-based approach to slowing or stopping the progression of a form of ALS, the debilitating and deadly disease for which there is no cure. Most people with ALS, or amyotrophic lateral sclerosis, die within 3 to 5 years of when symptoms appear, usually of respiratory failure. Also known as Lou Gehrig's disease, people with ALS experience muscle twitching and lose the ability to move their limbs, swallow, speak, and breathe. The newly approved drug, called Qalsody, is made by the Swiss company Biogen. The FDA fast-tracked the approval based on early trial results. The agency said in a news release that its decision was based on the demonstrated ability of the drug to reduce a protein in the blood that is a sign of degeneration of brain and nerve cells. While the drug was shown to impact the chemical process in the body linked to degeneration, there was no significant change in people's symptoms during the first 28 weeks that they took the drug, Biogen said in a news release. But the company noted that some patients did see improved functioning after starting treatment. 'I have observed the positive impact Qalsody has on slowing the progression of ALS in people with SOD1 mutations,' Timothy M. Miller, MD, PhD, researcher and co-director of the ALS Center at Washington University School of Medicine in St. Louis, said in a statement released by Biogen. 'The FDA's approval of Qalsody gives me hope that people living with this rare form of ALS could experience a reduction in decline in strength, clinical function, and respiratory function.'"—From www.MedScape.com

ANAPHYLAXIS

Parenteral Corticosteroids *see* Appendix L. Parenteral Corticosteroids
Oral Corticosteroids *see* Appendix K. Oral Corticosteroids

▷ *epinephrine* (G) 0.3-0.5 mg (0.3-0.5 ml of a 1:1,000 soln) SC q 20-30 minutes as needed up to 3 doses
Pediatric: <2 years: 0.05-0.1 ml; 2-6 years: 0.1 ml; ≥6-12 years: 0.2 ml; all: may repeat dose every 20-30 minutes as needed up to 3 doses; ≥12 years: same as adult

ANAPHYLAXIS EMERGENCY TREATMENT KITS
▷ *epinephrine* 0.3 ml IM or SC in the thigh; may repeat if needed
Pediatric: 0.01 mg/kg SC or IM in the thigh; may repeat if needed; <15 kg: not established; 15-30 kg: 0.15 mg; >30 kg: same as adult
    Adrenaclick *Auto-injector:* 0.15, 0.3 mg (1 mg/ml; 1, 2/carton) (sulfites)
    Auvi-Q *Auto-injector:* 0.15, 0.3 mg (1 mg/ml; 1/pck w. 1 non-active training device) (sulfites)
    EpiPen *Auto-injector:* 0.3 mg (*epi* 1:1,000, 0.3 ml) (1, 2/carton) (sulfites)
    EpiPen Jr *Auto-injector:* 0.15 mg (*epi* 1:2,000, 0.3 ml) (1, 2/carton) (sulfites)
    Symjepi *Prefilled syringe:* 0.3 mg (0.3 ml), single-dose, for manual injection
    Comment: Each **Symjepi** syringe is overfilled for stability purposes. More than half the solution remains in the syringe after use (and the syringe cannot be reused).
    Twinject *Auto-injector:* 0.15, 0.3 mg (epi 1:1,000) (1, 2/carton) (sulfites)
▷ *epinephrine* plus *chlorpheniramine epinephrine* 0.3 ml SC or IM plus 4 tabs *chlorpheniramine* by mouth
Pediatric: infants to 2 years: 0.05-0.1 ml SC or IM; ≥2-6 years: 0.15 ml SC or IM plus 1 tab chlor; ≥6-12 years: 0.2 ml SC or IM plus 2 tabs chlor; ≥12 years: same as adult
    Ana-Kit *Prefilled injector:* 0.3 ml epi 1:1,000 for self-injection plus 4 x chlor 2 mg chew tabs

ANEMIA: BETA THALASSEMIA-ASSOCIATED

ERYTHROID MATURATION AGENT (EMA)
Comment: Reblozyl *(luspatercept-aamt)* is a first-in-class erythroid maturation agent (EMA) indicated for the treatment of beta thalassemia-associated anemia in adult patients who require regular red blood cell (RBC) transfusions. **Reblozyl** is not indicated for use as a substitute for RBC transfusions in patients who require immediate correction of anemia.

▷ *luspatercept-aamt Recommended starting dose:* is 1 mg/kg SC once every 3 weeks into the upper arm, abdomen, or thigh; divide doses requiring >1.2 ml reconstituted volume into separate similar volume injections and inject into separate sites; if multiple injections are required, use a new syringe and needle for each injection; review hemoglobin (Hgb) results prior to each administration; if the patient does not achieve a reduction in RBC transfusion burden after at least 2 consecutive doses (6 weeks) at the 1 mg/kg starting dose, increase the **Reblozyl** dose to 1.25 mg/kg; do not increase the dose beyond the maximum dose of 1.25 mg/kg; if an RBC transfusion occurs prior to dosing, the pre-transfusion Hgb must be considered for dosing purposes; if a planned administration of **Reblozyl** is delayed or missed, administer **Reblozyl** as soon as possible and continue dosing as prescribed, with at least 3 weeks between doses; if the pre-dose Hgb is ≥11.5 gm/dL, and the Hgb level is not influenced by recent transfusion, delay dosing until the Hgb is ≤11 gm/dL; if the patient experiences a response followed by a lack of, or loss of, response to **Reblozyl**, initiate a search for causative factors (e.g., a bleeding event); if typical causes for a lack or loss of hematologic response are excluded, follow dosing recommendations therapy (see mfr pkg insert) for management of patients with an insufficient response to **Reblozyl**; if the patient does not experience a decrease in transfusion burden after 9 weeks of treatment (administration of 3 doses) at the maximum dose level or if unacceptable toxicity occurs at any time, *discontinue* **Reblozyl**
Pediatric: safety and efficacy not established

(continued)

Reblozyl *Vial:* 25, 75 mg, single-dose, pwdr for reconstitution and SC administration (see mfr pkg insert for reconstitution directions)

Comment: There is increased risk of thrombosis/thromboembolism in patients with beta thalassemia. Monitor patients receiving **Reblozyl** for signs and symptoms of thromboembolic events and institute treatment promptly. Monitor blood pressure (BP) during treatment and initiate antihypertensive treatment if necessary. The most common adverse reactions (incidence >10%) in patients with beta thalassemia have been headache, bone pain, arthralgia, fatigue, cough, abdominal pain, diarrhea, and dizziness. There are <u>no</u> available data on **Reblozyl** use in pregnant females to inform a drug-associated risk of major birth defects, miscarriage, <u>or</u> adverse maternal <u>or</u> fetal outcomes. In animal reproduction studies, administration of *luspatercept-aamt* in pregnancy during the period of organogenesis resulted in adverse developmental outcomes, including embryo/fetal mortality, alterations to growth, and structural abnormalities at exposures (based on area under the curve [AUC]) above those occurring at the maximum recommended human dose (MRHD). Advise pregnant females of the potential embryo/fetal risk. Advise females of reproductive potential of the potential risk of embryo/fetal toxicity and to use effective contraception. Advise patients <u>not</u> to breastfeed. *Luspatercept-aamt* has been detected in milk of lactating rats. When a drug is present in animal milk, it is likely that the drug will be present in human milk. There are <u>no</u> data on the presence of **Reblozyl** in human milk <u>or</u> effects on the breastfed infant. Because of the potential for serious adverse reactions, advise patients that breastfeeding is <u>not</u> recommended during treatment with **Reblozyl** and for 3 months after the last dose.

ANEMIA OF CHRONIC KIDNEY DISEASE/ANEMIA OF CHRONIC RENAL FAILURE

SELECTIVE MINERALOCORTICOID RECEPTOR ANTAGONIST (MRA)

▷ *finerenone* *Starting Dose:* 10 mg or 20 mg once daily (based on estimated glomerular filtration rate [eGFR] and serum potassium thresholds); May take with or without food; After 4 weeks, may increase to the target dose of 20 mg once daily (based on eGFR and serum potassium thresholds); *Child-Pugh Class A or B:* no dosage adjustment; *Child-Pugh Class B:* consider additional serum potassium monitoring; *Child-Pugh Class C:* avoid use

Pediatric: <18 years: Safety and efficacy <u>not</u> established; ≥18 years: same as adult

Kerendia *Tab:* 10, 20 mg film-coat

Comment: **Kerendia** is a non-steroidal, selective mineralocorticoid receptor antagonist (MRA) for the treatment of patients with chronic kidney disease (CKD) associated with type 2 diabetes (T2D). Adverse reactions occurring in ≥1% of patients on **Kerendia** and more frequently than placebo are hyperkalemia, hypotension, and hyponatremia. Contraindications to **Kerendia** use are concomitant use with strong CYP3A4 inhibitors and patients with adrenal insufficiency. Avoid concomitant use of Kerendia with grapefruit <u>or</u> grapefruit juice. Monitor serum potassium during drug initiation and dose adjustment of **Kerendia** <u>or</u> concomitant moderate <u>or</u> weak CYP3A4 inhibitors, and adjust **Kerendia** dose as appropriate. Avoid concomitant use of **Kerendia** with strong <u>or</u> moderate CYP3A4 Inducers. There are <u>no</u> available data on **Kerendia** use in pregnancy to evaluate for a drug-associated risk of major birth defects, miscarriage, <u>or</u> adverse maternal <u>or</u> fetal outcomes. Animal studies have demonstrated developmental toxicity at exposures about 4 times those expected in humans. Because of the potential risk to breastfed infants from exposure to **Kerendia**; avoid breastfeeding during treatment and for 1 day after treatment.

PHOSPHATE BINDER

▷ *ferric citrate* *Iron deficiency anemia in CKD <u>not</u> on dialysis:* starting dose is 1 tablet tid with meals, adjust dose as needed to achieve and maintain hemoglobin (Hgb) goal up to max 12 tabs/day; *Hyperphosphatemia in CKD on dialysis:* starting dose is 2 tabs orally tid with meals; adjust dose by 1 to 2 tabs as needed to maintain serum phosphorus at target levels, up to max 12 tabs/day; dose can be titrated at 1 week <u>or</u> longer intervals

Pediatric: <18 years: <u>not</u> recommended; ≥18 years: same as adult

Auryxia *Tab:* 210 mg *ferric iron* (equivalent to 1 gm *ferric citrate*)

Comment: **Auryxia** is a phosphate binder indicated for the control of serum phosphorus levels in patients ≥18 years of age with CKD on dialysis. Ferric iron binds dietary phosphate in the gastrointestinal (GI) tract and precipitates as ferric phosphate. This compound is insoluble and is excreted in the stool. **Auryxia** is also an iron replacement product indicated for the treatment of iron deficiency anemia in patients >18 years of age with CKD <u>not</u> on dialysis. Ferric iron is reduced from the ferric to the ferrous form by ferric reductase in the GI tract. After transport through the enterocytes into the blood, oxidized ferric iron circulates bound to the plasma protein transferrin, for incorporation into Hgb. **Auryxia** is contraindicated in iron overload syndromes (e.g., hemochromatosis). Monitor ferritin and TSAT. (NOTE: *Ferritin* is a blood protein that contains iron. Ferritin level is an indicator of how much iron is stored. If ferritin level is lower than normal, iron stores are low and, as such, the body is iron deficient.

Transferrin saturation [TSAT] is the ratio of serum iron to total iron-binding capacity (TIBC) and is considered an important biochemical marker of overall bodily iron status, which can be used to monitor response to ESA [erythropoiesis-stimulating agent] and/or iron therapy in CKD.) When clinically significant drug interactions are expected, consider separation of the timing of administration. Consider monitoring clinical responses or blood levels of the concomitant medication. The most common adverse reactions (incidence ≥5%) are discolored feces, diarrhea, constipation, nausea, vomiting, cough, abdominal pain, and hyperkalemia. There are no available data on **Auryxia** use in pregnancy to inform a drug-associated risk of major birth defects and miscarriage; however, an overdose of iron may carry a risk of spontaneous abortion, gestational diabetes, and fetal malformation. There are no human data regarding the effects of **Auryxia** on the breastfed infant. Accidental overdose of iron-containing products is a leading cause of fatal poisoning in children under 6 years of age. Keep this product out of reach of children. In case of accidental overdose, contact the poison control center immediately and transfer to emergency care.

ERYTHROPOIESIS STIMULATING AGENTS (ESAs)

▷ **darbepoetin alfa** (erythropoiesis stimulating protein) administer IV or SC every 1 to 2 weeks; do not increase more frequently than once per month; Not *currently receiving epoetin alfa:* initially 0.75 mcg/kg once weekly; adjust based on Hgb levels (target is not to exceed 12 gm/dL); reduce dose if Hgb increases more than 1 gm/dL in any 2-week period; suspend therapy if polycythemia occurs; *Converting from epoetin alfa and for dose titration:* see mfr pkg insert
Pediatric: <12 years: not recommended; ≥12 years: same as adult
   Aranesp *Vial:* 25, 40, 60, 100, 150, 200, 300, 500 mcg/ml (single-dose) for IV or SC administration (preservative-free, albumin [human] or polysorbate 80)
   Aranesp Singleject and **Aranesp Sureclick Singleject** *Prefilled syringe:* 25, 40, 60, 100, 150, 200, 300, 500 mcg (single-dose) for IV or SC administration (preservative-free, albumin [human] or polysorbate 80)
▷ **peginesatide** use the lowest effective dose; initiate when Hgb <10 gm/dL; do not increase dose more often than every 4 weeks; if Hgb rises rapidly (i.e., >1 gm/dL in 2 weeks or >2 gm/dL in 4 weeks), reduce dose by 25% or more; if Hgb approaches or exceeds 11 gm/dL, reduce or interrupt dose and then when Hgb decreases, resume dose at approximately 25% below previous dose; if Hgb does not increase by >1 gm/dL after 4 weeks, increase dose by 25%; if response is inadequate after a 12-week escalation period, use the lowest dose that will maintain Hgb sufficient to reduce need for RBC transfusion; discontinue if response does not improve; Not *currently on ESA:* initially 0.04 mg/kg as a single IV or SC dose once monthly; *Converting from epoetin alfa:* administer first dose 1 week after last **epoetin alfa**; *Converting from darbepoetin alfa:* administer first dose at next scheduled dose of **darbepoetin alfa**
Pediatric: <12 years: not established; ≥12 years: use the lowest effective dose
   Omontys *Vial, single-use:* 2, 3, 4, 5, 6 mg (0.5 ml) (preservative-free); *Vial, multiuse:* 10, 20 mg (2 ml) (preservatives); *Prefilled syringe:* 2, 3, 4, 5, 6 mg (0.5 ml) (preservative-free)

ERYTHROPOIETIN HUMAN, RECOMBINANT

▷ **epoetin alfa** individualize; initially 50-100 units/kg 3 x/week; IV (dialysis or non-dialysis) or SC (non-dialysis); usual max 200 units/kg 3 x weekly (dialysis) or 150 units/kg 3 x/week (non-dialysis); target hematocrit (Hct) is 30% to 36%
Pediatric: <1 month: not recommended; ≥1 month: individualize; *Dialysis:* initially 50 units/kg 3 x/week IV or SC; target Hct 30%-36%
   Epogen *Vial:* 2,000, 3,000, 4,000, 10,000, 40,000 units/ml (1 ml), single-use for IV or SC administration (albumin [human]; preservative-free)
   Epogen Multidose *Vial:* 10,000 units/ml (2 ml), 20,000 units/ml (1 ml) for IV or SC administration (albumin [human]; benzoyl alcohol)
   Procrit *Vial:* 2,000, 3,000, 4,000, 10,000, 40,000 units/ml (1 ml), single-use for IV or SC administration (albumin [human]) (preservative-free)
   Procrit Multidose *Vial:* 10,000 units/ml (2 ml), 20,000 units/ml (1 ml) for IV or SC administration (albumin [human]; benzoyl alcohol)
▷ **epoetin alfa-epbx** evaluate iron status before and during treatment and maintain iron repletion; correct or exclude other causes of anemia before initiating treatment; *Patients with CKD: initial dose (infants ≥1 month and children):* 50 units/kg 3 x weekly; *initial dose (≥18 years of age):* 50-100 units/kg 3 x weekly; individualize maintenance dose; IV route recommended for patients on hemodialysis; *Patients on zidovudine due to HIV infection:* 100 units/kg 3 x weekly; *Patients with cancer on chemotherapy:* 40,000 units once weekly or 150 units/kg 3 weekly (adults), 600 units/kg IV once weekly (pediatric patients >5 years); *Surgery patients:* 300 units/kg once daily for 15 days or 600 units/kg once weekly
   Retacrit *Vial:* 2,000, 3,000, 4,000, 10,000, 40,000 units/ml (1 ml), single-dose, for SC or IV infusion
   Comment: **Retacrit** *(epoetin alfa-epbx)* is the first FDA-approved biosimilar to **Epogen/Procrit** *(epoetin alfa)* for the SC or IV infusion treatment of anemia caused by CKD, chemotherapy, or *zidovudine* treatment for HIV infection. **Retacrit** is also approved for use before and after surgery to reduce the potential need for blood transfusions due to blood loss during surgery. Common reported adverse side effects with **Retacrit** include high blood pressure, joint pain, muscle spasm, fever, and dizziness. Contraindications to **Retacrit** include uncontrolled hypertension, pure red cell aplasia (PRCA) that begins after treatment with **Retacrit** or other erythropoietin protein drugs, and serious allergic reactions to **Retacrit** or other **epoetin alfa** products. *Boxed Warning:* ESAs increase the risk of myocardial infarction, stroke, venous thromboembolism, thrombosis of vascular access, and tumor progression or recurrence, and death (see mfr pkg insert for the full BBW). Therefore, use the lowest **Retacrit** dose

(continued)

sufficient to reduce the need for red blood cell (RBC) transfusions, and deep venous thrombosis (DVT) prophylaxis is recommended. The limited available data on *epoetin alfa* use in pregnancy are insufficient to determine a drug-associated risk of adverse developmental outcomes. There is no information regarding the presence of *epoetin alfa* products in human milk or effects on the breastfed infant. Safety and effectiveness in pediatric patients <1 month of age have not been established.

ORAL HYPOXIA-INDUCIBLE FACTOR PROLYL HYDROXYLASE INHIBITOR (HIF-PHI)

▷ *daprodustat* administer once daily without regard to the timing or type of dialysis; take with or without food; see mfr pkg insert for full prescribing information, for starting dosage based on hemoglobin level, liver function, and concomitant medications, for dose titration, and for monitoring recommendations; *Child-Pugh B*: reduce the starting dose; *Child-Pugh C*: not recommended; *Active malignancy*: Not recommended
Pediatric: safety and efficacy not established

Jesduvroq *Tab*: 1, 2, 4, 6, 8 mg
Comment: Jesduvroq is the first FDA-approved oral hypoxia-inducible factor prolyl hydroxylase inhibitor (HIF-PHI) indicated for the treatment of adult patients with anemia of CKD who have been on dialysis for at least 4 months. Jesduvroq is not indicated for use as a substitute for RBC transfusions in patients who require immediate correction of anemia or for the treatment of anemia of CKD in patients who are not on dialysis. Jesduvroq has not shown to improve quality of life, fatigue, or patient well-being.
Boxed Warning: Increased risk of death, myocardial infarction, stroke, venous thromboembolism, and thrombosis of vascular access. Jesduvroq increases the risk of thrombotic vascular events, including major adverse cardiovascular events (MACE). Targeting an Hgb level greater than 11 g/dL is expected to further increase the risk of death and arterial venous thrombotic events, as occurs with ESAs, which also increase erythropoietin levels. No trial has identified an Hgb target level, dose of Jesduvroq, or dosing strategy that does not increase these risks. Use the lowest dose of Jesduvroq sufficient to reduce the need for RBC transfusions. See mfr pkg insert for the full boxed warning. Jesduvroq is contraindicated in patients with uncontrolled hypertension and with concomitant use of strong CYP2C8 inhibitors (e.g., *gemfibrozil*). Risk of hospitalization for heart failure is increased in patients with a history of heart failure. Worsening hypertension, including hypertensive crisis, may occur; monitor blood pressure and adjust antihypertensive therapy as needed. Gastric or esophageal erosions and GI bleeding have been reported. Active malignancy: Jesduvroq may have unfavorable effects on cancer growth and therefore is not recommended in patients with active malignancy. The most common adverse reactions reported with Jesduvroq were hypertension, thrombotic vascular events, and abdominal pain. With concomitant moderate CYP2C8 inhibitors, reduce the starting dose of Jesduvroq. With concomitant CYP2C8 inducers, monitor hemoglobin and adjust the dose of Jesduvroq as appropriate. Jesduvroq may cause fetal harm. Available data with Jesduvroq use in human pregnancy are insufficient to establish a drug-associated risk of major birth defects, miscarriage, or adverse maternal or fetal outcomes. There are risks to the mother and the fetus associated with CKD. *Daprodustat* administered orally to pregnant animals during the period of organogenesis was associated with adverse fetal outcomes, including embryonic and fetal loss and reduced fetal weight, at doses that caused maternal toxicity and polycythemia. Advise pregnant patients of the potential risk to the fetus. Do not initiate Jesduvroq in pregnancy. If pregnancy is confirmed during treatment, discontinue Jesduvroq immediately. Exclude pregnancy prior to starting Jesduvroq and advise female and male patients of reproductive potential to use effective contraception. Breastfeeding is not recommended until 1 week after the final dose of Jesduvroq. To report suspected adverse reactions, contact GlaxoSmithKline at 1-888-825-5249 or FDA at 1-800-FDA-1088 or www.fda.gov/medwatch.

ANEMIA: FOLIC ACID DEFICIENCY

▷ *folic acid* (OTC) 0.4-1 mg once daily
Comment: *Folic acid (vitamin B9)* 400 mcg daily is recommended during pregnancy to prevent neural tube defects. Women who have had a baby with a neural tube defect should take 400 mcg every day, even when not planning to become pregnant, and if planning to become pregnant should take 4 mg daily during the month before becoming pregnant until at least the 12th week of pregnancy.

ANEMIA: HEMOLYTIC/ANEMIA: PYRUVATE KINASE (PK) DEFICIENCY

PYRUVATE KINASE (PK) ACTIVATOR

▷ *mitapivat* initially 5 mg bid, with or without food; swallow whole, do not break, crush, or chew; see the mfr pkg insert for full prescribing information, including dose titration and taper schedules
Pediatric: Safety and efficacy not established
Comment: Pyrukynd is a pyruvate kinase (PK) activator and is the first disease-modifying therapy indicated for the treatment of hemolytic anemia in adults with PK deficiency. Abruptly stopping and pausing Pyrukynd could worsen premature red blood cell destruction; see pkg insert for appropriate tapering for discontinuation. The most common side effects of Pyrukynd are decreases in estrone and estradiol in men, and increased urate, back pain, and joint stiffness. The effects of Pyrukynd on estrone and estradiol could not be reliably assessed in women due to normal changes in these hormones during the menstrual cycle

and use of hormonal contraception. Avoid concomitant use of **Pyrukynd** with strong CYP3A inhibitors and inducers. Do not titrate **Pyrukynd** beyond 20 mg bid with concomitant moderate CYP3A inducers. Consider alternatives that are not moderate CYP3A inducers; if there are no alternatives, adjust the **Pyrukynd** dose. Avoid concomitant use of **Pyrukynd** with substrates that have a narrow therapeutic index: sensitive CYP3A, CYP2B6, and CYP2C substrates, including hormonal contraceptives; UGT1A1 substrates; and P-gp substrates. Avoid use of **Pyrukynd** in patients with Child-Pugh B or C impairment. Consider maternal and fetal risk/benefit of **Pyrukynd** in females with untreated versus treated as it is known that untreated PK deficiency in pregnancy may precipitate acute hemolysis, preterm labor, miscarriage, and severe anemia requiring frequent transfusion. Additionally, preeclampsia and severe hypertension have been reported. Available data from clinical trials of **Pyrukynd** are insufficient to evaluate for a drug-associated risk of major birth defects, miscarriage, or other adverse maternal or fetal outcomes. In pre- and postnatal animal reproduction studies, *mitapivat* orally administered bid, including the period of organogenesis, was not teratogenic or otherwise harmful to fetal developmental outcomes at doses up to 13 and 3 times the maximum recommended human dose (MRHD). There are no data on the presence of **Pyrukynd** or its metabolites in human or animal milk or effects on the breastfed infant. Developmental and health benefits of breastfeeding should be considered along with the mother's clinical need for **Pyrukynd** and any potential adverse effects on the breastfed infant from **Pyrukynd** or from the underlying maternal condition.

ANEMIA: IRON DEFICIENCY (IDA)

Comment: Hemochromatosis and hemosiderosis are contraindications to iron therapy. **Iron** supplements are best absorbed when taken between meals and with **vitamin C-rich foods**. Excessive **iron** may be extremely hazardous to infants and young children. All vitamin and mineral supplements should be kept out of reach of children. Untreated iron deficiency anemia (IDA) in pregnancy is associated with adverse maternal outcomes such as postpartum anemia. Adverse pregnancy outcomes associated with IDA include increased risk for preterm delivery and low birth weight.

IRON AGENTS (ORAL FORMS)
▷ *ferrous gluconate* (G) 1 tab once daily
    Pediatric: <12 years: not recommended; ≥12 years: same as adult
    Fergon (OTC)
      Tab: iron 27 mg (240 mg as gluconate)
▷ *ferric maltol* 30 mg bid on an empty stomach (1 hour before or 2 hours after a meal); continue as long as necessary to replenish body iron stores; do not open, break, or chew
    Pediatric: safety and efficacy not established
    Accrufer *Cap:* 30 mg
    Comment: Accrufer *(ferric maltol)*, formerly **Feraccru**, is a non-salt formulation of ferric iron for the treatment of iron deficiency in adults. **Accrufer** is not absorbed systemically as an intact complex following oral administration. Maternal use in pregnancy is not expected to result in fetal exposure, and breastfeeding is not expected to result in exposure of the infant.
▷ *ferrous sulfate* (G)
    Feosol Tablets (OTC) 1 tab tid-qid pc and HS
    Pediatric: <6 years: use elixir; ≥6-12 years: 1 tab tid pc
      Tab: iron 65 mg (200 mg as sulfate)
    Feosol Capsules (OTC) 1-2 caps daily
    Pediatric: not recommended
      Cap: iron 50 mg (169 mg as sulfate) sust-rel
    Feosol Elixir (OTC) 5-10 ml tid between meals
    Pediatric: <1 year: not recommended; >1-11 years: 2.5-5 ml tid between meals; ≥12 years: same as adult
      Elix: iron 44 mg (220 mg as sulfate) per 5 ml
    Fer-In-Sol (OTC) 5 ml daily
    Pediatric: <4 years, use drops; ≥4 years: 5 ml once daily
      Syr: iron 18 mg (90 mg as sulfate) per 5 ml (480 ml)
    Fer-In-Sol Drops (OTC)
    Pediatric: <4 years: 0.6 ml daily; ≥4 years: use syrup
      Oral drops: iron 15 mg (75 mg as sulfate) per 5 ml (50 ml)

IRON AGENT (IV INFUSION)
▷ *ferric carboxymaltose* ≥*50 kg:* 750 mg via IV infusion in 2 doses separated by at least 7 days for a total cumulative dose of 1,500 mg; ≥*50 kg, Alternative dosing:* 15 mg/kg as a single treatment dose to a max of 1,000 mg; <*50 kg:* 15 mg/kg via IV infusion in two doses separated by at least 7 days; treatment may be repeated if IDA reoccurs
    Pediatric: <1 year: not recommended; ≥1 year, <50 kg: 15 mg/kg via IV infusion in two doses separated by at least 7 days; treatment may be repeated if IDA reoccurs; ≥1 year, ≥50 kg: same as adult

(continued)

Injectafer *Vial:* 100 mg/2 ml, 750 mg/15 ml, 1,000 mg/20 ml (50 mg/ml), single-dose
Comment: Injectafer is an iron replacement product indicated for the treatment of IDA in adults and pediatric patients ≥1 year of age who have either intolerance to oral iron or an unsatisfactory response to oral iron, and adult patients who have non-dialysis-dependent chronic kidney disease (CKD). Hypersensitivity reaction to Injectafer or any of its inactive components is the only contraindication to Injectafer. Observe for signs and symptoms of hypersensitivity during and after Injectafer administration for at least 30 minutes and until clinically stable following completion of each administration. Monitor serum phosphate levels in patients at risk for low serum phosphate who require a repeat course of treatment. Monitor patients closely for signs and symptoms of hypertension following each Injectafer administration. The most common adverse reactions in adult patients (>2%) have been nausea, hypertension, flushing, injection site reactions, erythema, hypophosphatemia, and dizziness. The most common adverse reactions in pediatric patients (≥4) have been hypophosphatemia, injection site reaction, rash, headache, and vomiting. There are risks to the fetus associated with untreated IDA in pregnancy (e.g., increased risk for preterm delivery and low birth weight), as well as risks to the fetus associated with maternal severe hypersensitivity reaction (e.g., circulatory failure [severe hypotension and shock, including in the context of anaphylactic reaction] may occur in pregnant patients receiving parenteral iron products [which may cause fetal bradycardia, especially during the second and third trimesters]). Published studies and available data from postmarketing reports are insufficient to assess the risk of major birth defects and miscarriage. Iron is present in human breast milk. Among the breastfed infants, adverse reactions included constipation and diarrhea, but none of the adverse reactions reported were considered related to *ferric carboxymaltose* exposure through breastfeeding. Developmental and health benefits of breastfeeding should be considered along with the mother's clinical need for Injectafer in addition to any potential adverse effects on the breastfed infant from the drug or from the underlying maternal condition.

▷ *ferumoxytol Recommended dose:* initially 510 mg via IV infusion followed by a second 510 mg IV infusion 3 to 8 days later; administer infusion undiluted at a rate of up to 1 ml/sec (30 mg/sec); the recommended dose may be readministered to patients with persistent or recurrent IDA
Pediatric:
Feraheme *Vial:* 510 mg/17 ml (30 mg/ml), single-use, elemental iron
Comment: Feraheme is an iron replacement product indicated for the treatment of IDA in adult patients with CKD. Monitor patients for signs and symptoms of hypersensitivity for at least 30 minutes following infusion administration. Feraheme infusion may cause hypotension; monitor for signs and symptoms of hypotension following the administration of Feraheme. Regularly monitor hematologic responses during Feraheme therapy; do not administer Feraheme to patients with iron overload. Feraheme can alter MRI studies. The most common adverse reactions (≥2%) following the administration of Feraheme have been diarrhea, nausea, dizziness, hypotension, constipation, and peripheral edema. There are no studies of Feraheme in human pregnancy. In animal studies, Feraheme caused decreased fetal weights and fetal malformations at maternally toxic doses of 13-15 times the human dose. Use Feraheme during pregnancy only if the potential benefit justifies the potential risk to the fetus. It is not known whether Feraheme is present in human milk. Because of the potential for adverse reaction in breastfeeding infants, a decision should be made whether to discontinue nursing or to avoid Feraheme, taking into account the importance of Feraheme to the mother and the known benefits of breastfeeding. To report suspected adverse reactions with Feraheme, contact AMAG Pharmaceuticals at 1-877-411-2510 or FDA at 1-800-FDA-1088 or www.fda.gov/medwatch.

ANEMIA: PERNICIOUS/MEGALOBLASTIC

Comment: Signs of **vitamin B12** deficiency include megaloblastic anemia, glossitis, paresthesias, ataxia, spastic motor weakness, and reduced mentation.
▷ *vitamin B12 (cyanocobalamin)* (G) 500 mcg intranasally once a week; may increase dose if serum B12 levels decline; adjust dose in 500 mcg increments
Nascobal Nasal Spray *Intranasal gel:* 500 mcg/0.1 ml (1.3 ml, 4 doses) (citric acid, benzalkonium chloride)
Comment: Nascobal Nasal Spray is indicated for maintenance of hematologic remission following IM B12 therapy without nervous system involvement. Must be primed before each use.

ANESTHESIA: PROCEDURAL SEDATION

▷ *remimazolam* individualize and titrate **Byfavo** to desired clinical effect; 2.5-5 mg IV over 1 minute; if necessary, administer supplemental doses of 1.25-2.5 mg IV over 15 seconds; wait at least 2 minutes before administration of any supplemental dose; may be administered only by a qualified healthcare provider who is trained in the administration of conscious sedation and who is not involved in the conduct of the diagnostic or therapeutic procedure, in an appropriate healthcare setting, equipped with supportive and resuscitative supplies and equipment

Pediatric: <18 years: not recommended; ≥18 years: same as adult

Byfavo *Vial:* 20 mg, single-patient, pwdr for reconstitution and intravenous push (IVP) administration

Comment: Byfavo *(remimazolam)* is an ultra-short-acting IV **benzodiazepine** sedative/anesthetic for the induction and maintenance of procedural sedation in adults undergoing procedures lasting 30 minutes or less. The administering personnel must be trained in the detection and management of airway obstruction, hypoventilation, and apnea, including the maintenance of a patent airway, supportive ventilation, and cardiovascular resuscitation. **Byfavo** has been associated with hypoxia, bradycardia, and hypotension. Continuously monitor vital signs during sedation and through the recovery period. Resuscitative drugs and age- and size-appropriate equipment for bag/valve/mask-assisted ventilation must be immediately available during administration of **Byfavo**. Concomitant use of benzodiazepines with opioid analgesics may result in profound sedation, respiratory depression, coma, and death. The sedative effect of IV **Byfavo** can be accentuated by concomitantly administered central nervous system (CNS) depressant medications, including other benzodiazepines and **propofol**. Continuously monitor patients for respiratory depression and depth of sedation. Sedating drugs, such as **Byfavo**, may cause confusion and oversedation in the elderly; elderly patients generally should be observed closely. *Severe Hepatic Impairment:* Reduced dosage may be indicated; titrate carefully to effect. Infants born to mothers using benzodiazepines during the later stages of pregnancy have been reported to experience symptoms of sedation. Although there are no data on the effects of **Byfavo** use in pregnant females, available data from published observational studies of pregnant females exposed to other benzodiazepines have not established a drug-associated risk of major birth defects, miscarriage, or adverse maternal or embryo/fetal outcomes. Breastfeeding females may pump and discard breast milk for 5 hours after treatment with **Byfavo**.

ANGIOFIBROMA, FACIAL, ASSOCIATED WITH TUBEROUS SCLEROSIS

mTOR INHIBITOR IMMUNOSUPPRESSANT

Comment: Mammalian target of rapamycin (mTOR) regulates cell proliferation, autophagy, and apoptosis by participating in multiple signaling pathways in the body. Studies have shown that the mTOR signaling pathway is also associated with cancer, arthritis, insulin resistance, osteoporosis, and other diseases. The mTOR signaling pathway, which is often activated in tumors, not only regulates gene transcription and protein synthesis to regulate cell proliferation and immune cell differentiation but also plays an important role in tumor metabolism. Therefore, the mTOR signaling pathway is a hot target in anti-tumor therapy research. In recent years, a variety of newly discovered mTOR inhibitors have entered clinical studies, and a variety of drugs have been shown to have high activity in combination with mTOR inhibitors.

▷ **sirolimus** apply to the skin of the face affected with angiofibroma bid; max 800 mg (2.5 cm)

Pediatric: <6 years: safety and efficacy not established; 6-11 years: apply to the skin of the face bid; max daily dose: 600 mg (2 cm); ≥12 years: same as adult

Hyftor Gel *Topical gel:* 0.2% (2 mg *sirolimus* per gm)

Comment: Hyftor topical gel is an mTOR inhibitor immunosuppressant indicated for the treatment of facial angiofibroma associated with tuberous sclerosis in adults and pediatric patients ≥6 years of age. Complete all age-appropriate vaccinations as recommended by current immunization guidelines prior to **Hyftor** initiation. Do not use with occlusive dressing. Oral **sirolimus** has been associated with hypersensitivity reactions, including anaphylactic/anaphylactoid reactions, angioedema, exfoliative dermatitis, and hypersensitivity vasculitis; discontinue **Hyftor** immediately if symptoms of hypersensitivity occur. Serious infections, including opportunistic infections and latent viral infections, such as progressive multifocal leukoencephalopathy, have been reported with oral **sirolimus**; discontinue **Hyftor** immediately if symptoms of infection occur. Oral **sirolimus** has been associated with malignancy, including lymphoma and skin cancer. Patients should minimize or avoid exposure to natural or artificial sunlight (tanning beds or UVA/B treatments) while using **Hyftor**. Oral **sirolimus** has been associated with increased serum cholesterol and triglycerides requiring treatment. Monitor for hyperlipidemia during treatment. Oral **sirolimus** has been associated with interstitial lung disease (ILD)/non-infectious pneumonitis (NIP), sometimes fatal; discontinue **sirolimus** if symptoms of ILD/NIP occur. During treatment with **Hyftor**, vaccinations may be less effective; avoid use of live vaccines during treatment. The most common adverse reactions (incidence ≥1%) have been dry skin, application site irritation, pruritus, acne, acneiform dermatitis, ocular hyperemia, skin hemorrhage, and skin irritation. During concomitant use of **Hyftor** with CYP3A4 inhibitors, monitor for **Hyftor** adverse reactions. During concomitant use of **Hyftor** with drugs that are both substrates and inhibitors of CYP3A, monitor for adverse reactions of the CYP3A substrate and inhibitor. Advise females of reproductive potential that, based on animal studies, oral sirolimus can cause fetal harm. Exclude pregnancy prior to initiating treatment with **Hyftor**. Use of effective contraception is recommended for females of reproductive potential prior to and throughout treatment and for 12 weeks after the final dose of **Hyftor**. Breastfeeding not recommended. Oral **sirolimus** has been associated with azoospermia and oligospermia. Advise males that **Hyftor** may impair fertility. To report suspected adverse reactions, contact Nobelpharma America at 1 (877) 375-0825 or FDA at 1-800-FDA-1088 or www.fda.gov/medwatch.

ANGINA PECTORIS: STABLE

▷ *aspirin* 325 mg (range 75-325 mg) once daily
  Comment: Daily *aspirin* dose is contingent upon whether the patient is also taking an anticoagulant or antiplatelet agent.

CALCIUM ANTAGONISTS

Comment: Calcium antagonists are contraindicated with history of ventricular arrhythmias, sick sinus syndrome (SSS), 2nd or 3rd degree heart block, cardiogenic shock, acute myocardial infarction, and pulmonary congestion.

▷ *amlodipine* (G) 5-10 mg daily
  Pediatric: <12 years: not recommended; ≥12 years: same as adult
    Norvasc *Tab:* 2.5, 5, 10 mg
▷ *amlodipine benzoate* recommended starting dose 5 mg orally once daily; max 10 mg once daily; small stature, fragile, or elderly patients, or patients with hepatic insufficiency may be started on 2.5 mg once daily
  Pediatric: <6 years: not studied; ≥6 years: starting dose: 2.5-5 mg once daily
    Katerzia *Oral susp:* 1 mg/ml (150 ml); keep refrigerated
    Comment: Katerzia *(amlodipine benzoate)* is a calcium channel blocker in an oral suspension formulation indicated for treatment of hypertension in adults and children ≥6 years of age to lower blood pressure. Lowering blood pressure reduces the risk of fatal and non-fatal cardiovascular events, primarily strokes and myocardial infarctions. **Katerzia** is also indicated for adult patients with coronary artery disease (CAD), chronic stable angina (CSA), vasospastic angina (Prinzmetal's or variant angina), and angiographically documented CAD in patients without heart failure or an ejection fraction <40%, at the same dose as for blood pressure management (2.5-10 mg once daily).
▷ *amlodipine besylate* *Recommended starting Dose:* 5 mg once daily; max 10 mg once daily; small, fragile, or elderly patients, or patients with hepatic insufficiency may be started on 2.5 mg once daily
  Pediatric: <6 years: safety and efficacy not established; ≥6 years: 2.5 (2.5 ml) to 5 mg (5 ml) once daily
    Norliqva *Oral soln:* 1 mg/ml (150 ml) (peppermint)
    Comment: Norliqva is an oral solution formulation of the approved calcium channel blocker (CCB) *amlodipine* indicated for the treatment of hypertension and angina in patients with CAD. The limited available data based on postmarketing reports with *amlodipine* use in human pregnancy are not sufficient to inform a drug-associated risk of major birth defects and miscarriage. There are risks to the mother and the fetus associated with poorly controlled hypertension in pregnancy. In animal reproduction studies, there was no evidence of adverse developmental effects when treated orally with *amlodipine maleate* during organogenesis at doses approximately 10 and 20 times the maximum recommended human dose (MRHD), respectively. However, litter size was significantly decreased (by about 50%) and the number of intrauterine deaths was significantly increased (about five fold). *Amlodipine* has been shown to prolong both the gestation period and the duration of labor at this dose. Limited available data from a published clinical lactation study report that *amlodipine* is present in human milk at an estimated median relative infant dose of 4.2%. No adverse effects of amlodipine on the breastfed infant have been observed.

▷ *diltiazem* (G)
  Pediatric: <12 years: not recommended; ≥12 years: same as adult
    Cardizem initially 30 mg qid; may increase gradually every 1-2 days; max 360 mg/day in divided doses
      Tab: 30, 60, 90, 120 mg
    Cardizem CD initially 120-180 mg daily; adjust at 1- to 2-week intervals; max 480 mg/day
      Cap: 120, 180, 240, 300, 360 mg ext-rel
    Cardizem LA initially 180-240 mg daily; titrate at 2 week intervals; max 540 mg/day
      Tab: 120, 180, 240, 300, 360, 420 mg ext-rel
    Cartia XT initially 180 mg or 240 mg once daily; max 540 mg once daily
      Cap: 120, 180, 240, 300 mg ext-rel
    Dilacor XR initially 180 mg or 240 mg once daily; max 540 mg once daily
      Cap: 180, 240 mg ext-rel
    Tiazac initially 120-180 mg daily; max 540 mg/day
      Cap: 120, 180, 240, 300, 360, 420 mg ext-rel
▷ *nicardipine* (G) initially 20 mg tid; adjust q 3 days; max 120 mg/day
  Pediatric: not recommended
    Cardene *Cap:* 20, 30 mg
▷ *nifedipine* (G)
  Pediatric: <12 years: not recommended; ≥12 years: same as adult
    Adalat CC initially 30 mg once daily; usual range 30-60 mg tid; max 90 mg/day
      Tab: 30, 60, 90 mg ext-rel
    Procardia initially 10 mg tid; titrate over 7-14 days: max 30 mg/dose and 180 mg/day in divided doses
      Cap: 10, 20 mg
    Procardia XL initially 30-60 mg daily; titrate over 7-14 days; max dose 90 mg/day
      Tab: 30, 60, 90 mg ext-rel

▷ *verapamil* (G)
  Pediatric: <12 years: <u>not</u> recommended; ≥12 years: same as adult
    Calan 80-120 mg tid; increase daily <u>or</u> weekly if needed
      Tab: 40, 80*, 120*mg
        Calan SR initially 120 mg once daily; increase weekly if needed
          Tab: 120, 180, 240 mg
        Covera HS initially 180 mg q HS; titrate in steps to 240 mg; then to 360 mg; then to 480 mg if needed
          Tab: 180, 240 mg ext-rel
        Isoptin SR initially 120-180 mg in the AM; may increase to 240 mg in the AM; then 180 mg q 12 hours
        <u>or</u> 240 mg in the AM and 120 mg in the PM; then 240 mg q 12 hours
          Tab: 120, 180*, 240*mg sust-rel

BETA-BLOCKERS

Comment: Beta-blockers are contraindicated with history of SSS, second- or third-degree heart block, cardiogenic shock, pulmonary congestion, asthma, moderate-to-severe chronic obstructive pulmonary disease (COPD) with FEV1 (forced expiratory volumn in1 second) <50%: of predicted, <u>and/or</u> patients on chronic bronchodilator treatment.
▷ *atenolol* (G) initially 25-50 mg daily; increase weekly if needed; max 200 mg daily
  Pediatric: <12 years: <u>not</u> recommended; ≥12 years: same as adult
    Tenormin *Tab:* 25, 50, 100 mg
▷ *metoprolol succinate*
  Pediatric: <12 years: <u>not</u> recommended; ≥12 years: same as adult
    Toprol-XL initially 100 mg in a single dose once daily; increase weekly if needed; max 400 mg/day
      Tab: 25*, 50*, 100*, 200*mg ext-rel
▷ *metoprolol tartrate*
  Pediatric: <12 years: <u>not</u> recommended; ≥12 years: same as adult
    Lopressor (G) initially 25-50 mg bid; increase weekly if needed; max 400 mg/day
      Tab: 25, 37.5, 50, 75, 100 mg
▷ *nadolol* (G) initially 40 mg daily; increase q 3-7 days; max 240 mg/day
  Pediatric: <u>not</u> recommended
    Corgard *Tab:* 20*, 40*, 80*, 120*, 160*mg
▷ *propranolol* (G)
  Pediatric: <12 years: <u>not</u> recommended; ≥12 years: same as adult
    Inderal LA initially 80 mg daily in a single dose; increase q 3-7 days; usual range 120-160 mg/day; max 320 mg/day in a single dose
      Cap: 60, 80, 120, 160 mg sust-rel
    InnoPran XL initially 80 mg q HS; max 120 mg/day
      Cap: 80, 120 mg ext-rel

NITRATES

Comment: Use a daily nitrate dosing schedule that provides a dose-free period of 14 hours <u>or</u> more to prevent tolerance. *Aspirin* and *acetaminophen* may relieve nitrate-induced headache. *Isosorbide* is <u>not</u> recommended for use in myocardial infarction (MI) <u>and/or</u> congestive heart failure (CHF). Nitrate use is a contraindication to using phosphodiesterase type 5 inhibitors: *sildenafil* (Viagra), *tadalafil* (Cialis), and *vardenafil* (Levitra).
▷ *isosorbide dinitrate*
  Pediatric: <12 years: <u>not</u> recommended; ≥12 years: same as adult
    Dilatrate-SR 40 mg once daily; max 160 mg/day
      Cap: 40 mg sust-rel
    Isordil Titradose initially 5-20 mg q 6 hours; maintenance 10-40 mg q 6 hours
      Tab: 5, 10, 20, 30, 40 mg
▷ *isosorbide mononitrate*
  Pediatric: <12 years: <u>not</u> recommended; ≥12 years: same as adult
    Imdur initially 30-60 mg q AM; may increase to 120 mg daily; max 240 mg/day
      Tab: 30*, 60*, 120 mg ext-rel
    Ismo 20 mg upon awakening; then 20 mg 7 hours later
      Tab: 20*mg
▷ *nitroglycerin* (G)
  Pediatric: <12 years: <u>not</u> recommended; ≥12 years: same as adult
    Nitro-Bid Ointment initially 1/2 inch q 8 hours; titrate in 1/2 inch increments
      Oint: 2% (20, 60 gm)
    Nitrodisc initially one 0.2 <u>to</u> 0.4 mg/Hr patch for 12-14 hours/day
      Transdermal disc: 0.2, 0.3, 0.4 mg/hour (30, 100/carton)
    Nitrolingual Pump Spray 1-2 sprays on <u>or</u> under tongue; max 3 sprays/15 minutes
      Spray: 0.4 mg/dose (14.5 gm, 200 doses)

(continued)

Nitromist 1-2 sprays at onset of attack, on or under the tongue while sitting; may repeat q 5 minutes as needed; max 3 sprays/15 minutes; may use prophylactically 5-10 minutes prior to exertion; do not inhale spray; do not rinse mouth for 5-10 minutes after use
> *Lingual aerosol spray:* 0.4 mg/actuation (230 metered sprays)

Nitrostat 1 tab SL; may repeat q 5 minutes x 3
> *SL tab:* 0.3 (1/100 gr), 0.4 (1/150 gr), 0.6 (1/4 gr) mg

Transderm-Nitro initially one 0.2 mg/hour or 0.4 mg/hour patch for 12-14 hours/day
> *Transdermal patch:* 0.1, 0.2, 0.4, 0.6, 0.8 mg/hour

NON-NITRATE PERIPHERAL VASODILATOR

▷ *hydralazine* (G) initially 10 mg qid x 2-4 days; then increase to 25 mg qid for the remainder of the first week; then increase to 50 mg qid; max 300 mg/day
Pediatric: <12 years: not recommended; ≥12 years: same as adult
> *Tab:* 10, 25, 50, 100 mg

NITRATE+PERIPHERAL VASODILATOR COMBINATION

▷ *isosorbide+hydralazine HCl* initially 1 tab tid; max 2 tabs tid
Pediatric: <12 years: not established; ≥12 years: same as adult
> **Bidil** *Tab:* isosorb 20 mg+hydral 37.5 mg

NON-NITRATE ANTIANGINAL

▷ *ranolazine* initially 500 mg bid; may increase to max 1 gm bid
Pediatric: <12 years: not recommended; ≥12 years: same as adult
> **Ranexa** *Tab:* 500, 1000 mg ext-rel
> **Comment:** Ranexa is indicated for the treatment of chronic angina that is inadequately controlled with other antianginals. Use with *amlodipine*, beta-blocker, or nitrate.

ANOREXIA/CACHEXIA

APPETITE STIMULANTS

▷ *cyproheptadine* (G) initially 4 mg tid prn; then adjust as needed; usual range 12-16 mg/day; max 32 mg/day
Pediatric: <2 years: not recommended; ≥2-6 years: 2 mg bid-tid prn; max 12 mg/day; 7-14 years: 4 mg bid-tid prn; max 16 mg/day; >14 years: same as adult
> **Periactin** *Tab:* cypro 4*mg; *Syr:* cypro 2 mg/5 ml

▷ *dronabinol* (cannabinoid) (III)
Pediatric: safety and efficacy not established; younger patients may be more sensitive to neurologic and psychoactive effects of *dronabinol;* **Syndros** contains dehydrated alcohol and 5.5% (w/w) propylene glycol; ethanol competitively inhibits the metabolism of propylene glycol, which may lead to elevated concentrations of propylene glycol; preterm neonates may be at increased risk of propylene glycol-associated adverse events due to diminished ability to metabolize it, thereby leading to accumulation; avoid use with preterm infants in the immediate postnatal period
> **Marinol** initially 2.5 mg bid before lunch and dinner; may reduce to 2.5 mg q HS or increase to 2.5 mg before lunch and 5 mg before dinner; max 20 mg/day in divided doses
>> *Cap:* 2.5, 5, 10 mg (sesame oil)
> **Syndros** take each dose with 6-8 oz water
> *Anorexia/cachexia associated with weight loss in patients with AIDS:* initially 2.1 mg bid 1 hour before lunch and dinner; if elderly, or severe or persistent central nervous system (CNS) effects occur, reduce dose to 2.1 mg once daily 1 hour before dinner or at bedtime; if tolerated, may gradually increase to 2.1 mg 1 hour before lunch and dinner or at bedtime as tolerated; max 8.4 mg bid;
> *Nausea/vomiting associated with chemotherapy:* recommended starting dosage is 4.2 mg/m^2, administered 1 to 3 hours prior to chemotherapy; then every 2 to 4 hours after chemotherapy for a total of 4-6 doses/day; administer the first dose on an empty stomach at least 30 minutes prior to eating; subsequent doses can be taken without regard to meals
> *Oral soln:* 5 mg/ml (50% w/w dehydrated alcohol, 5.5% w/w propylene glycol)

Comment: Dronabinol is contraindicated within 14 days before and 7 days after taking *disulfiram* or *metronidazole*. *Dronabinol* is highly protein-bound. Therefore, there is potential for displacement of other drugs from plasma proteins. Monitor for adverse reactions to concomitant narrow therapeutic index drugs (e.g., *warfarin, cyclosporine, amphotericin B*) when initiating or increasing the dosage of *dronabinol*. Delta-9-THC has been measured in the cord blood of some infants whose mothers reported prenatal use of cannabis, suggesting *dronabinol* may cross the placenta to the fetus during pregnancy. Effects of delta-9-THC on the fetus are not known. (NOTE: Delta-9 tetrahydrocannabinol [THC] and the less-potent delta-8 tetrahydrocannabinol [THC] are the psychoactive components of the cannabis sativa plant.) There are limited data on the presence of *dronabinol* in human milk and effects on the breastfed infant. The reported effects of inhaled cannabis transferred to the breastfeeding infant have been inconsistent and insufficient to establish causality. Because of the possible adverse effects from *dronabinol* on the breastfed infant, advise females with nausea/vomiting associated with cancer chemotherapy not to breastfeed during treatment with *dronabinol* and for 9 days after the last chemotherapy dose.

➤ *megestrol* (progestin) (G) 40 mg qid
  Pediatric: <12 years: not recommended; ≥12 years: same as adult
  Megace *Tab:* 20*, 40*mg
  Megace ES *Oral susp (concentrate):* 125 mg/ml, 625 mg/5 ml (5 oz) (lemon-lime)
  Megace Oral Suspension *Oral susp:* 40 mg/ml (8 oz), 820 mg/20 ml (lemon-lime)
  Megestrol Acetate Oral Suspension (G) 125 mg/ml
  Comment: *Megestrol* is indicated for the treatment of anorexia, cachexia, or an unexplained, significant weight loss in patients with a diagnosis of AIDS.

ANTHRAX (*BACILLUS ANTHRACIS*)

POST-EXPOSURE PROPHYLAXIS OF INHALATIONAL ANTHRAX AND TREATMENT OF INHALED AND CUTANEOUS ANTHRAX INFECTION

Comment: *Bacillus anthracis* spores are resistant to destruction, are easily spread by release into the air, and cause irreversible tissue damage and death. The most lethal form is inhalational anthrax. Even with the most aggressive treatment, the mortality rate is about 45%. People at risk are those who work in slaughterhouses, tanneries, and wood mills who are exposed to infected animals.

Comment: All 14 members of the Advisory Committee on Immunization Practices (ACIP) voted to approve the anthrax vaccine recommendations for 2018-2019 at their meeting. The recommendations to the committee sought to optimize the use of Anthrax Vaccine Adsorbed (AVA) in post-exposure prophylaxis (PEP) in the event of a wide-area release of *B. anthracis* spores. In this event, a mass vaccination effort would be undertaken requiring expedited administration of AVA. ACIP now recommends that the intramuscular administration may be used over the traditional subcutaneous approach if there are any operational or logistical challenges that delay effective vaccination. Another recommendation from ACIP would allow 2 full doses or 3 half-doses of AVA to be used to expand vaccine coverage for PEP in the event there is an inadequate vaccine supply. The committee also recommended that AbxPEP, an antimicrobial, be stopped 42 days after the first dose of AVA or 2 weeks after the last dose. The committee's recommendations will be used by the CDC to inform state and local health departments to better prepare for an emergency response to a wide-area release of *B. anthracis* spores. The committee's recommendations must be approved by the CDC's director before they are considered official recommendations.

Immune Globulin

➤ *bacillus anthracis immune globulin intravenous (human)* administer via IV infusion at a maximum rate of 2 ml/min; dose is weight-based as follows, but may be doubled in severe cases if weight >5 kg:
  Pediatric: <16 years: not established; 5-<10 kg: 1 vial; 10-<18 kg: 2 vials; 18-<25 kg: 3 vials; 25-<35 kg: 4 vials; 35-<50 kg: 5 vials; 50-<60 kg: 6 vials; ≥60 kg: 7 vials
  Anthrasil *Vial:* (60 units) sterile solution of purified human immune globulin g (IgG) containing polyclonal antibodies that target the anthrax toxins of *B. anthracis* for IV infusion (preservative-free)
  Comment: Anthrasil is indicated for the emergent treatment of inhaled anthrax, in combination with appropriate antibacterial agents.

MONOCLONAL ANTIBODIES

Comment: *Obiltoxaximab* and *raxibacumab* have no antibacterial activity; rather, they are monoclonal antibodies that neutralize toxins produced by *B. anthracis* by binding to the bacterium's protective antigen, preventing intracellular entry of key enzymatic toxin components. *Obiltoxaximab* (Anthim) and *raxibacumab* are indicated for the treatment of inhalational anthrax, in combination with appropriate antibacterial drugs, and for prophylaxis of inhalational anthrax when alternative therapies are unavailable or inappropriate. Vials must be refrigerated and protected from light. Do not shake the vials. Premedicate the patient with *diphenhydramine*.

➤ *obiltoxaximab* 16 mg/kg diluted in 0.9% NS via IV infusion over 90 minutes
  Pediatric: see mfr pkg insert for dosing based on kilograms body weight
  Anthim *Vial:* 600 mg in 6 ml (100 mg/ml), single-use, for dilution in 0.9% NS and IV infusion
➤ *raxibacumab* (G) 40 mg/kg diluted in 0.45% NS or 0.9% NS via IV infusion over 2 hours and 15 minutes; see mfr pkg insert for recommended volume of dilution according to weight-based dose
  Pediatric: ≤15 kg: 80 mg/kg; >15-50 kg: 60 mg/kg; >50 kg: same as adult
  Vial: 1700 mg/34 ml (50 mg/ml), single-use, for dilution and IV infusion

ANTIBACTERIAL AGENTS

➤ *ciprofloxacin* 500 mg (or 10-15 mg/kg/day) q 12 hours for 60 days (start as soon as possible after exposure)
  Pediatric: <18 years: 20-40 mg/kg/day divided q 12 hours; ≥18 years: same as adult
  Cipro (G) *Tab:* 250, 500, 750 mg; *Oral susp:* 250, 500 mg/5 ml (100 ml) (strawberry)
  Cipro XR *Tab:* 500, 1000 mg ext-rel
  ProQuin XR *Tab:* 500 mg ext-rel
  Comment: *Ciprofloxacin, a fluoroquinolone*, is usually contraindicated in patients <18 years of age and during pregnancy and lactation. Risk/benefit must be assessed in the case of anthrax.

(continued)

▶ *doxycycline* (G) 100 mg daily bid
  Pediatric: <8 years: usually contraindicated; ≥8 years, <100 lb: 2 mg/lb on the first day in 2 divided doses, followed by 1 mg/lb/day in a single or 2 divided doses; ≥8 years, ≥100 lb: same as adult;
  see Appendix BB.19. *doxycycline* (G) (Vibramycin Syrup/Suspension) *for dose by weight*
    Acticlate *Tab:* 75, 150**mg
    Adoxa *Tab:* 50, 75, 100, 150 mg ent-coat
    Doryx *Tab:* 50, 75, 100, 150, 200 mg del-rel
    Doxteric *Tab:* 50 mg del-rel
    Monodox *Cap:* 50, 75, 100 mg
    Oracea *Cap:* 40 mg del-rel
    Vibramycin *Tab:* 100 mg; *Cap:* 50, 100 mg; *Syr:* 50 mg/5 ml (raspberry-apple) (sulfites); *Oral susp:* 25 mg/5 ml (raspberry)
    Vibra-Tab *Tab:* 100 mg film-coat
  Comment: *Doxycycline,* a tetracycline, is usually contraindicated in patients <8 years of age and during pregnancy and lactation (discolors developing tooth enamel). Risk/benefit must be assessed in the case of anthrax.
▶ *minocycline* (G) 2 mg/lb on the first day in 2 divided doses, followed by 1 mg/lb q 12 hours x 9 more days; ≥8 years, >100 mg: 100 mg every 12 hours
  Pediatric: <8 years: usually not recommended; ≥8 years, <100 lb: same as adult
    Dynacin *Cap:* 50, 100 mg
    Minocin *Cap:* 50, 75, 100 mg; *Oral susp:* 50 mg/5 ml (60 ml) (custard) (sulfites, alcohol 5%)
  Comment: *Minocycline,* a tetracycline, is usually contraindicated in patients <8 years of age and during pregnancy and lactation (discolors developing tooth enamel). Risk/benefit must be assessed in the case of anthrax.

TREATMENT OF GASTROINTESTINAL AND OROPHARYNGEAL ANTHRAX

▶ *ciprofloxacin* 400 mg IV q 12 hours (start as soon as possible); then switch to 500 mg PO q 12 hours for a total of 60 days; infuse dose over 60 minutes
  Pediatric: <18 years: usually not recommended; 10-15 mg/kg IV q 12 hours (start as soon as possible); then switch to 10-15 mg/kg PO q 12 hours for 60 days
    Cipro (G) *Tab:* 250, 500, 750 mg; *Oral susp:* 250, 500 mg/5 ml (100 ml) (strawberry); *IV conc:* 10 mg/ml after dilution (20, 40 ml); *IV premix:* 2 mg/ml (100, 200 ml)
    Cipro XR *Tab:* 500, 1,000 mg ext-rel
    ProQuin XR *Tab:* 500 mg ext-rel
  Comment: *Ciprofloxacin, a fluoroquinolone,* is usually contraindicated in ptients <18 years of age and during pregnancy and lactation. Risk/benefit must be assessed in the case of anthrax.
▶ *doxycycline* (G) 100 mg daily bid
  Pediatric: <8 years: not recommended; ≥8 years, <100 lb: 2 mg/lb on the first day in 2 divided doses, followed by 1 mg/lb/day in a single or 2 divided doses; ≥8 years, ≥100 lb: same as adult;
  see Appendix BB.19. *doxycycline* (G) (Vibramycin Syrup/Suspension) *for dose by weight*
    Acticlate *Tab:* 75, 150**mg
    Adoxa *Tab:* 50, 75, 100, 150 mg ent-coat
    Doryx *Tab:* 50, 75, 100, 150, 200 mg del-rel
    Doxteric *Tab:* 50 mg del-rel
    Monodox *Cap:* 50, 75, 100 mg
    Oracea *Cap:* 40 mg del-rel
    Vibramycin *Tab:* 100 mg; *Cap:* 50, 100 mg; *Syr:* 50 mg/5 ml (raspberry-apple) (sulfites); *Oral susp:* 25 mg/5 ml (raspberry)
    Vibra-Tab *Tab:* 100 mg film-coat
  Comment: *Doxycycline, (GAD AND SAD) a tetracycline,* is usually contraindicated in patients <8 years of age and during pregnancy and lactation. Risk/benefit must be assessed in the case of anthrax.
▶ *minocycline* (G) 100 mg q 12 hours
  Pediatric: <8 years: usually not recommended; ≥8 years, <100 lb: 2 mg/lb on first day in 2 divided doses, followed by 1 mg/lb q 12 hours x 9 more days; ≥8 years, ≥100 lb: same as adult
    Dynacin *Cap:* 50, 100 mg
    Minocin *Cap:* 50, 75, 100 mg; *Oral susp:* 50 mg/5 ml (60 ml) (custard) (sulfites, alcohol 5%)
  Comment: *Minocycline, a tetracycline,* is usually contraindicated in patients <8 years of age and during pregnancy and lactation. Risk/benefit must be assessed in the case of anthrax.

ANXIETY DISORDER: GENERALIZED (GAD), ANXIETY DISORDER: SOCIAL (SAD)

FIRST-GENERATION ORAL ANTIHISTAMINES

▶ *diphenhydramine* (G) 25-50 mg q 6-8 hours; max 100 mg/day
  Pediatric: <2 years: not recommended; 2-6 years: 6.25 mg q 4-6 hours, max 37.5 mg/day; >6-12 years: 12.5-25 mg q 4-6 hours, max 150 mg/day; ≥12 years: same as adult
    Benadryl (OTC) *Chew tab:* 12.5 mg (grape) (phenylalanine); *Liq:* 12.5 mg/5 ml (4, 8 oz); *Cap:* 25 mg; *Tab:* 25 mg; *Dye-free soft gel:* 25 mg; *Dye-free liq:* 12.5 mg/5 ml (4, 8 oz)

▷ *hydroxyzine* (G) 50-100 mg qid; max 600 mg/day
  Pediatric: <6 years: 50 mg/day divided qid; ≥6 years: 50-100 mg/day divided qid
    Atarax *Tab:* 10, 25, 50, 100 mg; *Syr:* 10 mg/5 ml (alcohol 0.5%)
    Vistaril *Cap:* 25, 50, 100 mg; *Oral susp:* 25 mg/5 ml (4 oz) (lemon)
  Comment: *Hydroxyzine* is contraindicated in early pregnancy and in patients with a prolonged QT interval. It is not known whether this drug is excreted in human milk; therefore, *hydroxyzine* should not be given to nursing mothers.

AZAPIRONE
▷ *buspirone* initially 7.5 mg bid; may increase by 5 mg/day every 2 to 3 days; max 60 mg/day
  Pediatric: <6 years: not recommended; ≥6 years: same as adult
    BuSpar *Tab:* 5, 10, 15*, 30*mg

BENZODIAZEPINES
Comment: If possible when considering a benzodiazepine to treat anxiety, a short-acting benzodiazepine should be used only prn to avert intense anxiety and panic for the least time necessary while a different non-addictive antianxiety regimen (e.g., selective serotonin reuptake inhibitor (SSRI), serotonin-norepinephrine reuptake inhibitor (SNRI), tricyclic antidepressant (TCA), *buspirone*, and beta-blocker) is established and effective treatment goals achieved. Benzodiazepines have a high addiction potential when they are chronically used and are common drugs of abuse. *Benzodiazepine withdrawal syndrome* may include restlessness, agitation, anxiety, insomnia, tachycardia, tachypnea, and diaphoresis, and may be potentially life-threatening depending on the benzodiazepine and the length of use. Symptoms of withdrawal from short-acting benzodiazepines, such as *alprazolam* (Xanax), *oxazepam*, *lorazepam* (Ativan), and *triazolam* (Halcion), usually appear within 6-8 hours after the last dose and may continue 10-14 days. Symptoms of withdrawal from long-acting benzodiazepines, such as *diazepam* (Valium), *clonazepam* (Klonopin), and *chlordiazepoxide* (Librium), usually appear within 24-96 hours after the last dose and may continue from 3-4 weeks to 3 months. People who are heavily dependent on benzodiazepines may experience *protracted withdrawal syndrome* (PAWS), random periods of sharp withdrawal symptoms months after quitting. A closely monitored medical detoxification regimen may be required for a safe withdrawal and to prevent PAWS. Detoxification includes gradual tapering of the benzodiazepine along with other medications to manage the withdrawal symptoms.

Short-Acting Benzodiazepines
▷ *alprazolam* (IV)(G)
  Pediatric: <18 years: not recommended; ≥18 years: same as adult
    Niravam initially 0.25-0.5 mg tid; may titrate every 3-4 days; max 4 mg/day
      Tab: 0.25*, 0.5*, 1*, 2*mg orally-disint
    Xanax initially 0.25-0.5 mg tid; may titrate every 3-4 days; max 4 mg/day
      Tab: 0.25*, 0.5*, 1*, 2*mg
    Xanax XR initially 0.5-1 mg once daily, preferably in the AM; increase at intervals of at least 3 to 4 days by up to 1 mg/day; taper no faster than 0.5 mg every 3 days; max 10 mg/day; when switching from immediate-release *alprazolam*, give total daily dose of immediate-release once daily
      Tab: 0.5, 1, 2, 3 mg ext-rel
▷ *oxazepam* (IV)(G) 10-15 mg tid-qid for moderate symptoms; 15-30 mg tid-qid for severe symptoms
  Pediatric: <12 years: not recommended; ≥12 years: same as adult
  Cap: 10, 15, 30 mg

Intermediate-Acting Benzodiazepines
▷ *lorazepam* (IV)(G) 1-10 mg/day in 2 or 3 divided doses
  Pediatric: <12 years: not recommended; ≥12 years: same as adult
    Ativan *Tab:* 0.5, 1*, 2*mg
    Lorazepam Intensol *Oral conc:* 2 mg/ml (30 ml w. graduated dropper)

Long-Acting Benzodiazepines
▷ *chlordiazepoxide* (IV)(G)
  Pediatric: <6 years: not recommended; ≥6 years: 5 mg bid-qid; increase to 10 mg bid-tid
    Librium 5-10 mg tid to qid for moderate symptoms; 20-25 mg tid-qid for severe symptoms
      Cap: 5, 10, 25 mg
    Librium Injectable 50-100 mg IM or IV; then 25-50 mg IM tid-qid prn; max 300 mg/day
      Inj: 100 mg
▷ *chlordiazepoxide+clidinium* (IV) 1-2 caps tid-qid: max 8 caps/day
  Pediatric: not recommended
    Librax *Cap:* chlor 5 mg+clid 2.5 mg

(continued)

▷ *clonazepam* (IV)(G) initially 0.25 mg bid; increase to 1 mg/day after 3 days
  Pediatric: <18 years: <u>not</u> recommended; ≥18 years: same as adult
    Klonopin *Tab:* 0.5*, 1, 2 mg
    Klonopin Wafers dissolve in mouth with <u>or</u> without water
      Wafer: 0.125, 0.25, 0.5, 1, 2 mg orally-disint
▷ *clorazepate* (IV)(G) 30 mg/day in divided doses; max 60 mg/day
  Pediatric: <9 years: <u>not</u> recommended; ≥9 years: same as adult
    Tranxene *Tab:* 3.75, 7.5, 15 mg
    Tranxene SD do <u>not</u> use for initial therapy
      Tab: 22.5 mg ext-rel
    Tranxene SD Half Strength do <u>not</u> use for initial therapy
      Tab: 11.25 mg ext-rel
    Tranxene T-Tab *Tab:* 3.75*, 7.5*, 15*mg
▷ *diazepam* (IV)(G) 2-10 mg bid to qid
  Pediatric: <12 years: <u>not</u> recommended; ≥12 years: same as adult
    Diastat *Rectal gel delivery system:* 2.5 mg
    Diastat AcuDial *Rectal gel delivery system:* 10, 20 mg
    Valium *Tab:* 2*, 5*, 10*mg
    Valium Injectable *Vial:* 5 mg/ml (10 ml); *Amp:* 5 mg/ml (2 ml); *Prefilled syringe:* 5 mg/ml (5 ml)
    Valium Intensol Oral Solution *Conc oral soln:* 5 mg/ml (30 ml w. dropper) (alcohol 19%)
    Valium Oral Solution *Oral soln:* 5 mg/5 ml (500 ml) (wintergreen spice)

TRICYCLIC ANTIDEPRESSANTS (TCAs)
Comment: Co-administration of TCAs with SSRIs requires extreme caution.
▷ *amitriptyline* (G) 10-20 mg q HS
  Pediatric: <12 years: <u>not</u> recommended; ≥12 years: same as adult
    Tab: 10, 25, 50, 75, 100, 150 mg
▷ *amoxapine* initially 50 mg bid to tid; after 1 week may increase to 100 mg bid-tid; usual effective dose is
  200 to 300 mg/day; if total dose exceeds 300 mg/day, give in divided doses (max 400 mg/day); may give as a
  single bedtime dose (max 300 mg q HS)
  Pediatric: <12 years: <u>not</u> recommended; ≥12 years: same as adult
    Tab: 25, 50, 100, 150 mg
▷ *clomipramine* (G) initially 25 mg daily in divided doses; gradually increase to 100 mg during the first
  2 weeks; max 250 mg/day; total maintenance dose may be given at HS
  Pediatric: <10 years: <u>not</u> recommended; 10-<16 years: initially 25 mg daily in divided doses; gradually
  increase; max 3 mg/kg <u>or</u> 100 mg, whichever is smaller; ≥16 years: same as adult
    Anafranil *Cap:* 25, 50, 75 mg
▷ *desipramine* (G) 100-200 mg/day in single <u>or</u> divided doses; max 300 mg/day
  Pediatric: <12 years: <u>not</u> recommended; ≥12 years: same as adult
    Norpramin *Tab:* 10, 25, 50, 75, 100, 150 mg
▷ *doxepin* (G) usual optimum dose 75-150 mg/day; Elderly: lower initial dose and therapeutic dose; max
  single dose 150 mg; max 300 mg/day in divided doses
  Pediatric: <12 years: <u>not</u> recommended; ≥12 years: same as adult
    Sinequan *Cap:* 10, 25, 50, 75, 100, 150 mg; *Oral conc:* 10 mg/ml (4 oz w. dropper)
  Comment: Glaucoma, urinary retention, and bipolar disorder are contraindications to *doxepin*. Separate
  from monoamine oxidase inhibitors (MAOIs) by at least 14 days. Separate from *fluoxetine* by at least 5
  weeks. Avoid abrupt cessation. *Doxepin* is potentiated by CYP2D6 inhibitors (e.g., *cimetidine*, SSRIs,
  phenothiazines, type 1C antiarrhythmics).
▷ *imipramine* (G)
  Pediatric: <12 years: <u>not</u> recommended; ≥12 years: same as adult
  Tofranil initially 75 mg daily (max 200 mg); <u>Adolescents:</u> initially 30 to 40 mg once daily (max 100 mg/day);
  if maintenance dose exceeds 75 mg daily, may switch to Tofranil PM for divided <u>or</u> bedtime dose
    Tab: 10, 25, 50 mg
  Tofranil PM initially 75 mg daily 1 hour before HS; max 200 mg
    Cap: 75, 100, 125, 150 mg
▷ *nortriptyline* (G) initially 25 mg tid to qid; max 150 mg/day
  Pediatric: <12 years: <u>not</u> recommended; ≥12 years: same as adult
    Pamelor *Cap:* 10, 25, 50, 75 mg; *Oral soln:* 10 mg/5 ml (16 oz)
▷ *protriptyline* initially 5 mg tid; usual dose 15-40 mg/day in 3 to 4 divided doses; max 60 mg/day
  Pediatric: <12 years: <u>not</u> recommended; ≥12 years: same as adult
    Vivactil *Tab:* 5, 10 mg
▷ *trimipramine* initially 75 mg/day in divided doses; max 200 mg/day
  Pediatric: <12 years: <u>not</u> recommended; ≥12 years: same as adult
    Surmontil *Cap:* 25, 50, 100 mg

PHENOTHIAZINES
▷ *prochlorperazine* (G)
  Pediatric: <12 years: <u>not</u> recommended; ≥12 years: same as adult
    Compazine 5 mg tid to qid
      Tab: 5 mg; *Syr:* 5 mg/5 ml (4 oz) (fruit); *Rectal supp:* 2.5, 5, 25 mg
    Compazine Spansule 15 mg q AM <u>or</u> 10 mg q 12 hours
      Spansule: 10, 15 mg sust-rel
▷ *trifluoperazine* (G) 1-2 mg bid; max 6 mg/day; max 12 weeks
  Pediatric: <12 years: <u>not</u> recommended; ≥12 years: same as adult
    Stelazine *Tab:* 1, 2, 5, 10 mg

SELECTIVE SEROTONIN REUPTAKE INHIBITORS (SSRIs)
Comment: Co-administration of SSRIs with TCAs requires extreme caution. Concomitant use of MAOIs and SSRIs is absolutely contraindicated. Avoid St. John's wort and other serotonergic agents. A potentially fatal adverse event is *serotonin syndrome*, caused by serotonin excess. Milder symptoms require healthcare provider intervention to avert severe symptoms that can be rapidly fatal without urgent/emergent medical care. Symptoms include restlessness, agitation, confusion, tachycardia, hypertension, dilated pupils, muscle twitching, muscle rigidity, loss of muscle coordination, diaphoresis, diarrhea, headache, shivering, piloerection, hyperpyrexia, cardiac arrhythmias, seizures, loss of consciousness, coma, and death. Common symptoms of *serotonin discontinuation syndrome* include flu-like symptoms (nausea, vomiting, diarrhea, headaches, diaphoresis), sleep disturbances (insomnia, nightmares, constant sleepiness), mood disturbances (dysphoria, anxiety, agitation), cognitive disturbances (mental confusion, hyperarousal), and sensory and movement disturbances (imbalance, tremors, vertigo, dizziness, electric-shock-like sensations in the brain often described by sufferers as "brain zaps").
▷ *citalopram* (G) initially 20 mg once daily; may increase after week to 40 mg once daily; max 40 mg
  Pediatric: 12 years: <u>not</u> recommended; ≥12 years: same as adult
    Celexa *Tab:* 10, 20, 40 mg; *Oral soln:* 10 mg/5 ml (120 ml) (peppermint) (sugar-free, alcohol-free, parabens)
▷ *escitalopram* (G) initially 10 mg daily; may increase to 20 mg daily after 1 week; *Elderly* <u>or</u> *hepatic impairment:* 10 mg once daily
  Pediatric: <12 years: <u>not</u> recommended; 12-17 years: initially 10 mg once daily; may increase to 20 mg once daily after 3 weeks
    Lexapro *Tab:* 5, 10*, 20* mg
    Lexapro Oral Solution *Oral soln:* 1 mg/ml (240 ml) (peppermint) (parabens)
▷ *fluoxetine* (G)
    Prozac initially 20 mg daily; may increase after 1 week; doses >20 mg/day may be divided into AM and noon doses; max 80 mg/day
    Pediatric: <8 years: <u>not</u> recommended; 8-17 years: initially 10-20 mg once daily; start lower weight children at 10 mg once daily; if starting at 10 mg once daily, may increase after 1 week to 20 mg once daily
      Cap: 10, 20, 40 mg; *Tab:* 30*, 60* mg; *Oral soln:* 20 mg/5 ml (4 oz) (mint)
    Prozac Weekly following daily *fluoxetine* therapy at 20 mg/day x 13 weeks, may initiate **Prozac Weekly** 7 days after the last 20 mg *fluoxetine* dose
    Pediatric: <12 years: <u>not</u> recommended; ≥12 years: same as adult
      Cap: 90 mg ent-coat del-rel pellets
▷ *paroxetine maleate* (G)
  Pediatric: <12 years: <u>not</u> recommended; ≥12 years: same as adult
    Paxil initially 10-20 mg once daily in the AM; may increase by 10 mg/day at weekly intervals as needed; max 60 mg/day
      Tab: 10*, 20*, 30, 40 mg
    Paxil CR initially 12.5-25 mg once daily in the AM; may increase by 12.5 mg at weekly intervals as needed; max 62.5 mg/day
      Oral Tab: 12.5, 25, 37.5 mg ent-coat cont-rel
    Paxil Suspension initially 10-20 mg once daily in the AM; may increase by 10 mg/day at weekly intervals as needed; max 60 mg/day
      Oral susp: 10 mg/5 ml (250 ml) (orange)
▷ *paroxetine mesylate* (G) initially 7.5 mg once daily in the AM; may increase by 10 mg/day at weekly intervals as needed; max 60 mg/day
  Pediatric: <12 years: <u>not</u> recommended; ≥12 years: same as adult
    Brisdelle *Cap:* 7.5 mg
▷ *sertraline* initially 50 mg once daily; increase at 1 week intervals if needed; max 200 mg daily
  Pediatric: <6 years: <u>not</u> recommended; 6-12 years: initially 25 mg once daily, max 200 mg/day; 13-17 years: initially 50 mg daily, max 200 mg/day
    Zoloft *Tab:* 15*, 50*, 100* mg; *Oral conc:* 20 mg per ml (60 ml [dilute just before administering in 4 oz water, ginger ale, lemon-lime soda, lemonade, <u>or</u> orange juice]) (alcohol 12%)

SEROTONIN NOREPINEPHRINE REUPTAKE INHIBITORS (SNRIs)

▷ *desvenlafaxine* (**G**) swallow whole; initially 50 mg once daily; max 120 mg/day
  Pediatric: <18 years: <u>not</u> recommended; ≥18 years: same as adult
    Pristiq *Tab:* 50, 100 mg ext-rel
▷ *duloxetine* (**G**) swallow whole; initially 30 mg once daily x 1 week; then, increase to 60 mg once daily; max 120 mg/day
  Pediatric: <12 years: <u>not</u> recommended; ≥12 years: same as adult
    Cymbalta *Cap:* 20, 30, 40, 60 mg del-rel
▷ *venlafaxine* (**G**)
    Effexor initially 75 mg/day in 2-3 divided doses; may increase at 4-day intervals in 75 mg increments to 150 mg/day; max 225 mg/day
    Pediatric: <18 years: <u>not</u> recommended; ≥18 years: same as adult
      Tab: 37.5, 75, 150, 225 mg
    Effexor XR initially 75 mg q AM; may start at 37.5 mg daily x 4-7 days; then increase by increments of up to 75 mg/day at intervals of at least 4 days; usual max 375 mg/day
    Pediatric: <18 years: <u>not</u> recommended; ≥18 years: same as adult
      Tab: Cap: 37.5, 75, 150 mg ext-rel

COMBINATION AGENTS

▷ *chlordiazepoxide+amitriptyline* (**G**)
  Pediatric: <12 years: <u>not</u> recommended; ≥12 years: same as adult
    Limbitrol 3-4 tabs/day in divided doses
      Tab: chlor 5 mg+amit 12.5 mg
    Limbitrol DS 3-4 tabs/day in divided doses; max 6 tabs/day
      Tab: chlor 10 mg+amit 25 mg
▷ *perphenazine+amitriptyline* (**G**) 1 tab bid-qid
  Pediatric: <12 years: <u>not</u> recommended; ≥12 years: same as adult
    Tab: Etrafon 2-10 perph 2 mg+amit 10 mg
      Etrafon 2-25 perph 2 mg+amit 25 mg
      Etrafon 4-25 perph 4 mg+amit 25 mg

APHASIA, EXPRESSIVE: STROKE-INDUCED

Comment: Per the *New England Journal of Medicine*, a 52-year-old right-handed, woman who sustained an ischemic stroke 3 years prior had areas of infarction that included the left insula, putamen, and superior temporal gyrus. Her stroke resulted in expressive aphasia, leaving her with no intelligible words, but with intact full language comprehension. *Zolpidem* 10 mg was prescribed for insomnia. In repeated measures, it was found that the patient consistently demonstrated dramatic speech improvement, durable until HS, and return of the expressive aphasia in the AM. Subsequent single-photon emission computed tomography (SPECT) scanning of this patient indicated that *zolpidem* increases flow in the Broca area of the brain, an area intimately involved with speech. From these observations, the authors concluded that a select subgroup of patients with aphasia, perhaps with subcortical lesions and spared but hypometabolic cortical structures, might benefit from this treatment. It may be worth trying *zolpidem* in patients who have been labeled with otherwise refractory chronic expressive aphasia. This finding raises the question of whether this intervention could help patients earlier in the course, patients with milder disease, <u>and/or</u> patients with other ischemic central nervous system syndromes?

▷ *zolpidem* oral solution spray (imidazopyridine hypnotic) (**IV**)(**G**) 2 actuations (10 mg) immediately before bedtime; *Elderly, debilitated,* or *hepatic impairment:* 2 actuations (5 mg); max 2 actuations (10 mg)
  Pediatric: <18 years: <u>not</u> recommended; ≥18 years: same as adult
    ZolpiMist *Oral soln spray:* 5 mg/actuation (60 metered actuations) (cherry)
  Comment: The lowest dose of *zolpidem* in all forms is recommended for persons >50 years of age and women as drug elimination is slower than in men.
▷ *zolpidem* tabs (pyrazolopyrimidine hypnotic) (**IV**)(**G**) 5-10 mg <u>or</u> 6.25-12.5 ext-rel q HS prn; max 12.5 mg/day x 1 month; do <u>not</u> take if unable to sleep for at least 8 hours before required to be active again; delayed effect if taken with a meal
  Pediatric: <18 years: <u>not</u> recommended; ≥18 years: same as adult
    Ambien *Tab:* 5, 10 mg
    Ambien CR *Tab:* 6.25, 12.5 mg ext-rel
  Comment: The lowest dose of *zolpidem* in all forms is recommended for persons >50 years of age and women as drug elimination is slower than in men.
▷ *zolpidem* sublingual tabs (**IV**) (imidazopyridine hypnotic) dissolve 1 tab under the tongue; allow to disintegrate completely before swallowing; take <u>only</u> once per night and <u>only</u> if at least 4 hours of bedtime remain before planned time for awakening

Pediatric: <18 years: <u>not</u> recommended; ≥18 years: same adult
  Edluar *SL Tab:* 5, 10 mg
  Intermezzo *SL Tab:* 1.75, 3.5 mg
  Comment: Edluar is indicated for the treatment of insomnia when a middle-of-the-night awakening is followed by difficulty returning to sleep. The lowest dose of ***zolpidem*** in all forms is recommended for persons >50 years of age and women as drug elimination is slower than in men.

APHTHOUS STOMATITIS (MOUTH ULCER, CANKER SORE)

Comment: Aphthous ulcers are very painful sores with an inflamed base and non-viable tissue in the center that appears bacterial <u>or</u> viral. Although the sores are usually neither bacterial nor viral, herpetiform ulcers are most prevalent among the elderly. The sores may be single round/ovoid, <u>or</u> several may be coalesced to form larger lesions, and located under the lip, on the buccal membrane, and/or on the tongue. Poor oral hygiene <u>or</u> an underlying immunity impairment can predispose the patient to ulcer formation (e.g., chronic illness, chemotherapy, poor nutrition, vitamin and mineral deficiencies, allergies, local trauma, stress, tobacco use, and inflammatory bowel disease). They are frequently the result of local trauma (e.g., orthodontic ware, chipped tooth) <u>or</u> allergy/irritation to a toothpaste <u>or</u> mouthwash ingredient (e.g., sodium lauryl sulfate). Changing toothpaste and applying dental wax to sharp edges are recommended until dental care is accessed. Debridement of the non-viable tissue by the direct application of salt (osmotic pulling pressure) for a few minutes, thus leaving a healthy tissue crater, speeds healing. Relief of the offending source of tissue trauma and application of a 5 mg prednisone tablet directly to the debrided ulcer are other remedies with reported success. These sores usually first appear in childhood <u>or</u> adolescence. Family history may have a role in the formation of recurrent aphthous stomatitis (RAS). When cases tend to occur in the same family (est 25%–40% of the time), the ulcers are earlier and with greater severity.

ANTI-INFLAMMATORY AGENTS
▷ ***dexamethasone*** elixir 5 ml swish and spit q 12 hours
  Pediatric: <12 years: <u>not</u> recommended; ≥12 years: same as adult
    Elix: 0.5 mg/ml
▷ ***triamcinolone acetonide*** 0.1% dental paste (G) press (do <u>not</u> rub) a thin film onto the lesion at bedtime and, if needed, 2-3 x daily after meals; re-evaluate if no improvement in 7 days
  Pediatric: <12 years: <u>not</u> recommended; ≥12 years: same as adult
    Oralone *Dental paste:* 0.1% (5 gm)
▷ ***triamcinolone*** 1% in **Orabase** apply 1/4 inch to each ulcer bid-qid until ulcer heals
  Pediatric: <12 years: <u>not</u> recommended; ≥12 years: same as adult
    Kenalog in Orabase *Crm:* 1% (15, 60, 80 gm)

TOPICAL ANESTHETICS
▷ ***benzocaine*** topical gel (G) apply tid-qid
▷ ***benzocaine*** topical spray (G) 1 spray to painful area every 2 hours as needed; retain for 15 seconds, then spit
    Cepacol Spray (OTC), Chloraseptic Spray (OTC)
▷ ***lidocaine*** viscous soln (G) 15 ml gargle <u>or</u> swish, then spit; repeat after 3 hours; max 8 doses/day
  Pediatric: <3 years: <u>not</u> recommended; 3-11 years: 1.25 ml; apply with cotton-tipped applicator; may repeat after 3 hours; max 8 doses/day; ≥12 years: same as adult
    Xylocaine Viscous Solution *Viscous soln:* 2% (20, 100, 450 ml)
▷ ***triamcinolone*** (**Kenalog**) in **Orabase** apply with swab

DEBRIDING AGENT/CLEANSER
▷ ***carbamide peroxide 10%*** (OTC) apply 10 drops to the affected area; swish x 2-3 minutes, then spit; do <u>not</u> rinse; repeat treatment qid
  Pediatric: <3 years: <u>not</u> recommended; ≥3 years: same as adult
    Gly-Oxide *Liq:* 10% (50, 60 ml squeeze bottle w. applicator)

ANTI-INFECTIVES
▷ ***minocycline*** (G) swish and spit 10 ml susp (50 mg/5 ml) <u>or</u> 1 x 100 mg cap <u>or</u> 2 x 50 mg caps dissolved in 180 ml water, bid x 4-5 days
  Pediatric: <8 years: <u>not</u> recommended; ≥8 years: same as adult
    Dynacin *Cap:* 50, 100 mg
    Minocin *Cap:* 50, 75, 100 mg; *Oral susp:* 50 mg/5 ml (60 ml) (custard) (sulfites, alcohol 5%)
▷ ***tetracycline*** swish and spit 10 ml susp (125 mg/5 ml) <u>or</u> one 250 mg tab/cap dissolved in 180 ml water qid x 4-5 days
  Pediatric: <8 years: <u>not</u> recommended; ≥8 years: same as adult; *see* Appendix BB.31. *tetracycline* (G) (Sumycin Suspension) *for dose by weight*
    Achromycin V *Cap:* 250, 500 mg
    Sumycin *Tab:* 250, 500 mg; *Cap:* 250, 500 mg; *Oral susp:* 125 mg/5 ml (100, 200 ml) (fruit) (sulfites)

ASPERGILLOSIS, BLASTOMYCOSIS, HISTOPLASMOSIS

INVASIVE INFECTION

▷ *isavuconazonium* swallow cap whole; *Loading dose:* 372 mg q 8 hours x 6 doses (48 hours); *Maintenance:* 372 mg once daily starting 12-24 hours after last loading dose
Pediatric: <18 years: not established; ≥18 years: same as adult
  Cresemba *Cap:* 186 mg; *Vial:* 372 mg pwdr for reconstitution (7/blister pck) (preservative-free)
  Comment: Cresemba is indicated for the treatment of invasive aspergillus and mucormycosis in patients >18 years old who are at high risk due to being severely compromised.

▷ *itraconazole* take with food; do not break, crush, or chew; 130 mg (2 x 65 mg caps) once daily; if no obvious improvement or there is evidence of progressive fungal disease, the dose should be increased in 65 mg increments to a maximum of 260 mg/day (130 mg [2 x 65 mg capsules] bid); doses >130 mg/day should be administered in two divided doses; *Treatment of life-saving situations:* although clinical studies did not provide for a loading dose, it is recommended, based on pharmacokinetic data, that a loading dose should be used; a loading dose of 130 mg (2 x 65 mg capsules) tid (390 mg/day) is recommended to be administered for the first 3 days, followed by the appropriate recommended dosing based on indication; treatment should be continued for a minimum of 3 months and until clinical parameters and laboratory tests indicate that the active fungal infection has subsided; an inadequate period of treatment may lead to recurrence of active infection
  Tolsura *Gelcap:* 65 mg
  Comment: Tolsura is not interchangeable or substitutable with other *itraconazole* products. Tolsura is not indicated for the treatment of onychomycosis. Tolsura is an azole antifungal indicated for the treatment of blastomycosis (pulmonary and extrapulmonary), histoplasmosis (including chronic cavitary pulmonary disease and disseminated, non-meningeal histoplasmosis), and aspergillosis (pulmonary and extrapulmonary), in patients who are intolerant of or who are refractory to *amphotericin B* therapy). These serious infections most commonly occur in vulnerable or immunocompromised patients, for example, those with a history of cancer, transplants (solid organ or bone marrow), HIV/AIDS, or chronic rheumatic disorders, and are often associated with high mortality rates or long-term health issues. The most common adverse reactions (incidence ≥1%) are nausea, rash, vomiting, edema, headache, diarrhea, fatigue, fever, pruritus, hypertension, abnormal hepatic function, abdominal pain, dizziness, hypokalemia, anorexia, malaise, decreased libido, somnolence, albuminuria, and impotence. *Itraconazole* is mainly metabolized through CYP3A4.

▷ *posaconazole* (G) *Oral therapy:* take with food; swallow tab whole; *Day 1:* 300 mg bid; then 300 mg once daily x 13 days; *IV infusion therapy:* must be administered through an in-line filter over approximately 90 minutes via a central venous line. Never administer Noxafil as an IV bolus injection; *Loading dose:* a single 300 mg IV infusion; *Maintenance dose:* a single 300 mg IV infusion once daily for the duration of treatment (e.g., resolution of neutropenia or immunosuppression)
Pediatric: <13 years: not recommended; ≥13 years: same as adult
  Noxafil *Tab:* 100 mg ext-rel; *Oral susp:* 40 mg/ml (105 oz w. dosing spoon) (cherry); *Vial:* 300 mg/16.7 ml (18 mg/ml) soln for IV infusion
  Comment: Noxafil is indicated as prophylaxis for invasive aspergillus and candida infections in patients >13 years old who are at high risk due to being severely compromised.

▷ *voriconazole* (G) *PO:* <40 kg: 100 mg q 12 hours; may increase to 150 mg q 12 hours if inadequate response; >40 kg: 200 mg q 12 hours; may increase to 300 mg q 12 hours if inadequate response; *IV:* 6 mg/kg q 12 hours x 2 doses; then 4 mg/kg q 12 hours; max rate 3 mg/kg/hour over 1-2 hours
Pediatric: <12 years: not recommended; ≥12 years: same as adult
  Vfend *Tab:* 50, 200 mg
  Vfend I.V. for Injection *Vial:* 200 mg pwdr for reconstitution (preservative-free)
  Vfend *Oral susp:* 40 mg/ml pwdr for reconstitution (75 ml) (orange)

ASTHMA

Parenteral Corticosteroids *see* Appendix L. Parenteral Corticosteroids
Oral Corticosteroids *see* Appendix K. Oral Corticosteroids

EPINEPHRINE INHALATION AEROSOL (BRONCHODILATOR)

▷ *epinephrine inhalation aerosol* (OTC) shake and spray one time into the air prior to each inhalation; after 1 inhalation, wait 1 minute; if inadequate relief, may repeat; 1 to 2 inhalations constitute one dose; wait at least 4 hours between doses; max 8 inhalations/24 hours
Pediatric: <12 years: safety and efficacy not established; ≥12 years: same as adult
  Primatene MIST *Pump inh: 0.125 mg per inhalation spray* (160 sprays) (no sulfites; dehydrated alcohol 1%, hydrofluoroalkane [HFA-134a], polysorbate 80, thymol)
  Comment: Primatene Mist *(epinephrine inhalation aerosol)* is indicated for the temporary relief of mild symptoms of intermittent asthma (wheezing, chest tightness, shortness of breath) and is delivered by a metered-dose inhaler (MDI) with a non-chlorofluorocarbon (CFC) propellant. After every 20 sprays, the spray indicator resets (160, 140, 120…20, 0). The spray indicator cannot be manually reset.

INHALED RACEPINEPHRINE (BRONCHODILATOR)

Comment: Inhalation racemic epinephrine is indicated for urgent/emergent acute bronchospasm rescue (e.g., acute asthma attack, laryngospasm, croup, epiglottitis, acute inflammation causing airway obstruction). Inhalational racemic epinephrine is *only* recommended for use during pregnancy when there are no alternatives and benefit outweighs risk.

▷ *racepinephrine* (OTC)(G) for atomized (nebulizer) treatment

Pediatric: <4 years: not recommended; ≥4 years: same as adult

Asthmanefrin *Starter kit:* 10 x 0.5 ml vials 2.25% solution for atomized inhalation w. EZ Breathe Atomizer; *Refills:* 30 x 0.5 ml vials 2.25% solution for atomized inhalation

INHALED BETA-2 AGONISTS (BRONCHODILATORS)

▷ *albuterol sulfate* (G)

AccuNeb Inhalation Solution 1 unit-dose vial tid-qid prn by nebulizer; ages 2-12 years only; not for adult

Pediatric: <2 years: not recommended; 2-12 years: initially 0.63 mg or 1.25 mg tid-qid; 6-12 years: with severe asthma, or >40 kg, or 11-12 years: initially 1.25 mg tid-qid

Inhal soln: 0.63, 1.25 mg/3 ml (3 ml, 25/carton) (preservative-free)

Albuterol Inhalation Solution (G) not recommended for adults

Pediatric: <2 years: not recommended; ≥2 years: 1 vial via nebulizer over 5-15 minutes

Inhal soln: 0.63 mg/3 ml (0.021%); 1.25 mg/3 ml (0.042%) (25/carton)

Albuterol Inhalation Solution 0.5% (G) not recommended

Pediatric: <4 years: not recommended; ≥4 years: same as adult

Inhal soln: 0.083% (25/carton)

Albuterol Nebules (G) 2.5 mg (0.5 ml of 5% diluted to 3 ml with sterile NS or 3 ml of 0.083%) tid-qid

Pediatric: use <12 years: other forms; ≥12 years: same as adult

Inhal soln: 0.083% (25/carton)

ProAir Digihaler *Inhal pwdr* 117 mcg/actuation (0.65 gm, 200 inh)

Pediatric: <4 years: not established; ≥4 years: same as adult

Comment: **ProAir Digihaler** is the first and only digital inhaler with built-in sensors that detect inhaler use and measure inspiratory flow. The data are sent to the companion mobile app using Bluetooth wireless technology for patients and healthcare professionals to review over time. **ProAir Digihaler** is indicated for the treatment or prevention of bronchospasm in reversible obstructive airway disease and for the prevention of exercise-induced bronchospasm.

Proair HFA Inhaler 1-2 inhalations q 4-6 hours prn; 2 inhalations 15 minutes before exercise as prophylaxis for exercise-induced asthma (EIA)

Pediatric: <4 years: not established; ≥4 years: same as adult

Inhaler: 90 mcg/actuation (0.65 gm, 200 inh) (CFC-free)

Proair RespiClick 1-2 inhalations q 4-6 hours prn; 2 inhalations 15-30 minutes before exercise as prophylaxis for EIA

Pediatric: <12 years: not established; ≥12 years: same as adult

Inhaler: 90 mcg/actuation (8.5 gm, 200 inh)

Proventil HFA Inhaler 1-2 inhalations q 4-6 hours prn; 2 inhalations 15 minutes before exercise as prophylaxis for EIA

Pediatric: <4 years: use syrup; ≥4 years: same as adult

Inhaler: 90 mcg/actuation with a dose counter (6.7 gm, 200 inh)

Proventil Inhalation Solution 2.5 mg diluted to 3 ml with normal saline tid-qid prn by nebulizer

Pediatric: use syrup

Inhal soln: 0.5% (20 ml w. dropper); 0.083% (3 ml; 25/carton)

Ventolin Inhaler 2 inhalations q 4-6 hours prn; 2 inhalations 15 minutes before exercise as prophylaxis for EIA

Pediatric: <2 years: not recommended; 2-4 years: use syrup; ≥4 years: same as adult

Inhaler: 90 mcg/actuation (17 gm, 220 inh)

Ventolin Rotacaps 1-2 cap inhalations q 4-6 hours prn; 2 inhalations 15 minutes before exercise as prophylaxis for EIA

Pediatric: <4 years: not recommended; ≥4 years 1-2 caps q 4-6 hours prn

Rotacaps: 200 mcg/Rotacap dose (100 doses)

Ventolin 0.5% Inhalation Solution

Pediatric: <2 years: not recommended; ≥2 years: initially 0.1-0.15 mg/kg/dose tid-qid prn; 10-15 kg: 0.25 ml diluted to 3 ml with normal saline by nebulizer tid-qid prn; >15 kg: 0.5 ml diluted to 3 ml with normal saline by nebulizer tid-qid prn

Inhal soln: 20 ml w. dropper

Ventolin Nebules

Pediatric: <2 years: not recommended; ≥2 years: initially 0.1-0.15 mg/kg/ dose tid-qid prn; 10-15 kg: 1.25 mg or 1/2 nebule tid-qid prn; >15 kg: 2.5 mg or 1 nebule tid-qid prn

Inhal soln: 0.083% (3 ml; 25/carton)

(continued)

▷ *isoproterenol Rescue:* 1 inhalation prn; repeat if no relief in 2-5 minutes; *Maintenance:* 1-2 inhalations q 4-6 hours
Pediatric: <12 years: <u>not</u> recommended; ≥12 years: same as adult
    Medihaler-1SO *Inhaler:* 80 mcg/actuation (15 ml, 30 inh)
▷ *levalbuterol tartrate* (G) initially 0.63 mg tid q 6-8 hours prn by nebulizer; may increase to 1.25 mg tid at 6-8 hour intervals as needed
Pediatric: <12 years: <u>not</u> recommended; ≥12 years: same as adult
    Xopenex *Inhal soln:* 0.31, 0.63, 1.25 mg/3 ml (24/carton) (preservative-free)
    Xopenex HFA *Inh:* 45 mg (15 gm, 200 inh) (preservative-free)
    Xopenex Concentrate *Vial:* 1.25 mg/0.5 ml (30/carton) (preservative-free)
▷ *metaproterenol* (G)
    Alupent 2-3 inhalations tid-qid prn; max 12 inhalations/day
    Pediatric: <6 years: use syrup; ≥6 years: via nebulizer 0.1-0.2 ml diluted with normal saline to 3 ml, up to q 4 hours prn
        Inhaler: 0.65 mg/actuation (14 gm, 200 doses)
    Alupent Inhalation Solution 5-15 inhalations tid-qid prn; q 4 hours prn for acute attack
    Pediatric: <6 years: use syrup ≥6 years: via nebulizer 0.1-0.2 ml diluted with normal saline to 3 ml, up to q 4 hours prn
        Inhal soln: 5% (10, 30 ml w. dropper)
▷ *pirbuterol* 1-2 inhalations q 4-6 hours prn; max 12 inhalations/day
Pediatric: <12 years: <u>not</u> recommended; ≥12 years: same as adult
    Maxair *Autohaler:* 200 mcg/actuation (14 gm, 400 inh); *Inhaler:* 200 mcg/actuation (25.6 gm, 300 inh)
▷ *terbutaline* 2 inhalations q 4-6 hours prn
Pediatric: <12 years: <u>not</u> recommended; ≥12 years: same as adult
    Inhaler: 0.2 mg/actuation (10.5 gm, 300 inh)

INHALED ANTICHOLINERGICS
▷ *ipratropium bromide* (G)
Pediatric: <12 years: <u>not</u> established; ≥12 years: same as adult
    Atrovent 2 inhalations qid; additional inhalations as required; max 12 inhalations/day
    Inhaler: 18 mcg/actuation (14 gm, 200 inh)
    Atrovent Inhalation Solution 500 mcg tid-qid prn by nebulizer
    Inhal soln: 0.02% (500 mcg in 2.5 ml; 25/carton)

INHALED BETA-2 AGONIST+CORTICOSTEROID
▷ *albuterol+budesonide* administer 1-2 inhalations; max 6 doses (12 inhalations) per 24 hours
Pediatric: <18 years: safety and efficacy <u>not</u> established; ≥18 years: same as adult
    Airsupra *Metered pump inhaler:* 90 mcg/80 mcg inhalation aerosol per actuation
    Comment: **Airsupra** is a first-in-class, pressurized metered-dose inhaler (pMDI), fixed-dose combination of *albuterol* (short-acting beta-2-adrenergic agonist [SABA])+*budesonide* (inhaled corticosteroid [ICD]) rescue inhaler for as-needed use to reduce bronchoconstriction and risk of severe asthma exacerbations. The safety and tolerability of **Airsupra** in patients studied were consistent with the known profiles of the components, with the most common adverse events including headache, oral candidiasis, cough, and dysphonia.

INHALED CORTICOSTEROIDS
Comment: ICDs are <u>not</u> for primary (rescue) treatment of acute asthma attack. After every inhalation of a steroid <u>or</u> steroid-containing medication treatment, rinse mouth to reduce risk of oral candidiasis. ICDs are <u>not</u> for primary (rescue) treatment of acute asthma attack. For twice-daily dosing, allow 12 hours between doses.
▷ *beclomethasone dipropionate* (G) *Previously using <u>only</u> bronchodilators:* initiate 40-80 mcg bid, max 320 mcg bid; *Previously using ICD:* initiate 40-160 mcg bid, max 320 mcg/day; *Previously taking a systemic corticosteroid:* attempt to wean off the systemic drug after approximately 1 week after initiating; rinse mouth after use
Pediatric: <12 years: <u>not</u> recommended; ≥12 years: same as adult
    Qvar *Inhal aerosol:* 40, 80 mcg/metered dose actuation (8.7 gm, 120 inh) MDI (CFC-free)
▷ *budesonide*
    Pulmicort Flexhaler initially 180-360 mcg bid; max 360 mcg bid; rinse mouth after use
    Pediatric: <6 years: <u>not</u> recommended; ≥6 years: 1-2 inhalations bid
      Flexhaler: 90 mcg/actuation (60 inh), 180 mcg/actuation (120 inh)
    Pulmicort Respules (G) adults and ≥8 years: use flexhaler
    Pediatric: <12 months: <u>not</u> recommended; 12 months-8 years: *Previously using <u>only</u> bronchodilators:* initiate 0.5 mg/day once daily <u>or</u> in 2 divided doses, may start at 0.25 mg daily; *Previously using ICDs:* initiate 0.5 mg once daily <u>or</u> in 2 divided doses, max 1 mg/day; *Previously taking oral corticosteroids:* initiate 1 mg/day daily <u>or</u> in 2 divided doses; ≥8 years: use **Flexhaler**; rinse mouth after use
      Inhal susp: 0.25, 0.5, 1 mg/2 ml (30/carton)

➤ *ciclesonide* initially 80 mcg bid; max 320 mcg/day; rinse mouth after use; *Previously on ICD:* initially 80 mcg bid; *Previously on oral steroid:* 320 mg bid
    Pediatric: <12 years: not recommended; ≥12 years: same as adult
      Alvesco *Inhal aerosol:* 80, 160 mcg/actuation (6.1 gm, 60 inh)
➤ *flunisolide* rinse mouth after use
      AeroBid, AeroBid-M initially 2 inhalations bid; max 8 inhalations/day; rinse mouth after use
      Pediatric: <6 years: not recommended; 6-15 years: 2 inhalations bid; ≥15 years: same as adult
        Inhaler: 250 mcg/actuation (7 gm, 100 inh)
      Aerospan HFA initially 160 mcg bid; max 320 mcg bid
      Pediatric: <6 years: not recommended; 6-11 years: 80 mcg bid, max 160 mcg bid; ≥12 years: same as adult
        Inhaler: 80 mcg (5.1 gm, 60 doses; 80 mcg, 120 doses)
➤ *fluticasone furoate Currently* not *on ICD:* usually initiate at 100 mcg once daily at the same time each day; may increase to 200 mcg once daily if inadequate response after 2 weeks; max 200 mcg/day; rinse mouth after use
    Pediatric: <12 years: not established; ≥12 years: same as adult**Arnuity Ellipta** *Inhal:* 100, 200 mcg/dry pwdr per inhalation (30 doses)
      Comment: Arnuity Ellipta is not for primary treatment of status asthmaticus or acute asthma episodes. Arnuity Ellipta is contraindicated with severe hypersensitivity to milk proteins.
➤ *fluticasone propionate*
      ArmonAir 1 inhalation bid (12 hours apart); initially 55 mcg bid; *Previously using an ICD:* see mfr pkg insert; if insufficient response after 2 weeks, may increase the bid dose; max 232 mcg bid; after stability is achieved, titrate to lowest effective dose; do not use with spacer or volume-holding chamber
      Pediatric: <12 years: not established; ≥12 years: same as adult
        Inhaler: 55, 113, 232 mcg/actuation (60 inh)
      Flovent, Flovent HFA initially 88 mcg bid; *Previously using an ICD:* initially 88-220 mcg bid; *Previously taking an oral corticosteroid:* 880 mcg bid; rinse mouth after use
      Pediatric: <11 years: use **Flovent Diskus**; ≥12 years: same as adult
        Inhaler: 44 mcg/actuation (7.9 gm, 60 inh; 13 gm, 120 inh), 110 mcg/ actuation (13 gm, 120 inh), 220 mcg/actuation (13 gm, 120 inh)
      Flovent Diskus initially 100 mcg bid; max 500 mcg bid; *Previously using an ICD:* initially 100-250 mcg bid, max 500 mcg bid; *Previously taking an oral corticosteroid:* 1,000 mcg bid
      Pediatric: <4 years: not recommended; 4-11 years: initially 50 mcg bid, max 100 mcg bid, rinse mouth after use; ≥12 years: same as adult
        Diskus: 50, 100, 250 mcg/inh dry pwdr (60 blisters w. diskus)
➤ *mometasone furoate* 220-440 mcg once daily or bid; max 880 mcg/day; rinse mouth after use
      Asmanex HFA *Inhaler:* 100, 200 mcg/actuation (13 gm, 120 inh)
      Pediatric: <12 years: not established; ≥12 years: same as adult
      Asmanex Twisthaler *Inhaler:* 110 mcg/actuation (30 inh), 220 mcg/actuation (30, 60, 120 inh)
      Pediatric: <4 years: not recommended; 4-11 years: 110 mcg once daily in the PM; >12 years: may use **Asmanex HFA**; rinse mouth after use
➤ *triamcinolone*
      Azmacort 2 inhalations tid-qid or 4 inhalations bid; rinse mouth after use
      Pediatric: <6 years: not recommended; 6-12 years: 1-2 inhalations tid or 2-4 inhalations bid; >12 years: same as adult
        Inhaler: 100 mcg/actuation (20 gm, 240 inh)

LEUKOTRIENE RECEPTOR ANTAGONISTS (LRAs)
Comment: Leukotriene receptor antagonists (LRAs) are indicated for prophylaxis and chronic treatment, only. Not for primary (rescue) treatment of acute asthma attack.
➤ *montelukast* (G) 10 mg once daily in the PM; for exercise-induced asthma (EIA) take at least 2 hours before exercise; max 1 dose/day
    Pediatric: <12 months: not recommended; 12-23 months: one 4 mg granule pkt once daily; 2-5 years: one 4 mg chew tab or granule pkt once daily; 6-14 years: one 5 mg chew tab daily; ≥15 years: same as adult
      Singulair *Tab:* 10 mg
      Singulair Chewable *Chew tab:* 4, 5 mg (cherry) (phenylalanine)
      Singulair Oral Granules *Granules:* 4 mg/pkt; take within 15 minutes of opening pkt; may mix with applesauce, carrots, rice, or ice cream
➤ *zafirlukast* 20 mg bid, 1 hour ac or 2 hours pc
    Pediatric: <7 years: not recommended; 7-11 years: 10 mg bid 1 hour ac or 2 hours pc; ≥12 years: same as adult
      Accolate *Tab:* 10, 20 mg
➤ *zileuton* (G)
    Pediatric: <12 years: not recommended; ≥12 years: same as adult
      Zyflo 1 tab qid (total 2400 mg/day)
      Tab: 600 mg

(continued)

Zyflo CR 2 tabs bid (total 2400 mg/day)
Tab: 600 mg ext-rel

IMMUNOGLOBULIN E (IGE) BLOCKER (IMMUNOGLOBULIN G1K [IGG1K] MONOCLONAL ANTIBODY)

▷ *omalizumab* 150-375 mg SC every 2-4 weeks based on body weight and pretreatment serum total IgE level; max 150 mg/injection site; approved for patient self-administration after education by a qualified healthcare provider
Pediatric: <12 years: not recommended; 30-90 kg + IgE >30-100 IU/ml: 150 mg every 4 weeks; 90-150 kg + IgE >30-100 IU/ml or 30-90 kg + IgE >100-200 IU/ml or 30-60 kg + IgE >200-300 IU/ml: 300 mg every 4 weeks; >90-150 kg + IgE >100-200 IU/ml or >60-90 kg + IgE >200-300 IU/ml or 30-70 kg + IgE >300-400 IU/ml: 225 mg q 2 weeks; >90-150 kg + IgE >200-300 IU/ml or >70-90 kg + IgE >300-400 IU/ml or 30-70 kg + IgE >400-500 IU/ml or 30-60 kg + IgE >500-600 IU/ml or 30-60 kg + IgE >600-700 IU/ml: 375 mg every 2 weeks
Xolair *Vial:* 150 mg, single-dose, pwdr for SC injection after reconstitution; *Prefilled syringe:* 75 mg/0.5 ml, 150 mg/1 ml single-dose (preservative-free)

INHALED MAST CELL STABILIZERS (IMCSs) (PROPHYLAXIS)

Comment: Inhaled mast cell stabilizers (IMCS) are for prophylaxis and chronic treatment, only. Not for primary (rescue) treatment of acute asthma attack.
▷ *cromolyn sodium* (G)
Intal 2 inhalations qid; 2 inhalations up to 10-60 minutes before precipitant as prophylaxis; rinse mouth after use
Pediatric: <2 years: not recommended; 2-5 years: use inhal soln via nebulizer; >5 years: 2 inhalations qid via inhaler
Inhaler: 0.8 mg/actuation (8.1, 14.2 gm; 112, 200 inh)
Intal Inhalation Solution 20 mg by nebulizer qid; 20 mg up to 10-60 minutes before precipitant as prophylaxis
Pediatric: <2 years: not recommended; ≥2 years: same as adult
Inhal soln: 20 mg/2 ml (60, 120/carton)
▷ *nedocromil sodium*
Tilade 2 sprays qid; rinse mouth after use
Pediatric: <6 years: not recommended; ≥6 years: 2 sprays qid
Inhaler: 1.75 mg/spray (16.2 gm; 104 sprays)
Tilade Nebulizer Solution 0.5% 1 amp qid by nebulizer
Pediatric: <2 years: not recommended; ≥2 years: initially 1 amp qid by nebulizer; 2-5 years: initially 1 amp tid by nebulizer; ≥5 years: same as adult
Inhal soln: 11 mg/2.2 ml (2 ml; 60, 120/carton)

INHALED LONG-ACTING ANTICHOLINERGIC

▷ *tiotropium (as bromide monohydrate)* 2 inhalations once daily using inhalation device; do not swallow caps
Pediatric: <12 years: not recommended; ≥12 years: same as adult
Spiriva HandiHaler *Inhal device:* 18 mcg/cap pwdr for inhalation (5, 30, 90 caps w. inhalation device)
Spiriva Respimat *Inhal device:* 1.25, 2.5 mcg/actuation cartridge w. inhalation device (4 gm, 60 metered actuations) (benzalkonium chloride)
Comment: *Tiotropium* is for prophylaxis and chronic treatment, only. Not for primary (rescue) treatment of acute attack. Avoid getting powder in the eyes. Caution with narrow-angle glaucoma, benign prostatic hyperplasia (BPH), bladder neck obstruction, and pregnancy. Contraindicated with allergy to *atropine* or its derivatives (e.g., *ipratropium*).

INHALED ANTICHOLINERGIC+BETA-2 AGONIST

▷ *ipratropium bromide+albuterol sulfate* 2 inhalations qid
Pediatric: <12 years: not recommended; ≥12 years: same as adult
Combivent 2 inhalations qid; additional inhalations as required; max 12 inhalations/day
Inhaler: ipra 18 mcg+albu 90 mcg/actuation (14.7 gm, 200 inh)
Duoneb 1 vial via nebulizer 4-6 times daily prn
Inhal soln: ipra 0.5 mg (0.017%)+albu 2.5 mg (0.083%) per 3 ml (23/carton)

INHALED LONG-ACTING BETA-2 AGONIST (LABA)

Comment: Long-acting beta-2 agonist (LABA) agents are not for primary (rescue) treatment of acute asthma attack. For twice daily dosing, allow 12 hours between doses.

▷ *arformoterol* (G) 15 mcg bid via nebulizer
Pediatric: <12 years: not recommended; ≥12 years: same as adult
Brovana *Inhal soln:* 15 mcg/2 ml (2 ml; 30/carton)

Comment: *Arformoterol* is indicated for the treatment of chronic obstructive pulmonary disease (COPD) but is used off-label for the treatment of asthma. It is used for prophylaxis and chronic treatment, <u>only</u>. <u>Not</u> for primary (rescue) treatment of acute attack.

▷ *formoterol fumarate* **(G)**
  Foradil Aerolizer 12 mcg q 12 hours
  Pediatric: <5 years: <u>not</u> recommended; ≥5 years: same as adult
    Inhaler: 12 mcg/cap (12, 60 caps w. device)
  Perforomist 20 mcg q 12 hours
  Pediatric: <12 years: <u>not</u> recommended; ≥12 years: same as adult
    Inhal soln: 20 mcg/2 ml (60/carton)
Comment: *Formoterol* is for prophylaxis and chronic treatment, <u>only</u>. <u>Not</u> for primary (rescue) treatment of acute attack. Do <u>not</u> mix *formoterol* with other drugs. Use of *formoterol* is off-label for asthma.

▷ *olodaterol* 12 mcg q 12 hours
  Pediatric: <12 years: <u>not</u> established; ≥12 years: same as adult
    Striverdi Respimat
    Inhal soln: 2.5 mcg/cartridge (metered actuation) (40 gm, 60 metered actuations) (benzalkonium chloride)
    Comment: Striverdi Respimat is contraindicated in persons with asthma without concomitant use of long-term control medication.

▷ *salmeterol* **(G)** 2 inhalations q 12 hours prn; 2 inhalations at least 30-60 minutes before exercise as prophylaxis for EIA; do <u>not</u> use extra doses for exercise-induced bronchospasm if already using regular dose
  Pediatric: <4 years: <u>not</u> recommended; 4-<12 years: 1 inhalation q 12 hours prn; 1 inhalation at least 30-60 minutes before exercise as prophylaxis for EIA; do <u>not</u> use extra doses for exercise-induced bronchospasm if already using regular dose; ≥12 years: same as adult
    Serevent Diskus *Diskus (pwdr):* 50 mcg/actuation (60 doses/diskus)

INHALED CORTICOSTEROID+LABA

Comment: ICD and LABA agents are <u>not</u> for primary (rescue) treatment of acute asthma attack. For twice daily dosing, allow 12 hours between doses. After every inhalation of a steroid <u>or</u> steroid-containing medication treatment, rinse mouth to reduce risk of oral candidiasis.

▷ *budesonide+formoterol* **(G)** 1 inhalation bid; rinse mouth after use
  Pediatric: <12 years: <u>not</u> established; ≥12 years: same as adult
    Symbicort 80/4.5 *Inhaler:* bud 80 mcg+for 4.5 mcg
    Symbicort 160/4.5 *Inhaler:* bud 160 mcg+for 4.5 mcg
▷ *fluticasone propionate+salmeterol*
  Advair HFA <u>Not</u> *previously using inhaled steroid:* start with 2 inh 45/21 <u>or</u> 115/21 bid; if insufficient response after 2 weeks, use next higher strength; max 2 inh 230/50 bid; allow 12 hours between doses; *Already using inhaled steroid:* see mfr pkg insert
    Advair HFA 45/21 1 inhalation bid; rinse mouth after use
    Pediatric: <12 years: <u>not</u> recommended; ≥12 years: same as adult
      Inhaler: flu pro 45 mcg+sal 21 mcg/actuation (CFC-free)
    Advair HFA 115/21 1 inhalation bid; rinse mouth after use
    Pediatric: <12 years: <u>not</u> established; ≥12 years: same as adult
      Inhaler: flu pro 115 mcg+sal 21 mcg/actuation (CFC-free)
    Advair HFA 230/21 1 inhalation bid; rinse mouth after use
    Pediatric: <12 years: <u>not</u> established; ≥12 years: same as adult
      Inhaler: flu pro 230 mcg+sal 21 mcg/actuation (CFC-free)
    Advair Diskus (G) <u>Not</u> *previously using inhaled steroid:* start with 1 inh 100/50 bid; *Already using inhaled steroid:* see mfr pkg insert; rinse mouth after use
    Advair Diskus (G) 100/50 1 inhalation bid; rinse mouth after use
    Pediatric: <4 years: <u>not</u> recommended; 4-11 years: 1 bid; >11 years: 1 inhalation bid
      Diskus: flu pro 100 mcg+sal 50 mcg/actuation (60 blisters)
    Advair Diskus (G) 250/50 1 inhalation bid; rinse mouth after use
    Pediatric: <4 years: <u>not</u> recommended; 4-12 years: use 100/50 strength; >12 years: same as adult
      Diskus: flu pro 250 mcg+sal 50 mcg/actuation (60 blisters)
    Advair Diskus (G) 500/50 1 inhalation bid; rinse mouth after use
    Pediatric: <4 years: <u>not</u> recommended; 4-12 years: use 100/50 strength; >12 years: same as adult
      Diskus: flu pro 500 mcg+sal 50 mcg/actuation (60 blisters)
    AirDuo RespiClick pwdr for oral inhalation; <u>Not</u> *previously using an inhaled steroid:* 1 inh 55/14 bid; *Already using an inhaled steroid:* see mfr pkg insert; if insufficient response after 2 weeks, titrate with a higher strength; max inh 232/14 bid
    Pediatric: <12 years: <u>not</u> established; ≥12 years: same as adult
      AirDuo RespiClick 55/14 flu pro 55 mcg+sal (as xinafoate) 14 mcg dry pwdr/actuation (60 actuations)

(continued)

AirDuo RespiClick 113/14 flu pro 113 mcg+sal (as xinafoate) 14 mcg dry pwdr/actuation (60 actuations)

AirDuo RespiClick 232/14 flu pro 232 mcg+sal (as xinafoate) 14 mcg dry pwdr/actuation (60 actuations)

▷ *fluticasone furoate+vilanterol* 1 inhalation 100/25 once daily at the same time each day

Pediatric: <17 years: not established; ≥17 years: same as adult

Breo Ellipta 100/25 flu 100 mcg+vil 25 mcg dry pwdr per inhalation (30 doses)

Breo Ellipta 200/25 flu 200 mcg+vil 25 mcg dry pwdr per inhalation (30 doses)

Comment: Breo Ellipta is contraindicated with severe hypersensitivity to milk proteins.

▷ *mometasone furoate+formoterol fumarate* 2 inhalations bid; rinse mouth after use

Pediatric: <12 years: not established; ≥12 years: same as adult

Dulera 100/5 *Inhaler:* mom 100 mcg/for 5 mcg (HFA)

Dulera 200/5 *Inhaler:* mom 200 mcg/for 5 mcg (HFA)

Comment: Dulera is not a rescue inhaler.

INHALED ANTICHOLINERGIC+LABA

▷ *glycopyrrolate+formoterol fumarate* 2 inhalations bid (AM & PM)

Pediatric: <18 years: not established; ≥18 years: same as adult

Bevespi Aerosphere 9/4.8 *MDI:* gly 9 mcg+for 4.8 mcg/inhalation (10.7 gm, 120 inh)

INHALED CORTICOSTEROID+ANTICHOLINERGIC+LABA COMBINATION

▷ *fluticasone furoate+umeclidinium bromide+vilanterol trifenatate* 1 inhalation once daily

Pediatric: safety and efficacy not established

Trelegy Ellipta flutic 100 mcg/umec 62.5 mcg/vilan 25 mcg dry

Comment: Trelegy Ellipta is maintenance therapy for patients with asthma and/or COPD, who are receiving fixed-dose *furoate* and *vilanterol* for airflow obstruction and to reduce exacerbations, or receiving *umeclidinium* and a fixed-dose combination of *fluticasone furoate* and *vilanterol*. Trelegy Ellipta is the first FDA-approved once-daily single-dose inhaler that combines *fluticasone furoate*, a corticosteroid, *umeclidinium*, a long-acting muscarinic antagonist, and *vilanterol*, a long-acting beta-2 adrenergic agonist. Common adverse reactions reported with **Trelegy Ellipta** have included headache, back pain, dysgeusia, diarrhea, cough, oropharyngeal pain, and gastroenteritis. **Trelegy Ellipta** has been found to increase the risk of pneumonia in patients with COPD and increase the risk of asthma-related death. **Trelegy Ellipta** is not indicated for the treatment of acute bronchospasm.

ORAL BETA-2 AGONISTS (BRONCHODILATORS)

▷ *albuterol* (G)

Albuterol Syrup *Adult:* 2-4 mg tid-qid, may increase gradually, max 8 mg qid; *Elderly:* initially 2-3 mg tid-qid, may increase gradually, max 8 mg qid

Pediatric: <2 years: not recommended; ≥2-6 years: 0.1 mg/kg tid, initially max 2 mg tid, may increase gradually to 0.2 mg/kg tid, max 4 mg tid; >6-12 years: 2 mg tid-qid, may increase gradually, max 6 mg qid; ≥12 years: same as adult

Syr: 2 mg/5 ml

Proventil 2-4 mg tid-qid prn

Pediatric: <6 years: not recommended; ≥6 years: same as adult

Tab: 2, 4 mg

Proventil Repetabs 4-8 mg q 12 hours prn

Pediatric: use syrup

Repetab: 4 mg sust-rel

Proventil Syrup 5-10 ml tid-qid prn; may increase gradually; max 20 ml qid prn

Pediatric: <2 years: not recommended; ≥2-6 years: 0.1 mg/kg tid prn, max initially 5 ml tid prn, may increase gradually to 0.2 mg/kg tid prn, max 10 ml tid; >6-14 years: 5 ml tid-qid prn, may increase gradually, max 60 ml/day in divided doses; >14 years: same as adult

Syr: 2 mg/5 ml

Ventolin 2-4 mg tid-qid prn; may increase gradually; max 8 mg qid

Pediatric: <2 years: not recommended; ≥2-6 years: 0.1 mg/kg tid prn, max initially 2 mg tid prn, may increase gradually to 0.2 mg/kg tid, max 4 mg tid; >6-14 years: 2 mg tid-qid prn, may increase gradually, max 6 mg tid

Tab: 2, 4 mg; *Syr:* 2 mg/5 ml (strawberry)

VoSpire ER 4-8 mg q 12 hours prn; max 32 mg/day divided q 12 hours; swallow whole, do not crush or chew

Pediatric: <6 years: not recommended; ≥6-12 years: 4 mg q 12 hours; max 24 mg/day q 12 hours; >12 years: same as adult

Tab: 4, 8 mg ext-rel

▷ *metaproterenol* 20 mg tid-qid prn

Pediatric: <6 years: not recommended (doses of 1.3-2.6 mg/kg/day have been used); ≥6-9 years, <60 lb: 10 mg tid-qid prn; >9-12 years, ≥60 lb: 20 mg tid-qid prn; >12 years: same as adult

Alupent *Tab:* 10, 20 mg; *Syr:* 10 mg/5 ml

METHYLXANTHINES

Comment: Obtain serum *theophylline* level just before the 5th dose is administered. Therapeutic *theophylline* level is 10-20 mcg/ml.

▶ *theophylline* (G)

Theo-24 initially 300-400 mg once daily at HS; after 3 days, increase to 400-600 mg once daily at HS; max 600 mg/day

Pediatric: <45 kg: initially 12-14 mg/kg/day; max 300 mg/day; increase after 3 days to 16 mg/kg/day to max 400 mg, after 3 more days, increase to 30 mg/kg/day to max 600 mg/day; ≥45 kg: same as adult

   Cap: 100, 200, 300, 400 mg ext-rel

Theo-Dur initially 150 mg bid; increase to 200 mg bid after 3 days; then to 300 mg bid after 3 more days

Pediatric: <6 years: not recommended; 6-15 years: initially 12-14 mg/kg/day in 2 divided doses, max 300 mg/day; then increase to 16 mg/kg in 2 divided doses, max 400 mg/day; then to 20 mg/kg/day in 2 divided doses, max 600 mg/day; ≥15 years: same as adult

   Tab: 100, 200, 300 mg ext-rel

Theolair-SR

Pediatric: not recommended

   Tab: 200, 250, 300, 500 mg sust-rel

Uniphyl 400-600 mg daily with meals

Pediatric: not recommended

   Tab: 400*, 600*mg cont-rel

METHYLXANTHINE+EXPECTORANT COMBINATION

▶ *dyphylline+guaifenesin* 1 tab qid

Lufyllin GG *Tab:* dyphy 200 mg+guaif 200 mg; *Elix:* dyphy 100 mg+guaif 100 mg per 15 ml

JANUS KINASE (JAK) 1 INHIBITOR

▶ *abrocitinib* administer 100 mg once daily; do not break, crush, or chew; may be used with or without topical corticosteroid; if a dose is missed, administer the dose as soon as possible; if <12 hours before the next dose, skip the missed dose and resume dosing at the regular scheduled time; if response to treatment is inadequate after 12 weeks, consider increasing dose to 200 mg once daily; then, if response remains inadequate discontinue **Cibinqo**

Pediatric: Safety and efficacy not established

Cibinqo *Tab:* 50, 100, 200 mg film-coat

Comment: **Cibinqo** is a Janus kinase (JAK) 1 inhibitor indicated for the treatment of adults with refractory, moderate-to-severe atopic dermatitis, whose disease is not adequately controlled with other systemic drug products, including biologics, or when use of those therapies is inadvisable. **Cibinqo** is not approved for use in rheumatoid arthritis (RA). **Cibinqo** is not recommended for use in combination with other JAK inhibitors, biologic immunomodulators, or with other immunosuppressants. **Cibinqo** is contraindicated in patients taking antiplatelet therapies, *except* for low-dose aspirin (≤81 mg daily), during the first 3 months of treatment. **Cibinqo** initiation is not recommended in patients with active tuberculosis (TB). For patients with latent TB or those with a negative latent TB test who are at high risk for TB, start preventive therapy for latent TB *prior to* initiation of **Cibinqo**. **Cibinqo** initiation is not recommended in patients with active hepatitis B or hepatitis C. **Cibinqo** initiation is not recommended in patients with a platelet count <150,000/mm³, absolute lymphocyte count <500/mm³, absolute neutrophil count <1,000/mm³, or hemoglobin <8 gm/dL. Prior to initiating **Cibinqo**, complete all age-appropriate vaccinations as recommended by current immunization guidelines, including prophylactic herpes zoster vaccinations. Avoid vaccination with live vaccines immediately prior to, during, and immediately after **Cibinqo** therapy. Consider the benefits and risks for the individual patient prior to initiating or continuing therapy with **Cibinqo**, particularly in patients who are current or past smokers and patients with other cardiovascular risk factors. Patients should be informed about the symptoms of serious cardiovascular events and the steps to take if they occur. Discontinue **Cibinqo** in patients who have experienced a myocardial infarction or stroke. Avoid **Cibinqo** in patients who may be at increased risk of thrombosis. If symptoms of thrombosis occur, discontinue **Cibinqo** and evaluate and treat patients appropriately. There is a pregnancy exposure registry that monitors pregnancy outcomes in females exposed to **Cibinqo** during pregnancy. Pregnant patients exposed to **Cibinqo** and healthcare providers are encouraged to call 1-877-311-3770.

▶ *ruxolitinib* apply a thin layer bid to affected areas; max 20% body surface area (BSA); max: 60 gm per week

Pediatric: <12 years: safety and efficacy not established; ≥12 years: same as adult

Opzelura *Crm:* 1.5% (60 gm aluminum tube)

Comment: **Opzelura** cream is a JAK inhibitor indicated for topical short-term and non-continuous, chronic treatment of mild-to-moderate atopic dermatitis in non-immunocompromised patients >12 years of age whose disease is not adequately controlled with other topical prescription therapies or when those therapies are not advisable. Use of **Opzelura** in combination with therapeutic biologics, other JAK inhibitors, or potent immunosuppressants such as *azathioprine* or *cyclosporine* is not recommended. *Boxed Warning:* Serious infection, mortality, malignancy, major adverse cardiovascular

(continued)

events (MACE), and thrombosis. Serious infections leading to hospitalization or death, including TB and bacterial, invasive fungal, viral, and other opportunistic infections, have occurred in patients receiving JAK inhibitors for inflammatory conditions. A higher rate of all-cause mortality, including sudden cardiovascular death, has been observed in patients treated with JAK inhibitors for inflammatory conditions. Lymphoma and other malignancies have been observed in patients treated with JAK inhibitors for inflammatory conditions. A higher rate of MACE (including cardiovascular death, myocardial infarction, and stroke) has been observed in patients treated with JAK inhibitors for inflammatory conditions. Thrombosis, including deep venous thrombosis (DVT), pulmonary embolism (PE), and arterial thrombosis, some fatal, have occurred in patients treated with JAK inhibitors for inflammatory conditions (see mfr pck insert for full prescribing information and complete boxed warning). The most common adverse reactions (incidence ≥1%) have been nasopharyngitis, diarrhea, bronchitis, ear infection, increased eosinophil count, urticaria, folliculitis, tonsillitis, and rhinorrhea. Adverse reactions that occurred in trials 1 and 2 in <1% of subjects in the **Opzelura** group, and none in the vehicle group, were neutropenia, allergic conjunctivitis, pyrexia, seasonal allergy, herpes zoster, otitis externa, staphylococcal infection, and acneiform dermatitis. As serious bacterial, mycobacterial, fungal, and viral infections have occurred, monitor patients for infection and manage all infections appropriately and promptly. Non-melanoma skin cancers (i.e., basal cell and squamous cell carcinoma) have occurred. Perform periodic skin examinations during treatment and following treatment as appropriate. Thromboembolic events have occurred. Thrombocytopenia, anemia, and neutropenia have occurred; monitor CBC as clinically indicated. *Ruxolitinib* is known to be a substrate for cytochrome P450 3A4 (CYP3A4). Inhibitors of CYP3A4 may increase *ruxolitinib* systemic concentrations, whereas inducers of CYP3A4 may decrease *ruxolitinib* systemic concentrations. Available data from human pregnancies reported in clinical trials with **Opzelura** are not sufficient to evaluate a drug-associated risk of major birth defects, miscarriage, or other adverse maternal or fetal outcomes. In animal reproduction studies, oral administration of *ruxolitinib* during the period of organogenesis resulted in adverse developmental outcomes at doses associated with maternal toxicity. There is a pregnancy registry that monitors pregnancy outcomes in persons exposed to **Opzelura** during pregnancy. Pregnant persons exposed to **Opzelura** and healthcare providers should report **Opzelura** exposure by calling 1-855-463-3463. Advise patients not to breastfeed during treatment with **Opzelura** and for 4 weeks after the last dose.

INTERLEUKIN-4 RECEPTOR ALPHA ANTAGONIST

▷ *dupilumab* administer SC into the upper arm, abdomen, or thigh; rotate sites; initially 600 mg (2 x 300 mg injections at different sites), followed by 300 mg SC once every other week; may use with or without topical corticosteroids; may use with calcineurin inhibitors, but reserve only for problem areas (e.g., face, neck, intertriginous, and genital areas); avoid live vaccines
Pediatric: <12 years: not recommended; ≥12 years: same as adult
   Dupixent *Prefilled syringe:* 300 mg/2 ml (2/pck without needle) (preservative-free)
Comment: *Dupilumab* is a human monoclonal immunoglobulin G4 (IgG4) antibody that inhibits interleukin-4 (IL-4) and interleukin-13 (IL-13) signaling by specifically binding to the IL4Ra subunit shared by the IL-4 and IL-13 receptor complexes, thereby inhibiting the release of proinflammatory cytokines, chemokines, and immunoglobulin E (IgE). *Dupilumab* is indicated as an add-on maintenance therapy for patients ≥12 years of age with moderate-to-severe asthma with an eosinophilic subtype or with oral corticosteroid-dependent asthma.

▷ *dupilumab* administer SC into the upper arm, abdomen, or thigh; rotate sites; *Initial dose:* 400 mg (2 x 200 mg SC at different sites); then 200 mg SC every other week or *Initial dose:* 600 mg (2 x 300 mg SC at different sites); then 300 mg SC every other week (this dosing regimen is for patients requiring concomitant oral corticosteroids or with comorbid moderate-to-severe atopic dermatitis for which **Dupixent** is indicated)
Pediatric: <12 years: not recommended; ≥12 years: same as adult)
   Dupixent *Prefilled syringe:* 200 mg/1.14 ml, 300 mg/2 ml, single-dose (2/pck without needle) (preservative-free)
Comment: *Dupilumab* is a human monoclonal IgG4 antibody that inhibits IL-4 and IL-13 signaling by specifically binding to the IL4Ra subunit shared by the IL-4 and IL-13 receptor complexes, thereby inhibiting the release of proinflammatory cytokines, chemokines, and IgE. *Dupilumab* is indicated as an add-on maintenance therapy for patients ≥12 years of age with moderate-to-severe asthma with an eosinophilic subtype or with oral corticosteroid-dependent asthma. **Dupixent** is also indicated, at different dosing regimens, for patients ≥12 years of age with atopic dermatitis and adult patients with chronic rhinosinusitis with nasal polyposis (CRSwNP). Avoid live vaccines.

ASTHMA-COPD OVERLAP SYNDROME (ACOS)

Comment: An estimated 16% of patients with asthma or chronic obstructive pulmonary disease (COPD) have asthma–COPD overlap syndrome (ACOS), a poorly understood disease with an increasing morbidity and mortality. PROSPRO (Prospective Study to Evaluate Predictors of Clinical Effectiveness in Response to

Omalizumab), a 48-week, prospective, multicenter, observational study, included patients (n = 806) who were 12 years of age and older who were initiating *omalizumab* treatment for moderate-to-severe allergic asthma, including patients with comorbid COPD (n = 78). Researchers reported that *omalizumab* (**Xolair**) decreased asthma exacerbations and improved symptom control to a similar extent in patients with ACOS as seen in patients with asthma but no COPD. While patients with COPD typically experience annual declines in lung function, at least some of the ACOS patients in this study, which included one of the largest observational cohorts to date of patients with ACOS, showed preserved lung function after 48 weeks of *omalizumab* treatment (as demonstrated by improved postbronchodilator forced expiratory volumn in 1 second FEV1) at the end of the study), and the number of asthma exacerbations reduced from baseline through month 12 from 3 or more exacerbations in both ACOS and non-ACOS groups to 1.1 or less.

IMMUNOGLOBULIN E (IGE) BLOCKER (IMMUNOGLOBULIN G1K [IGG1K] MONOCLONAL ANTIBODY)

▷ *omalizumab* 150-375 mg SC every 2-4 weeks based on body weight and pretreatment serum total IgE level; max 150 mg/injection site; approved for patient self-administration after education by a qualified healthcare provider
Pediatric: <12 years: not recommended; 30-90 kg + IgE >30-100 IU/ml: 150 mg every 4 weeks; 90-150 kg + IgE >30-100 IU/ml or 30-90 kg + IgE >100-200 IU/ml or 30-60 kg + IgE >200-300 IU/ml: 300 mg every 4 weeks; >90-150 kg + IgE >100-200 IU/ml or >60-90 kg + IgE >200-300 IU/ml or 30-70 kg + IgE >300-400 IU/ml: 225 mg every 2 weeks; >90-150 kg + IgE >200-300 IU/ml or >70-90 kg + IgE >300-400 IU/ml or 30-70 kg + IgE >400-500 IU/ml or 30-60 kg + IgE >500-600 IU/ml or 30-60 kg + IgE >600-700 IU/ml: 375 mg every 2 weeks
Xolair *Vial:* 150 mg, single-dose, pwdr for SC injection after reconstitution; *Prefilled syringe:* 75 mg/0.5 ml, 150 mg/1 ml, single-dose (preservative-free)

INHALED CORTICOSTEROID+ANTICHOLINERGIC+LONG-ACTING BETA-2 AGONIST (LABA) COMBINATION

▷ *fluticasone furoate+umeclidinium bromide+vilanterol trifenatate* 1 inhalation once daily
Pediatric: not established
flutic 100 mcg/umec 62.5 mcg/vilan 25 mcg dry
Comment: Trelegy Ellipta is maintenance therapy for patients with asthma and/or COPD who are receiving fixed-dose *furoate* and *vilanterol* for airflow obstruction and to reduce exacerbations, or receiving *umeclidinium* and a fixed-dose combination of *fluticasone furoate* and *vilanterol*. **Trelegy Ellipta** is the first FDA-approved once-daily single-dose inhaler that combines *fluticasone furoate*, a corticosteroid, *umeclidinium*, a long-acting muscarinic antagonist, and *vilanterol*, a long-acting beta-2 adrenergic agonist. Common adverse reactions reported with **Trelegy Ellipta** have included headache, back pain, dysgeusia, diarrhea, cough, oropharyngeal pain, and gastroenteritis. **Trelegy Ellipta** has been found to increase the risk of pneumonia in patients with COPD and increase the risk of asthma-related death. **Trelegy Ellipta** is not indicated for the treatment of acute bronchospasm.

ASTHMA: SEVERE, EOSINOPHILIA; HYPEREOSINOPHILIA SYNDROMES (HES)

Comment: Currently available therapies for patients with severe eosinophilia asthma and hypereosinophilia syndromes (HES) include anti-immunoglobulin E (IgE) therapy (*omalizumab* [**Xolair**]); anti-interleukin monoclonal antibodies *mepolizumab* (**Nucala**), *reslizumab* (**Cinqair**), and *benralizumab* (**Fasenra**); and interleukin receptor antagonist *dupilumab* (**Dupixent**). The data on pregnancy exposure from the clinical trials are insufficient to inform on drug-associated risk. Monoclonal antibodies are transported across the placenta in a linear fashion as pregnancy progresses; therefore, potential effects on the fetus are likely to be greater during the 2nd and 3rd trimesters of pregnancy. Immunoglobulin G (IgG) is known to be present in human milk; however, the effects on the breastfed infant are unknown.

INTERLEUKIN-4 RECEPTOR ALPHA ANTAGONIST

▷ *dupilumab* administer SC into the upper arm, abdomen, or thigh; rotate sites; *Initial dose:* 400 mg (2 x 200 mg SC at different sites); then 200 mg SC every other week or *Initial dose:* 600 mg (2 x 300 mg SC at different sites); then 300 mg SC every other week (this dosing regimen is for patients requiring concomitant oral corticosteroids or with comorbid moderate-to-severe atopic dermatitis for which **Dupixent** is indicated)
Pediatric: <12 years: not recommended; ≥12 years: same as adult
Dupixent *Prefilled syringe:* 200 mg/1.14 ml, 300 mg/2 ml, single-dose (2/pck without needle) (preservative-free)
Comment: *Dupilumab* is a human monoclonal IgG4 antibody that inhibits interleukin-4 (IL-4) and interleukin-13 (IL-13) signaling by specifically binding to the IL4Ra subunit shared by the IL-4 and IL-13 receptor complexes, thereby inhibiting the release of proinflammatory cytokines, chemokines, and IgE. *Dupilumab* is indicated as an add-on maintenance therapy for patients ≥12 years of age with moderate-to-severe asthma with an eosinophilic subtype or with oral corticosteroid-dependent asthma. **Dupixent** is also indicated, at different dosing regimens, for patients ≥12 years of age with atopic dermatitis and adult patients with chronic rhinosinusitis with nasal polyposis (CRSwNP). Avoid live vaccines.

HUMANIZED INTERLEUKIN-5 ANTAGONIST MONOCLONAL ANTIBODY
Interleukin-5 Antagonist Monoclonal Antibody (Immunoglobulin G1 [IgG1] Kappa)

▶ *mepolizumab Adult:* Severe asthma: 100 mg SC once q 4 weeks;
CRSwNP: 100 mg SC once every 4 weeks;
Eosinophilic granulomatosis with polyangiitis (EGPA) and HES: 300 mg as 3 separate 100 mg SC injections once every 4 weeks
Pediatric: <6 years: safety and efficacy not established; severe asthma and with an eosinophilic phenotype in patients aged 6-11 years: 40 mg SC once q 4 weeks as an add-on maintenance treatment; may self-administer or the caregiver may administer (with healthcare provider approval); severe asthma in patients aged ≥12 years: 100 mg SC once q 4 weeks

Nucala *Vial:* 100 mg/ml, pwdr for reconstitution, single-dose; *Prefilled syringe:* 40 mg/0.4 ml, 100 mg/ml, single-dose; *Prefilled autoinjector:* 100 mg/ml, single-dose

Comment: Nucala is an interleukin-5 antagonist monoclonal antibody (IgG1 kappa) indicated for the treatment of severe eosinophilic asthma, EGPA (Churg–Strauss syndrome), HES, and CRSwNP. Nucala is not indicated for relief of acute bronchospasm or status asthmaticus. Hypersensitivity reactions (e.g., anaphylaxis, angioedema, bronchospasm, hypotension, urticaria, rash) have occurred after administration of **Nucala**; discontinue **Nucala** in the event of a hypersensitivity reaction. Herpes zoster (HZ) infections have occurred in patients receiving **Nucala**; consider vaccination if medically appropriate. Do not discontinue systemic or inhaled corticosteroids abruptly upon initiation of therapy with **Nucala**; decrease corticosteroids gradually, if appropriate. Treat patients with preexisting helminth infections before therapy with **Nucala**. If patients become infected while receiving treatment with **Nucala** and do not respond to antihelminth treatment, discontinue **Nucala** until the parasitic infection resolves. The most common adverse reactions (incidence ≥5%) are the following: *Asthma:* headache, injection site reaction, back pain, and fatigue; *CRSwNP:* oropharyngeal pain and arthralgia; *EGPA and HES:* similar to asthma. In pregnant females with poorly or moderately controlled asthma, evidence demonstrates that there is an increased risk of preeclampsia in the mother, and prematurity, low birth weight (LBW), and small for gestational age (SGA) in the neonate. The level of asthma control should be closely monitored in pregnant women and treatment adjusted as necessary to maintain optimal control. Data on pregnancy exposure are insufficient to inform on **Nucala**-associated risk. Monoclonal antibodies, such as *mepolizumab*, are transported across the placenta in a linear fashion as pregnancy progresses; therefore, potential effects on the fetus are likely to be greater during the 2nd and 3rd trimesters of pregnancy. There is a pregnancy exposure registry that monitors pregnancy outcomes in women with asthma exposed to **Nucala** during pregnancy. Healthcare providers can enroll patients or encourage patients to enroll themselves by calling 1-877-311-8972 or www.mothertobaby.org/asthma. *Mepolizumab* is a humanized monoclonal antibody (IgG1 kappa), and IgG is present in human milk in small amounts. Developmental and health benefits of breastfeeding should be considered along with the mother's clinical need for **Nucala** and any potential adverse effects on the breastfed infant from *mepolizumab* or from the underlying maternal condition.

Interleukin-5 Antagonist Monoclonal Antibody (Immunoglobulin G4 [IgG4] Kappa)

▶ *reslizumab* should be administered by a qualified healthcare professional and, in line with clinical practice, monitoring of patients after administration of biologic agents is recommended; recommended dose is 3 mg/kg once every 4 weeks via IV infusion over 20-50 minutes; do not administer as an intravenous push (IVP) or bolus
Pediatric: <18 years: not established; ≥18 years: same as adult

Cinqair *Vial:* 100 mg/10 ml (10 mg/ml) soln, single-use (preservative-free)

Comment: Cinqair is an interleukin-5 antagonist monoclonal antibody (IgG4 kappa). It is an add-on maintenance treatment for patients ≥18 years of age with severe asthma and with an eosinophilic phenotype. **Cinqair** is also indicated for the treatment of patients >18 years of age with EGPA. **Cinqair** is not for relief of acute bronchospasm or status asthmaticus. Hypersensitivity reactions (e.g., anaphylaxis, angioedema, bronchospasm, hypotension, urticaria, rash) have occurred after administration of **Cinqair**; discontinue **Cinqair** in the event of a hypersensitivity reaction. HZ infections have occurred in patients receiving **Cinqair**. Consider vaccination if medically appropriate. Do not discontinue systemic or inhaled corticosteroids abruptly upon initiation of therapy with **Cinqair**. Decrease corticosteroids gradually, if appropriate. Treat patients with preexisting parasitic helminth infections before therapy with **Cinqair**. If patients become infected while receiving treatment with **Cinqair** and do not respond to antihelminth treatment, discontinue **Cinqair** until parasitic infection resolves. The most common adverse reactions (incidence ≥5%) include headache, injection site reaction, back pain, and fatigue. Formal drug interaction trials have not been performed with **Cinqair**. Data on pregnancy exposure are insufficient to inform on drug-associated risk. Monoclonal antibodies, such as *reslizumab*, are transported across the placenta in a linear fashion as pregnancy progresses; therefore, potential effects on a fetus are likely to be greater during the second and third trimesters of pregnancy. There is a pregnancy exposure registry that monitors pregnancy outcomes in patients exposed to **Cinqair** during pregnancy. Healthcare providers can enroll patients or encourage patients to enroll themselves by calling 1-877-311-8972 or www.mothertobaby.org/

asthma. There is no information regarding the presence of *reslizumab* in human milk or effects on the breastfed infant.

IMMUNOGLOBULIN E (IGE) BLOCKER (IMMUNOGLOBULIN G1K [IGG1K] MONOCLONAL ANTIBODY)

▷ *omalizumab* 150-375 mg SC every 2-4 weeks based on body weight and pretreatment serum total IgE level; max 150 mg/injection site; approved for patient self-administration after education by a qualified healthcare provider
Pediatric: <12 years: not recommended; >12 years: 30-90 kg + IgE >30-100 IU/ml: 150 mg q 4 weeks; 90-150 kg + IgE >30-100 IU/ml or 30-90 kg + IgE >100-200 IU/ml or 30-60 kg + IgE >200-300 IU/ml: 300 mg every 4 weeks; >90-150 kg + IgE >100-200 IU/ml or >60-90 kg + IgE >200-300 IU/ml or 30-70 kg + IgE >300-400 IU/ml: 225 mg every 2 weeks; >90-150 kg + IgE >200-300 IU/ml or >70-90 kg + IgE >300-400 IU/ml or 30-70 kg + IgE >400-500 IU/ml or 30-60 kg + IgE >500-600 IU/ml or 30-60 kg + IgE >600-700 IU/ml: 375 mg every 2 weeks
  Xolair *Vial:* 150 mg, single-dose, pwdr for SC injection after reconstitution; *Prefilled syringe:* 75 mg/0.5 ml, 150 mg/1 ml, single-dose (preservative-free)

INTERLEUKIN-5 RECEPTOR ALPHA-DIRECTED CYTOLYTIC MONOCLONAL ANTIBODY (IGG1, KAPPA)

▷ *benralizumab* should be administered by a qualified healthcare professional and, in line with clinical practice, monitoring of patients after administration of biologic agents is recommended; recommended dose is 30 mg SC every 4 weeks for the first 3 doses; then once every 8 weeks thereafter; inject SC into the upper arm, abdomen, or thigh; store in refrigerator; do not freeze; prior to administration; warm **Fasenra** by leaving the carton at room temperature for about 30 minutes; administer within 24 hours or discard into sharps container
Pediatric: <12 years: not established; ≥12 years: same as adult
  Fasenra *Prefilled syringe:* 30 mg/ml soln, single-dose (preservative-free)
  Comment: *Benralizumab* is an interleukin-5 receptor alpha-directed cytolytic monoclonal antibody (IgG1, kappa) produced in Chinese hamster ovary cells by recombinant DNA technology. **Fasenra** is indicated as add-on maintenance treatment of patients with severe asthma ≥12 years of age, and with an eosinophilic phenotype. It is not for the treatment of other eosinophilic conditions: Discontinue systemic or inhaled corticosteroids abruptly upon initiation of therapy with **Fasenra**; decrease corticosteroids gradually, if appropriate. Treat patients with preexisting parasitic helminth infection before therapy with **Fasenra**. If patients become infected while receiving **Fasenra** and do not respond to antihelminth treatment, discontinue **Fasenra** until the parasitic infection resolves. The most common adverse reactions (incidence ≥5%) include headache and pharyngitis. No formal drug interaction studies have been conducted. The data on pregnancy exposure from the clinical trials are insufficient to inform on drug-associated risk. Monoclonal antibodies such as *benralizumab* are transported across the placenta during the 3rd trimester of pregnancy; therefore, potential effects on the fetus are likely to be greater during the 3rd trimester of pregnancy. In women with poorly or moderately controlled asthma, evidence demonstrates that there is an increased risk of preeclampsia in the mother and prematurity, LBW, and SGA in the neonate. The level of asthma control should be closely monitored in pregnant females and treatment adjusted as necessary to maintain optimal control. There is no information regarding the presence of *benralizumab* in human or animal milk, and the effects of *benralizumab* on the breastfed infant and on milk production are not known.

ATROPHIC VAGINITIS

Oral Estrogens *see Menopause*

VAGINAL ESTROGEN PREPARATIONS

▷ *estradiol* (G)
  Vagifem Vaginal Tablet 1 tab intravaginally daily x 2 weeks; then 1 tab intravaginally twice weekly
    Vag tab: 10 mcg (15 tabs w. applicators)
  Yuvafem Vaginal Tablet 1 tab intravaginally daily x 2 weeks; then 1 tab intravaginally twice weekly
    Vag tab: 10 mcg (15 tabs w. applicators)
▷ *estradiol* (G)
  Estrace Vaginal Cream 2-4 gm daily x 1-2 weeks; then gradually reduce to 1/2 initial dose x 1-2 weeks; then maintenance dose of 1 gm 1-3 x weekly
    Vag crm: 0.01% (1 oz tube w. calib applicator)
▷ *estrogens, conjugated*
  Premarin Cream 2 gm/day intravaginally
    Vag crm: 1.5 oz w. applicator marked in 1/2 gm increments to max of 2 gm
▷ *estropipate*
  Ogen Cream 2-4 gm intravaginally daily x 3 weeks; discontinue during the 4th week; continue in this cyclical pattern
    Vag crm: 1.5 mg/gm (42.5 gm w. calib applicator)

ATTENTION DEFICIT HYPERACTIVITY DISORDER (ADHD)

SELECTIVE NOREPINEPHRINE REUPTAKE INHIBITORS (SNRIs)

▶ *atomoxetine* (G) take one dose daily in the morning *or* in two divided doses in the morning and late afternoon *or* early evening; initially 40 mg/kg; increase after at least 3 days to 80 mg/kg; then after 2-4 weeks may increase to max 100 mg/day
Pediatric: <6 years: not recommended; ≥6 years, <70 kg: initially 0.5 mg/kg/day: increase after at least 3 days to 1.2 mg/kg/day, max 1.4 mg/kg/day *or* 100 mg/day (whichever is less); ≥6 years, >70 kg: same as adult
    Strattera *Cap:* 10, 18, 25, 40, 60, 80, 100 mg
    Comment: Strattera is not associated with stimulant *or* euphoric effects. May discontinue without tapering. Common adverse effects associated with *atomoxetine* in children and adolescents included upset stomach, decreased appetite, nausea *or* vomiting, dizziness, tiredness, and mood swings. For adult patients, the most common adverse side effects included constipation, dry mouth, nausea, decreased appetite, sexual side effects, problems passing urine, and dizziness. Other adverse effects associated with *atomoxetine* included severe liver damage and potential for serious cardiovascular events. In addition, *atomoxetine* increases the risk of suicidal ideation in children and adolescents. Healthcare providers should monitor patients taking this medication for clinical worsening, suicidality, and unusual changes in behavior, particularly within the first few months of initiation *or* during dose changes.

▶ *viloxazine*
Pediatric: <6 years: not established; 6-11 years: recommended starting dose is 100 mg once daily, may titrate in increments of 100 mg weekly to max of 400 mg once daily; 12-17 years: recommended starting dose is 200 mg once daily, may titrate after 1 week, by an increment of 200 mg to max of 400 mg once daily; capsules may be swallowed whole *or* opened and the entire contents sprinkled onto applesauce; do not bite, crush, *or* chew capsuled *or* capsule contents; *Hepatic impairment:* not recommended; *Severe renal impairment:* max 200 mg once daily
    Qelbree *Cap:* 100, 150, 200 mg ext-rel
    Comment: Qelbree *(viloxazine)* is a selective norepinephrine reuptake inhibitor (SNRI) for the treatment of attention deficit hyperactivity disorder (ADHD) in pediatric patients 6-17 years of age. The most commonly observed adverse reactions to **Qelbree** (≥5% and at least twice the rate of placebo) have been somnolence, decreased appetite, fatigue, nausea, vomiting, insomnia, and irritability. *Boxed Warning:* In clinical trials, higher rates of suicidal thoughts and behavior were reported in pediatric patients treated with **Qelbree** than in patients treated with placebo. Closely monitor for worsening and emergence of suicidal thoughts and behavior. Contraindications to **Qelbree** are (1) concomitant administration of monoamine oxidase inhibitors (MAOIs) *or* dosing within 14 days after discontinuing an MAOI and (2) concomitant administration of sensitive CYP1A2 substrates *or* CYP1A2 substrates with a narrow therapeutic range. Moderate sensitive CYP1A2 substrates are not recommended for co-administration with **Qelbree**; dose reduction may be warranted. **Qelbree** may cause maternal harm in pregnancy; discontinue when pregnancy is recognized. Available data from case series with *viloxazine* use in pregnant women are insufficient to determine a drug-associated risk of major birth defects, miscarriage, *or* adverse maternal outcomes. There is a pregnancy exposure registry that monitors pregnancy outcomes in women exposed to **Qelbree** during pregnancy. Healthcare providers are encouraged to register patients by calling the National Pregnancy Registry for Psychiatric Medications at 1-866-961-2388 *or* www.womensmentalhealth.org/preg. There are no data on the presence of *viloxazine* in human milk *or* effects on the breastfed infant. However, it is likely that *viloxazine* is present in human milk.

CENTRAL NERVOUS SYSTEM (CNS) STIMULANTS

▶ *amphetamine, mixed salts of single entity amphetamine* (II)(G)
    Adzenys ER initially 12.5 mg (10 ml) once daily in the morning; take with *or* without food; individualize the dosage according to the therapeutic needs and response
    Pediatric: <6 years: not recommended; 6-17 years: take with *or* without food; individualize the dosage according to the therapeutic needs and response; 6-12 years: initially 6.3 mg (5 ml) once daily in the morning, max dose 18.8 mg (15 ml); 13-17 years:12.5 mg (10 ml) once daily in the morning; ≥17 years: same as adult
        Oral susp: 125 mg/ml ext-rel (450 ml) (orange)
    Comment: Patients taking **Adderall XR** may be switched to **Adzenys ER** at the equivalent dose taken once daily; switching from any other amphetamine products (e.g., **Adderall** immediate-release), discontinue that treatment and titrate with **Adzenys ER** using the titration schedule (see mfr pkg insert). To avoid substitution errors and overdosage, do not substitute for other amphetamine products on a mg-per-mg basis due to different amphetamine salt compositions and differing pharmacokinetic profiles. No dosage adjustments for renal *or* hepatic insufficiency are provided in the manufacturer's labeling.
    Adzenys XR-ODT take with *or* without food; individualize the dosage according to the therapeutic needs and response; initially 12.5 mg once daily; max recommended dose 18.8 mg once daily
    Pediatric: <6 years: not recommended; ≥6 years: take with *or* without food, individualize the dosage according to the therapeutic needs and response; 6-12 years: initially 6.3 mg once daily in the morning; increase in increments of 3.1 mg *or* 6.3 mg at weekly intervals; max recommended dose 18.8 mg once daily; ≥13 years: 12.5 mg (10 ml) once daily in the morning

Comment: Patients taking **Adderall XR** may be switched to **Adzenys XR-ODT** at the equivalent dose taken once daily; switching from any other amphetamine products (e.g., **Adderall** immediate-release), discontinue that treatment and titrate with **Adzenys XR-ODT** using the titration schedule (see mfr pkg insert). To avoid substitution errors and overdosage, do not substitute for other amphetamine products on a mg-per-mg basis due to different amphetamine salt compositions and differing pharmacokinetic profiles. No dosage adjustments for renal or hepatic insufficiency are provided in the manufacturer's labeling.

Dyanavel XR <6 years: not recommended; ≥6 years: initially 2.5 mg or 5 mg once daily in the morning; may increase in increments of 2.5 mg to 5 mg/day every 4 to 7 days; max 20 mg/day; shake bottle prior to administration
> *Oral susp:* 2.5 mg/ml (464 ml) ext-rel
> *Tab:* 5*, 10*, 15*, 20*mg ext-rel

Evekeo <3 years: not recommended; ≥3-5 years: initially 2.5 mg once or twice daily at the same time(s) each day, may increase by 2.5 mg/day at weekly intervals, max 40 mg/day; >5 years: initially 5 mg once or twice daily at the same time(s) each day, may increase by 5 mg/day at weekly intervals; max 40 mg/day
> *Tab:* 5, 10 mg

Mydayis initially 12.5 mg once daily in the morning; may titrate at weekly intervals; max 50 mg/day
Pediatric: <13 years: not recommended; 13-17 years: initially 12.5 mg once daily in the morning, may titrate at weekly intervals to max 25 mg/day; >17 years: same as adult
> *Cap:* 12.5, 25, 37.5, 50 mg ext-rel

▷ *dexmethylphenidate* (II)(G) not indicated for adults
Focalin <6 years: not established; ≥6 years: initially 2.5 mg bid; allow at least 4 hours between doses; may increase at 1 week intervals; max 20 mg/day
> *Tab:* 2.5, 5, 10*mg (dye-free)

Focalin ER <6 years: not established; ≥6 years: initially 5 mg weekly; usual dose 10-30 mg/day
> *Cap:* 15, 30 mg ext-rel

Focalin XR <6 years: not established; ≥6 years: initially 5 mg weekly; usual dose 10-30 mg/day
> *Cap:* 5, 10, 15, 20, 25, 30, 35, 40 mg ext-rel

▷ *dextroamphetamine* (II) *Recommended starting dose*: 9 mg/9 hours; titrate dose in weekly increments of 4.5 mg up to a max of 18 mg/9 hours; apply 1 **Xelstrym** transdermal system 2 hours before an effect is needed and remove/discard within 9 hours; apply **Xelstrym** to the hip, upper arm, chest, upper back, or flank; remove and discard the previous patch and change the site of application when applying a new transdermal system; do not substitute for other amphetamine products on a milligram-per-milligram basis due to different amphetamine base compositions and differing pharmacokinetic profiles; *Severe renal impairment:* max recommended dose is 13.5 mg/9 hours; *End-stage renal disease (ESRD):* max recommended dose is 9 mg/9 hours
Pediatric: <6 years: safety and efficacy not established; 6–17 years: *Recommended starting dose:* 4.5 mg/9 hours, titrate dose in weekly increments of 4.5 mg up to a max of 18 mg/9 hours; ≥18 years: same as adult; apply 1 **Xelstrym** transdermal system 2 hours before an effect is needed and remove/discard within 9 hours; apply **Xelstrym** to the hip, upper arm, chest, upper back, or flank; remove and discard the previous patch and change the site of application when applying a new transdermal system; do not substitute for other amphetamine products on a milligram-per-milligram basis due to different amphetamine base compositions and differing pharmacokinetic profiles; *Severe renal impairment:* max recommended dose is 13.5 mg/9 hours; *ESRD:* max recommended dose is 9 mg/9 hours (NOTE: *dextroamphetamine* is not dialyzable)
Xelstrym *Transdermal system:* 4.5 mg/9 hours, 9 mg/9 hours, 13.5 mg/9 hours, 18 mg/9 hours
> **Comment:** On removal, fold the used transdermal system in half onto itself and dispose in compliance with local laws and regulations on drug disposal of central nervous system (CNS) stimulants.

Comment: Xelstrym transdermal system is a CNS stimulant indicated for the treatment of ADHD in adults and children >6 years of age. *Boxed Warning*: CNS stimulants, including **Xelstrym**, other amphetamine-containing products, and methylphenidate, have a high potential for abuse and dependence. Assess the risk of abuse prior to prescribing and monitor for signs of abuse and dependence while on therapy. **Xelstrym** is contraindicated in patients with known hypersensitivity to amphetamine products or other ingredients in **Xelstrym** and concomitant use with MAOIs or within 14 days of the last MAOI dose. The most common adverse reactions (incidence ≥5% and at a rate at least twice placebo) in adults treated with *lisdexamfetamine* have been decreased appetite, insomnia, dry mouth, diarrhea, nausea, and anxiety. The most common adverse reactions (incidence ≥2% and greater than the rate for placebo) in pediatric patients 6 to 17 years treated with **Xelstrym** have been decreased appetite, headache, insomnia, tic, abdominal pain, vomiting, nausea, irritability, increased blood pressure, and increased heart rate. Serious cardiovascular reactions, including sudden death, have been reported in association with CNS stimulant treatment at recommended doses in pediatric patients with structural cardiac abnormalities or other serious heart problems. In adults, sudden death, stroke, and myocardial infarction have been reported. Avoid **Xelstrym** use in patients with known structural cardiac abnormalities, cardiomyopathy, serious heart rhythm abnormalities, or coronary artery disease (CAD). Monitor the patient for increases in blood pressure and heart rate. Consider risk/benefit before **Xelstrym** use in patients in whom blood pressure increases may be problematic. Psychiatric

(continued)

adverse reaction may cause psychotic or manic symptoms in patients with no history or exacerbation of symptoms in patients with preexisting psychosis. Evaluate for bipolar disorder prior to initiating **Xelstrym**. Obtain height and weight measurements in pediatric patients at baseline and during treatment to monitor potential growth suppression. Stimulants are associated with peripheral vasculopathy, including Raynaud's phenomenon. Careful observation for digital changes is necessary during treatment with ADHD stimulants. There is increased risk of serotonin syndrome when **Xelstrym** is co-administered with serotonergic agents (e.g., selective serotonin reuptake inhibitors [SSRIs], selective norepinephrine reuptake inhibitors (SNRIs), triptans), but also during **Xelstrym** overdose situations. If it occurs, discontinue **Xelstrym** immediately and initiate supportive treatment. Use of **Xelstrym** may lead to contact sensitization; discontinue **Xelstrym** if contact sensitization is suspected. During wear time or immediately after removal of **Xelstrym**, local skin reactions may occur. Select a different application site each day.

▷ *dextroamphetamine sulfate (II)(G)* initially start with 10 mg daily; increase by 10 mg at weekly intervals if needed; may switch to daily dose with sust-rel spansules when titrated
  Pediatric: <3 years: not recommended; ≥3-5 years: 2.5 mg daily; may increase by 2.5 mg daily at weekly intervals if needed; 6-12 years: initially 5 mg once daily or bid; may increase by 5 mg/day at weekly intervals; usual max 40 mg/day; >12 years: initially 10 mg daily; may increase by 10 mg/day at weekly intervals to max of 40 mg/day
    Dexedrine *Tab:* 5*mg (tartrazine)
    Dexedrine Spansule *Cap:* 5, 10, 15 mg ext-rel
    Dextrostat *Tab:* 5, 10 mg (tartrazine)

▷ *dextroamphetamine saccharate+dextroamphetamine sulfate+amphetamine aspartate+amphetamine sulfate (II)(G)* not indicated for adults
    Adderall initially 10 mg daily; may increase weekly by 10 mg/day; usual max 60 mg/day in 2-3 divided doses; first dose on awakening; then q 4-6 hours prn
    Pediatric: <6 years: not indicated; ≥6-12 years: initially 5 mg daily; may increase by 5 mg/day at weekly intervals; >12 years: same as adult
      Tab: 5**, 7.5**, 10**, 12.5**, 15**, 20**, 30**mg
    Adderall XR 20 mg by mouth once daily in the AM; may increase by 10 mg/day at weekly intervals; max: 60 mg/day
    Pediatric: <6 years: not recommended; ≥ to a max of 6 years: initially 10 mg daily in the AM; may increase by 10 mg/day at weekly intervals, max 30 mg/day; 13-17 years: 10-20 mg by mouth daily in the AM; may increase by 10 mg/day at weekly intervals; max 40 mg/day; may sprinkle on apple sauce; do not chew
      Cap: 5, 10, 15, 20, 25, 30 mg ext-rel

▷ *lisdexamfetamine dimesylate (II)* 30 mg once daily in the AM; may increase by 10-20 mg/day at weekly intervals; max 70 mg/day
  Pediatric: <6 years: not recommended; ≥6 years: same as adult
    Vyvanse *Cap:* 20, 30, 40, 50, 60, 70 mg
    Comment: May dissolve **Vyvanse** capsule contents in water; take immediately.

▷ *methylphenidate (regular-acting) (II)(G)*
    Methylin, Methylin Chewable, Methylin Oral Solution usual dose 20-30 mg/day in 2-3 divided doses 30-45 minutes before a meal; max 60 mg/day
    Pediatric: <6 years: not recommended; ≥6 years: initially 5 mg bid ac (breakfast and lunch); may increase 5-10 mg/day at weekly intervals; max 60 mg/day
      Tab: 5, 10*, 20*mg; *Chew tab:* 2.5, 5, 10 mg (grape) (phenylalanine); *Oral soln:* 5, 10 mg/5 ml (grape)
    Ritalin 10-60 mg/day in 2-3 divided doses 30-45 minutes ac; max 60 mg/day
    Pediatric: <6 years: not recommended; ≥6 years: initially 5 mg bid ac (breakfast and lunch); may increase by 5-10 mg at weekly intervals as needed; max 60 mg/day
      Tab: 5, 10*, 20*mg

▷ *methylphenidate (long-acting) (G)(II)*
    Concerta initially 18 mg q AM; may increase in 18 mg increments as needed; max 54 mg/day; do not crush or chew
    Pediatric: <6 years: not recommended; ≥6-12 years: initially 18 mg daily; max 54 mg/day; ≥13-17 years: initially 18 mg daily; max 72 mg/day or 2 mg/kg, whichever is less
      Tab: 18, 27, 36, 54 mg sust-rel
    Cotempla XR-ODT (G) take consistently with or without food in the morning
    Pediatric: <6 years: not recommended; 6-17 years: initially 8.6 mg; may increase as needed and tolerated by 8.6 mg/day; daily dosage >51.8 mg is not recommended
      ODT: 8.6, 17.3, 25.9 mg ext-rel orally-disint
    Jornay PM 20 mg daily in the evening; adjust the timing of administration between 6:30 PM and 9:30 PM to optimize the tolerability and the efficacy the next morning and throughout the day; dose may be increased weekly in 20 mg per day increments; max 100 mg once daily; administer consistently either with or without food; swallow caps whole or open and sprinkle the entire dose onto applesauce
    Pediatric: <6 years: not established; ≥6 years: same as adult
      Cap: 20, 40, 60, 80, 100 mg del-rel/ext-rel
    Comment: Jornay PM is a proprietary drug therapy platform that consists of two functional film coatings. The first layer delays the initial drug release for up to 10 hours. The second layer helps control the release

rate of the active ingredient throughout the day. Do not substitute **Jornay PM** for other *methylphenidate* product on a milligram-per-milligram basis.

Metadate CD (G) 1 cap daily in the AM; may sprinkle on food; do not crush or chew

Pediatric: <6 years: not recommended; ≥6 years: initially 20 mg daily; may gradually increase by 20 mg/day at weekly intervals as needed; max 60 mg/day

    Cap: 10, 20, 30, 40, 50, 60 mg immed- and ext-rel beads

Metadate ER 1 tab daily in the AM; do not crush or chew

Pediatric: <6 years: not recommended; ≥6 years: use in place of regular-acting *methylphenidate* when the 8-hour dose of **Metadate-ER** corresponds to the titrated 8-hour dose of regular-acting *methylphenidate*

    Tab: 10, 20 mg ext-rel (dye-free)

QuilliChew ER (G) initially 1 x 10 mg chew tab once daily in the AM

Pediatric: <6 years: not recommended; initially 10 mg daily; may gradually increase by 20 mg/day at weekly intervals as needed; max 60 mg/day

    Chew tab: 20*, 30*40 mg ext-rel

Quillivant XR (G) initially 20 mg once daily in the AM, with or without food; may be titrated in increments of 10-20 mg/day at weekly intervals; daily doses above 60 mg have not been studied and are not recommended; shake the bottle vigorously for at least 10 seconds to ensure that the correct dose is administered

Pediatric: <6 years: not recommended; ≥6 years: same as adult

    Bottle: 5 mg/ml, 25 mg/5 ml pwdr for reconstitution; 300 mg (60 ml), 600 mg (120 ml), 750 mg (150 ml), 900 mg (180 ml)

Comment: Quillivant XR must be reconstituted by a pharmacist, not by the patient or the caregiver

Ritalin LA (G) 1 cap daily in the AM

Pediatric: <6 years: not recommended; ≥6 years: use in place of regular-acting *methylphenidate* when the 8-hour dose of **Ritalin LA** corresponds to the titrated 8-hour dose of regular-acting *methylphenidate*; max 60 mg/day

    Cap: 10, 20, 30, 40 mg ext-rel (immed- and ext-rel beads)

Ritalin SR 1 cap daily in the AM

Pediatric: <6 years: not recommended; ≥6 years: use in place of regular-acting *methylphenidate* when the 8-hour dose of **Ritalin SR** corresponds to the titrated 8-hour dose of regular-acting *methylphenidate*; max 60 mg/day

    Tab: 20 mg sust-rel (dye-free)

▷ *methylphenidate* transdermal patch (II)(G)

Pediatric: <6 years: not recommended; ≥6-17 years: initially 10 mg patch applied to hip 2 hours before desired effect daily in the AM; may increase by 5-10 mg at weekly intervals; max 60 mg/day; >17 years: not applicable

    Daytrana *Transdermal patch:* 10, 15, 20, 30 mg

▷ *serdexmethylphenidate+dexmethylphenidate Recommended starting dose:* 39.2 mg/7.8 mg once daily in the morning; after 1 week, dose may be increased to 52.3 mg/10.4 mg once daily; administer with or without food; swallow whole or open and sprinkle onto applesauce or add to water; do not substitute for other *methylphenidate* products on a milligram-per-milligram basis to avoid substitution errors and possible overdosage

Pediatric: <6 years: safety and efficacy not established; *6-12 years: Recommended starting dose:* 39.2 mg/7.8 mg once daily in the morning; after 1 week, dose may be increased to 52.3 mg/10.4 mg daily or decreased to 26.1 mg/5.2 mg daily, max 52.3 mg/10.4 mg once daily; *≥13 years:* same as adult

    Azstarys *Cap:* 26.1 mg/5.2 mg, 39.2 mg/7.8 mg, 52.3 mg/10.4 mg

    Comment: Azstarys is a CNS stimulant indicated for the treatment of ADHD in patients ≥6 years of age. *Boxed Warning: mfr pkg insert for complete boxed warning).* CNS stimulants, including **Azstarys**, other *methylphenidate*-containing products, and *amphetamines*, have a high potential for abuse and dependence. Assess the risk of abuse prior to prescribing and monitor for signs of abuse and dependence and diversion while on therapy. Based on accumulated data from other *methylphenidate* products, the most common (>5% and twice the rate of placebo) adverse reactions have been decreased appetite, insomnia, nausea, vomiting, dyspepsia, abdominal pain, decreased weight, anxiety, dizziness, irritability, affect lability, tachycardia, and increased blood pressure. Sudden death has been reported in association with CNS stimulant treatment at recommended doses in pediatric patients with structural cardiac abnormalities or other serious heart problems. In adults, sudden death, stroke, and myocardial infarction have been reported. Avoid use in patients with known structural cardiac abnormalities, cardiomyopathy, serious heart arrhythmias, or CAD. Monitor blood pressure and pulse. Consider the benefits and risks in patients in whom an increase in blood pressure or heart rate would be problematic. Use of stimulants may cause psychotic or manic symptoms in patients with no history or exacerbation of symptoms in patients with preexisting psychiatric illness. Evaluate for bipolar disorder prior to **Azstarys** use. Cases of painful and prolonged penile erections and priapism have been reported with *methylphenidate* products. Immediate medical attention should be sought if signs or symptoms of prolonged penile erections or priapism are observed. Stimulants used to treat ADHD are associated with peripheral vasculopathy, including

(continued)

Raynaud's phenomenon. Careful observation for digital changes is necessary during treatment with ADHD stimulants. Monitor height and weight at appropriate intervals in pediatric patients. There are no available data on **Azstarys** use in pregnant females to evaluate for a drug-associated risk of major birth defects, miscarriage, or other adverse maternal or fetal outcomes. Published studies and postmarketing reports on *methylphenidate* use during pregnancy have not identified a drug-associated risk of major birth defects, miscarriage, or adverse maternal or fetal outcomes. There is a pregnancy exposure registry that monitors pregnancy outcomes in women exposed to ADHD medications, including **Azstarys**, during pregnancy. Healthcare providers are encouraged to register patients by calling the National Pregnancy Registry for Psychostimulants at 1-866-961-2388. *Methylphenidate* is present in human milk. There are no reports of adverse effects on the breastfed infant. Long-term neurodevelopmental effects on infants from stimulant exposure are unknown. Monitor breastfeeding infants for adverse reactions, such as agitation, anorexia, and reduced weight gain. The developmental and health benefits of breastfeeding should be considered along with the mother's clinical need for **Azstarys** and any potential adverse effects on the breastfed infant from **Azstarys**.

CENTRAL ALPHA-2 AGONIST
▷ *guanfacine* (G)
  Pediatric: <6 years: not recommended; ≥6-17 years: initially 1 mg once daily, may increase by 1 mg/day at weekly intervals, usual max 4 mg/day; >17 years: not applicable
  Intuniv *Tab*: 1, 2, 3, 4 mg ext-rel
  Comment: Take **Intuniv** with water, milk, or other liquid. Do not take with a high-fat meal. Withdraw gradually by 1 mg every 3 to 7 days.

TRICYCLIC ANTIDEPRESSANTS (TCAS)
See Depression

OTHER AGENTS
▷ *clonidine* (G)
  Catapres 4-5 mcg/kg/day
  Pediatric: <12 years: not recommended; ≥12 years: same as adult
    Tab: 0.1*, 0.2*, 0.3*mg
  Catapres-TTS <12 years: not recommended; ≥12 years: initially 0.1 mg patch weekly; increase after 1-2 weeks if needed; max 0.6 mg/day
    Patch: 0.1, 0.2 mg/day (12/carton), 0.3 mg/day (4/carton)
  Kapvay not indicated for adults
  Pediatric: <6 years: not recommended; ≥6-12 years: initially 0.1 mg at bedtime x 1 week; then 0.1 mg bid x 1 week; then 0.1 mg AM and 0.2 mg PM x 1 week; then 0.2 mg bid; withdraw gradually by 0.1 mg/day at 3 to 7 day intervals
    Tab: 0.1, 0.2 mg ext-rel
  Nexiclon XR initially 0.18 mg (2 ml) suspension or 0.17 mg tab once daily; usual max 0.52 mg (6 ml suspension) once daily
  Pediatric: <12 years: not recommended; ≥12 years: same as adult
    Tab: 0.17, 0.26 mg ext-rel; Oral susp: 0.09 mg/ml ext-rel (4 oz)

AMINOKETONES (FOR THE TREATMENT OF ATTENTION DEFICIT HYPERACTIVITY DISORDER [ADHD])
▷ *bupropion HBr* (G) initially 100 mg bid for at least 3 days; may increase to 375 or 400 mg/day after several weeks; then after at least 3 more days, 450 mg in 4 divided doses; max 450 mg/day, 174 mg/single-dose
  Pediatric: <18 years: not recommended; ≥18 years: safety and effectiveness in the pediatric population not established; when considering the use of **Aplenzin** in a child or adolescent, balance the potential risks with the clinical need
  Aplenzin *Tab*: 174, 348, 522 mg
▷ *bupropion hcl* (G)
  Forfivo XL do not use for initial treatment; use immediate-release *bupropion* forms for initial titration; switch to **Forfivo XL** 450 mg once daily when total dose/day reaches 450 mg; may switch to **Forfivo XL** when total dose/day reaches 300 mg for 2 weeks and the patient needs 450 mg/day to reach therapeutic target; swallow whole, do not crush or chew
  Pediatric: <18 years: not recommended; >18 years: same as adult; safety and effectiveness of long-acting and extended-release *bupropion* in the pediatric population have not been established; when considering the use of **Forfivo XL** in a child or adolescent, balance the potential risks with the clinical need
    Tab: 450 mg ext-rel
  Wellbutrin initially 100 mg bid for at least 3 days; may increase to 375 or 400 mg/day after several weeks; then after at least 3 more days, 450 mg in 4 divided doses; max 450 mg/day, 150 mg/single-dose
  Pediatric: <12 years: not recommended; ≥12 years: same as adult
    Tab: 75, 100 mg
  Wellbutrin SR initially 150 mg in AM for at least 3 days; may increase to 150 mg bid if well tolerated; usual dose 300 mg/day; max 400 mg/day

Pediatric: <12 years: <u>not</u> recommended; ≥12 years: same as adult
> *Tab:* 100, 150 mg sust-rel
Wellbutrin XL initially 150 mg in AM for at least 3 days; increase to 150 mg bid if well tolerated; usual dose 300 mg/day; max 400 mg/day
Pediatric: <12 years: <u>not</u> recommended; ≥12 years: same as adult
> *Tab:* 150, 300 mg sust-rel

BACTERIAL ENDOCARDITIS: PROPHYLAXIS

Comment: Bacterial endocarditis prophylaxis is appropriate for persons with a history of infective endocarditis, persons with a prosthetic cardiac valve <u>or</u> prosthetic material used for valve repair, cardiac transplant patients who develop cardiac valvulopathy, congenital heart disease (CHD), unrepaired cyanotic CHD including palliative shunts and conduits, completely repaired congenital heart defect(s) with prosthetic material <u>or</u> device, whether placed by surgery <u>or</u> by catheter intervention, during the first 6 months after the procedure, repaired CHD with residual defects at the site <u>or</u> adjacent to the site of a prosthetic patch <u>or</u> prosthetic device (which may inhibit endothelialization), <u>or</u> any other condition deemed to place a patient at high risk.

DENTAL, ORAL, RESPIRATORY TRACT, ESOPHAGEAL PROCEDURES
▷ *amoxicillin* (G) 2 gm PO 30-60 minutes before procedure as a single dose <u>or</u> 3 gm 1 hour before procedure and 1.5 gm 6 hours later
Pediatric: 50 mg/kg as a single dose <u>or</u> 50 mg/kg (max 3 gm) 1 hour before procedure and (max 1.5 gm) 25 mg/kg 6 hours later; ≥40 kg: same as adult; *see* Appendix BB.3. *amoxicillin* (G) (Amoxil Suspension, Trimox Suspension) *for dose by weight*
> **Amoxil** *Cap:* 250, 500 mg; *Tab:* 875*mg; *Chew tab:* 125, 200, 250, 400 mg (cherry-banana-peppermint) (phenylalanine); *Oral susp:* 125, 250 mg/5 ml (80, 100, 150 ml) (strawberry); 200, 400 mg/5 ml (50, 75, 100 ml) (bubble gum); *Oral drops:* 50 mg/ml (30 ml) (bubble gum)
> **Trimox** *Tab:* 125, 250 mg; *Cap:* 250, 500 mg; *Oral susp:* 125, 250 mg/5 ml (80, 100, 150 ml) (raspberry-strawberry)
▷ *ampicillin* (G) 2 gm PO/IM/IV 30-60 minutes before procedure
Pediatric: <12 years: 50 mg/kg PO/IM/IV 30-60 minutes before procedure; ≥12 years: same as adult
> **Omnipen, Principen** *Cap:* 250, 500 mg; *Oral susp:* 125, 250 mg/5 ml (100, 150, 200 ml) (fruit)
> **Unasyn** *Vial:* 1.5, 3 gm
▷ *azithromycin* (G) 500 mg 30-60 minutes before procedure
Pediatric: <12 years: 15 mg/kg 30-60 minutes before procedure; max 500 mg; *see* Appendix BB.7.
azithromycin (G) (Zithromax Suspension, Zmax Suspension) *for dose by weight;* ≥12 years: same as adult
> **Zithromax** *Tab:* 250, 500, 600 mg; *Oral susp:* 100 mg/5 ml (15 ml); 200 mg/5 ml (15, 22.5, 30 ml) (cherry)
▷ *cefazolin* 1 gm IM/IV 30-60 minutes before procedure
Pediatric: <12 years: 25 mg/kg IM/IV 30-60 minutes before procedure; ≥12 years: same as adult
> **Ancef** *Vial:* 250, 500 mg; 1, 5 gm
> **Kefzol** *Vial:* 500 mg; 1 gm
▷ *ceftriaxone* (G) 1 gm IM/IV as a single dose
Pediatric: <12 years: 50 mg/kg IM/IV as a single dose; ≥12 years: same as adult
> **Rocephin** *Vial:* 250, 500 mg; 1, 2 gm
▷ *cephalexin* (G) 2 gm as a single dose 30-60 minutes before procedure
Pediatric: 50 mg/kg as a single dose 30-60 minutes before procedure; *see* Appendix BB.15. *cephalexin* (G) (Keflex Suspension) *for dose by weight*
> **Keflex** *Cap:* 250, 333, 500, 750 mg; *Oral susp:* 125, 250 mg/5 ml (100, 200 ml) (strawberry)
▷ *clarithromycin* (G) 500 mg <u>or</u> 500 mg ext-rel as a single dose 30-60 minutes before procedure
Pediatric: 15 mg/kg as a single dose 30-60 minutes before procedure; *see* Appendix BB.16. *clarithromycin* (G) (Biaxin Suspension) *for dose by weight*
> **Biaxin** *Tab:* 250, 500 mg
> **Biaxin Oral Suspension** *Oral susp:* 125, 250 mg/5 ml (50, 100 ml) (fruit punch)
> **Biaxin XL** *Tab:* 500 mg ext-rel
▷ *clindamycin* (G) 600 mg PO as a one-time single-dose <u>or</u> 300 mg 30-60 minutes before procedure and 150 mg 6 hours later; take with a full glass of water
Pediatric: <12 years: 20 mg/kg (max 300 mg) 1 hour before procedure and 10 mg/kg (max 150 mg) 6 hours later; take with a full glass of water; *see* Appendix BB.17. *clindamycin* (G) (Cleocin Pediatric Granules) *for dose by weight;* ≥12 years: same as adult
> **Cleocin (G)** *Cap:* 75 (tartrazine), 150 (tartrazine), 300 mg; *Vial:* 150 mg/ml (2, 4 ml) (benzyl alcohol)
> **Cleocin Pediatric Granules (G)** *Oral susp:* 75 mg/ml (100 ml) (cherry)
▷ *erythromycin estolate* (G) 1 gm 1 hour before procedure; then 500 mg 6 hours later
Pediatric: <12 years: 20 mg/kg 1 hour before procedure; then 10 mg/kg 6 hours later; *see* Appendix BB.20.
erythromycin estolate (G) (Ilosone Suspension) *for dose by weight;* ≥12 years: same as adult
> **Ilosone** *Pulvule:* 250 mg; *Tab:* 500 mg; *Liq:* 125, 250 mg/5 ml (100 ml)

(continued)

▷ *penicillin v potassium* (G) 2 gm 1 hour before procedure; then 1 gm 6 hours later or 2 gm 1 hour before procedure; then 1 gm q 6 hours x 8 doses
Pediatric: <12 years, <60 lb: 1 gm 1 hour before procedure; then 500 mg 6 hours later or 1 gm 1 hour before procedure; then 500 mg q 6 hours x 8 doses; *see* Appendix BB.29. *penicillin v potassium* (G) (Pen-Vee K Solution, Veetids Solution) *for dose by weight;* ≥12 years: same as adult
     Pen-Vee K *Tab:* 250, 500 mg; *Oral soln:* 125 mg/5 ml (100, 200 ml), 250 mg/5 ml (100, 150, 200 ml)

BACTERIAL VAGINOSIS (BV, *GARDNERELLA VAGINALIS*)

PROPHYLAXIS AND RESTORATION OF VAGINAL ACIDITY

▷ *acetic acid+oxyquinoline* one full applicator intravaginally bid for up to 30 days
Pediatric: <12 years: not recommended; ≥12 years: same as adult
     Relagard *Gel:* acet acid 0.9%+oxyq 0.025% (50 gm tube w. applicator)
Comment: The following treatment regimens for *bacterial vaginosis (BV)* are published in the **2021 CDC Sexually Transmitted Diseases Treatment Guidelines.** Treatment regimens are presented by generic drug name first, followed by information about brands and dose forms. BV is associated with adverse pregnancy outcomes, including premature rupture of the membranes, preterm labor, preterm birth, intra-amniotic infection, and postpartum endometritis. Therefore, treatment is recommended for all pregnant females with symptoms or positive screen.

RECOMMENDED REGIMENS

Regimen 1
▷ *metronidazole* 500 mg bid x 7 days or *metronidazole* ext-rel 750 mg once daily x 7 days

Regimen 2
▷ *metronidazole* gel 0.75% one applicatorful (5 gm) once daily x 5 days

Regimen 3
▷ *clindamycin* cream 2% one full applicatorful (5 gm) intravaginally once daily at bedtime x 5 days

ALTERNATE REGIMENS

Regimen 1
▷ *tinidazole* 2 gm once daily x 2 days

Regimen 2
▷ *tinidazole* 1 gm once daily x 5 days

Regimen 3
▷ *clindamycin* 300 mg bid x 7 days

Regimen 4
▷ *clindamycin* ovules 100 mg intravaginally once daily at bedtime x 3 days

Regimen 5
▷ *secnidazole* one 2 gm packet as a single dose

Drug Brands and Dose Forms

▷ *clindamycin*
     Cleocin (G) *Cap:* 75 (tartrazine), 150 (tartrazine), 300 mg
     Cleocin Pediatric Granules (G) *Oral susp:* 75 mg/5 ml (100 ml) (cherry)
     Cleocin Vaginal Cream *Vag crm:* 2% (21, 40 gm tubes w. applicator)
     Cleocin Vaginal Ovules *Vag supp:* 100 mg
▷ *metronidazole* Use in the 1st trimester of pregnancy is not recommended
     Flagyl *Tab:* 250*, 500*mg
     Flagyl 375 *Cap:* 375 mg
     Flagyl ER *Tab:* 750 mg ext-rel
     MetroGel-Vaginal, Vandazole *Vag gel:* 0.75% (70 gm w. applicator) (parabens)
     Nuvessa 1.3% one single-dose, prefilled disposable applicatorful, administered once intravaginally at bedtime
          Prefilled disposable applicator: 1.3% (65 mg/5 gm, 1 applicator/carton), single-dose
Comment: Nitroimidazole antimicrobials are indicated for the treatment of BV in females ≥12 years of age. Breastfeeding is not recommended; discontinue breastfeeding for 2 days after use. Concomitant use of *disulfiram*, or within 2 weeks of *disulfiram*, and concomitant use of alcohol are contraindications to *metronidazole* use.

▷ *secnidazole*

Solosec *Oral granules:* 2 gm/pkt

Comment: Solosec is a nitroimidazole antimicrobial. Do not dissolve **Solosec** in liquid. Sprinkle contents onto applesauce, yogurt, or pudding. Consume within 30 minutes without chewing or crunching. May follow with a glass of water. Potential adverse side effects are vulvovaginal pruritus, vulvovaginal candidiasis (VVC), headache, nausea, dysgeusia, vomiting, diarrhea, and abdominal pain. Whereas *metronidazole* and *tinidazole* are contraindicated during the 1st trimester of pregnancy, no adverse developmental outcomes have been found in animal reproductive studies and the labeling for *secnidazole* does not include a restriction for use in pregnancy. Breastfeeding is not recommended during and for 96 hours after dose; may pump and discard milk during this time period.

▷ *tinidazole*

Tindamax *Tab:* 250*, 500*mg

Comment: Other than for use in the treatment of *giardiasis* and *amebiasis* in pediatric patients >3 years of age, the safety and effectiveness of *tinidazole* in pediatric patients have not been established. *Tinidazole* is excreted in breast milk in concentrations similar to those seen in serum and can be detected in breast milk for up to 72 hours following administration. Interruption of breastfeeding is recommended during *tinidazole* therapy and for 3 days following the last dose.

TOPICAL LINCOSAMIDE ANTIBACTERIAL

▷ *clindamycin phosphate* administer 1 applicatorful (5 gm of gel containing 100 mg of *clindamycin*) once intravaginally as a single dose at any time of the day

Pediatric: <12 years: safety and efficacy not established; ≥12 years: same as adult

Xaciato *Vag Gel:* 2% (25 gm tube w. 1 single-dose, user-filled, disposable applicator)

Comment: Xaciato is a topical lincosamide antibacterial for the vaginally administered treatment of BV in female patients ≥12 years of age. **Xaciato** is contraindicated in patients with a history of hypersensitivity to *clindamycin* or *lincomycin*. *Clostridioides difficile*-associated diarrhea may develop; discontinue and evaluate if diarrhea occurs. The most common adverse reactions reported in >2% of patients and at a higher rate in the **Xaciato** group than in the placebo group were vulvovaginal candidiasis (VVC) and vulvovaginal discomfort (VVD). **Xaciato** is not compatible with and may weaken polyurethane condoms; therefore, use of polyurethane condoms is not recommended during and for 7 days following treatment with **Xaciato**. Advise patients to use latex or polyisoprene condoms for contraception during and for 7 days following treatment with **Xaciato**. **Xaciato** use has not been studied in human pregnancy. However, based on the low systemic absorption of **Xaciato** following the intravaginal route of administration in non-pregnant females, maternal use is not likely to result in significant fetal exposure to the drug. Available data from published observational studies, based on first-through-third trimester exposure to oral and IV *clindamycin*, did not identify consistent increases in the risk of miscarriage or other adverse maternal or fetal outcomes. Animal reproduction studies conducted during organogenesis (gestational days 6-21) showed no evidence of teratogenicity. Systemic absorption following intravaginal administration of *clindamycin* is low; therefore, transfer of *clindamycin* into breast milk is likely to be low and adverse effects on the breastfed infant are not expected. Developmental and health benefits of breastfeeding should be considered along with the mother's clinical need for *clindamycin* and any potential adverse effects on the breastfed infant from *clindamycin* or from the underlying maternal condition.

BALDNESS: MALE PATTERN

TYPE II 5-ALPHA-REDUCTASE SPECIFIC INHIBITOR

▷ *finasteride* (G) 1 mg daily

Propecia *Tab:* 1 mg

Comment: Pregnant females should not touch broken *finasteride* tabs. Use of **Propecia**, a 5-alpha reductase inhibitor, is associated with low but increased risk of high-grade prostate cancer.

PERIPHERAL VASODILATOR

▷ *minoxidil* topical soln (G) 1 ml from dropper or 6 sprays bid

Pediatric: <18 years: not recommended; ≥18 years: same as adult

Rogaine for Men (OTC) *Regular soln:* 2% (60 ml w. applicator) (alcohol 60%); *Extra-strength soln:* 5% (60 ml w. applicator) (alcohol 30%)

Rogaine for Women (OTC) *Regular soln:* 2% (60 ml w. applicator) (alcohol 60%); *Topical aerosol:* 5%

Comment: Do not use *minoxidil* on abraded or inflamed scalp.

BELL'S PALSY

▷ *prednisone* (G) 80 mg once daily x 3 days; then 60 mg daily x 3 days; then 40 mg daily x 3 days; then 20 mg x 1 dose; then discontinue

Pediatric: <18 years: oral suspension options by weight

Deltasone *Tab:* 2.5*, 5*, 10*, 20*, 50*mg

BENIGN ESSENTIAL TREMOR

ANTI-PARKINSON'S AGENT
▷ *amantadine* (G) 200 mg daily or 100 mg bid; 4 tsp of syrup once daily or 2 tsp bid
  Gocovri *Cap:* 68.5, 37 mg ext-rel
  Symmetrel *Tab:* 100 mg; *Syr:* 50 mg/5 ml (raspberry)

BETA-BLOCKER
▷ *propranolol* (G)
  Inderal initially 40 mg bid; usual range 160-240 mg/day
    Tab: 10*, 20*, 40*, 60*, 80*mg
  Inderal LA initially 80 mg once daily in a single dose; increase q 3-7 days; usual range 120-160 mg/day; max 320 mg/day in a single dose
    Cap: 60, 80, 120, 160 mg sust-rel
  InnoPran XL initially 80 mg q HS; max 120 mg/day
    Cap: 80, 120 mg ext-rel

BENIGN PROSTATIC HYPERPLASIA (BPH)

ALPHA-1 BLOCKERS
Comment: Educate the patient regarding potential side effect of hypotension, especially with the first dose. Usually start at the lowest dose and titrate upward.
▷ *doxazosin*
  Cardura initially 1 mg daily; may double dose every 1-2 weeks; max 8 mg/day
    Tab: 1*, 2*, 4*, 8*mg
  Cardura XL initially 4 mg once daily with breakfast; may titrate after 3-4 weeks; max 8 mg/day
    Tab: 4, 8 mg ext-rel
▷ *silodosin* (G) 8 mg once daily; *CrCl 30-50 ml/min:* 4 mg once daily
  Rapaflo *Cap:* 4, 8 mg
▷ *terazosin* (G) initially 1 mg q HS; titrate up to 10 mg once daily; max 20 mg/day
  Hytrin *Cap:* 1, 2, 5, 10 mg

ALPHA-1A BLOCKERS
▷ *alfuzosin* (G) 10 mg once daily taken immediately after the same meal each day
  UroXatral *Tab:* 10 mg ext-rel
▷ *tamsulosin* (G) initially 0.4 mg once daily; may increase to 0.8 mg daily after 2-4 weeks if needed
  Flomax *Cap:* 0.4 mg
  Comment: May take Flomax 0.4 mg plus Imitrex 0.5 mg once daily as combination therapy.

TYPE II 5-ALPHA-REDUCTASE INHIBITOR
Comment: Pregnant females and females of childbearing age should not handle *finasteride*. Monitor for potential side effects of decreased libido and/or impotence. Low, but increased risk of being diagnosed with high-grade prostate cancer.
▷ *finasteride* 5 mg once daily
  Proscar *Tab:* 5 mg

TYPES I AND II 5-ALPHA-REDUCTASE INHIBITOR
Comment: Pregnant females and females of childbearing age should not handle *dutasteride*. Monitor for potential side effects of decreased libido and/or impotence. Low, but increased risk of being diagnosed with high-grade prostate cancer.
▷ *dutasteride* (G) 0.5 mg once daily
  Avodart *Cap:* 0.5 mg
  Comment: May take Avodart 0.5 mg with Flomax 0.4 mg once daily as combination therapy.

TYPE I AND II 5-ALPHA-REDUCTASE INHIBITOR+ALPHA-1A BLOCKER
▷ *dutasteride+tamsulosin* (G) take 1 cap once daily after the same meal each day
  Jalyn *Cap:* duta 0.5 mg+tam 0.4 mg

PHOSPHODIESTERASE TYPE 5 (PDE5) INHIBITORS, CGMP-SPECIFIC
Comment: Oral phosphodiesterase type 5 (PDE5) inhibitors are contraindicated in patients taking nitrates. Caution with history of recent myocardial infarction (MI), stroke, life-threatening arrhythmia, hypotension, hypertension, cardiac failure, unstable angina, retinitis pigmentosa, CYP3A4 inhibitors (e.g., *cimetidine*, the azoles, *erythromycin*, grapefruit juice), protease inhibitors (e.g., *ritonavir*), CYP3A4 inducers (e.g., *rifampin*, *carbamazepine*, *phenytoin*, *phenobarbital*), alcohol, and antihypertensive agents. Side effects include headache, flushing, nasal congestion, rhinitis, dyspepsia, and diarrhea. (NOTE: Current good manufacturing

practice (cGMP) regulations, enforced by the FDA, provides for systems that assure proper design, monitoring, and control of manufacturing processes and facilities. Good manufacturing practice (GMP) requires manufacturers to ensure that their products are safe and effective. cGMP requires manufactures to employ technologies and systems that are up to date and comply with GMP regulations.

➤ *tadalafil* (G) 5 mg once daily at the same time each day; *CrCl 30-50 ml/min:* initially 2.5 mg; *CrCl <30 ml/min:* not recommended; *Concomitant alpha-blockers:* not recommended

Cialis *Tab:* 2.5, 5, 10, 20 mg

5-ALPHA-REDUCTASE INHIBITOR+PDE5 INHIBITOR

➤ *finasteride+tadalafil* administer 1 capsule once daily at approximately the same time every day, without food, for up to 26 weeks; take without food

Pediatric: <18 years: safety and efficacy not established; ≥18 years: same as adult

Entadfi *Cap:* 5 mg/5 mg

Comment: Entadfi is a fixed-dose combination of *finasteride* 5 mg (5α-reductase inhibitor)+*tadalafil* 5 mg (phosphodiesterase [DE5] inhibitor) indicated for the treatment of urinary tract symptoms caused by benign prostatic hyperplasia (BPH). Contraindications to Entadfi: (1) concomitant use with any form of organic nitrate, either regularly and/or intermittently (Entadfi can potentiate the hypotensive effect of nitrates); (2) concomitant use with guanylate cyclase (GC) stimulators (Entadfi may potentiate the hypotensive effects of GC stimulators); (3) known hypersensitivity to Entadfi or any of its components; and (4) pregnancy. Administer nitrates concomitantly only in life-threatening situations under close medical supervision. *Child-Pugh class A and B:* Use Entadfi with caution. *Child-Pugh Class C:* Use of Entadfi is not recommended. CrCl <50 ml/min or hemodialysis: Use of Entadfi is not recommended. Concomitant use of CYP3A4 inducers with Entadfi is not recommended as this drug combination can increase *tadalafil* exposure. Use alpha-blockers, antihypertensives, strong CYP3A4 inhibitors, and alcohol with caution due to the potential for symptomatic hypotension. Consider other urologic conditions prior to initiation of treatment for BPH. Carefully monitor patients with large residual urinary volume and/or severely diminished urinary flow for obstructive uropathy. Prostate cancer and BPH may coexist. Prostate-specific antigen (PSA) reduction by approximately 50% within 6 months of treatment can be seen, which can affect interpretation of serial and isolated PSA values. Evaluate any confirmed increase in PSA as it may signal the presence of prostate cancer (increased incidence of high-grade prostate cancer has been observed). There is risk to the male fetus from topical Entadfi exposure to pregnant females: Pregnant females should not handle crushed or open Entadfi capsules. Immediately discontinue Entadfi and initiate appropriate management of signs or symptoms of a hypersensitivity reaction. There is increased prolonged erection and priapism with Entadfi use. Use Entadfi with caution in patients predisposed to priapism. Advise patients to seek emergency treatment if an erection lasts more than 4 hours. Discontinue Entadfi in the event of a sudden loss of vision in one or both eyes; such an event may be a sign of non-arteritic anterior ischemic optic neuropathy (NAION). Use Entadfi with caution in patients at increased risk of NAION. Discontinue Entadfi for sudden hearing loss and evaluate/treat promptly. The most common adverse reactions associated with *finasteride* monotherapy (≥1%) in a 4-year study were impotence, decreased libido, decreased volume of ejaculate, breast enlargement, breast tenderness, and rash. The most common adverse reactions (≥2%) associated with *tadalafil* were headache, dyspepsia, back pain, myalgia, nasal congestion, flushing, and pain in limb. Treatment with *finasteride* for 24 weeks to evaluate semen parameters in healthy male volunteers revealed no clinically meaningful effects on sperm concentration, mobility, morphology, or pH. A 0.6 ml (22.1%) median decrease in ejaculate volume with a concomitant reduction in total sperm per ejaculate was observed. These parameters remained within the normal range and were reversible upon discontinuation of therapy, with an average time to return to baseline of 84 weeks. Based on the data from 3 studies in adult males, *tadalafil* decreased sperm concentrations in the study of 10 mg *tadalafil* for 6 months and the study of 20 mg tadalafil for 9 months. This effect was not seen in the study of 20 mg *tadalafil* taken for 6 months. There was no adverse effect of *tadalafil* 10 mg or 20 mg on mean concentrations of testosterone, luteinizing (LH) hormone, or follicle stimulating hormone (FSH). The clinical significance of the decreased sperm concentrations in the two studies is unknown. No overall differences in safety or efficacy of *finasteride* or *tadalafil* have been observed between patients ≥65 years of age and younger adult patients. To report suspected adverse reactions, contact Veru at www.verupharma.com or FDA at 1-800-FDA-1088 or http://www.fda.gov/medwatch.

BETA THALASSEMIA

➤ *betibeglogene autotemcel* see mfr pkg insert for full prescribing information including proper product storage, handling, preparation, and administration to adults and children

Zynteglo *Cell suspension for IV infusion;* Zynteglo is composed of up to four infusion bags which contain 2.0-20 × 10^6 cells/ml suspended in cryopreservation solution; each infusion bag contains approximately 20 ml of Zynteglo; a single dose of Zynteglo contains a minimum of 5.0 × 10^6 CD34+ cells per kilogram of body weight, suspended in cryopreservation solution; see mfr pkg insert for proper storage and handling

(continued)

Comment: Zynteglo is a one-time autologous hematopoietic stem cell-based gene therapy indicated for the treatment of adult and pediatric patients with beta thalassemia (also known as beta thalassemia major or Cooley's anemia) who require regular red blood cell (RBC) transfusions. Beta thalassemia is caused by a change in the beta-globin gene, which causes the body to produce reduced or no beta-globin. **Zynteglo** is made specifically for each patient, using the patient's own blood stem cells and adds functional copies of the beta-globin gene to those cells. This may allow the patient to produce sufficient hemoglobin to stop receiving regular transfusions. On the day of treatment, **Zynteglo** may cause increased heart rate and/or abdominal pain. **Zynteglo** may cause the following side effects following treatment for up to 6 months: decreased platelets, decreased WBCs, and pain in the arms or legs. Patients should be monitored at least yearly for at least 15 years for any blood changes. Potential adverse events requiring immediate medical care include severe headache, unusual stomach or back pain, or abnormal bruising, epistaxis, hematuria, hematochezia, hemoptysis, or hematemesis. There is a potential risk of blood cancer associated with this treatment; however, no cases have been seen in clinical studies. If the patient is diagnosed with a cancer, the treating physician should contact Bluebird Bio at 1-833-999-6378. There are no data on the use of **Zynteglo** in human or animal pregnancy or lactation. The risks of myeloablative chemotherapy agents during pregnancy should be considered. **Zynteglo** should not be administered to females who are pregnant. Exclude pregnancy prior to starting treatment with **Zynteglo**. Ensure a negative serum pregnancy test before mobilization and exclude pregnancy again before initiating conditioning procedures and drug product administration. Advise patients to consult their physician if they plan to become pregnant after receiving this product. Males with female partners of reproductive potential should be advised to use effective contraception from the start of mobilization and for at least 6 months after the drug product administration. Appraise patients of the risks associated with conditioning agents. Advise patients to cryopreserve semen or ova if appropriate before treatment due to the risk of infertility with myeloablative conditioning. **Zynteglo** is not recommended for females who are breastfeeding. Benefit to the mother should outweigh risk to the breastfeeding infant.

BILE ACID DEFICIENCY

BILE ACID
➤ **ursodiol**
Dissolution of radiolucent non-calcified gallstones <20 mm diameter: 8-10 mg/kg/day in 2-3 divided doses;
Prevention: 13-15 mg/kg/day in 4 divided doses
Pediatric: <12 years: not recommended; ≥12 years: same as adult
   Actigall *Cap:* 300 mg
Comment: *Ursodiol* decreases the amount of cholesterol produced by the liver and absorbed by the intestines. It helps break down cholesterol that has formed into stones in the gallbladder. *Ursodiol* increases bile flow in patients with primary biliary cirrhosis. It is used to treat small gallstones in people who cannot have cholecystectomy surgery and to prevent gallstones in overweight patients undergoing rapid weight loss. *Ursodiol* is not for treating gallstones that are calcified.

BINGE EATING DISORDER

CENTRAL NERVOUS SYSTEM (CNS) STIMULANT
➤ **lisdexamfetamine dimesylate** (II) swallow whole or may open and mix/dissolve contents of cap in yogurt, water, and orange juice and take immediately; 30 mg once daily in the AM; may adjust in increments of 20 mg at weekly intervals; target dose 50-70 mg/day; max 70 mg/day; *GFR 15-<30 ml/min:* max 50 mg/day; *GFR <15 ml/min, end-stage renal disease (ESRD):* max 30 mg/day
Pediatric: <18 years: not established; ≥18 years: same as adult
   Vyvanse *Cap:* 10, 20, 30, 40, 50, 60, 70 mg
   Comment: Vyvanse is not approved or recommended for weight loss treatment of obesity.

BIPOLAR DISORDER

Comment: Bipolar I disorder is characterized by one or more manic episodes that last at least a week or require hospitalization. Severe mania may manifest symptoms of psychosis. Bipolar II disorder is characterized by one or more depressive episodes accompanied by at least one hypomanic episode. When one parent has bipolar disorder, the risk to each child developing the disorder is estimated to be 15%–30%. When both parents have the disorder, the risk to each child increases to 50%-75%. Symptoms of mood disorders may be difficult to diagnose in children and adolescents because they can be mistaken for age-appropriate emotions and behaviors or overlap with symptoms of other conditions such as attention deficit hyperactivity disorder (ADHD). However, since anxiety and depression in children may be precursors to bipolar disorder, these behaviors should be carefully monitored and evaluated. The cornerstone of treatment for bipolar disorder is mood stabilizers (**lithium** and **valproate**). Common adjunctive agents include antiepileptics, antipsychotics, and combination agents. Mounting evidence suggests that antidepressants are not effective in the treatment of bipolar depression. A major study funded by the National Institute of Mental Health (NIMH) showed that adding an antidepressant to a mood stabilizer was no more effective in treating bipolar depression than using a mood stabilizer alone. Another NIMH study found that antidepressants work no better than placebo. If antidepressants are used at all, they should be combined with a mood stabilizer, such as *lithium* or *valproic acid*. Antidepressants, without a concomitant mood stabilizer, can increase the frequency of mood cycling and trigger a manic episode. Many experts believe that, over time, antidepressant use as monotherapy (i.e., without a mood stabilizer) in people with bipolar disorder has a mood de-stabilizing effect, increasing the frequency of manic and depressive episodes. Drugs and conditions that can mimic bipolar disorder include thyroid disorders, corticosteroids, antidepressants, adrenal disorders (e.g., Addison's disease, Cushing's syndrome), antianxiety drugs, drugs for Parkinson's disease, vitamin B12 deficiency, and neurologic disorders (e.g., epilepsy, multiple sclerosis).

MOOD STABILIZERS
Lithium Salts Mood Stabilizer

▷ *lithium carbonate* (G) swallow whole; *Usual maintenance:* 900-1,200 mg/day in 2-3 divided doses
Pediatric: <12 years: not recommended; ≥12 years: same as adult
   Lithobid *Tab:* 300 mg slow-rel
Comment: Signs and symptoms of *lithium* toxicity can occur below 2 mEq/L and include blurred vision, tinnitus, weakness, dizziness, nausea, abdominal pain, vomiting, and diarrhea, to (severe) hand tremors, ataxia, muscle twitches, nystagmus, seizures, slurred speech, decreased level of consciousness, coma, and death.

Valproate Mood Stabilizer

▷ *divalproex sodium* (G) take once daily; swallow ext-rel form whole; initially 25 mg/kg/day in divided doses; max 60 mg/kg/day; *Elderly:* reduce initial dose and titrate slowly
Pediatric: <12 years: not recommended; ≥12 years: same as adult
   Depakene *Cap:* 250 mg; *Syr:* 250 mg/5 ml (16 oz)
      Depakote *Tab:* 125, 250 mg
      Depakote ER *Tab:* 250, 500 mg ext-rel
      Depakote Sprinkle *Cap:* 125 mg

ANTIEPILEPTICS

▷ *carbamazepine* ext-rel oral forms should be swallowed whole; may open caps and sprinkle on applesauce (do not crush or chew beads); initially 400 mg/day in 2 divided doses; adjust in increments of 200 mg/day; max 1.6 gm/day; *Elderly:* reduce initial dose and titrate slowly; oral doses are preferred; IV administration is recommended when the patient is unable to swallow an oral form (see **Carnexiv**)
Pediatric: <12 years: not recommended; ≥12 years: same as adult
      Carbatrol (G) *Cap:* 200, 300 mg ext-rel
      Carnexiv *Vial:* 10 mg/ml (20 ml)
      Comment: The total daily dose of **Carnexiv** is 70% of the total daily oral *carbamazepine* dose (see mfr pkg insert for dosage conversion table). The total daily dose should be equally divided into four 30-minute infusions, separated by 6 hours. Must be diluted prior to administration. Patients should be switched back to oral *carbamazepine* at their previous total daily oral dose and frequency of administration as soon as clinically appropriate. The use of **Carnexiv** for more than 7 consecutive days has not been studied.
      Equetro (G) *Cap:* 100, 200, 300 mg ext-rel
      Tegretol (G) *Tab:* 200*mg; *Chew tab:* 100*mg; *Oral susp:* 100 mg/5 ml (450 ml; citrus-vanilla)
      Tegretol XR (G) *Tab:* 100, 200, 400 mg ext-rel
   Comment: *Carbamazepine* is indicated in mixed episodes in bipolar I disorder.
▷ *lamotrigine* (G) Not *taking an enzyme-inducing antiepileptic drug (EIAED) (e.g., phenytoin, carbamazepine, phenobarbital, primidone, valproic acid):* 25 mg once daily x 2 weeks; then 50 mg once daily x 2 weeks; then 100 mg once daily x 2 weeks; then target dose 200 mg once daily; *Concomitant valproic acid:* 25 mg every other day x 2 weeks; then 25 mg once daily x 2 weeks; then 50 mg once daily x 1 week; then target dose 100 mg once daily; *Concomitant EIAED,* not *valproic acid:* 50 mg once daily x 2 weeks; then 100 mg daily in divided doses; then increase weekly by 100 mg in divided doses to target dose 400 mg/day in divided doses daily
Pediatric: <12 years: not recommended; ≥12 years: same as adult
      Lamictal *Tab:* 25*, 100*, 150*, 200*mg
      Lamictal Chewable Dispersible Tab *Chew tab:* 2, 5, 25, 50 mg (black current)
      Lamictal ODT *ODT:* 25, 50, 100, 200 mg
      Lamictal XR *Tab:* 25, 50, 100, 200 mg ext-rel
   Comment: *Lamotrigine* is indicated for maintenance treatment of bipolar I disorder. See mfr pkg insert for drug interactions, interactions with contraceptives and hormone replacement therapy, and discontinuation protocol.

ANTIPSYCHOTICS

Comment: Common side effects of antipsychotic drugs include drowsiness, weight gain, sexual dysfunction, dry mouth, constipation, and blurred vision. *Neuroleptic malignant syndrome* (NMS) and *tardive dyskinesia* (TD) are adverse side effects (ASEs) most often associated with the older antipsychotic drugs. Risk is decreased with the newer "atypical" antipsychotic drugs. However, these syndromes can develop, although much less commonly, after relatively brief treatment periods at low doses. Given these considerations, antipsychotic drugs should be prescribed in a manner that is most likely to minimize the occurrence. NMS, a potentially fatal symptom complex, is characterized by hyperpyrexia, muscle rigidity, altered mental status, and evidence of autonomic instability (irregular pulse or blood pressure, tachycardia, diaphoresis, and cardiac dysrhythmia). Additional signs may include elevated creatine phosphokinase (CPK), myoglobinuria (rhabdomyolysis), and acute renal failure (ARF). TD is a syndrome consisting of potentially irreversible, involuntary, dyskinetic movements that can develop in patients with antipsychotic drugs. Characteristics include repetitive involuntary movements, usually of the jaw, lips, and tongue, such as grimacing, sticking out the tongue, and smacking the lips. Some affected people also experience involuntary movement of the extremities or difficulty breathing. The syndrome may remit, partially or completely, if antipsychotic treatment is withdrawn. If signs and symptoms of NMS and/or TD appear in a patient, management should include immediate discontinuation of antipsychotic drugs and other drugs not essential to concurrent therapy, intensive symptomatic treatment, medical monitoring, and treatment of any concomitant serious medical problems. The risk of developing NMS and/or TD and the likelihood that either syndrome will become irreversible are believed to increase as the duration of treatment and the total cumulative dose of antipsychotic drugs administered to the patient increase. The first and only FDA-approved treatment for TD is *valbenazine* (**Ingrezza**) (*see* Tardive Dyskinesia)

▶ *aripiprazole* (G) initially 15 mg once daily; may increase to max 30 mg/day
   Pediatric: <10 years: not recommended; ≥10-17 years: initially 2 mg/day in a single dose for 2 days; then increase to 5 mg/day in a single dose for 2 days; then increase to target dose of 10 mg/day in a single dose; may increase by 5 mg/day at weekly intervals as needed to max 30 mg/day
   Abilify *Tab:* 2, 5, 10, 15, 20, 30 mg
   Abilify Discmelt *Tab:* 15 mg orally-disint (vanilla) (phenylalanine)
   Abilify Maintena *Vial:* 300, 400 mg ext-rel pwdr for IM injection reconstitution; 300, 400 mg single dose prefilled dual-chamber syringes w. supplies
   Comment: Abilify is indicated for acute and maintenance treatment of mixed episodes in bipolar I disorder, as monotherapy or as adjunct to *lithium* or *valproic acid.*
   asenapine (C)(G) allow SL tab to dissolve on tongue; do not split, crush, chew, or swallow; do not eat or drink for 10 minutes after administration; *Monotherapy:* 10 mg bid; *Adjunctive therapy:* 5 mg bid; may increase to max 10 mg bid
   Pediatric: <10 years: not established; 10-17 years: *Monotherapy:* initially 2.5 mg bid; may increase to 5 mg bid after 3 days; then to 10 mg bid after 3 more days; max 10 mg bid
   Saphris *SL tab:* 2, 5, 5, 10 mg (black cherry)
   Comment: Saphris is indicated for acute treatment of manic or mixed episodes in bipolar I disorder, as monotherapy or as adjunct to *lithium* or *valproic acid.*

▶ *cariprazine* (G) *Recommended starting dose:* 1.5 mg daily; *Max recommended daily dose:* 6 mg (doses above 6 mg daily do not confer significant benefit, but increase the risk of dose-related adverse reactions)
   Pediatric: Safety and efficacy not established
   Vraylar *Cap:* 1.5, 3, 4.5, 6 mg
   Comment: Vraylar is an atypical antipsychotic for the treatment of schizophrenia and bipolar disorder, and as an adjunct for major depressive disorder (MDD) in adults. The most common adverse reactions in the treatment of schizophrenia (incidence ≥5% and at least twice the rate of placebo) have been extrapyramidal symptoms (EPS) and akathisia. Due to Vraylar's long half-life, monitor patients for adverse reactions for several weeks after starting Vraylar and with each dose change. *Boxed Warning:* Elderly patients with dementia-related psychosis treated with antipsychotic drugs are at an increased risk of death. Vraylar is not approved for the treatment of patients with dementia-related psychosis. Antidepressants increased the risk of suicidal thoughts and behaviors in pediatric and young adult patients. Closely monitor all antidepressant-treated patients for clinical worsening and emergence of suicidal thoughts and behaviors. When taken with strong CYP3A4 inhibitors, reduce Vraylar dose by half. Concomitant use of Vraylar with CYP3A4 inducers is not recommended. See the mfr pkg insert for full prescribing information and complete black-box warning. Monitor patients for hyperglycemia and diabetes mellitus, dyslipidemia, and weight gain. Monitor for leukopenia, neutropenia, and agranulocytosis; perform complete blood counts (CBCs) in patients with preexisting low white blood cell (WBC) count or history of leukopenia or neutropenia and consider discontinuing Vraylar if a clinically significant decline in WBC occurs in the absence of other causative factors. Monitor patients for orthostatic hypotension and syncope. Monitor heart rate and blood pressure and warn patients with known cardiovascular or cerebrovascular disease and risk of dehydration or syncope. Use Vraylar cautiously in patients with a history of seizures or with conditions that lower the seizure threshold. Due to potential for cognitive and motor impairment, advise patients to use caution when operating machinery (e.g., driving a motor vehicle). Safety and effectiveness of Vraylar have not been established in pediatric patients. Based on animal data, Vraylar may cause fetal harm; advise females of reproductive

potential of fetal risk and to use effective contraception. Lactation studies have not been conducted to assess the presence of *cariprazine* in human milk or effects on the breastfed infant. However, *cariprazine* is present in rat milk. Development and health benefits of breastfeeding should be considered along with the mother's clinical need for **Vraylar** and any potential adverse effects on the breastfed infant from **Vraylar** or from the underlying maternal condition.

▷ *lumateperone* 42 mg once daily; no titration required; take with or without food
Pediatric: safety and efficacy not established

Caplyta *Cap:* 42 mg

Comment: Caplyta *(lumateperone)* is the first-in-class atypical antipsychotic for the treatment of schizophrenia in adults. **Caplyta** is also indicated for the treatment of adult patients with depressive episodes associated with bipolar disorder (i.e., bipolar depression) as monotherapy and as adjunctive therapy with a mood stabilizer (such as *lithium* or *valproate*). **Caplyta** is not approved for the treatment of patients with dementia-related psychosis due to increased incidence of cerebrovascular adverse reactions (e.g., stroke, transient ischemic attack [TIA]) and death in these patients. Avoid **Caplyta** use with moderate-to-severe hepatic impairment. Avoid use with concomitant CYP3A4 inducers and moderate or strong CYP3A4 inhibitors. Discontinue **Caplyta** immediately and monitor the patient closely if signs of neuroleptic malignant syndrome (NMS) develop. Manage signs of tardive dyskinesia (TD) with discontinuation if clinically appropriate. Monitor for hyperglycemia/diabetes mellitus, dyslipidemia, and weight gain. Leukopenia, neutropenia, and agranulocytosis may develop; therefore, monitor CBC—especially in patients with preexisting low WBC or history of leukopenia or neutropenia. Consider discontinuing **Caplyta** if clinically significant decline in WBC occurs in the absence of other causative factors. Orthostatic hypotension and syncope may occur; therefore, monitor HR and BP and warn patients with known cardiovascular or cerebrovascular disease, and caution to avoid dehydration. Use caution in patients with a history of seizure or with conditions that lower seizure threshold. There is potential for cognitive and motor impairment; therefore, advise caution when operating hazardous equipment or machinery and monitor as appropriate. The most common adverse reactions reported in clinical trials (incidence >5% and >2 x placebo) have been somnolence/sedation, dizziness, nausea, and dry mouth. Based on findings from animal studies, *lumateperone* may impair male and female fertility. There is risk to the mother from untreated schizophrenia or untreated bipolar depression, including increased risk of relapse, hospitalization, and suicide, and schizophrenia is associated with increased adverse perinatal outcomes, including preterm birth. It is not known if this is a direct result of the illness or other comorbid factors. Extrapyramidal and/or withdrawal symptoms, including agitation, hypertonia, hypotonia, tremor, somnolence, respiratory distress, and feeding disorder, have been reported in neonates who were exposed to antipsychotic drugs during the 3rd trimester of pregnancy. These symptoms have varied in severity. Developmental and health benefits of breastfeeding should be considered along with the mother's clinical need for **Caplyta** and any potential adverse effects on the breastfed infant from **Caplyta** or from the underlying maternal condition. Use of effective contraception during treatment with **Caplyta** is advisable. There is a pregnancy exposure registry that monitors pregnancy outcomes in women exposed to atypical antipsychotics, including **Caplyta**, during pregnancy. Healthcare providers are encouraged to register patients by contacting the National Pregnancy Registry for Atypical Antipsychotics at 1-866-961-2388 or online at http://womensmentalhealth.org/clinical-and-research-programs/pregnancyregistry/. There are published reports of sedation, failure to thrive, jitteriness, and EPS (tremors and abnormal muscle movements) in breastfed infants exposed to antipsychotics. Based on findings of toxicity in animal studies and the potential for serious adverse reactions in the breastfed infant, breastfeeding is not recommended during treatment with **Caplyta**.

▷ *lurasidone* (G) initially 20 mg once daily; usual range 20 to max 120 mg/day; take with food; *CrCl <50 ml/min, moderate hepatic impairment (Child-Pugh 7-9):* max 80 mg/day; *Child-Pugh 10-15):* max 40 mg/day
Pediatric: <10 years: not established; 10-17 years: initially 20 mg once daily; may titrate up to max 80 mg/day; >17 years: same as adult

Latuda *Tab:* 20, 40, 60, 80, 120 mg

Comment: Latuda is indicated for major depressive episodes associated with bipolar I disorder as monotherapy and as adjunctive therapy with *lithium* or *valproic* acid. Contraindicated with concomitant strong CYP3A4 inhibitors (e.g., *ketoconazole, voriconazole, clarithromycin, ritonavir*) and inducers (e.g., *phenytoin, carbamazepine, rifampin, St. John's wort*); see mfr pkg insert if the patient is taking moderate CYP3A4 inhibitors (e.g., *diltiazem, atazanavir, erythromycin, fluconazole, verapamil*). The efficacy of **Latuda** in the treatment of mania associated with bipolar disorder has not been established.

▷ *quetiapine fumarate* (G)

Seroquel initially 25 mg bid, titrate every 2nd or 3rd day in increments of 25 to 50 mg bid-tid; usual maintenance 400-600 mg/day in 2-3 divided doses
Pediatric: <10 years: not recommended; ≥10-17 years: initially 25 mg bid, titrate every 2nd or 3rd day in increments of 25-50 mg bid-tid; max 600 mg/day in 2-3 divided doses

Tab: 25, 50, 100, 200, 300, 400 mg

Seroquel XR swallow whole; administer once daily in the PM; *Day 1:* 50 mg; *Day 2:* 100 mg; *Day 3:* 200 mg; *Day 4:* 300 mg; usual range 400-600 mg/day

(continued)

Pediatric: <18 years: not recommended; ≥18 years: same as adult

> *Tab:* 50, 150, 200, 300, 400 mg ext-rel

▶ **risperidone** (Oral Forms) *Tab:* initially 2-3 mg once daily; may adjust at 24-hour intervals by 1 mg/day; usual range 1-6 mg/day; max 6 mg/day; *Oral soln:* do not take with cola or tea; *M-tab:* dissolve on the tongue with or without fluid; *Consta:* administer deep IM in the deltoid or gluteal; give with oral **risperidone** or other antipsychotic x 3 weeks; then stop oral form; 25 mg IM every 2 weeks; max 50 mg every 2 weeks

Risperdal

Pediatric: <5 years: not established; 5-10 years: initially 0.5 mg once daily at the same time each day, adjust at 24-hour intervals by 0.5-1 mg to target dose of 1-2.5 mg/day; usual range 1-6 mg/day; max 6 mg/day; >10 years: same as adult

> *Tab:* 0.25, 0.5, 1, 2, 3, 4 mg; *Oral soln:* 1 mg/ml (100 ml)

Risperdal M-Tab

Pediatric: <10 years: not established; ≥10 years: same as adult

> *Tab:* 0.5, 1, 2, 3, 4 mg orally-disint (phenylalanine)

Comment: Risperdal tabs, oral solution, and M-tabs are indicated for the short-term monotherapy of acute mania or mixed episodes associated with bipolar I disorder, or in combination with **lithium** or **valproic acid** in adults

▶ **risperidone** (Parenteral Forms)

Comment: Risperdal Consta was the first-in-class long-acting parenteral formulation of **risperidone** for administration every 2 weeks. Rykindo is the second-in-class. For patients who have never taken oral **risperidone**, tolerability should be established with oral **risperidone** prior to initiating treatment with Risperdal Consta or Rykindo. Administer by deep IM deltoid or gluteal injection. Do not administer by any other route. Each injection should be administered by a qualified healthcare professional only. A starting dose of 12.5 mg may be appropriate for some patients. Patients not responding may benefit from 37.5 mg or 50 mg. *Dose titration:* should not be made more frequently than every 4 weeks. *Max Dose:* 50 mg once every 2 weeks. *Renal or Hepatic Impairment:* Titrate with oral **risperidone** up to at least 2 mg prior to initiating Risperdal Consta or Rykindo. **Risperidone** is thought to work through a combination of dopamine type 2 (D_2) and serotonin type 2 ($5HT_2$) receptor antagonism. Warnings and precautions associated with parenteral risperidone include cerebrovascular adverse reactions in elderly patients with dementia-related psychosis, neuroleptic malignant syndrome (NMS), tardive dyskinesia (TD), metabolic changes, hyperprolactinemia, orthostatic hypotension and syncope, low WBC count, potential for cognitive and motor impairment, and seizures. Concomitant strong CYP2D6 inhibitors (e.g., **fluoxetine, paroxetine**) increase **risperidone** plasma concentration. Concomitant strong CYP3A4 inducers (e.g., **carbamazepine**) decrease plasma concentrations of **risperidone**. See the mfr pkg insert for full prescribing information, including storage, preparation, warnings, precautions, and potential adverse events, for **Risperdal Consta or Rykindo,** prior to use. Based on the pharmacologic action of **risperidone** (D2 receptor antagonism), treatment with **Risperdal Consta or Rykindo** may result in an increase in serum prolactin levels, which may lead to a reversible reduction in fertility in females of reproductive potential. There is a risk to the mother from untreated schizophrenia or bipolar I disorder, including increased risk of relapse, hospitalization, and suicide. Schizophrenia and bipolar I disorder are associated with increased adverse perinatal outcomes, including preterm birth. It is not known if this is a direct result of the illness or other comorbid factors. Available data from published epidemiologic studies of pregnant patients exposed to **risperidone** have not established a drug-associated risk of major birth defects, miscarriage, or adverse maternal or fetal outcomes. **Risperidone** has been detected in the plasma of adult subjects up to 6 weeks after a single dose of **Risperdal Consta or Rykindo.** The clinical significance of an injection of **risperidone** administered before or during pregnancy is unknown. There is a pregnancy exposure registry that monitors pregnancy outcomes in women exposed to atypical antipsychotics during pregnancy. Healthcare providers are encouraged to register patients by contacting the National Pregnancy Registry for Atypical Antipsychotics at 866-961-2388 or online at http://womensmentalhealth.org/clinicaland-research-programs/pregnancyregistry/. Extrapyramidal and/or withdrawal symptoms (including agitation, hypertonia, hypotonia, tremor, somnolence, respiratory distress, and feeding disorder) have been reported in neonates who were exposed to antipsychosis drugs, including **risperidone**, during the third trimester of pregnancy. These symptoms varied in severity. Monitor neonates for extrapyramidal and/or withdrawal symptoms and manage symptoms appropriately. Some neonates recovered within hours or days without specific treatment; others required prolonged hospitalization. Limited data from published literature report the presence of **risperidone** and its metabolite, 9-hydroxyrisperidone, in human breast milk. Infants exposed to **Risperdal Consta or Rykindo** through breast milk should be monitored for excess sedation, failure to thrive, jitteriness, and EPS (tremors and abnormal muscle movements). Developmental and health benefits of breastfeeding should be considered along with the mother's clinical need for **Risperdal Consta or Rykindo** and any potential adverse effects on the breastfed infant from **Risperdal Consta or Rykindo** or from the mother's underlying condition.

Pediatric: <18 years: safety and efficacy not established; ≥18 years: same as adult

> **Risperdal Consta** Vial: 12.5, 25, 37.5, 50 mg pwdr for reconstitution, single-use, w. diluent and supplies
> **Rykindo** Vial: 12.5, 25, 37.5, 50 mg, long-acting ext-rel, susp for IM injection

▶ **ziprasidone** (G) *Adult:* take with food; initially 40 mg bid; on day 2, may increase to 60-80 mg bid; *Elderly:* lower initial dose and titrate slowly

Pediatric: <12 years: <u>not</u> recommended; ≥12 years: same as adult

    Geodon *Cap:* 20, 40, 60, 80 mg

    Comment: Geodon is indicated for acute and maintenance treatment of mixed episodes in bipolar I disorder, as monotherapy <u>or</u> as adjunct to *lithium* <u>or</u> *valproic acid.*

COMBINATION AGENTS
Thienobenzodiazepine+Selective Serotonin Reuptake Inhibitor (SSRI) Combinations

▷ *olanzapine+fluoxetine* initially 1 x 6/25 cap once daily in the PM; titrate; max 1 x 12/50 cap once daily in the PM

    Pediatric: <10 years: <u>not</u> recommended; 10-17 years: initially 1 x 3/25 cap once daily in the PM; max 1 x 12/50 cap once daily in the PM

    Symbyax

        Cap: **Symbyax 3/25** olan 3 mg+fluo 25 mg

            Symbyax 6/25 olan 6 mg+fluo 25 mg

            Symbyax 6/50 olan 6 mg+fluo 50 mg

            Symbyax 12/25 olan 12 mg+fluo 25 mg

            Symbyax 12/50 olan 12 mg+fluo 50 mg

    Comment: Symbyax is indicated for the treatment of depressive episode associated with bipolar I disorder and treatment-resistant depression (TRD).

BITE: CAT

TETANUS PROPHYLAXIS

▷ *tetanus toxoid* vaccine 0.5 ml IM x 1 dose if previously immunized; *see* **Tetanus** for patients <u>not</u> previously immunized

    Vial: 5 Lf units/0.5 ml (0.5, 5 ml); *Prefilled syringe:* 5 Lf units/0.5 ml (0.5 ml)

ANTI-INFECTIVES

▷ *amoxicillin+clavulanate* (G)

    Augmentin 500 mg tid <u>or</u> 875 mg bid x 10 days

    Pediatric: 40-45 mg/kg/day divided tid x 10 days <u>or</u> 90 mg/kg/day divided bid x 10 days; *see* Appendix BB.4. *amoxicillin+clavulanate* (G) (Augmentin Suspension) *for dose by weight*

    Tab: 250, 500, 875 mg; *Chew tab:* 125, 250 mg (lemon-lime); 200, 400 mg (cherry-banana) (phenylalanine); *Oral susp:* 125 mg/5 ml (banana), 250 mg/5 ml (75, 100, 150 ml) (orange); 200, 400 mg/5 ml (50, 75, 100 ml) (orange) (phenylalanine)

    Augmentin ES-600 <u>not</u> recommended for adults

    Pediatric: <3 months: <u>not</u> recommended; ≥3 months, <40 kg: 90 mg/kg/day in 2 divided doses x 10 days; ≥40 kg: <u>not</u> recommended

    Oral susp: 42.9 mg/5 ml (50, 75, 100, 125, 150, 200 ml) (strawberry cream) (phenylalanine)

    Augmentin XR 2 tabs q 12 hours x 10 days

    Pediatric: <16 years: use other forms; ≥16 years: same as adult

    Tab: 1,000*mg ext-rel

▷ *doxycycline* (G) 100 mg bid day 1; then 100 mg daily x 10 days

    Pediatric: <8 years: <u>not</u> recommended ≥8 years, <100 lb: 2 mg/lb on first day in 2 divided doses, followed by 1 mg/lb/day in 1-2 divided doses; *see* Appendix BB.19. *doxycycline* (G) (Vibramycin Syrup/Suspension) for dose by weight; ≥8 years, ≥100 lb: same as adult

    Acticlate *Tab:* 75, 150**mg

    Adoxa *Tab:* 50, 75, 100, 150 mg ent-coat

    Doryx *Tab:* 50, 75, 100, 150, 200 mg del-rel

    Doxteric *Tab:* 50 mg del-rel

    Monodox *Cap:* 50, 75, 100 mg

    Oracea *Cap:* 40 mg del-rel

    Vibramycin *Tab:* 100 mg; *Cap:* 50, 100 mg; *Syr:* 50 mg/5 ml (raspberry-apple) (sulfites); *Oral susp:* 25 mg/5 ml (raspberry)

    Vibra-Tab *Tab:* 100 mg film-coat

▷ *penicillin v potassium* (G) 500 mg PO qid x 3 days

    Pediatric: <12 years: 15-50 mg/kg/day in 3-6 divided doses x 3 days; *see* Appendix BB.29. *penicillin v potassium* (G) (Pen-Vee K Solution, Veetids Solution) *for dose by weight;* ≥12 years: same as adult

    Pen-Vee K *Tab:* 250, 500 mg; *Oral soln:* 125 mg/5 ml (100, 200 ml), 250 mg/5 ml (100, 150, 200 ml)

BITE: DOG

TETANUS PROPHYLAXIS

▷ *tetanus toxoid* vaccine 0.5 ml IM x 1 dose if previously immunized; *see* **Tetanus** for patients <u>not</u> previously immunized

    Vial: 5 Lf units/0.5 ml (0.5, 5 ml); *Prefilled syringe:* 5 Lf units/0.5 ml (0.5 ml)

ANTI-INFECTIVES

▷ *amoxicillin+clavulanate* (G)
    Augmentin 500 mg tid <u>or</u> 875 mg bid x 10 days
    Pediatric: 40-45 mg/kg/day divided tid x 10 days <u>or</u> 90 mg/kg/day divided bid x 10 days; *see* Appendix
    BB.4. *amoxicillin+clavulanate* (G) (Augmentin Suspension) *for dose by weight*
    Tab: 250, 500, 875 mg; *Chew tab:* 125, 250 mg (lemon-lime), 200, 400 mg (cherry-banana)
    (phenylalanine); *Oral susp:* 125 mg/5 ml (banana), 250 mg/5 ml (75, 100, 150 ml) (orange); 200, 400
    mg/5 ml (50, 75, 100 ml) (orange) (phenylalanine)
    Augmentin ES-600 <u>not</u> recommended for adults
    Pediatric: <3 months: <u>not</u> recommended; ≥3 months, <40 kg: 90 mg/kg/day in 2 divided doses x 10 days;
    ≥40 kg: <u>not</u> recommended
      Oral susp: 42.9 mg/5 ml (50, 75, 100, 125, 150, 200 ml) (strawberry cream) (phenylalanine)
    Augmentin XR 2 tabs q 12 hours x 10 days
    Pediatric: <16 years: use other forms; ≥16 years: same as adult
      Tab: 1,000*mg ext-rel
▷ *clindamycin* administer with fluoroquinolone in adult and trimethoprim+sulfamethoxazole [TMP-SMX] in
  children 300 mg qid x 10 days
    Pediatric: 8-16 mg/kg/day in 3-4 divided doses x 10 days; *see* Appendix BB.17. *clindamycin* (G) (Cleocin
    Pediatric Granules) *for dose by weight*
    Cleocin (G) *Cap:* 75 (tartrazine), 150 (tartrazine), 300 mg
    Cleocin Pediatric Granules (G) *Oral susp:* 75 mg/5 ml (100 ml) (cherry)
▷ *doxycycline* (G) 100 mg bid
    Pediatric: <8 years: <u>not</u> recommended ≥8 years, <100 lb: 2 mg/lb on the first day in 2 divided doses, followed
    by 1 mg/lb/day in 1-2 divided doses; ≥8 years, ≥100 lb: same as adult; *see* Appendix BB.19. *doxycycline* (G)
    (Vibramycin Syrup/Suspension) *for dose by weight*
    Acticlate *Tab:* 75, 150**mg
    Adoxa *Tab:* 50, 75, 100, 150 mg ent-coat
    Doryx *Tab:* 50, 75, 100, 150, 200 mg del-rel
    Doxteric *Tab:* 50 mg del-rel
    Monodox *Cap:* 50, 75, 100 mg
    Oracea *Cap:* 40 mg del-rel
    Vibramycin *Tab:* 100 mg; *Cap:* 50, 100 mg; *Syr:* 50 mg/5 ml (raspberry-apple) (sulfites); *Oral susp:* 25
    mg/5 ml (raspberry)
    Vibra-Tab *Tab:* 100 mg film-coat
▷ *penicillin v potassium* (G) 500 mg PO qid x 3 days
    Pediatric: 50 mg/kg/day in 4 divided doses x 3 days; ≥12 years: same as adult; *see* Appendix BB.29. *penicillin*
    v potassium (G) (Pen-Vee K Solution, Veetids Solution) *for dose by weight*
    Pen-Vee K *Tab:* 250, 500 mg; *Oral soln:* 125 mg/5 ml (100, 200 ml), 250 mg/5 ml (100, 150, 200 ml)

BITE: HUMAN

TETANUS PROPHYLAXIS

▷ *tetanus toxoid* vaccine 0.5 ml IM x 1 dose if previously immunized; *see* **Tetanus** for patients <u>not</u> previously
  immunized
    Vial: 5 Lf units/0.5 ml (0.5, 5 ml); *Prefilled syringe:* 5 Lf units/0.5 ml (0.5 ml)

ANTI-INFECTIVES

▷ *amoxicillin+clavulanate* (G)
    Augmentin 500 mg tid <u>or</u> 875 mg bid x 10 days
    Pediatric: 40-45 mg/kg/day divided tid x 10 days <u>or</u> 90 mg/kg/day divided bid x 10 days; *see* Appendix
    BB.4. *amoxicillin+clavulanate* (G) (Augmentin Suspension) *for dose by weight*
    Tab: 250, 500, 875 mg; *Chew tab:* 125, 250 mg (lemon-lime); 200, 400 mg (cherry-banana)
    (phenylalanine); *Oral susp:* 125 mg/5 ml (banana), 250 mg/5 ml (75, 100, 150 ml) (orange); 200, 400
    mg/5 ml (50, 75, 100 ml) (orange) (phenylalanine)
    Augmentin ES-600 <u>not</u> recommended for adults
    Pediatric: <3 months: <u>not</u> recommended; ≥3 months, <40 kg: 90 mg/kg/day in 2 divided doses x 10 days;
    ≥40 kg: <u>not</u> recommended
    Oral susp: 42.9 mg/5 ml (50, 75, 100, 125, 150, 200 ml) (strawberry cream) (phenylalanine)
    Augmentin XR 2 tabs q 12 hours x 10 days
    Pediatric: <16 years: use other forms; ≥16 years: same as adult
    Tab: 1,000*mg ext-rel
▷ *cefoxitin* 80-160 mg/kg/day IM in 3-4 divided doses x 10 days; max 12 gm/day
  Pediatric: <3 months: <u>not</u> recommended; ≥3 months: same as adult
    Mefoxin Injectable *Vial:* 1, 2 g
▷ *ciprofloxacin* 500 mg bid x 10 days

Pediatric: <18 years: <u>not</u> recommended; ≥18 years: same as adult
> **Cipro (G)** *Tab:* 250, 500, 750 mg; *Oral susp:* 250, 500 mg/5 ml (100 ml) (strawberry)
> **Cipro XR** *Tab:* 500, 1,000 mg ext-rel
> **ProQuin XR** *Tab:* 500 mg ext-rel
➤ ***erythromycin base*** (G) 250 mg qid x 10 days
Pediatric: <45 kg: 30-40 mg/kg/day in 4 divided doses x 10 days; ≥45 kg: same as adult
> **Ery-Tab** *Tab:* 250, 333, 500 mg ent-coat
> **PCE** *Tab:* 333, 500 mg
➤ ***erythromycin ethylsuccinate*** (G) 400 mg qid x 10 days
Pediatric: 30-50 mg/kg/day in 4 divided doses x 10 days; may double dose with severe infection; max 100 mg/kg/day; *see* Appendix BB.21. *erythromycin ethylsuccinate* (G) (E.E.S. Suspension, EryPed Drops/Suspension) *for dose by weight*
> **EryPed** *Oral susp:* 200 mg/5 ml (100, 200 ml) (fruit); 400 mg/5 ml (60, 100, 200 ml) (banana); *Oral drops:* 200, 400 mg/5 ml (50 ml) (fruit); *Chew tab:* 200 mg wafer (fruit)
> **E.E.S.** *Oral susp:* 200, 400 mg/5 ml (100 ml) (fruit)
> **E.E.S. Granules** *Oral susp:* 200 mg/5 ml (100, 200 ml) (cherry)
> **E.E.S. 400 Tablets** *Tab:* 400 mg
➤ ***trimethoprim+sulfamethoxazole (TMP-SMX)*(G)** bid x 10 days
Pediatric: <2 months: <u>not</u> recommended; ≥2 months: 40 mg/kg/day of ***sulfamethoxazole*** in 2 divided doses bid x 10 days; *see Appendix BB.33. trimethoprim+sulfamethoxazole* (G) (Bactrim Suspension, Septra Suspension) *for dose by weight*
> **Bactrim, Septra** 2 tabs bid x 10 days
> *Tab:* trim 80 mg+sulfa 400 mg*
> **Bactrim DS, Septra DS** 1 tab bid x 10 days
> *Tab:* trim 160 mg+sulfa 800 mg*
> **Bactrim Pediatric Suspension, Septra Pediatric Suspension**
> *Oral susp:* trim 40 mg+sulfa 200 mg per 5 ml (100 ml) (cherry) (alcohol 0.3%)

BLEPHARITIS

OPHTHALMIC AGENTS
➤ ***erythromycin*** ophthalmic ointment apply 1/2 inch bid-qid x 14 days; then q HS x 10 days
Pediatric: same as adult
> **Ilotycin** *Oint:* 5 mg/gm (1/2 oz)
➤ ***polymyxin b+bacitracin*** ophthalmic ointment apply 1/2 inch bid-qid x 14 days; then q HS
Pediatric: same as adult
> **Polysporin** *Oint:* poly b 10,000 U+baci 500 U (3.75 gm)
➤ ***polymyxin b+bacitracin+neomycin*** ophthalmic ointment apply 1/2 inch bid-qid x 14 days; then q HS
Pediatric: same as adult
> **Neosporin** *Oint:* poly b 10,000 U+baci 400 U+neo 3.5 mg/gm (3.75 gm)
➤ ***sodium sulfacetamide***
> **Bleph-10 Ophthalmic Solution** 2 drops q 4 hours x 7-14 days
> *Pediatric:* <2 years: <u>not</u> recommended; ≥2 years: 1-2 drops q 2-3 hours during the day x 7-14 days
> *Ophth soln:* 10% (2.5, 5, 15 ml) (benzalkonium chloride)
> **Bleph-10 Ophthalmic Ointment** apply 1/2 inch qid and HS x 7-14 days
> *Pediatric:* <2 years: <u>not</u> recommended; ≥2 years: same as adult
> *Ophth oint:* 10% (3.5 gm) (phenylmercuric acetate)

SYSTEMIC AGENTS
➤ ***tetracycline*** (G) 250 mg qid x 7 days
Pediatric: <8 years: <u>not</u> recommended; ≥8 years, <100 lb: 25-50 mg/kg/day in 2-4 divided doses x 7-10 days; ≥100 lb: same as adult; *see* Appendix BB.31. *tetracycline* (G) (Sumycin Suspension) *for dose by weight*
> **Achromycin V** *Cap:* 250, 500 mg
> **Sumycin** *Tab:* 250, 500 mg; *Cap:* 250, 500 mg; *Oral susp:* 125 mg/5 ml (100, 200 ml) (fruit) (sulfites)

BLEPHAROPTOSIS, ACQUIRED (DROOPY EYELID)

DIRECT-ACTING ALPHA-ADRENERGIC RECEPTOR AGONIST
➤ ***oxymetazoline hydrochloride ophthalmic solution, 0.1%*** instill 1 drop into 1 <u>or</u> both ptotic eye(s) once daily
Pediatric: <u>not</u> established
> **Upneeq** *Ophth soln:* 0.1% (0.3 ml; 15, 30 single-patient-use containers in a foil pouch within a child-resistant zipper bag/carton)

(continued)

Comment: Upneeq *(oxymetazoline hydrochloride ophthalmic solution, 0.1%)* is a novel, once-daily ophthalmic formulation of *oxymetazoline*. The most common adverse reactions (incidence 1%-5%) have been punctate keratitis, conjunctival hyperemia, dry eye, blurred vision, instillation site pain, eye irritation, and headache. Alpha-adrenergic agonists as a class may impact blood pressure. Advise patients with cardiovascular disease, orthostatic hypotension, and/or uncontrolled hypertension or hypotension to seek medical care if their condition worsens. Use with caution in patients with cerebral or coronary insufficiency or Sjögren's syndrome and advise patients to seek medical care if signs and symptoms of potentiation of vascular insufficiency develop. Advise patients to seek immediate medical care if pain, redness, blurred vision, and photophobia occur (signs and symptoms of acute angle closure). There are no available data on Upneeq in pregnant females to inform a drug-associated risk of major birth defects and miscarriage. No clinical data are available to assess the amount of *oxymetazoline* present in human breast milk post-dose. Developmental and health benefits of breastfeeding should be considered along with the mother's clinical need for Upneeq and any potential adverse effects on the breastfed infant.

BOWEL RESECTION WITH PRIMARY ANASTOMOSIS

▷ *alvimopan* administer 12 mg 30 minutes to 5 hours prior to surgery; then 12 mg bid for up to 7 days; max 15 doses
Pediatric: <18 years: not established; ≥18 years: same as adult
Entereg *Cap:* 12 mg
Comment: Entereg is a peripherally acting μ-opioid receptor antagonist indicated to accelerate the time to upper and lower gastrointestinal recovery following partial large or small bowel resection surgery with primary anastomosis. Therapeutic doses of opioids for more than 7 consecutive days prior to Entereg is contraindicated. A higher number of myocardial infarctions were reported in patients treated with *alvimopan* 0.5 mg bid compared with placebo in a 12-month study of patients treated with opioids for chronic pain, although a causal relationship has not been established. Entereg is not recommended for patients with severe hepatic impairment and end-stage renal disease (ESRD). Dosage adjustment is not required in patients with mild-to-severe renal impairment but they should be monitored for adverse effects. The most common adverse reactions (incidence ≥3%) in patients undergoing bowel resection were anemia, dyspepsia, hypokalemia, back pain, and urinary retention. Entereg is available only for short-term (15 doses) use in hospitalized patients, and only hospitals that have registered in and met all of the requirements for the ENTEREG Access Support and Education (E.A.S.E.) program may use Entereg.

BRONCHIOLITIS

Inhaled Beta-2 Agonists (Bronchodilators) *see Asthma*
Oral Beta-2 Agonists (Bronchodilators) *see Asthma*
Inhaled Corticosteroids *see Asthma*
Parenteral Corticosteroids *see* Appendix L. Parenteral Corticosteroids
Oral Corticosteroids *see* Appendix K. Oral Corticosteroids

BRONCHITIS: ACUTE AND ACUTE EXACERBATION OF CHRONIC BRONCHITIS (AECB)

Comment: Antibiotics are seldom needed for the treatment of acute bronchitis because the etiology is usually viral.
Inhaled Beta-2 Agonists (Bronchodilators) *see Asthma*
Oral Beta-2 Agonists (Bronchodilators) *see Asthma*
Decongestants *see* Appendix Z. Drugs for the Management of Allergy, Cough, and Cold Symptoms online at https://connect.springerpub.com/content/reference-book/978-0-8261-7935-7/back-matter/part02/back-matter/bmatter27
Expectorants *see* Appendix Z. Drugs for the Management of Allergy, Cough, and Cold Symptoms online at https://connect.springerpub.com/content/reference-book/978-0-8261-7935-7/back-matter/part02/back-matter/bmatter27
Antitussives *see* Appendix Z. Drugs for the Management of Allergy, Cough, and Cold Symptoms online at https://connect.springerpub.com/content/reference-book/978-0-8261-7935-7/back-matter/part02/back-matter/bmatter27

ANTI-INFECTIVES FOR SECONDARY BACTERIAL INFECTION

▷ *amoxicillin* (G) 500-875 mg bid or 250-500 mg tid x 10 days
Pediatric: <40 kg (88 lb): 20-40 mg/kg/day in 3 divided doses x 10 days or 25-45 mg/kg/day in 2 divided doses x 10 days; ≥40 kg: same as adult; *see* Appendix BB.3. *amoxicillin* (G) (Amoxil Suspension, Trimox Suspension) *for dose by weight*

Amoxil *Cap:* 250, 500 mg; *Tab:* 875*mg; *Chew tab:* 125, 200, 250, 400 mg (cherry-banana-peppermint) (phenylalanine); *Oral susp:* 125, 250 mg/5 ml (80, 100, 150 ml) (strawberry); 200, 400 mg/5 ml (50, 75, 100 ml) (bubble gum); *Oral drops:* 50 mg/ml (30 ml) (bubble gum)

Moxatag *Tab:* 775 mg ext-rel

Trimox *Tab:* 125, 250 mg; *Cap:* 250, 500 mg; *Oral susp:* 125, 250 mg/5 ml (80, 100, 150 ml) (raspberry-strawberry)

➤ *amoxicillin+clavulanate* (G)

Augmentin 500 mg tid or 875 mg bid x 7-10 days
Pediatric: 40-45 mg/kg/day divided tid x 10 days or 90 mg/kg/day divided bid x 10 days; *see* Appendix BB.4. *amoxicillin+clavulanate* (G) (Augmentin Suspension) *for dose by weight*
Tab: 250, 500, 875 mg; *Chew tab:* 125, 250 mg (lemon-lime); 200, 400 mg (cherry-banana) (phenylalanine); *Oral susp:* 125 mg/5 ml (banana), 250 mg/5 ml (75, 100, 150 ml) (orange); 200, 400 mg/5 ml (50, 75, 100 ml) (orange) (phenylalanine)
Augmentin ES-600 not recommended for adults
Pediatric: <3 months: not recommended; ≥3 months, <40 kg: 90 mg/kg/day in 2 divided doses x 7-10 days; ≥40 kg: not recommended
Oral susp: 42.9 mg/5 ml (50, 75, 100, 125, 150, 200 ml) (strawberry cream) (phenylalanine)
Augmentin XR 2 tabs q 12 hours x 7-10 days
Pediatric: <16 years: use other forms; ≥16 years: same as adult
Tab: 1,000*mg ext-rel

➤ *ampicillin* 250-500 mg qid x 10 days
Pediatric: not recommended for bronchitis in children
Omnipen, Principen *Cap:* 250, 500 mg; *Oral susp:* 125, 250 mg/5 ml (100, 150, 200 ml) (fruit)

➤ *azithromycin* (G) 500 mg x 1 dose on day 1, then 250 mg daily on days 2-5 or 500 mg once daily x 3 days or 2 gm in a single dose
Pediatric: not recommended for bronchitis in children
Zithromax *Tab:* 250, 500, 600 mg; *Oral susp:* 100 mg/5 ml (15 ml); 200 mg/5 ml (15, 22.5, 30 ml) (cherry); *Pkt:* 1 gm for reconstitution (cherry-banana)
Zithromax Tri-Pak *Tab:* 3 x 500 mg tabs/pck
Zithromax Z-Pak *Tab:* 6 x 250 mg tabs/pck
Zmax *Oral susp:* 2 gm ext-rel for reconstitution (cherry-banana) (148 mg Na⁺)

➤ *cefaclor* (G)

Ceclor 250 mg tid or 375 mg bid 3-10 days
Pediatric: <1 month: not recommended; 1 month-12 years: 20-40 mg/kg divided bid or q 12 hours x 3-10 days; max 1 gm/day; *see* Appendix BB.8. *cefaclor* (G) (Ceclor Suspension) *for dose by weight;* >12 years: same as adult
Tab: 500 mg; *Cap:* 250, 500 mg; *Susp:* 125 mg/5 ml (75, 150 ml) (strawberry), 187 mg/5 ml (50, 100 ml) (strawberry), 250 mg/5 ml (75, 150 ml) (strawberry), 375 mg/5 ml (50, 100 ml) (strawberry)
Ceclor Extended Release 375-500 mg bid x 3-10 days
Pediatric: <16 years: ext-rel not recommended; ≥16 years: same as adult
Tab: 375, 500 mg ext-rel

➤ *cefadroxil* 1-2 gm in 1-2 divided doses x 10 days
Pediatric: 30 mg/kg/day in 2 divided doses x 10 days; *see* Appendix BB.9. *cefadroxil* (G) (Duricef Suspension) *for dose by weight*
Duricef *Tab:* 1 gm; *Cap:* 500 mg; *Oral susp:* 250 mg/5 ml (100 ml); 500 mg/5 ml (75, 100 ml) (orange-pineapple)

➤ *cefdinir* 300 mg bid x 5-10 days or 600 mg daily x 10 days
Pediatric: <6 months: not recommended; 6 months-12 years: 14 mg/kg/day in 1-2 divided doses x 10 days; ≥12 years: same as adult; *see* Appendix BB.10. *cefdinir* (G) (Omnicef Suspension) *for dose by weight*
Omnicef *Cap:* 300 mg; *Oral susp:* 125 mg/5 ml (60, 100 ml) (strawberry)

➤ *cefditoren pivoxil* 400 mg bid x 10 days
Pediatric: <12 years: not recommended; ≥12 years: same as adult
Spectracef *Tab:* 200 mg
Comment: Spectracef is contraindicated with milk protein allergy or carnitine deficiency.

➤ *cefixime* (G)
Pediatric: <6 months: not recommended; ≥6 months-12 years, <50 kg: 8 mg/kg/day in 1-2 divided doses x 10 days; ≥12 years, >50 kg: same as adult; *see* Appendix BB.11. *cefixime* (G) (Suprax Oral Suspension) *for dose by weight*
Suprax *Tab:* 400 mg; *Cap:* 400 mg; *Oral susp:* 100, 200, 500 mg/5 ml (50, 75, 100 ml) (strawberry)

➤ *cefpodoxime proxetil* 200 mg bid x 10 days
Pediatric: <2 months: not recommended; ≥2 months-12 years: 10 mg/kg/day (max 400 mg/dose) or 5 mg/kg/day bid (max 200 mg/dose) x 10 days; >12 years: same as adult; *see* Appendix BB.12. *cefpodoxime proxetil* (C) (Vantin Suspension) *for dose by weight*
Vantin *Tab:* 100, 200 mg; *Oral susp:* 50, 100 mg/5 ml (50, 75, 100 mg) (lemon creme)

(continued)

▷ *cefprozil* 500 mg q 12 hours x 10 days
  Pediatric: <2 years: not recommended; 2-12 years: 15 mg/kg q 12 hours x 10 days; *see* Appendix BB.13.
  cefprozil (G) (Cefzil Suspension) *for dose by weight;* >12 years: same as adult
      Cefzil *Tab:* 250, 500 mg; *Oral susp:* 125, 250 mg/5 ml (50, 75, 100 ml) (bubble gum) (phenylalanine)
▷ *ceftibuten* 400 mg daily x 10 days
  Pediatric: 9 mg/kg daily x 10 days; max 400 mg/day; *see* Appendix BB.14. *ceftibuten* (G) (Cedax Suspension)
  for dose by weight
      Cedax *Cap:* 400 mg; *Oral susp:* 90 mg/5 ml (30, 60, 90, 120 ml); 180 mg/5 ml (30, 60, 120 ml) (cherry)
▷ *ceftriaxone* (G) 1-2 gm IM daily continued 2 days after signs of infection have disappeared; max 4 gm/day
  Pediatric: 50 mg/kg IM daily and continued 2 days after clinical stability
      Rocephin *Vial:* 250, 500 mg; 1, 2 gm
▷ *cephalexin* (G) 250-500 mg qid or 500 mg bid x 10 days
  Pediatric: 25-50 mg/kg/day in 4 divided doses x 10 days; ≥12 years: same as adult; *see* Appendix BB.15.
  cephalexin (G) (Keflex Suspension) *for dose by weight*
      Keflex *Cap:* 250, 333, 500, 750 mg; *Oral susp:* 125, 250 mg/5 ml (100, 200 ml) (strawberry)
▷ *clarithromycin* (G) 500 mg bid or 500 mg ext-rel once daily x 7 days
  Pediatric: <6 months: not recommended; ≥6 months: 7.5 mg/kg bid x 7 days; *see* Appendix BB.17.
  clindamycin (G) (Cleocin Pediatric Granules) *for dose by weight;* ≥12 years: same as adult
      Biaxin *Tab:* 250, 500 mg
      Biaxin Oral Suspension *Oral susp:* 125, 250 mg/5 ml (50, 100 ml) (fruit-punch)
      Biaxin XL *Tab:* 500 mg ext-rel
▷ *dirithromycin* (G) 500 mg daily x 7 days
  Pediatric: <12 years: not recommended; ≥12 years: same as adult
      Dynabac *Tab:* 250 mg
▷ *doxycycline* (G) 100 mg bid x 10 days
  Pediatric: <8 years: not recommended; ≥8 years, <100 lb: 2 mg/lb on the first day in 2 divided doses,
  followed by 1 mg/lb/day in 1-2 divided doses; ≥8 years, ≥100 lb: same as adult; *see* Appendix BB.19.
  doxycycline (G) (Vibramycin Syrup/Suspension) *for dose by weight*
      Acticlate *Tab:* 75, 150**mg
      Adoxa *Tab:* 50, 75, 100, 150 mg ent-coat
      Doryx *Tab:* 50, 75, 100, 150, 200 mg del-rel
      Doxteric *Tab:* 50 mg del-rel
      Monodox *Cap:* 50, 75, 100 mg
      Oracea *Cap:* 40 mg del-rel
      Vibramycin *Tab:* 100 mg; *Cap:* 50, 100 mg; *Syr:* 50 mg/5 ml (raspberry-apple) (sulfites); *Oral susp:* 25
      mg/5 ml (raspberry)
      Vibra-Tab *Tab:* 100 mg film-coat
▷ *erythromycin ethylsuccinate* (G) 400 mg qid x 7 days
  Pediatric: 30-50 mg/kg/day in 4 divided doses x 7 days; may double dose with severe infection; max 100
  mg/kg/day; *see* Appendix BB.21. erythromycin ethylsuccinate (G) (E.E.S. Suspension, Ery-Ped Drops/
  Suspension) *for dose by weight*
      EryPed *Oral susp:* 200 mg/5 ml (100, 200 ml) (fruit), 400 mg/5 ml (60, 100, 200 ml) (banana); *Oral*
      drops: 200, 400 mg/5 ml (50 ml) (fruit); *Chew tab:* 200 mg wafer (fruit)
      E.E.S. *Oral susp:* 200, 400 mg/5 ml (100 ml) (fruit)
      E.E.S. Granules *Oral susp:* 200 mg/5 ml (100, 200 ml) (cherry)
      E.E.S. 400 Tablets *Tab:* 400 mg
▷ *gemifloxacin* 320 mg daily x 5 days
  Pediatric: <18 years: not recommended; ≥18 years: same as adult
      Factive *Tab:* 320*mg
▷ *levofloxacin* Uncomplicated: 500 mg daily x 7 days; *Complicated:* 750 mg daily x 7 days
  Pediatric: <18 years: not recommended; ≥18 years: same as adult
      Levaquin *Tab:* 250, 500, 750 mg
▷ *loracarbef* 200-400 mg bid x 7 days
  Pediatric: 30 mg/kg/day in 2 divided doses x 7 days; ≥12 years: same as adult; *see* Appendix BB.27. *loracarbef*
  (G) (Lorabid Suspension) *for dose by weight*
      Lorabid *Pulvule:* 200, 400 mg; *Oral susp:* 100 mg/5 ml (50, 100 ml); 200 mg/5 ml (50, 75, 100 ml)
      (strawberry bubble gum)
▷ *moxifloxacin* (G) 400 mg daily x 5 days
  Pediatric: <18 years: not recommended; ≥18 years: same as adult
      Avelox *Tab:* 400 mg; *IV soln:* 400 mg/250 mg (latex-free, preservative-free)
▷ *ofloxacin* (G) 400 mg bid x 10 days
  Pediatric: <18 years: not recommended; ≥18 years: same as adult
      Floxin *Tab:* 200, 300, 400 mg
▷ *telithromycin* 800 mg once daily x 7-10 days; *Severe renal impairment including dialysis:* 600 mg once daily;
  Severe renal impairment with coexisting hepatic impairment: 400 mg once daily

Pediatric: <18 years: <u>not</u> recommended; ≥18 years: same as adult

    Ketek *Tab:* 400, 500 mg

Comment: *Telithromycin* is a ketolide indicated for the treatment of mild-to-moderate community acquired pneumonia (CAP). Fatal acute liver injury has been reported; discontinue immediately if signs and symptoms of hepatitis occur. There is increased risk for ventricular arrhythmias, including ventricular tachycardia and *torsades de pointes* with fatal outcomes; avoid use in patients with known QT prolongation, hypokalemia, and with class IA and III antiarrhythmics. Fatalities with *colchicine*, rhabdomyolysis with HMG-CoA reductase inhibitors (statins), and hypotension with calcium channel blockers (CCBs) have been reported; therefore, avoid concomitant use. Monitor for toxicity and consider dose reduction of the concomitant medication if concomitant use is unavoidable. Evaluate for *Clostridioides difficile* if diarrhea occurs. Contraindications include myasthenia gravis, concomitant **cisapride** <u>or</u> **pimozide**, and history of hepatitis <u>or</u> jaundice with any macrolide.

▶ *tetracycline* **(G)** 250-500 mg qid x 7 days

Pediatric: <8 years: <u>not</u> recommended; ≥8 years, <100 lb: 25-50 mg/kg/day in 2-4 divided doses x 7 days; ≥8 years, ≥100 lb: same as adult; *see* Appendix BB.31. *tetracycline* (G) (Sumycin Suspension) *for dose by weight*

    Achromycin V *Cap:* 250, 500 mg

    Sumycin *Tab:* 250, 500 mg; *Cap:* 250, 500 mg; *Oral susp:* 125 mg/5 ml (100, 200 ml) (fruit) (sulfites)

▶ *trimethoprim+sulfamethoxazole (TMP-SMX)* **(G)** bid x 10 days

Pediatric: <2 months: <u>not</u> recommended; ≥2 months: 40 mg/kg/day of *sulfamethoxazole* in 2 divided doses bid x 10 days; *see* Appendix BB.33. *trimethoprim+sulfamethoxazole* (G) (Bactrim Suspension, Septra Suspension) *for dose by weight;* ≥12 years: same as adult

    Bactrim, Septra 2 tabs bid x 10 days

      Tab: trim 80 mg+sulfa 400 mg*

    Bactrim DS, Septra DS 1 tab bid x 10 days

      Tab: trim 160 mg+sulfa 800 mg*

    Bactrim Pediatric Suspension, Septra Pediatric Suspension

      Oral susp: trim 40 mg+sulfa 200 mg per 5 ml (100 ml) (cherry) (alcohol 0.3%)

BRONCHITIS: CHRONIC/CHRONIC OBSTRUCTIVE PULMONARY DISEASE (COPD)

Oral Beta-2 Agonists (Bronchodilators) *see Asthma*
Inhaled Corticosteroids *see Asthma*
Parenteral Corticosteroids *see* Appendix L. Parenteral Corticosteroids
Oral Corticosteroids *see* Appendix K. Oral Corticosteroids
Inhaled Beta-2 Agonists (Bronchodilators) *see Asthma*

LONG-ACTING INHALED BETA-2 AGONIST (LABA)

▶ *indacaterol* inhale contents of one 75 mcg cap daily

Pediatric: <12 years: <u>not</u> recommended; ≥12 years: same as adult

    Arcapta Neohaler *Neohaler Device/Cap:* 75 mcg pwdr for inhalation (5 blister cards, 6 caps/card)

Comment: Remove cap from blister cap immediately before use. For oral inhalation with **Neohaler** device <u>only</u>. **Indacaterol** is indicated for the long-term maintenance treatment of bronchoconstriction in patients with chronic obstructive pulmonary disease (COPD). <u>Not</u> indicated for treating asthma, for primary treatment of acute symptoms, <u>or</u> for acute deterioration of COPD.

▶ *indacaterol+glycopyrrolate* inhale the contents of one cap bid

Pediatric: <18 years: <u>not</u> recommended; ≥18 years: same as adult

    Utibron Neohaler *Neohaler Device/Cap:* inda 27.5 mcg+glyco 15.6 mcg pwdr for inhalation (1, 10 blister cards, 6 caps/card)

▶ *olodaterol* 12 mcg q 12 hours

Pediatric: <12 years: <u>not</u> recommended; ≥12 years: same as adult

    Striverdi Respimat *Inhal soln:* 2.5 mcg/cartridge (metered actuation) (40 gm, 60 metered actuations) (benzalkonium chloride)

▶ *salmeterol* **(G)** 1 inhalation q 12 hours

Pediatric: <4 years: <u>not</u> recommended; ≥4 years: same as adult

    Serevent Diskus *Diskus (pwdr):* 50 mcg/actuation (60 doses/diskus)

INHALED ANTICHOLINERGICS

▶ *glycopyrrolate inhalation solution*

    Lonhala Magnair administer the contents of 1 vial via Magnair handset

      Vial: 25 mcg/ml (1 ml) unit dose for use with Magnair handset; *Starter kit:* 60 unit-dose vials w. Magnair handset; *Refill kit:* 60 unit-dose vials w. Magnair handset

Comment: For oral inhalation <u>only</u>. Do <u>not</u> swallow **Lonhala** solution. <u>Only</u> use **Lonhala** vials with **Magnair**. Do <u>not</u> initiate in acutely deteriorating COPD <u>or</u> to treat acute symptoms. If paradoxical bronchospasm occurs, discontinue **Lonhala Magnair** immediately and institute alternative therapy. Worsening of narrow-angle glaucoma may occur; use with caution in patients with narrow-angle

(continued)

glaucoma and instruct patients to contact a physician immediately if symptoms occur. Worsening of urinary retention may occur. Use with caution in patients with prostatic hyperplasia (benign prostatic hyperplasia [BPH]) or bladder neck obstruction (BNO) and instruct patients to consult a physician immediately if symptoms occur. Avoid administration with other anticholinergic drugs. Consider risk versus benefit in patients with severe renal impairment. The most common adverse reactions (incidence ≥2.0%) are dyspnea and urinary tract infection. There are no adequate and well-controlled studies in pregnancy. **Lonhala Magnair** should only be used during pregnancy if the expected benefit to the patient outweighs the potential risk to the fetus. There are no data on the presence of *glycopyrrolate* or its metabolites in human milk or effects on the breastfed infant. The developmental and health benefits of breastfeeding should be considered along with the mother's clinical need for **Lonhala Magnair** and any potential adverse effects on the breastfed infant from **Lonhala Magnair** or from the underlying maternal condition.

Seebri Neohaler inhale the contents of 1 capsule bid at the same time of day, AM and PM, using the Neohaler; do not swallow caps
> *Pediatric:* not indicated
>> *Inhal cap:* 15.6 mcg (60/blister pck) dry pwdr for inhalation w. 1 Neohaler device (lactose)

▷ *ipratropium bromide* (G)
> *Pediatric:* <12 years: not recommended; ≥12 years: same as adult
>> **Atrovent** 2 inhalations qid; max 12 inhalations/day
>>> *Inhaler:* 14 gm (200 inh)
>> **Atrovent Inhalation Solution** 500 mcg by nebulizer tid-qid
>>> *Inhal soln:* 0.02% (2.5 ml)
> **Comment:** *Ipratropium bromide* is contraindicated with severe hypersensitivity to milk proteins.

▷ *umeclidinium* 1 inhalation once daily at the same time each day
> *Pediatric:* <12 years: not recommended; ≥12 years: same as adult
>> **Incruse Ellipta** *Inhal pwdr:* 62.5 mcg/inhalation (30 doses) (lactose)
>> **Comment:** Incruse Ellipta is contraindicated with allergy to *atropine* or its derivatives.

INHALED LONG-ACTING ANTICHOLINERGICS (LAA) (ANTIMUSCARINICS)

Comment: Inhaled long-acting anticholinergics (LAA) are for prophylaxis and chronic treatment, only. Not for primary (rescue) treatment of acute attack. Avoid getting powder in the eyes. Caution with narrow-angle glaucoma, BPH, BNO, and pregnancy. Contraindicated with allergy to atropine or its derivatives (e.g., *ipratropium*). Avoid other anticholinergic agents.

▷ *aclidinium bromide* 1 inhalation bid using inhaler
> *Pediatric:* <12 years: not recommended; ≥12 years: same as adult
>> **Tudorza Pressair** *Inhal device:* 400 mcg/actuation (60 doses per inhalation device)

▷ *glycopyrrolate inhalation solution* administer the contents of 1 vial bid at the same time of day, AM and PM, via the **Magnair** neb inhal device; do not swallow solution; do not use **Magnair** with any other medicine; length of treatment is 2-3 minutes; do not use 2 vials/treatment or more than 2 vials/day
> *Pediatric:* not indicated
>> **Lonhala Magnair** *Vial:* 25 mcg/ml (1 ml) unit dose for use with **Magnair** handset; *Starter kit:* 60 unit-dose vials w. **Magnair** handset; *Refill kit:* 60 unit-dose vials (low-density polyethylene [LDPE]) w. **Magnair** handset (preservative-free)
>> **Comment:** Lonhala Magnair is the first nebulizing long-acting muscarinic antagonist (LAMA) approved for the treatment of COPD in the United States. Its approval was based on data from clinical trials in the Glycopyrrolate for Obstructive Lung Disease via Electronic Nebulizer (GOLDEN) program, including GOLDEN-3 and GOLDEN-4, two phase 3, 12-week, randomized, double-blind, placebo-controlled, parallel-group, multicenter studies. Do not initiate **Lonhala Magnair** in acutely deteriorating COPD or to treat acute symptoms. If paradoxical bronchospasm occurs, discontinue **Lonhala Magnair** immediately and institute alternative therapy. Worsening of narrow-angle glaucoma may occur; use with caution in patients with narrow-angle glaucoma and instruct patients to contact a physician immediately if symptoms occur. Worsening of urinary retention may occur. Use with caution in patients with prostatic hyperplasia (BPH) or BNO and instruct patients to seek medical care immediately if symptoms occur. Avoid administration with other anticholinergic drugs. Consider risk versus benefit in patients with severe renal impairment. The most common adverse reactions (incidence ≥2.0%) have been dyspnea and urinary tract infection. There are no adequate and well-controlled studies in pregnancy. **Lonhala Magnair** should only be used during pregnancy if the expected benefit to the patient outweighs the potential risk to the fetus. There are no data on the presence of *glycopyrrolate* or its metabolites in human milk or effects on the breastfed infant. The developmental and health benefits of breastfeeding should be considered along with the mother's clinical need for **Lonhala Magnair** and any potential adverse effects on the breastfed infant from **Lonhala Magnair** or from the underlying maternal condition.

▷ *revefenacin inhalation solution* administer the contents of 1 vial via nebulizer once daily at the same time of day; do not swallow solution; do not use more than 1 vial/day; do not use **Yupelri** with any other medicine
> *Pediatric:* not indicated
>> **Yupelri** *Vial:* 175 mcg/3 ml (3 ml) unit-dose solution for nebulizer

Comment: Yupelri is the first and only LAMA solution for once-daily nebulized administration. **Yupelri** is indicated for maintenance treatment of moderate-to-severe COPD. Do not initiate **Yupelri** in acutely deteriorating COPD or to treat acute symptoms. If paradoxical bronchospasm occurs, discontinue **Yupelri** immediately and institute alternative therapy. Worsening of narrow-angle glaucoma may occur; use with caution in patients with narrow-angle glaucoma and instruct patients to contact a healthcare provider immediately if symptoms occur. Use with caution in patients with prostatic hyperplasia or BNO and instruct patients to contact a healthcare provider immediately if symptoms occur. May interact additively with other concomitantly used anticholinergic medications; avoid administration of **Yupelri** with other anticholinergic-containing drugs. Co-administration of **Yupelri** with OATP1B1 and OATP1B3 inhibitors (e.g., *rifampicin, cyclosporine*) may lead to an increase in exposure of the active metabolite; co-administration with **Yupelri** is not recommended. Avoid use of **Yupelri** in patients with hepatic impairment. The most common adverse reactions (incidence ≥2%) include cough, nasopharyngitis, upper respiratory tract infection, headache, and back pain. There are no adequate and well-controlled studies with **Yupelri** in pregnancy and no information regarding the presence of *revefenacin* in human milk or effects on the breastfed infant.

▷ **tiotropium (as bromide monohydrate)** 1 inhalation daily using inhaler; do not swallow caps
Pediatric: <12 years: not recommended; ≥12 years: same as adult
　Spiriva HandiHaler *Inhal device:* 18 mcg/cap (5, 30, 90 caps w. inhalation device)

INHALED LAMA AND LABA COMBINATION

▷ **aclidinium bromide+formoterol fumarate** one breath-actuated oral inhalation bid (morning and evening)
　Duaklir Pressair *Inhal pwdr:* aclid brom 400 mcg+foro fum 12 mcg per actuation (30, 60 single-use metered doses/Pressair inhaler); remove the Pressair inhaler from the storage bag immediately before use and store the Pressair inhaler inside the sealed bag; discard the bag (and the desiccant sachet inside) and the Pressair inhaler after the marking "0" with a red background is visible in the middle of the dose indicator, when the device is empty and locks out, or 2 months after the date the sealed bag that the inhaler comes in was open, whichever comes first.
　Comment: Duaklir Pressair *(aclidinium bromide+formoterol fumarate)* is a LAMA and long-acting beta-2 agonist (LABA) fixed-dose combination maintenance bronchodilator for the treatment of COPD. **Duaklir Pressair** is not indicated for relief of acute bronchospasm or treatment of asthma. There are no adequate and well-controlled studies of **Duaklir Pressair** or its individual components in pregnancy to inform drug-associated embryo/fetal risks, and there are no available data on presence in human milk or effects on the breastfed infant.

▷ **ipratropium/albuterol** 1 inhalation qid; max 6 inhalations/day
Pediatric: <12 years: not established; ≥12 years: same as adult
　Combivent Respimat *Inhal soln:* ipra 20 mcg+alb 100 mcg per inhalation (4 gm, 120 inhal)
　Comment: Combivent Respimat is contraindicated with *atropine* allergy.

▷ **tiotropium+olodaterol** 2 inhalations once daily at the same time each day; max 2 inhalations/day
Pediatric: <12 years: not recommended; ≥12 years: same as adult
　Stiolto Respimat *Inhal soln:* tio 2.5 mcg+olo 2.5 mcg per actuation (4 gm, 60 inh) (benzalkonium chloride)
　Comment: Stiolto Respimat is not for treatment of asthma, acute bronchospasm, or acutely deteriorating COPD.

▷ **umeclidinium+vilanterol** 1 inhalation once daily at the same time each day
Pediatric: <12 years: not recommended; ≥12 years: same as adult
　Anoro Ellipta *Inhal soln:* ume 62.5 mcg+vila 25 mcg per inhalation (30 doses)
　Comment: Anoro Ellipta is contraindicated with severe hypersensitivity to milk proteins.

INHALED CORTICOSTEROID+LABA COMBINATION

▷ **fluticasone furoate+vilanterol** 1 inhalation 100/25 once daily at the same time each day
Pediatric: <17 years: not recommended; ≥17 years: same as adult
　Breo Ellipta 100/25 *Inhal pwdr:* flu 100 mcg+vil 25 mcg dry pwdr per inhalation (30 doses)
　Breo Ellipta 200/25 *Inhal pwdr:* flu 200 mcg+vil 25 mcg dry pwdr per inhalation (30 doses)
　Comment: Breo Ellipta is contraindicated with severe hypersensitivity to milk proteins.

INHALED CORTICOSTEROID+ANTICHOLINERGIC+LABA COMBINATION

▷ **budesonide+glycopyrrolate +formoterol fumarate** one inhalation bid
　Breztri Aerosphere *Metered Dose Inhal:* fixed-dose aerosol containing budes 160 mcg+glyco 9 mcg+fom fum 4.8 mcg per inhalation
　Comment: Breztri Aerosphere is maintenance therapy for patients with COPD. **Breztri** is not indicated for relief of acute bronchospasm or for treatment of asthma. The most common adverse reactions (incidence ≥2%) have been upper respiratory infection (URI), pneumonia, back pain, oral candidiasis, influenza, muscle spasm, urinary tract infection, cough, sinusitis, and diarrhea. If paradoxical bronchospasm occurs, discontinue **Breztri Aerosphere** and institute alternative therapy. Use with caution in patients with convulsive disorders, thyrotoxicosis, diabetes mellitus, and ketoacidosis. Be alert for hypokalemia and hyperglycemia. Use with caution in patients with cardiovascular disorders because

(continued)

of beta-adrenergic stimulation. Assess for decrease in bone mineral density initially and periodically thereafter. Glaucoma and cataracts may occur with long-term use of inhaled corticosteroids. Worsening of narrow-angle glaucoma may occur; use with caution in patients with narrow-angle glaucoma and instruct patients to contact a healthcare provider immediately if symptoms occur. Consider referral to an ophthalmologist in patients who develop ocular symptoms or who use **Breztri Aerosphere** long term. Worsening of urinary retention may occur; use with caution in patients with prostatic hyperplasia or BNO and instruct patients to contact a healthcare provider immediately if symptoms occur. *Candida albicans* infection of the mouth and pharynx may occur; advise patients to rinse mouth with water without swallowing after inhalation. Potential worsening of infections (e.g., existing tuberculosis; fungal, bacterial, viral, or parasitic infection; ocular herpes simplex); use with caution in patients with these infections. More serious or even fatal course of chickenpox or measles can occur in susceptible patients. There is risk of impaired adrenal function when transferring from systemic corticosteroids. Taper patients slowly from systemic corticosteroids if transferring to **Breztri Aerosphere**. Hypercorticism and adrenal suppression may occur with very high doses or at the regular dose in susceptible persons. *Budesonide* and *formoterol fumarate* systemic exposure may increase in patients with severe hepatic impairment. In patients with severe renal impairment, use should be considered only if the potential benefit of the treatment outweighs the risk.

▷ *fluticasone furoate+umeclidinium+vilanterol* one inhalation once daily
   Trelegy Ellipta flutic furo 100 mcg+umec 62.5 mcg+vilan 25 mcg dry pwdr
   Comment: Trelegy Ellipta is maintenance therapy for patients with COPD, including chronic bronchitis and emphysema, who are receiving fixed-dose *furoate* and *vilanterol* for airflow obstruction and to reduce exacerbations, or receiving *umeclidinium* and a fixed-dose combination of *fluticasone furoate* and *vilanterol*. Trelegy Ellipta is the first FDA-approved once-daily single-dose inhaler that combines *fluticasone furoate*, a corticosteroid, *umeclidinium*, a LAMA, and *vilanterol*, a long-acting beta-2 adrenergic agonist. Common adverse reactions reported with **Trelegy Ellipta** included headache, back pain, dysgeusia, diarrhea, cough, oropharyngeal pain, and gastroenteritis. **Trelegy Ellipta** has been found to increase the risk of pneumonia in patients with COPD and increase the risk of asthma-related death in patients with asthma. **Trelegy Ellipta** is not indicated for treatment of acute bronchospasm.

METHYLXANTHINES
Comment: Check serum theophylline level just before the fifth dose is administered. Therapeutic theophylline level is 10-20 mcg/ml.

▷ *theophylline* (G)
   Theo-24 initially 300-400 mg once daily at HS; after 3 days, increase to 400-600 mg once daily at HS; max 600 mg/day
   Pediatric: <45 kg: initially 12-14 mg/kg/day; max 300 mg/day; increase after 3 days to 16 mg/kg/day to max 400 mg; after 3 more days, increase to 30 mg/kg/day to max 600 mg/day; ≥45 kg: same as adult
      Cap: 100, 200, 300, 400 mg ext-rel
   Theo-Dur initially 150 mg bid; increase to 200 mg bid after 3 days; then increase to 300 mg bid after 3 more days
   Pediatric: <6 years: not recommended; ≥6-15 years: initially 12-14 mg/kg/day in 2 divided doses; max 300 mg/day; then increase to 16 mg/kg in 2 divided doses; max 400 mg/day; then to 20 mg/kg/day in 2 divided doses; max 600 mg/day
      Tab: 100, 200, 300 mg ext-rel
   Theolair-SR
   Pediatric: <12 years: not recommended; ≥12 years: same as adult
   Tab: 200, 250, 300, 500 mg sust-rel
   Uniphyl 400-600 mg daily with meals
   Pediatric: <12 years: not recommended; ≥12 years: same as adult
      Tab: 400*, 600*mg cont-rel

METHYLXANTHINE+EXPECTORANT COMBINATION
▷ *dyphylline+guaifenesin*
   Lufyllin GG 1 tab qid or 15-30 ml qid
      Tab: dyphy 200 mg+guaif 200 mg; *Elix:* dyphy 100 mg+guaif 100 mg per 15 ml

SELECTIVE PHOSPHODIESTERASE 4 (PDE4) INHIBITOR
▷ *roflumilast* (G) 500 mcg once daily
   Pediatric: <12 years: not recommended; ≥12 years: same as adult
      Daliresp *Tab:* 500 mcg
   Comment: *Roflumilast* is indicated to reduce the risk of COPD exacerbations in severe COPD patients with chronic bronchitis and a history of exacerbations.

LONG-ACTING MUSCARINIC ANTAGONISTS (LAMA)
▷ *glycopyrrolate*
Comment: There are no data on the safety of *glycopyrrolate* use in pregnancy or presence of *glycopyrrolate* or its metabolites in human milk or effects on the breastfed infant.

Lonhala Magnair inhale the contents of 1 vial bid at the same time of day, AM and PM, via Magnair neb inhal device; do not swallow solution; do not use **Magnair** with any other medicine; length of treatment is 2-3 minutes; do not use 2 vials/treatment or more than 2 vials/day
Pediatric: not indicated for use in children
Neb soln: Vial: 25 mcg/1 ml single-dose for administration with Magnair neb inhal device; *Starter kit:* 30-day supply 2 vials/pouch, 30 foil pouches/carton and one complete Magnair Nebulizer System; *Refill kit:* 2 vials/pouch, 30 foil pouches/carton and one complete Magnair refill handset
Comment: Lonhala Magnair is the first nebulizing LAMA approved for the treatment of COPD in the United States. Its approval was based on data from clinical trials in the GOLDEN program, including GOLDEN-3 and GOLDEN-4, two phase 3, 12-week, randomized, double-blind, placebo-controlled, parallel-group, multicenter studies.
Seebri Neohaler inhale the contents of 1 capsule bid at the same time of day, AM and PM, using the Neohaler; do not swallow caps
Pediatric: not indicated for use in children
    Inhal cap: 15.6 mcg (60/blister pck) dry pwdr for inhalation w. one Neohaler device (lactose)

BULIMIA NERVOSA

SELECTIVE SEROTONIN REUPTAKE INHIBITOR (SSRI)
▷ *fluoxetine* (G)
    Prozac initially 20 mg daily; may increase after 1 week; doses >20 mg/day may be divided into AM and noon doses; usual daily dose 60 mg; max 80 mg/day
    Pediatric: <8 years: not recommended; 8-17 years: initially 10-20 mg/day; start lower weight children at 10 mg/day; if starting at 10 mg daily, may increase after 1 week to 20 mg daily; >17 years: same as adult
        Cap: 10, 20, 40 mg; *Tab:* 30*, 60*mg; *Oral soln:* 20 mg/5 ml (4 oz) (mint)
    Prozac Weekly following daily *fluoxetine* therapy at 20 mg/day for 13 weeks, may initiate **Prozac Weekly** 7 days after the last 20 mg *fluoxetine* dose
    Pediatric: <12 years: not recommended; ≥12 years: same as adult
        Cap: 90 mg ent-coat del-rel pellets

BURN: MAJOR

▷ *anacaulase-bcdb*
    Pediatric: safety and efficacy not established
    NexoBrid *Topical gel:* 8.8%; supplied as (1) one vial of 2 gm lyophilized pwdr (containing *anacaulase-bcdb* 1.94 gm) plus one jar of gel vehicle 20 gm (co-packaged per carton); (2) one vial of 5 gm lyophilized pwdr (containing *anacaulase-bcdb* 4.85 gm) plus one jar of gel vehicle 50 gm (co-packaged per carton)
    Comment: NexoBrid is a concentrate of proteolytic enzymes indicated for removal of eschar in adults with deep partial- and severe full-thickness thermal burns in adults (bromelain-based enzymatic debridement). The active substance in NexoBrid is a mixture of enzymes extracted from the stem of the pineapple plant. This mixture of enzymes acts as a debriding agent, a substance used to remove dead tissue (eschar from areas of the skin, such as burn wounds, by dissolving the burn wound eschar). NexoBrid is approved in the European Union and other international markets and has been designated as an orphan biologic drug in the United States, European Union, and other international markets. The safety and effectiveness of NexoBrid have not been established for the treatment of chemical or electrical burns; burns on the face, perineum, or genitalia; burns on the feet of patients with diabetes mellitus or on the feet of patients with occlusive vascular disease; circumferential burns; and burns in patients with significant cardiopulmonary disease, including inhalation injury. NexoBrid is not recommended for the treatment of burn wounds where medical devices or vital structures could become exposed during eschar removal. NexoBrid is not recommended for wounds contaminated with radioactive and other hazardous substances to avoid unforeseeable reactions with the product and an increased risk of spreading the noxious substance. NexoBrid is contraindicated in patients with known hypersensitivity to *anacaulase-bcdb*, bromelain (a component of *anacaulase-bcdb*), pineapples, or to any other components, and known hypersensitivity to papayas or papain due to the risk of cross-sensitivity. The most common adverse reactions (>10%) have been pruritus and pyrexia. Clinical studies of NexoBrid did not include a sufficient number of subjects 65 years of age and older to determine whether they respond differently from younger adult subjects. NexoBrid is not recommended for the treatment of burn wounds where medical devices or vital structures could become exposed during eschar removal. Serious hypersensitivity reactions, including anaphylaxis, have been reported with postmarketing use of *anacaulase-bcdb*. Avoid use of NexoBrid in patients with uncontrolled disorders of coagulation. Use with caution in patients on anticoagulant therapy or other drugs affecting coagulation, and in patients with low platelet counts and increased risk of bleeding from other causes. Monitor patients for possible signs of coagulation abnormalities and

(continued)

signs of bleeding. Manage pain as appropriate for an extensive dressing change of burn wounds. At least 15 minutes prior to **NexoBrid**-related procedures, ensure adequate pain control measures are in place. There are no available data on **NexoBrid** use in pregnancy to evaluate for a drug-associated risk of major birth defects, miscarriage, or other adverse maternal or fetal outcomes. No significant developmental toxicities were observed in animal studies. There are no data on the presence of *anacaulase-bcdb* in either human or animal milk or effects on the breastfed infant. The developmental and health benefits of breastfeeding should be considered along with the mother's clinical need for **NexoBrid** and any potential adverse effects on the breastfed infant from **NexoBrid** or from the underlying maternal condition.

BURN: MINOR

▷ *silver sulfadiazine* (G) apply topically to burn 1-2 x daily
   Pediatric: <12 years: not recommended; ≥12 years: same as adult
      Silvadene *Crm:* 1% (20, 50, 85, 400, 1,000 gm jar; 20 gm tube)
   Comment: *Silver sulfadiazine* is contradicted in sulfa allergy.

TOPICAL AND TRANSDERMAL ANESTHETICS
Comment: *Lidocaine* should not be applied to non-intact skin.
▷ *lidocaine* cream apply to affected area bid prn
   Pediatric: <12 years: not recommended; ≥12 years: same as adult
      LidaMantle *Crm:* 3% (1, 2 oz)
      Lidoderm *Crm:* 3% (85 gm)
      ZTlido topical system 1% (30/carton)
      Comment: Compared to Lidoderm (*lidocaine* patch 5%), which contains 700 mg/patch, ZTlido only requires 35 mg per topical system to achieve the same therapeutic dose.
▷ *lidocaine* lotion apply to affected area bid prn
   Pediatric: <12 years: not recommended; ≥12 years: same as adult
      LidaMantle *Lotn:* 3% (177 ml)
▷ *lidocaine 5% patch* (G) apply up to 3 patches at one time for up to 12 hours/24-hour period (12 hours on/12 hours off); patches may be cut into smaller sizes before removal of the release liner; do not reuse
   Pediatric: <12 years: not recommended; ≥12 years: same as adult
      Lidoderm *Patch:* 5% (10 × 14 cm; 30/carton)
▷ *lidocaine+dexamethasone*
   Pediatric: <12 years: not recommended; ≥12 years: same as adult
      Decadron Phosphate With Xylocaine *Lotn:* dexa 4 mg+lido 10 mg per ml (5 ml)
▷ *lidocaine+hydrocortisone* (G) apply to affected area bid prn
   Pediatric: <12 years: not recommended; ≥12 years: same as adult
      LidaMantle HC *Crm:* lido 3%+hydro 0.5% (1, 3 oz); *Lotn:* (177 ml)
▷ *lidocaine 2.5%+prilocaine 2.5%* apply sparingly to the burn bid-tid prn
   Pediatric: <12 years: not recommended; ≥12 years: same as adult
      Emla Cream 5, 30 gm/tube

BURSITIS

Acetaminophen for IV Infusion *see Pain*
NSAIDs *see* NSAIDs online at https://connect.springerpub.com/content/reference-book/978-0-8261-7935-7/back-matter/part02/back-matter/bmatter10
Opioid Analgesics *see Pain*
Topical and Transdermal Analgesics *see Pain*
Parenteral Corticosteroids *see* Appendix L. Parenteral Corticosteroids
Oral Corticosteroids *see* Appendix K. Oral Corticosteroids
Topical Analgesic and Anesthetic Agents *see* Appendix H. Anesthetic Agents for Local Infiltration and Dermal/Mucosal Membrane Application online at https://connect.springerpub.com/content/reference-book/978-0-8261-7935-7/back-matter/part02/back-matter/bmatter9

CANCER: BASAL CELL CARCINOMA (BCC)

PROGRAMMED DEATH RECEPTOR-1 (PD-1)-BLOCKING ANTIBODY
▷ *cemiplimab-rwlc* 350 mg as IV infusion over 30 minutes every 3 weeks
   Pediatric: safety and efficacy not established
      Libtayo *Vial:* 350 mg/7 ml (50 mg/ml), single-dose, soln for dilution and IV infusion
      Comment: Libtayo is indicated for the treatment of (1) patients with locally advanced basal cell carcinoma (laBCC) previously treated with a hedgehog pathway inhibitor or for whom a hedgehog pathway inhibitor

is not appropriate and (2) patients with metastatic basal cell carcinoma (mBCC) previously treated with a hedgehog pathway inhibitor or for whom a hedgehog pathway inhibitor is not appropriate. The most common adverse reactions (incidence ≥15%) have been musculoskeletal pain, fatigue, rash, and diarrhea. The most common grade 3-4 laboratory abnormalities (incidence ≥2%) have been lymphopenia, hyponatremia, hypophosphatemia, increased aspartate aminotransferase, anemia, and hyperkalemia. For infusion-related reactions, interrupt, slow the rate of infusion, or permanently discontinue based on severity of the reaction. Immune-mediated adverse reactions, which may be severe or fatal, can occur in any organ system or tissue, including the following: immune-mediated pneumonitis, immune-mediated colitis, immune-mediated hepatitis, immune-mediated endocrinopathies, immune-mediated dermatologic adverse reactions, immune-mediated nephritis and renal dysfunction, and solid organ transplant rejection. Monitor for early identification and management. Evaluate liver enzymes, creatinine, and thyroid function at baseline and periodically during treatment. Withhold or permanently discontinue **Libtayo** based on the severity of reaction. Fatal and other serious complications can occur in patients who receive allogeneic hematopoietic stem cell transplantation (HSCT) before or after being treated with a programmed death receptor-1 (PD-1)/programmed death-ligand 1 (PD-L1)-blocking antibody. Based on its mechanism of action, **Libtayo** can cause embryo/fetal harm when administered to a pregnant female. Animal studies have demonstrated that inhibition of the PD-1/PD-L1 pathway can lead to increased risk of immune-mediated rejection of the developing fetus, resulting in fetal death. Advise women of the potential risk and advise males and females of reproductive potential to use effective contraception during treatment with **Libtayo** and for at least 4 months after the last dose. There is no information regarding the presence of *cemiplimab-rwlc* in human milk or its effects on the breastfed infant. Because of the potential for serious adverse reactions in breastfed infants, advise mothers not to breastfeed during treatment and for at least 4 months after the last dose.

CANCER: BLADDER, UROTHELIAL CARCINOMA

NECTIN-4-DIRECTED ANTIBODY AND MICROTUBULE INHIBITOR CONJUGATE

▷ *enfortumab vedotin-ejfv* 1.25 mg/kg (max 125 mg) via IV infusion over 30 minutes on days 1, 8, and 15 of a 28-day cycle until disease progression or unacceptable toxicity; for IV infusion only; do not administer as an IV push or bolus; do not mix with, or administer as an infusion with, other medicinal products; *Moderate/Severe hepatic impairment:* avoid use

Padcev Vial: 20, 30 mg, single-dose, pwdr for reconstitution, dilution, and IV infusion

Comment: **Padcev** is indicated for the treatment of adult patients with locally advanced or metastatic urothelial cancer who have previously received a programmed death receptor-1 (PD-1) or programmed death-ligand 1 (PD-L1) inhibitor, and a platinum-containing chemotherapy in the neoadjuvant/adjuvant, locally advanced or metastatic setting. This indication is approved under accelerated approval based on tumor response rate. Continued approval for this indication may be contingent upon verification and description of clinical benefit in confirmatory trials. Concomitant use of strong CYP3A4 inhibitors with **Padcev** may increase the exposure to monomethyl auristatin E (MMAE). The most common adverse reactions (incidence ≥20%) have been fatigue, peripheral neuropathy, decreased appetite, rash, alopecia, nausea, dysgeusia, diarrhea, dry eye, pruritus, and dry skin. Diabetic ketoacidosis (DKA) may occur in patients with and without preexisting diabetes mellitus, which may be fatal. Closely monitor blood glucose (BG) levels in patients with or at risk of diabetes mellitus or hyperglycemia. Withhold **Padcev** if BG >250 mg/dL. Monitor patients for new or worsening peripheral neuropathy and consider dose interruption, dose reduction, or discontinuation of **Padcev** as appropriate. Consider prophylactic artificial tears for dry eyes and treatment with ophthalmic topical steroids after an ophthalmic exam. Monitor for ocular disorders, including vision changes, and consider dose interruption or dose reduction of **Padcev** when symptomatic ocular disorders occur. Skin reactions may occur; if severe, withhold **Padcev** until improvement or resolution. Ensure adequate venous access prior to beginning the infusion and monitor the infusion site. Stop the infusion immediately for suspected extravasation. **Padcev** can cause embryo/fetal harm; therefore, advise women to use effective contraception. Because of the potential for serious adverse reactions in the breastfed infant, advise women not to breastfeed during treatment with **Padcev** and for at least 3 weeks after the last dose.

HUMAN PD-1 (PROGRAMMED DEATH RECEPTOR-1)-BLOCKING ANTIBODY

▷ *pembrolizumab* administer 200 mg via IV infusion once every 3 weeks or 400 mg via IV infusion once every 6 weeks until disease progression, unacceptable toxicity, or for **Keytruda** up to 24 months; administer **Keytruda** prior to chemotherapy when given on the same day

Pediatric: safety and efficacy not established

Keytruda Vial: 100 mg/4 ml (25 mg/ml) single-dose, soln for dilution and IV infusion

Comment: **Keytruda** is a PD-1-blocking antibody indicated for the treatment of multiple cancers, including patients with urothelial carcinoma. **Keytruda**, in combination with *enfortumab vedotin*, is indicated for the treatment of adult patients with locally advanced or metastatic urothelial carcinoma who are not eligible for *cisplatin*-containing chemotherapy. This indication is approved under accelerated approval based on tumor response rate and durability of response. Continued approval

(continued)

for this indication may be contingent upon verification and description of clinical benefit in the confirmatory trials. **Keytruda**, as a single agent, is indicated for the treatment of patients with locally advanced or metastatic urothelial carcinoma (1) who are not eligible for any platinum-containing chemotherapy or (2) who have disease progression during or following platinum-containing chemotherapy or within 12 months of neoadjuvant or adjuvant treatment with platinum-containing chemotherapy. **Keytruda**, as a single agent, is also indicated for the treatment of patients with Bacillus Calmette-Guerin (BCG)-unresponsive, high-risk, non-muscle invasive bladder cancer (NMIBC) with carcinoma in situ (CIS) with or without papillary tumors who are ineligible for or have elected not to undergo cystectomy. **Keytruda** can cause fetal harm. Exclude pregnancy prior to initiating treatment with Keytruda. Advise females of reproductive potential of the embryo/fetal risk and to use effective contraception and for 4 months after the last **Keytruda** dose. Advise mothers not to breastfeed during treatment and for 4 months after the last **Keytruda** dose. See mfr pkg insert for full prescribing information including storage, preparation, warnings, precautions, drug-drug interactions, and adverse reactions.

CANCER: BREAST

NON-STEROIDAL ANTI-ESTROGEN AGENTS
▷ *fulvestrant* (G) 250 mg IM once monthly; administer 2.5 ml IM in each buttock concurrently
    Faslodex *Prefilled syringe:* 50 mg/ml (2 x 2.5 ml, 1 x 5 ml)
▷ *letrozole* (G) 2.5 mg daily
    Femara *Tab:* 2.5 mg film-coat

PROGRAMMED DEATH RECEPTOR-1 (PD-1)-BLOCKING ANTIBODY
▷ *pembrolizumab administer* 200 mg via IV infusion over 30 minutes once every 3 weeks or 400 mg via IV infusion once every 6 weeks until disease progression, unacceptable toxicity, or for **Keytruda** up to 24 months; administer **Keytruda** prior to chemotherapy when given on the same day
Pediatric: safety and efficacy not established
    Keytruda *Vial:* 100 mg/4 ml (25 mg/ml), single-dose, soln for dilution and IV infusion
    Comment: Keytruda is a programmed death receptor-1 (PD-1)-blocking antibody indicated for the treatment of multiple cancers, including patients with breast cancer. **Keytruda** is indicated for the treatment of patients with high-risk, early-stage, triple-negative breast cancer (TNBC) in combination with chemotherapy as neoadjuvant treatment, and then continued as a single agent as adjuvant treatment after surgery. **Keytruda**, in combination with chemotherapy, is indicated for the treatment of patients with locally recurrent unresectable or metastatic TNBC whose tumors express programmed death-ligand 1 (PD-L1) (combined positive score [CPS] ≥10) as determined by an FDA-approved test. **Keytruda** can cause fetal harm. Exclude pregnancy prior to initiating treatment with **Keytruda**. Advise females of reproductive potential of the embryo/fetal risk and to use effective contraception. Advise mothers not to breastfeed during treatment and for 4 months after the last **Keytruda** dose. See mfr pkg insert for full prescribing information including storage, preparation, warnings, precautions, drug-drug interactions, and adverse reactions.

KINASE INHIBITORS
▷ *abemaciclib Starting dose in combination with fulvestrant or an aromatase inhibitor:* 150 mg bid; *Starting dose as monotherapy:* 200 mg bid; dosing interruption and/or dose reductions may be required based on individual safety and tolerability
Pediatric: <18 years: not recommended; >18 years: same as adult
    Verzenio *Tab:* 50, 100, 150, 200 mg
    Comment: Verzenio, a kinase inhibitor, has been approved for use in early breast cancer for certain patients. One expert has described the drug as the first advance for this patient population in 20 years. *Abemaciclib* had already been approved for use in the treatment of hormone receptor (HR)-positive, human epidermal growth factor receptor 2 (HER2)-negative advanced or metastatic breast cancer. Now it is also approved for use in HR-positive, HER2-negative early breast cancer for patients who have high-risk, node-positive disease and whose tumors have a Ki-67 score of ≥20%, as determined by a U.S. FDA-approved test. The FDA also approved the Ki-67 IHC MIB-1 pharmDx (Dako Omnis) assay for use. **Verzenio** is indicated (1) in combination with endocrine therapy (*tamoxifen* or an *aromatase inhibitor*) for the adjuvant treatment of adult patients with HR-positive, HER2-negative, node-positive, early breast cancer at high risk of recurrence and a Ki-67 score ≥20% as determined by an FDA-approved test; (2) in combination with an *aromatase inhibitor* as initial endocrine-based therapy for the treatment of postmenopausal women, and men, with HR-positive, HER2-negative advanced or metastatic breast cancer; (3) in combination with *fulvestrant* for the treatment of adult patients with HR-positive, HER2-negative advanced or metastatic breast cancer with disease progression following endocrine therapy; and (4) as monotherapy for the treatment of adult patients with HR-positive, HER2-negative

advanced or metastatic breast cancer with disease progression following endocrine therapy and prior chemotherapy in the metastatic setting. The most common adverse reactions (incidence ≥20%) have been diarrhea, neutropenia, nausea, abdominal pain, infections, fatigue, anemia, leukopenia, decreased appetite, vomiting, headache, alopecia, and thrombocytopenia. **Verzenio** can cause severe cases of diarrhea, associated with dehydration and infection. Instruct patients at the first sign of loose stools to initiate antidiarrheal therapy and increase oral fluids. Neutropenia may occur. Monitor complete blood counts (CBCs) prior to the start of **Verzenio** therapy, every 2 weeks for the first 2 months, monthly for the next 2 months, and as clinically indicated. Interstitial lung disease (ILD) and/or pneumonitis can occur. Severe and fatal cases of ILD/pneumonitis have been reported. Monitor for clinical symptoms or radiologic changes indicative of ILD/pneumonitis. Permanently discontinue **Verzenio** in all patients with grade 3 or 4 ILD or pneumonitis. Hepatotoxicity can occur. Increases in serum transaminase levels have been observed. Obtain liver function tests (LFTs) before initiating treatment with **Verzenio** and monitor LFTs every 2 weeks for the first 2 months, and monthly for the next 2 months, and as clinically indicated. Venous thromboembolism can occur: Monitor patients for signs and symptoms of thrombosis and pulmonary embolism (PE) and treat as medically appropriate. Avoid concomitant use of *ketoconazole* with CYP3A inhibitors. Reduce the **Verzenio** dose with concomitant use of other strong and moderate CYP3A inhibitors. Avoid concomitant use of strong and moderate CYP3A inducers with **Verzenio**. There are no available human data informing the drug-associated risk in human pregnancy. However, based on findings in animal studies and its mechanism of action, **Verzenio** is embryo toxic in human pregnancy. In animal reproduction studies, administration of *abemaciclib* during organogenesis is teratogenic and causes decreased fetal weight at maternal exposures similar to human clinical exposure based on area under the curve (AUC) at the maximum recommended human dose. Advise pregnant women of the potential risk to the fetus. Exclude pregnancy prior to initiating treatment with **Verzenio**. Advise patients of reproductive potential of risk to the fetus and to use effective contraception. Advise not to breastfeed during treatment with **Verzenio** and for at least 3 weeks after the last dose. **Verzenio** may impair fertility in males of reproductive potential. To report suspected adverse reactions, contact Eli Lilly at 1-800-LillyRx (1-800-545-5979) or FDA at 1-800-FDA-1088 or www.fda.gov/medwatch.

▷ *alpelisib* recommended dose is 300 mg (2 x 150 mg tablets) as a single dose once daily; take with food
   Pediatric: safety and efficacy not established
   Piqray *Tab:* 50, 150, 200 mg film-coat
   Comment: Piqray *(alpelisib)* is a kinase inhibitor indicated in combination with fulvestrant for the treatment of postmenopausal women, and men, with HR-positive, HER2-negative, PIK3CA-mutated, advanced, or metastatic breast cancer as detected by an FDA-approved test following progression on or after an endocrine-based regimen. Piqray is the first FDA-approved PI3K inhibitor for breast cancer treatment. The most common adverse reactions, including laboratory abnormalities (all grades, incidence ≥20%), have been increased sGLU and sCr, decreased lymphocyte count, increased GGT and ALT, decreased hemoglobin, increased lipase, stomatitis, loss of appetite, nausea, vomiting, diarrhea, weight loss, fatigue, decreased calcium, prolonged aPTT, and alopecia. For adverse reactions, consider dose interruption, dose reduction, or discontinuation. For a severe hypersensitivity reaction, permanently discontinue Piqray and promptly initiate appropriate treatment. Severe cases of pneumonitis and ILD have been reported. Do not initiate treatment in patients with a history of SJS, EM, or toxic epidermal necrolysis (TEN), and permanently discontinue Piqray if SJS, EM, or TEN is confirmed. Safety of Piqray in patients with type 1 or uncontrolled type 2 diabetes has not been established. Before initiating treatment, test fasting plasma glucose (FPG) and HbA1c, and optimize sGLU. Avoid co-administration of Piqray with strong CYP3A4 inducers and breast cancer resistance protein (BCRP) inhibitors. Closely monitor when Piqray is co-administered with CYP2C9 substrates as these drugs may reduce Piqray activity. Piqray is used in combination with *fulvestrant*. Exclude pregnancy prior to initiating treatment with Piqray and *fulvestrant* and advise females of reproductive potential to use effective contraception during treatment and for 1 week after the last dose. Advise male patients with female partners of reproductive potential to use condoms and effective contraception during treatment and for 1 week after the last dose. There are no data on the presence of *alpelisib* in human milk or effects on the breastfed infant. Advise lactating women to not breastfeed during treatment with Piqray and for 1 week after the last dose.

▷ *lapatinib ditosylate* (G) *Recommended dose:* Tykerb: 1,250 mg (5 tablets) once daily on days 1 through 21 continuously; take *in combination* with *capecitabine* 2,000 mg/m²/day (administered in 2 doses approximately 12 hours apart) on days 1 through 14 in a repeating 21-day cycle; Tykerb should be taken at least 1 hour before or 1 hour after a meal; *capecitabine* should be taken with food or within 30 minutes after food; Tykerb should be taken as a single dose once daily; do not divide daily doses of Tykerb; modify dose for cardiac and other toxicities, severe hepatic impairment, and CYP3A4 drug interactions
   Pediatric: safety and efficacy not established
   Tykerb *Tab:* 250 mg
   Comment: Tykerb is a kinase inhibitor indicated in combination with *capecitabine* for treatment of patients with advanced or metastatic breast cancer whose tumors overexpress HER2 and who have received prior therapy including an *anthracycline*, a taxane, and a *trastuzumab*. The most common (incidence >20%) adverse reactions during treatment with Tykerb plus *capecitabine* have been

(continued)

diarrhea, palmar-plantar erythrodysesthesia, nausea, rash, vomiting, and fatigue. Decreases in left ventricular ejection fraction (LVEF) have been reported. Confirm normal LVEF before starting Tykerb and continue evaluations during treatment. Tykerb dose reduction in patients with severe hepatic impairment should be considered. Diarrhea, including severe diarrhea, has been reported during treatment; manage with antidiarrheal agents and replace fluids and electrolytes if severe. *Lapatinib* prolongs the QT interval in some patients; consider ECG and electrolyte monitoring. Tykerb is likely to increase exposure to concomitantly administered drugs which are metabolized by CYP3A4 or CYP2C8; avoid strong CYP3A4 inhibitors. If unavoidable, consider dose reduction of Tykerb in patients co-administered a strong CYP3A4 inhibitor. Avoid strong CYP3A4 inducers. If unavoidable, consider gradual dose increase of Tykerb in patients co-administered a strong CYP3A4 inducer. There are no adequate and well-controlled studies with Tykerb in human pregnancy. However, animal studies have demonstrated serious adverse developmental effects on the fetus and spontaneous abortion. Exclude pregnancy prior to starting treatment with Tykerb. Females of reproductive potential should be advised of the risks to the fetus and to use effective contraception as it is not advisable to become pregnant during treatment with Tykerb. If the patient does become pregnant during treatment with Tykerb, immediately discontinue the drug. It is not known whether *lapatinib* is excreted in human milk. Because of the potential for serious adverse effects on breastfed infants from Tykerb, a decision should be made whether to discontinue breastfeeding or discontinue Tykerb, considering the importance of the drug to the mother. To report suspected adverse reactions, contact GlaxoSmithKline at 888-825-5249 or FDA at 1-800-FDA-1088 or www.fda.gov/medwatch.

▷ *sodium neratinib*
Antidiarrheal prophylaxis: initiate **loperamide** with the first dose of **Nerlynx** and continue during the first 56 days of treatment; after day 56, use **loperamide** to maintain 1-2 bowel movements per day
Extended adjuvant treatment of early-stage breast cancer: 240 mg (6 tablets) once daily, with food, continuously until disease recurrence for up to 1 year
Advanced or metastatic breast cancer: 240 mg (6 tablets) once daily with food on days 1-21 of a 21-day cycle plus *capecitabine* (750 mg/m² bid) on days 1-14 of a 21-day cycle until disease progression or unacceptable toxicity; dose interruptions and/or dose reductions are recommended based on individual safety and tolerability
Hepatic impairment: reduce starting dose to 80 mg
Pediatric: safety and efficacy not established
    Nerlynx *Tab:* 40 mg
    Comment: Nerlynx *(neratinib)* is a tyrosine kinase inhibitor (TKI) indicated (1) as a single agent for the extended adjuvant treatment of adult patients with early stage HER2-positive breast cancer, to follow adjuvant trastuzumab-based therapy; and (2) in combination with *capecitabine* treatment of adult patients with advanced or metastatic HER2-positive breast cancer who have received two or more prior anti-HER2-based regimens in the metastatic setting. The most common adverse reactions (incidence ≥5%) have been (1) *Nerlynx as a single agent:* diarrhea, nausea, abdominal pain, fatigue, vomiting, rash, stomatitis, decreased appetite, muscle spasms, dyspepsia, increased aspartate aminotransferase (AST) or ALT, nail disorder, dry skin, abdominal distention, epistaxis, decreased weight, and urinary tract infection; and (2) *Nerlynx in combination with capecitabine:* diarrhea, nausea, vomiting, decreased appetite, constipation, fatigue/asthenia, decreased weight, dizziness, back pain, arthralgia, urinary tract infection, upper respiratory tract infection, abdominal distention, renal impairment, and muscle spasms.
▷ *tucatinib* 300 mg bid; *Severe hepatic impairment:* 200 mg bid; take with or without food
Pediatric: safety and efficacy not established
    Tukysa *Tab:* 50, 150 mg
    Comment: Tukysa *(tucatinib)* is a potent TKI for the treatment of patients with locally advanced or metastatic HER2-positive breast cancer. The most common adverse reactions (incidence ≥20%) have been diarrhea, palmar-plantar erythrodysesthesia, nausea, fatigue, hepatotoxicity, vomiting, stomatitis, decreased appetite, abdominal pain, headache, anemia, and rash. Severe diarrhea, including dehydration, acute kidney injury, and death have been reported. Administer antidiarrheal treatment as clinically indicated. Severe hepatotoxicity has been reported. Monitor ALT, AST, and bilirubin prior to starting Tukysa, every 3 weeks during treatment and as clinically indicated. Based on adverse reaction severity, interrupt dose and then restart at reduced dose, or permanently discontinue Tukysa as indicated. Avoid concomitant use of strong CYP3A inducers or moderate CYP2C8 inducers. Avoid concomitant use of strong CYP2C8 inhibitors; reduce Tukysa dose if concomitant use cannot be avoided. Avoid concomitant use of Tukysa with CYP3A substrates, where minimal concentration changes may lead to serious or life-threatening toxicities. Consider reducing the dose of P-gp substrates, where minimal concentration changes may lead to serious or life-threatening toxicities. Tukysa can cause fetal harm. Advise patients of potential risk to the fetus and to use effective contraception. Advise not to breastfeed and for at least 1 week after last Tukysa dose. Refer to the respective *trastuzumab* and *capecitabine* mfr pkg inserts for adverse reactions, drug interactions, and pregnancy, contraception, and breastfeeding information.

POLY(ADP-RIBOSE) POLYMERASE (PARP) INHIBITOR

▷ *olaparib* 400 mg bid; with or without food; continue treatment until disease progression or unacceptable toxicity; *Adverse side effects (ASEs):* consider dose interruption or dose reduction; *CrCl 31-50 ml/min:* 300 mg bid
Pediatric: safety and efficacy not established
  Lynparza *Tab:* 100, 150 mg; *Cap:* 50 mg
  Comment: Lynparza is indicated for the treatment of adult patients with deleterious or suspected deleterious gBRCAm, HER2-negative metastatic breast cancer who have been treated with chemotherapy in the neoadjuvant, adjuvant, or metastatic setting. Patients with HR-positive breast cancer should have been treated with a prior endocrine therapy or be considered inappropriate for endocrine therapy. Select patients for therapy based on an FDA-approved companion diagnostic for **Lynparza.** Myelodysplastic syndrome/acute myeloid leukemia (MDS/AML) has occurred in <1.5% of patients exposed to **Lynparza** monotherapy and the majority of events had a fatal outcome. Monitor patients for hematologic toxicity at baseline and monthly thereafter. Discontinue if MDS/AML is confirmed. Pneumonitis has occurred in <1% of patients exposed to **Lynparza** and some cases have been fatal. Interrupt treatment if pneumonitis is suspected and discontinue if pneumonitis is confirmed. Avoid concomitant use of strong or moderate CYP3A inhibitors. If the inhibitor cannot be avoided, reduce the dose. Avoid concomitant use of strong or moderate CYP3A inducers as decreased efficacy can occur. The most common adverse reactions (incidence ≥20%) in clinical trials have been anemia, nausea, fatigue (including asthenia), vomiting, nasopharyngitis/upper respiratory tract infection/influenza, diarrhea, arthralgia/myalgia, dysgeusia, headache, dyspepsia, decreased appetite, constipation, and stomatitis. The most common laboratory abnormalities (incidence ≥25%) have been decrease in hemoglobin, increase mean corpuscular volume (MCV), decrease in lymphocytes, decrease in leukocytes, decrease in absolute neutrophil count, increase in serum creatinine, and decrease in platelets. **Lynparza** can cause embryo/fetal harm. Exclude pregnancy prior to initiation and advise females of reproductive potential to use effective contraception during and for 6 months after the last dose. Males with female partners should use effective contraception and not donate sperm during and for 3 months after last dose. Advise women not to breastfeed during and for 1 month after the last dose.

▷ *talazoparib* recommended dose 1 mg once daily if unacceptable toxicity occurs; for adverse reactions, consider dose interruption or dose reduction; *CrCl 30-59 ml/min:* 0.75 mg once daily without food; treat until disease progression
Pediatric: <18 years: not recommended; >18 years: same as adult
  Talzenna *Cap:* 0.25, 1 mg
  Comment: Talzenna *(talazoparib)* is a poly(ADP-ribose) polymerase (PARP) inhibitor indicated for the treatment of adult patients with deleterious or suspected deleterious germline BRCA-mutated (gBRCAm) HER2-negative, locally advanced or metastatic breast cancer. Select patients for therapy based on an FDA-approved companion diagnostic for **Talzenna.** The most common (incidence ≥20%) adverse reactions of any grade were fatigue, anemia, nausea, neutropenia, headache, thrombocytopenia, vomiting, alopecia, diarrhea, and decreased appetite. The most common laboratory abnormalities (incidence ≥25%) were *decreases* in hemoglobin, platelets, neutrophils, lymphocytes, leukocytes, and calcium and *increases* in glucose, alanine aminotransferase, aspartate aminotransferase, and alkaline phosphatase. Reduce **Talzenna** dose with certain P-gp inhibitors. Monitor for potential increased adverse reactions with concomitant BCRP inhibitors. There are no available data on **Talzenna** use in pregnant females to inform drug-associated embryo/fetal risk. However, animal studies have demonstrated embryo/fetal harm. Breastfeeding is not advisable.

HER2/NEU RECEPTOR ANTAGONISTS

▷ *margetuximab-cmkb Initial dose:* 15 mg/kg via IV infusion over 120 minutes; then 15 mg/kg via IV infusion over a minimum of 30 minutes every 3 weeks
  Margenza *Vial:* 250 mg/10 ml (25 mg/ml), single-dose
  Comment: Margenza *(margetuximab-cmkb)* is indicated, in combination with chemotherapy, for the treatment of adult patients with metastatic HER2-positive breast cancer who have received two or more prior anti-HER2 regimens, at least one of which was for metastatic disease. **Margenza** is an Fc-engineered, monoclonal antibody that targets the HER2 oncoprotein. HER2 is expressed by tumor cells in breast, gastroesophageal, and other solid tumors. Similar to *trastuzumab, margetuximab-cmkb* inhibits tumor cell proliferation, reduces shedding of the HER2 extracellular domain, and mediates antibody-dependent cellular cytotoxicity (ADCC). The most common adverse drug reactions (incidence ≥10%) with **Margenza,** in combination with chemotherapy, have beeen fatigue/asthenia, nausea, diarrhea, vomiting, constipation, headache, pyrexia, alopecia, abdominal pain, peripheral neuropathy, arthralgia/myalgia, cough, decreased appetite, dyspnea, infusion-related reactions (IRRs), palmar-plantar erythrodysesthesia, and extremity pain. **Margenza** can cause IRRs. Symptoms may include fever, chills, arthralgia, cough, dizziness, fatigue, nausea, vomiting, headache, diaphoresis, tachycardia, hypotension, pruritus, rash, urticaria, and dyspnea. Monitor patients during and after **Margenza** infusion. Have medications and emergency equipment to treat IRRs available for immediate use. In patients experiencing mild-to-moderate IRRs, decrease rate of infusion and consider premedications, including

(continued)

antihistamines, corticosteroids, and antipyretics. Monitor patients until symptoms completely resolve. Interrupt **Margenza** infusion in patients experiencing dyspnea or clinically significant hypotension and intervene with supportive medical therapy as needed. Permanently discontinue **Margenza** in all patients with severe or life-threatening IRRs. **Margenza** use may lead to reductions in LVEF. Evaluate cardiac function prior to and during treatment. **Margenza** has not been studied in patients with a pretreatment LVEF value of <50%, a history of myocardial infarction or unstable angina within 6 months, or congestive heart failure (CHF) New York Heart Association (NYHA) class II-IV. Withhold **Margenza** for ≥16% absolute decrease in LVEF from pretreatment values or LVEF below institutional limits of normal (or 50% if no limits available) and ≥10% absolute decrease in LVEF from pretreatment values. Permanently discontinue **Margenza** if LVEF decline persists greater than 8 weeks or dosing is interrupted more than 3 times due to LVEF decline. Evaluate cardiac function within 4 weeks prior to, and every 3 months during, and upon completion of treatment. Conduct thorough cardiac assessment, including history, physical examination, and determination of LVEF by echocardiogram or multigated acquisition (MUGA) scan. Monitor cardiac function every 4 weeks if **Margenza** is withheld for significant left ventricular cardiac dysfunction. Based on findings in animal studies and mechanism of action, **Margenza** can cause fetal harm when administered to a pregnant female. Postmarketing studies of other HER2-directed antibodies during pregnancy resulted in cases of oligohydramnios and oligohydramnios sequence manifesting as pulmonary hypoplasia, skeletal abnormalities, and neonatal death. Exclude pregnancy prior to initiation of **Margenza**. Advise pregnant females and females of reproductive potential that exposure to **Margenza** during pregnancy, or within 4 months prior to conception, can result in embryo/fetal harm. Advise women of reproductive potential to use effective contraception during treatment and for 4 months following the last dose of **Margenza**. Advise not to breastfeed.

Trastuzumab Products

Comment: Exposure to *trastuzumab* products during pregnancy can result in embryo/fetal toxicity, including oligohydramnios, in some cases complicated by pulmonary hypoplasia and neonatal death. Exclude pregnancy prior to initiation. Advise patients of these risks and the need for effective contraception. There is no information regarding the presence of *trastuzumab* products in human milk or effects on the breastfed infant. Treatment with a *trastuzumab* product can result in subclinical and clinical cardiac failure manifesting as CHF and decreased LVEF, with the greatest risk when administered concurrently with anthracyclines. Evaluate cardiac function prior to and during treatment. Discontinue for cardiomyopathy, anaphylaxis, angioedema, interstitial pneumonitis, or acute respiratory distress syndrome (ARDS). Monitor patient for exacerbation of chemotherapy-induced neutropenia (CIN). Do not substitute a *trastuzumab* product for or with **Kadcyla** *(ado-trastuzumab emtansine)*. *Adjuvant Breast Cancer Treatment ASEs:* The most common (incidence ≥5%) are headache, diarrhea, nausea, and chills. *Metastatic Breast Cancer Treatment ASEs:* The most common (incidence ≥10%) are fever, chills, headache, infection, CHF, insomnia, cough, and rash.

Dosing of *Trastuzumab* Products:
Adjuvant treatment of HER2-overexpressing breast cancer: Administer initial dose of 4 mg/kg over 90 minutes via IV infusion; then 2 mg/kg over 30 minutes via IV infusion once weekly x 12 weeks (with **paclitaxel** or **docetaxel**) or x 18 weeks (with **docetaxel** and **carboplatin**); then 1 week after the last weekly dose of the *trastuzumab* product, administer 6 mg/kg via IV infusion over 30-90 minutes once every 3 weeks to complete a total of 52 weeks of therapy
or
Administer initial dose of 8 mg/kg over 90 minutes via IV infusion; then 6 mg/kg over 30-90 minutes via IV infusion once every 3 weeks x 52 weeks
Treatment of metastatic HER2-overexpressing breast cancer: Administer initial dose of 4 mg/kg over 90 minutes via IV infusion; then once weekly doses of 2 mg/kg via 30 minute IV infusions

▷ *trastuzumab*
  Herceptin for Injection *Vial:* 150 mg, single-dose; 420 mg multidose, pwdr for reconstitution, dilution, and IV infusion
▷ *trastuzumab-anns*
  Kanjinti *Vial:* 420 mg, multidose (21 mg/ml) pwdr for reconstitution, dilution, and IV infusion
  Comment: Kanjinti is biosimilar to Herceptin *(trastuzumab)*. See Trastuzumab Products above for prescribing information.
▷ *trastuzumab-dkst*
  Ogivri for Injection *Vial:* 420 mg, multidose pwdr for reconstitution, dilution, and IV infusion
  Comment: Ogivri is biosimilar to Herceptin *(trastuzumab)*. See Trastuzumab Products above for prescribing information.
▷ *trastuzumab-dttb*
  Ontruzant for Injection *Vial:* 150 mg single-dose; 420 mg multidose; pwdr for reconstitution, dilution, and IV infusion
  Comment: Ontruzant is biosimilar to Herceptin *(trastuzumab)*. See Trastuzumab Products above for prescribing information.

▷ *trastuzumab-pkrb*
　　Herzuma *Vial:* 420 mg, multidose, pwdr for reconstitution, dilution, and IV infusion
　　Comment: Herzuma is biosimilar to **Herceptin** *(trastuzumab)*. See **Trastuzumab Products** above for prescribing information.
▷ *trastuzumab-qyyp*
　　Adjuvant treatment of HER2-overexpressing breast cancer:
　　　　Administer either:
　　　　Initial dose of 4 mg/kg via IV infusion over 90 minutes; then 2 mg/kg via IV infusion over 30 minutes once weekly x 12 weeks (with *paclitaxel* or *docetaxel*) or 18 weeks (with *docetaxel* and *carboplatin*); 1 week after the last weekly dose of **Trazimera**, administer 6 mg/kg via IV infusion over 30-90 minutes once every 3 weeks to complete a total of 52 weeks of therapy
　　　　　　or
　　　　Initial dose of 8 mg/kg via IV infusion over 90 minutes; then 6 mg/kg via IV infusion over 30-90 minutes once every 3 weeks for a total of 52 weeks of therapy
　　Metastatic HER2-overexpressing breast cancer:
　　　　Initial dose of 4 mg/kg via IV infusion over 90 minutes, followed by subsequent once weekly doses of 2 mg/kg via IV infusions over 30 minutes
　　Metastatic HER2-overexpressing gastric cancer:
　　　　Initial dose of 8 mg/kg via IV infusion over 90 minutes, followed by 6 mg/kg via IV infusion over 30-90 minutes once every 3 weeks
　　Pediatric: safety and efficacy not established
　　　　Trazimera *Vial:* 420 mg, multidose, pwdr for reconstitution and IV infusion
　　Comment: Trazimera is biosimilar to **Herceptin (*trastuzumab*)** indicated for the treatment of HER2-overexpressing breast cancer and the treatment of HER2-overexpressing metastatic gastric or gastroesophageal junction adenocarcinoma. Do not substitute **Trazimera** *(trastuzumab-qyyp)* for or with ***ado-trastuzumab emtansine***. *Trastuzumab* products can cause embryo/fetal harm when administered during pregnancy. Exclude pregnancy prior to initiating treatment with **Trazimera** and advise females of reproductive potential to use effective contraception during treatment and for 7 months following the last dose.

HER2/NEU RECEPTOR ANTAGONIST+ENDOGLYCOSIDASE COMBINATION
▷ *trastuzumab*+hyaluronidase
　　Pediatric: safety and efficacy not established
　　　　Herceptin Hylecta administer a single-dose (600/10,000 in 5 ml) SC over 3–5 minutes once every 3 weeks
　　　　Vial: trastuzumab 600 mg+hyaluronidase 10,000 units/5 ml, single-dose soln
　　Comment: Herceptin Hylecta *(trastuzumab+hyaluronidase-oysk)* is a combination of the approved HER2/neu receptor antagonist *trastuzumab* (Herceptin) and *recombinant human hyaluronidase PH20* (an enzyme that helps to deliver *trastuzumab* under the skin) indicated for the treatment of HER2-overexpressing breast cancer. **Herceptin Hylecta** has different dosage and administration instructions than IV *trastuzumab* products. Do not administer **Herceptin Hylecta** intravenously. Do not substitute **Herceptin Hylecta** for or with *ado-trastuzumab emtansine* or any other *trastuzumab* product. The most common ASEs in the treatment of adjuvant breast cancer (incidence ≥10%) are fatigue, arthralgia, diarrhea, injection site reaction, upper respiratory tract infection, rash, myalgia, nausea, headache, edema, flushing, pyrexia, cough, and pain in extremity. The most common ASEs in the treatment of metastatic breast cancer are based on IV *trastuzumab*) are fever, chills, headache, infection, CHF, insomnia, cough, and rash (incidence ≥10%). Exposure to **Herceptin Hylecta** during pregnancy can result in embryo/fetal toxicity (oligohydramnios, in some cases complicated by pulmonary hypoplasia and neonatal death). Exclude pregnancy prior to initiation and advise patients of these risks and the need for effective contraception. There is no information regarding the presence of *trastuzumab* or hyaluronidase in human milk or effects on the breastfed infant (consider the *trastuzumab* washout period is 7 months).

HER2-DIRECTED ANTIBODY+TOPOISOMERASE INHIBITOR CONJUGATE
▷ *fam-trastuzumab deruxtecan-nxki Recommended dose:* 5.4 mg/kg via IV infusion once every 3 weeks (21-day cycle) until disease progression or unacceptable toxicity
　　Enhertu *Vial:* 100 mg pwdr, single-dose, for reconstitution and IV infusion
　　Comment: Enhertu *(fam-trastuzumab deruxtecan-nxki)* is an HER2-directed antibody and topoisomerase inhibitor conjugate indicated for the treatment of adult patients with unresectable or metastatic HER2-positive breast cancer who have received two or more prior anti-HER2-based regimens in the metastatic setting. This indication is approved under accelerated approval based on tumor response rate and duration of response. Continued approval for this indication may be contingent upon verification and description of clinical benefit in a confirmatory trial. Do not substitute **Enhertu** for or with *trastuzumab* or *ado-trastuzumab emtansine*. For IV infusion only. Do not administer as an IV push or bolus. Do not use Sodium Chloride Injection, USP. Management of adverse reactions

(continued)

to Enhertu (ILD, neutropenia, or left ventricular dysfunction) may require temporary interruption, dose reduction, or discontinuation. Neutropenia may develop. Monitor CBC prior to initiation of and prior to each dose of Enhertu and as clinically indicated. Manage through treatment interruption or dose reduction. Assess LVEF prior to initiation of Enhertu and at regular intervals during treatment as clinically indicated and manage through treatment interruption or discontinuation. Permanently discontinue Enhertu in patients with symptomatic CHF. ILD and pneumonitis, including fatal cases, have been reported with Enhertu. Monitor for, and promptly investigate, signs and symptoms including cough, dyspnea, fever, and other new or worsening respiratory symptoms. Permanently discontinue Enhertu in all patients with grade 2 or higher ILD/pneumonitis. Advise patients of the risk and to immediately report symptoms. Exclude pregnancy prior to initiation of Enhertu as exposure to Enhertu during pregnancy can cause embryo/fetal harm. Advise patients of these risks and the need for effective contraception. There are no data regarding the presence of *fam-trastuzumab deruxtecan-nxki* in human milk or effects on the breastfed infant. Because of the potential for serious adverse reactions in the breastfed infant, advise women not to breastfeed during treatment with Enhertu and for 7 months after the last dose.

TROP-2-DIRECTED ANTIBODY+TOPOISOMERASE INHIBITOR CONJUGATE

▶ *sacituzumab govitecan-hziy* 10 mg/kg via IV infusion once weekly on days 1 and 8 of continuous 21-day treatment cycles until disease progression or unacceptable toxicity; monitor patients during the infusion and for at least 30 minutes after completion of infusion; treatment interruption and/or dose reduction may be needed to manage adverse reactions

Pediatric: safety and efficacy not established

Trodelvy *Vial:* 180 mg, single-dose, pwdr for reconstitution, dilution, and IV infusion

Comment: Trodelvy *(sacituzumab govitecan-hziy)* is a Trop-2-directed antibody and topoisomerase inhibitor conjugate indicated for the treatment of adult patients with metastatic triple-negative breast cancer (mTNBC) who have received at least two prior therapies for metastatic disease. This indication is approved under accelerated approval based on tumor response rate and duration of response. Continued approval for this indication may be contingent upon verification and description of clinical benefit in confirmatory trials. Do not substitute Trodelvy for or use with other drugs containing irinotecan or its active metabolite SN-38. For IV infusion only. Avoid concomitant use of Trodelvy with uridine diphosphate glucuronosyltransferase 1A1 (UGT1A1) inhibitors or inducers. Do not administer as an IV push or bolus. Premedication for prevention of infusion reactions and prevention of chemotherapy-induced nausea and vomiting is recommended. The most common adverse reactions (incidence >25%) in patients with mTNBC are nausea, neutropenia, diarrhea, fatigue, anemia, vomiting, alopecia, constipation, rash, decreased appetite, and abdominal pain. Hypersensitivity reactions including severe anaphylactic reactions have been observed. Monitor patients for IRRs and permanently discontinue Trodelvy if a severe or life-threatening reaction occurs. Use antiemetic preventive treatment and withhold Trodelvy for patients with grade 3 nausea or grade 3-4 vomiting at the time of scheduled treatment. Patients who are homozygous for the UGT1A1*28 allele are at increased risk for neutropenia following initiation of Trodelvy treatment. Trodelvy can cause embryo/fetal harm. Advise females of potential embryo/fetal risk and to use effective contraception during treatment and for 6 months after the last dose. Because of the potential for genotoxicity, advise male patients with female partners of reproductive potential to use effective contraception during treatment and for 3 months after the last dose. Advise females not to breastfeed during treatment and for 1 month after the last dose.

NON-STEROIDAL ANTI-ESTROGEN

▶ *tamoxifen citrate* Ductal carcinoma in situ (DCIS): 20 mg once daily x 5 years; *Reduction in breast cancer incidence in high-risk women:* 20 mg once daily x 5 years

Tab: 10, 20 mg

Comment: *Tamoxifen citrate* is an orally administered non-steroidal antiestrogen. *Tamoxifen* is effective in the treatment of metastatic breast cancer in women and men. In females with DCIS, following breast surgery and radiation, *Tamoxifen* is indicated to reduce the risk of developing invasive breast cancer. *Tamoxifen* is indicated to reduce the incidence of breast cancer in females at high risk for breast cancer (high risk is defined as women at least 35 years of age with a 5-year predicted risk of breast cancer ≥1.67%, as calculated by the Gail Model). For premenopausal women with metastatic breast cancer, *tamoxifen* is an alternative to oophorectomy or ovarian irradiation. Available evidence indicates that patients whose tumors are estrogen receptor-positive are more likely to benefit from *tamoxifen* therapy. *Tamoxifen* is indicated for the treatment of node-positive breast cancer in women following total mastectomy or segmental mastectomy, axillary dissection, and breast irradiation. In some *tamoxifen* adjuvant studies, most of the benefits to date have been in the subgroup with four or more positive axillary nodes. *Tamoxifen* is indicated for treatment of axillary node-negative breast cancer in women following total mastectomy or segmental mastectomy, axillary dissection, and breast irradiation. *Tamoxifen* has demonstrated effectiveness in the palliative treatment of male breast cancer. *Tamoxifen* reduces the occurrence of contralateral breast cancer in patients receiving adjuvant *tamoxifen* therapy for breast cancer. Reduction in recurrence and mortality has been greater in studies using *tamoxifen* for about 5 years than in those that used *tamoxifen* for a shorter period of therapy. Serious and life-threatening events associated with *tamoxifen* in the risk reduction setting (women at high risk for cancer and women with DCIS) include uterine malignancies, stroke, and PE. The benefits of *tamoxifen* outweigh its risks in women already diagnosed with breast cancer. The effects of age, gender, and race on the pharmacokinetics of *tamoxifen* have not been determined. The safety and efficacy of *tamoxifen* in girls aged 2–10 years with McCune–Albright syndrome and precocious puberty have not been studied beyond 1 year of treatment. The effects of reduced liver function on the metabolism and pharmacokinetics of *tamoxifen* have not been determined. *In vitro* studies have shown that *erythromycin, cyclosporin, nifedipine,* and *diltiazem* competitively inhibited the formation of N-desmethyltamoxifen. The clinical significance of these *in vitro* studies is unknown. *Tamoxifen* is contraindicated in females who require concomitant coumarin-type anticoagulant therapy or in females with a history of deep vein thrombosis (DVT) or PE. *Tamoxifen* may cause fetal harm in pregnancy. Patients should be advised not to become pregnant while taking *tamoxifen* or within 2 months of discontinuation and should use barrier or non-hormonal contraceptive measures. *Tamoxifen* does not cause infertility. Patients should be apprised of the potential risks to the fetus, including the potential long-term risk of a DES-like syndrome. (NOTE: Diethylstilbestrol syndrome (DES syndrome) refers to developmental or health problems caused by exposure to DES before birth (*in utero*), such as reproductive tract differences, infertility, and an increased risk for certain cancers. For sexually active patients of childbearing potential, *tamoxifen* should be initiated during menstruation. In patients with menstrual irregularity, a negative B-HCG immediately prior to the initiation of therapy is sufficient. *Tamoxifen* has been reported to inhibit lactation. There are no data that address whether *tamoxifen* is excreted into human milk or effects on the breastfed infant. Due to the potential for serious adverse reactions in breastfed, patients taking *tamoxifen* should not breastfeed. Although adverse reactions to *tamoxifen* are relatively mild and rarely severe enough to require discontinuation, loss of libido and impotence resulting in male discontinuation has been reported. In oligospermic males treated with *tamoxifen,* luteinizing hormone (LH), follicle-stimulating hormone (FSH), testosterone, and estrogen levels were elevated. However, no significant clinical changes have been reported.

SELECTIVE ESTROGEN RECEPTOR DOWN REGULATORS (SERMs)

▷ *elacestrant Recommended dose:* 345 mg, once daily; take with food; *Child-Pugh B:* reduce dose; *Child-Pugh C:* avoid use
Pediatric: Safety and efficacy not established
  Orserdu *Tab:* 86, 345 mg
  Comment: Orserdu is an estrogen receptor antagonist indicated for the treatment of postmenopausal women or adult men with ER-positive, HER2-negative, ESR1-mutated advanced or metastatic breast cancer with disease progression following at least one line of endocrine therapy. Select patients for the treatment with Orserdu based on the presence of ESR1 mutations. Orserdu may cause hypercholesterolemia and hypertriglyceridemia. Monitor lipid profile prior to starting treatment and periodically thereafter. Avoid concomitant use of strong and moderate CYP3A4 inducers and inhibitors with Orserdu. The most common (>10%) adverse reactions, including laboratory abnormalities, have been musculoskeletal pain, nausea, increased cholesterol, increased AST, increased triglycerides, fatigue, decreased hemoglobin, vomiting, increased ALT, decreased sodium, increased creatinine, decreased appetite, diarrhea, headache, constipation, abdominal pain, hot flashes, and dyspepsia. Based on findings in animal studies and its mechanism of action, Orserdu is embryo/fetal toxic. There are no available human data on Orserdu use in human pregnancy to inform the drug-associated risk. However, in animal reproduction and development studies, oral administration of *elacestrant* during organogenesis caused embryo/fetal mortality and structural abnormalities at maternal exposures below the recommended dose based on AUC. Exclude pregnancy prior to initiating Orserdu treatment. Inform pregnant patients of the risk to the fetus. Advise patients of reproductive potential to use effective contraception during treatment and for 1 week after the last dose. Advise mothers not to breastfeed during treatment and for 1 week after the last dose. Advise males and females of reproductive potential that Orserdu may impair fertility. To report suspected adverse reactions, contact Stemline Therapeutics at 1-877-332-7961 or FDA at 1-800-FDA-1088 or www.fda.gov/medwatch.

▷ *toremifene* (G) 60 mg once daily
  Fareston *Tab:* 60 mg
  Comment: Fareston *(toremifene)* is an estrogen agonist/antagonist indicated for the treatment of metastatic breast cancer in postmenopausal women with estrogen-receptor positive or unknown tumors. The most common adverse reactions are hot flashes, sweating, nausea, and vaginal discharge. Fetal harm may occur when administered to a pregnant woman. Women should be advised not to become pregnant when taking Fareston. Females of childbearing potential should use effective non-hormonal contraception during Fareston therapy. Discontinue drug or nursing taking into account the importance of the drug to the mother.

CANCER: CERVICAL

VASCULAR ENDOTHELIAL GROWTH FACTOR (VEGF) INHIBITOR

▶ *bevacizumab-adcd Regimen for persistent, recurrent, or metastatic cervical cancer:* 15 mg/kg every 3 weeks with *paclitaxel* and *cisplatin, or paclitaxel* and *topotecan.* Withhold for at least 28 days prior to elective surgery; do not administer **Vegzelma** for 28 days following major surgery and until adequate wound healing; store refrigerated at 2°C-8°C (36°F-46°F) in the original carton until time of use to protect from light; do not freeze or shake the vial or carton; see mfr pkg insert for full prescribing information including proper preparation and administration instructions and dosage modifications for adverse reactions
Pediatric: <18 years: safety and efficacy not established; ≥18 years: same as adult
  Vegzelma *Vial:* 100 mg/4 ml (25 mg/ml) or 400 mg/16 ml (25 mg/ml), single-dose, soln for dilution and IV infusion
  Comment: Vegzelma is a vascular endothelial growth factor (VEGF) inhibitor biosimilar to **Avastin** indicated for the treatment of multiple types of cancer, including colorectal cancer, non-small cell lung cancer, glioblastoma, renal cell carcinoma, cervical cancer, and epithelial ovarian, fallopian tube, or primary peritoneal cancer. *Bevacizumab* products increase the risk of ovarian failure and may impair fertility. Inform females of reproductive potential of the risk of ovarian failure prior to the first dose of **Vegzelma.** The long-term effects of *bevacizumab* products on fertility are not known. *Bevacizumab* products may cause fetal harm when administered to a pregnant female. Advise females of reproductive potential to use effective contraception during treatment with **Vegzelma** and for 6 months after the last dose. No data are available regarding the presence of *bevacizumab* products in human milk or effects on the breastfed infant. Because of the potential for serious adverse reactions in breastfed infants, advise mothers not to breastfeed during treatment with **Vegzelma** and for 6 months after the last dose. See mfr pkg insert for full prescription information.
▶ *bevacizumab-bvzr* administer 15 mg/kg every 3 weeks via IV infusion with *paclitaxel* and *cisplatin* or *paclitaxel* and *topotecan*; do not administer **Zirabev** for 28 days following major surgery and until the surgical wound is fully healed
  Zirabev *Vial:* 100 mg/4 ml (25 mg/ml), 400 mg/16 ml (25 mg/ml), single-dose
  Comment: Zirabev is biosimilar to **Avastin** *(bevacizumab)* with indications for the treatment of multiple types of cancer with *paclitaxel* and *cisplatin* or *paclitaxel* and *topotecan.*

PROGRAMMED DEATH RECEPTOR-1 (PD-1)-BLOCKING ANTIBODY

▶ *pembrolizumab* administer 200 mg via IV infusion over 30 minutes once q 3 weeks or 400 mg via IV infusion over 30 minutes once q 6 weeks until disease progression, unacceptable toxicity, or for **Keytruda** up to 24 months; administer **Keytruda** prior to chemotherapy with or without *bevacizumab* when given on the same day
Pediatric: safety and efficacy not established
  Keytruda *Vial:* 100 mg/4 ml (25 mg/ml), single-dose, soln for dilution and IV infusion
  Comment: Keytruda is a programmed death receptor-1 (PD-1)-blocking antibody indicated for treatment of multiple cancers, including cervical cancer. **Keytruda**, in combination with chemotherapy, with or without *bevacizumab*, is indicated for the treatment of patients with persistent, recurrent, or metastatic cervical cancer whose tumors express programmed death-ligand 1 (PD-L1; combined positive score [CPS] ≥1) as determined by an FDA-approved test. **Keytruda**, as a single agent, is indicated for the treatment of patients with recurrent or metastatic cervical cancer with disease progression on or after chemotherapy whose tumors express PD-L1 (CPS ≥1) as determined by an FDA-approved test. **Keytruda** can cause fetal harm. Exclude pregnancy prior to initiating treatment with **Keytruda**. Advise females of reproductive potential of the embryo/fetal risk and to use effective contraception during treatment and for 4 months after the last **Keytruda** dose. Advise mothers not to breastfeed during treatment and for 4 months after the last **Keytruda** dose. See mfr pkg insert for full prescribing information including storage, preparation, warnings, precautions, drug-drug interactions, and adverse reactions.

CANCER: COLORECTAL

PROGRAMMED DEATH RECEPTOR-1 (PD-1) BLOCKING ANTIBODY

▶ *pembrolizumab* administer 200 mg via IV infusion over 30 minutes once every 3 weeks or 400 mg via IV infusion over 30 minutes once every 6 weeks until disease progression, unacceptable toxicity, or for **Keytruda** up to 24 months
Pediatric: safety and efficacy not established
  Keytruda *Vial:* 100 mg/4 ml (25 mg/ml), single-dose, soln for dilution and IV infusion
  Comment: Keytruda is a programmed death receptor-1 (PD-1)-blocking antibody indicated for the treatment of multiple cancers, including unresectable or metastatic MSI-H or mismatch repair deficient (dMMR) colorectal cancer (CRC) as determined by an FDA-approved test. (NOTE: MSI-H and dMMR are biomarkers for unresectable or metastatic solid tumors. MSI-H, which stands for microsatellite instability-high, refers to a piece of genetic coding and means there is a lot of instability in the tumor. MSI status is an indicator of how the cancer will behave and helps guide treatment decisions.) **Keytruda**

can cause fetal harm. Exclude pregnancy prior to initiating treatment with **Keytruda**. Advise females of reproductive potential of the embryo/fetal risk and to use effective contraception during treatment and for 4 months after the last **Keytruda** dose. Advise mothers not to breastfeed during treatment and for 4 months after the last **Keytruda** dose. See mfr pkg insert for full prescribing information including storage, preparation, warnings, precautions, drug-drug interactions, and adverse reactions.

VASCULAR ENDOTHELIAL GROWTH FACTOR (VEGF) INHIBITOR

▶ *bevacizumab-adcd Regimen for persistent, recurrent, or metastatic cervical cancer:* 15 mg/kg q 3 weeks with **paclitaxel** and **cisplatin**, or **paclitaxel** and **topotecan**. Withhold for at least 28 days prior to elective surgery; do not administer **Vegzelma** for 28 days following major surgery and until adequate wound healing; store refrigerated at 2°C-8°C (36°F-46°F) in the original carton until time of use to protect from light; do not freeze or shake the vial or carton; see mfr pkg insert for full prescribing information including proper preparation and administration instructions and dosage modifications for adverse reactions
Pediatric: <18 years: safety and efficacy not established; ≥18 years: same as adult
Vegzelma *Vial:* 100 mg/4 ml (25 mg/ml) or 400 mg/16 ml (25 mg/ml), single-dose, soln for dilution and IV infusion
Comment: Vegzelma is a vascular endothelial growth factor (VEGF) inhibitor biosimilar to **Avastin** indicated for the treatment of multiple types of cancer, including colorectal cancer, non-small cell lung cancer, glioblastoma, renal cell carcinoma, cervical cancer, and epithelial ovarian, fallopian tube, or primary peritoneal cancer. *Bevacizumab* products increase the risk of ovarian failure and may impair fertility. Inform females of reproductive potential of the risk of ovarian failure prior to the first dose of **Vegzelma**. The long-term effects of *bevacizumab* products on fertility are not known. *Bevacizumab* products may cause fetal harm when administered to a pregnant female. Advise females of reproductive potential to use effective contraception during treatment with **Vegzelma** and for 6 months after the last dose. No data are available regarding the presence of *bevacizumab* products in human milk or effects on the breastfed infant. Because of the potential for serious adverse reactions in breastfed infants, advise mothers not to breastfeed during treatment with **Vegzelma** and for 6 months after the last dose. See mfr pkg insert for full prescription information.

▶ *bevacizumab-bvzr Option 1:* 5 mg/kg via IV infusion q 2 weeks with bolus-IFL; *Option 2:* 10 mg/kg via IV infusion q 2 weeks with FOLFOX4; *Option 3:* 5 mg/kg via IV infusion q 2 weeks or 7.5 mg/kg q 3 weeks with *fluoropyrimidine-irinotecan-* or *fluoropyrimidine-oxaliplatin*-based chemotherapy, after progression on a first-line *bevacizumab* product-containing regimen; do not administer **Zirabev** for 28 days following major surgery and until surgical wound is fully healed
Zirabev *Vial:* 100 mg/4 ml (25 mg/ml), 400 mg/16 ml (25 mg/ml), single-dose
Comment: Zirabev is biosimilar to **Avastin** *(bevacizumab)* with indications for the treatment of multiple types of cancer, including metastatic colorectal cancer, non-small cell lung cancer, glioblastoma, metastatic renal cell carcinoma, and cervical cancer, using diagnosis-specific dosing regimens. **Zirabev** is used to treat metastatic colorectal cancer, as a first- or second-line treatment, in combination with IV fluorouracil-based chemotherapy. **Zirabev** is also used to treat metastatic colorectal cancer, in combination with *fluoropyrimidine-irinotecan-* or *fluoropyrimidine-oxaliplatin*-based chemotherapy, for second-line treatment in patients who have progressed on a first-line *bevacizumab* product-containing regimen. **Zirabev** is not indicated for adjuvant treatment of colon cancer.

CANCER: ENDOMETRIAL CARCINOMA

PROGRAMMED DEATH RECEPTOR-1 (PD-1)-BLOCKING ANTIBODY

▶ *dostarlimab-gxly Doses 1 through 4:* 500 mg via IV infusion q 3 weeks; *Beginning 3 weeks after dose 4 (dose 5 onwards):* 1,000 mg via IV infusion q 6 weeks
Pediatric: safety and efficacy not established
Jemperli *Vial:* 500 mg/10 ml (50 mg/ml), single-dose, soln for dilution and IV infusion
Comment: Jemperli is indicated for the treatment of adult patients with mismatch repair deficient (dMMR) recurrent or advanced endometrial cancer, as determined by an FDA-approved test, that has progressed on or following prior treatment with a platinum-containing regimen. The most common adverse reactions (incidence ≥20%) have been fatigue/asthenia, nausea, including the following: immune-mediated pneumonitis, immune-mediated colitis, immune-mediated hepatitis, immune-mediated endocrinopathies, immune-mediated nephritis, and immune-mediated, dermatologic adverse reactions. Monitor for signs and symptoms of immune-mediated adverse reactions. Evaluate clinical chemistries, including liver and thyroid function, at baseline and periodically during treatment. Withhold or permanently discontinue **Jemperli** and administer corticosteroids based on the severity of reaction. For infusion-related reactions, interrupt, slow the rate of infusion, or permanently discontinue **Jemperli** based on severity of reaction. Follow patients closely for evidence of transplant-related complications of allogeneic hematopoietic stem cell transplantation (HSCT) after programmed death receptor-1 (PD-1)/programmed death-ligand 1 (PD-L1)-blocking antibody and intervene promptly. Based on its mechanism of action, **Jemperli** can cause fetal harm when administered in human pregnancy. Animal studies have demonstrated that inhibition of the PD-1/PD-L1 pathway can lead to

(continued)

increased risk of immune-mediated rejection of the developing fetus, resulting in fetal death. Human immunoglobulins (IgG4) are known to cross the placental barrier; therefore, *dostarlimab-gxly* has the potential to be transmitted from the mother to the developing fetus. Exclude pregnancy prior to starting treatment with **Jemperli**. Advise females of reproductive potential of the potential risk to the fetus and to use effective contraception during treatment and for 4 months after the last dose. Mothers are advised not to breastfeed; because of the potential for serious adverse reactions in a breastfed infant, advise women not to breastfeed during treatment and for 4 months after the last dose of **Jemperli**. To report suspected adverse reactions, contact GlaxoSmithKline at 1-888-825-5249 or FDA at 1-800-FDA-1088 or www.fda.gov/medwatch.

▷ *pembrolizumab* administer 200 mg via IV infusion over 30 minutes once q 3 weeks or 400 mg via IV infusion over 30 minutes once q 6 weeks until disease progression, unacceptable toxicity, or for **Keytruda** up to 24 months; administer **Keytruda** prior to chemotherapy when given on the same day
Pediatric: safety and efficacy not established
    Keytruda *Vial:* 100 mg/4 ml (25 mg/ml), single-dose, soln for dilution and IV infusion
    Comment: Keytruda is a programmed death receptor-1 (PD-1)-blocking antibody indicated for treatment of multiple cancers, including endometrial carcinoma (EC). **Keytruda**, in combination with *lenvatinib*, is indicated for treatment of patients with advanced EC that is mismatch repair proficient (pMMR) as determined by an FDA-approved test or not MSI-H, who have disease progression following prior systemic therapy in any setting and are not candidates for curative surgery or radiation. **Keytruda**, as a single agent, is indicated for treatment of patients with advanced EC that is MSI-H or dMMR, as determined by an FDA-approved test, who have disease progression following prior systemic therapy in any setting and are not candidates for curative surgery or radiation. **Keytruda** can cause fetal harm. Exclude pregnancy prior to initiating treatment with **Keytruda**. Advise females of reproductive potential of the embryo/fetal risk and to use effective contraception during treatment and for 4 months after the last **Keytruda** dose. Advise mothers not to breastfeed during treatment and for 4 months after the last **Keytruda** dose. See mfr pkg insert for full prescribing information including storage, preparation, warnings, precautions, drug-drug interactions, and adverse reactions.

CANCER: EPITHELIAL, EPITHELIOID SARCOMA

METHYLTRANSFERASE INHIBITOR

▷ *tazemetostat* 800 mg bid, with or without food, until disease progression or unacceptable toxicity; swallow tablets whole; if a dose is missed or vomiting occurs, do not take an additional dose, but continue with the next scheduled dose
    Tazverik *Tab:* 200 mg, film-coat
    Comment: Tazverik *(tazemetostat)* is indicated for the treatment of adults and pediatric patients ≥16 years of age with metastatic or locally advanced epithelioid sarcoma not eligible for complete resection. This indication is approved under accelerated approval based on overall response rate and duration of response. Continued approval for this indication may be contingent upon verification and description of clinical benefit in a confirmatory trial. Increases the risk of developing secondary malignancies, including T cell lymphoblastic lymphoma, myelodysplastic syndrome, and acute myeloid leukemia. The most common (incidence ≥20%) adverse reactions are pain, fatigue, nausea, decreased appetite, vomiting, and constipation. Recommended dose reductions of **Tazverik** for a first adverse reaction is 600 mg bid and for a second adverse reaction is 400 mg bid. Permanently discontinue **Tazverik** in patients who are unable to tolerate 400 mg bid. Avoid co-administration of strong and moderate CYP3A inhibitors with **Tazverik**. Reduce the dose of **Tazverik** if co-administration of moderate CYP3A inhibitors cannot be avoided. Avoid co-administration of **Tazverik** with strong and moderate CYP3A inducers. **Tazverik** can cause embryo/fetal harm; therefore, advise patients of potential risk and to use effective non-hormonal contraception. Breastfeeding is not recommended during treatment and for 1 week after the last dose.

CANCER: FALLOPIAN TUBE

POLY(ADP-RIBOSE) POLYMERASE (PARP) INHIBITOR

▷ *niraparib tosylate* 300 mg (3 × 100 mg) once daily, with or without food; continue treatment until disease progression or unacceptable adverse reaction; for adverse reactions, consider interruption of treatment, dose reduction, or dose discontinuation
Pediatric: safety and efficacy not established
    Zejula *Cap:* 100 mg
    Comment: Zejula *(niraparib)* is indicated for the maintenance treatment of adult patients with recurrent epithelial ovarian, fallopian tube, or primary peritoneal cancer who are in a complete or partial response to platinum-based chemotherapy and for late-line treatment of recurrent ovarian cancer. The most common adverse reactions (incidence ≥10%) have been anemia, thrombocytopenia, neutropenia, leukopenia, hypertension, palpitations, nausea, vomiting, abdominal pain/distention, diarrhea, constipation, mucositis/stomatitis, dry mouth, fatigue/asthenia, dyspepsia, decreased appetite, urinary tract infection, aspartate

aminotransferase (AST)/alanine aminotransferase (ALT) elevation, back pain, myalgia, arthralgia, headache, dizziness, dysgeusia, insomnia, anxiety, nasopharyngitis, dyspnea, cough, and rash. Monitor complete blood count (CBC) weekly for the first month, then monthly for the next 11 months, and then periodically thereafter. Monitor blood pressure (BP) and heart rate (HR) monthly for the first year and periodically thereafter. Manage BP and HR with appropriate medication as indicated and adjust the **Zejula** dose if necessary. Because myelodysplastic syndrome/acute myeloid leukemia (MDS/AML) has occurred in patients exposed to **Zejula,** with some cases being fatal, monitor patients for hematologic toxicity and discontinue **Zejula** if MDS/AML is confirmed. **Zejula** can cause embryo/fetal toxicity; therefore, advise females of reproductive potential of the potential risk and to use effective contraception. Advise women <u>not</u> to breastfeed during treatment with **Zejula** and for 1 month after receiving the final dose.

▷ *olaparib* 300 mg bid; with <u>or</u> without food; see the mfr pkg insert for recommended duration of treatment; CrCl: 31-50 ml/min: 200 mg bid
   Pediatric: safety and efficacy <u>not</u> established
   Lynparza *Tab:* 100, 150 mg
   Comment: **Lynparza** is a first-class poly(ADP-ribose) polymerase (PARP) inhibitor indicated for
   (1) maintenance treatment of adult patients with deleterious <u>or</u> suspected deleterious germline <u>or</u> somatic BRCA-mutated advanced epithelial ovarian, fallopian tube, <u>or</u> primary peritoneal cancer who are in complete <u>or</u> partial response to first-line platinum-based chemotherapy; select patients for therapy based on an FDA-approved companion diagnostic for **Lynparza**;
   (2) maintenance treatment of adult patients with recurrent epithelial ovarian, fallopian tube, <u>or</u> primary peritoneal cancer who are in complete <u>or</u> partial response to platinum-based chemotherapy;
   (3) treatment of adult patients with deleterious <u>or</u> suspected deleterious germline BRCA-mutated (gBRCAm) advanced ovarian cancer who have been treated with three <u>or</u> more prior lines of chemotherapy; select patients for therapy based on an FDA-approved companion diagnostic for **Lynparza**;
   (4) first-line maintenance treatment with *bevacizumab* for HRD-positive advanced ovarian cancer; and
   (5) treatment of adult patients with deleterious <u>or</u> suspected deleterious germline <u>or</u> somatic homologous recombination repair (HRR) gene-mutated metastatic castration-resistant prostate cancer (mCRPC) who have progressed following prior treatment with *enzalutamide* <u>or</u> *abiraterone;* select patients for therapy based on an FDA-approved companion diagnostic for **Lynparza**.
   The most common adverse reactions (incidence ≥10%) in clinical trials have been nausea, fatigue (including asthenia), vomiting, abdominal pain, anemia, diarrhea, dizziness, neutropenia, leukopenia, nasopharyngitis/upper respiratory tract infection/influenza, respiratory tract infection, arthralgia/myalgia, dysgeusia, headache, dyspepsia, decreased appetite, constipation, stomatitis, dyspnea, and thrombocytopenia. Avoid concomitant use of strong <u>or</u> moderate CYP3A inhibitors. If the inhibitor cannot be avoided, reduce the **Lynparza** dose. Avoid concomitant use of strong <u>or</u> moderate CYP3A inducers as decreased **Lynparza** efficacy can occur. The most common adverse reactions (incidence ≥20%) in clinical trials have been anemia, nausea, fatigue (including asthenia), vomiting, nasopharyngitis/upper respiratory tract infection/influenza, diarrhea, arthralgia/myalgia, dysgeusia, headache, dyspepsia, decreased appetite, constipation, and stomatitis. The most common laboratory abnormalities (incidence ≥25%) have been decrease in hemoglobin, increase MCV, decrease in lymphocytes, decrease in leukocytes, decrease in absolute neutrophil count, increase in serum creatinine, and decrease in platelets. **Lynparza** can cause embryo/fetal harm. Exclude pregnancy prior to initiation and advise females of reproductive potential to use effective contraception during and for 6 months after the last dose. Males with female partners should use effective contraception and <u>not</u> donate sperm during and for 3 months after the last dose. Advise women <u>not</u> to breastfeed during and for 1 month after the last dose.

FOLATE RECEPTOR ALPHA (FRα)-DIRECTED ANTIBODY <u>AND</u> MICROTUBULE INHIBITOR CONJUGATE

▷ *mirvetuximab soravtansine-gynx* 6 mg/kg adjusted ideal body weight administered via IV infusion q 3 weeks until disease progression <u>or</u> unacceptable toxicity; administer **Elahere** as IV infusion <u>only</u> after dilution in D5W (Alert: **Elahere** is incompatible with normal saline); premedicate with a corticosteroid antihistamine, antipyretic, antiemetic, ophthalmic steroid, and lubricating eye drops; store **Elahere** vials upright in a refrigerator at 2°C-8°C (36°F-46°F) in the original carton to protect from light until the time of preparation; do <u>not</u> freeze <u>or</u> shake; **Elahere** is a hazardous drug; see mfr pkg insert for special handling and disposal procedures
   Pediatric: Safety and efficacy <u>not</u> established
   Elahere *Vial:* 100 mg/20 ml (5 mg/ml), single-dose, soln for dilution and IV infusion
   Comment: **Elahere** is a folate receptor alpha (FRα)-directed antibody and microtubule inhibitor conjugate indicated for the treatment of adult patients with FRα-positive, platinum-resistant epithelial ovarian, fallopian tube, <u>or</u> primary peritoneal cancer who have received one to three prior systemic treatment regimens. These indications are approved under accelerated approval based on tumor response rate and durability of response. Continued approval for this indication may be contingent upon verification and description of clinical benefit in a confirmatory trial. *Boxed Warning:* **Elahere** can cause severe ocular toxicities, including visual impairment, keratopathy, dry eye, photophobia, eye pain, and uveitis. Conduct an ophthalmic exam, including visual acuity and slit lamp exam, prior to initiation of

(continued)

Elahere, every other cycle for the first eight cycles and as clinically indicated. Administer prophylactic artificial tears and ophthalmic steroid. Withhold **Elahere** for ocular toxicities until improvement and resume at the same or reduced dose. Discontinue **Elahere** for grade 4 ocular toxicities. Withhold **Elahere** for persistent or recurrent grade 2 pneumonitis and consider dose reduction. Permanently discontinue **Elahere** for grade 3 or 4 pneumonitis. Monitor patients for new or worsening peripheral neuropathy. Withhold dose, pause dose, slow the rate of infusion, or permanently discontinue **Elahere** based on the severity of peripheral neuropathy. The most common (≥20 %) adverse reactions, including laboratory abnormalities, have been vision impairment, fatigue, increased aspartate aminotransferase, nausea, increased alanine aminotransferase, keratopathy, abdominal pain, decreased lymphocytes, peripheral neuropathy, diarrhea, decreased albumin, constipation, increased alkaline phosphatase, dry eye, decreased magnesium, decreased leukocytes, decreased neutrophils, and decreased hemoglobin. *Child-Pugh Class B or C:* Avoid use. Closely monitor patients for adverse reactions if taking strong CYP3A4 inhibitors. **Elahere** is embryo/fetal toxic. Human immunoglobulin G (IgG) is known to cross the placental barrier; therefore, **Elahere** has the potential to be transmitted from the mother to the developing fetus. The cytotoxic component, DM4, disrupts microtubule function, is genotoxic, and can be toxic to actively dividing cells, suggesting it has the potential to cause embryotoxicity and teratogenicity. Advise patients of the potential risk to the fetus and to use effective contraception. There are no data on the presence of *mirvetuximab soravtansine-gynx* in human milk or effects on the breastfed infant. Because of the potential for serious adverse reactions in the breastfed infant, advise mothers **not** to breastfeed during treatment with **Elahere** and for 1 month after the last dose.

VASCULAR ENDOTHELIAL GROWTH (VEGF) INHIBITOR

▶ *bevacizumab-adcd Regimens for epithelial ovarian, fallopian tube, and primary peritoneal cancer:* Stage III or IV epithelial ovarian, fallopian tube, or primary peritoneal cancer following initial surgical resection: 15 mg/kg q 3 weeks with *carboplatin* and *paclitaxel* for up to 6 cycles, followed by 15 mg/kg q 3 weeks as a single agent, for a total of up to 22 cycles; platinum-resistant recurrent epithelial ovarian, fallopian tube, or primary peritoneal cancer: 10 mg/kg q 2 weeks with *paclitaxel*, pegylated liposomal *doxorubicin*, or *topotecan* given every week; 15 mg/kg q 3 weeks with *topotecan* given q 3 weeks as a single agent; platinum-sensitive recurrent epithelial ovarian, fallopian tube, or primary peritoneal cancer: 15 mg/kg q 3 weeks with *carboplatin* and *gemcitabine* for 6-10 cycles, followed by 15 mg/kg q 3 weeks as a single agent; 15 mg/kg q 3 weeks with *carboplatin* and *paclitaxel* for 6-8 cycles in combination with **carboplatin** and *paclitaxel* or *carboplatin* and *gemcitabine*, followed by 15 mg/kg q 3 weeks with *carboplatin* and *gemcitabine* for 6-10 cycles, followed by 15 mg/kg q 3 weeks as a single agent; do **not** administer **Vegzelma** for 28 days following major surgery and until adequate wound healing; store refrigerated at 2°C-8°C (36°F-46°F) in the original carton until time of use to protect from light; do **not** freeze or shake the vial or carton; see mfr pkg insert for full prescribing information including proper preparation and administration instructions and dosage modifications for adverse reactions

Pediatric: <18 years: safety and efficacy **not** established; ≥18 years: same as adult

    Vegzelma *Vial:* 100 mg/4 ml (25 mg/ml) or 400 mg/16 ml (25 mg/ml), single-dose, soln for dilution and IV infusion

    Comment: Vegzelma is a vascular endothelial growth factor (VEGF) inhibitor biosimilar to **Avastin** indicated for treatment of multiple types of cancer, including colorectal cancer, non-small cell lung cancer, glioblastoma, renal cell carcinoma, cervical cancer, and epithelial ovarian, fallopian tube, or primary peritoneal cancer. *Bevacizumab* products increase the risk of ovarian failure and may impair fertility. Inform females of reproductive potential of the risk of ovarian failure prior to the first dose of **Vegzelma**. The long-term effects of *bevacizumab* products on fertility are **not** known. *Bevacizumab* products may cause fetal harm when administered to a pregnant female. Advise females of reproductive potential to use effective contraception during treatment with **Vegzelma** and for 6 months after the last dose. **No** data are available regarding the presence of *bevacizumab* products in human milk or effects on the breastfed infant. Because of the potential for serious adverse reactions in breastfed infants, advise mothers **not** to breastfeed during treatment with **Vegzelma** and for 6 months after the last dose. See mfr pkg insert for full prescription information.

CANCER: GASTRIC/GASTROESOPHAGEAL/ESOPHAGEAL

PROGRAMMED DEATH RECEPTOR-1 (PD-1)-BLOCKING ANTIBODY

▶ *pembrolizumab* administer via IV infusion over 30 minutes, either 200 mg once every 3 weeks or 400 mg once every 6 weeks, until disease progression, unacceptable toxicity, or for **Keytruda** up to 24 months; administer **Keytruda** prior to chemotherapy when given on the same day

Pediatric: safety and efficacy **not** established

    Keytruda *Vial:* 100 mg/4 ml (25 mg/ml), single-dose, soln for dilution and IV infusion

    Comment: Keytruda is a programmed death receptor-1 (PD-1)-blocking antibody indicated for the treatment of multiple cancers. **Keytruda**, in combination with *trastuzumab*, fluoropyrimidine- and platinum-containing chemotherapy, is indicated for the first-line treatment of patients with locally advanced unresectable or metastatic human epidermal growth factor receptor 2 (HER2)-positive gastric or gastroesophageal junction (GEJ) adenocarcinoma. This indication is approved under accelerated approval based on tumor response rate and durability of response. Continued approval of this indication may be contingent upon verification and description of clinical benefit in confirmatory trials. **Keytruda** is also indicated for the treatment of patients with locally advanced or metastatic esophageal or GEJ (tumors with epicenter 1–5 cm above the GEJ) carcinoma that is not amenable to surgical resection or definitive chemoradiation, either (1) in combination with platinum- and fluoropyrimidine-based chemotherapy or (2) as a single agent after one or more prior lines of systemic therapy for patients with tumors of squamous cell histology that express programmed death-ligand 1 (PD-L1; CPS ≥10) as determined by a Food and Drug Administration (FDA)-approved test. **Keytruda** can cause fetal harm. Exclude pregnancy prior to initiating treatment with **Keytruda**. Advise females of reproductive potential of the embryo/fetal risk and to use effective contraception during treatment and for 4 months after the last **Keytruda** dose. Advise mothers not to breastfeed during treatment and for 4 months after the last **Keytruda** dose. See mfr pkg insert for full prescribing information including storage, preparation, warnings, precautions, drug-drug interactions, and adverse reactions.

CANCER: GASTROINTESTINAL STROMAL TUMOR (GIST)

KINASE INHIBITOR

▶ *avapritinib* 300 mg once daily, on an empty stomach, at least 1 hour before or 2 hours after a meal
Ayvakit *Tab:* 100, 200, 300 mg
Comment: Ayvakit *(avapritinib)* is a kinase inhibitor indicated for the treatment of adults with unresectable or metastatic gastrointestinal stromal tumor (GIST) harboring a platelet-derived growth factor receptor alpha (PDGFRA) exon 18 mutation, including PDGFRA D842V mutations. Avoid co-administration of **Ayvakit** with strong and moderate CYP3A inhibitors; if co-administration with a moderate inhibitor cannot be avoided, reduce the dose of **Ayvakit**. Avoid co-administration of **Ayvakit** with strong and moderate CYP3A inducers. Central nervous system (CNS) adverse reactions include cognitive impairment, dizziness, sleep disorders, mood disorders, speech disorders, and hallucinations. Depending on the severity, continue **Ayvakit** at the same dose, withhold and then resume at the same or reduced dose upon improvement, or permanently discontinue **Ayvakit**. The most common adverse reactions (incidence ≥20%) have been edema, nausea, fatigue/asthenia, cognitive impairment, vomiting, decreased appetite, diarrhea, hair color changes, increased lacrimation, abdominal pain, constipation, rash, and dizziness. **Ayvakit** can cause embryo/fetal harm. Exclude pregnancy prior to initiating **Ayvakit**. Advise females of reproductive potential of the potential risk and to use effective contraception. Breastfeeding is not recommended during treatment and for 2 weeks following the last **Ayvakit** dose.

▶ *ripretinib* 150 mg once daily, with or without food
Pediatric: safety and efficacy not established
Qinlock *Tab:* 50 mg
Comment: Qinlock *(ripretinib)* is a broad-spectrum KIT and PDGFRα inhibitor for the treatment of adult patients with advanced GIST who have received prior treatment with three or more kinase inhibitors, including *imatinib*. The most common adverse reactions (incidence ≥20%) have been alopecia, fatigue, nausea, abdominal pain, constipation, myalgia, diarrhea, decreased appetite, palmar-plantar erythrodysesthesia, and vomiting. The most common grade 3 or 4 laboratory abnormalities (incidence ≥4%) have been increased lipase and decreased phosphate. Based on severity, withhold **Qinlock** and resume at the same or reduced dose in the occurrence of palmar-plantar erythrodysesthesia syndrome (PPES). Monitor for new primary cutaneous malignancies when initiating **Qinlock** and routinely during treatment. Do not initiate **Qinlock** in patients with uncontrolled hypertension and monitor blood pressure during treatment. Assess ejection fraction by echocardiogram or multigated acquisition (MUGA) scan prior to initiating **Qinlock** and during treatment, as clinically indicated. Permanently discontinue for grade 3 or 4 left ventricular systolic dysfunction. There is risk of impaired wound healing with **Qinlock**. Therefore, withhold **Qinlock** for at least 1 week prior to elective surgery and do not administer for at least 2 weeks after major surgery and until adequate wound healing. Safe resumption of **Qinlock** after resolution of wound healing complications has not been established. Monitor more frequently for adverse reactions when co-administered with strong CYP3A inhibitors. Avoid concomitant use of strong CYP3A inducers. **Qinlock** can cause fetal harm. There are no available data on **Qinlock** use in pregnant females to inform drug-associated risk. Exclude pregnancy prior to initiating **Qinlock** and advise females of reproductive potential of the possible risk to the fetus and to use effective contraception. There are no data on the presence of *ripretinib* or its metabolites in human milk or effects on the breastfed infant. Because of the potential for serious adverse embryo/fetal effects, advise women not to breastfeed during treatment with **Retevmo** and for 1 week after the final dose.

▶ *sunitinib malate* recommended dose of **Sutent** for GIST is 50 mg once daily, on a schedule of 4 weeks on treatment, followed by 2 weeks off (i.e., schedule 4/2) until disease progression or unacceptable toxicity; take with or without food
Pediatric: safety and efficacy not established
Sutent *Cap:* 12.5, 25, 50 mg

(continued)

Comment: Sutent is a kinase inhibitor indicated for the treatment of adult patients with GIST after disease progression on or intolerance to *imatinib mesylate*. The most common adverse reactions (incidence ≥25%) have been fatigue/asthenia, diarrhea, mucositis/stomatitis, nausea, decreased appetite/anorexia, vomiting, abdominal pain, hand-foot syndrome, hypertension, bleeding events, dysgeusia/altered taste, dyspepsia, and thrombocytopenia. Consider dose reduction of Sutent when administered with strong CYP3A4 inhibitors. Consider dose increase of Sutent when administered with strong CYP3A4 inducers. Fatal liver failure has been observed. Monitor liver function tests at baseline, during each cycle and as clinically indicated. Interrupt Sutent for grade 3 hepatotoxicity until resolution to grade ≤1 or baseline and resume Sutent at a reduced dose; discontinue if no resolution. Discontinue Sutent in patients with grade 4 hepatoxicity and in patients who have subsequent severe changes in liver function tests or other signs and symptoms of liver failure. Myocardial ischemia, myocardial infarction, heart failure, cardiomyopathy, and decreased left ventricular ejection fraction (LVEF) to below the lower limit of normal (LLN), including death, have occurred. Monitor for signs and symptoms of congestive heart failure and consider monitoring LVEF at baseline and periodically during treatment. Discontinue Sutent for clinical manifestations of congestive heart failure. Interrupt and/or reduce dose for decreased LVEF. Monitor patients at higher risk of developing QT interval prolongation and torsade de pointes. Consider monitoring ECGs and electrolytes. Monitor blood pressure at baseline and as clinically indicated. Initiate and/or adjust antihypertensive therapy as appropriate. Interrupt Sutent for grade 3 hypertension until resolution to grade ≤1 or baseline, then resume Sutent at a reduced dose. Discontinue Sutent for grade 4 hypertension. Tumor-related hemorrhage and viscus perforation, both with fatal events, have occurred. Obtain serial complete blood counts (CBCs) and physical examinations. Interrupt Sutent for grade 3 or 4 hemorrhagic events until resolution to grade ≤1 or baseline, then resume at a reduced dose and discontinue Sutent if no resolution. Tumor lysis syndrome (TLS), some fatal, has been reported; monitor and treat as clinically indicated. Thrombotic microangiopathy (TMA), including thrombotic thrombocytopenic purpura (TTP) and hemolytic uremic syndrome (HUS), sometimes leading to renal failure or a fatal outcome, has been reported; discontinue Sutent for TMA. Monitor urine protein. Interrupt Sutent treatment for 24-hour urine protein of 3 or more grams; discontinue for repeat episodes of 24-hour urine protein of 3 or more grams despite dose reductions or nephrotic syndrome. Necrotizing fasciitis, erythema multiforme, Stevens-Johnson syndrome (SJS), and toxic epidermal necrolysis (TEN), some fatal, have occurred; discontinue Sutent for any of these events. Reversible posterior leukoencephalopathy syndrome (RPLS), some fatal, has been reported. Monitor for signs and symptoms of RPLS. Withhold Sutent until resolution. Monitor thyroid function at baseline, periodically during treatment, and as clinically indicated. Initiate and/or adjust therapy for thyroid dysfunction as appropriate. Monitor patients for hypoglycemia regularly and assess if antidiabetic drug dose modifications are required. Osteonecrosis of the jaw (ONJ) has occurred. Withhold Sutent for at least 3 weeks prior to invasive dental procedures and monitor ONJ until complete resolution. Withhold Sutent for at least 3 weeks prior to elective surgery and do not administer Sutent for at least 2 weeks following major surgery and until adequate wound healing. Safety of resuming Sutent treatment after resolution of wound healing complications has not been established. There are no available data in human pregnancy to inform a drug-associated risk to the fetus. In animal developmental and reproductive toxicology studies, oral administration of *sunitinib* throughout organogenesis resulted in teratogenicity (embryo lethality, craniofacial and skeletal malformations). Based on animal reproduction studies and its mechanism of action, Sutent can cause fetal harm when administered in human pregnancy. Exclude pregnancy prior to initiating treatment with Sutent. Advise females of reproductive potential to use effective contraception during treatment with Sutent and for at least 4 weeks after the last dose. Advise males with female partners of reproductive potential to use effective contraception during treatment with Sutent and for 7 weeks after the last dose. Based on findings in animal studies, Sutent may impair male and female fertility. There is no information regarding the presence of *sunitinib* and its metabolites in human milk. *Sunitinib* and its metabolites were excreted in animal milk at concentrations up to 12-fold higher than in plasma. Because of the potential for serious adverse reactions in breastfed infants, advise mothers not to breastfeed during treatment and for at least 4 weeks after the last Sutent dose. To report suspected adverse reactions, contact Pfizer at 800-438-1985 or FDA at 800-FDA-1088 or www.fda.gov/medwatch.

CANCER: GLIOBLASTOMA MULTIFORME

VASCULAR ENDOTHELIAL GROWTH FACTOR (VEGF) INHIBITOR

▷ *bevacizumab-adcd Regimen for recurrent glioblastoma:* 10 mg/kg q 2 weeks; do not administer Vegzelma for at least 28 days prior to elective surgery; do not administer Vegzelma for 28 days following major surgery and until adequate wound healing; store refrigerated at 2°C-8°C (36°F-46°F) in the original carton until time of use to protect from light; do not freeze or shake the vial or carton; see mfr pkg insert for full prescribing information including proper preparation and administration instructions and dosage modifications for adverse reactions

Pediatric: <18 years: safety and efficacy not established; ≥18 years: same as adult

    Vegzelma *Vial:* 100 mg/4 ml (25 mg/ml) or 400 mg/16 ml (25 mg/ml), single-dose, soln for dilution and IV infusion

Comment: Vegzelma is a vascular endothelial growth factor (VEGF) inhibitor biosimilar to **Avastin** indicated for the treatment of multiple types of cancer, including colorectal cancer, non-small cell lung cancer, glioblastoma, renal cell carcinoma, cervical cancer, and epithelial ovarian, fallopian tube, or primary peritoneal cancer. **Bevacizumab** products increase the risk of ovarian failure and may impair fertility. Inform females of reproductive potential of the risk of ovarian failure prior to the first dose of **Vegzelma**. The long-term effects of **bevacizumab** products on fertility are not known. **Bevacizumab** products may cause fetal harm when administered to a pregnant female. Advise females of reproductive potential to use effective contraception during treatment with **Vegzelma** and for 6 months after the last dose. No data are available regarding the presence of **bevacizumab** products in human milk or effects on the breastfed infant. Because of the potential for serious adverse reactions in breastfed infants, advise mothers not to breastfeed during treatment with **Vegzelma** and for 6 months after the last dose. See mfr pkg insert for full prescription information.

▶ *bevacizumab-bvzr* 10 mg/kg via IV infusion q 2 weeks; do not administer **Zirabev** for 28 days following major surgery and until the surgical wound is fully healed

    Zirabev *Vial:* 100 mg/4 ml (25 mg/ml), 400 mg/16 ml (25 mg/ml), single-dose

    Comment: Zirabev is biosimilar to **Avastin** *(bevacizumab)* with indications for the treatment of multiple types of cancer, including metastatic colorectal cancer, non-small cell lung cancer, glioblastoma, metastatic renal cell carcinoma, and cervical cancer, using diagnosis-specific dosing regimens. See mfr pkg insert for prescribing information.

CANCER: KIDNEY, RENAL CELL CARCINOMA (RCC)

KINASE INHIBITOR

▶ *sorafenib* (G) 400 mg (2 x 200 mg) bid, without food

    Nexavar *Tab:* 200 mg

    Comment: Nexavar is indicated for the treatment of advanced renal cell carcinoma (RCC). The most common adverse reactions (incidence ≥20%) have been diarrhea, fatigue, infection, alopecia, hand-foot skin reaction, rash, weight loss, decreased appetite, nausea, gastrointestinal and abdominal pain, hypertension, and hemorrhage. **Nexavar** in combination with **carboplatin** and **paclitaxel** is contraindicated in patients with squamous cell lung cancer. Avoid strong CYP3A4 inducers. Monitor ECG (for QT prolongation) and electrolytes in patients at increased risk for ventricular arrhythmias. Consider temporary or permanent discontinuation of **Nexavar** in the event of a cardiovascular event. Discontinue **Nexavar** if needed in the event of bleeding. Monitor the patient for hypertension, weekly during the first 6 weeks and periodically thereafter. Interrupt and/or decrease **Nexavar** for severe or persistent dermal reaction, and immediately discontinue **Nexavar** if Stevens-Johnson syndrome (SJS) or toxic epidermal necrolysis (TEN) is suspected. Discontinue **Nexavar** in the event of gastrointestinal perforation. **Nexavar** may cause hepatotoxicity; monitor liver function tests regularly and discontinue for unexplained transaminase elevation. Monitor thyroid stimulating hormone (TSH) monthly and adjust thyroid replacement therapy in patients with thyroid cancer. **Nexavar** may cause embryo/fetal harm; exclude pregnancy prior to initiating **Nexavar** and advise females and males of reproductive potential to use effective contraception. Advise women not to breastfeed.

▶ *sunitinib malate* recommended dose of **Sutent** for advanced (RCC) is 50 mg once daily, on a schedule of 4 weeks on treatment, followed by 2 weeks off (i.e., schedule 4/2) until disease progression or unacceptable toxicity; recommended dose of **Sutent** for the adjuvant treatment of RCC is 50 mg once daily, on a schedule of 4 weeks on treatment, followed by 2 weeks off (i.e., schedule 4/2), for nine 6-week cycles; **Sutent** may be taken with or without food

Pediatric: safety and efficacy not established

    Sutent *Cap:* 12.5, 25, 50 mg

    Comment: Sutent is a kinase inhibitor indicated as monotherapy for the treatment of adult patients with advanced RCC. **Sutent** is also indicated for the adjuvant treatment of adult patients at high risk of recurrent RCC following nephrectomy. The most common adverse reactions (incidence ≥25%) have been fatigue/asthenia, diarrhea, mucositis/stomatitis, nausea, decreased appetite/anorexia, vomiting, abdominal pain, hand-foot syndrome, hypertension, bleeding events, dysgeusia/altered taste, dyspepsia, and thrombocytopenia. Consider dose reduction of **Sutent** when administered with strong CYP3A4 inhibitors. Consider dose increase of **Sutent** when administered with strong CYP3A4 inducers. Fatal liver failure has been observed. Monitor liver function tests at baseline, during each cycle, and as clinically indicated. Interrupt **Sutent** for grade 3 hepatotoxicity until resolution to grade ≤1 or baseline and resume **Sutent** at a reduced dose; discontinue if no resolution. Discontinue **Sutent** in patients with grade 4 hepatoxicity and in patients who have subsequent severe changes in liver function tests or other signs and symptoms of liver failure. Myocardial ischemia, myocardial infarction, heart failure, cardiomyopathy, and decreased left ventricular ejection fraction (LVEF) to below the lower limit of normal (LLN), including death, have occurred. Monitor for signs and symptoms of congestive heart failure and consider monitoring LVEF at baseline and periodically during treatment. Discontinue **Sutent** for clinical manifestations of congestive heart failure. Interrupt and/or reduce dose for decreased LVEF.

(continued)

Monitor patients at higher risk of developing QT interval prolongation and torsade de pointes. Consider monitoring ECGs and electrolytes. Monitor blood pressure at baseline and as clinically indicated. Initiate and/or adjust antihypertensive therapy as appropriate. Interrupt **Sutent** for grade 3 hypertension until resolution to grade ≤1 or baseline, then resume **Sutent** at a reduced dose. Discontinue **Sutent** for grade 4 hypertension. Tumor-related hemorrhage and viscus perforation, both with fatal events, have occurred. Obtain serial complete blood counts (CBCs) and physical examinations. Interrupt **Sutent** for grade 3 or 4 hemorrhagic events until resolution to grade ≤1 or baseline, then resume at a reduced dose and discontinue **Sutent** if no resolution. Tumor lysis syndrome (TLS), some fatal, has been reported; monitor and treat as clinically indicated. Thrombotic microangiopathy (TMA), including thrombotic thrombocytopenic purpura (TTP) and hemolytic uremic syndrome (HUS), sometimes leading to renal failure or a fatal outcome, has been reported; discontinue **Sutent** for TMA. Monitor urine protein. Interrupt **Sutent** treatment for 24-hour urine protein of 3 or more grams; discontinue for repeat episodes of 24-hour urine protein of 3 or more grams despite dose reductions or nephrotic syndrome. Necrotizing fasciitis, erythema multiforme, SJS, and TEN, some fatal, have occurred; discontinue **Sutent** for any of these events. Reversible posterior leukoencephalopathy syndrome (RPLS), some fatal, has been reported. Monitor for signs and symptoms of RPLS. Withhold **Sutent** until resolution. Monitor thyroid function at baseline, periodically during treatment, and as clinically indicated. Initiate and/or adjust therapy for thyroid dysfunction as appropriate. Monitor patients for hypoglycemia regularly and assess if antidiabetic drug dose modifications are required. Osteonecrosis of the jaw (ONJ) has occurred. Withhold **Sutent** for at least 3 weeks prior to invasive dental procedures and monitor ONJ until complete resolution. Withhold **Sutent** for at least 3 weeks prior to elective surgery and do not administer **Sutent** for at least 2 weeks following major surgery and until adequate wound healing. Safety of resuming **Sutent** treatment after resolution of wound healing complications has not been established. There are no available data in human pregnancy to inform a drug-associated risk to the fetus. In animal developmental and reproductive toxicology studies, oral administration of *sunitinib* throughout organogenesis resulted in teratogenicity (embryo lethality, craniofacial and skeletal malformations). Based on animal reproduction studies and its mechanism of action, **Sutent** can cause fetal harm when administered in human pregnancy. Exclude pregnancy prior to initiating treatment with **Sutent**. Advise females of reproductive potential to use effective contraception during treatment with **Sutent** and for at least 4 weeks after the last dose. Advise males with female partners of reproductive potential to use effective contraception during treatment with **Sutent** and for 7 weeks after the last dose. Based on findings in animal studies, **Sutent** may impair male and female fertility. There is no information regarding the presence of *sunitinib* and its metabolites in human milk. *Sunitinib* and its metabolites were excreted in animal milk at concentrations up to 12-fold higher than in plasma. Because of the potential for serious adverse reactions in breastfed infants, advise mothers not to breastfeed during treatment and for at least 4 weeks after the last **Sutent** dose. To report suspected adverse reactions, contact Pfizer at 800-438-1985 or FDA at 800-FDA-1088 or www.fda.gov/medwatch.

VASCULAR ENDOTHELIAL GROWTH FACTOR (VEGF) INHIBITOR

▷ **bevacizumab-adcd** *Regimen for metastatic RCC:* 10 mg/kg q 2 weeks with **interferon alfa**; withhold for at least 28 days prior to elective surgery; do not administer **Vegzelma** for 28 days following major surgery and until adequate wound healing; store refrigerated at 2°C-8°C (36°F-46°F) in the original carton until time of use to protect from light; do not freeze or shake the vial or carton; see mfr pkg insert for full prescribing information including proper preparation and administration instructions and dosage modifications for adverse reactions

Pediatric: <18 years: safety and efficacy not established; ≥18 years: same as adult

Vegzelma *Vial:* 100 mg/4 ml (25 mg/ml) or 400 mg/16 ml (25 mg/ml), single-dose, soln for dilution and IV infusion

Comment: **Vegzelma** is a vascular endothelial growth factor (VEGF) inhibitor biosimilar to **Avastin** indicated for the treatment of multiple types of cancer, including colorectal cancer, non-small cell lung cancer, glioblastoma, RCC, cervical cancer, and epithelial ovarian, fallopian tube, or primary peritoneal cancer. **Bevacizumab** products increase the risk of ovarian failure and may impair fertility. Inform females of reproductive potential of the risk of ovarian failure prior to the first dose of **Vegzelma**. The long-term effects of **bevacizumab** products on fertility are not known. **Bevacizumab** products may cause fetal harm when administered to a pregnant female. Advise females of reproductive potential to use effective contraception during treatment with **Vegzelma** and for 6 months after the last dose. No data are available regarding the presence of **bevacizumab** products in human milk or effects on the breastfed infant. Because of the potential for serious adverse reactions in breastfed infants, advise mothers not to breastfeed during treatment with **Vegzelma** and for 6 months after the last dose. See mfr pkg insert for full prescription information.

▷ **bevacizumab-bvzr** 10 mg/kg via IV infusion q 2 weeks with **interferon alfa**; do not administer **Zirabev** for 28 days following major surgery and until the surgical wound is fully healed

Zirabev *Vial:* 100 mg/4 ml (25 mg/ml), 400 mg/16 ml (25 mg/ml), single-dose

Comment: **Zirabev** is biosimilar to **Avastin** (*bevacizumab*) with indications for the treatment of multiple types of cancer, including metastatic colorectal cancer, non-small cell lung cancer, glioblastoma, metastatic RCC, and cervical cancer, using diagnosis-specific dosing regimens. **Zirabev** is used to treat recurrent glioblastoma in adults. **Zirabev** is used to treat metastatic RCC in combination with **interferon alfa**.

PROGRAMMED DEATH LIGAND-1 (PD-L1)-BLOCKING ANTIBODY

▷ *avelumab* 800 mg via IV infusion over 60 minutes q 2 weeks; premedicate for the first 4 infusions and subsequently as needed

Pediatric: <12 years: not established; ≥12 years: same as adult

Bavencio *Vial:* 200 mg/10 ml (20 mg/ml), single-dose, solution for IV infusion

Comment: Bavencio *(avelumab)* is indicated for the treatment of patients with metastatic MCC. The most common adverse reactions (>20%) in patients treated for MCC have been fatigue, musculoskeletal pain, diarrhea, nausea, infusion-related reaction, rash, decreased appetite, and peripheral edema. Withhold Bavencio for moderate immune-mediated pneumonitis; permanently discontinue for severe, life-threatening, or recurrent moderate pneumonitis. Monitor liver function tests for hepatotoxicity and immune-mediated hepatitis. Withhold Bavencio for moderate hepatitis; permanently discontinue for severe or life-threatening hepatitis. Withhold Bavencio for moderate or severe immune-mediated colitis and permanently discontinue for life-threatening or recurrent severe colitis. For immune-mediated endocrinopathies, withhold Bavencio for severe or life-threatening endocrinopathies. Monitor renal function. Withhold Bavencio for moderate or severe nephritis and renal dysfunction and permanently discontinue for life-threatening nephritis or renal dysfunction. For infusion-related reactions, interrupt Bavencio or slow the rate of infusion for mild or moderate infusion-related reactions. Stop the infusion, and permanently discontinue Bavencio, for severe or life-threatening infusion-related reactions. Optimize management of cardiovascular risk factors. Bavencio can cause embryo/fetal harm. Advise females of reproductive potential of embryo/fetal risk potential and to use effective contraception. There is no information regarding the presence of *avelumab* in human milk or effects on the breastfed infant. Advise not to breastfeed.

▷ *pembrolizumab* administer 200 mg via IV infusion over 30 minutes once q 3 weeks or 400 mg via IV infusion over 30 minutes once q 6 weeks until disease progression, unacceptable toxicity, or for Keytruda up to 24 months; administer Keytruda in combination with *axitinib* 5 mg orally bid or in combination with *lenvatinib* 20 mg orally once daily

Pediatric: safety and efficacy not established

Keytruda *Vial:* 100 mg/4 ml (25 mg/ml), single-dose, soln for dilution and IV infusion

Comment: Keytruda is a programmed death receptor-1 (PD-1)-blocking antibody indicated for the treatment of multiple cancers, including RCC. Keytruda, in combination with *axitinib*, is indicated for the first-line treatment of adult patients with advanced RCC. Keytruda, in combination with *lenvatinib*, is indicated for the first-line treatment of adult patients with advanced RCC. Keytruda is indicated for the adjuvant treatment of patients with RCC at intermediate-high or high risk of recurrence following nephrectomy, or following nephrectomy and resection of metastatic lesions. Keytruda can cause fetal harm. Advise females of reproductive potential of the embryo/fetal risk and to use effective contraception. Advise mothers not to breastfeed during treatment and for 4 months after the last Keytruda dose. See mfr pkg insert for full prescribing information including storage, preparation, warnings, precautions, drug-drug interactions, and adverse reactions.

▷ *selpercatinib* <50 kg: 120 mg bid; >50 kg: 160 mg bid; reduce dose in patients with severe hepatic impairment

Pediatric: <12 years: not established; ≥12 years: same as adult

Retevmo *hgc:* 40, 80 mg

Comment: Retevmo *(selpercatinib)* is a kinase inhibitor indicated for adult patients with metastatic RET fusion-positive non-small cell lung cancer; adult and pediatric patients ≥12 years of age with advanced or metastatic RET-mutant medullary thyroid cancer (MTC) who require systemic therapy; and adult and pediatric patients ≥12 years of age with advanced or metastatic RET fusion-positive thyroid cancer who require systemic therapy and who are radioactive iodine-refractory (if radioactive iodine is appropriate). The most common adverse reactions (incidence ≥25%), including laboratory abnormalities, have been increased aspartate aminotransferase (AST), increased alanine aminotransferase (ALT), increased glucose, decreased leukocytes, decreased albumin, decreased calcium, dry mouth, diarrhea, increased creatinine, increased alkaline phosphatase, hypertension, fatigue, edema, decreased platelets, increased total cholesterol, rash, decreased sodium, and constipation. Monitor ALT and AST prior to initiating Retevmo, every 2 weeks during the first 3 months, then monthly thereafter, and as clinically indicated. Do not initiate Retevmo in patients with uncontrolled hypertension; optimize blood pressure prior to initiating Retevmo and monitor blood pressure after 1 week, at least monthly thereafter and as clinically indicated. Monitor patients who are at significant risk of developing QTc prolongation. Assess QT interval, electrolytes, and TSH at baseline and periodically during treatment. Monitor QT interval more frequently when Retevmo is concomitantly administered with strong and moderate CYP3A inhibitors or drugs known to prolong QTc interval. Permanently discontinue Retevmo in patients with severe or life-threatening hemorrhage. Withhold Retevmo and initiate corticosteroids in the occurrence of any hypersensitivity reaction and, upon resolution, resume at a reduced dose and increase dose by one dose level each week until reaching the dose taken prior to onset of hypersensitivity. Continue steroids until the patient reaches target dose of Retevmo and then taper. Withhold Retevmo for at least 7 days prior to elective surgery. Do not administer for at least 2 weeks following major surgery and until adequate

(continued)

wound healing. The safety of resumption of **Retevmo** after resolution of wound healing complications has not been established. Avoid co-administration with proton pump inhibitors (PPIs); if co-administration cannot be avoided, take **Retevmo** with food (with PPI) or modify its administration time (with H2 receptor antagonist or locally acting antacid). Avoid co-administration with strong and moderate CYP3A inhibitors; if co-administration cannot be avoided, reduce the **Retevmo** dose. Avoid co-administration with strong and moderate CYP3A inducers. Avoid co-administration with CYP2C8 and CYP3A substrates; if co-administration cannot be avoided, modify the substrate dosage as recommended in its product labeling. Based on findings from animal studies and its mechanism of action, **Retevmo** can cause fetal harm. There are no available data on **Retevmo** use in pregnant women to inform drug-associated risk. Therefore, exclude pregnancy prior to initiating **Retevmo** and advise females of reproductive potential of the possible risk to the fetus and to use effective contraception. There are no data on the presence of *selpercatinib* or its metabolites in human milk or effects on the breastfed infant. Because of the potential for serious adverse embryo/fetal effects, advise women not to breastfeed during treatment with **Retevmo** and for 1 week after the final dose.

CANCER: LEUKEMIA

ORAL NUCLEOSIDE METABOLIC INHIBITOR

▶ *azacytidine* 300 mg orally once daily on days 1 through 14 of each 28-day cycle; administer an antiemetic before each dose for at least the first 2 cycles

Onureg *Tab:* 200, 300 mg

Comment: Onureg *(azacitidine)* is an oral form of *azacytidine* indicated for the continued treatment of adult patients with acute myeloid leukemia (AML) who have achieved first complete remission (CR) or complete remission with incomplete blood count recovery (CRi) following intensive induction chemotherapy and are not able to complete intensive curative therapy. The indications and dosing regimen for **Onureg** differ from that of IV or SC forms of *azacytidine*; do not substitute **Onureg** for IV or SC forms. Monitor complete blood counts every other week for the first 2 cycles and prior to the start of each cycle thereafter. Increase monitoring to every other week for the 2 cycles after any dose reduction. Withhold and then resume at the same or reduced dose or discontinue **Onureg** based on severity. **Onureg** can cause fetal harm; advise patients of the potential embryo/fetal risk and to use effective contraception. Advise not to breastfeed during treatment and for 1 week after the last dose.

CHRONIC LYMPHOCYTIC LEUKEMIA (CLL)

▶ *zanubrutinib* 160 mg (2 x 80 mg) bid or 320 mg (4 x 80 mg) once daily; swallow whole with water, with or without food; do not open, break, or chew capsules; *Child-Pugh Class C:* reduce dose; manage toxicity with dose reduction treatment interruption or discontinuation
Pediatric: safety and efficacy not established

Brukinsa *Cap:* 80 mg

Comment: Brukinsa is a kinase inhibitor (KI) indicated for the treatment of: (1) mantle cell lymphoma (MCL) who have received at least one prior therapy. (This indication is approved under accelerated approval based on overall response rate. Continued approval for this indication may be contingent upon verification and description of clinical benefit in a confirmatory; (2) marginal zone lymphoma (MZL); (3) relapsed or refractory marginal zone lymphoma (MZL) who have received at least one anti–CD20-based regimen; (4) chronic lymphocytic leukemia (CLL) or small lymphocytic lymphoma (SLL); and (5) Waldenström macroglobulinemia (WM). There are no contraindications to the use of **Brukinsa**. Monitor for bleeding and manage appropriately. Monitor patients for signs and symptoms of infection, including opportunistic infections, and treat as needed. Monitor CBCs for cytopenias during treatment. Other malignancies have developed, including skin cancers and non-skin carcinomas; advise patients to use sun protection. Monitor for signs and symptoms of cardiac arrhythmias and manage appropriately. Modify **Brukinsa** dose with moderate or strong CYP3A inhibitors. Avoid co-administration with strong or moderate CYP3A inducers. Dose adjustment may be recommended with moderate CYP3A inducers. The most common adverse reactions (≥30%), including laboratory abnormalities, are decreased neutrophil count, upper respiratory tract infection, decreased platelet count, hemorrhage, and musculoskeletal pain. **Brukinsa** is embryo/fetal toxic; it can cause fetal harm. Advise patients of reproductive potential of potential risk to the fetus and to use effective contraception. Advise not to breastfeed.

ASPARAGINE SPECIFIC ENZYME

▶ *asparaginase erwinia chrysanthemi (recombinant)-rywn* there are two **Rylaze** regimens that can be used to replace a long-acting asparaginase product: *administered q 48 hours:* 25 mg/m² IM every 48 hours; *administered Monday/Wednesday/Friday:* 25 mg/m² IM on Monday morning and Wednesday morning and 50 mg/m² IM on Friday afternoon

Rylaze *Vial:* 10 mg/0.5 ml soln, single-dose (preservative-free)

Comment: Rylaze is an asparagine-specific enzyme indicated as a component of a multiagent chemotherapeutic regimen for the treatment of acute lymphoblastic leukemia (ALL) and lymphoblastic lymphoma (LBL) in adult and pediatric patients ≥1 month of age who have developed hypersensitivity to *Escherichia coli*-derived asparaginase. The most common adverse reactions (incidence >20%) are abnormal liver test, nausea, musculoskeletal pain, infection, fatigue, headache, febrile neutropenia, pyrexia, hemorrhage, stomatitis, abdominal pain, decreased appetite, drug hypersensitivity, hyperglycemia, diarrhea, pancreatitis, and hypokalemia. **Rylaze** is contraindicated in patients with a history of (1) serious hypersensitivity reactions to **Rylaze**, including anaphylaxis; (2) serious pancreatitis during previous L-asparaginase therapy; (3) serious thrombosis during previous L-asparaginase therapy; and (4) serious hemorrhagic events during previous L-asparaginase therapy. Discontinue **Rylaze** for serious hypersensitivity reaction. Monitor for symptoms of pancreatitis and discontinue **Rylaze** if symptoms occur. Discontinue **Rylaze** for severe or life-threatening thrombosis and provide anticoagulation therapy as indicated. Discontinue **Rylaze** for severe or life-threatening hemorrhage. Monitor for hepatotoxicity and discontinue **Rylaze** for grade 4 increases in bilirubin. **Rylaze** is embryo/fetal toxic. Advise pregnant women of the potential risk to the fetus and advise females of reproductive potential to inform their healthcare provider of a known or suspected pregnancy. Exclude pregnancy prior to initiating treatment with **Rylaze**. Advise females of reproductive potential to use effective non-hormonal contraception during treatment with **Rylaze** and for 3 months after the last dose. Advise women not to breastfeed during treatment with **Rylaze** and for 1 week after the last dose.

CD20-DIRECTED CYTOLYTIC ANTIBODY

➤ *ofatumumab* dilute and administer each dose as an IV infusion; do not administer as an intravenous push (IVP) or bolus; protect vials from light; refrigerate between 2°C and 8°C (36° to 46°F); do not freeze; premedicate patients 30 minutes to 2 hours prior to each infusion with oral *acetaminophen* 1,000 mg (or equivalent), oral or IV antihistamine (*cetirizine* 10 mg or equivalent), and IV corticosteroid (*prednisolone* 100 mg or equivalent); see mfr pkg insert for routine rates of infusion and grade-based guidance in the setting of infusion reaction

Infusion Dose and Schedule (see mfr pkg insert for dose modifications following an infusion reaction)
• Total of 12 doses
• Dose 1: 300 mg (3 vials), followed 1 week later by
• Doses 2 through 8: each dose 2,000 mg (20 vials) once weekly x 7 doses (7 weeks), followed 4 weeks later by
• Doses 9 through 12: each dose 2,000 mg (20 vials) once every 4 weeks x 4 doses (16 weeks)
Preparation of Solution
300 mg Dose
• Withdraw and discard 15 ml from a 1,000 ml polyolefin bag of 0.9% NaCl, USP
• Withdraw 5 ml from each of 3 vials of **Arzerra** and add to the bag
• Mix diluted solution by gentle inversion; do not shake
2,000 mg Dose
• Withdraw and discard 100 ml from a 1,000 ml bag of 0.9% NaCl, USP
• Withdraw 5 ml from each of 20 vials of **Arzerra** and add to the bag
• Mix diluted solution by gentle inversion; do not shake
Administration Instructions
• Do not mix **Arzerra** with, or administer as an infusion with, other medicinal products
• Administer using an infusion pump, the in-line filter provided with the product, and a polyvinyl chloride (PVC) administration set
• Flush the IV line with 0.9% NaCl Injection, USP before and after each dose
• Start infusion within 12 hours of preparation
• Discard prepared solution after 24 hours
Pediatric: safety and efficacy not established

    Arzerra *Vial:* 100 mg/5 ml (20 mg/ml), single-use soln (3, 10 vials/carton with 2 filters) (preservative-free; latex-free)

    Comment: Arzerra is a CD20-directed cytolytic monoclonal antibody indicated for treatment of patients with CLL refractory to *fludarabine* and *alemtuzumab*. The effectiveness of **Arzerra** is based on the demonstration of durable objective responses. No data demonstrate an improvement in disease-related symptoms or increased survival with **Arzerra**. Monitor blood counts at regular intervals for neutropenia and thrombocytopenia. Increase the frequency of monitoring in patients who develop Grade 3 or 4 cytopenias. Monitor neurologic function and discontinue **Arzerra** if progressive multifocal leukoencephalopathy (PML) is suspected. Screen high-risk patients for hepatitis B (HBV) prior to treatment initiation with **Arzerra**. Discontinue **Arzerra** in patients who develop viral hepatitis or reactivation of viral hepatitis. The most common adverse reactions (≥10%) have been neutropenia, pneumonia, pyrexia, cough, diarrhea, anemia, fatigue, dyspnea, rash, nausea, bronchitis, and upper respiratory tract infections. **Arzerra** can cause serious infusion reactions manifesting as bronchospasm, dyspnea, laryngeal edema, pulmonary edema, flushing, hypertension, hypotension, syncope, cardiac ischemia/infarction, back pain, abdominal pain, pyrexia, rash, urticaria, and angioedema. Infusion reactions occur more frequently with the first 2 infusions. Premedicate with an IV corticosteroid (as appropriate), an oral analgesic, and an oral or IV antihistamine. Monitor patients closely during infusions and interrupt infusion of any severity if an infusion reaction occurs. Institute medical

(continued)

management for severe infusion reactions, including angina or other signs and symptoms of myocardial ischemia. In a study of patients with moderate-to-severe chronic obstructive pulmonary disease (COPD), an indication for which **Arzerra** is <u>not</u> approved, 2 of 5 patients developed Grade 3 bronchospasm during the infusion. Do <u>not</u> administer live viral vaccines to patients who have recently received **Arzerra**. There are no adequate or well-controlled studies of *ofatumumab* in human pregnancy. A reproductive animal study where pregnant females received *ofatumumab* at doses up to 3.5 times the recommended human dose did <u>not</u> demonstrate maternal toxicity or teratogenicity. *Ofatumumab* crossed the placental barrier, and fetuses exhibited depletion of peripheral B cells and decreased spleen and placental weights. **Arzerra** should be used during pregnancy only if the potential benefit to the mother justifies the potential risk to the fetus. Published data suggest that breastfeeding does <u>not</u> result in substantial absorption of maternal antibodies into fetal circulation. Developmental and health benefits of breastfeeding should be considered along with the mother's clinical need for **Arzerra** and any potential adverse effects on the breastfed infant from **Arzerra** or from the mother's underlying condition. To report suspected adverse reactions, contact GlaxoSmithKline at 1-888-825-5249 or FDA at 1-800-FDA-1088 or www.fda.gov/medwatch.

▷ *rituximab Recommended dose:* 375 mg/m² via IV infusion the day prior to the initiation of *fludarabine* and *cyclophosphamide* (FC) chemotherapy; then 500 mg/m² on Day 1 of cycles 2 through 6 (every 28 days); *First infusion:* initiate at 50 mg/hour; in the absence of infusion toxicity, increase infusion rate by 50 mg/hour increments every 30 minutes, to a max of 400 mg/hour; *Subsequent infusions: standard infusion:* initiate at 100 mg/hour; in the absence of infusion toxicity, increase by 100 mg/hour increments at 30-minute intervals, to a max of 400 mg/hour; patients who have clinically significant cardiovascular disease or who have a circulating lymphocyte count ≥5,000/mm³ before Cycle 2 should <u>not</u> be administered a 90-minute infusion; interrupt the infusion or slow the infusion rate for infusion-related reactions; continue the infusion at one-half the previous rate upon improvement of symptoms; **Rituxan** should <u>only</u> be administered by a qualified healthcare professional with appropriate medical support to manage severe infusion-related reactions that can be fatal if they occur

Pediatric: safety and efficacy <u>not</u> established

    Rituxan *Vial:* 100 mg/10 ml (10 mg/ml), 500 mg/50 ml (10 mg/ml), single-dose, soln for dilution and IV infusion (preservative-free)

    Comment: **Rituxan** is indicated for the treatment of adult patients with previously untreated <u>and</u> previously treated CD20-positive CLL in combination with *fludarabine* <u>and</u> *cyclophosphamide*. The most common adverse common reactions (incidence >25%) have been infusion-related reactions and neutropenia. For tumor lysis syndrome (TLS), administer aggressive IV hydration and antihyperuricemic agents, and monitor renal function. Monitor for infections; withhold **Rituxan** and institute appropriate anti-infective therapy. For cardiac adverse reactions, discontinue **Rituxan** infusions in case of serious or life-threatening events. Discontinue **Rituxan** in patients with rising serum creatinine or oliguria. Bowel obstruction and perforation can occur; consider and evaluate for abdominal pain, vomiting, or related symptoms. Live virus vaccinations prior to or during **Rituxan** treatment is <u>not</u> recommended. **Rituxan** is embryo/fetal toxic. Advise males and females of reproductive potential of the potential embryo/fetal risk and to use appropriate contraception. Advise women <u>not</u> to breastfeed during treatment and for at least 6 months after the last dose.

▷ *rituximab-arrx First Cycle:* 375 mg/m²; then, *Cycles 2 through 6:* 500 mg/m² in combination with *fludarabine* and *phosphamide* (FC) administered every 28 days; administer <u>all</u> doses of **Riabni** in combination with glucocorticoids; **Riabni** should <u>only</u> be administered by a qualified healthcare professional with appropriate medical support to manage severe infusion-related reactions that can be fatal

    Riabni *Vial:* 100 mg/10 ml (10 mg/ml), 500 mg/50 ml (10 mg/ml) soln, single-dose

    Comment: **Riabni** *(rituximab-arrx)* is a biosimilar to **Rituxan** indicated for previously untreated and previously treated CD20-positive CLL in combination with *fludarabine* and *cyclophosphamide* (FC). The most common adverse reactions in clinical trials with CLL (incidence ≥25%) have been infusion-related reactions and neutropenia. Monitor renal function. Discontinue **Riabni** in patients with rising serum creatinine or oliguria. If TLS is suspected, administer aggressive IV hydration and antihyperuricemic agents. If infection occurs, withhold **Riabni** and institute appropriate antiinfective therapy. Bowel obstruction and perforation can occur; evaluate for abdominal pain, vomiting, and related symptoms. Live virus vaccine administration prior to or during treatment with **Riabni** is <u>not</u> recommended. **Riabni** can cause embryo/fetal harm. Advise females of reproductive potential of embryo/fetal risk and to use effective contraception. Advise <u>not</u> to breastfeed.

CD20-DIRECTED CYTOLYTIC ANTIBODY+ENDOGLYCOSIDASE

▷ *rituximab+hyaluronidase human* administer 1,600 mg/26,800 units (*rituximab* 1,400 mg and *hyaluronidase human* 23,400 units) SC on Day 1 of Cycles 2 through 6 (every 28 days) for a total of 5 cycles <u>following</u> a single IV dose on Day 1, Cycle 1 (i.e., 6 cycles in total); *Premedicate:* with *acetaminophen* and antihistamine before each dose; consider premedication with glucocorticoids; **Rituxan Hycela** should <u>only</u> be administered by a qualified healthcare professional with appropriate medical support to manage severe infusion-related reactions that can be fatal if they occur

    Rituxan Hycela *Vial: rituximab* 1,400 mg + *hyaluronidase human* 23,400 units per 11.7 ml (120 mg/2,000 units/ml), single dose, soln for dilution and IV infusion; *rituximab* 1,600 mg + *hyaluronidase human* 26,800 units per 13.4 ml (120 mg/2,000 units/ml), single dose, soln for dilution and IV infusion

Comment: Rituxan Hycela is a fixed two-drug combination indicated for the treatment of CLL. The most common adverse reactions (incidence ≥20%) have been infections, neutropenia, nausea, thrombocytopenia, pyrexia, vomiting, and injection site erythema. There is risk of renal toxicity when **Rituxan Hycela** is used in combination with **cisplatin**. Local cutaneous reactions may occur more than 24 hours after administration. Interrupt **Rituxan Hycela** injections if severe reaction develops and administer aggressive IV hydration and antihyperuricemic agents, and monitor renal function. Monitor for infections; withhold and institute appropriate anti-infective therapy as appropriate. With cardiac adverse reactions, discontinue in case of serious or life-threatening events. Discontinue in patients with rising serum creatinine or oliguria. Bowel obstruction and perforation may occur; consider and evaluate for abdominal pain, vomiting, or related symptoms. Live virus vaccinations prior to or during treatment not recommended. **Rituxan Hycela** is embryo/fetal toxic. Advise males and females of reproductive potential of the potential embryo/fetal risk and to use effective contraception. Advise women not to breastfeed during treatment and for at least 6 months after the last dose.

CANCER: LIVER, HEPATOCELLULAR CARCINOMA (HCC)

KINASE INHIBITOR

▶ **sorafenib (G)** 400 mg (2 x 200 mg) bid, without food
  Nexavar *Tab:* 200 mg
  Comment: Nexavar is indicated for the treatment of unresectable hepatocellular carcinoma (uHCC). The most common adverse reactions (incidence ≥20%) have been diarrhea, fatigue, infection, alopecia, hand-foot skin reaction, rash, weight loss, decreased appetite, nausea, gastrointestinal and abdominal pain, hypertension, and hemorrhage. **Nexavar** in combination with **carboplatin** and **paclitaxel** is contraindicated in patients with squamous cell lung cancer. Avoid strong CYP3A4 inducers. Monitor ECG (for QT prolongation) and electrolytes in patients at increased risk for ventricular arrhythmias. Consider temporary or permanent discontinuation of **Nexavar** in the event of a cardiovascular event. Discontinue **Nexavar** if needed in the event of bleeding. Monitor the patient for hypertension, weekly during the first 6 weeks and periodically thereafter. Interrupt and/or decrease **Nexavar** for severe or persistent dermal reaction, and immediately discontinue **Nexavar** if Stevens-Johnson syndrome (SJS) and toxic epidermal necrolysis (TEN) is suspected. Discontinue **Nexavar** in the event of gastrointestinal perforation. **Nexavar** may cause hepatotoxicity; monitor liver function tests regularly and discontinue for unexplained transaminase elevation. Monitor thyroid stimulating hormone (TSH) monthly and adjust thyroid replacement therapy in patients with thyroid cancer. **Nexavar** may cause embryo/fetal harm; exclude pregnancy prior to initiating **Nexavar** and advise females and males of reproductive potential to use effective contraception. Advise women not to breastfeed.

PROGRAMMED DEATH RECEPTOR-1 (PD-1)-BLOCKING ANTIBODY

▶ **pembrolizumab** administer 200 mg via IV infusion over 30 minutes once every 3 weeks or 400 mg via IV infusion over 30 minutes once every 6 weeks until disease progression, unacceptable toxicity, or for Keytruda up to 24 months
  Pediatric: safety and efficacy not established
  Keytruda *Vial:* 100 mg/4 ml (25 mg/ml), single-dose, soln for dilution and IV infusion
  Comment: Keytruda is a programmed death receptor-1 (PD-1)-blocking antibody indicated for treatment of multiple cancers, including patients with hepatocellular carcinoma (HCC) who have been previously treated with **sorafenib**. This indication is approved under accelerated approval based on tumor response rate and durability of response. Continued approval for this indication may be contingent upon verification and description of clinical benefit in confirmatory trials. **Keytruda** can cause fetal harm. Exclude pregnancy prior to initiating treatment with **Keytruda**. Advise females of reproductive potential of the embryo/fetal risk and to use effective contraception during treatment and for 4 weeks after the last **Keytruda** dose. Advise mothers not to breastfeed during treatment and for 4 months after the last **Keytruda** dose. See mfr pkg insert for full prescribing information including storage, preparation, warnings, precautions, drug-drug interactions, and adverse reactions.

CYTOTOXIC T-LYMPHOCYTE-ASSOCIATED ANTIGEN 4 (CTLA-4) BLOCKING ANTIBODY

▶ **tremelimumab-actl** *Dose preparation:* store **Imjudo** vials in a refrigerator at 2°C to 8°C (36°F to 46°F) in original carton to protect from light; do not freeze; do not shake; withdraw the required dose (volume) from the vial(s) of **Imjudo** and transfer into the IV fluid bag containing 0.9% NaCl, USP or 5% Dextrose Injection, USP; mix diluted solution by gentle inversion; do not shake the solution; the maximum final concentration of the diluted solution should not exceed 10 mg/ml; the total volume of diluent for use with each dose and patient weight is presented in the table below; discard partially used or empty vial(s) of **Imjudo**; **Imjudo** does not contain a preservative; administer the infusion solution immediately once prepared; if the infusion solution is not administered immediately and needs to be stored, the total time from preparation to the start of administration should not exceed 24 hours in a refrigerator at 2°C to 8°C (36°F to 46°F) or 24 hours at room temperature up to 30°C (86°F).

(continued)

Dose	Weight	Total Solution
300 mg	≥30 kg	150 ml
4 mg/kg	<30 kg	80 ml
75 mg	≥30 kg	150 ml
1 mg/kg	<30 kg	80 ml

Treatment: administer **Imjudo** via infusion over 60 minutes after dilution;
Weight ≥30 kg: Administer **Imjudo** 300 mg, as a single dose, in combination with *durvalumab* 1,500 mg at cycle 1/day 1, followed by *durvalumab* as a single agent once every 4 weeks;
Weight <30 kg: administer **Imjudo** 4 mg/kg, as a single dose, in combination with *durvalumab* 20 mg/kg on Cycle 1/Day 1, followed by *durvalumab* as a single agent once every 4 weeks; see mfr pkg insert for full prescribing information, including dose modifications for adverse reactions
Pediatric: safety and efficacy not established
    Imjudo *Vial:* 25 mg/1.25 ml (20 mg/ml), 300 mg/15 ml (20 mg/ml), single-dose, solution for dilution and IV infusion (preservative-free)
    Comment: Imjudo is a cytotoxic T-lymphocyte-associated antigen 4 (CTLA-4)-blocking antibody indicated in combination with *durvalumab*, for the treatment of adult patients with uHCC. Immune-mediated adverse reactions, which may be severe or fatal, can occur in any organ system or tissue, including the following: immune-mediated pneumonitis, immune-mediated colitis, immune-mediated hepatitis, immune-mediated endocrinopathies, immune-mediated dermatologic adverse reactions, immune-mediated nephritis with renal dysfunction, and immune-mediated pancreatitis. Monitor for early identification and management of an immune-mediated adverse reaction. Evaluate liver enzymes, creatinine, adrenocorticotropic hormone level, and thyroid function at baseline and before each dose. Withhold or permanently discontinue **Imjudo** based on severity and type of reaction. For infusion-related reactions, interrupt, slow the rate of infusion, or permanently discontinue treatment based on the severity of the reaction. The most common adverse reactions (incidence ≥20%) of patients with uHCC have been rash, diarrhea, fatigue, pruritus, musculoskeletal pain, and abdominal pain. The most common laboratory abnormalities (incidence ≥40%) in patients with uHCC have been increased aspartate aminotransferase (AST) and alanine aminotransferase (ALT), decreased hemoglobin, decreased sodium, increased bilirubin, increased alkaline phosphatase, and decreased lymphocytes. Human immunoglobulin G2 (IgG2) is known to cross the placental barrier; therefore, **Imjudo** has the potential to be transmitted from the mother to the developing fetus. There are no available data on the use of **Imjudo** in human pregnancy. However, based on findings from animal studies and the drug's mechanism of action, **Imjudo** is embryo/fetal toxic. CTLA-4 blockade is associated with increased risk of immune-mediated rejection of the developing fetus and fetal death. Therefore, advise females of reproductive potential of the potential risk to the fetus. Exclude pregnancy prior to initiating treatment, and advise females of reproductive potential to use effective contraception with **Imjudo.** There are no data on the presence of ***tremelimumab-actl*** in human milk or effects on the breastfed infant. Maternal immunoglobulin G (IgG) is known to be present in human milk. The effects of local gastrointestinal exposure and limited systemic exposure in the breastfed infant to **Imjudo** are unknown. Because of the potential for serious adverse reactions, advise women not to breastfeed during treatment with **Imjudo** and for 3 months after the last **Imjudo** dose. To report suspected adverse reactions, contact AstraZeneca at 800-236-9933 or FDA at 800-FDA-1088 or www.fda.gov/medwatch.

ALKYLATING AGENT
Comment: Treanda is contraindicated in patients with a history of a hypersensitivity reaction to *bendamustine*; reactions have included anaphylaxis and anaphylactoid reactions. Consider alternative concomitant therapies that are not CYP1A2 inducers or inhibitors during treatment. Do not use in patients with CrCl 3 × the upper limit of normal (ULN). Monitor the patient for myelosuppression; delay or reduce dose and restart treatment based on absolute neutrophil count (ANC) and platelet count recovery. Monitor for fever and other signs of infection or reactivation of infection and treat promptly. Monitor the patient for progressive multifocal leukoencephalopathy (PML) (new or worsening neurologic, cognitive, or behavioral signs or symptoms suggestive of PML). Premedicate in subsequent cycles for milder reactions. Tumor lysis syndrome (TLS) may lead to acute renal failure and death; anticipate and use supportive measures in patients at high risk. Discontinue for severe skin reactions; cases of SJS, drug reaction with eosinophilia and systemic symptoms (DRESS), and TEN, some fatal, have been reported. Monitor liver chemistry tests prior to and during treatment. Premalignant and malignant diseases have been reported. Take precautions to avoid extravasation, including monitoring the IV infusion site during and after administration. **Treanda** can cause fetal harm; advise females of reproductive potential of the potential risk to the fetus and to use an effective method of contraception. Advise not to breastfeed. **Treanda** may impair fertility.

ISOCITRATE DEHYDROGENASE-1 (IDH1) INHIBITOR

▶ *olutasidenib Recommend:* 150 mg bid, until disease progression or unacceptable toxicity; take on an empty stomach at least 1 hour before or 2 hours after a meal

Pediatric: safety and efficacy not established

Rezlidhia *Cap:* 150 mg

Comment: Rezlidhia *(olutasidenib)* is an isocitrate dehydrogenase-1 (IDH1) inhibitor indicated for the treatment of adult patients with relapsed or refractory acute myeloid leukemia (AML) with a susceptible IDH1 mutation as detected by an FDA-approved test. Avoid concomitant use of strong or moderate CYP3A inducers. Avoid concomitant use of sensitive CYP3A substrates (monitor if unavoidable). Monitor liver function tests during treatment with **Rezlidhia**. If hepatotoxicity occurs, interrupt and reduce or discontinue **Rezlidhia**. *Boxed Warning:* Differentiation syndrome, which can be fatal, can occur with **Rezlidhia** treatment. If differentiation syndrome is suspected, withhold **Rezlidhia** and initiate corticosteroids and hemodynamic monitoring until symptom resolution. The most common (>20%) adverse reactions, including laboratory abnormalities, are increased AST, increased ALT, decreased potassium, decreased sodium, increased alkaline phosphatase, nausea, increased creatinine, fatigue/malaise, arthralgia, constipation, increased lymphocytes, increased bilirubin, leukocytosis, increased uric acid, dyspnea, pyrexia, rash, increased lipase, mucositis, diarrhea, and transaminitis. There are no available data on human use of **Rezlidhia** in pregnancy to evaluate for a drug-associated risk. However, in embryo/fetal development studies, oral *olutasidenib* resulted in embryo/fetal death and altered fetal growth and development. Advise pregnant women of the potential risk to the fetus and advise the use of effective contraceptive during treatment with **Rezlidhia**. There are no data on the presence of *olutasidenib* or its metabolites in human milk or effects on the breastfed infant. Because of the potential for adverse reactions in the breastfed infant, advise patients not to breastfeed during treatment with **Rezlidhia** and for 2 weeks after the last dose.

IRREVERSIBLE TYROSINE KINASE INHIBITOR (ITKI)

▶ *futibatinib* confirm the presence of a fibroblast growth factor receptor 2 (FGFR2) gene fusion or other rearrangement prior to initiation of treatment with **Lytgobi**; *recommended dose:* 20 mg (5 x 4 mg tablets) once daily until disease progression or unacceptable toxicity occurs; swallow whole, do not cut or crush tablets; take with or without food

Pediatric: safety and efficacy not established

Lytgobi *Tab:* 4 mg film-coat; *20 mg daily dose* (1 blister card containing a 7-day supply [35 tablets]/carton); *16 mg daily dose* (1 blister card containing a 7-day supply [28 tablets]); *12 mg daily dose* (1 blister card containing a 7-day supply [21 tablets]/carton)

Comment: Lytgobi is an irreversible tyrosine kinase inhibitor of FGFR1, 2, 3, and 4 for treatment of intrahepatic cholangiocarcinoma harboring FGFR2 gene fusions or other rearrangements and for previously treated, unresectable, locally advanced or metastatic cholangiocarcinoma. This indication is approved under accelerated approval based on overall response rate and duration of response. Continued approval for this indication may be contingent upon verification and description of clinical benefit in a confirmatory trial(s). The most common (incidence ≥20%) adverse reactions have been nail toxicity, musculoskeletal pain, constipation, diarrhea, fatigue, dry mouth, alopecia, stomatitis, abdominal pain, dry skin, arthralgia, dysgeusia, dry eye, nausea, decreased appetite, urinary tract infection (UTI), palmar-plantar erythrodysesthesia syndrome, and vomiting. The most common laboratory abnormalities (incidence ≥20%) have been increased phosphate, increased creatinine, decreased hemoglobin, increased glucose, increased calcium, decreased sodium, decreased phosphate, increased ALT, increased alkaline phosphatase, decreased lymphocytes, increased AST, decreased platelets, increased activated partial thromboplastin time, decreased leukocytes, decreased albumin, decreased neutrophils, increased creatine kinase, increased bilirubin, decreased glucose, increased prothrombin international normalized ratio (INR), and decreased potassium. **Lytgobi** can cause retinal pigment epithelial detachment (RPED). A comprehensive ophthalmologic examination, including optical coherence tomography (OCT), should be performed prior to initiation of therapy, every 2 months for the first 6 months, and every 3 months thereafter, and urgently at any time for visual symptoms. Increases in phosphate levels can cause hyperphosphatemia, leading to soft tissue mineralization, calcinosis, non-uremic calciphylaxis, and vascular calcification. Monitor for hyperphosphatemia and withhold, reduce the dose, or permanently discontinue **Lytgobi** based on duration and severity of hyperphosphatemia. Avoid co-administration of dual P-gp and strong CYP3A inhibitors, and avoid co-administration of dual P-gp and strong CYP3A inducers, when taking **Lytgobi**. Based on findings in animal studies and its mechanism of action, **Lytgobi** can cause fetal harm (malformations or loss of pregnancy) when administered in human pregnancy. Exclude pregnancy prior to initiating treatment with **Lytgobi**. Advise females of reproductive potential of the potential risk to the fetus and to use effective contraception during treatment and for 1 week after the last dose. There are no data on the presence of *futibatinib* or its metabolites in human milk or effects on the breastfed infant. Because of the potential for serious adverse reactions from **Lytgobi** in breastfed infants, advise mothers not to breastfeed during treatment and for 1 week after the last dose. To report suspected adverse reactions, contact Taiho Oncology at 844-878-2446 or FDA at 800-FDA-1088 or http://www.fda.gov/medwatch.

CANCER: LUNG

See Mesothelioma

CISPLATIN NEUTRALIZING AGENT

▶ *sodium thiosulfate* not indicated for adults
  Pediatric: <1 month: safety and efficacy not established; ≥1 month: *Recommended Dose:* based on body surface area (BSA) according to actual body weight (see dosing table below); *Administer* via IV infusion over 15 minutes starting 6 hours after completion of *cisplatin* infusion; *Multi-Day Cisplatin Regimens:* Administer 6 hours after each *cisplatin* infusion, but at least 10 hours before the next *cisplatin* infusion; Do not start if less than 10 hours before starting the next *cisplatin* infusion; Store at 20°C to 25°C (68°F to 77°F); Excursions are permitted between 15°C and 30°C (59°F to 86°F)

Pedmark Dose by Weight	
Weight	Dose
<5 kg	10 g/m²
<5 kg to 10 kg	15 g/m²
>10 kg	20 g/m²

  Pedmark *Vial:* 12.5 gm/100 ml (125 mg/ml), single-use, for IV infusion
  Comment: **Pedmark** is indicated to reduce the risk of ototoxicity associated with *cisplatin* in pediatric patients ≥1 month of age with localized, non-metastatic solid tumors. **Pedmark** is not recommended for treatment of patients <1 year of age due to increased risk of hypernatremia. **Pedmark** is not indicated for treatment of pediatric patients <1 month of age (due to increased risk of hypernatremia) or pediatric patients with metastatic cancer. **Pedmark** may not reduce the risk of ototoxicity when administered following longer *cisplatin* infusions because irreversible ototoxicity may have already occurred. The most common adverse reactions (≥25% with difference between arms of >5% compared to *cisplatin* alone) in SIOPEL 6 are vomiting, nausea, decreased hemoglobin, and hypernatremia. The most common adverse reaction (≥25% with difference between arms of >5% compared to *cisplatin* alone) in COG ACCL0431 is hypokalemia. History of severe hypersensitivity to *sodium thiosulfate* or any components is the only contraindication. For signs and symptoms of hypersensitivity reaction, immediately discontinue **Pedmark** and institute appropriate care. Administer premedications before each subsequent dose. **Pedmark** may contain sodium sulfite; patients with sulfite sensitivity may have hypersensitivity reactions. Monitor serum sodium and potassium at baseline and as clinically indicated; monitor more closely if glomerular filtration rate (GFR) falls below 60 ml/min/1.73 m². Withhold **Pedmark** with serum sodium >145 mmol/L. For nausea and vomiting, administer antiemetics prior to each dose administration. There are no available data on **Pedmark** to evaluate for drug-associated risk in human pregnancy or lactation. In animal studies, *sodium thiosulfate* was not embryotoxic or teratogenic. Additionally, an intravenous pharmacokinetic study in gravid animals indicated that *sodium thiosulfate* does not cross the placenta. **Pedmark** is administered following *cisplatin* infusions, which can cause embryo/fetal harm. There are no available data on the presence of *sodium thiosulfate* in human milk or effects on the breastfed infant. Refer to *cisplatin* mfr pkg insert for additional information. To report suspected adverse reactions, contact Fennec Pharmaceuticals at 1-833-336-6321 or FDA at 1-800-FDA-1088 or www.fda.gov/medwatch.

VASCULAR ENDOTHELIAL GROWTH FACTOR (VEGF) INHIBITOR

▶ *bevacizumab-adcd Regimen for first-line non-squamous non-small cell lung cancer:* 15 mg/kg every 3 weeks with *carboplatin* and *paclitaxel;* Withhold for at least 28 days prior to elective surgery; Do not administer Vegzelma for 28 days following major surgery and until adequate wound healing; Store refrigerated at 2°C to 8°C (36°F to 46°F) in the original carton until time of use to protect from light; Do not freeze or shake the vial or carton; See mfr pkg insert for full prescribing information, including proper preparation and administration instructions and dosage modifications for adverse reactions
  Pediatric: <18 years: Safety and efficacy not established; ≥18 years: same as adult
  Vegzelma *Vial:* 100 mg/4 ml (25 mg/ml) or 400 mg/16 ml (25 mg/ml), single-dose, soln for dilution and IV infusion
  Comment: **Vegzelma** is a vascular endothelial growth factor (VEGF) inhibitor biosimilar to **Avastin** indicated for the treatment of multiple types of cancer, including colorectal cancer, NSCLC, glioblastoma, renal cell carcinoma, cervical cancer, and epithelial ovarian, fallopian tube, or primary peritoneal cancer. *Bevacizumab* products increase the risk of ovarian failure and may impair fertility. Inform females of reproductive potential of the risk of ovarian failure prior to the first dose of **Vegzelma**. Long-term effects of *bevacizumab* products on fertility are not known. *Bevacizumab* products may cause fetal harm when administered to a pregnant female. Advise females of reproductive potential to use effective contraception during treatment with **Vegzelma** and for 6 months after the last dose. No data are available regarding the presence of *bevacizumab* products in human milk or effects on

the breastfed infant. Because of the potential for serious adverse reactions in breastfed infants, advise mothers <u>not</u> to breastfeed during treatment with **Vegzelma** and for 6 months after the last dose. See mfr pkg insert for full prescription information.

➤ *bevacizumab-bvzr* administer 15 mg/kg via IV infusion every 3 weeks <u>with</u> *carboplatin* <u>and</u> *paclitaxel*; do <u>not</u> administer **Zirabev** for 28 days following major surgery and until surgical wound is fully healed
Zirabev *Vial:* 100 mg/4 ml (25 mg/ml), 400 mg/16 ml (25 mg/ml), single-dose
Comment: Zirabev is biosimilar to **Avastin** *(bevacizumab)* with indications for treatment of multiple types of cancer, including NSCLC, using diagnosis-specific dosing regimens. See mfr pkg insert for prescribing information. **Zirabev** is used, in combination with *carboplatin* and *paclitaxel*, for first-line treatment of unresectable, locally advanced, recurrent <u>or</u> metastatic non-squamous NSCLC.

KINASE INHIBITORS

➤ *brigatinib* 90 mg once daily x 7 days; then increase to 180 mg once daily; take with <u>or</u> without food; if a dose is missed <u>or</u> if the patient vomits after taking a dose, do <u>not</u> to repeat the dose, take the next dose at the regular time
Pediatric: safety and efficacy <u>not</u> established
Alunbrig *Tab:* 30, 90, 180 mg film-coat
Comment: Alunbrig is an anaplastic lymphoma kinase (ALK) inhibitor for the treatment of patients with ALK-positive metastatic NSCLC as detected by an FDA-approved test. The most common adverse reactions (incidence ≥25%) with **Alunbrig** have been diarrhea, fatigue, nausea, rash, cough, myalgia, headache, hypertension, vomiting, and dyspnea. Withhold **Alunbrig**, then consider dose reduction <u>or</u> permanent discontinuation, based on occurrence <u>and/or</u> severity of physiologic changes. Assess fasting serum glucose prior to starting **Alunbrig** and regularly during treatment. Monitor for new <u>or</u> worsening respiratory symptoms, particularly during the first week of treatment. Withhold **Alunbrig** for new <u>or</u> worsening respiratory symptoms and promptly evaluate for interstitial lung disease (ILD)/pneumonitis. Monitor BP after 2 weeks and then at least monthly during treatment. Monitor heart rate regularly during treatment. Monitor creatine phosphokinase (CPK) regularly during treatment and occurrence of muscle pain <u>or</u> weakness. Monitor lipase and amylase levels regularly during treatment. Monitor for hepatic impairment <u>or</u> renal impairment. **Alunbrig** can cause fetal harm. Exclude pregnancy in females of reproductive potential prior to initiating **Alunbrig**. Advise females of reproductive potential of the potential embryo/fetal risk and to use a non-hormonal method of effective contraception during treatment and for at least 4 months after the last dose. Advise <u>not</u> to breastfeed during treatment with **Alunbrig** and for 1 week after the last dose.

➤ *capmatinib* 400 mg bid with <u>or</u> without food
Pediatric: safety and efficacy <u>not</u> established
Tabrecta *Tab:* 150, 200 mg
Comment: Tabrecta *(capmatinib)* is indicated for the treatment of adult patients with metastatic NSCLC, whose tumors have a mutation that leads to mesenchymal-epithelial transition (MET) exon 14 skipping, as detected by an FDA-approved test. The most common adverse reactions (incidence ≥20%) have been peripheral edema, nausea, fatigue, vomiting, dyspnea, and decreased appetite. Monitor for new <u>or</u> worsening pulmonary symptoms indicative of ILD/pneumonitis. Permanently discontinue **Tabrecta** in patients with ILD/pneumonitis. Monitor liver function tests. In the event of hepatotoxicity, withhold, reduce dose, <u>or</u> permanently discontinue **Tabrecta** based on severity. **Tabrecta** may cause photosensitivity reactions. Advise patients to limit direct ultraviolet (UV) exposure. **Tabrecta** can cause embryo/fetal harm. Advise patients of reproductive potential to use effective contraception. Advise <u>not</u> to breastfeed.

➤ *pralsetinib* 400 mg once daily; Take on an empty stomach (no food for at least 2 hours before and at least 1 hour after taking the dose)
Pediatric: safety and efficacy <u>not</u> established
Gavreto *Cap:* 100 mg
Comment: Gavreto is an oral selective rearranged during transfection (RET) kinase inhibitor for the treatment of adult patients with metastatic RET fusion-positive NSCLC as detected by an FDA-approved test. This indication is approved under accelerated approval based on overall response rate and duration of response. Continued approval for this indication may be contingent upon verification and description of clinical benefit in confirmatory trial(s). See the mfr pkg insert for prescribing information. There are <u>no</u> available data on **Gavreto** use in pregnant females to inform drug-associated risk. Based on findings from animal studies and its mechanism of action, **Gavreto** can cause embryo/fetal harm when administered to a pregnant female. There are <u>no</u> data on the presence of *pralsetinib* <u>or</u> its metabolites in human milk <u>or</u> their effects on the breastfed infant. Because of the potential for serious adverse reactions in breastfed children, advise women <u>not</u> to breastfeed during treatment with **Gavreto** and for 1 week after the final dose.

➤ *selpercatinib* *<50 kg:* 120 mg bid; *>50 kg:* 160 mg bid; reduce dose in patients with severe hepatic impairment
Pediatric: <12 years: safety and efficacy <u>not</u> established; ≥12 years: same as adult
Retevmo *hgc:* 40, 80 mg

(continued)

Comment: Retevmo is a kinase inhibitor indicated for adult patients with metastatic RET fusion-positive NSCLC; adult and pediatric patients ≥12 years of age with advanced or metastatic RET-mutant medullary thyroid cancer (MTC) who require systemic therapy; and adult and pediatric patients ≥12 years of age with advanced or metastatic RET fusion-positive thyroid cancer who require systemic therapy and who are radioactive iodine-refractory (if radioactive iodine is appropriate). The most common adverse reactions (incidence ≥25%), including laboratory abnormalities, have been increased aspartate aminotransferase (AST), increased alanine aminotransferase (ALT), increased glucose, decreased leukocytes, decreased albumin, decreased calcium, dry mouth, diarrhea, increased creatinine, increased alkaline phosphatase, hypertension, fatigue, edema, decreased platelets, increased total cholesterol, rash, decreased sodium, and constipation. Monitor ALT and AST prior to initiating Retevmo, every 2 weeks during the first 3 months, then monthly thereafter and as clinically indicated. Do not initiate Retevmo in patients with uncontrolled hypertension; optimize BP prior to initiating Retevmo and monitor BP after 1 week, at least monthly thereafter, and as clinically indicated. Monitor patients who are at significant risk of developing QTc prolongation. Assess QT interval, electrolytes, and thyroid stimulating hormone (TSH) at baseline and periodically during treatment. Monitor QT interval more frequently when Retevmo is concomitantly administered with strong and moderate CYP3A inhibitors or drugs known to prolong QTc interval. Permanently discontinue Retevmo in patients with severe or life-threatening hemorrhage. Withhold Retevmo and initiate corticosteroids in the occurrence of any hypersensitivity reaction and, upon resolution, resume at a reduced dose and increase dose by 1 dose level each week until reaching the dose taken prior to the onset of hypersensitivity. Continue steroids until the patient reaches target dose of Retevmo and then taper. Withhold Retevmo for at least 7 days prior to elective surgery. Do not administer for at least 2 weeks following major surgery and until adequate wound healing. The safety of resumption of Retevmo after resolution of wound healing complications has not been established. Avoid co-administration with proton pump inhibitors (PPIs); if co-administration cannot be avoided, take Retevmo with food (with PPI) or modify its administration time (with H2 receptor antagonist or locally acting antacid). Avoid co-administration with strong and moderate CYP3A inhibitors; if co-administration cannot be avoided, reduce the Retevmo dose. Avoid co-administration with strong and moderate CYP3A inducers. Avoid co-administration with CYP2C8 and CYP3A substrates; if co-administration cannot be avoided, modify the substrate dosage as recommended in its product labeling. Based on findings from animal studies and its mechanism of action, Retevmo can cause fetal harm. There are no available data on Retevmo use in pregnant women to inform drug-associated risk. Therefore, exclude pregnancy in females of reproductive potential prior to initiating Retevmo and advise females of reproductive potential of the possible risk to the fetus and to use effective contraception. There are no data on the presence of *selpercatinib* or its metabolites in human milk or effects on the breastfed infant. Because of the potential for serious adverse embryo/fetal effects, advise women not to breastfeed during treatment with Retevmo and for 1 week after the final dose.

▷ **tepotinib** *Recommended dose:* 450 mg once daily with food until disease progression or unacceptable toxicity
Tepmetko *Tab:* 225 mg
Comment: Tepmetko is the first and only oral MET inhibitor for the treatment of patients with metastatic NSCLC harboring MET exon 14 skipping alterations. The most common adverse reactions (incidence ≥20%) have been edema, fatigue, nausea, diarrhea, musculoskeletal pain, and dyspnea. The most common Grade 3 to 4 laboratory abnormalities (incidence ≥2%) have been decreased lymphocytes, decreased albumin, decreased sodium, increased gamma-glutamyltransferase, increased amylase, increased ALT, increased AST, and decreased hemoglobin. Avoid concomitant use of dual strong CYP3A inhibitors and P-gp inhibitors. Avoid concomitant use of certain P-gp substrates where minimal concentration changes may lead to serious or life-threatening toxicity. Immediately withhold Tepmetko in patients with suspected ILD/Pneumonitis. Permanently discontinue Tepmetko in patients diagnosed with ILD/pneumonitis of any severity. Monitor liver function tests and withhold, dose reduce, or permanently discontinue Tepmetko based on severity. Tepmetko is embryo/fetal toxic. Advise patients of reproductive potential of the risk and to use effective contraception. Advise not to breastfeed.

▷ **trilaciclib** administer 240 mg/m² via IV infusion over 30 minutes; complete infusion within 4 hours prior to the start of chemotherapy on each chemotherapy day
Cosela *Vial:* 300 mg pwdr, single-dose, for reconstitution, dilution, and IV infusion
Comment: *Trilaciclib* is a kinase inhibitor indicated to decrease the incidence of chemotherapy-induced myelosuppression in adult patients when administered prior to a platinum/etoposide-containing regimen or topotecan-containing regimen for extensive-stage small cell lung cancer (SCLC). The most common adverse reactions (incidence ≥10%) have been fatigue, hypocalcemia, hypokalemia, hypophosphatemia, increased aspartate aminotransferase, headache, and pneumonia. Monitor for signs and symptoms of injection site reactions, including phlebitis and thrombophlebitis, and acute drug hypersensitivity reactions, including edema (facial, eye, and tongue), urticaria, pruritus, and anaphylactic reactions. Withhold Cosela for moderate reactions. Stop infusion and permanently discontinue Cosela for severe or life-threatening reactions. Patients should be monitored for pulmonary symptoms indicative of ILD/pneumonitis. Interrupt and evaluate patients with new or worsening symptoms and permanently discontinue Cosela in patients with recurrent symptomatic or severe/life-threatening ILD/pneumonitis. Cosela is embryo/fetal toxic. Advise patients of reproductive potential to use effective contraception. Advise mothers not to breastfeed.

TYROSINE KINASE INHIBITOR (TKI)

▶ **gefitinib** (G) *Recommended dose:* 250 mg once daily with or without food
  Pediatric: safety and efficacy not established
  Iressa *Tab:* 250 mg
  Comment: Iressa is a tyrosine kinase inhibitor indicated for the first-line treatment of patients with metastatic NSCLC whose tumors have epidermal growth factor receptor (EGFR) exon 19 deletions or exon 21 (L858R) substitution mutations as detected by an FDA-approved test. Safety and efficacy of Iressa have not been established in patients whose tumors have EGFR mutations other than exon 19 deletions or exon 21 (L858R) substitution mutations. The most commonly reported adverse drug reactions (incidence >20% of the patients and greater than placebo) have been skin reactions and diarrhea. ILD has occurred in patients taking Iressa. Withhold Iressa for worsening of respiratory symptoms and discontinue if ILD is confirmed. Hepatotoxicity has occurred with Iressa. Obtain periodic liver function testing. Withhold Iressa for Grade 2 or higher for ALT and/or AST elevations and discontinue for severe hepatic impairment. Discontinue Iressa if a gastrointestinal perforation occurs. Withhold Iressa for Grade 3 or higher diarrhea. Withhold Iressa for signs and symptoms of severe or worsening ocular disorders, including keratitis, and discontinue for persistent ulcerative keratitis. Withhold Iressa for Grade 3 or higher skin reactions or exfoliative conditions. Iressa can cause fetal harm. In animal reproductive studies, oral administration of *gefitinib* from organogenesis through weaning resulted in fetotoxicity and neonatal death at doses below the recommended human dose. Advise pregnant females and females of reproductive potential of the potential hazard to the fetus and risk of pregnancy loss. Advise females of reproductive potential to use effective contraception. Exclude pregnancy prior to initiating treatment with Iressa. It is advisable to retest monthly during treatment as well. Studies indicate that *gefitinib* and its metabolites are present in animal milk at a concentration higher than those in maternal plasma. Because of the potential for serious adverse reactions in breastfeeding infants, breastfeeding is not recommended. Advise mothers to discontinue breastfeeding during treatment with Iressa and for 2 weeks after the last dose. To report suspected adverse reactions, contact AstraZeneca at 800-236-9933 or FDA at 1-800-FDA-1088 or www.fda.gov/medwatch.

FOLATE ANALOG METABOLIC INHIBITOR

▶ **pemetrexed** (G) for injection *Recommended dose, administered as a single agent or with cisplatin, in patients with CrCl ≥45 ml/min:* 500 mg/m² via IV infusion over 10 minutes on Day 1 of each 21-day cycle; *Initiate Folic Acid:* 400-1,000 mcg orally once daily beginning 7 days prior to the first dose and continue until 21 days after the last dose; *Administer vitamin B12:* 1 mg IM 1 week prior to the first dose and every 3 cycles thereafter; *Administer dexamethasone:* 4 mg orally bid the day before, the day of, and the day after Pemfexy administration
  Pediatric: safety and efficacy not established
  Pemfexy *Vial:* 500 mg/20 ml (25 mg/ml), single dose, for dilution and IV infusion
  Comment: Pemfexy is a branded alternative to Alimta for the treatment of non-squamous NSCLC and malignant pleural mesothelioma. Pemfexy is indicated (1) in combination with *cisplatin* for the initial treatment of patients with locally advanced or metastatic non-squamous NSCLC, (2) as a single agent for the maintenance treatment of patients with locally advanced or metastatic non-squamous NSCLC whose disease has not progressed after 4 cycles of *platinum-based first-line chemotherapy*, and (3) as a single agent for the treatment of patients with recurrent, metastatic non-squamous NSCLC after prior chemotherapy. Pemfexy is not indicated for the treatment of patients with squamous cell non-small cell lung cancer (NSCLC). Pemfexy can cause severe bone marrow suppression resulting in cytopenia and an increased risk of infection. Do not administer Pemfexy when the absolute neutrophil count is less than 1,500 cells/mm³ and platelets are <100,000 cells/mm³. Initiate supplementation with oral folic acid and vitamin B12 IM to reduce the severity of hematologic and gastrointestinal toxicity. Pemfexy can cause severe, and sometimes fatal, renal failure. Do not administer when CrCl <45 ml/min. Permanently discontinue for severe and life-threatening bullous, blistering, or exfoliating skin toxicity. Withhold for acute onset of new or progressive unexplained pulmonary symptoms and permanently discontinue if interstitial pneumonitis is confirmed. Radiation recall can occur in patients who received radiation weeks to years previously; permanently discontinue for signs of radiation recall. The most common adverse reactions (incidence ≥20%) of *pemetrexed* when administered as a single agent have been fatigue, nausea, and anorexia. The most common adverse reactions (incidence ≥20%) of *pemetrexed* when administered with *cisplatin* have been vomiting, neutropenia, anemia, stomatitis/pharyngitis, thrombocytopenia, and constipation. Pemfexy is embryo/fetal toxic. Advise males and females of reproductive potential of the potential risk and to use effective contraception. Advise not to breastfeed.

PROGRAMMED DEATH RECEPTOR-1 (PD-1)-BLOCKING ANTIBODY

▶ **cemiplimab-rwlc** 350 mg via infusion over 30 minutes every 3 weeks
  Pediatric: safety and efficacy not established
  Libtayo *Vial:* 350 mg/7 ml (50 mg/ml), single-dose, soln for dilution and IV infusion
  Comment: Libtayo is indicated for the first-line treatment of patients with NSCLC whose tumors have high programmed death-ligand 1 (PD-L1) expression (Tumor Proportion Score [TPS] ≥ 50%) as determined by an FDA-approved test, with no EGFR, ALK, or ROS1 aberrations, and is (1) locally

(continued)

advanced, where patients are not candidates for surgical resection or definitive chemoradiation, or (2) metastatic. The most common adverse reactions (incidence ≥15%) have been musculoskeletal pain, fatigue, rash, and diarrhea. The most common Grade 3-4 laboratory abnormalities (incidence ≥2%) have been lymphopenia, hyponatremia, hypophosphatemia, increased AST, anemia, and hyperkalemia. For infusion-related reactions (IRRs), interrupt, slow the rate of infusion, or permanently discontinue based on severity of the reaction. Immune-mediated adverse reactions, which may be severe or fatal, can occur in any organ system or tissue, including the following: immune-mediated pneumonitis, immune-mediated colitis, immune-mediated hepatitis, immune-mediated endocrinopathies, immune-mediated dermatologic adverse reactions, immune-mediated nephritis and renal dysfunction, and solid organ transplant rejection. Monitor for early identification and management. Evaluate liver enzymes, creatinine, and thyroid function at baseline and periodically during treatment. Withhold or permanently discontinue Libtayo based on the severity of reaction. Fatal and other serious complications can occur in patients who receive allogeneic hematopoietic stem cell transplantation (HSCT) before or after being treated with a programmed death receptor-1 (PD-1)/PD-L1-blocking antibody. Based on its mechanism of action, Libtayo can cause embryo/fetal harm when administered to a pregnant female. Animal studies have demonstrated that inhibition of the PD-1/PD-L1 pathway can lead to increased risk of immune-mediated rejection of the developing fetus, resulting in fetal death. Advise women of the potential risk and advise males and females of reproductive potential to use effective contraception during treatment with Libtayo and for at least 4 months after the last dose. There is no information regarding the presence of cemiplimab-rwlc in human milk or its effects on the breastfed infant. Because of the potential for serious adverse reactions in breastfed infants, advise mothers not to breastfeed during treatment and for at least 4 months after the last dose.

▷ *pembrolizumab* 200 mg via IV infusion every 3 weeks or 400 mg via IV infusion every 6 weeks
  Keytruda 100 mg/4 ml (25 mg/ml) soln, single-dose
  Comment: Keytruda *(pembrolizumab)* is indicated for the treatment of multiple cancers, including (1) metastatic SCLC with disease progression on or after *platinum*-based chemotherapy and at least one other prior line of therapy (this indication is approved under accelerated approval based on tumor response rate and durability of response; continued approval for this indication may be contingent upon verification and description of clinical benefit in confirmatory trials); (2) in combination with *pemetrexed* and *platinum* chemotherapy, for the first-line treatment of metastatic NSCLC, with no EGFR or ALK genomic tumor aberrations; (3) in combination with *carboplatin* and either *paclitaxel* or *paclitaxel* protein-bound as a single agent, for treatment of patients with metastatic NSCLC whose tumors express PD-L1 (TPS ≥1%) as determined by an FDA-approved test; (4) as a single agent, for the first-line treatment of patients with NSCLC expressing PD-L1 (TPS ≥1%) as determined by an FDA-approved test, with no EGFR or ALK genomic tumor aberrations, metastatic or stage III where patients are not candidates for surgical resection or definitive chemoradiation; and (5) as a single agent, indicated for the treatment of metastatic NSCLC with tumors that express PD-L1 (TPS ≥1%) as determined by an FDA-approved test, with disease progression on or after *platinum*-containing chemotherapy; patients with EGFR or ALK genomic tumor aberrations should have disease progression on FDA-approved therapy for these aberrations prior to receiving **Keytruda**. **Keytruda** can cause fetal harm. Advise females of the potential embryo/fetal risk and to use effective method of contraception. Advise not to breastfeed. See mfr pkg insert for full prescribing information.

CYTOTOXIC T-LYMPHOCYTE-ASSOCIATED ANTIGEN 4 (CTLA-4)-BLOCKING ANTIBODY

▷ *tremelimumab-actl* Dose Preparation: Store **Imjudo** vials in a refrigerator at 2°C to 8°C (36°F to 46°F) in original carton to protect from light. Do not freeze. Do not shake. Withdraw the required dose (volume) from the vial(s) of **Imjudo** and transfer into the IV fluid bag containing 0.9% NaCl, USP or 5% Dextrose Injection, USP. Mix diluted solution by gentle inversion. Do not shake the solution. The maximum final concentration of the diluted solution should not exceed 10 mg/ml. The total volume of diluent for use with each dose and patient weight is presented in the table below. Discard partially used or empty vial(s) of **Imjudo**. **Imjudo** does not contain a preservative. Administer the infusion solution immediately once prepared. If the infusion solution is not administered immediately and needs to be stored, the total time from preparation to the start of administration should not exceed 24 hours in a refrigerator at 2°C to 8°C (36°F to 46°F) or 24 hours at room temperature up to 30°C (86°F).

Dose	Weight	Total Solution
300 mg	≥30 kg	150 ml
4 mg/kg	<30 kg	80 ml
75 mg	≥30 kg	150 ml
1 mg/kg	<30 kg	80 ml

Treatment: Administer **Imjudo** as IV infusion over 60 minutes after dilution; *Weight ≥30 kg: First,* administer **Imjudo** 75 mg as a single dose once every 3 weeks, in combination with *durvalumab* 1,500 mg and platinum-based chemotherapy for 4 cycles; *Then, administer durvalumab* 1,500 mg every 4 weeks as a single agent with histology-based pemetrexed therapy every 4 weeks; *Then, administer* a fifth dose of **Imjudo** 75 mg in combination with *durvalumab* dose 6 at week 16; *Weight <30 kg: First, administer* **Imjudo** 1 mg/kg as a single dose once every 3 weeks, in combination with *durvalumab* 20 mg/kg and platinum-based chemotherapy for 4 cycles; *Then, administer durvalumab* 20 mg/kg every 4 weeks as a single agent with histology-based pemetrexed therapy every 4 weeks; *Then, administer* a fifth dose of **Imjudo** 1 mg/kg in combination with *durvalumab* dose 6 at week 16 See mfr pkg insert for full prescribing information, including dose modifications for adverse reactions.

Pediatric: safety and efficacy not established

    Imjudo *Vial:* 25 mg/1.25 ml (20 mg/ml), 300 mg/15 ml (20 mg/ml), single-dose, soln for dilution and IV infusion (preservative-free)

    Comment: **Imjudo** is a cytotoxic T-lymphocyte-associated antigen 4 (CTLA-4)-blocking antibody indicated in combination with *durvalumab* and platinum-based chemotherapy for the treatment of adult patients with metastatic NSCLC with no sensitizing EGFR mutation or ALK genomic tumor aberrations. Immune-mediated adverse reactions, which may be severe or fatal, can occur in any organ system or tissue, including the following: immune-mediated pneumonitis, immune-mediated colitis, immune-mediated hepatitis, immune-mediated endocrinopathies, immune-mediated dermatologic adverse reactions, immune-mediated nephritis with renal dysfunction, and immune-mediated pancreatitis. Monitor for early identification and management for an immune-mediated adverse reaction. Evaluate liver enzymes, creatinine, adrenocorticotropic hormone level, and thyroid function at baseline and before each dose. Withhold or permanently discontinue **Imjudo** based on severity and type of reaction. For IRRs, interrupt, slow the rate of infusion, or permanently discontinue treatment based on the severity of the reaction. The most common adverse reactions (incidence ≥20%) in patients with metastatic NSCLC have been nausea, fatigue, musculoskeletal pain, decreased appetite, rash, and diarrhea. Human immunoglobulin G2 (IgG2) is known to cross the placental barrier; therefore, **Imjudo** has the potential to be transmitted from the mother to the developing fetus. There are no available data on the use of **Imjudo** in human pregnancy. However, based on findings from animal studies and the drug's mechanism of action, **Imjudo** is embryo/fetal toxic. CTLA-4 blockade is associated with increased risk of immune-mediated rejection of the developing fetus and fetal death. Therefore, advise females of reproductive potential of the potential risk to the fetus, exclude pregnancy prior to initiating treatment, and advise females of reproductive potential to use effective contraception with **Imjudo**. There are no data on the presence of *tremelimumab-actl* in human milk or effects on the breastfed infant. Maternal immunoglobulin G (IgG) is known to be present in human milk. The effects of local gastrointestinal exposure and limited systemic exposure in the breastfed infant to **Imjudo** are unknown. Because of the potential for serious adverse reactions, advise women not to breastfeed during treatment with **Imjudo** and for 3 months after the last **Imjudo** dose. To report suspected adverse reactions, contact AstraZeneca at 800-236-9933 or FDA at 800-FDA-1088 or www.fda.gov/medwatch.

BISPECIFIC EGFR-DIRECTED AND MET RECEPTOR-DIRECTED ANTIBODY

▶ *amivantamab-vmjw* Recommended dose is based on baseline body weight; refer to the weight-based dosing table; *Administer* pre-medications as recommended; *Administer* via a peripheral IV line on Week 1 and Week 2; *Then administer* x 4 weeks, with the initial dose as a split infusion in Week 1 on Day 1 and Day 2; *Then, administer* every 2 weeks starting at Week 5; *Body Weight at Baseline Recommended Dose:* <80 kg: 1,050 mg (3 vials); ≥80 kg: 1400 mg (4 vials)

Pediatric: safety and efficacy not established

    Rybrevant *Vial:* 350 mg/7 ml (50 mg/ml), single-dose, soln for dilution and IV infusion (preservative-free)

    Comment: **Rybrevant** is a bispecific EGFR-directed and MET receptor-directed antibody indicated for the treatment of adult patients with locally advanced or metastatic NSCLC with EGFR exon 20 insertion mutations, as detected by an FDA-approved test, whose disease has progressed on or after platinum-based chemotherapy, and the first targeted treatment for NSCLC with EGFR exon 20 insertion mutations. This indication is approved under accelerated approval based on overall response rate and duration of response. Continued approval for this indication may be contingent upon verification and description of clinical benefit in confirmatory trials. the first targeted treatment for non-small cell lung cancer (NSCLC) with epidermal growth factor receptor (EGFR) exon 20 insertion mutations. **Rybrevant** is indicated for treatment of adult patients with locally advanced or metastatic NSCLC with EGFR exon 20 insertion mutations. Interrupt infusion at the first sign of an IRR. Reduce infusion rate, reduce dose, or permanently discontinue **Rybrevant** based on IRR severity. Monitor closely for new or worsening adverse symptoms. Immediately withhold **Rybrevant** in patients with suspected ILD/pneumonitis and permanently discontinue if ILD/pneumonitis is confirmed. **Rybrevant** may cause rash, including acneiform dermatitis and toxic epidermal necrolysis (TEN). Withhold, reduce dose, or permanently discontinue **Rybrevant** based on severity. **Rybrevant** can cause ocular toxicity, including keratitis, dry eye symptoms, conjunctival redness, blurred vision, visual impairment, ocular itching, and uveitis; promptly refer patients with worsening eye symptoms to an ophthalmologist. The most common adverse reactions (≥20%) have been rash, IRRs, paronychia, musculoskeletal pain, dyspnea, nausea, fatigue, edema, stomatitis, cough, constipation, and vomiting. The most common Grade 3 or

(continued)

4 laboratory abnormalities (≥2%) have been decreased lymphocytes, decreased albumin, decreased phosphate, decreased potassium, increased alkaline phosphatase, increased glucose, increased gamma-glutamyl transferase, and decreased sodium. Based on animal models, **Rybrevant** is embryo/fetal toxic and hence can cause fetal harm. There are no available data on the use of **Rybrevant** in human pregnancy. However, disruption or depletion of EGFR in animal models has resulted in impairment of embryo/fetal development, including effects on placental, lung, cardiac, skin, and neural development. The absence of EGFR or MET signaling has resulted in embryo lethality, malformations, and postnatal death in animals. Exclude pregnancy in females of reproductive potential prior to initiating **Rybrevant** and advise females of reproductive potential of the potential risk to the fetus and to use effective contraception during treatment and for 3 months after the final dose. There are no data on the presence of *amivantamab-vmjw* in human milk or effects on the breastfed infant. Because of the potential for serious adverse reactions from **Rybrevant** in breastfed infants, advise mothers not to breastfeed during treatment and for 3 months after the final dose.

RAS GTPase INHIBITOR

▷ *adagrasib* Recommended dose: 600 mg bid; swallow whole with or without food
Pediatric: safety and efficacy not established
    Krazati *Tab:* 200 mg film-coat
    Comment: Krazati is an inhibitor of the RAS GTPase family indicated for the treatment of adult patients with *KRAS* G12C-mutated locally advanced or metastatic NSCLC, as determined by an FDA-approved test, who have received at least one prior systemic therapy. This indication is approved under accelerated approval based on objective response rate (ORR) and duration of response (DOR). Continued approval for this indication may be contingent upon verification and description of a clinical benefit in a confirmatory trial(s). The most common (incidence ≥25%) adverse reactions were nausea, diarrhea, vomiting, fatigue, musculoskeletal pain, hepatotoxicity, renal impairment, edema, dyspnea, and decreased appetite. The most common Grade 3 or 4 (incidence ≥2%) laboratory abnormalities were decreased lymphocytes, decreased hemoglobin, increased ALT, increased AST, hypokalemia, hyponatremia, increased lipase, decreased leukocytes, decreased neutrophils, and increased alkaline phosphatase. *Gastrointestinal Adverse Reactions:* Monitor patients for diarrhea, nausea, and vomiting and provide supportive care as needed. Withhold, reduce the dose, or permanently discontinue based on severity. Avoid concomitant use of **Krazati** with other products with a known potential to prolong the QTc interval. Monitor ECG and electrolytes in patients at risk and in patients taking medications known to prolong the QT interval. Withhold, reduce the dose, or permanently discontinue based on severity. Monitor liver laboratory tests prior to the start of **Krazati** and monthly for 3 months after and as clinically indicated. Reduce the dose, withhold, or permanently discontinue based on severity. Monitor for new or worsening respiratory symptoms. Withhold **Krazati** for suspected ILD/pneumonitis and permanently discontinue if no other potential causes of ILD/pneumonitis are identified. Avoid concomitant use of strong CYP3A4 inducers with **Krazati**. Avoid concomitant use of strong CYP3A4 inhibitors until *adagrasib* concentrations have reached steady state. Avoid concomitant use of sensitive CYP3A4 substrates with **Krazati**. Avoid concomitant use of sensitive CYP2C9 or CYP2D6 substrates or P-gp substrates where minimal concentration changes may lead to serious adverse reactions. Avoid concomitant use of drugs that prolong the QT interval with **Krazati**. In animal embryo/fetal development studies, *adagrasib* administered during the period of organogenesis induced maternal toxicity and skeletal malformations at 2 times the recommended dose of 600 mg bid based on BSA. Advise females of reproductive potential to use effective contraception during treatment with **Krazati** and for at least 4 weeks after the last dose. Exclude pregnancy in females of reproductive potential prior to initiating treatment with **Krazati**. Advise females of reproductive potential to use effective contraception during treatment with **Sutent** and for at least 4 weeks after the last dose. There are no data on the presence of *adagrasib* or its metabolites in human milk or effects on the breastfed infant. Because of the potential for serious adverse reactions in breastfed infants, advise women not to breastfeed during treatment with **Krazati** and for 1 week after the last dose. Based on findings from animal studies, **Krazati** may impair fertility in females and males of reproductive potential. To report suspected adverse reactions, contact Mirati Therapeutics at 844-MIRATI-1 (844-647-2841) or FDA at 800-FDA-1088 or www.fda.gov/medwatch.

CANCER: LYMPHOMA

HUMAN PROGRAMMED DEATH RECEPTOR-1 (PD-1)-BLOCKING ANTIBODY

▷ *pembrolizumab* Administer 400 mg via IV infusion over 30 minutes every 6 weeks
Pediatric: Administer 2 mg/kg (up to a maximum of 200 mg) via IV infusion over 30 minutes once every 3 weeks until disease progression, unacceptable toxicity, or up to 24 months
    Keytruda *Vial:* 100 mg/4 ml (25 mg/ml), single-dose, soln for dilution and IV infusion
    Comment: Keytruda is a programmed death receptor-1 (PD-1)-blocking antibody indicated for the treatment of multiple cancers, including classical Hodgkin lymphoma (cHL) and primary mediastinal large B-cell lymphoma (PMBCL). The adult indications and dosing regimen are approved for cHL

and PMBCL under accelerated approval based on pharmacokinetic data, the relationship of exposure to efficacy, and the relationship of exposure to safety. Continued approval for this dosage may be contingent upon verification and description of clinical benefit in confirmatory trials. **Keytruda** can cause fetal harm. Exclude pregnancy in females of reproductive potential prior to initiating **Keytruda**. Advise females of reproductive potential of the embryo/fetal risk and to use effective contraception during treatment and for 4 months after the last Keytruda dose. Advise mothers not to breastfeed during treatment and for 4 months after the last **Keytruda** dose. See mfr pkg insert for full prescribing information, including storage, preparation, warnings, precautions, drug–drug interactions, and adverse reactions.

BRUTON'S TYROSINE KINASE (BTK) INHIBITOR

▷ *zanubrutinib* 160 mg (2 x 80 mg) bid or 320 mg (4 x 80 mg) once daily; swallow whole with water, with or without food; Do not open, break, or chew capsules; *Child-Pugh Class C:* reduce dose; manage toxicity with dose reduction, treatment interruption, or discontinuation
Pediatric: safety and efficacy not established

Brukinsa *Cap:* 80 mg

Comment: Brukinsa is a Bruton's tyrosine kinase (BTK) inhibitor indicated for the treatment of patients with mantle cell lymphoma (MCL) who have received at least one prior therapy. This indication is approved under accelerated approval based on overall response rate. Continued approval for this indication may be contingent upon verification and description of clinical benefit in a confirmatory trial. Patients with relapsed or refractory marginal zone lymphoma (MZL) who have received at least one anti–CD20-based regimen; patients with chronic lymphocytic leukemia (CLL) or small lymphocytic lymphoma (SLL), and patients with Waldenström's macroglobulinemia (WM). There are no contraindications to the use of **Brukinsa**. Monitor for bleeding and manage appropriately. Monitor patients for signs and symptoms of infection, including opportunistic infections, and treat as needed. Monitor complete blood counts (CBCs) for cytopenias during treatment. Other malignancies have developed, including skin cancers and non-skin carcinomas; advise patients to use sun protection. Monitor for signs and symptoms of cardiac arrhythmias and manage appropriately. Modify **Brukinsa** dose with moderate or strong CYP3A inhibitors. Avoid co-administration with strong or moderate CYP3A inducers. Dose adjustment may be recommended with moderate CYP3A inducers. The most common adverse reactions (incidence ≥20%), including laboratory abnormalities, are decreased neutrophil count, upper respiratory tract infection, decreased platelet count, hemorrhage, and musculoskeletal pain. **Brukinsa** can cause fetal harm. Exclude pregnancy prior to initiating treatment with **Brukinsa**. Advise females and males of reproductive potential of risk to the fetus and to use effective contraception during treatment and for at least 1 week after the last dose. Advise mothers not to breastfeed during treatment with *Brukinsa* and for 2 weeks after the last dose. To report suspected adverse reactions, contact BeiGene at 877-828-5596 or FDA at 800-FDA-1088 or www.fda.gov/medwatch.

CD19-DIRECTED ANTIBODY AND ALKYLATING AGENT CONJUGATE

▷ *loncastuximab tesirine-lpyl* 0.15 mg/kg *via IV infusion* over 30 minutes on Day 1 of each 3-week cycle for the first 2 cycles; then 0.075 mg/kg *via IV infusion* over 30 minutes every 3 weeks for subsequent cycles; *Premedicate:* with *dexamethasone* 4 mg orally or IV bid for 3 days beginning the day before each infusion
Pediatric: safety and efficacy not established

Zynlonta *Vial:* 10 mg, single-dose, pwdr for reconstitution, dilution, and IV infusion

Comment: Zynlonta is indicated for the treatment of adult patients with relapsed or refractory large B-cell lymphoma after two or more lines of systemic therapy, including diffuse large B-cell lymphoma (DLBCL) not otherwise specified, DLBCL arising from low-grade lymphoma, and high-grade B-cell lymphoma. The most common (incidence ≥20%) adverse reactions, including laboratory abnormalities, are thrombocytopenia, increased gamma-glutamyltransferase, neutropenia, anemia, hyperglycemia, transaminase elevation, fatigue, hypoalbuminemia, rash, edema, nausea, and musculoskeletal pain. Monitor patients for the development of pleural effusion, pericardial effusion, ascites, peripheral edema, and general edema; consider diagnostic imaging when symptoms develop or worsen. Monitor for myelosuppression. Withhold, reduce, or discontinue **Zynlonta** based on severity. Monitor for infection and treat promptly. Monitor patients for new or worsening cutaneous reactions, including photosensitivity reactions; dermatologic consultation should be considered. **Zynlonta** is embryo/fetal toxic. Advise males and females of reproductive potential of the potential risk and to use effective contraception. Advise not to breastfeed during treatment and for 3 months after the last dose.

BISPECIFIC CD20-DIRECTED CD3 T-CELL ENGAGER

▷ *epcoritamab-bysp* For SC injection only; Patients should be hospitalized for 24 hours after administration of Cycle 1, Day 15, 48 mg SC injection; Administer pre-medications and prophylaxis as recommended; Doses of 0.16 mg and 0.8 mg require dilution prior to administration; See mfr pkg insert for full prescribing information including instructions on pre-medication, prophylaxis, preparation, and administration (see dosing table below)

(continued)

Epkinly Dosing Table			
Treatment Cycle*	Treatment Day	Epkinly Dose	
Cycle 1	1	Step-up Dose 1	0.16 mg
	8	Step-up Dose 2	0.8 mg
	15	First Full Dose	48 mg
	22	48 mg	
Cycles 2 and 3	1, 8, 15, 22	48 mg	
Cycles 4 to 9	1 and 15	48 mg	
Cycles 10 and continuing	1	48 mg	

*Cycle = 28 days

Pediatric: safety and efficacy not established

Epkinly *Vial:* 4 mg/0.8 ml, single-dose, soln for dilution and SC injection; 48 mg/0.8 ml, single-dose, soln for SC injection (preservative-free)

Comment: **Epkinly** is a bispecific CD20-directed CD3 T-cell engager indicated for the treatment of adult patients with relapsed or refractory DLBCL, not otherwise specified, including DLBCL arising from indolent lymphoma, and high-grade B-cell lymphoma after two or more lines of systemic therapy. This indication is approved under accelerated approval based on response rate and durability of response. Continued approval for this indication may be contingent upon verification and description of clinical benefit in a confirmatory trial(s). **Epkinly** can cause serious or fatal infections; monitor patients for signs or symptoms of infection, including opportunistic infections, and treat appropriately. **Epkinly** can cause cytopenia; monitor CBCs during treatment. The most common (incidence ≥20%) adverse reactions have been cytokine release syndrome (CRS), fatigue, musculoskeletal pain, injection site reactions, pyrexia, abdominal pain, nausea, and diarrhea. The most common Grade 3 to 4 laboratory abnormalities (incidence ≥10%) have been decreased lymphocyte count, decreased neutrophil count, decreased white blood cell (WBC) count, decreased hemoglobin, and decreased platelets. There are no available data on the use of **Epkinly** in human pregnancy to evaluate for a drug-associated risk, and no animal reproductive or developmental toxicity studies have been conducted with *epcoritamab-bysp*. However, *epcoritamab-bysp* causes T-cell activation and cytokine release; immune activation may compromise pregnancy maintenance. Additionally, based on expression of CD20 on B-cells and the finding of B-cell depletion in non-pregnant animals, *epcoritamab-bysp* can cause B-cell lymphocytopenia in infants exposed to *epcoritamab-bysp* in utero. Human immunoglobulin G (IgG) is known to cross the placenta. For these reasons, **Epkinly** has the potential to be transmitted from the mother to the developing fetus. Advise females of the potential risk to the fetus. Exclude pregnancy prior to initiating treatment with **Epkinly**. Advise females of reproductive potential to use effective contraception during treatment and for 4 months after the last dose of **Epkinly**. There is no information regarding the presence of *epcoritamab-bysp* in human milk, the effect on the breastfed child, or milk production. Because maternal IgG is present in human milk and there is potential for *epcoritamab-bysp* absorption leading to serious adverse reactions in a breastfed infant, advise mothers not to breastfeed during treatment with **Epkinly** and for 4 months after the last dose. To report suspected adverse reactions, contact Genmab US at 855-4GENMAB (855-443-6622) or FDA at 800-FDA-1088 or www.fda.gov/medwatch.

CHIMERIC ANTIGEN RECEPTOR (CAR) T-CELL THERAPY

▷ *lisocabtagene maraleucel* dosing is based on the number of chimeric antigen receptor (CAR)-positive viable T-cells: 50-110 × 10⁶ CAR-positive viable T-cells (consisting of CD8 and CD4 components); administer via IV infusion only; do not use a leukodepleting filter; *Before the infusion:* confirm availability of *tocilizumab*; administer a lymphodepleting regimen of *fludarabine* and *cyclophosphamide*; premedicate with *acetaminophen* and an H1 antihistamine; for autologous use only; must be administered in a certified healthcare facility

Pediatric: safety and efficacy not established

Breyanzi *Vial:* 50 to 110 × 10⁶ CAR-positive viable T-cells/5 ml (1.5-70 × 10⁶ CAR-positive viable T-cells/ml), single-dose, cell suspension for IV infusion; a single dose contains 50-110 × 10⁶ CAR-positive viable T-cells consisting of 1:1 CAR-positive viable T-cells of the CD8 and CD4 components, with each component supplied separately in 1-4 single-dose 5 ml vials.

Comment: **Breyanzi** is a CD19-directed genetically modified autologous T-cell immunotherapy indicated for the treatment of adult patients with relapsed or refractory large B-cell lymphoma after two or more lines of systemic therapy, including DLBCL not otherwise specified (including DLBCL arising from indolent lymphoma), high-grade B-cell lymphoma, PMBCL, and follicular lymphoma grade 3B. The most common non-laboratory adverse reactions (incidence ≥20%) have been fatigue, CRS, musculoskeletal pain, nausea, headache, encephalopathy, infections (pathogen unspecified), decreased appetite, diarrhea, hypotension, tachycardia, dizziness, cough, constipation, abdominal pain, vomiting, and edema. Monitor for hypersensitivity reactions during infusion. Monitor patients for signs and symptoms of infection; treat appropriately. Patients may exhibit grade 3 or higher cytopenias for several weeks following **Breyanzi** infusion. Monitor CBCs. Monitor and consider immunoglobulin replacement therapy. In the event that a secondary malignancy occurs after treatment with **Breyanzi**, contact Bristol Myers Squibb at 1-888-805-4555. Advise patients to refrain from driving and engaging in hazardous occupations or activities, such as operating heavy or potentially dangerous machinery for at least 8 weeks after administration. There are no available data with **Breyanzi** use in pregnant females. No animal reproductive and developmental toxicity studies have been conducted with **Breyanzi** to assess whether it can cause embryo/fetal harm. It is not known if **Breyanzi** has the potential to be transferred to the fetus. Based on the mechanism of action, if the transduced cells cross the placenta, they may cause fetal toxicity, including B-cell lymphocytopenia and hypogammaglobulinemia. Therefore, **Breyanzi** is not recommended for females who are pregnant. Pregnancy after **Breyanzi** infusion should be discussed with the treating physician. There is no information regarding the presence of **Breyanzi** in human milk or effect on the breastfed infant. The developmental and health benefits of breastfeeding should be considered along with the mother's clinical need for **Breyanzi** and any potential adverse effects on the breastfed infant from **Breyanzi** or from the underlying maternal condition.

FOLATE ANALOG METABOLIC INHIBITOR

▶ *pemetrexed* (G) for injection *Recommended dose, administered as a single agent or with* **cisplatin**, *in patients with CrCl ≥45 ml/min: 500 mg/m² via IV infusion over 10 minutes on Day 1 of each 21-day cycle; Initiate Folic Acid: 400-1,000 mcg orally once daily beginning 7 days prior to the first dose and continue until 21 days after the last dose; Administer vitamin B12: 1 mg IM 1 week prior to the first dose and every 3 cycles thereafter; Administer* **dexamethasone**: *4 mg orally bid the day before, the day of, and the day after* Pemfexy administration
Pediatric: safety and efficacy not established
Pemfexy *Vial:* 500 mg/20 ml (25 mg/ml), single dose, for dilution and IV infusion
Comment: Pemfexy is a branded alternative to **Alimta** for the treatment of non-squamous non-small cell lung cancer (NSCLC) and malignant pleural mesothelioma. **Pemfexy** is indicated (1) in combination with **cisplatin** for the initial treatment of patients with locally advanced or metastatic non-squamous NSCLC; (2) as a single agent for the maintenance treatment of patients with locally advanced or metastatic non-squamous NSCLC whose disease has not progressed after 4 cycles of *platinum-based first-line chemotherapy*; and (3) as a single agent for the treatment of patients with recurrent, metastatic non-squamous NSCLC after prior chemotherapy. **Pemfexy** is not indicated for the treatment of patients with squamous cell NSCLC. **Pemfexy** can cause severe bone marrow suppression resulting in cytopenia and an increased risk of infection. Do not administer **Pemfexy** when the absolute neutrophil count is less than 1,500 cells/mm³ and platelets are <100,000 cells/mm³. Initiate supplementation with oral folic acid and vitamin B$_{12}$ IM to reduce the severity of hematologic and gastrointestinal toxicity. **Pemfexy** can cause severe, and sometimes fatal, renal failure. Do not administer when CrCl <45 ml/min. Permanently discontinue for severe and life-threatening bullous, blistering, or exfoliating skin toxicity. Withhold for acute onset of new or progressive unexplained pulmonary symptoms and permanently discontinue if interstitial pneumonitis is confirmed. Radiation recall can occur in patients who received radiation weeks to years previously; permanently discontinue for signs of radiation recall. The most common adverse reactions (incidence ≥20%) of *pemetrexed* when administered as a single agent have been fatigue, nausea, and anorexia. The most common adverse reactions (incidence ≥20%) of *pemetrexed* when administered with *cisplatin* have been vomiting, neutropenia, anemia, stomatitis/pharyngitis, thrombocytopenia, and constipation. **Pemfexy** is embryo/fetal toxic. Advise males and females of reproductive potential of the potential risk and to use effective contraception. Advise not to breastfeed.

CD20-DIRECTED CYTOLYTIC ANTIBODY

▶ *rituximab* Rituxan should only be administered by a qualified healthcare professional with appropriate medical support to manage severe infusion-related reactions that can be fatal if they occur
Recommended Dose: 375 mg/m² via IV infusion according to the following schedules:
- Relapsed or Refractory, Low-Grade or Follicular, CD20-Positive, or B-Cell NHL: Administer once weekly x 4 or 8 doses
- Retreatment for Relapsed or Refractory, Low-Grade or Follicular, CD20-Positive, B-Cell NHL: Administer once weekly x 4 doses
- Previously Untreated, Follicular, CD20-Positive, B-Cell NHL: Administer on Day 1 of each cycle of chemotherapy for up to 8 doses in patients with complete or partial response, initiate **Rituxan** maintenance 8 weeks following completion of a *rituximab* product in combination with chemotherapy; Administer **Rituxan** as a single agent every 8 weeks x 12 doses
- Non-progressing, Low-Grade, CD20-Positive, B-Cell NHL, after first-line *cyclophosphamide, vincristine,* and *prednisone* (CVP) chemotherapy--Following completion of 6 to 8 cycles of CVP chemotherapy, administer **Rituxan** once weekly x 4 doses at 6-month intervals to a maximum of 16 doses
- Diffuse Large B-Cell NHL: Administer on Day 1 of each cycle of chemotherapy for up to 8 infusions

(continued)

- As a component of **Zevalin** therapeutic regimen for treatment of NHL, 1 infuse 250 mg/m² in accordance with the **Zevalin** mfr pkg insert (refer to the **Zevalin** mfr pkg insert for full prescribing information regarding the **Zevalin** therapeutic regimen)

Rituxan should <u>only</u> be administered by a qualified healthcare professional with appropriate medical support to manage severe infusion-related reactions that can be fatal if they occur

Recommended Infusion Rate:
- *First Infusion:* initiate at 50 mg/hr; in the absence of infusion toxicity, increase infusion rate by 50 mg/hr increments every 30 minutes, to max 400 mg/hr
- *Subsequent Infusions: Standard Infusion:* initiate at 100 mg/hr; in the absence of infusion toxicity, increase by 100 mg/hr increments at 30-minute intervals, to max 400 mg/hr
- *Previously Untreated Follicular Non-Hodgekin's Lymphona (NHL) and Difuse Large B Cell Lymphoma (DLBCL):* If patients did <u>not</u> experience a Grade 3 <u>or</u> 4 infusion-related adverse event during Cycle 1, a 90-minute infusion can be administered in Cycle 2 with a glucocorticoid-containing chemotherapy regimen; initiate at a rate of 20% of the total dose given in the first 30 minutes and the remaining 80% of the total dose given over the next 60 minutes; If the 90-minute infusion is tolerated in Cycle 2, the same rate can be used when administering the remainder of the treatment regimen (through Cycle 6 <u>or</u> 8)
- Patients who have clinically significant cardiovascular disease <u>or</u> who have a circulating lymphocyte count ≥5,000/mm³ before Cycle 2 should <u>not</u> be administered a 90-minute infusion
- *Infusion-RelatedRreaction:* interrupt the infusion <u>or</u> slow the infusion rate for a severe reaction; continue the infusion at one-half the previous rate upon improvement of symptoms

Pediatric: safety and efficacy <u>not</u> established

Rituxan *Vial:* 100 mg/10 ml (10 mg/ml), 500 mg/50 ml (10 mg/ml), single-dose, soln for dilution and IV infusion (preservative-free)

Comment: Rituxan is indicated for the treatment of adult patients with (1) relapsed <u>or</u> refractory, low-grade <u>or</u> follicular, CD20-positive B-cell NHL, as a single agent therapy, (2) previously untreated follicular, CD20-positive, B-cell NHL, in combination with first line chemotherapy, <u>and</u> in patients achieving a complete <u>or</u> partial response to a *rituximab* product in combination with chemotherapy, as single-agent maintenance therapy, (3) non-progressing (including stable disease), low-grade, CD20-positive, B-cell NHL, as a single agent <u>after</u> first-line CVP chemotherapy, and (4) previously untreated diffuse large B-cell, CD20-positive NHL in combination with *cyclophosphamide, doxorubicin, vincristine,* and *prednisone* (CHOP) <u>or</u> other anthracycline-based chemotherapy regimen. In CLL patients older than 70 years of age, exploratory analyses suggest no benefit with the addition of **Rituxan** to *udarabine* and *cyclophosphamide* (FC) chemotherapy; The most adverse common reactions (incidence >25%) have been infusion-related reactions, fever, lymphopenia, chills, infection, and asthenia. For tumor lysis syndrome (TLS), administer aggressive IV hydration and antihyperuricemic agents, and monitor renal function. Monitor for infections; withhold **Rituxan** and institute appropriate anti-infective therapy. For cardiac adverse reactions, discontinue **Rituxan** infusions in case of serious <u>or</u> life-threatening events. Discontinue **Rituxan** in patients with rising serum creatinine <u>or</u> oliguria. Bowel obstruction and perforation can occur; consider and evaluate for abdominal pain, vomiting, <u>or</u> related symptoms. Live virus vaccinations prior to <u>or</u> during **Rituxan** treatment is <u>not</u> recommended. **Rituxan** is embryo/fetal toxic. Advise males and females of reproductive potential of the potential embryo/fetal risk and to use effective contraception. Advise women <u>not</u> to breastfeed during treatment and for at least 6 months after the last dose.

CD20-DIRECTED CYTOLYTIC ANTIBODY+ENDOGLYCOSIDASE

▶ *rituximab+hyaluronidase human* Administer 1,400 mg/23,400 units (*rituximab* 1,400 mg and *hyaluronidase human* 23,400 units) SC according to recommended schedule; *Premedicate:* with *acetaminophen* and antihistamine before each dose and consider premedication with glucocorticoids; Patients <u>must</u> receive at least one full dose of a *rituximab* product via IV infusion before receiving **Rituxan Hycela** via SC injection; **Rituxan Hycela** should <u>only</u> be administered by a qualified healthcare professional with appropriate medical support to manage severe infusion-related reactions that can be fatal if they occur; administer via SC injection only:
- Relapsed <u>or</u> Refractory, Follicular Lymphoma: administer once weekly x 3 <u>or</u> 7 weeks following a full dose of a *rituximab* product by IV infusion at week 1 (i.e., 4 <u>or</u> 8 weeks in total)
- Retreatment for Relapsed <u>or</u> Refractory, Follicular Lymphoma: administer once weekly x 3 weeks following a full dose of a *rituximab* product by IV infusion at week 1 (i.e., 4 weeks in total)
- Previously untreated, Follicular Lymphoma: administer on Day 1 of Cycles 2–8 of chemotherapy (every 21 days), for up to 7 cycles following a full dose of a *rituximab* product by IV infusion on Day 1 of Cycle 1 of chemotherapy (i.e., up to 8 cycles in total); for patients with complete <u>or</u> partial response: initiate maintenance treatment 8 weeks following completion of **Rituxan Hycela** in combination with chemotherapy; administer **Rituxan Hycela** as a single agent every 8 weeks x 12 doses
- Non-progressing, Follicular Lymphoma after first-line CVP chemotherapy: following completion of six to eight cycles of CVP chemotherapy and a full dose of a *rituximab* product by IV infusion at week 1, administer once weekly x 3 weeks (i.e., 4 weeks in total) at 6-month intervals to a max of 16 doses

– DLBCL: administer **Rituxan Hycela** 1,400 mg/23,400 units via SC injection on Day 1 of Cycles 2–8 of CHOP chemotherapy for up to 7 cycles, following a full dose of a *rituximab* product via IV infusion at Day 1, Cycle 1 of CHOP chemotherapy (i.e., up to 6 to 8 cycles in total)

Rituxan Hycela *Vial:* *rituximab* 1,400 mg+*hyaluronidase human* 23,400 units per 11.7 ml (120 mg/2,000 units/ml), single-dose, soln for dilution and IV infusion; *rituximab* 1,600 mg +*hyaluronidase human* 26,800 units per 13.4 ml (120 mg/2,000 units/ml), single-dose, soln for dilution and IV infusion
Comment: Rituxan Hycela is a fixed 2-drug combination indicated for the treatment of (1) relapsed or refractory follicular lymphoma as a single agent, (2) previously untreated follicular lymphoma in combination with first-line chemotherapy and, in patients achieving a complete or partial response to *rituximab* in combination with chemotherapy, as single-agent maintenance therapy, (3) non-progressing (including stable disease) follicular lymphoma as a single agent after first-line CVP chemotherapy; and (4) previously untreated DLBCL in combination with CHOP or other anthracycline-based chemotherapy regimens. The most common adverse reactions (incidence ≥20%) have been infections, neutropenia, nausea, constipation, cough, and fatigue in follicular lymphoma, and infections, neutropenia, alopecia, nausea, and anemia in DLBCL. There is risk of renal toxicity when **Rituxan Hycela** is used in combination with *cisplatin*. Local cutaneous reactions may occur more than 24 hours after administration. Interrupt **Rituxan Hycela** injections if severe reaction develops and administer aggressive IV hydration and antihyperuricemic agents, and monitor renal function. Monitor for infections; withhold and institute appropriate anti-infective therapy as appropriate. With cardiac adverse reactions, discontinue in case of serious or life-threatening events. Discontinue in patients with rising serum creatinine or oliguria. Bowel obstruction and perforation may occur; consider and evaluate for abdominal pain, vomiting, or related symptoms. Live virus vaccinations prior to or during treatment are not recommended. **Rituxan Hycela** is embryo/fetal toxic. Advise males and females of reproductive potential of the potential embryo/fetal risk and to use effective contraception. Advise women not to breastfeed during treatment and for at least 6 months after the last dose.

▷ *rituximab-arrx* 375 mg/m² via IV infusion; administer all doses of **Riabni** in combination with glucocorticoids; **Riabni** should only be administered by a qualified healthcare professional with appropriate medical support to manage severe infusion-related reactions that can be fatal
Pediatric: safety and efficacy not established

Riabni *Vial:* 100 mg/10 ml (10 mg/ml), 500 mg/50 ml (10 mg/ml), soln for dilution and IV infusion, single-dose
Comment: Riabni *(rituximab-arrx)* is a biosimilar to **Rituxan** indicated for the treatment of adult patients with: (1) relapsed or refractory, low-grade or follicular, CD20-positive B-cell NHL as a single agent; (2) previously untreated follicular, CD20-positive, B-cell NHL in combination with first-line chemotherapy and, in patients achieving a complete or partial response to a *rituximab* product in combination with chemotherapy, as single-agent maintenance therapy; (3) non-progressing (including stable disease), low-grade, CD20-positive, B-cell NHL as a single agent after first-line CVP chemotherapy; and (4) previously untreated diffuse large B-cell, CD20-positive NHL in combination with CHOP or other anthracycline-based chemotherapy regimens. The most common adverse reactions in clinical trials with NHL (incidence ≥25%) have been infusion-related reactions, fever, lymphopenia, chills, infection, and asthenia. Monitor renal function. Discontinue **Riabni** in patients with rising serum creatinine or oliguria. If TLS is suspected, administer aggressive IV hydration and antihyperuricemic agents. If infection occurs, withhold **Riabni** and institute appropriate anti-infective therapy. Bowel obstruction and perforation can occur; evaluate for abdominal pain, vomiting, and related symptoms. Live virus vaccine administration prior to or during treatment with **Riabni** is not recommended. **Riabni** can cause embryo/fetal harm. Advise males and females of reproductive potential of embryo/fetal risk and to use effective contraception. Advise not to breastfeed.

BISPECIFIC CD20-DIRECTED CD3 T-CELL ENGAGER

▷ *mosunetuzumab-axgb* *Premedicate:* to reduce risk of CRS and infusion-related reactions; administer only as an IV infusion; *Recommended stepped-up dosing schedule:* Cycle 1, Day 1: 1 mg; Cycle 1, Day 8: 2 mg; Cycle 1, Day 15: 60 mg; Cycle 2, Day 1: 60 mg; Cycle 3+, Day 1: 30 mg; See mfr pkg insert for instructions on preparation and administration
Pediatric: safety and efficacy not established

Lunsumio *Vial:* 1 mg/ml (1 ml), 30 mg/30 ml (30 ml), single-dose for dilution and IV infusion
Comment: Lunsumio is a first-in-class bispecific CD20-directed CD3 T-cell engager for the treatment of relapsed or refractory follicular lymphoma in adults. This FDA indication is approved under accelerated approval based on response rate. Continued approval for this indication may be contingent upon verification and description of clinical benefit in a confirmatory trial(s). CRS, including serious or life-threatening reactions, can occur in patients receiving **Lunsumio**. Initiate treatment with the **Lunsumio** stepped-up dosing schedule to reduce the risk of CRS. Withhold **Lunsumio** until CRS resolves or permanently discontinue based on severity. The most common adverse reactions (≥20%) are CRS, fatigue, rash, pyrexia, and headache. The most common Grade 3 to 4 laboratory abnormalities (incidence ≥10%) have been decreased lymphocyte count, decreased phosphate, increased glucose, decreased neutrophil count, increased uric acid, decreased WBC count, decreased hemoglobin, and decreased

(continued)

platelets. **Lunsumio** can cause serious neurologic toxicity, including immune effector cell-associated neurotoxicity syndrome (ICANS); monitor and withhold or permanently discontinue based on severity. **Lunsumio** can cause serious or fatal infection; monitor patients for signs and symptoms of infection, including opportunistic infections, and treat as needed. Monitor CBCs for cytopenias during treatment. **Lunsumio** can cause serious tumor flare reactions; monitor patients at risk of complications of tumor flare. **Lunsumio** is embryo/fetal toxic; advise females of reproductive potential of fetal risk and to use effective contraception. Advise not to breastfeed.

CD30-DIRECTED ANTIBODY-DRUG CONJUGATE (ADC)

▶ *brentuximab vedotin* Recommended dose: 1.8 mg/kg administered only via IV infusion over 30 minutes every 3 weeks; Continue treatment until a max of 16 cycles, disease progression, or unacceptable toxicity *Pediatric:* safety and efficacy not established

    Adcetris *Vial:* 50 mg, single use, cake or pwdr for reconstitution, dilution, and IV infusion (preservative-free)

    Comment: Adcetris *(brentuximab vedotin)* is a CD30-directed antibody-drug conjugate (ADC) used for the treatment of (1) Hodgkin's lymphoma, after failure of autologous stem cell transplant (ASCT) or after failure of at least two prior multiagent chemotherapy regimens in patients who are not ASCT candidates, (2) systemic anaplastic large cell lymphoma, after failure of ASCT or after failure of at least two prior multiagent chemotherapy regimens in patients who are not ASCT candidates, and (3) systemic anaplastic large cell lymphoma after failure of at least one prior multiagent chemotherapy regimen. These indications are based on response rate. There are no data available demonstrating improvement in patient-reported outcomes or survival with **Adcetris**. The most common adverse reactions (incidence ≥20%) are neutropenia, peripheral sensory neuropathy, fatigue, nausea, anemia, upper respiratory tract infection, diarrhea, pyrexia, rash, thrombocytopenia, cough, and vomiting. Monitor patients for neuropathy and institute dose modifications accordingly. If an infusion reaction occurs, the infusion should be interrupted and appropriate medical management instituted. If anaphylaxis occurs, the infusion should be discontinued immediately and appropriate medical management instituted. Monitor CBCs prior to each dose of **Adcetris**. If Grade 3 or 4 neutropenia develops, manage by dose delays, reductions, or discontinuation. Patients with rapidly proliferating tumor and high tumor burden are at risk of TLS and these patients should be monitored closely and appropriate measures taken. If Stevens-Johnson syndrome (SJS) occurs, discontinue **Adcetris** and administer appropriate medical therapy. A fatal case of progressive multifocal leukoencephalopathy (PML) has been reported in a patient who received 4 chemotherapy regimens prior to receiving **Adcetris**. Patients who are receiving strong CYP3A4 inhibitors concomitantly with **Adcetris** should be closely monitored for adverse reactions. Based on its mechanism of action and findings in animal studies, **Adcetris** can cause fetal harm when administered in human pregnancy. **Adcetris** exposure during organogenesis has demonstrated embryo/fetal toxicities, including postimplantation loss and deformities. Females of reproductive potential should be advised of the risk to the fetus and to use effective contraception. It is not known whether *brentuximab vedotin* is excreted in human milk; however, because of the potential for serious adverse reactions in breastfeeding infants from **Adcetris**, a decision should be made whether to discontinue breastfeeding or to discontinue **Adcetris**, taking into account the importance of the drug to the mother. To report suspected adverse reactions, contact Seattle Genetics at 855-473-2436 or FDA at 800-FDA-1088 or www.fda.gov/medwatch.

RETINOID X RECEPTOR (RXR) ACTIVATOR

▶ *bexarotene* soft gelcap (sGC)/*bexarotene* 1% topical gel (G)

    Comment: Targretin soft gelcap (sgc) and **Targretin** 1% topical gel contain *bexarotene*. *Bexarotene* is a member of a subclass of retinoids that selectively activate retinoid X receptors (RXRs). These retinoid receptors have biologic activity distinct from that of retinoic acid receptors (RARs). *Bexarotene* selectively binds and activates RXR subtypes (RXRα, RXRβ, RXRγ). RXRs can form heterodimers with various receptor partners, such as RARs, vitamin D receptors, thyroid receptors, and peroxisome proliferator activator receptors (PPARs). Once activated, these receptors function as transcription factors that regulate the expression of genes that control cellular differentiation and proliferation. *Bexarotene* inhibits the growth in vitro of some tumor cell lines of hematopoietic and squamous cell origin. *Bexarotene* also induces tumor regression *in vivo* in some animal models. The exact mechanism of action of *bexarotene* in the treatment of cutaneous T-cell lymphoma (CTCL) is unknown. **Targretin** is indicated for the treatment of cutaneous manifestations of CTCL in patients who are refractory to at least one prior systemic therapy, patients with cutaneous CTCL (Stage IA and IB) lesions who have refractory or persistent disease after other therapies, or who have not tolerated other therapies. **Targretin** should be used with caution in patients with a known hypersensitivity to *bexarotene* and/or to other retinoids. No clinical instances of cross-reactivity have been noted. In clinical studies, patients were advised to limit vitamin A intake to ≤15,000 IU/day. Because of the relationship of *bexarotene* to vitamin A, patients should be advised to limit vitamin A supplements to avoid potential additive toxic effects. Retinoids as a class have been associated with photosensitivity. In vitro assays indicate that *bexarotene* is a potential photosensitizing agent. There were no reports of photosensitivity in patients in the clinical studies. However, patients should be advised to minimize exposure to sunlight and artificial UV light during use of **Targretin**. On the basis of the metabolism of *bexarotene* by cytochrome P450 3A4, concomitant *ketoconazole, itraconazole, erythromycin* and grapefruit juice could increase *bexarotene* plasma concentrations. Similarly, based on data that *gemfibrozil* increases *bexarotene* concentrations following oral *bexarotene* administration, concomitant *gemfibrozil* could potentially increase *bexarotene* plasma concentrations with topical *bexarotene* administration. However, due to the low systemic exposure to *bexarotene* after low-to-moderately intense gel regimens, increases that occur are unlikely to be of sufficient magnitude to result in adverse effects. Because *bexarotene* is embryo/fetal toxic, neither **Targretin** gelcaps nor **Targretin** topical gel should be used by females who are pregnant and for 1 month after the last day of use. Negative pregnancy status should be verified (via serum beta-human chorionic gonadotropin, [beta-hCG] with a sensitivity of at least 50 mlU/L) within 1 week of starting **Targretin** oral or topical therapy and repeated monthly to confirm absence of pregnancy. Females of reproductive potential must use effective contraception continuously starting 1 month before beginning treatment with **Targretin** gelcaps or topical gel until 1 month after the last day of use. It is recommended that two reliable forms of contraception be used together. It is not known whether *bexarotene* is excreted in human milk. Because of the potential for serious adverse reactions in breastfeeding infants from *bexarotene* exposure, a decision should be made whether to discontinue breastfeeding or to discontinue use of the drug, taking into account the importance of the drug to the mother.

Pediatric: safety and efficacy not established

Targretin *Topical gel:* 1% (60 gm/tube) (dehydrated ethanol)

Comment: Do not use concomitantly with the oral form due to risk of drug toxicity. Initially, apply to lesions once every other day for the first week; then, increase application frequency at weekly intervals to once daily, then bid, then tid, and finally qid; If application site toxicity occurs, the application frequency can be reduced. Should severe irritation occur, application can be temporarily discontinued for a few days until the symptoms subside; Apply sufficient gel to cover each lesion with a generous coating (do not apply gel to unaffected skin); Allow the gel to dry before covering with clothing (do not apply occlusive dressings). Treatment should be continued as long as the patient is deriving benefit.

Targretin *Gelcaps:* 75 mg (100 gelcaps/bottle)

Comment: Do not use the oral and topical forms of **Targretin** concomitantly due to risk of drug toxicity. **Targretin** gelcaps dosage is based on body surface area (BSA) calculation. The recommended initial dose of oral **Targretin** is 300 mg/m²/day (see table below). **Targretin** gelcaps should be taken as a single oral daily dose with a meal.

Starting Dose: 300 mg/m²/day		
BSA (m²)	Dose	# Caps
0.88 to 1.12	300 mg	4
1.13 to 1.37	375 mg	5
1.38 to 1.62	450 mg	6
1.63 to 1.87	525 mg	7
1.88 to 2.12	600 mg	8
2.13 to 2.37	675 mg	9
2.38 to 2.62	750 mg	10

Dose Modification Guidelines: **Targretin** gelcaps may be adjusted to 200 mg/m²/day, then to 100 mg/m²/day, or temporarily suspended, if necessitated by toxicity. When toxicity is controlled, doses may be carefully readjusted upward. If there is no tumor response after 8 weeks of treatment and if the initial dose of 300 mg/m²/day is well tolerated, the dose may be escalated to 400 mg/m²/day with careful monitoring. *Duration of Therapy:* In clinical trials in CTCL, **Targretin** gelcaps were administered for up to 97 weeks. **Targretin** capsules should be continued as long as the patient is deriving benefit. Caution should be used when administering **Targretin** gelcaps in patients using insulin, agents enhancing insulin secretion (e.g., sulfonylureas), or insulin-sensitizers (e.g., *troglitazone*). Based on the mechanism of action, **Targretin** gelcaps could enhance the action of these agents, resulting in hypoglycemia. Hypoglycemia has not been associated with the use of **Targretin** gelcaps as monotherapy. Blood lipid determinations should be performed and fasting triglycerides should be normal or normalized with appropriate intervention prior to initiation of therapy with **Targretin** gelcaps. Hyperlipidemia usually occurs within the initial 2 to 4 weeks. Therefore, weekly lipid determinations are recommended during this interval. Subsequently, in patients not hyperlipidemic, determinations can be performed less frequently. Monitor patients for leukopenia, liver function test (LFT) abnormalities, and thyroid axis alterations. A WBC count with differential should be obtained at baseline and periodically during treatment. Baseline LFTs should be obtained and carefully monitored after 1, 2, and 4 weeks of treatment. If stable, monitor periodically during treatment. Baseline thyroid function tests should be obtained and then monitored during treatment as indicated. Adverse events leading to dose reduction or study drug discontinuation in at least two patients were hyperlipemia, neutropenia/leukopenia, diarrhea, fatigue/lethargy, hypothyroidism, headache, LFT abnormalities, rash, pancreatitis, nausea, anemia, allergic reaction, muscle spasm, pneumonia, and confusion.

CANCER: MELANOMA

PROGRAMMED DEATH RECEPTOR-1 (PD-1)-BLOCKING ANTIBODY

▶ **pembrolizumab** *Unresectable or Metastatic: Administer* 200 mg via IV infusion over 30 minutes once every 3 weeks or 400 mg via IV infusion over 30 minutes once every 6 weeks until disease progression or unacceptable toxicity; *Stage IIB, IIC, or III following Complete Resection: Administer* 200 mg via IV infusion over 30 minutes once every 3 weeks or 400 mg via IV infusion over 30 minutes once every 6 weeks until disease recurrence, unacceptable toxicity, or up to 12 months
Pediatric: <12 years: safety and efficacy not established; ≥12 years, *Stage IIB, IIC, or III following Complete Resection:* same as adult

Keytruda *Vial:* 100 mg/4 ml (25 mg/ml), single-dose, soln for dilution and IV infusion
Comment: Keytruda is a programmed death receptor-1 (PD-1)-blocking antibody indicated for the treatment of multiple cancers, including melanoma. **Keytruda** is indicated for the treatment of patients with unresectable or metastatic melanoma. **Keytruda** is also indicated for the adjuvant treatment of adult and pediatric (≥12 years of age) patients with stage IIB, IIC, or III melanoma following complete resection. **Keytruda** can cause fetal harm. Exclude pregnancy prior to initiating treatment with **Keytruda**. Advise females of reproductive potential of the embryo/fetal risk and to use effective contraception during treatment and for 4 months after the last **Keytruda** dose. Advise mothers not to breastfeed. See mfr pkg insert for full prescribing information, including storage, preparation, warnings, precautions, drug-drug interactions, and adverse reactions.

PD-1-BLOCKING AND LYMPHOCYTE ACTIVATION GENE-3 (LAG-3)-BLOCKING ANTIBODY

▶ **nivolumab+relatlimab-rmbw** *Administer* **nivolumab** 480 mg and *relatlimab* 160 mg (2 x **Opdualag** 240/80 vials), via IV infusion over 30 minutes, every 4 weeks; Do not shake. Store **Opdualag** refrigerated at 2°C to 8°C (36°F-46°F) in the original carton to protect from light until time of use; Do not freeze; See mfr pkg insert for storage, preparation, and administration
Pediatric: <12 years, <40 kg: safety and efficacy not established; ≥12 years, ≥40 kg: same as adult

Opdualag *Vial:* **nivolumab** 240 mg and *relatlimab* 80 mg per 20 ml (12 mg and 4 mg per ml, respectively), soln, single-dose
Comment: Opdualag is a fixed-dose combination of *nivolumab*, a PD-1-blocking antibody and *relatlimab*, a lymphocyte activation gene-3 (LAG-3)-blocking antibody, indicated for the treatment of unresectable or metastatic melanoma. The most common adverse reactions (≥20%) have been musculoskeletal pain, fatigue, rash, pruritus, and diarrhea. The most common laboratory abnormalities (≥20%) are decreased hemoglobin, decreased lymphocytes, increased aspartate aminotransferase (AST), increased alanine aminotransferase (ALT), and decreased sodium. Immune-mediated adverse reactions, which may be severe or fatal, can occur in any organ system or tissue, including the following: immune-mediated pneumonitis, immune-mediated colitis, immune-mediated hepatitis, immune-mediated endocrinopathies, immune-mediated dermatologic adverse reactions, immune-mediated nephritis with renal dysfunction, and immune-mediated myocarditis. Monitor for early identification and management. Evaluate liver enzymes, creatinine, and thyroid function at baseline and periodically during treatment. Withhold or permanently discontinue based on severity and type of reaction. In the event of an infusion-related reaction, interrupt the infusion, slow the rate, or permanently discontinue **Opdualag** based on reaction severity. Fatal and other serious complications can occur in patients who receive allogeneic hematopoietic stem cell transplantation (HSCT) before or after being treated with a PD-1/programmed death-ligand 1 (PD-L1)-blocking antibody. There are no available data on **Opdualag** in human pregnancy to evaluate a drug-associated risk. However, based on findings in animal studies and mechanism of action, **Opdualag** can cause fetal harm when administered in human pregnancy. Administration of *nivolumab* from the onset of organogenesis through delivery resulted in increased abortion and premature infant death. Human immunoglobulin G4 (IgG4) is known to cross the placenta; therefore, *nivolumab* and *relatlimab* have the potential to be transmitted from the mother to the developing fetus. The effects of **Opdualag** are likely to be greater during the 2nd and 3rd trimesters of pregnancy. One function of the PD-1/PD-L1 pathway is to preserve pregnancy by maintaining immune tolerance to the fetus. In animal studies, effects of *nivolumab* on prenatal and postnatal development were evaluated in animals receiving *nivolumab* twice weekly from the onset of organogenesis through delivery at exposure levels of between 9 and 42 times higher than those observed at the clinical dose of 3 mg/kg (based on area under the curve [AUC]). *Nivolumab* administration resulted in a non-dose-related increase in spontaneous abortion and increased neonatal death. In surviving infants (18 of 32 compared to 11 of 16 vehicle-exposed infants) treated with *nivolumab*, there were no apparent malformations and no adverse effects on neurobehavioral, immunologic, or clinical pathology parameters throughout the 6-month postnatal period. There are no available animal data on *relatlimab*. The effects of a murine surrogate anti-LAG-3 antibody were evaluated in animal studies using syngeneic and allogeneic breeding models. When anti-LAG-3 antibodies were administered beginning on gestation day 6, there were no maternal or developmental effects in either syngeneic or allogeneic breedings. Exclude pregnancy in females of reproductive potential prior to initiating **Opdualag**. If a pregnancy is confirmed, do not initiate **Opdualag** treatment. Advise females of reproductive potential to use effective contraception during treatment and for at least 5 months following the last dose of **Opdualag**. If a pregnancy is suspected during treatment with **Opdualag**, discontinue **Opdualag** immediately. There are no data on the presence

of *nivolumab* and *relatlimab* in human milk or effects on the breastfed infant. Because *nivolumab* and *relatlimab* may be excreted in human milk and because of the potential for serious adverse reactions in the breastfed infant, advise mothers not to breastfeed during treatment with **Opdualag** and for at least 5 months after the last dose. To report suspected adverse reactions, contact Bristol Myers Squibb at 1-800-721-5072 or FDA at 1-800-FDA-1088 or www.fda.gov/medwatch.

JANUS KINASE (JAK) INHIBITOR

▶ *dabrafenib Recommended dose:* 150 mg (2 x 75 mg capsules) bid; Take dose at least 1 hour before or at least 2 hours after a meal

Pediatric: **Tafinlar** is only indicated in pediatrics for the treatment of solid tumors and low-grade glioma (LGG)

Tafinlar *Cap:* 50, 75 mg; *Tab for oral susp:* 10 mg

Comment: **Tafinlar** is a kinase inhibitor indicated (1) as a single agent for the treatment of patients with unresectable or metastatic melanoma with BRAF V600E mutation as detected by an FDA-approved test (2) in combination with *trametinib* for the treatment of patients with unresectable or metastatic melanoma with BRAF V600E or V600K mutations as detected by an FDA-approved test, and (3) as adjuvant treatment of patients with melanoma with BRAF V600E or V600K mutations, as detected by an FDA-approved test, and involvement of lymph node(s), following complete resection. New primary malignancies, cutaneous and non-cutaneous, can occur when **Tafinlar** is administered as a single agent or with *trametinib*. Monitor patients for new malignancies prior to and while on therapy and following discontinuation of treatment. Increased cell proliferation can occur with BRAF inhibitors. Major hemorrhagic events can occur in patients receiving **Tafinlar** with *trametinib*; monitor for signs and symptoms of bleeding. Assess left ventricular ejection fraction (LVEF) before treatment with **Tafinlar** and *trametinib* after one month of treatment, then every 2 to 3 months thereafter. Uveitis can occur with **Tafinlar**; perform ophthalmologic evaluation for any visual disturbances. Incidence and severity of pyrexia are increased with **Tafinlar** and *trametinib*. Monitor for skin toxicities. Discontinue for intolerable Grade 2 or Grade 3 or 4 rash not improving within 3 weeks despite interruption of **Tafinlar**. Permanently discontinue for severe cutaneous adverse reaction (SCAR). Monitor serum glucose levels in patients with preexisting diabetes or hyperglycemia. For patients with glucose-6-phosphate dehydrogenase deficiency (G6PD), closely monitor for hemolytic anemia. The most common adverse reactions (incidence ≥20%) with **Tafinlar** as a single agent have been hyperkeratosis, headache, pyrexia, arthralgia, papilloma, alopecia, and palmar-plantar erythrodysesthesia syndrome. The most common adverse reactions (incidence ≥20%) for **Tafinlar**, in combination with *trametinib*, include: Unresectable or metastatic melanoma: pyrexia, rash, chills, headache, arthralgia, and cough; Adjuvant treatment of melanoma: pyrexia, fatigue, nausea, headache, rash, chills, diarrhea, vomiting, arthralgia, and myalgia.

Avoid concurrent administration of **Tafinlar** with strong inhibitors of CYP3A4 or CYP2C8. Concomitant use of **Tafinlar** with agents that are sensitive substrates of CYP3A4, CYP2C8, CYP2C9, CYP2C19, or CYP2B6 may result in loss of efficacy of these agents. **Tafinlar** is embryo/fetal toxic. Exclude pregnancy in females of reproductive potential prior to initiating **Tafinlar**. Advise females of reproductive potential of potential risk to the fetus and to use an effective non-hormonal method of contraception during treatment and for 2 weeks after the last dose. Counsel patients that **Tafinlar** can render hormonal contraceptives ineffective. Advise mothers not to breastfeed during treatment with **Tafinlar** and for 2 weeks following the last dose. Advise females and males of reproductive potential that **Tafinlar** may impair fertility. To report suspected adverse reactions, contact Novartis Pharmaceuticals Corporation at 888-669-6682 or FDA at 800-FDA-1088 or www.fda.gov/medwatch.

▶ *trametinib Recommended dose*: 2 mg once daily at least 1 hour before or at least 2 hours after a meal; Confirm the presence of BRAF V600E or V600K mutation in tumor specimens prior to initiation of treatment

Pediatric: safety and efficacy not established

Mekinist *Tab:* 0.5, 1, 2 mg film-coat

Comment: **Mekinist** is a kinase inhibitor indicated for the treatment of patients with unresectable or metastatic melanoma with BRAF V600E or V600K mutations as detected by an FDA-approved test. **Mekinist** is not indicated for the treatment of patients who have received prior BRAF inhibitor therapy. The most common adverse reactions (incidence ≥20%) reported with **Mekinist** have been rash, diarrhea, and lymphedema. No formal clinical study has been conducted to evaluate the effect of hepatic impairment on the pharmacokinetics of *trametinib*. No dose adjustment is recommended in patients with mild hepatic impairment (Child-Pugh Class A) based on a population pharmacokinetic analysis. The appropriate dose of **Mekinist** has not been established in patients with moderate or severe hepatic impairment (Child-Pugh Class B or C). No formal clinical study has been conducted to evaluate the effect of renal impairment on the pharmacokinetics of **trametinib**. No dose adjustment is recommended in patients with mild or moderate renal impairment based on a population pharmacokinetic analysis. The appropriate dose of **Mekinist** has not been established in patients with severe renal impairment. Monitor patients for cardiomyopathy; reassess LVEF after one month of treatment and evaluate approximately every 2 to 3 months thereafter. Monitor patients for retinal pigment epithelial detachment

(continued)

(RPED). Conduct an ophthalmologic evaluation for any visual disturbances. Withhold **Mekinist** if RPED is diagnosed and discontinue **Mekinist** if no improvement after 3 weeks. Discontinue **Mekinist** if retinal vein occlusion (RVO) occurs. Withhold Mekinist for new or progressive unexplained pulmonary symptoms or findings, such as cough, dyspnea, hypoxia, or infiltrates. Permanently discontinue **Mekinist** for treatment-related interstitial lung disease (ILD) or pneumonitis. Monitor for skin toxicities and for secondary infections. Discontinue **Mekinist** for intolerable Grade 2, or Grade 3 or 4 rash not improving within 3 weeks despite interruption of the drug. *Trametinib* was embryotoxic and abortifacient in animal studies. Accordingly, *Mekinist* can cause fetal harm when administered in human pregnancy. Advise females of reproductive potential of potential risk to the fetus. Males and females of reproductive potential should be advised to use highly effective contraception during treatment and for 4 months after the end of treatment with **Mekinist**. Breastfeeding is not recommended. A decision should be made whether to discontinue the drug or discontinue breastfeeding taking into account the importance of the drug to the mother. *Trametinib* may impair fertility in female patients. To report suspected adverse reactions, contact GlaxoSmithKline at 1-888-825-5249 or FDA at 1-800-FDA-1088 or www.fda.gov/medwatch.

HUMAN PD-1-BLOCKING ANTIBODY

▷ *nivolumab* Administer 3 mg/kg via IV infusion over 60 minutes once every 2 weeks
   Pediatric: safety and efficacy not established
   Opdivo *Vial:* 40 mg/4 ml (10 mg/ml), 100 mg/10 ml (10 mg/ml), single-use, soln for dilution and IV infusion
   Comment: **Opdivo** is a PD-1-blocking antibody indicated for the treatment of patients with unresectable or metastatic melanoma and disease progression following *ipilimumab* and, if BRAF V600 mutation-positive, a BRAF inhibitor. This indication is approved under accelerated approval based on tumor response rate and durability of response. Continued approval for this indication may be contingent upon verification and description of clinical benefit in confirmatory trials. The most common adverse reaction (incidence ≥20%) in patients with melanoma has been rash. For immune-mediated adverse reactions, administer corticosteroids based on the severity of the reaction. Withhold **Opdivo** for moderate and permanently discontinue for severe or life-threatening pneumonitis. Withhold **Opdivo** for moderate or severe immune-mediated colitis and permanently discontinue **Opdivo** for life-threatening colitis. For immune-mediated hepatitis, withhold **Opdivo** for moderate and permanently discontinue for severe or life-threatening transaminase or total bilirubin elevation. Withhold **Opdivo** for moderate or severe and permanently discontinue for life-threatening serum creatinine elevation. For immune-mediated hypothyroidism or hyperthyroidism, initiate thyroid hormone replacement as needed. Based on its mechanism of action and data from animal studies, **Opdivo** can cause fetal harm. *Nivolumab* is an IgG4 and human IgG4 is known to cross the placental barrier; therefore, *nivolumab* has the potential to be transmitted from the mother to the developing fetus. The effects of **Opdivo** are likely to be greater during the 2nd and 3rd trimesters of pregnancy. Exclude pregnancy in females of reproductive potential prior to initiating **Opdivo**. Advise females of reproductive potential of the embryo/fetal risk and to use effective contraception during treatment and for 5 months after the last **Opdivo** dose. Advise mothers not to breastfeed during treatment and for 5 months after the last **Opdivo** dose. See mfr pkg insert for full prescribing information, including storage, preparation, warnings, precautions, drug-drug interactions, and adverse reactions. To report suspected adverse reactions, contact Bristol Myers Squibb at 800-721-5072 or FDA at 800-FDA-1088 or www.fda.gov/medwatch.

CD38-DIRECTED CYTOLYTIC ANTIBODY AND HYALURONIDASE

▷ *daratumumab+hyaluronidase* Pre-medicate with a corticosteroid, acetaminophen, and a histamine-1 receptor antagonist; *Recommended Dose:* 1,800 mg *daratumumab* + 30,000 units *hyaluronidase* administered SC into the abdomen over approximately 3 to 5 minutes according to the recommended schedule
   Pediatric: safety and efficacy not established
   Darzalex Faspro *Vial:* 1,800 mg *daratumumab* + 30,000 units *hyaluronidase* per 15 ml (120 mg + 2,000 units/ml), single-dose, soln for SC infusion
   Comment: **Darzalex Faspro** is a combination of *daratumumab*, a CD38-directed cytolytic antibody, and *hyaluronidase*, an endoglycosidase, for the treatment of adult patients with multiple myeloma: (1) in combination with *bortezomib*, *melphalan*, and *prednisone* in newly diagnosed patients who are ineligible for autologous stem cell transplant; (2) in combination with *lenalidomide* and *dexamethasone* in newly diagnosed patients who are ineligible for autologous stem cell transplant and in patients with relapsed or refractory multiple myeloma who have received at least one prior therapy; (3) in combination with *bortezomib* and *dexamethasone* in patients who have received at least one prior therapy; and (4) as monotherapy in patients who have received at least three prior lines of therapy, including a proteasome inhibitor (PI) and an immunomodulatory agent, or who are double-refractory to a PI and an immunomodulatory agent. The most common adverse reaction (incidence ≥20%) with **Darzalex Faspro** monotherapy is upper respiratory tracts infection. The most common adverse reactions (incidence ≥20%) with D-VMP are upper respiratory tract infection, constipation, nausea, fatigue, pyrexia, peripheral sensory neuropathy, diarrhea, cough, insomnia, vomiting, and back pain. The

most common adverse reactions (incidence ≥20%) with D-Rd are fatigue, diarrhea, upper respiratory tract infection, muscle spasms, constipation, pyrexia, pneumonia, and dyspnea. The most common hematology laboratory abnormalities (incidence ≥40%) with **Darzalex Faspro** are decreased leukocytes, decreased lymphocytes, decreased neutrophils, decreased platelets, and decreased hemoglobin. The only contraindication to **Darzalex Faspro** is patient history of severe hypersensitivity to **daratumumab** or any of the components of the formulation. Permanently discontinue **Darzalex Faspro** for life-threatening reactions. Neutropenia can occur; monitor complete blood cell counts (CBCs) periodically during treatment. Monitor patients with neutropenia for signs of infection. Consider withholding **Darzalex Faspro** to allow recovery of neutrophils. Thrombocytopenia can occur; monitor CBCs periodically during treatment. Consider withholding **Darzalex Faspro** to allow recovery of platelets. **Darzalex Faspro** interferes with cross-matching and red blood cell antibody screening. Type and screen patients prior to starting treatment and inform blood banks that a patient has received **Darzalex Faspro**. **Darzalex Faspro** is embryo/fetal toxic and therefore can cause fetal harm. The assessment of associated risks with **daratumumab** products is based on the mechanism of action and data from target antigen CD38 knockout animal models. Advise pregnant females of the potential risk to the fetus and advise females of reproductive potential to use effective contraception. Exclude pregnancy before initiating treatment with **Darzalex Faspro**. Because of the potential for serious adverse reactions in the breastfed infant when **Darzalex Faspro** is administered with **lenalidomide** and **dexamethasone**, advise mothers not to breastfeed during treatment with **Darzalex Faspro** and for 3 months after the last dose. Refer to **lenalidomide** prescribing information for additional information. To report suspected adverse reactions, contact Janssen Biotech at 800-526-7736 (800-JANSSEN) or FDA at 800-FDA-1088 or www.fda.gov/medwatch.

CANCER: MERKEL CELL CARCINOMA

PROGRAMMED DEATH RECEPTOR-1 (PD-1)-BLOCKING ANTIBODY

▷ *pembrolizumab* Administer 200 mg via IV infusion over 30 minutes once every 3 weeks or 400 mg via IV infusion over 30 minutes every 6 weeks until disease progression, unacceptable toxicity, or up to 24 months *Pediatric:* 2 mg/kg (up to a maximum of 200 mg) via IV infusion once every 3 weeks until disease progression, unacceptable toxicity, or up to 24 months

    Keytruda *Vial:* 100 mg/4 ml (25 mg/ml) single-dose, soln for dilution and IV infusion

    Comment: Keytruda is a programmed death receptor-1 (PD-1)-blocking antibody indicated for the treatment of multiple cancers, including adult and pediatric patients with recurrent locally advanced or metastatic Merkel cell carcinoma. This indication is approved under accelerated approval based on tumor response rate and durability of response. Continued approval for this indication may be contingent upon verification and description of clinical benefit in the confirmatory trials. **Keytruda** can cause fetal harm. Advise females of the potential embryo/fetal risk and to use effective contraception. Advise not to breastfeed. See mfr pkg insert for full prescribing information.

▷ *retifanlimab-dlwr* Recommended dose: 500 mg via IV infusion over 30 minutes once q 4 weeks until disease progression, unacceptable toxicity, or up to 24 months *Pediatric:* safety and efficacy not established

    Zynyz *Vial:* 500 mg/20 ml (25 mg/ml), single-dose, soln for dilution and IV infusion

    Comment: Zynyz is a programmed death receptor-1 (PD-1)-blocking antibody indicated for the treatment of adult patients with metastatic or recurrent locally advanced Merkel cell carcinoma. This indication is approved under accelerated approval based on tumor response rate and duration of response. Continued approval for this indication may be contingent upon verification and description of clinical benefit in confirmatory trials. The most common (incidence ≥10%) adverse reactions have been fatigue, musculoskeletal pain, pruritus, diarrhea, rash, pyrexia, and nausea. Immune-mediated adverse reactions, which may be severe or fatal, can occur in any organ system or tissue, including the following: immune-mediated pneumonitis, immune-mediated colitis, immune-mediated hepatitis, immune-mediated endocrinopathies, immune-mediated nephritis with renal dysfunction, and immune-mediated dermatologic adverse reactions, and solid organ transplant rejection. Monitor for early identification and manage as appropriate. Evaluate liver enzymes, creatinine, and thyroid function at baseline and periodically during treatment. Withhold or permanently discontinue **Zynyz** and administer corticosteroids based on the severity of reaction. Fatal and other serious complications can occur in patients who receive allogeneic hematopoietic stem cell transplantation (HSCT) before or after being treated with a PD-1/programmed death-ligand 1 (PD-L1)-blocking antibody. See mfr pkg insert for full prescribing information, including storage, preparation, and dose adjustments based on signs and symptoms of adverse effects. Based on its mechanism of action, **Zynyz** is embryo/fetal toxic in human pregnancy. Human immunoglobulin G4 (IgG4) are known to cross the placenta; therefore, **retifanlimab-dlwr** has the potential to be transmitted from the mother to the developing fetus. Animal studies have demonstrated that inhibition of the PD-1/PD-L1 pathway can lead to increased risk of immune-mediated rejection of the developing fetus, resulting in fetal death. Advise women of the potential risk of serious harm to the fetus. Exclude pregnancy prior to starting treatment with **Zynyz**. Advise females of reproductive potential to use effective contraception during treatment and for 4 months after the last dose. There is no information regarding the presence of

(continued)

retifanlimab-dlwr in human milk or its effects on the breastfed infant. Maternal immunoglobulin G (IgG) is known to be present in human milk. The effects of local gastrointestinal exposure and limited systemic exposure in the breastfed infant to **Zynyz** are unknown. Because of the potential for serious adverse reactions in breastfed infants, advise mothers not to breastfeed during treatment and for 4 months after the last dose of **Zynyz**. To report suspected adverse reactions, contact Incyte Corporation at 855-463-3463 or FDA at 800-FDA-1088 or www.fda.gov/medwatch.

CANCER: MESOTHELIOMA

KINASE INHIBITOR

▷ *capmatinib* 400 mg bid with or without food
    Tabrecta *Tab:* 150, 200 mg
    Comment: Tabrecta *(capmatinib)* is a kinase inhibitor indicated for the treatment of adult patients with metastatic non-small cell lung cancer (NSCLC) whose tumors have a mutation that leads to mesenchymal-epithelial transition (MET) exon 14 skipping as detected by a Food and Drug Administration (FDA)-approved test. The most common adverse reactions (incidence ≥20%) have been peripheral edema, nausea, fatigue, vomiting, dyspnea, and decreased appetite. Monitor for new or worsening pulmonary symptoms indicative of interstitial lung disease (ILD)/pneumonitis. Permanently discontinue **Tabrecta** in patients with ILD/pneumonitis. Monitor liver function tests. In the event of hepatotoxicity, withhold, reduce dose, or permanently discontinue **Tabrecta** based on severity. **Tabrecta** may cause photosensitivity reactions. Advise patients to limit direct UV exposure. **Tabrecta** can cause embryo/fetal harm. Advise patients of reproductive potential to use effective contraception. Advise not to breastfeed.

CANCER: MULTIPLE MYELOMA, MYELODYSPLASTIC SYNDROME

PROTEASOME INHIBITOR

▷ *carfilzomib* see mfr pkg insert for recommended dosing regimens
    Pediatric: safety and efficacy not established
    Kyprolis *Vial:* 10, 30, 60 mg, single-dose, pwdr for reconstitution, dilution, and IV infusion
    Comment: Kyprolis *(carfilzomib)* is indicated for the treatment of patients with relapsed or refractory multiple myeloma (1) who have received one to three lines of therapy in combination with *dexamethasone* or with *lenalidomide* plus *dexamethasone* or with *daratumumab* plus *dexamethasone* or (2) as a single agent for the treatment of patients with relapsed or refractory multiple myeloma who have received one or more lines of therapy. The most common adverse reactions (incidence 20%) in patients treated with **Kyprolis** (1) in the combination therapy trials have been anemia, diarrhea, fatigue, hypertension, pyrexia, upper respiratory infection (URI), thrombocytopenia, cough, dyspnea, and insomnia; and (2) in monotherapy trials have been fatigue, thrombocytopenia, nausea, pyrexia, dyspnea, diarrhea, headache, cough, and peripheral edema. See the mfr pkg insert for full prescribing information.

CD38-DIRECTED CYTOLYTIC ANTIBODY AND HYALURONIDASE

▷ *daratumumab+hyaluronidase* premedicate with a corticosteroid, acetaminophen, and a histamine-1 receptor antagonist; *Recommended dose:* 1,800 mg *daratumumab* + 30,000 units *hyaluronidase* administered SC into the abdomen over approximately 3-5 minutes according to the recommended schedule
    Pediatric: safety and efficacy not established
    Darzalex Faspro *Vial:* 1,800 mg *daratumumab* + 30,000 units *hyaluronidase* per 15 ml (120 mg + 2,000 units/ml), single-dose, soln for SC infusion
    Comment: Darzalex Faspro is a combination of *daratumumab*, a CD38-directed cytolytic antibody, and *hyaluronidase*, an endoglycosidase, for the treatment of adult patients with multiple myeloma: (1) in combination with *bortezomib*, *melphalan*, and *prednisone* in newly diagnosed patients who are ineligible for autologous stem cell transplant; (2) in combination with *lenalidomide* and *dexamethasone* in newly diagnosed patients who are ineligible for autologous stem cell transplant and in patients with relapsed or refractory multiple myeloma who have received at least one prior therapy; (3) in combination with *bortezomib* and *dexamethasone* in patients who have received at least one prior therapy; and (4) as monotherapy in patients who have received at least three prior lines of therapy, including a proteasome inhibitor (PI) and an immunomodulatory agent, or who are double-refractory to a PI and an immunomodulatory agent. The most common adverse reaction (incidence ≥20%) with **Darzalex Faspro** monotherapy is upper respiratory tracts infection. The most common adverse reactions (incidence ≥20%) with D-VMP are upper respiratory tract infection, constipation, nausea, fatigue, pyrexia, peripheral sensory neuropathy, diarrhea, cough, insomnia, vomiting, and back pain. The most common adverse reactions (incidence ≥20%) with D-Rd are fatigue, diarrhea, upper respiratory tract infection, muscle spasms, constipation, pyrexia, pneumonia, and dyspnea. The most common

hematology laboratory abnormalities (incidence ≥40%) with **Darzalex Faspro** are decreased leukocytes, decreased lymphocytes, decreased neutrophils, decreased platelets, and decreased hemoglobin. The only contraindication to **Darzalex Faspro** is patient history of severe hypersensitivity to *daratumumab* or any of the components of the formulation. Permanently discontinue **Darzalex Faspro** for life-threatening reactions. Neutropenia can occur; monitor complete blood cell counts (CBCs) periodically during treatment. Monitor patients with neutropenia for signs of infection. Consider withholding **Darzalex Faspro** to allow recovery of neutrophils. Thrombocytopenia can occur; monitor CBCs periodically during treatment. Consider withholding **Darzalex Faspro** to allow recovery of platelets. **Darzalex Faspro** interferes with cross-matching and red blood cell antibody screening. Type and screen patients prior to starting treatment and inform blood banks that a patient has received **Darzalex Faspro**. **Darzalex Faspro** is embryo/fetal toxic and therefore can cause fetal harm. The assessment of associated risks with *daratumumab* products is based on the mechanism of action and data from target antigen CD38 knockout animal models. Advise pregnant females of the potential risk to the fetus and advise females of reproductive potential to use effective contraception. Exclude pregnancy before initiating treatment with **Darzalex Faspro**. Because of the potential for serious adverse reactions in the breastfed infant when **Darzalex Faspro** is administered with *lenalidomide* and *dexamethasone*, advise mothers not to breastfeed during treatment with **Darzalex Faspro** and for 3 months after the last dose. Refer to *lenalidomide* prescribing information for additional information. To report suspected adverse reactions, contact Janssen Biotech at 800-526-7736 (800-JANSSEN) or FDA at 800-FDA1088 or www.fda.gov/medwatch.

B-CELL MATURATION ANTIGEN (BCMA)-DIRECTED ANTIBODY AND MICROTUBULE INHIBITOR CONJUGATE

▷ *belantamab mafodotin-blmf* 2.5 mg/kg via IV infusion over 30 minutes once q 3 weeks

Blenrep *Vial:* 100 mg, single-dose, pwdr for reconstitution, dilution, and IV infusion

Comment: Blenrep is indicated for the treatment of adult patients with relapsed or refractory multiple myeloma who have received at least four prior therapies, including an anti-CD38 monoclonal antibody, a PI, and an immunomodulatory agent. This indication is approved under accelerated approval based on response rate. Continued approval for this indication may be contingent upon verification and description of clinical benefit in confirmatory trial(s). The most common adverse reactions (incidence ≥20%) are keratopathy (corneal epithelium change on eye exam), decreased visual acuity, nausea, blurred vision, pyrexia, infusion-related reactions, and fatigue. The most common grade 3 or 4 laboratory abnormalities (incidence ≥5%) are decreased platelets, lymphocytes, hemoglobin, and neutrophils, and increased creatinine and gamma-glutamyl transferase. Obtain a baseline CBC prior to initiating therapy with **Blenrep** and during therapy as clinically indicated. Monitor patients for infusion-related reactions; interrupt and then reduce the rate or permanently discontinue based on the severity. **Blenrep** can cause embryo/fetal harm; advise females of reproductive potential of the potential risk and to use effective contraception. Advise not to breastfeed

ANTICANCER PEPTIDE-DRUG CONJUGATE

▷ *melphalan flufenamide Recommended dose:* 40 mg via IV infusion over 30 minutes on day 1 of each 28-day treatment cycle, in combination with *dexamethasone*

Pediatric: safety and efficacy not established

Pepaxto *Vial:* 20 mg, single-dose, pwdr for reconstitution, dilution, and IV infusion

Comment: Pepaxto is an alkylating drug indicated, in combination with *dexamethasone,* for the treatment of adult patients with relapsed or refractory multiple myeloma who have received at least four prior lines of therapy and whose disease is refractory to at least one PI, one immunomodulatory agent, and one CD38-directed monoclonal antibody. The most common adverse reactions (incidence >20%) have been fatigue, nausea, diarrhea, pyrexia, and respiratory tract infection. The most common laboratory abnormalities (incidence ≥50%) have been decreased leukocytes, decreased platelets, decreased lymphocytes, decreased neutrophils, decreased hemoglobin, and decreased creatinine increase. Monitor these labs at baseline, during treatment, and as clinically indicated. **Pepaxto** is a genotoxic drug with risk of embryo/fetal harm. Advise females and males of reproductive potential for drug-associated embryo/fetal toxicity. Advise the use of effective contraception for 6 months after the last dose (females) and 3 months after the last dose (males). Breastfeeding is not recommended during treatment and for 1 week after the last dose.

THALIDOMIDE ANALOG

▷ *lenalidomide* see the mfr pkg insert for full prescribing information, including routine dosage treatment duration according to patient characteristics, dose modifications, and specific laboratory values to monitor

Pediatric: <18 years: safety and efficacy not established; >18 years: same as adult

Revlimid: *Cap:* 2.5, 5, 10, 15, 20, 25 mg

Comment: Revlimid, a *thalidomide* analog, is an immunomodulatory agent with antiangiogenic properties indicated for the treatment of patients ≥18 years of age with transfusion-dependent anemia due to low- or intermediate-risk myelodysplastic syndromes (MDS) associated with a deletion 5q cytogenetic abnormality with or without additional cytogenetic abnormalities. **Revlimid** is contraindicated for use during pregnancy. *Thalidomide* is a known human teratogen that causes life-threatening human birth defects or embryo/fetal

(continued)

death. **Revlimid** is only available under a restricted distribution program called "RevAssist." Only prescribers and pharmacists registered with the program are able to prescribe and dispense the product. **Revlimid** may only be dispensed to patients who are registered and meet all the conditions of the RevAssist program. Expanded information about **Revlimid** and the RevAssist program is available at www.REVLIMID.com or by calling Celgene Corporation at 888-4CELGEN. **Revlimid** is associated with significant neutropenia and thrombocytopenia in patients with del 5q MDS. Patients on therapy should have their CBCs monitored weekly for the first 8 weeks of therapy and at least monthly thereafter. Patients may require dose interruption and/or reduction. Patients may require use of blood product support and/or growth factors. This drug has demonstrated a significantly increased risk of deep vein thrombosis (DVT) and pulmonary embolism (PE) in patients with multiple myeloma who were treated with **Revlimid** combination therapy. Patients and physicians are advised to be observant for the signs and symptoms of thromboembolism. Patients should be instructed to seek medical care if they develop symptoms such as shortness of breath, chest pain, or arm or leg swelling. It is not known whether prophylactic anticoagulation or antiplatelet therapy prescribed in conjunction with **Revlimid** may lessen the potential for venous thromboembolic events. The decision to take prophylactic measures should be done carefully after an assessment of an individual patient's underlying risk factors. **Revlimid** is known to be substantially excreted by the kidney, and the risk of toxic reactions to this drug may be greater in patients with impaired renal function. Because elderly patients are more likely to have decreased renal function, care should be taken in dose selection, and it would be prudent to monitor renal function. If pregnancy does occur during treatment, the drug should be immediately discontinued. Under these conditions, the patient should be referred to an obstetrician/gynecologist experienced in reproductive toxicity for further evaluation and counseling. Any suspected fetal exposure to **Revlimid** should be reported to Celgene Corporation at 888-4CELGEN (888-423-5436) or the FDA via the MedWatch program at 800-FDA-1088. It is not known whether **Revlimid** is excreted in human milk. Because of the potential for adverse reactions in breastfed infants from *lenalidomide*, a decision should be made whether to discontinue breastfeeding or to discontinue **Revlimid**, taking into account the importance of the drug to the mother.

CANCER: OVARIAN

VASCULAR ENDOTHELIAL GROWTH FACTOR (VEGF) INHIBITOR

▷ *bevacizumab-adcd*
  Regimens for Epithelial Ovarian, Fallopian Tube and Primary Peritoneal Cancer:
  (1) Stage III or IV epithelial ovarian, fallopian tube, or primary peritoneal cancer following initial surgical resection: 15 mg/kg every 3 weeks with *carboplatin* and *paclitaxel* for up to 6 cycles, followed by 15 mg/kg every 3 weeks as a single agent, for a total of up to 22 cycles
  (2) Platinum-resistant recurrent epithelial ovarian, fallopian tube, or primary peritoneal cancer: 10 mg/kg every 2 weeks with *paclitaxel*, pegylated liposomal *doxorubicin*, or *topotecan* given every week; 15 mg/kg every 3 weeks with *topotecan* given every 3 weeks as a single agent
  (3) Platinum-sensitive recurrent epithelial ovarian, fallopian tube, or primary peritoneal cancer: 15 mg/kg every 3 weeks with *carboplatin* and *gemcitabine* for 6-10 cycles, followed by 15 mg/kg every 3 weeks as a single agent; 15 mg/kg every 3 weeks with *carboplatin* and *paclitaxel* for 6-8 cycles in combination with *carboplatin* and *paclitaxel* or *carboplatin* and *gemcitabine*, followed by 15 mg/kg every 3 weeks with *carboplatin* and *gemcitabine* for 6-10 cycles, followed by 15 mg/kg every 3 weeks as a single agent
  Do not administer **Vegzelma** for 28 days following major surgery and until adequate wound healing; store refrigerated at 2°C-8°C (36°F-46°F) in the original carton until time of use to protect from light; do not freeze or shake the vial or carton; see mfr pkg insert for full prescribing information, including proper preparation and administration instructions and dosage modifications for adverse reactions
  Pediatric: <18 years: safety and efficacy not established; ≥18 years: same as adult
    Vegzelma *Vial:* 100 mg/4 ml (25 mg/ml) or 400 mg/16 ml (25 mg/ml), single-dose, soln for dilution and IV infusion
    Comment: **Vegzelma** is a vascular endothelial growth factor (VEGF) inhibitor biosimilar to **Avastin** indicated for the treatment of multiple types of cancer, including colorectal cancer, non-small cell lung cancer, glioblastoma, renal cell carcinoma, cervical cancer, and epithelial ovarian, fallopian tube, or primary peritoneal cancer. *Bevacizumab* products increase the risk of ovarian failure and may impair fertility. Inform females of reproductive potential of the risk of ovarian failure prior to the first dose of **Vegzelma**. The long-term effects of *bevacizumab* products on fertility are not known. *Bevacizumab* products may cause fetal harm when administered to a pregnant female. Advise females of reproductive potential to use effective contraception during treatment with **Vegzelma** and for 6 months after the last dose. No data are available regarding the presence of *bevacizumab* products in human milk or effects on the breastfed infant. Because of the potential for serious adverse reactions in breastfed infants, advise mothers not to breastfeed during treatment with **Vegzelma** and for 6 months after the last dose. See mfr pkg insert for full prescription information.

POLY(ADP-RIBOSE) POLYMERASE (PARP) INHIBITOR

▷ *niraparib tosylate* 300 mg (3 x 100 mg) once daily, with or without food; continue treatment until disease progression or unacceptable adverse reaction; for adverse reactions, consider interruption of treatment, dose reduction, or dose discontinuation

Pediatric: safety and efficacy not established

Zejula *Cap:* 100 mg

Comment: Zejula *(niraparib)* is indicated for the maintenance treatment of adult patients with recurrent epithelial ovarian, fallopian tube, or primary peritoneal cancer who are in complete or partial response to platinum-based chemotherapy, and for late-line treatment of recurrent ovarian cancer. The most common adverse reactions (incidence ≥10%) have been anemia, thrombocytopenia, neutropenia, leukopenia, hypertension, palpitations, nausea, vomiting, abdominal pain/distention, diarrhea, constipation, mucositis/stomatitis, dry mouth, fatigue/asthenia, dyspepsia, decreased appetite, urinary tract infection, aspartate aminotransferase (AST)/alanine aminotransferase (ALT) elevation, back pain, myalgia, arthralgia, headache, dizziness, dysgeusia, insomnia, anxiety, nasopharyngitis, dyspnea, cough, and rash. Monitor complete blood count (CBC) weekly for the first month, then monthly for the next 11 months, and then periodically thereafter. Monitor blood pressure (BP) and heart rate (HR) monthly for the first year and periodically thereafter. Manage BP and HR with appropriate medication as indicated and adjust the **Zejula** dose if necessary. Because myelodysplastic syndrome/acute myeloid leukemia (MDS/AML) has occurred in patients exposed to **Zejula,** with some cases being fatal, monitor patients for hematologic toxicity and discontinue **Zejula** if MDS/AML is confirmed. **Zejula** can cause embryo/fetal toxicity; therefore, advise females of reproductive potential of the potential risk and to use effective contraception. Advise women not to breastfeed during treatment with **Zejula** and for 1 month after receiving the final dose.

▶ *rucaparib* 600 mg bid with or without food

Pediatric: not established

Rubraca *Tab:* 200, 250, 300 mg

Comment: Rubraca *(rucaparib)* is indicated for maintenance treatment of adult patients with recurrent epithelial ovarian, fallopian tube, and primary peritoneal cancer who are in complete or partial response to platinum-based chemotherapy and for treatment of adult patients with a deleterious BRCA mutation (germline and/or somatic)-associated epithelial ovarian, fallopian tube, or primary peritoneal cancer who have been treated with two or more chemotherapies. Select patients for therapy based on an FDA-approved companion diagnostic for **Rubraca.** Continue treatment until disease progression or unacceptable toxicity. For adverse reactions, consider interruption of treatment or dose reduction. The most common adverse reactions (incidence ≥20%) have been nausea, fatigue (including asthenia), vomiting, anemia, dysgeusia, AST/ALT elevation, constipation, decreased appetite, diarrhea, thrombocytopenia, neutropenia, stomatitis, nasopharyngitis/upper respiratory infection (URI), rash, abdominal pain/distention, and dyspnea. The most common adverse reactions (incidence ≥20%) among patients with BRCA-mutated metastatic castration-resistant prostate cancer (mCRPC) have been fatigue (including asthenia), nausea, anemia, increased ALT/AST, decreased appetite, rash, constipation, thrombocytopenia, vomiting, and diarrhea. MDS and AML have occurred in patients exposed to **Rubraca,** and some cases have been fatal. Monitor patients for hematologic toxicity at baseline and monthly thereafter. Discontinue **Rubraca** if MDS/AML is confirmed. Adjust the dosage of CYP1A2, CYP3A, CYP2C9, and CYP2C19 substrates if clinically indicated. **Rubraca** can cause embryo/fetal harm. Advise females of the potential embryo/fetal risk and to use effective contraception. Advise females not to breastfeed.

FOLATE RECEPTOR ALPHA (FRα)-DIRECTED ANTIBODY AND MICROTUBULE INHIBITOR CONJUGATE

▶ *mirvetuximab soravtansine-gynx* 6 mg/kg adjusted ideal body weight administered via IV infusion every 3 weeks until disease progression or unacceptable toxicity; administer **Elahere** as IV infusion only after dilution in D5W (Alert: **Elahere** is incompatible with normal saline); premedicate with a corticosteroid antihistamine, antipyretic, antiemetic, ophthalmic steroid, and lubricating eye drops; store **Elahere** vials upright in a refrigerator at 2°C-8°C (36°F-46°F) in the original carton to protect from light until the time of preparation; do not freeze or shake; **Elahere** is a hazardous drug; see mfr pkg insert for special handling and disposal procedures

Pediatric: safety and efficacy not established

Elahere *Vial:* 100 mg/20 ml (5 mg/ml), single-dose, soln for dilution and IV infusion

Comment: Elahere is a folate receptor alpha (FRα)-directed antibody and microtubule inhibitor conjugate indicated for the treatment of adult patients with FRα-positive, platinum-resistant epithelial ovarian, fallopian tube, or primary peritoneal cancer who have received one to three prior systemic treatment regimens. These indications are approved under accelerated approval based on tumor response rate and durability of response. Continued approval for this indication may be contingent upon verification and description of clinical benefit in a confirmatory trial. *Black Box Warning:* **Elahere** can cause severe ocular toxicities, including visual impairment, keratopathy, dry eye, photophobia, eye pain, and uveitis. Conduct an ophthalmic exam, including visual acuity and slit lamp exam, prior to initiation of **Elahere,** every other cycle for the first eight cycles and as clinically indicated. Administer prophylactic artificial tears and ophthalmic steroid. Withhold **Elahere** for ocular toxicities until improvement and resume at the same or reduced dose. Discontinue **Elahere** for grade 4 ocular toxicities. Withhold **Elahere** for persistent or recurrent grade 2 pneumonitis and consider dose reduction. Permanently discontinue **Elahere** for grade 3 or 4 pneumonitis. Monitor patients for new or worsening peripheral neuropathy. Withhold dose, pause dose, slow the rate of infusion, or permanently discontinue **Elahere** based on the severity of peripheral

(continued)

neuropathy. The most common (≥20%) adverse reactions, including laboratory abnormalities, have been vision impairment, fatigue, increased AST, nausea, increased ALT, keratopathy, abdominal pain, decreased lymphocytes, peripheral neuropathy, diarrhea, decreased albumin, constipation, increased alkaline phosphatase, dry eye, decreased magnesium, decreased leukocytes, decreased neutrophils, and decreased hemoglobin. *Child-Pugh Class B or C:* Avoid use. Closely monitor patients for adverse reactions if taking strong CYP3A4 inhibitors. **Elahere** is embryo/fetal toxic. Human immunoglobulin G (IgG) is known to cross the placental barrier; therefore, **Elahere** has the potential to be transmitted from the mother to the developing fetus. The cytotoxic component, DM4, disrupts microtubule function, is genotoxic, and can be toxic to actively dividing cells, suggesting it has the potential to cause embryotoxicity and teratogenicity. Advise patients of the potential risk to the fetus and to use effective contraception. There are no data on the presence of ***mirvetuximab soravtansine-gynx*** in human milk or effects on the breastfed infant. Because of the potential for serious adverse reactions in the breastfed infant, advise mothers not to breastfeed during treatment with **Elahere** and for 1 month after the last dose.

CANCER: PANCREATIC

CISPLATIN NEUTRALIZING AGENT

▶ *sodium thiosulfate*
Pediatric: <1 month: safety and efficacy not established; ≥1 month: *Recommended dose:* based on body surface area (BSA) according to actual body weight (see dosing table); administer via IV infusion over 15 minutes starting 6 hours after completion of *cisplatin* infusion; *Multi-day cisplatin regimens:* administer 6 hours after each *cisplatin* infusion, but at least 10 hours before the next *cisplatin* infusion; do not start if less than 10 hours before starting the next *cisplatin* infusion; store at 20°C-25°C (68°F-77°F); excursions are permitted between 15°C and 30°C (59°F-86°F).

Pedmark Dose by Weight	
Weight	Dose
<5 kg	10 g/m²
<5-10 kg	15 g/m²
>10 kg	20 g/m²

Pedmark *Vial:* 12.5 gm/100 ml (125 mg/ml), single-use, for IV infusion
Comment: **Pedmark** is indicated to reduce the risk of ototoxicity associated with *cisplatin* in pediatric patients ≥1 month of age with localized, non-metastatic solid tumors. **Pedmark** is not recommended for treatment of patients <1 year of age due to increased risk of hypernatremia. **Pedmark** is not indicated for treatment of pediatric patients <1 month of age (due to increased risk of hypernatremia) or pediatric patients with metastatic cancer. **Pedmark** may not reduce the risk of ototoxicity when administered following longer *cisplatin* infusions because irreversible ototoxicity may have already occurred. The most common adverse reactions (≥25% with difference between arms of >5% compared to *cisplatin* alone) in SIOPEL 6 are vomiting, nausea, decreased hemoglobin, and hypernatremia. The most common adverse reaction (≥25% with difference between arms of >5% compared to *cisplatin* alone) in COG ACCL0431 is hypokalemia. History of severe hypersensitivity to ***sodium thiosulfate*** or any components are the only contraindication. For signs and symptoms of hypersensitivity reaction, immediately discontinue **Pedmark** and institute appropriate care. Administer premedications before each subsequent dose. **Pedmark** may contain sodium sulfite; patients with sulfite sensitivity may have hypersensitivity reactions. Monitor serum sodium and potassium at baseline and as clinically indicated; monitor more closely if glomerular filtration rate (GFR) falls below 60 ml/min/1.73m². Withhold **Pedmark** with serum sodium >145 mmol/L. For nausea and vomiting, administer antiemetics prior to each dose administration. There are no available data on **Pedmark** to evaluate for drug-associated risk in human pregnancy or lactation. In animal studies, sodium thiosulfate was not embryotoxic or teratogenic. Additionally, an intravenous pharmacokinetic study in gravid animals indicated that sodium thiosulfate does not cross the placenta. **Pedmark** is administered following *cisplatin* infusions, which can cause embryo/fetal harm. There are no available data on the presence of sodium thiosulfate in human milk or effects on the breastfed infant. Refer to *cisplatin* mfr pkg insert for additional information. To report suspected adverse reactions, contact Fennec Pharmaceuticals at 1-833-336-6321 or FDA at 1-800-FDA-1088 or www.fda.gov/medwatch.

POLY(ADP-RIBOSE) POLYMERASE (PARP) INHIBITOR

▶ *olaparib* 300 mg bid, with or without food; see the mfr pkg insert for recommended duration of treatment; *CrCl: 31-50 ml/min:* 200 mg bid
Pediatric: not studied
Lynparza *Tab:* 100, 150 mg
Comment: Lynparza is indicated for the maintenance treatment of adult patients with deleterious or suspected deleterious gBRCAm metastatic pancreatic adenocarcinoma whose disease has not progressed on at least 16 weeks of a first-line platinum-based chemotherapy regimen. Select patients

for therapy based on an FDA-approved companion diagnostic for **Lynparza**. The most common adverse reactions (incidence ≥10%) in clinical trials have been nausea, fatigue (including asthenia), vomiting, abdominal pain, anemia, diarrhea, dizziness, neutropenia, leukopenia, nasopharyngitis/ upper respiratory tract infection/influenza, respiratory tract infection, arthralgia/myalgia, dysgeusia, headache, dyspepsia, decreased appetite, constipation, stomatitis, dyspnea, and thrombocytopenia. Avoid concomitant use of strong <u>or</u> moderate CYP3A inhibitors. If the inhibitor cannot be avoided, reduce the **Lynparza** dose. Avoid concomitant use of strong <u>or</u> moderate CYP3A inducers as decreased **Lynparza** efficacy can occur. The most common adverse reactions (incidence ≥20%) in clinical trials have been anemia, nausea, fatigue (including asthenia), vomiting, nasopharyngitis/ upper respiratory tract infection/influenza, diarrhea, arthralgia/myalgia, dysgeusia, headache, dyspepsia, decreased appetite, constipation, and stomatitis. The most common laboratory abnormalities (incidence ≥25%) have been decrease in hemoglobin, increase in MCV, decrease in lymphocytes, decrease in leukocytes, decrease in absolute neutrophil count, increase in serum creatinine, and decrease in platelets. **Lynparza** can cause embryo/fetal harm. Exclude pregnancy prior to initiation and advise females of reproductive potential to use effective contraception during and for 6 months after the last dose. Males with female partners should use effective contraception and <u>not</u> donate sperm during and for 3 months after the last dose. Advise women <u>not</u> to breastfeed during and for 1 month after the last dose.

CANCER: PERITONEAL

POLY(ADP-RIBOSE) POLYMERASE (PARP) INHIBITOR

▷ **niraparib tosylate** 300 mg (3 x 100 mg) once daily, with <u>or</u> without food; continue treatment until disease progression <u>or</u> unacceptable adverse reaction; for adverse reactions, consider interruption of treatment, dose reduction, <u>or</u> dose discontinuation
Pediatric: safety and efficacy <u>not</u> established

    Zejula *Cap:* 100 mg

    Comment: Zejula *(niraparib)* is indicated for the maintenance treatment of adult patients with recurrent epithelial ovarian, fallopian tube, <u>or</u> primary peritoneal cancer who are in complete <u>or</u> partial response to platinum-based chemotherapy, and for late-line treatment of recurrent ovarian cancer. The most common adverse reactions (incidence ≥10%) have been anemia, thrombocytopenia, neutropenia, leukopenia, hypertension, palpitations, nausea, vomiting, abdominal pain/distention, diarrhea, constipation, mucositis/ stomatitis, dry mouth, fatigue/asthenia, dyspepsia, decreased appetite, urinary tract infection, aspartate aminotransferase (AST)/alanine aminotransferase (ALT) elevation, back pain, myalgia, arthralgia, headache, dizziness, dysgeusia, insomnia, anxiety, nasopharyngitis, dyspnea, cough, and rash. Monitor complete blood count (CBC) weekly for the first month, then monthly for the next 11 months, and then periodically thereafter. Monitor blood pressure (BP) and heart rate (HR) monthly for the first year and periodically thereafter. Manage BP and HR with appropriate medication as indicated and adjust the **Zejula** dose if necessary. Because myelodysplastic syndrome/acute myeloid leukemia (MDS/AML) has occurred in patients exposed to **Zejula,** with some cases being fatal, monitor patients for hematologic toxicity and discontinue **Zejula** if MDS/AML is confirmed. **Zejula** can cause embryo/fetal toxicity; therefore, advise females of reproductive potential of the potential risk and to use effective contraception. Advise women <u>not</u> to breastfeed during treatment with **Zejula** and for 1 month after receiving the final dose.

▷ **olaparib** 300 mg bid, with <u>or</u> without food; see the mfr pkg insert for recommended duration of treatment; *CrCl: 31-50 ml/min:* 200 mg bid
Pediatric: <u>not</u> established

    Lynparza *Tab:* 100, 150 mg

    Comment: Lynparza is a first-class poly(ADP-ribose) polymerase (PARP) inhibitor indicated for (1) maintenance treatment of adult patients with deleterious <u>or</u> suspected deleterious germline <u>or</u> somatic BRCA-mutated advanced epithelial ovarian, fallopian tube, <u>or</u> primary peritoneal cancer who are in complete <u>or</u> partial response to first-line platinum-based chemotherapy; select patients for therapy based on an FDA-approved companion diagnostic for **Lynparza**; (2) maintenance treatment of adult patients with recurrent epithelial ovarian, fallopian tube, <u>or</u> primary peritoneal cancer who are in complete <u>or</u> partial response to platinum-based chemotherapy; (3) treatment of adult patients with deleterious <u>or</u> suspected deleterious germline BRCA-mutated (gBRCAm) advanced ovarian cancer who have been treated with three <u>or</u> more prior lines of chemotherapy; select patients for therapy based on an FDA-approved companion diagnostic for **Lynparza**; (4) first-line maintenance treatment with *bevacizumab* for HRD-positive advanced ovarian cancer; and (5) treatment of adult patients with deleterious <u>or</u> suspected deleterious germline <u>or</u> somatic homologous recombination repair (HRR) gene-mutated metastatic castration-resistant prostate cancer (mCRPC) who have progressed following prior treatment with *enzalutamide* <u>or</u> *abiraterone*; select patients for therapy based on an FDA-approved companion diagnostic for **Lynparza**. The most common adverse reactions (incidence ≥10%) in clinical trials have been nausea, fatigue (including asthenia), vomiting, abdominal pain, anemia, diarrhea, dizziness, neutropenia, leukopenia, nasopharyngitis/upper respiratory tract infection/influenza, respiratory tract infection, arthralgia/myalgia, dysgeusia, headache, dyspepsia, decreased appetite, constipation, stomatitis, dyspnea, and thrombocytopenia. Avoid concomitant

(continued)

use of strong or moderate CYP3A inhibitors. If the inhibitor cannot be avoided, reduce the **Lynparza** dose. Avoid concomitant use of strong or moderate CYP3A inducers as decreased **Lynparza** efficacy can occur. The most common adverse reactions (incidence ≥20%) in clinical trials have been anemia, nausea, fatigue (including asthenia), vomiting, nasopharyngitis/upper respiratory tract infection/influenza, diarrhea, arthralgia/myalgia, dysgeusia, headache, dyspepsia, decreased appetite, constipation, and stomatitis. The most common laboratory abnormalities (incidence ≥25%) have been decrease in hemoglobin, increase in MCV, decrease in lymphocytes, decrease in leukocytes, decrease in absolute neutrophil count, increase in serum creatinine, and decrease in platelets. **Lynparza** can cause embryo/fetal harm. Exclude pregnancy prior to initiation and advise females of reproductive potential to use effective contraception during and for 6 months after the last dose. Males with female partners should use effective contraception and not donate sperm during and for 3 months after the last dose. Advise women not to breastfeed during and for 1 month after the last dose.

▷ *rucaparib* 600 mg bid, with or without food
Pediatric: not established
    Rubraca *Tab:* 200, 250, 300 mg
    Comment: Rubraca *(rucaparib)* is indicated for maintenance treatment of adult patients with recurrent epithelial ovarian, fallopian tube, and primary peritoneal cancer who are in complete or partial response to platinum-based chemotherapy and treatment of adult patients with a deleterious BRCA mutation (germline and/or somatic)-associated epithelial ovarian, fallopian tube, or primary peritoneal cancer who have been treated with two or more chemotherapies. Select patients for therapy based on an FDA-approved companion diagnostic for **Rubraca**. Continue treatment until disease progression or unacceptable toxicity. For adverse reactions, consider interruption of treatment or dose reduction. The most common adverse reactions (incidence ≥20%) have been nausea, fatigue (including asthenia), vomiting, anemia, dysgeusia, AST/ALT elevation, constipation, decreased appetite, diarrhea, thrombocytopenia, neutropenia, stomatitis, nasopharyngitis/upper respiratory infection (URI), rash, abdominal pain/distention, and dyspnea. The most common adverse reactions (incidence ≥20%) among patients with BRCA-mutated mCRPC have been fatigue (including asthenia), nausea, anemia, increased ALT/AST, decreased appetite, rash, constipation, thrombocytopenia, vomiting, and diarrhea. MDS and AML have occurred in patients exposed to **Rubraca**, and some cases have been fatal. Monitor patients for hematologic toxicity at baseline and monthly thereafter. Discontinue **Rubraca** if MDS/AML is confirmed. Adjust the dosage of CYP1A2, CYP3A, CYP2C9, and CYP2C19 substrates if clinically indicated. **Rubraca** can cause embryo/fetal harm. Advise females of the potential embryo/fetal risk and to use effective contraception. Advise females not to breastfeed.

FOLATE RECEPTOR ALPHA (FRα)-DIRECTED ANTIBODY AND MICROTUBULE INHIBITOR CONJUGATE

▷ *mirvetuximab soravtansine-gynx* 6 mg/kg adjusted ideal body weight administered via IV infusion every 3 weeks until disease progression or unacceptable toxicity; administer **Elahere** as IV infusion only after dilution in D5W (Alert: **Elahere** is incompatible with normal saline); premedicate with a corticosteroid antihistamine, antipyretic, antiemetic, ophthalmic steroid, and lubricating eye drops; store **Elahere** vials upright in a refrigerator at 2°C-8°C (36°F-46°F) in the original carton to protect from light until the time of preparation; do not freeze or shake; **Elahere** is a hazardous drug; see mfr pkg insert for special handling and disposal procedures
Pediatric: safety and efficacy not established
    Elahere *Vial:* 100 mg/20 ml (5 mg/ml), single-dose, soln for dilution and IV infusion
    Comment: Elahere is a folate receptor alpha (FRα)-directed antibody and microtubule inhibitor conjugate indicated for the treatment of adult patients with FRα-positive, platinum-resistant epithelial ovarian, fallopian tube, or primary peritoneal cancer who have received one to three prior systemic treatment regimens. These indications are approved under accelerated approval based on tumor response rate and durability of response. Continued approval for this indication may be contingent upon verification and description of clinical benefit in a confirmatory trial. *Black Box Warning:* **Elahere** can cause severe ocular toxicities, including visual impairment, keratopathy, dry eye, photophobia, eye pain, and uveitis. Conduct an ophthalmic exam, including visual acuity and slit lamp exam, prior to initiation of **Elahere**, every other cycle for the first eight cycles and as clinically indicated. Administer prophylactic artificial tears and ophthalmic steroid. Withhold **Elahere** for ocular toxicities until improvement and resume at the same or reduced dose. Discontinue **Elahere** for grade 4 ocular toxicities. Withhold **Elahere** for persistent or recurrent grade 2 pneumonitis and consider dose reduction. Permanently discontinue **Elahere** for grade 3 or 4 pneumonitis. Monitor patients for new or worsening peripheral neuropathy. Withhold dose, pause dose, slow the rate of infusion, or permanently discontinue **Elahere** based on the severity of peripheral neuropathy. The most common (≥20%) adverse reactions, including laboratory abnormalities, have been vision impairment, fatigue, increased AST, nausea, increased ALT, keratopathy, abdominal pain, decreased lymphocytes, peripheral neuropathy, diarrhea, decreased albumin, constipation, increased alkaline phosphatase, dry eye, decreased magnesium, decreased leukocytes, decreased neutrophils, and decreased hemoglobin. *Child-Pugh Class B or C:* Avoid use. Closely monitor patients for adverse reactions if taking strong CYP3A4 inhibitors. **Elahere** is embryo/fetal toxic. Human immunoglobulin G (IgG) is known to cross the placental barrier; therefore, **Elahere** has the potential to be transmitted from the mother to the developing fetus. The cytotoxic component, DM4, disrupts

microtubule function, is genotoxic, and can be toxic to actively dividing cells, suggesting it has the potential to cause embryotoxicity and teratogenicity. Advise patients of the potential risk to the fetus and to use effective contraception. There are no data on the presence of *mirvetuximab soravtansine-gynx* in human milk or effects on the breastfed infant. Because of the potential for serious adverse reactions in the breastfed infant, advise mothers not to breastfeed during treatment with **Elahere** and for 1 month after the last dose.

VASCULAR ENDOTHELIAL VASCULAR (VEGF) INHIBITOR

▷ *bevacizumab-adcd*
  Regimens for Epithelial Ovarian, Fallopian Tube and Primary Peritoneal Cancer:
  (1) Stage III or IV epithelial ovarian, fallopian tube, or primary peritoneal cancer following initial surgical resection: 15 mg/kg every 3 weeks with *carboplatin* and *paclitaxel* for up to 6 cycles, followed by 15 mg/kg every 3 weeks as a single agent, for a total of up to 22 cycles
  (2) Platinum-resistant recurrent epithelial ovarian, fallopian tube, or primary peritoneal cancer: 10 mg/kg every 2 weeks with *paclitaxel*, pegylated liposomal *doxorubicin*, or *topotecan* given every week; 15 mg/kg every 3 weeks with *topotecan* given every 3 weeks as a single agent
  (3) Platinum-sensitive recurrent epithelial ovarian, fallopian tube, or primary peritoneal cancer: 15 mg/kg every 3 weeks with *carboplatin* and *gemcitabine* for 6-10 cycles, followed by 15 mg/kg every 3 weeks as a single agent; 15 mg/kg every 3 weeks with *carboplatin* and *paclitaxel* for 6-8 cycles in combination with *carboplatin* and *paclitaxel* or *carboplatin* and *gemcitabine*, followed by 15 mg/kg every 3 weeks with *carboplatin* and *gemcitabine* for 6-10 cycles followed by 15 mg/kg every 3 weeks as a single agent
  Do not administer **Vegzelma** for 28 days following major surgery and until adequate wound healing; store refrigerated at 2°C-8°C (36°F-46°F) in the original carton until time of use to protect from light; do not freeze or shake the vial or carton; see mfr pkg insert for full prescribing information, including proper preparation and administration instructions and dosage modifications for adverse reactions
  Pediatric: <18 years: safety and efficacy not established; ≥18 years: same as adult
    Vegzelma *Vial:* 100 mg/4 ml (25 mg/ml) or 400 mg/16 ml (25 mg/ml), single-dose, soln for dilution and IV infusion
    Comment: Vegzelma is a vascular endothelial growth factor (VEGF) inhibitor biosimilar to **Avastin** indicated for the treatment of multiple types of cancer, including colorectal cancer, non-small cell lung cancer, glioblastoma, renal cell carcinoma, cervical cancer, and epithelial ovarian, fallopian tube, or primary peritoneal cancer. *Bevacizumab* products increase the risk of ovarian failure and may impair fertility. Inform females of reproductive potential of the risk of ovarian failure prior to the first dose of **Vegzelma**. The long-term effects of *bevacizumab* products on fertility are not known. *Bevacizumab* products may cause fetal harm when administered to a pregnant female. Advise females of reproductive potential to use effective contraception during treatment with **Vegzelma** and for 6 months after the last dose. No data are available regarding the presence of *bevacizumab* products in human milk or effects on the breastfed infant. Because of the potential for serious adverse reactions in breastfed infants, advise mothers not to breastfeed during treatment with **Vegzelma** and for 6 months after the last dose. See mfr pkg insert for full prescription information.

CANCER: PROSTATE

GONADOTROPIN-RELEASING HORMONE (GnRH) RECEPTOR ANTAGONIST

▷ *degarelix acetate* (G) *Initial dose:* administer 240 mg (2 x 120 mg) as two single 3 ml SC injections; reconstitute each vial with 3 ml of Sterile Water for Injection; 3 ml is withdrawn to deliver 120 mg *degarelix acetate* at a concentration of 40 mg/ml; *Maintenance dose:* 80 mg (4 ml) SC once every 28 days; reconstitute the vial with 4.2 ml of Sterile Water for Injection; 4 ml is withdrawn to deliver 80 mg *degarelix acetate* at a concentration of 20 mg/ml
    Firmagon *Vial:* 80, 120 mg, single-dose, pwdr for reconstitution and SC injection (mannitol)
    Comment: Firmagon is a gonadotropin-releasing hormone (GnRH) receptor antagonist indicated for treatment of patients with advanced prostate cancer. The most commonly observed adverse reactions (incidence ≥10%) during therapy with *degarelix acetate* have included injection site reactions (e.g., pain, erythema, swelling, or induration), hot flashes, increased weight, and increases in serum levels of transaminases and gamma-glutamyltransferase (GGT). *Degarelix acetate* can cause fetal harm when administered to pregnant females. Long-term androgen deprivation therapy prolongs the QT interval. Physicians should consider whether the benefits of androgen deprivation therapy outweigh the potential risks in patients with congenital long QT syndrome, electrolyte abnormalities, or congestive heart failure and in patients taking class IA (e.g., *quinidine, procainamide*) or class III (e.g., *amiodarone, sotalol*) antiarrhythmic medications. Therapy with **Firmagon** results in suppression of the pituitary gonadal system. Results of diagnostic tests of the pituitary gonadotropic and gonadal functions conducted during and after **Firmagon** may be affected. The therapeutic effect of **Firmagon** should be monitored by measuring serum concentrations of prostate-specific antigen (PSA) periodically. If PSA increases, serum concentrations of testosterone should be measured. Decreased bone density has been reported in the medical literature in men who have had orchiectomy or who have been treated with a GnRH agonist. It can be anticipated that long periods of medical castration in men will result in decreased bone density. *Degarelix* is not a substrate for the

(continued)

human CYP450 system. *Degarelix* is not an inducer or inhibitor of the CYP450 system in vitro. Therefore, clinically significant CYP450 pharmacokinetic drug–drug interactions are unlikely. There is no need to adjust the dose for the elderly or for patients with mild or moderate impaired liver or kidney function. Patients with severe liver or kidney dysfunction have not been studied and caution is therefore warranted. To report suspected adverse reactions, contact Ferring at 1-888-FERRING (1-888-337-7464) or FDA at 1 800-FDA-1088 or www.fda.gov/medwatch.

▷ *leuprolide mesylate* 42 mg SC every 6 months; see mfr pkg insert for instructions on the preparation and administration of the injectable emulsion
Pediatric: safety and efficacy not established

    Camcevi *Prefilled syringe:* 42 mg emul
    Comment: Camcevi is a ready-to-use, 6-month depot formulation of the approved GnRH agonist *leuprolide* indicated for the treatment of adult patients with advanced prostate cancer. Transient worsening of bone pain, ureteral obstruction, spinal cord compression, or the occurrence of additional signs and of prostate cancer may develop during the first few weeks of treatment. Hyperglycemia and an increased risk of developing diabetes have been reported in men receiving GnRH agonists. Increased risk of myocardial infarction, sudden cardiac death, and stroke has been reported in men receiving GnRH agonists. Androgen deprivation therapy may prolong the QT interval. Consider periodic monitoring of ECGs and electrolytes. Patients may be at risk of convulsions. The most common (>10%) adverse reactions have been hot flashes, hypertension, injection site reactions, upper respiratory tract infections, musculoskeletal pain, fatigue, and pain in extremity. Based on findings in animals and mechanism of action, **Camcevi** may impair fertility in males of reproductive potential. To report suspected adverse reactions, contact Foresee Pharmaceuticals at 1-302-366-1785 or FDA at 1-800-FDA-1088 or www.fda.gov/medwatch.

▷ *relugolix Loading dose:* 360 mg on day 1; then 120 mg once daily ongoing; take at approximately the same time each day; if treatment is interrupted for >7 days, resume administration with a 360 mg loading dose on the first day, followed by 120 mg once daily; take with or without food; swallow whole, do not crush or chew

    Orgovyx *Tab:* 120 mg
    Comment: Orgovyx *(relugolix)* is an oral GnRH receptor antagonist indicated for the treatment of adult patients with advanced prostate cancer. The most common adverse reactions (incidence ≥10%) and laboratory abnormalities (incidence ≥15%) have been hot flashes, increased glucose, increased triglycerides, musculoskeletal pain, decreased hemoglobin, increased alanine aminotransferase (ALT), fatigue, increased aspartate aminotransferase (AST), constipation, and diarrhea. Androgen deprivation therapy may prolong the QT interval. Avoid co-administration of **Orgovyx** with P-gp inhibitors. If unavoidable, take **Orgovyx** first, separate dosing by at least 6 hours, and monitor patients more frequently for adverse reactions. Avoid co-administration of P-gp and strong CYP3A inducers. If unavoidable, increase the **Orgovyx** dose to 240 mg once daily. **Orgovyx** can cause fetal harm. Based on findings in animals and mechanism of action, **Orgovyx** can cause embryo/fetal harm and loss of pregnancy when administered to a pregnant female. There are no human data on the use of **Orgovyx** in pregnant females to inform the drug-associated risk. Advise males with female partners of reproductive potential to use effective contraception.

CYP17 INHIBITOR (G)

▷ *abiraterone acetate*
    Comment: Patients receiving treatment with *abiraterone acetate* should also receive a GnRH analog concurrently or should have had a bilateral orchiectomy. Avoid concomitant strong CYP3A4 inducers; if a strong CYP3A4 must be co-administered, increase the *abiraterone acetate* dosing frequency. Avoid co-administration of *abiraterone acetate* with CYP2D6 substrates that have a narrow therapeutic index; if an alternative treatment cannot be used, exercise caution and consider a dose reduction of the CYP2D6 substrate. Hepatotoxicity can be severe and fatal. Do not initiate *abiraterone acetate* in patients with baseline severe hepatic impairment (Child-Pugh Class C). *Abiraterone acetate* should be discontinued if patients develop severe hepatotoxicity. Monitor liver function and modify, interrupt, or discontinue *abiraterone acetate* dosing as recommended. Advise males with female partners of reproductive potential to use effective contraception during treatment and for 3 weeks after the last dose. Based on animal studies, *abiraterone acetate* may impair reproductive function and fertility in males of reproductive potential.

    Yonsa 500 mg (4 x 125 mg tabs) administered once daily (in combination with *methylprednisolone* 4 mg administered orally bid); take with or without food; swallow whole with water, do not crush or chew
      Tab: 125 mg
    Comment: Yonsa is an ultramicrosize formulation of the oral CYP17 inhibitor *abiraterone acetate* (FDA-approved as Zytiga) used in combination with *methylprednisolone* for the treatment of metastatic castration-resistant prostate cancer (CRPC). The most common adverse side effects (incidence ≥10%) are fatigue, joint swelling or discomfort, edema, hot flashes, diarrhea, vomiting, cough, hypertension, dyspnea, urinary tract infection (UTI), and confusion. The most common laboratory abnormalities (incidence >20%) are anemia, elevated alkaline phosphatase, hypertriglyceridemia, lymphopenia, hypercholesterolemia, hyperglycemia, elevated AST and ALT, hyperkalemia, and hypophosphatemia. Monitor for signs and symptoms of mineralocorticoid excess and adrenocortical insufficiency and treat as appropriate.

Zytiga *CRPC:* 1,000 mg (4 x 250 mg or 2 x 500 mg tabs) administered once daily (in combination with **prednisone** 5 mg administered orally bid); *Castration-sensitive prostate cancer (CSPC):* 1,000 mg (4 x 250 mg or 2 x 500 mg tabs) administered once daily (in combination with **prednisone** 5 mg administered orally once daily); take on an empty stomach, at least 1 hour before or 2 hours after a meal; swallow whole with water; do not crush or chew

    Tab: 250, 500 mg

Comment: Zytiga (*abiraterone acetate*) is an oral CYP17 inhibitor used in combination with **prednisone** for the treatment of metastatic CRPC and metastatic high-risk CSPC. The most common adverse reactions (incidence ≥10%) are fatigue, arthralgia, hypertension, nausea, edema, hypokalemia, hot flashes, diarrhea, vomiting, upper respiratory infection, cough, and headache. The most common laboratory abnormalities (incidence ≥20%) are anemia, elevated alkaline phosphatase, hypertriglyceridemia, lymphopenia, hypercholesterolemia, hyperglycemia, and hypokalemia. Monitor for signs and symptoms of mineralocorticoid excess and adrenocortical insufficiency and treat as appropriate.

ANDROGEN RECEPTOR INHIBITOR (ARI)

▷ *apalutamide* administer 240 mg (4 x 60 mg tablets) once daily; swallow tablets whole, do not crush or chew; take with or without food.

    Erleada *Tab:* 60 mg

    Comment: Erleada (*apalutamide*) is the first FDA-approved treatment for non-metastatic, castration-resistant prostate cancer (nmCRPC). Patients should also receive a GnRH analog concurrently or should have had bilateral orchiectomy. Concomitant use of **Erleada** with medications that are sensitive substrates of CYP3A4, CYP2C19, CYP2C9, UGT, P-gp, BCRP, or OATP1B1 may result in loss of activity of these medications. The most common adverse reactions (incidence ≥10%) have been fatigue, hypertension, rash, diarrhea, nausea, decreased weight, arthralgia, fall, hot flashes, decreased appetite, fracture, and peripheral edema. Falls (16%) and fractures (12%) have occurred in patients receiving **Erleada**. Evaluate patients for fall and fracture risk, and treat patients with bone-targeted agents according to established guidelines. Seizure has occurred in 0.2% of patients receiving **Erleada**. Permanently discontinue **Erleada** in patients who develop a seizure during treatment. Advise males with female partners of reproductive potential to use effective contraception.

▷ *darolutamide* 600 mg (2 x 300 mg tablets) bid; *Moderate hepatic impairment:* 300 mg bid; *Severe renal impairment (not on hemodialysis):* 300 mg bid; swallow whole, do not crush or chew; take with food

    Nubeqa *Tab:* 300 mg

    Comment: Nubeqa (*darolutamide*) is an androgen receptor inhibitor (ARi) indicated for the treatment of nmCRPC. Patients taking **Nubeqa** should also receive a GnRH analog concurrently or should have had bilateral orchiectomy. When **Nubeqa** is taken in combination with P-gp and strong CYP3A inhibitors, monitor patients more frequently for **Nubeqa** adverse reactions. Avoid concomitant use of P-gp and strong or moderate CYP3A inducers. Avoid concomitant use with drugs that are BCRP substrates where possible; if used together, monitor patients more frequently for adverse reactions and consider dose reduction of the BCRP substrate drug. The most common adverse reactions (incidence ≥2%) have been fatigue, pain in extremity, and rash. **Nubeqa** can cause embryo/fetal harm and loss of pregnancy. Advise males with female partners of reproductive potential to use effective contraception.

POLY(ADP-RIBOSE) POLYMERASE (PARP) INHIBITORS

▷ *niraparib tosylate* 300 mg (3 x 100 mg) once daily, with or without food

    Pediatric: safety and efficacy not established

    Zejula *Cap:* 100 mg

    Comment: Zejula (*niraparib*) is indicated for the maintenance treatment of adult patients with recurrent epithelial ovarian, fallopian tube, or primary peritoneal cancer who are in complete or partial response to platinum-based chemotherapy, and for late-line treatment of recurrent ovarian cancer. Continue treatment until disease progression or unacceptable adverse reaction; for adverse reactions, consider interruption of treatment, dose reduction, or dose discontinuation. The most common adverse reactions (incidence ≥10%) have been anemia, thrombocytopenia, neutropenia, leukopenia, hypertension, palpitations, nausea, vomiting, abdominal pain/distention, diarrhea, constipation, mucositis/stomatitis, dry mouth, fatigue/asthenia, dyspepsia, decreased appetite, UTI, AST/ALT elevation, back pain, myalgia, arthralgia, headache, dizziness, dysgeusia, insomnia, anxiety, nasopharyngitis, dyspnea, cough, and rash. Monitor complete blood count (CBC) weekly for the first month, then monthly for the next 11 months, and then periodically thereafter. Monitor blood pressure (BP) and heart rate (HR) monthly for the first year and periodically thereafter. Manage BP and HR with appropriate medication as indicated and adjust the **Zejula** dose if necessary. Because myelodysplastic syndrome (MDS) and acute myeloid leukemia (AML) have occurred in patients exposed to **Zejula**, with some cases being fatal, monitor patients for hematologic toxicity and discontinue **Zejula** if MDS/AML is confirmed. **Zejula** can cause embryo/fetal toxicity; therefore, advise females of reproductive potential of the potential risk and to use effective contraception. Advise women not to breastfeed during treatment with **Zejula** and for 1 month after receiving the final dose.

(continued)

▷ *rucaparib* 600 mg bid, with or without food
   Pediatric: safety and efficacy not established
   Rubraca *Tab:* 200, 250, 300 mg
   Comment: Rubraca *(rucaparib)* is indicated for the treatment of adult patients with a deleterious BRCA mutation (germline and/or somatic)-associated metastatic CRPC who have been treated with androgen receptor-directed therapy and a taxane-based chemotherapy. This indication is approved under accelerated approval based on objective response rate and duration of response. Continued approval for this indication may be contingent upon verification and description of clinical benefit in confirmatory trials. Patients receiving **Rubraca** for metastatic CRPC should also receive a GnRH analog concurrently or should have had bilateral orchiectomy. Continue treatment until disease progression or unacceptable toxicity. For adverse reactions, consider interruption of treatment or dose reduction. The most common adverse reactions (incidence ≥20%) among patients with BRCA-mutated metastatic CRPC have been fatigue (including asthenia), nausea, anemia, increased ALT/AST, decreased appetite, rash, constipation, thrombocytopenia, vomiting, and diarrhea. MDS and AML have occurred in patients exposed to **Rubraca**, and some cases have been fatal. Monitor patients for hematologic toxicity at baseline and monthly thereafter. Discontinue **Rubraca** if MDS/AML is confirmed. Adjust the dosage of CYP1A2, CYP3A, CYP2C9, and CYP2C19 substrates if clinically indicated.

MICROTUBULE INHIBITOR

▷ *cabazitaxel* (G) *Recommended dose:* 25 mg/m² administered once every 3 weeks as a 60-minute IV infusion in combination with oral *prednisone* 10 mg administered once daily throughout **Jevtana** treatment; **Jevtana** requires two dilutions prior to administration; use the entire contents of the accompanying diluent to achieve a concentration of 10 mg/ml; PVC equipment should not be used; *Premedication regimen:* administer 30 minutes before each dose of **Jevtana**: (1) antihistamine (*dexchlorpheniramine* 5 mg or *diphenhydramine* 25 mg or equivalent antihistamine); (2) corticosteroid (*dexamethasone* 8 mg or equivalent steroid); and (3) H2 antagonist (*ranitidine* 50 mg or equivalent H2 antagonist); antiemetic prophylaxis (oral or IV) is recommended as needed; see mfr pkg insert for full prescribing information, including dosing modifications
   Pediatric: safety and efficacy not established
   Jevtana *Vial:* 60 mg/1.5 ml, single-dose w. diluent (5.7 ml), for further dilution and IV infusion (polysorbate 80)
   Comment: Jevtana is a microtubule inhibitor indicated in combination with prednisone for treatment of patients with hormone-refractory metastatic prostate cancer previously treated with a *docetaxel*-containing treatment regimen. The most common all-grades adverse reactions (incidence ≥10%) have been neutropenia, anemia, leukopenia, thrombocytopenia, diarrhea, fatigue, nausea, vomiting, constipation, asthenia, abdominal pain, hematuria, back pain, anorexia, peripheral neuropathy, pyrexia, dyspnea, dysgeusia, cough, arthralgia, and alopecia. Contraindications to Jevtana include (1) neutrophil count ≤1,500/mm³ or (2) history of severe hypersensitivity to Jevtana or polysorbate 80. Neutropenic deaths have been reported. Monitor blood counts frequently to determine if initiation of granulocyte colonystimulating factor (G-CSF) and/or dosage modification is needed. Primary prophylaxis with G-CSF should be considered in patients with high-risk clinical features. Severe hypersensitivity reactions can occur. Premedicate with corticosteroids and H2 antagonists. Discontinue infusion immediately if hypersensitivity is observed and treat as indicated. Gastrointestinal symptoms (nausea, vomiting, and diarrhea may occur): Mortality related to diarrhea has been reported. Rehydrate and treat with antiemetics and antidiarrheals as needed. If the patient is experiencing grade ≥3 diarrhea, the Jevtana dosage should be modified. Renal failure, including cases with fatal outcomes, has been reported; identify the cause and manage aggressively. Patients ≥65 years of age were more likely to experience fatal outcomes not related to disease progression and certain adverse reactions, including neutropenia and febrile neutropenia; monitor closely. Patients with impaired hepatic function were excluded from the randomized clinical trial. Hepatic impairment is likely to increase the *cabazitaxel* concentrations. Jevtana should not be given to patients with hepatic impairment. Jevtana crosses the placenta and can cause fetal harm when administered to a pregnant woman. (5.7) (8.1) Jevtana can cause fetal harm when administered to a pregnant female. *Cabazitaxel* is embryotoxic, fetotoxic, and abortifacient. Because of the potential for serious adverse reactions in nursing infants from Jevtana, a decision should be made whether to discontinue breastfeeding or to discontinue the drug, taking into account the importance of the drug to the mother.
   To report suspected adverse reactions, contact sanofi-aventis U.S. LLC at 1-800-633-1610 or FDA at 1-800-FDA-1088 or www.fda.gov/medwatch.

CANCER: SQUAMOUS CELL CARCINOMA (SCC)

PROGRAMMED DEATH RECEPTOR-1 (PD-1)-BLOCKING ANTIBODY

▷ *cemiplimab-rwlc* 350 mg as IV infusion over 30 minutes q 3 weeks
   Pediatric: safety and efficacy not established
   Libtayo *Vial:* 350 mg/7 ml (50 mg/ml), single-dose, soln for dilution and IV infusion
   Comment: Libtayo is indicated for the treatment of patients with metastatic cutaneous squamous cell carcinoma (mCSCC) or locally advanced CSCC (laCSCC) who are not candidates for curative

surgery or curative radiation. The most common adverse reactions (incidence ≥15%) have been musculoskeletal pain, fatigue, rash, and diarrhea. The most common grade 3-4 laboratory abnormalities (incidence ≥2%) have been lymphopenia, hyponatremia, hypophosphatemia, increased aspartate aminotransferase, anemia, and hyperkalemia. For infusion-related reactions, interrupt, slow the rate of infusion, or permanently discontinue based on severity of the reaction. Immune-mediated adverse reactions, which may be severe or fatal, can occur in any organ system or tissue, including the following: immune-mediated pneumonitis, immune-mediated colitis, immune-mediated hepatitis, immune-mediated endocrinopathies, immune-mediated dermatologic adverse reactions, immune-mediated nephritis and renal dysfunction, and solid organ transplant rejection. Monitor for early identification and management. Evaluate liver enzymes, creatinine, and thyroid function at baseline and periodically during treatment. Withhold or permanently discontinue **Libtayo** based on the severity of reaction. Fatal and other serious complications can occur in patients who receive allogeneic hematopoietic stem cell transplantation (HSCT) before or after being treated with a programmed death receptor-1 (PD-1)/ programmed death-ligand 1 (PD-L1)-blocking antibody. Based on its mechanism of action, **Libtayo** can cause embryo/fetal harm when administered to a pregnant female. Animal studies have demonstrated that inhibition of the PD-1/PD-L1 pathway can lead to increased risk of immune-mediated rejection of the developing fetus, resulting in fetal death. Advise women of the potential risk and advise males and females of reproductive potential to use effective contraception during treatment with **Libtayo** and for at least 4 months after the last dose. There is no information regarding the presence of *cemiplimab-rwlc* in human milk or its effects on the breastfed infant. Because of the potential for serious adverse reactions in breastfed infants, advise mothers not to breastfeed during treatment and for at least 4 months after the last dose.

▷ *pembrolizumab* administer 200 mg via IV infusion over 30 minutes once every 3 weeks or 400 mg via IV infusion over 30 minutes once every 6 weeks until disease progression, unacceptable toxicity, or for **Keytruda** up to 24 months; administer **Keytruda** prior to chemotherapy when given on the same day
Pediatric: safety and efficacy not established
    Keytruda *Vial:* 100 mg/4 ml (25 mg/ml), single-dose, soln for dilution and IV infusion
    Comment: Keytruda is a PD-1-blocking antibody indicated for the treatment of multiple cancers, including cutaneous squamous cell carcinoma (cSCC) and head and neck squamous cell carcinoma (HNSCC). **Keytruda**, in combination with platinum and fluorouracil (FU), is indicated for the first-line treatment of patients with metastatic or with unresectable, recurrent HNSCC. **Keytruda**, as a single agent, is indicated for the first-line treatment of patients with metastatic or with unresectable, recurrent HNSCC whose tumors express PD-L1 (Combined Positive Score [CPS] ≥1) as determined by an FDA-approved test. **Keytruda**, as a single agent, is also indicated for treatment of patients with recurrent or metastatic cSCC or HNSCC with disease progression on or after platinum-containing chemotherapy. **Keytruda** can cause fetal harm. Exclude pregnancy prior to initiating treatment with Keytruda. Advise females of reproductive potential of the embryo/fetal risk and to use effective contraception. Advise mothers not to breastfeed during treatment and for 4 months after the last **Keytruda** dose. See mfr pkg insert for full prescribing information, including storage, preparation, warnings, precautions, drug-drug interactions, and adverse reactions.

CANCER: THYROID CARCINOMA

KINASE INHIBITOR

▷ *selpercatinib* <*50 kg:* 120 mg bid; >*50 kg:* 160 mg bid; reduce dose in patients with severe hepatic impairment
Pediatric: <12 years: not established; ≥12 years: same as adult
    Retevmo *hgc:* 40, 80 mg
    Comment: Retevmo *(selpercatinib)* is a kinase inhibitor indicated for adult patients with metastatic RET (rearranged during transfection) fusion-positive non-small cell lung cancer; adult and pediatric patients ≥12 years of age with advanced or metastatic RET-mutant medullary thyroid cancer (MTC) who require systemic therapy; and adult and pediatric patients ≥12 years of age with advanced or metastatic RET fusion-positive thyroid cancer who require systemic therapy and who are radioactive iodine-refractory (if radioactive iodine is appropriate). The most common adverse reactions, including laboratory abnormalities (incidence ≥25%), have been increased aspartate aminotransferase (AST), increased alanine aminotransferase (ALT), increased glucose, decreased leukocytes, decreased albumin, decreased calcium, dry mouth, diarrhea, increased creatinine, increased alkaline phosphatase, hypertension, fatigue, edema, decreased platelets, increased total cholesterol, rash, decreased sodium, and constipation. Monitor ALT and AST prior to initiating **Retevmo**, every 2 weeks during the first 3 months, then monthly thereafter, and as clinically indicated. Do not initiate **Retevmo** in patients with uncontrolled hypertension; optimize blood pressure (BP) prior to initiating **Retevmo** and monitor BP after 1 week, at least monthly thereafter, and as clinically indicated. Monitor patients who are at significant risk of developing QTc prolongation. Assess QT interval, electrolytes, and thyroid stimulating hormone (TSH) at baseline and periodically during treatment. Monitor QT interval more

(continued)

frequently when **Retevmo** is concomitantly administered with strong and moderate CYP3A inhibitors or drugs known to prolong QTc interval. Permanently discontinue **Retevmo** in patients with severe or life-threatening hemorrhage. Withhold **Retevmo** and initiate corticosteroids in the occurrence of any hypersensitivity reaction and, upon resolution, resume at a reduced dose and increase dose by one dose level each week until reaching the dose taken prior to onset of hypersensitivity. Continue steroids until the patient reaches target dose of **Retevmo** and then taper. Withhold **Retevmo** for at least 7 days prior to elective surgery. Do not administer for at least 2 weeks following major surgery and until adequate wound healing. The safety of resumption of **Retevmo** after resolution of wound healing complications has not been established. Avoid co-administration with proton pump inhibitors (PPIs); if co-administration cannot be avoided, take **Retevmo** with food (with PPI) or modify its administration time (with H2 receptor antagonist or locally acting antacid). Avoid co-administration with strong and moderate CYP3A inhibitors; if co-administration cannot be avoided, reduce the **Retevmo** dose. Avoid co-administration with strong and moderate CYP3A inducers. Avoid co-administration with CYP2C8 and CYP3A substrates; if co-administration cannot be avoided, modify the substrate dosage as recommended in its product labeling. Based on findings from animal studies and its mechanism of action, **Retevmo** can cause fetal harm. There are no available data on **Retevmo** use in pregnant women to inform drug-associated risk. Therefore, exclude pregnancy in females of reproductive potential prior to initiating **Retevmo** and advise females of reproductive potential of the possible risk to the fetus and to use effective contraception. There are no data on the presence of *selpercatinib* or its metabolites in human milk or effects on the breastfed infant. Because of the potential for serious adverse embryo/fetal effects, advise women not to breastfeed during treatment with **Retevmo** and for 1 week after the final dose.

▷ *sorafenib* (G) 400 mg (2 x 200 mg) bid, without food
   Nexavar *Tab:* 200 mg
   Comment: Nexavar is indicated for the treatment of locally recurrent or metastatic, progressive, differentiated thyroid carcinoma refractory to radioactive iodine treatment. The most common adverse reactions (incidence ≥20%) have been diarrhea, fatigue, infection, alopecia, hand-foot skin reaction, rash, weight loss, decreased appetite, nausea, gastrointestinal and abdominal pain, hypertension, and hemorrhage. **Nexavar** in combination with *carboplatin* and *paclitaxel* is contraindicated in patients with squamous cell lung cancer. Avoid strong CYP3A4 inducers. Monitor ECG (for QT prolongation) and electrolytes in patients at increased risk for ventricular arrhythmias. Consider temporary or permanent discontinuation of **Nexavar** in the event of a cardiovascular event. Discontinue **Nexavar** if needed in the event of bleeding. Monitor the patient for hypertension, weekly during the first 6 weeks, and periodically thereafter. Interrupt and/or decrease **Nexavar** for severe or persistent dermal reaction, and immediately discontinue **Nexavar** if Stevens-Johnson syndrome or toxic epidermal necrolysis is suspected. Discontinue **Nexavar** in the event of gastrointestinal perforation. **Nexavar** may cause hepatotoxicity; monitor liver function tests regularly and discontinue for unexplained transaminase elevation. Monitor TSH monthly and adjust thyroid replacement therapy in patients with thyroid cancer. **Nexavar** may cause embryo/fetal harm; exclude pregnancy prior to initiating **Nexavar** and advise females and males of reproductive potential to use effective contraception. Advise women not to breastfeed.

CANCER: TUMOR, SOLID

CISPLATIN NEUTRALIZING AGENT
▷ *sodium thiosulfate*
   Pediatric: <1 month: safety and efficacy not established; ≥1 month: *Recommended dose:* based on body surface area (BSA) according to actual body weight (see dosing table); administer via IV infusion over 15 minutes starting 6 hours after completion of *cisplatin* infusion; *Multi-day cisplatin regimens:* administer 6 hours after each *cisplatin* infusion, but at least 10 hours before the next *cisplatin* infusion; do not start if less than 10 hours before starting the next *cisplatin* infusion; store at 20°C-25°C (68°F-77°F); excursions are permitted between 15°C and 30°C (59°F-86°F).

Pedmark Dose by Weight	
Weight	Dose
<5 kg	10 g/m²
<5 kg-10 kg	15 g/m²
>10 kg	20 g/m²

Pedmark *Vial:* 12.5 gm/100 ml (125 mg/ml), single-use, for IV infusion
Comment: Pedmark is indicated to reduce the risk of ototoxicity associated with *cisplatin* in pediatric patients ≥1 month of age with localized, non-metastatic solid tumors. **Pedmark** is not recommended for treatment of patients <1 year of age due to increased risk of hypernatremia. **Pedmark** is not indicated for treatment of pediatric patients <1 month of age (due to increased risk of hypernatremia)

or pediatric patients with metastatic cancer. **Pedmark** may not reduce the risk of ototoxicity when administered following longer *cisplatin* infusions because irreversible ototoxicity may have already occurred. The most common adverse reactions (≥25% with difference between arms of >5% compared to *cisplatin* alone) in SIOPEL 6 are vomiting, nausea, decreased hemoglobin, and hypernatremia. The most common adverse reaction (≥25% with difference between arms of >5% compared to *cisplatin* alone) in COG ACCL0431 is hypokalemia. History of severe hypersensitivity to *sodium thiosulfate* or any components is the only contraindication. For signs and symptoms of hypersensitivity reaction, immediately discontinue **Pedmark** and institute appropriate care. Administer premedications before each subsequent dose. **Pedmark** may contain sodium sulfite; patients with sulfite sensitivity may have hypersensitivity reactions. Monitor serum sodium and potassium at baseline and as clinically indicated; Monitor more closely if glomerular filtration rate (GFR) falls below 60 ml/min/1.73 m². Withhold **Pedmark** with serum sodium >145 mmol/L. For nausea and vomiting, administer antiemetics prior to each dose administration. There are no available data on **Pedmark** to evaluate for drug-associated risk in human pregnancy or lactation. In animal studies, sodium thiosulfate was not embryotoxic or teratogenic. Additionally, an intravenous pharmacokinetic study in gravid animals indicated that sodium thiosulfate does not cross the placenta. **Pedmark** is administered following *cisplatin* infusions, which can cause embryo/fetal harm. There are no available data on the presence of sodium thiosulfate in human milk or effects on the breastfed infant. Refer to *cisplatin* mfr pkg insert for additional information. To report suspected adverse reactions, contact Fennec Pharmaceuticals at 1-833-336-6321 or FDA at 1-800-FDA-1088 or www.fda.gov/medwatch.

PROGRAMMED DEATH RECEPTOR-1 (PD-1)-BLOCKING ANTIBODY

▶ *pembrolizumab* administer 200 mg via IV infusion over 30 minutes once every 3 weeks or 400 mg via IV infusion over 30 minutes once every 6 weeks until disease progression, unacceptable toxicity, or for **Keytruda** up to 24 months; administer **Keytruda** prior to chemotherapy when given on the same day *Pediatric:* 2 mg/kg every 3 weeks (up to a max of 200 mg) until disease progression, unacceptable toxicity, or up to 24 months; *Limitations of use:* the safety and effectiveness of **Keytruda** in pediatric patients with tumor mutational burden-high (TMB-H) central nervous system cancers have not been established

Keytruda *Vial:* 100 mg/4 ml (25 mg/ml), single-dose, soln for dilution and IV infusion
Comment: Keytruda is a programmed death receptor-1 (PD-1)-blocking antibody indicated for treatment of multiple cancers, including adult and pediatric patients with (1) unresectable or metastatic TMB-H (≥10 mutations/megabase [mut/Mb]) solid tumors, (2) unresectable or metastatic microsatellite instability-high (MSI-H), or (3) mismatch repair deficient (dMMR) solid tumor. There are three requirements: an FDA-approved diagnostic test, disease progressed following prior treatment, and no satisfactory alternative treatment options. These indications are approved under accelerated approval based on tumor response rate and durability of response. Continued approval for these indications may be contingent upon verification and description of clinical benefit in confirmatory trials. **Keytruda** can cause fetal harm. Exclude pregnancy prior to initiating treatment with **Keytruda**. Advise females of reproductive potential of the embryo/fetal risk and to use effective contraception during treatment and for 4 months after the last **Keytruda** dose. Advise mothers not to breastfeed during treatment and for 4 months after the last **Keytruda** dose. See mfr pkg insert for full prescribing information, including storage, preparation, warnings, precautions, drug-drug interactions, and adverse reactions.

CANCER: UROTHELIAL CARCINOMA

KINASE INHIBITOR

▶ *erdafitinib* recommended initial dosage is 8 mg orally once daily with a dose increase to 9 mg daily if criteria are met; swallow whole with or without food; prior to initiation of treatment, confirm the presence of FGFR genetic alterations in tumor specimens and confirm negative pregnancy
Pediatric: safety and efficacy not established

Balversa *Tab:* 3, 4, 5 mg
Comment: Balversa (*erdafitinib*) is a kinase inhibitor indicated for the treatment of adult patients with locally advanced or metastatic urothelial carcinoma that has susceptible FGFR3 or FGFR2 genetic alterations and progressed during or following at least one line of prior platinum-containing chemotherapy, including within 12 months of neoadjuvant or adjuvant platinum-containing chemotherapy. **Balversa** can cause central serous retinopathy/retinal pigment epithelial detachment (CSR/RPED). Perform monthly ophthalmologic examinations during the first 4 months of treatment, every 3 months afterwards, and at any time for visual symptoms. Withhold **Balversa** when CSR/RPED occurs and permanently discontinue if it does not resolve within 4 weeks or if grade 4 in severity. Increases in phosphate levels are a pharmacodynamic effect of **Balversa**. Monitor for hyperphosphatemia and manage with dose modifications when required. *Drug Interaction Precautions:* Avoid concomitant use of agents that can alter serum phosphate levels before the initial dose modification period. Avoid concomitant use of strong CYP2C9 or CYP3A4 inducers and consider alternative agents or monitor closely for adverse reactions. Increase **Balversa** dose up to 9 mg with concomitant use of moderate CYP2C9 or CYP3A4 inducers. Avoid concomitant use of

(continued)

CYP3A4 substrates with narrow therapeutic indices. Consider alternative agents or consider reducing the dose of OCT2 substrates based on tolerability; separate **Balversa** administration by at least 6 hours before or after administration of P-gp substrates with narrow therapeutic indices. **Balversa** can cause fetal harm; advise females of reproductive potential, and their male partners, to use effective contraception during treatment with **Balversa** and for 1 month after the last dose. There are no data on the presence of *erdafitinib* in human milk or effects on the breastfed infant; advise mothers not to breastfeed.

PROGRAMMED DEATH RECEPTOR-1 (PD-1)-BLOCKING ANTIBODY

▷ *pembrolizumab* administer 200 mg via IV infusion over 30 minutes once every 3 weeks or 400 mg via IV infusion over 30 minutes once every 6 weeks

Keytruda Vial: 100 mg/4 ml (25 mg/ml), single-dose, soln for dilution and IV infusion
Comment: Keytruda is indicated for treatment of multiple cancers, including urothelial carcinoma. Keytruda can cause fetal harm. Advise females of the potential embryo/fetal risk and to use effective contraception. Advise mothers not to breastfeed. See mfr pkg insert for full prescribing information.

NECTIN-4 DIRECTED ANTIBODY-DRUG CONJUGATE (ADC)

▷ *enfortumab vedotin-ejfv* 1.25 mg/kg (up to a max of 125 mg) administered as IV infusion over 30 minutes on days 1, 8, and 15 of a 28-day cycle until disease progression or unacceptable toxicity; for IV infusion only; do not administer as an IV push or bolus; do not mix with or administer as an infusion with other medicinal products
Pediatric: safety and efficacy not established

Padcev *Vial:* 20, 30 mg pwdr for reconstitution, dilution, and IV infusion, single-dose
Comment: Padcev is indicated for the treatment of patients with locally advanced or metastatic urothelial cancer. The most common adverse reactions, including laboratory abnormalities (≥20%), have included rash, increased aspartate aminotransferase (AST), increased glucose, increased creatinine, fatigue, peripheral neuropathy, decreased lymphocytes, alopecia, decreased appetite, decreased hemoglobin, diarrhea, decreased sodium, nausea, pruritus, decreased phosphate dysgeusia, increased alanine aminotransferase (ALT), anemia, decreased albumin, decreased neutrophils, increased urate, increased lipase, decreased platelets, decreased weight, and dry skin. *Child-Pugh Class B or C:* Avoid use of Padcev. Use of dual P-gp and strong CYP3A4 inhibitors with Padcev may increase exposure to monomethyl auristatin E (MMAE). Diabetic ketoacidosis (DKA) may occur in patients with and without preexisting diabetes mellitus, which may be fatal. Closely monitor blood glucose levels in patients with, or at risk for, diabetes mellitus or hyperglycemia. Withhold Padcev if blood glucose is >250 mg/dL. Severe, life-threatening, or fatal pneumonitis may occur; withhold Padcev for persistent or recurrent grade 2 pneumonitis and consider dose reduction. Permanently discontinue Padcev for grade 3 or 4 pneumonitis. Monitor patients for new or worsening peripheral neuropathy and consider dose interruption, dose reduction, or discontinuation of Padcev. Ocular disorders, including vision changes, may occur; monitor patients for signs or symptoms of ocular disorders. Consider prophylactic artificial tears for dry eyes and treatment with ophthalmic topical steroids after an ophthalmic exam. Consider dose interruption or dose reduction of Padcev when symptomatic ocular disorders occur. Ensure adequate venous access prior to administration. Monitor the infusion site during Padcev administration and stop the infusion immediately for suspected infusion site extravasation. Padcev is embryo/fetal toxic. Advise females of reproductive potential of the potential fetal risk and to use effective contraception. Advise not to breastfeed.

CANDIDIASIS: ABDOMEN, BLADDER, ESOPHAGUS, KIDNEY

▷ *voriconazole* (G) *PO:* <40 kg: 100 mg q 12 hours; may increase to 150 mg q 12 hours if inadequate response; ≥40 kg: 200 mg q 12 hours; may increase to 300 mg q 12 hours if inadequate; *IV:* 6 mg/kg q 12 hours x 2 doses; then 4 mg/kg q 12 hour; max rate 3 mg/kg/hour over 1-2 hours
Pediatric: <12 years: not recommended; ≥12 years: same as adult
Vfend *Tab:* 50, 200 mg
Vfend I.V. for Injection *Vial:* 200 mg pwdr for reconstitution (preservative-free)
Vfend *Oral susp:* 40 mg/ml pwdr for reconstitution (75 ml) (orange)

CANDIDIASIS: ORAL (THRUSH)

ORAL ANTIFUNGALS

▷ *clotrimazole* Prophylaxis: 1 troche dissolved in mouth tid; *Treatment:* 1 troche dissolved in mouth 5 x/day x 10-14 days
Pediatric: <3 years: not recommended; ≥3 years: same as adult
Mycelex Troches *Troche:* 10 mg

▷ *fluconazole* 200 mg x 1 dose first day; then 100 mg once daily x 13 days
    Pediatric: >2 weeks: 6 mg/kg x 1 day; Then 3 mg/kg/day for at least 3 weeks; *see* Appendix BB.23. *fluconazole*
    (Diflucan Suspension) *for dose by weight*
      Diflucan *Tab:* 50, 100, 150, 200 mg; *Oral susp:* 10, 40 mg/ml (35 ml) (orange) (sucrose)
▷ *gentian violet* (G) apply to oral mucosa with a cotton swab tid x 3 days
▷ *itraconazole* (G) 200 mg daily x 7-14 days
    Pediatric: 5 mg/kg daily x 7-14 days; max 200 mg/day; *see* Appendix BB.26. *itraconazole* (Sporanox
    Solution) *for dose by weight*
      Sporanox *Oral soln:* 10 mg/ml (150 ml) (cherry-caramel)
▷ *miconazole* 1 buccal tab once daily x 14 days; apply to upper gum region; hold in place 30 seconds; do not
    crush, chew, or swallow
    Pediatric: <16 years: not recommended; ≥16 years: same as adult
      Oravig *Buccal tab:* 50 mg (14/pck)
▷ *nystatin* (G)
      Mycostatin 1-2 pastilles dissolved slowly in mouth 4-5 x/day x 10-14 days; max 14 days
      Pediatric: same as adult
        Pastille: 200,000 units (30 pastilles/pck)
      Mycostatin Suspension 4-6 ml qid, swish and swallow
      Pediatric: infants: 1 ml in each cheek qid after feedings; older children: same as adult
        Oral susp: 100,000 units/ml (60 ml w. dropper)

INVASIVE INFECTION

▷ *posaconazole* (G) *Oral Therapy:* take with food; 100 mg bid on day 1; then 100 mg once daily x 13 days;
    refractory, 400 mg bid x 13 days; *IV Infusion Therapy:* must be administered through an in-line filter over
    approximately 90 minutes via a central venous line. Never administer **Noxafil** as an IV bolus injection;
    Loading Dose: a single 300 mg IV infusion; *Maintenance Dose:* a single 300 mg IV infusion once daily;
    duration of therapy is based on recovery from neutropenia or immunosuppression
    Pediatric: <13 years: not recommended; ≥13 years: same as adult
      Noxafil *Tab:* 100 mg ext-rel; *Oral susp:* 40 mg/ml (105 ml) (cherry); *Vial:* 300 mg/16.7 ml (18 mg/ml),
      soln for IV infusion
      Comment: Noxafil is indicated as prophylaxis for invasive aspergillus and candida infections in patients
      >13 years old who are at high risk due to being severely compromised.

CANDIDIASIS: SKIN

TOPICAL ANTIFUNGALS

▷ *butenafine* (G) apply bid x 1 week or once daily x 4 weeks
    Pediatric: <12 years: not recommended; ≥12 years: same as adult
      Lotrimin Ultra (OTC) *Crm:* 1% (12, 24 gm)
      Mentax *Crm:* 1% (15, 30 gm)
    Comment: *Butenafine* is a benzylamine, not an azole. Fungicidal activity continues for at least 5 weeks after
    the last application.
▷ *ciclopirox*
      Loprox Cream apply bid; max 4 weeks
      Pediatric: <10 years: not recommended; ≥10 years: same as adult
        Crm: 0.77% (15, 30, 90 gm)
      Loprox Lotion apply bid; max 4 weeks
      Pediatric: <10 years: not recommended; ≥10 years: same as adult
        Lotn: 0.77% (30, 60 ml)
      Loprox Gel apply bid; max 4 weeks
      Pediatric: <16 years: not recommended; ≥16 years: same as adult
        Gel: 0.77% (30, 45 gm)
▷ *clotrimazole* apply bid x 7 days
    Pediatric: <12 years: not recommended; ≥12 years: same as adult
      Lotrimin *Crm:* 1% (15, 30, 45 gm)
      Lotrimin AF (OTC) *Crm:* 1% (12 gm); *Lotn:* 1% (10 ml); *Soln:* 1% (10 ml)
▷ *econazole* apply bid x 14 days
    Pediatric: <12 years: not recommended; ≥12 years: same as adult
      Spectazole *Crm:* 1% (15, 30, 85 gm)
▷ *ketoconazole* apply once daily x 14 days
    Pediatric: <12 years: not recommended; ≥12 years: same as adult
      Nizoral Cream *Crm:* 2% (15, 30, 60 gm)

(continued)

▷ *miconazole* 2% apply once daily x 2 weeks
  Pediatric: <12 years: not recommended; ≥12 years: same as adult
    Lotrimin AF Spray Liquid (OTC) *Spray liq:* 2% (113 gm) (alcohol 17%)
    Lotrimin AF Spray Powder (OTC) *Spray pwdr:* 2% (90 gm) (alcohol 10%)
    Monistat-Derm *Crm:* 2% (1, 3 oz); *Spray liq:* 2% (3.5 oz); *Spray pwdr:* 2% (3 oz)
▷ *nystatin* dust affected skin freely bid-tid
    Nystop Powder *Pwdr:* 100,000 U/gm (15 gm)

ORAL ANTIFUNGALS
▷ *amphotericin b*
    Fungizone *Oral susp:* 100 mg/ml (24 ml w. dropper)
▷ *ketoconazole* 400 mg once daily x 1-2 weeks
  Pediatric: <2 years: not recommended; ≥2 years: 3.3-6.6 mg/kg once daily
    Nizoral *Tab:* 200 mg

INVASIVE INFECTION
▷ *posaconazole* (G) *Oral Therapy:* take with food; 100 mg bid on day 1; then 100 mg once daily x
  13 days; refractory, 400 mg bid x 13 days; *IV Infusion Therapy:* must be administered through an
  in-line filter over approximately 90 minutes via a central venous line. Never administer **Noxafil**
  as an IV bolus injection; *Loading Dose:* a single 300 mg IV infusion; *Maintenance Dose:* a single
  300 mg IV infusion once daily; duration of therapy is based on recovery from neutropenia or
  immunosuppression
  Pediatric: <13 years: not recommended; ≥13 years: same as adult
    Noxafil *Tab:* 100 mg ext-rel; *Oral susp:* 40 mg/ml (105 ml) (cherry); *Vial:* 300 mg/16.7 ml (18 mg/ml),
    soln for IV infusion
    Comment: Noxafil is indicated as prophylaxis for invasive aspergillus and candida infections in patients
    >13 years old who are at high risk due to being severely compromised.

CANDIDIASIS: VULVOVAGINAL (VVC, MONILIASIS)

PROPHYLAXIS
▷ *acetic acid+oxyquinoline* 1 full applicator intravaginally bid for up to 30 days
  Pediatric: <12 years: not recommended; ≥12 years: same as adult
    Relagard *Gel:* acetic acid 0.9%+oxyquin 0.025% (50 gm tube w. applicator)

Comment: The following treatment regimens for vulvovaginal candidiasis (VVC) are published in the
2021 CDC Sexually Transmitted Diseases Treatment Guidelines. Treatment regimens are presented
by generic drug name first, followed by information about brands and dose forms. Complicated
VVC (recurrent, severe, non-albicans, or women with uncontrolled diabetes, debilitation, or
immunosuppression) may require more intensive treatment and/or longer duration of treatment. VVC
frequently occurs during pregnancy. Only topical azole therapies, applied for 7 days, are recommended
during pregnancy.

Rx ORAL AGENTS
▷ *fluconazole* 150 mg in a single dose; complicated VVC, 150 mg x 3 doses on days 1, 4, and 7 or weekly x
  6 months
▷ *ibrexafungerp* *Treatment of VVC: Single treatment:* 300 mg (2 x 150 mg tabs) administered approximately
  12 hours apart (i.e., 2 tabs in the morning and 2 tabs in the evening) for a total of 600 mg (4 x 150 mg
  tabs) for a single day; *Treatment of recurrent vulvovaginal candidiasis (RVVC):* 300 mg (2 x 150 mg tabs)
  administered approximately 12 hours apart (i.e., 2 tabs in the morning and 2 tabs in the evening) for a total
  of 600 mg (4 x 150 mg tabs) for a single day and repeat once monthly for 6 months; May be taken with or
  without food
  Pediatric: Premenarchal: safety and efficacy not established; *Postmenarchal:* same as adult
    Brexafemme *Tab:* 150 mg
    Comment: Brexafemme is a first-in-class, non-azole, triterpenoid antifungal agent indicated for the
    treatment of adult and postmenarchal pediatric females with VVC and for reduction in the incidence
    of RVVC. The most frequently reported adverse reactions in patients treated for active VCC (incidence
    ≥2%) have been diarrhea, nausea, abdominal pain, dizziness, and vomiting. The most frequently
    reported adverse reactions in patients treated for reduction in the incidence of RVVC (incidence
    ≥2%) have been headache, abdominal pain, diarrhea, nausea, urinary tract infection, and fatigue.
    Concomitant use of strong CYP3A *inhibitors* increases the exposure of *ibrexafungerp*; therefore, reduce
    the dose of **Brexafemme** with concomitant use of a strong CYP3A inhibitor to 150 mg bid on each
    treatment day. Concomitant use of strong and moderate CYP3A *inducers* may significantly reduce
    the exposure of *ibrexafungerp*; therefore, avoid concomitant administration of **Brexafemme** with

strong or moderate CYP3A inducers. *Boxed Warning:* **Brexafemme** is contraindicated in pregnancy because it may cause fetal harm based on findings from animal reproductive studies. For females of reproductive potential, verify that the patient is <u>not</u> pregnant prior to initiating treatment. Reassessing pregnancy status prior to each dose is recommended when **Brexafemme** is used monthly for 6 months for reduction in the incidence of RVVC. Advise females of reproductive potential to use effective contraception during treatment throughout the 6-month treatment and for 4 days after the last dose. There is a pregnancy safety study for **Brexafemme**. If **Brexafemme** is inadvertently administered during pregnancy <u>or</u> if pregnancy is detected within 4 days after a patient receives **Brexafemme**, pregnant females exposed to **Brexafemme** and healthcare providers should report pregnancies to SCYNEXIS, Inc. at 1-888-982-SCYX (7299). There are no data on the presence of *ibrexafungerp* in human milk <u>or</u> effects on the breastfed infant.

▷ *secnidazole*
   Solosec *Oral granules:* 2 gm/pkt
   Comment: Solosec is a nitroimidazole antimicrobial. Do <u>not</u> dissolve **Solosec** in liquid. Sprinkle contents onto applesauce, yogurt, <u>or</u> pudding. Consume within 30 minutes without chewing <u>or</u> crunching; may follow with a glass of water. Potential adverse side effects are vulvovaginal pruritus, VVC, headache, nausea, dysgeusia, vomiting, diarrhea, and abdominal pain. Whereas *metronidazole* and *tinidazole* are contraindicated during the 1st trimester of pregnancy, no adverse developmental outcomes have been found in animal reproductive studies, and the labeling for *secnidazole* does <u>not</u> include a restriction for use in pregnancy. Breastfeeding is <u>not</u> recommended during and for 96 hours after dose; may pump and discard milk during this time period.

Rx INTRAVAGINAL AGENTS
Regimen 1
▷ *butoconazole* 2% cream (bioadhesive product) 5 gm intravaginally in a single dose

Regimen 2
▷ *nystatin* 100,000-unit vaginal tablet once daily x 14 days

Regimen 3
▷ *terconazole* 0.4% cream 5 gm intravaginally once daily x 7 days

Regimen 4
▷ *terconazole* 0.8% cream 5 gm intravaginally once daily x 3 days

Regimen 5
▷ *terconazole* 80 mg vaginal suppository intravaginally once daily x 3 days

OTC INTRAVAGINAL AGENTS
Regimen 1
▷ *butoconazole* 2% cream 5 gm intravaginally once daily x 3 days

Regimen 2
▷ *clotrimazole* 1% cream intravaginally once daily x 7-14 days

Regimen 3
▷ *clotrimazole* 2% cream intravaginally once daily x 3 days

Regimen 4
▷ *miconazole* 2% cream intravaginally once daily x 7 days

Regimen 5
▷ *miconazole* 4% cream intravaginally once daily x 3 days

Regimen 6
▷ *miconazole* 100 mg vaginal suppository intravaginally once daily x 7 days

Regimen 7
▷ *miconazole* 200 mg vaginal suppository intravaginally once daily x 3 days

Regimen 8
▷ *miconazole* 1,200 mg vaginal suppository intravaginally in a single application

Regimen 9
▷ *tioconazole* 6.5% ointment 5 gm intravaginally in a single application

DRUG BRANDS AND DOSE FORMS
▷ *butoconazole* cream 2%
    Gynazole-12% Vaginal Cream *Prefilled vag applicator:* 5 g
    Femstat-3 Vaginal Cream (OTC) *Vag crm:* 2% (20 gm w. 3 applicators); *Prefilled vag applicator:* 5 gm (3/pck)
▷ *clotrimazole* (OTC)
    Gyne-Lotrimin Vaginal Cream (OTC) *Vag crm:* 1% (45 gm w. applicator)
    Gyne-Lotrimin Vaginal Suppository (OTC) *Vag supp:* 100 mg (7/pck)
    Gyne-Lotrimin 3 Vaginal Suppository (OTC) *Vag supp:* 200 mg (3/pck)
    Gyne-Lotrimin Combination Pack (OTC) *Combination pck:* 7-100 mg supp with 7 gm 1% cream
    Gyne-Lotrimin 3 Combination Pack (OTC) *Combination pck:* 200 mg supp (7/pck) plus 1% cream (7 gm)
    Mycelex-G Vaginal Cream *Vag crm:* 1% (45, 90 gm w. applicator)
    Mycelex-G Vaginal Tab 1 *Tab:* 500 mg (1/pck)
    Mycelex Twin Pack *Twin pck:* 500 mg tab (7/pck) with 1% crm (7 gm)
    Mycelex-7 Vaginal Cream (OTC) *Vag crm:* 1% (45 gm w. applicator)
    Mycelex-7 Vaginal Inserts (OTC) *Vag insert:* 100 mg insert (7/pck)
    Mycelex-7 Combination Pack (OTC) *Combination pck:* 100 mg inserts (7/pck) plus 1% crm (7 gm)
▷ *fluconazole*
    Diflucan *Tab:* 50, 100, 150, 200 mg; *Oral susp:* 10, 40 mg/ml (35 ml) (orange)
▷ *miconazole*
    Monistat-3 Combination Pack (OTC) *Combination pck:* 200 mg supp (3/pck) plus 2% crm (9 gm)
    Monistat-7 Combination Pack (OTC) *Combination pck:* 100 mg supp (7/pck) plus 2% crm (9 gm)
    Monistat-7 Vaginal Cream (OTC) *Vag crm:* 2% (45 gm w. applicator)
    Monistat-7 Vaginal Suppositories (OTC) *Vag supp:* 100 mg (7/pck)
    Monistat-3 Vaginal Suppositories (OTC) *Vag supp:* 200 mg (3/pck)
▷ *nystatin*
    Mycostatin *Vag tab:* 100,000 U (1/pck)
▷ *terconazole*
    Terazol-3 Vaginal Cream *Vag crm:* 0.8% (20 gm w. applicator)
    Terazol-3 Vaginal Suppositories *Vag supp:* 80 mg supp (3/pck)
    Terazol-7 Vaginal Cream *Vag crm:* 0.4% (45 gm w. applicator)
▷ *tioconazole*
    1-Day (OTC) *Vag oint:* 6.5% (prefilled applicator x 1)
    Monistat 1 Vaginal Ointment (OTC) *Vag oint:* 6.5% (prefilled applicator x 1)
    Vagistat-1 Vaginal Ointment (OTC) *Vag oint:* 6.5% (prefilled applicator x 1)

INVASIVE INFECTION
▷ *posaconazole* (G) *Oral Therapy:* take with food; 100 mg bid on day 1; then 100 mg once daily x 13 days; refractory, 400 mg bid x 13 days; *IV Infusion Therapy:* must be administered through an in-line filter over approximately 90 minutes via a central venous line; Never administer **Noxafil** as an IV bolus injection; *Loading Dose:* a single 300 mg IV infusion; *Maintenance Dose:* a single 300 mg IV infusion once daily; duration of therapy is based on recovery from neutropenia or immunosuppression
Pediatric: <13 years: not recommended; ≥13 years: same as adult
    Noxafil *Tab:* 100 mg ext-rel; *Oral susp:* 40 mg/ml (105 ml) (cherry); *Vial:* 300 mg/16.7 ml (18 mg/ml), soln for IV infusion
    Comment: Noxafil is indicated as prophylaxis for invasive aspergillus and candida infections in patients >13 years old who are at high risk due to being severely compromised.

CANNABINOID HYPEREMESIS SYNDROME (CHS)

Comment: Cannabinoid hyperemesis syndrome (CHS) is indicated by recurrent episodes of refractory nausea and vomiting with vague diffuse abdominal pain (accompanied by compulsive, frequent hot baths or showers for relief of abdominal pain; these behaviors are thought to be learned through their cyclical periods of emesis) in the setting of chronic cannabis use (at least weekly for >2 years). The nausea and vomiting typically do not respond to antiemetic medications. 5HT3 (e.g., *ondansetron*), D2 (e.g., *prochlorperazine*), H1 (e.g., *promethazine*), or neurokinin-1 (NK-1) receptor antagonists (e.g., *aprepitant*) can be tried, but these therapies often are ineffective. The recovery phase can last weeks to months despite continued cannabis use prior to returning to the hyperemetic phase. Symptoms are worse in the morning, with normal bowel habits, and with negative evaluation, including laboratory, radiography, and endoscopy. Resolution requires cannabis cessation from 1 to 3 months. Returning to cannabis use often results in the return of CHS.

PHENOTHIAZINES

▷ *chlorpromazine* (G) 10-25 mg PO q 4 hours prn or 50-100 mg rectally q 6-8 hours prn
  Pediatric: <6 months: not recommended; ≥6 months: 0.25 mg/lb orally q 4-6 hours prn or 0.5 mg/lb rectally q 6-8 hours prn
    Thorazine *Tab:* 10, 25, 50, 100, 200 mg; *Spansule:* 30, 75, 150 mg sust-rel; *Syr:* 10 mg/5 ml (4 oz) (orange custard); *Conc:* 30 mg/ml (4 oz), 100 mg/ml (2, 8 oz); *Supp:* 25, 100 mg

▷ *perphenazine* 5 mg IM (may repeat in 6 hours) or 8-16 mg/day PO in divided doses; max 15 mg/day IM; max 24 mg/day PO
  Pediatric: <12 years: not recommended; ≥12 years: same as adult
    Trilafon *Tab:* 2, 4, 8, 16 mg; *Oral conc:* 16 mg/5 ml (118 ml); *Amp:* 5 mg/ml (1 ml)

▷ *prochlorperazine* (G) 5-10 mg tid-qid prn; usual max 40 mg/day
    Compazine
    Pediatric: <2 years or <20 lb: not recommended; 20-29 lb: 2.5 mg daily bid prn; max 7.5 mg/day; 30-39 lb: 2.5 mg bid-tid prn, max 10 mg/day; 40-85 lb: 2.5 mg tid or 5 mg bid prn; max 15 mg/day
    Tab: 5, 10 mg; *Syr:* 5 mg/5 ml (4 oz) (fruit)
    Compazine Suppository 25 mg rectally bid prn; usual max 50 mg/day
    Pediatric: <2 years or <20 lb: not recommended; 20-29 lb: 2.5 mg daily-bid prn; max 7.5; mg/day; 30-39 lb: 2.5 mg bid-tid prn; max 10 mg/day; 40-85 lb: 2.5 mg tid or 5 mg bid prn; max 15 mg/day
    Rectal supp: 2.5, 5, 25 mg
    Compazine Injectable 5-10 mg tid or qid prn
    Pediatric: <2 years or <20 lb: not recommended; ≥2 years or ≥20 lb: 0.06 mg/kg x 1 dose
    Vial: 5 mg/ml (2, 10 ml)
    Compazine Spansule 15 mg q AM prn or 10 mg q 12 hours prn; usual max 40 mg/day
    Pediatric: <12 years: not recommended; ≥12 years: same as adult
    Spansule: 10, 15 mg sust-rel

▷ *promethazine* (G) 25 mg PO or rectally q 4-6 hours prn
  Pediatric: <2 years: not recommended; ≥2 years: 0.5 mg/lb or 6.25-25 mg q 4-6 hours prn
    Phenergan *Tab:* 12.5*, 25*, 50 mg; *Plain syr:* 6.25 mg/5 ml; *Fortis syr:* 25 mg/5 ml; *Rectal supp:* 12.5, 25, 50 mg

Comment: *Promethazine* is contraindicated in children with uncomplicated nausea, dehydration, Reye's syndrome, history of sleep apnea, asthma, and lower respiratory disorders. *Promethazine* lowers the seizure threshold in children and may cause cholestatic jaundice, anticholinergic effects, extrapyramidal effects, and potentially fatal respiratory depression.

SUBSTANCE P/NEUROKININ 1 RECEPTOR ANTAGONIST

▷ *aprepitant* (G) administer with 5HT-3 receptor antagonist; *Day 1:* 125 mg x 1 dose; *starting Day 2:* 80 mg once daily in the morning
  Pediatric: <6 months: years: not recommended; ≥6 months: use oral suspension (see mfr pkg insert for dose by weight
    Emend *Cap:* 40, 80, 125 mg (2 x 80 mg bifold pck; 1 x 25 mg/2 x 80 mg trifold pck); *Oral susp:* 125 mg pwdr for oral suspension, single-dose pouch w. dispenser; *Vial:* 150 mg pwdr for reconstitution and IV infusion

SEROTONIN (5HT-3) RECEPTOR ANTAGONISTS

▷ *dolasetron* Administer 100 mg IV over 30 seconds; max 100 mg/dose
  Pediatric: <2 years: not recommended; 2-16 years: 1.8 mg/kg; >16 years: same as adult
    Anzemet *Tab:* 50, 100 mg; *Amp:* 12.5 mg/0.625 ml; *Prefilled carpuject syringe:* 12.5 mg (0.625 ml); *Vial:* 100 mg/5 ml (single-use); *Vial:* 500 mg/25 ml (multidose)

▷ *granisetron*
    Kytril *Administer* IV over 30 seconds; max 1 dose/week
    Pediatric: <2 years: not recommended; ≥2 years: 10 mcg/kg
      Tab: 1 mg; *Oral soln:* 2 mg/10 ml (30 ml) (orange); *Vial:* 1 mg/ml (1 ml single-dose) (preservative-free); 1 mg/ml (4 ml multidose) (benzyl alcohol)
    Sancuso apply 1 patch; remove 24 hours (minimum) to 7 days (maximum)
    Transdermal patch: 3.1 mg/day

▷ *granisetron extended-release injection* Administer SC over 20-30 seconds (due to drug viscosity) on Day 1 of chemotherapy and not more frequently than once every 7 days; *CrCl 30-59 ml/min:* repeat dose no more than every 14th day; *CrCl <30 ml/min:* not recommended; for patients receiving moderately emetogenic chemotherapy (MEC), the recommended *dexamethasone* dosage is 8 mg IV on Day 1; For patients receiving *anthracycline* and *cyclophosphamide* (AC) combination chemotherapy regimens, the recommended *dexamethasone* dosage is 20 mg IV on Day 1, followed by 8 mg PO bid on Days 2, 3, and 4; if Sustol is administered with an NK-1 receptor antagonist, see that drug's mfr pkg insert for the recommended *dexamethasone* dosing
  Pediatric: <12 years: not established; ≥12 years: same as adult
    Sustol *Syringe:* 10 mg/0.4 ml ext-rel; prefilled single-dose/kit

(continued)

Comment: At least 60 minutes prior to administration, remove the **Sustol** kit from refrigeration; activate a warming pouch and wrap the syringe in the warming pouch for 5–6 minutes to warm it to room temperature.

▷ *ondansetron* **(G)** Oral Forms: 8 mg q 8 hours x 2 doses; then 8 mg q 12 hours
  Pediatric: <4 years: not recommended; 4-11 years: 4 mg q 4 hours x 3 doses; then 4 mg q 8 hours
    Zofran *Tab:* 4, 8, 24 mg
    Zofran ODT *ODT:* 4, 8 mg (strawberry) (phenylalanine)
    Zofran Oral Solution *Oral soln:* 4 mg/5 ml (50 ml) (strawberry) (phenylalanine); *Parenteral form:* see mfr pkg insert
    Zofran Injection *Vial:* 2 mg/ml (2 ml single-dose), 2 mg/ml (20 ml muti-dose), 32 mg/50 ml (50 ml multidose); *Prefilled syringe:* 4 mg/2 ml, single-use (24/carton)
    Zuplenz Oral Soluble Film: 4, 8 mg oral-dis (10/carton) (peppermint)
    Comment: The FDA has issued an updated warning against *ondansetron* use in pregnancy. *Ondansetron* is a 5-HT3 receptor antagonist approved by the FDA for preventing nausea and vomiting related to cancer chemotherapy and surgery. However, it has been used "off label" to treat the nausea and vomiting of pregnancy. The FDA has cautioned against the use of *ondansetron* in pregnancy in light of studies of *ondansetron* in early pregnancy and associated with congenital cardiac malformations and oral clefts (i.e., cleft lip and cleft palate). Further, there are potential maternal risks in pregnancy with electrolyte imbalance caused by severe nausea and vomiting (as with hyperemesis gravidarum). These risks include *serotonin syndrome* (a triad of cognitive and behavioral changes including confusion, agitation, autonomic instability, and neuromuscular changes). Therefore, *ondansetron* should not be taken during pregnancy.
▷ *palonosetron* **(G)** administer 0.25 mg IV over 30 seconds; max 1 dose/week
  Pediatric: <1 month: not recommended; 1 month to 17 years: 20 mcg/kg; max 1.5 mg/single dose; infuse over 15 minutes
    Aloxi *Vial (single-use):* 0.075 mg/1.5 ml; 0.25 mg/5 ml (mannitol)

CARCINOID SYNDROME DIARRHEA (CSD)

TRYPTOPHAN HYDROXYLASE
▷ *telotristat* take with food; 250 mg tid
  Pediatric: <12 years: not established; ≥12 years: same as adult
    Xermelo *Tab:* 250 mg (4 x 7 daily dose pcks/carton)
    Comment: Take **Xermelo** in combination with somatostatin analog (SSA) therapy to treat patients inadequately controlled by SSA therapy. Breastfeeding females should monitor the infant for constipation.

CARDIOMYOPATHY OF TRANSTHYRETIN-MEDIATED AMYLOIDOSIS

TRANSTHYRETIN STABILIZERS
Comment: *Tafamidis* (Vyndamax) and *tafamidis meglumine* (Vyndaqel) are transthyretin stabilizers indicated for the treatment of cardiomyopathy of wild-type or hereditary transthyretin-mediated amyloidosis in adults to reduce cardiovascular mortality and cardiovascular-related hospitalization. **Vyndamax** and **Vyndaqel** are not interchangeable or substitutable on a mg-per-mg basis. Although there are no contraindications to these drugs, animal studies have demonstrated potential for embryo/fetal harm. Consider pregnancy planning and prevention for females of reproductive potential. There are no available data on the presence of *tafamidis* in human milk or effects on the breastfed infant. Based on findings from animal studies, which suggest potential for serious adverse reactions in the breastfed infant, breastfeeding is not recommended during treatment. Safety and efficacy of *tafamidis* have not been established in pediatric patients. No dosage adjustment is required in patients ≥65 years of age.

▷ *tafamidis* 61 mg once daily
    Vyndamax *Cap:* 61 mg
▷ *tafamidis meglumine* 80 mg (4 x 20 mg) once daily
    Vyndaqel *Cap:* 20 mg

CARPAL TUNNEL SYNDROME (CTS)

Acetaminophen for IV Infusion *see Pain*
NSAIDs *see* NSAIDs online at https://connect.springerpub.com/content/reference-book/978-0-8261-7935-7/back-matter/part02/back-matter/bmatter10
Opioid Analgesics *see Pain*
Topical and Transdermal Analgesics *see Pain*
Parenteral Corticosteroids *see* Appendix L. Parenteral Corticosteroids
Oral Corticosteroids *see* Appendix K. Oral Corticosteroids

Topical Analgesic and Anesthetic Agents *see* Appendix H. Anesthetic Agents for Local Infiltration and Dermal/Mucosal Membrane Application online at https://connect.springerpub.com/content/reference-book/978-0-8261-7935-7/back-matter/part02/back-matter/bmatter9

CAT SCRATCH FEVER (*BARTONELLA* INFECTION)

Comment: Cat scratch fever is usually self-limited. Treatment should be limited to severe or debilitating cases.

ANTI-INFECTIVES

➤ *azithromycin* (G) 500 mg x 1 dose on Day 1, then 250 mg daily on Days 2-5 or 500 mg daily x 3 days or Zmax 2 gm in a single dose
  Pediatric: 12 mg/kg/day x 5 days; max 500 mg/day; *see* Appendix BB.7. azithromycin (G) (Zithromax Suspension, Zmax Suspension) *for dose by weight*
    Zithromax *Tab:* 250, 500, 600 mg; *Oral susp:* 100 mg/5 ml (15 ml), 200 mg/5 ml (15, 22.5, 30 ml) (cherry); *Pkt:* 1 gm for reconstitution (cherry-banana)
    Zithromax Tri-Pak *Tab:* 3 x 500 mg tabs/pck
    Zithromax Z-Pak *Tab:* 6 x 250 mg tabs/pck
    Zmax *Oral susp:* 2 gm ext-rel for reconstitution (cherry-banana) (148 mg Na⁺)

➤ *doxycycline* (G) 100 mg daily bid
  Pediatric: <8 years: not recommended ≥8 years, <100 lb: 2 mg/lb on first day in 2 divided doses, followed by 1 mg/lb/day in 1-2 divided doses; ≥8 years, ≥100 lb: same as adult; *see* Appendix BB.19. doxycycline (Vibramycin Syrup/Suspension) *for dose by weight*
    Acticlate *Tab:* 75, 150**mg
    Adoxa *Tab:* 50, 75, 100, 150 mg ent-coat
    Doryx *Tab:* 50, 75, 100, 150, 200 mg del-rel
    Doxteric *Tab:* 50 mg del-rel
    Monodox *Cap:* 50, 75, 100 mg
    Oracea *Cap:* 40 mg del-rel
    Vibramycin *Tab:* 100 mg; *Cap:* 50, 100 mg; *Syr:* 50 mg/5 ml (raspberry-apple) (sulfites); *Oral susp:* 25 mg/5 ml (raspberry)
    Vibra-Tab *Tab:* 100 mg film-coat

➤ *erythromycin base* (G) 500-1,000 mg qid x 4 weeks
  Pediatric: <45 kg: 30-50 mg in 2-4 divided doses x 4 weeks; ≥45 kg: same as adult
    Ery-Tab *Tab:* 250, 333, 500 mg ent-coat
    PCE *Tab:* 333, 500 mg

➤ *erythromycin ethylsuccinate* (G) 400 mg qid x 4 weeks
  Pediatric: 30-50 mg/kg/day in 4 divided doses x 4 weeks; may double dose with severe infection; max 100 mg/kg/day; *see* Appendix BB.21. erythromycin ethylsuccinate (E.E.S. Suspension, EryPed Drops/Suspension) *for dose by weight*
    EryPed *Oral susp:* 200 mg/5 ml (100, 200 ml) (fruit), 400 mg/5 ml (60, 100, 200 ml) (banana); *Oral drops:* 200, 400 mg/5 ml (50 ml) (fruit); *Chew tab:* 200 mg wafer (fruit)
    E.E.S. *Oral susp:* 200, 400 mg/5 ml (100 ml) (fruit)
    E.E.S. Granules *Oral susp:* 200 mg/5 ml (100, 200 ml) (cherry)
    E.E.S. 400 Tablets *Tab:* 400 mg

➤ *trimethoprim+sulfamethoxazole* (TMP-SMX)(G) bid x 10 days
  Pediatric: <2 months: not recommended; ≥2 months: 40 mg/kg/day of *sulfamethoxazole* in 2 divided doses bid x 10 days; *see* Appendix BB.33. trimethoprim+sulfamethoxazole (G) (Bactrim Suspension, Septra Suspension) *for dose by weight*
    Bactrim, Septra 2 tabs bid x 10 days
      Tab: trim 80 mg+sulfa 400 mg*
    Bactrim DS, Septra DS 1 tab bid x 10 days
      Tab: trim 160 mg+sulfa 800 mg*
    Bactrim Pediatric Suspension, Septra Pediatric Suspension
      Oral susp: trim 40 mg+sulfa 200 mg per 5 ml (100 ml) (cherry) (alcohol 0.3%)
Comment: Sulfonamides are contraindicated in the 1st trimester of pregnancy, the final month of pregnancy, and infants <8 weeks of age. *CrCl 15-30 ml/min:* reduce dose by 1/2; *CrCl <15 ml/min:* not recommended. Contraindicated with glucose-6-phosphate dehydrogenase deficiency (G6PD). A high fluid intake is indicated during sulfonamide therapy to avoid crystallization in the kidneys.

CELLULITE

COLLAGENASE CLOSTRIDIUM HISTOLYTICUM-AAES

➤ *collagenase clostridium histolyticum-aaes* a treatment area is defined as a single buttock receiving up to 12 injections, 0.3 ml each (up to a total of 3.6 ml); a treatment visit may consist of up to 2 treatment areas;

(continued)

treatment visits should be repeated every 21 days for 3 treatment visits; reconstitute **QWO** lyophilized powder with the supplied diluent prior to use; inject 0.84 mg per treatment area as 12 SC injections (0.3 ml administered as three 0.1 ml aliquots per injection)
Pediatric: not established

> **QWO** Vial: 0.92, 1.84 mg, single dose, pwdr for reconstitution with provided diluent
> **Comment:** QWO *(collagenase clostridium histolyticum-aaes)* is a combination of bacterial collagenases indicated for the treatment of moderate-to-severe cellulite in the buttocks of adult women. The most common adverse reactions (incidence ≥1%) have been related to the injection site (bruising, pain, nodule, pruritus, erythema, discoloration, swelling, and warmth). Injection site bruising occurs frequently after **QWO** administration. Use with caution in patients with bleeding abnormalities or who are currently being treated with antiplatelet (except those taking ≤150 mg *aspirin* daily) or anticoagulant therapy. Serious hypersensitivity reactions, including anaphylaxis, may occur with *collagenase clostridium histolyticum.* If a serious hypersensitivity reaction occurs, initiate appropriate therapy. **QWO** must not be substituted for other injectable collagenase products. **QWO** is not indicated for the treatment of Peyronie's disease or Dupuytren's contracture. Following SC injection, the systemic concentrations for **QWO** have been below the bioanalytical assay limit of quantification. There are no available data on *collagenase clostridium histolyticum* use in pregnant women to evaluate for a drug-associated risk of major birth defects, miscarriage or adverse maternal or fetal outcomes. There are no data on the presence of *collagenase clostridium histolyticum* in human milk or effects on the breastfed infant.

CELLULITIS, ACUTE BACTERIAL SKIN AND SKIN STRUCTURE INFECTION (ABSSSI)

Comment: Duration of treatment should be 10-30 days. Obtain culture from site. Consider blood cultures.

ANTI-INFECTIVES

▷ *amoxicillin* **(G)** 500-875 mg bid or 250-500 mg tid x 10 days
Pediatric: <40 kg (88 lb): 20-40 mg/kg/day in 3 divided doses x 10 days or 25-45 mg/kg/day in 2 divided doses x 10 days; ≥40 kg: same as adult; *see Appendix BB.3. amoxicillin* (G) (Amoxil Suspension, Trimox Suspension) *for dose by weight*
> **Amoxil** *Cap:* 250, 500 mg; *Tab:* 875*mg; *Chew tab:* 125, 200, 250, 400 mg (cherry-banana-peppermint) (phenylalanine); *Oral susp:* 125, 250 mg/5 ml (80, 100, 150 ml) (strawberry); 200, 400 mg/5 ml (50, 75, 100 ml) (bubble gum); *Oral drops:* 50 mg/ml (30 ml) (bubble gum)
> **Moxatag** *Tab:* 775 mg ext-rel
> **Trimox** *Tab:* 125, 250 mg; *Cap:* 250, 500 mg; *Oral susp:* 125, 250 mg/5 ml (80, 100, 150 ml) (raspberry-strawberry)

▷ *amoxicillin+clavulanate* **(G)**
> **Augmentin** 500 mg tid or 875 mg bid x 7-10 days
> *Pediatric:* 40-45 mg/kg/day divided tid x 10 days or 90 mg/kg/day divided bid x 10 days see Appendix BB.4. *amoxicillin+clavulanate* (G) (Augmentin Suspension) *for dose by weight*
> *Tab:* 250, 500, 875 mg; *Chew tab:* 125, 250 mg (lemon-lime); 200, 400 mg (cherry-banana) (phenylalanine); *Oral susp:* 125 mg/5 ml (banana), 250 mg/5 ml (75, 100, 150 ml) (orange); 200, 400 mg/5 ml (50, 75, 100 ml) (orange) (phenylalanine)
> **Augmentin ES-600** not recommended for adults
> *Pediatric:* <3 months: not recommended; ≥3 months, <40 kg: 90 mg/kg/day in 2 divided doses x 7-10 days; ≥40 kg: not recommended
> *Oral susp:* 42.9 mg/5 ml (50, 75, 100, 125, 150, 200 ml) (strawberry cream) (phenylalanine)
> **Augmentin XR** 2 tabs q 12 hours x 7-10 days
> *Pediatric:* <16 years: use other forms; ≥16 years: same as adult
> > *Tab:* 1,000*mg ext-rel

▷ *azithromycin* **(G)** 500 mg x 1 dose on day 1, then 250 mg daily on days 2-5 or 500 mg daily x 3 days or **Zmax** 2 gm in a single dose
Pediatric: 12 mg/kg/day x 5 days; max 500 mg/day; *see Appendix BB.7. azithromycin* (G) (Zithromax Suspension, Zmax Suspension) *for dose by weight*
> **Zithromax** *Tab:* 250, 500, 600 mg; *Oral susp:* 100 mg/5 ml (15 ml); 200 mg/5 ml (15, 22.5, 30 ml) (cherry); *Pkt:* 1 gm for reconstitution (cherry-banana)
> **Zithromax Tri-Pak** *Tab:* 3 x 500 mg tabs/pck
> **Zithromax Z-Pak** *Tab:* 6 x 250 mg tabs/pck
> **Zmax** *Oral susp:* 2 gm ext-rel for reconstitution (cherry-banana) (148 mg Na⁺)

▷ *cefaclor* **(G)**
> **Ceclor** 250 mg tid or 375 mg bid 3-10 days
> *Pediatric:* <1 month: not recommended; 1 month-12 years: 20-40 mg/kg divided bid or q 12 hours x 3-10 days; max 1 gm/day; see Appendix BB.8. *cefaclor* (G) (Ceclor Suspension) for *dose by weight*; >12 years: same as adult
> *Tab:* 500 mg; *Cap:* 250, 500 mg; *Susp:* 125 mg/5 ml (75, 150 ml) (strawberry), 187 mg/5 ml (50, 100 ml) (strawberry), 250 mg/5 ml (75, 150 ml) (strawberry), 375 mg/5 ml (50, 100 ml) (strawberry)
> **Ceclor Extended Release** 375-500 mg bid x 3-10 days

Pediatric: <16 years: ext-rel <u>not</u> recommended; ≥16 years: same as adult

　　Tab: 375, 500 mg ext-rel

▷ *cefpodoxime proxetil* 400 mg bid x 7-14 days

Pediatric: <2 months: <u>not</u> recommended; ≥2 months-12 years: 10 mg/kg/day (max 400 mg/dose) <u>or</u> 5 mg/kg/day bid (max 200 mg/dose) x 7-14 days; *see Appendix BB.12. Cefpodoxime Proxetil* (G) (Vantin Suspension) *for dose by weight;* >12 years: same as adult

　　Vantin *Tab:* 100, 200 mg; *Oral susp:* 50, 100 mg/5 ml (50, 75, 100 mg) (lemon creme)

▷ *cefprozil* 500 mg q 12 hours x 10 days

Pediatric: <2 years: <u>not</u> recommended; 2-12 years: 15 mg/kg q 12 hours x 10 days; *see Appendix BB.13. cefprozil* (G) *(Cefzil Suspension) for dose by weight;* >12 years: same as adult

　　Cefzil *Tab:* 250, 500 mg; *Oral susp:* 125, 250 mg/5 ml (50, 75, 100 ml) (bubble gum) (phenylalanine)

▷ *ceftaroline fosamil* administer 600 mg once every 12 hours, by IV infusion over 5-60 minutes, x 5-14 days

Pediatric: <18 years: <u>not</u> established; ≥18 years: same as adult

　　Teflaro *Vial:* 400, 600 mg pwdr for reconstitution, single-use (10/carton)

　　Comment: Teflaro is indicated for the treatment of adults with acute bacterial skin and skin structures infection (ABSSSI).

▷ *ceftriaxone* (G) 1-2 gm daily x 5-14 days IM; max 4 gm daily

Pediatric: 50-75 mg/kg IM in 1-2 divided doses x 5-14 days; max 2 gm/day

　　Rocephin *Vial:* 250, 500 mg; 1, 2 gm

▷ *cephalexin* (G) 500 mg bid x 10 days

Pediatric: 25-50 mg/kg/day in 4 divided doses x 10 days; *see Appendix BB.15. cephalexin (Keflex Suspension) for dose by weight*

　　Keflex *Cap:* 250, 333, 500, 750 mg; *Oral susp:* 125, 250 mg/5 ml (100, 200 ml) (strawberry)

▷ *clarithromycin* (G) 500 mg q 12 hours <u>or</u> 500 mg ext-rel once daily x 10 days

Pediatric: <6 months: <u>not</u> recommended; ≥6 months: 7.5 mg/kg bid x 10 days; *see Appendix BB.16. clarithromycin* (G) (Biaxin Suspension) *for dose by weight*

　　Biaxin *Tab:* 250, 500 mg

　　Biaxin Oral Suspension *Oral susp:* 125, 250 mg/5 ml (50, 100 ml) (fruit punch)

　　Biaxin XL *Tab:* 500 mg ext-rel

SECOND-GENERATION LIPOGLYCOPEPTIDE

▷ *dalbavancin* administer via IV infusion over 30 minutes; *CrCl* ≥30 ml/min: single-dose regimen: administer a single 1,500 mg dose; *two-dose regimen:* administer a single 1,000 mg dose on day 1, followed by a single 500 mg dose 1 week (7 days) later; *CrCl* <30 ml/min, <u>not</u> on regular hemodialysis: single-dose regimen: administer a single 1,125 mg dose; *two-dose regimen:* administer a single 750 mg dose on day 1, followed by a single 375 mg (1 vial) dose 1 week (7 days) later

Pediatric: administer via IV infusion over 30 minutes; *CrCl* <30 ml/min: <u>not</u> recommended; *CrCl* ≥30 ml/min: Birth-<6 years: administer 22.5 mg/kg (max 1,500 mg) as a single dose; 6-<18 years: administer 18 mg/kg (max 1,500 mg) as a single dose; ≥18 years: same as adult

　　Dalvance *Vial:* 500 mg pwdr for reconstitution, dilution, and IV infusion, single-dose

　　Comment: Dalvance is a second-generation lipoglycopeptide antibiotic for the treatment of adult patients with complicated skin and skin structure infections (ABSSSI) caused by designated susceptible strains of gram-positive microorganisms, including those caused by methicillin-resistant *Staphylococcus aureus* (MRSA). The most common adverse reactions occurring in >4% of adult patients treated with Dalvance have been nausea, headache, and diarrhea. The most common adverse reaction that has occurred in >1% of pediatric patients has been pyrexia. Serious hypersensitivity (anaphylactic) and skin reactions have been reported in patients treated with Dalvance. If an allergic reaction occurs, discontinue treatment with Dalvance and institute appropriate treatment. Carefully monitor patients with known hypersensitivity to glycopeptides. Rapid IV infusion of Dalvance can cause flushing of the upper body, urticaria, pruritus, rash, and/or back pain. Stopping <u>or</u> slowing the infusion may result in cessation of these reactions. Alanine aminotransferase (ALT) elevations with Dalvance treatment have been reported in clinical trials. *Clostridioides difficile*-associated diarrhea (CDAD) has been reported with nearly all systemic antibacterial agents, including Dalvance; evaluate if diarrhea occurs. Safety and effectiveness of Dalvance in the treatment of ABSSSI have been established in pediatric patients aged birth to <18 years. Use of Dalvance for this indication is supported by evidence from adequate and well-controlled studies in adults with additional pharmacokinetic and safety data in pediatric patients aged birth to <18 years. There are <u>no</u> adequate and well-controlled studies with Dalvance use in pregnant females to evaluate for a drug-associated risk of major birth defects, miscarriage, <u>or</u> adverse developmental outcomes. There are <u>no</u> data on the presence of *dalbavancin* <u>or</u> its metabolite in human milk <u>or</u> effects on the breastfed infant. The developmental and health benefits of breastfeeding should be considered along with the mother's clinical need for Dalvance and any potential adverse effects on the breastfed infant from Dalvance <u>or</u> from the underlying maternal condition.

▷ *delafloxacin* *IV infusion:* administer 300 mg every 12 hours over 60 minutes x 5-14 days; *Tablet:* 450 mg every 12 hours x 5-14 days; dosage for patients with renal impairment is based on estimated glomerular filtration rate (eGFR; see mfr pkg insert)

Pediatric: <18 years: <u>not</u> recommended; ≥18 years: same as adult

　　Baxdela *Tab:* 450 mg; *Vial:* 300 mg pwdr for reconstitution and IV infusion

(continued)

Comment: Baxdela, a fluoroquinolone, is indicated for the treatment of acute bacterial skin and skin structure infections (ABSSSI) caused by designated susceptible bacteria. Fluoroquinolones have been associated with disabling and potentially irreversible serious adverse reactions that have occurred together, including tendinitis and tendon rupture, peripheral neuropathy, and central nervous system effects. Discontinue **Baxdela** immediately and avoid the use of fluoroquinolones, including **Baxdela,** in patients who experience any of these serious adverse reactions. Fluoroquinolones may exacerbate muscle weakness in patients with myasthenia gravis. Therefore, avoid **Baxdela** in patients with known history of myasthenia gravis. The most common adverse reactions are nausea, diarrhea, headache, transaminase elevations, and vomiting. Closely monitor serum creatinine in patients with severe renal impairment (eGFR 15-29 ml/min/1.73 m²) receiving IV *delafloxacin.* If SCr level increases occur, consider changing to oral *delafloxacin.* Discontinue **Baxdela** if eGFR decreases to <15 ml/min/1.73 m². The limited available data with **Baxdela** use in pregnant females are insufficient to inform a drug-associated risk of major birth defects and miscarriages. There are no data available on the presence of *delafloxacin* in human milk or effects on the breastfed infant.

▷ *dicloxacillin* **(G)** 500 mg q 6 hours x 10 days
  Pediatric: 12.5-25 mg/kg/day in 4 divided doses x 10 days; *see Appendix BB.18. dicloxacillin* (G) (Dynapen Suspension) *for dose by weight*
     Dynapen Cap: 125, 250, 500 mg; *Oral susp:* 62.5 mg/5 ml (80, 100, 200 ml)
▷ *dirithromycin* **(G)** 500 mg once daily x 5-7 days
  Pediatric: <12 years: not recommended; ≥12 years: same as adult
     Dynabac Tab: 250 mg
▷ *erythromycin base* **(G)** 250 mg qid or 333 mg tid or 500 mg bid x 7-10 days; then taper to the lowest effective dose
  Pediatric: <45 kg: 30-50 mg in 2-4 divided doses x 7-10 days; ≥45 kg: same as adult
     Ery-Tab Tab: 250, 333, 500 mg ent-coat
     PCE Tab: 333, 500 mg
▷ *erythromycin ethylsuccinate* **(G)** 400 mg qid x 7-10 days
  Pediatric: 30-50 mg/kg/day in 4 divided doses x 7-10 days; may double dose with severe infection; max 100 mg/kg/day; *see Appendix BB.21. erythromycin ethylsuccinate* (G) (E.E.S. Suspension, EryPed Drops/ Suspension) *for dose by weight*
     EryPed Oral susp: 200 mg/5 ml (100, 200 ml) (fruit); 400 mg/5 ml (60, 100, 200 ml) (banana); *Oral drops:* 200, 400 mg/5 ml (50 ml) (fruit); *Chew tab:* 200 mg wafer (fruit)
     E.E.S. Oral susp: 200, 400 mg/5 ml (100 ml) (fruit)
     E.E.S. Granules Oral susp: 200 mg/5 ml (100, 200 ml) (cherry)
     E.E.S. 400 Tablets Tab: 400 mg
▷ *linezolid* **(G)** 600 mg q 12 hours x 10-14 days
  Pediatric: <5 years: 10 mg/kg q 8 hours x 10-14 days; 5-11 years: 10 mg/kg q 12 hours x 10-14 days; >11 years: same as adult
     Zyvox Tab: 400, 600 mg; *Oral susp:* 100 mg/5 ml (150 ml) (orange) (phenylalanine)
  Comment: *Linezolid* is indicated for treatment of susceptible vancomycin-resistant *Enterococcus faecium* infections of skin and skin structures, including diabetic foot without osteomyelitis.
▷ *loracarbef* 200 mg bid x 10 days
  Pediatric: 15 mg/kg/day in 2 divided doses x 10 days; *see Appendix BB.27. loracarbef* (G) (Lorabid Suspension) *for dose by weight*
     Lorabid Pulvule: 200, 400 mg; *Oral susp:* 100 mg/5 ml (50, 100 ml), 200 mg/5 ml (50, 75, 100 ml) (strawberry bubble gum)
▷ *moxifloxacin* **(G)** 400 mg once daily x 5 days
  Pediatric: <18 years: recommended; ≥18 years: same as adult
     Avelox Tab: 400 mg; *IV soln:* 400 mg/250 ml (latex-free, preservative-free)
▷ *omadacycline before* oral dosing, fast x at least 4 hours and then take tablets with water; *after* oral dosing, no food or drink (except water) x 2 hours and no dairy products, antacids, or multivitamins x 4 hours; total treatment duration 7-14 days
  OPTION 1, Loading Dose, Day 1: 200 mg via IV infusion over 60 minutes or 100 mg via IV infusion over 30 minutes twice; *Maintenance:* 100 mg via IV infusion over 30 minutes once daily or 300 mg orally once daily
  OPTION 2 (tablets only), Day 1 and Day 2: 450 mg orally once daily; then reduce dose to 300 mg orally once daily
  Pediatric: <18 years: not recommended; ≥18 years: same as adult
     Nuzyra Tab: 150 mg; *Vial:* 100 mg single-dose for reconstitution, dilution, and IV infusion
  Comment: Nuzyra *(omadacycline)* is an aminomethylcycline tetracycline antibiotic for treatment of community-acquired bacterial pneumonia (CABP) and ABSSSI. The most common adverse reactions (incidence ≥2%) are nausea, vomiting, infusion site reactions, increased ALT, increased aspartate aminotransferase (AST), increased gamma-glutamyltransferase (GGT), hypertension, headache, diarrhea, insomnia, and constipation. Like other tetracycline-class antibacterial drugs, **Nuzyra** may cause discoloration of deciduous teeth and reversible inhibition of bone growth when administered during the 2nd and 3rd trimesters of pregnancy. The limited available data of **Nuzyra** use in pregnancy are insufficient to inform drug-associated risk of major birth defects and miscarriages. There is no information on the presence of *omadacycline* in human milk or effects on the breastfed infant.

➤ *oritavancin* see mfr pkg insert for dose preparation and administration
Pediatric: <18 years: safety and efficacy not established; ≥18 years: same as adult
  Kimyrsa *Administer* 1,200 mg (1 vial) as a single dose via IV infusion over 1 hour; carefully follow the mfr pkg insert for full preparation, dilution, and infusion information
    Vial: 1,200 mg, single-dose, pwdr for reconstitution, dilution, and IV infusion
  Orbactiv *Administer* 1,200 mg (3 vials) as a single dose via IV infusion over 3 hours; carefully follow the mfr pkg insert for full preparation, dilution, and infusion information
    Vial: 400 mg, single-dose, pwdr for reconstitution, dilution, and IV infusion
Comment: *Oritavancin* is a lipoglycopeptide antibacterial agent indicated for the treatment of adult patients with ABSSSI caused or suspected to be caused by susceptible isolates of designated gram-positive microorganisms. There are two *oritavancin* products: **Kimyrsa** and **Orbactiv**. These have *differences* in dose strength, duration of infusion, and preparation instructions, including reconstitution and dilution instructions and compatible diluents. Use of IV administered unfractionated *heparin sodium* is contraindicated for 120 hours (5 days) after *oritavancin* administration. *Oritavancin* has been shown to artificially prolong activated partial thromboplastin time (aPTT) for up to 120 hours, and may prolong prothrtombin time/partial thromboplastin time (PT/PTT) and international normalized ratio (INR) for up to 12 hours and activated clotting time (ACT) for up to 24 hours. For patients who require aPTT monitoring within 120 hours of *oritavancin* dosing, consider a non-phospholipid-dependent coagulation test such as a Factor Xa (chromogenic) assay or an alternative anticoagulant not requiring aPTT. *Oritavancin* has been shown to artificially prolong PT/INR for up to 12 hours when administered concomitantly with *warfarin*; patients should be monitored for bleeding. Serious hypersensitivity reactions, including anaphylaxis, have been reported with the use of *oritavancin* products; discontinue infusion if signs of acute hypersensitivity occur. Carefully monitor patients with known hypersensitivity to glycopeptides. Infusion-related reactions have been reported with the glycopeptide class of antimicrobial agents. Stopping or slowing the infusion results in cessation of these reactions. CDAD may develop; evaluate patients if diarrhea occurs. Institute appropriate alternate antibacterial therapy in patients with confirmed or suspected osteomyelitis. The most common adverse reactions (incidence ≥3%) in patients treated with *oritavancin* products have been headache, nausea, vomiting, limb and subcutaneous abscesses, and diarrhea. There are no available data on *oritavancin* use in pregnant females to evaluate for a drug-associated risk of major birth defects, miscarriage, or adverse maternal or embryo/fetal outcomes. In animal reproduction studies, no effects on embryo/fetal development or survival were observed throughout organogenesis. There are no data on the presence of *oritavancin* in human milk or the effects on the breastfed infant. In animal studies, *oritavancin* is present in breast milk. Developmental and health benefits of breastfeeding should be considered along with the mother's clinical need for *oritavancin* and any potential adverse effects on the breastfed infant from *oritavancin* or from the underlying maternal condition.

➤ *penicillin v potassium* 250-500 mg q 6 hours x 5-7 days
Pediatric: <12 years: see Appendix BB.29. penicillin v potassium (G) (Pen-Vee K Solution, Veetids Solution) for dose by weight; >12 years: same as adult
  Pen-Vee K *Tab:* 250, 500 mg; *Oral soln:* 125 mg/5 ml (100, 200 ml), 250 mg/5 ml (100, 150, 200 ml)

➤ *tedizolid phosphate* administer 200 mg once daily x 6 days, via PO or IV infusion over 1 hour
Pediatric: <18 years: not established; ≥18 years: same as adult
  Sivextro *Tab:* 200 mg (6/blister pck)
  Comment: **Sivextro** is indicated for the treatment of adults with acute bacterial skin and skin structures infection (ABSSSI).

➤ *tigecycline* (G) 100 mg as a single dose; then 50 mg q 12 hours x 5-14 days; with severe hepatic impairment (Child-Pugh Class C), 100 mg as a single dose; then 25 mg q 12 hours
Pediatric: <18 years: not recommended; ≥18 years: same as adult
  Tygacil *Vial:* 50 mg pwdr for reconstitution and IV infusion (preservative-free)
  Comment: **Tygacil** is contraindicated in pregnancy and lactation (discolors developing tooth enamel). A side effect may be photosensitivity (photophobia). Do not give with antacids, calcium supplements, milk or other dairy, or within 2 hours of taking another drug.

CERUMEN IMPACTION

OTIC ANALGESIC

➤ *antipyrine+benzocaine+zinc acetate dihydrate* otic fill ear canal with solution; then moisten cotton plug with solution and insert into the meatus; may repeat every 1-2 hours prn
Pediatric: same as adult
  Otozin *Otic soln:* antipyr 5.4%+benz 1%+zinc 1% per ml (10 ml w. dropper)

CERUMENOLYTICS

➤ *triethanolamine* (OTC)(G) fill ear canal and insert cotton plug for 15-30 minutes before irrigating with warm water
  Cerumenex *Soln:* 10% (6, 12 ml)

➤ *carbamide peroxide* (OTC) (G) instill 5-10 drops in the ear canal; keep drops in ear several minutes; then irrigate with warm water; repeat bid for up to 4 days
  Debrox *Soln:* 15, 30 ml squeeze bottle w. applicator

CHAGAS DISEASE (AMERICAN TRYPANOSOMIASIS)

Comment: Chagas disease is a protozoal parasite (*Trypanosoma cruzi*) infection with increasing prevalence in the United States attributed to immigration from *T. cruzi*-endemic areas of South and Central Latin America. Approximately 300,000 persons in the United States have chronic Chagas disease, and up to 30% of them will develop clinically evident cardiovascular and/or gastrointestinal (GI) disease. Chagas disease is one of the five neglected parasitic infections (NPIs) targeted by the Centers for Disease Control and Prevention (CDC) for public health action. It is transmitted by the bite of the triatomine bug ("kissing bug"), which feeds on human blood, maternal–fetus vertical transmission, blood transfusion, consumption of contaminated food, and organ donation. A clinical marker is Romaña sign (periorbital swelling), chagoma (skin nodule), and schizotrypanides (non-pruritic morbilliform rash). Only two antiparasitic drugs, **benznidazole** and **nifurtimox**, have demonstrated effectiveness in altering the progression of this chronic disease. These drugs are not FDA approved and are available only from CDC under investigational protocols. Treatment is indicated for all cases of acute or reactivated Chagas disease and for chronic *T. cruzi* infection in children ≤18. Congenital infections are considered acute disease. Treatment is strongly recommended up to 50 years old with chronic infection who do not already have advanced Chagas cardiomyopathy. For adults older than 50 years with chronic *T. cruzi* infection, the decision to treat with antiparasitic drugs should be individualized, weighing the potential benefits and risks for the patient. Patients taking either of these drugs should have complete blood count (CBC) and comprehensive metabolic panel (CMP) at the start of treatment and then bi-monthly for the duration of treatment to monitor for rare bone marrow suppression. Contraindications to treatment include severe hepatic and/or renal disease. As safety for infants exposed through breastfeeding has not been documented, withholding treatment while breastfeeding is also recommended. For emergencies (e.g., acute Chagas disease with severe manifestations, Chagas disease in a newborn, or Chagas disease in an immunocompromised person) outside of regular business hours, call the CDC Emergency Operations Center (770-488-7100) and ask for the person on call for parasitic diseases. For more detailed information about screening, assessment, and treatment of this public health threat, see McDonald, J, & Mattingly, J. (November, 2016). Chagas disease: Creeping into family practice in the United States, *Clinician Reviews*, pp. 38-45, or call 404-718-4745 or email questions to chagas@cdc.gov.

ANTIPARASITIC AGENTS

▷ **benznidazole (G)** Take do with a meal to avoid GI upset; <2 years: not established; 2-12 years: 5-7.5 mg/kg/day divided bid x 60 days; >12 years: not established
Comment: Common side effects of **benznidazole** are allergic dermatitis, peripheral neuropathy, insomnia, and anorexia with weight loss. **Benznidazole** is contraindicated in patients who have taken **disulfiram** within the previous 2 weeks due to the potential for a psychotic reaction. Alcohol beverages and any product containing propylene glycol are contraindicated from 2 weeks before initiating the first dose of **benznidazole**, throughout treatment, and the first 3 days after the last dose of **benznidazole** to prevent a **disulfiram**-like reaction (e.g., flushing, headache, abdominal cramping, and nausea/vomiting).

▷ **nifurtimox (G)** Take dose with a meal to avoid GI upset; ≤10 years: 15-20 mg/kg/day divided tid-qid x 90 days; 11-16 years: 12.5-15 mg/kg/day divided tid-qid x 90 days; ≥17 years: 8-10 mg/kg/day divided tid-qid x 90 days
Comment: Common side effects of **nifurtimox** are anorexia and weight loss, nausea, vomiting, polyneuropathy, headache, and dizziness or vertigo. **Nifurtimox** is contraindicated in patients who have taken **disulfiram** within the previous 2 weeks due to the potential for a psychotic reaction. Alcohol beverages and any product containing propylene glycol are contraindicated from 2 weeks before initiating the first dose of **nifurtimox**, throughout treatment, and the first 3 days after the last dose of **nifurtimox** to prevent a **disulfiram**-like reaction (e.g., flushing, headache, abdominal cramping, and nausea/vomiting).
　Lampit *Weight-based dosing:* ≥40 kg: 8-10 mg/kg divided tid x 60 days; <40 kg: 10-20 mg/kg divided tid x 60 days; take with food; obtain a pregnancy test in females of reproductive potential prior to initiating treatment
　　Tab: 30*, 120*mg
　Comment: Lampit is a nitrofuran antiprotozoal indicated in pediatric patients (term newborn to <18 years of age and weighing at least 2.5 kg) for the treatment of Chagas disease (*American Trypanosomiasis*) caused by *T. cruzi*. The most frequently reported adverse reactions (incidence ≥5%) have been vomiting, abdominal pain, headache, decreased appetite, nausea, pyrexia, and rash. *Renal and/or Hepatic Impairment:* Administer under close medical supervision.

CHANCROID

ANTI-INFECTIVES

▷ **azithromycin (G)** 500 mg x 1 dose on day 1, then 250 mg daily on days 2-5 or 500 mg daily x 3 days or **Zmax** 2 gm in a single dose
　Pediatric: 12 mg/kg/day x 5 days; max 500 mg/day; *see Appendix BB.7. azithromycin (G) (Zithromax Suspension, Zmax Suspension) for dose by weight*

      Zithromax *Tab:* 250, 500, 600 mg; *Oral susp:* 100 mg/5 ml (15 ml), 200 mg/5 ml (15, 22.5, 30 ml) (cherry); *Pkt:* 1 gm for reconstitution (cherry-banana)

      Zithromax Tri-Pak *Tab:* 3 x 500 mg tabs/pck

      Zithromax Z-Pak *Tab:* 6 x 250 mg tabs/pck

      Zmax *Oral susp:* 2 gm ext-rel for reconstitution (cherry-banana) (148 mg Na⁺)

➢ *ceftriaxone* (G) 250 mg IM in a single dose

    Pediatric: <45 kg: 125 mg IM in a single dose; ≥45 kg: same as adult

      Rocephin *Vial:* 250, 500 mg; 1, 2 gm

➢ *ciprofloxacin* 500 mg bid x 3 days

    Pediatric: <18 years: <u>not</u> recommended; ≥18 years: same as adult

      Cipro *Tab:* 250, 500, 750 mg; *Oral susp:* 250, 500 mg/5 ml (100 ml) (strawberry)

      Cipro XR *Tab:* 500, 1,000 mg ext-rel

      ProQuin XR *Tab:* 500 mg ext-rel

➢ *erythromycin base* (G) 500 mg qid x 7 days

    Pediatric: 30-50 mg/kg/day divided bid-qid; max 100 mg/kg/day

      Ery-Tab *Tab:* 250, 333, 500 mg ent-coat

      PCE *Tab:* 333, 500 mg

➢ *erythromycin ethylsuccinate* (G) 400 mg qid x 7 days

    Pediatric: 30-50 mg/kg/day in 4 divided doses x 7 days; may double dose with severe infection; max 100 mg/kg/day; *see Appendix BB.21. erythromycin ethylsuccinate* (G) (E.E.S. Suspension, EryPed Drops/ Suspension) *for dose by weight*

      EryPed *Oral susp:* 200 mg/5 ml (100, 200 ml) (fruit), 400 mg/5 ml (60, 100, 200 ml) (banana); *Oral drops:* 200, 400 mg/5 ml (50 ml) (fruit); *Chew tab:* 200 mg wafer (fruit)

      E.E.S. *Oral susp:* 200, 400 mg/5 ml (100 ml) (fruit)

      E.E.S. Granules *Oral susp:* 200 mg/5 ml (100, 200 ml) (cherry)

      E.E.S. 400 Tablets *Tab:* 400 mg

CHEMOTHERAPY-INDUCED NAUSEA/VOMITING (CINV)

PHENOTHIAZINES

➢ *chlorpromazine* (G) 10-25 mg PO q 4 hours prn <u>or</u> 50-100 mg rectally q 6-8 hours prn

    Pediatric: <6 months: <u>not</u> recommended; ≥6 months: 0.25 mg/lb orally q 4-6 hours prn <u>or</u> 0.5 mg/lb rectally q 6-8 hours prn; >12 years: same as adult

      Thorazine *Tab:* 10, 25, 50, 100, 200 mg; *Spansule:* 30, 75, 150 mg sust-rel; *Syr:* 10 mg/5 ml (4 oz; orange custard); *Conc:* 30 mg/ml (4 oz), 100 mg/ml (2, 8 oz); *Supp:* 25, 100 mg

➢ *perphenazine* 5 mg IM (may repeat in 6 hours) <u>or</u> 8-16 mg/day PO in divided doses; max 15 mg/day IM; max 24 mg/day PO

    Pediatric: <12 years: <u>not</u> recommended; ≥12 years: same as adult

      Trilafon *Tab:* 2, 4, 8, 16 mg; *Oral conc:* 16 mg/5 ml (118 ml); *Amp:* 5 mg/ml (1 ml)

➢ *prochlorperazine* (G) 5-10 mg tid-qid prn; usual max 40 mg/day

      Compazine

    Pediatric: <2 years <u>or</u> <20 lb: <u>not</u> recommended; 20-29 lb: 2.5 mg daily bid prn; max 7.5 mg/day; 30-39 lb: 2.5 mg bid-tid prn; max 10 mg/day; 40-85 lb: 2.5 mg tid <u>or</u> 5 mg bid prn; max 15 mg/day; >85 lb: same as adult

      Tab: 5, 10 mg; *Syr:* 5 mg/5 ml (4 oz) (fruit)

      Compazine Suppository 25 mg rectally bid prn; usual max 50 mg/day

    Pediatric: <2 years <u>or</u> <20 lb: <u>not</u> recommended; 20-29 lb: 2.5 mg daily-bid prn; max 7.5; mg/day; 30-39 lb: 2.5 mg bid-tid prn; max 10 mg/day; 40-85 lb: 2.5 mg tid <u>or</u> 5 mg bid prn; max 15 mg/day; >85 lb: same as adult

      Rectal supp: 2.5, 5, 25 mg

      Compazine Injectable 5-10 mg tid <u>or</u> qid prn

    Pediatric: <2 years <u>or</u> <20 lb: <u>not</u> recommended; ≥2 years <u>or</u> ≥20 lb: 0.06 mg/kg x 1 dose; >12 years: same as adult

      Vial: 5 mg/ml (2, 10 ml)

      Compazine Spansule 15 mg q AM prn <u>or</u> 10 mg q 12 hours prn; usual max 40 mg/day

    Pediatric: <12 years: <u>not</u> recommended; ≥12 years: same as adult

      Spansule: 10, 15 mg sust-rel

➢ *promethazine* (G) 25 mg PO <u>or</u> rectally q 4-6 hours prn

    Pediatric: <2 years: <u>not</u> recommended; ≥2 years: 0.5 mg/lb <u>or</u> 6.25-25 mg every 4-6 hours prn; >12 years: same as adult

      Phenergan *Tab:* 12.5*, 25*, 50 mg; *Plain syr:* 6.25 mg/5 ml; *Fortis syr:* 25 mg/5 ml; *Rectal supp:* 12.5, 25, 50 mg

Comment: *Promethazine* is contraindicated in children with uncomplicated nausea, dehydration, Reye's syndrome, history of sleep apnea, asthma, and lower respiratory disorders in children. *Promethazine* lowers the seizure threshold in children and may cause cholestatic jaundice, anticholinergic effects, extrapyramidal effects, and potentially fatal respiratory depression.

SUBSTANCE P/NEUROKININ-1 (NK-1) RECEPTOR ANTAGONIST

▶ *aprepitant* (G) administer with corticosteroid and 5-HT3 receptor antagonist; *Day 1 of chemotherapy cycle:* 125 mg 1 hour prior to chemotherapy; *Days 2 and 3:* 80 mg in the morning
Pediatric: <6 months: years: not recommended; ≥6 months-12 years: use oral suspension (see mfr pkg insert for dose by weight); >12 years: same as adult
   Emend *Cap:* 40, 80, 125 mg (2 x 80 mg bifold pck; 1 x 25 mg/2 x 80 mg trifold pck); *Oral susp:* 125 mg pwdr for oral suspension, single-dose pouch w. dispenser; *Vial:* 150 mg pwdr for reconstitution and IV infusion

SUBSTANCE P/NK-1 RECEPTOR ANTAGONIST AND SEROTONIN-3 (5-HT3) RECEPTOR ANTAGONIST COMBINATION

▶ *fosnetupitant+palonosetron*
   Comment: Akynzeo capsules and Akynzeo for Injection are indicated in combination with *dexamethasone* for the prevention of acute and delayed nausea and vomiting associated with initial and repeat courses of cancer chemotherapy. The most common adverse reactions (incidence ≥3%) are headache, asthenia, dyspepsia, fatigue, constipation, and erythema. Avoid concomitant CYP3A4 substrates for 1 week; if not avoidable, consider dose reduction of the CYP3A4 substrate because inhibition of CYP3A4 by *netupitant* can result in increased plasma concentrations of the concomitant drug for 6 days after single dosage administration of Akynzeo. CYP3A4 inducers (e.g., *rifampin*) decrease plasma concentrations of *netupitant.*
   Pediatric: <18 years: not recommended; ≥18 years: same as adult
      Akynzeo administer a single dose approximately 1 hour prior to the start of chemotherapy, with or without food, with concurrent administration of *dexamethasone* 12 mg; on days 2-4, omit *dexamethasone*
         Cap: netu 300 mg+palo 0.5 mg
      Akynzeo for Injection reconstitute in 50 ml of D₅0.9% NaCl and administer via IV infusion over 30 minutes starting approximately 30 minutes prior to the start of chemotherapy with concurrent administration of *dexamethasone* 12 mg; on days 2-4, decrease *dexamethasone* to 8 mg each day
         Vial: fosn 235 mg+palo 0.25 mg single-dose pwdr for reconstitution and IV infusion

5-HT3 RECEPTOR ANTAGONISTS

Comment: The selective 5-HT3 receptor antagonists are indicated for prevention of nausea and vomiting associated with moderately to highly emetogenic chemotherapy.
▶ *dolasetron* Administer 100 mg IV over 30 seconds, 30 minutes prior to administration of chemotherapy or 2 hours before surgery; Max 100 mg/dose
   Pediatric: <2 years: not recommended; 2-16 years: 1.8 mg/kg; >16 years: same as adult
      Anzemet *Tab:* 50, 100 mg; *Amp:* 12.5 mg(0.625) ml; *Prefilled carpuject syringe:* 12.5 mg (0.625 ml); *Vial:* 100 mg/5 ml (single-use); *Vial:* 500 mg/25 ml (multi-dose)
▶ *granisetron*
      Kytril *Administer* 10 mcg/kg as a single dose; administer IV over 30 seconds, 30 minutes prior to administration of chemotherapy; max 1 dose/week
      Pediatric: <2 years: not recommended; ≥2 years: same as adult
         Tab: 1 mg; *Oral soln:* 2 mg/10 ml (30 ml; orange); *Vial:* 1 mg/ml (1 ml, single-dose) (preservative-free); 1 mg/ml (4 ml multidose) (benzyl alcohol)
      Sancuso apply 1 patch 24-48 hours before chemo; remove 24 hours (minimum) to 7 days (maximum) after completion of treatment
      Pediatric: <2 years: not recommended; ≥2 years: same as adult
         Transdermal patch: 3.1 mg/day
▶ *granisetron extended release injection* Administer SC over 20-30 seconds (due to drug viscosity) on Day 1 of chemotherapy and not more frequently than once every 7 days; *CrCl 30-59 ml/min:* repeat dose no more than every 14th day; *CrCl <30 ml/min:* not recommended; for patients receiving minimum effective concentration (MEC), the recommended *dexamethasone* dosage is 8 mg IV on Day 1; for patients receiving AC combination chemotherapy regimens, the recommended *dexamethasone* dosage is 20 mg IV on Day 1, followed by 8 mg PO bid on Days 2, 3, and 4; if Sustol is administered with an neurokinin-1 (NK-1) receptor antagonist, see that drug's mfr pkg insert for the recommended *dexamethasone* dosing
   Pediatric: <18 years: not recommended; ≥18 years: same as adult
      Sustol *Syringe:* 10 mg/0.4 ml ext-rel; prefilled single-dose/kit
      Comment: At least 60 minutes prior to administration, remove the Sustol kit from refrigeration; activate a warming pouch and wrap the syringe in the warming pouch for 5-6 minutes to warm it to room temperature.
▶ *ondansetron* (G) Oral Forms: *Highly Emetogenic Chemotherapy:* 24 mg x 1 dose 30 minutes prior to start of single-day chemotherapy; *Moderately Emetogenic Chemotherapy:* 8 mg q 8 hours x 2 doses beginning 30 minutes prior to start of chemotherapy; then 8 mg q 12 hours x 1-2 days following
   Pediatric: <4 years: not recommended; 4-11 years: *Moderately emetogenic chemotherapy:* 4 mg q 4 hours x 3 doses beginning 30 minutes prior to start; then 4 mg q 8 hours x 1-2 days following

Zofran *Tab:* 4, 8, 24 mg
Zofran ODT *ODT:* 4, 8 mg (strawberry) (phenylalanine)
Zofran Oral Solution *Oral soln:* 4 mg/5 ml (50 ml) (strawberry) (phenylalanine); *Parenteral form:* see mfr pkg insert
Zofran Injection *Vial:* 2 mg/ml (2 ml, single-dose), 2 mg/ml (20 ml, multidose), 32 mg/50 ml (50 ml multidose); *Prefilled syringe:* 4 mg/2 ml, single-use (24/carton)
Zuplenz Oral Soluble Film: 4, 8 mg oral-dis (10/carton) (peppermint)
Comment: The FDA has issued a warning against *ondansetron* use in pregnancy. *Ondansetron* is a 5-HT3 receptor antagonist approved by the FDA to prevent nausea and vomiting related to cancer chemotherapy and surgery. However, it has been used "off label" to treat the nausea and vomiting of pregnancy. The FDA has cautioned against the use of *ondansetron* in pregnancy in light of studies of *ondansetron* in early pregnancy and associated with congenital cardiac malformations and oral clefts (i.e., cleft lip and cleft palate). Further, there are potential maternal risks in pregnancy with electrolyte imbalance caused by severe nausea and vomiting (as with hyperemesis gravidarum). These risks include *serotonin syndrome* (a triad of cognitive and behavioral changes including confusion, agitation, autonomic instability, and neuromuscular changes). Therefore, *ondansetron* should <u>not</u> be taken during pregnancy.

▷ *palonosetron* (G) *Chemotherapy:* administer 0.25 mg IV over 30 seconds, 30 minutes prior to administration of chemo; max 1 dose/week <u>or</u> 1 cap 1 hour before chemo; *Postop:* administer 0.075 mg IV over 10 seconds immediately before induction of anesthesia
Pediatric: <1 month: <u>not</u> recommended; 1 month-17 years: 20 mcg/kg; max 1.5 mg single-dose; infuse over 15 minutes beginning 30 minutes prior to administration of chemo
Aloxi *Vial (single-use):* 0.075 mg/1.5 ml; 0.25 mg/5 ml (mannitol)

CANNABINOIDS

▷ *dronabinol* (III) Initially 5 mg/m^2 administer 1-3 hours before chemotherapy; Then q 2-4 hours prn; Max 4-6 doses/day, 15 mg/m^2
Pediatric: <18 years: <u>not</u> recommended; ≥18 years: same as adult
Marinol *Cap:* 2.5, 5, 10 mg (sesame seed oil)
▷ *nabilone* (II) 1-2 mg bid; max 6 mg/day in 3 divided doses; initially 1-3 hours before chemotherapy; may give 1-2 mg the night before chemo; may continue 48 hours after each chemo cycle
Pediatric: <18 years: <u>not</u> recommended; ≥18 years: same as adult
Cesamet *Cap:* 1 mg (sesame seed oil)

CHICKENPOX (VARICELLA)

PROPHYLAXIS
▷ *Varicella virus* vaccine, live, attenuated
Varivax 0.5 ml SC; repeat 4-8 weeks later
Pediatric: <12 months: <u>not</u> recommended; 12 months-12 years: 1 dose of 0.5 ml SC; repeat 4-6 weeks later
Vial: 1350 PFU/0.5 ml single-dose w. diluent (preservative-free)
Comment: Administer **Varivax** SC in the deltoid for adults and children.

IMMUNE GLOBULIN
▷ *immune globulin (human)* administer via IM injection <u>only</u> (<u>never</u> IV); ensure adequate hydration prior to administration
Household and Institutional Varicella Case Contacts: promptly administer 0.6-1.2 ml/kg IM as a single dose (if Varicella-Zoster Immune Globulin [Human] is unavailable)
Planned Travel to Varicella Endemic Area: administer 0.6-1.2 ml/kg as a single dose at least 6 days prior to travel (if Varicella-Zoster Immune Globulin (Human) is unavailable
Pediatric: 0.25 ml/kg IM (0.5 ml/kg in immunocompromised children)
GamaSTAN S/D *Vial:* 2, 10 ml single-dose
Comment: GamaSTAN S/D is the <u>only</u> *gamma globulin* product FDA-approved for measles and HAV post-exposure prophylaxis (PEP). **GamaSTAN S/D** is also FDA-approved for varicella PEP. Other **GamaSTAN S/D** indications: to prevent <u>or</u> modify measles in a susceptible person exposed fewer than 6 days previously; to modify varicella; and to modify rubella in exposed females who will <u>not</u> consider a therapeutic abortion. **GamaSTAN S/D** is <u>not</u> indicated for routine prophylaxis <u>or</u> treatment of viral hepatitis B, rubella, poliomyelitis, mumps, <u>or</u> varicella. Contraindications to **GamaSTAN S/D** include persons with cancer, chronic liver disease, and persons allergic to *gamma globulin*, the HAV vaccine, <u>or</u> a component of the HAV vaccine. Dosage is higher for HAV PEP than for measles and varicella PEP based on recently observed decreasing concentrations of HAV antibodies in **GamaSTAN S/D**, attributed to the decreasing prevalence of previous HAV infection among plasma donors.

TREATMENT
Antipyretics *see Fever*
Infants and young children: No aspirin

ORAL ANTIPRURITICS

▷ *diphenhydramine* (OTC)(G) 25-50 mg q 6-8 hours; max 100 mg/day
  Pediatric: <2 years: <u>not</u> recommended; 2-6 years: 6.25 mg q 4-6 hours, max 37.5 mg/day; >6-12 years: 12.5-25 mg q 4-6 hours, max 150 mg/day; >12 years: same as adult
    Benadryl (OTC) *Chew tab:* 12.5 mg (grape; phenylalanine); *Liq:* 12.5 mg/5 ml (4, 8 oz); *Cap:* 25 mg; *Tab:* 25 mg; *Dye-free soft gel:* 25 mg; *Dye-free liq:* 12.5 mg/5 ml (4, 8 oz)

▷ *hydroxyzine* (G) 50-100 mg qid; max 600 mg/day
  Pediatric: <6 years: 50 mg/day divided qid; ≥6 years: 50-100 mg/day divided qid
    Atarax *Tab:* 10, 25, 50, 100 mg; *Syr:* 10 mg/5 ml (alcohol 0.5%)
    Vistaril *Cap:* 25, 50, 100 mg; *Oral susp:* 25 mg/5 ml (4 oz) (lemon)

ANTIVIRALS

▷ *acyclovir* (G) 800 mg qid x 5 days
  Pediatric: <2 years: <u>not</u> recommended; ≥2 years, <40 kg: 20 mg/kg qid x 5 days; ≥2 years, >40 kg: 800 mg qid x 5 days; *see Appendix BB.1. ayclovir* (Zovirax Suspension) *for dose by weight*
    Zovirax *Cap:* 200 mg; *Tab:* 400, 800 mg
    Zovirax Oral Suspension *Oral susp:* 200 mg/5 ml (banana)

CHIKUNGUNYA VIRUS/CHIKUNGUNYA-RELATED ARTHRITIS

Comment: Chikungunya is a mosquito-borne viral disease first described during an outbreak in southern Tanzania in 1952. It is an RNA virus that belongs to the alphavirus genus of the family Togaviridae. The name "chikungunya" derives from a word in the Kimakonde language, meaning "to become contorted," and describes the stooped appearance of sufferers with joint pain (arthralgia). Acute infection with *chikungunya virus* is associated with fever, rash, headache, and muscle and joint pain, with outbreaks having been reported in Africa, Asia, the Indian and Pacific Ocean islands, and Europe. In 2013, for the first time the virus was first detected in the Caribbean region, and more than 1.2 million peoples in the Americas have now been infected. After transmission by an *Aedes aegypti* <u>or</u> *Aedes albopictus* mosquito bite, *chikungunya virus* undergoes local replication and then dissemination to lymphoid tissue," the researchers explained. Viremia is detectable for <u>only</u> 5 to 12 days, but animal studies have indicated that the virus can be found in lymphoid organs, joints, and muscles for several months and that viral RNA can be detected in muscle, liver, and spleen for long periods. However, it is <u>not</u> known whether the remnants of the virus actually persist in humans and if so whether this can be causatively linked with chronic arthritis, which has implications for treatment. With no evidence of viral persistence, potential mechanisms for arthritis included epigenetic changes to host DNA, as has been observed with *Epstein Barr virus* infection, modification of macrophages, and molecular mimicry. There is currently <u>no</u> cure and <u>no</u> standard treatment for acute *chikungunya virus* infection <u>or</u> chikungunya-related arthritis. However, various immunosuppressants such as **methotrexate** (MTX) and **hydroxychloroquine** and biologics such as **adalimumab** (Humira) and **etanercept** (Enbrel) have been tried, despite concerns of renewed viral replication in the synovium and relapse of systemic viral infection. However, no relapses have been reported, and the lack of evidence of viral persistence in the joint seen in this analysis may provide some reassurance that treatment with immunosuppressant antirheumatic medications 2 years after infection is a viable option.

CHLAMYDIA TRACHOMATIS

Comment: The following treatment regimens for *Chlamydia trachomatis* are published in the **2021 CDC Sexually Transmitted Diseases Treatment Guidelines**. Treatment regimens are presented by generic drug name first, followed by information about brands and dose forms. Treat all sexual contacts. Patients who are HIV-positive should receive the same treatment as those who are HIV-negative. Sexual abuse must be considered a cause of chlamydial infection in preadolescent children, although perinatally transmitted *C. trachomatis* infections of the nasopharynx, urogenital tract, and rectum may persist for >1 year.

RECOMMENDED REGIMENS: ADOLESCENT AND >18 YEARS, NON-PREGNANT
Regimen 1

▷ *azithromycin* 1 gm in a single dose

Regimen 2

▷ *doxycycline* 100 mg bid x 7 days

ALTERNATIVE REGIMENS: ADOLESCENT AND ADULT, NON-PREGNANT
Regimen 1

▷ *erythromycin base* 500 mg qid x 7 days

Regimen 2

▷ *erythromycin ethylsuccinate* 800 mg qid x 7 days

Regimen 3
▷ *levofloxacin* 500 mg once daily x 7 days

Regimen 4
▷ *ofloxacin* 300 mg bid x 7 days

RECOMMENDED REGIMENS: PREGNANCY
Regimen 1
▷ *azithromycin* 1 gm in a single dose

Regimen 2
▷ *amoxicillin* 500 mg tid x 7 days

ALTERNATE REGIMENS: PREGNANCY
Regimen 1
▷ *erythromycin base* 500 mg qid x 7 days

Regimen 2
▷ *erythromycin base* 250 mg qid x 14 days

Regimen 3
▷ *erythromycin ethylsuccinate* 800 mg qid x 7 days

Regimen 4
▷ *erythromycin ethylsuccinate* 400 mg qid x 14 days

ALTERNATE REGIMENS: CHILDREN (>8 YEARS)
Regimen 1
▷ *azithromycin* 1 gm in a single dose

Regimen 2
▷ *doxycycline* 100 mg bid x 7 days

ALTERNATE REGIMEN: CHILDREN (>45 KG; <8 YEARS)
Regimen 1
▷ *azithromycin* 1 gm in a single dose

ALTERNATE REGIMENS: INFANTS
Regimen 1
▷ *erythromycin base* 50 mg/kg/day in divided doses qid x 14 days

Regimen 2
▷ *erythromycin ethylsuccinate* 50 mg/kg/day divided qid x 14 days

DRUG BRANDS AND DOSE FORMS
▷ *azithromycin* (G) 500 mg x 1 dose on day 1, then 250 mg daily on days 2-5 <u>or</u> 500 mg daily x 3 days <u>or</u> Zmax 2 gm in a single dose
   Pediatric: 12 mg/kg/day x 5 days; max 500 mg/day; *see Appendix BB.7. azithromycin* (G) (Zithromax Suspension, Zmax Suspension) *for dose by weight*
      Zithromax *Tab:* 250, 500, 600 mg; *Oral susp:* 100 mg/5 ml (15 ml), 200 mg/5 ml (15, 22.5, 30 ml) (cherry); *Pkt:* 1 gm for reconstitution (cherry-banana)
      Zithromax Tri-Pak *Tab:* 3 x 500 mg tabs/pck
      Zithromax Z-Pak *Tab:* 6 x 250 mg tabs/pck
      Zmax *Oral susp:* 2 gm ext-rel for reconstitution (cherry-banana) (148 mg Na⁺)
▷ *doxycycline* (G)
      Acticlate *Tab:* 75, 150**mg
      Adoxa *Tab:* 50, 75, 100, 150 mg ent-coat
      Doryx *Tab:* 50, 75, 100, 150, 200 mg del-rel
      Doxteric *Tab:* 50 mg del-rel
      Monodox *Cap:* 50, 75, 100 mg
      Oracea *Cap:* 40 mg del-rel
      Vibramycin *Tab:* 100 mg; *Cap:* 50, 100 mg; *Syr:* 50 mg/5 ml (raspberry-apple) (sulfites); *Oral susp:* 25 mg/5 ml (raspberry)
      Vibra-Tab *Tab:* 100 mg film-coat

(*continued*)

▷ *erythromycin base* (G)
    Ery-Tab *Tab:* 250, 333, 500 mg ent-coat
    PCE *Tab:* 333, 500 mg
▷ *erythromycin ethylsuccinate* (G)
    EryPed *Oral susp:* 200 mg/5 ml (100, 200 ml) (fruit), 400 mg/5 ml (60, 100, 200 ml) (banana); *Oral drops:* 200, 400 mg/5 ml (50 ml) (fruit); *Chew tab:* 200 mg wafer (fruit)
    E.E.S. *Oral susp:* 200, 400 mg/5 ml (100 ml) (fruit)
    E.E.S. Granules *Oral susp:* 200 mg/5 ml (100, 200 ml) (cherry)
    E.E.S. 400 Tablets *Tab:* 400 mg
▷ *levofloxacin*
    Levaquin *Tab:* 250, 500, 750 mg
▷ *ofloxacin* (G)
    Floxin *Tab:* 200, 300, 400 mg

CHOLANGITIS, PRIMARY BILIARY (PBC)

Comment: Monitor intensity of pruritis and administer antihistamines as appropriate for dermal pruritis. Ocaliva (*obeticholic acid*), a farnesoid X receptor (FXR) agonist, is indicated for the treatment of primary biliary cholangitis (PBC), in combination with *ursodeoxycholic acid* (UDCA), in adults with an inadequate response to UDCA, or as monotherapy in adults unable to tolerate UDCA. This indication is approved under accelerated approval based on a reduction in alkaline phosphatase (ALP). An improvement in survival or disease-related symptoms has not been established. Continued approval for this indication may be contingent upon verification and description of clinical benefit in confirmatory trials.

FARNESOID X RECEPTOR (FXR) AGONIST

▷ *obeticholic acid* initially 5 mg once daily (this lower starting dose is recommended to reduce pruritis); then after 3 months of treatment, if an adequate reduction in ALP and/or total bilirubin is not achieved, and if the patient is tolerating the drug, increase the dose to 10 mg once daily; take with or without food
Pediatric: <18 years: not recommended; ≥18 years: same as adult
    Ocaliva *Tab:* 5, 10 mg
    Comment: Ocaliva is contraindicated in patients with complete biliary obstruction. If this complication develops, discontinue Ocaliva. Because PBC management strategies include bile acid binding resin (e.g., *cholestyramine, colestipol, or colesevelam*), concurrent use with *obeticholic acid* should be separated by at least 4 hours. Concurrent use of *obeticholic acid* and *warfarin* may reduce the international normalized ratio (INR); monitor INR and adjust the *warfarin* dose as necessary. Monitor concentrations of CYP1A2 substrates with a narrow therapeutic index (e.g., *theophylline* and *tizanidine*) as *obeticholic acid* is a CYP1A2 inhibitor. Reduce the dose of Ocaliva in patients with moderate or severe hepatic impairment, and monitor liver function tests (LFTs) and lipid levels (especially reduction in high-density lipoprotein [HDL]).

URSODEOXYCHOLIC ACID (UDCA)

▷ *ursodeoxycholic acid* (UDCA) (G) in the first 3 months of treatment, the total daily dose should be divided tid (morning, midday, evening); as liver function values improve, the total daily dose may be taken once a day at bedtime (see mfr pkg insert for dose table based on kilogram weight); monitor hepatic function every 4 weeks for the first 3 months; then monitor hepatic function once every 3 months
Pediatric: same as adult
    Ursofalk *Tab:* 500 mg film-coat; *Cap:* 250 mg; *Oral susp:* 250 mg/5 ml
    Comment: *Ursodeoxycholic acid* (UDCA) is indicated for dissolution of cholesterol gallstones that are radiolucent (not visible on plain x-ray), ≤15 mm, and the gall bladder must still be functioning despite the gallstones.

BILE ACID BINDING RESINS

Comment: This drug class may produce or severely worsen preexisting constipation. The dosage should be increased gradually in patients to minimize the risk of developing fecal impaction. Increased fluid and fiber intake should be encouraged to alleviate constipation, and a stool softener may occasionally be indicated. If the initial dose is well tolerated, the dose may be increased as needed by 1 dose/day (at monthly intervals) with periodic monitoring of serum lipoproteins. If constipation worsens or the desired therapeutic response is not achieved at 1 to 6 doses/day, combination therapy or alternate therapy should be considered. Bile acid sequestrants may decrease absorption of fat-soluble vitamins. Use caution in patients susceptible to fat-soluble vitamin deficiencies.

▷ *cholestyramine* (G) *Starting Dose:* 1 packet or 1 scoopful of powder once daily for 5-7 days; Then, increase to bid with monitoring of constipation and of serum lipoproteins, at least twice, 4 to 6 weeks apart; empty one packet into a glass or cup; add 1/2 to 1 cup (4 to 8 ounces) of water, fruit juice, or diet soft drink; stir well and drink immediately; do not swallow dry form; Take with meals

Pediatric: 240 mg/kg/day of anhydrous cholestyramine resin in two to three divided doses, normally not to exceed 8 gm/day, with dose titration based on response and tolerance

> **Prevalite** *Pwdr:* 4 gm/pkt, 4 gm/scoopful (1 level tsp) for oral suspension

▶ **colestipol (G)** *Starting Dose Tabs:* 2 gm once or twice daily; then increases should occur at 1- or 2-month intervals; usual dose is 2-16 gm/day given once daily or in divided doses; *Starting Dose Granules:* 1 packet or 1 scoopful (1 level tsp) of granules once daily for 5-7 days, increasing to bid with monitoring of constipation and of serum lipoproteins, at least twice, 4-6 weeks apart; empty 1 packet or 1 scoopful (1 level tsp) of granules into a glass or cup; add 1/2 to 1 cup (4-8 oz) of water, fruit juice, or diet soft drink; stir well and drink immediately; do not swallow dry form; take with meals

Pediatric: <12 years: not established; ≥12 years: same as adult

> **Colestid** *Tab:* 1 gm; *Granules:* 5 gm/pkt, 5 gm/scoopful (1 level tsp) for oral suspension
> **Flavored Colestid** *Granules:* 5 gm/pkt, 5 gm/scoopful (1 level tsp) for oral suspension (orange)

▶ **colesevelam (G)**

> **WelChol** recommended dose is 6 tablets once daily or 3 tablets bid; Take with a meal and liquid

Pediatric: <10 years: not recommended; ≥10 years: same as adult

> *Tab:* 625 mg

> **WelChol for Oral Suspension** recommended dose is one 3.75 gm packet once daily or one 1.875 gm packet bid; empty 1 packet into a glass or cup; add 1/2 to 1 cup (4-8 oz) of water, fruit juice, or diet soft drink; stir well and drink immediately; do not swallow dry form; take with meals

Pediatric: <12 years: not established; ≥12 years: same as adult

> *Pwdr:* 3.75 gm/pkt (30 pkt/carton), 1.875 gm/pkt (60 pkt/carton) for oral suspension

Comment: WelChol is indicated as adjunctive therapy to improve glycemic control in adults with type 2 diabetes. It can be added to ***metformin***, sulfonylureas, or insulin alone or in combination with other antidiabetic agents.

CHOLELITHIASIS

▶ *ursodeoxycholic acid* (UDCA) **(G)** in the first 3 months of treatment, the total daily dose should be divided tid (morning, midday, evening); as liver function values improve, the total daily dose may be taken once a day at bedtime (see mfr pkg insert for dose table based on kilogram weight); monitor hepatic function every 4 weeks for the first 3 months; then monitor hepatic function once every 3 months

Pediatric: same as adult

> **Ursofalk** *Tab:* 500 mg film-coat; *Cap:* 250 mg; *Oral susp:* 250 mg/5 ml

Comment: *Ursodeoxycholic acid* (UDCA) is indicated for dissolution of gallstones that are radiolucent (not visible on plain x-ray), ≤15 mm, and the gall bladder must still be functioning despite the gallstones

▶ *ursodiol* 8-10 mg/kg/day in 2-3 divided doses

Pediatric: <12 years: not recommended; ≥12 years: same as adult

> **Actigall** *Cap:* 300 mg

> **Comment:** Actigall is indicated for dissolution of radiolucent, non-calciferous, gallstones <20 mm in diameter and for prevention of gallstones during rapid weight loss.

BILE ACID BINDING RESINS

Comment: This drug class may produce or severely worsen preexisting constipation. The dosage should be increased gradually in patients to minimize the risk of developing fecal impaction. Increased fluid and fiber intake should be encouraged to alleviate constipation, and a stool softener may occasionally be indicated. If the initial dose is well tolerated, the dose may be increased as needed by 1 dose/day (at monthly intervals) with periodic monitoring of serum lipoproteins. If constipation worsens or the desired therapeutic response is not achieved at 1-6 doses/day, combination therapy or alternate therapy should be considered. Bile acid sequestrants may decrease absorption of fat-soluble vitamins. Use caution in patients susceptible to fat-soluble vitamin deficiencies.

▶ *cholestyramine* **(G)** *Starting Dose:* 1 packet or 1 scoopful of powder once daily for 5 to 7 days; then increase to bid with monitoring of constipation and of serum lipoproteins, at least twice, 4 to 6 weeks apart; empty 1 packet into a glass or cup; add 1/2 to 1 cup (4-8 oz) of water, fruit juice, or diet soft drink; stir well and drink immediately; Do not swallow dry form; Take with meals

Pediatric: <12 years: 240 mg/kg/day of anhydrous cholestyramine resin in 2-3 divided doses, normally not to exceed 8 gm/day, with dose titration based on response and tolerance

> **Prevalite** *Pwdr:* 4 gm/pkt, 4 gm/scoopful (1 level tsp) for oral suspension

▶ *colestipol* **(G)** *Starting Dose Tabs:* 2 gm once or twice daily; then increases should occur at 1- or 2-month intervals; usual dose is 2–16 gm/day given once daily or in divided doses; *Starting Dose Granules:* 1 packet or 1 scoopful (1 level tsp) of granules once daily for 5-7 days, increasing to bid with monitoring of constipation and of serum lipoproteins, at least twice, 4-6 weeks apart; empty 1 packet or 1 scoopful (1 level tsp) of granules into a glass or cup; add 1/2 to 1 cup (4-8 oz) of water, fruit juice, or diet soft drink; stir well and drink immediately; do not swallow dry form; take with meals

Pediatric: <12 years: not established; ≥12 years: same as adult

> **Colestid** *Tab:* 1 gm; *Granules:* 5 gm/pkt, 5 gm/scoopful (1 level tsp) for oral suspension
> **Flavored Colestid** *Granules:* 5 gm/pkt, 5 gm/scoopful (1 level tsp) for oral suspension (orange)

(continued)

▷ *colesevelam* (G)

WelChol recommended dose is 6 tablets once daily <u>or</u> 3 tablets bid; take with a meal and liquid
Pediatric: <10 years: <u>not</u> recommended; ≥10 years: same as adult
  Tab: 625 mg
WelChol for Oral Suspension recommended dose is one 3.75 gm packet once daily <u>or</u> one 1.875 gm packet
bid; empty 1 packet into a glass <u>or</u> cup; add 1/2 to 1 cup (4-8 oz) of water, fruit juice, <u>or</u> diet soft drink; stir
well and drink immediately; do <u>not</u> swallow dry form; take with meals
Pediatric: <12 years: <u>not</u> established; ≥12 years: same as adult
  Pwdr: 3.75 gm/pkt (30 pkt/carton), 1.875 gm/pkt (60 pkt/carton) for oral suspension
Comment: WelChol is indicated as adjunctive therapy to improve glycemic control in adults with type 2 diabetes.
It can be added to **metformin**, sulfonylureas, <u>or</u> insulin alone <u>or</u> in combination with other antidiabetic agents.

CHOLESTASIS

ILEAL BILE ACID TRANSPORTER (IBAT) INHIBITOR

▷ *odevixibat* Recommended Dose: 40 mcg/kg once daily in the morning with a meal; If there is <u>no</u>
improvement in pruritus after 3 months, the dose may be increased in 40 mcg/kg increments up to 120 mcg/
kg once daily, <u>not</u> to exceed a total daily dose of 6 mg; For patients taking bile acid binding resins, take **Bylvay**
at least 4 hours before <u>or</u> 4 hours after taking a bile acid binding resin; bile acid binding resins may bind
odevixibat in the gut, which may reduce **Bylvay** efficacy. *Capsules:* Do <u>not</u> crush <u>or</u> chew capsules; Swallow
capsules whole with a glass of water; Alternatively, for patients unable to swallow the capsules whole, **Bylvay**
capsules may be opened and sprinkled and mixed with a small amount of soft food; follow directions for
oral pellets to prepare and administer such a mixture *Oral Pellets:* Mix the contents of the shell containing
oral pellet(s) into soft food; Do <u>not</u> mix **Bylvay** in liquids; Do <u>not</u> swallow the shell containing oral pellets;
Patients who are exclusively on liquid food should <u>not</u> use **Bylvay**; Place a small amount of soft food (up to 30
ml [2 tbsp] of apple sauce, oatmeal, banana <u>or</u> carrot puree, chocolate <u>or</u> rice pudding) in a bowl; Keep food
at <u>or</u> below room temperature; Open the shell containing the oral pellet(s) and empty the contents into the
bowl of soft food; Gently tap the oral pellet shell to ensure that all contents have been dispersed; If the dose
requires more than one shell of oral pellets, repeat the process; Gently mix until the pellets are well dispersed
and administer the entire dose immediately; Follow the dose with water; Do <u>not</u> store mixture for future use
Pediatric: <3 months: safety and efficacy <u>not</u> established; >3 months: same as adult
  Bylvay *Caps:* 400, 1200 mcg; *Oral Pellets:* 200, 600 mcg
  Comment: Bylvay is an ileal bile acid transporter (IBAT) inhibitor indicated for the treatment of pruritus
  in patients ≥3 months of age with progressive familial intrahepatic cholestasis (PFIC). **Bylvay** may <u>not</u>
  be effective in PFIC type 2 patients with ABCB11 gene variants resulting in non-functional <u>or</u> complete
  absence of bile salt export pump protein (BSEP-3). (Note: The ABCB11 gene provides instructions for
  making a protein called the bile salt export pump (BSEP), which is found in the liver.) The most common
  adverse reactions (incidence >2%) have been liver test abnormalities, diarrhea, abdominal pain, vomiting,
  and fat-soluble vitamin (FSV) deficiency. Obtain baseline liver tests and monitor during treatment; dose
  reduction <u>or</u> treatment interruption may be required if abnormalities occur. For persistent <u>or</u> recurrent liver
  test abnormalities, consider treatment discontinuation. If diarrhea occurs, treat dehydration. Treatment
  interruption <u>or</u> discontinuation may be required for persistent diarrhea. FSV deficiency may occur. Obtain
  baseline levels and monitor during treatment. Supplement FSVs if deficiency is observed. If FSV deficiency
  persists <u>or</u> worsens despite FSV supplementation, discontinue treatment. Based on animal data, **Bylvay** may
  cause fetal cardiac malformations. Exclude pregnancy prior to initiating treatment with **Bylvay** and advise
  females of reproductive potential of the risk to the fetus and to use effective contraception during treatment
  with **Bylvay**. There are no data on the presence of *odevixibat* in human milk <u>or</u> effects on the breastfed
  infant. Monitor FSV levels and increase FSV intake if FSV deficiency is observed during lactation. The
  developmental and health benefits of breastfeeding should be considered along with the mother's clinical
  need for **Bylvay** and any potential adverse effects on the breastfed infant from **Bylvay** <u>or</u> from the underlying
  maternal condition.
  Swallow the capsule whole with a glass of water. Alternatively, for patients unable to swallow the capsules
  whole, **Bylvay** capsules may be opened and sprinkled and mixed with a small amount of soft food. Follow
  directions above for oral pellets to prepare and administer such a mixture.

CHOLERA (*VIBRIO CHOLERAE*)

Comment: On June 10, 2016, the FDA approved the first vaccine for the prevention of cholera caused by
serogroup O1 (the most predominant cause of cholera globally [WHO]) in adults age 18-64 years traveling
to cholera-affected areas (https://www.drugs.com/newdrugs/fda-approves-vaxchora-cholera-vaccine-live-
oral-prevent-cholera-travelers-4396.html). Vaxchora (R) is the <u>only</u> FDA-approved vaccine for the prevention
of cholera. The bacterium *Vibrio cholerae* is acquired by ingesting contaminated water <u>or</u> food and causes
nausea, vomiting, and watery diarrhea that may be mild to severe. Profuse fluid loss may cause life-threatening
dehydration if antibiotics and fluid replacement are <u>not</u> initiated promptly.

VACCINE PROPHYLAXIS

▷ *Vibrio cholerae* vaccine

Vaxchora Reconstitute the buffer component in 100 ml purified bottled water; Then add the active component (lyophilized V. cholerae CVD 103-HgR); the total dose after reconstitution is 100 ml; Instruct the patient to avoid eating or drinking fluids for 60 minutes before and after ingestion of the dose

Comment: Vaxchora is a live attenuated vaccine that is taken as a single oral dose at least 10 days before travel to a cholera-affected area and at least 10 days before starting antimalarial prophylaxis. Diminished immune response when taken concomitantly with *chloroquine*. Avoid concomitant administration with systemic antibiotics since these agents may be active against the vaccine strain. Do not administer to patients who have received an oral or parenteral antibiotic within 14 days prior to vaccination. **Vaxchora** may be shed in the stool of recipients for at least 7 days. There is potential for transmission of the vaccine strain to non-vaccinated and immunocompromised close contacts. The CDC and several health professional organizations state that vaccines given to a nursing mother do not affect the safety of breastfeeding for mothers or infants and that breastfeeding is not a contraindication to cholera vaccine. **Vaxchora** is not absorbed systemically, and maternal use is not expected to result in fetal exposure to the drug. The **Vaxchora** pregnancy exposure registry for reporting adverse events is 800-533-5899. There are 0 disease interactions, but at least 165 drug-drug interactions with **Vaxchora** (see mfr pkg insert).

TREATMENT

Comment: The first-line treatment for *V. cholerae* is oral rehydration therapy (ORT) and IV fluid replacement as indicated. Antibiotic therapy may shorten the duration and severity of symptoms but is optional in other than severe cases. Although *doxycycline* is contraindicated in pregnancy and in children under 7 years of age, the benefits may outweigh the risks (WHO, CDC, UNICEF). Although *ciprofloxacin* is contraindicated in children under 18 years of age, the benefits may outweigh the risks (WHO, CDC, UNICEF). Cholera is not transmitted from person to person, but rather via the fecal–oral route. Therefore, chemoprophylaxis is not usually required with strict hand hygiene and sanitation measures and avoidance of contaminated food and water. Drugs and dosages for chemoprophylaxis are the same as for treatment.

NON-PREGNANT FEMALES ≥15 YEARS
Regimen 1

▷ *doxycycline* (G) 300 mg in a single dose
    Acticlate *Tab:* 75, 150**mg
    Adoxa *Tab:* 50, 75, 100, 150 mg ent-coat
    Doryx *Tab:* 50, 75, 100, 150, 200 mg del-rel
    Doxteric *Tab:* 50 mg del-rel
    Monodox *Cap:* 50, 75, 100 mg
    Oracea *Cap:* 40 mg del-rel
    Vibramycin *Tab:* 100 mg; *Cap:* 50, 100 mg; *Syr:* 50 mg/ml (raspberry-apple) (sulfites); *Oral susp:* 25 mg/5 ml (raspberry)
    Vibra-Tab *Tab:* 100 mg film-coat

Regimen 2

▷ *azithromycin* (G) 1,000 mg in a single dose
    Zithromax *Tab:* 250, 500, 600 mg
    Zmax *Oral susp:* 2 gm ext-rel for reconstitution (cherry-banana) (148 mg Na$^+$)
    or
▷ *ciprofloxacin* (G) 1,000 mg in a single dose
    Cipro *Tab:* 250, 500, 750 mg;
    Cipro XR *Tab:* 500, 1,000 mg ext-rel
    ProQuin XR *Tab:* 500 mg ext-rel

PREGNANT FEMALES ≥15 YEARS

▷ *azithromycin* (G) 1,000 mg in a single dose
    Zithromax *Tab:* 250, 500, 600 mg
    Zmax *Oral susp:* 2 gm ext-rel for reconstitution (cherry-banana) (148 mg Na$^+$)
    or
▷ *erythromycin* (G) 500 mg q 6 hours x 3 days
    E.E.S. 400 Tablets *Tab:* 400 mg
    Ery-Tab *Tab:* 250, 333, 500 mg ent-coat
    PCE *Tab:* 333, 500 mg

CHILDREN 3-15 YEARS WHO CAN SWALLOW TABLETS
Regimen 1

▷ *erythromycin* (G) 12.5 mg/kg q 6 hours x 3 days
    E.E.S. 400 Tablets *Tab:* 400 mg
    Ery-Tab *Tab:* 250, 333, 500 mg ent-coat

(continued)

PCE *Tab:* 333, 500 mg
or
▷ *azithromycin* (G) 20 mg/kg in a single dose; max 1 gm
Zithromax *Tab:* 250, 500, 600 mg
Zmax *Oral susp:* 2 gm ext-rel for reconstitution (cherry-banana) (148 mg Na⁺)

Regimen 2
▷ *ciprofloxacin* (G) <18 years usually not recommended; *erythromycin* or *azithromycin* preferred; consider risk/benefit; 20 mg/kg in a single dose
Cipro *Tab:* 250, 500, 750 mg;
Cipro XR *Tab:* 500, 1,000 mg ext-rel
ProQuin XR *Tab:* 500 mg ext-rel
or
▷ *doxycycline* (G) <8 years usually not recommended; *erythromycin* or *azithromycin* preferred; consider risk benefit; >8 years: 2-4 mg/kg in a single dose
Acticlate *Tab:* 75, 150**mg
Adoxa *Tab:* 50, 75, 100, 150 mg ent-coat
Doryx *Tab:* 50, 75, 100, 150, 200 mg del-rel
Doxteric *Tab:* 50 mg del-rel
Monodox *Cap:* 50, 75, 100 mg
Oracea *Cap:* 40 mg del-rel
Vibramycin *Tab:* 100 mg; *Cap:* 50, 100 mg; *Syr:* 50 mg/ml (raspberry-apple) (sulfites); *Oral susp:* 25 mg/5 ml (raspberry)
Vibra-Tab *Tab:* 100 mg film-coat

CHILDREN <3 YEARS
Regimen 1
▷ *erythromycin ethylsuccinate* (G) 12.5 mg/kg q 6 hours x 3 days; use suspension
E.E.S. *Oral susp:* 200, 400 mg/5 ml (100 ml) (fruit)
E.E.S. Granules *Oral susp:* 200 mg/5 ml (100, 200 ml) (cherry, fruit); *Chew tab:* 200 mg wafer (fruit)
EryPed *Oral susp:* 200 mg/5 ml (100, 200 ml) (fruit, 400 mg/5 ml (60, 100, 200 ml) (banana); *Oral drops:* 200, 400 mg/5 ml (50 ml) (fruit); *Chew tab:* 200 mg wafer (fruit)
or
▷ *azithromycin* (G) 20 mg/kg in a single dose; max 1 gm; use suspension
Zithromax *Tab:* 250, 500, 600 mg; *Oral susp:* 100 mg/5 ml (15 ml), 200 mg/5 ml (15, 22.5, 30 ml) (cherry)
Zmax *Oral susp:* 2 gm ext-rel for reconstitution (cherry-banana) (148 mg Na⁺)

Regimen 2
▷ *ciprofloxacin* (G) <18 years: usually not recommended; *erythromycin* or *azithromycin* preferred; consider risk benefit; 20 mg/kg in a single dose; use suspension
Cipro *Oral susp:* 250, 500 mg/5 ml (100 ml) (strawberry)
or
▷ *doxycycline* (G) <8 years: usually not recommended; *erythromycin* or *azithromycin* preferred; consider risk benefit; 2-4 mg/kg in a single dose; use suspension or syrup
Vibramycin *Syr:* 50 mg/5 ml (raspberry-apple) (sulfites); *Oral susp:* 25 mg/5 ml (raspberry)

CLOSTRIDIOIDES DIFFICILE INFECTION (CDI)/PSEUDOMEMBRANOUS COLITIS

Comment: Acid-suppressing drugs including proton pump inhibitors (PPIs), third- and fourth-generation cephalosporins, carbapenems, and *piperacillin-tazobactam* significantly increase the risk of hospital-onset *Clostridioides difficile* infection (CDI), according to the results of a recent study. Patients who received tetracyclines, macrolides, or *clindamycin* had lower risk of developing hospital-onset CDI.

MACROLIDE ANTIBACTERIAL AGENT
▷ *fidaxomicin* 200 mg bid x 10 days with or without food
Pediatric: <18 years: not established; ≥18 years: same as adult
Dificid *Tab:* 200 mg film-coat
Comment: Dificid is a macrolide antibacterial agent FDA-approved for treatment of *C. difficile*–associated diarrhea (CDAD). **Dificid** should not be used for treatment of systemic infections. Only use **Dificid** for infection proven or strongly suspected to be caused by *C. difficile*. Prescribing **Dificid** in the absence of a proven or strongly suspected *C. difficile* infection is unlikely to provide benefit to the patient and increases the risk of development of drug-resistant bacteria. Acute hypersensitivity reactions, including dyspnea, rash pruritus, and angioedema of the mouth, throat, and face, have been reported with *fidaxomicin*. If a severe hypersensitivity reaction occurs, **Dificid** should be discontinued and

appropriate therapy should be instituted. The most common adverse reactions reported in clinical trials are nausea (11%), vomiting (7%), abdominal pain (6%), gastrointestinal hemorrhage (4%), anemia (2%), and neutropenia (2%). Among patients receiving **Dificid**, 5.9% withdrew from trials as a result of adverse reactions. Vomiting was the primary adverse reaction leading to discontinuation of dosing (incidence of 0.5% for both **Dificid** and *vancomycin* patients). No dose adjustment is recommended for patients ≥65 years of age. No dose adjustment is recommended for patients with renal impairment. No dosage adjustments are recommended when co-administering *fidaxomicin* with substrates of P-gp or CYP enzymes. The impact of hepatic impairment on the pharmacokinetics of *fidaxomicin* has not been evaluated; however, because *fidaxomicin* and its active metabolite (OP-1118) do not appear to undergo significant hepatic metabolism, elimination of *fidaxomicin* and OP-1118 is not expected to be significantly affected by hepatic impairment. There are no adequate and well-controlled studies in pregnancy; **Dificid** should be used during pregnancy only if clearly needed. It is not known whether *fidaxomicin* is excreted in human milk.

GLYCOPEPTIDE ANTIBACTERIAL AGENTS

▷ *vancomycin hcl capsule* (G) 500 mg to 2 gm in 3-4 doses x 7-10 days; max 2 gm/day
    Pediatric: 40 mg/kg/day in 3-4 doses x 7-10 days; max 2 gm/day; use caps or oral solution as appropriate
        Vancocin *Cap:* 125, 250 mg

▷ *vancomycin hcl (Oral Solution)* (G) see mfr pkg insert for preparation and important administration information; <18 years: *CDAD and Staphylococcus enterocolitis:* 40 mg/kg orally in 3 or 4 divided doses x 7-10 days; total daily dosage max 2 gm; ≥18 years: *CDAD* 125 mg orally 4 qid x 10 days; *S. enterocolitis:* 500 mg to 2 gm orally in 3-4 divided doses x 7-10 days
    Firvanq *Kit w. pwdr for oral soln:* 25, 50 mg/ml (150, 300 ml) equivalent to 3.75, 7.5, 10.5, or 15 gm *vancomycin hcl*, plus grape-flavored diluent

Comment: *Vancomycin hcl*, a glycopeptide antibacterial agent, is FDA-approved for treatment of CDAD and enterocolitis caused by *S. aureus*, including methicillin-resistant strains (MRSA). *Vancomycin hcl* should be used only to treat or prevent infections that are proven or strongly suspected to be caused by susceptible bacteria. Orally administered *vancomycin hcl* is not effective for treatment of other types of infections. Prescribing *vancomycin hcl* in the absence of a proven or strongly suspected bacterial infection is unlikely to provide benefit to the patient and increases the risk of the development of drug-resistant bacteria. Nephrotoxicity has occurred following oral *vancomycin hcl* therapy and can occur either during or after completion of therapy. The risk is increased in geriatric patients. Monitor renal function. Ototoxicity has occurred in patients receiving *vancomycin hcl*. Assessment of auditory function may be appropriate in some instances. The most common adverse reactions (incidence ≥10%) have been nausea (17%), abdominal pain (15%), and hypokalemia (13%). There are no available data on **Firvanq** use in the 1st trimester of pregnancy to inform a drug-associated risk of major birth defects or miscarriage. Available published data on *vancomycin hcl* use in pregnancy during the 2nd and 3rd trimesters have not shown an association with adverse pregnancy-related outcomes. There are insufficient data to inform the levels of *vancomycin hcl* in human milk. However, systemic absorption of *vancomycin hcl* following oral administration is expected to be minimal. There are no data on the effects of **Firvanq** on the breastfed infant.

HUMAN IMMUNOGLOBULIN G1 (IGG1) MONOCLONAL ANTIBODY

Comment: *Bezlotoxumab* is a human immunoglobulin G1 (IgG1) monoclonal antibody that inhibits the binding of *C. difficile* toxin B, preventing its effects on mammalian cells. *Bezlotoxumab* does not bind to *C. difficile* toxin A. *Bezlotoxumab* is indicated to reduce the recurrence of CDI in patients who are receiving antibacterial drug treatment of CDI and are at high risk for CDI recurrence. CDI recurrence is defined as a new episode of diarrhea associated with a positive stool test for toxigenic *C. difficile* following a clinical cure of the presenting CDI episode. It is not indicated for the primary treatment of CDI infection. It is to be used only in conjunction with appropriate primary drug treatment of CDI. Patients at high risk for CDI recurrence, studied in clinical trials establishing efficacy, include those ≥65 years of age, with a history of CDI in the previous 6 months, immunocompromised state, severe CDI at presentation, and *C. difficile* ribotype 027.

▷ *bezlotoxumab* administer a single dose of 10 mg/kg via IV infusion over 60 minutes
    Pediatric: <18 years: not established; ≥18 years: same as adult
        Zinplava *Vial:* 1,000 mg/40 ml (40 ml, 25 mg/ml), single-use

MICROBIOTA-BASED LIVE BIOTHERAPEUTIC

▷ *fecal microbiota, live-jslm* Treatment is administered rectally 24 to 72 hours after the last dose of antibiotics for the treatment of recurrent CDI; The patient is instructed to empty bladder and bowel before the procedure, if possible; Position the patient in left side-lying left or knee-chest position with buttocks elevated; The administration tube attached to the **Rebyota** bag is positioned in the rectum and the bag is raised to allow the contents to be delivered by gravity; The bag should not be squeezed; The patient should remain in the same position for up to 15 minutes to minimize any cramping
    Pediatric: <18 years: safety and efficacy not established; ≥18 years: same as adult
        Rebyota 150 ml, single-dose, for rectal instillation (1 box w. 6 cartons, each carton w. with one dose and one administration set)

(continued)

Comment: Rebyota is a first-in-class microbiota-based live biotherapeutic indicated for the prevention of recurrence of CDI following antibiotic treatment for recurrent CDI. **Rebyota** is not indicated for the first occurrence of *C. diff.* Safety and efficacy of **Rebyota** were studied in the largest clinical trial program in the field of microbiome-based therapeutics, including five clinical trials with more than 1,000 participants. The most common side effects may include stomach pain (8.9%), diarrhea (7.2%), bloating (3.9%), gas (3.3%), and nausea (3.3%). **Rebyota** is not indicated for treatment of CDI. **Rebyota** is a fecal transplant product manufactured from human fecal matter donated by screened individuals. It works by facilitating restoration of the gut. **Rebyota** is administered rectally 24 to 72 hours after the last dose of antibiotics for treatment of recurrent CDI. **Rebyota** should be stored in an ultracold freezer at −60°C to −90°C (−76°F to −130°F). Alternatively, store in a refrigerator at 2°C to 8°C (36°F to 46°F) for up to 5 days (including thaw time). Do not thaw using a heat source such as a microwave or hot water. Store the administration set at 10°C to 34°C (50°F to 93°F). Do not store the administration set in the freezer. Before using, **Rebyota** must be thawed completely in a refrigerator at 2°C to 8°C (36°F to 46°F) for approximately 24 hours. Do not refreeze **Rebyota** after thawing. Because **Rebyota** is manufactured from human fecal matter, it may carry a risk of transmitting infectious agents and may contain food allergens. Dispose of all components in medical waste. Appropriate medical treatment must be immediately available in the event of an acute anaphylactic reaction. Any infection suspected by a physician possibly to have been transmitted by the product should be reported by the physician or other healthcare provider to Ferring Pharmaceuticals Inc. at 1-888-FERRING (1-888-337-7464). **Rebyota** is not absorbed systemically following rectal administration, and maternal use is not expected to result in fetal exposure to the drug. Breastfeeding is not expected to result in exposure of the infant to **Rebyota**.

REFERENCE

Khanna, S, Assi, M, Lee, C, *et al.* Efficacy and safety of RBX2660 in PUNCH CD3, a Phase III, randomized, double-blind, placebo-controlled trial with a Bayesian primary analysis for the prevention of recurrent *Clostridioides difficile* infection. Drugs (2022). Available at: https://doi.org/10.1007/s40265-022-01797-x.

▷ *fecal microbiota, spores, live-brpk* Take four capsules by mouth as a single dose once daily for 3 consecutive days; Take each dose (4 capsules) on an empty stomach prior to the first meal of the day; *Prior to taking the first dose:* Complete antibacterial treatment for CDI 2 to 4 days before initiating treatment with **Vowst**; Antibacterials should not be administered concurrently with **Vowst** (**Vowst** is not a treatment for CDI); In clinical studies, participants with impaired kidney function received polyethylene glycol electrolyte solution (250 ml GoLYTELY, not approved for this use).

Pediatric: <18 years: safety and efficacy not established; ≥18 years: same as adult

Vowst 12 capsules/bottle

Comment: Vowst is the first orally administered microbiota-based therapy to prevent the recurrence of CDI in adults 18 years of age and older following antibacterial treatment for recurrent CDI. **Vowst** is a bacterial spore suspension in capsules for oral administration. It contains purified bacterial spores of multiple *Firmicute* species obtained from the stool of healthy human donors. The approval was supported by data from the multicenter, randomized, placebo-controlled ECOSPOR III study (ClinicalTrials.gov Identifier: NCT03183128), which included adults with a confirmed diagnosis of recurrent CDI who had a total of at least 3 episodes of CDI within 12 months. The application was granted priority review, breakthrough therapy and orphan designations. **Vowst** contains live bacteria and is manufactured from human fecal matter that has been donated by qualified individuals. Although the donors and donated stool are tested for a panel of transmissible pathogens, **Vowst** may carry a risk of transmitting infectious agents. It is also possible for **Vowst** to contain food allergens; the potential for **Vowst** to cause adverse reactions due to food allergens is unknown. The safety of **Vowst** was evaluated in a randomized, double-blind, placebo-controlled clinical study and an open-label clinical study conducted in the United States and Canada. The participants had recurrent CDI, were 48 to 96 hours postantibacterial treatment, and their symptoms were controlled. Across both studies, 346 individuals ≥18 years of age with recurrent CDI received all scheduled doses of **Vowst**. In an analysis among 90 **Vowst** recipients, when compared to 92 placebo recipients, the most commonly reported side effects by **Vowst** recipients, which occurred at a greater frequency than reported by placebo recipients, were abdominal bloating, fatigue, constipation, chills, and diarrhea. Effectiveness of **Vowst** was evaluated in the randomized, placebo-controlled clinical study in which 89 participants received **Vowst** and 93 participants received placebo. Through 8 weeks after treatment, CDI recurrence in **Vowst**-treated participants was lower compared to placebo-treated participants (12.4% compared to 39.8%). The most common adverse reactions reported were abdominal distension (31.1%), fatigue (22.2%), constipation (14.4%), chills (11.1%), and diarrhea (10.0%). There are no data on use of **Vowst** in human pregnancy. Developmental toxicity studies in animals have not been conducted with **Vowst**. It is not known whether **Vowst** is excreted in human milk. Data are not available to assess the effects of **Vowst** on the breastfed infant. Developmental and health benefits of breastfeeding should be considered, along with the mother's clinical need for **Vowst** and any other potential adverse effects on the breastfed infant from **Vowst** or from the underlying maternal condition. To report suspected adverse reactions, contact Aimmune Therapeutics at 833-246-2566 or FDA at 800-FDA-1088 or www.fda.gov/medwatch.

COLD AGGLUTININ DISEASE (CAD)

CLASSICAL COMPLEMENT INHIBITOR

▷ *sutimlimab-jome* vaccinate against encapsulated bacteria at least two weeks prior to treatment; Administer **Enjaymo** via IV infusion once weekly for 2 weeks; then increase administration to every 2 weeks; *Dose is weight-based: Wt:* 39 kg to <75 kg: 6,500 mg via IV infusion; *Wt:* ≥75 kg: 7,500 mg via IV infusion; *Preparation/Infusion:* Withdraw the calculated volume of **Enjaymo** from the appropriate number of vials based on the recommended dosage; dilute the calculated volume with 0.9% NaCl Injection, USP to a total volume of 500 ml; Administer **Enjaymo** infusion solution only through a 0.2 micron in-line filter with a polyethersulfone (PES) membrane; Administer the infusion over 1 to 2 hours depending on the patient's body weight (refer to Table below); Prime the infusion tubing with the dosing solution immediately before infusion and flush immediately following completion of the infusion with a sufficient quantity (approximately 20 ml) of 0.9% NaCl Injection, USP; if the **Enjaymo** infusion solution is not used immediately, store refrigerated at 36°F to 46°F (2°C to 8°C); once removed from refrigeration, allow the **Enjaymo** infusion solution to adjust to room temperature 68°F to 77°F (20°C to 25°C) and administer within 8 hours; Total time from the time of preparation, including refrigeration, adjustment to room temperature, and the expected infusion time should not exceed 36 hours; In-line infusion warmers may be used; However, not exceed a temperature of 40°C (104°F); Store **Enjaymo** vials refrigerated at 36°F to 46°F (2°C to 8°C) in the original carton to protect from light; Do not shake; Do not shak; Discard unused portion; See mfr pkg insert for full prescribing information including reference tables for infusing undiluted and diluted **Enjaymo**.

Pediatric: safety and efficacy not established

  Enjaymo *Vial:* 1,100 mg/22 ml (50 mg/ml), single-dose (preservative-free) due to hemolysis in adults with cold agglutinin disease (CAD)

  Enjaymo is a classical complement inhibitor indicated to decrease the need for red blood cell (RBC) transfusion due to hemolysis in adults with cold agglutinin disease (CAD). There is a risk of recurrent hemolysis after **Enjaymo** discontinuation; monitor patients for signs and symptoms of hemolysis if treatment with **Enjaymo** is interrupted. **Enjaymo** is contraindicated in patients with known hypersensitivity to *sutimlimab-jome* or any of the inactive ingredients. The most common adverse reactions (incidence ≥10%) are respiratory tract infection, viral infection, diarrhea, dyspepsia, cough, arthralgia, arthritis, and peripheral edema. Ensure patients are vaccinated against encapsulated bacteria. Monitor patients for early signs and symptoms of infections. Monitor patients for infusion-related reactions, interrupt if a reaction occurs, and institute appropriate medical management as needed. There is risk of autoimmune disease with **Enjaymo**; monitor patients for signs and symptoms and manage medically as appropriate. There are no available data on **Enjaymo** use in human pregnancy to evaluate for a drug-associated risk of major birth defects, miscarriage, or adverse maternal or fetal outcomes. Human immunoglobulin G (IgG) antibodies are known to cross the placental barrier; therefore, *sutimlimab-jome* may be transmitted from the mother to the developing fetus. In animal reproduction studies, IV administration of *sutimlimab-jome* during organogenesis at doses 2 to 3 times the maximum recommended human doses did not result in adverse effects on pregnancy or offspring development. Further, no effects on reproductive and developmental parameters were observed in maternal animals or offspring, respectively. There are no data on the presence of *sutimlimab-jome* in human milk or effects on the breastfed infant. Maternal IgG is known to be present in human milk. The effects of local gastrointestinal exposure and limited systemic exposure in the breastfed infant to *sutimlimab-jome* are unknown. No conclusions can be drawn regarding whether or not **Enjaymo** is safe for use during breastfeeding. Developmental and health benefits of breastfeeding should be considered along with the mother's clinical need for **Enjaymo** and any potential adverse effects on the breastfed infant from **Enjaymo** or from the underlying maternal condition. To report suspected adverse reactions, contact Bioverativ USA (A Sanofi Company) at 800-745-4447 or FDA at 800-FDA-1088 or www.fda.gov/medwatch.

COLIC: INFANTILE

▷ *hyoscyamine* (G)

  Levsin Drops

    Pediatric: Wt: 3-4 kg: 4 drops q 4 hours prn; max 24 drops/day; *Wt:* 5 kg: 5 drops q 4 hours prn; max 30 drops/day; *Wt:* 7 kg: 6 drops q 4 hours prn, max 36 drops/day; *Wt:* 10 kg: 8 drops q 4 hours prn, max 40 drops/day *Oral drops:* 0.125 mg/ml (15 ml) (orange) (alcohol 5%)

▷ *simethicone*

  Mylicon Drops (OTC) *Oral drops:* 40 mg/0.6 ml (30 ml) with calibrated dropper (dye-free)

    Pediatric: <2 years, <24 lb: 0.3 ml; >2 years, >24 lb: 0.6 ml; shake well before using; *Administer* after meals and at bedtime; max 12 doses/day

COLONOSCOPY PREP/COLON CLEANSE

▷ *polyethylene glycol 3350 with electrolytes* 2 doses of **Plenvu** are required for a complete preparation for colonoscopy, using a One-Day or Two-Day dosing regimen; reconstitute in water prior to ingestion; additional clear liquids must be consumed after each dose for both dosing regimens; Do not take oral medications within 1 hour of starting each dose; For complete information on dosing, preparation, and administration, see mfr pkg insert
One-Day Regimen: Dose 1 the morning of the colonoscopy (approximately 3 am to 7 am) and Dose 2 (pouch A and B) a minimum of 2 hours after the start of Dose 1
Two-Day Regimen: Dose 1 the evening before the colonoscopy (approximately 4 pm to 8 pm) and Dose 2 (pouch A and B) the next morning approximately 12 hours after the start of Dose 1
    Plenvu for Oral Solution *Oral soln*: polyethylene glycol 3350 (140 gm), sodium ascorbate (48.11 gm), sodium sulfate (9 gm), ascorbic acid (7.54 gm), sodium chloride (5.2 gm), and potassium chloride (2.2 gm); *Dose 1*: PEG 3350 (100 gm), sodium sulfate (9 gm), sodium chloride (2 gm), potassium chloride (1 gm); *Dose 2, Pouch A*: PEG 3350 (40 gm), sodium chloride (3.2 gm), potassium chloride (1.2 gm); *Dose 2, Pouch B*: sodium ascorbate (48.11 gm), ascorbic acid (7.54 gm)
    Comment: **Plenvu for Oral Solution** before a colonoscopy procedure is a lower volume, polyethylene glycol-based osmotic laxative indicated for cleansing of the colon as a preparation for colonoscopy in adults. Correct fluid and electrolyte abnormalities before treatment with **Plenvu.** Patients with glucose-6-phosphate dehydrogenase deficiency (G6PD) should use it with caution. **Plenvu** contains phenylalanine; there is risk for patients with phenylketonuria (PKA). The most common adverse reactions (incidence ≥2%) are nausea, vomiting, dehydration, and abdominal pain/discomfort.
▷ *sodium picosulfate+magnesium oxide+citric acid* (G) reconstitute pwdr with cold water right before use; two dosing regimen options—each requires two separate dosing times; *Split Dose Method* (preferred): *Administer the* 1st dose during evening before the colonoscopy and 2nd dose the next day during the morning prior to the colonoscopy; *Day Before Method* (alternative, if split dose is not appropriate): *Administer* the 1st dose during the afternoon or early evening before the colonoscopy and the 2nd dose 6 hours later during evening before colonoscopy; additional clear liquids (no solid food or milk) must be consumed after every dose in both dosing regimens
Pediatric: <18 years: not recommended; ≥18 years: same as adult
    Prepopik *Pwdr*: sod picos 10 mg+mag oxide 3.5 gm+anhy cit acid 12 gm/pkt pwdr for oral solution (2 pkts)
    Comment: **Prepopik** is a combination of sodium picosulfate, a stimulant laxative, and magnesium oxide and anhydrous citric acid, which form magnesium citrate, an osmotic laxative, indicated for cleansing of the colon as a preparation for colonoscopy in adults. Rule out diagnosis of suspected gastrointestinal (GI) obstruction or perforation diagnosis before administration. **Prepopik** should be used during pregnancy only if clearly needed. **Prepopik** is contraindicated with severely reduced renal function (creatinine clearance (CrCl)< 30 ml/min), GI obstruction or ileus, bowel perforation, toxic colitis or toxic megacolon, and gastric retention for any reason.

COMMON COLD (VIRAL UPPER RESPIRATORY INFECTION, URI)

Drugs for the Management of Allergy, Cough, and Cold Symptoms *see* Appendix Z. Drugs for the Management of Allergy, Cough, and Cold Symptoms online at https://connect.springerpub.com/content/reference-book/978-0-8261-7935-7/back-matter/part02/back-matter/bmatter27
Oral Decongestants *see* Appendix Z. Drugs for the Management of Allergy, Cough, and Cold Symptoms online at https://connect.springerpub.com/content/reference-book/978-0-8261-7935-7/back-matter/part02/back-matter/bmatter27
Oral Expectorants *see* Appendix Z. Drugs for the Management of Allergy, Cough, and Cold Symptoms online at https://connect.springerpub.com/content/reference-book/978-0-8261-7935-7/back-matter/part02/back-matter/bmatter27
Oral Antitussives *see* Appendix Z. Drugs for the Management of Allergy, Cough, and Cold Symptoms online at https://connect.springerpub.com/content/reference-book/978-0-8261-7935-7/back-matter/part02/back-matter/bmatter27
Oral Antipyretic-Analgesics *see Fever*

NASAL SALINE DROPS & SPRAYS

Comment: Homemade saline nose drops: 1/4 tsp salt added to 8 oz boiled water, then cool water.
▷ *saline* nasal spray (G)
    Afrin Saline Mist w. Eucalyptol and Menthol (OTC) 2-6 sprays in each nostril prn
    Pediatric: 1 month-2 years: 1-2 sprays in each nostril prn; >2-12 years: 1-4 sprays in each nostril prn; >12 years: same as adult
        Squeeze bottle: 45 ml
    Afrin Moisturizing Saline Mist (OTC) 2-6 sprays in each nostril prn

Pediatric: 1 month-2 years: 1-2 sprays in each nostril prn; 2-12 years: 1-4 sprays in each nostril prn; >12 years: same as adult
  Squeeze bottle: 45 ml
Ocean Mist (OTC) 2-6 sprays in each nostril prn
Pediatric: 1 month-2 years: 1-2 sprays in each nostril prn; >2-12 years: 1-4 sprays in each nostril prn; >12 years: same as adult
  Squeeze bottle: saline 0.65% (45 ml) (alcohol-free)
Pediamist (OTC) 2-6 sprays in each nostril prn
Pediatric: 1 month-2 years: 1-2 sprays in each nostril prn; >2-12 years: 1-4 sprays in each nostril prn; >12 years: same as adult
  Squeeze bottle: saline 0.5% (15 ml) (alcohol-free)

NASAL SYMPATHOMIMETICS
▷ *oxymetazoline* (OTC)
  4-Hour Formulation: 2-3 drops <u>or</u> sprays in each nostril q 10-12 hours prn; max 2 doses/day; max duration 5 days
  Pediatric: <6 years: <u>not</u> recommended; ≥6 years: same as adult
    Afrin 4-Hour
  12-Hour Formulation: 2-3 drops <u>or</u> sprays q 4 hours prn; max duration 5 days
  Pediatric: <12 years: <u>not</u> recommended; ≥12 years: same as adult
    Afrin 12-Hour Extra Moisturizing Nasal Spray
    Afrin 12-Hour Nasal Spray Pump Mist
    Afrin 12-Hour Original Nasal spray
    Afrin 12-Hour Original Nose Drops
    Afrin 12-Hour Severe Congestion Nasal Spray
    Afrin 12-Hour Sinus Nasal Spray
      Nasal spray: 0.05% (45 ml); *Nasal drops:* 0.05% (45 ml)
    Afrin 4-Hour Nasal Spray
    Neo-Synephrine 12-Hour Nasal Spray
    Neo-Synephrine 12-Hour Extra Moisturizing Nasal Spray
      Nasal spray: 0.05% (15 ml)
▷ *phenylephrine*
    Afrin Allergy Nasal Spray (OTC) 2-3 sprays in each nostril q 4 hours prn; max duration 5 days
    Pediatric: <12 years: <u>not</u> recommended; ≥12 years: same as adult
      Nasal spray: 0.5% (15 ml)
    Afrin Nasal Decongestant Children's Pump Mist (OTC)
    Pediatric: <6 years: <u>not</u> recommended; ≥6 years: 2-3 sprays in each nostril q 4 hours prn; max duration 5 days
      Nasal spray: 0.25% (15 ml)
    Neo-Synephrine Extra Strength (OTC) 2-3 sprays <u>or</u> drops in each nostril q 4 hours prn; max duration 5 days
    Pediatric: <12 years: <u>not</u> recommended; ≥12 years: same as adult
      Nasal spray: 0.1% (15 ml); *Nasal drops:* 0.1% (15 ml)
    Neo-Synephrine Mild Formula (OTC) 2-3 sprays <u>or</u> drops in each nostril q 4 hours prn; max duration 5 days
    Pediatric: <6 years: <u>not</u> recommended; ≥6 years: same as adult
      Nasal spray: 0.25% (15 ml)
    Neo-Synephrine Regular Strength (OTC) 2-3 sprays <u>or</u> drops in each nostril q 4 hours prn; max duration 5 days
    Pediatric: <12 years: <u>not</u> recommended; ≥12 years: same as adult
      Nasal spray: 0.5% (15 ml); *Nasal drops:* 0.5% (15 ml)
▷ *tetrahydrozoline*
    Tyzine 2-4 drops <u>or</u> 3-4 sprays in each nostril q 3-8 hours prn; max duration 5 days
    Pediatric: <6 years: <u>not</u> recommended; ≥6 years: same as adult
      Nasal spray: 0.1% (15 ml); *Nasal drops:* 0.1% (30 ml)
    Tyzine Pediatric Nasal Drops 2-3 sprays <u>or</u> drops in each nostril q 3-6 hours prn
      Nasal drops: 0.05% (15 ml)

CONJUNCTIVITIS/BLEPHAROCONJUNCTIVITIS: BACTERIAL

OPHTHALMIC ANTI-INFECTIVES
▷ *azithromycin* (G) ophthalmic solution (G) 1 drop to affected eye(s) bid x 2 days; then 1 drop once daily for the next 5 days
  Pediatric: <1 year: <u>not</u> recommended; ≥1 year: same as adult
    AzaSite Ophthalmic Solution *Ophth susp:* 1% (2.5 ml) (benzalkonium chloride)

(continued)

► **bacitracin** ophthalmic ointment **(G)** apply 1/2 inch ribbon to the lower conjunctival sac of affected eye(s) 1-3 x daily x 7 days
  Pediatric: same as adult
    Bacitracin Ophthalmic Ointment *Ophth oint:* 500 units/gm (3.5 gm)
► **besifloxacin** ophthalmic solution 1 drop to affected eye(s) tid x 7 days
  Pediatric: <1 year: <u>not</u> recommended; ≥1 year: same as adult
    Besivance Ophthalmic Solution *Ophth susp:* 0.6% (5 ml) (benzalkonium chloride)
► **ciprofloxacin** ophthalmic ointment apply 1/2 inch ribbon to the lower conjunctival sac of affected eye(s) tid x 2 days; then bid x 5 days
  Pediatric: <2 years: <u>not</u> recommended; ≥2 years: same as adult
    Ciloxan Ophthalmic Ointment *Ophth oint:* 0.3% (3.5 gm)
► **ciprofloxacin** ophthalmic solution 1-2 drops to affected eye(s) q 2 hours while awake x 2 days; then q 4 hours while awake x 5 days
  Pediatric: <1 years: <u>not</u> recommended; ≥1 year: same as adult
    Ciloxan Ophthalmic Solution *Ophth soln:* 0.3% (2.5, 5, 10 ml) (benzalkonium chloride)
► **erythromycin** ophthalmic ointment apply 1/2 inch ribbon to the lower conjunctival sac of affected eye(s) up to 6 x/day
  Pediatric: same as adult
    Ilotycin Ophthalmic Ointment *Ophth oint:* 5 mg/gm (1/8 oz)
► **gatifloxacin** ophthalmic solution
  Pediatric: <1 years: <u>not</u> recommended; ≥1 year: same as adult
    Zymar Ophthalmic Solution initially 1 drop to affected eye(s) q 2 hours while awake up to 8 x a day for 2 days; then 1 drop qid while awake × 5 more days
      Ophth soln: 0.3% (5 ml) (benzalkonium chloride)
    Zymaxid Ophthalmic Solution (G) initially 1 drop to affected eye(s) q 2 hours while awake up to 8 x a day on day 1; then 1 drop bid-qid while awake on days 2-7
      Ophth soln: 0.5% (2.5 ml) (benzalkonium chloride)
► **gentamicin sulfate** ophthalmic ointment **(G)** apply 1/2 inch ribbon to the lower conjunctival sac of affected eye(s) bid-tid
  Pediatric: same as adult
    Garamycin Ophthalmic Ointment *Ophth oint:* 3 mg/gm (3.5 gm) (preservative-free formulation available)
    Genoptic Ophthalmic Ointment *Ophth oint:* 3 mg/gm (3.5 gm)
    Gentacidin Ophthalmic Ointment *Ophth oint:* 3 mg/gm (3.5 gm)
► **gentamicin sulfate** ophthalmic solution **(G)** 1-2 drops to affected eye(s) q 4 hours x 7-14 days; max 2 drops q 1 hour
  Pediatric: same as adult
    Garamycin Ophthalmic Solution *Ophth soln:* 0.3% (5 ml) (benzalkonium chloride)
    Genoptic Ophthalmic Solution *Ophth soln:* 0.3% (3, 5 ml)
► **levofloxacin** ophthalmic solution 1-2 drops to affected eye(s) q 2 hours while awake on days 1 and 2 (max 8 x/day); then 1-2 drops q 4 hours while awake on days 3-7; max 4 x/day
  Pediatric: <1 years: <u>not</u> recommended; ≥1 years: same as adult
    Quixin Ophthalmic Solution *Ophth soln:* 0.5% (2.5, 5 ml) (benzalkonium chloride)
► **moxifloxacin** ophthalmic solution **(G)** 1 drop to affected eye(s) tid x 7 days
  Pediatric: <1 years: <u>not</u> recommended; ≥1 year: same as adult
    Moxeza Ophthalmic Solution (G) *Ophth soln:* 0.5% (3 ml)
    Vigamox Ophthalmic Solution *Ophth soln:* 0.5% (3 ml)
► **ofloxacin** ophthalmic solution 1-2 drops to affected eye(s) q 2-4 hours x 2 days; then qid x 5 days
  Pediatric: <1 years: <u>not</u> recommended; ≥1 year: same as adult
    Ocuflox Ophthalmic Solution *Ophth soln:* 0.3% (5, 10 ml) (benzalkonium chloride)
► **sulfacetamide** ophthalmic solution and ointment
    Bleph-10 Ophthalmic Solution 1-2 drops to affected eye(s) q 2-3 hours x 7-10 days
      Pediatric: <2 months: <u>not</u> recommended; ≥2 months: 1-2 drops q 2-3 hours during the day x 7-10 days
        Ophth soln: 10% (2.5, 5, 15 ml) (benzalkonium chloride)
    Bleph-10 Ophthalmic Ointment apply 1/2 inch ribbon to the lower conjunctival sac of affected eye(s) q 3-4 hours and HS x 7-10 days
      Pediatric: <2 years: <u>not</u> recommended; ≥2 years: same as adult
        Ophth oint: 10% (3.5 gm) (phenylmercuric acetate)
    Cetamide Ophthalmic Solution initially 1-2 drops to affected eye(s) q 2-3 hours; then increase dosing interval as condition improves
      Pediatric: <2 years: <u>not</u> recommended; ≥2 years: same as adult
        Ophth soln: 15% (5, 15 ml)
    Isopto Cetamide Ophthalmic Ointment initially 1/2 inch ribbon in lower conjunctival sac of affected eye(s) q 3-4 hours; then increase dosing interval as condition improves
      Pediatric: <2 years: <u>not</u> recommended; ≥2 years: same as adult
        Ophth oint: 10% (3.5 gm)

Isopto Cetamide Ophthalmic Solution initially 1-2 drops to affected eye(s) q 2-3 hours; then increase dosing interval as condition improves
Pediatric: <2 years: <u>not</u> recommended; ≥2 years: same as adult
  Ophth soln: 15% (5, 15 ml)
▷ *tobramycin*
Tobrex Ophthalmic Solution 1-2 drops to affected eye(s) q 4 hours
Pediatric: same as adult
  Ophth soln: 0.3% (5 ml) (benzalkonium chloride)
Tobrex Ophthalmic Ointment apply 1/2 inch ribbon to the lower conjunctival sac of affected eye(s) bid-tid
Pediatric: same as adult
  Ophth oint: 0.3% (3.5 gm) (chlorobutanol)

OPHTHALMIC ANTI-INFECTIVE COMBINATIONS

▷ *polymyxin b sulfate+bacitracin* ophthalmic ointment apply 1/2 inch ribbon to the lower conjunctival sac of affected eye(s) q 3-4 hours x 7-10 days
Pediatric: same as adult
Polysporin Ophthalmic Ointment *Ophth oint:* poly b 10,000 U+bac 500 U (3.75 gm)
▷ *polymyxin b sulfate+bacitracin zinc+neomycin sulfate* ophthalmic ointment apply 1/2 inch ribbon to the lower conjunctival sac of affected eye(s) q 3-4 hours x 7-10 days
Pediatric: same as adult
Neosporin Ophthalmic Ointment *Ophth oint:* poly b 10,000 U+bac 400 U+neo 3.5 mg/gm (3.75 gm)
▷ *polymyxin b sulfate+gramicidin+neomycin* ophthalmic solution 1-2 drops to affected eye(s) q 1 hour x 2-3 doses; then 1-2 drops bid-qid x 7-10 days
Pediatric: <12 years: <u>not</u> recommended; ≥12 years: same as adult
Neosporin Ophthalmic Solution *Ophth soln:* poly b 10,000 U+grami 0.025 mg+neo 1.7 mg/gm (10 ml)
▷ *trimethoprim+polymyxin b sulfate* ophthalmic solution 1 drop to affected eye(s) q 3 hours x 7-10 days; max 6 doses/day
Pediatric: <2 years: <u>not</u> recommended; ≥2 years: same as adult
Polytrim *Ophth soln:* trim 1 mg+poly b 10,000 U/ml (10 ml) (benzalkonium chloride)

OPHTHALMIC ANTI-INFECTIVE+STEROID COMBINATIONS

Comment: Ophthalmic corticosteroids are contraindicated after removal of a corneal foreign body, epithelial herpes simplex keratitis, varicella, other viral infections of the cornea <u>or</u> conjunctiva, fungal ocular infections, and mycobacterial ocular infections. Limit ophthalmic steroid use to 2-3 days if possible; usual max 2 weeks. With prolonged <u>or</u> frequent use, there is risk of corneal and scleral thinning and cataract formation.
▷ *gentamicin sulfate+prednisolone acetate* ophthalmic suspension
Pediatric: <12 years: <u>not</u> recommended; ≥12 years: same as adult
Pred-G Ophthalmic Suspension 1 drop to affected eye(s) bid-qid; max 20 ml/therapeutic course
  Ophth susp: gent 0.3%+pred 1%/ml (2, 5, 10 ml) (benzalkonium chloride)
Pred-G Ophthalmic Ointment apply 1/2 inch ribbon to the lower conjunctival sac of affected eye(s) once daily-tid; max 8 gm/therapeutic course
  Ophth oint: gent 0.3%+pred 0.6%/gm (3.5 gm)
▷ *neomycin sulfate+polymyxin b sulfate+dexamethasone* ophthalmic suspension
Pediatric: <12 years: <u>not</u> recommended; ≥12 years: same as adult
Maxitrol Ophthalmic Suspension 1-2 drops to affected eye(s) q 1 hour (severe infection) <u>or</u> qid (mild to moderate infection)
  Ophth susp: neo 0.35%+poly b 10,000 U+dexa 1%/ml (5 ml) (benzalkonium chloride)
Maxitrol Ophthalmic Ointment apply 1/2 inch ribbon to the lower conjunctival sac of affected eye(s) q 1 hour (severe infection) <u>or</u> qid (mild to moderate infection)
  Ophth oint: neo 0.35%+poly b 10,000 U+dexa 0.1%/gm (3.5 gm)
▷ *neomycin sulfate+polymyxin b sulfate+prednisolone acetate ophthalmic suspension*
Pediatric: <12 years: <u>not</u> recommended; ≥12 years: same as adult
Poly-Pred Ophthalmic Suspension 1-2 drops to affected eye(s) q 3-4 hours; more often as necessary; max 20 ml/therapeutic course
  Ophth susp: neo 0.35%+poly b 10,000 U+pred 0.5%/ml (10 ml)
▷ *polymyxin b sulfate+neomycin sulfate+hydrocortisone* ophthalmic suspension
Pediatric: <12 years: <u>not</u> recommended; ≥12 years: same as adult
Cortisporin Ophthalmic Suspension 1-2 drops to affected eye(s) tid-qid; more often if necessary; max 20 ml/therapeutic course
  Ophth susp: poly b 10,000 U+neo 0.35%+hydro 1%/ml (7.5 ml) (thimerosal)
▷ *polymyxin b sulfate+neomycin sulfate+bacitracin zinc+hydrocortisone* ophthalmic ointment
Pediatric: <12 years: <u>not</u> recommended; ≥12 years: same as adult
Cortisporin Ophthalmic Ointment apply 1/2 inch ribbon to the lower conjunctival sac of affected eye(s) tid-qid; more often if necessary; max 8 gm/therapeutic course
  Ophth oint: poly b 10,000 U+neo 0.35%+bac 400 U+hydro 1%/gm (3.5 gm)

(continued)

▷ **sulfacetamide sodium+fluorometholone** suspension 1 drop to affected eye(s) qid; max 20 ml/therapeutic course
  Pediatric: <12 years: <u>not</u> recommended; ≥12 years: same as adult
    FML-S *Ophth susp:* sulfa 10%+fluoro 0.1%+ml (5, 10, 15 ml) (benzalkonium chloride)
▷ **sulfacetamide sodium+prednisolone acetate** ophthalmic suspension and ointment
  Pediatric: <6 years: <u>not</u> recommended; ≥6 years: same as adult
    Blephamide Liquifilm 2 drops to affected eye(s) qid and HS
      Ophth susp: sulfa10%+pred 0.2%/ml (5, 10 ml) (benzalkonium chloride)
    Blephamide S.O.P. Ophthalmic Ointment apply 1/2 inch ribbon to the lower conjunctival sac of affected eye(s) tid-qid
      Ophth oint: sulfa 10%+pred 0.2%/gm (3.5 gm) (benzalkonium chloride)
▷ **sulfacetamide sodium+prednisolone sodium phosphate** ophthalmic solution 2 drops to affected eye(s) every 4 hours
  Pediatric: <6 years: <u>not</u> recommended; ≥6 years: same as adult
    Vasocidin Ophthalmic Solution *Ophth soln:* sulfa 10%+pred 0.25%/ml (5, 10 ml)
▷ **tobramycin+dexamethasone** ophthalmic solution and ointment
    TobraDex Ophthalmic Solution 1-2 drops to affected eye(s) q 2-6 hours x 24-48 hours; then 4-6 hours; reduce frequency of dose as condition improves; max 20 ml per therapeutic course
    Pediatric: ≤2 years: <u>not</u> recommended; ≥2 years: 1-2 drops q 4-6 hours; may start with 1-2 drops q 2 hours first 1-2 days
      Ophth susp: tobra 0.3%+dexa 0.1%/ml (2.5, 5 ml) (benzalkonium chloride)
    TobraDex Ophthalmic Ointment apply 1/2 inch ribbon to the lower conjunctival sac of affected eye(s) tid-qid; may use at bedtime in conjunction with daytime drops; max 8 gm/therapeutic course
    Pediatric: <2 years: <u>not</u> recommended; ≥2 years: apply 1/2 inch ribbon to lower conjunctival sac tid-qid
      Ophth oint: tobra 0.3%/dexa 0.1%/gm (3.5 gm) (chlorobutanol chloride)
    TobraDex ST 1-2 drops to affected eye(s) q 2-6 hours x 24-48 hours; then 4-6 hours; reduce frequency of dose as condition improves; max 20 ml per therapeutic course
    Pediatric: <12 years: <u>not</u> recommended; ≥12 years: same as adult
      Ophth susp: tobra 0.3%/dexa 0.5%/ml (2.5, 5, 10 ml) (benzalkonium chloride)
▷ **tobramycin+loteprednol etabonate** ophthalmic suspension
  Pediatric: <12 years: <u>not</u> recommended; ≥12 years: same as adult
    Zylet 1-2 drops to affected eye(s) q 1-2 hours first 24-48 hours; reduce frequency of dose to q 4-6 hours as condition improves; max 20 ml per therapeutic course
      Ophth susp: tobra 0.3%+lote etab 0.5%/ml (2.5, 5, 10 ml) (benzalkonium chloride)

CONJUNCTIVITIS: CHLAMYDIAL

Comment: A chlamydial etiology should be considered for all infants aged ≤30 days who have conjunctivitis, especially if the mother has a history of chlamydia infection. Topical antibiotic therapy alone is inadequate for treatment of *ophthalmia neonatorum* caused by chlamydia and is unnecessary when systemic treatment is administered.

RECOMMENDED FIRST-LINE REGIMEN
▷ **erythromycin base** (G) 250 mg qid x 14 days <u>or</u> 500 mg qid x 7 days
  Pediatric: <45 kg: 50 mg/kg/day in 4 divided doses x 14 days; ≥45 kg: same as adult
    Ery-Tab *Tab:* 250, 333, 500 mg ent-coat
    PCE *Tab:* 333, 500 mg
    or
▷ **erythromycin ethylsuccinate** (G) 400 mg qid x 14 days <u>or</u> 800 mg qid x 7 days
  Pediatric: 50 mg/kg/day in 4 divided doses x 7 days; max 100 mg/kg/day; *see Appendix BB.21: erythromycin ethylsuccinate* (G) (E.E.S. Suspension, EryPed Drops/Suspension) *for dose by weight*
    EryPed *Oral susp:* 200 mg/5 ml (100, 200 ml) (fruit), 400 mg/5 ml (60, 100, 200 ml) (banana); *Oral drops:* 200, 400 mg/5 ml (50 ml) (fruit); *Chew tab:* 200 mg wafer (fruit)
    E.E.S. *Oral susp:* 200, 400 mg/5 ml (100 ml) (fruit)
    E.E.S. Granules *Oral susp:* 200 mg/5 ml (100, 200 ml) (cherry)
    E.E.S. 400 Tablets *Tab:* 400 mg

ALTERNATE REGIMEN
▷ **azithromycin** (G) 500 mg x 1 dose on day 1; then 250 mg once daily on days 2-5 <u>or</u> 500 mg daily x 3 days <u>or</u> 2 gm in a single dose
  Pediatric: 20 mg/kg in a single dose once daily x 3 days
    Zithromax *Tab:* 250, 500, 600 mg; *Oral susp:* 100 mg/5 ml (15 ml), 200 mg/5 ml (15, 22.5, 30 ml) (cherry); *Pkt:* 1 gm for reconstitution (cherry-banana)
    Zithromax Tri-Pak *Tab:* 3 x 500 mg tabs/pck
    Zithromax Z-Pak *Tab:* 6 x 250 mg tabs/pck
    Zmax *Oral susp:* 2 gm ext-rel for reconstitution (cherry-banana) (148 mg Na$^+$)

CONJUNCTIVITIS: FUNGAL

▶ *natamycin* ophthalmic suspension 1 drop q 1-2 hours x 3-4 days; then 1 drop q 6 hours; treat for 14-21 days; withdraw dose gradually at 4- to 7-day intervals
Pediatric: <1 year: not recommended; ≥1 year: same as adult
Natacyn Ophthalmic Suspension *Ophth susp:* 0.5% (15 ml) (benzalkonium chloride)

CONJUNCTIVITIS: GONOCOCCAL

RECOMMENDED REGIMENS
Regimen 1

▶ *ceftriaxone* (G) 250 mg IM x 1 dose
Pediatric: <45 kg: 50 mg/kg IM x 1 dose; max 125 mg IM
Rocephin *Vial:* 250, 500 mg; 1, 2 gm

Regimen 2

▶ *erythromycin base* (G) 250 mg qid x 10-14 days
Pediatric: <45 kg: 50 mg/kg/day in 4 divided doses x 10-14 days; ≥45 kg: same as adult
Ery-Tab *Tab:* 250, 333, 500 mg ent-coat
PCE *Tab:* 333, 500 mg
▶ *erythromycin ethylsuccinate* (G) 400 mg qid x 14 days or 800 mg qid x 7 days
Pediatric: 50 mg/kg/day in 4 divided doses x 7 days; max 100 mg/kg/day; *see Appendix BB.21. erythromycin ethylsuccinate* (G) (E.E.S. Suspension, EryPed Drops/Suspension) *for dose by weight*
EryPed *Oral susp:* 200 mg/5 ml (100, 200 ml) (fruit), 400 mg/5 ml (60, 100, 200 ml) (banana); *Oral drops:* 200, 400 mg/5 ml (50 ml) (fruit); *Chew tab:* 200 mg wafer (fruit)
E.E.S. *Oral susp:* 200, 400 mg/5 ml (100 ml) (fruit)
E.E.S. Granules *Oral susp:* 200 mg/5 ml (100, 200 ml) (cherry)
E.E.S. 400 Tablets *Tab:* 400 mg

ALTERNATE REGIMEN

▶ *azithromycin* (G) 500 mg x 1 dose on day 1; then 250 mg once daily on days 2-5 or 500 mg daily x 3 days or 2 gm in a single dose
Pediatric: not recommended for bronchitis in children
Zithromax *Tab:* 250, 500, 600 mg; *Oral susp:* 100 mg/5 ml (15 ml), 200 mg/5 ml (15, 22.5, 30 ml) (cherry); Pkt: 1 gm for reconstitution (cherry-banana)
Zithromax Tri-Pak *Tab:* 3 x 500 mg tabs/pck
Zithromax Z-Pak *Tab:* 6 x 250 mg tabs/pck
Zmax *Oral susp:* 2 gm ext-rel for reconstitution (cherry-banana) (148 mg Na$^+$)

CONJUNCTIVITIS/KERATITIS/KERATOCONJUNCTIVITIS: ALLERGIC (VERNAL)

Oral Antihistamines *see* Appendix Z. Drugs for the Management of Allergy, Cough, and Cold Symptoms online at https://connect.springerpub.com/content/reference-book/978-0-8261-7935-7/back-matter/part02/back-matter/bmatter27

OPHTHALMIC CORTICOSTEROIDS
Comment: Concomitant contact lens wear is contraindicated during therapy. Ophthalmic steroids are contraindicated with ocular, fungal, mycobacterial, viral (except herpes zoster), and untreated bacterial infection. Ophthalmic steroids may mask or exacerbate infection, and may increase intraocular pressure, optic nerve damage, cataract formation, or corneal perforation. Limit ophthalmic steroid use to 2-3 days if possible; usual max 2 weeks. With prolonged or frequent use, there is risk of corneal and scleral thinning and cataract formation.
▶ *dexamethasone* initially 1-2 drops hourly during the day and q 2 hours at night; then prolong dosing interval to 4-6 hours as condition improves
Pediatric: <12 years: not recommended; ≥12 years: same as adult
Maxidex *Ophth susp:* 0.1% (5, 15 ml) (benzalkonium chloride)
▶ *dexamethasone phosphate* initially 1-2 drops hourly during the day and q 2 hours at night; then 1 drop q 4-8 hours or more as condition improves
Pediatric: <12 years: not recommended; ≥12 years: same as adult
Decadron *Ophth soln:* 0.1% (5 ml) (sulfites)
▶ *fluorometholone* 1 drop bid-qid or 1/2 inch of ointment 1-3 x/day; may increase dose frequency during the initial 24-48 hours
Pediatric: <2 years: not recommended; ≥2 years: same as adult
FML *Ophth susp:* 0.1% (5, 10, 15 ml) (benzalkonium chloride)
FML Forte *Ophth susp:* 0.25% (5, 10, 15 ml) (benzalkonium chloride)
FML S.O.P. Ointment *Ophth oint:* 0.1% (3.5 gm)

(continued)

➤ *fluorometholone acetate* initially 2 drops q 2 hours during the first 24-48 hours; then 1-2 drops qid as condition improves
  Pediatric: <12 years: <u>not</u> recommended; ≥12 years: same as adult
    Flarex *Ophth susp:* 0.1% (2.5, 5 ml) (benzalkonium chloride)
➤ *loteprednol etabonate* (G)
  Pediatric: <12 years: <u>not</u> recommended; ≥12 years: same as adult
    Alrex 1 drop qid
      Ophth susp: 0.2% (5, 10 ml) (benzalkonium chloride)
    Lotemax 1-2 drops qid
      Ophth susp: 0.5% (5, 10, 15 ml) (benzalkonium chloride)
➤ *medrysone* 1 drop up to q 4 hours
  Pediatric: <12 years: <u>not</u> recommended; ≥12 years: same as adult
    HMS *Ophth susp:* 1% (5, 10 ml) (benzalkonium chloride)
➤ *rimexolone* initially 1-2 drops hourly while awake x 1 week; then 1 drop every 2 hours while awake x 1 week; then taper as condition improves
  Pediatric: <12 years: <u>not</u> recommended; ≥12 years: same as adult
    Vexol *Ophth susp:* 0.1% (5, 10 ml) (benzalkonium chloride)
➤ *prednisolone acetate* (G)
  Pediatric: <12 years: <u>not</u> recommended; ≥12 years: same as adult
    Econopred 2 drops qid
      Ophth susp: 0.125% (5, 10 ml)
    Econopred Plus 2 drops qid
      Ophth susp: 1% (5, 10 ml)
    Pred Forte initially 2 drops hourly x 24-48 hours; then 1-2 drops bid-qid
      Ophth susp: 1% (1, 5, 10, 15 ml) (benzalkonium chloride, sulfites)
    Pred Mild initially 2 drops hourly x 24-48 hours; then 1-2 drops bid-qid
      Ophth susp: 0.12% (5, 10 ml) (benzalkonium chloride)
➤ *prednisolone sodium phosphate* initially 1-2 drops hourly during the day and q 2 hours at night; then 1 drop q 4 hours; then 1 drop tid-qid as condition improves
  Pediatric: <12 years: <u>not</u> recommended; ≥12 years: same as adult
    Inflamase Forte *Ophth soln:* 1% (5, 10, 15 ml) (benzalkonium chloride)
    Inflamase Mild *Ophth soln:* 1/8% (5, 10 ml) (benzalkonium chloride)

OPHTHALMIC H1 ANTAGONISTS (ANTIHISTAMINES)
Comment: May insert contact lens 10 minutes after administration of ophthalmic antihistamine.
➤ *cetirizine* 1 drop bid prn
  Pediatric: <2 years: <u>not</u> established; ≥2 years: same as adult
    Zerviate *Ophth soln:* 0.24%/ml (5 ml [7.5 ml bottle]; 7.5 ml [10 ml bottle])
➤ *emedastine* 1 drop qid prn
  Pediatric: <3 years: <u>not</u> recommended; ≥3 years: same as adult
    Emadine *Ophth soln:* 0.05% (5 ml) (benzalkonium chloride)
➤ *levocabastine* 1 drop qid prn
  Pediatric: <12 years: <u>not</u> recommended; ≥12 years: same as adult
    Livostin *Ophth susp:* 0.05% (2.5, 5, 10 ml) (benzalkonium chloride)

OPHTHALMIC MAST CELL STABILIZERS
Comment: Concomitant contact lens wear is contraindicated during treatment.
➤ *cromolyn sodium* 1-2 drops 4-6 x/day at regular intervals
  Pediatric: <4 years: <u>not</u> recommended; ≥4 years: same as adult
    Crolom *Ophth soln:* 4% (10 ml) (benzalkonium chloride)
➤ *lodoxamide tromethamine* 1-2 drops qid up to 3 months
  Pediatric: <2 years: <u>not</u> recommended; ≥2 years: same as adult
    Alomide *Ophth soln:* 1% (10 ml) (benzalkonium chloride)
➤ *nedocromil* 1-2 drops bid
  Pediatric: <3 years: <u>not</u> recommended; ≥3 years: same as adult
    Alocril *Ophth soln:* 2% (5 ml) (benzalkonium chloride)
➤ *pemirolast potassium* 1-2 drops qid
  Pediatric: <3 years: <u>not</u> recommended; ≥3 years: same as adult
    Alamast *Ophth soln:* 0.1% (10 ml) (lauralkonium chloride)

OPHTHALMIC ANTIHISTAMINE+MAST CELL STABILIZER COMBINATIONS
➤ *alcaftadine* 1 drop each eye daily (G)
  Pediatric: <2 years: <u>not</u> recommended; ≥2 years: same as adult
    Lastacaft *Ophth soln:* 0.25% (6 ml) (benzalkonium chloride)
Comment: May insert contact lens 10 minutes after ophthalmic administration.

▷ *azelastine* 1 drop each eye bid
　　Pediatric: <3 years: <u>not</u> recommended; ≥3 years: same as adult
　　　　Optivar *Ophth soln:* 0.05% (6 ml) (benzalkonium chloride)
　　Comment: May insert contact lens 10 minutes after ophthalmic administration.
▷ *bepotastine besilate* (G) 1 drop each eye bid
　　Pediatric: <2 years: <u>not</u> recommended; ≥2 years: same as adult
　　　　Bepreve *Ophth soln:* 1.5% (10 ml) (benzalkonium chloride)
　　Comment: May insert contact lens 10 minutes after ophthalmic administration.
▷ *epinastine* (G) 1 drop each eye bid
　　Pediatric: <3 years: <u>not</u> recommended; ≥3 years: same as adult
　　　　Elestat *Ophth soln:* 0.05% (5 ml) (benzalkonium chloride)
　　Comment: May insert contact lens 10 minutes after administration.
▷ *ketotifen fumarate* 1 drop each eye q 8-12 hours
　　Pediatric: <3 years: <u>not</u> recommended; ≥3 years: same as adult
　　　　Alaway (OTC) *Ophth soln:* 0.025% (10 ml) (benzalkonium chloride)
　　　　Claritin Eye (OTC) *Ophth soln:* 0.025% (5 ml) (benzalkonium chloride)
　　　　Refresh Eye Itch Relief (OTC) *Ophth soln:* 0.025% (5 ml) (benzalkonium chloride)
　　　　Zaditor (OTC) *Ophth soln:* 0.025% (5 ml) (benzalkonium chloride)
　　　　Zyrtec Itchy Eye (OTC) *Ophth soln:* 0.025% (5 ml) (benzalkonium chloride)
　　Comment: May insert contact lens 10 minutes after administration.
▷ *olopatadine* (G) 1 drop each eye bid
　　Pediatric: <3 years: <u>not</u> recommended; ≥3 years: same as adult
　　　　Pataday *Ophth soln:* 0.2% (2.5 ml) (benzalkonium chloride)
　　　　Patanol *Ophth soln:* 0.1% (5 ml) (benzalkonium chloride)
　　　　Pazeo *Ophth soln:* 0.7% (2.5 ml) (benzalkonium chloride)
　　Comment: May insert contact lens 10 minutes after administration.

OPHTHALMIC VASOCONSTRICTORS
Comment: Concomitant contact lens wear is contraindicated during treatment.
▷ *naphazoline* 1-2 drops each eye qid prn
　　Pediatric: <12 years: <u>not</u> recommended; ≥12 years: same as adult
　　　　Vasocon-A *Ophth soln:* 0.1% (15 ml) (benzalkonium chloride)
▷ *oxymetazoline* (OTC) 1-2 drops each eye qid prn
　　Pediatric: <6 years: <u>not</u> recommended; ≥6 years: same as adult
　　　　Visine L-R *Ophth soln:* 0.025% (15, 30 ml)
▷ *tetrahydrozoline* (OTC)(G) 1-2 drops each eye qid prn
　　Pediatric: <6 years: <u>not</u> recommended; ≥6 years: same as adult
　　　　Visine *Ophth soln:* 0.05% (15, 22.5, 30 ml)

OPHTHALMIC VASOCONSTRICTOR+MOISTURIZER COMBINATION
Comment: Concomitant contact lens wear is contraindicated during treatment.
▷ *tetrahydrozoline+polyethylene glycol 400+povidone+dextran 70* (OTC) 1-2 drops each eye qid prn
　　Pediatric: <6 years: <u>not</u> recommended; ≥6 years: same as adult
　　　　Advanced Relief Visine *Ophth soln:* tetra 0.025%+poly 1%+pov 1%+dex 0.1% (15, 30 ml)

OPHTHALMIC VASOCONSTRICTOR+ASTRINGENT COMBINATION
Comment: Concomitant contact lens wear is contraindicated during treatment.
▷ *tetrahydrozoline+zinc sulfate* (OTC) 1-2 drops each eye qid prn
　　Pediatric: <6 years: <u>not</u> recommended; ≥6 years: same as adult
　　　　Visine AC *Ophth soln:* tetra 0.025%+zinc 0.05% (15, 30 ml)

OPHTHALMIC VASOCONSTRICTOR+ANTIHISTAMINE COMBINATIONS
Comment: Concomitant contact lens wear is contraindicated during treatment.
▷ *naphazoline+pheniramine* 1-2 drops each eye qid
　　Pediatric: <6 years: <u>not</u> recommended; ≥6 years: same as adult
　　　　Naphcon-A (OTC) *Ophth soln:* naph 0.025%+phen 0.3% (15 ml) (benzalkonium chloride)

OPHTHALMIC NONSTEROIDAL ANTI-INFLAMMATORY DRUGS (NSAIDs)
Comment: Concomitant contact lens wear is contraindicated during treatment.

▷ *bromfenac* (G) 1 drop affected eye(s) bid
　　　　Bromday Ophthalmic Solution *Ophth soln:* 0.09% (2.5 ml in 7.5 ml dropper bottle; 7.5 ml in 10 ml dropper bottle)
　　　　Xibrom Ophthalmic Solution *Ophth soln:* 0.09% (2.5 ml in 7.5 ml dropper bottle; 7.5 ml in 10 ml dropper bottle)

(continued)

▷ *diclofenac* 1 drop affected eye(s) qid
  Pediatric: <12 years: not recommended; ≥12 years: same as adult
    Voltaren Ophthalmic Solution *Ophth soln:* 0.1% (2.5, 5 ml)
▷ *ketorolac tromethamine* 1 drop affected eye(s) qid; max x 4 days
  Pediatric: <3 years: not recommended; ≥3 years: same as adult
    Acular *Ophth soln:* 0.5% (3, 5, 10 ml) (benzalkonium chloride)
    Acular LS *Ophth soln:* 0.4% (5 ml) (benzalkonium chloride)
    Acular PF *Ophth soln:* 0.5% (0.4 ml; 12 single-use vials/carton) (preservative-free)
▷ *nepafenac* 1 drop affected eye(s) tid
  Pediatric: <10 years: not recommended; ≥10 years: same as adult
    Nevanac Ophthalmic Suspension *Ophth susp:* 0.1% (3 ml) (benzalkonium chloride)

CALCINEURIN INHIBITOR IMMUNOSUPPRESSANT

▷ *cyclosporine* administration: instill 1 drop in each affected eye 4 x/day (morning, noon, afternoon, and evening)
  Pediatric: <4 years: safety and efficacy not established; ≥4 years: same as adult
  Verkazia *Vial:* 0.1% (0.3 ml, 1 mg/ml), single-dose, ophthalmic emulsion, 5 vials per aluminum pouch, 6, 12, 24 pouches per box
  Comment: Verkazia is a calcineurin inhibitor immunosuppressant indicated for the treatment of vernal keratoconjunctivitis (VKC) in children and adults. There are no adequate and well-controlled studies of **Verkazia** administration in pregnant patients to inform a drug-associated risk. Oral administration of *cyclosporine* in animal studies did not produce teratogenicity at clinically relevant doses. The most common adverse reactions following use of **Verkazia** were eye pain (12%) and eye pruritis (8%). There is no information regarding the presence of *cyclosporine* in human milk following topical administration or effect of **Verkazia** on the breastfed infant.

CONJUNCTIVITIS: VIRAL

Comment: For prevention of secondary bacterial infection, see agents listed under bacterial conjunctivitis. Ophthalmic corticosteroids are contraindicated with herpes simplex, keratitis, varicella, and other viral infections of the cornea.
▷ *trifluridine* ophthalmic suspension 1 drop q 2 hours while awake; max 9 drops/day; after re-epithelialization, 1 drop every 4 hours x 7 days (at least 5 drops/day); max 21 days of therapy
  Pediatric: <6 years: not recommended; ≥6 years: same as adult
    Viroptic Ophthalmic Solution *Ophth soln:* 1% (7.5 ml) (thimerosal)

CONSTIPATION: CHRONIC IDIOPATHIC (CIC)

GUANYLATE CYCLASE-C AGONISTS

Comment: Guanylate cyclase-C agonists increase intestinal fluid, and intestinal transit time may induce diarrhea and bloating and therefore are contraindicated with known or suspected mechanical gastrointestinal (GI) obstruction.

▷ *linaclotide* (G) 145 mcg orally once daily or 72 mcg orally once daily based on individual presentation or tolerability; take on an empty stomach at least 30 minutes before the first meal of the day; swallow whole, do not crush or chew cap or cap contents; may open cap and administer with applesauce or water (e.g., nasogastric tube [NGT], percutaneous endoscopic gastrostomy [PEG] tube)
  Pediatric: ≤18 years: not established (<6 years: contraindicated; 6-18 years: avoid); >18 years: same as adult
    Linzess *Cap:* 72, 145, 290 mcg
  Comment: *Linaclotide* and its active metabolite are negligibly absorbed systemically following oral administration, and maternal use is not expected to result in fetal exposure to the drug. There is no information regarding the presence of *plecanatide* in human milk or its effects on the breastfed infant.
▷ *plecanatide* take one tab once daily; if necessary, may crush and administer with applesauce or water (e.g., NGT, PEG tube)
  Pediatric: ≤18 years: not established (<6 years: contraindicated; 6-18 years: avoid); >18 years: same as adult
    Trulance *Tab:* 3 mg
  Comment: Suspend *plecanatide* dosing and rehydrate if severe diarrhea occurs. The most common adverse reactions in chronic idiopathic constipation (CIC) are sinusitis, upper respiratory infection (URI), diarrhea, abdominal distension and tenderness, flatulence, and increased liver enzymes. *Plecanatide* and its active metabolite are negligibly absorbed systemically following oral administration, and maternal use is not expected to result in fetal exposure to the drug. There is no information regarding the presence of *plecanatide* in human milk or its effects on the breastfed infant.

CHLORIDE CHANNEL ACTIVATOR

▷ *lubiprostone* (G) one 24 mcg cap bid with food and water; swallow whole, do not break apart or chew
 Pediatric: <18 years: not recommended; ≥18 years: same as adult
  Amitiza *Cap:* 8, 24 mcg
  Comment: Amitiza increases intestinal fluid and intestinal transit time. Suspend dosing and rehydrate if severe diarrhea occurs. **Amitiza** is contraindicated with known or suspected mechanical GI obstruction. The most common adverse reactions in CIC are nausea, diarrhea, headache, abdominal pain, abdominal distension, and flatulence.

Selective Serotonin Type 4 (5-HT4) Receptor Agonist

▷ *prucalopride* 2 mg once daily; *CrCl <30 ml/min:* 1 mg once daily; *end-stage renal disease (ESRD):* avoid
 Pediatric: <18 years: not established; ≥18 years: same as adult
  Motegrity *Tab:* 1, 2 mg film-coat
  Comment: Motegrity *(prucalopride)* is a selective serotonin type 4 (5-HT4) receptor agonist for treatment of CIC in adults. *Prucalopride* is a prokinetic agent that stimulates colonic peristalsis (high-amplitude propagating contractions [HAPCs]), which increases bowel motility. The most common adverse reactions (incidence ≥2%) have been headache, abdominal pain, nausea, diarrhea, abdominal distension, dizziness, vomiting, flatulence, and fatigue. Contraindications include intestinal perforation or obstruction due to structural or functional disorder of the gut wall, obstructive ileus, severe inflammatory conditions of the intestinal tract such as Crohn's disease, ulcerative colitis, and toxic megacolon/megarectum. Monitor patients for persistent worsening of depression and emergence of suicidal thoughts and behavior. Instruct patients to discontinue **Motegrity** immediately and contact their healthcare provider if their depression is persistently worse, or they experience emerging suicidal thoughts or behaviors. Available data from case reports with *prucalopride* use in pregnancy are insufficient to identify any drug-associated risks of miscarriage, major birth defects, or adverse maternal or fetal outcomes. *Prucalopride* is present in breast milk. There are no data on the effects of *Prucalopride* on the breastfed infant.

CONSTIPATION: OCCASIONAL, INTERMITTENT

BULK-FORMING AGENTS

▷ *calcium polycarbophil* 2 tabs once daily to qid
 Pediatric: <6 years: not recommended; 6-12 years: 1 tab once daily to qid
  FiberCon (OTC) *Cplt:* 625 mg
  Konsyl Fiber Tablets (OTC) *Tab:* 625 mg
▷ *methylcellulose*
  Citrucel 1 heaping tbsp in 8 oz cold water tid
  Pediatric: <6 years: not recommended; 6-12 years: 1/2 adult dose
   Oral pwdr: 16, 24, 30 oz and single-dose pkts (orange)
  Citrucel Sugar-Free 1 heaping tbsp in 8 oz cold water tid
  Pediatric: <6 years: not recommended; 6-12 years: 1/2 adult dose
   Oral pwdr: 16, 24, 30 oz and single-dose pkts (orange) (sugar-free, phenylalanine)
▷ *psyllium husk*
 Pediatric: <6 years: not recommended; 6-12 years: 1/2 adult dose in 8 oz liquid tid
  Metamucil (OTC) wafer or cap or 1 pkt or 1 rounded tsp (1 rounded tbsp for sugar-containing form) in 8 oz liquid tid
   Cap: psyllium husk 5.2 gm (100, 150/carton); *Wafer:* psyllium husk 3.4 gm/rounded tsp (24/carton) (apple crisp, cinnamon spice); *Plain and flavored pwdr:* 3.4 gm/rounded tsp (15, 20, 24, 29, 30, 36, 44, 48 oz); *Efferv sugar-free flav pkts:* 3.4 gm/pkt (30/carton) (phenylalanine)
▷ *psyllium* hydrophilic mucilloid 2 rounded tsp in 8 oz water qid
 Pediatric: <6 years: not recommended; 6-12 years: 1 rounded tsp in 8 oz liquid tid
  Konsyl (OTC) *Pwdr:* 6 gm/rounded tsp (10.6, 15.9 oz); *Pwdr pkt:* 6 gm/ rounded tsp (30/carton)
  Konsyl-D (OTC) *Pwdr:* 3.4 gm/rounded tsp (11.5, 17.59 oz); *Pwdr pkt:* 3.4 gm/rounded tsp (30/carton)
  Konsyl Easy Mix Formula (OTC) *Pwdr:* 3.4 gm/rounded tsp (8 oz) (sugar-free, low sodium)
  Konsyl Orange (OTC) *Pwdr:* 3.4 gm/rounded tsp (19 oz); *Pwdr pkt:* 3.4 gm/rounded tsp (30/carton)
  Konsyl Orange SF (OTC) *Pwdr:* 3.5 gm/rounded tsp (15 oz) (phenylalanine); *Pwdr pkt:* 3.5 gm/rounded tsp (30/carton) (phenylalanine)

STOOL SOFTENERS

▷ *docusate sodium* (OTC) 50-200 mg/day
 Pediatric: <3 years: 10-40 mg/day; 3-6 years: 20-60 mg/day; >6 years: 40-120 mg/day
  Cap: 50, 100 mg; *Liq:* 10 mg/ml (30 ml w. dropper); *Syr:* 20 mg/5 ml (8 oz) (alcohol ≤1%)
  Dialose 1 tab q HS

(continued)

Pediatric: <6 years: <u>not</u> recommended; ≥6 years: same as adult
  Tab: 100 mg
Surfak (OTC) 240 mg/day
Pediatric: <12 years: <u>not</u> recommended; ≥12 years: same as adult
  Cap: 240 mg
▷ *docusate* enema
  DocuSol Kids (OTC) <2 years: <u>not</u> established; 2-12 years: 1 x 5 ml mini-enema
  Mini-enema: 100 mg/5 ml (5 ml, 5/box)
  Comment: Results of one mini-enema are usually seen within 5-15 minutes.

OSMOTIC LAXATIVES
▷ *lactulose* **(G)** take 10-20 gm dissolved in 4 oz water once daily prn; max 40 gm/day
  Pediatric: <12 years: <u>not</u> recommended; ≥12 years: same as adult
    Kristalose *Crystals for oral soln:* 10, 20 gm single-dose pkts (30/carton)
▷ *magnesium citrate* **(G)** 1 full bottle (120-300 ml) once daily prn
  Pediatric: <2 years: <u>not</u> recommended; 2-6 years: 4-12 ml once daily prn; ≥6-12 years: 50-100 ml once daily prn
    Citrate of Magnesia (OTC) *Oral soln:* 300 ml
▷ *magnesium hydroxide* 30-60 ml/day in a single <u>or</u> divided doses prn
  Pediatric: 2-5 years: 5-15 ml/day in a single <u>or</u> divided doses; 6-11 years: 15-30 ml/day in a single <u>or</u> divided doses; ≥12 years: same as adult
    Milk of Magnesia *Liq:* 390 mg/5 ml (10, 15, 20, 30, 100, 120, 180, 360, 720 ml)
▷ *polyethylene glycol (PEG)* **(OTC)(G)** 1 tbsp (17 gm) dissolved in 4-8 oz water per day for up to max 7 days; may need 2-4 days for results
  Pediatric: ≤17: <12 years: <u>not</u> recommended; ≥12 years: same as adult
    GlycoLax Powder for Oral Solution *Oral pwdr:* 7, 14, 30, and 45 dose bottles w. 17 gm dosing cup (gluten-free, sugar-free); 17 gm single-dose pkts (20/carton)
    MiraLAX Powder for Oral Solution *Oral pwdr:* 7, 14, 30, and 45 dose bottles w. 17 gm dosing cup (gluten-free, sugar-free)
    Polyethylene Glycol 3350 Powder for Oral Solution (G) *Oral pwdr:* 3350 gm w. dosing cup; 17 gm/scoop
  Comment: *PEG* is an osmotic indicated for occasional constipation without affecting glucose and electrolyte levels. Contraindicated with suspected <u>or</u> known bowel obstruction.

STIMULANTS
▷ *bisacodyl* 2-3 tabs <u>or</u> 1 suppository bid prn
  Dulcolax, Gentlax *Tab:* 5 mg; *Rectal supp:* 10 mg
  Pediatric: <12 years: 1/2 suppository once daily prn; 6-12 years: 1 tablet <u>or</u> 1/2 suppository once daily prn; >12 years: same as adult
  Senokot (OTC) initially 2-4 tabs <u>or</u> 1 level tsp at HS prn; max 4 tabs <u>or</u> 2 tsp bid
  Pediatric: <2 years: <u>not</u> recommended; 2-6 years: 1/4 tab <u>or</u> 1/2 tsp once daily prn; max 1 tab <u>or</u> 1/2 tsp bid; 6-12 years: 1 tab <u>or</u> 1/2 tsp once daily prn; max 2 tabs <u>or</u> 1 tsp once daily
    Tab: 8.6*mg; *Granules:* 15 mg/tsp (2, 6, 12 oz) (cocoa)
  Senokot Syrup (OTC) initially 10-15 ml at HS prn; max 15 ml bid
  Pediatric: use **Childrens Syrup**
    Syr: 8.8 mg/5 ml (2, 8 oz) (chocolate) (alcohol-free)
  Senokot Childrens Syrup (OTC)
  Pediatric: <2 years: <u>not</u> recommended; 2-6 years: 2.5-3.75 ml once daily prn; max 3.75 ml bid prn; ≥6-12 years: 5-7.5 ml once daily prn; max 7.5 ml bid
    Syr: 8.8 mg/5 ml (2.5 oz) (chocolate) (alcohol-free)
  SenokotXtra (OTC) 1 tab at HS prn; max 2 tabs bid
  Pediatric: <2 years: <u>not</u> recommended; 2-6 years: use **Childrens Syrup**; 6-12 years: 1/2 tab once daily at HS; max 1 tab bid
    Tab: 17*mg

BULK FORMING AGENT+STIMULANT COMBINATIONS
▷ *psyllium+senna*
  Perdiem (OTC) 1-2 rounded tsp swallowed with 8 oz cool liquid once daily to bid
  Pediatric: <7 years: <u>not</u> recommended; 7-11 years: 1 rounded tsp swallowed with 8 oz cool liquid once daily-bid; ≥12 years: same as adult
    Canister: 8.8, 14 oz; *Individual pkt:* 6 gm (6/pck)
  SennaPrompt (OTC) initially 2-5 caps bid
  Pediatric: <12 years: <u>not</u> recommended; ≥12 years: same as adult
    Cap: psyl 500 mg+senna 9 mg

STOOL SOFTENER+STIMULANT COMBINATIONS
▷ *docusate+casanthranol*
  Doxidan (OTC) 1-3 caps/day; max 1 week
  Pediatric: <2 years: <u>not</u> recommended; ≥2 years: 1 cap/day
    Cap: doc 60 mg+cas 30 mg

Peri-Colace (OTC) 1-2 caps <u>or</u> 15-30 ml q HS; max 2 caps <u>or</u> 30 ml bid <u>or</u> 3 caps q HS
Pediatric: 5-15 ml q HS
Cap: doc 100 mg+cas 30 mg; *Syr:* doc 60 mg+cas 30 mg per 15 ml (8, 16 oz)
▷ *docusate+senna* concentrate
Senokot S (OTC) 2 tabs q HS; max 4 tabs bid
Pediatric: <2 years: <u>not</u> recommended; 2-6 years: 1/2 tab daily; max 1 tab bid; >6-12 years: 1 tab daily; max 2 tabs bid
Tab: doc 50 mg+senna 8.6 mg

ENEMAS AND SUPPOSITORIES

▷ *glycerin* suppository (OTC) 1 adult suppository
Pediatric: <6 years: 1 pediatric suppository; ≥6 years: 1 adult suppository
▷ *docusate* enema
Pediatric: <2 years: <u>not</u> established; 2-12 years: 1 x 5 ml mini-enema
DocuSol Kids (OTC) *Mini-enema:* 100 mg/5 ml (5 ml, 5/box)
Comment: Results of one mini-enema are usually seen within 5-15 minutes.
▷ *sodium biphosphate+sodium phosphate* enema (OTC)
Fleets Adult 59-118 ml rectally
Enema: sod biphos 19 gm+sod phos 7 gm (59, 118 ml w. applicator)
Fleets Pediatric 59 ml rectally
Enema: sod biphos 19 gm+sod phos 7 gm (59 ml w. applicator)

CORNEAL EDEMA

▷ *sodium chloride* (G)
Pediatric: same as adult 1-2 drops <u>or</u> 1 inch ribbon q 3-4 hours prn; reduce frequency as edema subsides
Various (OTC)
Ophth soln: 2, 5% (15, 30 ml); *Ophth oint:* 5% (3.5 gm)

CORNEAL ULCERATION

ANTIBACTERIAL OPHTHALMIC SOLUTION/OINTMENT
See *Conjunctivitis/Blepharoconjunctivitis: Bacterial*

COSTOCHONDRITIS (CHEST WALL SYNDROME)

Acetaminophen for IV Infusion *see Pain*
NSAIDs *see* Appendix I. NSAIDs online at https://connect.springerpub.com/content/reference-book/978-0-8261-7935-7/back-matter/part02/back-matter/bmatter10
Opioid Analgesics *see Pain*
Topical and Transdermal Analgesics *see Pain*
Parenteral Corticosteroids *see* Appendix L. Parenteral Corticosteroids
Oral Corticosteroids *see* Appendix K. Oral Corticosteroids
Topical Analgesic and Anesthetic Agents *see* Appendix H. Anesthetic Agents for Local Infiltration and Dermal/Mucosal Membrane Application online at https://connect.springerpub.com/content/reference-book/978-0-8261-7935-7/back-matter/part02/back-matter/bmatter9

COVID-19 (*CORONAVIRUS*)

Centers for Disease Control and Prevention (CDC), Media Release, April 19, 2023—Following FDA regulatory action, CDC announced simplified COVID-19 vaccine recommendations, allowing for more flexibility for people at higher risk who want the option of added protection from additional COVID-19 vaccine doses. The CDC's Advisory Committee on Immunization Practices (ACIP) expressed support for these new recommendations, which are delineated below:

(1) CDC's new recommendations allow an additional updated (bivalent) vaccine dose for adults ages 65 years of age and older and additional doses for people who are immunocompromised. This allows more flexibility for healthcare providers to administer additional doses to immunocompromised patients as needed.

(2) Monovalent (original) mRNA COVID-19 vaccines are no longer be recommended for use in the United States.

(3) CDC recommends that everyone ages 6 years of age and older receive an updated (bivalent) mRNA [Pfizer-BioNTech or Moderna] COVID-19 vaccine, regardless of whether they previously completed their (monovalent) primary series.

(continued)

(4) Individuals ages 6 years of age and older who have already received an updated (bivalent) mRNA vaccine do not need to take any action unless they are 65 years of age or older or are immunocompromised.
(5) For young children, multiple doses continue to be recommended and will vary by age, vaccine, and which vaccines were previously received.

Recommendations for use of monovalent Novavax or Johnson & Johnson's Janssen COVID-19 vaccines are not affected by these changes. Alternatives to mRNA COVID-19 vaccines remain available for people who cannot or will not receive an mRNA vaccine.

The monovalent COVID-19 vaccines have a component of, or a component that corresponds to, the original strain of the virus that causes COVID-19. The bivalent COVID-19 vaccines have two mRNA components: one of which corresponds to the original strain of the virus that is broadly protective against COVID-19 and the other corresponds to the omicron variant BA.4 and BA.5 lineages to provide better protection against COVID-19 caused by the omicron variant. The monovalent Moderna and Pfizer-BioNTech COVID-19 vaccines are no longer authorized for use in the U.S. because the available data indicate that the bivalent Pfizer-BioNTech and Moderna COVID-19 vaccines provide improved protection against severe illness, hospitalization and death due to COVID-19 caused by currently circulating variants.

CDC and ACIP will continue to monitor COVID-19 disease levels and vaccine effectiveness in the months ahead and look forward to additional discussion around potential updates.

TREATMENT
SARS-CoV-2 Nucleotide Analog RNA Polymerase Inhibitor

▶ **remdesivir** *Loading Dose on Day 1:* 200 mg via IV infusion; *Maintenance:* 100 mg via IV infusion once daily starting Day 2; administer each infusion over 30-120 minutes; *Patients* not *requiring invasive mechanical ventilation* and/or *extracorporeal membrane oxygenation (ECMO):* the total treatment duration is 5 days; If no clinical improvement, treatment may be extended for up to 5 additional days for total treatment duration up to 10 days; *Patients requiring invasive mechanical ventilation* and/or *ECMO:* treatment duration is 10 days; *Estimated glomerular filtration rate (eGFR) <30 ml/min:* not recommended; *Dose Preparation/ administration:* see mfr pkg insert for full prescribing information
Pediatric: <28 days, <3 kg: safety and efficacy not established; ≥28 days, ≥3 kg to <40 kg: The only approved dose form and route of administration for these pediatric patients is **Veklury** for injection (supplied as 100 mg lyophilized powder for reconstitution with sterile water for injection, dilution in 250 ml 0.9% NaCl, and administration via IV infusion); Recommended dosage for these pediatric patients is a single loading dose of 5 mg/kg via IV infusion on Day 1, followed by once-daily maintenance doses of 2.5 mg/kg starting Day 2; Recommended total treatment duration for hospitalized patients requiring invasive mechanical ventilation and/or ECMO is 10 days; Treatment duration for hospitalized patients not requiring invasive mechanical ventilation and/or ECMO is 5 days (if a patient does not demonstrate clinical improvement, treatment may be extended for up to 5 additional days for a treatment duration of up to 10 days; ≥40 kg: same as adult
    Veklury Vial: 100 mg, single-dose, pwdr, for reconstitution, dilution, and IV infusion; 100 mg/20 ml (5 mg/ml), single-dose, soln for dilution and IV infusion (preservative-free)
    Comment: **Veklury** is a SARS-CoV-2 nucleotide analog RNA polymerase inhibitor indicated for treatment of COVID-19. **Veklury** is the first and only approved treatment for pediatric patients under 12 years of age. *Remdesivir* is indicated for patients with COVID-19 requiring hospitalization. **Veklury** should only be administered in a hospital or in a healthcare setting capable of providing acute care comparable to inpatient hospital care. Co-administration of **Veklury** and *chloroquine phosphate* or *hydroxychloroquine sulfate* is not recommended based on cell culture data demonstrating an antagonistic effect of chloroquine on the intracellular metabolic activation and antiviral activity of **Veklury**. In all patients, before initiating **Veklury** and during treatment as clinically appropriate, perform renal and hepatic laboratory testing and assess prothrombin time. The most common adverse reactions (incidence ≥5%, all grades) are nausea and increased alanine aminotransferase (ALT) and aspartate aminotransferase (AST). Consider discontinuing **Veklury** if ALT levels increase to >10 times the upper limit of normal (>a 10 x ULN). Discontinue **Veklury** if ALT elevation is accompanied by signs or symptoms of liver inflammation. Hypersensitivity reactions have been observed during and following administration of **Veklury**. Slower infusion rates, with a maximum infusion time of up to 120 minutes, can be considered to potentially prevent signs and symptoms of hypersensitivity. If signs and symptoms of a clinically significant hypersensitivity reaction occur, immediately discontinue administration of **Veklury** and initiate appropriate treatment. Available data from published case reports and compassionate use of *remdesivir* in pregnant females are insufficient to evaluate for a drug-associated risk of major birth defects, miscarriage, or adverse maternal or fetal outcomes. In non-clinical reproductive toxicity studies, *remdesivir* demonstrated no adverse effect on embryo/fetal development when administered to pregnant animals at systemic exposures (area under the curve (AUC)) of the predominant circulating metabolite of *remdesivir* (GS-441524) that were four times the exposure in humans at the recommended human dose (RHD). There are no available data on the presence of *remdesivir* in human milk or effects on the breastfed infant.

▷ *nirmatrelvir+ritonavir* co-administer *nirmatrelvir* 300 mg (2 x 150 mg tabs) plus *ritonavir* 100 mg (1 x 100 mg tab) together (3 tabs) bid x 5 days; take with or without food; swallow whole, do not crush, chew, or break tablets; if a dose of **Paxlovid** is missed within 8 hours of the time it is usually taken, take it as soon as possible and resume the normal dosing schedule; if a dose is missed by more than 8 hours, do not take the missed dose and instead take the next dose at the regularly scheduled time; do not double the dose to make up for a missed dose; *nirmatrelvir* must be co-administered with *ritonavir*; failure to correctly co-administer *nirmatrelvir* with *ritonavir* may result in plasma levels of *nirmatrelvir* that are insufficient to achieve the desired therapeutic effect

Pediatric: <12 years, <40 kg: safety and efficacy not established; ≥12 years, ≥40 kg: same as adult

Paxlovid *Tab:* *nirmatrelvir* 150 mg (20 tabs) plus ritonavir 150 mg (10 tabs) co-packaged in 5 daily blister cards

Comment: **Paxlovid** has emergency use authorization (EUA) for the treatment of mild-to-moderate COVID-19 in patients ≥12 years of age, weighing at least 40 kg (88 lb), with positive results of direct SARS-CoV-2 testing, and who are at high risk for progression to severe COVID-19, including hospitalization or death. **Paxlovid** should be initiated as soon as possible after diagnosis of COVID-19 and within 5 days of symptom onset. *eGFR* ≥30-<60 ml/min: reduce **Paxlovid** dose to *nirmatrelvir* 150 mg and *ritonavir* 100 mg twice daily x 5 days; *eGFR <30 ml/min:* **Paxlovid** not recommended; *Child-Pugh Class C:* **Paxlovid** is not recommended. *Nirmatrelvir* and *ritonavir* are CYP3A substrates; therefore, drugs that induce CYP3A may *decrease* **Paxlovid** plasma concentrations, decreasing **Paxlovid**'s efficacy. Co-administration of **Paxlovid** with drugs highly dependent on CYP3A for clearance and for which elevated plasma concentrations are associated with serious and/or life-threatening events is contraindicated (for a complete list of drugs that should not be taken in combination with **Paxlovid**, refer to the *Paxlovid Fact Sheet for Healthcare Providers*). No dosage adjustment is required when co-administered with other products containing *ritonavir* or *cobicistat*. Patients on *ritonavir-* or *cobicistat*-containing HIV or hepatitis C virus (HCV) regimens should continue their treatment as indicated. Potential side effects of **Paxlovid** include impaired sense of taste, diarrhea, elevated blood pressure, muscle aches, and generally feeling unwell. Females of childbearing potential should use effective contraception during therapy. *Ritonavir* may reduce the efficacy of combined hormonal contraceptives; patients of childbearing potential using these products should be advised to use an effective alternative contraceptive method or an additional barrier method of contraception during therapy. *Ritonavir* is excreted in breast milk. No information is available on use of *nirmatrelvir* during breastfeeding. Developmental and health benefits of breastfeeding should be considered along with the mother's clinical need for **Paxlovid** in addition to any potential effects on the breastfed infant from the drug or from the underlying maternal condition.

CYTOMEGALOVIRUS (CMV) DNA TERMINASE COMPLEX INHIBITOR

Comment: *Letermovir* is a cytomegalovirus (CMV) DNA terminase complex inhibitor indicated for prophylaxis of CMV infection and disease in adult CMV-seropositive recipients [R+] of an allogeneic hematopoietic stem cell transplant (HSCT).

▷ *cidofovir* administer via IV infusion over 1 hour; pretreat with oral *probenecid* (2 gm, 3 hours prior to starting the *cidofovir* infusion; and 1 gm, 2 and 8 hours after the infusion is ended) and 1 liter of IV NaCl should be infused immediately before each dose of *cidofovir* (a 2nd liter of NaCl should also be infused either during or; after each dose of *cidofovir* if a fluid load is tolerable); *Induction:* 5 mg/kg once weekly for 2 consecutive weeks; *Maintenance:* 5 mg/kg once every 2 weeks; reduce to 3 mg/kg if serum creatinine (sCr) increases 0.3-0.4 mg/dL above baseline; discontinue if sCr increases to >0.5 mg/dL above baseline or if >3+ proteinuria develops

Pediatric: <12 years: not recommended; >12 years: same as adult

Vistide *Vial:* 75 mg/ml (5 ml) (preservative-free)

Comment: *Cidofovir* is a nucleoside analog indicated for treatment of AIDS-related CMV retinitis.

▷ *letermovir* administer dose orally or as an IV infusion over 1 hour; dose is 480 mg once daily through 100 days posttransplant; if co-administered with *cyclosporine*, decrease the *letermovir* dose to 240 mg once daily

Pediatric: <18 years: not recommended; ≥18 years: same as adult

Prevymis *Tab:* 240, 450 mg; *Vial:* 240 mg/12 ml (20 mg/ml), 480 mg/24 ml (20 mg/ml), single-dose

Comment: Closely monitor sCr levels in patients with CrCl <50 ml/min using **Prevymis** injection for IV infusion. **Prevymis** is not recommended for patients with severe (Child-Pugh Class C) hepatic impairment. **Prevymis** is contraindicated with *pimozide*, ergot alkaloids, and *pitavastatin* and *simvastatin* when co-administered with *cyclosporine*. The most common adverse events (10%) have been nausea, diarrhea, vomiting, peripheral edema, cough, headache, fatigue, and abdominal pain. No adequate human data are available to inform whether **Prevymis** poses a risk to pregnancy outcomes. It is not known whether *letermovir* is present in human breast milk or effects the breastfed infant.

▷ *valganciclovir* (G) Take with food; *Induction:* 900 mg bid x 21 days; *Maintenance:* 900 mg daily; *CrCl <60 ml/min:* Reduce dose (see mfr pkg insert); *Hemodialysis or CrCl <10 ml/min:* Not recommended (use *ganciclovir*)

Pediatric: <4 months: not recommended; 4 months-16 years: see mfr pkg insert for dosing calculation equation

Valcyte *Tab:* 450 mg (preservative-free); *Oral pwdr for reconstitution:* 50 mg/ml (tutti-frutti)

JANUS KINASE (JAK) INHIBITOR

▷ *baricitinib Recommended dose:* 4 mg once daily; Take with or without food; for 14 days or until hospital discharge, whichever occurs first; An alternative method of oral administration may be used for patients unable to swallow tablets
Pediatric: Safety and efficacy not established

Olumiant *Tab:* 1, 2, 4 mg film-coat

Comment: Olumiant is a Janus kinase (JAK) inhibitor indicated for the treatment of COVID-19 in hospitalized adults requiring supplemental oxygen, non-invasive or invasive mechanical ventilation, or extracorporeal membrane oxygenation (ECMO). See the mfr pkg insert for full prescribing information, including a boxed warning regarding serious infections, mortality, malignancy, major adverse cardiovascular events (MACE), and thrombosis. The most common adverse reactions (incidence >1%) have included upper respiratory infection, nausea, herpes simplex, and herpes zoster. See the mfr pkg insert for full prescribing information, including a boxed warning regarding serious infections, mortality, malignancy, major adverse cardiovascular events (MACE), and thrombosis. See mfr pkg insert for other warnings, precautions, adverse reactions, dose modifications, drug interactions, laboratory abnormalities (cytopenias), hepatic and renal impairment, carcinogenesis, mutagenesis, and fertility impairment. Advise patients of the potential benefits and risks of treatment with Olumiant and advise patients to read the FDA-approved patient labeling (Medication Guide). Limited data on Olumiant use in human pregnancy are not sufficient to inform a drug-associated risk of major birth defects or miscarriage. Pregnancy status should be determined prior to initiating treatment with Olumiant. Females of reproductive potential should be informed of the risks to the fetus and advised to use effective contraception during treatment. Because of the potential for serious adverse reactions in breastfed infants, advise Olumiant-treated mothers not to breastfeed. Report pregnancies to Eli Lilly at 1-800-LillyRx (1-800-545-5979). To report suspected adverse reactions, contact Eli Lilly at 1-800-LillyRx (1-800-545-5979) or FDA at 1-800-FDA-1088 or www.fda.gov/medwatch.

HUMANIZED INTERLEUKIN-6 (IL-6) RECEPTOR-INHIBITING MONOCLONAL ANTIBODY

▷ *tocilizumab Administer* 8 mg per kg via a 60-minute IV infusion; Do not administer as a bolus or IV push; See mfr pkg insert for instructions on preparation and administration
Pediatric: Safety and efficacy not established

Actemra *Vial:* 80 mg/4 ml (20 mg/ml), 200 mg/10 ml (20 mg/ml), 400 mg/20 ml (20 mg/ml), single-dose, for further dilution and IV infusion; *Prefilled ACTPen autoinjector:* 162 mg/0.9 ml, single-dose, for SC administration

Comment: Actemra is a humanized interleukin-6 (IL-6) receptor-inhibiting monoclonal antibody with indications for the treatment of rheumatoid arthritis (RA), systemic juvenile idiopathic arthritis (SJIA), polyarticular juvenile idiopathic arthritis (PJIA), giant cell arteritis (GCA), CAR T-cell-induced severe or life-threatening cytokine release syndrome (CRS), systemic sclerosis-associated interstitial lung disease (ILD), and for hospitalized adult patients with COVID-19. Monitor patients for dose-related laboratory changes, including elevated liver function tests (LFTs), neutropenia, and thrombocytopenia. Actemra should not be initiated in patients with an absolute neutrophil count (ANC) below 2,000 per mm³, platelet count below 100,000 per mm³, or who have ALT or AST above 1.5 times the ULN. Registration in the Pregnancy Exposure Registry (1-877-311-8972) is encouraged for monitoring pregnancy outcomes in women exposed to Actemra during pregnancy. The limited available data with Actemra in pregnant females are not sufficient to determine whether there is a drug-associated risk of major birth defects and miscarriage. Monoclonal antibodies, such as *tocilizumab*, are actively transported across the placenta during the third trimester of pregnancy and may affect immune response in the infant exposed *in utero*. It is not known whether *tocilizumab* passes into breast milk; therefore, breastfeeding is not recommended while using Actemra.

CRAMPS: ABDOMINAL, INTESTINAL

ANTISPASMODIC-ANTICHOLINERGIC AGENTS

▷ *dicyclomine* (G) initially 20 mg bid-qid; may increase to 40 mg qid PO; usual IM dose 80 mg/day divided qid; do not use IM route for more than 1-2 days
Pediatric: <12 years: not recommended; ≥12 years: same as adult

Bentyl *Tab:* 20 mg; *Cap:* 10 mg; *Syr:* 10 mg/5 ml (16 oz); *Vial:* 10 mg/ml (10 ml); *Amp:* 10 mg/ml (2 ml)
▷ *methscopolamine bromide* 1 tab q 6 hours prn
Pediatric: <12 years: not recommended; ≥12 years: same as adult

Pamine *Tab:* 2.5 mg
Pamine Forte *Tab:* 5 mg

ANTICHOLINERGICS

▷ *hyoscyamine* (G)
Anaspaz 1-2 tabs q 4 hours prn; max 12 tabs/day

Pediatric: <2 years: not recommended; 2-12 years: 0.0625-0.125 mg q 4 hours prn; max 0.75 mg/day; ≥12 years: same as adult
> *Tab:* 0.125*mg
Levbid 1-2 tabs q 12 hours prn; max 4 tabs/day
Pediatric: <12 years: not recommended; ≥12 years: same as adult
> *Tab:* 0.375*mg ext-rel
Levsin 1-2 tabs q 4 hours prn; max 12 tabs/day
Pediatric: <6 years: not recommended; ≥6-12 years: 1 tab q 4 hours prn
> *Tab:* 0.125*mg
Levsinex SL 1-2 tabs q 4 hours SL or PO; max 12 tabs/day
Pediatric: 2-12 years: 1 tab SL or PO q 4 hours; max 6 tabs/day
> *Tab:* 0.125 mg sublingual
Levsinex Timecaps 1-2 caps q 12 hours; may adjust to 1 cap q 8 hours
Pediatric: 2-12 years: 1 cap q 12 hours; max 2 caps/day
> *Cap:* 0.375 mg time-rel
NuLev dissolve 1-2 tabs on tongue, with or without water, q 4 hours prn; max 12 tabs/day
Pediatric: <2 years: not recommended; 2-12 years: dissolve 1 tab on tongue, with or without water, q 4 hours prn; max 6 tabs/day; >12 years: same as adult
> *ODT:* 0.125 mg (mint) (phenylalanine)

▷ *simethicone* (G) 0.3 ml qid pc and HS
> **Mylicon Drops (OTC)** *Oral drops:* 40 mg/0.6 ml (30 ml)

▷ *phenobarbital+hyoscyamine+atropine+scopolamine* (IV)(G)
> **Donnatal** 1-2 tabs ac and HS
> *Pediatric:* <12 years: not recommended; ≥12 years: same as adult
>> *Tab:* pheno 16.2 mg+hyo 0.1037 mg+atro 0.0194 mg+scop 0.0065 mg
> **Donnatal Elixir** 1-2 tsp ac and HS
> *Pediatric:* 20 lb: 1 ml q 4 hours or 1.5 ml q 6 hours; 30 lb: 1.5 ml q 4 hours or 2 ml q 6 hours; 50 lb: 1/2 tsp q 4 hours or 3/4 tsp q 6 hours; 75 lb: 3/4 tsp q 4 hours or 1 tsp q 6 hours; 100 lb: 1 tsp q 4 hours or 1 tsp q 6 hours
>> *Elix:* pheno 16.2 mg+hyo 0.1037 mg+atro 0.0194 mg+scop 0.0065 mg per 5 ml (4, 16 oz)
> **Donnatal Extentabs** 1 tab q 12 hours
> *Pediatric:* <12 years: not recommended; ≥12 years: same as adult
>> *Tab:* pheno 48.6 mg+hyo 0.3111 mg+atro 0.0582 mg+scop 0.0195 mg ext-rel

ANTICHOLINERGIC+SEDATIVE COMBINATION
▷ *chlordiazepoxide+clidinium* (IV) 1-2 caps ac and HS; max 8 caps/day
> *Pediatric:* <12 years: not recommended; ≥12 years: same as adult
>> **Librax** *Cap:* chlor 5 mg+clid 2.5 mg

CROHN'S DISEASE

Parenteral Corticosteroids *see* Appendix L. Parenteral Corticosteroids
Oral Corticosteroids *see* Appendix K. Oral Corticosteroids

Comment: Standard treatment regimen for active disease (flare) is antibiotic, antispasmodic, and bowel rest, progress to clear liquids, then progress to high-fiber diet. Long-term management of chronic disease includes salicylates, immune modulators, and tumor necrosis factor (TNF) blockers.

ORAL ANTI-INFECTIVES
▷ *metronidazole* (G) 500 mg tid or 750 mg bid; max 8 weeks
> *Pediatric:* 35-50 mg/kg/day in 3 divided doses x 10 days
>> **Flagyl** *Tab:* 250*, 500*mg
>> **Flagyl 375** *Cap:* 375 mg
>> **Flagyl ER** *Tab:* 750 mg ext-rel

SALICYLATES
▷ *mesalamine* (G)
> **Asacol** 800 mg tid x 6 weeks; maintenance 1.6 gm/day in divided doses; swallow whole, do not crush or chew
> *Pediatric:* <12 years: not recommended; ≥12 years: same as adult
>> *Tab:* 400 mg del-rel
> **Comment:** 2 x **Asacol** 400 mg tabs are not bioequivalent to 1 x **Asacol HD** 800 mg tab.
> **Asacol HD** 1,600 mg tid x 6 weeks; swallow whole, do not crush or chew
> *Pediatric:* <12 years: not recommended; ≥12 years: same as adult
>> *Tab:* 800 mg del-rel
> **Comment:** 1 x **Asacol HD** 800 mg tab is not bioequivalent to 2 x **Asacol** 400 mg tabs
> **Canasa** 1 gm qid for up to 8 weeks

(continued)

Pediatric: <12 years: <u>not</u> recommended; ≥12 years: same as adult
   Rectal supp: 1 gm del-rel (30, 42/pck)
Delzicol *Treatment:* 800 mg tid x 6 weeks; *Maintenance:* 1.6 gm/day in 2-4 divided doses daily; Swallow
whole, Do <u>not</u> crush <u>or</u> chew
Pediatric: <5 years: <u>not</u> established; ≥5 years: same as adult
   Cap: 400 mg del-rel
Comment: 2 x **Delzicol** 400 mg caps are <u>not</u> bioequivalent to 1 x ***mesalamine*** 800 mg del-rel tab
Lialda 2.4-4.8 gm daily in a single dose for up to 8 weeks; swallow whole, do <u>not</u> crush <u>or</u> chew
Pediatric: <18 years: <u>not</u> recommended; ≥18 years: same as adult
   Tab: 1.2 gm del-rel
Pentasa 1 gm qid for up to 8 weeks; swallow whole, do <u>not</u> crush <u>or</u> chew
Pediatric: <12 years: <u>not</u> recommended; ≥12 years: same as adult
   Cap: 250 mg cont-rel
Rowasa Enema 4 gm rectally by enema q HS; retain for 8 hours x 3-6 weeks
Pediatric: <12 years: <u>not</u> recommended; ≥12 years: same as adult
   Enema: 4 gm/60 ml (7, 14, 28/pck; kit, 7, 14, 28/pck w. wipes)
Rowasa Suppository 1 suppository rectally bid x 3-6 weeks; retain for 1-3 hours <u>or</u> longer
   Rectal supp: 500 mg
Sulfite-Free Rowasa Rectal Suspension 4 gm rectally by enema q HS; retain for 8 hours x 3-6 weeks
   Enema: 4 gm/60 ml (7, 14, 28/pck; kit, 7, 14, 28/pck w. wipes)
▷ *olsalazine*
   Dipentum 1 gm/day in 2 divided doses; max 2 gm/day
     Cap: 250 mg
   Comment: Indicated in persons who cannot tolerate ***sulfasalazine***.
▷ *sulfasalazine* (G)
   Azulfidine initially 1-2 gm/day; increase to 3-4 gm/day in divided doses pc until clinical symptoms
   controlled; maintenance 2 gm/day; max 4 gm/day
   Pediatric: <2 years: <u>not</u> recommended; 2-16 years: initially 40-60 mg/kg/day in 3-6 divided doses; max 2
   gm/day
     Tab: 500*mg
   Azulfidine EN initially 500 mg in the PM x 7 days; then 500 mg bid x 7 days; then 500 mg in the AM
   and 1 gm in the PM x 7 days; then 1 gm bid; max 4 gm/day
   Pediatric: <12 years: <u>not</u> recommended; ≥12 years: same as adult
     Tab: 500 mg ent-coat
▷ *budesonide micronized* (G)
  Pediatric: <12 years: <u>not</u> recommended; ≥12 years: same as adult
   Entocort EC *Treatment:* 9 mg once daily in the AM for up to 8 weeks; may repeat an 8-week course;
   Maintenance of remission: 6 mg once daily for up to 3 months
     Cap: 3 mg ent-coat ext-rel granules
   Comment: Taper other systemic steroids when transferring to **Entocort EC**. When corticosteroids
   are used chronically, systemic effects such as hypercorticism and adrenal suppression may occur.
   Corticosteroids can reduce the response of the hypothalamus-pituitary-adrenal (HPA) axis to stress.
   In situations where patients are subject to surgery <u>or</u> other stress situations, supplementation with a
   systemic corticosteroid is recommended. General precautions concerning corticosteroids should be
   followed.

PURINE ANTIMETABOLITE IMMUNOSUPPRESSANT
▷ *azathioprine* (G)
   Imuran *Tab:* 50*mg; *Injectable:* 100 mg
   Comment: **Imuran** is usually administered on a daily basis. The initial dose should be approximately 1.0
   mg/kg (50-100 mg) as a single dose <u>or</u> divided bid. Dose may be increased beginning at 6-8 weeks, and
   thereafter at 4-week intervals, if there are no serious toxicities and if initial response is unsatisfactory.
   Dose increments should be 0.5 mg/kg/day, up to max 2.5 mg/kg per day. Therapeutic response usually
   occurs after 6-8 weeks of treatment. An adequate trial should be a minimum of 12 weeks. Patients <u>not</u>
   improved after 12 weeks can be considered refractory. **Imuran** may be continued long term in patients
   with clinical response, but patients should be monitored carefully and gradual dosage reduction should
   be attempted to reduce risk of toxicities. Maintenance therapy should be at the lowest effective dose, and
   the dose given can be lowered decrementally with changes of 0.5 mg/kg <u>or</u> approximately 25 mg daily
   every 4 weeks while other therapy is kept constant. The optimum duration of maintenance **Imuran** has
   <u>not</u> been determined. **Imuran** can be discontinued abruptly, but delayed effects are possible.

TUMOR NECROSIS FACTOR (TNF) BLOCKERS
▷ *adalimumab* *Day 1:* 160 mg SC (single dose <u>or</u> split over 2 consecutive days); *Day 15:* 80 mg SC; *Starting
day 29:* 40 mg SC every other week; Administer SC in the abdomen <u>or</u> thigh and rotate sites

Pediatric: <17 kg (37 lb): <u>not</u> recommended; 17 kg (37 lb) to <40 kg (<88 lb): *Day 1:* 80 mg SC; *Day 15:* 40 mg SC; *Starting Day 29:* 20 mg every other week; >40 kg (>88 lb): *Day 1:* 160 mg SC (single dose <u>or</u> split over 2 consecutive days); *Day 15:* 80 mg SC; *Starting Day 29:* 40 mg SC every other week

    Humira *Prefilled pen (Humira Pen):* 40 mg/0.4 ml, 40 mg/0.8 ml, 80 mg/0.8 ml, single-dose; *Prefilled glass syringe:* 10 mg/0.1 ml, 10 mg/0.2 ml, 20 mg/0.2 ml, 20 mg/0.4 ml, 40 mg/0.4 ml. 40 mg/0.8 ml, 80 mg/0.8 ml, single-dose; *Vial:* 40 mg/0.8 ml, single dose, institutional use only (preservative-free)

Comment: May use with corticosteroids, salicylates, nonsteroidal anti-inflammatory drugs (NSAIDs), <u>or</u> analgesics.

▷ *adalimumab-aacf* Administer: 160 mg SC on Day 1 (may split dose over 2 consecutive days); then 80 mg SC on Day 15; then 40 mg SC every other week starting on Day 29; Discontinue in patients without evidence of clinical remission by 8 weeks (Day 57)

Pediatric: <6 years: <u>not</u> recommended; ≥6 years, ≥40 kg (88 lb): same as adult

    Idacio *Prefilled pen (Idacio Pen):* 40 mg/0.8 ml, single-dose; *Prefilled glass syringe:* 40 mg/0.8 ml, single dose

    Comment: Idacio is biosimilar to **Humira** *(adalimumab)*.

▷ *adalimumab-adaz* First Dose (Day 1): 160 mg SC (4 x 40 mg injections in 1 day <u>or</u> 2 x 40 mg injections per day x 2 consecutive days); *Second dose 2 weeks later (Day 15):* 80 mg SC; Then, *2 weeks later (Day 29)* begin a maintenance dose of 40 mg SC every other week

Pediatric: <18 years: <u>not</u> recommended; ≥18 years: same as adult

    Hyrimoz *Prefilled syringe:* 40 mg/0.8 ml single-dose (preservative-free)

    Comment: Hyrimoz is biosimilar to **Humira** *(adalimumab)*.

▷ *adalimumab-adbm* First Dose (day 1): 160 mg SC (4 x 40 mg injections in 1 day <u>or</u> 2 x 40 mg injections per day for 2 consecutive days); *Second dose 2 weeks later (Day 15):* 80 mg SC; Then, *2 weeks later (Day 29),* begin a maintenance dose of 40 mg SC every other week

Pediatric: <18 years: <u>not</u> recommended; ≥18 years: same as adult

    Cyltezo *Prefilled syringe:* 40 mg/0.8 ml single-dose (preservative-free)

    Comment: Cyltezo is biosimilar to **Humira** *(adalimumab)*.

▷ *adalimumab-afzb* 40 mg SC every other week; Some patients with rheumatoid arthritis (RA) <u>not</u> receiving *methotrexate (MTX)* may benefit from increasing the frequency to 40 mg SC every week

    Abrilada *Prefilled pen:* 40 mg/0.8 ml, single-dose; *Prefilled syringe:* 40 mg/0.8 ml, 20 mg/0.4 ml, 10 mg/0.2 ml, single-dose; *Vial:* 40 mg/0.8 ml, single-use (for institutional use only) (preservative-free)

    Comment: Abrilada is biosimilar to **Humira** *(adalimumab)*.

▷ *adalimumab-bwwd* Initial Dose (Day 1): 160 mg SC; *Second dose 2 weeks later (Day 15):* 80 mg SC; Then, *2 weeks later (Day 29),* begin maintenance dose of 40 mg every other week

    Hadlima *Prefilled autoinjector:* 40 mg/0.8 ml, single-dose (Hadlima PushTouch); *Prefilled syringe:* 40 mg/0.8 ml, single-dose

    Comment: Hadlima is biosimilar to **Humira** *(adalimumab)*.

▷ *certolizumab* 400 mg SC (2 x 200 mg inj at two different sites on day 1); then 400 mg SC at weeks 2 and 4; maintenance 400 mg SC every 4 weeks; administer in the abdomen <u>or</u> thigh and rotate sites

Pediatric: <12 years: <u>not</u> recommended; ≥12 years: same as adult

    Cimzia *Vial:* 200 mg (2/pck); *Prefilled syringe:* 200 mg/ml single-dose (2/pck; 2, 6/starter pck) (preservative-free)

▷ *infliximab* must be refrigerated at 2°C to 8°C (36°F to 46°F); administer dose IV over a period of <u>not</u> less than 2 hours; do <u>not</u> use beyond the expiration date as this product contains no preservative; 5 mg/kg at 0, 2, and 6 weeks, then every 8 weeks

Pediatric: <6 years: safety and efficacy <u>not</u> established; ≥6-17 years: 5 mg/kg at 0, 2, and 6 weeks, then every 8 weeks; ≥18 years: same as adult

    Remicade *Vial:* 100 mg for reconstitution to 10 ml administration volume, single-dose pwdr (preservative-free)

    Comment: Remicade is indicated to reduce signs and symptoms and induce and maintain clinical remission in adults and children ≥6 years of age with moderately to severely active disease who have had an inadequate response to conventional therapy <u>and</u> reduce the number of draining enterocutaneous and rectovaginal fistulas and maintain fistula closure in adults with fistulizing disease. Common adverse effects associated with **Remicade** included abdominal pain, headache, pharyngitis, sinusitis, and upper respiratory infections (URIs). In addition, **Remicade** might increase the risk of serious infections, including tuberculosis, bacterial sepsis, and invasive fungal infections. Available data from published literature on the use of *infliximab* products during pregnancy have <u>not</u> reported a clear association with *infliximab* products and adverse pregnancy outcomes. *Infliximab* products cross the placenta, and infants exposed *in utero* should <u>not</u> be administered live vaccines for at least 6 months after birth. Otherwise, the infant may be at increased risk of infection, including disseminated infection, which can become fatal. Available information is insufficient to inform the amount of *infliximab* products present in human milk <u>or</u> effects on the breastfed infant.

▷ *infliximab-abda*

    Renflexis *Vial:* 100 mg pwdr for reconstitution to 10 ml administration volume, single-dose

    Comment: Renflexis is biosimilar to **Remicade** *(infliximab)*.

(continued)

▷ **infliximab-axxq** *Initially*: 5 mg/kg via IV infusion at 0, 2, and 6 weeks; *Maintenance*: 5 mg/kg via IV infusion every 8 weeks
Pediatric: <6 years: not studied; ≥6 years: same as adult
> Avsola *Vial*: 100 mg pwdr in a 20 ml single-dose vial, for reconstitution, dilution, and IV infusion
> **Comment**: Avsola is biosimilar to **Remicade** *(infliximab)*.

▷ *infliximab-qbtx*
> Ixifi *Vial*: 100 pwdr mg for reconstitution to 10 ml administration volume, single-dose
> **Comment**: Ixifi is biosimilar to **Remicade** *(infliximab)*.

INTERLEUKIN-23 ANTAGONIST

▷ *risankizumab-rzaa* **Recommended**: Obtain liver enzymes and bilirubin level prior to initiating treatment; *Recommended Induction Dose*: 600 mg via IV infusion over at least 1 hour at Week 0, Week 4, and Week 8; *Recommended Maintenance*: 180 mg or 360 mg SC at Week 12, and every 8 weeks thereafter; Use the lowest effective dosage to maintain therapeutic response. Do not freeze; Do not shake; Keep in the original cartons to protect from light; No natural rubber latex
Pediatric: safety and efficacy not established
> Skyrizi *Single-dose preservative-free soln for IV infusion: Vial*: 600 mg/10 ml (60 mg/ml); *single-dose preservative-free soln for SC injection: Prefilled pen*: 150 mg/ml (1 ml); *Prefilled syringe*: 75 mg/0.83 ml (150 mg/ml), 180 mg/1.2 ml (150 mg/ml) (Note: prefilled pen and prefilled syringe have a fixed 27-gauge 1/2 inch needle with needle guard); *Prefilled cartridge*: 360 mg/2.4 ml (150 mg/ml) (Note: prefilled cartridge is supplied with an on-body injector device)
> **Comment**: Skyrizi is an interleukin-23 antagonist indicated for the treatment of moderate-to-severe plaque psoriasis in adults who are candidates for systemic therapy or phototherapy, active psoriatic arthritis in adults, and moderately to severely active Crohn's disease in adults. Reported adverse side effects (incidence >3%) have been: *Induction*: URI, headache, and arthralgia; *Maintenance*: arthralgia, abdominal pain, injection site reactions, anemia, pyrexia, back pain, arthropathy, and urinary tract infection (UTI). **Skyrizi** is contraindicated in patients with a history of serious hypersensitivity reaction to *risankizumab-rzaa* or any of the excipients. Serious hypersensitivity reactions, including anaphylaxis, may occur. **Skyrizi** may increase the risk of infection; instruct patients to seek medical advice if signs or symptoms of clinically important infection occur and, if such an infection develops, do not administer **Skyrizi** until the infection resolves. Evaluate for tuberculosis prior to initiating treatment. Drug-induced liver injury during induction has been reported. Monitor liver enzymes and bilirubin levels at baseline and, during induction, up to at least 12 weeks of treatment; thereafter, monitor according to routine patient management. Avoid use of live vaccines. Available pharmacovigilance and clinical trial data with *risankizumab-rzaa* use in pregnancy are insufficient to establish a drug-associated risk of major birth defects, miscarriage, or other adverse maternal or fetal outcomes. Although there are no data on *risankizumab-rzaa*, monoclonal antibodies can be actively transported across the placenta, and **Skyrizi** may cause immunosuppression in the infant exposed *in utero*. Transport of endogenous immunoglobulin G (IgG) antibodies across the placenta increases as pregnancy progresses and peaks during the third trimester. Because *risankizumab-rzaa* may interfere with immune response to infection, risks and benefits should be considered prior to administering live vaccines to infants exposed to **Skyrizi** *in utero*. There are insufficient data regarding infant serum levels of *risankizumab-rzaa* at birth and the duration of persistence of *risankizumab-rzaa* in infant serum after birth. Although a specific time frame to delay live virus immunizations in infants exposed *in utero* is unknown, a minimum of 5 months after birth should be considered because of the half-life of **Skyrizi**. (NOTE: Published data suggest that the risk of adverse pregnancy outcomes in females with inflammatory bowel disease [IBD] is associated with increased disease activity with adverse pregnancy outcomes, including preterm delivery [<37 weeks' gestation], low birthweight [<2,500 gm] infants, and small for gestational age [SGA] at birth). Advise females of reproductive potential of potential fetal risk and recommend effective contraception during treatment. There is a pregnancy exposure registry that monitors outcomes in women who become pregnant while treated with **Skyrizi**. Patients should be encouraged to enroll by calling 1-877-302-2161 or visiting http://glowpregnancyregistry.com. There are no data on the presence of *risankizumab-rzaa* in human milk or effects on the breastfed infant. However, endogenous maternal IgG and monoclonal antibodies are transferred in human milk. The effects of local gastrointestinal exposure and limited systemic exposure in the breastfed infant to *risankizumab-rzaa* are unknown. Developmental and health benefits of breastfeeding should be considered along with the mother's clinical need for **Skyrizi** and any potential adverse effects on the breastfed infant from **Skyrizi** or from the underlying maternal condition.

INTERLEUKIN-12+INTERLEUKIN-23 ANTAGONIST

▷ *ustekinumab* **Recommened Dose**: Wt: *<100 kg (<220 lbs)*: 45 mg SC initially and and repeat 4 weeks later, followed by 45 mg SC every 12 weeks; *Wt: >100 kg (>220 lbs)*: 90 mg SC initially and repeat 4 weeks later, followed by 90 mg SC every 12 weeks
Pediatric: <18 years: not recommended; ≥18 years: same as adult
> Stelara *Prefilled sytinge*: 45 mg/0.5 ml, single-use; *Vial*: 45 mg/0.5 ml, 90 mg/ml, single-use (preservative-free)

INTEGRIN RECEPTOR ANTAGONIST (IMMUNOMODULATOR)

► *natalizumab* administer by IV infusion over 1 hour; monitor during and for 1 hour postinfusion; 300 mg every 4 weeks; discontinue after 12 weeks if no therapeutic response or if unable to taper off chronic concomitant steroids within 6 months; may continue aminosalicylates
Pediatric: <18 years: not established; ≥18 years: same as adult
  Tysabri *Vial:* 300 mg single-dose, soln after dilution for IV infusion (preservative-free)
  Stelara *Prefilled syringe:* 45 mg/0.5 ml, single-dose; *Vial:* 45 mg/0.5 ml, 90 mg/ml, single-dose, 130 mg/26 ml, single-dose (preservative-free)

► *vedolizumab* administer by IV infusion over 30 minutes; 300 mg at weeks 0, 2, and 6; then once every 8 weeks
Pediatric: <18 years: not established; ≥18 years: same as adult
  Entyvio *Vial:* 300 mg (20 ml), single-dose, pwdr for IV infusion after reconstitution (preservative-free)

JANUS KINASE (JAK) INHIBITOR

► *upadacitinib* 15 mg once daily; may be used as monotherapy or in combination with *MTX* or other nonbiologic Disease-modifying antirheumatic drugs (DMARDs); avoid initiation or interrupt Rinvoq if absolute lymphocyte count is <500 cells/mm³, absolute neutrophil count is <1,000 cells/mm³, or hemoglobin (Hgb) is <8 gm/dL.
Pediatric: <18 years: not established; ≥18 years: same as adult
  Rinvoq Extended-Release Tablets *Tab:* 15 mg ext-rel
  Comment: Rinvoq *(upadacitinib)* is a Janus kinase (JAK) inhibitor for the treatment of adult patients with moderate-to-severe active Crohn's disease who have had an inadequate response or intolerance to *MTX*. Use of Rinvoq in combination with other JAK inhibitors, biologic DMARDs, or with potent immunosuppressants such as *azathioprine* and *cyclosporine* is not recommended. Use of Rinvoq in patients with severe hepatic impairment (Child-Pugh Class C) is not recommended. Co-administration of Rinvoq with strong CYP3A4 inducers (e.g., *rifampin*) is not recommended. Use with caution in patients receiving chronic treatment with strong CYP3A4 inhibitors (e.g., *ketoconazole*). Avoid use of Rinvoq with live vaccines. Serious infections leading to hospitalization or death, including tuberculosis and bacterial, invasive fungal, viral, and other opportunistic infections, have occurred in patients receiving Rinvoq. Avoid use of Rinvoq in patients with active, serious infection, including localized infection. If a serious infection develops, interrupt Rinvoq until the infection is controlled. Prior to starting Rinvoq, test for latent tuberculosis; if the test is positive, start treatment for tuberculosis. Monitor all patients for active tuberculosis during treatment, even if the initial latent tuberculosis test is negative. Lymphoma and other malignancies have been observed in patients treated with Rinvoq. Thrombosis, including deep vein thrombosis, pulmonary embolism, and arterial thrombosis, has occurred in patients treated with JAK inhibitors used to treat inflammatory conditions. Consider risk/benefit prior to initiating Rinvoq in patients with a known malignancy and patients who may be at increased risk of thrombosis or gastrointestinal perforation. Monitor for potential changes in lymphocytes, neutrophils, Hgb, liver enzymes, and lipids. Rinvoq may cause embryo/fetal toxicity; therefore, advise females of reproductive potential to use effective contraception during treatment and for 4 weeks following the final dose. Advise lactating women that breastfeeding is not recommended during treatment with *upadacitinib* and for 6 days (approximately 10 half-lives) after the last dose.

CRYPTOSPORIDIOSIS (*CRYPTOSPORIDIUM PARVUM*)

► *nitazoxanide* (G) 500 mg by mouth q 12 hours x 3 days
Pediatric: 12-47 months: 5 ml q 12 hours x 3 days; 4-11 years: 10 ml q 12 hours x 3 days; ≥12 years: same as adult
  Alinia *Oral susp:* 100 mg/5 ml (60 ml)
  Comment: Alinia is an antiprotozoal for the treatment of diarrhea due to *Giardia lamblia* or *Cryptosporidium parvum*.

CUSHING'S SYNDROME

CORTISOL RECEPTOR BLOCKER

► *mifepristone* administer once daily with a meal; initially 300 mg once daily; may increase in 300 mg increments to a maximum of 1,200 mg once daily based on clinical response and tolerability; Do not exceed 20 mg/kg/day; *Renal impairment:* do not exceed 600 mg once daily; *Mild-to-Moderate Hepatic Impairment:* do not exceed 600 mg once daily; *Severe Hepatic Impairment:* Do not use
Pediatric: safety and efficacy not established
  Korlym *Tab:* 300 mg film-coat
  Comment: Korlym *(mifepristone)* is a cortisol receptor blocker indicated to control hyperglycemia secondary to hypercortisolism in adult patients with endogenous Cushing's syndrome who have type 2

(continued)

diabetes mellitus or glucose intolerance and have failed surgery or are not candidates for surgery. The most common adverse reactions in Cushing's syndrome (incidence ≥20%) have been nausea, fatigue, headache, decreased blood potassium, arthralgia, vomiting, peripheral edema, hypertension, dizziness, decreased appetite, and endometrial hypertrophy. Closely monitor patients for signs and symptoms of adrenal insufficiency. Correct hypokalemia prior to treatment and monitor potassium during treatment. Women may experience endometrial thickening or unexpected vaginal bleeding. Use with caution if the patient also has a hemorrhagic disorder or is on anticoagulant therapy. Avoid use with QT interval-prolonging drugs and patients with potassium channel variants resulting in a long QT interval. Administer drugs that are metabolized by CYP3A at the lowest dose when used with **Korlym**. Limit *mifepristone* dose to 900 mg/day when used with strong CYP3A inhibitors. Do not use **Korlym** with CYP3A inducers. Use the lowest dose of CYP2C8/2C9 substrates when used with **Korlym**. Use caution when **Korlym** is used concomitantly with *bupropion* and *efavirenz*. Contraindications to **Korlym** include: taking drugs metabolized by CYP3A (e.g., *simvastatin*, *lovastatin*), and CYP3A substrates with narrow therapeutic ranges; receiving systemic corticosteroids for life-saving purposes; and history of unexplained vaginal bleeding or endometrial hyperplasia with atypia or endometrial carcinoma. *Mifepristone* has potent antiprogestational effects and will result in termination of pregnancy. Pregnancy must, therefore, be excluded before initiation of treatment with **Korlym** and if treatment is interrupted for more than 14 days in females of reproductive potential. **Korlym** interferes with the effectiveness of hormonal contraceptives; therefore, recommend non-hormonal contraception for the duration of treatment and for 1 month after the last dose. *Mifepristone* is present in human milk; however, there are no data on the amount of *mifepristone* in human milk or effects on the breastfed infant. Developmental and health benefits of breastfeeding should be considered along with the mother's clinical need for **Korlym** and any potential adverse effects on the breastfed infant from **Korlym** or from the underlying maternal condition. To minimize exposure to a breastfed infant, women who discontinue or interrupt **Korlym** treatment may consider pumping and discarding milk during treatment and for 18-21 days (5-6 half-lives) after the last dose before breastfeeding.

SOMATOSTATIN ANALOG

▶ *pasireotide* initially 0.6 mg or 0.9 mg SC bid; recommended dose range is 0.3 mg to 0.9 mg SC bid; titrate dosage based on treatment response (i.e., clinically meaningful reduction in 24-hour urinary free cortisol [UFC] and/or improvements in signs and symptoms of disease) and tolerability; *Child-Pugh Class B:* initially 0.3 mg SC bid; max: 0.6 mg bid; *Child-Pugh Class C:* avoid use
Pediatric: safety and efficacy not established
   Signifor *Amp:* 0.3 mg/ml (1 ml), 0.6 mg/ml (1ml), 0.9 mg/ml (1ml), single-dose

   Comment: Signifor is a somatostatin analog indicated for treatment of adult patients with Cushing's disease for whom pituitary surgery is not an option or has not been curative. *Testing Prior to Dosing:* fasting plasma glucose (FPG), hemoglobin A1c (HbA1c), liver function tests, ECG, gallbladder ultrasound, and serum potassium and magnesium levels. The most common adverse reactions (incidence ≥20%) in patients have been diarrhea, nausea, hyperglycemia, cholelithiasis, headache, abdominal pain, fatigue, and diabetes mellitus. Decreases in circulating levels of cortisol may occur resulting in biochemical and/or clinical hypocortisolism; **Signifor** dose reduction or interruption and/or adding a low-dose short-term glucocorticoid may be necessary. Hyperglycemia and diabetes occur with initiation of **Signifor**; therefore, intensive glucose monitoring is recommended and may require initiation or adjustment of antidiabetic treatment per standard of care. Bradycardia and QT prolongation can occur with **Signifor**; use with caution in at-risk patients and monitor ECG prior to and during treatment. Evaluate liver function tests (LFTs) prior to and during treatment. Cholelithiasis and complications of cholelithiasis may occur; monitor periodically and discontinue **Signifor** if complications of cholelithiasis are suspected. Use **Signifor** with caution in patients who are at significant risk of developing QTc prolongation. Consider additional monitoring with concomitant use of *cyclosporine*. With concomitant *bromocriptine*, consider *bromocriptine* dose reduction. The limited data with **Signifor** use in pregnant females are insufficient to inform a drug-associated risk of major birth defects and miscarriage. In embryo/fetal animal development studies, findings indicating developmental delay were observed with SC administration of *pasireotide* during organogenesis at doses less than the exposure in humans at the highest recommended dose. The reduction or normalization of serum cortisol levels in female patients with Cushing's disease treated with *pasireotide* may lead to improved fertility; therefore, females and males of reproductive potential should be advised of the potential for an unintended pregnancy. There is no information available on the presence of **Signifor** in human milk or effects of the drug on the breastfed infant. Developmental and health benefits of breastfeeding should be considered along with the mother's clinical need for **Signifor** and any potential adverse effects on the breastfed infant from **Signifor** or from the underlying maternal condition.

CORTISOL SYNTHESIS INHIBITOR

▶ *levoketoconazole Initial dose:* 150 mg bid, with or without food; titrate dose by 150 mg daily, no more frequently than every 2-3 weeks; Max 1,200 mg/day administered as 600 mg bid; Obtain baseline liver and ECG tests and correct hypokalemia and hypomagnesemia before initiating treatment; For additional recommendations on titration and monitoring for efficacy, see the mfr pkg insert; For recommendations on safety monitoring and dose modifications for hepatoxicity, QT prolongation, and hypocortisolism, see the mfr pkg insert

Pediatric: <18 years: safety and efficacy not established; ≥18 years: same as adult

Recorlev *Tab:* 150 mg film-coat

Comment: Recorlev is a cortisol synthesis inhibitor indicated for the treatment of endogenous hypercortisolemia in adult patients with Cushing's syndrome for whom surgery is not an option or has not been curative. **Recorlev** is not approved for the treatment of fungal infections. *Boxed Warning:* **Recorlev** is associated with serious hepatotoxicity. Cases of hepatotoxicity with fatal outcome or requiring liver transplantation have been reported with oral *ketoconazole*—some patients had no obvious risk factors for liver disease. Evaluate liver enzymes prior to and during treatment. **Recorlev** is associated with dose-related QT interval prolongation. QT interval prolongation may result in life-threatening ventricular dysrhythmias such as torsades de pointes. Perform ECG prior to and during treatment. Use of **Recorlev** is contraindicated for use in: (1) Patients with hepatic cirrhosis, acute liver disease or poorly controlled chronic liver disease, baseline aspartate aminotransferase (AST) or alanine aminotransferase (ALT) >3 the upper limit of normal (ULN), recurrent symptomatic cholelithiasis, history of drug-induced liver injury due to *ketoconazole* or any azole antifungal therapy that required discontinuation of treatment, or extensive metastatic liver disease; (2) Patients taking drugs that cause QT prolongation associated with ventricular arrythmias, including torsades de pointes; (3) Prolonged QTcF interval >470 msec at baseline, history of torsades de pointes, ventricular tachycardia (VT), ventricular fibrillation (VF), or prolonged QT syndrome; (4) Patients with hypersensitivity to *levoketoconazole, ketoconazole,* or any excipient in **Recorlev**; (5) Patients taking drugs that are sensitive substrates of CYP3A4 or CYP3A4 and P-gp. (Note: Consult approved product labeling for drugs that are substrates of CYP3A4, P-gp, OCT2, and MATE prior to initiating **Recorlev**). Hypocortisolism has been reported with **Recorlev**. Monitor patients for hypocortisolism; dosage reduction or interruption may be necessary. Hypersensitivity to **Recorlev** has been reported and anaphylaxis has been reported with oral *ketoconazole*. **Recorlev** may lower serum testosterone in men and women; inform male patients to report associated symptoms, which may include gynecomastia, impotence, and oligospermia. These manifestations of decreased testosterone have been shown to be reversible when treatment is discontinued. There are no available data on *ketoconazole* use during pregnancy to inform the risk of miscarriage. Available published data from case series and case-control studies on the use of the racemic *ketoconazole* during pregnancy are insufficient to determine a drug-associated risk of major birth defects. However, in animal reproduction studies, embryotoxic effects were observed. Fetal malformations were observed following oral dosing of racemic *ketoconazole* during the period of organogenesis. Active Cushing's syndrome during pregnancy has been associated with an increased risk of maternal and fetal morbidity and mortality (including gestational diabetes, gestational hypertension, preeclampsia, maternal death, miscarriage, intrauterine fetal demise, preterm birth, and neonatal death). Therefore, advise pregnant women of the potential risk to the fetus and consider whether the benefits of treatment with **Recorlev** outweigh the risks and advise females of reproductive potential to consider use of effective contraception. Advise mothers not to breastfeed during treatment and for 1 day after the final dose of **Recorlev**.

▷ *osilodrostat* initially 2 mg bid, with or without food; titrate dose by 1-2 mg bid, no more frequently than every 2 weeks based on rate of cortisol changes, individual tolerability, and improvement in signs and symptoms; max 30 mg bid; *Child-Pugh Class B:* initially 1 mg bid; *Child-Pugh Class C:* initially 1 mg once daily in the evening

Pediatric: safety and efficacy not established

Isturisa *Tab:* 1, 5, 10 mg

Comment: Isturisa is a cortisol synthesis inhibitor indicated for treatment of adult patients with Cushing's disease. Correct hypokalemia and hypomagnesemia and obtain baseline ECG prior to starting **Isturisa**. The most common adverse reactions (incidence >20%) have been adrenal insufficiency, fatigue, nausea, headache, and edema. Monitor patients closely for hypocortisolism and potentially life-threatening adrenal insufficiency. Dosage reduction or interruption may be necessary; ECG is required for all patients; use with caution in patients with risk factors for QTc prolongation. Monitor patients for elevations in adrenal hormone precursors and androgens. Monitor for hypokalemia, worsening of hypertension, edema, and hirsutism. Reduce the dose of **Isturisa** by half with concomitant use of a strong CYP3A4 inhibitor. An increase in **Isturisa** dose may be needed if **Isturisa** is used concomitantly with strong CYP3A4 and CYP2B6 inducers. A reduction in **Isturisa** dosage may be needed if strong CYP3A4 and CYP2B6 inducers are discontinued while using **Isturisa**. There are no available data on *osilodrostat* use in pregnant females to evaluate for a drug-associated risk of major birth defects, miscarriage, or adverse maternal or fetal outcomes. There are risks to the mother and fetus associated with active Cushing's syndrome during pregnancy. Breastfeeding is not recommended during treatment with **Isturisa** and for at least 1 week after the last dose.

CYCLOSPORIASIS (*CYCLOSPORA CAYETANENSIS*)

Comment: The CDC, state and local health departments, and the U.S. FDA have issued a Health Alert Network advisory after an increase in reported cases of cyclosporiasis, an intestinal illness caused by the parasite *Cyclospora cayetanensis*. Clinicians should consider a diagnosis of cyclosporiasis in patients who experience prolonged or remitting-relapsing diarrhea. Since May 1, 2017, 206 cases have been identified, more than twice the 88 cases reported from May 1 to August 3, 2016. Most laboratories in the United States do not routinely test for *Cyclospora*, even when a stool sample has been tested for parasites, so providers must specifically order the test. Several stool specimens may be required because *Cyclospora* oocysts may be shed intermittently and at low levels, even in persons with profuse diarrhea. Symptoms include watery diarrhea, which can be profuse, anorexia, fatigue, weight loss, nausea, flatulence, stomach cramps, myalgia, vomiting, and low-grade fever. Symptoms begin from 2 days to more than 2 weeks (average 7 days) after ingestion of the parasite. *Cyclospora* is food- and waterborne; it is not transmitted directly from person to person. The recommended treatment is *trimethoprim-sulfamethoxazole (TMP/SMX)*. There are no effective alternatives for people who are allergic to or who cannot tolerate *TMP/SMX*; observation and symptomatic care are recommended for these patients. If untreated, illness may last for a few days to a month or longer.

➤ *trimethoprim+sulfamethoxazole (TMP-SMX)*(G) bid × 10 days
  Pediatric: <2 months: not recommended; ≥2 months: 40 mg/kg/day of *sulfamethoxazole* in 2 divided doses x 10 days; *see Appendix BB.33: trimethoprim+sulfamethoxazole* (G) (Bactrim Suspension, Septra Suspension) *for dose by weight*
      Bactrim, Septra 2 tabs bid x 10 days
      Tab: trim 80 mg+sulfa 400 mg*
      Bactrim DS, Septra DS 1 tab bid x 10 days
      Tab: trim 160 mg+sulfa 800 mg*
      Bactrim Pediatric Suspension, Septra Pediatric Suspension
      Oral susp: trim 40 mg+sulfa 200 mg per 5 ml (100 ml) (cherry) (alcohol 0.3%)

CYSTIC FIBROSIS (CF)

➤ *acetylcysteine* (G) Administer via face mask, mouthpiece, tracheostomy T-piece, mist tent, or croupette;
  Routine tracheostomy care: 1-2 ml of a 10%-20% solution may be administered by direct instillation into the tracheostomy every 1-4 hours
  Pediatric: same as adult
      Mucomyst *Vial:* 10, 20% (4, 10, 30 ml) soln for inhalation
      Comment: Mucomyst is a mucolytic. For inhalation, the 10% concentration may be used undiluted; the 20% concentration should be diluted with sterile water or normal saline (either for injection or inhalation).

CYSTIC FIBROSIS TRANSMEMBRANE CONDUCTANCE REGULATOR (CFTR) POTENTIATOR

➤ *ivacaftor* 150 mg q 12 hours; administer with fat-containing food (e.g., eggs, butter, peanut butter, cheese pizza); avoid food and juices containing grapefruit or Seville oranges
  Pediatric: <6 months, <7 kg: not recommended; 6 months-<6 years, 7-<14 kg: 1 x 50 mg pkt oral granules mixed with 1 tsp (5 ml) soft food or liquid every 12 hours with fat-containing food; 6 months-<6 years, ≥14 kg: 1 x 75 mg pkt oral granules mixed with 1 tsp (5 ml) soft food or liquid every 12 hours with fat-containing food; ≥6 years: same as adult
      Kalydeco *Tab:* 150 mg film-coat; *Oral granules:* 50, 75 mg unit dose pkts (56 pkt/carton)
      Comment: Ivacaftor is indicated for the treatment of cystic fibrosis (CF) in patients who have a G551D co-mutation in the cystic fibrosis transmembrane conductance regulator (CFTR) gene. If the patient's genotype is unknown, an FDA-cleared CF mutation test should be used to detect the presence of the G551D mutation. **Kalydeco** is not effective in patients with CF who are homozygous for the F508del mutation in the CFTR gene. Transaminases (alanine aminotransferase [ALT] and aspartate aminotransferase [AST]) should be assessed prior to initiating **Kalydeco**, every 3 months during the first year of treatment, and annually thereafter. Patients who develop increased transaminase levels should be closely monitored until the abnormalities resolve. Dosing should be interrupted in patients with ALT or AST greater than 5 times the upper limit of normal (ULN). Following resolution of transaminase elevations, consider the benefits and risks of resuming **Kalydeco**. Concomitant use with strong CYP3A inducers (e.g., *rifampin*, St. John's wort) substantially decreases exposure of **Kalydeco** (which may diminish effectiveness); therefore, co-administration is not recommended. Reduce dose to 150 mg twice weekly when co-administered with strong CYP3A inhibitors (e.g., *ketoconazole*). Reduce dose to 150 mg once daily when co-administered with moderate CYP3A inhibitors. Caution is recommended in patients with severe renal impairment (CrCl ≤30 ml/min) or end-stage renal disease (ESRD). No dose adjustment is necessary for patients with mild hepatic impairment (Child-Pugh Class A). A reduced dose of 150 mg once daily is recommended in patients with moderate hepatic impairment (Child-Pugh Class B). No studies have been conducted in patients with severe hepatic impairment (Child-Pugh Class C). The most commonly reported adverse reactions are headache, sore throat, nasopharyngitis, upper respiratory infection (URI), nasal congestion, abdominal pain, nausea, diarrhea, dizziness, and rash. Excretion of **Kalydeco** into human milk is probable.

CFTR POTENTIATOR COMBINATIONS

▷ *lumacaftor+ivacaftor* <6 years: not recommended; 6-11 years: 2 x 100/125 tabs q 12 hours; ≥12 years: 2 x 200/125 tabs q 12 hours

Orkambi *Tab:* luma 100 mg+iva 125 mg; luma 200 mg+iva 125 mg film-coat

Comment: Orkambi is indicated for the treatment of CF in patients ≥6 years of age who are homozygous for the F508del mutation in the CFTR gene. The efficacy and safety of **Orkambi** have not been established in patients with CF other than those homozygous for the F508del mutation. If the patient's genotype is unknown, an FDA-cleared CF mutation test should be used to detect the presence of the F508del mutation on both alleles of the CFTR gene. Reduce the dose of **Orkambi** in patients with moderate-to-severe hepatic impairment. In patients with advanced liver disease, use with caution and only if the benefits are expected to outweigh the risks. When initiating **Orkambi** in patients taking strong CYP3A inhibitors, reduce the dose of **Orkambi** for the first week of treatment. There are limited and incomplete human data from clinical trials and postmarketing reports on use of **Orkambi** or its individual components in pregnancy to inform a drug-associated risk. There is no information regarding the presence of *lumacaftor* or *ivacaftor* in human milk or effects on the breastfed infant.

▷ *tezacaftor+ivacaftor* **plus** *ivacaftor* <12 years: safety and efficacy not established; ≥12 years: 1 x 100/150 fixed-dose tab in the morning and 1 x 150 mg *ivacaftor* tab in the evening, approximately 12 hours later; Take with fat-containing food; Avoid grapefruit and Seville oranges

Symdeko *Tab:* teza 100 mg+iva 150 mg, fixed-dose combination *plus* Tab: iva 150 mg (4-week supply/carton)

Comment: Symdeko is indicated for the treatment of the underlying cause of CF in patients ≥12 years of age who have two copies of the F508del mutation in the CFTR gene or who have ≥1 mutation that is responsive to *tezacaftor+ivacaftor*. If the patient's genotype is unknown, an FDA-cleared CF mutation test should be used to detect the presence of a CFTR mutation, followed by verification with bidirectional sequencing when recommended by the mutation test instructions for use. Reduce dose with moderate-to-severe hepatic impairment. Reduce dose when co-administered with drugs that are moderate or strong CYP3A inhibitors. There are limited and incomplete human data from clinical trials and postmarketing reports on the use of **Symdeko** in pregnancy to inform a drug-associated risk. There is no information regarding the presence of *tezacaftor* or *ivacaftor* in human milk or effects on the breastfed infant.

▷ *elexacaftor+ivacaftor+tezacaftor* **plus** *ivacaftor* See mfr pkg insert for morning and evening doses based on age and weight; Take morning and evening doses 12 hours apart; Take each dose with fat-containing food; avoid food- and drinks-containing grapefruit

Pediatric: <2 years: safety and efficacy not established; ≥2 years: refer to the mfr pkg insert for the age- and weight-based dosing table

Trikafta *Tab:* elexa 50 mg+iva 37.5 mg+teza 25 mg plus iva 75 mg; elexa 100 mg+iva 75 mg+teza 50 mg plus iva 150 mg, co-packaged blister packs sealed in a wallet (4 wallets/carton)

Comment: Trikafta *(elexacaftor+ivacaftor+tezacaftor)* is a fixed-triple combination regimen for the treatment of cystic fibrosis (CF) in adult and pediatric patients ≥2 years of age who have at least one copy of the F508del mutation in the CFTR gene. If the patient's genotype is unknown, an FDA-cleared CF mutation test should be used to confirm the presence of at least one F508del mutation. Liver function should be assessed prior to initiation of **Trikafta**. Monitor liver function tests (LFTs) every 3 months during the first year of treatment and annually thereafter. In patients with a history of hepatobiliary disease or elevated LFTs, more frequent monitoring should be considered. *Moderate Hepatic Impairment:* It is not recommended unless benefit exceeds risk (if used, reduce dose and monitor LFTs closely). *Severe Hepatic Impairment:* **Trikafta** should not be used. Dosing should be interrupted in patients with ALT or AST >5 × the ULN or ALT or AST >3 × the ULN with bilirubin >2 × the ULN. Following resolution of transaminase elevations, consider the benefits and risks of resuming treatment. Reduce dose when co-administered with drugs that are moderate or strong CYP3A inhibitors. Concomitant use with strong CYP3A inducers (e.g., *rifampin*, St. John's wort) significantly decreases *ivacaftor* exposure and expected to decrease *elexacaftor* and *tezacaftor* exposure, which may reduce **Trikafta** efficacy, and therefore co-administration is not recommended. Non-congenital lens opacities/cataracts have been reported in pediatric patients treated with *ivacaftor*-containing regimens. Baseline and follow-up examinations are recommended in pediatric patients initiating **Trikafta** treatment. There are limited and incomplete human data from clinical trials on the use of **Trikafta** or its individual components, *elexacaftor, tezacaftor,* and *ivacaftor,* in pregnant females to inform a drug-associated risk. There is no information regarding the presence of *elexacaftor, tezacaftor,* or ivacaftor in human milk or effects on the breastfed infant. The most common adverse drug reactions to **Trikafta** (incidence ≥5% of patients and at a frequency higher than placebo by ≥1%) have been headache, upper respiratory tract infection, abdominal pain, diarrhea, rash, increased aminotransferase, nasal congestion, increased phosphokinase, increased AST, rhinorrhea, rhinitis, influenza, sinusitis, and increased blood bilirubin.

URSODEOXYCHOLIC ACID (UDCA)

Comment: *Ursodeoxycholic acid (UDCA)* is indicated for liver disease associated with CF in children 6-18 years of age.

(continued)

➤ *ursodeoxycholic acid (UDCA)* (G) in the first 3 months of treatment, the total daily dose should be divided tid (morning, midday, evening); as liver function values improve, the total daily dose may be taken once a day at bedtime (see mfr pkg insert for dose table based on kilogram weight); monitor hepatic function every 4 weeks for the first 3 months; then monitor hepatic function once every 3 months
Pediatric: 6-18 years: same as adult
    Ursofalk *Tab:* 500 mg film-coat; *Cap:* 250 mg; *Oral susp:* 250 mg/5 ml
Comment: *UDCA* is indicated for dissolution of cholesterol gallstones that are radiolucent (not visible on plain X-ray), <15 mm, and the gall bladder must still be functioning despite the gallstones.

ANTI-INFECTIVE

➤ *ciprofloxacin* (G) <18 years: 20-40 mg/kg/day divided q 12 hours; ≥18 years: 500 mg bid x 7-10 days; max 1.5 gm/day
    Cipro *Tab:* 250, 500, 750 mg; *Oral susp:* 250, 500 mg/5 ml (100 ml) (strawberry)
    Cipro XR *Tab:* 500, 1,000 mg ext-rel
    ProQuin XR *Tab:* 500 mg ext-rel

MONOBACTAM ANTIBACTERIAL AGENT

➤ *aztreonam for inhalation solution* Administer one dose (one single-use vial and one ampule of diluent) tid for 28 days (followed by 28 days off **Cayston** therapy); Doses should be administered at least 4 hours apart; patients should use a bronchodilator before administration of a treatment with **Cayston**; Administer doses immediately after reconstitution; Administer doses only with the Altera Nebulizer System; do not administer treatments with any other type of nebulizer
Pediatric: <7 years: safety and efficacy not established; ≥7 years: same as adult (dose is not adjusted for age or weight)
    Cayston *Vial:* 75 mg pwdr for reconstitution and diluent (0.17% sodium chloride), 1 ml/ampule, single-dose, co-packaged soln for nebulized inhalation
Comment: **Cayston** is a monobactam antibacterial indicated to improve respiratory symptoms in patients with *Pseudomonas aeruginosa* infection. To reduce the development of drug-resistant bacteria and maintain the effectiveness of **Cayston** and other antibacterial drugs, **Cayston** should be used only to treat patients with CF known to have *P. aeruginosa* in the lungs. Safety and effectiveness have not been established in pediatric patients younger than 7 years of age, patients with FEV1 <25% or >75% predicted, or patients colonized with *Burkholderia cepacia.* (Note: Forced expiratory volume (FEV1) calculates the amount of air that a person can force out of their lungs in 1 second. FEV1 values that are lower than average suggest the presence of COPD.) Do not administer **Cayston** to patients allergic to *aztreonam.* Allergic reaction to **Cayston** was seen in clinical trials. Stop treatment if an allergic reaction occurs. Use caution when **Cayston** is administered to patients with a known allergic reaction to beta-lactams (such as penicillins, cephalosporins, and/or carbapenems) since cross-reactivity may occur. Bronchospasm has been reported with **Cayston.** Stop treatment if chest tightness develops during nebulizer use. Common adverse reactions (incidence >5%) occurring more frequently in **Cayston**-treated patients are cough, nasal congestion, wheezing, pharyngolaryngeal pain, pyrexia, chest discomfort, abdominal pain, and vomiting. **Cayston** should be used during pregnancy only if clearly needed. Use of **Cayston** during breastfeeding is unlikely to pose a risk to infants. To report suspected adverse reactions, contact Gilead Sciences at 800-GILEAD5, option 3, or FDA at 800-FDA-1088 or www.fda.gov/medwatch.

CYSTINURIA

➤ *tiopronin* (G) recommended initial dosage in adult patients is 800 mg/day (in clinical studies, the average dosage was about 1,000 mg/day; avoid doses >50 mg/kg/day; administer in 3 divided doses at the same times each day, at least 1 hour before or 2 hours after meals; measure urinary cystine 1 month after initiation of **Thiola/Thiola EC** and every 3 months thereafter; **Thiola EC** should be swallowed whole (do not break, crush, or chew)
Pediatric: <20 kg: not established; ≥20 kg: recommended initial dosage is 15 mg/kg/day; administer in 3 divided doses at the same time each day, at least 1 hour before or 2 hours after meals; measure urinary cystine 1 month after initiation of **Thiola/Thiola EC** and every 3 months thereafter; **Thiola EC** should be swallowed whole (do not break, crush, or chew)
    Thiola *Tab:* 100 mg
    Thiola EC *Tab:* 100, 300 mg del-rel
Comment: Oral *tiopronin* undergoes a thiol-disulfide exchange with cystine to form a water-soluble mixed disulfide complex. Thus, the amount of sparingly soluble cystine is reduced. By reducing urinary cystine concentrations below the solubility limit, **tiopronin** helps reduce cystine stone formation. **Thiola** and **Thiola EC** are a reducing and complexing thiol indicated for inhibition of cystine stone formation in patients with cystinuria, in combination with high fluid intake, alkali, and diet modification, in adults and pediatric patients weighing ≥20 kg with severe homozygous cystinuria who are not responsive to these measures alone. Proteinuria, including nephrotic syndrome, and membranous nephropathy have been reported with *tiopronin* use. Pediatric patients receiving greater than 50 mg/kg of *tiopronin* per day may be at increased

risk for proteinuria. The most common adverse reactions (incidence ≥10%) have been nausea, diarrhea or soft stools, oral ulcers, rash, fatigue, fever, arthralgia, proteinuria, and emesis. Choose dose carefully and monitor renal function in the elderly. Available published case report data with *tiopronin* have not identified a drug-associated risk of major birth defects, miscarriage, or adverse maternal or fetal outcomes. Renal stones in pregnancy may result in adverse pregnancy outcomes. Breastfeeding is not recommended.

CYTOMEGALOVIRUS (CMV): POSTTRANSPLANT

CYTOMEGALOVIRUS (CMV) pUL97 KINASE INHIBITOR

▶ *maribavir* 400 mg (2 x 200 mg) bid, with or without food
Pediatric: <12 years, <35 kg: safety and efficacy not established; ≥12 years, ≥35 kg: same as adult
Livtencity *Tab:* 200 mg

Comment: Livtencity is a cytomegalovirus (CMV) pUL97 kinase inhibitor indicated for the treatment of adults and pediatric patients ≥12 years of age and weighing at least 35 kg with posttransplant CMV infection/disease that is refractory to treatment (with or without genotypic resistance) with *ganciclovir, valganciclovir, cidofovir,* or *foscarnet.* The most common adverse events (all grades, >10%) in subjects treated with **Livtencity** have been taste disturbance, nausea, diarrhea, vomiting, and fatigue. **Livtencity** may antagonize the antiviral activity of *ganciclovir* and *valganciclovir;* co-administration is not recommended. Virologic failure can occur during and after treatment with **Livtencity**; monitor CMV DNA levels and check for resistance if the patient does not respond to treatment. Some *maribavir* pUL97 resistance-associated substitutions confer cross-resistance to *ganciclovir* and *valganciclovir.* The concomitant use of **Livtencity** and certain drugs may result in potentially significant drug interactions, some of which may lead to reduced therapeutic effect of **Livtencity** or adverse reactions of concomitant drugs. **Livtencity** has the potential to increase the drug concentrations of immunosuppressant drugs that are CYP3A4 and/or P-gp substrates, where minimal concentration changes may lead to serious adverse events (including *tacrolimus, cyclosporine, sirolimus,* and *everolimus*). Frequently monitor immune-suppressant drug levels throughout treatment with **Livtencity**, especially following initiation and after discontinuation of **Livtencity** and adjust the dose, as needed. Refer to the mfr pkg insert for full prescribing information for important drug interactions with **Livtencity**. Co-administration with strong CYP3A4 inducers is not recommended. Refer to the mfr pkg insert for full prescribing information for dosage modification when co-administered with certain anticonvulsants. No adequate human data are available to establish whether **Livtencity** poses a risk to pregnancy outcomes. In animal reproduction studies, embryo/fetal survival was at *maribavir* exposures less than those observed in humans at the recommended human dose (RHD). In a combined fertility and embryo/fetal development animal study, *maribavir* was administered to males and females in oral doses of 100, 200, or 400 mg/kg/day. Females were dosed for 15 consecutive days prior to pairing, throughout pairing, and up to gestation day (GD) 17, while males were dosed 29 days prior to mating and throughout mating. A decrease in the number of viable fetuses and increase in early resorptions and postimplantation losses were observed at ≥100 mg/kg/day (exposures approximately half the human exposure at the RHD). Intermittent reduced body weight gain was observed in pregnant animals at ≥200 mg/kg/day. *Maribavir* had no effect on embryo/fetal growth or development at dose levels up to 400 mg/kg/day, at exposures similar to those observed in humans at the RHD. It is not known whether *maribavir* or its metabolites are present in human or animal milk or effects on the breastfed infant. Developmental and health benefits of breastfeeding should be considered along with the mother's clinical need for **Livtencity** and any potential adverse effects to the breastfed infant.

Comment: *Cidofovir* and *valganciclovir* are nucleoside analogs and prodrugs of *ganciclovir* indicated for treatment of AIDS-related CMV retinitis and prevention of CMV disease in adult kidney, heart, and kidney-pancreas transplant patients at high risk, and for prevention of CMV disease in pediatric kidney and heart transplant patients at high risk. *Letermovir* is a CMV DNA terminase complex inhibitor indicated for prophylaxis of CMV infection and disease in adult CMV-seropositive recipients [R+] of an allogeneic hematopoietic stem cell transplant (HSCT).

▶ *cidofovir* administer via IV infusion over 1 hour; pretreat with oral *probenecid* (2 gm, 3 hours prior to starting the *cidofovir* infusion; and 1 gm, 2 and 8 hours after the infusion is ended) and 1 liter of IV NaCl should be infused immediately before each dose of *cidofovir* (a second liter of NaCl should also be infused either during or after each dose of *cidofovir* if a fluid load is tolerable); *Induction:* 5 mg/kg once weekly for 2 consecutive weeks; *Maintenance:* 5 mg/kg once every 2 weeks; reduce to 3 mg/kg if serum creatinine (sCr) increases 0.3-0.4 mg/dL above baseline; discontinue if sCr increases to >0.5 mg/dL above baseline or if >3+ proteinuria develops
Pediatric: <12 years: not recommended; ≥12 years: same as adult
Vistide *Vial:* 75 mg/ml (5 ml) (preservative-free)

Comment: *Cidofovir* is a nucleoside analog indicated for treatment of AIDS related CMV retinitis.

▶ *valganciclovir* (G) take with food; *Induction:* 900 mg bid x 21 days; *Maintenance:* 900 mg daily; *CrCl <60 ml/min:* reduce dose (see mfr pkg insert); Hemodialysis or *CrCl <10 ml/min:* not recommended (use *ganciclovir*)
Pediatric: <4 months: not recommended; 4 months-16 years: see mfr pkg insert for dosing calculation equation
Valcyte *Tab:* 450 mg (preservative-free); *Oral pwdr for reconstitution:* 50 mg/ml (tutti-frutti)

CMV DNA TERMINASE COMPLEX INHIBITOR

Comment: *Letermovir* is a CMV DNA terminase complex inhibitor indicated for prophylaxis of CMV infection and disease in adult CMV-seropositive recipients [R+] of an HSCT.

▷ *cidofovir* administer via IV infusion over 1 hour; pretreat with oral *probenecid* (2 gm, 3 hours prior to starting the *cidofovir* infusion; and 1 gm, 2 and 8 hours after the infusion is ended) and 1 liter of IV NaCl should be infused immediately before each dose of **cidofovir** (a second liter of NaCl should also be infused either during or after each dose of *cidofovir* if a fluid load is tolerable); *Induction:* 5 mg/kg once weekly for 2 consecutive weeks; *Maintenance:* 5 mg/kg once every 2 weeks; reduce to 3 mg/kg if sCr increases 0.3-0.4 mg/dL above baseline; discontinue if sCr increases to >0.5 mg/dL above baseline or if >3+ proteinuria develops
Pediatric: <12 years: not recommended; >12 years: same as adult
Vistide *Vial:* 75 mg/ml (5 ml) (preservative-free)
Comment: *Cidofovir* is a nucleoside analog indicated for treatment of AIDS-related CMV retinitis.

▷ *letermovir* administer dose orally or via IV infusion over 1 hour; dose is 480 mg once daily through 100 days posttransplant; if co-administered with *cyclosporine*, decrease the *letermovir* dose to 240 mg once daily
Pediatric: <18 years: not recommended; ≥18 years: same as adult
Prevymis *Tab:* 240, 450 mg; *Vial:* 240 mg/12 ml (20 mg/ml), 480 mg/24 ml (20 mg/ml), single-dose
Comment: Closely monitor sCr levels in patients with CrCl <50 ml/min using **Prevymis** injection for IV infusion. **Prevymis** is not recommended for patients with severe (Child-Pugh Class C) hepatic impairment. **Prevymis** is contraindicated with *pimozide*, ergot alkaloids, and *pitavastatin* and *simvastatin* when co-administered with *cyclosporine*. The most common adverse events (10%) have been nausea, diarrhea, vomiting, peripheral edema, cough, headache, fatigue, and abdominal pain. No adequate human data are available to inform whether **Prevymis** poses a risk to pregnancy outcomes. It is not known whether *letermovir* is present in human breast milk or has effects on the breastfed infant.

▷ *valganciclovir* (G) take with food; *Induction:* 900 mg bid x 21 days; *Maintenance:* 900 mg daily; CrCl <60 ml/min: reduce dose (see mfr pkg insert); hemodialysis or CrCl <10 ml/min not recommended (use ganciclovir)
Pediatric: <4 months: not recommended; 4 months-16 years: see mfr pkg insert for dosing calculation equation
Valcyte *Tab:* 450 mg (preservative-free); *Oral pwdr for reconstitution:* 50 mg/ml (tutti-frutti)

CYTOMEGALOVIRUS (CMV): RETINITIS

Comment: *Cidofovir and valganciclovir* are nucleoside analogs and prodrugs of *ganciclovir* indicated for the treatment of AIDS-related cytomegalovirus (CMV) retinitis and prevention of CMV disease in adult kidney, heart, and kidney-pancreas transplant patients at high risk, and for prevention of CMV disease in pediatric kidney and heart transplant patients at high risk. *Letermovir* is a CMV DNA terminase complex inhibitor indicated for prophylaxis of CMV infection and disease in adult CMV-seropositive recipients [R+] of an allogeneic hematopoietic stem cell transplant (HSCT).

▷ *cidofovir* Administer via IV infusion over 1 hour; Pretreat with oral *probenecid* (2 gm, 3 hours prior to starting the *cidofovir* infusion; and 1 gm, 2 and 8 hours after the infusion is ended) and 1 liter of IV NaCl should be infused immediately before each dose of *cidofovir* (a second liter of NaCl should also be infused either during or after each dose of *cidofovir* if a fluid load is tolerable); *Induction:* 5 mg/kg once weekly for 2 consecutive weeks; *Maintenance:* 5 mg/kg once every 2 weeks; reduce to 3 mg/kg if serum creatinine (sCr) increases 0.3-0.4 mg/dL above baseline; discontinue if sCr increases to >0.5 mg/dL above baseline or if >3+ proteinuria develops
Pediatric: <12 years: not recommended; ≥12 years: same as adult
Vistide *Vial:* 75 mg/ml (5 ml) (preservative-free)
Comment: *Cidofovir* is a nucleoside analog indicated for treatment of AIDS-related CMV retinitis.

▷ *valganciclovir* (G) take with food; *Induction:* 900 mg bid × 21 days; *Maintenance:* 900 mg daily; *creatinine clearance (CrCl) <60 ml/min:* reduce dose (see mfr pkg insert); *Hemodialysis or CrCl <10 ml/min:* not recommended (use *ganciclovir*)
Pediatric: <4 months: not recommended; 4 months-16 years: see mfr pkg insert for dosing calculation equation
Valcyte *Tab:* 450 mg (preservative-free); *Oral pwdr for reconstitution:* 50 mg/ml (tutti-frutti)

CMV DNA TERMINASE COMPLEX INHIBITOR

Comment: *Letermovir* is a CMV DNA terminase complex inhibitor indicated for prophylaxis of CMV infection and disease in adult CMV-seropositive recipients [R+] of an allogeneic hemato-poietic stem cell transplant (HSCT).

▷ *cidofovir* administer via IV infusion over 1 hour; pretreat with oral *probenecid* (2 gm, 3 hours prior to starting the *cidofovir* infusion; and 1 gm, 2 and 8 hours after the infusion is ended) and 1 liter of IV NaCl should be infused immediately before each dose of *cidofovir* (a second liter of NaCl should also be infused either during or after each dose of *cidofovir* if a fluid load is tolerable); *Induction:* 5 mg/kg once weekly for 2

consecutive weeks; *Maintenance:* 5 mg/kg once every 2 weeks; reduce to 3 mg/kg if sCr increases 0.3-0.4 mg/dL above baseline; discontinue if sCr increases to >0.5 mg/dL above baseline or if >3+ proteinuria develops
Pediatric: <12 years: not recommended; >12 years: same as adult
> Vistide *Vial:* 75 mg/ml (5 ml) (preservative-free)

Comment: *Cidofovir* is a nucleoside analog indicated for treatment of AIDS-related cytomegalovirus (CMV) retinitis.

➤ *letermovir* Administer dose orally or as IV infusion over 1 hour; dose is 480 mg once daily through 100 days posttransplant; if co-administered with *cyclosporine*, decrease the *letermovir* dose to 240 mg once daily
Pediatric: <18 years: not recommended; ≥18 years: same as adult
> Prevymis *Tab:* 240, 450 mg; *Vial:* 240 mg/12 ml (20 mg/ml), 480 mg/24 ml (20 mg/ml), single-dose
> **Comment:** Closely monitor serum creatinine (sCr) levels in patients with creatinine clearance (CrCl) <50 ml/min using **Prevymis** injection for IV infusion. **Prevymis** is not recommended for patients with severe (Child-Pugh Class C) hepatic impairment. **Prevymis** is contraindicated with *pimozide*, ergot alkaloids, and *pitavastatin* and *simvastatin* when co-administered with *cyclosporine*. The most common adverse events (10%) have been nausea, diarrhea, vomiting, peripheral edema, cough, headache, fatigue, and abdominal pain. No adequate human data are available to inform whether **Prevymis** poses a risk to pregnancy outcomes. It is not known whether *letermovir* is present in human breast milk or has effects on the breastfed infant.

➤ *valganciclovir* **(G)** Take with food; *Induction:* 900 mg bid x 21 days; *Maintenance:* 900 mg daily; *CrCl <60 ml/min:* reduce dose (see mfr pkg insert); *Hemodialysis or CrCl <10 ml/min:* not recommended (use *ganciclovir*)
Pediatric: <4 months: not recommended; 4 months-16 years: see mfr pkg insert for dosing calculation equation
> Valcyte *Tab:* 450 mg (preservative-free); *Oral pwdr for reconstitution:* 50 mg/ml (tutti-frutti)

DEEP VEIN THROMBOSIS (DVT) PROPHYLAXIS

Anticoagulation Therapy *see* Appendix S. Anticoagulants

DEHYDRATION

ORAL REHYDRATION AND ELECTROLYTE REPLACEMENT THERAPY
➤ *oral electrolyte replacement* **(OTC)(G)**
> Kao Lectrolyte 1 pkt dissolved in 8 oz water q 3-4 hours
> *Pediatric:* <2 years: not indicated
>> *Pkt:* sodium 12 mEq+potassium 5 mEq+chloride 10 mEq+citrate 7 mEq+ dextrose 5 gm+calories 22 per 6.2 gm
> Pedialyte
> *Pediatric:* <2 years: as desired and as tolerated; ≥2 years: 1-2 liters/day
>> *Oral soln:* dextrose 20 gm+fructose 5 gm+sodium 25 mEq+potassium 20 mEq+chloride 35 mEq+citrate 30 mEq+calories 100 per liter (8 oz, 1 liter)
> Pedialyte Freezer Pops
> *Pediatric:* as desired and as tolerated
>> *Pops:* dextrose 1.6 gm+sodium 2.8 mEq+potassium 1.25 mEq+chloride 2.2 mEq+citrate 1.88 mEq+calories 6.25 per 62.5 ml (2.1 fl oz) pop

DELIRIUM: END-OF-LIFE

Comment: "Ultimately ... it is essential for clinicians to focus on the humanness of medicine; to keep dying patients comfortable and as awake as they and their families would like them to be so they can make the last few hours or days of life meaningful; and to make reasonable efforts not to cloud their sensorium unless essential to alleviate patient pain or other severe symptoms" (Pandharipande & Ely, 2017). In a preliminary randomized control study, Hui et al. (2017) demonstrated that adding the benzodiazepine *lorazepam* to background *haloperidol* therapy significantly reduced agitated delirium at 8 hours compared with *haloperidol* alone in patients admitted to an acute palliative care unit with advanced cancer and a very short life expectancy. Moreover, most of the effects the combination had on delirium were achieved in the first 30 minutes following administration (Hui, et al., 2017).

REFERENCES
Hui, D., Frisbee-Hume, S., Wilson, A., Dibaj, S. S., Nguyen, T., De La Cruz, M., … Bruera, E. (2017). Effect of lorazepam with haloperidol vs haloperidol alone on agitated delirium in patients with advanced cancer receiving palliative care. *Journal of the American Medical Association, 318*(11), 1047–1056. doi:10.1001/jama.2017.11468
Pandharipande, P. P., & Ely, E. W. (2017). Humanizing the treatment of hyperactive delirium in the last days of life. *Journal of the American Medical Association, 318*(11), 1014–1015. doi:10.1001/jama.2017.11466

BENZODIAZEPINE: INTERMEDIATE-ACTING

▷ *lorazepam* (IV) (G) 1-10 mg/day in 2-3 divided doses
  Pediatric: <12 years: not recommended; ≥12 years: same as adult
      Ativan *Tab:* 0.5, 1*, 2*mg
      Lorazepam Intensol *Oral conc:* 2 mg/ml (30 ml w. graduated dropper)

ANTIPSYCHOSIS AGENTS

▷ *haloperidol* (G)
  Oral Route of Administration: Moderate Symptomology: 0.5 to 2 mg orally 2 to 3 times a day; *Severe Symptomology:* 3 to 5 mg orally 2 to 3 x/day; Initial doses of up to 100 mg/day have been necessary in some severely resistant cases; *Maintenance:* after achieving a satisfactory response, the dose should be adjusted as practical to achieve optimum control
  Parenteral Route of Administration: Prompt control of acute agitation: 2 to 5 mg IM every 4 to 8 hours; *Maintenance:* frequency of IM administration should be determined by patient response and may be given as often as every hour; max: 20 mg/day
      Haldol *Tab:* 0.5*, 1*, 2*, 5*, 10*, 20*mg
      Haldol Lactate *Vial:* 5 mg for IM injection, single-dose
▷ *mesoridazine* initially 25 mg tid; max 300 mg/day
      Serentil *Tab:* 10, 25, 50, 100 mg; *Conc:* 25 mg/ml (118 ml)
▷ *olanzapine* initially 2.5-10 mg daily; increase to 10 mg/day within a few days; then by 5 mg/day at weekly intervals; max 20 mg/day
      Zyprexa *Tab:* 2.5, 5, 7.5, 10 mg
      Zyprexa Zydis *ODT:* 5, 10, 15, 20 mg (phenylalanine)
▷ *quetiapine fumarate* (G)
      Seroquel initially 25 mg bid, titrate every 2nd or 3rd day in increments of 25-50 mg bid-tid; usual maintenance 400-600 mg/day in 2-3 divided doses
          Tab: 25, 50, 100, 200, 300, 400 mg
      Seroquel XR administer once daily in the PM; *Day 1:* 50 mg; *Day 2:* 100 mg; *Day 3:* 200 mg; *Day 4:* 300 mg; usual range 400-600 mg/day
          Tab: 50, 150, 200, 300, 400 mg ext-rel
▷ *risperidone* 0.5 mg bid x 1 day; adjust in increments of 0.5 mg bid; usual range 0.5-5 mg/day
      Risperdal *Tab:* 1, 2, 3, 4 mg; *Oral soln:* 1 mg/ml (100 ml)
      Risperdal M-Tab *Tab:* 0.5, 1, 2 mg
▷ *thioridazine* (G) 10-25 mg bid
      Mellaril *Tab:* 10, 15, 25, 50, 100, 150, 200 mg; *Oral susp:* 25 mg/5 ml, 100 mg/5 ml; *Oral conc:* 30 mg/ml, 100 mg/ml (4 oz)

DEMENTIA

Alzheimer's Disease *see Alzheimer's Disease*
Antidepressants *see Depression*
Hypnotics/Sedatives *see Insomnia*

ANTIPSYCHOTICS

Comment: Underlying cause should be explored, accurately diagnosed, and addressed. All antipsychotic agents are associated with increased risk of mortality in elderly patients with dementia-related psychosis (Black Box Warning.) The American Psychological Association (APA) recommends that non-emergency antipsychotic medication should only be used for treatment of agitation or psychosis in patients with dementia when symptoms are severe, are dangerous, and/or cause significant distress to the patient. The APA recommends that before non-emergency treatment with an antipsychotic is initiated in patients with dementia, the potential risks and benefits are discussed with the patient and the patient's surrogate decision-maker with input from the family or others involved with the patient. *Haloperidol injection* is not approved for the treatment of patients with dementia-related psychosis.

▷ *haloperidol* (G) 0.5-1 mg q HS
      Haldol *Tab:* 0.5, 1, 2, 5, 10, 20 mg
▷ *mesoridazine* initially 25 mg tid; max 300 mg/day
      Serentil *Tab:* 10, 25, 50, 100 mg; *Conc:* 25 mg/ml (118 ml)
▷ *olanzapine* initially 2.5-10 mg daily; increase to 10 mg/day within a few days; then by 5 mg/day at weekly intervals; max 20 mg/day
      Zyprexa *Tab:* 2.5, 5, 7.5, 10 mg
      Zyprexa Zydis *ODT:* 5, 10, 15, 20 mg (phenylalanine)
▷ *quetiapine fumarate* (G)
      Seroquel initially 25 mg bid, titrate every 2nd or 3rd day in increments of 25-50 mg bid-tid; usual maintenance 400-600 mg/day in 2-3 divided doses
          Tab: 25, 50, 100, 200, 300, 400 mg

Seroquel XR administer once daily in the PM; *Day 1:* 50 mg; *Day 2:* 100 mg; *Day 3:* 200 mg; *Day 4:* 300 mg; usual range 400-600 mg/day
    Tab: 50, 150, 200, 300, 400 mg ext-rel

▷ *risperidone* 0.5 mg bid x 1 day; adjust in increments of 0.5 mg bid; usual range 0.5-5 mg/day
    Risperdal *Tab:* 1, 2, 3, 4 mg; *Oral soln:* 1 mg/ml (100 ml)
    Risperdal M-Tab *Tab:* 0.5, 1, 2 mg

▷ *thioridazine* (G) 10-25 mg bid
    Mellaril *Tab:* 10, 15, 25, 50, 100, 150, 200 mg; *Oral susp:* 25 mg/5 ml, 100 mg/5 ml; *Oral conc:* 30 mg/ml, 100 mg/ml (4 oz)

DENGUE FEVER (DENGUE VIRUS)

Comment: Dengue is the most common arthropod-borne viral (arboviral) illness in humans. The CDC reports that cases of dengue in returning U.S. travelers have increased steadily during the past 20 years, and dengue has become the leading cause of acute febrile illness in U.S. travelers returning from the Caribbean, South America, and Asia. Dengue is transmitted by mosquitoes of the genus *Aedes*, which are widely distributed in subtropical and tropical areas of the world. A small percentage of persons who have previously been infected by one dengue serotype develop bleeding and endothelial leak upon infection with another dengue serotype. This syndrome is termed "dengue hemorrhagic fever." Dengue fever is typically a self-limited disease, with a mortality rate of less than 1%. When treated, dengue hemorrhagic fever has a mortality rate of 2%-5%, but when left untreated the mortality rate is as high as 50%. Supportive care with analgesics, fluid replacement, and bed rest is usually sufficient. Acetaminophen may be used to treat fever and relieve other symptoms. *Aspirin*, nonsteroidal anti-inflammatory drugs (NSAIDs), and corticosteroids should be avoided. Management of severe dengue requires careful attention to fluid management and proactive treatment of hemorrhage. Single-dose methylprednisolone showed no mortality benefit in the treatment of dengue shock syndrome in a prospective, randomized, double-blind, placebo-controlled trial. **There is no specific antiviral treatment currently available for dengue fever.** Because lack of immunity to a single dengue strain is the major risk factor for dengue hemorrhagic fever and dengue shock syndrome, a vaccine must provide high levels of immunity to all **four dengue strains** to be clinically useful.

A live attenuated tetravalent vaccine against dengue was effective against all four serotypes of the virus and well tolerated among children, according to researchers. Interim results from a phase 2 study showed that children at four study sites in dengue-endemic areas of Asia and Latin America who received the vaccine all had significantly higher levels of antibody titers 18 months later. The vaccine (TAK-003 or TDV) comprised a molecularly cloned attenuated strain of dengue serotype 2 (DENV-2) and engineered strains of dengue serotypes 1, 3, and 4 (DENV-1, DENV-3, and DENV-4). Prior phase 1 and phase 2 data found the vaccine was well tolerated and immunogenic against all four dengue serotypes. The trial will take 48 months to complete. The trial is ongoing at three sites in the Dominican Republic (n = 535), Panama (n = 935), and the Philippines (n = 330). Participants are "healthy" children, ages 2 to 17 years, randomized into three groups plus a placebo group. A phase 3 efficacy trial for the vaccine, entitled Tetravalent Immunization against Dengue Efficacy Study (TIDES), is currently being conducted in eight dengue-endemic countries.

In 2019, **Dengvaxia** was approved external icon by the U.S. FDA in the United States for use in children 9 to 16 years old living in an area where dengue is common (the U.S. territories of American Samoa, Puerto Rico, and the U.S. Virgin Islands), with laboratory-confirmed prior dengue virus infection. *CYD-TDV*, sold under the brand name **Dengvaxia**, is a live attenuated tetravalent chimeric vaccine made using recombinant DNA technology by replacing the PrM (premembrane) and E (envelope) structural genes of the yellow fever attenuated 17D strain vaccine with those from the four dengue serotypes. In 2016, a partially effective vaccine for dengue fever (*CYD-TDV*, **Dengvaxia**) became commercially available in 11 countries: Mexico, the Philippines, Indonesia, Brazil, El Salvador, Costa Rica, Paraguay, Guatemala, Peru, Thailand, and Singapore. WHO recommends that countries should consider vaccination with *CYD-TDV* only if the risk of severe dengue in seronegative individuals can be minimized either through prevaccination screening or recent documentation of high seroprevalence rates in the area (at least 80% by age 9 years). In 2017, the manufacturer (Sanofi Pasteur) recommended that the vaccine only be used in people who have previously had a dengue infection, as outcomes may be worsened in those who have not been previously infected. **WHO** updated its recommendations regarding the use of **Dengvaxia** in 2018 based on the evidence that seronegative vaccine recipients have an excess risk of severe dengue compared with unvaccinated seronegative individuals.

REFERENCES

Sáez-Llorens, X., Tricou, V., Yu, D., Rivera, L., Jimeno, J., Villarreal, A. C., . . . Wallace, D. (2018). Immunogenicity and safety of one versus two doses of tetravalent dengue vaccine in healthy children aged 2–17 years in Asia and Latin America: 18-month interim data from a phase 2, randomised, placebo-controlled study. *The Lancet: Infectious Diseases, 18*(2), 162–170. doi:10.1016/s1473-3099(17)30632-1

Tricou, V., Sáez-Llorens, X., Yu, D., Rivera, L., Borkowski, A., & Wallace, D. (2017, November 6). *Progress in development of Takeda's tetravalent dengue vaccine candidate.* Paper presented at the 66th annual meeting of the American Society of Tropical Medicine & Hygiene, Baltimore, MD. Retrieved from http://www.abstractsonline.com/pp8/#!/4395/presentation/1438

Yoon, I.-K., & Thomas, S. J. (2018). Encouraging results but questions remain for dengue vaccine. *The Lancet: Infectious Diseases, 18*(2), 125–126. doi:10.1016/s1473-3099(17)30634-5

(continued)

The following is taken from the most recent (2019) U.S. FDA-approved Dengvaxia label (mfr pkg insert):

▷ **Dengue virus vaccine** Following reconstitution, administer 0.5 ml SC as a 3-dose series; administer at 0, 6, and 12 months (i.e., 6 months apart); See limitations and restrictions in the comment below and the mfr pkg insert for full prescribing information
Pediatric: <9 years: safety and efficacy not established; ≥9 years: same as adult; see limitations and restrictions in the comment below and the mfr pkg insert for full prescribing information
    Dengvaxia *Vial:* pwdr for reconstitution with the supplied diluent to 0.5 ml suspension for SC injection
    Comment: Dengvaxia is a vaccine indicated for the prevention of dengue disease caused by dengue virus serotypes 1, 2, 3, and 4. **Dengvaxia** is approved for use in individuals 9 through 16 years of age with laboratory-confirmed previous dengue infection and living in endemic areas. Previous dengue infection can be assessed through a medical record of a previous laboratory-confirmed dengue infection or through serologic testing prior to vaccination. Endemic areas include Puerto Rico, American Samoa, U.S. Virgin Islands, Federated States of Micronesia, Republic of Marshall Islands, and the Republic of Palau. Safety and effectiveness of **Dengvaxia** have not been established in individuals living in dengue non-endemic areas who travel to dengue-endemic areas. **Dengvaxia** is not approved for use in individuals not previously infected by any dengue virus serotype or for whom this information is unknown. In persons not previously infected by the dengue virus, an increased risk of severe dengue disease can occur following vaccination with **Dengvaxia** and subsequent infection with any dengue virus serotype. **Dengvaxia** is contraindicated in persons with a history of severe allergic reaction to a previous dose of **Dengvaxia** or to any component of **Dengvaxia** and immunocompromised individuals. There is no FDA-cleared test available to determine a previous dengue infection. False-negative tuberculin purified protein derivative (PPD) test results may occur within 1 month following vaccination with **Dengvaxia**. The most frequently reported adverse reactions, regardless of the dengue serostatus prior to vaccination, have been headache (40%), injection site pain (32%), malaise (25%), asthenia (25%), and myalgia (29%). Pregnant females are at increased risk of complications associated with dengue infection compared to non-pregnant females. Pregnant females with dengue infection may be at increased risk for adverse pregnancy outcomes, including preterm labor and delivery. Vertical transmission of dengue virus from mothers with viremia at delivery to their infants has been reported. However, no specific studies of **Dengvaxia** have been performed among pregnant women; available data in pregnant females are not sufficient to determine the effects of **Dengvaxia** on pregnancy, embryo/fetal development, parturition, and postnatal development. A limited number of cases of inadvertent exposure during pregnancy were reported during clinical studies. Isolated adverse pregnancy outcomes (e.g., stillbirth, intrauterine death, spontaneous abortion, blighted ovum) have been observed for these exposed pregnancies, with similar frequency and nature in the vaccinated individuals compared to the control group, and with risk factors identified for all cases. Vaccine viremia can occur 7 to 14 days after vaccination with a duration of <7 days. The potential for transmission of the vaccine virus from the mother to the infant *in utero* is unknown. The potential for transmission of the vaccine virus from the mother to the infant through breast milk is unknown. Developmental and health benefits of breastfeeding should be considered along with the mother's clinical need for **Dengvaxia** and any potential adverse effects on the breastfed child from **Dengvaxia** or from the underlying maternal condition. For preventive vaccines, the underlying condition is susceptibility to disease prevented by the vaccine. Females who receive **Dengvaxia** during pregnancy are encouraged to contact directly or have their healthcare professional contact Sanofi Pasteur at 1-800-822-2463 (1-800-VACCINE) to enroll in or obtain information about the registry. To report suspected adverse reactions, contact the Pharmacovigilance Department, Sanofi Pasteur, Discovery Drive, Swiftwater, PA 18370 at 1-800-822-2463 (1-800-VACCINE) or VAERS at https://vaers.hhs.gov/esub/index.jsp

DENTAL ABSCESS

ANTI-INFECTIVES
▷ *amoxicillin+clavulanate* (G)
    Augmentin 500 mg tid or 875 mg bid x 7-10 days
    Pediatric: 40-45 mg/kg/day divided tid x 10 days or 90 mg/kg/day divided bid x 10 days; *see Appendix BB.4. amoxicillin+clavulanate* (G) (Augmentin Suspension) *for dose by weight*
        Tab: 250, 500, 875 mg; *Chew tab:* 125, 250 mg (lemon-lime); 200, 400 mg (cherry-banana) (phenylalanine); *Oral susp:* 125 mg/5 ml (banana); 250 mg/5 ml (75, 100, 150 ml) (orange); 200, 400 mg/5 ml (50, 75, 100 ml) (orange) (phenylalanine)
    Augmentin ES-600 not recommended for adults
    Pediatric: <3 months: not recommended; ≥3 months, <40 kg: 90 mg/kg/day in 2 divided doses x 7-10 days; ≥40 kg: not recommended
        Oral susp: 42.9 mg/5 ml (50, 75, 100, 125, 150, 200 ml) (strawberry cream) (phenylalanine)
    Augmentin XR 2 tabs q 12 hours x 7-10 days
    Pediatric: <16 years: use other forms; ≥16 years: same as adult
        Tab: 1,000*mg ext-rel

▷ *clindamycin* (Administer with a fluoroquinolone in adults and *trimethoprim-sulfamethoxazole (TMP-SMX)* in children) 300 mg qid x 10 days
Pediatric: 8-16 mg/kg/day in 3-4 divided doses x 10 days
    Cleocin (G) *Cap:* 75 (tartrazine), 150 (tartrazine), 300 mg
    Cleocin Pediatric Granules (G) *Oral susp:* 75 mg/5 ml (100 ml) (cherry)
▷ *erythromycin base* (G) 500 mg q 6 hours x 10 days
Pediatric: 30-40 mg/kg/day in 4 divided doses x 10 days
    Ery-Tab *Tab:* 250, 333, 500 mg ent-coat
    PCE *Tab:* 333, 500 mg
▷ *erythromycin ethylsuccinate* (G) 400 mg qid x 7 days
Pediatric: 30-50 mg/kg/day in 4 divided doses x 7 days; may double dose with severe infection; max 100 mg/kg/day; *see Appendix BB.21: erythromycin ethylsuccinate (G) (E.E.S. Suspension, EryPed Drops/Suspension) for dose by weight*
    EryPed *Oral susp:* 200 mg/5 ml (100, 200 ml) (fruit); 400 mg/5 ml (60, 100, 200 ml) (banana); *Oral drops:* 200, 400 mg/5 ml (50 ml) (fruit); *Chew tab:* 200 mg wafer (fruit)
    E.E.S. *Oral susp:* 200, 400 mg/5 ml (100 ml) (fruit)
    E.E.S. Granules *Oral susp:* 200 mg/5 ml (100, 200 ml) (cherry)
    E.E.S. 400 Tablets *Tab:* 400 mg
▷ *penicillin v potassium* 250-500 mg q 6 hours x 5-7 days
Pediatric: <12 years: 25-50 mg/kg/day divided q 6 hours x 5-7 days; *see Appendix BB.29. penicillin v potassium (G) (Pen-Vee K Solution, Veetids Solution) for dose by weight;* ≥12 years: same as adult
    Pen-Vee K *Tab:* 250, 500 mg; *Oral soln:* 125 mg/5 ml (100, 200 ml), 250 mg/5 ml (100, 150, 200 ml)

DENTURE IRRITATION

DEBRIDING AGENT/CLEANSER
▷ *carbamide peroxide 10%* (OTC) apply 10 drops to affected area; swish x 2-3 minutes, then spit; do **not** rinse; repeat treatment qid
Pediatric: with adult supervision **only**
    Gly-Oxide *Liq:* 10% (15, 60 ml, squeeze bottle w. applicator)

DEPRESSION/MAJOR DEPRESSIVE DISORDER (MDD)

Comment: Antidepressant monotherapy should be avoided until any presence of (hypo)mania **or** positive family history of bipolar spectrum disorder has been ruled out as antidepressant monotherapy can induce mania in the bipolar patient. Abrupt withdrawal **or** interruption of treatment with an antidepressant medication is sometimes associated with an antidepressant discontinuation syndrome, which may be mediated by gradually tapering the drug over a period of 2 weeks **or** longer, depending on the dose strength and length of treatment. Common symptoms of antidepressant withdrawal include flu-like symptoms, insomnia, nausea, imbalance, sensory disturbances, and hyperarousal. These medications include selective serotonin reuptake inhibitors (SSRIs), tricyclic antidepressants (TCAs), monoamine oxidase inhibitors (MAOIs), and atypical agents such as *venlafaxine* (Effexor), *mirtazapine* (Remeron), *trazodone* (Desyrel), and *duloxetine* (Cymbalta). Common symptoms of the *serotonin discontinuation syndrome* include flu-like symptoms (nausea, vomiting, diarrhea, headaches, sweating), sleep disturbances (insomnia, nightmares, constant sleepiness), mood disturbances (dysphoria, anxiety, agitation) cognitive disturbances (mental confusion, hyperarousal), sensory and movement disturbances (imbalance, tremors, vertigo, dizziness), and electric-shock-like sensations in the brain, often described by sufferers as "brain zaps."

SELECTIVE SEROTONIN REUPTAKE INHIBITORS (SSRIs)
Comment: Co-administration of SSRIs with TCAs requires extreme caution. Concomitant use of MAOIs and SSRIs is absolutely contraindicated. Avoid St. John's wort and other serotonergic agents. A potentially fatal adverse event is *serotonin syndrome*, caused by serotonin excess. Milder symptoms require healthcare provider intervention to avert severe symptoms, which can be rapidly fatal without urgent/emergent medical care. Symptoms include restlessness, agitation, confusion, tachycardia, hypertension, dilated pupils, muscle twitching, muscle rigidity, loss of muscle coordination, diaphoresis, diarrhea, headache, shivering, piloerection, hyperpyrexia, cardiac arrhythmias, seizures, loss of consciousness, coma, and death. Common symptoms of the *serotonin discontinuation syndrome* include flu-like symptoms (nausea, vomiting, diarrhea, headaches, sweating), sleep disturbances (insomnia, nightmares, constant sleepiness), mood disturbances (dysphoria, anxiety, agitation), cognitive disturbances (mental confusion, hyperarousal, hallucinations), sensory and movement disturbances (imbalance, tremors, vertigo, dizziness), and electric-shock-like sensations in the brain, often described by sufferers as "brain zaps."
▷ *citalopram* (G) Initially 20 mg daily; May increase after 1 week to 40 mg; Max 40 mg
Pediatric: <12 years: **not** recommended; ≥12 years: same as adult
    Celexa *Tab:* 10, 20, 40 mg; *Oral soln:* 10 mg/5 ml (120 ml) (peppermint) (sugar-free, alcohol-free, parabens)

(continued)

▷ *escitalopram* (G) Initially 10 mg daily; May increase to 20 mg daily after 1 week; *Elderly or Hepatic Impairment*: 10 mg once daily
 Pediatric: <12 years: <u>not</u> recommended; 12-17 years: initially 10 mg daily; may increase to 20 mg daily after 3 weeks
    Lexapro *Tab*: 5, 10*, 20*mg
    Lexapro Oral Solution *Oral soln*: 1 mg/ml (240 ml) (peppermint) (parabens)
▷ *fluoxetine* (G)
    Prozac Initially 20 mg daily; May increase after 1 week; Doses >20 mg/day should be divided into AM and noon doses; Max 80 mg/day
    Pediatric: <8 years: <u>not</u> recommended; 8-17 years: initially 10 mg/day, may increase after 1 week to 20 mg/day, range 20-60 mg/day; range for lower weight children, 20-30 mg/day; >17 years: same as adult
        Cap: 10, 20, 40 mg; *Tab*: 30*, 60*mg; *Oral soln*: 20 mg/5 ml (4 oz) (mint)
    Prozac Weekly Following daily *fluoxetine* therapy at 20 mg/day for 13 weeks, may initiate **Prozac Weekly** 7 days after the last 20 mg *fluoxetine* dose
    Pediatric: <12 years: <u>not</u> recommended; ≥12 years: same as adult
        Cap: 90 mg ent-coat del-rel pellets
▷ *levomilnacipran* Swallow whole; Initially 20 mg once daily for 2 days; Then increase to 40 mg once daily; May increase dose in 40 mg increments at intervals of ≥2 days; Max 120 mg once daily; *CrCl 30-59 ml/min*: Max 80 mg once daily; *CrCl 15-29 ml/min*: Max 40 mg once daily
    Pediatric: <12 years: <u>not</u> recommended; ≥12 years: same as adult
        Fetzima *Cap*: 20, 40, 80, 120 mg ext-rel
▷ *paroxetine maleate* (G)
    Pediatric: <12 years: <u>not</u> recommended; ≥12 years: same as adult
    Paxil Initially 20 mg daily in AM; May increase by 10 mg/day at weekly intervals as needed; Max 60 mg/day
        Tab: 10*, 20*, 30, 40 mg
    Paxil CR Initially 25 mg daily in AM; May increase by 12.5 mg at weekly intervals as needed; Max 62.5 mg/day
        Tab: 12.5, 25, 37.5 mg cont-rel ent-coat
    Paxil Oral Suspension Initially 20 mg daily in AM; May increase by 10 mg/day at weekly intervals as needed; Max 60 mg/day
        Oral susp: 10 mg/5 ml (250 ml) (orange)
▷ *paroxetine mesylate* (G) Initially 7.5 mg daily in AM; May increase by 10 mg/day at weekly intervals as needed; Max 60 mg/day
    Pediatric: <12 years: <u>not</u> established; ≥12 years: same as adult
        Brisdelle *Cap*: 7.5 mg
▷ *sertraline* (G) Initially 50 mg daily; Increase at 1-week intervals if needed; Max 200 mg daily; Dilute oral concentrate immediately prior to administration in 4 oz water, ginger ale, lemon-lime soda, lemonade, <u>or</u> orange juice
    Pediatric: <6 years: <u>not</u> recommended; 6-12 years: initially 25 mg daily; max 200 mg/day; 13-17 years: initially 50 mg daily, max 200 mg/day; >17 years: same as adult
    Zoloft *Tab*: 25*, 50*, 100*mg; *Oral conc*: 20 mg per ml (60 ml) (alcohol 12%)

SEROTONIN NOREPINEPHRINE REUPTAKE INHIBITORS (SNRIs)
▷ *desvenlafaxine* (G) Swallow whole; Initially 50 mg once daily; Max 120 mg/day
    Pediatric: <12 years: <u>not</u> recommended; ≥12 years: same as adult
    Pristiq *Tab*: 50, 100 mg ext-rel
▷ *duloxetine* (G) Swallow whole; initially 30 mg once daily x 1 week; Then increase to 60 mg once daily; Max 120 mg/day
    Pediatric: <12 years: <u>not</u> recommended; ≥12 years: same as adult
    Cymbalta *Cap*: 20, 30, 40, 60 mg del-rel
▷ *levomilnacipran* Swallow whole; Initially 20 mg once daily for 2 days; Then increase to 40 mg once daily; May increase dose in 40 mg increments at intervals of ≥2 days; Max 120 mg once daily; *CrCl 30-59 ml/min*: max 80 mg once daily; *CrCl 15-29 ml/min*: max 40 mg once daily
    Pediatric: <12 years: <u>not</u> recommended; ≥12 years: same as adult
    Fetzima *Cap*: 20, 40, 80, 120 mg ext-rel
▷ *venlafaxine* (G)
    Effexor Initially 75 mg/day in 2-3 divided doses; May increase at 4-day intervals in 75 mg increments to 150 mg/day; Max 225 mg/day
    Pediatric: <18 years: <u>not</u> recommended; ≥18 years: same as adult
        Tab: 37.5, 75, 150, 225 mg
    Effexor XR Initially 75 mg q AM; May start at 37.5 mg daily x 4-7 days; Then increase by increments of up to 75 mg/day at intervals of at least 4 days; Usual max 375 mg/day
    Pediatric: <18 years: <u>not</u> recommended; ≥18 years: same as adult
        Tab/Cap: 37.5, 75, 150 mg ext-rel
▷ *vortioxetine* (G) Initially 10 mg once daily; Max 30 mg/day
    Pediatric: <18 years: <u>not</u> established; ≥18 years: same as adult
    Trintellix *Tab*: 5, 10, 15, 20 mg

SSRI+5HT-14 RECEPTOR PARTIAL AGONIST COMBINATION
➤ *vilazodone* (G) Take with food; Initially 10 mg once daily x 7 days; Then 20 mg once daily x 7 days; Then 40 mg once daily
   Pediatric: <18 years: not established; ≥18 years: same as adult
      Viibryd *Tab:* 10, 20, 40 mg

THIENOBENZODIAZEPINE+SSRI COMBINATION
➤ *olanzapine+fluoxetine* Initially one 6/25 cap in the PM; Titrate; Max one 18/75 cap once daily in the PM
   Pediatric: <10 years: not established; ≥10 years: same as adult
      Symbyax
      Cap: **Symbyax 3/25** olan 3 mg+fluo 25 mg
                Symbyax 6/25 olan 6 mg+fluo 25 mg
                Symbyax 6/50 olan 6 mg+fluo 50 mg
                Symbyax 12/25 olan 12 mg+fluo 25 mg
                Symbyax 12/50 olan 12 mg+fluo 50 mg
   Comment: Symbyax is a thienobenzodiazepine-SSRI indicated for the treatment of depressive episodes associated with bipolar depression disorder and treatment-resistant depression (TRD).

TRICYCLIC ANTIDEPRESSANTS (TCAs)
Comment: Co-administration of TCAs with SSRIs requires extreme caution.
➤ *amitriptyline* (G) Initially 75 mg/day in divided doses or 50-100 mg in a single dose at HS; Max 300 mg/day
   Pediatric: <12 years: not recommended; ≥12 years: same as adult
      Tab: 10, 25, 50, 75, 100, 150 mg
➤ *amoxapine* Initially 50 mg bid-tid; After 1 week may increase to 100 mg bid-tid; Usual effective dose 200-300 mg/day; If total dose exceeds 300 mg/day, give in divided doses (max 400 mg/day); May give as a single bedtime dose (Max 300 mg q HS)
   Pediatric: <12 years: not recommended; ≥12 years: same as adult
      Tab: 25, 50, 100, 150 mg
➤ *desipramine* (G) 100-200 mg/day in single or divided doses; Max 300 mg/day
   Pediatric: <12 years: not recommended; ≥12 years: same as adult
      Norpramin *Tab:* 10, 25, 50, 75, 100, 150 mg
➤ *doxepin* (G) 75 mg/day; Max 150 mg/day
   Pediatric: <12 years: not recommended; ≥12 years: same as adult
      Cap: 10, 25, 50, 75, 100, 150 mg; *Oral conc:* 10 mg/ml (4 oz w. dropper)
➤ *imipramine* (G)
   Pediatric: <12 years: not recommended; ≥12 years: same as adult
      Tofranil Initially 75 mg daily (Max 200 mg); Adolescents initially 30-40 mg daily (Max 100 mg/day); If maintenance dose exceeds 75 mg daily, may switch to **Tofranil PM** for divided or bedtime dose
         Tab: 10, 25, 50 mg
      Tofranil PM Initially 75 mg daily 1 hour before HS; Max 200 mg
         Cap: 75, 100, 125, 150 mg
      Tofranil Injection 50 mg IM; lower dose for adolescents; Switch to oral form as soon as possible
         Amp: 25 mg/2 ml (2 ml)
➤ *nortriptyline* (G) Initially 25 mg tid-qid; Max 150 mg/day
   Pediatric: <12 years: not recommended; ≥12 years: same as adult
      Pamelor *Cap:* 10, 25, 50, 75 mg; *Oral soln:* 10 mg/5 ml (16 oz)
➤ *protriptyline* Initially 5 mg tid; Usual dose 15-40 mg/day in 3-4 divided doses; Max 60 mg/day
   Pediatric: <12 years: not recommended; ≥12 years: same as adult
      Vivactil *Tab:* 5, 10 mg
➤ *trimipramine* Initially 75 mg/day in divided doses; Max 200 mg/day
   Pediatric: not recommended
      Surmontil *Cap:* 25, 50, 100 mg

AMINOKETONES
➤ *bupropion HBr* (G)
   Pediatric: safety and efficacy of *bupropion* in the pediatric population have not been established; When considering the use of **bupropion** in a child or adolescent, balance the potential risks with the clinical need
      Aplenzin Initially 100 mg bid for at least 3 days; may increase to 375 or 400 mg/day after several weeks; Then after at least 3 more days, 450 mg in 4 divided doses; Max 450 mg/day, 174 mg/single-dose
         Tab: 174, 348, 522 mg
➤ *bupropion HCl* (G)
   Pediatric: safety and efficacy of *bupropion* in the pediatric population not established; When considering the use of **bupropion** in a child or adolescent, balance the potential risks with the clinical need
      Forfivo XL Do not use for initial treatment; Use immediate-release *bupropion* forms for initial titration; Switch to **Forfivo XL** 450 mg once daily when total dose/day reaches 450 mg; May switch to **Forfivo XL**

(continued)

when total dose/day reaches 300 mg for 2 weeks and the patient needs 450 mg/day to reach therapeutic target; Swallow whole, Do not crush or chew
> *Tab:* 450 mg ext-rel

Wellbutrin Initially 100 mg bid for at least 3 days; May increase to 375 or 400 mg/day after several weeks; Then after at least 3 more days, 450 mg in 4 divided doses; Max 450 mg/day, 150 mg/single dose
> *Tab:* 75, 100 mg

Wellbutrin SR Initially 150 mg in AM for at least 3 days; increase to 150 mg bid if well tolerated; Usual dose 300 mg/day; max 400 mg/day
> *Tab:* 100, 150 mg sust-rel

Wellbutrin XL Initially 150 mg in AM for at least 3 days; Increase to 150 mg bid if well tolerated; Usual dose 300 mg/day; Max 450 mg/day
> *Tab:* 150, 300 mg sust-rel

MONOAMINE OXIDASE INHIBITORS (MAOIS)

Comment: Many drug and food interactions with this class of drugs; use cautiously. These should be reserved for refractory depression that has not responded to other classes of antidepressants. Concomitant use of MAOIs and SSRIs is an absolute contraindication. See mfr pkg insert for drug and food interactions.

▷ *isocarboxazid* (G) Initially 10 mg bid; Increase by 10 mg every 2-4 days up to 40 mg/day; May increase by 20 mg/week to max 60 mg/day divided bid-qid
Pediatric: <16 years: not recommended; ≥16 years: same as adult
> **Marplan** *Tab:* 10 mg

▷ *phenelzine* (G) Initially 15 mg tid; Max 90 mg/day
Pediatric: <16 years: not recommended; ≥16 years: same as adult
> **Nardil** *Tab:* 15 mg

▷ *selegiline* Initially 10 mg tid; Max 60 mg/day
> **Emsam** *Transdermal patch:* 6 mg/24 hours, 9 mg/24 hours, 12 mg/24 hours
> **Comment:** With the Emsam transdermal patch 6 mg/24 hours dose, the dietary restrictions commonly required when using non-selective MAOIs are not necessary.

▷ *tranylcypromine* Initially 10 mg tid; May increase in 10 mg/day every 1-3 weeks; Max 60 mg/day
> **Parnate** *Tab:* 10 mg

TETRACYCLICS

▷ *maprotiline* (G) Initially 75 mg/day for 2 weeks; Then change gradually as needed in 25 mg increments; max 225 mg/day
Pediatric: <18 years: not recommended; ≥18 years: same as adult
> **Ludiomil** *Tab:* 25, 50, 75 mg

▷ *mirtazapine* Initially 15 mg q HS; increase at intervals of 1-2 weeks; Usual range 15-45 mg/day; Max 45 mg/day
Pediatric: <12 years: not recommended; ≥12 years: same as adult
> **Remeron** *Tab:* 15*, 30*, 45*mg
> **Remeron SolTab** *ODT:* 15, 30, 45 mg (orange) (phenylalanine)

▷ *chlordiazepoxide+amitriptyline* (IV)
Pediatric: <12 years: not recommended; ≥12 years: same as adult
> **Limbitrol** 3-4 tabs in divided doses
> > *Tab:* chlor 5 mg+amit 12.5 mg
> **Limbitrol DS** 3-4 tabs in divided doses; Max 6 tabs/day
> > *Tab:* chlor 10 mg+amit 25 mg

▷ *trazodone* (G) initially 150 mg/day in divided doses with food; increase by 50 mg/day q 3-4 days; max 400 mg/day in divided doses
Pediatric: <18 years: not recommended; ≥18 years: same as adult
> **Oleptro** *Tab:* 50, 100*, 150*, 200, 250, 300 mg

ATYPICAL ANTIPSYCHOTICS

▷ *aripiprazole* (G) Initially 15 mg daily; May increase to max 30 mg/day
Pediatric: <10 years: not recommended; 10-17 years: initially 2 mg/day for 2 days; then increase to 5 mg/day for 2 days; then increase to target dose of 10 mg/day; may increase by 5 mg/day at 1-week intervals as needed to a max of 30 mg/day
> **Abilify** *Tab:* 2, 5, 10, 15, 20, 30 mg
> **Abilify Discmelt** *Tab:* 15 mg orally disintegrating (vanilla) (phenylalanine)
> **Abilify Maintena** *Vial:* 300, 400 mg ext-rel pwdr for IM injection after reconstitution; 300, 400 mg single-dose prefilled dual-chamber syringes w. supplies
> **Comment:** Abilify is indicated for acute and maintenance treatment of manic or mixed episodes in bipolar I disorder, as monotherapy or as an adjunct to **lithium** or **valproate**, as adjunct to antidepressants for major depressive disorder (MDD), and for irritability associated with autistic disorder.

▷ *brexpiprazole* Administer once daily with or without food; *Starting Dose:* 0.5 to 1 mg once daily; *Recommended Maintenance Dose:* 2 mg once daily; Max 3 mg once daily; Dosage increases should occur at weekly intervals based on the patient's clinical response and tolerability; For patients with moderate, severe, or end-stage renal impairment (CrCl 60 ml/min), the max recommended dose is 2 mg once daily; For patients with moderate to severe hepatic impairment (Child-Pugh score ≥7), the max recommended dose is 2 mg once daily

Pediatric: Safety and efficacy not established

Rexulti *Tab:* 0.25, 0.5, 1, 2, 3, 4 mg

Comment: Rexulti is an atypical antipsychotic indicated for the treatment of MDD, schizophrenia, and agitation associated with dementia due to Alzheimer's disease. The most common adverse reactions (incidence ≥5% and at least twice the rate for placebo) were weight gain and akathisia. If co-administered with strong CYP2D6 or CYP3A4 inhibitors, administer half of the usual dose of **Rexulti**. If co-administered with strong/moderate CYP2D6 inhibitors and strong/moderate CYP3A4 inhibitors, administer 1/4 of the usual **Rexulti** dose. If the patient is a known CYP2D6 poor metabolizer and is taking a strong/moderate CYP3A4 inhibitor, administer 1/4 of the usual **Rexulti** dose. If co-administered with strong CYP3A4 inducers, double the usual dose of **Rexulti** and further adjust the **Rexulti** dose based on clinical response. **Rexulti** may be administered without dosage adjustment in patients with MDD when co-administered with strong CYP2D6 inhibitors (e.g., *paroxetine, fluoxetine*). Closely monitor patients for signs and symptoms of neuroleptic malignant syndrome (NMS); if this occurs, immediately discontinue **Rexulti** and treat as appropriate. The **Rexulti** drug label (mfr pkg insert) contains a boxed warning that elderly patients with dementia-related psychosis treated with antipsychotic drugs are at an increased risk of death. Therefore, use of **Rexulti** in these patients is contraindicated. Closely monitor patients for signs and symptoms of tardive dyskinesia (TD). If this occurs, discontinue **Rexulti** if clinically appropriate. Monitor patients for metabolic changes (such as hyperglycemia/diabetes mellitus, dyslipidemia, and weight gain). Leukopenia, neutropenia, and agranulocytosis may develop. Obtain complete blood counts (CBCs) in patients with preexisting low white blood cell count (WBC) or history of leukopenia or neutropenia. Consider discontinuing **Rexulti** if a clinically significant decline in WBC occurs in the absence of other causative factor. Advise patients and caregivers that orthostatic hypotension and/or syncope may occur; monitor heart rate (HR) and blood pressure (BP), especially patients with known cardiovascular or cerebrovascular disease, and avoid dehydration. Use **Rexulti** cautiously in patients with a history of seizures or with conditions that lower the seizure threshold. Adequate and well-controlled studies have not been conducted with **Rexulti** in human pregnancy to inform drug-associated risks. In animal reproduction studies, no teratogenicity was observed with oral administration of *brexpiprazole* during organogenesis at doses up to 73 and 146 times, respectively, of the maximum recommended human dose (MRHD) of 4 mg/day on a mg/m² basis. However, when administered *brexpiprazole* during the period of organogenesis through lactation, the number of perinatal deaths of pups was increased at 73 times the MRHD. Extrapyramidal and/or withdrawal symptoms, including agitation, hypertonia, hypotonia, tremor, somnolence, respiratory distress, and feeding disorder, have been reported in neonates whose mothers were exposed to antipsychotic drugs during the 3rd of pregnancy. These symptoms have varied in severity. Some neonates recovered within hours or days without specific treatment; others required prolonged hospitalization. Monitor neonates for extrapyramidal and/or withdrawal symptoms and manage symptoms appropriately. There is a pregnancy exposure registry that monitors pregnancy outcomes in women exposed to **Rexulti** during pregnancy. For more information contact the National Pregnancy Registry for Atypical Antipsychotics at 866-961-2388 or visit http://womensmentalhealth.org/clinical-and-research-programs/pregnancyregistry/. Lactation studies have not been conducted to assess the presence of *brexpiprazole* in human milk or effects of *brexpiprazole* on the breastfed infant. However, *brexpiprazole* is present in animal milk. Developmental and health benefits of breastfeeding should be considered along with the mother's clinical need for **Rexulti** and any potential adverse effects on the breastfed infant from **Rexulti** or from the underlying maternal condition. To report suspected adverse reactions, contact Otsuka America Pharmaceutical at 800-438-9927 or FDA at 800-FDA-1088 or www.fda.gov/medwatch.

▶ *cariprazine Bipolar Depression: Recommended starting dose:* 1.5 mg daily; Max recommended daily dose: 3 mg; *Bipolar Mania: Recommended Starting Dose:* 1.5 mg daily; *Max Recommended Daily Dose:* 6 mg (doses above 6 mg daily do not confer significant benefit, but increase the risk of dose-related adverse reactions)

Pediatric: safety and efficacy not established

Vraylar *Cap:* 1.5, 3, 4.5, 6 mg

Comment: Vraylar is an atypical antipsychotic for the treatment of schizophrenia, bipolar disorder (BPD), and as an adjunct for major depressive disorder (MDD) in adults. The most common adverse reactions in the treatment of *bipolar mania* (incidence ≥5% and at least twice the rate of placebo) have been extrapyramidal symptoms (EPS), akathisia, dyspepsia, vomiting, somnolence, and restlessness. The most common adverse reactions in the treatment of *bipolar depression* (incidence ≥5% and at least twice the rate of placebo) have been nausea, akathisia, restlessness, and EPS. Due to **Vraylar's** long half-life, monitor patients for adverse reactions for several weeks after starting **Vraylar** and with each dose change. *Boxed Warning:* Elderly patients with dementia-related psychosis treated with antipsychotic drugs are at an increased risk of death. **Vraylar** is not approved for the treatment of patients with dementia-related psychosis. Antidepressants increased the risk of suicidal thoughts and behaviors in pediatric and young adult patients. Closely monitor all antidepressant-treated patients for clinical worsening and emergence of suicidal thoughts and behaviors. When taken with strong CYP3A4 inhibitors, reduce **Vraylar** dose by

(continued)

half. Concomitant use of **Vraylar** with CYP3A4 inducers is not recommended. See the mfr pkg insert for full prescribing information and complete black box warning. Monitor patients for hyperglycemia and diabetes mellitus, dyslipidemia, and weight gain. Monitor for leukopenia, neutropenia, and agranulocytosis; perform CBCs in patients with preexisting low WBCs or history of leukopenia or neutropenia and consider discontinuing **Vraylar** if a clinically significant decline in WBC occurs in the absence of other causative factors. Monitor patients for orthostatic hypotension and syncope. Monitor HR and BP and warn patients with known cardiovascular or cerebrovascular disease and risk of dehydration or syncope. Use **Vraylar** cautiously in patients with a history of seizures or with conditions that lower the seizure threshold. Due to potential for cognitive and motor impairment, advise patients to use caution when operating machinery (e.g., driving a motor vehicle). Based on animal data, **Vraylar** may cause fetal harm; advise females of reproductive potential of fetal risk and to use effective contraception. Lactation studies have not been conducted to assess the presence of *cariprazine* in human milk or effects on the breastfed infant. However, *cariprazine* is present in animal milk. Development and health benefits of breastfeeding should be considered along with the mother's clinical need for **Vraylar** and any potential adverse effects on the breastfed infant from **Vraylar** or from the underlying maternal condition.

DEPRESSION: POSTPARTUM

NEUROACTIVE STEROID GAMMA-AMINOBUTYRIC ACID A (GABA$_A$) RECEPTOR-POSITIVE ALLOSTERIC MODULATOR

▶ *brexanolone* (IV) *Administer* as a continuous IV infusion over 60 hours (2½ days) by a qualified healthcare provider making infusion rate adjustments according to the 60-hour (2½ day) schedule below; Patients are at risk for excessive sedation or sudden loss of consciousness and must be continuously monitored, including continuous pulse oximetry for SpO2 monitoring; The healthcare provider must be available on site for the duration of the infusion and intervene as necessary with appropriate supportive care; The diluted product in the infusion bag can be used at room temperature for up to 12 hours; If the diluted product is not used immediately after dilution, store under refrigerated conditions for up to 96 hours
Pediatric: safety and effectiveness in children not established

> *Zulresso Vial:* 100 mg/20 ml (5 mg/ml, 20 ml), single-dose for dilution and IV infusion (preservative-free)
> **Comment:** **Zulresso** *(brexanolone)* is a gamma-aminobutyric acid A (GABA$_A$) receptor-positive allosteric modulator indicated for the treatment of postpartum depression (PPD) in adults. Avoid use in patients with end-stage renal disease (ESRD). The most common adverse reactions (incidence ≥5%) have been sedation/somnolence, dry mouth, loss of consciousness, and flushing/hot flashing. Assess the patient for newly emergent suicidal thoughts and behaviors. Consider changing the therapeutic regimen, including discontinuing **Zulresso**, in patients whose PPD becomes worse or who experience emergent suicidal thoughts and behaviors. Patients must be accompanied during interactions with their child(ren). May cause fetal harm. *Brexanolone* is transferred to breast milk in nursing mothers. Assess risk/benefit of breastfeeding along with the mother's clinical need for **Zulresso** and any potential adverse effects on the breastfed infant from **Zulresso** and the underlying maternal condition. **Zulresso** is available only through a restricted Risk Evaluation and Mitigation Strategy (REMS) Program. The pregnancy exposure registry monitors pregnancy outcomes in women exposed to antidepressants during pregnancy. Healthcare providers are encouraged to register patients by calling the National Pregnancy Registry for Antidepressants at 1-844-405-6185 or https://womensmentalhealth.org/research/pregnancyregistry/antidepressants/.

DEPRESSION: TREATMENT-RESISTANT (TRD)

NON-COMPETITIVE N-METHYL D-ASPARTATE (NMDA) RECEPTOR ANTAGONIST

▶ *esketamine* nasal spray (III) *Administer* intranasally under the supervision of a qualified healthcare provider in an approved setting; Assess blood pressure (BP) prior to and after administration; Allow each spray to absorb; Do not blow nose; During and after **Spravato** administration at each treatment session, observe the patient for at least 2 hours until the patient is safe to leave; Evidence of therapeutic benefit should be evaluated at the end of the induction phase to determine need for continued treatment; Administer **Spravato** in conjunction with an oral antidepressant as follows:

Induction Phase	Weeks 1 to 4 Administer twice weekly	Dose Day 1 starting dose: 56 mg Subsequent doses: 56 mg or 84 mg
Maintenance Phase	Weeks 5 to 8 Administer once weekly Week 9 and after Administer every 2 weeks or once weekly	56 mg or 84 mg 56 mg or 84 mg

Spravato *Nasal spray:* 28 mg/device (1 device=2 sprays=total 28 mg; 2 devices=4 sprays=56 mg; 3 devices=6 sprays=84 mg)

> **Comment: Spravato***(esketamine)* is a rapid-acting, nasal spray formulation of a non-competitive N-methyl D-aspartate (NMDA) receptor antagonist indicated, in conjunction with an oral antidepressant, for use in adults with treatment-resistant depression (TRD). Contraindications include aneurysm, vascular disease (including thoracic and abdominal aorta, intracranial and peripheral arterial vessels, and arteriovenous malformation), and intracerebral hemorrhage. Patients with cardiovascular and cerebrovascular conditions and risk factors may be at an increased risk of associated adverse effects. Risk factors during a treatment include sedation and dissociation. Risk factors following a treatment are impaired attention, judgment, thinking, reaction speed, and motor skills. The patient should <u>not</u> drive <u>or</u> operate machinery until the next day after a restful sleep. There is potential for abuse/misuse with **Spravato** as a schedule III (CIII) drug. Consider risk versus benefit prior to initiation of treatment in patients at higher risk and monitor for signs and symptoms of abuse/misuse. There is increased risk of suicidal thoughts and behaviors in pediatric and young adult patients taking antidepressants. Therefore, closely monitor all antidepressant-treated patients for clinical worsening and emergence of suicidal thoughts and behaviors. **Spravato** may cause embryo/fetal toxicity. Consider pregnancy planning and prevention in females of reproductive potential. Breastfeeding is <u>not</u> recommended. **Spravato** is <u>only</u> available through the restricted **Spravato** Risk Evaluation and Mitigation Strategy (REMS) Program. Healthcare settings must be certified in the program and ensure that **Spravato** is <u>only</u> dispensed in healthcare settings and administered to patients who are enrolled in the program. Pharmacies must be certified in the REMS program and must <u>only</u> dispense **Spravato** to healthcare settings that are certified in the program. Further information, including a list of certified pharmacies, is available at www. SPRAVATOrems.com <u>or</u> 1-855-382-6022.

DERMATITIS: ATOPIC (ECZEMA)

Parenteral Corticosteroids *see* Appendix L. Parenteral Corticosteroids
Oral Corticosteroids *see* Appendix K. Oral Corticosteroids
Topical Corticosteroids *see* Appendix J: Topical Corticosteroids by Potency

PHOSPHODIESTERASE 4 INHIBITOR
▷ *crisaborole 2%* apply sparingly bid; max 4 weeks
  Pediatric: <2 years: <u>not</u> recommended; ≥2 years: same as adult
    Eucrisa *Oint:* 2% (60 gm)

MOISTURIZING AGENTS
Aquaphor Healing Ointment (OTC) *Oint:* 1.75, 3.5, 14 oz (alcohol)
Eucerin Daily Sun Defense (OTC) *Lotn:* 6 oz (fragrance-free)
Comment: Eucerin Daily Sun Defense is a moisturizer with SPF-15 sunscreen.
Eucerin Facial Lotion (OTC) *Lotn:* 4 oz
Eucerin Light Lotion (OTC) *Lotn:* 8 oz
Eucerin Lotion (OTC) *Lotn:* 8, 16 oz
Eucerin Original Creme (OTC) *Crm:* 2, 4, 16 oz (alcohol)
Eucerin Plus Creme (OTC) *Crm:* 4 oz
Eucerin Plus Lotion (OTC) *Lotn:* 6, 12 oz
Eucerin Protective Lotion (OTC) *Lotn:* 4 oz (alcohol)
Comment: Eucerin Protective Lotion is a moisturizer with SPF-25 sunscreen.
Lac-Hydrin Cream (OTC) *Crm:* 280, 385 gm
Lac-Hydrin Lotion (OTC) *Lotn:* 25, 400 gm
Lubriderm Dry Skin Scented (OTC) *Lotn:* 6, 10, 16, 32 oz
Lubriderm Dry Skin Unscented (OTC) *Lotn:* 3.3, 6, 10, 16 oz (fragrance-free)
Lubriderm Sensitive Skin Lotion (OTC) *Lotn:* 3.3, 6, 10, 16 oz (lanolin-free)
Lubriderm Dry Skin (OTC) *Lotn (scented):* 2.5, 6, 10, 16 oz;
  Lotn (fragrance-free): 1, 2.5, 6, 10, 16 oz
Lubriderm Bath 1-2 capfuls in bath <u>or</u> rub onto wet skin as needed, then rinse
  Oil: 8 oz
Moisturel (OTC) apply as needed
  Crm: 4, 16 oz; *Lotn:* 8, 12 oz; *Clnsr:* 8.75 oz

OATMEAL COLLOIDS
Aveeno (OTC) add to bath as needed
  Regular: 1.5 oz (8/pck); *Moisturizing:* 0.75 oz (8/pck)
Aveeno Oil (OTC) add to bath as needed
  Oil: 8 oz
Aveeno Moisturizing (OTC) apply as needed
  Lotn: 2.5, 8, 12 oz; *Crm:* 4 oz

(continued)

Aveeno Cleansing Bar (OTC) *Bar:* 3 oz
Aveeno Gentle Skin Cleanser (OTC) *Liq clnsr:* 6 oz

TOPICAL OIL

▷ *fluocinolone acetonide* 0.01% topical oil
Pediatric: <6 years: <u>not</u> recommended; ≥6 years: apply sparingly bid for up to 4 weeks
  Derma-Smoothe/FS Topical Oil apply sparingly tid
    Topical oil: 0.01% (4 oz) (peanut oil)

TOPICAL STEROIDS

Comment: Topical steroids should be applied sparingly and for the shortest time necessary. Do <u>not</u> use in the diaper area. Do <u>not</u> use an occlusive dressing. Systemic absorption of topical corticosteroids can induce reversible hypothalamic-pituitary-adrenal (HPA) axis suppression with the potential for clinical corticosteroid insufficiency.

▷ *desonide* 0.05% topical gel (G) apply sparingly bid-tid; max 4 weeks
Pediatric: <3 months: <u>not</u> recommended; ≥3 months: same as adult
  Desonate *Gel:* 0.05% (60 gm) (89% purified water; fragrance-free, surfactant-free, alcohol-free)

SECOND-GENERATION ORAL ANTIHISTAMINES

Comment: The following drugs are second-generation antihistamines. As such they are minimally sedating, much less so than the first-generation antihistamines. All antihistamines are excreted into breast milk.

▷ *cetirizine* (OTC) (G) initially 5-10 mg once daily; 5 mg once daily; *>65 years:* use with caution
Pediatric: <6 years: <u>not</u> recommended; ≥6 years: same as adult
  cetirizine Cap: 10 mg
  Children's Zyrtec Chewable *Chew tab:* 5, 10 mg (grape)
  Children's Zyrtec Allergy Syrup *Syr:* 1 mg/ml (4 oz) (grape, bubble gum) (sugar-free, dye-free)
  Zyrtec *Tab:* 10 mg
  Zyrtec Hives Relief *Tab:* 10 mg
  Zyrtec Liquid Gels *Liq gel:* 10 mg

▷ *desloratadine*
  Clarinex 1/2-1 tab once daily
  Pediatric: <6 years: <u>not</u> recommended; ≥6 years: same as adult
    Tab: 5 mg
  Clarinex RediTabs 5 mg once daily
  Pediatric: <6 years: <u>not</u> recommended; 6-12 years: 2.5 mg once daily; ≥12 years: same as adult
    ODT: 2.5, 5 mg (tutti-frutti) (phenylalanine)
  Clarinex Syrup 5 mg (10 ml) once daily
  Pediatric: <6 months: <u>not</u> recommended; 6-11 months: 1 mg (2 ml) once daily; 1-5 years: 1.25 mg (2.5 ml) once daily; 6-11 years: 2.5 mg (5 ml) once daily; ≥12 years: same as adult
    Syr: 0.5 mg per ml (4 oz) (tutti-frutti) (phenylalanine)
  Desloratadine ODT 1 tab once daily
  Pediatric: <6 years: <u>not</u> recommended; 6-11 years: 1/2 tab once daily; ≥12 years: same as adult
    ODT: 5 mg

▷ *fexofenadine* (OTC)(G) 60 mg once daily-bid <u>or</u> 180 mg once daily; *CrCl <90 ml/min:* 60 mg once daily
Pediatric: <6 months: <u>not</u> recommended; 6 months-2 years: 15 mg bid; *CrCl ≤90 ml/min:* 15 mg once daily; 2-11 years: 30 mg bid; *CrCl ≤90 ml/min:* 30 mg once daily; ≥12 years: same as adult
  Allegra *Tab:* 30, 60, 180 mg film-coat
  Allegra Allergy *Tab:* 60, 180 mg film-coat
  Allegra ODT *ODT:* 30 mg (phenylalanine)
  Allegra Oral Suspension *Oral susp:* 30 mg/5 ml (6 mg/ml) (4 oz)

▷ *levocetirizine* (OTC)(G) administer dose in the PM; *Seasonal Allergic Rhinitis:* <2 years: <u>not</u> recommended; may start at ≥2 years; *Chronic Idiopathic Urticaria (CIU), Perennial Allergic Rhinitis:* <6 months: <u>not</u> recommended; may start at ≥ 6 months; *Dosing by Age:* 6 months to 5 years: max 1.25 mg once daily; 6-11 years: max 2.5 mg once daily; ≥12 years: 2.5-5 mg once daily; *Renal Dysfunction:* <12 years: contraindicated; *Renal Dysfunction:* ≥12 years: *CrCl 50-80 ml/min:* 2.5 mg once daily; *CrCl 30-50 ml/min:* 2.5 mg every other day; *CrCl 10-30 ml/min:* 2.5 mg twice weekly (every 3-4 days); *CrCl <10 ml/min, end-stage renal disease (ESRD), or Hemodialysis:* contraindicated
  Children's Xyzal Allergy 24HR *Oral Soln:* 0.5 mg/ml (150 ml)
  Xyzal Allergy 24HR *Tab:* 5*mg

▷ *loratadine* (OTC)(G) 5 mg bid <u>or</u> 10 mg once daily; *Hepatic <u>or</u> Renal Insufficiency:* see mfr pkg insert
Pediatric: <2 years: <u>not</u> recommended; 2-5 years: 5 mg once daily; ≥6 years: same as adult
  Children's Claritin Chewables *Chew tab:* 5 mg (grape) (phenylalanine)
  Children's Claritin Syrup 1 mg/ml (4 oz) (fruit) (sugar-free, alcohol-free, dye-free; sodium 6 mg/5 ml)
  Claritin *Tab:* 10 mg
  Claritin Hives Relief *Tab:* 10 mg
  Claritin Liqui-Gels *Liq gel:* 10 mg

Claritin RediTabs 12 Hours *ODT:* 5 mg (mint)
Claritin RediTabs 24 Hours *ODT:* 10 mg (mint)

FIRST-GENERATION ANTIHISTAMINES

▷ *diphenhydramine* (G) 25-50 mg q 6-8 hours; max 100 mg/day
Pediatric: <2 years: not recommended; 2-6 years: 6.25 mg q 4-6 hours; max 37.5 mg/day; >6-12 years: 12.5-25 mg q 4-6 hours; max 150 mg/day; >12 years: same as adult
   Benadryl (OTC) *Chew tab:* 12.5 mg (grape) (phenylalanine); *Liq:* 12.5 mg/5 ml (4, 8 oz); *Cap:* 25 mg; *Tab:* 25 mg; *Dye-free soft gel:* 25 mg; *Dye-free liq:* 12.5 mg/5 ml (4, 8 oz)
▷ *diphenhydramine injectable* (G) 25-50 mg IM immediately; then q 6 hours prn
Pediatric: <12 years: see mfr pkg insert: 1.25 mg/kg up to 25 mg IM x 1 dose; then q 6 hours prn; ≥12 years: same as adult
   Benadryl Injectable *Vial:* 50 mg/ml (1 ml single-use), 50 mg/ml (10 ml multidose); *Amp:* 10 mg/ml (1 ml); *Prefilled syringe:* 50 mg/ml (1 ml)
▷ *hydroxyzine* (G) 50 mg/day divided qid prn; 50-100 mg/day divided qid prn
Pediatric: <6 years: 50 mg/day divided qid prn; ≥6 years: same as adult
   Atarax *Tab:* 10, 25, 50, 100 mg; *Syr:* 10 mg/5 ml (alcohol 0.5%)
   Vistaril *Cap:* 25, 50, 100 mg; *Oral susp:* 25 mg/5 ml (4 oz) (lemon)
Comment: *Hydroxyzine* is contraindicated in early pregnancy and in patients with a prolonged QT interval. It is not known whether this drug is excreted in human milk; therefore, *hydroxyzine* should not be given to nursing mothers.

TOPICAL ANALGESICS

▷ *capsaicin* cream (G) apply tid-qid prn
Pediatric: <2 years: not recommended; ≥2 years: apply sparingly tid-qid prn
   Axsain *Crm:* 0.075% (1, 2 oz)
   Capsin (OTC) *Lotn:* 0.025, 0.075% (59 ml)
   Capzasin-HP (OTC) *Crm:* 0.075% (1.5 oz); *Lotn:* 0.075% (2 oz)
   Capzasin-P (OTC) *Crm:* 0.025% (1.5 oz); *Lotn:* 0.025% (2 oz)
   Dolorac *Crm:* 0.025% (28 gm)
   Double Cap (OTC) *Crm:* 0.05% (2 oz)
   R-Gel *Gel:* 0.025% (15, 30 gm)
   Zostrix (OTC) *Crm:* 0.025% (0.7, 1.5, 3 oz)
   Zostrix HP (OTC) *Emol crm:* 0.075% (1, 2 oz)

TOPICAL AND TRANSDERMAL ANALGESICS

▷ *capsaicin* 8% patch apply up to 4 patches for one 60-minute application to clean dry skin; may prep area with topical anesthetic; wear non-latex gloves; patches may be cut to size/shape; treatment may be repeated every 3 months
Pediatric: <18 years: not recommended; ≥18 years: same as adult
   Qutenza *Patch:* 8% (1,640 mcg/cm, 179 mg) (1 or 2 patches w. 1-50 gm tube cleansing gel/carton)
▷ *diclofenac sodium* apply qid prn to intact skin; *Pregnancy:* not recommended ≥30 weeks;
Pediatric: <12 years: safety and efficacy not established; ≥12 years: same as adult
   Pennsaid 1.5% in 10 drop increments, dispense and rub into front, side, and back of knee: usually; 40 drops (40 mg) qid
      Topical soln: 1.5% (150 ml)
   Pennsaid 2% apply 2 pump actuations (40 mg) and rub into front, side, and back of knee bid
      Topical soln: 2% (20 mg/pump actuation, 112 gm)
   Solaraze Gel massage into clean skin bid prn
      Gel: 3% (50 gm) (benzyl alcohol)
   Voltaren Gel (G)(OTC) apply qid prn to intact skin
      Gel: 1% (100 gm)
Comment: *Diclofenac* is contraindicated with *aspirin* allergy. As with other nonsteroidal anti-inflammatory drugs (NSAIDs), it should be avoided in late pregnancy (≥30 weeks) because it may cause premature closure of the ductus arteriosus.
▷ *doxepin* (G) cream apply to affected area qid at intervals of at least 3-4 hours; max 8 days
Pediatric: <12 years: not recommended; >12 years: same as adult
   Prudoxin *Crm:* 5% (45 gm)
   Zonalon *Crm:* 5% (30, 45 gm)
▷ *pimecrolimus* 1% cream (G) <2 years: not recommended; ≥2 years: apply to affected area bid; do not apply an occlusive dressing
   Elidel *Crm:* 1% (30, 60, 100 gm)
Comment: *Pimecrolimus* is indicated for short-term and intermittent long-term use. Discontinue use when resolution occurs. Contraindicated if the patient is immunosuppressed. Change to the 0.1% preparation or if secondary bacterial infection is present.

(continued)

▷ *trolamine salicylate* apply tid-qid
  Pediatric: <2 years: <u>not</u> recommended; ≥2 years: same as adult
    Mobisyl Creme *Crm:* 10% (100 gm)

TOPICAL AND TRANSDERMAL ANESTHETICS

Comment: *Lidocaine* should <u>not</u> be applied to non-intact skin.
▷ *lidocaine* cream apply to affected area bid prn
  Pediatric: <12 years: <u>not</u> recommended; ≥12 years: same as adult
    LidaMantle *Crm:* 3% (1, 2 oz)
    Lidoderm *Crm:* 3% (85 gm)
    ZTlido *lidocaine* topical system 1% (30/carton)
    Comment: Compared to **Lidoderm** (*lidocaine* patch 5%), which contains 700 mg/patch, **ZTlido** requires only 35 mg per topical system to achieve the same therapeutic dose.
▷ *lidocaine* lotion apply to affected area bid prn
  Pediatric: <12 years: <u>not</u> recommended; ≥12 years: same as adult
    LidaMantle *Lotn:* 3% (177 ml)
▷ *lidocaine* 5% patch **(G)** apply up to 3 patches at one time for up to 12 hours/24-hour period (12 hours on/12 hours off); patches may be cut into smaller sizes before removal of the release liner; do <u>not</u> reuse
  Pediatric: <12 years: <u>not</u> recommended; ≥12 years: same as adult
    Lidoderm *Patch:* 5% (10 × 14 cm; 30/carton)
▷ *lidocaine+dexamethasone*
  Pediatric: <12 years: <u>not</u> recommended; ≥12 years: same as adult
    Decadron Phosphate with Xylocaine *Lotn:* dexa 4 mg+lido 10 mg per ml (5 ml)
▷ *lidocaine+hydrocortisone* **(G)** apply to affected area bid prn
  Pediatric: <12 years: <u>not</u> recommended; ≥12 years: same as adult
    LidaMantle HC *Crm:* lido 3%+hydro 0.5% (1, 3 oz); *Lotn:* (177 ml)
▷ *lidocaine* 2.5%+*prilocaine* 2.5% apply sparingly to the burn bid-tid prn
  Pediatric: <12 years: <u>not</u> recommended; ≥12 years: same as adult
    Emla Cream 5, 30 gm/tube

JANUS KINASE (JAK) 1 INHIBITOR

▷ *abrocitinib* Administer 100 mg once daily; Do not break, crush, <u>or</u> chew; may be used with <u>or</u> without topical corticosteroid; If a dose is missed, administer the dose as soon as possible; if <12 hours before the next dose, skip the missed dose and resume dosing at the regular scheduled time; If response to treatment is inadequate after 12 weeks, consider increasing dose to 200 mg once daily; then, if response remains inadequate discontinue Cibingo
  Pediatric: Safety and efficacy <u>not</u> established
    Cibinqo *Tab:* 50, 100, 200 mg film-coat
    Comment: Cibinqo is a Janus kinase (JAK) 1 inhibitor indicated for the treatment of adults with refractory, moderate-to-severe atopic dermatitis, whose disease is <u>not</u> adequately controlled with other systemic drug products, including biologics, <u>or</u> when use of those therapies is inadvisable. **Cibinqo** is not approved for use in RA. **Cibinqo** is <u>not</u> recommended for use in combination with other JAK inhibitors, biologic immunomodulators, <u>or</u> with other immunosuppressants. **Cibinqo** is contraindicated in patients taking antiplatelet therapies, *except* for low-dose aspirin (≤81 mg daily), during the first 3 months of treatment. **Cibinqo** initiation is <u>not</u> recommended in patients with active TB. For patients with latent TB <u>or</u> those with a negative latent TB test who are at high risk for TB, start preventive therapy for latent TB *prior* to initiation of **Cibinqo**. **Cibinqo** initiation is <u>not</u> recommended in patients with active hepatitis B or hepatitis C. **Cibinqo** initiation is <u>not</u> recommended in patients with a platelet count <150,000/mm^3, absolute lymphocyte count <500/mm^3, absolute neutrophil count <1,000/mm^3, <u>or</u> hemoglobin <8 gm/dL. Prior to initiating **Cibinqo**, complete all age-appropriate vaccinations as recommended by current immunization guidelines including prophylactic herpes zoster vaccinations. Avoid vaccination 7 with live vaccines immediately prior to, during, and immediately after **Cibinqo** therapy. Consider the benefits and risks for the individual patient prior to initiating or continuing therapy with **Cibinqo**, particularly in patients who are current <u>or</u> past smokers and patients with other cardiovascular risk factors. Patients should be informed about the symptoms of serious cardiovascular events and the steps to take if they occur. Discontinue **Cibinqo** in patients that have experienced a myocardial infarction or stroke. Avoid **Cibinqo** in patients who may be at increased risk of thrombosis. If symptoms of thrombosis occur, discontinue **Cibinqo** and evaluate and treat patients appropriately. There is a pregnancy exposure registry that monitors pregnancy outcomes in females exposed to **Cibinqo** during pregnancy. Pregnant patients exposed to **Cibinqo**, and healthcare providers, are encouraged to call 1-877-311-3770.
▷ *ruxolitinib* Apply a thin layer twice daily to affected areas; Max 20% body surface area (BSA); Max: 60 gm per week
  Pediatric: <12 years: Safety and efficacy not established; ≥12 years: same as adult
    Opzelura *Crm:* 1.5% (60 gm aluminum tube)

Comment: Opzelura cream is a Janus kinase (JAK) inhibitor indicated, for topical short-term and non-continuous, chronic treatment of mild-to-moderate atopic dermatitis in non-immunocompromised patients >12 years of age whose disease is not adequately controlled with other topical prescription therapies or when those therapies are not advisable. Use of **Opzelura** in combination with therapeutic biologics, other JAK inhibitors or potent immunosuppressants such as *azathioprine* or *cyclosporine* is not recommended. BBW: Serious Infection, Mortality, Malignancy, Major Adverse Cardiovascular Events (MACE), and Thrombosis. Serious infections leading to hospitalization or death, including tuberculosis and bacterial, invasive fungal, viral, and other opportunistic infections, have occurred in patients receiving JAKIs for inflammatory conditions. Higher rate of all-cause mortality, including sudden cardiovascular death, have been observed in patients treated with JAKIs for inflammatory conditions. Lymphoma and other malignancies have been observed in patients treated with JAKIs for inflammatory conditions. A higher rate of MACE (including cardiovascular death, myocardial infarction, and stroke) has been observed in patients treated with JAKIs for inflammatory conditions. Thrombosis, including deep venous thrombosis (DVT), pulmonary embolism (PE), and arterial thrombosis, some fatal, have occurred in patients treated with JAKIs for inflammatory conditions (See mfr pck insert for full prescribing information and complete boxed warning). The most common adverse reactions (incidence ≥1%) have been nasopharyngitis, diarrhea, bronchitis, ear infection, eosinophil count increased, urticaria, folliculitis, tonsillitis, and rhinorrhea. Adverse reactions that occurred in Trials 1 and 2 in <1% of subjects in the **Opzelura** group, and none in the vehicle group, were neutropenia, allergic conjunctivitis, pyrexia, seasonal allergy, herpes zoster, otitis externa, Staphylococcal infection, and acneiform dermatitis. As serious bacterial, mycobacterial, fungal and viral infections have occurred, monitor patients for infection and manage all infections appropriately and promptly. Non-melanoma skin cancers (i.e., basal cell and squamous cell carcinoma have occurred. Perform periodic skin examinations during treatment and following treatment as appropriate. Thromboembolic events have occurred. Thrombocytopenia, anemia and neutropenia have occurred; monitor CBC as clinically indicated. *Ruxolitinib* is known to be a substrate for cytochrome P450 3A4 (CYP3A4). Inhibitors of CYP3A4 may increase *ruxolitinib* systemic concentrations whereas inducers of CYP3A4 may decrease *ruxolitinib* systemic concentrations. Available data from human pregnancies reported in clinical trials with **Opzelura** are not sufficient to evaluate a drug-associated risk for major birth defects, miscarriage, or other adverse maternal or fetal outcomes. In animal reproduction studies, oral administration of *ruxolitinib* during the period of organogenesis resulted in adverse developmental outcomes at doses associated with maternal toxicity. There will be a pregnancy registry that monitors pregnancy outcomes in pregnant persons exposed to **Opzelura** during pregnancy. Pregnant persons exposed to **Opzelura** and healthcare providers should report **Opzelura** exposure by calling 1-855-463-3463. Advise patients not to breastfeed during treatment with **Opzelura** and for four week after the last dose.

INTERLEUKIN-4 RECEPTOR ALPHA ANTAGONIST

▷ *dupilumab* administer SC into the upper arm, abdomen, or thigh; rotate sites; *Initial Dose:* 600 mg (2 x 300 mg SC in different injection sites), then 300 mg SC once every other week; may use with or without topical corticosteroids; may use with calcineurin inhibitors, but reserve only for problem areas (e.g., face, neck, intertriginous, and genital areas); avoid live vaccines
Pediatric: <12 years: not recommended; ≥12 years: <60 kg: *Initial Dose:* 400 mg (2 x 200 mg SC in different injection sites; then 200 mg SC once every other week; ≥60 kg: same as adult
   Dupixent *Prefilled syringe:* 200 mg/1.14 ml, 300 mg/2 ml, single-dose (2/pck without needle) (preservative-free)
Comment: Dupilumab is a human monoclonal immunoglobulin G4 (IgG4) antibody that inhibits interleukin-4 (IL-4) and interleukin-13 (IL-13) signaling by specifically binding to the IL4Ra subunit shared by the IL-4 and IL-13 receptor complexes, thereby inhibiting the release of proinflammatory cytokines, chemokines, and IgE. **Dupixent** is indicated for the treatment of moderate-to-severe atopic dermatitis when the disease is not adequately controlled with topical prescription therapies or when those therapies are not advisable. **Dupixent** can be used with or without topical corticosteroids. **Dupilumab** is also indicated as an add-on maintenance therapy, at different dosing regimens, for patients ≥12 years of age with moderate-to-severe asthma with an eosinophilic subtype or with oral corticosteroid-dependent asthma. Avoid live vaccines.

DERMATITIS: CONTACT

Topical Corticosteroids *see* Appendix J: Topical Corticosteroids by Potency
Parenteral Corticosteroids *see* Appendix L. Parenteral Corticosteroids
Oral Corticosteroids *see* Appendix K. Oral Corticosteroids
OTC Diphenhydramine Cream

PROPHYLAXIS

▷ *bentoquatam* apply as a wet film to exposed skin at least 15 minutes prior to possible contact; reapply at least q 4 hours; remove with soap and water
Pediatric: <6 years: not recommended; ≥6 years: same as adult
   IvyBlock (OTC) *Soln:* 120 ml
Comment: Provides protection against genus *Rhus* (poison ivy, oak, and sumac).

TREATMENT
Oatmeal Colloids

    Aveeno (OTC) add to bath as needed
      Regular: 1.5 oz (8/pck); *Moisturizing*: 0.75 oz (8/pck)
    Aveeno Oil (OTC) add to bath as needed
      Oil: 8 oz
    Aveeno Moisturizing (OTC) apply as needed
      Lotn: 2.5, 8, 12 oz; *Crm*: 4 oz
    Aveeno Cleansing Bar (OTC) *Bar*: 3 oz
    Aveeno Gentle Skin Cleanser (OTC) *Liq clnsr*: 6 oz

SECOND-GENERATION ORAL ANTIHISTAMINES
Comment: The following drugs are second-generation antihistamines. As such they are minimally sedating, much less so than the first-generation antihistamines. All antihistamines are excreted into breast milk.

▷ *cetirizine* (OTC)(G) initially 5-10 mg once daily; 5 mg once daily; *≥65 years*: use with caution
  Pediatric: <6 years: <u>not</u> recommended; ≥6 years: same as adult
    cetirizine Cap: 10 mg
    Children's Zyrtec Chewable *Chew tab*: 5, 10 mg (grape)
    Children's Zyrtec Allergy Syrup *Syr*: 1 mg/ml (4 oz) (grape, bubble gum) (sugar-free, dye-free)
    Zyrtec *Tab*: 10 mg
    Zyrtec Hives Relief *Tab*: 10 mg
    Zyrtec Liquid Gels *Liq gel*: 10 mg

▷ *desloratadine*
    Clarinex 1/2-1 tab once daily
  Pediatric: <6 years: <u>not</u> recommended; ≥6 years: same as adult
    Tab: 5 mg
    Clarinex RediTabs 5 mg once daily
  Pediatric: <6 years: <u>not</u> recommended; 6-12 years: 2.5 mg once daily; ≥12 years: same as adult
    ODT: 2.5, 5 mg (tutti-frutti) (phenylalanine)
    Clarinex Syrup 5 mg (10 ml) once daily
  Pediatric: <6 months: <u>not</u> recommended; 6-11 months: 1 mg (2 ml) once daily; 1-5 years: 1.25 mg (2.5 ml) once daily; 6-11 years: 2.5 mg (5 ml) once daily; ≥12 years: same as adult
    Syr: 0.5 mg per ml (4 oz) (tutti-frutti) (phenylalanine)
    Desloratadine ODT 1 tab once daily
  Pediatric: <6 years: <u>not</u> recommended; 6-11 years: 1/2 tab once daily; ≥12 years: same as adult
    ODT: 5 mg

▷ *fexofenadine* (OTC)(G) 60 mg once daily-bid <u>or</u> 180 mg once daily; *CrCl <90 ml/min*: 60 mg once daily
  Pediatric: <6 months: <u>not</u> recommended; 6 months-2 years: 15 mg bid; *CrCl ≤90 ml/min*: 15 mg once daily; 2-11 years: 30 mg bid; *CrCl ≤90 ml/min*: 30 mg once daily; ≥12 years: same as adult
    Allegra *Tab*: 30, 60, 180 mg film-coat
    Allegra Allergy *Tab*: 60, 180 mg film-coat
    Allegra ODT *ODT*: 30 mg (phenylalanine)
    Allegra Oral Suspension *Oral susp*: 30 mg/5 ml (6 mg/ml) (4 oz)

▷ *levocetirizine* (OTC)(G) administer dose in the PM; *Seasonal Allergic Rhinitis*: <2 years: <u>not</u> recommended; may start at ≥2 years; *Chronic Idiopathic Urticaria (CIU), Perennial Allergic Rhinitis*: <6 months: <u>not</u> recommended; may start at ≥ 6 months; *Dosing by Age*: 6 months to 5 years: max 1.25 mg once daily; 6-11 years: max 2.5 mg once daily; ≥12 years: 2.5-5 mg once daily; *Renal Dysfunction*: <12 years: contraindicated; *Renal Dysfunction, ≥12 years*: CrCl 50-80 ml/min: 2.5 mg once daily; CrCl 30-50 ml/min: 2.5 mg every other day; CrCl: 10-30 ml/min: 2.5 mg twice weekly (every 3-4 days); *CrCl <10 ml/min, end-stage renal disease (ESRD), or Hemodialysis*: contraindicated
    Children's Xyzal Allergy 24HR *Oral Soln*: 0.5 mg/ml (150 ml)
    Xyzal Allergy 24HR *Tab*: 5*mg

▷ *loratadine* (OTC)(G) 5 mg bid <u>or</u> 10 mg once daily; *Hepatic <u>or</u> Renal Insufficiency*: see mfr pkg insert
  Pediatric: <2 years: <u>not</u> recommended; 2-5 years: 5 mg once daily; ≥6 years: same as adult
    Children's Claritin Chewables *Chew tab*: 5 mg (grape) (phenylalanine)
    Children's Claritin Syrup 1 mg/ml (4 oz) (fruit) (sugar-free, alcohol-free, dye-free; sodium 6 mg/5 ml)
    Claritin *Tab*: 10 mg
    Claritin Hives Relief *Tab*: 10 mg
    Claritin Liqui-Gels *Liq gel*: 10 mg
    Claritin RediTabs 12 Hours *ODT*: 5 mg (mint)
    Claritin RediTabs 24 Hours *ODT*: 10 mg (mint)

FIRST-GENERATION ORAL ANTIHISTAMINES
▷ *diphenhydramine* (G) 25-50 mg q 6-8 hours; max 100 mg/day
  Pediatric: <2 years: <u>not</u> recommended; 2-6 years: 6.25 mg q 4-6 hours; max 37.5 mg/day; >6-12 years: 12.5-25 mg q 4-6 hours, max 150 mg/day; >12 years: same as adult
    Benadryl (OTC) *Chew tab*: 12.5 mg (grape) (phenylalanine); *Liq*: 12.5 mg/5 ml (4, 8 oz); *Cap*: 25 mg; *Tab*: 25 mg; *Dye-free soft gel*: 25 mg; *Dye-free liq*: 12.5 mg/5 ml (4, 8 oz)

▶ *hydroxyzine* (G) 50 mg/day divided qid prn; 50-100 mg/day divided qid prn
  Pediatric: <6 years: 50 mg/day divided qid prn; ≥6 years: same as adult
    Atarax *Tab:* 10, 25, 50, 100 mg; *Syr:* 10 mg/5 ml (alcohol 0.5%)
    Vistaril *Cap:* 25, 50, 100 mg; *Oral susp:* 25 mg/5 ml (4 oz) (lemon)
  Comment: *Hydroxyzine* is contraindicated in early pregnancy and in patients with a prolonged QT interval.
  It is not known whether this drug is excreted in human milk; therefore, *hydroxyzine* should not be given to
  nursing mothers.

FIRST-GENERATION PARENTERAL ANTIHISTAMINE

▶ *diphenhydramine* injectable (G) 25-50 mg IM immediately; then q 6 hours prn
  Pediatric: <12 years: see mfr pkg insert: 1.25 mg/kg up to 25 mg IM x 1 dose; then q 6 hours prn; ≥12 years:
  same as adult
    Benadryl Injectable *Vial:* 50 mg/ml (1 ml single-use); 50 mg/ml (10 ml multidose); *Amp:* 10 mg/ml
    (1 ml); *Prefilled syringe:* 50 mg/ml (1 ml)

DERMATITIS: GENUS *RHUS* (POISON OAK, POISON IVY, POISON SUMAC)

Topical Corticosteroids *see* Appendix J: Topical Corticosteroids by Potency
Parenteral Corticosteroids *see* Appendix L. Parenteral Corticosteroids
Oral Corticosteroids *see* Appendix K. Oral Corticosteroids
OTC Calamine Lotion
OTC Diphenhydramine Cream

PROPHYLAXIS

▶ *bentoquatam* <6 years: not recommended; ≥6 years: apply as a wet film to exposed skin at least 15 minutes
  prior to possible contact; reapply at least q 4 hours; remove with soap and water
    IvyBlock (OTC) *Soln:* 120 ml
  Comment: Provides protection against genus *Rhus* (poison oak, poison ivy, and poison sumac).

TREATMENT
Oatmeal Colloids
Aveeno (OTC) add to bath as needed
  Regular: 1.5 oz (8/pck); *Moisturizing:* 0.75 oz (8/pck)
Aveeno Oil (OTC) add to bath as needed
  Oil: 8 oz
Aveeno Moisturizing (OTC) apply as needed
  Lotn: 2.5, 8, 12 oz; *Crm:* 4 oz
Aveeno Cleansing Bar (OTC) *Bar:* 3 oz
Aveeno Gentle Skin Cleanser (OTC) *Liq clnsr:* 6 oz

SECOND-GENERATION ORAL ANTIHISTAMINES
Comment: The following drugs are second-generation antihistamines. As such they are minimally
sedating, much less so than the first-generation antihistamines. All antihistamines are excreted into breast milk.
▶ *cetirizine* (OTC)(G) initially 5-10 mg once daily; maintenance: 5 mg once daily; ≥65 years: use with caution
  Pediatric: <6 years: not recommended; ≥6 years: same as adult
    cetirizine *Cap:* 10 mg
    Children's Zyrtec Chewable *Chew tab:* 5, 10 mg (grape)
    Children's Zyrtec Allergy Syrup *Syr:* 1 mg/ml (4 oz) (grape, bubble gum) (sugar-free, dye-free)
    Zyrtec *Tab:* 10 mg
    Zyrtec Hives Relief *Tab:* 10 mg
    Zyrtec Liquid Gels *Liq gel:* 10 mg
▶ *desloratadine*
    Clarinex 1/2-1 tab once daily
    Pediatric: <6 years: not recommended; ≥6 years: same as adult
      Tab: 5 mg
    Clarinex RediTabs 5 mg once daily
    Pediatric: <6 years: not recommended; 6-12 years: 2.5 mg once daily; ≥12 years: same as adult
      ODT: 2.5, 5 mg (tutti-frutti) (phenylalanine)
    Clarinex Syrup 5 mg (10 ml) once daily
    Pediatric: <6 months: not recommended; 6-11 months: 1 mg (2 ml) once daily; 1-5 years: 1.25 mg
    (2.5 ml) once daily; 6-11 years: 2.5 mg (5 ml) once daily; ≥12 years: same as adult
      Syr: 0.5 mg per ml (4 oz) (tutti-frutti) (phenylalanine)
    Desloratadine ODT 1 tab once daily
    Pediatric: <6 years: not recommended; 6-11 years: 1/2 tab once daily; ≥12 years: same as adult
      ODT: 5 mg

(continued)

▷ *fexofenadine* (OTC)(G) 60 mg once daily-bid or 180 mg once daily; *CrCl <90 ml/min:* 60 mg once daily
  Pediatric: <6 months: not recommended; 6 months-2 years: 15 mg bid; *CrCl ≤90 m/min:* 15 mg once daily;
  2-11 years: 30 mg bid; *CrCl ≤90 m/min:* 30 mg once daily; ≥12 years: same as adult
    Allegra *Tab:* 30, 60, 180 mg film-coat
    Allegra Allergy *Tab:* 60, 180 mg film-coat
    Allegra ODT *ODT:* 30 mg (phenylalanine)
    Allegra Oral Suspension *Oral susp:* 30 mg/5 ml (6 mg/ml) (4 oz)
▷ *levocetirizine* (OTC)(G) administer dose in the PM; *Seasonal Allergic Rhinitis:* <2 years: not recommended;
  may start at ≥2 years; *Chronic Idiopathic Urticaria (CIU), Perennial Allergic Rhinitis:* <6 months: not
  recommended; may start at ≥ 6 months; *Dosing by Age:* 6 months-5 years: max 1.25 mg once daily; 6-11
  years: max 2.5 mg once daily; ≥12 years: 2.5-5 mg once daily; *Renal dysfunction, <12 years:* contraindicated;
  Renal dysfunction, ≥12 years: CrCl 50-80 ml/min: 2.5 mg once daily; CrCl 30-50 ml/min: 2.5 mg every
  other day; CrCl: 10-30 ml/min: 2.5 mg twice weekly (every 3-4 days); CrCl <10 ml/min, ESRD or
  hemodialysis: contraindicated
    Children's Xyzal Allergy 24HR *Oral Soln:* 0.5 mg/ml (150 ml)
    Xyzal Allergy 24HR *Tab:* 5*mg
▷ *loratadine* (OTC)(G) 5 mg bid or 10 mg once daily; *Hepatic or Renal Insufficiency:* see mfr pkg insert
  Pediatric: <2 years: not recommended; 2-5 years: 5 mg once daily; ≥6 years: same as adult
    Children's Claritin Chewables *Chew tab:* 5 mg (grape) (phenylalanine)
    Children's Claritin Syrup 1 mg/ml (4 oz) (fruit) (sugar-free, alcohol-free, dye-free, sodium 6 mg/5 ml)
    Claritin *Tab:* 10 mg
    Claritin Hives Relief *Tab:* 10 mg
    Claritin Liqui-Gels *Liq gel:* 10 mg
    Claritin RediTabs 12 Hours *ODT:* 5 mg (mint)
    Claritin RediTabs 24 Hours *ODT:* 10 mg (mint)

FIRST-GENERATION ANTIHISTAMINES

▷ *diphenhydramine* (G) 25-50 mg q 6-8 hours; max 100 mg/day
  Pediatric: <2 years: not recommended; 2-6 years: 6.25 mg q 4-6 hours; max 37.5 mg/day; >6-12 years:
  12.5-25 mg q 4-6 hours; max 150 mg/day; >12 years: same as adult
    Benadryl (OTC) *Chew tab:* 12.5 mg (grape) (phenylalanine); *Liq:* 12.5 mg/5 ml (4, 8 oz); *Cap:* 25 mg;
    Tab: 25 mg; *Dye-free soft gel:* 25 mg; *Dye-free liq:* 12.5 mg/5 ml (4, 8 oz)
▷ *diphenhydramine* injectable (G) 25-50 mg IM immediately; then q 6 hours prn
  Pediatric: <12 years: see mfr pkg insert: 1.25 mg/kg up to 25 mg IM x 1 dose; then q 6 hours prn; ≥12 years:
  same as adult
    Benadryl Injectable *Vial:* 50 mg/ml (1 ml single-use), 50 mg/ml (10 ml multidose); *Amp:* 10 mg/ml
    (1 ml); *Prefilled syringe:* 50 mg/ml (1 ml)
▷ *hydroxyzine* (G) 50 mg/day divided qid prn; 50-100 mg/day divided qid prn
  Pediatric: <6 years: 50 mg/day divided qid prn; ≥6 years: same as adult
    Atarax *Tab:* 10, 25, 50, 100 mg; *Syr:* 10 mg/5 ml (alcohol 0.5%)
    Vistaril *Cap:* 25, 50, 100 mg; *Oral susp:* 25 mg/5 ml (4 oz) (lemon)
  Comment: *Hydroxyzine* is contraindicated in early pregnancy and in patients with a prolonged QT interval.
  It is not known whether this drug is excreted in human milk; therefore, *hydroxyzine* should not be given to
  nursing mothers.

DERMATITIS: SEBORRHEIC

ANTIFUNGAL SHAMPOOS AND TOPICAL AGENTS

▷ *chloroxine* shampoo massage onto wet scalp; wait 3 minutes, rinse, repeat, and rinse thoroughly; use twice
  weekly
  Pediatric: <12 years: not recommended; ≥12 years: same as adult
    Capitrol Shampoo *Shampoo:* 2% (4 oz)
▷ *ciclopirox* apply gel once daily or apply cream or lotion bid, x 4 weeks, or shampoo twice weekly; massage
  shampoo onto wet scalp; wait 3 minutes, rinse, repeat, and rinse thoroughly; shampoo twice weekly
    Loprox Cream
      Pediatric: <10 years: not recommended; ≥10 years: same as adult
      Crm: 0.77% (15, 30, 90 gm)
    Loprox Gel
      Pediatric: <16 years: not recommended; ≥16 years: same as adult
      Gel: 0.77% (30, 45 gm)
    Loprox Lotion
      Pediatric: <10 years: not recommended; ≥10 years: same as adult
      Lotn: 0.77% (30, 60 ml)
    Loprox Shampoo *Shampoo:* 1% (120 ml)

▷ *coal tar* (G)
　　Pediatric: same as adult
　　　　Scytera (OTC) apply once daily-qid; use lowest effective dose
　　　　　　Foam: 2%
　　　　T/Gel Shampoo Extra Strength (OTC) use every other day; max 4 x/week; massage into wet scalp for 5 minutes; rinse; repeat;
　　　　Shampoo: 1%
　　　　T/Gel Shampoo Original Formula (OTC) use every other day; max 7 x/week; massage into wet scalp for 5 minutes; rinse; repeat
　　　　　　Shampoo: 0.5%
　　　　T/Gel Shampoo Stubborn Itch Control (OTC) use every other day; max 7 x/week; massage into wet scalp for 5 minutes; rinse; repeat
　　　　　　Shampoo: 0.5%
▷ *fluocinolone acetonide*
　　　　Derma-Smoothe/FS Shampoo apply up to 1 oz to scalp daily, lather, and leave on x 5 minutes, then rinse twice
　　　　Pediatric: <12 years: not recommended; ≥12 years: same as adult
　　　　　　Shampoo: 0.01% (4 oz)
　　　　Derma-Smoothe/FS Topical Oil *fluocinolone acetonide* 0.01% topical oil apply sparingly tid; for scalp psoriasis, wet or dampen hair or scalp, then apply a thin film, massage well, cover with a shower cap and leave on for at least 4 hours or overnight, then wash hair with regular shampoo and rinse
　　　　Pediatric: <6 years: not recommended; ≥6 years: apply sparingly bid for up to 4 weeks
　　　　　　Topical oil: 0.01% (4 oz) (peanut oil)
▷ *ketoconazole* apply cream or gel once daily x 4 week or apply up to 1 oz shampoo to scalp daily, lather, leave on x 5 minutes, then rinse twice
　　Pediatric: <12 years: not recommended; ≥12 years: same as adult
　　　　Nizoral Cream *Crm:* 2% (15, 30, 60 gm)
　　　　Nizoral Shampoo *Shampoo:* 2% (4 oz)
　　　　Xolegel *Gel:* 2% (45 gm)
　　　　Xolegel Duo *Kit:* **Xolegel** *Gel:* 2% (45 gm) + **Xolex** *Shampoo:* 2% (4 oz)
▷ *selenium sulfide* massage cream into scalp twice weekly x 2 weeks or massage into wet scalp, wait 2-3 minutes, rinse; repeat twice weekly x 2 weeks; may continue treatment with lotion of shampoo 1-2 x weekly as needed
　　Pediatric: <12 years: not recommended; ≥12 years: same as adult
　　　　Exsel Shampoo *Shampoo:* 2.5% (4 oz)
　　　　Selsun Rx *Lotn:* 2.5% (4 oz)
　　　　Selsun Shampoo *Shampoo:* 1% (120, 210, 240, 330 ml), 2.5% (120 ml)
▷ *sodium sulfacetamide+sulfur*
　　　　Clenia Emollient Cream apply daily tid
　　　　　　Emol crm: sod sulfa 10%+sulfur 5% (10 oz)
　　　　Clenia Foaming Wash wash 1-2 x/day
　　　　　　Wash: sod sulfa 10%+sulfur 5% (6, 12 oz)
　　　　Rosula Gel apply daily tid
　　　　　　Gel: sod sulfa 10%+sulfur 5% (45 ml)
　　　　Rosula Lotion apply daily tid
　　　　　　Lotn: sod sulfa 10%+sulfur 5% (45 ml) (alcohol-free)
　　　　Rosula Wash wash bid
　　　　　　Clnsr: sod sulfa 10%+sulfur 5% (335 ml)

TOPICAL STEROID

▷ *betamethasone valerate* 0.12% foam (G) apply bid in AM and PM; invert can and dispense a small amount of foam onto a clean saucer or other cool surface (do not apply directly to hand) and massage a small amount into affected area until foam disappears
　　Pediatric: <12 years: not recommended; ≥12 years: same as adult
　　　　Luxiq *Foam:* 100 gm

OXIDIZING AGENT

▷ *hydrogen peroxide 40%* apply 4 times to targeted lesion(s) approximately 1 minute apart during a single session; repeat if lesions have not cleared after 3 weeks; treatments must be applied by a qualified healthcare provider
　　Pediatric: not applicable
　　　　Eskata *Pen applicator:* 1.5, 2.2 ml/pen (1, 3, 12/carton)
　　Comment: Not for oral, ophthalmic, or intravaginal use. Avoid open or infected seborrheic keratoses, lesions within the orbital rim, eyes, and mucous membranes. The most common adverse reactions include erythema (99%), stinging (97%), edema (91%), scaling (90%), crusting (81%), and pruritus (58%).

DIABETIC MACULAR EDEMA, RETINOPATHY, MACULAR DEGENERATION

VASCULAR ENDOTHELIAL GROWTH FACTOR (VEGF) INHIBITOR

Comment: Diabetic retinopathy is the leading cause of blindness among working-age adults in the United States **Lucentis** *(ranibizumab)* is <u>only</u> one FDA-approved drug for the treatment of diabetic retinopathy. Additional labeled indications include treatment of diabetic macular edema (DME), treatment of neovascular (wet) age-related macular degeneration (AMD), treatment of macular edema following retinal vein occlusion (RVO), and treatment of myopic choroidal neovascularization (mCNV).

▶ *aflibercept intravitreal injection* 2 mg (0.05 ml) administered by intravitreal injection, with a 30-gauge x ½-inch injection needle, every 4 weeks (monthly) for the first 3 months, followed by 2 mg (0.05 ml) via intravitreal injection once every 8 weeks (2 months); although **Eylea** may be dosed as frequently as 2 mg every 4 weeks (monthly), additional efficacy has <u>not</u> been demonstrated; *AMD:* although <u>not</u> as effective as the every 8-week dosing regimen, patients with AMD may also be treated with 1 dose every 12 weeks after 1 year of effective therapy; must <u>only</u> be administered by a qualified physician
Pediatric: <18 years: <u>not</u> established; ≥18 years: same as adult
   Eylea *(aflibercept)* Injection *Vial:* 2 mg/0.05 ml, single-dose; *Prefilled syringe:* 2 mg/0.05 ml, single-dose
   Comment: Eylea *(aflibercept)* is indicated for the treatment of patients with neovascular (wet) AMD, macular edema following RVO, DME, and diabetic retinopathy. It is designed to block the growth of new blood vessels and decrease the ability of fluid to pass through blood vessels (vascular permeability) in the eye by blocking vascular endothelial growth factor (VEGF)-A and placental growth factor (PLGF), two growth factors involved in angiogenesis.

▶ *brolucizumab-dbll* administration via intravitreal injection by a qualified healthcare provider; recommended dose is 6 mg (0.05 ml of 120 mg/ml solution) once monthly (approximately every 25-31 days) for the first 3 doses; then 6 mg (0.05 ml) dose every 8-12 weeks; refrigerate at 2 to 8°C (36 to 46°F). do <u>not</u> freeze; prior to use, the unopened glass vial of **Beovu** may be kept at room temperature, 20 to 25°C (68 to 77°F) for up to 24 hours; store vial in the outer carton to protect from light
Pediatric: <18 years: <u>not</u> established; ≥18 years: same as adult
   Beovu *Vial:* 6 mg/0.05 ml (120 mg/ml), single-dose, with one sterile 5-micron blunt filter needle (18-gauge x 1½ inch, 1.2 mm x 40 mm)
   Comment: Beovu *(brolucizumab-dbll)* is a human VEGF inhibitor indicated for the treatment of neovascular (wet) AMD. Endophthalmitis and retinal detachments may occur following intravitreal injections. Patients should be instructed to report any symptoms suggestive of endophthalmitis <u>or</u> retinal detachment without delay. Increases in intraocular pressure (IOP) have occurred within 30 minutes of an intravitreal injection. There is a potential risk of an arterial thromboembolic event (ATE) following intravitreal use of VEGF inhibitors. Contraindications include ocular <u>or</u> periocular infection, active intraocular inflammation, and hypersensitivity. The most common adverse reactions (≥5%) reported in patients receiving **Beovu** have been blurred vision (10%), cataract (7%), conjunctival hemorrhage (6%), eye pain (5%), and vitreous floaters (5%). There are <u>no</u> adequate and well-controlled studies of **Beovu** administration in pregnancy. There is <u>no</u> information regarding the presence of *brolucizumab* in human milk <u>or</u> effects on the breastfed infant.

▶ *ranibizumab*
Pediatric: <18 years: <u>not</u> established; ≥18 years: same as adult
   Diabetic retinopathy: intravitreal: 0.3 mg once a month (approximately every 28 days)
   DME: intravitreal: 0.3 mg once a month (approximately every 28 days); in clinical trials, monthly doses of 0.5 mg were also studied
   Neovascular (wet) AMD: intravitreal: 0.5 mg once a month (approximately every 28 days); frequency may be reduced (e.g., 4-5 injections over 9 months) after the first 3 injections <u>or</u> may be reduced after the first 4 injections to once every 3 months if monthly injections are <u>not</u> feasible (NOTE: A regimen averaging 4 to 5 doses over 9 months is expected to maintain visual acuity and an every 3-month dosing regimen has reportedly resulted in a 5 letter (1 line) loss of visual acuity over 9 months, as compared to monthly dosing, which may result in an additional 1 to 2 letter gain)
   Macular edema following RVO: intravitreal: 0.5 mg once a month (approximately every 28 days)
   mCNV: intravitreal: 0.5 mg once a month (approximately every 28 days) for up to 3 months; may retreat if necessary
   Lucentis *Prefilled syringe:* 0.3 mg/0.05 ml (0.05 ml), 0.5 mg/0.05 ml (0.05 ml), single-use for intravitreal injection (preservative free); *Vial:* 10 mg/ml (**Lucentis** 0.5 mg), 6 mg/ml solution (**Lucentis** 0.3 mg), single-use; a 5-micron sterile filter needle (19 gauge x 1½ inch) is required for preparation, but <u>not</u> included; keep refrigerated; do <u>not</u> freeze; protect vial from light; see mfr pkg insert for other precautions

Comment: *Ranibizumab* is a recombinant humanized monoclonal antibody fragment that binds to and inhibits human VEGF-A. **Lucentis** inhibits VEGF from binding to its receptors and thereby suppressing neovascularization and slowing vision loss. Contraindications include ocular <u>or</u> periocular infection and active intraocular inflammation. For ophthalmic intravitreal injection <u>only</u>. Each vial <u>or</u> prefilled syringe should <u>only</u> be used for the treatment of a single eye. If the contralateral eye requires treatment, a new vial <u>or</u> prefilled syringe should be used, and the sterile field, syringe, gloves, drapes, eyelid speculum, filter, and injection needles should be changed before **Lucentis** is administered to the other eye. Adequate anesthesia and a topical broad-spectrum antimicrobial agent should be administered prior to the procedure. Refer to manufacturer labeling for additional detailed information. Based on its mechanism of action, adverse effects on pregnancy would be expected. Information related to use in pregnancy is limited. The intravitreal injection procedure should be carried out under controlled aseptic conditions, which include the use of sterile gloves, a sterile drape, and a sterile eyelid speculum (or equivalent). Adequate anesthesia and a broad-spectrum microbicide should be given prior to the injection. Prior to and 30 minutes following the intravitreal injection, patients should be monitored for elevation in IOP using tonometry. Each prefilled syringe or vial should only be used for the treatment of a single eye. If the contralateral eye requires treatment, a new prefilled syringe or vial should be used, and the sterile field, syringe, gloves, drapes, eyelid speculum, filter needle (vial only), and injection needles should be changed.

▷ *ranibizumab-nuna* for intravitreal injection only by a trained and qualified healthcare provider in an appropriate healthcare setting; recommended adult treatment schedule by indication is as follows:
Pediatric: safety and efficacy not established
Neovascular (wet) AMD: intravitreal injection: 0.5 mg (0.05 ml) once a month (approximately every 28 days); although not as effective, patients may be treated with 3 monthly doses followed by less frequent dosing with regular assessment; although not as effective, patients may also be treated with 1 dose every 3 months after 4 monthly doses
Macular edema following RVO: intravitreal injection: 0.5 mg (0.05 ml) once a month (approximately every 28 days)
mCNV: intravitreal injection: 0.5 mg (0.05 ml) once a month (approximately 28 days) for up to 3 months; patients may be re-treated if needed
　　Byooviz *Vial:* 0.05 ml (10 mg/ml), single-dose, soln for intravitreal injection
　　Comment: Byooviz *(ranibizumab-nuna)* is the first biosimilar to Lucentis *(ranibizumab).*

HUMANIZED BISPECIFIC ANTI-BODY

▷ *faricimab-svoa* each vial should only be used for the treatment of a single eye; patients should be assessed frequently
Neovascular (wet) AMD recommended dose: 6 mg (0.05 ml of 120 mg/ml soln) via intravitreal injection every 4 weeks (approximately every 28 ± 7 days, monthly) for the first 4 doses, followed by optical coherence tomography and visual acuity evaluations 8 and 12 weeks later to inform whether to give a 6 mg dose via intravitreal injection on one of the following three regimens: (1) Weeks 28, and 44, (2) Weeks 24, 36, and 48, or (3) Weeks 20, 28, 36, and 44; although additional efficacy was not demonstrated in most patients dosed every 4 weeks compared to every 8 weeks, some patients may need every 4-week (monthly) dosing after the first 4 doses
DME recommended dose: one of two regimens: (1) 6 mg (0.05 ml of 120 mg/ml soln) via intravitreal injection every 4 weeks (approximately every 28 days ± 7 days, monthly) for at least 4 doses; if after at least 4 doses resolution of edema based on the central subfield thickness (CST) of the macula as measured by optical coherence tomography is achieved, then the interval of dosing may be modified by extensions of up to 4-week interval increments or reductions of up to 8-week interval increments based on CST and visual acuity evaluations through week 52; or (2) 6 mg dose administered every 4 weeks for the first 6 doses, followed by 6 mg dose via intravitreal injection at intervals of every 8 weeks (2 months) over the next 28 weeks; although additional efficacy was not demonstrated in most patients when dosed every 4 weeks compared to every 8 weeks, some patients may need every 4-week (monthly) dosing after the first 4 doses
Pediatric: safety and efficacy not established
　　Vabysmo *Vial:* 120 mg/ml, single-dose, soln for intravitreal injection
　　Comment: Vabysmo is a humanized bispecific antibody that works by inhibiting the angiopoietin-2 (Ang-2) and VEGF-A pathways. Blocking both pathways is expected to stabilize blood vessels and potentially improve vision outcomes in patients with retinal conditions. Vabysmo is indicated for the treatment of wet, or neovascular, AMD and DME. Vabysmo is contraindicated in patients with active intraocular inflammation and in those with ocular or periocular infections. The product is administered via intravitreal injection, which has been associated with endophthalmitis and retinal detachments, increased intraocular pressure (IOP), and thromboembolic events. Contraindications to treatment with Vabysmo are ocular or periocular infection, active intraocular inflammation, or hypersensitivity. There are no adequate and well-controlled studies of Vabysmo administration in pregnancy. However, based on the mechanism of action of VEGF and Ang-2 inhibitors, there is a potential risk to female reproductive capacity and to embryo/fetal development. Vabysmo should not be used during pregnancy unless the potential benefit to the patient outweighs the potential risk to the fetus. Females of reproductive potential are advised to use effective contraception prior to the initial dose, during treatment and for at least 3 months following the last dose of Vabysmo. There is no information regarding the presence of *faricimab* in human milk or effects on the breastfed infant. Developmental and health benefits of breastfeeding should be considered along with the mother's clinical need for Vabysmo and any potential adverse effects on the breastfed infant from Vabysmo.

INTRAVITREAL IMPLANT

▷ *fluocinolone acetonide* surgical intravitreal injection is administered by a qualified healthcare provider under sterile conditions in the office/clinic/hospital setting; the implant is a 36-month sustained-release system

(continued)

Yutiq 0.18 mg non-bioerodible intravitreal implant, single-dose, preloaded applicator w. 25 g needle, for ophthalmic intravitreal injection

Comment: Yutiq is indicated for the treatment of macular edema, diabetic macular edema (DME), and chronic noninfectious posterior uveitis. Placement of a Yutiq intravitreal implant is contraindicated with active infection (e.g., ocular herpes simplex, acute blepharoconjunctivitis) or glaucoma. Use of Yutiq may increase risk of cataract development and postprocedure blurring of vision, which should clear within 4 weeks. Avoid driving and hazardous activity until vision returns to baseline. If both eyes require treatment, the implants should be placed on separate dates to decrease risk of infection in both eyes.

DIABETIC PERIPHERAL NEUROPATHY (DPN)

Other Oral Analgesics *see Pain*

NUTRITIONAL SUPPLEMENT

▷ **L-methylfolate calcium (as** Metafolin)+pyridoxal 5-phosphate+methylcobalamin 1 cap bid or 2 caps once daily
Pediatric: <12 years: not recommended; ≥12 years: same as adult
  Metanx *Cap:* meta 3 mg+pyr 35 mg+methyl 2 mg
  Comment: Metanx is indicated as adjunct treatment for patients with endothelial cell dysfunction who have loss of protective sensation and neuropathic pain associated with diabetic peripheral neuropathy.

ORAL ANALGESICS

▷ *acetaminophen* (G) *see Fever*
▷ *aspirin* (G) *see Fever*
▷ *tramadol* (IV)(G)
  Rybix ODT initially 100 mg once daily; may increase by 100 mg every 5 days; max 300 mg/day; *CrCl <30 ml/min or severe hepatic impairment:* not recommended; *Cirrhosis:* max 50 mg q 12 hours
  Pediatric: <18 years: not recommended; ≥18 years: same as adult
    ODT: 50 mg (mint) (phenylalanine)
  Ryzolt initially 100 mg once daily; may increase by 100 mg every 5 days; max 300 mg/day; *CrCl <30 ml/min or severe hepatic impairment:* not recommended
  Pediatric: <18 years: not recommended; ≥18 years: same as adult
    Tab: 100, 200, 300 mg ext-rel
  Ultram 50-100 mg q 4-6 hours prn; max 400 mg/day; *CrCl <30 ml/min,* max 100 mg q 12 hours; cirrhosis, max 50 mg q 12 hours
  Pediatric: <18 years: not recommended; ≥18 years: same as adult
    Tab: 50*mg
  Ultram ER initially 100 mg once daily; may increase by 100 mg every 5 days; max 300 mg/day; *CrCl <30 ml/min or severe hepatic impairment:* not recommended
    Pediatric: <18 years: not recommended; ≥18 years: same as adult
    Tab: 100, 200, 300 mg ext-rel
▷ *tramadol+acetaminophen* (IV)(G) 2 tabs q 4-6 hours; max 8 tabs/day x 5 days; *CrCl <30 ml/min:* max 2 tabs q 12 hours; max 4 tabs/day x 5 days
  Pediatric: <18 years: not recommended; ≥18 years: same as adult
    Ultracet *Tab:* tram 37.5+acet 325 mg

TOPICAL ANALGESICS

▷ *capsaicin* cream (G) apply tid-qid after lesions have healed
  Pediatric: <2 years: not recommended; ≥2 years: same as adult
    Axsain *Crm:* 0.075% (1, 2 oz)
    Capsin *Lotn:* 0.025, 0.075% (59 ml)
    Capzasin-HP (OTC) *Crm:* 0.075% (1.5 oz), 0.025% (45, 90 gm); *Lotn:* 0.075% (2 oz), 0.025% (45, 90 gm)
    Capzasin-P (OTC) *Crm:* 0.025% (1.5 oz); *Lotn:* 0.025% (2 oz)
    Capsaicin-HP (OTC) *Crm:* 0.075% (1.5 oz); *Lotn:* 0.075% (2 oz); *Crm:* 0.025%
    Dolorac *Crm:* 0.025% (28 gm)
    Double Cap (OTC) *Crm:* 0.05% (2 oz)
    R-Gel *Gel:* 0.025% (15, 30 gm)
    Zostrix (OTC) *Crm:* 0.025% (0.7, 1.5, 3 oz)
    Zostrix HP *Emol crm:* 0.075% (1, 2 oz)
▷ *capsaicin* 8% patch apply up to 4 patches for one 60-minute application to clean dry skin; may prep area with topical anesthetic; wear non-latex gloves; patches may be cut to size/shape; treatment may be repeated every 3 months
  Pediatric: <18 years: not recommended; ≥18 years: same as adult
    Qutenza *Patch:* 8% 1,640 mcg/cm (179 mg) (1 or 2 patches w. 1-50 gm tube cleansing gel/carton)
▷ *diclofenac sodium* (C; D ≥30 wks) apply qid prn to intact skin; pregnancy: not recommended ≥30 weeks
  Pediatric: <12 years: not established; ≥12 years: same as adult

Pennsaid 1.5% in 10 drop increments, dispense and rub into front, side, and back of knee; usually 40 drops (40 mg) qid
> *Topical soln:* 1.5% (150 ml)

Pennsaid 2% apply 2 pump actuations (40 mg) and rub into front, side, and back of knee bid
> *Topical soln:* 2% (20 mg/pump actuation, 112 gm)

Solaraze Gel massage in to clean skin bid prn
> *Gel:* 3% (50 gm) (benzyl alcohol)

Voltaren Gel (G)(OTC) apply qid prn to intact skin
> *Gel:* 1% (100 gm)

Comment: *Diclofenac* is contraindicated with **aspirin** allergy. As with other NSAIDs, should be avoided in late pregnancy (≥30 weeks) because it may cause premature closure of the ductus arteriosus.

▷ *doxepin* **(G)** cream apply to affected area qid at intervals of at least 3-4 hours; max 8 days
> *Pediatric:* <12 years: not recommended; ≥12 years: same as adult
> **Prudoxin** *Crm:* 5% (45 gm)
> **Zonalon** *Crm:* 5% (30, 45 gm)

▷ *pimecrolimus* 1% cream **(G)** <2 years: not recommended; ≥2 years: apply to affected area bid; do not apply an occlusive dressing
> **Elidel** *Crm:* 1% (30, 60, 100 gm)

Comment: *Pimecrolimus* is indicated for short-term and intermittent long-term use. Discontinue use when resolution occurs. Contraindicated if the patient is immunosuppressed. Change to the 0.1% preparation or if secondary bacterial infection is present.

▷ *trolamine salicylate* apply tid-qid
> *Pediatric:* <2 years: not recommended; ≥2 years: same as adult
> **Mobisyl Creme** *Crm:* 10% (100 gm)

TOPICAL AND TRANSDERMAL ANESTHETICS

Comment: *Lidocaine* should not be applied to non-intact skin.

▷ *lidocaine* cream apply to affected area bid prn
> *Pediatric:* <12 years: not recommended; ≥12 years: same as adult
> **LidaMantle** *Crm:* 3% (1, 2 oz)
> **Lidoderm** *Crm:* 3% (85 gm)
> **ZTlido** *lidocaine* topical system 1% (30/carton)
> **Comment:** Compared to **Lidoderm** (*lidocaine* patch 5%), which contains 700 mg/patch, **ZTlido** only requires 35 mg per topical system to achieve the same therapeutic dose.

▷ *lidocaine* lotion apply to affected area bid prn
> *Pediatric:* <12 years: not recommended; ≥12 years: same as adult
> **LidaMantle** *Lotn:* 3% (177 ml)

▷ *lidocaine* 5% patch **(G)** apply up to 3 patches at one time for up to 12 hours/24-hour period (12 hours on/12 hours off); patches may be cut into smaller sizes before removal of the release liner; do not reuse
> *Pediatric:* <12 years: not recommended; ≥12 years: same as adult
> **Lidoderm** *Patch:* 5% (10x14 cm; 30/carton)

▷ *lidocaine+dexamethasone*
> *Pediatric:* <12 years: not recommended; ≥12 years: same as adult
> **Decadron Phosphate with Xylocaine** *Lotn:* dexa 4 mg+lido 10 mg per ml (5 ml)

▷ *lidocaine+hydrocortisone* **(G)** apply to affected area bid prn
> *Pediatric:* <12 years: not recommended; ≥12 years: same as adult
> **LidaMantle HC** *Crm:* lido 3%+hydro 0.5% (1, 3 oz); *Lotn:* (177 ml)

▷ *lidocaine* 2.5%+*prilocaine* 2.5% apply sparingly to the burn bid-tid prn
> *Pediatric:* <12 years: not recommended; ≥12 years: same as adult
> **Emla Cream** 5, 30 gm/tube

ANTICONVULSANTS
Gamma Aminobutyric Acid Analog

Comment: The gabapentinoids (*gabapentin* [Gralise, Neurontin, Horizant] and *pregabalin* [Lyrica]) have respiratory depression risk potential. Therefore, when coprescribed with other central nervous system (CNS) depressant agents, initiate the gabapentinoid at the lowest possible dose and monitor the patient for respiratory depression (especially elders and patients with compromised pulmonary function). Side effects include fatigue, somnolence/sedation, dizziness, vertigo, feeling drunk, headache, nausea, and dry mouth. To discontinue a gabapentinoid, withdraw gradually over 1 week or longer.

▷ *gabapentin*
> *Pediatric:* <3 years: not recommended; 3-12 years: initially 10-15 mg/kg/day in 3 divided doses; max 12 hours between doses, titrate over 3 days; 3-4 years: titrate to 40 mg/kg/day; 5-12 years: titrate to 25-35 mg/kg/day; max 50 mg/kg/day

(continued)

Gralise Day 1: 300 mg; Day: 2: 600 mg; Days 3-6: 900 mg; Days 7-10: 1,200 mg; Days 11-14: 1,500 mg; then titrate on Days 11-14; Day 15: begin 1,800 mg; take entire dose once daily with the evening meal; do not crush, split, or chew

Tab: 300, 600 mg

Neurontin (G) *Tab:* 600*, 800*mg; *Cap:* 100, 300, 400 mg; *Oral soln:* 250 mg/5 ml (480 ml) (strawberry-anise)

▷ *gabapentin enacarbil* 600 mg once daily at about 5:00 PM; if dose is not taken at recommended time, next dose should be taken the following day; swallow whole; take with food; *CrCl 30-59 ml/min:* Day 1: 600mg; Day 3: begin 600 mg every day; *CrCl <30 ml/min:* or on hemodialysis: not recommended

Pediatric: <12 years: not recommended; ≥12 years: same as adult

Horizant *Tab:* 300, 600 mg ext-rel

▷ *pregabalin (GABA analog)* (G)(V)

Pediatric: <12 years: not recommended; ≥12 years: same as adult

Lyrica initially 50 mg tid; may titrate to 100 mg tid within 1 week; max 600 mg divided tid; discontinue over 1 week

Cap: 25, 50, 75, 100, 150, 200, 225, 300 mg; *Oral soln:* 20 mg/ml

Lyrica CR usual dose: 165 mg once daily; may increase to 330 mg/day within 1 week; max 660 mg/day

Tab: 82.5, 165, 330 mg ext-rel

TRICYCLIC ANTIDEPRESSANTS (TCAs)

Comment: Co-administration of tricyclic antidepressants (TCAs) with selective serotonin reuptake (SSRIs) requires extreme caution.

▷ *amitriptyline* (G) titrate to achieve pain relief; max 300 mg/day

Pediatric: <12 years: not recommended; ≥12 years: same as adult

Tab: 10, 25, 50, 75, 100, 150 mg

▷ *amoxapine* titrate to achieve pain relief; if total dose exceeds 300 mg/day, give in divided doses; max 400 mg/day

Pediatric: <12 years: not recommended; ≥12 years: same as adult

Tab: 25, 50, 100, 150 mg

▷ *desipramine* (G) titrate to achieve pain relief; max 300 mg/day

Pediatric: <12 years: not recommended; ≥12 years: same as adult

Norpramin *Tab:* 10, 25, 50, 75, 100, 150 mg

▷ *doxepin* (G) titrate to achieve pain relief; max 150 mg/day

Pediatric: <12 years: not recommended; ≥12 years: same as adult

Cap: 10, 25, 50, 75, 100, 150 mg; *Oral conc:* 10 mg/ml (4 oz w. dropper)

▷ *imipramine* (G)

Pediatric: <12 years: not recommended; ≥12 years: same as adult

Tofranil titrate to achieve pain relief; max 200 mg/day; adolescents max 100 mg/day; if maintenance dose exceeds 75 mg/day, may switch to **Tofranil PM** at bedtime

Tab: 10, 25, 50 mg

Tofranil PM titrate to achieve pain relief; initially 75 mg at HS; max 200 mg at HS

Cap: 75, 100, 125, 150 mg

Tofranil Injection 50 mg IM; lower dose for adolescents; switch to oral form as soon as possible

Amp: 25 mg/2 ml (2 ml)

▷ *nortriptyline* (G) titrate to achieve pain relief; initially 10-25 mg tid-qid; max 150 mg/day; lower doses for elderly and adolescents

Pediatric: <12 years: not recommended; ≥12 years: same as adult

Pamelor titrate to achieve pain relief; max 150 mg/day

Cap: 10, 25, 50, 75 mg; *Oral soln:* 10 mg/5 ml (16 oz)

▷ *protriptyline* titrate to achieve pain relief; initially 5 mg tid; max 60 mg/day

Pediatric: <12 years: not recommended; ≥12 years: same as adult

Vivactil *Tab:* 5, 10 mg

▷ *trimipramine* titrate to achieve pain relief; max 200 mg/day

Pediatric: <12 years: not recommended; ≥12 years: same as adult

Surmontil *Cap:* 25, 50, 100 mg

DIAPER RASH

Topical Corticosteroids *see* Appendix J: Topical Corticosteroids by Potency

Comment: Low-to-intermediate potency topical corticosteroids are indicated if inflammation is present.

BARRIER AGENTS

▷ *aloe+vitamin e+zinc oxide* ointment apply at each diaper change after thoroughly cleansing skin

Balmex *Oint:* 2, 4 oz tube; 16 oz jar

▷ *vitamin a and e* (G) ointment apply at each diaper change after thoroughly cleansing skin
  A&D Ointment *Oint:* 1.5, 4 oz
▷ *zinc oxide* (G) cream and ointment apply at each diaper change after thoroughly cleansing the skin
  A&D Ointment with Zinc Oxide *Oint:* 10% (1.5, 4 oz)
  Desitin *Oint:* 40% (1, 2, 4, 9 oz)
  Desitin Cream *Crm:* 10% (2, 4 oz)

TOPICAL ANTIFUNGALS

Comment: Use if caused by *Candida albicans.*
▷ *butenafine* (G) apply bid x 1 week <u>or</u> once daily x 4 weeks
  Pediatric: <12 years: <u>not</u> recommended; ≥12 years: same as adult
  Lotrimin Ultra (OTC) *Crm:* 1% (12, 24 gm)
  Mentax *Crm:* 1% (15, 30 gm)
  Comment: *Butenafine* is a benzylamine, <u>not</u> an azole. Fungicidal activity continues for at least 5 weeks after last application.
▷ *clotrimazole* apply to affected area bid x 7 days
  Pediatric: same as adult
  Lotrimin (OTC) *Crm:* 1% (15, 30, 45 gm)
  Lotrimin AF (OTC) *Crm:* 1% (12 gm); *Lotn:* 1% (10 ml); *Soln:* 1% (10 ml)
▷ *econazole* apply bid x 7 days
  Spectazole *Crm:* 1% (15, 30, 85 gm)
▷ *ketoconazole* (G)
  Nizoral Cream *Crm:* 2% (15, 30, 60 gm)
▷ *miconazole* 2% (G) apply bid x 7 days
  Pediatric: same as adult
  Lotrimin AF Spray Liquid (OTC) *Spray liq:* 2% (113 gm) (alcohol 17%)
  Lotrimin AF Spray Powder (OTC) *Spray pwdr:* 2% (90 gm) (alcohol 10%)
  Monistat-Derm *Crm:* 2% (1, 3 oz); *Spray liq:* 2% (3.5 oz); *Spray pwdr:* 2% (3 oz)
▷ *nystatin* (G) apply bid x 7 days
  Mycostatin *Crm:* 100,000 U/gm (15, 30 gm)

COMBINATION AGENT

▷ *clotrimazole+betamethasone* (G) cream apply bid x 7 days
  Lotrisone *Crm:* 15, 45 gm

DIARRHEA: ACUTE

▷ *attapulgite*
  Donnagel (OTC) 30 ml after each loose stool; max 7 doses/day x 2 days
  Pediatric: <3 years: <u>not</u> recommended; 3-6 years: 7.5 ml; >6-12 years: 15 ml; >12 years: same as adult
    Liq: 600 mg/15 ml (120, 240 ml)
  Donnagel Chewable Tab (OTC) 2 tabs after each loose stool; max 14 tabs/day
  Pediatric: <3 years: <u>not</u> recommended; 3-6 years: 1/2 tab after each loose stool; max 7 doses/day; >6-12 years: 1 tab after each loose stool; max 7 tabs/day
    Chew tab: 600 mg
  Kaopectate (OTC) 30 ml after each loose stool; max 7 doses/day x 2 days
  Pediatric: <3 years: <u>not</u> recommended; 3-6 years: 7.5 ml after each loose stool; >6-12 years: 15 ml after each loose stool; >12 years: same as adult
    Liq: 600 mg/15 ml (120, 240 ml)
▷ *bismuth subsalicylate* (G)
  Pepto-Bismol (OTC) 2 tabs <u>or</u> 30 ml q 30-60 minutes as needed; max 8 doses/day
  Pediatric: <3 years (14-18 lb): 2.5 ml q 4 hours; max 6 doses/day; <3 years (18-28 lb): 5 ml q 4 hours; max 6 doses/day; 3-6 years: 1/3 tab <u>or</u> 5 ml q 30-60 minutes; max 8 doses/day; >6-9 years: 2/3 tab <u>or</u> 10 ml q 30-60 minutes prn, max 8 doses/day; >9-12 years: 1 tab <u>or</u> 15 ml q 30-60 minutes; max 8 doses/day
    Chew tab: 262 mg; *Liq:* 262 mg/15 ml (4, 8, 12, 16 oz)
  Pepto-Bismol Maximum Strength (OTC) 30 ml q 60 minutes; max 4 doses/day
  Pediatric: <3 years: <u>not</u> recommended; 3-6 years: 5 ml q 60 minutes; max 4 doses/day; >6-9 years: 10 ml q 60 minutes; max 4 doses/day; >9-12 years: 15 ml q 60 minutes; max 4 doses/day
    Liq: 525 mg/15 ml (4, 8, 12, 16 oz)
▷ *calcium polycarbophil*
  Pediatric: <6 years: <u>not</u> recommended; 6-12 years: 1 tab daily qid; >12 years: same as adult
  Fibercon (OTC) 2 tabs daily qid
    Cplt: 625 mg

(continued)

▷ *crofelemer* 2 tabs once daily; swallow whole with or without food; do not crush or chew
  Pediatric: <12 years: not established; ≥12 years: same as adult
    Mytesi *Tab:* 125 mg del-rel
    Comment: *Crofelemer* is indicated for the symptomatic relief of non-infectious diarrhea in adult patients with HIV/AIDS on antiretroviral therapy.
▷ *difenoxin+atropine*
  Pediatric: <2 years: not recommended; ≥2 years: same as adult
    Motofen 2 tabs, then 1 tab after each loose stool or 1 tab q 3-4 hours as needed; max 8 tab/day x 2 days
    Tab: dif 1 mg+atro 0.025 mg
▷ *diphenoxylate+atropine* (V)(G)
  Pediatric: <2 years: not recommended; 2-12 years: initially 0.3-0.4 mg/kg/day in 4 divided doses; >12 years: same as adult
    Lomotil 2 tabs or 10 ml qid until diarrhea is controlled
    Tab: diphen 2.5 mg+atrop 0.025 mg; *Liq:* diphen 2.5 mg+atrop 0.025 mg per 5 ml (2 oz)
▷ *loperamide* (OTC)(G)
    Imodium 4 mg initially, then 2 mg after each loose stool; max 16 mg/day x 2 days
    Pediatric: <5 years: not recommended; ≥5 years: same as adult
      Cap: 2 mg
    Imodium A-D 4 mg initially, then 2 mg after each loose stool; usual max 8 mg/day x 2 days
    Pediatric: <2 years: not recommended; 2-5 years (24-47 lb): 1 mg up to tid x 2 days; 6-8 years (48-59 lb): 2 mg initially, then 1 mg after each loose stool; max 4 mg/day x 2 days; 9-11 years (60-95 lb): 2 mg initially, then 1 mg after each loose stool; max 6 mg/day x 2 days
      Cplt: 2 mg; *Liq:* 1 mg/5 ml (2, 4 oz) (cherry-mint) (alcohol 0.5%)
▷ *loperamide+simethicone* (OTC)(G)
    Imodium Advanced 2 tabs chewed after loose stool, then 1 after the next loose stool; max 4 tabs/day
    Pediatric: 6-8 years: chew 1 tab after loose stool, then chew 1/2 tab after next loose stool; 9-11 years: chew 1 tab after loose stool, then chew 1/2 tab after next loose stool; max 3 tabs/day; ≥12 years: same as adult
      Chew tab: loper 2 mg+simeth 125 mg (vanilla-mint)

ORAL REHYDRATION AND ELECTROLYTE REPLACEMENT THERAPY
▷ *oral electrolyte replacement* (OTC)
    CeraLyte 50 dissolve in 8 oz water
    Pediatric: <4 years: not indicated; ≥4 years, same as adult
      Pkt: sodium 50 mEq+potassium 20 mEq+chloride 40 mEq+citrate 30 mEq+rice syrup solids 40 gm+calories 190 per liter (mixed berry) (gluten-free)
    CeraLyte 70 dissolved in 8 oz water
    Pediatric: <4 years: not indicated; ≥4 years: same as adult
      Pkt: sodium 70 mEq+potassium 20 mEq+chloride 60 mEq+citrate 30 mEq+rice syrup solids 40 gm+calories 165 per liter (natural, lemon) (gluten-free)
    Kao Lectrolyte 1 pkt dissolved in 8 oz water q 3-4 hours
    Pediatric: <2 years: not indicated; ≥2 years: same as adult
      Pkt: sodium 12 mEq+potassium 5 mEq+chloride 10 mEq+citrate 7 mEq+ dextrose 5 gm+calories 22 per 6.2 gm
    Pedialyte
    Pediatric: <2 years: as desired and as tolerated; ≥2 years: 1-2 liters/day
      Oral soln: dextrose 20 gm+fructose 5 gm+sodium 25 mEq+potassium 20 mEq+chloride 35 mEq+citrate 30 mEq+calories 100 per liter (8 oz to 1 lite/day 1 liter)
    Pedialyte Freezer Pops
    Pediatric: as desired and as tolerated
      Pops: dextrose 1.6 gm+sodium 2.8 mEq+potassium 1.25 mEq+chloride 2.2 mEq+citrate 1.88 mEq+calories 6.25 per 6.25 ml pop (8 oz, 1 liter)

DIARRHEA: CARCINOID SYNDROME (CSD)

TRYPTOPHAN HYDROXYLASE
▷ *telotristat* take with food; 250 mg tid
  Pediatric: <18 years: not established; ≥18 years: same as adult
    Xermelo *Tab:* 250 mg (4 x 7 daily dose pcks/carton)
    Comment: Take Xermelo, in combination with somatostatin analog (SSA) therapy, to treat patients inadequately controlled by SSA therapy. Breastfeeding females should monitor the infant for constipation. End-stage renal disease (ESRD) requiring dialysis has not been studied.

DIARRHEA: CHRONIC

▷ *cholestyramine*
Questran Powder for Oral Suspension initially 1 pkt or scoop daily; usual maintenance 2-4 pkts or scoops daily in 2 doses; max 6 pkts or scoops daily
Oral pwdr: 9 gm pkts; 9 gm equal to 4 gm *anhydrous cholestyramine resin* (60/pck); *Bulk can:* 378 gm w. scoop
Questran Light initially 1 pkt or scoop daily; usual maintenance 2-4 pkts or scoops daily in 2 doses
Light: 5 gm pkts; 5 gm is equal to 4 gm *anhydrous cholestyramine resin* (60/pck); *Bulk can:* 210 gm w. scoop
Comment: Use *cholestyramine* only if diarrhea is due to bile salt malabsorption.
▷ *crofelemer* 2 tabs once daily; swallow whole with or without food; do not crush or chew
Pediatric: <12 years: not established; ≥12 years: same as adult
Mytesi *Tab:* 125 mg del-rel
Comment: *crofelemer* is indicated for the symptomatic relief of non-infectious diarrhea in adult patients with HIV/AIDS on antiretroviral therapy.
▷ *difenoxin+atropine* 2 tabs, then 1 tab after each loose stool or 1 tab q 3-4 hours prn; max 8 tab/day x 2 days
Pediatric: <2 years: not recommended; ≥2 years: same as adult
Motofen *Tab:* dif 1 mg+atrop 0.025 mg
▷ *diphenoxylate+atropine* (V)(G)
Pediatric: <2 years: not recommended; 2-12 years: initially 0.3-0.4 mg/kg/day in 4 divided doses; >12 years: same as adult
Lomotil 5-20 mg/day in divided doses
Tab: diphen 2.5 mg+atrop 0.025 mg; *Liq:* diphen 2.5 mg+atrop 0.025 mg per 5 ml (2 oz w. dropper)
▷ *attapulgite* (G)
Donnagel (OTC) 30 ml after each loose stool; max 7 doses/day
Pediatric: <2 years: not recommended; 2-6: 7.5 ml after each loose stool; >6 years: same as adult
Liq: 600 mg/15 ml (120, 240 ml)
Donnagel Chewable Tab 2 tabs after each loose stool; max 14 tabs/day
Pediatric: <3 years: not recommended; 3-6 years: 1/2 tab after each stool; max 7 doses/day; >6-12 years: 1 tab after each loose stool; max 7 tabs/day; >12 years: same as adult
▷ *loperamide* (OTC)(G)
Imodium (OTC) 4-16 mg/day in divided doses
Pediatric: <5 years: not recommended; ≥5 years: same as adult
Cap: 2 mg
Imodium A-D (OTC) 4-16 mg/day in divided doses
Pediatric: <2 years: not recommended; 2-5 years (24-47 lb): 1 mg up to tid x 2 days; 6-8 years (48-59 lb): 2 mg initially, then 1 mg after each loose stool; max 4 mg/day x 2 days; 9-11 years (60-95 lb): 2 mg initially, then 1 mg after each loose stool; max 6 mg/day x 2 days; ≥12 years: same as adult
Cplt: 2 mg; *Liq:* 1 mg/5 ml (2, 4 oz)
▷ *loperamide+simethicone* (OTC)(G)
Imodium Advanced 2 tabs chewed after loose stool, then 1 after the next loose stool; max 4 tabs/day
Pediatric: 6-8 years: chew 1 tab after loose stool, then chew 1/2 tab after next loose stool; 9-11 years: chew 1 tab after loose stool, then chew 1/2 tab after next loose stool; max 3 tabs/day
Chew tab: loper 2 mg+simeth 125 mg

DIARRHEA: TRAVELER'S

Comment: Traveler's diarrhea is the most common travel-related illness, affecting an estimated 10%-40% of travelers worldwide each year. Traveler's diarrhea is defined by having ≥3 unformed stools in 24 hours in a person who is traveling. It is caused by a variety of pathogens, but most commonly bacteria found in food and water. The highest risk destinations are in most of Asia as well as the Middle East, Africa, Mexico, and Central and South America.

ANTI-INFECTIVES
▷ *ciprofloxacin* 500 mg bid x 3 days
Pediatric: <18 years: not recommended; ≥18 years: same as adult
Cipro (G) *Tab:* 250, 500, 750 mg; *Oral susp:* 250, 500 mg/5 ml (100 ml) (strawberry)
Cipro XR *Tab:* 500, 1,000 mg ext-rel
ProQuin XR *Tab:* 500 mg ext-rel
▷ *rifamycin* take 388 mg (2 x 194 mg tabs) bid x 3 days; may be taken with or without food; swallow whole, do not crush, break, or chew; contraindicated with concomitant alcohol; discontinue if diarrhea worsens or persists more than 24 hours; not for use if diarrhea is accompanied by fever or blood in the stool or if causative organism other than *Escherichia coli* is suspected
Pediatric: <18 years: not recommended; ≥18 years: same as adult
Aemcolo *Tab:* 194 mg del-rel

(continued)

Comment: FDA-approved in November 2018, **Aemcolo** *(rifamycin)* is an antibacterial drug indicated for the treatment of adult patients with traveler's diarrhea caused by noninvasive strains of *E. coli*, not complicated by fever or blood in the stool. **Aemcolo** is a broad-spectrum, semisynthetic, orally administered, minimally absorbed antibiotic. Mechanism of action is inhibition of bacterial DNA-dependent RNA synthesis. **Aemcolo** has the potential to be used for the treatment of other bacterial infections of the colon, such as infectious colitis, *Clostridioides difficile*-associated disease, diverticulitis, and also as supportive treatment of inflammatory bowel diseases and hepatic encephalopathy. **Aemcolo** should not be used in patients with a known hypersensitivity to *rifamycin* or any of the other *rifamycin*-class antimicrobial agents (e.g., *rifaximin*). The most common adverse reactions (incidence > 2%) have been headache and constipation. There are no available data on **Aemcolo** use in pregnancy to inform any drug-associated risks of major birth defects, miscarriage, or adverse maternal or fetal outcomes. Systemic absorption of **Aemcolo** in humans is negligible; however, there is no information regarding the presence of **Aemcolo** in human milk and the effects on the breastfed infant.

▷ *rifaximin* 200 mg tid x 3 days; discontinue if diarrhea worsens or persists more than 24 hours; not for use if diarrhea is accompanied by fever or blood in the stool or if causative organism other than *E. coli* is suspected
Pediatric: <12 years: not recommended; ≥12 years: same as adult
Xifaxan *Tab:* 200 mg
▷ *trimethoprim+sulfamethoxazole (TMP-SMX)* **(G)** bid x 10 days
Pediatric: <2 months: not recommended; ≥2 months: 40 mg/kg/day of *sulfamethoxazole* in 2 divided doses x 10 days; *see Appendix BB.33: trimethoprim+ sulfamethoxazole* (Bactrim Suspension, Septra Suspension) *for dose by weight*
  Bactrim, Septra 2 tabs bid x 10 days
   Tab: trim 80 mg+sulfa 400 mg*
  Bactrim DS, Septra DS 1 tab bid x 10 days
   Tab: trim 160 mg+sulfa 800 mg*
  Bactrim Pediatric Suspension, Septra Pediatric Suspension
   Oral susp: trim 40 mg+sulfa 200 mg per 5 ml (100 ml) (cherry) (alcohol 0.3%)

DIGITALIS TOXICITY

Comment: The digitalis therapeutic index is narrow, 0.8-1.2 ng/ml. Whether acute or chronic toxicity, the patient should be treated in the emergency department and/or admitted to inpatient service for continued monitoring and care. Signs and symptoms of digitalis toxicity include loss of appetite, nausea, vomiting, abdominal pain, diarrhea, visual disturbances (diplopia, blurred, or yellow vision, yellow-green halos around lights and other visual images, spots, blind spots), decreased urine output, generalized edema, orthopnea, confusion, delirium, decreased consciousness, potentially lethal cardiac arrhythmias (ranging from ventricular tachycardia [VT] and ventricular fibrillation [VF] to sinoatrial heart block atrioventricular block [AVB]). Treatment measures include repeated doses of charcoal via nasogastric (NG) tube administered after gastric lavage for acute ingestion (methods to induce vomiting are usually discouraged because vomiting can worsen bradyarrhythmias) and digitalis binders. Monitoring includes serial ECGs, serum digitalis level, chemistries, potassium (hyperkalemia), magnesium (hypomagnesemia), blood urea nitrogen (BUN), and creatinine.

DIGOXIN BINDER
▷ *digoxin (immune fab [ovine])*
  Digibind contents of 1 vial of **Digibind** neutralizes 0.5 mg digoxin; dose based on the amount of *digoxin* or *digitoxin* to be neutralized; see mfr pkg insert
  Pediatric: see mfr pkg insert
   Vial: 38 mg
  Digifab dose is based on the amount of *digoxin* or *digitoxin* to be neutralized (see mfr pkg insert for dosage; contents of 1 vial neutralizes 0.5 mg digoxin.
  Pediatric: see mfr pkg insert
   Vial: 40 mg for IV injection after reconstitution (preservative-free)

DIPHTHERIA (*CORYNEBACTERIUM DIPHTHERIAE*)

Prophylaxis *see Childhood Immunizations*
Immunization Series see *Childhood Immunizations*

POST-EXPOSURE PROPHYLAXIS FOR NON-IMMUNIZED PERSONS
▷ *erythromycin base* **(G)** 500 mg qid x 14 days
Pediatric: <45 kg: 50 mg/kg/day in 4 divided doses x 14 days; ≥45 kg: same as adult
  Ery-Tab *Tab:* 250, 333, 500 mg ent-coat
  PCE *Tab:* 333, 500 mg

▷ *erythromycin ethylsuccinate* (G) 400 mg qid x 14 days
Pediatric: 30-50 mg/kg/day in 4 divided doses x 14 days; may double dose with severe infection; max 100 mg/kg/day; *see* Appendix BB.21: *erythromycin ethylsuccinate* (E.E.S. Suspension, EryPed Drops/Suspension) *for dose by weight*

    EryPed *Oral susp:* 200 mg/5 ml (100, 200 ml) (fruit), 400 mg/5 ml (60, 100, 200 ml) (banana); *Oral drops:* 200, 400 mg/5 ml (50 ml) (fruit); *Chew tab:* 200 mg wafer (fruit)
    E.E.S. *Oral susp:* 200, 400 mg/5 ml (100 ml) (fruit)
    E.E.S. Granules *Oral susp:* 200 mg/5 ml (100, 200 ml) (cherry)
    E.E.S. 400 Tablets *Tab:* 400 mg

COMBINATION VACCINES

▷ Pentacel (DTaP-IPV/Hib) is commercially available as a kit containing single-dose vial of fixed-combination vaccine containing diphtheria, tetanus, pertussis, and poliovirus antigens (DTaP-IPV vaccine) and single-dose vial of lyophilized Hib vaccine (PRP-T; ActHIB). Prior to administration, reconstitute vial of lyophilized PRP-T (ActHIB) vaccine by adding the entire content of a vial of DTaP-IPV vaccine in the kit according to manufacturer's instructions to provide a combination vaccine containing diphtheria, tetanus, pertussis, IPV, and Hib antigens. Gently swirl until cloudy, uniform, white to off-white (yellow tinge) suspension is obtained. Administer IM immediately after reconstitution. Pentacel is approved for use as a four-dose series in children 6 weeks through 4 years of age (prior to fifth birthday). Pentacel is to be administered as a four-dose series at 2, 4, 6, and 15-18 months of age. The first dose may be given as early as 6 weeks of age. Four doses of Pentacel constitute a primary immunization course against pertussis. Three doses of Pentacel constitute an immunization course against diphtheria, tetanus, *Haemophilus influenzae* type b invasive disease, and poliomyelitis; the fourth dose is a booster for diphtheria, tetanus, *H. influenzae* type b invasive disease, and poliomyelitis immunizations. See mfr pkg insert for full prescribing information, including product storage, preparation, administration, contraindications, warnings, and precautions.

▷ Vaxelis *Vial:* 0.5 ml susp, single-dose; *Prefilled syringe:* 0.5 ml susp, single-dose (preservative-free)
Comment: Vaxelis is a single fixed-dose combination of six vaccines: diphtheria, tetanus toxoid, acellular pertussis, inactivated poliovirus, *Haemophilus* b conjugate, and hepatitis B. The 3-dose immunization series consists of a 0.5 ml IM injection administered at 2, 4, and 6 months of age. See mfr pkg insert for full prescribing information, including product storage, preparation, administration, contraindications, warnings, and precautions.

POST-EXPOSURE PROPHYLAXIS FOR IMMUNIZED PERSONS

▷ *Diphtheria* immunization booster

DIVERTICULITIS

ANTI-INFECTIVES

▷ *amoxicillin* (G) 500 mg q 8 hours or 875 mg q 12 hours x 7 days
    Amoxil *Cap:* 250, 500 mg; *Tab:* 875*mg; *Chew tab:* 125, 200, 250, 400 mg (cherry-banana-peppermint) (phenylalanine); *Oral susp:* 125, 250 mg/5 ml (80, 100, 150 ml) (strawberry); 200, 400 mg/5 ml (50, 75, 100 ml) (bubble gum); *Oral drops:* 50 mg/ml (30 ml) (bubble gum)
    Moxatag *Tab:* 775 mg ext-rel
    Trimox *Tab:* 125, 250 mg; *Cap:* 250, 500 mg; *Oral susp:* 125, 250 mg/5 ml (80, 100, 150 ml) (raspberry-strawberry)

▷ *amoxicillin+clavulanate* (G)
    Augmentin 500 mg tid or 875 mg bid x 7-10 days
    Pediatric: 40-45 mg/kg/day divided tid x 10 days or 90 mg/kg/day divided bid x 10 days; *see* Appendix BB.4. *amoxicillin+clavulanate* (G) (Augmentin Suspension) *for dose by weight*
        Tab: 250, 500, 875 mg; *Chew tab:* 125, 250 mg (lemon-lime); 200, 400 mg (cherry-banana) (phenylalanine); *Oral susp:* 125 mg/5 ml (banana), 250 mg/5 ml (75, 100, 150 ml) (orange), 200, 400 mg/5 ml (50, 75, 100 ml) (orange) (phenylalanine)
    Augmentin ES-600 not recommended for adults
    Pediatric: <3 months: not recommended; ≥3 months, <40 kg: 90 mg/kg/day in 2 divided doses x 7-10 days; ≥40 kg: not recommended
        Oral susp: 42.9 mg/5 ml (50, 75, 100, 125, 150, 200 ml) (strawberry cream) (phenylalanine)
    Augmentin XR 2 tabs q 12 hours x 7-10 days
    Pediatric: <16 years: use other forms; ≥16 years: same as adult
        Tab: 1,000*mg ext-rel

▷ *ciprofloxacin* 500 mg bid x 7 days
    Cipro (G) *Tab:* 250, 500, 750 mg; *Oral susp:* 250, 500 mg/5 ml (100 ml) (strawberry)
    Cipro XR *Tab:* 500, 1,000 mg ext-rel
    ProQuin XR *Tab:* 500 mg ext-rel

(continued)

▷ *metronidazole* (G) 250-500 mg q 8 hours or 750 mg q 12 hours x 7 days
    Flagyl *Tab:* 250*, 500*mg
    Flagyl **375** *Cap:* 375 mg
    Flagyl ER *Tab:* 750 mg ext-rel
▷ *trimethoprim+sulfamethoxazole (TMP-SMX)* (G) bid x 7 days
    Bactrim, Septra 2 tabs bid x 7 days
      Tab: trim 80 mg+sulfa 400 mg*
    Bactrim DS, Septra DS 1 tab bid x 7 days
      Tab: trim 160 mg+sulfa 800 mg*
    Bactrim Pediatric Suspension, Septra Pediatric Suspension 20 ml bid x 7 days
      Oral susp: trim 40 mg+sulfa 200 mg per 5 ml (100 ml) (cherry) (alcohol 0.3%)

DIVERTICULOSIS

BULK-PRODUCING AGENTS
See Constipation

DROOLING

ANTICHOLINERGIC
▷ glycopyrrolate
    Pediatric: <3 years: safety and efficacy not established; 3-16 years: initiate dose at 0.02 mg/kg tid; titrate in increments of 0.02 mg/kg every 5-7 days, based on therapeutic response and adverse reactions; max 0.1 mg/kg tid; do not exceed 1.5 to 3 mg per dose based on weight; administer at least 1 hour before or 2 hours after meals
    Cuvposa *Oral soln:* 1 mg/5 ml (16 oz)(cherry)
    Comment: Cuvposa is an anticholinergic indicated to reduce chronic severe drooling in patients 3-16 years of age with neurologic conditions associated with problem drooling (e.g., cerebral palsy). Constipation or intestinal pseudo-obstruction may present as abdominal distention, pain, nausea, or vomiting. Assess patients for constipation, particularly within 4-5 days of initial dosing and after a dose increase. Incomplete mechanical intestinal obstruction may present as diarrhea. If obstruction is suspected, discontinue Cuvposa and evaluate. To reduce risk of heat prostration, avoid high ambient temperatures. **Glycopyrrolate** can increase the serum levels of *digoxin* tablets; monitor patients and consider use of alternative *digoxin* dose form. Effects of *glycopyrrolate* may be increased with concomitant administration of *amantadine*; consider decreasing the dose of *glycopyrrolate* during concomitant use. *Glycopyrrolate* may increase the serum levels of *atenolol* or *metformin*; consider dose reduction when used with *glycopyrrolate*. *Glycopyrrolate* may decrease serum levels of *haloperidol* or *levodopa*; consider a dose increase when used with *glycopyrrolate*. Use **Cuvposa** with caution in patients with renal impairment. Use of **Cuvposa** is contraindicated with medical conditions that preclude anticholinergic therapy. Use of solid oral dose forms of potassium chloride are contraindicated with concomitant **Cuvposa**. It is not known whether *glycopyrrolate* can cause fetal harm when administered in human pregnancy or can affect reproduction capacity. **Cuvposa** should be given to a pregnant female only if clearly needed.

DRY EYE DISEASE/SYNDROME (KERATOCONJUNCTIVITIS SICCA)

▷ *lifitegrast* (G) instill 1 drop in each eye bid q 12 hours; use 1 single-use container to dose both eyes and discard unused portion; contacts may be reinserted after 15 minutes
    Pediatric: <17 years: not recommended; ≥17 years: same as adult
    Xiidra *Ophth soln* 5% (50 mg/ml) (foil pouch containing 5 low-density polyethylene 0.2 ml single-use containers, 60 single-use containers/carton) (preservative-free)
    Comment: The exact mechanism of action of *lifitegrast* in dry eye disease is not known. However, it is known that *lifitegrast* binds to the integrin lymphocyte function-associated antigen-1 (LFA-1), a cell surface protein found on leukocytes, and blocks the interaction of LFA-1 with its cognate ligand intercellular adhesion molecule-1 (ICAM-1). ICAM-1 may be overexpressed in corneal and conjunctival tissues in dry eye disease. LFA-1/ICAM-1 interaction can contribute to the formation of an immunologic synapse resulting in T-cell activation and migration to target tissues. *In vitro* studies demonstrated that *lifitegrast* may inhibit T-cell adhesion to ICAM-1 in a human T-cell line and may inhibit secretion of inflammatory cytokines in human peripheral blood mononuclear cells.

SELECTIVE CHOLINERGIC AGONIST
▷ *varenicline* 1 spray in each nostril bid approximately 12 hours apart; prime with 7 actuations before initial use; re-prime with 1 actuation if not used for ≥5 days; do not shake
    Pediatric: safety and efficacy not established
    Tyrvaya 0.03 mg (0.05 ml) per actuation (60 sprays/bottle [each bottle delivers 1 spray in each nostril bid x 15 days], 2 spray bottles/carton)
    Comment: Tyrvaya is a nasally administered selective cholinergic agonist for the treatment of the signs and symptoms of dry eye disease. There are no contraindications to Tyrvaya use. The most common adverse

reaction reported in 82% of patients has been sneezing. Events reported in 5%-16% of patients have been cough, throat irritation, and instillation site (nose) irritation. There are no available data on **Tyrvaya** use in pregnancy to inform any drug-associated risks. In animal reproduction studies, *varenicline* did not produce malformations at clinically relevant doses. There are no data on the presence of *varenicline* in human milk, the effects on the breastfed infant, or the effects on milk production. In animal studies, *varenicline* was present in milk of lactating rats. However, due to species-specific differences in lactation physiology, animal data may not reliably predict drug levels in human milk. Lack of clinical data during lactation precludes a clear determination of the risk of **Tyrvaya** to an infant during lactation; however, the developmental and health benefits of breastfeeding should be considered along with the mother's clinical need for **Tyrvaya** and any potential adverse effects on the breastfed infant from **Tyrvaya**.

OPHTHALMIC IMMUNOMODULATOR/ANTI-INFLAMMATORY
Comment: Ophthalmic immunomodulators are contraindicated with active ocular infection. Allow at least 15 minutes between doses of artificial tears. May reinsert contact lenses 15 minutes after treatment.

▷ *cyclosporine* using 1 single-use disposable vial, instill 1 drop in each eye bid q 12 hours
  Pediatric: <16 years: not recommended; ≥16 years: same as adult
    Cequa *Ophth soln:* 0.09% single-use vials (0.25 ml, 6 pouches, 10 vials/pouch per carton) (preservative-free)
    Comment: **Cequa** ophthalmic solution is a calcineurin inhibitor immune-suppressant indicated to increase tear production in patients with keratoconjunctivitis sicca. It is the first cyclosporine product to utilize nanomicellar technology, facilitating the drug molecule to penetrate the eye's aqueous layer and preventing the release of active lipophilic molecule prior to penetration.
    Restasis (G) *Ophth emul:* 0.05% (0.4 ml) (preservative-free)

OCULAR LUBRICANTS
Comment: Remove contact lens prior to using an ocular lubricant.
▷ *dextran 70+hypromellose* 1-2 drops prn
  Pediatric: same as adult
    Bion Tears (OTC) *Ophth soln:* single-use containers (28/pck) (preservative-free)
▷ *hydroxypropyl cellulose* apply 1/2 inch ribbon or 1 insert in each inferior cul-de-sac 1-2 x/day prn
  Pediatric: same as adult
    Lacrisert *Ophth inserts:* 5 mg (60/pck) (preservative-free)
    Hypotears Ophthalmic Ointment (OTC) *Ophth oint:* 1% (3.5 gm) (preservative-free)
    Comment: Place insert in the inferior cul-de-sac of the eye, beneath the base of the tarsus, not in apposition to the cornea nor beneath the eyelid at the level of the tarsal plate.
▷ *hydroxypropyl methylcellulose* 1-2 drops prn
  Pediatric: same as adult
    GenTeal Mild, GenTeal Moderate (OTC) *Ophth soln:* (15 ml) (perborate)
    GenTeal Severe (OTC) *Ophth soln:* (15 ml) (carbopol 980, perborate)
▷ *petrolatum+mineral oil* apply 1/2 inch ribbon prn
  Pediatric: same as adult
    Hypotears Ophthalmic Ointment (OTC) *Ophth oint:* 1% (3.5 gm) (benzalkonium chloride, alcohol 1%)
    Hypotears PF Ophthalmic Ointment (OTC) *Ophth oint:* 1% (3.5 gm) (preservative-free, alcohol 1%)
    Lacri-Lube (OTC) *Ophth oint:* 1% (3.5, 7 gm)
    Lacri-Lube NP (OTC) *Ophth oint:* 1% (0.7 gm, 24/pck) (preservative-free)
▷ *petrolatum+lanolin+mineral oil* apply 1/4 inch ribbon prn
  Pediatric: same as adult
    Duratears Naturale (OTC) *Ophth oint:* 3.5 gm (preservative-free)
▷ *polyethylene glycol+glycerin+hydroxypropyl methylcellulose* 1-2 drops prn
  Pediatric: same as adult
    Visine Tears (OTC) *Ophth soln:* 1% (15, 30 ml)
▷ *polyethylene glycol* 400 0.4%+*propylene glycol* 0.3% 1-2 drops prn
  Pediatric: same as adult
    Systane (OTC) *Ophth soln:* (15, 30, 40 ml) (polyquaternium-1, zinc chloride); *Vial:* 0.01 oz (28) (preservative-free)
    Systane Ultra (OTC) *Ophth soln:* (10, 20 ml) (aminomethylpropanol, polyquaternium-1, sorbitol; zinc chloride); *Vial:* 0.01 oz (24) (preservative-free)
▷ *polyvinyl alcohol* 1-2 drops prn
  Pediatric: same as adult
    Hypotears (OTC) *Ophth soln:* 1% (15, 30 ml)
    Hypotears PF (OTC) 1-2 drops q 3-4 hours prn
      Ophth soln: 1% (0.02 oz single-use containers, 30/pck) (preservative-free)
▷ *propylene glycol* 0.6% 1-2 drops prn
  Pediatric: same as adult
    Systane Balance (OTC) *Ophth soln:* (10 ml) (polyquaternium-1)

CORTICOSTEROID

▷ *loteprednol etabonate ophthalmic suspension 0.25%* shake for 2-3 seconds before using; instill 1-2 drops into each eye 4 qid; max 2 weeks
Pediatric: safety and efficacy <u>not</u> established
    Eysuvis *Ophth susp:* 2.5 mg/ml (8.3 ml) (benzalkonium chloride)
    Comment: Eysuvis a corticosteroid indicated for the short-term treatment of the signs and symptoms of dry eye disease. As with other ophthalmic corticosteroids, **Eysuvis** is contraindicated in most viral diseases of the cornea and conjunctiva, including epithelial herpes simplex keratitis (dendritic keratitis), vaccinia, and varicella, and also mycobacterial infection of the eye and fungal diseases of ocular structures. The most common adverse reaction (incidence 5%) following the use of **Eysuvis** for 2 weeks has been instillation site pain. Potential complications of prolonged ophthalmic corticosteroid use include delayed healing, corneal perforation, intraocular pressure (IOP) increase, glaucoma with damage to the optic nerve, defects in visual acuity, and cataract formation.

SEMIFLUORINATED ALKANE

▷ *perfluorohexyloctane* instill 1 drop in each eye 4 qid; remove contact lenses before using **Miebo** and wait for at least 30 minutes before reinserting
Pediatric: <18 years: safety and efficacy <u>not</u> established; ≥18 years: same as adult
    Miebo *Ophth soln: perfluorohexyloctane* 100%
    Comment: Miebo is a semifluorinated alkane indicated for the treatment of the signs and symptoms of dry eye disease (DED). **Miebo** is the first and only FDA-approved treatment for DED that directly targets tear evaporation. *Perfluorohexyloctane*, a semifluorinated alkane, works to stabilize the tear film on the surface of the eye, stopping the tears from evaporating and preventing drying of the eyes. *Perfluorohexyloctane* forms a monolayer at the air–liquid interface of the tear film which can be expected to reduce evaporation. The exact mechanism of action for **Miebo** in DED is <u>not</u> known. The FDA approval of **Miebo** was based on results from two 57-day, multicenter, randomized, double-masked, saline-controlled studies, GOBI and MOJAVE, which enrolled a total of 1,217 patients with a history of DED and clinical signs of meibomian gland dysfunction (MGD), a major cause of DED development and disease progression. An estimated 86% of people with DED have excessive tear evaporation whereby MGD is the major contributor. In the GOBI and MOJAVE phase 3 pivotal studies, **Miebo** met both primary sign and symptom efficacy endpoints. The two primary endpoints were change from baseline at week 8 (day 57 ± 2) in total corneal fluorescein staining (tCFS) and eye dryness Visual Analog Scale (VAS) score. Patients experienced relief of symptoms as early as day 15 and through day 57, with statistically significant reduction in VAS eye dryness score favoring **Miebo** observed in both studies. Additionally, at days 15 and day 57, a significant reduction in tCFS favoring **Miebo** was observed in both studies. The most common adverse reactions experienced with **Miebo** were blurred vision (1.3-3%) and eye redness (1-3%). To report suspected adverse reactions, contact Bausch & Lomb at 800-553-5340 <u>or</u> FDA at 800-FDA-1088 <u>or</u> www.fda.gov/medwatch.

DUCHENNE MUSCULAR DYSTROPHY (DMD)

CORTICOSTEROID

▷ *deflazacort* 0.9 mg/kg/day administered once daily; take with <u>or</u> without food; may crush and mix with applesauce (then take immediately)
Pediatric: <2 years: <u>not</u> established; ≥2 years: same as adult
    Emflaza *Tab:* 6, 18, 30, 36 mg; *Oral susp:* 22.75 mg/ml (13 ml)
    Comment: Emflaza is the first and <u>only</u> FDA-approved corticosteroid indicated for Duchenne muscular dystrophy (DMD) to decrease inflammation and reduce the activity of the immune system. The side effects caused by **Emflaza** are similar to those experienced with other corticosteroids. The most common side effects include facial puffiness (cushingoid appearance), weight gain, increased appetite, upper respiratory tract infection, cough, extraordinary daytime urinary frequency (pollakiuria), hirsutism, and central obesity. Other side effects that are less common include problems with endocrine function, increased susceptibility to infection, elevation in blood pressure, risk of gastrointestinal perforation, serious skin rashes, behavioral and mood changes, decrease in the density of the bones, and vision problems such as cataracts. Patients receiving immunosuppressive doses of corticosteroids should <u>not</u> be given live <u>or</u> live attenuated vaccines (LAVs). Moderate <u>or</u> strong CYP3A4 inhibitors give one-third of the recommended dosage of **Emflaza**. Avoid use of moderate <u>or</u> strong CYP3A4 inducers with **Emflaza** as they may reduce efficacy. Dosage must be decreased gradually if the drug has been administered for more than a few days. Use <u>only</u> the oral dispenser provided with the product. After withdrawing the appropriate dose into the oral dispenser, slowly add the oral suspension into 3-4 oz of juice <u>or</u> milk and mix well and the dose should then be administered immediately. Do <u>not</u> administer with grapefruit. Discard any unused **Emflaza** oral suspension remaining after 1 month of first opening the bottle.

ANTISENSE OLIGONUCLEOTIDE

▷ *casimersen* administer 30 mg/kg once weekly as IV infusion over 35-60 minutes via an in-line 0.2 micron filter
Pediatric: same as adult

Amondys 45 *Vial:* 100 mg/2 ml (50 mg/ml), single-dose, soln for dilution in 0.9% NS and IV infusion (preservative-free)

Comment: Amondys 45 is indicated for patients who have genetic mutations that are amenable to skipping exon 45 of the Duchenne gene.

▷ *eteplirsen* 30 mg/kg via IV infusion over 35-60 minutes once weekly

Pediatric: same as adult

Exondys 51 *Vial:* 100 mg/2 ml, 500 mg/10 ml (50 mg/ml), single-dose, for dilution and IV infusion

Comment: Exondys is indicated for patients who have a confirmed mutation of the dystrophin gene amenable to exon 51 skipping, which affects about 13% of patients with DMD. There are no controlled data to inform safety in human pregnancy, lactation, or effects on the breastfed infant.

▷ *viltolarsen* 80 mg/kg via IV infusion over 60 minutes once weekly; obtain serum cystatin C, urine dipstick, and urine protein-to-creatinine ratio before starting; if the volume of **Viltepso** required is less than 100 ml, dilution in 0.9% NS is required

Viltepso *Vial:* 250 mg/5 ml (50 mg/ml), single-dose (preservative-free)

Comment: Viltepso is indicated for the treatment of DMD in patients who have a confirmed mutation of the DMD gene that is amenable to exon 53 skipping. This indication is approved under accelerated approval based on an increase in dystrophin production in skeletal muscle observed in patients treated with **Viltepso**. Continued approval for this indication may be contingent upon verification and description of clinical benefit in a confirmatory trial. Based on animal data, it may cause kidney toxicity. Kidney function should be monitored; creatinine may not be a reliable measure of renal function in DMD patients. The most common adverse reactions (incidence ≥15%) have been upper respiratory infection, injection site reaction, cough, and pyrexia. There are no controlled data to inform safety in human pregnancy, lactation, or effects on the breastfed infant.

PHOSPHORODIAMIDATE MORPHOLINO OLIGOMER

▷ *golodirsen* 30 mg/kg via IV infusion over 35-60 minutes once weekly; measure glomerular filtration rate (GFR) prior to initiating treatment

Vyondys 53 *Vial:* 100 mg/2 ml (50 mg/ml), single-dose, for reconstitution, dilution, and IV infusion

Comment: Vyondys 53 (*golodirsen*) is a phosphorodiamidate morpholino oligomer for the treatment of DMD in patients with a confirmed mutation amenable to exon 53 skipping. This indication is approved under accelerated approval based on an increase dystrophin production in skeletal muscle observed in patients treated with **Vyondys 53**. Continued approval for this indication may be contingent upon verification of a clinical benefit in confirmatory trials. Renal function should be monitored. Creatinine may not be a reliable measure of renal function in DMD patients. Measure GFR prior to initiating treatment. The most common adverse reactions (incidence ≥20%) have been pyrexia, fall, abdominal pain, nausea, vomiting, and nasopharyngitis. There are no human or animal data available to assess the use of **Vyondys 53** during pregnancy, presence of *golodirsen* in human milk, or effects on the breastfed infant.

DUST MITE ALLERGY

ALLERGEN EXTRACT

▷ *dermatophagoides farinae+dermatophagoides pteronyssinus allergen extract* 1 tab SL daily; dissolves in 10 seconds; do not swallow for at least 1 minute; the *first dose* should be administered under the supervision of a physician with experience in the diagnosis and treatment of allergic diseases and the patient should be observed in the office for at least 30 minutes; prescribe autoinjectable epinephrine, instruct and train patients on its appropriate use, and instruct patients to seek immediate medical care upon its use

Pediatric: <18 years: not recommended; ≥18 years: same as adult

Odactra *SL tab:* 12 SQ-HDM

Comment: Odactra can cause life-threatening allergic reactions, such as anaphylaxis and severe laryngopharyngeal restriction. **Odactra** may not be suitable for patients with certain underlying medical conditions that may reduce their ability to survive a serious allergic reaction. **Odactra** may not be suitable for patients who may be unresponsive to epinephrine or inhaled bronchodilators, such as those taking beta-blockers. Contraindications to **Odactra** include severe, unstable, or uncontrolled asthma; history of any severe systemic allergic reaction or any severe local reaction to sublingual allergen immunotherapy; and history of eosinophilic esophagitis. The most common solicited adverse reactions reported in ≥10% of subjects treated with **Odactra** were throat irritation/tickle, itching in the mouth, itching in the ear, swelling of the uvula/back of the mouth, swelling of the lips, swelling of the tongue, nausea, tongue pain, throat swelling, tongue ulcer/sore on the tongue, stomach pain, mouth ulcer/sore in the mouth, and taste alteration/food tastes different. Available data on **Odactra** are insufficient to inform associated risks in pregnancy or effects on the breastfed infant.

DYSFUNCTIONAL UTERINE BLEEDING (DUB)

NSAIDs *see* Appendix I. NSAIDs online at https://connect.springerpub.com/content/reference-book/978-0-8261-7935-7/back-matter/part02/back-matter/bmatter10
Opioid Analgesics *see* **Pain**
Oral and Injectable Progesterone-Only Contraceptives
Combined Oral Contraceptives

▷ *medroxyprogesterone acetate* 10 mg daily x 10-13 days
   Provera *Tab:* 2.5, 5, 10 mg
▷ *combined oral contraceptive* with 35 mcg estrogen equivalent

DYSHIDROSIS (DYSHIDROTIC ECZEMA, POMPHOLYX)

Topical Corticosteroids *see* Appendix J: Topical Corticosteroids by Potency
Comment: Intermediate-to-high potency ophthalmic steroid treatment is indicated for dyshidrosis.

DYSLIPIDEMIA (HYPERCHOLESTEROLEMIA, HYPERLIPIDEMIA, MIXED DYSLIPIDEMIA)

Comment: As recommended by the American Heart, Lung, and Blood Institute, children and adolescents should be screened for dyslipidemia once between 9 and 11 years of age and once between 17 and 21 years of age.

OMEGA 3-FATTY ACID ETHYL ESTERS
Comment: Vascepa, Lovaza, and Epanova are indicated for the treatment of triglyceride (TG) ≥500 mg/dL.

▷ *icosapent ethyl (omega 3-fatty acid ethyl ester of EPA)* (G) 2 caps bid with food; max 4 gm/day; swallow whole, do not crush or chew
   Pediatric: <18 years: not recommended; ≥18 years: same as adult
      Vascepa *sgc:* 0.5, 1 gm (alpha-tocopherol 4 mg/cap)
▷ *omega 3-acid ethyl esters* (G) 2 gm bid or 4 gm once daily; swallow whole, do not crush or chew
   Pediatric: <18 years: not recommended; ≥18 years: same as adult
      Lovaza *Soft gelcap:* 1 gm (alpha-tocopherol 4 mg/cap)
      Epanova *Gelcap:* 1 gm

MICROSOMAL TRIGLYCERIDE-TRANSFER PROTEIN (MTP) INHIBITOR
▷ *lomitapide mesylate* 10 mg daily
   Pediatric: <12 years: not established; ≥12 years: same as adult
      Juxtapid *Cap:* 5, 10, 20 mg
      Comment: Juxtapid is an adjunct to low-fat diet and other lipid-lowering treatments, including low-density lipoprotein (LDL) apheresis where available, to reduce low-density lipoprotein cholesterol (LDL-C), total cholesterol (TC), apo-B, and non-high-density lipoprotein cholesterol (HDL-C) in patients with homozygous familial hypercholesterolemia (HoFH); not for patients with hypercholesterolemia who do not have HoFH.

OLIGONUCLEOTIDE INHIBITOR OF APO B-100 SYNTHESIS
▷ *mipomersen* administer 200 mg SC once weekly, on the same day, in the upper arm, abdomen, or thigh; administer first injection under appropriate professional supervision
   Pediatric: <12 years: not established; ≥12 years: same as adult
      Kynamro *Vial/Prefilled syringe:* 200 mg mg/ml soln for SC inj single-use vial (preservative-free)
      Comment: Kynamro is an adjunct to low-fat diet and other lipid-lowering treatments to reduce LDL-C, apo-B, TC, and non-HDL-C in patients with HoFH.

CHOLESTEROL ABSORPTION INHIBITOR
▷ *ezetimibe* (G) 10 mg daily
   Pediatric: <10 years: not recommended; ≥10 years: same as adult
      Zetia *Tab:* 10 mg
      Comment: *Ezetimibe* is contraindicated with concomitant statins in liver disease, persistent elevations in serum transaminase, pregnancy, and nursing mothers. Concomitant fibrates are not recommended. **Zetia** is potentiated by *fenofibrate, gemfibrozil,* and possibly *cyclosporine.* Separate dosing of bile acid sequestrants is required; take *ezetimibe* at least 2 hours before or 4 hours after.

ANGIOPOIETIN-LIKE 3 (ANGPTL3) INHIBITOR
▷ *evinacumab-dgnb* administer 15 mg/kg via IV infusion over 60 minutes every 4 weeks; administer infusion through an IV line containing a sterile, in-line or add-on, 0.2-micron to 5-micron filter; do not mix other medications or administer other medications concomitantly via the same infusion line

Evkeeza *Vial:* 345 mg/2.3 ml (150 mg/ml), 1,200 mg/8 ml (150 mg/ml) soln, single-dose, for dilution and IV infusion

Comment: Evkeeza is a first-in-class angiopoietin-like 3 (ANGPTL3) inhibitor indicated as an adjunct to other LDL-C lowering therapies for the treatment of adult and pediatric patients, ≥5 years of age, with HoFH. HoFH is an ultra-rare inherited condition that affects approximately 1,300 people in the United States and is the most severe form of familial hypercholesterolemia (FH). HoFH occurs when two copies of the FH-causing genes are inherited, one from each parent, resulting in dangerously high levels (usually >400 mg/dL) of LDL-C. Those living with HoFH are at risk of premature atherosclerotic disease and cardiac events even in their teenage years. Many patients are not diagnosed or are only diagnosed later in life. Common adverse reactions (incidence ≥5%) have been nasopharyngitis, influenza-like illness, dizziness, rhinorrhea, and nausea. Serious hypersensitivity reactions have occurred with Evkeeza in clinical trials. If a serious hypersensitivity reaction occurs, discontinue the infusion, treat according to standard-of-care, and monitor until signs and symptoms resolve. Based on animal studies, Evkeeza is embryo/fetal toxic. Advise patients of reproductive potential of the risk and to use reliable contraception during treatment and for at least 5 months following the last dose. There are no data on the presence of *evinacumab-dgnb* in human milk or effects on the breastfed infant. Developmental and health benefits of breastfeeding should be considered along with the mother's clinical need for Evkeeza and any potential adverse effects on the breastfed infant or from the underlying maternal condition.

PROPROTEIN CONVERTASE SUBTILISIN KEXIN TYPE 9 (PCSK9) INHIBITOR

Comment: Proprotein convertase subtilisin kexin type 9 (PCSK9) inhibitors are an adjunct to maximally tolerated statin therapy in persons who require additional lowering of LDL-C. There is currently no information regarding the use of PCSK9 inhibitors in pregnancy or the presence of PCSK9 inhibitors in human milk.

▷ *alirocumab* administer SC in the upper outer arm, abdomen, or thigh; initially 75 mg SC once every 2 weeks; measure LDL 4-8 weeks after initiation or titration; if inadequate response, may increase to 150 mg SC every 2 weeks or 300 mg SC once monthly

Pediatric: <18 years: not established; ≥18 years: same as adult

Praluent *Soln for SC inj:* 75, 150 mg/ml, single-use, prefilled syringe (preservative-free)

Comment: The FDA has approved a new once-monthly 300 mg dosing option for Praluent injection for the treatment of patients with high LDL-C. The drug is indicated as an adjunct to diet and other treatments for HoFH for patients with heterozygous familial hypercholesterolemia (HeFH) or clinical atherosclerotic cardiovascular disease (ASCVD) who require additional LDL lowering. The most common side effects of Praluent include injection site reactions, symptoms of the common cold, and flu-like symptoms. Each 150 mg pen delivers the dose over 20 seconds. A 300 mg once monthly dose = administration of 2 x 150 mg pens. Praluent is contraindicated in the 2nd and 3rd trimester of pregnancy.

▷ *evolocumab* administer SC in the upper outer arm, elbow, or thigh; measure LDL 4-8 weeks after initiation; *HeFH or primary hyperlipidemia:* 140 mg SC once every 2 weeks or 420 mg once monthly; *HoFH:* 420 mg once monthly

Pediatric: HeFH, primary hyperlipidemia: not established; HoFH: <10 years: not established; ≥10 years: same as adult

Repatha *Soln for SC inj:* single-use, prefilled syringe; 140 mg/syringe; single-use prefilled SureClick autoinjector (140 mg/syringe preservative-free)

Comment: To administer 420 mg of Repatha, administer 150 mg SC x 3 within 30 minutes. Repatha is contraindicated in pregnancy.

SMALL INTERFERING RNA (SIRNA) DIRECTED TO PCSK9 MRNA

▷ *inclisiran* administration by a healthcare professional only; *initially,* 284 mg SC (in combination with maximally tolerated statin therapy); repeat at 3 months; then continue every 6 months thereafter; inject SC into the upper arm, abdomen, or thigh; rotate sites; do not inject in areas of active skin disease or injury, such as sunburns, skin rashes, inflammation, or skin infections

Pediatric: safety and efficacy not established

Leqvio *Prefilled syringe:* 284 mg/1.5 ml (189 mg/ml), single dose soln

Comment: Leqvio is a small interfering RNA (siRNA) directed to PCSK9 (proprotein convertase subtilisin kexin type 9) mRNA indicated as an adjunct to diet and maximally tolerated statin therapy for treatment of adults with heterozygous familial hypercholesterolemia (HeFH) or clinical atherosclerotic cardiovascular disease (ASCVD who require additional lowering of low-density lipoprotein cholesterol (LDL-C). There are no available data on the use of Leqvio in pregnancy to evaluate for a drug-associated risk of major birth defects, miscarriage, or adverse maternal or fetal outcomes. However, discontinuation of Leqvio is recommended when pregnancy is recognized. There is no information on the presence of *inclisiran* in human milk or effects on the breastfed infant.

ADENOSINE TRIPHOSPHATE-CITRATE LYASE (ACL) INHIBITOR

▷ *bempedoic acid* take 1 tablet once daily, with or without food

Pediatric: safety and efficacy not established

Nexletol *Tab:* 180mg

(continued)

Comment: Nexletol *(bempedoic acid)* is a first-in-class adenosine triphosphate-citrate lyase (ACL) inhibitor for the treatment of adults with HeFH or established ASCVD who require additional lowering of LDL-cholesterol. The most common (incidence ≥2%) adverse reactions have been upper respiratory tract infection, muscle spasms, hyperuricemia, back pain, abdominal pain or discomfort, bronchitis, pain in extremity, anemia, and elevated liver enzymes. Avoid concomitant use of **Nexletol** with *simvastatin* dose greater than 20 mg. Avoid concomitant use of **Nexletol** with *pravastatin* dose greater than 40 mg. Elevations in serum uric acid have occurred. Assess uric acid levels periodically as clinically indicated. Monitor for signs and symptoms of hyperuricemia, and initiate treatment with urate-lowering drugs as appropriate. Tendon rupture has occurred. Discontinue **Nexletol** at the first sign of tendon rupture. Avoid **Nexletol** in patients who have a history of tendon disorders or tendon rupture. Discontinue **Nexletol** when pregnancy is recognized unless the benefits of therapy outweigh the potential risks to the fetus. **Nexletol** decreases cholesterol synthesis and possibly the synthesis of other biologically active substances derived from cholesterol and may cause harm to the breastfed infant; therefore, breastfeeding is not recommended during treatment with **Nexletol**.

HMG-COA REDUCTASE INHIBITORS (STATINS)

Comment: The statins decrease TC, LDL-C, TG, and apo-B, and increase HDL-C. Before initiating and at 4-6 weeks, 3 months, and 6 months of therapy, check fasting lipid profile and liver function tests (LFTs). Side effects include myopathy and increased liver enzymes. Relative contraindications include concomitant use of cyclosporine, a macrolide antibiotic, various oral antifungal agents, and CYP450 inhibitors. An absolute contraindication is active or chronic liver disease.

▷ *atorvastatin* **(G)** initially 10 mg daily; usual range 10-80 mg/day
  Pediatric: <10 years: not recommended; ≥10 years (female postmenarche): same as adult
    Lipitor *Tab:* 10, 20, 40, 80 mg
▷ *fluvastatin* **(G)** initially 20-40 mg q HS; usual range 20-80 mg/day
  Pediatric: <18 years: not recommended; ≥18 years: same as adult
    Lescol *Cap:* 20, 40 mg
    Lescol XL *Tab:* 80 mg ext-rel
▷ *lovastatin*
    Mevacor initially 20 mg daily at evening meal; may increase at 4-week intervals; max 80 mg/day in single or divided doses; if concomitant fibrates, *niacin,* or *CrCl <30 ml/min,* usual max 20 mg/day
  Pediatric: <10 years: not recommended; 10-17 years: initially 10-20 mg daily at evening meal; may increase at 4-week intervals; max 40 mg daily
    Tab: 10, 20, 40 mg
    Altoprev initially 20 mg daily at evening meal; may increase at 4-week intervals; max 60 mg/day; if concomitant fibrates, or *niacin;* >1 gm/day, usual max 40 mg/day; if concomitant *cyclosporine, amiodarone,* or *verapamil,* or *CrCl <30 ml/min,* usual max 20 mg/day
  Pediatric: <20 years: not recommended
    Tab: 10, 20, 40, 60 mg ext-rel
▷ *pitavastatin* **(G)** initially 2 mg q HS; may increase to 4 mg after 4 weeks; max 4 mg/day; if concomitant *erythromycin* or *CrCl <60 ml/min;* 1 mg/day with usual max 2 mg/day; if concomitant rifampin, max 2 mg once daily
  Pediatric: <12 years: not established; ≥12 years: same as adult
    Livalo *Tab:* 1, 2, 4 mg
    Nikita *Tab:* 1, 2, 4 mg
    Zypitamag *Tab:* 1, 2, 4 mg
▷ *pravastatin* initially 10-20 mg q HS; usual range 10-40 mg/day; may start at 40 mg/day
  Pediatric: <8 years: not recommended; 8-13 years: 20 mg daily; 14-18 years: 40 mg daily
    Pravachol *Tab:* 10, 20, 40, 80 mg
▷ *rosuvastatin* **(G)** initially 10-20 mg q HS; usual range 5-40 mg/day; adjust at 4-week intervals
  Pediatric: <10 years: not recommended; 10-17 years: 5-20 mg/day; max 20 mg/day
    Crestor *Tab:* 5, 10, 20, 40 mg
▷ *simvastatin* initially 20 mg q PM; usual range 5-80 mg/day; adjust at 4-week intervals
  Pediatric: <10 years: not recommended; ≥10 years (female postmenarche): same as adult
    Zocor *Tab:* 5, 10, 20, 40, 80 mg

CHOLESTEROL ABSORPTION INHIBITOR+HMG-COA REDUCTASE INHIBITOR COMBINATIONS

▷ *ezetimibe+atorvastatin* **(G)** take once daily in the PM; may start at 10/40; swallow whole, do not cut, crush, or chew
  Pediatric: <17 years: not recommended; ≥17 years: same as adult
    Tab: **Liptruzet 10/10** ezet 10 mg+atorva 10 mg
         Liptruzet 10/20 ezet 10 mg+atorva 20 mg
         Liptruzet 10/40 ezet 10 mg+atorva 40 mg
         Liptruzet 10/80 ezet 10 mg+atorva 80 mg
▷ *ezetimibe+rosuvastatin* take once daily in the PM; may start at 10/40; swallow whole, do not cut, crush, or chew
  Pediatric: safety and efficacy not established
    Tab: **Roszet 5/10** rosuva 5 mg+ezet 10 mg

Roszet 10/10 rosuva10 mg+ezet 10 mg
Roszet 20/20 rosuva 20 mg+ezet 10 mg
Roszet 40/40 rosuva 40 mg +ezet 10 mg

▷ *ezetimibe+simvastatin* (G) take once daily in the PM; may start at 10/40; swallow whole, do not cut, crush, or chew
Pediatric: <17 years: not recommended; ≥17 years: same as adult
  Tab: **Vytorin 10/10** ezet 10 mg+simva 10 mg
       Vytorin 10/20 ezet 10 mg+simva 20 mg
       Vytorin 10/40 ezet 10 mg+simva 40 mg
       Vytorin 10/80 ezet 10 mg+simva 80 mg
Comment: These agents decrease TC, LDL-C, and TG, and increase HDL-C. They are indicated when the primary problem is very high TG level. Side effects include epigastric discomfort, dyspepsia, abdominal pain, cholelithiasis, myopathy, and neutropenia. Before initiating, and at 4-6 weeks, 3 months, and 6 months of therapy, check fasting complete blood count (CBC), lipid profile, LFT, and serum creatinine. Absolute contraindications include severe renal disease and severe hepatic disease.

ISOBUTYRIC ACID DERIVATIVES

▷ *gemfibrozil* (G) 600 mg bid 30 minutes before AM and PM meal
Pediatric: <12 years: not recommended; ≥12 years: same as adult
  Lopid *Tab*: 600*mg

FIBRATES (FIBRIC ACID DERIVATIVES)

▷ *fenofibrate* (G) take with meals; adjust at 4- to 8-week intervals; discontinue if inadequate response after 2 months; lowest dose or contraindicated with renal impairment and the elderly
Pediatric: <12 years: not recommended; ≥12 years: same as adult
  Antara 43-130 mg daily; max 130 mg/day
    Cap: 43, 87, 130 mg
  Fenoglide 40-120 mg daily; max 120 mg/day
    Tab: 40, 120 mg
  FibriCor 30-105 mg daily; max 105 mg/day
    Tab: 30, 105 mg
  TriCor 48-145 mg daily; max 145 mg/day
    Tab: 48, 145 mg
  TriLipix 45-135 mg daily; max 135 mg/day
    Cap: 45, 135 mg del-rel
  Lipofen 50-150 mg daily; max 150 mg/day
    Cap: 50, 150 mg
  Lofibra 67-200 mg daily; max 200 mg/day
    Tab: 67, 134, 200 mg

NICOTINIC ACID DERIVATIVES

Comment: Nicotinic acid derivatives decrease TC, LDL-C, and TG, and increase HDL-C. Before initiating and at 4-6 weeks, 3 months, and 6 months of therapy, check fasting lipid profile, LFT, glucose, and uric acid. Side effects include hyperglycemia, upper gastrointestinal (GI) distress, hyperuricemia, hepatotoxicity, and significant transient skin flushing. Take with food and take *aspirin* 325 mg 30 minutes before *niacin* dose to decrease flushing. *Relative contraindications:* diabetes, hyperuricemia (gout), and PUD; *Absolute contraindications:* severe gout and chronic liver disease.

▷ *niacin*
  Niaspan (G) 375 mg daily for 1st week, then 500 mg daily for 2nd week, then 750 mg daily for 3rd week, then 1 gm daily for weeks 4-7; may increase by 500 mg q 4 weeks; usual range 1-2 gm/day; max 2 gm/day
  Pediatric: <21 years: not recommended; ≥21 years: same as adult
    Tab: 500, 750, 1,000 mg ext-rel
  Slo-Niacin one 250 or 500 mg tab q AM or HS or one-half 750 mg tab q AM or HS
  Pediatric: <12 years: not recommended; ≥12 years: same as adult
    Tab: 250, 500, 750 mg cont-rel

BILE ACID SEQUESTRANTS

Comment: Bile acid sequestrants decrease total cholesterol and LDL-C, and increase HDL-C, but have no effect on triglycerides. A relative contraindication is TG ≥200 mg/dL and an absolute contraindication is TG ≥400 mg/dL. Before initiating and at 4-6 weeks, 3 months, and 6 months of therapy, check fasting lipid profile. Side effects include sandy taste in mouth, abdominal gas, abdominal cramping, and constipation. These agents decrease the absorption of many other drugs.

▷ *cholestyramine*
  Pediatric: see mfr pkg insert

(continued)

Questran Powder for Oral Suspension initially 1 pkt or scoop daily; usual maintenance 2-4 pkts or scoops daily in 2 divided doses; max 6 pkts or scoops daily
> *Pwdr:* 9 gm pkts; 9 gm equals 4 gm anhydrous *cholestyramine* resin for reconstitution (60/pck); *Bulk can:* 378 gm w. scoop

Questran Light initially 1 pkt or scoop daily; usual maintenance 2-4 pkts or scoops daily in 2 doses
> *Light:* 5 gm pkts; 5 gm equals 4 gm anhydrous *cholestyramine* resin (60/pck): *Bulk can:* 210 gm w. scoop

▷ *colesevelam* (G)
WelChol recommended dose is 6 tablets once daily or 3 tablets bid; take with a meal and liquid
Pediatric: <10 years: not recommended; ≥10 years: same as adult
> *Tab:* 625 mg

WelChol for Oral Suspension recommended dose is one 3.75 gm packet once daily or one 1.875 gm packet bid; empty 1 packet into a glass or cup; add 1/2 to 1 cup (4-8 oz) of water, fruit juice, or diet soft drink; stir well and drink immediately; do not swallow dry form; take with meals
Pediatric: <12 years: not established; ≥12 years: same as adult
> *Pwdr:* 3.75 gm/pkt (30 pkt/carton), 1.875 gm/pkt (60 pkt/carton) for oral suspension

Comment: WelChol is indicated as adjunctive therapy to improve glycemic control in adults with type 2 diabetes. It can be added to *metformin*, sulfonylureas, or insulin alone or in combination with other antidiabetic agents.

▷ *colestipol*
Comment: *Colestipol* lowers LDL and TC.
Pediatric: <12 years: not recommended; ≥12 years: same as adult
> **Colestid** *Tabs:* 2-16 gm daily in a single or divided doses; *Granules:* 5-30 gm daily in a single or divided dose
>> *Tabs:* 1 gm (120); *Granules:* unflavored: 5 gm pkt (30, 90/carton); unflavored bulk: 300, 500 gm w. scoop; orange-flavored: 7.5 gm pkt (60/carton) (aspartame); orange-flavored bulk: 450 gm w. scoop (aspartame); flavored: 7.5 gm pkt; flavored bulk: 450 gm w. scoop

> **Colestid Tab** initially 2 gm bid; increase by 2 gm bid at 1- to 2-month intervals; usual maintenance 2-16 gm/day
>> *Tab:* 1 gm

ANTILIPID COMBINATIONS
Zetia Nicotinic Acid Derivative+HMG-CoA Reductase Inhibitors Combinations
Comment: Nicotinic acid derivatives decrease TC, LDL-C, and TG, and increase HDL-C. Before initiating and at 4-6 weeks, 3 months, and 6 months of therapy, check fasting lipid profile, LFT, glucose, and uric acid. Side effects include hyperglycemia, upper GI distress, hyperuricemia, hepatotoxicity, and significant transient skin flushing. Take with food and take *aspirin* 325 mg 30 minutes before *niacin* dose to decrease flushing. *Relative Contraindications:* Diabetes, hyperuricemia (gout), and PUD. *Absolute contraindications:* severe gout and chronic liver disease.

▷ *niacin+lovastatin*
Pediatric: <18 years: not recommended; ≥18 years: same as adult
> **Advicor** swallow whole at bedtime with a low-fat snack; may pretreat with aspirin; start at lowest niacin dose; may titrate niacin by no more than 500 mg/day every 4 weeks; max 2,000/40 daily
>> *Tab:* **Advicor 500/20** nia 500 mg ext-rel+lova 20 mg
>> **Advicor 750/20** nia 750 mg ext-rel+lova 20 mg
>> **Advicor 1000/20** nia 1000 mg ext-rel+lova 20 mg
>> **Advicor 1000/40** nia 1000 mg ext-rel+lova 40 mg

▷ *niacin+simvastatin*
Pediatric: <18 years: not recommended; ≥18 years: same as adult
> **Simcor** swallow whole at bedtime with a low-fat snack; may pretreat with *aspirin*; to reduce niacin reaction; start at lowest *niacin* dose; may titrate *niacin* by no more than 500 mg/day every 4 weeks; max 2,000/40 daily; take *aspirin* 325 mg 30 minutes before dose to decrease niacin flushing
>> *Tab:* **Simcor 500/20** nia 500 mg ext-rel+simva 20 mg
>> **Simcor 750/20** nia 750 mg ext-rel+simva 20 mg
>> **Simcor 1000/20** nia 1000 mg ext-rel+simva 20 mg
>> **Simcor 500/40** nia 500 mg ext-rel+simva 40 mg
>> **Simcor 1000/40** nia 1000 mg ext-rel+simva 40 mg

ANTIHYPERTENSIVE+ANTILIPID COMBINATIONS
Calcium Channel Blocker+HMG-CoA Reductase Inhibitor (Statin) Combinations
▷ *amlodipine+atorvastatin* (G)
> **Caduet** select according to blood pressure and lipid values; titrate *amlodipine* over 7-14 days; titrate atorvastatin according to monitored lipid values; max amlodipine 10 mg/day and max atorvastatin 80 mg/day; refer to contraindications and precautions for calcium channel blocker (CCB) and statin therapy

Pediatric: <10 years: not recommended; ≥10 years (female, postmenarche): same as adult
Tab: **Caduet 5/10** amlo 5 mg+ator 10 mg
    Caduet 5/20 amlo 5 mg+ator 20 mg
    Caduet 5/40 amlo 5 mg+ator 40 mg
    Caduet 5/80 amlo 5 mg+ator 80 mg
    Caduet 10/10 amlo 10 mg+ator 10 mg
    Caduet 10/20 amlo 10 mg+ator 20 mg
    Caduet 10/40 amlo 10 mg+ator 40 mg
    Caduet 10/80 amlo 10 mg+ator 80 mg

DYSMENORRHEA: PRIMARY

NSAIDs *see* Appendix I. NSAIDs online at https://connect.springerpub.com/content/reference-book/978-0-8261-7935-7/back-matter/part02/back-matter/bmatter10
Opioid Analgesics *see Pain*
Combined Oral Contraceptives *see* Appendix G. Contraceptives

BENZENEACETIC ACID DERIVATIVE

➤ *diclofenac* take on empty stomach; 35 mg tid; *Hepatic impairment*: use lowest dose
  Pediatric: <18 years: not recommended; ≥18 years: same as adult
    Zorvolex *Gelcap*: 18, 35 mg
➤ *diclofenac sodium*
  Pediatric: <18 years: not recommended; ≥18 years: same as adult
    Voltaren 50 mg bid to qid or 75 mg bid or 25 mg qid with an additional 25 mg at HS if necessary
      Tab: 25, 50, 75 mg ent-coat
    Voltaren XR 100 mg once daily; rarely, 100 mg bid may be used
      Tab: 100 mg ext-rel
Comment: *Diclofenac* is contraindicated with *aspirin* allergy. As with other NSAIDs, should be avoided in late pregnancy (≥30 weeks) because it may cause premature closure of the ductus arteriosus.

FENAMATE

Comment: Avoid *aspirin* with a fenamate.
➤ *mefenamic acid* 500 mg once; then 250 mg q 6 hours for up to 2-3 days; take with food
  Pediatric: <14 years: not recommended; ≥14 years: same as adult
    Ponstel *Cap*: 250 mg

COX-2 INHIBITORS

Comment: Cox-2 inhibitors are contraindicated with history of asthma, urticaria, and allergic-type reactions to *aspirin*, other NSAIDs, and sulfonamides, third trimester of pregnancy, and coronary artery bypass graft (CABG) surgery.
➤ *celecoxib* (G) 400 mg x 1 dose; then 200 mg more on the first day if needed; then 400 mg daily-bid; max 800 mg/day
  Pediatric: <18 years: not recommended; ≥18 years: same as adult
    Celebrex *Cap*: 50, 100, 200, 400 mg
➤ *meloxicam* (G)
    Mobic <2 years, <60 kg: not recommended; ≥2 years, >60 kg: 0.125 mg/kg, max 7.5 mg once daily; ≥18 years: initially 7.5 mg once daily, max 15 mg once daily; *Hemodialysis*: max 7.5 mg/day
      Tab: 7.5, 15 mg; *Oral susp*: 7.5 mg/5 ml (100 ml) (raspberry)
    Vivlodex <18 years: not established; ≥18 years: initially 5 mg once daily; may increase to max 10 mg/day; *Hemodialysis*: max 5 mg/day
      Cap: 5, 10 mg
➤ *meloxicam injection* administer 30 mg via IV bolus once daily; administer dose over 15 seconds; monitor analgesic response and administer a short-acting, non-NSAID, immediate-release analgesic if response is inadequate; patients must be well hydrated before **Anjeso** administration; use **Anjeso** for the shortest duration consistent with individual patient treatment goals
Pediatric: safety and efficacy not established
    Anjeso *Vial*: 30 mg/ml (1 ml), single dose
    Comment: Anjeso *(meloxicam)* is an NSAID injection indicated for use in adults for the management of moderate-to-severe pain, alone or in combination with non-NSAID analgesics. Because of delayed onset of analgesia, **Anjeso** as monotherapy is not recommended for use when rapid onset of analgesia is required. The most common adverse reactions (incidence ≥2%) in controlled clinical trials have included constipation, increased gamma-glutamyltransferase (GGT), and anemia. Use of NSAIDs during the third trimester of pregnancy increases the risk of premature closure of the fetal ductus arteriosus; therefore, avoid **Anjeso** use after 30 weeks' gestation. There are no human data available on whether *meloxicam* is present in human milk or on the effects on breastfed infants. NSAIDs are associated with reversible infertility. Consider withdrawal of **Anjeso** in women who have difficulties conceiving. **Anjeso** may also compromise fertility in males of reproductive potential; it is not known if this effect on male fertility is reversible.

DYSPAREUNIA (POSTMENOPAUSAL PAINFUL INTERCOURSE)

Oral and Transdermal Hormonal Therapy *see Menopause*

NON-HORMONAL THERAPY

➤ *prasterone (dehydroepiandrosterone [DHEA])* insert 1 tab intravaginally daily at bedtime
   Intrarosa *Vaginal inserts:* 6.5 mg (20 tabs+28 applicators/carton)
   Comment: Intrarosa is the first local (intravaginal) non-estrogen drug approved for moderate-to-severe dyspareunia. **Prasterone** is an active endogenous steroid converted into active androgens and/or estrogens.

HORMONAL THERAPY

Comment: Estrogen-alone therapy should not be used for the prevention of cardiovascular disease or dementia. The Women's Health Initiative (WHI) estrogen-alone substudy reported increased risks of stroke and deep vein thrombosis (DVT). The WHI Memory Study (WHIMS) estrogen-alone ancillary study of WHI reported an increased risk of probable dementia in postmenopausal women 65 years of age and older. *Contraindications:* undiagnosed abnormal genital bleeding, known or suspected estrogen-dependent neoplasia (e.g., breast cancer), active DVT, pulmonary embolism (PE), or history of these conditions; active arterial thromboembolic disease (e.g., stroke, acute myocardial infarction [AMI]), or history of these conditions; known or suspected pregnancy; and severe hepatic impairment (Child-Pugh Class C).

➤ *estradiol* (G)
   Imvexxy administer 1 vaginal insert once daily x 2 weeks; then 1 vaginal insert twice weekly x 2 weeks (e.g., Monday/Thursday); consider the addition of a progestin with intact uterus
   Vag inserts: 4, 10 mcg (8, 18/pck) applicator-free
   Comment: Imvexxy is the only product in its class that is available in a 4 mcg and 10 mcg dose. The 4-mcg dose is currently the lowest approved dose of vaginal estradiol available. **Imvexxy** is a bioidentical vaginal estrogen product that offers a fraction of the estrogen contained in the average doses of other products on the market.
   Yuvafem Vaginal Tablet insert one 10 mcg or 25 mcg vaginal tablet once daily x 2 weeks; then twice weekly x 2 weeks (e.g., Tuesday/Friday); consider the addition of a progestin with intact uterus
      Vag tab: 10, 25 mcg (8, 18/blister pck with applicator)

ESTROGEN AGONIST-ANTAGONIST

➤ *ospemifene* take 1 tab daily
   Osphena *Tab:* 60 mg
   Comment: *Ospemifene* is an estrogen agonist-antagonist with tissue selective effects. In the endometrium, **Osphena** has estrogen agonistic effects. There is an increased risk of endometrial cancer in a woman with a uterus who uses unopposed estrogens. Adding a progestin to estrogen therapy reduces the risk of endometrial hyperplasia, which may be a precursor to endometrial cancer. Estrogen-alone therapy has an increased risk of stroke and deep vein thrombosis (DVT). **Osphena** 60 mg had cerebral thromboembolic and hemorrhagic stroke incidence rates of 0.72 and 1.45 per thousand women, respectively, versus 1.04 and 0 per thousand women, respectively, in the placebo group. For DVT, the incidence rate for **Osphena** 60 mg is 1.45 per thousand women versus 1.04 per thousand women in placebo. Do not use estrogen or estrogen agonist/antagonist concomitantly with **Osphena**. *Fluconazole* increases serum concentration of **Osphena**. *Rifampin* decreases serum concentration of **Osphena**.

EBOLA ZAIRE DISEASE (ZAIRE EBOLAVIRUS)

PROPHYLAXIS

Comment: There are six species of *Ebolavirus* (formerly known as Ebola hemorrhagic fever). *Zaire ebolavirus* is one of four *Ebolavirus* species that can cause a potentially fatal human disease. The most recent outbreaks of Ebola in West Africa (2014-2016) and Democratic Republic of the Congo (2018-2019) were caused by *Zaire ebolavirus*. Until recently, there were no approved vaccines or treatments for *Zaire ebolavirus* infection, with supportive care and treatment for medical complications the only available options. The first Ebola vaccine was approved by the FDA on December 19, 2019. **Ervebo** *(Ebola Zaire Vaccine, Live)* is used for prevention of disease caused by *Zaire ebolavirus* in adults. **Ervebo** does not protect against other species of *Ebolavirus*. The first Ebola treatment, **Inmazeb** *(atoltivimab, maftivimab,* and *odesivimab-ebgn),* was approved by the FDA on October 14, 2020 for treatment *Zaire ebolavirus* in adults and children, including newborns of mothers who have tested positive for the virus. A second treatment, **Ebanga** *(ansuvimab-zykl),* was granted orphan drug designation and breakthrough therapy designation on December 21, 2020.

➤ *ebola zaire vaccine, live* administer 1 ml IM once as a single dose
   Pediatric: <18 years: not established; ≥18 years: same as adult
      Ervebo *Vial:* 1 ml, single-dose

Comment: Ervebo *(ebola zaire vaccine, live)* is a vaccine indicated for the prevention of disease caused by *Zaire ebolavirus* in individuals ≥18 years of age. The duration of protection conferred by **Ervebo** is unknown. **Ervebo** does not protect against other species of *Ebolavirus* or *Marburgvirus*. Effectiveness of the vaccine when administered concurrently with antiviral medication, immune globulin (IG), and/or blood or plasma transfusions is unknown. Anaphylaxis has been observed following administration of **Ervebo**; appropriate medical treatment and supervision must be available. Vaccinated individuals should continue to adhere to infection control practices to prevent *Zaire ebolavirus* infection and transmission. Vaccine virus RNA has been detected in blood, saliva, urine, and fluid from skin vesicles of vaccinated adults; transmission of vaccine virus is a theoretical possibility. The most common injection-site adverse events have been injection-site pain (70%), swelling (17%), and redness (12%). The most common systemic adverse reactions have been headache (37%), feverishness (34%), muscle pain (33%), fatigue (19%), joint pain (18%), nausea (8%), arthritis (5%), rash (4%), and abnormal sweating (3%). There are no adequate and well-controlled studies of **Ervebo** in pregnancy, and human data available from clinical trials with **Ervebo** are insufficient to establish the presence or absence of vaccine-associated risk during pregnancy. The decision to vaccinate a woman who is pregnant should consider the woman's risk of exposure to *Zaire ebolavirus*. Human data are not available to assess the impact of **Ervebo** on presence in breast milk or effects on the breastfed infant. The developmental and health benefits of breastfeeding should be considered along with the mother's clinical need for **Ervebo** and any potential adverse effects on the breastfed infant from **Ervebo** or from the underlying maternal condition.

TREATMENT

➤ *atoltivimab+maftivimab+odesivimab* recommended dose of **Inmazeb** is 50 mg of *atoltivimab*, 50 mg of *maftivimab*, and 50 mg of *odesivimab* per kilogram diluted and administered as a single IV infusion; prior to administration, **Inmazeb** must be further diluted in an IV PVC infusion bag (N containing 0.9% NS or D5W or lactated Ringer's; for neonates, **Inmazeb** should be diluted in D5W; total infusion volume is based on the patient's weight; (NOTE: PVC IV bags are designed for parenteral nutrition, packaging of rehydration solutions [e.g., sodium chloride, glucose, lactated Ringer's solution, etc.), and certain antibiotics and analgesics); see mfr pkg insert for full prescribing information, and information on preparation (mix by gentle inversion; do not shake), **Inmazeb** volume per kilogram of body weight (3 ml per kg), total infusion volume (ml) after dilution, and infusion time; the IV infusion must be prepared and administered under the supervision of a qualified healthcare provider

    Inmazeb *Vial:* atolti 241.7 mg+mafti 241.7 mg+odesi 241.7 mg per 14.5 ml (atolti 16.67 mg+mafti 16.67 mg+odesi 16.67 mg per ml), single-dose (preservative-free)

    Comment: Inmazeb *(atoltivimab+maftivimab+odesivimab)* is a monoclonal antibody combination indicated for the treatment of *Zaire ebolavirus* infection in adults and children, including newborns of mothers who have tested positive for the virus. Efficacy of **Inmazeb** has not been established for other species of the *Ebolavirus* and *Marburgvirus* genera. *Zaire ebolavirus* can change over time, and factors such as emergence of resistance or changes in viral virulence could diminish the clinical benefit of antiviral drugs. Consider available information on drug susceptibility patterns for circulating *Zaire ebolavirus* strains when deciding whether to use **Inmazeb**. No vaccine interaction studies have been performed. **Inmazeb** may reduce efficacy of the live vaccine. The interval between live vaccination following initiation of **Inmazeb** therapy should be in accordance with current vaccination guidelines. The most common adverse events (incidence ≥20%) have been pyrexia, chills, tachycardia, tachypnea, and vomiting. Hypersensitivity reactions including infusion-associated events have been reported, including acute, life-threatening reactions during and after the infusion. In the case of severe or life-threatening hypersensitivity reactions, discontinue the **Inmazeb** immediately and administer appropriate emergency care. Available data are insufficient to evaluate for a drug-associated risk of major birth defects, miscarriage, or adverse maternal/fetal outcome. Maternal, fetal, and neonatal outcomes are poor among pregnant women infected with *Zaire ebolavirus*, with the majority of pregnancies resulting in maternal death with miscarriage, stillbirth, or neonatal death. Treatment should not be withheld due to pregnancy. There are no data on the presence of *atoltivimab*, *maftivimab*, and *odesivimab-ebgn* in human or animal milk or effects on the breastfed infant. Females infected with *Zaire ebolavirus* should be instructed not to breastfeed due to the potential for *Zaire ebolavirus* transmission.

➤ *ansuvimab-zykl* 50 mg/kg reconstituted, further diluted, and administered as a single IV infusion over 60 minutes; see mfr pkg insert for further instructions on preparation, dilution, and administration
Pediatric: same as adult

    Ebanga *Vial:* 400 mg, single-dose, pwdr for reconstitution, dilution, and IV infusion

    Comment: Ebanga *(ansuvimab-zykl)* is a *Zaire ebolavirus* glycoprotein (EBOV GP)-directed human monoclonal antibody indicated for treatment of infection caused by *Zaire ebolavirus* in adult and pediatric patients, including neonates born to a mother who is RT-PCR-positive for *Zaire ebolavirus* infection. The efficacy of **Ebanga** has not been established for other species of the *Ebolavirus* and *Marburgvirus* genera. *Zaire ebolavirus* can change over time, and factors such as emergence of resistance or changes in viral virulence could diminish the clinical benefit of antiviral drugs. Consider available information on drug susceptibility patterns for circulating *Zaire ebolavirus* strains when deciding whether to use **Ebanga**. The most frequently reported adverse events (incidence ≥5%) after administration of **Ebanga** have been pyrexia, tachycardia, diarrhea, vomiting, hypotension, tachypnea, and chills. Hypersensitivity reactions including infusion-associated events have been reported with

(continued)

Ebanga. These may include acute, life-threatening reactions during and after the infusion. Monitor patients, and in the case of severe or life-threatening hypersensitivity reactions discontinue the administration of **Ebanga** immediately and administer appropriate emergency care. No vaccine interaction studies have been performed. **Ebanga** may reduce the efficacy of the live vaccine. The interval between administration of **Ebanga** therapy and live vaccination should be in accordance with current vaccination guidelines. Maternal, fetal, and neonatal outcomes are poor among pregnant women infected with *Zaire ebolavirus*. The majority of such pregnancies result in maternal death with miscarriage, stillbirth, or neonatal death. Treatment should not be withheld due to pregnancy. Monoclonal antibodies, such as **Ebanga**, are transported across the placenta; therefore, **Ebanga** has the potential to be transferred from the mother to the developing fetus. Females infected with *Zaire ebolavirus* should be instructed not to breastfed due to the potential for *Zaire ebolavirus* transmission.

EDEMA

THIAZIDE DIURETICS
▷ *chlorthalidone* (G) initially 30-60 mg daily or 60 mg on alternate days; max 90-120 mg/day
  Thalitone *Tab:* 15 mg
▷ *chlorothiazide* (G) 0.5-1 gm/day in a single or divided doses; max 2 gm/day
  Pediatric: <6 months: up to 15 mg/lb/day in 2 divided doses; ≥6 months: 10 mg/lb/day in 2 divided doses; max 375 mg/day
    Diuril *Tab:* 250*, 500*mg; *Oral susp:* 250 mg/5 ml (237 ml)
▷ *hydrochlorothiazide* (G)
  Pediatric: <12 years: not recommended; ≥12 years: same as adult
    Esidrix 25-200 mg daily
      Tab: 25, 50, 100 mg
    Microzide 12.5 mg daily; usual max 50 mg/day
      Cap: 12.5 mg
▷ *hydroflumethiazide* 50-200 mg/day in a single or 2 divided doses
  Pediatric: <12 years: not recommended; ≥12 years: same as adult
    Saluron *Tab:* 50 mg
▷ *methyclothiazide+deserpidine* initially 2.5 mg daily; max 5 mg daily
  Pediatric: <12 years: not recommended; ≥12 years: same as adult
    Enduronyl *Tab:* methy 5 mg+deser 0.25 mg*
    Enduronyl Forte *Tab:* methy 5 mg+deser 0.5 mg*
▷ *polythiazide* 1-4 mg daily
  Pediatric: <12 years: not recommended; ≥12 years: same as adult
    Renese *Tab:* 1, 2, 4 mg

POTASSIUM-SPARING DIURETICS
▷ *amiloride* (G) initially 5 mg; may increase to 10 mg; max 20 mg
  Pediatric: <12 years: not recommended; ≥12 years: same as adult
    Tab: 5 mg
▷ *spironolactone* initially 25-200 mg in a single or divided doses; titrate at 2-week intervals
  Pediatric: <12 years: not recommended; ≥12 years: same as adult
    Aldactone (G) *Tab:* 25, 50*, 100*mg
    CaroSpir *Oral susp:* 25 mg/5 ml (118, 473 ml) (banana)
▷ *triamterene* 100 mg bid; max 300 mg
  Pediatric: <12 years: not recommended; ≥12 years: same as adult
    Dyrenium *Cap:* 50, 100 mg

LOOP DIURETICS
▷ *bumetanide* (G) 0.5-2 mg daily; *Tab:* 5 mg; may repeat at 4 to 5 hour intervals; max 10 mg/day
  Pediatric: <18 years: not recommended; ≥18 years: same as adult
    Tab: 1*mg
  Comment: *Bumetanide* is contraindicated with sulfa drug allergy.
▷ *ethacrynic acid* (G) initially 50-100 mg once daily to bid; max 400 mg/day
  Pediatric: infants: not recommended; ≥1 month: initially 25 mg/day, then adjust dose in 25 mg increments
    Edecrin *Tab:* 25, 50 mg
▷ *ethacrynate sodium* for IV injection (G) administer smallest dose required to produce gradual weight loss (about 1-2 lb per day); onset of diuresis usually occurs at 50-100 mg in children ≥12 years; after diuresis has been achieved, the minimally effective dose (usually 50-200 mg/day) may be administered on a continuous or intermittent dosage schedule; dose titrations are usually in 25-50 mg increments to avoid derangement electrolyte and water excretion; the patient should be weighed under standard conditions before and during administration of *ethacrynate sodium*; the following schedule may be helpful in determining the lowest effective dose: Day 1: 50 mg once daily after a meal; Day 2: 50 mg bid after meals, if necessary; Day 3: 100 mg in the morning and 50-100 mg following the afternoon or evening meal, depending upon response to

the morning dose; a few patients may require initial and maintenance doses as high as 200 mg bid; these higher doses, which should be achieved gradually, are most often required in patients with severe, refractory edema

Pediatric: <1 month: not recommended; ≥1 month-12 years: use the smallest effective dose; initially 25 mg; then careful stepwise increments in dosage of 25 mg to achieve effective maintenance

> **Sodium Edecrin** *Vial:* 50 mg single-dose

Comment: *Ethacrynate sodium* is more potent than more commonly used loop and thiazide diuretics. Treatment of the edema associated with congestive heart failure, cirrhosis of the liver, and renal disease, including nephrotic syndrome; short-term management of ascites due to malignancy, idiopathic edema, and lymphedema; and short-term management of hospitalized pediatric patients, other than infants, with congenital heart disease or nephrotic syndrome. IV **Sodium Edecrin** is indicated when a rapid onset of diuresis is desired (e.g., in acute pulmonary edema or when gastrointestinal absorption is impaired or oral medication is not practical).

➤ *furosemide* (G) initially 20-80 mg as a single dose
Pediatric: <12 years: not recommended; ≥12 years: same as adult
> **Lasix** *Tab:* 20, 40*, 80 mg; *Oral soln:* 10 mg/ml (2, 4 oz w. dropper)
Comment: *Furosemide* is contraindicated with sulfa drug allergy.

➤ *torsemide* (G) 5 mg daily; may increase to 10 mg daily
Pediatric: <12 years: not recommended; ≥12 years: same as adult
> **Demadex** *Tab:* 5*, 10*, 20*, 100*mg

➤ *torsemide (reformulated) Recommended initial dose:* 20 mg orally once daily; titrate dose by approximately doubling until desired diuretic response is obtained; doses >200 mg have not been studied
Pediatric: safety and efficacy not established
> **Soaanz** *Tab:* 20, 40, 60 mg film-coat

Comment: **Soaanz** is a reformulated loop diuretic indicated for the treatment of edema associated with heart failure or renal disease in adults. **Soaanz** is contraindicated with hypersensitivity to **Soaanz**, anuria, and hepatic coma. Taking concomitant NSAIDs reduces the diuretic, natriuretic, and antihypertensive effects and increases risk of renal impairment. Concomitant use with CYP2C9 inhibitors can decrease *torsemide* clearance. *Torsemide* may affect the efficacy and safety of sensitive CYP2C9 substrates or of substrates with a narrow therapeutic range, such as *warfarin* or *phenytoin*. Concomitant *colestyramine* decreases exposure of **Soaanz**. Co-administered organic anion drugs (e.g., *probenecid*) may decrease the diuretic activity of **Soaanz**. Like other diuretics, **torsemide** reduces the renal clearance of lithium, inducing a high risk of *lithium* toxicity. Monitor *lithium* levels periodically when **Soaanz** is co-administered. Renin-angiotensin inhibitors (i.e., angiotensin converting enzyme inhibitors [ACEIs] and angiotensin receptor blockers [ARBs]) increase risk of hypotension and renal impairment. Radiocontrast agents increase risk of renal toxicity. Corticosteroids and adrenocorticotropic hormone (ACTH) increase risk of hypokalemia. Monitor serum glucose and labs for electrolyte and metabolic derangements. Monitor patients for signs and symptoms of ototoxicity. Tinnitus and hearing loss (usually reversible) have been observed with loop diuretics, including **torsemide**. Higher than recommended doses, severe renal impairment, and hypoproteinemia appear to increase the risk of ototoxicity. Loop diuretics increase the ototoxic potential of other ototoxic drugs, including *aminoglycoside* antibiotics (e.g., *gentamycin*) and *ethacrynic acid*; avoid concomitant use with **Soaanz**. There are no available data on use of **Soaanz** in pregnant women and the risk of major birth defects or miscarriage. Diuretics can suppress lactation. There are no data regarding the presence of *torsemide* in human milk or the effects of *torsemide* on the breastfed infant.

OTHER DIURETICS

➤ *indapamide* initially 1.25 mg daily; may titrate every 4 weeks if needed; max 5 mg/day
Pediatric: <12 years: not recommended; ≥12 years: same as adult
> **Lozol** *Tab:* 1.25, 2.5 mg
Comment: *Indapamide* is contraindicated with sulfa drug allergy.

➤ *metolazone*
Pediatric: <12 years: not recommended; ≥12 years: same as adult
> **Mykrox** initially 0.5 mg q AM; max 1 mg/day
> *Tab:* 0.5 mg
> **Zaroxolyn** 2.5-5 mg once daily
> *Tab:* 2.5, 5, 10 mg
Comment: *Metolazone* is contraindicated with sulfa drug allergy.

DIURETIC COMBINATIONS

➤ *amiloride+hydrochlorothiazide* (G) initially 1 tab daily; may increase to 2 tabs/day in a single or divided doses
Pediatric: <12 years: not recommended; ≥12 years: same as adult
> **Moduretic** *Tab:* amil 5 mg+hctz 50 mg*

➤ *spironolactone+hydrochlorothiazide* (G) usual maintenance is 100 mg each of *spironolactone* and *hydrochlorothiazide* daily, in a single-dose or in divided doses; range 25-200 mg of each component daily depending on the response to the initial titration

(continued)

Pediatric: <12 years: <u>not</u> recommended; ≥12 years: same as adult

> **Aldactazide**
>> *Tab:* **Aldactazide 25** *Tab:* spiro 25 mg+hctz 25 mg
>> **Aldactazide 50** *Tab:* spiro 50 mg+hctz 50 mg

▷ *triamterene+hydrochlorothiazide* (G)

Pediatric: <12 years: <u>not</u> recommended; ≥12 years: same as adult

> **Dyazide** 1-2 caps once daily
>> *Cap:* triam 37.5 mg+hctz 25 mg
>
> **Maxzide** 1 tab once daily
>> *Tab:* triam 75 mg+hctz 50 mg*
>
> **Maxzide-25** 1-2 tabs once daily
>> *Tab:* triam 37.5 mg+hctz 25 mg*

EMPHYSEMA

Inhaled Corticosteroids *see Asthma*
Parenteral Corticosteroids *see* Appendix L. Parenteral Corticosteroids
Oral Corticosteroids *see* Appendix K. Oral Corticosteroids
Inhaled Beta-2 Agonists (Bronchodilators) *see Asthma*
Oral Beta-2 Agonists (Bronchodilators) *see Asthma*

METHYLXANTHINES
see Asthma

LONG-ACTING INHALED BETA-2 AGONIST (LABA)
▷ *indacaterol*

> **Arcapta Neohaler** inhale contents of one 75 mcg cap once daily
>> *Neohaler Device/Cap:* 75 mcg (5 blister cards, 6 caps/card)
>
> **Comment:** Remove cap from blister cap immediately before use. For oral inhalation with Neohaler device <u>only</u>. Arcapta Neohaler is indicated for the long-term maintenance treatment of bronchoconstriction in persons with chronic obstructive pulmonary disease (COPD). It is <u>not</u> indicated for treatment of asthma, for primary treatment of acute symptoms, <u>or</u> for acute deterioration of COPD.

▷ *olodaterol* 12 mcg q 12 hours

> **Striverdi Respimat** *Inhal soln:* 2.5 mcg/cartridge (metered actuation) (40 gm, 60 metered actuations) (benzalkonium chloride)

CORTICOSTEROID+INHALED LABA
▷ *fluticasone furoate/vilanterol* 1 inhalation 100/25 <u>or</u> 200/25 once daily at the same time each day

> **Breo Ellipta 100/25** *Inhal pwdr:* flu 100 mcg+vil 25 mcg dry pwdr per inhal (30 doses)
> **Breo Ellipta 200/25** *Inhal pwdr:* flu 200 mcg+vil 25 mcg dry pwdr per inhal (30 doses)
> **Comment:** Breo Ellipta is contraindicated with severe hypersensitivity to milk proteins.

INHALED ANTICHOLINERGICS (ANTIMUSCARINICS)
▷ *glycopyrrolate inhalation solution* inhale the contents of 1 capsule bid at the same time of day, AM and PM, using the Neohaler; do <u>not</u> swallow caps

Pediatric: <u>not</u> indicated

> **Seebri Neohaler** *Inhal cap:* 15.6 mcg (60/blister pck) dry pwdr for inhalation w. 1 Neohaler device (lactose)

▷ *ipratropium* (G)

> **Atrovent** 2 inhalations qid; max 12 inhalations/day
>> *Inhaler:* 14 gm (200 inh)
>
> **Atrovent Inhaled Solution** 500 mcg by nebulizer tid to qid
>> *Inhal soln:* 0.02%; 500 mcg (2.5 ml)

INHALED LONG-ACTING MUSCARINIC ANTAGONISTS (LAMAs)
Comment: Inhaled long-acting muscarinic antagonists (LAMAs) are indicated for prophylaxis and chronic treatment, <u>only</u>. Not for primary (rescue) treatment of acute attack. Avoid getting powder/nebulizer solution in the eyes. Caution with narrow-angle glaucoma, benign prostatic hyperplasia (BPH), bladder neck obstruction (BNO), and pregnancy. Contraindicated with allergy to atropine <u>or</u> its derivatives (e.g., **ipratropium**). Avoid other anticholinergic agents.

▷ *aclidinium bromide* 1 inhalation bid using inhaler

> **Tudorza Pressair** *Inhal device:* 400 mcg/actuation (60 doses per inhalation device)

▷ *glycopyrrolate inhalation solution* administer the contents of 1 vial bid at the same time of day, AM and PM, via the **Magnair** neb inhal device; do <u>not</u> swallow solution; do <u>not</u> use **Magnair** with any other medicine; length of treatment is 2-3 minutes; do <u>not</u> use 2 vials/treatment <u>or</u> more than 2 vials/day

Pediatric: <18 years: <u>not</u> indicated

Lonhala Magnair *Vial:* 25 mcg/ml (1 ml) unit dose for use with **Magnair** handset; *Starter kit:* 60 unit-dose vials w. **Magnair** handset; *Refill kit:* 60 unit-dose vials (low-density polyethylene [LDPE]) w. **Magnair** handset (preservative-free)

Comment: **Lonhala Magnair** is the first nebulizing LAMA approved for the treatment of COPD in the United States. Its approval was based on data from clinical trials in the Glycopyrrolate for Obstructive Lung Disease via Electronic Nebulizer (GOLDEN) program, including GOLDEN-3 and GOLDEN-4, two phase 3, 12-week, randomized, double-blind, placebo-controlled, parallel-group, multicenter study. Do not initiate **Lonhala Magnair** in acutely deteriorating COPD or to treat acute symptoms. If paradoxical bronchospasm occurs, discontinue **Lonhala Magnair** immediately and institute alternative therapy. Worsening of narrow-angle glaucoma may occur; use with caution in patients with narrow-angle glaucoma and instruct patients to contact a physician immediately if symptoms occur. Worsening of urinary retention may occur. Use with caution in patients with BPH or BNO and instruct patients to seek medical care immediately if symptoms occur. Avoid administration with other anticholinergic drugs. Consider risk versus benefit in patients with severe renal impairment. Most common adverse reactions (incidence ≥2.0%) have been dyspnea and urinary tract infection. There are no adequate and well-controlled studies in pregnancy. **Lonhala Magnair** should only be used during pregnancy if the expected benefit to the patient outweighs the potential risk to the fetus. There are no data on the presence of *glycopyrrolate* or its metabolites in human milk or effects on the breastfed infant. The developmental and health benefits of breastfeeding should be considered along with the mother's clinical need for **Lonhala Magnair** and any potential adverse effects on the breastfed infant from **Lonhala Magnair** or from the underlying maternal condition.

➤ *revefenacin inhalation solution* administer the contents of 1 vial via nebulizer once daily at the same time of day; do not swallow solution; do not use more than 1 vial/day; do not use **Yupelri** with any other medicine *Pediatric:* not indicated

Yupelri *Vial:* 175 mcg/3 ml (3 ml) unit-dose solution for nebulizer

Comment: **Yupelri** is the first and only LAMA solution for once-daily nebulized administration. **Yupelri** is indicated for maintenance treatment of moderate-to-severe COPD. Do not initiate **Yupelri** in acutely deteriorating COPD or to treat acute symptoms. If paradoxical bronchospasm occurs, discontinue **Yupelri** immediately and institute alternative therapy. Worsening of narrow-angle glaucoma may occur; use with caution in patients with narrow-angle glaucoma and instruct patients to contact a healthcare provider immediately if symptoms occur. Use with caution in patients with BPH or BNO and instruct patients to contact a healthcare provider immediately if symptoms occur. May interact additively with other concomitantly used anticholinergic medications; avoid administration of **Yupelri** with other anticholinergic-containing drugs. Co-administration of **Yupelri** with OATP1B1 and OATP1B3 inhibitors (e.g., *rifampicin, cyclosporine*) may lead to an increase in exposure of the active metabolite; co-administration with **Yupelri** is not recommended. Avoid use of **Yupelri** in patients with hepatic impairment. The most common adverse reactions (incidence ≥2%) include cough, nasopharyngitis, upper respiratory tract infection, headache, and back pain. There are no adequate and well-controlled studies with **Yupelri** in pregnancy and no information regarding the presence of *revefenacin* in human milk or effects on the breastfed infant.

➤ *tiotropium (as bromide monohydrate)* (G) 2 inhalations once daily using inhalation device; do not swallow caps

Spiriva HandiHaler *Inhal device:* 18 mcg/cap pwdr for inhalation (5, 30, 90 caps w. inhalation device)
Spiriva Respimat *Inhal device:* 1.25, 2.5 mcg/actuation cartridge w. inhalation device (4 gm, 60 metered actuations) (benzalkonium chloride)

Comment: *Tiotropium* is for prophylaxis and chronic treatment, only. Not for primary (rescue) treatment of acute attack. Avoid getting powder in the eyes. Caution with narrow-angle glaucoma, BPH, BNO, and pregnancy. Contraindicated with allergy to *atropine* or its derivatives (e.g., *ipratropium*).

➤ *umeclidinium* 1 inhalation once daily at the same time each day
Incruse Ellipta *Inhal pwdr:* 62.5 mcg/inhalation (30 doses) (lactose)
Comment: **Incruse Ellipta** is contraindicated with allergy to atropine or its derivatives.

INHALED BRONCHODILATOR+ANTICHOLINERGIC COMBINATION

➤ *ipratropium/albuterol* 2 inhalations qid; max 12 inhalations/day
Combivent MDI *Inhaler:* 14.7 gm (200 inh)

INHALED ANTICHOLINERGIC+LABA COMBINATIONS

➤ *indacaterol+glycopyrrolate*
Utibron Neohaler inhale the contents of 1 capsule 2 bid at the same time of day, AM and PM, using the Neohaler; do not swallow caps
Inhal cap: indac 27.5 mcg+glycop 15.6 mcg per cap (60/blister pck) dry pwdr for inhalation w. 1 Neohaler device (lactose)

➤ *ipratropium+albuterol* 1 inhalation qid; max 6 inhalations/day
Combivent Respimat *Inhal soln:* ipra 20 mcg+alb 100 mcg per inhal (4 gm, 120 inhal)
Comment: When the labeled number of metered actuations (120) has been dispensed from the **Combivent Respimat** inhaler, the locking mechanism engages and no more actuations can be dispensed. **Combivent Respimat** is contraindicated with atropine allergy.

(continued)

▷ *tiotropium+olodaterol* 2 inhalations once daily at the same time each day; max 2 inhalations/day
    Stiolto Respimat *Inhal soln:* tio 2.5 mcg+olo 2.5 mcg per actuation (4 gm, 60 inh) (benzalkonium chloride)
    Comment: Stiolto Respimat is not for treating asthma, for relief of acute bronchospasm, or acutely deteriorating COPD.
▷ *umeclidinium+vilanterol* 1 inhalation once daily at the same time each day
    Anoro Ellipta *Inhal soln:* ume 62.5 mcg+vila 25 mcg per inhal (30 doses)
    Comment: Anoro Ellipta is contraindicated with severe hypersensitivity to milk proteins.

INHALED CORTICOSTEROID+ANTICHOLINERGIC+LABA COMBINATION

▷ *fluticasone furoate+umeclidinium+vilanterol* 1 inhalation once daily
    Trelegy Ellipta flutic furo 100 mcg+umec 62.5 mcg+vilan 25 mcg dry pwdr
    Comment: Trelegy Ellipta is maintenance therapy for patients with COPD, including chronic bronchitis and emphysema, who are receiving fixed-dose *furoate* and *vilanterol* for airflow obstruction and to reduce exacerbations, or receiving *umeclidinium* and a fixed-dose combination of *fluticasone furoate* and *vilanterol*. **Trelegy Ellipta** is the first FDA-approved, once-daily, single-dose inhaler that combines *fluticasone furoate*, a corticosteroid, *umeclidinium*, a LAMA, and *vilanterol*, a long-acting beta-2-adrenergic agonist. Common adverse reactions reported with **Trelegy Ellipta** included headache, back pain, dysgeusia, diarrhea, cough, oropharyngeal pain, and gastroenteritis. **Trelegy Ellipta** has been found to increase the risk of pneumonia in patients with COPD and increase the risk of asthma-related death in patients with asthma. **Trelegy Ellipta** is not indicated for the treatment of asthma or acute bronchospasm.

METHYLXANTHINES
see Asthma

METHYLXANTHINE+EXPECTORANT COMBINATION

▷ *dyphylline+guaifenesin*
    Pediatric: <12 years: not recommended; ≥12 years: same as adult
    Lufyllin GG 1 tab qid
      Tab: dyph 200 mg+guaif 200 mg
    Lufyllin GG Elixir 30 ml qid
      Elix: dyph 100 mg+guaif 100 mg per 15 ml (16 oz)

OTHER METHYLXANTHINE COMBINATION

▷ *theophylline+potassium iodide+ephedrine+phenobarbital* (II) 1 tab tid-qid prn; add an additional dose q HS as needed
    Pediatric: <6 years: not recommended; ≥6-12 years: 1/2 tab tid
    Quadrinal *Tab:* theo 130 mg+pot iod 320 mg+ephed 24 mg+phenol 24 mg

ENCOPRESIS

INITIAL BOWEL EVACUATION

▷ *mineral oil* 1 oz x 1 day
    Comment: Mineral oil can inhibit absorption of the fat-soluble vitamins (A, D, E, and K).
▷ *bisacodyl* 1 suppository daily prn
    Pediatric: <12 years: 1/2 suppository daily prn
    Dulcolax *Rectal supp:* 10 mg
▷ *glycerin* suppository 1 adult suppository
    Pediatric: <6 years: 1 pediatric suppository; ≥6 years: same as adult

MAINTENANCE

▷ *mineral oil* 5-15 ml once daily
    Comment: Mineral oil can inhibit absorption of the fat-soluble vitamins (A, D, E, and K).

ENDOMETRIOSIS

Acetaminophen for IV Infusion *see Pain*
NSAIDs *see* Appendix I. NSAIDs online at https://connect.springerpub.com/content/reference-book/978-0-8261-7935-7/back-matter/part02/back-matter/bmatter10
Opioid Analgesics *see Pain*
Other Contraceptives *see* Appendix G. Contraceptives
▷ *medroxyprogesterone* 30 mg daily
    Provera *Tab:* 2.5, 5, 10 mg
▷ *medroxyprogesterone acetate* injectable 100-400 mg IM monthly
    Depo-Provera *Injectable:* 300 mg/ml (2.5, 10 ml)

▷ *norethindrone acetate* initially 5 mg daily x 2 weeks; then increase by 2.5 mg/day every 2 weeks up to 15 mg/day maintenance dose; then continue for 6 to 9 months unless breakthrough bleeding is intolerable
    Aygestin *Tab:* 5*mg

GONADOTROPIN-RELEASING HORMONE (GNRH) RECEPTOR ANTAGONIST

▷ *elagolix Normal to mildly impaired hepatic function:* 150 mg once daily for up to 24 months <u>or</u> 200 mg bid for up to 6 months; *Moderate hepatic impairment:* 150 mg once daily for up to 6 months
    Pediatric: <18 years: <u>not</u> recommended; ≥18 years: same as adult
    Orilissa *Tab:* 150, 200 mg
    Comment: Orilissa *(elagolix)* is an orally administered gonadotropin-releasing hormone (GnRH) receptor antagonist for the management of moderate-to-severe pain associated with endometriosis. Contraindications are severe hepatic impairment, pregnancy, concomitant strong organic anion transporting polypeptide (OATP) 1B1 inhibitors, and osteoporosis. Assess bone mineral density (BMD) in women with additional risk factors for bone loss; dose- and duration-dependent decreases in BMD may occur that may <u>not</u> be completely reversible. Due to potential for reduced efficacy with estrogen-containing contraceptives, use non-hormonal contraception during treatment and for 1 week after discontinuing Orilissa. Orilissa may alter menstrual bleeding, which may reduce the ability to recognize pregnancy. Test if pregnancy is suspected and discontinue if pregnancy is confirmed. Dose-dependent elevations in serum alanine aminotransferase (ALT) may occur; counsel patients on signs and symptoms of liver injury. Counsel patients about potential for suicidal ideation and mood disorders and advise to seek medical attention for suicidal ideation, suicidal behavior, new-onset <u>or</u> worsening depression, anxiety, <u>or</u> other mood changes. The most common adverse reactions (incidence >5%) in clinical trials included hot flashes and night sweats, headache, nausea, insomnia, amenorrhea, anxiety, arthralgia, depression-related adverse reactions, and mood changes.

Gonadotropin-Releasing Hormone Analogs (GnRHa)

Comment: These agonists can have unpleasant side effects (e.g., hot flashes, vaginal dryness, bone loss, changes in mood).
▷ *goserelin (GnRH analog)* implant implant SC into upper abdominal wall; 1 SC implant q 28 days for up to 6 months; retreatment <u>not</u> recommended
    Pediatric: <18 years: <u>not</u> recommended; ≥18 years: same as adult
    Zoladex SC implant in syringe: 3.6 mg
▷ *leuprolide acetate (GnRH analog)*
    Pediatric: <18 years: <u>not</u> recommended; ≥18 years: same as adult
    Lupron Depot 3.75 mg 3.75 mg SC monthly for up to 6 months; may repeat one 6-month cycle
    Syringe: 3.75 mg (single-dose depo susp for SC injection)
    Lupron Depot-3 Month 22.5 mg SC q 3 months (84 days); max 2 injections
    Syringe: 22.5 mg (single-dose depo susp for IM injection)
    Comment: Do <u>not</u> split doses.
▷ *nafarelin acetate* 1 spray (200 mcg) into one nostril q AM, then 1 spray (200 mcg) into the other nostril q PM x 6 months; if no response after 2 months, may increase to 2 sprays (400 mcg) bid
    Pediatric: <18 years: <u>not</u> recommended; ≥18 years: same as adult
    Synarel *Nasal spray:* 2 mg/ml (10 ml)
    Comment: Start *nafarelin acetate* (Synarel) on the 3rd <u>or</u> 4th day of the menstrual period <u>or</u> after a negative pregnancy test.

Synthetic Steroid Derived From Ethisterone

▷ *danazol* start on 3rd <u>or</u> 4th day of menstrual period <u>or</u> after a negative pregnancy test; initially 400 mg bid; gradual downward titration of dosage may be considered dependent upon patient response; mild cases may respond to 100-200 mg bid
    Pediatric: <18 years: <u>not</u> recommended; ≥18 years: same as adult
    Danocrine *Cap:* 50, 100, 200 mg
    Comment: *Danazol* is a synthetic steroid derived from ethisterone. It suppresses the pituitary-ovarian axis. This suppression is probably a combination of depressed hypothalamic-pituitary response to lowered *estrogen* production, the alteration of sex steroid metabolism, and interaction of *danazol* with sex hormone receptors. The <u>only</u> other demonstrable hormonal effects are weak androgenic activity and depression of both follicle-stimulating hormone (FSH) and luteinizing hormone (LH) output. Recent evidence suggests a direct inhibitory effect at gonadal sites and a binding of Danocrine to receptors of gonadal steroids at target organs. In addition, Danocrine has been shown to significantly decrease immunoglobulin G (IgG), immunoglobulin M (IgM), and immunoglobulin A (IgA) levels, as well as phospholipid and IgG isotope autoantibodies, in patients with endometriosis and associated elevations of autoantibodies, suggesting this could be another mechanism by which it facilitates regression of endometrial lesions. Danocrine alters the normal and ectopic endometrial tissue so that it becomes inactive and atrophic. Complete resolution of endometrial lesions occurs in the majority of cases. Changes in the menstrual pattern may occur. Generally, the pituitary-suppressive action of Danocrine is reversible. Ovulation and cyclic bleeding usually return within 60 to 90 days when therapy with Danocrine is discontinued. Danocrine is also used to treat

(continued)

fibrocystic breast disease (reduces breast tissue nodularity and breast pain) and hereditary angioedema (to prevent attacks). Contraindications include pregnancy, breastfeeding, active or history of thromboembolic disease/event, porphyria, undiagnosed abnormal genital bleeding, androgen-dependent tumor, and markedly impaired hepatic, renal, or cardiac function.

ORAL GNRH RECEPTOR ANTAGONIST+ESTROGEN+PROGESTIN COMBINATION

▶ *relugolix+estradiol+norethindrone acetate* exclude pregnancy and discontinue hormonal contraceptives prior to initiation of treatment; take 1 tablet once daily; take a missed dose as soon as possible the same day; then resume regular dosing the next day at the usual time; if concomitant use of oral P-glycoprotein (P-gp) inhibitors is unavoidable, take the **Myfembree** dose 6 hours before taking the P-gp inhibitor; use of **Myfembree** should be limited to 24 months due to the risk of continued bone loss, which may not be reversible
Pediatric: safety and efficacy not established

> **Myfembree** *Tab*: fixed-dose combination of *relugolix* 40 mg+*estradiol* 1 mg+*norethindrone* acetate 0.5 mg, film-coat
> **Comment:** Myfembree is a fixed-dose combination of *relugolix* (GnRH receptor antagonist), *estradiol* (estrogen), and *norethindrone acetate* (progesterone) indicated for the management of heavy menstrual bleeding associated with uterine leiomyomas (fibroid tumors) and endometriosis in premenopausal females. In patients with heavy menstrual bleeding associated with uterine fibroids, the most common adverse reactions (incidence ≥3%) have been vasomotor symptoms, uterine bleeding, alopecia, and decreased libido. In patients with moderate-to-severe pain associated with endometriosis, the most common adverse reactions (incidence ≥3%) have been headache, vasomotor symptoms, mood disorders, abnormal uterine bleeding, nausea, toothache, back pain, decreased sexual desire and arousal, arthralgia, fatigue, and dizziness. *Black Box Warning*: Estrogen and progestin combinations, including **Myfembree**, increase the risk of thrombotic or thromboembolic disorders, especially in females at increased risk for these events. **Myfembree** is contraindicated in women with current or a history of thrombotic or thromboembolic disorders and in females at increased risk for these events, including females >35 years of age who smoke or females with uncontrolled hypertension. Other contraindications are pregnancy, known osteoporosis, current or history of breast cancer or other hormone-sensitive malignancy, known hepatic impairment or disease, undiagnosed abnormal uterine bleeding, and known hypersensitivity to components of **Myfembree** (see mfr pkg insert for complete boxed warning). Discontinue **Myfembree** if an arterial or venous thrombotic, cardiovascular, or cerebrovascular event occurs. Discontinue **Myfembree** if there is sudden unexplained partial or complete loss of vision, proptosis, diplopia, papilledema, or retinal vascular lesion, and evaluate for retinal vein thrombosis immediately. Baseline bone marrow density assessment is recommended in all patients receiving treatment with **Myfembree**. In patients with heavy menstrual bleeding associated with uterine fibroids, periodic BMD assessments are recommended. In patients with moderate-to-severe pain associated with endometriosis, annual BMD assessments are recommended. Assess risk–benefit to patients with additional risk factors for bone loss. Advise patients to seek medical attention for new-onset or worsening depression, anxiety, or other mood changes, or suicidal ideation. Monitor transaminase for elevation and other signs and symptoms of liver injury and inform patients regarding the signs and symptoms. Do not use **Myfembree** in patients with uncontrolled hypertension. For patients with well-controlled hypertension, continue to monitor blood pressure and stop **Myfembree** if blood pressure rises significantly. **Myfembree** may cause a change in menstrual bleeding pattern and reduced ability to recognize pregnancy. Inform patients that **Myfembree** can cause early pregnancy loss and advise using an effective form of non-hormonal contraception during treatment and for 1 week after discontinuing **Myfembree**. Perform testing if pregnancy is suspected and discontinue **Myfembree** if pregnancy is confirmed. Advise patients to seek medical attention for severe uterine bleeding, which could signal miscarriage or uterine fibroid prolapse or expulsion. Immediately discontinue **Myfembree** if a hypersensitivity reaction occurs. Epidemiologic studies and meta-analyses have not found an increased risk of genital or non-genital birth defects (including cardiac anomalies and limb reduction defects) following exposure to estrogens and progestins before conception or during early pregnancy. In animal studies, exposure to *relugolix* during organogenesis showed no fetal malformations were present at any dose level; however, exposure to *relugolix* resulted in spontaneous abortion and total litter loss at *relugolix* exposures about half those at the maximum recommended human dose (MRHD) of 40 mg. Therefore, **Myfembree** is contraindicated in pregnancy. There is a pregnancy exposure registry that monitors pregnancy outcomes in females exposed to **Myfembree** during pregnancy. Pregnant females exposed to **Myfembree** and healthcare providers are encouraged to call the Myfembree Pregnancy Exposure Registry at 1-855-428-0707. There are no data on the presence of *relugolix* or its metabolites in human milk or effects on the breastfed infant. However, *relugolix* has been detected in lactating animals. When a drug is present in animal milk, it is likely that the drug will be present in human milk. Detectable amounts of estrogen and progestin have been identified in the breast milk of patients receiving estrogen plus progestin therapy and can reduce milk production in breastfeeding patients. This reduction can occur at any time but is less likely to occur once breastfeeding is well established. Developmental and health benefits of breastfeeding should be considered along with the mother's clinical need for **Myfembree** and any potential adverse effects on the breastfed infant from **Myfembree** or from the underlying maternal condition.

ENURESIS: PRIMARY, NOCTURNAL

VASOPRESSIN

▶ *desmopressin acetate*

DDAVP usual dosage 0.2 mg before bedtime

Pediatric: <6 years: <u>not</u> recommended; ≥6 years: same as adult

Tab: 0.1*, 0.2*mg

DDAVP Rhinal Tube 10 mcg <u>or</u> 0.1 ml of soln each nostril (20 mcg total dose) before bedtime

Pediatric: <6 years: <u>not</u> recommended; ≥6 years: same as adult

Nasal spray: 10 mcg/actuation (5 ml, 50 sprays); *Rhinal tube:* 0.1 mg/ml (2.5 ml)

TRICYCLIC ANTIDEPRESSANTS (TCAs)

Comment: Co-administration of selective serotonin reuptake inhibitors (SSRIs) and tricyclic antidepressant (TCAs) requires extreme caution.

▶ *amitriptyline* (G) initially 10 mg before bedtime; use lowest effective dose

Pediatric: <12 years: <u>not</u> recommended; ≥12 years: same as adult

Tab: 10, 25, 50, 75, 100, 150 mg

Pediatric: <12 years: <u>not</u> recommended; ≥12 years: same as adult

▶ *amoxapine* initially 25 mg before bedtime; use lowest effective dose

Tab: 25, 50, 100, 150 mg

▶ *clomipramine* (G) initially 25 mg before bedtime; use lowest effective dose

Pediatric: <10 years: <u>not</u> recommended; ≥10 years: same as adult

Anafranil *Cap:* 25, 50, 75 mg

▶ *desipramine* (G) initially 25 mg before bedtime; use lowest effective dose

Pediatric: <12 years: <u>not</u> recommended; ≥12 years: same as adult

Norpramin *Tab:* 10, 25, 50, 75, 100, 150 mg

▶ *doxepin* (G) initially 10 mg before bedtime; use lowest effective dose

Pediatric: <12 years: <u>not</u> recommended; ≥12 years: same as adult

Cap: 10, 25, 50, 75, 100, 150 mg; *Oral conc:* 10 mg/ml (4 oz w. dropper)

▶ *imipramine* (G) initially 10 mg before bedtime; use lowest effective dose

Pediatric: <12 years: <u>not</u> recommended; ≥12 years: same as adult

Tofranil initially 10 mg at bedtime; use lowest effective dose; if bedtime dose exceeds 75 mg daily, may switch to **Tofranil PM**

Tab: 10, 25, 50 mg

Tofranil PM initially 75 mg before bedtime; use lowest effective dose

Cap: 75, 100, 125, 150 mg

▶ *nortriptyline* (G)

Pediatric: <12 years: <u>not</u> recommended; ≥12 years: initially 10 mg before bedtime; use lowest effective dose

Pamelor *Cap:* 10, 25, 50, 75 mg; *Oral soln:* 10 mg/5 ml (16 oz)

▶ *protriptyline* initially 5 mg before bedtime; use lowest effective dose

Pediatric: <12 years: <u>not</u> recommended; ≥12 years: same as adult

Vivactil *Tab:* 5, 10 mg

▶ *trimipramine* initially 25 mg before bedtime; use lowest effective dose

Pediatric: <12 years: <u>not</u> recommended; ≥12 years: same ad adult

Surmontil *Cap:* 25, 50, 100 mg

EOSINOPHILIC GRANULOMATOSIS WITH POLYANGIITIS (EGPA) (FORMERLY CHURG-STRAUSS SYNDROME)

Comment: Eosinophilic granulomatosis with polyangiitis (EGPA) is a rare autoimmune disease that causes vasculitis, an inflammation in the wall of the blood vessels of the body. EGPA is characterized by asthma, high levels of eosinophils, and inflammation of small- to medium-sized blood vessels affecting organ systems, including the lungs, gastrointestinal (GI) tract, skin, heart, and nervous system. **Nucala** *(mepolizumab)* is the first FDA-approved therapy specifically to treat EGPA. This expanded indication of **Nucala** meets a critical and previously unmet need for EGPA patients. It is notable that patients taking **Nucala** in clinical trials reported a significant improvement in their symptoms. The FDA granted this application Priority Review and Orphan Drug designation.

INTERLEUKIN-5 ANTAGONIST MONOCLONAL ANTIBODY (IGG1 KAPPA)

▶ *mepolizumab Adult:* Severe asthma: 100 mg SC once every 4 weeks; Chronic rhinosinusitis with nasal polyps (CRSwNP) 100 mg SC once every 4 weeks; EGPA and hypereosinophilic syndrome (HES): 300 mg as three separate 100 mg SC injections once every 4 weeks

Pediatric: <6 years: safety and efficacy <u>not</u> established; Severe asthma and with an eosinophilic phenotype in patients aged 6-11 years: 40 mg SC once q 4 weeks as an add-on maintenance treatment; may

(continued)

self-administer or caregiver may administer (with healthcare professional approval); Severe asthma in patients aged ≥12 years: 100 mg SC once every 4 weeks

Nucala *Vial:* 100 mg/ml, pwdr for reconstitution, single-dose; *Prefilled syringe:* 40 mg/0.4ml, 100 mg/ml, single-dose; *Prefilled autoinjector:* 100 mg/ml, single-dose

Comment: Nucala is an interleukin-5 antagonist monoclonal antibody (immunoglobulin G1 [IgG1] kappa) indicated for the treatment of severe eosinophilic asthma, EGPA (Churg-Strauss syndrome), HES, and CRSwNP. **Nucala** is not indicated for relief of acute bronchospasm or status asthmaticus. Hypersensitivity reactions (e.g., anaphylaxis, angioedema, bronchospasm, hypotension, urticaria, rash) have occurred after administration of **Nucala**; discontinue **Nucala** in the event of a hypersensitivity reaction. Herpes zoster (HZ) infections have occurred in patients receiving **Nucala**; consider vaccination if medically appropriate. Do not discontinue systemic or inhaled corticosteroids abruptly upon initiation of therapy with **Nucala**; decrease corticosteroids gradually, if appropriate. Treat patients with preexisting helminth infections before therapy with **Nucala**. If patients become infected while receiving treatment with **Nucala** and do not respond to antihelminth treatment, discontinue **Nucala** until the parasitic infection resolves. The most common adverse reactions (incidence ≥5%) are the following: *asthma:* headache, injection site reaction, back pain, and fatigue; *CRSwNP:* oropharyngeal pain and arthralgia; *EGPA and HES:* similar to asthma. In pregnant females with poorly or moderately controlled asthma, evidence demonstrates that there is an increased risk of preeclampsia in the mother, and prematurity, low birth weight (LBW), and small for gestational age (SGA) in the neonate. The level of asthma control should be closely monitored in pregnant women and treatment adjusted as necessary to maintain optimal control. Data on pregnancy exposure are insufficient to inform on **Nucala**-associated risk. Monoclonal antibodies, such as *mepolizumab*, are transported across the placenta in a linear fashion as pregnancy progresses; therefore, potential effects on the fetus are likely to be greater during the 2nd and 3rd trimesters of pregnancy. There is a pregnancy exposure registry that monitors pregnancy outcomes in women with asthma exposed to **Nucala** during pregnancy. Healthcare providers can enroll patients or encourage patients to enroll themselves by calling 1-877-311-8972 or www.mothertobaby.org/asthma. *Mepolizumab* is a humanized monoclonal antibody (IgG1 kappa), and immunoglobulin G (IgG) is present in human milk in small amounts. Developmental and health benefits of breastfeeding should be considered along with the mother's clinical need for **Nucala** and any potential adverse effects on the breastfed infant from *mepolizumab* or from the underlying maternal condition.

EPICONDYLITIS

NSAIDs *see* Appendix I. NSAIDs online at https://connect.springerpub.com/content/reference-book/978-0-8261-7935-7/back-matter/part02/back-matter/bmatter10
Opioid Analgesics *see* **Pain**
Topical and Transdermal Analgesics *see* **Pain**
Parenteral Corticosteroids *see* Appendix L. Parenteral Corticosteroids
Oral Corticosteroids *see* Appendix K. Oral Corticosteroids
Topical Analgesic and Anesthetic Agents *see* Appendix H. Anesthetic Agents for Local Infiltration and Dermal/Mucosal Membrane Application online at https://connect.springerpub.com/content/reference-book/978-0-8261-7935-7/back-matter/part02/back-matter/bmatter9

EPIDIDYMITIS

Comment: The following treatment regimens for epididymitis are published in the **2021 CDC Transmitted Diseases Treatment Guidelines**. Treatment regimens are presented by generic drug name first, followed by information about brands and dose forms. Empiric treatment requires concomitant treatment of chlamydia. Treat all sexual contacts. Patients who are HIV-positive should receive the same treatment as those who are HIV-negative.

RECOMMENDED REGIMEN
Regimen 1
➤ *ceftriaxone* (G) 250 mg IM in a single dose
    plus
➤ *doxycycline* (G) 100 mg bid x 10 days

RECOMMENDED REGIMENS: LIKELY CAUSED BY ENTERIC ORGANISMS
Regimen 1
➤ *levofloxacin* 500 mg daily x 10 days

Regimen 2
➤ *ofloxacin* (G) 300 mg bid x 10 day

DRUG BRANDS AND DOSE FORMS

▷ *ceftriaxone* (G)
  Rocephin *Vial:* 250, 500 mg; 1, 2 gm
▷ *doxycycline* (G)
  Acticlate *Tab:* 75, 150**mg
  Adoxa *Tab:* 50, 75, 100, 150 mg ent-coat
  Doryx *Tab:* 50, 75, 100, 150, 200 mg del-rel
  Doxteric *Tab:* 50 mg del-rel
  Monodox *Cap:* 50, 75, 100 mg
  Oracea *Cap:* 40 mg del-rel
  Vibramycin *Tab:* 100 mg; *Cap:* 50, 100 mg; *Syr:* 50 mg/5 ml (raspberry-apple) (sulfites); *Oral susp:* 25 mg/5 ml (raspberry)
  Vibra-Tab *Tab:* 100 mg film-coat
▷ *levofloxacin*
  Levaquin *Tab:* 250, 500, 750 mg; *Oral soln:* 25 mg/ml (480 ml) (benzyl alcohol)
▷ *ofloxacin* (G)
  Floxin *Tab:* 200, 300, 400 mg

ERECTILE DYSFUNCTION (ED)

Comment: Due to a degree of cardiac risk with sexual activity, consider the cardiovascular status of the patient before instituting therapeutic measures for erectile dysfunction.

PHOSPHODIESTERASE TYPE 5 (PDE5) INHIBITORS, CGMP-SPECIFIC

Comment: Oral phosphodiesterase type 5 (PDE5) inhibitors (**Cialis, Levitra, Staxyn, Viagra**) are contraindicated in patients taking nitrates. Caution with history of recent myocardial infarction (MI), stroke, life-threatening arrhythmia, hypotension, hypertension, cardiac failure, unstable angina, retinitis pigmentosa, CYP3A4 inhibitors (e.g., *cimetidine*, the azoles, *erythromycin*, grapefruit juice), protease inhibitors (e.g., *ritonavir*), CYP3A4 inducers (e.g., *rifampin, carbamazepine, phenytoin, phenobarbital*), alcohol, and antihypertensive agents. Side effects include headache, flushing, nasal congestion, rhinitis, dyspepsia, and diarrhea. Use with caution in patients with anatomical deformation of the penis (e.g., angulation, cavernosal fibrosis, or Peyronie's disease) or in patients who have conditions which may predispose them to priapism (e.g., sickle cell anemia, multiple myeloma, or leukemia). In the event of an erection that persists longer than 4 hours, the patient should seek immediate medical assistance. If priapism (painful erection greater than 6 hours in duration) is not treated immediately, penile tissue damage and permanent loss of potency could result.

▷ *avanafil* initially 100 mg taken 30 minutes prior to sexual activity; may decrease to 50 mg or increase to 200 mg based on response; max 1 administration/day
  Stendra *Tab:* 50, 100, 200 mg
▷ *sildenafil citrate* (G) 1 dose about 1 hour (range 30 minutes to 4 hours) before sexual activity; usual initial dose 50 mg; may decrease to 25 mg or increase to max 100 mg/dose based on response; max 1 administration/day
  Viagra *Tab:* 25, 50, 100 mg
▷ *tadalafil* (G) initially 10 mg prior to sexual activity up to once daily; may decrease to 5 mg or increase to 20 mg based on response; max 1 administration/day; effect may last 36 hours
  Cialis *Tab:* 2.5, 5, 10, 20 mg
▷ *vardenafil* initially 10 mg taken 60 minutes prior to sexual activity; may decrease to 5 mg or increase to 20 mg based on response; max 1 administration/day
  Levitra *Tab:* 2.5, 5, 10, 20 mg film-coat
  Comment: Levitra is not interchangeable with **Staxyn**.
▷ *vardenafil (as HCl)* (G) dissolve 1 tab on tongue 60 minutes prior to sexual activity; max once daily
  Staxyn *Tab:* 10 mg orally disintegrating (peppermint) (phenylalanine)
  Comment: Staxyn is not interchangeable with **Levitra**.
▷ *alprostadil urethral suppository* initially 125 or 250 mcg inserted in the urethra after urination; adjust dose in stepwise manner on separate occasions; max 2 administrations/day
  Muse *Urethral supp:* 125, 250, 500, 1,000 mcg
Comment: Contraindicated with urethral stricture, balanitis, severe hypospadias and curvature, urethritis, predisposition to venous thrombosis, and hyperviscosity syndrome. Extreme caution with anticoagulant therapy (e.g., warfarin, heparin). Potential for hypotension and/or syncope.
▷ *alprostadil injection* inject over 5-10 seconds into the dorsal lateral aspect of the proximal third of the penis; avoid visible veins; rotate injection sites and sides; if no initial response, may give next higher dose within 1 hour; if partial response, give next higher dose after 24 hours; max 60 mcg and 3 self-injections/week; allow at least 24 hours between doses; reduce dose if erection lasts >1 hour
  Caverject *Vial:* 5, 10, 20, 40 mcg/vial (pwdr for reconstitution w. diluent)

(continued)

Caverject Impulse *Cartridge:* 10, 20 mcg (2 cartridge starter and refill pcks)
Edex *Vial:* 5, 10, 20, 40 mcg (6/pck); *Syringe:* 5, 10, 20, 40 mcg (4/pck); *Cartridge:* 10, 20, 40 mcg (2 cartridge starter and refill pcks)
Comment: Determine dose of injectable prostaglandins in the office. Contraindicated with predisposition to priapism, penile angulation, cavernosal fibrosis, Peyronie's disease, and penile implant. Extreme caution with anticoagulant therapy (e.g., **warfarin, heparin**).

ERYSIPELAS

Comment: Erysipelas is most commonly due to GABHS (group A beta-hemolytic *Streptococcus*).

TREATMENT OF CHOICE

▷ *penicillin v potassium* 250-500 mg q 6 hours x 10 days
Pediatric: 25-50 mg/kg/day divided q 6 hours x 10 days; *see* Appendix BB.29. *penicillin v potassium* (Pen-Vee K Solution, Veetids Solution) *for dose by weight*
Pen-Vee K *Tab:* 250, 500 mg; *Oral soln:* 125 mg/5 ml (100, 200 ml), 250 mg/5 ml (100, 150, 200 ml)

TREATMENT IF PENICILLIN-ALLERGIC

▷ *erythromycin base* (G) 250 mg q 6 hours x 10 days
Pediatric: 30-40 mg/kg/day divided q 6 hours x 10 days; >40 kg: same as adult
Ery-Tab *Tab:* 250, 333, 500 mg ent-coat
PCE *Tab:* 333, 500 mg
▷ *erythromycin ethylsuccinate* (G) 400 mg qid x 7 days
Pediatric: 30-50 mg/kg/day in 4 divided doses x 7 days; may double dose with severe infection; max 100 mg/ kg/day; *see* Appendix BB.21: *erythromycin ethylsuccinate* (E.E.S. Suspension, EryPed Drops/Suspension) *for dose by weight*
EryPed *Oral susp:* 200 mg/5 ml (100, 200 ml) (fruit), 400 mg/5 ml (60, 100, 200 ml) (banana); *Oral drops:* 200, 400 mg/5 ml (50 ml) (fruit); *Chew tab:* 200 mg wafer (fruit)
E.E.S. *Oral susp:* 200, 400 mg/5 ml (100 ml) (fruit)
E.E.S. Granules *Oral susp:* 200 mg/5 ml (100, 200 ml) (cherry)
E.E.S. 400 Tablets *Tab:* 400 mg

ERYTHROPOIETIC PROTOPORPHYRIA (EPP)

SELECTIVE AGONIST OF THE MELANOCORTIN 1 RECEPTOR (MC1R)

▷ *afamelanotide* administer a single implant SC, 3-4 cm above the anterior suprailiac crest, every 2 months using an SFM Implantation Cannula or other implantation devices that have been determined by the manufacturer to be suitable for implantation of **Scenesse;** should be administered by a qualified healthcare professional who is proficient in the subcutaneous implantation procedure and has completed training prior to administration; monitor the patient for 30 minutes following implant administration
Pediatric: safety and efficacy <u>not</u> established
Scenesse *Sub Cu implant:* 16 mg (<u>not</u> supplied with an implant device)
Comment: Scenesse *(afamelanotide)* is a selective agonist of the melanocortin 1 receptor (MC1R) for prevention of phototoxicity in adult patients with erythropoietic protoporphyria (EPP). Maintain sun and light protection measures during treatment with **Scenesse** to prevent phototoxic reactions related to EPP. The most common adverse reactions (incidence >2%) have been implant site reaction, nausea, oropharyngeal pain, cough, fatigue, dizziness, skin hyperpigmentation, somnolence, melanocytic nevus, respiratory tract infection, non-acute porphyria, and skin irritation. **Scenesse** may induce darkening of preexisting nevi and ephelides due to its pharmacologic effect. A regular full body skin examination is recommended twice yearly to monitor all nevi and other skin abnormalities. There are <u>no</u> data on **Scenesse** use in pregnancy to evaluate for any drug-associated risk of major birth defects, miscarriage, <u>or</u> adverse maternal <u>or</u> embryo/fetal outcomes. There are <u>no</u> data on the presence of *afamelanotide* <u>or</u> any of its metabolites in human <u>or</u> animal milk <u>or</u> effects on the breastfed infant.

ESOPHAGITIS, EROSIVE

Antacids *see GERD*
H2 Antagonists *see GERD*
Proton Pump Inhibitors *see GERD*
▷ *sucralfate* (G) *Active ulcer:* 1 gm qid; *Maintenance:* 1 gm bid
Carafate *Tab:* 1*gm; *Oral susp:* 1 gm/10 ml (14 oz)

EXOCRINE PANCREAS INSUFFICIENCY (EPI)/PANCREATIC ENZYME DEFICIENCY

Comment: Seen in chronic pancreatitis, postpancreatectomy, cystic fibrosis, post-gastrointestinal (GI) tract bypass surgery (Whipple procedure), and ductal obstruction from neoplasia. May sprinkle cap; however, do not crush or chew cap or tab. May mix with applesauce or other acidic food; follow with water or juice. Do not let any drug remain in mouth. Take dose with (not before or after) each meal and snack (half dose with snacks). Base dose on lipase units; adjust per diet and clinical response (i.e., steatorrhea). Pancrelipase products are interchangeable. Contraindicated with pork protein hypersensitivity.

PANCRELIPASE PRODUCTS
▷ *pancreatic enzymes*

Creon 500 units/kg per meal; max 2,500 units/kg per meal or <10,000 units/kg per day or <4,000 units/ gm fat ingested per day

Pediatric: <12 months: 2,000-4,000 units per 120 ml formula or per breastfeeding (do not mix directly into formula or breast milk); 12 months to 4 years: 1,000 units/kg per meal; max 2,500 units/kg per meal; <10,000 units/kg per day; >4 years: same as adult

Cap: **Creon 3000** lip 3,000 units+pro 9,500 units+amyl 15,000 units del-rel
    Creon 6000 lip 6,000 units+pro 19,000 units+amyl 30,000 units del-rel
    Creon 12000 lip 12,000 units+pro 38,000 units+amyl 60,000 units del-rel
    Creon 24000 lip 24,000 units+pro 76,000 units+amyl 120,000 units del-rel
    Creon 36000 lip 36,000 units+pro 114,000 units+amyl 180,000 units del-rel

Cotazym 1-3 tabs just prior to each meal or snack

Pediatric: <12 years: not recommended; ≥12 years: same as adult

Tab: **Cotazym** lip 1,000 units+pro 12,500 units+amyl 12,500 units del-rel
    Cotazym-S lip 5,000 units+pro 20,000 units+amyl 20,000 units del-rel

Donnazyme 1-3 caps just prior to each meal or snack

Pediatric: <12 years: not recommended; ≥12 years: same as adult

Cap: **Donnazyme** lip 5,000 units+pro 20,000 units+amyl 20,000 units del-rel

Ku-Zyme 1-2 caps just prior to each meal or snack

Pediatric: <12 years: not recommended; ≥12 years: same as adult

Cap: **Ku-Zyme:** lip 12,000 units+pro 15,000 units+amyl 15,000 units del-rel

Kutrase 1-2 caps just prior to each meal or snack

Pediatric: <12 years: not recommended; ≥12 years: same as adult

Cap: **Kutrase:** lip 12,000 units+pro 30,000 units+amyl 30,000 units del-rel

Pancreaze 2,500 lipase units/kg per meal or <10,000 lipase units/kg per day or <4,000 lipase units/gm fat ingested per day

Pediatric: <12 months: 2,000-4,000 lipase units per 120 ml formula or per breastfeeding; >12 months to <4 years 1,000 lipase units/kg per meal; ≥4 years: 500 lipase units/kg per meal; max: adult dose

Cap: **Pancreaze 4200** lip 4,200 units+pro 10,000 units+amyl 17,500 units ec-microtabs
    Pancreaze 10500 lip 10,500 units+pro 25,000 units+amyl 43,750 units ec-microtabs
    Pancreaze 16800 lip 16,800 units+pro 40,000 units+amyl 70,000 units ec-microtabs
    Pancreaze 21000 lip 21,000 units+pro 37,000 units+amyl 61,000 units ec-microtabs

Pertzye *12 months to 4 years and ≥8 kg:* initially 1,000 lipase units/kg per meal; *≥4 years and ≥16 kg:* initially 500 lipase units/kg per meal; *Both:* 2,500 lipase units/kg per meal or <10,000 units/kg per day or <4,000 lipase units/gm fat ingested per day

Cap: **Pertzye 8000** lip 8,000 units+pro 28,750 units+amyl 30,250 units del-rel
    Pertzye 16000 lip 16,000 units+pro 57,500 units+amyl 65,000 units del-rel

Ultrase 1-3 tabs just prior to each meal or snack

Pediatric: same as adult

Cap: **Ultrase** lip 4,500 units+pro 20,000 units+amyl 25,000 units del-rel
    Ultrase MT lip 12,000 units+pro 39,000 units+amyl 39,000 units del-rel
    Ultrase MT 18 lip 18,000 units+pro 58,500 units+amyl 58,500 units del-rel
    Ultrase MT 20 lip 20,000 units+pro 65,000 units+amyl 65,000 units del-rel

Viokace initially 500 lipase units/kg per meal; max 2,500 lipase units/kg per meal, or <10,000 lipase units/ kg per meal, or <4,000 units/gm fat ingested per day

Pediatric: same as adult

Tab: **Viokace 8000** lip 8,000 units+pro 30,000 units+amyl 30,000 units
    Viokace 16000 lip 16,000 units+pro 60,000 units amyl 60,000 units
    Viokace 10440 lip 10,440 units+pro 39,150 units amyl 39,150 units
    Viokace 20880 lip 20,880 units+pro 78,300 units amyl 78,300 units

Comment: Viokace 10440 and Viokace 20880 should be taken with a daily proton pump inhibitor.

Viokace Powder 1/4 tsp (0.7 gm) with meals

Viokace Powder lip 16,800 units+pro 70,000 units+amyl 70,000 units per 1/4 tsp (8 oz)

Zenpep initially 500 lipase units/kg per meal; max 2,500 lipase units/kg per meal or <10,000 units/kg per day or <4,000 units/gm fat ingested per day

Pediatric: Infants-12 months: infants may be given 3,000 lipase units (1 capsule) per 120 ml of formula or per breastfeeding; do not mix capsule contents directly into formula or breast milk prior to administration; Children ≥12 months to <4 years: enzyme dosing should begin with 1,000 lipase units/kg of body weight

(continued)

per meal to a maximum of 2,500 lipase units/kg of body weight per meal (or ≤10,000 lipase units/kg/day), or <4,000 lipase units/gm fat ingested per day; Children ≥4 years: same as adult

> *Cap:* **Zenpep 3000** lip 3,000 units+pro 10,000 units+amyl 14,000 units del-rel
> **Zenpep 5000** lip 5,000 units+pro 17,000 units+amyl 24,000 units del-rel
> **Zenpep 10000** lip 10,000 units+pro 32,000 units+amyl 42,000 units del-rel
> **Zenpep 15000** lip 15,000 units+pro 47,000 units+amyl 63,000 units del-rel
> **Zenpep 20000** lip 20,000 units+pro 63,000 units+amyl 84,000 units del-rel
> **Zenpep 25000** lip 25,000 units+pro 79,000 units+amyl 105,000 units del-rel
> **Zenpep 40000** lip 40,000 units+pro 126,000 units+amyl 168,000 units del-rel

Comment: Zenpep is not interchangeable with any other pancrelipase product. Dosing should not exceed the recommended maximum dosage set forth by the Cystic Fibrosis Foundation Consensus Conferences Guidelines. **Zenpep** should be swallowed whole. For infants or patients unable to swallow intact capsules, the contents may be sprinkled on soft acidic food, e.g., applesauce.

Zymase 1-3 caps just prior to each meal or snack
Pediatric: <12 years: not recommended; ≥12 years: same as adult

> *Cap:* **Zymase** lip 12,000 units+pro 24,000 units+amyl 24,000 units del-rel

EXTRAPYRAMIDAL SIDE EFFECTS (EPS)

➤ *amantadine*

Gocovri *Initially:* 137 mg once daily at bedtime; after 1 week, increase to 274 mg once daily at bedtime; swallow whole; may sprinkle contents on soft food; take with or without food; avoid use with alcohol; a lower dose is recommended for patients with moderate or severe renal impairment; contraindicated with end-stage renal disease (ESRD)

Cap: 68.5, 137 mg ext-rel

Comment: Gocovri is a chronosynchronous *amantadine* therapy indicated for the treatment of dyskinesia in patients with Parkinson's disease receiving *levodopa*-based therapy, with or without concomitant dopaminergic medications, as adjunctive treatment to *levodopa/carbidopa* in patients with Parkinson's disease experiencing "off" episodes. The most commonly observed adverse reactions (incidence ≥10%) have been hallucination, dizziness, dry mouth, peripheral edema, constipation, fall, and orthostatic hypotension. Advise patients prior to treatment about the potential to fall asleep during activities of daily living (ADLs); discontinue if this occurs. Monitor patients for depressed mood, depression, or suicidal ideation or behavior. Patients with major psychotic disorder should ordinarily not be treated with **Gocovri**; observe patients for the occurrence of hallucinations throughout treatment, especially at initiation and after dose increases. Monitor patients for dizziness and orthostatic hypotension, especially after starting **Gocovri** and after dose increases. Avoid sudden discontinuation, which can result in withdrawal-emergent hyperpyrexia and confusion. Impulse control and compulsive behaviors may occur, such as gambling urges, sexual urges, and uncontrolled spending; consider dose reduction or discontinuation if any occur. Increased risk of anticholinergic effects may require reduction of **Gocovri** or dose of the anticholinergic drug(s). Excretion of *amantadine* increases with acidic urine, resulting in possible accumulation with urine change toward alkaline. Live attenuated vaccines (LAVs) are not recommended during treatment with **Gocovri**. Concomitant use of alcohol is not recommended due to increased potential for central nervous system (CNS) effects. There are no adequate data on embryo/fetal risk associated with use of *amantadine* in pregnant females. Animal studies suggest a potential risk for fetal harm with *amantadine*. *Amantadine* is excreted in human milk, but amounts have not been quantified. There is no information on the risk to the breastfed infant.

Osmolex ER *Tab:* 129, 193, 258 mg ext-rel

Comment: Osmolex ER is not interchangeable with other *amantadine* immediate- or extended-release products. The most common adverse reactions (incidence ≥5%) are nausea, dizziness/lightheadedness, and insomnia. **Osmolex ER** is contraindicated in patients with ESRD. Advise patients prior to treatment about potential for falling asleep during ADLs and somnolence and discontinue **Osmolex ER** if it occurs. Monitor patients for depressed mood, depression, and suicidal ideation or behavior. Patients with major psychotic disorder should ordinarily not be treated with **Osmolex ER**; observe patients throughout treatment for the occurrence of hallucinations, especially at initiation and after dose increases. Monitor patients for dizziness and orthostatic hypotension, especially after starting **Osmolex ER** or increasing the dose. Avoid sudden withdrawal/discontinuation due to risk of withdrawal-emergent hyperpyrexia and confusion. Monitor patients for development of impulse control/compulsive behaviors. Ask patients about increased gambling urges, sexual urges, uncontrolled spending, or other urges, and consider dose reduction or discontinuation if any occur. Increased risk of anticholinergic effects may require reduction of **Osmolex ER** or dose of the anticholinergic drug(s). Excretion of *amantadine* increases with acidic urine, resulting in possible accumulation with urine change toward alkaline. Live Attenuated Influenza Vaccines (LAVs) are not recommended during treatment with **Osmolex ER**. Concomitant use of alcohol is not recommended due to increased potential for CNS effects. There are no adequate data on the developmental risk associated with use of *amantadine* in pregnant females. Animal studies suggest a potential risk for fetal harm with *amantadine*. *Amantadine* is excreted in human milk, but amounts have not been quantified. There is no information on the risk to the breastfed infant.

EYE PAIN

OPHTHALMIC NONSTEROIDAL ANTI-INFLAMMATORY DRUGS (NSAIDS)
Comment: Concomitant contact lens wear is contraindicated during therapy. Etiology of eye pain must be known prior to use of ophthalmic nonsteroidal anti-inflammatory drugs (NSAIDs).
▷ *diclofenac* 1 drop affected eye qid
  Pediatric: <12 years: <u>not</u> recommended; ≥12 years: same as adult
    Voltaren Ophthalmic Solution *Ophth soln:* 0.1% (2.5, 5 ml)
▷ *ketorolac tromethamine* 1 drop affected eye qid for up to 4 days
  Pediatric: <3 years: <u>not</u> recommended; ≥3 years: same as adult
    Acular *Ophth soln:* 0.5% (3, 5, 10 ml) (benzalkonium chloride)
    Acular LS *Ophth soln:* 0.4% (5 ml) (benzalkonium chloride)
    Acular PF *Ophth soln:* 0.5% (0.4 ml; 12 single-use vials/carton) (preservative-free)
▷ *nepafenac* 1 drop affected eye tid
  Pediatric: <10 years: <u>not</u> recommended; ≥10 years: same as adult
    Nevanac Ophthalmic Suspension *Ophth susp:* 0.1% (3 ml) (benzalkonium chloride)

OPHTHALMIC STEROIDS
Comment: Ophthalmic steroids are contraindicated with mycobacterial, fungal, <u>and</u> viral infections. Effectiveness of treatment should be assessed after 2 days. The corticosteroid should be tapered and treatment concluded within 14 days if possible due to risk of corneal <u>and/or</u> scleral thinning with prolonged use.
▷ *difluprednate* (G) 1 drop affected eye qid; *Postop pain:* beginning 24 hours after surgery, 1 drop affected eye qid; continue for 2 weeks postop; then bid x 1 week; then taper until resolved
  Pediatric: <12 years: <u>not</u> recommended; ≥12 years: same as adult
    Durezol Ophthalmic Solution *Ophth emul:* 0.05% (5 ml)
▷ *etabonate* 1 drop affected eye qid
  Pediatric: <12 years: <u>not</u> recommended; ≥12 years: same as adult
    Alrex Ophthalmic Solution *Ophth emul:* 0.2% (5 ml) (benzalkonium chloride)
▷ *loteprednol etabonate 1%* 1-2 drops affected eye bid
  Pediatric: <12 years: <u>not</u> established; ≥12 years: same as adult
    Inveltys *Ophth soln:* 1% (5 ml) (benzalkonium chloride)
    Comment: Inveltys is indicated for postop inflammation and pain following ocular surgery beginning the day after surgery and continuing throughout the first 2 weeks of the postoperative period.

FACIAL HAIR: EXCESSIVE/UNWANTED

TOPICAL HAIR GROWTH RETARDANT
▷ *eflornithine* 13.9% cream apply a thin layer to affected areas of the face and under the chin bid at least 8 hours apart; rub in thoroughly; do <u>not</u> wash treated area for at least 4 hours following application
  Pediatric: <12 years: <u>not</u> recommended; ≥12 years: same as adult
    Vaniqa *Crm:* 13.9% (30, 60 gm)
    Comment: After **Vaniqa** dries, may apply cosmetics <u>or</u> sunscreen. Hair removal techniques may be continued as needed.

FECAL ODOR

▷ *bismuth subgallate powder* (OTC) 1-2 tabs tid with meals
    Devrom *Chew tab:* 200 mg; *Cap:* 200 mg
    Comment: Devrom is an internal (oral) deodorant for control of odors from ileostomy <u>or</u> colostomy drainage <u>or</u> fecal incontinence.

FEVER (PYREXIA)

ACETAMINOPHEN FOR IV INFUSION
▷ *acetaminophen* injectable (G) administer by IV infusion over 15 minutes; 1,000 mg q 6 hours prn <u>or</u> 650 mg q 4 hours prn; max 4,000 mg/day
  Pediatric: <2 years: <u>not</u> recommended; 2-13 years <50 kg: 15 mg/kg q 6 hours prn <u>or</u> 12.5 mg/kg q 4 hours prn; max 750 mg/single dose; max 75 mg/kg per day
    Ofirmev *Vial:* 10 mg/ml (100 ml) (preservative-free)
    Comment: The **Ofirmev** vial is intended for single use. If any portion is withdrawn from the vial, use within 6 hours. Discard the unused portion. For pediatric patients, withdraw the intended dose and administer via syringe pump. Do <u>not</u> ad-mix **Ofirmev** with any other drugs. **Ofirmev** is physically incompatible with diazepam and chlorpromazine hydrochloride.

(continued)

▷ *acetaminophen* (G)

Children's Tylenol (OTC) 10-20 mg/kg q 4-6 hours prn
Oral susp: 80 mg/tsp
4-11 months (12-17 lb): 1/2 tsp q 4 hours prn; 12-23 months (18-23 lb): 3/4 tsp q 4 hours prn; 2-3 years (24-35 lb): 1 tsp q 4 hours prn; 4-5 years (36-47 lb): 1 tsp q 4 hours prn; 6-8 years (48-59 lb): 2 tsp q 4 hours prn; 9-10 years (60-71 lb): 2 tsp q 4 hours prn; 11 years (72-95 lb): 3 tsp q 4 hours prn; all ages: max 5 doses/day
Elix: 160 mg/5 ml (2, 4 oz)
Chew tab: 80 mg
2-3 years (24-35 lb): 2 tabs q 4 hours prn; 4-5 years (36-47 lb): 3 tabs q 4 hours prn; 6-8 years (48-59 lb): 4 tabs q 4 hours prn; 9-10 years (60-71 lb): 5 tabs q 4 hours prn; 11 years (72-95 lb): 6 tabs q 4 hours prn; all ages: max 5 doses/day
Junior strength:
6-8 years: 2 tabs q 4 hours prn; 9-10 years: 2 tabs q 4 hours prn; 11 years: 3 tabs q 4 hours prn; 12 years: 4 tabs q 4 hours prn; all ages: max 5 doses/day
Chew tab: 160 mg
Junior cplt: 160 mg
Infant's drops and suspension: 80 mg/0.8 ml (1/2, 1 oz)
<3 months: 0.4 ml q 4 hours prn; 4-11 months: 0.8 ml q 4 hours prn; 12-23 months: 1.2 ml q 4 hours prn; 2-3 years (24-35 lb): 1.6 ml q 4 hours prn; 4-5 years (36-47 lb): 2.4 ml q 4 hours prn; all ages: max 5 doses/day
Extra Strength Tylenol (OTC) 1 gm q 4-6 hours prn; max 4 gm/day
Pediatric: <12 years: not recommended; ≥12 years: same as adult
Tab/Cplt/Gel tab/Gelcap: 500 mg; *Liq:* 500 mg/15 ml (8 oz)
FeverAll Extra Strength Tylenol (OTC)
Pediatric: <3 months: not recommended; 3-36 months: 80 mg q 4 hours prn; 3-6 years: 120 mg q 4 hours prn; ≥6 years: 325 mg q 4 hours prn; *Rectal supp:* 80, 120, 325 mg (6/carton)
Maximum Strength Tylenol Sore Throat (OTC) 500-1,000 mg q 4-6 hours prn
Pediatric: <12 years: not recommended; ≥12 years: same as adult
Liq: 1,000 mg/30 ml (8 oz)
Tylenol (OTC) 650 mg q 4-6 hours; max 4 gm/day
Pediatric: <6 years: not recommended; 6-11 years: 325 mg q 4-6 hours prn; max 1.625 gm/day; ≥12 years: same as adult

▷ *aspirin* (G)

Bayer (OTC) 325-650 mg q 4 hours prn; max 5 doses/day
Pediatric: <12 years: not recommended; ≥12 years: same as adult
Tab/Cplt: 325 mg ext-rel
Extra Strength Bayer (OTC) 500 mg-1 gm q 4-6 hours prn; max 4 gm/day
Pediatric: <12 years: not recommended; ≥12 years: same as adult
Cplt: 500 mg
Extended-Release Bayer 8 Hour (OTC) 650-1,300 mg q 8 hours prn
Pediatric: <12 years: not recommended; ≥12 years: same as adult
Cplt: 650 mg ext-rel

▷ *aspirin+caffeine* (G)

Anacin (OTC) 800 mg q 4 hours prn; max 4 gm/day
Pediatric: <6 years: not recommended; 6-12 years: 400 mg q 4 hours prn; max 2 gm/day; ≥12 years: same as adult
Tab/Cplt: 400 mg
Anacin Maximum Strength (OTC) 1 gm tid-qid
Pediatric: <12 years: not recommended; ≥12 years: same as adult
Tab: 500 mg

▷ *aspirin+antacid* (G)

Extra Strength Bayer Plus (OTC) 500 mg-1 gm q 4-6 hours prn; usual max 4 gm/day
Pediatric: <12 years: not recommended; ≥12 years: same as adult
Cplt: 500 mg aspirin+calcium carbonate
Bufferin (OTC) 650 mg q 4 hours; max 3.9 mg/day
Pediatric: <12 years: not recommended; ≥12 years: same as adult
Tab: 325 mg aspirin+calcium carbonate+magnesium carbonate+magnesium oxide

▷ *ibuprofen* (G)

Comment: *Ibuprofen* is contraindicated in children <6 months of age.
Children's Advil (OTC), ElixSure IB (OTC), Motrin (OTC), PediaCare (OTC), PediaProfen (OTC)
Pediatric: 5-10 mg/kg q 6-8 hours, max 40 mg/kg/day; <24 lb (<2 years): individualize; 24-35 lb (2-3 years): 5 ml q 6-8 hours prn; 36-47 lb (4-5 years): 7.5 ml q 6-8 hours prn; 48-59 lb (6-8 years): 10 ml or 2 tabs q 6-8 hours prn; 60-71 lb (9-10 years): 12.5 ml or 2 tabs q 6-8 hours prn; 72-95 lb (11 years): 15 ml or 3 tabs q 6-8 hours prn
Oral susp: 100 mg/5 ml (2, 4 oz) (berry); *Junior tabs:* 100 mg

Children's Motrin Drops (OTC), PediaCare Drops (OTC)
Pediatric: <24 lb (<2 years): individualize; 24-35 lb (2-3 years): 2.5 ml q 6-8 hours prn
   Oral drops: 50 mg/1.25 ml (15 ml) (berry)
Children's Motrin Chewables and Caplets (OTC)
Pediatric: 48-59 lb (6-8 years): 200 mg q 6-8 hours prn; 60-71 lb (9-10 years): 250 mg q 6-8 hours prn;
72-95 lb (11 years): 300 mg q 6-8 hours prn; ≥12 years: same as adult
   Chew tab: 100*mg (citrus; phenylalanine); *Cplt:* 100 mg
Motrin (OTC) 400 mg q 6 hours prn
Pediatric: <6 months: <u>not</u> recommended; ≥6 months, fever <102.5°F: 5 mg/kg q 6-8 hours prn; >6
months, fever >102.5°F: 10 mg/kg q 6-8 hours prn; all ages: max 40 mg/kg/day
   Tab: 400 mg; *Cplt:* 100*mg; *Chew tab:* 50*, 100*mg (citrus; phenylalanine); *Oral susp:* 100 mg/5 ml (4,
16 oz) (berry); *Oral drops:* 40 mg/ml (15 ml) (berry)
Advil (OTC), Motrin IB (OTC), Nuprin (OTC) 200-400 mg q 4-6 hours; max 1.2 gm/day
Pediatric: <12 years: <u>not</u> recommended; ≥12 years: same as adult
   Tab/Cplt/Gelcap: 200 mg
▷ *naproxen* (G)
Pediatric: <2 years: <u>not</u> recommended; ≥2 years: 2.5-5 mg/kg bid-tid; max: 15 mg/kg/day
   Aleve (OTC) 400 mg x 1 dose; then 200 mg q 8-12 hours prn; max 10 days
     Tab/Cplt/Gelcap: 200 mg
   Anaprox 550 mg x 1 dose; then 550 mg q 12 hours <u>or</u> 275 mg q 6-8 hours prn; max 1.375 gm first day
   and 1.1 gm/day thereafter
     Tab: 275 mg
   Anaprox DS 1 tab bid
     Tab: 550 mg
   EC-Naprosyn 375 <u>or</u> 500 mg bid prn; may increase dose up to max 1,500 mg/day as tolerated
     Tab: 375, 500 mg del-rel
   Naprelan 1 gm daily <u>or</u> 1.5 gm daily for limited time; max 1 gm/day thereafter
     Tab: 375, 500 mg
   Naprosyn initially 500 mg; then 500 mg q 12 hours <u>or</u> 250 mg q 6-8 hours prn; max 1.25 gm first day
   and 1 gm/day thereafter
     Tab: 250, 375, 500 mg; *Oral susp:* 125 mg/5 ml (473 ml) (pineapple-orange)

FIBROCYSTIC BREAST DISEASE

Contraceptives *see* Appendix G. Contraceptives
▷ *spironolactone* 10 mg bid premenstrually
   Aldactone (G) *Tab:* 25, 50*, 100*mg
   CaroSpir *Oral susp:* 25 mg/5 ml (118, 473 ml) (banana)
▷ *vitamin E* 400-600 IU daily
▷ *vitamin B6* 50-100 mg daily

Synthetic Steroid Derived From Ethisterone

▷ *danazol* start on 3rd <u>or</u> 4th day of menstrual period <u>or</u> after a negative pregnancy test; 50-200 mg bid x 2-6
months
Pediatric: <18 years: <u>not</u> recommended; ≥18 years: same as adult
   Danocrine *Cap:* 50, 100, 200 mg
Comment: *Danazol* is a synthetic steroid derived from ethisterone. It suppresses the pituitary-ovarian axis.
This suppression is probably a combination of depressed hypothalamic-pituitary response to lowered
estrogen production, the alteration of sex steroid metabolism, and interaction of *danazol* with sex hormone
receptors. The <u>only</u> other demonstrable hormonal effects are weak androgenic activity and depression of
both follicle-stimulating hormone (FSH) and luteinizing hormone (LH) output. Recent evidence suggests a
direct inhibitory effect at gonadal sites and a binding of **Danocrine** to receptors of gonadal steroids at target
organs. In addition, **Danocrine** has been shown to significantly decrease IgG, IgM, and IgA levels, as well as
phospholipid and IgG isotope autoantibodies, in patients with endometriosis and associated elevations of
autoantibodies, suggesting this could be another mechanism by which it facilitates regression of fibrocystic
breast disease. **Danocrine** usually produces partial-to-complete disappearance of breast tissue nodularity
and complete relief of pain and tenderness. Changes in the menstrual pattern may occur. Generally, the
pituitary-suppressive action of **Danocrine** is reversible. Ovulation and cyclic bleeding usually return within
60 to 90 days when therapy with **Danocrine** is discontinued. **Danocrine** is also used to treat endometriosis
(to relieve associated abdominal pain) and hereditary angioedema (to prevent attacks). Contraindications
include pregnancy, breastfeeding, active <u>or</u> history of thromboembolic disease/event, porphyria,
undiagnosed abnormal genital bleeding, androgen-dependent tumor, and markedly impaired hepatic, renal,
<u>or</u> cardiac function.

FIBROMYALGIA

Acetaminophen for IV Infusion *see* **Pain**
NSAIDs *see* Appendix I. NSAIDs online at https://connect.springerpub.com/content/reference-book/978-0-8261-7935-7/back-matter/part02/back-matter/bmatter10
Opioid Analgesics *see* **Pain**
Topical and Transdermal Analgesics *see* **Pain**
Parenteral Corticosteroids *see* Appendix L. Parenteral Corticosteroids
Oral Corticosteroids *see* Appendix K. Oral Corticosteroids
Topical Analgesic and Anesthetic Agents *see* Appendix H. Anesthetic Agents for Local Infiltration and Dermal/Mucosal Membrane Application online at https://connect.springerpub.com/content/reference-book/978-0-8261-7935-7/back-matter/part02/back-matter/bmatter9

SEROTONIN NOREPINEPHRINE REUPTAKE INHIBITORS (SNRIs)
▷ *duloxetine* (G) swallow whole; initially 30 mg once daily x 1 week; then increase to 60 mg once daily; max 120 mg/day
  Pediatric: <12 years: not recommended; ≥12 years: same as adult
     Cymbalta *Cap:* 20, 30, 60 mg ent-coat pellets
▷ *milnacipran* (G) *Day 1:* 12.5 mg once; *Days 2-3:* 12.5 mg bid; *Days 4-7:* 25 mg bid; max 100 mg bid
  Pediatric: <17 years: not recommended; ≥17 years: same as adult
     Savella *Tab:* 12.5, 25, 50, 100 mg

GAMMA-AMINOBUTYRIC ACID ANALOGS
Comment: The gabapentinoids (*gabapentin* [Gralise, Neurontin, Horizant] and *pregabalin* [Lyrica]) have respiratory depression risk potential. Therefore, when coprescribed with other central nervous system (CNS) depressant agents, initiate the gabapentinoid at the lowest possible dose and monitor the patient for respiratory depression (especially elders and patients with compromised pulmonary function). Side effects include fatigue, somnolence/sedation, dizziness, vertigo, feeling drunk, headache, nausea, and dry mouth. To discontinue a gabapentinoid, withdraw gradually over 1 week or longer.

▷ *gabapentin* initially 300 mg on day 1; then 600 mg on day 2; then 900 mg on days 3-6; then 1,200 mg on days 7-10; then 1,500 mg on days 11-14; titrate up to 1,800 mg on day 15; take entire dose once daily with the evening meal; do not crush, split, or chew
  Pediatric: <3 years: not recommended; 3-12 years: initially 10-15 mg/kg/day in 3 divided doses, max 12 hours between doses, titrate over 3 days; 3-4 years: titrate to 40 mg/kg/day; 5-12 years: titrate to 25-35 mg/kg/day, max 50 mg/kg/day; >12 years: same as adult
     Gralise *Tab:* 300, 600 mg
     Neurontin (G) 100 mg daily x 1 day; then 100 mg bid x 1 day; then 100 mg tid continuously or 300 mg bid; max 900 mg tid
     Tab: 600*, 800*mg; *Cap:* 100, 300, 400 mg; *Oral soln:* 250 mg/5 ml (480 ml) (strawberry-anise)
▷ *gabapentin enacarbil* 600 mg once daily at about 5:00 PM; if dose not taken at recommended time, next dose should be taken the following day; swallow whole; take with food; *CrCl 30-59 ml/min:* 600 mg on Day 1, Day 3, and every day thereafter; *CrCl <30 ml/min:* or on hemodialysis: not recommended
  Pediatric: <12 years: not recommended; ≥12 years: same as adult
     Horizant *Tab:* 300, 600 mg ext-rel
▷ *pregabalin (GABA analog)* (G)(V)
  Pediatric: <18 years: not recommended; ≥18 years: same as adult
     Lyrica initially 50 mg tid; may titrate to 100 mg tid within 1 week; max 600 mg divided tid; discontinue over 1 week
        Cap: 25, 50, 75, 100, 150, 200, 225, 300 mg; *Oral soln:* 20 mg/ml
     Lyrica CR usual dose 165 mg once daily; may increase to 330 mg/day within 1 week; max 660 mg/day
        Tab: 82.5, 165, 330 mg ext-rel

OTHER AGENTS
▷ *amitriptyline* (G) 20 mg q HS; may increase gradually to max 50 mg q HS
  Pediatric: <12 years: not recommended; ≥12 years: same as adult
     Tab: 10, 25, 50, 75, 100, 150 mg
▷ *cyclobenzaprine* (G) 10 mg tid; usual range 20-40 mg/day in divided doses; max 60 mg/day x 2-3 weeks or 15 mg ext-rel once daily; max 30 mg ext-rel/day x 2-3 weeks
  Pediatric: <15 years: not recommended; ≥15 years: same as adult
     Amrix *Cap:* 15, 30 mg ext-rel
     Fexmid *Tab:* 7.5 mg
     Flexeril *Tab:* 5, 10 mg
▷ *eszopiclone* (IV)(G) (pyrrolopyrazine) 1-3 mg; max 3 mg/day x 1 month; do not take if unable to sleep for at least 8 hours before required to be active again; delayed effect if taken with a meal

Pediatric: <18 years: not recommended; ≥18 years: same as adult
  Lunesta *Tab:* 1, 2, 3 mg

▶ ***flurazepam*** (IV)(G) 15 mg q HS; may increase to 30 mg q HS
Pediatric: <18 years: not recommended; ≥18 years: same as adult
  Dalmane *Cap:* 15, 30 mg

▶ ***trazodone*** (G) 50 mg q HS
Pediatric: <18 years: not recommended; ≥18 years: same as adult
  Desyrel *Tab:* 50, 100, 150, 300 mg

▶ ***triazolam*** (IV)(G) 0.125 mg q HS; may increase gradually to 0.5 mg
Pediatric: <18 years: not recommended; ≥18 years: same as adult
  Halcion *Tab:* 0.125, 0.25*mg

▶ ***zaleplon*** (IV) (imidazopyridine) 5-10 mg at HS or after going to bed if unable to sleep; do not take if unable to sleep for at least 4 hours before required to be active again; max 20 mg/day x 1 month; delayed effect if taken with a meal
Pediatric: <12 years: not recommended; ≥12 years: same as adult
  Sonata *Cap:* 5, 10 mg (tartrazine)
  Comment: Sonata is indicated for the treatment of insomnia when a middle-of the-night awakening is followed by difficulty returning to sleep.

▶ ***zolpidem*** oral solution spray (IV)(G) (imidazopyridine hypnotic) 2 actuations (10 mg) immediately before bedtime; *Elderly, debilitated, or hepatic impairment:* 2 actuations (5 mg); max 2 actuations (10 mg)
Pediatric: <18 years: not recommended; ≥18 years: same as adult
  ZolpiMist *Oral soln spray:* 5 mg/actuation (60 metered actuations) (cherry)
Comment: The lowest dose of ***zolpidem*** in all forms is recommended for persons >50 years of age and women as drug elimination is slower than in men.

▶ ***zolpidem*** tabs (IV)(G) (pyrazolopyrimidine hypnotic) 5-10 mg or 6.25-12.5 ext-rel q HS prn; max 12.5 mg/day x 1 month; do not take if unable to sleep for at least 8 hours before required to be active again; delayed effect if taken with a meal
Pediatric: <18 years: not recommended; ≥18 years: same as adult
  Ambien *Tab:* 5, 10 mg
  Ambien CR *Tab:* 6.25, 12.5 mg ext-rel
Comment: The lowest dose of ***zolpidem*** in all forms is recommended for persons >50 years of age and women as drug elimination is slower than in men.

▶ ***zolpidem*** sublingual tabs (imidazopyridine hypnotic) (IV) dissolve 1 tab under the tongue; allow to disintegrate completely before swallowing; take only once per night and only if at least 4 hours of bedtime remain before planned time for awakening
Pediatric: <18 years: not recommended; ≥18 years: same as adult
  Edluar *SL Tab:* 5, 10 mg
  Intermezzo *SL Tab:* 1.75, 3.5 mg
  Comment: Intermezzo is indicated for the treatment of insomnia when a middle-of-the-night awakening is followed by difficulty returning to sleep. The lowest dose of ***zolpidem*** in all forms is recommended for persons >50 years of age and women as drug elimination is slower than in men.

FIFTH DISEASE (*ERYTHEMA INFECTIOSUM*)

Antipyretics *see* ***Fever***

FLATULENCE

▶ ***simethicone*** (G)
  Gas-X (OTC) 2-4 tabs pc and HS prn
    Tab: 40, 80, 125 mg; *Cap:* 125 mg
  Mylicon (OTC) 2-4 tabs pc and HS prn
    Tab: 40, 80, 125 mg; *Cap:* 125 mg
  Phazyme-95 1-2 tabs with each meal and HS prn
    Tab: 95 mg
  Phazyme Infant Oral Drops
  Pediatric: <2 years: 0.3 ml qid pc and HS prn; 2-12 years: 0.6 ml qid pc and HS prn; >12 years: 1.2 ml qid pc and HS prn
    Oral drops: 40 mg/0.6 ml (15, 30 ml w. calibrated dropper) (orange) (alcohol-free)
  Maximum Strength Phazyme 1-2 caps with each meal and HS prn
    Cap: 125 mg

FLUORIDATION, WATER, <0.6 PPM

▷ *fluoride* (G)

    Luride

    Pediatric: Water fluoridation 0.3-0.6 ppm: <3 years: use drops; 3-6 years: 0.25 mg daily; 7-16 years: 0.5 mg daily; *Water fluoridation <0.3 ppm:* <3 years: use drops; 6 months-3 years: 0.25 mg daily; 4-6 years: 0.5 mg daily; 7-16 years: 1 mg daily

        Chew tab: 0.25, 0.5, 1 mg (sugar-free)

    Luride Drops

    Pediatric: Water fluoridation 0.3-0.6 ppm: 6 months-3 years: 0.25 ml once daily; 4-6 years: 0.5 ml once daily; 7-16 years: 1 ml once daily; *Water fluoridation <0.3 ppm:* 6 months-3 years: 0.5 ml once daily; 4-6 years: 1 ml once daily; 7-16 years: 2 ml daily

        Oral drops: 0.5 mg/ml (50 ml) (sugar-free)

COMBINATION AGENTS

▷ *fluoride+vitamin a+vitamin d+vitamin c* (G)

    Pediatric: Water fluoridation 0.3-0.6 ppm: <3 years: <u>not</u> recommended; 3-6 years: 0.25 mg fluoride/day; 7-16 years: 0.5 mg fluoride/day; *Water fluoridation <0.3 ppm:* <6 months: <u>not</u> recommended; 6 months-3 years: 0.25 mg fluoride/day; 4-6 years: 0.5 mg fluoride/day; 7-16 years: 1 mg fluoride/day

    Tri-Vi-Flor Drops

        Oral drops: fluoride 0.25 mg+vit a 1,500 u+vit d 400 u+vit c 35 mg per ml (50 ml)

        Oral drops: fluoride 0.5 mg+vit a 1,500 u+vit d 400 u+vit c 35 mg per ml (50 ml)

▷ *fluoride+vitamin a+vitamin d+vitamin c+iron*

    Pediatric: Water fluoridation 0.3-0.6 ppm: <3 years: <u>not</u> recommended; 3-6 years: 0.25 mg fluoride/day; 7-16 years: 0.5 mg fluoride/day; *Water fluoridation <0.3 ppm:* <6 months: <u>not</u> recommended; 6 months-3 years: 0.25 mg fluoride/day; 4-6 years: 0.5 mg fluoride/day; 7-16 years: 1 mg fluoride/day

    Tri-Vi-Flor w. Iron Drops

        Oral drops: fluoride 0.25 mg+vit a 1500 u+vit d 400 u+vit c 35 mg+iron 10 mg per ml (50 ml)

FOLLICULITIS BARBAE

Topical Corticosteroids *see* Appendix J: Topical Corticosteroids by Potency

TOPICAL AGENTS

▷ *benzoyl peroxide* apply after shaving; may discolor clothing and linens

    Benzac W initially apply to affected area once daily; increase to bid-tid as tolerated

        Gel: 2.5, 5, 10% (60 gm)

    Benzac W Wash wash affected area bid

        Wash: 5% (4, 8 oz), 10% (8 oz)

    Benzagel apply to affected area one <u>or</u> more times a day

        Gel: 5, 10% (1.5, 3 oz) (alcohol 14%)

    Benzagel Wash wash affected area bid

        Gel: 10% (6 oz)

    Desquam X₅ wash affected area bid

        Wash: 5% (5 oz)

    Desquam X₁₀ wash affected area bid

        Wash: 10% (5 oz)

    Triaz apply to affected area daily bid

        Lotn: 3, 6, 9% (bottle), 3% (tube); *Pads:* 3, 6, 9% (jar)

    ZoDerm apply once <u>or</u> twice daily

        Gel: 4.5, 6.5, 8.5% (125 ml); *Crm:* 4.5, 6.5, 8.5% (125 ml); *Clnsr:* 4.5, 6.5, 8.5% (400 ml)

▷ *clindamycin* topical apply bid

    Pediatric: same as adult

        Cleocin T *Pad:* 1% (60/pck; alcohol 50%); *Lotn:* 1% (60 ml); *Gel:* 1% (30, 60 gm); *Soln w. applicator:* 1% (30, 60 ml) (alcohol 50%)

        Clindagel *Gel:* 1% (42, 77 gm)

        Clindets *Pad:* 1% (60/pck)

        Evoclin *Foam:* 1% (50, 100 gm) (alcohol)

▷ *clindamycin+benzoyl peroxide* topical (G)

    Pediatric: <12 years: <u>not</u> recommended; ≥12 years: same as adult

    Acanya apply once daily-bid

        Gel: clin 1.2%+benz 2.5% (50 gm)

    BenzaClin apply bid

        Gel: clin 1%+benz 5% (25, 50 gm)

    Duac apply daily in the evening

        Gel: clin 1%+benz 5% (45 gm)

Onexton Gel apply once daily
  Gel: clin 1.2%+benz 3.75% (50 gm pump) (alcohol-free) (preservative-free)
➤ *dapsone* topical **(G)** apply bid
  Pediatric: <12 years: <u>not</u> recommended; ≥12 years: same as adult
    Aczone *Gel:* 5% (30 gm)
➤ *tazarotene* **(G)** apply daily at HS
  Pediatric: <12 years: <u>not</u> recommended; ≥12 years: same as adult
    Avage Cream *Crm:* 0.1% (30 gm)
    Tazorac Cream *Crm:* 0.05, 0.1% (15, 30, 60 gm)
    Tazorac Gel *Gel:* 0.05, 0.1% (30, 100 gm)
➤ *tretinoin* **(G)** apply q HS
  Pediatric: <12 years: <u>not</u> recommended; ≥12 years: same as adult
    Atralin Gel *Gel:* 0.05% (45 gm)
    Avita *Crm:* 0.025% (20, 45 gm); *Gel:* 0.025% (20, 45 gm)
    Renova *Crm:* 0.02% (40 gm); 0.05% (40, 60 gm)
    Retin-A Cream *Crm:* 0.025, 0.05, 0.1% (20, 45 gm)
    Retin-A Gel *Gel:* 0.01, 0.025% (15, 45 gm) (alcohol 90%)
    Retin-A Liquid *Soln:* 0.05% (alcohol 55%)
    Retin-A Micro Gel *Gel:* 0.04, 0.08, 0.1% (20, 45 gm)
    Tretin-X Cream *Crm:* 0.075% (35 gm) (parabens-free, alcohol-free, propylene glycol-free)
    Retin-A Micro *Microspheres:* 0.04, 0.1% (20, 45 gm)

FOREIGN BODY: ESOPHAGUS

➤ *glucagon* 0.02 mg/kg IV <u>or</u> IM with serial x-rays; max 1 mg
  Glucagon (rDNA origin <u>or</u> beef/pork derived)
    Vial: 1 mg/ml w. diluent
  Comment: *Glucagon* facilitates passage of foreign body from esophagus into stomach.

FOREIGN BODY: EYE

➤ *proparacaine* 1-2 drops to anesthetize surface of the eye; then flush with normal saline
    Ophthaine *Ophth soln:* 0.5% (15 ml)
  Comment: *Proparacaine* facilitates the search, location, and removal of foreign body and examination of the cornea.

GASTRITIS/DYSPEPSIA

Antacids *see GERD*
H2 Antagonists *see GERD*

GASTRITIS-RELATED NAUSEA/VOMITING

OTC ANTIEMETIC
➤ *phosphorylated carbohydrate* solution **(G)** 1-2 tbsp q 15 minutes until nausea subsides; max 5 doses/day
  Pediatric: 1-2 tsp q 15 minutes until nausea subsides; max 5 doses/day
    Emetrol (OTC) *Soln:* dextrose 1.87 gm+fructose 1.87 gm+phosphoric acid 21.5 mg per 5 ml (4, 8, 16 oz)

Rx ANTIEMETICS
➤ *ondansetron* **(G)** 8 mg q 8 hours x 2 doses; then 8 mg q 12 hours
  Pediatric: <4 years: <u>not</u> recommended; 4-11 years: 4 mg q 4 hours x 3 doses; then 4 mg q 8 hours
    Zofran *Tab:* 4, 8, 24 mg
    Zofran ODT *ODT:* 4, 8 mg (strawberry) (phenylalanine)
    Zofran Oral Solution *Oral soln:* 4 mg/5 ml (50 ml) (strawberry) (phenylalanine); *Parenteral form:* see mfr pkg insert
    Zofran Injection *Vial:* 2 mg/ml (2 ml single-dose), 2 mg/ml (20 ml multidose), 32 mg/50 ml (50 ml multidose); *Prefilled syringe:* 4 mg/2 ml, single-use (24/carton)
    Zuplenz Oral Soluble Film: 4, 8 mg oral-dis (10/carton) (peppermint)
  Comment: The FDA has issued an updated warning against *ondansetron* use in pregnancy. *Ondansetron* is a 5-HT3 receptor antagonist approved by the FDA for preventing nausea and vomiting related to cancer chemotherapy and surgery. However, it has been used "off label" to treat the nausea and vomiting of pregnancy. The FDA has cautioned against the use of *ondansetron* in pregnancy in light of studies of *ondansetron* in early pregnancy and associated with congenital cardiac malformations and oral clefts (i.e., cleft lip and cleft palate). Further, there are potential maternal risks in pregnancy with electrolyte imbalance caused by severe nausea and vomiting (as with hyperemesis gravidarum). These risks include *serotonin syndrome* (a triad of cognitive and behavioral changes including confusion, agitation, autonomic instability, and neuromuscular changes). Therefore, *ondansetron* should <u>not</u> be taken during pregnancy.

(continued)

▷ *promethazine* (G) 25 mg PO or rectally q 4-6 hours prn
   Pediatric: <2 years: not recommended; ≥2 years: 0.5 mg/lb or 6.25-25 mg q 4-6 hours prn
     Phenergan *Tab:* 12.5*, 25*, 50 mg; *Plain syr:* 6.25 mg/5 ml; *Fortis syr:* 25 mg/5 ml; *Rectal supp:* 12.5, 25,
     50 mg
   Comment: *Promethazine* is contraindicated in children with uncomplicated nausea, dehydration, Reye's
syndrome, history of sleep apnea, asthma, and lower respiratory disorders. *Promethazine* lowers the seizure
threshold in children and may cause cholestatic jaundice, anticholinergic effects, extrapyramidal effects, and
potentially fatal respiratory depression.

GASTROESOPHAGEAL REFLUX (GER), GASTROESOPHAGEAL REFLUX DISEASE (GERD), IDIOPATHIC GASTRIC ACID HYPERSECRETION (IGAH)

Comment: Precipitators of gastric reflux include narcotics, benzodiazepines, calcium antagonists, alcohol,
nicotine, chocolate, and peppermint. Issues associated with H2 secretion and gastrointestinal (GI) health
(e.g., chronic remitting gastritis, Barrett's esophagitis, peptic ulcer disease [PUD]]), other organ system
impairments (e.g., cardiovascular disease [CVD], metabolic syndrome, hepatitis, autoimmune and immune
deficiency disorders, renal insufficiency), iatrogenic consequences of treatments (e.g., steroids, NSAIDs,
immune modulators), advanced age, and lifestyle (dietary habits and general nutritional health). Risk/benefit
discussions with patients can be challenging, but are necessary for informed decision-making and prudent
prescribing.

ANTACIDS
Comment: Antacids with *aluminum hydroxide* may potentiate constipation. Antacids with *magnesium
hydroxide* may potentiate diarrhea.
▷ *aluminum hydroxide*
   AlternaGEL (OTC) 5-10 ml between meals and HS prn; max 90 ml/day
   Pediatric: <12 years: not recommended; ≥12 years: same as adult
     Liq: 500 mg/5 ml (5, 12 oz)
   Amphojel (OTC) 10 ml 5-6 x/day between meals and HS prn; max 60 ml/day
   Pediatric: <12 years: not recommended; ≥12 years: same as adult
     Oral susp: 320 mg/5 ml (12 oz)
   Amphojel Tab (OTC) 600 mg 5-6 x a day between meals and HS prn; max 3.6 gm/day
   Pediatric: <12 years: not recommended; ≥12 years: same as adult
     Tab: 300, 600 mg
▷ *aluminum hydroxide+magnesium hydroxide* (OTC) (G)
   Maalox 10-20 ml qid and HS prn
   Pediatric: <12 years: not recommended; ≥12 years: same as adult
     Oral susp: alum 225 mg+mag 200 mg per 5 ml (5, 12, 26 oz) (mint, lemon, cherry)
   Maalox Therapeutic Concentrate 10-20 ml qid pc and HS prn
   Pediatric: <12 years: not recommended; ≥12 years: same as adult
     Oral susp: alum 600 mg+mag 300 mg per 5 ml (12 oz) (mint)
▷ *aluminum hydroxide+magnesium hydroxide+simethicone* (OTC)(G)
   Maalox Plus 10-20 ml qid pc and HS prn
   Pediatric: <12 years: not recommended; ≥12 years: same as adult
     Tab: alum 200 mg+mag 200 mg+sim 25 mg
   Extra Strength Maalox Plus 10-20 ml qid pc and HS prn
   Pediatric: <12 years: not recommended; ≥12 years: same as adult
     Tab: alum 350 mg+mag 350 mg+sim 30 mg
     Oral susp: alum 500 mg+mag 450 mg+sim 40 mg per 5 ml (5, 12, 26 oz)
   Extra Strength Maalox Plus Tab 1-3 tabs qid pc and HS prn
   Pediatric: <12 years: not recommended; ≥12 years: same as adult
     Tab: alum 350 mg+mag 350 mg+sim 30 mg
   Mylanta 10-20 ml between meals and HS prn
   Pediatric: <12 years: not recommended; ≥12 years: same as adult
     Liq: alum 200 mg+mag 200 mg+sim 20 mg per 5 ml (5, 12, 24 oz)
   Mylanta Double Strength 10-20 ml between meals and HS prn
   Pediatric: <12 years: not recommended; ≥12 years: same as adult
     Liq: alum 700 mg+mag 400 mg+sim 40 mg per 5 ml (5, 12, 24 oz)
▷ *aluminum hydroxide+magnesium carbonate* (OTC) (G)
   Maalox HRF 10-20 ml qid pc and HS prn
   Pediatric: <12 years: not recommended; ≥12 years: same as adults
     Oral susp: alum 280 mg+mag 350 mg per 10 ml (10 oz)
▷ *aluminum hydroxide+magnesium trisilicate* (G)
   Gaviscon chew 2-4 tabs qid pc and HS prn
   Pediatric: <12 years: not recommended; ≥12 years: same as adult
     Tab: alum 80 mg+mag 20 mg

Gaviscon Liquid 15-30 ml qid pc and HS prn
Pediatric: <12 years: not recommended; ≥12 years: same as adult
  Liq: alum 95 mg+mag 359 mg per 15 ml (6, 12 oz)
Gaviscon Extra Strength 2-4 tabs qid pc and HS prn
Pediatric: <12 years: not recommended; ≥12 years: same as adult
  Tab: alum 160 mg+mag 105 mg
Gaviscon Extra Strength Liquid 10-20 ml qid prn
Pediatric: <12 years: not recommended; ≥12 years: same as adult
  Liq: alum 508 mg+mag 475 mg per 10 ml (12 oz)
▷ *aluminum hydroxide+magnesium hydroxide+simethicone* (OTC)(G)
Maalox Maximum Strength 10-20 ml qid prn; max 60 ml/day
Pediatric: <12 years: not recommended; ≥12 years: same as adult
  Oral susp: alum 500 mg+mag 450 mg+sim 40 mg per 5 ml (5, 12, 26 oz) (mint, cherry)
▷ *calcium carbonate* (OTC)(G)
Children's Mylanta Tab
Pediatric: <2 years: not recommended; 2-5 years (24-47 lb): 1 tab as needed up to tid; 6-11 years (48-95 lb): 2 tabs as needed up to tid
  Tab: 400 mg
Children's Mylanta
Pediatric: <2 years: not recommended; 2-5 years (24-47 lb): 1 tab as needed up to tid; 6-11 years (48-95 lb): 2 tabs as needed up to tid
  Liq: 400 mg/5 ml (4 oz)
Maalox Tab chew 2-4 tabs prn; max 12 tabs/day
Pediatric: <12 years: not recommended; ≥12 years: same as adult
  Chew tab: 600 mg (wild berry, lemon, wintergreen) (phenylalanine)
Maalox Maximum Strength Tab 1-2 tabs prn; max 8 tabs/day
Pediatric: <12 years: not recommended; ≥12 years: same as adult
  Tab: 1 gm (wild berry, lemon, wintergreen; phenylalanine)
Rolaids Extra Strength 1-2 tabs dissolved in mouth or chewed q 1 hour prn; max 8 tabs/day
  Tab: 1,000 mg
Tums 1-2 tabs dissolved in mouth or chewed q 1 hour prn; max 16 tabs/day
  Tab: 500 mg
Tums E-X 1-2 tabs dissolved in mouth or chewed q 1 hour prn; max 16 tabs/day
  Tab: 750 mg
▷ *calcium carbonate+magnesium hydroxide*
Mylanta Tab 2-4 tabs between meals and HS prn
Pediatric: <12 years: not recommended; ≥12 years: same as adult
  Tab: calib 350 mg+mag 150 mg
Mylanta DS Tab 2-4 tabs between meals and HS prn
Pediatric: <12 years: not recommended; ≥12 years: same as adult
  Tab: calib 700 mg+mag 300 mg
Rolaids Sodium-Free 1-2 tabs dissolved in mouth or chewed q 1 hour as needed
  Tab: calib 317 mg+mag 64 mg
▷ *calcium carbonate+magnesium carbonate*
Mylanta Gel Caps (OTC) 2-4 caps prn
  Gelcap: calib 550 mg+mag 125 mg
▷ *dihydroxyaluminum*
Rolaids (OTC) 1-2 tabs dissolved in mouth or chewed q 1 hour prn; max 24 tabs/day
  Tab: 334 mg

H2 ANTAGONISTS
▷ *cimetidine* (OTC)(G) 800 mg bid or 400 mg qid; max 12 weeks
Pediatric: <16 years: not recommended; ≥16 years: same as adult
Tagamet 800 mg bid or 400 mg qid; max 12 weeks
  Tab: 200, 300, 400*, 800*mg
Tagamet HB *Prophylaxis:* 1 tab ac; *Treatment:* 1 tab bid
  Tab: 200 mg
Tagamet HB Oral Suspension *Prophylaxis:* 1-3 tsp ac; *Treatment:* 1 tsp bid
  Oral susp: 200 mg/20 ml (12 oz)
Tagamet Liquid *Liq:* 300 mg/5 ml (mint-peach) (alcohol 2.8%)
▷ *famotidine* (OTC)(G)
Pediatric: 0.5 mg/kg/day q HS prn or in 2 divided doses; max 40 mg/day
Maximum Strength Pepcid AC 1 tab ac
  Tab: 20 mg

(continued)

Pepcid 20-40 mg bid; max 6 weeks
Tab: 20, 40 mg; *Oral susp:* 40 mg/5 ml (50 ml)
Pepcid AC 1 tab ac; max 2 doses/day
   Tab/Rapid dissolving tab: 10 mg
Pepcid Complete (OTC) 1 tab ac; max 2 doses/day
   Tab: fam 10 mg+CaCO$_2$ 800 mg+mag hydroxide 165 mg
Pepcid RPD *Tab:* 20, 40 mg rapid dissolve
▷ *nizatidine* (OTC)(G) 150 mg bid <u>or</u> 300 mg once daily
   Pediatric: <12 years: <u>not</u> recommended; ≥12 years: same as adult
   Axid *Cap:* 150, 300 mg; *Oral soln:* 15 mg/ml (480 ml) (bubble gum)
▷ *ranitidine* (OTC)(G)
   Pediatric: <1 month: <u>not</u> recommended; 1 month to 16 years: 2-4 mg/kg/day in 2 divided doses; max 300
   mg/day; *duodenal/gastric ulcer:* 2-4 mg/kg/day divided bid; max 300 mg/day; *erosive esophagitis:* 5-10 mg/
   kg/day divided bid; max 300 mg/day; 20 lb, 9 kg: 0.6 ml; 30 lb, 13.6 kg: 0.9 ml; 40 lb, 18.2 kg: 1.2 ml; 50 lb,
   22.7 kg: 1.5 ml; 60 lb, 27.3 kg: 1.8 ml; 70 lb, 31.8 kg: 2.1 ml
   Zantac 150 mg bid <u>or</u> 300 mg q HS
      Tab: 150, 300 mg
   Zantac 75 1 tab ac
      Tab: 75 mg
   Zantac EFFERdose dissolve 25 mg tab in 5 ml water and dissolve 150 mg tab in 6-8 oz water
      Efferdose: 25, 150 mg effervescent
   Zantac Syrup *Syr:* 15 mg/ml (peppermint) (alcohol 7.5%)
▷ *ranitidine bismuth citrate* 400 mg bid
   Pediatric: <12 years: <u>not</u> recommended; ≥12 years: same as adult
   Tritec *Tab:* 400 mg

PROTON PUMP INHIBITORS (PPIs)

Comment: A study of 144,032 incident users of acid suppression therapy, including 125,596 proton pump
inhibitor (PPI) users and 18,436 histamine H2 receptor antagonist users were followed over 5 years. The
researchers reported PPI users had an increased risk of having an eGFR <60 ml/min/1.73m², incident CKD,
eGFR decline over 30%, and end-stage renal disease (ESRD) <u>or</u> eGFR decline over 50%, as compared with
those taking H2 blockers. They concluded "reliance on antecedent acute kidney injury (AKI) as a warning sign
to guard against the risk of CKD among PPI users is <u>not</u> sufficient as a sole mitigation strategy." Further, timely
PPI discontinuation is warranted if there is a first AKI to avoid progression to CKD.

Comment: Practice guidelines from the American Gastroenterological Association (AGA) address risks and
recommendations for prescribing PPI therapy based on an extensive review of the literature. PPI use may
increase the risk of fracture, vitamin B12 deficiency, hypomagnesemia, iron deficiency anemia, small intestinal
bacterial overgrowth (SIBO), *Clostridium difficile* infection, kidney disease, CVD, pneumonias, and dementia.
Healthcare providers are advised to discuss the risks/benefits of PPI therapy with respect to each individual
patient's situation.

▷ *dexlansoprazole* (G) 30-60 mg daily for up to 4 weeks
   Pediatric: <18 years: <u>not</u> recommended; ≥18 years: same as adult
   Dexilant *Cap:* 30, 60 mg ent-coat del-rel granules; may open and sprinkle on applesauce; do <u>not</u> crush <u>or</u>
   chew granules
   Dexilant SoluTab *Tab:* 30 mg del-rel orally disint
▷ *esomeprazole* (OTC)(G) 20-40 mg once daily; max 8 weeks; take 1 hour before food; swallow whole <u>or</u> mix
   granules with food <u>or</u> juice and take immediately; do <u>not</u> crush <u>or</u> chew granules
   Pediatric: <1 month: <u>not</u> established; 1 month-<1 year, 3-5 kg: 2.5 mg; 5-7.5 kg: 5 mg; 7.5-12 kg: 10 mg; 1-11
   years, <20 kg: 10 mg; ≥20 kg: 10-20 mg; 12-17 years: 20 mg; max 8 weeks; >17 years: same as adult
   Nexium *Cap:* 20, 40 mg ent-coat del-rel pellets
   Nexium for Oral Suspension *Oral susp:* 10, 20, 40 mg ent-coat del-rel granules/pkt; mix in 2 tbsp water
   and drink immediately; 30 pkt/carton
▷ *lansoprazole* (OTC)(G) 15-30 mg daily for up to 8 weeks; may repeat course; take before eating
   Pediatric: <1 year: <u>not</u> recommended; 1-11 years, <30 kg: 15 mg once daily; >11 years: same as adult
   Prevacid *Cap:* 15, 30 mg ent-coat del-rel granules; swallow whole <u>or</u> mix granules with food <u>or</u> juice and
   take immediately; do <u>not</u> crush <u>or</u> chew granules; follow with water
   Prevacid for Oral Suspension *Oral susp:* 15, 30 mg ent-coat del-rel granules/pkt; mix in 2 tbsp water and
   drink immediately; 30 pkt/carton (strawberry)
   Prevacid SoluTab *ODT:* 15, 30 mg (strawberry) (phenylalanine)
   Prevacid 24HR 15 mg ent-coat del-rel granules; swallow whole <u>or</u> mix granules with food <u>or</u> juice and
   take immediately; do <u>not</u> crush <u>or</u> chew granules; follow with water
▷ *omeprazole* (OTC)(G) 20-40 mg daily for 14 days; may repeat course in 4 months; take before eating;
   swallow whole <u>or</u> mix granules with applesauce and take immediately; do <u>not</u> crush <u>or</u> chew granules;
   follow with water

Pediatric: <18 years: <u>not</u> recommended; ≥18 years: same as adult

   Prilosec *Cap:* 10, 20, 40 mg ent-coat del-rel granules

   Pediatric: <1 year: <u>not</u> recommended; ≥1 year, 5 to <10 kg: 5 mg daily; 10 to <20 kg: 10 mg daily; ≥20 kg: same as adult

   Prilosec OTC *Tab:* 20 mg del-rel (regular, wildberry, strawberry)

   Pediatric: <18 years: <u>not</u> recommended; ≥18 years: same as adult

➢ **pantoprazole (G)** 40 mg daily

   Pediatric: <12 years: <u>not</u> recommended; ≥12 years: same as adult

   Protonix *Tab:* 40 mg ent-coat del-rel

   Protonix for Oral Suspension *Oral susp:* 40 mg ent-coat del-rel granules/pkt; mix in 1 tsp apple juice for 5 seconds <u>or</u> sprinkle on 1 tsp apple sauce, and swallow immediately; do <u>not</u> mix in water <u>or</u> any other liquid <u>or</u> food; take approximately 30 minutes prior to a meal; 30 pkt/carton

➢ **rabeprazole (OTC)(G)** *Tab:* 20 mg daily after breakfast; do <u>not</u> crush <u>or</u> chew; *Cap:* open cap and sprinkle contents on a small amount of soft food <u>or</u> liquid

   Pediatric: <1 year: <u>not</u> recommended; 1-11 years, <15 kg: 5 mg once daily for up to 12 weeks; ≥12 years, ≥15 kg: same as adult

   AcipHex *Tab:* 20 mg ent-coat del-rel

   AcipHex Sprinkle *Cap:* 5, 10 mg del-rel

PPI+SODIUM BICARBONATE COMBINATION

➢ **omeprazole+sodium bicarbonate (G)** 20 mg daily; do <u>not</u> crush <u>or</u> chew; max 8 weeks

   Pediatric: <18 years: <u>not</u> recommended; ≥18 years: same as adult

   Zegerid *Cap:* omep 20 mg+sod bicarb 1,100 mg; omep 40 mg+sod bicarb 1,100 mg

   Zegerid OTC (OTC) *Cap:* omep 20 mg+sod bicarb 1,100 mg

   Zegerid for Oral Suspension *Pwdr for oral susp:* omep 20 mg+sod bicarb 1,680 mg; omep 40 mg+sod bicarb 1,680 mg (30 pkt/carton)

PROMOTILITY AGENT

➢ **metoclopramide (G)** 10-15 mg qid 30 minutes ac and HS prn; up to 20 mg prior to provoking situation; max 12 weeks per therapeutic course

   Pediatric: <18 years: <u>not</u> recommended; ≥18 years: same as adult

   Metozolv ODT *ODT:* 5, 10 mg (mint)

   Reglan *Tab:* 5*, 10 mg; *Syr:* 5 mg/5 ml

   Reglan ODT *ODT:* 5, 10 mg (orange)

Comment: *Metoclopramide* is contraindicated when stimulation of GI motility may be dangerous. Observe for tardive dyskinesia and parkinsonism. Avoid concomitant drugs which may cause an extrapyramidal reaction (e.g., phenothiazines, *haloperidol*).

GAUCHER DISEASE TYPE 1

Comment: Gaucher disease type 1 (GD1) is the most common form of Gaucher disease. Like other types of Gaucher disease, GD1 is caused when insufficient glucocerebrosidase (GBA), an enzyme that breaks down glucocerebroside, is produced. Fat-filled Gaucher cells build up in areas like the spleen, liver, and bone marrow. Unlike types 2 and 3, GD1 does <u>not</u> usually involve the central nervous system. Symptoms of GD1 include enlarged spleen and liver, low blood cell counts, bleeding problems, and bone disease. Symptoms can range from mild to severe and may appear anytime from childhood to adulthood. Gaucher disease is caused by mutations in the GBA gene and is inherited as an autosomal-recessive gene. Treatments may include enzyme replacement therapy <u>or</u> medications that affect the making of fatty molecules (substrate reduction therapy). Patients with GD1 are usually able to live a normal lifespan. GD2 is universally fatal within 2 years. Patients with GD3 have a life expectancy of 20-40 years.

GLUCOSYLCERAMIDE SYNTHASE INHIBITORS

➢ **eliglustat tartrate (G)** select patients using an FDA-cleared test for determining CYP2D6 genotype; *CYP2D6 extensive metabolizers (EMs) and intermediate metabolizers (IMs):* 84 mg orally bid; *CYP2D6 poor metabolizers (PMs):* 84 mg once daily; swallow capsules whole; do <u>not</u> crush, dissolve, <u>or</u> open capsules; avoid eating grapefruit <u>or</u> drinking grapefruit juice; *Moderate-to-severe renal impairment:* <u>not</u> recommended; *Hepatic impairment:* <u>not</u> recommended

   Pediatric: safety and efficacy <u>not</u> established

   Cerdelga *Cap:* 84 mg

   Comment: **Cerdelga** is a glucosylceramide synthase inhibitor indicated for the long-term treatment of adult patients with GD1 who are CYP2D6 EMs, IMs, <u>or</u> PMs as detected by an FDA-cleared test. CYP2D6 ultra-rapid metabolizers may <u>not</u> achieve adequate concentrations of **Cerdelga** to achieve a therapeutic effect. A specific dosage cannot be recommended for CYP2D6 indeterminate metabolizers. Contraindications to **Cerdelga** are (1) CYP2D6 EMs and IMs taking a strong <u>or</u> moderate CYP2D6 inhibitor with a strong <u>or</u>

(continued)

moderate CYP3A inhibitor and (2) CYP2D6 IMs and PMs taking a strong CYP3A inhibitor. **Cerdelga** is not recommended in patients with preexisting cardiac disease, long QT syndrome, and concomitant use of class IA and Class III antiarrhythmics. *Eliglustat* is a CYP2D6 and CYP3A substrate. Co-administration of **Cerdelga** with drugs that inhibit CYP2D6 and CYP3A may significantly increase the exposure to *eliglustat* and result in prolongation of the PR, QTc, and/or QRS cardiac interval, which could result in cardiac arrhythmias. Consider potential drug interactions prior to and during therapy. CYP2D6 IMs and PMs taking moderate CYP3A inhibitors is not recommended. CYP2D6 PMs taking weak CYP3A inhibitors is not recommended. For CYP2D6 EMs and IMs taking strong or moderate CYP2D6 inhibitors and CYP2D6 EMs taking strong or moderate CYP3A inhibitors, reduce the **Cerdelga** dosage to 84 mg once daily. *Eliglustat* is an inhibitor of P-glycoprotein (P-gp) and CYP2D6. Co-administration with drugs that are substrates for P-gp or CYP2D6 may result in increased concentrations of the other drug. See the mfr pkg insert for full prescribing information and for a list of clinically significant drug interactions. The most common adverse reactions (incidence ≥10%) have been fatigue, headache, nausea, diarrhea, back pain, pain in extremities, and upper abdominal pain. Females with GD1 have an increased risk of spontaneous abortion, especially if disease symptoms are not treated and controlled preconception and during pregnancy. Pregnancy may exacerbate existing GD1 symptoms or result in new disease manifestations. GD1 manifestations may lead to adverse pregnancy outcomes, including hepatosplenomegaly, which can interfere with the normal growth of a pregnancy, and thrombocytopenia, which can lead to increased bleeding and possible hemorrhage. Animal studies have not ruled out adverse effects of **Cerdelga** on the developing fetus. Advise females of reproductive potential of the risk to the fetus and advise using effective contraception. Establish pregnancy status prior to initiating treatment. It is not known whether **Cerdelga** is present in human milk. Because of the potential for serious adverse reactions in breastfed infants from **Cerdelga**, a decision should be made whether to discontinue nursing or discontinue the drug, taking into account the importance of the drug to the mother. To report suspected adverse reactions, contact Genzyme Corporation at 800-745-4447 or FDA at 1-800-FDA-1088 or www.fda.gov/medwatch.

▸ *miglustat* (G) 100 mg tid at regular intervals; may reduce dose to 100 mg to once daily or bid in some patients due to tremor or diarrhea; *CrCl 50-70 ml/min:* start dose at 100 mg bid; *CrCl 30-50 ml/min:* 100 mg once daily; *CrCl <30 ml/min:* not recommended

 Zavesca *Cap* 100 mg

 Comment: Zavesca *(miglustat)* is a glucosylceramide synthase inhibitor indicated as monotherapy for the treatment of adult patients with mild/moderate GD1 for whom enzyme replacement therapy is not a therapeutic option. The most common adverse reactions (incidence ≥5%) are diarrhea, weight loss, stomach pain, gas, nausea, vomiting, headache, including migraine, tremor, leg cramps, dizziness, weakness, vision problems, thrombocytopenia, muscle cramps, back pain, constipation, dry mouth, heaviness in arms and legs, memory loss, unsteady walking, anorexia, indigestion, paresthesia, stomach bloating, stomach pain not related to food, and menstrual changes. Based on animal data, it may cause fetal harm. Discontinue **Zavesca** or breastfeeding based on the importance of the drug to the mother.

▸ *penicillamine* administer on an empty stomach, at least 1 hour before meals or 2 hours after meals, and at least 1 hour apart from any other drug, food, milk, antacid, and zinc- or iron-containing preparation; dosage must be individualized and may require adjustment during the course of treatment; initially, a single daily dose of 125-250 mg; then increase at 1 to 3 month intervals by 125-250 mg/day as patient response and tolerance indicate; if a satisfactory remission of symptoms is achieved, the dose associated with the remission should be continued as the patient's maintenance therapy; if there is no improvement and there are no signs of potentially serious toxicity after 2-3 months of treatment with doses of 500-750 mg/day, increase by 250 mg/day at 2 to 3 month intervals until a satisfactory remission occurs or signs of toxicity develop; if there is no discernible improvement after 3-4 months of treatment with 1,000-1,500 mg/day, discontinue **Cuprimine**; changes in maintenance dosage levels may not be reflected clinically or in the erythrocyte sedimentation rate (ESR) for 2-3 months after each dosage adjustment

 Cuprimine *Cap:* 125, 250 mg

 Depen: 250 mg

Comment: Taking *penicillamine* on an empty stomach permits maximum absorption and reduces the likelihood of inactivation by metal binding in the gastrointestinal (GI) tract. Optimal dosage can be determined by measurement of urinary copper excretion and determination of free copper in the serum. The urine must be collected in copper-free glassware and should be quantitatively analyzed for copper before and soon after initiation of therapy with **Cuprimine**. Determination of 24-hour urinary copper excretion is of greatest value in the first week of therapy with *penicillamine*. In the absence of any drug reaction, a dose between 0.75 and 1.5 gm that results in an initial 24-hour cupriuresis of over 2 mg should be continued for about 3 months, by which time the most reliable method of monitoring maintenance treatment is the determination of free copper in the serum. This equals the difference between quantitatively determined total copper and ceruloplasmin-copper. Adequately treated patients will usually have less than 10 mcg free copper/dL of serum. It is seldom necessary to exceed a dosage of 2 gm/day. In patients who cannot tolerate as much as 1 gm/day initially, initiating dosage with 250 mg/day and increasing gradually to the requisite amount gives closer control of the effects of the drug and may help reduce the incidence of adverse reactions. If the patient is intolerant to therapy with **Cuprimine**, an alternative treatment is *trientine* (Syprine). The use of *penicillamine* has been associated with fatalities due to certain diseases such as aplastic anemia, agranulocytosis, thrombocytopenia, Goodpasture's syndrome, and myasthenia gravis. Because of the potential for serious hematologic and renal adverse reactions to occur at any time, routine urinalysis, white and differential blood cell count, hemoglobin, and direct platelet count must be checked twice weekly, together with monitoring of the patient's skin, lymph nodes, and body temperature, during the first month of therapy, every 2 weeks for the next 5 months, and monthly thereafter. Patients should be instructed to report promptly the development of signs and symptoms of granulocytopenia and/or thrombocytopenia, such as fever, sore throat, chills, bruising, or bleeding; the above laboratory studies should then be promptly repeated.

▷ *trientine* (G) recommended initial dose is 500-750 mg/day for pediatric patients and 750-1250 mg/day for adults given in divided doses 2, 3, or 4 x/day; may be increased to max 2,000 mg/day for adults or 1,500 mg/day for patients ≤12 years of age; the daily dose of **Syprine** should be increased only when the clinical response is not adequate or the concentration of free serum copper is persistently above 20 mcg/dL; optimal long-term maintenance dose should be determined at 6 to 12 month intervals; administer on an empty stomach, at least 1 hour before meals or 2 hours after meals and at least 1 hour apart from any other drug, food, or milk; swallow whole with water; do not open the cap or chew the contents

    Syprine *Cap* 250 mg

    Comment: **Syprine** is indicated for the treatment of patients with Wilson's disease who are intolerant of *penicillamine*. Clinical experience with **Syprine** is limited and alternate dosing regimens have not been well characterized; all endpoints in determining an individual patient's dose have not been well defined. **Syprine** and *penicillamine* cannot be considered interchangeable. **Syprine** should be used when continued treatment with *penicillamine* is no longer possible because of intolerable or life-endangering side effects. Unlike *penicillamine*, **Syprine** is not recommended in cystinuria or rheumatoid arthritis. The absence of a sulfhydryl moiety renders it incapable of binding cystine and therefore it is of no use in cystinuria. In 15 patients with rheumatoid arthritis, **Syprine** was reported not to be effective in improving any clinical or biochemical parameter after 12 weeks of treatment. The most reliable index for monitoring treatment is the determination of free copper in the serum, which equals the difference between quantitatively determined total copper and ceruloplasmin-copper. Adequately treated patients will usually have less than 10 mcg free copper/dL of serum. Therapy may be monitored with a 24-hour urinary copper analysis periodically (i.e., every 6-12 months). Urine must be collected in copper-free glassware. Since a low copper diet should keep copper absorption down to <1 mg a day, the patient probably will be in the desired state of negative copper balance if 0.5 to 1 mg of copper is present in a 24-hour collection of urine. In general, mineral supplements should not be used since they may block the absorption of **Syprine**. However, iron deficiency may develop, especially in children and menstruating or pregnant females, or as a result of the low copper diet recommended for Wilson's disease. If necessary, iron may be given in short courses, but since iron and **Syprine** each inhibit absorption of the other, 2 hours should elapse between administration of **Syprine** and iron. *Trientine* was teratogenic in animals at doses similar to the human dose. The frequencies of both resorptions and fetal abnormalities, including hemorrhage and edema, increased while fetal copper levels decreased when *trientine* was given in the maternal diets. There are no adequate and well-controlled studies in pregnant females. **Syprine** should be used during pregnancy only if the potential benefit justifies the potential risk to the fetus. It is not known whether this drug is excreted in human milk. Caution should be exercised when **Syprine** is administered to a nursing mother. Clinical studies of **Syprine** did not include sufficient numbers of subjects ≥65 years of age to determine whether they respond differently from younger subjects. Other reported clinical experience is insufficient to determine differences in responses between the elderly and younger patients. In general, dose selection should be cautious, usually starting at the low end of the dosing range, reflecting the greater frequency of decreased hepatic, renal, or cardiac function, and of concomitant disease or other drug therapy. Clinical experience with **Syprine** has been limited. The following adverse reactions have been reported in a clinical study in patients with Wilson's disease who were on therapy with *trientine:* iron deficiency and systemic lupus erythematosus. In addition, the following adverse reactions have been reported in marketed use: dystonia, muscular spasm, and myasthenia gravis.

GIANT CELL ARTERITIS (GCA)/TEMPORAL ARTERITIS

Acetaminophen for IV Infusion *see Pain*
NSAIDs *see* Appendix I. NSAIDs online at https://connect.springerpub.com/content/reference-book/978-0-8261-7935-7/back-matter/part02/back-matter/bmatter10
Opioid Analgesics *see Pain*
Topical and Transdermal Analgesics *see Pain*
Parenteral Corticosteroids *see* Appendix L. Parenteral Corticosteroids
Oral Corticosteroids *see* Appendix K. Oral Corticosteroids

Comment: Giant cell arteritis (GCA), or temporal arteritis, is a systemic inflammatory vasculitis of unknown etiology that occurs in persons ≥50 years of age (median age of onset is 75 years) and can result in a wide variety of systemic, neurologic, and ophthalmologic complications. GCA is the most common form of systemic vasculitis in adults. Other names for GCA include arteritis cranialis, Horton's disease, granulomatous arteritis, and arteritis of the aged. GCA typically affects the superficial temporal arteries— hence the term temporal arteritis. In addition, GCA most commonly affects the ophthalmic, occipital,

(continued)

vertebral, posterior ciliary, and proximal vertebral arteries. It has also been shown to involve medium- and large-sized vessels, including the aorta and the carotid, subclavian, and iliac arteries. Common early symptoms include headache and visual difficulties. Potential consequences include blindness and aortic aneurysms. Newly recognized GCA should be considered a true neuro-ophthalmic emergency. Prompt initiation of treatment may prevent blindness and other potentially irreversible ischemic sequelae. Corticosteroids are the mainstay of therapy. In steroid-resistant cases, drugs such as *cyclosporine*, *azathioprine*, or *methotrexate* (*MTX*) may be used as steroid-sparing agents. GCA is the most common systemic vasculitis affecting elderly patients.

INTERLEUKIN-6 RECEPTOR ANTAGONIST

▷ *tocilizumab* <*100 kg:* 162 mg SC every other week on the same day followed by an increase according to clinical response; ≥*100 kg:* 162 mg SC once weekly on the same day; SC injections may be self-administered

Actemra *Vial:* 80 mg/4 ml, 200 mg/10 ml, 400 mg/20 ml, single-use, for IV infusion after dilution; *Prefilled syringe:* 162 mg (0.9 ml, single-dose); *Prefilled ACTPen autoinjector:* 162 mg/0.9 ml, single-dose, for SC administration

Comment: Actemra received FDA approval in May 2017 to treat GCA. This is the first FDA-approved drug specifically for the treatment of this form of vasculitis. *Tocilizumab* is an interleukin-6 receptor-alpha inhibitor also indicated for use in moderate-to-severe rheumatoid arthritis (RA) that has not responded to conventional therapy and some subtypes of juvenile idiopathic arthritis (JIA). Actemra may be used alone or in combination with *MTX*, and in RA other disease-modifying antirheumatic drugs (DMARDs) may be used. Monitor patient for dose-related laboratory changes including elevated liver function tests (LFTs), neutropenia, and thrombocytopenia. Actemra should not be initiated in patients with an absolute neutrophil count (ANC) <2,000/mm³, platelet count <100,000/mm³, or who have alanine aminotransferase (ALT) or aspartate aminotransferase (AST) above 1.5 times the upper limit of normal (ULN). Registration in the Pregnancy Exposure Registry (1-877-311-8972) is encouraged for monitoring pregnancy outcomes in women exposed to Actemra during pregnancy. The limited available data with Actemra in pregnant females are not sufficient to determine whether there is a drug-associated risk of major birth defects and miscarriage. Monoclonal antibodies, such as *tocilizumab*, are actively transported across the placenta during the 3rd trimester of pregnancy and may affect immune response in the infant exposed *in utero*. It is not known whether *tocilizumab* passes into breast milk; therefore, breastfeeding is not recommended while using Actemra.

GIARDIASIS (*GIARDIA LAMBLIA*)

▷ *metronidazole* (G) 250 mg tid x 5-10 days
Pediatric: 35-50 mg/kg/day in 3 divided doses x 10 days
Flagyl *Tab:* 250*, 500*mg
Flagyl 375 *Cap:* 375 mg
Flagyl ER *Tab:* 750 mg ext-rel

▷ *tinidazole* 2 gm in a single dose; take with food
Pediatric: <3 years: not recommended; ≥3 years: 50 mg/kg daily in a single dose; take with food; max 2 gm
Tindamax *Tab:* 250*, 500*mg

Comment: Other than for use in the treatment of *giardiasis* and *amebiasis* in pediatric patients older than 3 years of age, the safety and effectiveness of *tinidazole* in pediatric patients have not been established. *Tinidazole* is excreted in breast milk in concentrations similar to those seen in serum and can be detected in breast milk for up to 72 hours following administration. Interruption of breastfeeding is recommended during *tinidazole* therapy and for 3 days following the last dose.

▷ *nitazoxanide* (G) 500 mg q 12 hours x 3 days; take with food
Pediatric: <1 year: not recommended; 1-3 years: 100 mg q 12 hours x 3 days; 4-11 years: 200 mg q 12 hours x 3 days; ≥12 years: same as adult
Alinia *Tab:* 500 mg; *Oral susp:* 100 mg/5 ml (60 ml)

Comment: Alinia is an antiprotozoal for the treatment of diarrhea due to *Giardia lamblia* or *Cryptosporidium parvum*.

GINGIVITIS/PERIODONTITIS

ANTI-INFECTIVE ORAL RINSES

Comment: Oral treatments should be preceded by brushing and flossing the teeth. Avoid foods and liquids for 2-3 hours after a treatment

▷ *chlorhexidine gluconate* (G) swish 15 ml undiluted for 30 seconds bid; do not swallow; do not rinse mouth after treatment
Peridex, PerioGard *Oral soln:* 0.12% (480 ml)

GLAUCOMA: OPEN-ANGLE/OCULAR HYPERTENSION

Comment: Other ophthalmic medications should <u>not</u> be administered within 5-10 minutes of administering an ophthalmic antiglaucoma medication. Contact lenses should be removed prior to instillation of antiglaucoma medications and may be replaced 15 minutes later. Interactions with ophthalmic antiglaucoma agents include monoamine oxidase inhibitors (MAOIs), central nervous system (CNS) depressants, beta-blockers, tricyclic antidepressants, and hypoglycemics. Choices for medical treatment in progressive cases include **betaxolol** eye drops, which have a beneficial effect on optic nerve blood flow in addition to intraocular pressure (IOP) reduction. Other beta-blockers and adrenergic drugs (such as **dipivefrine**) should better be avoided due to the probability of nocturnal systemic hypotension and optic nerve hypoperfusion (e.g., in patients with untreated obstructive sleep apnea). Prostaglandin derivatives tend to have greater IOP-lowering effect which may be of overriding consideration. **Dorzolamide-timolol** fixed combination is a safe and effective IOP-lowering agent in patients with normal tension glaucoma (NTG). **Brimonidine** significantly improved retinal vascular autoregulation in NTG patients.

OPHTHALMIC ALPHA-2 ADRENERGIC RECEPTOR AGONISTS
Comment: Ophthalmic alpha-2 agonists are contraindicated with concomitant MAOI use. Cautious use with CNS depressants, beta-blockers (ocular and systemic), antihypertensives, cardiac glycosides, and tricyclic antidepressants.
➤ **apraclonidine** ophthalmic solution 1-2 drops affected eye tid
  Pediatric: <12 years: <u>not</u> recommended; ≥12 years: same as adult
    Iopidine *Ophth soln:* 0.5% (5 ml) (benzalkonium chloride)
➤ **brimonidine tartrate** ophthalmic solution **(G)** 1 drop affected eye q 8 hours
  Pediatric: <2 years: <u>not</u> recommended; ≥2 years: 1 drop affected eye q 8 hours
    Alphagan P *Ophth soln:* 0.1, 0.15% (5, 10, 15 ml) (purite)

OPHTHALMIC CARBONIC ANHYDRASE INHIBITORS
Comment: Ophthalmic carbonic anhydrase inhibitors are contraindicated in patients with sulfa allergy.
➤ **brinzolamide (G)** ophthalmic suspension 1 drop affected eye tid
  Pediatric: <12 years: <u>not</u> recommended; ≥12 years: same as adult
    Azopt *Ophth susp:* 1% (2.5, 5, 10, 15 ml) (benzalkonium chloride)
➤ **dorzolamide** ophthalmic solution **(G)** 1 drop affected eye tid
  Pediatric: same as adult
    Trusopt *Ophth soln:* 2% (10 ml) (benzalkonium chloride)

OPHTHALMIC ALPHA-2 ADRENERGIC RECEPTOR AGONIST+CARBONIC ANHYDRASE INHIBITOR
➤ **brimonidine+brinzolamide** 1 drop affected eye tid
  Pediatric: <12 years: <u>not</u> recommended; ≥12 years: same as adult
    Simbrinza *Ophth soln:* brim 1% mg+brinz 0.2% per ml (10 ml)

OPHTHALMIC CHOLINERGICS (MIOTICS)
➤ **carbachol+hydroxypropyl methylcellulose** ophthalmic solution 2 drops affected eye tid
  Pediatric: <12 years: <u>not</u> recommended; ≥12 years: same as adult
    Isopto Carbachol *Ophth soln:* carb 0.75% <u>or</u> 2.25%+hydroxy 1% (15 ml); carb 1.5% <u>or</u> 3%+hydroxy 1% (15, 30 ml) (benzalkonium chloride)
➤ **pilocarpine (G)**
  Pediatric: <12 years: <u>not</u> recommended; ≥12 years: same as adult
    Isopto Carpine 2 drops affected eye tid-qid
      Ophth soln: 1, 2, 4% (15 ml) (benzalkonium chloride)
    Ocusert Pilo change ophthalmic insert once weekly
      Ophth inserts: 20 mcg/hour (8/pck)
    Pilocar Ophthalmic Solution 1-2 drops affected eye 1 to 6 x/day
      Ophth soln: 0.5, 1, 2, 3, 4, 6, 8% (15 ml)
    Pilopine HS apply 1/2 inch ribbon in lower conjunctival sac q HS
    Ophth gel: 4% (4 gm)

OPHTHALMIC CHOLINESTERASE INHIBITORS
➤ **demecarium bromide** ophthalmic solution 1-2 drops affected eye q 12-48 hours
  Pediatric: <12 years: <u>not</u> recommended; ≥12 years: same as adult
    Humorsol Ocumeter *Ophth soln:* 0.125, 0.25% (5 ml)
➤ **echothiophate iodide** ophthalmic solution initially 1 drop of 0.03% affected eye bid; then increase strength as needed
  Pediatric: <12 years: <u>not</u> recommended; ≥12 years: same as adult
    Phospholine Iodide *Ophth soln:* 0.03, 0.06, 0.125, 0.25% (5 ml)

(continued)

OPHTHALMIC CARDIOSELECTIVE BETA-BLOCKERS

Comment: Ophthalmic beta-blockers are generally contraindicated in severe chronic obstructive pulmonary disease (COPD), history of or current bronchial asthma, sinus bradycardia, 2nd or 3rd degree AV block.

▷ *betaxolol* ophthalmic solution **(G)** 1-2 drops affected eye bid
  Pediatric: <12 years: not recommended; ≥12 years: same as adult
    Betoptic *Ophth soln:* 0.5% (5, 10, 15 ml) (benzalkonium chloride)
    Betoptic S *Ophth soln:* 0.25% (2.5, 5, 10, 15 ml) (benzalkonium chloride)

OPHTHALMIC BETA-BLOCKERS (NON-CARDIOSELECTIVE)

Comment: Ophthalmic beta-blockers are generally contraindicated in severe COPD, history of or current bronchial asthma, sinus bradycardia, 2nd or 3rd degree AV block.

▷ *carteolol* ophthalmic solution **(G)** 1 drop affected eye bid
  Pediatric: <12 years: not recommended; ≥12 years: same as adult
    Ocupress *Ophth soln:* 1% (5, 10, 15 ml) (benzalkonium chloride)
▷ *levobunolol* ophthalmic solution 1-2 drops affected eye bid
  Pediatric: <12 years: not recommended; ≥12 years: same as adult
    Betagan *Ophth soln:* 0.5% (5, 10, 15 ml) (benzalkonium chloride)
▷ *metipranolol* ophthalmic solution **(G)** 1 drop affected eye bid
  Pediatric: <12 years: not recommended; ≥12 years: same as adult
    OptiPranolol *Ophth soln:* 0.3% (5, 10 ml) (benzalkonium chloride)
▷ *timolol* ophthalmic solution and gel **(G)**
  Pediatric: <12 years: not recommended; ≥12 years: same as adult
    Betimol 1 drop affected eye bid
      Ophth soln: 0.25, 0.5% (5, 10, 15 ml) (benzalkonium chloride)
    Istalol 1 drop affected eye daily
      Ophth soln: 0.5% (2.5, 5 ml) (preservative-free)
    Timoptic 1 drop affected eye bid
      Ophth soln: 0.25, 0.5% (5, 10, 15 ml) (benzalkonium chloride)
    Timoptic Ocudose 1 drop bid
      Ophth soln: 0.25, 0.5% (0.2 ml/dose, 60 dose) (preservative-free)
    Timoptic-XE 1 drop affected eye bid
      Ophth gel: 0.25, 0.5% (2.5, 5 ml) (preservative-free)

OPHTHALMIC ALPHA-2 ADRENERGIC RECEPTOR AGONIST+NON-CARDIOSELECTIVE BETA-BLOCKER COMBINATION

Comment: Generally contraindicated in severe COPD, history of or current bronchial asthma, sinus bradycardia, and 2nd or 3rd degree AV block.

▷ *brimonidine tartrate+timolol* ophthalmic solution **(G)** 1 drop affected eye bid
  Pediatric: <2 years: not recommended; ≥2 years: same as adult
    Combigan *Ophth soln:* brimo 0.2%+timo 0.5% (5, 10, 15 ml) (benzalkonium chloride)

OPHTHALMIC PROSTAMIDE ANALOGS

▷ *bimatoprost* ophthalmic solution **(G)** 1 drop q affected eye HS
  Pediatric: <16 years: not recommended; ≥16 years: same as adult
    Lumigan *Ophth soln:* 0.01, 0.03% (2.5, 5, 7.5 ml) (benzalkonium chloride)
▷ *latanoprost* ophthalmic solution 1 drop affected eye q HS
  Pediatric: <12 years: not recommended; ≥12 years: same as adult
    Xalatan *Ophth soln:* 0.005% (2.5 ml) (benzalkonium chloride)
▷ *tafluprost* ophthalmic solution **(G)** 1 drop affected eye q HS
  Pediatric: <12 years: not recommended; ≥12 years: same as adult
    Zioptan *Ophth soln:* 0.0015% (0.3 ml single-use, 30-60/carton) (preservative-free)
▷ *travoprost* ophthalmic solution **(G)** 1 drop affected eye q HS
  Pediatric: <16 years: not recommended; ≥16 years: same as adult
    Travatan *Ophth soln:* 0.004% (2.5, 5 ml) (benzalkonium chloride)
    Travatan Z *Ophth soln:* 0.004% (2.5, 5 ml) (boric acid, propylene glycol, sorbitol, zinc chloride)

PROSTAGLANDIN F$_{2\alpha}$ ANALOG

▷ *latanoprost* 1 drop in the affected eye(s) in the evening
    Xelpros *Ophth emul:* 0.005% (2.5 ml) (potassium sorbate 0.47%)
    Comment: *Latanoprost* can cause pigmentation of the iris, periorbital tissue (eyelid), and eyelashes (iris pigmentation likely to be permanent) and gradual changes to eyelashes, including increased length, thickness, and number of lashes (usually reversible).

PROSTAGLANDIN ANALOG (WITH NITRIC OXIDE METABOLITE)

▷ *latanoprostene bunod* ophthalmic solution ≤16 years: not recommended (due to potential safety concerns related to increased pigmentation following long-term chronic use); >16 years: 1 drop affected eye once daily

Vyzulta *Ophth soln:* 0.024% (5 ml) (benzalkonium chloride)

Comment: **Vyzulta** is a prostaglandin analog with nitric oxide as one of its metabolites. **Vyzulta** exerts a dual mechanism of action through latanoprost acid and butanediol mononitrate, working in the uveoscleral pathway and Schlemm's canal. The most common ocular adverse reactions with incidence ≥2% are conjunctival hyperemia (6%), eye irritation (4%), eye pain (3%), and instillation site pain (2%). There may be increased pigmentation of the iris and periorbital tissue. Iris pigmentation is likely to be permanent. There may be gradual changes to eyelashes, including increased length, increased thickness, and number of eyelashes, which are usually reversible upon discontinuation of treatment. There are no available human data for the use of **Vyzulta** during pregnancy to inform any drug-associated risks. There are no data on the presence of **Vyzulta** in human milk or effects on the breastfed infant.

OPHTHALMIC RHO KINASE INHIBITOR

▷ *netarsudil* ophthalmic solution 1 drop affected eye once daily in the PM
Pediatric: <18 years: not established; ≥18 years: same as adult
Rhopressa *Ophth soln:* 0.02% (0.2 mg/ml, 2.5 ml) (benzalkonium chloride)

OPHTHALMIC RHO KINASE INHIBITOR+PROSTAGLANDIN F2α ANALOG COMBINATION

▷ *netarsudil+latanoprost* ophthalmic solution 1 drop in the affected eye(s) once daily in the evening
Pediatric: safety and efficacy not established
Rocklatan *Ophth soln:* netar 0.2 mg (0.02%)+latan 0.05 mg (0.005%) per ml (2.5 ml)
Comment: **Rocklatan** *(netarsudil and latanoprost ophthalmic solution)* is a fixed-dose combination ophthalmic solution of the Rho kinase inhibitor *netarsudil* (Rhopressa) and the prostaglandin analog *latanoprost* (Xalatan) indicated to reduce elevated IOP in patients with open-angle glaucoma or ocular hypertension. Inform patients that pigmentation of the iris, periorbital tissue (eyelid), and eyelashes can occur. Iris pigmentation is likely to be permanent. Gradual changes to eyelashes, including increased length, thickness, and number of lashes, can occur, which are usually reversible. *In vitro* studies have shown that precipitation occurs when eye drops containing thimerosal are mixed with *latanoprost* 0.005%. If such drugs are used, they should be administered at least 5 minutes apart. The most common adverse reaction is conjunctival hyperemia (incidence 59%). Other common adverse reactions have been instillation site pain (20%), corneal verticillata (15%), and conjunctival hemorrhage (11%). No overall differences in safety or effectiveness have been observed between elderly and other adult patients.

OPHTHALMIC SYMPATHOMIMETICS

Comment: Contraindicated in narrow-angle glaucoma. Use with caution in cardiovascular disease, hypertension, hyperthyroidism, diabetes, and asthma.
▷ *dipivefrin* ophthalmic solution 1 drop affected eye q 12 hours
Propine *Ophth soln:* 0.1% (5, 10, 15 ml) (benzalkonium chloride)

OPHTHALMIC CARBONIC ANHYDRASE INHIBITOR+NON-CARDIOSELECTIVE BETA-BLOCKER

▷ *dorzolamide+timolol* ophthalmic solution 1 drop affected eye bid
Pediatric: <12 years: not recommended; ≥12 years: same as adult
Cosopt *Ophth soln:* dorz 2%+tim 0.5% (10 ml) (benzalkonium chloride)
Cosopt PF *Ophth soln:* dorz 2%+tim 0.5% (10 ml) (preservative-free)

OPHTHALMIC SYNTHETIC DOCOSANOID

▷ *unoprostone isopropyl* ophthalmic solution 1 drop affected eye bid
Pediatric: <12 years: not recommended; ≥12 years: same as adult
Rescula *Ophth soln:* 0.15% (5 ml) (benzalkonium chloride)

ORAL CARBONIC ANHYDRASE INHIBITORS

▷ *acetazolamide* 250-1000 mg/day in divided doses or 500 mg bid sust-rel tabs; max 1 gm/day
Pediatric: <12 years: not recommended; ≥12 years: same as adult
Diamox *Tab:* 125*, 250*mg
Diamox Sequels *Tab:* 500 mg sust-rel
▷ *methazolamide* (G) 50-100 mg bid-tid
Pediatric: <12 years: not recommended; ≥12 years: same as adult
Neptazane *Tab:* 25, 50 mg
Comment: Administer ophthalmic osmotic and miotic agents concomitantly.

GONORRHEA (*NEISSERIA GONORRHOEAE*)

Comment: The following treatment regimens for *Neisseria gonorrhoeae* are published in the **2021 CDC Transmitted Diseases Treatment Guidelines**. Treatment regimens are presented by generic drug name first, followed by information about brands and dose forms. Empiric treatment requires concomitant treatment of chlamydia. Treat all sexual contacts. Patients who are HIV-positive should receive the same treatment as those who are HIV-negative. Sexual abuse must be considered a cause of gonococcal infection in preadolescent children.

RECOMMENDED REGIMENS, ≥12 YEARS: UNCOMPLICATED INFECTIONS OF THE CERVIX, URETHRA, AND RECTUM
Regimen 1
> *ceftriaxone* 250 mg IM in a single dose
>> plus
> *azithromycin* 1 gm in a single dose

Regimen 2
> *ceftriaxone* 250 mg IM in a single dose
>> plus
> *doxycycline* 100 mg bid x 7 days

RECOMMENDED REGIMENS, ≥12 YEARS: UNCOMPLICATED INFECTIONS OF THE PHARYNX
Regimen 1
> *ceftriaxone* 250 mg IM in a single dose
>> plus
> *azithromycin* 1 gm in a single dose

Regimen 2
> *ceftriaxone* 250 mg IM in a single dose
>> plus
> *doxycycline* 100 mg bid x 7 days

RECOMMENDED REGIMENS, CHILDREN ≥45 KG, ≥8 YEARS: UNCOMPLICATED INFECTIONS OF THE CERVIX, URETHRA, AND RECTUM
Regimen 1
> *ceftriaxone* 250 mg IM in a single dose
>> plus
> *azithromycin* 1 gm in a single dose

RECOMMENDED REGIMEN: CHILDREN >45 KG
Regimen 1
> *ceftriaxone* 250 mg IM in a single dose

RECOMMENDED REGIMEN: CHILDREN >45 KG WHO HAVE GONOCOCCAL BACTEREMIA OR GONOCOCCAL ARTHRITIS
Regimen 1
> *ceftriaxone* 50 mg/kg IM or IV in a single dose daily x 7 days

RECOMMENDED REGIMENS, CHILDREN <45 KG, <8 YEARS: UNCOMPLICATED GONOCOCCAL VULVOVAGINITIS, CERVICITIS, URETHRITIS, PHARYNGITIS, OR PROCTITIS
Regimen 1
> *ceftriaxone* 250 mg IM in a single dose

RECOMMENDED REGIMEN, CHILDREN <45 KG, <8 YEARS: GONOCOCCAL BACTEREMIA OR ARTHRITIS
Regimen 1
> *ceftriaxone* 50 mg/kg (max dose 1 gm) IM or IV in a single dose daily x 7 days

DRUG BRANDS AND DOSE FORMS
> *azithromycin* (G)
>> **Zithromax** *Tab:* 250, 500, 600 mg; *Oral susp:* 100 mg/5 ml (15 ml), 200 mg/5 ml (15, 22.5, 30 ml) (cherry); *Pkt:* 1 gm for reconstitution (cherry-banana)
>> **Zithromax Tri-Pak** *Tab:* 3 x 500 mg tabs/pck
>> **Zithromax Z-Pak** *Tab:* 6 x 250 mg tabs/pck
>> **Zmax** *Oral susp:* 2 gm ext-rel for reconstitution (cherry-banana) (148 mg Na⁺)

▷ *ceftriaxone* (G)
    Rocephin *Vial:* 250, 500 mg; 1, 2 gm
▷ *doxycycline* (G)
    Acticlate *Tab:* 75, 150**mg
    Adoxa *Tab:* 50, 75, 100, 150 mg ent-coat
    Doryx *Tab:* 50, 75, 100, 150, 200 mg del-rel
    Doxteric *Tab:* 50 mg del-rel
    Monodox *Cap:* 50, 75, 100 mg
    Oracea *Cap:* 40 mg del-rel
    Vibramycin *Tab:* 100 mg; *Cap:* 50, 100 mg; *Syr:* 50 mg/5 ml (raspberry-apple) (sulfites); *Oral susp:* 25 mg/5 ml (raspberry)
    Vibra-Tab *Tab:* 100 mg film-coat

ALTERNATE THERAPY

▷ *azithromycin* (G) 2 gm x 1 dose
  Pediatric: <u>not</u> recommended for the treatment of gonorrhea in children
    Zithromax *Tab:* 250, 500, 600 mg; *Oral susp:* 100 mg/5 ml (15 ml), 200 mg/5 ml (15, 22.5, 30 ml) (cherry); *Pkt:* 1 gm for reconstitution (cherry-banana)
    Zithromax Tri-Pak *Tab:* 3 x 500 mg tabs/pck
    Zithromax Z-Pak *Tab:* 6 x 250 mg tabs/pck
    Zmax *Oral susp:* 2 gm ext-rel for reconstitution (cherry-banana) (148 mg Na$^+$)
▷ *cefotaxime* 500 mg IM x 1 dose
    Claforan *Vial:* 500 mg; 1, 2 gm
▷ *cefotetan* 1 gm IM x 1 dose
  Pediatric: <12 years: <u>not</u> recommended; ≥12 years: same as adult
    Cefotan *Vial:* 1, 2 gm
▷ *cefoxitin* 2 gm IM x 1 dose
  Pediatric: <3 months: <u>not</u> recommended; ≥3 months: same as adult
    Mefoxin *Vial:* 1, 2 gm
      plus
▷ *probenecid* (G)
    Benemid 1 gm 30 minutes before *cefoxitin*
    Pediatric: <2 years: <u>not</u> recommended; 2-14 years: 25 mg/kg 30 minutes before *cefoxitin*; ≥14 years: same as adult
    Tab: 500*mg; *Cap:* 500 mg
▷ *cefpodoxime proxetil* 200 mg x 1 dose
  Pediatric: <2 months: <u>not</u> recommended; 2 months-12 years: 10 mg/kg/day (max 400 mg/dose) <u>or</u> 5 mg/kg/day bid (max 200 mg/dose)
    Vantin *Tab:* 100, 200 mg; *Oral susp:* 50, 100 mg/5 ml (50, 75, 100 mg) (lemon creme)
▷ *ceftizoxime* 1 gm IM x 1 dose
  Pediatric: <6 months: <u>not</u> recommended; ≥6 months: same as adult
    Cefizox *Vial:* 500 mg; 1, 2, 10 g
▷ *demeclocycline* 600 mg initially, followed by 300 mg q 12 hours x 4 days (total 3 gm)
  Pediatric: <8 years: <u>not</u> recommended; ≥8 years: same as adult
    Declomycin *Tab:* 300 mg
▷ *enoxacin* 400 mg x 1 dose
  Pediatric: <18 years: <u>not</u> recommended; ≥18 years: same as adult
    Penetrex *Tab:* 200, 400 mg
▷ *imipramine* 400 mg x 1 dose
  Pediatric: <18 years: <u>not</u> recommended; ≥18 years: same as adult
    Maxaquin *Tab:* 400 mg
▷ *norfloxacin* 800 mg x 1 dose
  Pediatric: <18 years: <u>not</u> recommended; ≥18 years: same as adult
    Noroxin *Tab:* 400 mg
▷ *spectinomycin* 2 gm IM x 1 dose
  Pediatric: 40 mg/kg IM x 1 dose
    Trobicin *Vial:* 2 gm

GOUT (HYPERURICEMIA)

see Pseudogout
Acetaminophen for IV Infusion *see Pain*
NSAIDs *see* Appendix I. NSAIDs online at https://connect.springerpub.com/content/reference-book/978-0-8261-7935-7/back-matter/part02/back-matter/bmatter10
Opioid Analgesics *see Pain*

(continued)

Topical and Transdermal Analgesics *see* **Pain**
Parenteral Corticosteroids *see* Appendix L. Parenteral Corticosteroids
Oral Corticosteroids *see* Appendix K. Oral Corticosteroids

XANTHINE OXIDASE INHIBITORS (PROPHYLAXIS)

▸ *allopurinol* (G) initially 100 mg daily; increase by 100 mg weekly; max 800 mg/day and 300 mg/dose; usual range for mild symptoms 200-300 mg/day; for severe symptoms 400-600 mg/day; take with food
Pediatric: <6 years: max 150 mg/day; 6-10 years: max 400 mg/day, max single dose 300 mg; >10 years: same as adult
  Zyloprim *Tab:* 100*, 300*mg
  Comment: Do not take *allopurinol* concurrent with *colchicine*. Gout flares may occur after initiation of urate-lowering therapy, such as *allopurinol*, due to changing serum uric acid (sUA) concentrations resulting in mobilization of urate from tissue deposits. If a gout flare occurs during treatment, *allopurinol* does not need to be discontinued. Manage the flare concurrently, as appropriate for the individual patient. The correct dose and frequency of dosage for maintaining the sUA concentration within the normal range is best determined by using the sUA concentration as an index. *Allopurinol* is not recommended for the treatment of asymptomatic hyperuricemia. Discontinue *allopurinol* when the potential for overproduction of uric acid is no longer present.

ACUTE ATTACK

▸ *colchicine* (G) 0.6-1.2 mg at first sign of attack; then 0.6 mg every hour or 1.2 mg every 2 hours until pain relief; then consider 0.6 mg/day or every other day for maintenance
Pediatric: <12 years: not recommended; ≥12 years: same as adult
  Colcrys *Tab:* 0.6 mg
  Gloperba *Oral soln:* 0.6 mg/5 ml (150 ml) (cherry odor)
  Mitigare *Cap:* 0.6 mg
  Comment: Do not take *colchicine* concurrently with *allopurinol*.
▸ *febuxostat* (G) initially 40 mg daily; after 2 weeks, may increase to 80 mg daily
Pediatric: <18 years: not recommended; ≥18 years: same as adult
  Uloric *Tab:* 40, 80 mg
  Comment: Gout flare prophylaxis with *colchicine* or a nonsteroidal anti-inflammatory drug (NSAID) is recommended on initiation of *febuxostat* (**Uloric**) and up to 6 months. In a recent report of research, gout patients with established cardiovascular (CV) disease treated with **Uloric** had a higher rate of CV death as compared to those treated with *allopurinol*. Therefore, the FDA issued a new *boxed warning* to consider the risks and benefits of **Uloric** when deciding to prescribe or continue patients on **Uloric**. Further, **Uloric** should only be used in patients who have an inadequate response to a maximally titrated dose of *allopurinol*, who are intolerant to *allopurinol*, or for whom treatment with *allopurinol* is not advisable.

PEGYLATED URIC ACID-SPECIFIC ENZYME

▸ *pegloticase* premedicate with antihistamine and corticosteroid; 8 mg once every 2 weeks; administer IV infusion after dilution over at least 2 hours; observe at least 1 hour postinfusion
Pediatric: <18 years: not recommended; ≥18 years: same as adult
  Krystexxa *Vial:* 8 mg/ml (1 ml), single-use pwdr for IV infusion after dilution
  Comment: Slow rate, or stop and restart at lower rate, if infusion reaction occurs (e.g., **Krystexxa** is contraindicated with glucose-6-phosphate dehydrogenase deficiency (G6PD); screen patients of African or Mediterranean descent). **Krystexxa** is not for the treatment of asymptomatic hyperuricemia.

URICOSURIC AGENT

▸ *probenecid* (G) 250 mg bid x 1 week; maintenance 500 mg bid
Pediatric: <18 years: not recommended; ≥18 years: same as adult
    Tab: 500*mg; *Cap:* 500 mg
  Comment: Avoid concomitant use of *probenecid* and salicylates.

URICOSURIC+ANTI-INFLAMMATORY COMBINATIONS

▸ *probenecid+colchicine* (G) 1 tab once daily x 1 week; then 1 tab bid thereafter
Pediatric: <18 years: not recommended; ≥18 years: same as adult
    Tab: prob 500 mg+colch 0.5 mg
  Comment: *Probenecid+colchicine* is contraindicated in the treatment of acute gout attack, patients with blood dyscrasias, and patients with uric acid kidney stones. Concomitant salicylates antagonize the uricosuric effects.
▸ *sulfinpyrazone* initially 200-400 mg bid; may gradually increase to 800 mg bid
Pediatric: <18 years: not recommended; ≥18 years: same as adult
  Anturane *Cap:* 100, 200 mg
  Comment: Goal is sUA <6.5 mg/dL.

XANTHINE OXIDASE INHIBITOR

▸ *febuxostat* 40 mg once daily x 2 weeks; if sUA is not <6 mg/dL, may increase to 80 mg once daily
Pediatric: <18 years: not established; ≥18 years: same as adult
  Uloric *Tab:* 40, 80 mg

Comment: Gout flare prophylaxis with *colchicine* or NSAID is recommended on initiation of *febuxostat* **Uloric** and up to 6 months. In a recent report of research, gout patients with established cardiovascular disease (CVD) treated with *febuxostat* (**Uloric**) had a higher rate of CV death as compared with those treated with *allopurinol*. Therefore, the FDA issued a new *boxed warning* to consider the risks and benefits of **Uloric** when deciding to prescribe or continue patients on **Uloric**. Further, **Uloric** should only be used in patients who have an inadequate response to a maximally titrated dose of *allopurinol*, who are intolerant to *allopurinol*, or for whom treatment with *allopurinol* is not advisable.

XANTHINE OXIDASE INHIBITOR+URATE INHIBITOR COMBINATION

▷ *allopurinol+lesinurad* take 1 tab once daily

Pediatric: <18 years: not established; ≥18 years: same as adult

Duzallo *Tab:* 200/200, 300/200 mg

Comment: The U.S. FDA recently approved **Duzallo** for treatment of hyperuricemia associated with gout in patients who have not achieved target sUA levels with *allopurinol* alone. **Duzallo** is the first drug to combine *allopurinol*, the current standard of care for hyperuricemia associated with gout, and *lesinurad*, the most recent FDA-approved treatment for this condition. The fixed-dose combination addresses the overproduction and underexcretion of sUA. Patients with asymptomatic hyperuricemia are not recommended to receive **Duzallo**. Common adverse reactions associated with **Duzallo** include headache, influenza, higher levels of blood creatinine, and heart burn. In addition, **Duzallo** has a boxed warning for the risk of acute renal failure associated with *lesinurad*. There are no available human data on use of **Duzallo** or *lesinurad* in pregnancy to inform a drug-associated risk of adverse developmental outcomes. Limited published data on *allopurinol* use in pregnancy do not demonstrate a clear pattern or increase in frequency of adverse development outcomes. There is no information regarding the presence of **Duzallo** or *lesinurad* in human milk or the effects on the breastfed infant. Based on information from a single case report, *allopurinol* and its active metabolite, *oxypurinol*, were detected in the milk of a mother at 5 weeks postpartum. The effect of *allopurinol* on the breastfed infant is unknown. *CrCl 45 to <60 ml/min:* adjust the *allopurinol* to a medically appropriate dose (200 mg). CrCl <45: *allopurinol* not recommended. Max *lesinurad* is 200 mg/day. In clinical trials evaluating the safety and efficacy of this combined therapy among adult patients with gout who failed to achieve target sUA levels on *allopurinol* alone, **Duzallo** was found to nearly double the number of patients who achieved target sUA at 6 months, the mean sUA was reduced to less than 6 mg/dL by 1 month, and this level was maintained through 12 months.

SELECTIVE URIC ACID REABSORPTION INHIBITOR (SURI)

▷ *lesinurad* 200 mg once daily in combination with a xanthine oxidase inhibitor (XOI)

Pediatric: <18 years: not established; ≥18 years: same as adult

Zurampic *Tab:* 200 mg

Comment: **Zurampic** inhibits URAT1, a urate transporter, which is responsible for the majority of renal absorption of uric acid and OAT4, organic anion transporter, a uric acid transporter involved in diuretic-induced hyperuricemia. Do not use as monotherapy. Use in combination with an XOI, such as *allopurinol* or *febuxostat*, to reduce the production of uric acid. Do not initiate if CrCl <45 ml/min, ESRD, dialysis, or kidney transplant.

GOUTY ARTHRITIS

Gout Management Drugs *see Gout (Hyperuricemia)*
Acetaminophen for IV Infusion *see Pain*
NSAIDs *see Appendix I.* NSAIDs online at https://connect.springerpub.com/content/reference-book/978-0-8261-7935-7/back-matter/part02/back-matter/bmatter10
Opioid Analgesics *see Pain*
Topical & Transdermal Analgesics *see Pain*
Parenteral Corticosteroids *see Appendix L. Parenteral Corticosteroids*
Oral Corticosteroids *see Appendix K. Oral Corticosteroids*
Topical Analgesic and Anesthetic Agents *see Appendix H. Anesthetic Agents for Local Infiltration and Dermal/Mucosal Membrane Application* online at https://connect.springerpub.com/content/reference-book/978-0-8261-7935-7/back-matter/part02/back-matter/bmatter9

TOPICAL AND TRANSDERMAL ANALGESICS

▷ *capsaicin* (G) apply tid-qid prn to intact skin

Pediatric: <2 years: not recommended; ≥2 years: same as adult

Axsain *Crm:* 0.075% (1, 2 oz)

Capsin *Lotn:* 0.025, 0.075% (59 ml)

Capzasin-HP (OTC) *Crm:* 0.075% (1.5 oz), 0.025% (45, 90 gm); *Lotn:* 0.075% (2 oz), 0.025% (45, 90 gm)

Capzasin-P (OTC) *Crm:* 0.025% (1.5 oz); *Lotn:* 0.025% (2 oz)

(continued)

Dolorac *Crm:* 0.025% (28 gm)
Double Cap (OTC) *Crm:* 0.05% (2 oz)
R-Gel *Gel:* 0.025% (15, 30 gm)
Zostrix (OTC) *Crm:* 0.025% (0.7, 1.5, 3 oz)
Zostrix HP (OTC) *Emol crm:* 0.075% (1, 2 oz)

▷ *capsaicin* 8% patch apply up to 4 patches for one 60-minute application to clean dry skin; may prep area with topical anesthetic; wear non-latex gloves; patches may be cut to size/shape; treatment may be repeated every 3 months
Pediatric: <18 years: not recommended; ≥18 years: same as adult
Qutenza *Patch:* 8% 1,640 mcg/cm (179 mg) (1 or 2 patches w. 1-50 gm tube cleansing gel/carton)

▷ *diclofenac sodium* apply qid prn to intact skin
Pediatric: <12 years: not established; ≥12 years: same as adult
Pennsaid 1.5% in 10 drop increments, dispense and rub into front, side, and back of knee: usually 40 drops (40 mg) qid
Topical soln: 1.5% (150 ml)
Pennsaid 2% apply 2 pump actuations (40 mg) and rub into front, side, and back of knee bid
Topical soln: 2% (20 mg/pump actuation, 112 gm)
Solaraze Gel massage into clean skin bid prn
Gel: 3% (50 gm) (benzyl alcohol)
Voltaren Gel (OTC)(G) apply qid prn to intact skin
Gel: 1% (100 gm)

Comment: *Diclofenac* is contraindicated with **aspirin** allergy. As with other nonsteroidal anti-inflammatory drugs (NSAIDs), should be avoided in late pregnancy (≥30 weeks) because it may cause premature closure of the ductus arteriosus.

▷ *doxepin* (G) cream apply to affected area qid at intervals of at least 3-4 hours; max 8 days
Pediatric: <12 years: not recommended; >12 years: same as adult
Prudoxin *Crm:* 5% (45 gm)
Zonalon *Crm:* 5% (30, 45 gm)

▷ *pimecrolimus* 1% cream (G) <2 years: not recommended; ≥2 years: apply to affected area bid; do not apply an occlusive dressing
Elidel *Crm:* 1% (30, 60, 100 gm)

Comment: *Pimecrolimus* is indicated for short-term and intermittent long-term use. Discontinue use when resolution occurs. Contraindicated if the patient is immunosuppressed. Change to the 0.1% preparation or if secondary bacterial infection is present.

▷ *trolamine salicylate* apply tid-qid
Pediatric: <2 years: not recommended; ≥2 years: same as adult
Mobisyl Creme *Crm:* 10% (100 gm)

TOPICAL AND TRANSDERMAL ANESTHETICS

Comment: *Lidocaine* should not be applied to non-intact skin.

▷ *lidocaine* cream apply to affected area bid prn
Pediatric: <12 years: not recommended; ≥12 years: same as adult
LidaMantle *Crm:* 3% (1, 2 oz)
Lidoderm *Crm:* 3% (85 gm)
ZTlido *lidocaine* topical system 1% (30/carton)
Comment: Compared to Lidoderm (*lidocaine* patch 5%), which contains 700 mg/patch, ZTlido requires 35 mg per topical system to achieve the same therapeutic dose.

▷ *lidocaine* lotion apply to affected area bid prn
Pediatric: <12 years: not recommended; ≥12 years: same as adult
LidaMantle *Lotn:* 3% (177 ml)

▷ *lidocaine* 5% patch (G) apply up to 3 patches at one time for up to 12 hours/24-hour period (12 hours on/12 hours off); patches may be cut into smaller sizes before removal of the release liner; do not reuse
Pediatric: <12 years: not recommended; ≥12 years: same as adult
Lidoderm *Patch:* 5% (10x14 cm; 30/carton)

▷ *lidocaine+dexamethasone*
Pediatric: <12 years: not recommended; ≥12 years: same as adult
Decadron Phosphate with Xylocaine *Lotn:* dexa 4 mg+lido 10 mg per ml (5 ml)

▷ *lidocaine+hydrocortisone* (G) apply to affected area bid prn
Pediatric: <12 years: not recommended; ≥12 years: same as adult
LidaMantle HC *Crm:* lido 3%+hydro 0.5% (1, 3 oz); *Lotn:* (177 ml)

▷ *lidocaine* 2.5%+*prilocaine* 2.5% apply sparingly to the burn bid-tid prn
Pediatric: <12 years: not recommended; ≥12 years: same as adult
Emla Cream 5, 30 gm/tube

ORAL SALICYLATE

➤ *indomethacin* initially 25 mg bid-tid; increase as needed at weekly intervals by 25-50 mg/day; max 200 mg/day
Pediatric: <14 years: usually not recommended; ≤2-14 years, if risk warranted: 1-2 mg/kg/day in divided doses; max 3-4 mg/kg/day (or 150-200 mg/day, whichever is less); ≤14 years: ER cap not recommended; >14 years: same as adult
Cap: 25, 50 mg; *Susp:* 25 mg/5 ml (pineapple-coconut, mint; alcohol 1%); *Supp:* 50 mg; *ER Cap:* 75 mg ext-rel
Comment: *Indomethacin* is indicated only for acute painful flares. Administer with food and/or antacids. Use lowest effective dose for shortest duration.

NONSTEROIDAL ANTI-INFLAMMATORY DRUG (NSAID) PLUS PROTON PUMP INHIBITOR (PPI)

➤ *esomeprazole+naproxen* (G) 1 tab bid; use lowest effective dose for the shortest duration; swallow whole; take at least 30 minutes before a meal
Pediatric: <18 years: not recommended; ≥18 years: same as adult
Vimovo *Tab:* nap 375 mg+eso 20 mg ext-rel; nap 500 mg+eso 20 mg ext-rel

COX-2 INHIBITORS

Comment: Cox-2 inhibitors are contraindicated with history of asthma, urticaria, and allergic-type reactions to *aspirin*, other NSAIDs, and sulfonamides, 3rd trimester of pregnancy, and coronary artery bypass graft (CABG) surgery.
➤ *celecoxib* (G) 100-400 mg bid; max 800 mg/day
Pediatric: <18 years: not recommended; ≥18 years: same as adult
Celebrex *Cap:* 50, 100, 200, 400 mg
➤ *meloxicam* (G)
Mobic initially 7.5 mg once daily; max 15 mg once daily; *Hemodialysis:* max 7.5 mg/day
Pediatric: <2 years, <60 kg: not recommended; ≥2 years, >60 kg-12 years: 0.125 mg/kg, max 7.5 mg once daily; ≥12 years: same as adult
Tab: 7.5, 15 mg; *Oral susp:* 7.5 mg/5 ml (100 ml) (raspberry)
Vivlodex initially 5 mg qd; may increase to max 10 mg/day; *Hemodialysis:* max 5 mg/day
Cap: 5, 10 mg

GRAFT VERSUS HOST DISEASE (GVHD)

KINASE INHIBITOR

➤ *belumosudil* 200 mg once daily with food
Pediatric: <12 years: safety and efficacy not established; ≥12 years: same as adult
Rezurock *Tab:* 200 mg
Comment: Rezurock is a kinase inhibitor indicated for the treatment of adult and pediatric patients 12 years and older with chronic graft versus host disease (GVHD) after failure of at least two prior lines of systemic therapy. The most common (incidence ≥20%) adverse reactions, including laboratory abnormalities, have been infections, asthenia, nausea, diarrhea, dyspnea, cough, edema, hemorrhage, abdominal pain, musculoskeletal pain, headache, decreased phosphate, increased gamma glutamyltransferase (GGT), decreased lymphocytes, and hypertension. When Rezurock is co-administered with strong CYP3A inducers, increase the Rezurock dose to 200 mg bid. When Rezurock is co-administered with proton pump inhibitors (PPIs), increase the Rezurock dose to 200 mg bid. Rezurock is embryo/fetal toxic. Advise females of reproductive potential of the potential fetal risk and to use effective contraception. Advise mothers not to breastfeed during treatment and for at least 1 week after the last dose. To report suspected adverse reactions, contact Kadmon Pharmaceuticals at 1-877-377-7862 or FDA at 1-800-FDA-1088 or www.fda.gov/medwatch.
➤ *ruxolitinib* initially 5 mg bid; therapeutic dose should be individualized based on safety and efficacy; *Renal impairment:* reduce starting dose or avoid use; *Hepatic impairment:* reduce starting dose or avoid use
Pediatric: <12 years: not established; ≥12 years: same as adult
Jakafi *Tab:* 5, 10, 15, 20, 25 mg
Comment: Jakafi *(ruxolitinib)* is approved for the treatment of steroid-refractory acute GVHD, myelofibrosis, and polycythemia vera. Manage thrombocytopenia, anemia, and neutropenia with dose reduction, or treatment interruption, or transfusion. Serious infections should be resolved before starting therapy with Jakafi. Assess patients for signs and symptoms of infection during Jakafi therapy and initiate appropriate treatment promptly. Manage symptom exacerbation following interruption or discontinuation of Jakafi with supportive care and then consider resuming treatment with Jakafi. There is risk of non-melanoma skin cancer (NMSC) with Jakafi use; perform periodic skin examinations. Assess lipid levels 8-12 weeks from start of Jakafi therapy and treat as appropriate. Avoid use of Jakafi with *fluconazole* doses greater than 200 mg except in patients with GVHD. With acute GVHD, the most common hematologic adverse reactions (incidence >50%) are anemia, thrombocytopenia, and neutropenia, and the most common nonhematologic adverse reactions (incidence >50%) have been infections and edema. There are no studies with the use of Jakafi in pregnant females to inform drug-associated risks. No data are available regarding the presence of *ruxolitinib* in human milk or the effects on the breastfed infant. Patients should be advised to discontinue breastfeeding during treatment with Jakafi and for 2 weeks after the final dose.

SOLUBLE FUSION PROTEIN

▶ **abatacept** *Preparation/Administration/Storage:* reconstitute each vial with 10 ml sterile H_2O for Injection, USP; use only the silicone-free disposable syringe provided with each vial and an 18-21 gauge needle; do not shake; gently rotate the vial with gentle swirling until the contents are completely dissolved; if the **Orencia** powder is accidentally reconstituted using a siliconized syringe, discard the dose; if the silicone-free syringe is dropped or otherwise contaminated, obtain a silicone-free syringe from stock; the reconstituted **Orencia** solution must be further diluted to 100 ml as follows: from a 100 ml infusion bag or bottle of 0.9% NaCl Injection, USP, withdraw a volume equal to the volume of the reconstituted **Orencia** vials (for 2 vials remove 20 ml, for 3 vials remove 30 ml, for 4 vials remove 40 ml); slowly transfer the reconstituted **Orencia** solution from each vial into the infusion bag or bottle using the same silicone-free disposable syringe provided with each vial; gently mix; the concentration of the fully diluted **Orencia** solution in the infusion bag or bottle will be approximately 5, 7.5, or 10 mg, respectively, of *abatacept* per milliliter of infusion solution, depending on whether 2, 3, or 4 vials of **Orencia** are used; any unused portion in the vials must be immediately discarded; the entire, fully diluted **Orencia** solution should be administered over a period of 30 minutes and must be administered with a sterile infusion set and a sterile, non-pyogenic, low-protein-binding filter (pore size 0.2-1.2 μm); the infusion of the fully diluted **Orencia** solution in the infusion bag must be completed within 24 hours of reconstitution of the **Orencia** vials; the fully diluted **Orencia** solution (the infusion bag) may be stored at room temperature or refrigerated at 2°C to 8°C (36°F to 46°F) before use; **Orencia** should not be infused concomitantly in the same IV line with other agents (no physical or biochemical compatibility studies have been conducted to evaluate the co-administration of **Orencia** with other agents); **Orencia** lyophilized powder must be refrigerated at 2°C to 8°C (36°F to 46°F); do not use beyond the expiration date; protect the vials from light by storing in the original package until time of use

Orencia Dosing Table		
Weight	Dose	# Vials
<60 kg	500 mg	2
60-100 kg	750 mg	3
>100 kg	1 gm	4

Pediatric: <2 years: safety and efficacy not established; 2-6 years: see the Orencia Dosing Table
   Orencia *Vial:* 250 mg pwdr for reconstitution (250 mg/10 ml reconstituted), dilution, and IV infusion (preservative-free) (silicone-free); co-packaged with a silicone-free syringe (NOTE: Additional silicone-free syringes can be ordered by contacting Bristol-Meyers-Squibb at 1-800-ORENCIA)
Comment: Orencia is a soluble fusion protein that consists of the extracellular domain of human cytotoxic T-lymphocyte associated antigen 4 (CTLA-4) linked to the modified Fc (hinge, CH2, and CH3 domains) portion of human immunoglobulin G1 (IgG1). *Abatacept* is produced by recombinant DNA technology in a mammalian cell expression system. **Orencia** is indicated for prophylaxis (prevention) of acute GVHD, a condition that occurs when donor bone marrow or stem cells attack the graft recipient, in combination with a calcineurin inhibitor and *methotrexate*. **Orencia** may be used in adults and pediatric patients ≥2 years of age undergoing hematopoietic stem cell transplantation (i.e., bone marrow transplantation or stem cell transplantation) from a matched or 1 allele-mismatched unrelated donor. **Orencia** is the first FDA-approved drug for acute GVHD prevention and incorporates real-world evidence (RWE) as one component of the determination of clinical effectiveness. RWE is clinical evidence regarding the usage and potential benefits, or risks, of a medical product derived from analysis of real-world data (i.e., data relating to patient health status and/or delivery of healthcare routinely collected data from a variety of sources, including registry data). There are significant ongoing efforts at the FDA to incorporate use of high-quality RWE to support regulatory decision-making. The most common side effects of **Orencia** for prevention of acute GVHD include anemia, hypertension, cytomegalovirus (CMV) reactivation/CMV infection, fever, pneumonia, nosebleed, decreased levels of specific white blood cells (WBCs) (CD4 lymphocytes), increased levels of magnesium in the blood, and acute kidney injury (AKI). Patients who receive **Orencia** should be monitored for Epstein-Barr virus reactivation in accordance with institutional practices and receive preventive medication for Epstein-Barr virus infection before starting treatment and for 6 months post-transplantation. Patients should also be monitored for CMV infection/reactivation for 6 months posttransplant. **Orencia** should not be administered to patients with known hypersensitivity to **Orencia** or any of its components. Concomitant use of **Orencia** with other potent immunosuppressants (e.g., biologic disease-modifying antirheumatic drugs [DMARDS], Janus kinase [JAK] inhibitors) is not recommended. There are no adequate and well-controlled studies in human pregnancy. *Abatacept* was found not to be teratogenic in animal studies at doses up to 300 mg/kg and up to 200 mg/kg daily (29-fold a human 10 mg/kg dose based on area under the curve [AUC] in animals). Animals treated with *abatacept* every 3 days during early gestation throughout the lactation period showed no adverse effects in the offspring at doses up to 45 mg/kg (3-fold a human 10 mg/kg dose based on AUC). At a dose of 12,200 mg/kg (11-fold a human 10 mg/kg dose based on AUC), alterations of immune function consisted of a nine fold increase in the T-cell-dependent antibody response in female pups and inflammation of the thyroid in 1 female

pup out of 10 males and 10 females evaluated. Whether these findings indicate a risk of development of autoimmune diseases in humans exposed *in utero* to **abatacept** has not been determined. *Abatacept* was shown to cross the placenta. Because animal reproduction studies are not always predictive of human response, **Orencia** should be used during pregnancy only if clearly needed. *Abatacept* has been shown to be present in animal milk. It is not known whether *abatacept* is excreted in human milk or absorbed systemically after ingestion. Because many drugs are excreted in human milk and because of the potential for serious adverse reactions in nursing infants from **Orencia**, possibly including effects on the developing immune system, a decision should be made whether to discontinue nursing or to discontinue the drug, taking into account the importance of the drug to the mother.

GRANULOMATOSIS, WEGENER'S GRANULOMATOSIS

Comment: Wegener's granulomatosis is granulomatosis with polyangiitis (GPA).

CD20-DIRECTED CYTOLYTIC ANTIBODY

▶ *rituximab* Induction: 375 mg/m² via IV infusion once weekly x 4 weeks, in combination with glucocorticoids; *follow-up, patients who have achieved disease control with induction treatment, in combination with glucocorticoids:* two 500 mg IV infusions separated by 2 weeks, followed by one 500 mg IV infusion every 6 months thereafter, based on clinical evaluation; **Rituxan** should only be administered by a qualified healthcare professional with appropriate medical support to manage severe infusion-related reactions that can be fatal if they occur

Pediatric: <2 years: safety and efficacy not established; ≥2 years: *Induction:* 375 mg/m² via IV infusion once weekly x 4 weeks, in combination with glucocorticoids; *Follow up, patients who have achieved disease control with induction treatment, in combination with glucocorticoids:* two 250 mg/m² via IV infusions separated by 2 weeks, followed by one 250 mg/m² via IV infusion every 6 months thereafter, based on clinical evaluation; **Rituxan** should only be administered by a qualified healthcare professional with appropriate medical support to manage severe infusion-related reactions that can be fatal if they occur

Rituxan *Vial:* 100 mg/10 ml (10 mg/ml), 500 mg/50 ml (10 mg/ml), single-dose, soln for dilution and IV infusion (preservative-free)

Comment: Rituxan is indicated for the treatment of Wegener's granulomatosis, in combination with glucocorticoids, for adults and pediatric patients ≥2 years of age. The most adverse common reactions (incidence ≥15%) in clinical trials have been infections, nausea, diarrhea, headache, muscle spasms, anemia, peripheral edema, and infusion-related reactions. For tumor lysis syndrome (TLS), administer aggressive IV hydration and antihyperuricemic agents, and monitor renal function. Monitor for infections; withhold **Rituxan** and institute appropriate anti-infective therapy. For cardiac adverse reactions, discontinue infusions in case of serious or life-threatening events. Discontinue **Rituxan** in patients with rising serum creatinine or oliguria. Bowel obstruction and perforation can occur; consider and evaluate for abdominal pain, vomiting, or related symptoms. Live virus vaccinations prior to or during **Rituxan** treatment is not recommended. **Rituxan** is embryo/fetal toxic. Advise males and females of reproductive potential of the potential risk and to use effective contraception. Advise women not to breastfeed during treatment and for at least 6 months after the last dose.

▶ *rituximab-arrx* Induction: 375 mg/m² once weekly x 4 weeks; then if disease control achieved, 500 mg via IV infusion x 2 doses separated by two weeks; then 500 mg via IV infusion once every 6 months based on clinical evaluation; administer all doses of **Riabni** in combination with glucocorticoids; **Riabni** should only be administered by a qualified healthcare professional with appropriate medical support to manage severe infusion-related reactions that can be fatal

Pediatric: safety and efficacy not established

Riabni *Vial:* 100 mg/10 ml (10 mg/ml), 500 mg/50 ml (10 mg/ml) soln, single-dose

Comment: Riabni *(rituximab-arrx)* is a biosimilar to **Rituxan** indicated for the treatment of adult patients with GPA (Wegener's Granulomatosis) in combination with glucocorticoids. The most common adverse reactions in clinical trials with GPA (incidence ≥15%) have been infections, nausea, diarrhea, headache, muscle spasms, anemia, peripheral edema, and infusion-related reactions. Monitor renal function. Discontinue **Riabni** in patients with rising serum creatinine or oliguria. If TLS is suspected, administer aggressive IV hydration and antihyperuricemic agents. If infection occurs, withhold **Riabni** and institute appropriate anti-infective therapy. Bowel obstruction and perforation can occur; evaluate for abdominal pain, vomiting, and related symptoms. Live virus vaccine administration prior to or during treatment with **Riabni** is not recommended. **Riabni** can cause embryo/fetal harm. Advise females of reproductive potential of embryo/fetal risk and to use effective contraception. Advise not to breastfeed.

GRANULOMA INGUINALE (DONOVANOSIS)

Comment: The following treatment regimens are published in the **2021 CDC Sexually Transmitted Diseases Treatment Guidelines**. Treatment regimens are for adults only; consult a specialist for the treatment of patients less than 18 years of age. Treatment regimens are presented by generic drug name first, followed by information about brands and dose forms. Persons who have sexual contact with a patient who has had granuloma inguinale within the past 60 days before onset of the patient's symptoms should be examined and offered therapy. Patients who are HIV-positive should receive the same treatment as those who are HIV-negative; however, the addition of a parenteral aminoglycoside (e.g., *gentamicin*) can also be considered.

RECOMMENDED REGIMEN
▷ *doxycycline* 100 mg bid x at least 3 weeks and until all lesions have completely healed

ALTERNATE REGIMENS
▷ *azithromycin* 1 gm once weekly for at least 3 weeks and until all lesions have completely healed
▷ *ciprofloxacin* 750 mg bid x at least 3 weeks and until all lesions have completely healed
▷ *erythromycin base* 500 mg qid x 14 days or *erythromycin ethylsuccinate* 400 mg qid x 14 days
▷ *trimethoprim+sulfamethoxazole* take 1 double-strength (160/800) dose bid x at least 3 weeks and until all lesions have completely healed

DRUG BRANDS AND DOSE FORMS
▷ *azithromycin* (G)
> **Zithromax** *Tab:* 250, 500, 600 mg; *Oral susp:* 100 mg/5 ml (15 ml), 200 mg/5 ml (15, 22.5, 30 ml) (cherry); *Pkt:* 1 gm for reconstitution (cherry-banana)
> **Zithromax Tri-Pak** *Tab:* 3 x 500 mg tabs/pck
> **Zithromax Z-Pak** *Tab:* 6 x 250 mg tabs/pck
> **Zmax** *Oral susp:* 2 gm ext-rel for reconstitution (cherry-banana) (148 mg Na$^+$)
▷ *ciprofloxacin*
> **Cipro (G)** *Tab:* 250, 500, 750 mg; *Oral susp:* 250, 500 mg/5 ml (100 ml) (strawberry)
> **Cipro XR** *Tab:* 500, 1,000 mg ext-rel
> **ProQuin XR** *Tab:* 500 mg ext-rel
▷ *doxycycline* (G)
> **Acticlate** *Tab:* 75, 150**mg
> **Adoxa** *Tab:* 50, 75, 100, 150 mg ent-coat
> **Doryx** *Tab:* 50, 75, 100, 150, 200 mg del-rel
> **Doxteric** *Tab:* 50 mg del-rel
> **Monodox** *Cap:* 50, 75, 100 mg
> **Oracea** *Cap:* 40 mg del-rel
> **Vibramycin** *Tab:* 100 mg; *Cap:* 50, 100 mg; *Syr:* 50 mg/5 ml (raspberry-apple) (sulfites); *Oral susp:* 25 mg/5 ml (raspberry)
> **Vibra-Tab** *Tab:* 100 mg film-coat
▷ *erythromycin base* (G)
> **Ery-Tab** *Tab:* 250, 333, 500 mg ent-coat
> **PCE** *Tab:* 333, 500 mg
▷ *erythromycin ethylsuccinate* (G)
> **EryPed** *Oral susp:* 200 mg/5 ml (100, 200 ml) (fruit), 400 mg/5 ml (60, 100, 200 ml) (banana); *Oral drops:* 200, 400 mg/5 ml (50 ml) (fruit); *Chew tab:* 200 mg wafer (fruit)
> **E.E.S.** *Oral susp:* 200, 400 mg/5 ml (100 ml) (fruit)
> **E.E.S. Granules** *Oral susp:* 200 mg/5 ml (100, 200 ml) (cherry)
> **E.E.S. 400 Tablets** *Tab:* 400 mg
▷ *trimethoprim+sulfamethoxazole (TMP-SMX)*(G)
> **Bactrim, Septra**
> *Tab:* trim 80 mg+sulfa 400 mg*
> **Bactrim DS, Septra DS**
> *Tab:* trim 160 mg+sulfa 800 mg*
> **Bactrim Pediatric Suspension, Septra Pediatric Suspension**
> *Oral susp:* trim 40 mg+sulfa 200 mg per 5 ml (100 ml) (cherry) (alcohol 0.3%)

GROWTH FAILURE

Comment: Administer growth hormones (GH) by SC injection into the thigh, buttocks, or abdomen. Rotate sites with each dose. Contraindicated in children with fused epiphyses or evidence of neoplasia.
▷ *mecasermin* (recombinant human insulin-like growth factor-1 [rhIGF-1])
> **Increlex** see mfr pkg insert
> *Vial:* 10 mg/ml (benzyl alcohol)
> **Comment:** Increlex is indicated for growth failure in children with severe primary IGF-1 deficiency (primary IGFD) or in those with GH gene deletion who have developed neutralizing antibodies to GH.
▷ *somatropin* (rDNA origin)
> **Genotropin** initially not more than 0.04 mg/kg/week divided into 6-7 doses; may increase at 4 to 8 week intervals; max 0.08 mg/kg/week divided into 6-7 doses
> *Pediatric:* usually 0.16-0.024 mg/kg/week divided into 6-7 doses

Intramix device: 1.5 mg (1.3 mg/ml after reconstitution), 5.8 mg (5 mg/ml after reconstitution) (two-chamber cartridge w. diluent); *Pen* or *Intramix device:* 5.8 mg (5 mg/ml after reconstitution), 13.8 mg (512 mg/ml after reconstitution) (two-chamber cartridge w. diluent)

Genotropin MiniQuick initially not more than 0.04 mg/kg/week divided into 6-7 doses; may increase at 4 to 8 week intervals; max 0.08 mg/kg/week divided into 6-7 doses
Pediatric: usually 0.16-0.024 mg/kg/week divided into 6-7 doses
   MiniQuick: 0.2, 0.4, 0.6, 0.8, 1, 1.2, 1.4, 1.6, 1.8, 2 mg/0.25 ml (pwdr for SC injection after reconstitution) (2-chamber cartridge w. diluent)

Humatrope
Pediatric: initially 0.18 mg/kg/week IM or SC divided into equal doses given either on 3 alternate days or 6 x a week; max 0.3 mg/kg/week
   Vial: 5 mg w. 5 ml diluent

Norditropin
Pediatric: 0.024-0.034 mg/kg SC 6-7 x/week
   Vial: 4 mg (12 IU), 8 mg (24 IU); *Cartridge for inj:* 5, 10, 15 mg/1.5 ml; *FlexPro prefilled pen:* 5, 10, 15 mg/1.5 ml; *NordiFlex prefilled pen:* 5, 10, 15 mg/1.5 ml; 30 mg/3 ml

Nutropin
Pediatric: 0.7 mg/kg/week SC in divided daily doses
   Vial: 5, 10 mg/vial w. diluent

Nutropin AQ *<35 years:* initially not more than 0.006 mg/kg SC daily; may increase to max 0.025 mg/kg SC daily; *≥35 years:* initially not more than 0.006 mg/kg SC daily; may increase to max 0.0125 mg/kg SC daily
Pediatric: Prepubertal: up to 0.043 mg/kg SC daily; *Pubertal:* up to 0.1 mg/kg SC daily; *Turner syndrome:* up to 0.0375 mg/kg/week divided into equal doses 3-7 x/week
   Vial: 5 mg/ml (2 ml)

Nutropin Depot 1.5 mg/kg SC monthly on the same day each month; max 22.5 mg/inj; divide injection if >22.5 mg
Pediatric: same as adult
   Vial: 13.5, 18, 22.5 mg/vial (pwdr for injection after reconstitution; single-use w. diluent and needle)

Omnitrope 0.16-0.24 mg/kg/week SC divided 3-7 x/week
   Vial: 5.8 mg

Omnitrope Pen 5 0.16-0.24 mg/kg/week SC divided 3-7 x/week
   Cartridge for inj: 5 mg/1.5 ml

Omnitrope Pen 10 0.16-0.24 mg/kg/week SC divided 3-7 x/week
   Cartridge for inj: 10 mg/1.5 ml

Saizen (G) 0.18 mg/kg/week IM or SC divided 3-7 x/week
   Vial: 5 mg (pwdr for SC injection w. diluent)

Serostim 0.1 mg/kg SC once daily at HS; max 6 mg
   Vial: 5, 4, 6, 8.8 mg (pwdr for SC injection w. diluent) (benzyl alcohol)

GROWTH HORMONE DEFICIENCY (GHD)

HUMAN GROWTH HORMONE ANALOG

▷ **somapacitan-beco** inject SC into the abdomen or thigh with regular rotation of injection sites to avoid lipohypertrophy/Lipoatrophy; *Initially:* 1.5 mg SC once weekly for the treatment-naïve patients and patients switching from daily growth hormone (GH); *Titration:* increase the weekly dose every 2 to 4 weeks by approximately 0.5-1.5 mg until the desired response has been achieved based on clinical response and serum insulin-like growth factor 1 (IGF-1) concentrations; max recommended dose is 8 mg SC once weekly; see mfr pkg insert for full prescribing information and for dosage recommendations in patients aged 65 years and older, patients with hepatic impairment, and females receiving oral estrogen
Pediatric: administer 5, 10, 15 mg SC once weekly in the abdomen or thigh (NOTE: Risks in pediatric patients associated with GH use include sudden death in pediatric patients with Prader–Willi syndrome, increased risk of second neoplasm in pediatric cancer survivors treated with radiation to the brain and/or head, slipped capital femoral epiphysis; progression of preexisting scoliosis, and pancreatitis.) **April 2023**—The FDA has approved a new indication for **Sogroya** injection 5 mg, 10 mg, or 15 mg for treatment of children aged ≥2.5 years of age who have growth failure due to inadequate secretion of endogenous GH. With this new pediatric indication, **Sogroya** became the first and only once-weekly subcutaneously administered GH treatment for both children and adults. FDA approval of the new indication for children with growth hormone deficiency (GHD) is based on data from the phase 3 REAL4 study. In the study, 200 treatment-naïve patients aged 2.5-11 years of age with GHD were either given once-weekly **Sogroya** (n=132) or daily *somatropin* (n=68) for 52 weeks. The results showed that **Sogroya** was comparable to daily *somatropin* for the primary endpoint of annualized height velocity (11.2 cm/year vs. 11.7 cm/year, respectively). Adverse reactions in the REAL4 study occurring in >5% of patients included nasopharyngitis, headache, pyrexia, pain in extremity, and injection site reactions. —From www.Drugs.com

(continued)

Sogroya *Prefilled pen:* 10 mg/1.5 ml (6.7 mg/ml)

Comment: Sogroya *(somapacitan-beco)* is indicated for replacement of endogenous GH in adults with GHD. Adverse reactions (incidence 2%) have been back pain, arthralgia, dyspepsia, sleep disorder, dizziness, tonsillitis, peripheral edema, vomiting, adrenal insufficiency, hypertension, blood creatine phosphokinase increase, weight increase, and anemia. There are no available data on **Sogroya** use in pregnant females. However, published studies with short-acting recombinant growth hormone (rhGH) use in pregnant females over several decades have not identified any drug-associated risk of major birth defects, miscarriage, or adverse maternal or fetal outcomes. In animal reproduction studies, subcutaneously administered *somapacitan-beco* was not teratogenic during organogenesis at doses approximately 12 times the clinical exposure at the maximum recommended human dose (MRHD) of 8 mg/week. No adverse developmental outcomes were observed in a pre- and postnatal development study with administration of *somapacitan-beco* to pregnant rats from organogenesis through lactation at approximately 275 times the clinical exposure at the MRHD. Available published data describing administration of short-acting rhGH to lactating females for 7 days reported that short-acting rhGH did not increase the normal breastmilk concentration of GH and no adverse effects were reported in breastfed infants. Developmental and health benefits of breastfeeding should be considered along with the mother's clinical need for **Sogroya** and any potential adverse effects on the breastfed infant from **Sogroya** or from the underlying maternal condition. There is no information on the presence of *somapacitan-beco* in human milk or effects on the breastfed infant. Risks in pediatric patients associated with GH use include sudden death in pediatric patients with Prader–Willi syndrome, increased risk of second neoplasm in pediatric cancer survivors treated with radiation to the brain and/or head, slipped capital femoral epiphysis, progression of preexisting scoliosis, and pancreatitis.

HAEMOPHILUS INFLUENZAE B (HIB)

COMBINATION VACCINES

➤ **Pentacel** (DTaP-IPV/Hib) is commercially available as a kit containing single-dose vial of fixed-combination vaccine containing diphtheria, tetanus, pertussis, and poliovirus antigens (DTaP-IPV vaccine) and single-dose vial of lyophilized Hib vaccine (PRP-T; ActHIB). Prior to administration, reconstitute vial of lyophilized PRP-T (ActHIB) vaccine by adding the entire content of the vial of DTaP-IPV vaccine in the kit according to manufacturer's instructions to provide a combination vaccine containing diphtheria, tetanus, pertussis, IPV, and Hib antigens. Gently swirl until cloudy, uniform, white to off-white (yellow tinge) suspension is obtained. Administer IM immediately after reconstitution. **Pentacel** is approved for use as a four-dose series in children 6 weeks through 4 years of age (prior to the fifth birthday). **Pentacel** is to be administered as a 4-dose series at 2, 4, 6, and 15-18 months of age. The first dose may be given as early as 6 weeks of age. Four doses of **Pentacel** constitute a primary immunization course against pertussis. Three doses of **Pentacel** constitute an immunization course against diphtheria, tetanus, *Haemophilus influenzae* type b invasive disease, and poliomyelitis; the fourth dose is a booster for diphtheria, tetanus, *H. influenzae* type b invasive disease, and poliomyelitis immunizations. See mfr pkg insert for full prescribing information, including product storage, preparation, administration, contraindications, warnings, and precautions.

➤ **Vaxelis** *Vial:* 0.5 ml susp, single-dose; *Prefilled syringe:* 0.5 ml susp, single-dose (preservative-free)

Comment: Vaxelis is a single-dose combination of six vaccines: diphtheria, tetanus toxoid, acellular pertussis, inactivated poliovirus, *Haemophilus* b conjugate, and hepatitis B. The 3-dose immunization series consists of a 0.5 ml IM injection, administered at 2, 4, and 6 months of age. See mfr pkg insert for full prescribing information, including product storage, preparation, administration, contraindications, warnings, and precautions.

HAND, FOOT, AND MOUTH DISEASE (*COXSACKIEVIRUS*)

NSAIDs *see* Appendix I. NSAIDs online at https://connect.springerpub.com/content/reference-book/978-0-8261-7935-7/back-matter/part02/back-matter/bmatter10

Opioid Analgesics *see* **Pain**

OTC Throat Lozenges

OTC Cough Drops and Cough Syrup

Comment: Hand, foot, and mouth disease occurs most commonly in children <10 years of age. Although adults are susceptible, most have built up natural immunity. The causative organism, *Coxsackievirus*, is transmitted via droplet spread (coughing and/or sneezing) and contact with contaminated objects and surfaces (same as influenza). Clinical signs and symptoms are typically relatively mild and include fever, sore throat, feeling generally unwell, malaise, headache, and poor appetite. Red spots, some painful blister-like lesions, most often appear on the tongue and roof of the mouth, palms of the hands, and soles of the feet (but not necessarily all three), and are often faint or sparse. Lesions, which are not pruritic, may also be noted on the dorsal surfaces of the hands/fingers and feet/toes. Medical treatment, per se, is not required. Treatment at home is with age/weight-dosed *ibuprofen* or *acetaminophen* for relief of sore throat, lesion pain, and fever. Other comfort measures include salt water gargles, throat lozenges, cough drops or cough syrup, and fluids. The disease typically resolves in 7-10 days.

HANSEN'S DISEASE (LEPROMATOUS LEPROSY, *MYCOBACTERIUM LEPRAE*)

Comment: The microorganism, *Mycobacterium leprae*, was discovered by Dr. Gerhard Armauer Hansen in 1874, a Norwegian physician who was searching for the unknown bacteria in the skin nodules of lepers. Hansen's disease is treated with a combination of antibiotics. Typically two or three antibiotics are used at the same time. These are *dapsone* with *rifampicin*, and *clofazimine* is added for some types of the disease. These drugs must never be used alone as monotherapy for leprosy. *Paucibacillary Form:* 2 antibiotics are used at the same time, daily *dapsone* and *rifampicin* once per month. *Multibacillary Form:* Daily *clofazimine* is added to *rifampicin* and *dapsone*. This multidrug treatment (MDT) strategy helps prevent the development of antibiotic resistance by the bacteria, which may otherwise occur due to the length of treatment. Treatment usually lasts between 1 and 2 years. The illness can be cured if treatment is completed as prescribed. A single dose of combination therapy has been used to cure single-lesion paucibacillary leprosy: *rifampicin* 600 mg, *ofloxacin* 400 mg, and *minocycline* 100 mg. The child with a single lesion takes half the adult dose of the 3 medications. WHO has designed blister pack medication kits for both paucibacillary leprosy and for multibacillary leprosy. Each kit contains medication for 28 days. The blister pack medication kit for single-lesion paucibacillary leprosy contains the necessary medication for the one-time administration of the 3 medications.

ANTIMYCOBACTERIALS
➤ *clofazimine* (G) should be administered with meals or milk
  Dapsone-sensitive lepromatous leprosy: 100 mg daily as part of a combination regimen for at least 2 years
  Dapsone-resistant lepromatous leprosy: 100 mg daily in combination with one or more other agents for 3 years
  Leprosy complicated by erythema nodosum leprosum: 100-200 mg daily for up to 3 months; taper dose to 100 mg as quickly as possible
  Pediatric: Safety and effectiveness in pediatric patients not established
     Soft gelcap: 50 mg
Comment: *Clofazimine* is sometimes given with other medicines for leprosy. When *clofazimine* is used to treat disease flares, it may be given with a cortisone-like medicine. *Clofazimine* may deposit in the intestinal mucosa, causing intestinal disturbances, including abdominal obstruction, bleeding, splenic infarction, and death. Reduce dose or discontinue *clofazimine* if the patient complains of pain in the abdomen or other gastrointestinal symptoms. QT prolongation and torsade de pointes may occur with *clofazimine*. Concomitant use with other QT-prolonging drugs or *bedaquiline* may cause additive QT prolongation. Monitor ECGs and discontinue *clofazimine* if significant ventricular arrhythmia or QTcF interval ≥500 msec develops. Advise patients that skin and body fluid discoloration frequently occurs. Depression and suicide due to skin discoloration may occurs. monitor patients for psychological effects of skin discoloration. The most common adverse reactions reported in 40-50% of patients are skin and body fluid discoloration, abdominal and epigastric pain, diarrhea, nausea, vomiting, and gastrointestinal intolerance. No dose adjustment of *clofazimine* is needed for HIV-infected patients. *Severe Renal Impairment:* Use with caution. *Hepatic Impairment:* Avoid. Monitor for toxicities when used concomitantly with substrates of CYP3A4/5. It may take up to 6 months before the full benefit of *clofazimine* is seen. Sexually active females of reproductive potential should have a negative pregnancy test prior to starting treatment. There are no studies of *clofazimine* use in pregnant females and few cases of *clofazimine* use during pregnancy have been reported in the literature. These reports indicate that the skin of infants born to women who had received *clofazimine* during pregnancy was deeply pigmented at birth; therefore, *clofazimine* should be used during pregnancy only if the potential benefit justifies the risk to the fetus. *Clofazimine* is excreted in human milk. Skin discoloration has been observed in breastfed infants of mothers receiving *clofazimine*. There are no adequate studies in women for determining infant risk when using this medication during breastfeeding; therefore, weigh the potential benefits against the potential risks before taking this medication while breastfeeding. In some areas, *clofazimine* is considered an investigational new drug (IND) that must be prescribed by a registered investigator; providers are encouraged to request investigator status by calling the National Hansen's Disease Program (NHDP) at 1-800-642-2477.

SULFONE
➤ *dapsone* topical (G) apply to affected area bid
  Pediatric: <12 years: not recommended; ≥12 years: same as adult
     Aczone *Gel:* 5, 7.5% (30, 60, 90 gm tube)
➤ *rifampin* (G) 600 mg orally once daily x 12 months
  Pediatric: <12 years: not recommended; ≥12 years: same as adult
     Rifadin, Rimactane *Cap:* 150, 300 mg

ALTERNATE DRUGS
Comment: *Ofloxacin* may be substituted for *clofazimine*. *Clarithromycin* may be substituted for any of the drugs. *Minocycline* may be substituted for *dapsone* in patients intolerant of *dapsone* and may also be used to substitute *clofazimine*; however, anti-inflammatory activity is not as substantial as with *clofazimine*.

(continued)

▷ *clarithromycin* (G) 500 mg/day
    Biaxin *Tab:* 250, 500 mg
    Biaxin Oral Suspension *Oral susp:* 125, 250 mg/5 ml (50, 100 ml) (fruit punch)
    Biaxin XL *Tab:* 500 mg ext-rel
▷ *ofloxacin* (G) 400 mg/day
    Pediatric: <18 years: not recommended; ≥18 years: same as adult
    Floxin *Tab:* 200, 300, 400 mg
▷ *minocycline* (G) 4 mg/kg once; then 2 mg/kg (max 100 mg) q 12 hours; *Renal impairment (CrCl*
  <80 ml/min): max 200 mg/day
    Pediatric: <8 years: not recommended, ≥8 years: same as adult
    Dynacin *Cap:* 50, 100 mg
    Minocin *Cap:* 50, 75, 100 mg; *Oral susp:* 50 mg/5 ml (60 ml) (custard) (sulfites, alcohol 5%); *Vial:* 100
    mg, single-dose, pwdr for reconstitution, dilution, and IV infusion and IM injection

HEADACHE: MIGRAINE, CLUSTER, VASCULAR

ERGOTAMINE AGENTS
Comment: Do not use an ergotamine-type drug within 24 hours of any triptan or other 5-HT agonist.
▷ *dihydroergotamine mesylate* (G)
    DHE 45 1 mg SC, IM, or IV; may repeat at 1 hour intervals; max 3 mg/day SC or IM/day; max 2 mg IV/
    day; max 6 mg/week
    Pediatric: <12 years: not recommended; ≥12 years: same as adult
      Amp: 1 mg/ml (1 ml)
    Migranal 1 spray in each nostril; may repeat 15 minutes later; max 6 sprays/day and 8 sprays/week
    Pediatric: <12 years: not recommended; ≥12 years: same as adult
      Nasal spray: 4 mg/ml; 0.5 mg/spray (caffeine)
▷ *ergotamine* (G) 1 tab SL at onset of attack; then q 30 minutes as needed; max 3 tabs/day and 5 tabs/week
    Tab: 2 mg
▷ *ergotamine+caffeine* (G)
    Pediatric: <12 years: not recommended; ≥12 years: same as adult
    Cafergot 2 tabs at onset of attack; then 1 tab every 1/2 hour if needed; max 6 tabs/attack and 10 tabs/
    week
      Tab: ergot 1 mg+caf 100 mg
    Cafergot Suppository 1 suppository rectally at onset of headache; may repeat x 1 after 1 hour; max 2/
    attack, 5/week
      Rectal supp: ergot 2 mg+caf 100 mg

5-HT RECEPTOR AGONISTS
Comment: Contraindications to 5-HT receptor agonists include cardiovascular disease, ischemic heart disease, cerebral vascular syndromes, peripheral vascular disease, uncontrolled hypertension, hemiplegic, or basilar migraine. Do not use any triptan within 24 hours of ergot-type drugs or other 5-HT1A agonists, or within 2 weeks of taking an MAOI.
▷ *almotriptan* (G) 6.25 or 12.5 mg; may repeat once after 2 hours; max 2 doses/day
    Pediatric: <12 years: not recommended; ≥12 years: same as adult
    Axert *Tab:* 6.25 mg (6/card), 12.5 mg (12/card)
  Comment: *Almotriptan* is indicated for patients 12-17 years of age with a past medical history (PMHx) of
  migraine headache lasting ≥4 hours untreated.
▷ *eletriptan* (G) 20 or 40 mg; may repeat once after 2 hours; max 80 mg/day
  Pediatric: <18 years: not recommended; ≥18 years: same as adult
    Relpax *Tab:* 20, 40 mg
▷ *frovatriptan* (G) 2.5 mg with fluids; may repeat once after 2 hours; max 7.5 mg/day
  Pediatric: <18 years: not recommended; ≥18 years: same as adult
    Frova *Tab:* 2.5 mg
▷ *naratriptan* 1 or 2.5 mg with fluids; may repeat once after 4 hours; max 5 mg/day
  Pediatric: <18 years: not recommended; ≥18 years: same as adult
    Amerge *Tab:* 1, 2.5 mg
▷ *rizatriptan*
    Maxalt initially 5 or 10 mg; may repeat in 2 hours if needed; max 30 mg/day
    Pediatric: <18 years: safety and efficacy not established; ≥18 years: same as adult
      Tab: 5, 10 mg
    Maxalt-MLT initially 5 or 10 mg; may repeat in 2 hours if needed; max 30 mg/day
    Pediatric: <18 years: safety and efficacy not established; ≥18 years: same as adult
      MLT: 5, 10 mg
    RizaFilm place 1 film on top of tongue; separate repeat doses by at least 2 hours; max 30 mg cumulative
    dosage in a 24-hour period

Pediatric: <12 years, <40 kg: safety and efficacy not established; ≥12-17 years, ≥40 kg: place 1 film on top of tongue; do not dose repeat within 24 hours

Oral film: 10 mg

▷ **sumatriptan (G)**
Pediatric: <18 years: not recommended; ≥18 years: same as adult

Alsuma 6 mg SC to the upper arm or lateral thigh only; may repeat after 1 hour if needed; max 2 doses/day
Prefilled syringe: 6 mg/0.5 ml (2/pck with autoinjector)

Imitrex Injectable 4-6 mg SC; may repeat after 1 hour if needed; max 2 doses/day
Prefilled syringe: 4, 6 mg/0.5 ml (2/pck with or without autoinjector)

Imitrex Nasal Spray (G) 5-20 mg intranasally; may repeat once after 2 hours if needed; max 40 mg/day
Nasal spray: 5, 20 mg/spray (single-dose)

Imitrex Tab 25-200 mg x 1 dose; may be repeated at intervals of at least 2 hours; max 200 mg/day
Tab: 25, 50, 100 mg rapid-rel

Imitrex STATdose Pen 6 mg/0.5 mg SC; may repeat once after 2 hours if needed; max 2 doses/day
Prefilled needle-free autoinjector delivery system: 6 mg/0.5 ml (6/pck)

Onzetra Xsail each disposable white nosepiece contains half a dose of medication (11 mg of **sumatriptan**); a full dose is 22 mg; do not use more than 2 nosepieces per dose; attach the mouthpiece and 1 nasal piece; then press the white button on the delivery device to pierce the capsule in the nasal piece, then insert the nasal piece into one nostril and blow into the mouthpiece to deliver the nasal powder in the contents of 1 capsule (11 mg); repeat in the opposite nostril for a total single 22 mg dose
Cap: 11 mg nasal pwdr; *Kit:* nosepieces (2), capsules (2), reusable breath-powered delivery device (1)

Sumavel DosePro 6 mg SC to the upper arm or lateral thigh only; may repeat after 1 hour if needed; max 2 doses/day
Prefilled needle-free delivery system: 6 mg/0.5 ml (6/pck)

Tosymra 10 mg (1 nasal spray); max 3 nasal sprays (30 mg)/24 hours; separate doses by at least 1 hour
Nasal spray: 10 mg/spray ready-to-use, single-dose, disposable unit (6 units/carton)

Zembrace SymTouch administer 3 mg SC at onset of headache; may repeat hourly; max 12 mg/24 hours
Pediatric: <18 years: not recommended; ≥18 years: same as adult
Autoinjector: 3 mg/0.5 ml (prefilled single-dose disposable autoinjector)

▷ **zolmitriptan** initially 2.5 mg; may repeat after 2 hours if needed; max 10 mg/day
Pediatric: <18 years: not recommended; ≥18 years: same as adult

Zomig (G) *Tab:* 2.5*, 5 mg

Zomig Nasal Spray *Nasal spray:* 5 mg/spray single-dose (6/carton)

Zomig-ZMT *ODT:* 2.5 mg (6 tabs), 5*mg (3 tabs) (orange) (phenylalanine)

Comment: Do not use any *triptan* within 24 hours of ergotamine-type drugs or other 5-HT agonists, or within 2 weeks of taking an MAOI.

SEROTONIN (5-HT) 1F RECEPTOR AGONIST

▷ **lasmiditan** 50, 100, or 200 mg taken orally, as needed; max 1 dose/24 hours
Pediatric: safety and efficacy not established

Reyvow *Tab:* 50, 100 mg

Comment: Reyvow *(lasmiditan)* is the first serotonin (5-HT) 1F receptor agonist indicated for the acute treatment of migraine with or without aura in adults. Advise patients not to drive or operate machinery until at least 8 hours after taking a dose of Reyvow. Patients who cannot follow this advice should not take Reyvow; these patients may not be able to assess their own driving competence and the degree of impairment caused by Reyvow. Reyvow has not been studied in patients with severe hepatic impairment (Child-Pugh Class C) and its use in these patients is not recommended. Reyvow may further lower heart rate when administered with heart rate-lowering drugs. Avoid concomitant use with P-glycoprotein (P-gp) and breast cancer resistance protein (BCRP) substrates. Reyvow may cause central nervous system (CNS) depression and should be used with caution if used in combination with alcohol or other CNS depressants. A reaction consistent with *serotonin syndrome* has been reported in patients treated with Reyvow. Discontinue Reyvow if symptoms of serotonin syndrome occur. If medication overuse headache (MOH) develops, detoxification may be necessary. The most common adverse reactions (incidence ≥5% and greater than the placebo) have been dizziness, fatigue, paresthesia, and sedation. In animal studies, adverse effects on development (increased incidence of fetal abnormalities, increased embryo/fetal and offspring mortality, decreased fetal body weight) occurred at maternal exposures less or greater than those observed clinically. There are no adequate data on developmental risk associated with Reyvow use in pregnant females. There are no data on the presence of *lasmiditan* in human milk or effects of *lasmiditan* on the breastfed infant. Developmental and health benefits of breastfeeding should be considered along with the mother's clinical need for Reyvow and any potential adverse effects on the breastfed infant from Reyvow or from the underlying maternal condition.

NONSTEROIDAL ANTI-INFLAMMATORY

▷ **celecoxib** 120 mg (4.8 ml) with or without food; max 120 mg/24 hours; limit use to the fewest number of days per month; *Moderate hepatic impairment (Child-Pugh Class B):* max 60 mg (2.4 ml); *Poor metabolizers of CYP2C9 substrates:* max 60 mg (2.4 ml); *Severe renal impairment:* avoid

Pediatric: safety and efficacy <u>not</u> established; disseminated intravascular coagulation (DIC) has occurred in pediatric patients

    Elyxyb *Oral soln:* 120 mg/4.8 ml (25 mg/ml), single-dose glass bottles (9 bottles/carton)

    Comment: Elyxyb *(celecoxib)* is an oral solution formulation of the nonsteroidal anti-inflammatory drug *celecoxib* (first approved under the brand name **Celebrex**) indicated for the acute treatment of migraine with <u>or</u> without aura in adults. **Elyxyb** is <u>not</u> indicated for the preventive treatment of migraine. Avoid use in pregnancy starting at 30 weeks' gestation (due to risk of premature closure of fetal ductus arteriosus). Limited data from 3 published reports that included a total of 12 breastfeeding women showed low levels of *celecoxib* in breast milk.

5-HT IB+ID RECEPTOR AGONIST+NONSTEROIDAL ANTI-INFLAMMATORY DRUG (NSAID) COMBINATION

▷ *sumatriptan+naproxen* (G)

    Pediatric: <18 years: <u>not</u> recommended; ≥18 years: same as adult

        Treximet initially 1 tab; may repeat after 2 hours; max 2 doses/day

          Tab: suma 85 mg+naprox 500 mg (9/blister card)

    Comment: Do <u>not</u> use *sumatriptan* within 24 hours of ergot-type drugs <u>or</u> other 5-HT agonists <u>or</u> within 2 weeks of taking an MAOI.

OTHER ANALGESICS

▷ *acetaminophen+aspirin+caffeine* (G)

    Excedrin Migraine (OTC) 2 tabs q 6 hours prn; max 8 tabs/day x 2 days

    Pediatric: <18 years: <u>not</u> recommended; ≥18 years: same as adult

        Tab: acet 250 mg+asp 250 mg+caf 65 mg

▷ *celecoxib* 120 mg (4.8 ml) with <u>or</u> without food; max 120 mg/24 hours; limit use to the fewest number of days per month; *Moderate hepatic impairment (Child-Pugh Class B):* max 60 mg (2.4 ml); *Poor metabolizers of CYP2C9 substrates:* max 60 mg (2.4 ml); *Severe renal impairment:* avoid

    Pediatric: safety and efficacy <u>not</u> established; disseminated intravascular coagulation (DIC) has occurred in pediatric patients

    Elyxyb *Oral soln:* 120 mg/4.8 ml (25 mg/ml), single-dose glass bottles (9 bottles/carton)

    Comment: Elyxyb *(celecoxib)* is an oral solution formulation of the nonsteroidal anti-inflammatory drug *celecoxib* (first approved under the brand name **Celebrex**) indicated for the acute treatment of migraine with <u>or</u> without aura in adults. **Elyxyb** is <u>not</u> indicated for the preventive treatment of migraine. Avoid use in pregnancy starting at 30 weeks' gestation (due to risk of premature closure of fetal ductus arteriosus). Limited data from three published reports that included a total of 12 breastfeeding women showed low levels of *celecoxib* in breast milk.

▷ *diclofenac potassium powder for oral solution* (C; D ≥30 weeks) empty the contents of 1 pkt into a cup containing 1-2 oz <u>or</u> 2-4 tbsp (30-60 ml) of water, mix well, and drink immediately; water <u>only</u>, no other liquids; take on an empty stomach; use the closest effective dose for the shortest duration of time; safety and effectiveness of a 2nd dose have <u>not</u> been established

    Pediatric: <18 years: <u>not</u> established; ≥18 years: same as adult

    Cambia *Pwdr for oral soln:* 50 mg/pkt (3 pkts/set, conjoined with a perforated border)

    Comment: Cambia is <u>not</u> indicated for migraine prophylaxis. May <u>not</u> be bioequivalent with other *diclofenac* forms (e.g., *diclofenac sodium* ent-coat tabs, *diclofenac sodium* ext-rel tabs, *diclofenac potassium* immed-rel tabs) even if the mg strength is the same; therefore, it is <u>not</u> possible to convert dosing from any other *diclofenac* formulation to **Cambia**. **Cambia** is contraindicated in the setting of coronary artery bypass graft. Use of **Cambia** should <u>not</u> be considered with hepatic impairment, gastric/duodenal ulcer, starting at 30 weeks' gestation (risk of premature closure of the ductus arteriosus in the fetus), concomitant nonsteroidal anti-inflammatory drugs (NSAIDs), selective serotonin reuptake inhibitors (SSRIs), anticoagulants/antiplatelets, and any risk factor for potential bleeding.

▷ *ibuprofen+acetaminophen*

    Advil Dual Action (OTC) *Cplt:* fixed-dose combination of *ibuprofen* 125 mg (NSAID, antipyretic, analgesic) and *acetaminophen* 250 mg (antipyretic, analgesic)

▷ *isometheptene mucate+dichloralphenazone+acetaminophen* (IV)

    Midrin 2 caps initially; then 1 cap q 1 hour until relieved; max 5 caps/12 hours

    Pediatric: <12 years: <u>not</u> recommended; ≥12 years: same as adult

        Cap: iso 65 mg+dichlor 100 mg+acet 325 mg

CALCITONIN GENE-RELATED PEPTIDE (CGRP) RECEPTOR ANTAGONIST

Comment: The calcitonin gene-related peptide (CGRP) receptor antagonists are a class of drugs that block the activity of CGRP as prophylaxis against migraine attacks.

▷ *atogepant Recommended:* 10, 30, <u>or</u> 60 mg taken orally once daily with <u>or</u> without food; *Mild <u>or</u> Moderate renal impairment:* no dosage adjustment required; *Severe renal impairment (CrCl 15-29 ml/min) <u>or</u> end-stage renal disease (ESRD; CrCl <15 ml/min):* max 10 mg once daily; *ESRD undergoing intermittent dialysis:* take 10 mg after dialysis; *Mild <u>or</u> moderate hepatic impairment:* no dose adjustment required; *Severe hepatic impairment:* avoid use

Pediatric: safety and efficacy not established

Qulipta *Tab:* 10, 30, 60 mg

Comment: Qulipta is an oral CGRP receptor antagonist indicated for the preventive treatment of episodic migraine in adults. The most common adverse reactions (at least 4% and greater than placebo) have been nausea, constipation, and fatigue. Taken with concomitant strong CYP3A4 inhibitors, limit daily dose to 10 mg. Taken with concomitant strong or moderate CYP3A4 inducers, daily dose 30 mg or 60 mg. Taken with concomitant organic ion transporting polypeptide (OATP) inhibitors, limit daily dose of **Qulipta** to 10 mg or 30 mg. Based on animal data, *atogepant* may cause fetal harm. Advise females of reproductive potential of potential fetal risk and recommend effective contraception during treatment. There are no data on the presence of *atogepant* in human milk or effects on the breastfed infant. The developmental and health benefits of breastfeeding should be considered along with the mother's clinical need for **Qulipta** and any potential adverse effects on the breastfed infant from **Qulipta** or from the underlying maternal condition.

▶ *erenumab-aooe* administer by SC injection only in the upper arm, abdomen, or thigh; recommended dose is 70 mg SC once monthly; some patients may benefit from a dosage of 140 mg SC once monthly (i.e., two consecutive injections of 70 mg each); the needle shield within the white cap of the prefilled autoinjector and the gray needle cap of the prefilled syringe contains dry natural rubber (a derivative of latex) which may cause allergic reactions in individuals sensitive to latex

Pediatric: <18 years: not recommended; ≥18 years: same as adult

Aimovig *Autoinjector:* 70 mg/ml (1 ml), prefilled single-dose, SureClick

Comment: The most common adverse side effects are injection site reaction and constipation. There are no adequate data on the developmental risk associated with the use of **Aimovig** in pregnant females. There are no data on the presence of *erenumab-aooe* in human milk or effects on the breastfed infant. Safety and effectiveness in pediatric patients have not been established.

▶ *fremanezumab-vfrm* administer by SC injection only in the upper arm, abdomen, or thigh; recommended dose is 225 mg SC once monthly or 675 mg SC once every 3 months (3 x 225 mg SC doses once quarterly)

Pediatric: <18 years: not recommended; ≥18 years: same as adult

Ajovy *Prefilled syringe:* 225 mg/1.5 ml (1.5 ml) solution, single-dose; *Autoinjector:* 225 mg/1.5 ml (1.5 ml) solution, single-dose

Comment: The most common adverse side effects are injection site reaction and constipation. There are no adequate data on the developmental risk associated with the use of **Ajovy** in pregnant females. There are no data on the presence of *fremanezumab-vfrm* in human milk or effects on the breastfed infant. Safety and effectiveness in pediatric patients have not been established.

▶ *galcanezumab-gnlm* administer by SC injection only in the back of the upper arm, abdomen, thigh, or buttocks; *Loading dose:* 240 mg (2 x 120 mg) SC; *Maintenance:* 120 mg SC once monthly

Pediatric: <18 years: not recommended; ≥18 years: same as adult

Emgality *Prefilled pen/Prefilled syringe:* 120 mg/ml (1 ml) solution, single-dose

Comment: The most common adverse side effect (incidence ≥2%) is injection site reaction. There are no adequate data on the developmental risk associated with the use of **Emgality** in pregnant females. There are no data on the presence of *fremanezumab-vfrm* in human milk or effects on the breastfed infant. Safety and effectiveness in pediatric patients have not been established.

▶ *rimegepant* 75 mg; max 75 mg/24 hours; safety of treating more than 15 migraines in a 30-day period has not been established

Pediatric: safety and efficacy not established

Nurtec ODT *Tab:* 75 mg oral-disint

Comment: Nurtec ODT *(rimegepant)* is a CGRP receptor antagonist for the acute treatment of migraine with or without aura. **Nurtec ODT** is not indicated for the preventive treatment of migraine. Avoid use in patients with severe hepatic impairment (Child-Pugh Class C). Avoid concomitant administration of **Nurtec ODT** with strong CYP3A4 inhibitors. When administered with a moderate CYP3A4 inhibitor, avoid another dose of **Nurtec ODT** for the next 48 hours. Avoid concomitant administration of **Nurtec ODT** with strong and moderate CYP3A inducers and inhibitors of P-gp or BCRP. There are no adequate data on embryo/fetal risk associated with the use of **Nurtec ODT** in pregnancy. However, in animal studies, oral administration of *rimegepant* during organogenesis resulted in decreased fetal body weight and increased incidence of fetal variations at exposures greater than those used clinically and which were associated with maternal toxicity. There are no data on the presence of *rimegepant* or its metabolites in human or animal milk or effects of *rimegepant* on the breastfed infant. The developmental and health benefits of breastfeeding should be considered along with the mother's clinical need for **Nurtec ODT** and any potential adverse effects on the breastfed infant from **Nurtec ODT** or from the underlying maternal condition.

▶ *ubrogepant* 50 or 100 mg; if needed, a second dose may be administered at least 2 hours after the initial dose; max 200 mg/24 hours; *severe hepatic or severe renal impairment:* 50 mg; if needed, a second 50 mg dose may be administered at least 2 hours after the initial dose; max 100 mg/24 hours

Ubrelvy *Tab:* 50, 100 mg

Comment: Ubrelvy *(ubrogepant)* is a potent, orally administered CGRP receptor antagonist for the acute treatment of migraine with or without aura. **Ubrelvy** is not indicated for the preventive treatment of migraine. **Ubrelvy** is contraindicated with concomitant use of strong CYP3A4 inhibitors. Strong

(continued)

CYP3A4 inducers should be avoided as concomitant use will result in reduction of *ubrogepant* exposure. For additional dose modifications for moderate or weak CYP3A4 inhibitors and inducers or BCRP and/ or P-gp only inhibitors, refer to the mfr pkg insert. The most common adverse reactions (incidence ≥2%) have been nausea and somnolence. There are no adequate data on the developmental risks associated with the use of **Ubrelvy** in pregnant females. However, animal studies have demonstrated adverse effects on embryo/fetal development and increased embryo/fetal mortality following administration of *ubrogepant* during pregnancy. There are no data on the presence of *ubrogepant* in human milk or effects on the breastfed infant.

▷ *zavegepant* Recommended dose: 10 mg administered as a single spray in one nostril, as needed; max 10 mg (1 spray)/24 hours; safety of treating more than 8 migraines in a 30-day period has not been established
Pediatric: Safety and efficacy not established
   Zavzpret *Nasal spray:* 10 mg/spray, ready-to-use, unit-dose, disposable device (6 units/carton)
   Comment: Zavzpret is a CGRP receptor antagonist nasal spray for the acute treatment of migraine with or without aura in adults. **Zavzpret** is not indicated for the preventive treatment of migraine. The most common adverse reactions (at least 2% and greater than placebo) have been taste disorders, nausea, nasal discomfort, and vomiting. If a serious hypersensitivity reaction occurs, discontinue **Zavzpret** and initiate appropriate therapy. Hypersensitivity reactions, including facial swelling and urticaria, have occurred with **Zavzpret**. Avoid concomitant use with drugs that inhibit and drugs that induce OATP1B3 or NTCP transporters. Avoid use of intranasal decongestants; if unavoidable, administer intranasal decongestants at least 1 hour after **Zavzpret** administration. Avoid use in patients with severe hepatic impairment *(Child-Pugh Class C)*. Avoid use in patients with CrCl <30 ml/min. There are no adequate human or animal data on the developmental risk associated with the use of **Zavzpret** in pregnancy. There are no data on the presence of *zavegepant* or its metabolites in human milk or effects of *zavegepant* on the breastfed infant. Developmental and health benefits of breastfeeding should be considered along with the mother's clinical need for **Zavzpret** and any potential adverse effects on the breastfed infant from **Zavzpret** or from the underlying maternal condition. To report suspected adverse reactions, contact Pfizer at 1-800-438-1985 or FDA at 1-800-FDA-1088 or www.fda.gov/medwatch.

ANTICONVULSANTS

▷ *divalproex sodium* Delayed-release: initially 250 mg bid, titrate weekly to usual max 500 mg bid; *Extended-release*: initially 500 mg once daily; may increase after 1 week to 1 gm once daily
Pediatric: <10 years: not recommended; ≥10 years: same as adult
   Depakene *Cap:* 250 mg del-rel; *Syr:* 250 mg/5 ml (16 oz)
   Depakote *Tab:* 125, 250, 500 mg del-rel
   Depakote ER *Tab:* 250, 500 mg ext-rel
   Depakote Sprinkle *Cap:* 125 mg del-rel
▷ *topiramate* (G) initially 25 mg daily in the PM and titrate up daily as tolerated; then 25 mg bid; then 25 mg in the AM and 50 mg in the PM; then 50 mg bid
Pediatric: <12 years: not recommended; ≥12 years: same as adult
   Eprontia *Oral soln:* 25 mg/ml
   Topamax *Tab:* 25, 50, 100, 200 mg
   Topamax Sprinkle Caps *Cap:* 15, 25 mg
   Trokendi XR *Cap:* 25, 50, 100, 200 mg ext-rel
   Qudexy XR *Cap:* 25, 50, 100, 150, 200 mg ext-rel
▷ *topiramate* initial dose, titration, and recommended maintenance dose vary by indication and age group; see mfr pkg insert for full prescribing information, including recommended dosage and dosing considerations in patients with renal impairment, geriatric patients, and patients undergoing hemodialysis
Pediatric: Seizure: <2 years: safety and efficacy not established; ≥2 years: see dosing tables below

Monotherapy Titration Schedule for Adults and Pediatric Patients ≥10 Years of age		
	Morning Dose	Evening Dose
Week 1	25 mg	25 mg
Week 2	50 mg	50 mg
Week 3	75 mg	75 mg
Week 4	100 mg	100 mg
Week 5	150 mg	150 mg
Week 6	200 mg	200 mg

Monotherapy Target Total Maintenance Dosing for Patients 2-9 Years of age		
Weight	Total Daily Minimum	Maximum Maintenance
Up to 11 kg	150 mg	250 mg
12 to 22 kg	200 mg	300 mg
23 to 31 kg	200 mg	350 mg
32 to 38 kg	250 mg	350 mg
>38 kg	250 mg	400 mg

Migraine Prophylaxis: dose and titration rate should be guided by clinical outcomes. If required, longer intervals between dose adjustments can be used. Recommended total daily dose is 100 mg administered in 2 divided doses. The recommended titration rate for **Eprontia** for the preventive treatment of migraine is as follows: *<12 years:* not *established;* ≥*12 years:* see dosing table below.

Preventive Treatment of Migraine Dose Titration Schedule for Patients ≥12 Years of age		
Week	Morning Dose	Evening Dose
1	None	25 mg
2	25 mg	25 mg
3	25 mg	50 mg
4	50 mg	50 mg

BETA-BLOCKERS
▷ *atenolol* (G) initially 25 mg bid; max 150 mg/day in divided doses
  Pediatric: <12 years: not recommended; ≥12 years: same as adult
    Tenormin *Tab:* 25, 50, 100 mg
▷ *metoprolol succinate*
  Pediatric: <12 years: not recommended; ≥12 years: same as adult
    Toprol-XL initially 25-100 mg in a single dose daily; increase weekly if needed; max 400 mg/day
      Tab: 25*, 50*, 100*, 200*mg ext-rel
▷ *metoprolol tartrate*
  Pediatric: <12 years: not recommended; ≥12 years: same as adult
    Lopressor (G) initially 25-50 mg bid; increase weekly if needed; max 400 mg/day
      Tab: 25, 37.5, 50, 75, 100 mg
▷ *nadolol* (G) initially 20 mg daily; max 240 mg/day in divided doses
  Pediatric: <12 years: not recommended; ≥12 years: same as adult
    Corgard *Tab:* 20*, 40*, 80*, 120*, 160*mg
▷ *propranolol* (G)
  Pediatric: <12 years: not recommended; ≥12 years: same as adult
    Inderal initially 10 mg bid; usual range 160-320 mg/day in divided doses
      Tab: 10*, 20*, 40*, 60*, 80*mg
    Inderal LA initially 80 mg daily in a single dose; increase q 3-7 days; usual range 120-160 mg/day; max 320 mg/day in a single dose
      Cap: 60, 80, 120, 160 mg sust-rel
    InnoPran XL initially 80 mg q HS; max 120 mg/day
      Cap: 80, 120 mg ext-rel
▷ *timolol* (G) initially 5 mg bid; max 60 mg/day in divided doses
  Pediatric: <12 years: not recommended; ≥12 years: same as adult
    Blocadren *Tab:* 5, 10*, 20*mg

CALCIUM ANTAGONISTS
▷ *diltiazem* (G)
  Pediatric: <12 years: not recommended; ≥12 years: same as adult
    Cardizem initially 30 mg qid; may increase gradually every 1-2 days; max 360 mg/day in divided doses
      Tab: 30, 60, 90, 120 mg
    Cardizem CD initially 120-180 mg once daily; adjust at 1- to 2-week intervals; max 480 mg/day
      Cap: 120, 180, 240, 300, 360 mg ext-rel

(continued)

Cardizem LA initially 180-240 mg once daily; titrate at 2-week intervals; max 540 mg/day
    Tab: 120, 180, 240, 300, 360, 420 mg ext-rel
Cardizem SR initially 60-120 mg bid; adjust at 2-week intervals; max 360 mg/day
    Cap: 60, 90, 120 mg sust-rel

▷ *nifedipine* (G)
  Pediatric: <12 years: <u>not</u> recommended; ≥12 years: same as adult
    Adalat initially 10 mg tid; usual range 10-20 mg tid; max 180 mg/day
      Cap: 10, 20 mg
    Procardia initially 10 mg tid; titrate over 7-14 days: max 30 mg/dose and 180 mg/day in divided doses
      Cap: 10, 20 mg
    Procardia XL initially 30-60 mg daily; titrate over 7-14 days; max 90 mg/day in divided doses

▷ *verapamil* (G)
  Pediatric: <12 years: <u>not</u> recommended; ≥12 years: same as adult
    Calan 80-120 mg tid; increase daily <u>or</u> weekly if needed
      Tab: 40, 80*, 120*mg
    Covera HS initially 180 mg q HS; titrate in steps to 240 mg; then to 360 mg; then to 480 mg if needed
      Tab: 180, 240 mg ext-rel
    Isoptin initially 80-120 mg tid
      Tab: 40, 80, 120 mg
    Isoptin SR initially 120-180 mg in the AM; may increase to 240 mg in the AM; then 180 mg q 12 hours <u>or</u> 240 mg in the AM and 120 mg in the PM; then 240 mg q 12 hours
      Tab: 120, 180*, 240*mg sust-rel

TRICYCLIC ANTIDEPRESSANTS (TCAs)

Comment: Co-administration of tricyclic antidepressants (TCAs) with SSRIs requires extreme caution.

▷ *amitriptyline* (G) 10-20 mg q HS
  Pediatric: <12 years: <u>not</u> recommended; ≥12 years: same as adult
    Tab: 10, 25, 50, 75, 100, 150 mg

▷ *doxepin* (G) 10-200 mg q HS
  Pediatric: <12 years: <u>not</u> recommended; ≥12 years: same as adult
    Cap: 10, 25, 50, 75, 100, 150 mg; *Oral conc:* 10 mg/ml (4 oz w. dropper)

▷ *imipramine* (G) 10-200 mg q HS
    Tofranil 25-50 mg; max 200 mg/day; if maintenance dose exceeds 75 mg daily, may switch to **Tofranil PM**
    Pediatric: <6 years: <u>not</u> recommended; 6-12 years: initially 25 mg; >12 years: 50 mg max 2.5 mg/kg/day
      Tab: 10, 25, 50 mg
    Tofranil PM initially 75 mg once daily 1 hour before HS; max 200 mg
      Cap: 75, 100, 125, 150 mg

▷ *nortriptyline* (G) 10-150 mg q HS
  Pediatric: <12 years: <u>not</u> recommended; ≥12 years: same as adult
    Pamelor *Cap:* 10, 25, 50, 75 mg; *Oral soln:* 10 mg/5 ml (16 oz)

SELECTIVE SEROTONIN REUPTAKE INHIBITORS (SSRIs)

Comment: Co-administration of SSRIs with TCAs requires extreme caution. Concomitant use of MAOIs and SSRIs is absolutely contraindicated. Avoid other serotonergic drugs. A potentially fatal adverse event is *serotonin syndrome*, caused by serotonin excess. Milder symptoms require healthcare provider intervention to avert severe symptoms which can be rapidly fatal without urgent/emergent medical care. Symptoms include restlessness, agitation, confusion, hallucinations, tachycardia, hypertension, dilated pupils, muscle twitching, muscle rigidity, loss of muscle coordination, diaphoresis, diarrhea, headache, shivering, piloerection, hyperpyrexia, cardiac arrhythmias, seizures, loss of consciousness, coma, and death. Abrupt withdrawal <u>or</u> interruption of treatment with an antidepressant medication is sometimes associated with an antidepressant discontinuation syndrome, which may be mediated by gradually tapering the drug over a period of 2 weeks <u>or</u> longer, depending on the dose strength and length of treatment. Common symptoms of the *serotonin discontinuation syndrome* include flu-like symptoms (nausea, vomiting, diarrhea, headaches, sweating), sleep disturbances (insomnia, nightmares, constant sleepiness), mood disturbances (dysphoria, anxiety, agitation), cognitive disturbances (mental confusion, hyperarousal), sensory and movement disturbances (imbalance, tremors, vertigo, dizziness), and electric-shock-like sensations in the brain, often described by sufferers as "brain zaps."

▷ *fluoxetine* (G)
    Prozac initially 20 mg daily; may increase after 1 week; doses >20 mg/day may be divided into AM and noon doses; max 80 mg/day
    Pediatric: <8 years: <u>not</u> recommended; 8-17 years: initially 10-20 mg/day; start lower weight children at 10 mg/day; if starting at 10 mg daily, may increase after 1 week to 20 mg once daily
      Cap: 10, 20, 40 mg; *Tab:* 30*, 60*mg; *Oral soln:* 20 mg/5 ml (4 oz) (mint)
    Prozac Weekly following daily *fluoxetine* therapy at 20 mg/day for 13 weeks, may initiate **Prozac Weekly** 7 days after the last 20 mg *fluoxetine* dose

Pediatric: <12 years: <u>not</u> recommended; ≥12 years: same as adult
    Cap: 90 mg ent-coat del-rel pellets

OTHER AGENT

▷ *methysergide maleate* 4-8 mg daily in divided doses with food; max 8 mg/day; max 6-month treatment course; wean off over the last 2-3 weeks of treatment course; separate treatment courses by a 3 to 4 week drug-free interval
Pediatric: <18 years: <u>not</u> recommended; ≥18 years: same as adult
    Sansert *Tab:* 2 mg
Comment: *Methysergide maleate* is indicated for the prevention <u>or</u> reduction of intensity and frequency of vascular headaches. It is contraindicated in pregnancy due to its oxytocic actions. *Methysergide maleate* is a semisynthetic compound structurally related to ergotamine and thus it may appear in breast milk. Ergot alkaloids have been reported to cause nausea, vomiting, diarrhea, and weakness in the nursing infant and suppression of prolactin secretion and lactation in the mother.

MAGNESIUM SUPPLEMENTS

▷ *magnesium*
    Slow-Mag 2 tabs daily
        Tab: 64 mg (as chloride)+110 mg (as carbonate)
▷ *magnesium oxide*
    Mag-Ox 400 1-2 tabs daily
        Tab: 400 mg

HEADACHE: TENSION (MUSCLE CONTRACTION)

Acetaminophen for IV Infusion *see Pain*
NSAIDs *see* Appendix I. NSAIDs online at https://connect.springerpub.com/content/reference-book/978-0-8261-7935-7/back-matter/part02/back-matter/bmatter10
Opioid Analgesics *see Pain*
Topical and Transdermal Analgesics *see Pain*
Parenteral Corticosteroids *see* Appendix L. Parenteral Corticosteroids
Oral Corticosteroids *see* Appendix K. Oral Corticosteroids
Topical Analgesic and Anesthetic Agents *see* Appendix H. Anesthetic Agents for Local Infiltration and Dermal/Mucosal Membrane Application online at https://connect.springerpub.com/content/reference-book/978-0-8261-7935-7/back-matter/part02/back-matter/bmatter9

ORAL ANALGESIC COMBINATIONS

▷ *butalbital+acetaminophen* (G)
Pediatric: <12 years: <u>not</u> recommended; ≥12 years: same as adult
    Phrenilin 1-2 tabs q 4 hours prn; max 6 tabs/day
        Tab: but 50 mg+acet 325 mg
    Phrenilin Forte 1 tab <u>or</u> cap q 4 hours prn; max 6 caps/day
        Cap/Tab: but 50 mg+acet 650 mg
▷*butalbital+acetaminophen+caffeine* (G)
Pediatric: <12 years: <u>not</u> recommended; ≥12 years: same as adult
    Fioricet 1-2 tabs q 4 hours prn; max 6/day
        Tab: but 50 mg+acet 325 mg+caf 40 mg
    Zebutal 1 cap q 4 hours prn; max 5/day
        Cap: but 50 mg+acet 500 mg+caf 40 mg
▷ *butalbital+acetaminophen+codeine+caffeine* (III) (G)
Pediatric: <18 years: <u>not</u> recommended; ≥18 years: same as adult
    Fioricet with Codeine 1-2 tabs at onset q 4 hours prn; max 6 tabs/day
        Tab: but 50 mg+acet 325 mg+cod 30 mg+caf 40 mg
▷ *butalbital+aspirin+caffeine* (III)(G)
Pediatric: <12 years: <u>not</u> recommended; ≥12 years: same as adult
    Fiorinal 1-2 tabs <u>or</u> caps q 4 hours prn; max 6 caps/tabs/day
        Tab/Cap: but 50 mg+asa 325 mg+caf 40 mg
▷ *butalbital+aspirin+codeine+caffeine* (III)(G)
Pediatric: 18 years: <u>not</u> recommended; ≥18 years: same as adult
    Fiorinal with Codeine 1-2 caps q 4 hours prn; max 6 caps/day
        Cap: but 50 mg+asp 325 mg+cod 30 mg+caf 40 mg
▷ *butorphanol tartrate* (IV)(G) initially 1 spray (1 mg) in one nostril and may repeat after 60-90 minutes (*elderly* after 90-120 minutes) in opposite nostril if needed <u>or</u> 1 spray in each nostril and may repeat q 3-4 hours prn
Pediatric: <18 years: <u>not</u> recommended; ≥18 years: same as adult
    Butorphanol Nasal Spray *Nasal spray:* 1 mg/actuation (10 mg/ml, 2.5 ml)
    Stadol Nasal Spray *Nasal spray:* 10 mg/ml, 1 mg/actuation (10 mg/ml, 2.5 ml)

(continued)

➢ **tramadol (IV)(G)** initially 100 mg once daily; may increase by 100 mg every 5 days; max 300 mg/day; *CrCl <30 ml/min* or *severe hepatic impairment*: not recommended; *Cirrhosis*: max 50 mg q 12 hours
  Pediatric: <18 years: not recommended; ≥18 years: same as adult
    Rybix ODT *ODT*: 50 mg (mint) (phenylalanine)
    Ryzolt *Tab*: 100, 200, 300 mg ext-rel
    Ultram *Tab*: 50*mg
    Ultram ER *Tab*: 100, 200, 300 mg ext-rel
➢ **tramadol+acetaminophen (IV)(G)** 2 tabs q 4-6 hours prn; max 8 tabs/day; 5 days; *CrCl <30 ml/min*: max 2 tabs q 12 hours; max 4 tabs/day x 5 days; *Cirrhosis or other liver disease*: contraindicated
  Pediatric: <18 years: not recommended; ≥18 years: same as adult
    Ultracet *Tab*: tram 37.5+acet 325 mg

TRICYCLIC ANTIDEPRESSANTS (TCAs)
Comment: Co-administration of tricyclic antidepressants (TCAs) with selective serotonin reuptake inhibitors (SSRIs) requires extreme caution.
➢ **amitriptyline (G)** 50-100 mg/day
  Pediatric: <12 years: not recommended; ≥12 years: same as adult
    Tab: 10, 25, 50, 75, 100, 150 mg
➢ **desipramine (G)** 50-100 mg bid
  Pediatric: <12 years: not recommended; ≥12 years: same as adult
    Norpramin *Tab*: 10, 25, 50, 75, 100, 150 mg
➢ **imipramine (G)**
  Pediatric: <12 years: not recommended; ≥12 years: same as adult
    Tofranil initially 75 mg daily (max 200 mg); adolescents initially 30-40 mg daily (max 100 mg/day); if maintenance dose exceeds 75 mg daily, may switch to **Tofranil PM** for divided or bedtime dosing
    Tab: 10, 25, 50 mg
    Tofranil PM initially 75 mg once daily 1 hour before HS; max 200 mg
      Cap: 75, 100, 125, 150 mg
    Tofranil Injection 50 mg IM; lower dose for adolescents; switch to oral form as soon as possible
      Amp: 25 mg/2 ml (2 ml)
➢ **nortriptyline (G)** 25-50 mg/day
  Pediatric: <12 years: not recommended; ≥12 years: same as adult
    Pamelor *Cap*: 10, 25, 50, 75 mg; *Oral soln*: 10 mg/5 ml (16 oz)

MAGNESIUM SUPPLEMENTS
➢ *magnesium*
    Slow-Mag 2 tabs daily
      Tab: 64 mg (as chloride)/110 mg (as carbonate)
➢ *magnesium oxide*
    Mag-Ox 400 1-2 tabs daily
      Tab: 400 mg

HEART FAILURE (HF)

HEART FAILURE AND DIABETES
Comment: About 6.7 million Americans suffer from heart failure (HF), with the prevalence expected to rise to 8.0 million by 2030. HF is the leading cause of hospitalizations for individuals aged 65 and older, triggering approximately 1.3 million hospitalizations a year. Patients with HF are at the highest risk of a HF event in the first 30 days postdischarge, with 7% dying and 25% being rehospitalized within 1 month. sodium-glucose co-transporter 2 (SGLT2) is responsible for glucose reabsorption by the kidney and sodium-glucose co-transporter 1 (SGLT1) is responsible for glucose absorption in the gastrointestinal tract. The SGLT inhibitor class was recommended as first-line treatment for HF by the American Heart Association (AHA), the American College of Cardiology (ACC), and the Heart Failure Society of America (HFSA) in their joint 2022 AHA/ACC/HFSA Guideline for the Management of Heart Failure. An April 2023 ACC expert consensus statement highlighted the benefit of SGLT inhibitors as part of Guideline-Directed Medical Therapy (GDMT) in patients with HF with preserved ejection fraction (HFpEF). According to the ACC expert consensus statement, SGLT2 inhibitors should be initiated in all individuals with HFpEF who are stable during hospitalization and have no patient population contraindications.
HF in the presence of type 2 diabetes mellitus (T2DM) has a 5-year survival rate on par with some of the worst diseases, such as lung cancer, because diabetes makes the pathophysiology of HF worse. Diabetes amplifies the neurohormonal response to HF, so it drives progressive HF and increases the risk for sudden death. **As left ventricular function decreases, patients with diabetes have heightened activation of the renin–angiotensin system (RAS).** They have increased left ventricular hypertrophy, and they have increased sympathetic nervous system (SNS) activation. The following is a "four Ds" framework that clinicians can use to improve prognosis in these patients: (1) *loop diuretics* to get the patient out of congestive cardiac syndrome as quickly as possible; (2) *disease modification* with beta-blockers and angiotensin-converting enzyme inhibitors (ACEIs), to the maximal

dose tolerated, the mainstays of treatment for patients with HF (ACEIs protect these patients against cardiac myocyte cell death and vasoconstriction and beta-blockers protect against the activation of the SNS); (3) *consider device therapy* (including defibrillators and resynchronization therapy); and (4) *optimize diabetes management.*

SODIUM-GLUCOSE CO-TRANSPORTER 2 (SGLT-2) INHIBITOR

▷ *dapagliflozin* (G) *Recommended starting dose:* 5 mg once daily, taken in the morning, with or without food; may increase dose to 10 mg once daily in patients tolerating **Farxiga** who require additional glycemic control; assess renal function before initiating **Farxiga**; do not initiate **Farxiga** if eGFR is <60 ml/min/1.73 m²; discontinue **Farxiga** if eGFR falls persistently <60 ml/min/1.73 m²
  Pediatric: <18 years: safety and efficacy not established; ≥18 years: same as adult
    Farxiga *Tab:* 5, 10 mg film-coat
    Comment: Farxiga *(dapagliflozin)* is an SGLT2 inhibitor indicated for the treatment of T2DM and to reduce the risk of hospitalization from HF, and chronic kidney disease (CKD). **Farxiga** is not for the treatment of type 1 diabetes mellitus (T1DM) or diabetic ketoacidosis.

▷ *sotagliflozin* correct volume status before starting **Inpefa** at 200 mg once daily and titrate to 400 mg as tolerated; in patients with decompensated HF, begin dosing when patients are hemodynamically stable; withhold **Inpefa** at least 3 days, if possible, prior to major surgery or procedures associated with prolonged fasting
  Pediatric: <18 years: safety and efficacy not established; ≥18 years: same as adult
    Inpefa *Tab:* 200, 400 mg
    Comment: Inpefa is an SGLT2 and SGLT1 inhibitor indicated to reduce the risk of cardiovascular death, hospitalization for HF, and urgent HF visit in adults with HF or T2DM, CKD, and other cardiovascular risk factors. The broad label encompasses HF patients across the full range of left ventricular ejection fraction (LVEF), including preserved ejection fraction and reduced ejection fraction, and for patients with or without diabetes. The approval is based on two randomized, double-blind, placebo-controlled phase 3 cardiovascular outcomes studies of **Inpefa** in patients with HF or at risk of HF. Together, SOLOIST-WHF (Worsening Heart Failure) and SCORED enrolled almost 12,000 patients. Results from SOLOIST-WHF showed that **Inpefa** significantly reduced the risk of the composite of hospitalizations for HF, urgent visits for HF, and cardiovascular death by 33% compared with placebo in patients who had been recently hospitalized for worsening HF. The most common adverse reactions (incidence ≥5%) are urinary tract infection, volume depletion, diarrhea, and hypoglycemia. There is a higher incidence of adverse reactions to **Inpefa** in the setting of volume depletion. Monitor for volume depletion, including hypotension and/or lethargy. Monitor for signs and symptoms of urosepsis and pyelonephritis and treat promptly. Monitor for signs and symptoms of hypoglycemia with concomitant use of insulin and insulin secretagogues; lowering of the insulin dose or insulin secretagogue dose may be required. There is risk of developing necrotizing fasciitis of the perineum (Fournier's gangrene). Monitor for pain, tenderness, erythema, or swelling in the genital/perineal area, along with fever or malaise; discontinue **Inpefa** and treat this complication urgently. Genital mycotic infection may occur; monitor and treat as appropriate. Monitor *digoxin* levels and *lithium* levels. *Sotagliflozin* exposure is reduced if taken with concomitant uridine 5'-diphospho-glucuronosyltransferase inducers (e.g., *rifampin*); monitor clinical status. Based on animal data showing renal effects, **Inpefa** is not recommended during the 2nd and 3rd trimesters of pregnancy. Pregnant females with congestive HF are at increased risk for preterm birth. Clinical classification of heart disease may worsen with pregnancy and lead to maternal death. Since human kidney maturation occurs *in utero* and during the first 2 years of life when lactational exposure may occur, there may be risk to the developing human kidney. Because of the potential for serious adverse reactions in the breastfed infant, advise mothers that breastfeeding is not recommended while taking **Inpefa**. To report suspected adverse reactions, contact Lexicon at 855-330-2573 or FDA at 800-FDA-1088 or www.fda.gov/medwatch.

ANGIOTENSIN-CONVERTING ENZYME INHIBITORS (ACEIs)

▷ *captopril* (G) initially 25 mg tid; after 1-2 weeks may increase to 50 mg tid; max 450 mg/day
  Pediatric: <12 years: not recommended; ≥12 years: same as adult
    Capoten *Tab:* 12.5*, 25*, 50*, 100*mg
▷ *enalapril* (G) initially 5 mg daily; usual dosage range 10-40 mg/day; max 40 mg/day
  Pediatric: <12 years: not recommended; ≥12 years: same as adult
    Epaned Oral Solution *Oral soln:* 1 mg/ml (150 ml) (mixed berry)
    Vasotec *Tab:* 2.5*, 5*, 10, 20 mg
▷ *fosinopril* (G) initially 10 mg daily, usual maintenance 20-40 mg/day in a single or divided doses
  Pediatric: <6 years, <50 kg: not recommended; 6-12 years, ≥50 kg: 5-10 mg daily; ≥12 years: same as adult
    Monopril *Tab:* 10*, 20, 40 mg
▷ *lisinopril* initially 5 mg daily
    Prinivil initially 10 mg daily; usual range 20-40 mg/day
    Pediatric: <12 years: not recommended; ≥12 years: same as adult
      Tab: 5*, 10*, 20*, 40 mg
    Qbrelis Oral Solution administer as a single dose once daily

(continued)

Pediatric: <6 years, glomerular filtration rate (GFR) <30 ml/min: not recommended; ≥6 years, GFR >30 ml/min: initially 0.07 mg/kg, max 5 mg; adjust according to BP up to a max of 0.61 mg/kg (40 mg) once daily

> *Oral soln:* 1 mg/ml (150 ml)

Zestril initially 10 mg daily; usual range 20-40 mg/day
Pediatric: <12 years: not recommended; ≥12 years: same as adult

> *Tab:* 2.5, 5*, 10, 20, 30, 40 mg

▷ *quinapril* initially 5 mg bid; increase weekly to 10-20 mg bid
Pediatric: <12 years: not recommended; ≥12 years: same as adult

Accupril *Tab:* 5*, 10, 20, 40 mg

▷ *ramipril* initially 2.5 mg bid; usual maintenance 5 mg bid
Pediatric: <12 years: not recommended; ≥12 years: same as adult

Altace *Tab/Cap:* 1.25, 2.5, 5, 10 mg

▷ *trandolapril* initially 1 mg daily; titrate to dose of 4 mg daily as tolerated
Pediatric: <12 years: not recommended; ≥12 years: same as adult

Mavik *Tab:* 1*, 2, 4 mg

BETA-BLOCKERS (CARDIOSELECTIVE)

▷ *carvedilol* (G)

Coreg initially 3.125 mg bid; may increase at 1 to 2 week intervals to 12.5 mg bid; usual max 50 mg bid
Pediatric: <18 years: not recommended; ≥18 years: same as adult

> *Tab:* 3.125, 6.25, 12.5, 25 mg

Coreg CR initially 10 mg once daily x 2 weeks; may double dose at 2 week intervals; max 80 mg once daily; may open caps and sprinkle on food
Pediatric: <18 years: not recommended; ≥18 years: same as adult

> *Cap:* 10, 20, 40, 80 mg cont-rel

▷ *metoprolol succinate*
Pediatric: <12 years: not recommended; ≥12 years: same as adult

Toprol-XL initially 12.5-25 mg in a single dose daily; increase weekly if needed; reduce if symptomatic bradycardia occurs; max 400 mg/day

> *Tab:* 25*, 50*, 100*, 200*mg ext-rel

▷ *metoprolol tartrate*
Pediatric: <12 years: not recommended; ≥12 years: same as adult

Lopressor (G) initially 25-50 mg bid; increase weekly if needed; max 400 mg/day

> *Tab:* 25, 37.5, 50, 75, 100 mg

ANGIOTENSIN II RECEPTOR BLOCKERS (ARBs)

▷ *valsartan* (G) initially 40 mg bid; increase to 160 mg bid as tolerated or 320 mg daily after 2-4 weeks; usual range 80-320 mg/day
Pediatric: <12 years: not recommended; ≥12 years: same as adult

Diovan *Tab:* 40*, 80, 160, 320 mg
Prexxartan Oral Solution *Oral soln:* 20 mg/5 ml, 80 mg/20 ml (120, 473 ml; 20 ml unit-dose cup)

NEPRILYSIN INHIBITOR+ARB COMBINATION

▷ *sacubitril+valsartan* (G) initially 49/51 bid; double dose after 2-4 weeks; maintenance 97/103 bid; *GFR <30 ml/min or moderate hepatic impairment:* initially 24/26 bid; double dose every 2-4 weeks to target maintenance 97/103 bid
Pediatric: <12 years: not established; ≥12 years: same as adult

Entresto
> *Tab:* **Entresto 24/26:** sacu 24 mg+val 26 mg
> **Entresto 49/51:** sacu 49 mg+val 51 mg
> **Entresto 97/103:** sacu 97 mg+val 103 mg

ALDOSTERONE RECEPTOR BLOCKER

▷ *eplerenone* initially 25 mg once daily; titrate within 4 weeks to 50 mg once daily; adjust dose based on serum K^+
Pediatric: <12 years: not recommended; ≥12 years: same as adult

Inspra *Tab:* 25, 50 mg
Comment: Inspra is contraindicated with concomitant potent CYP3A4 inhibitors. Risk of hyperkalemia with concomitant ACEI or angiotensin II receptor blocker (ARB). Monitor serum potassium at baseline, 1 week, and 1 month. Caution with serum creatinine (Cr) >2 mg/dL (male) or >1.8 mg/dL (female) and/or CrCl <50 ml/min and diabetes mellitus (DM) with proteinuria.

THIAZIDE DIURETICS

Comment: Monitor hydration status, blood pressure, urine output, and serum K^+.

▷ *chlorothiazide* (G) 0.5-1 gm/day in single or divided doses; max 2 gm/day
Pediatric: <6 months: up to 15 mg/lb/day in 2 divided doses; ≥6 months: 10 mg/lb/day in 2 divided doses

Diuril *Tab:* 250*, 500*mg; *Oral susp:* 250 mg/5 ml (237 ml)

▷ *hydrochlorothiazide* (G)
  Pediatric: <12 years: not recommended; ≥12 years: same as adult
    Esidrix 25-100 mg once daily
      Tab: 25, 50, 100 mg
    Microzide 12.5 mg daily; usual max 50 mg/day
      Cap: 12.5 mg
▷ *methyclothiazide+deserpidine* initially 2.5 mg once daily; max 5 mg once daily
  Pediatric: <12 years: not recommended; ≥12 years: same as adult
    Enduronyl *Tab:* methy 5 mg+deser 0.25 mg*
    Enduronyl Forte *Tab:* methy 5 mg+deser 0.5 mg*
▷ *polythiazide* 2-4 mg once daily
  Pediatric: <12 years: not recommended; ≥12 years: same as adult
    Renese *Tab:* 1, 2, 4 mg

POTASSIUM-SPARING DIURETICS

Comment: Monitor hydration status, blood pressure, urine output, and serum K^+.
▷ *amiloride* initially 5 mg once daily; may increase to 10 mg; max 20 mg
  Pediatric: <12 years: not recommended; ≥12 years: same as adult
    Midamor *Tab:* 5 mg
▷ *spironolactone* initially 50-100 mg in a single or divided doses; titrate at 2 week intervals
  Pediatric: <12 years: not established; ≥12 years: same as adult
    Aldactone (G) *Tab:* 25, 50*, 100*mg
    CaroSpir *Oral susp:* 25 mg/5 ml (118, 473 ml) (banana)

LOOP DIURETICS

Comment: Monitor hydration status, blood pressure, urine output, and serum K^+.
▷ *bumetanide* (G) 0.5-2 mg as a single dose; may repeat at 4 to 5 hour intervals; max 10 mg/day
  Pediatric: <18 years: not recommended; ≥18 years: same as adult
    Bumex *Tab:* 0.5*, 1*, 2*mg
  Comment: *Bumetanide* is contraindicated with sulfa drug allergy.
▷ *ethacrynic acid* (G) initially 50-200 mg once daily
  Pediatric: infants: not recommended; >1 month: initially 25 mg/day; then adjust dose in 25 mg increments
    Edecrin *Tab:* 25, 50 mg
▷ *ethacrynate sodium* (G) for IV injection
    Sodium Edecrin *Vial:* 50 mg single-dose
  Comment: **Sodium Edecrin** is more potent than more commonly used loop and thiazide diuretics.
▷ *furosemide*
  Comment: *Furosemide* may cause fluid, electrolyte, and metabolic abnormalities such as hypovolemia, hypokalemia, azotemia, hyponatremia, hypochloremic alkalosis, hypomagnesemia, hypocalcemia, hyperglycemia, or hyperuricemia, particularly in patients receiving higher doses, patients with inadequate oral electrolyte intake, and in elderly patients. Excessive diuresis may cause dehydration and blood volume reduction with circulatory collapse and possibly vascular thrombosis and embolism, particularly in elderly patients. Monitor the patient's serum electrolytes, CO_2, blood urea nitrogen (BUN), creatinine, glucose, and uric acid. Monitor the patient for dehydration and azotemia. Monitor the patient for symptoms of urinary retention. Avoid concomitant *ethacrynic acid* with *furosemide* as the risk of ototoxicity is increased. Avoid concomitant salicylates with *furosemide* as this combination increases risk of salicylate toxicity. Concomitant *cisplatin* and nephrotoxic drugs with *furosemide* potentiates risk of ototoxicity and nephrotoxicity. Concomitant *furosemide* and *lithium* potentiates the risk of *lithium* toxicity. Concomitant renin-angiotensin inhibitors increases the risk of hypotension and renal failure. Concomitant *furosemide* and adrenergic-blocking drugs can potentiate the action of the adrenergic-blocking drugs. Drugs undergoing renal tubular secretion can potentiate *furosemide* toxicity.
    Furoscix the single-use, on-body, infusor is preprogramed to deliver 30 mg of **Furoscix** over the first hour, then 12.5 mg per hour for the subsequent 4 hours; **Furoscix** is not for chronic use and should be replaced with oral diuretics as soon as practical
    Prefilled cartridge: 80 mg/10 ml (8 mg/ml, 10 ml), single-dose, soln co-packaged with a single-use on-body infusor
    Comment: **Furoscix** is a diuretic indicated for at-home treatment of congestion due to fluid overload in adults with New York Heart Association (NYHA) Class II/III chronic HF. The most common adverse reactions during treatment with the **Furoscix Infusor** were administration site and skin reactions: erythema, bruising, edema, and infusion site pain. **Furoscix** is contraindicated in patients with anuria, patients with a history of hypersensitivity to *furosemide* or medical adhesives, and/or patients with hepatic cirrhosis or ascites
    Lasix initially 40 mg bid
      Tab: 20, 40*, 80 mg; *Oral soln:* 10 mg/ml (2, 4 oz w. dropper)
▷ *torsemide* 5 mg once daily; may increase to 10 mg daily
  Pediatric: <12 years: not recommended; ≥12 years: same as adult
    Demadex *Tab:* 5*, 10*, 20*, 100*mg

(continued)

▷ *torsemide (reformulated)* Recommended initial dose: 20 mg orally once daily; titrate dose by approximately doubling until desired diuretic response is obtained; doses >200 mg have not been studied
Pediatric: safety and efficacy not established
  Soaanz *Tab:* 20, 40, 60 mg film-coat
  Comment: Soaanz is a reformulated loop diuretic indicated for the treatment of edema associated with HF or renal disease in adults. Soaanz is contraindicated with hypersensitivity to Soaanz, anuria, and hepatic coma. Taking concomitant NSAIDs reduces the diuretic, natriuretic, and antihypertensive effects and increases risk of renal impairment. Concomitant use with CYP2C9 inhibitors can decrease *torsemide* clearance. *Torsemide* may affect the efficacy and safety of sensitive CYP2C9 substrates or of substrates with a narrow therapeutic range, such as *warfarin* or *phenytoin*. Concomitant *colestyramine* decreases exposure of Soaanz. Co-administered organic anion drugs (e.g., *probenecid*) may decrease the diuretic activity of Soaanz. Like other diuretics, *torsemide* reduces the renal clearance of *lithium*, inducing a high risk of *lithium* toxicity. Monitor *lithium* levels periodically when Soaanz is co-administered. Renin-angiotensin inhibitors (ACEIs, ARBs) increase risk of hypotension and renal impairment. Radiocontrast agents increase risk of renal toxicity. Corticosteroids and ACTH increase risk of hypokalemia.

OTHER DIURETICS
Comment: Monitor hydration status, blood pressure, urine output, and serum K⁺.
▷ *indapamide* initially 1.25 mg once daily; may titrate dosage upward every 4 weeks if needed; max 5 mg/day
  Lozol *Tab:* 1.25, 2.5 mg
  Comment: *Indapamide* is contraindicated with sulfa drug allergy.
▷ *metolazone* 2.5-5 mg once daily
  Pediatric: <12 years: not recommended; ≥12 years: same as adult
  Zaroxolyn *Tab:* 2.5, 5, 10 mg
  Comment: *Metolazone* is contraindicated with sulfa drug allergy.

DIURETIC COMBINATIONS
Comment: Monitor hydration status, blood pressure, urine output, and serum K⁺.
▷ *amiloride+hydrochlorothiazide* (G) initially 1 tab once daily; may increase to 2 tabs/day in a single or divided doses
  Pediatric: <12 years: not recommended; ≥12 years: same as adult
  Moduretic *Tab:* amil 5 mg+hctz 50 mg*
▷ *spironolactone+hydrochlorothiazide* (G)
  Pediatric: <12 years: not recommended; ≥12 years: same as adult
  Aldactazide 25 usual maintenance 50-100 mg in a single or divided doses
    Tab: spiro 25 mg+hctz 25 mg
  Aldactazide 50 usual maintenance 50-100 mg in a single or divided doses
    Tab: spiro 50 mg+hctz 50 mg
▷ *triamterene+hydrochlorothiazide* (G)
  Pediatric: <12 years: not recommended; ≥12 years: same as adult
  Dyazide 1-2 caps daily
    Cap: triam 37.5 mg+hctz 25 mg
  Maxzide 1 tab once daily
    Tab: triam 75 mg+hctz 50 mg*
  Maxzide-25 1-2 tabs once daily
    Tab: triam 37.5 mg+hctz 25 mg*

NITRATE+PERIPHERAL VASODILATOR COMBINATION
▷ *isosorbide dinitrate+hydralazine* initially 1 tab tid; may reduce to 1/2 tab tid if not tolerated; titrate as tolerated after 3-5 days; max 2 tabs tid
  Pediatric: <12 years: not recommended; ≥12 years: same as adult
  BiDil *Tab:* isosor 20 mg+hydral 37.5 mg
  Comment: BiDil is an adjunct to standard therapy in self-identified black persons to improve survival, to prolong time to hospitalization for HF, and to improve patient-reported functional status.

CARDIAC GLYCOSIDES
Comment: In selecting a digoxin dosing regimen, it is important to consider factors that affect *digoxin* blood levels (e.g., body weight, age, renal function, concomitant drugs) since *digoxin* has a very narrow therapeutic index (i.e., toxic levels of *digoxin* are only slightly higher than therapeutic levels). Therapeutic serum level of digoxin is 0.8-2 mcg/ml. Dosing can be initiated either with a loading dose followed by maintenance dosing if rapid titration is desired or initiated with maintenance dosing without a loading dose. Parenteral administration of *digoxin* should be used only when the need for rapid digitalization is urgent or when the drug cannot be taken orally. IM injection can lead to severe pain at the injection site and thus IV administration is preferred. If the drug must be administered by the IM route, it should be injected deep into the muscle followed by massage. For adults, no more than 500 mcg of parenteral *digoxin* (Lanoxin Injection)

should be injected into a single site. For pediatric patients, no more than 200 mcg of *digoxin* (Lanoxin Injection Pediatric) should be injected into a single site. Administer IV *digoxin* dose over a period of 5 minutes or longer and avoid bolus administration to prevent systemic and coronary vasoconstriction. Mixing of Lanoxin Injection and Lanoxin Injection Pediatric with other drugs in the same container or simultaneous administration in the same IV line is not recommended. Lanoxin Injection and Lanoxin Injection Pediatric can be administered undiluted or diluted with a 4-fold or greater volume of Sterile Water for Injection, 0.9% Sodium Chloride for Injection, or D5W. The use of less than a fourfold volume of diluent could lead to precipitation of the *digoxin*. Immediate use of the diluted product is recommended. Lanoxin (*digoxin*) is a positive inotrope, negative chronotrope, and negative dromotrope. Therefore, monitor the patient for bradycardia and hypotension. The classic features of digitalis toxicity are nausea, vomiting, abdominal pain, headache, dizziness, confusion, delirium, visual disturbance (blurred or yellow vision), and symptomatic/unstable bradycardia and/or hypotension. For more information on the use of *digoxin* in pediatric HF, see Jain, S & Vaidyanathan, B. Digoxin in management of heart failure in children: Should it be continued or relegated to the history books? *Ann Pediatr Cardiol*. Jul-Dec 2009: 2(2):149–152.

▷ *digoxin* (G) *Loading dose:* 1-1.5 mg IM, IV, or PO in divided doses over 1-3 days; *Maintenance:* 0.125-0.5 mg/day
Pediatric: Total oral pediatric digitalizing dose (in 24 hours): <2 years: 40-50 mcg/kg; 2-10 years: 30-40 mcg/kg; >10 years: 0.75-1.5 mg; *Daily oral pediatric maintenance (single dose once daily):* <2 years: 10-12 mcg/kg; 2-10 years: 8-10 mcg/kg; >10 years: 0.125–0.5 mg; max: 0.125-0.5 mg; <10 years: use elixir or parenteral form

    Lanoxicap *Cap:* 0.05, 0.1, 0.2 mg soln-filled (alcohol)
    Lanoxin *Tab:* 0.0625, 0.125*, 0.1875, 0.25*mg; *Elix:* 0.05 mg/ml (2 oz w. dropper) (lime) (alcohol 10%)
    Lanoxin Injection *Amp:* 0.25 mg/ml (2 ml)
    Lanoxin Injection Pediatric *Amp:* 0.1 mg/ml (1 ml)

HYPERPOLARIZATION-ACTIVATED CYCLIC NUCLEOTIDE-GATED CHANNEL BLOCKER

▷ *ivabradine* (G) initially 5 mg bid with food; assess after 2 weeks and adjust dose to achieve a resting heart rate of 50-60 bpm; thereafter, adjust dose as needed based on resting heart rate and tolerability; max 7.5 mg bid; in patients with a history of conduction defects or for whom bradycardia could lead to hemodynamic compromise, initiate at 2.5 mg bid before increasing the dose based on heart rate
Pediatric: <18 years: not established; ≥18 years: same as adult
    Corlanor *Tab:* 5, 7.5 mg
    Comment: Corlanor is indicated to reduce the risk of hospitalization for worsening HF in patients with stable, symptomatic, chronic HF with LVEF ≤35%, who are in sinus rhythm with resting heart rate ≤70 bpm, and either are on maximally tolerated doses of beta-blockers or have a contraindication to beta-blocker use. Corlanor is contraindicated with acute decompensated heart failure, BP <90/50, sick sinus syndrome (SSS), sinoatrial block, and 3rd degree AV block (unless the patient has a functioning demand pacemaker). Corlanor may cause fetal toxicity when administered to pregnant females based on embryo/fetal toxicity and cardiac teratogenic to effects observed in animal studies. Therefore, females should be advised to use effective contraception when taking this drug.

SOLUBLE GUANYLATE CYCLASE (SGC) STIMULATOR

▷ *vericiguat* initially 2.5 mg orally once daily with food; then double the dose approximately every 2 weeks; target maintenance 10 mg once daily; tablets may be crushed and mixed with water for patients who have difficulty swallowing
    Verquvo *Tab:* 2.5, 5, 10 mg film-coat
    Comment: Verquvo is indicated to reduce the risk of cardiovascular death and HF hospitalization following a hospitalization for HF or need for outpatient IV diuretics in adults with symptomatic chronic HF and ejection fraction less than 45%. The most common adverse reactions reported (incidence ≥5%) have been hypotension and anemia. Verquvo is contraindicated in pregnancy. Exclude pregnancy before the start of treatment. Advise females of reproductive potential to use effective forms of contraception during treatment and for 1 month after discontinuation. Breastfeeding is not recommended.

HELICOBACTER PYLORI INFECTION

ERADICATION REGIMENS

Comment: There are many H2 receptor blocker-based and proton pump inhibitor (PPI)-based treatment regimens suggested in professional literature for the eradication of the *Helicobacter pylori* organism and subsequent ulcer healing. Generally, regimens range from 10 to 14 days for eradication and 2-6 more weeks of continued gastric acid suppression. A 3 to 4 antibiotic combination may increase treatment effectiveness and decrease the likelihood of resistant strain emergence. Empirical treatment is not recommended. Diagnosis should be confirmed before treatment is started. Antibiotic choices include *doxycycline, tetracycline, amoxicillin, amoxicillin+clavulanate, clarithromycin, clindamycin,* and *metronidazole.* Follow-up visits are recommended at 2 and 6 weeks to evaluate treatment outcomes.

Regimen 1

▷ Helidac Therapy (G) *bismuth subsalicylate* 525 mg qid + *tetracycline* 500 mg qid + *metronidazole* 250 mg qid x 14 days
Pediatric: <12 years: <u>not</u> recommended; ≥12 years: same as adult
Pack: bismuth subsalicylate Chew tab: 262.4 mg (112/pck); *tetracycline* Cap: 500 mg (56/pck); *metronidazole* Tab: 250 mg (56/pck)

Regimen 2

▷ PrevPac (G) *amoxicillin* 500 mg 2 caps bid + *lansoprazole* 30 mg bid + *clarithromycin* 500 mg bid x 14 days (1 card per day)
Pediatric: <12 years: <u>not</u> recommended; ≥12 years: same as adult
Kit: lansoprazole Cap: 30 mg (2/card); *amoxicillin* Cap: 500 mg (4/card); *clarithromycin* Tab: 500 mg (2/card) (14 daily cards/carton)

Regimen 3

▷ Pylera (G) take 3 caps qid after meals and at bedtime x 10 days; take with 8 oz water <u>plus</u> *omeprazole* 20 mg bid, with breakfast and dinner, for 10 days
Pediatric: <12 years: <u>not</u> recommended; ≥12 years: same as adult
Cap: bismuth subsalicylate 140 mg+*tetracycline* 125 mg+*metronidazole* 125 mg (120 caps)
Comment: *Omeprazole* is <u>not</u> included with **Pylera.**

Regimen 4

▷ Omeclamox-Pak *omeprazole* 20 mg bid + *amoxicillin* 1,000 mg bid + *clarithromycin* 500 mg bid x 10 days
Kit: omeprazole Cap: 20 mg (2/pck); *amoxicillin* Cap: 500 mg (4/pck); *clarithromycin* Tab: 500 mg (2/pck) (10 pcks/carton)

Regimen 5

▷ *omeprazole* 40 mg daily + *clarithromycin* 500 mg tid x 2 weeks; then continue *omeprazole* 10-40 mg daily x 6 more weeks

Regimen 6

▷ *lansoprazole* 30 mg tid + *amoxicillin* 1 gm tid x 10 days; then continue *lansoprazole* 15-30 mg daily x 6 more weeks

Regimen 7

▷ *omeprazole* 40 mg daily + *amoxicillin* 1 gm bid + *clarithromycin* 500 mg bid x 10 days; then continue *omeprazole* 10-40 mg daily x 6 more weeks

Regimen 8

▷ *bismuth subsalicylate* 525 mg qid + *metronidazole* 250 mg qid + *tetracycline* 500 mg qid + H₂ receptor agonist x 2 weeks; then continue H₂ receptor agonist x 6 more weeks

Regimen 9

▷ (<u>not</u> for use in 1st; B in 2nd, 3rd) *bismuth subsalicylate* 525 mg qid + *metronidazole* 250 mg qid + *amoxicillin* 500 mg qid + H₂ receptor agonist x 2 weeks; then continue H₂ receptor agonist x 6 more weeks

Regimen 10

▷ *ranitidine bismuth citrate* 400 mg bid + *clarithromycin* 500 mg bid x 2 weeks; then continue *ranitidine bismuth citrate* 400 mg bid x 2 more weeks

Regimen 11

▷ *omeprazole* 20 mg <u>or</u> *lansoprazole* 30 mg q AM + *bismuth subsalicylate* 524 mg qid + *metronidazole* 500 mg tid + *tetracycline* 500 mg qid x 2 weeks; then continue *omeprazole* 20 mg <u>or</u> *lansoprazole* 30 mg q AM for 6 more weeks

Regimen 12

▷ Talicia administer 4 capsules as a single dose every 8 hours x 14 days; take with food; swallow whole with a full glass of water, do <u>not</u> crush <u>or</u> chew; do <u>not</u> take with alcohol
Cap: (fixed dose combination) *omeprazole magnesium* 10 mg+*amoxicillin* 250 mg+*rifabutin* 12.5 mg del-rel

HEMOLYTIC UREMIC SYNDROME: ATYPICAL (aHUS)

COMPLEMENT INHIBITORS

▷ *eculizumab* dilute to a final admixture concentration of 5 mg/ml using the following steps: (1) withdraw the required amount of **Soliris** from the vial into a sterile syringe, (2) transfer the dose to an infusion bag, (3) add IV fluid equal to the drug volume (0.9% NaCl <u>or</u> 0.45% NaCl <u>or</u> D5W <u>or</u> Ringer's lactate); the final admixed

Soliris 5 mg/ml infusion volume is 300 mg dose (60 ml), 600 mg dose (120 ml), 900 mg dose (180 ml), and 1,200 mg dose (240 ml); administer a 900 mg IV infusion once weekly for the first 4 weeks; then 1,200 mg IV infusion for the 5th dose 1 week after the 4th dose; then 1,200 mg IV infusion once every 2 weeks thereafter *Pediatric:* <18 years: >40 kg: 900 mg IV infusion once weekly x 4 doses; then 1,200 mg at week 5; then 1,200 mg once every 2 weeks thereafter; 30-<40 kg: 600 mg IV infusion once weekly x 2 doses; then 900 mg IV infusion at week 3; then 900 mg IV infusion once every 2 weeks thereafter; 20-<30 kg: 600 mg IV infusion once weekly x 2 doses; then 600 mg IV infusion at week 3; then 600 mg IV infusion once every 2 weeks thereafter; 5-<10 kg: 300 mg IV infusion x 1 dose; then 300 mg IV infusion at week 2; then 300 mg IV infusion once every 3 weeks thereafter; <5 kg: not established

> Soliris *Vial:* 300 mg (10 mg/ml, 30 ml), single-use, concentrated solution for IV infusion (preservative-free)

Comment: Soliris *(eculizumab)* is a complement inhibitor indicated for treatment of patients with paroxysmal nocturnal hemoglobinuria (PNH) to reduce hemolysis and patients with atypical hemolytic uremic syndrome (aHUS) to inhibit complement-mediated thrombotic acetylcholine receptor (AchR) antibody positive. **Soliris** should be administered at the above recommended dosage regimen time points or within 2 days of each time point. Supplemental dosing of **Soliris** is required in the setting of concomitant support with plasmapheresis (PI) or plasma exchange (PE) or fresh frozen plasma (FFP) infusion (see mfr pkg insert for supplemental dosing). **Soliris** is not indicated for the treatment of patients with Shiga toxin *Escherichia coli*-related hemolytic uremic syndrome (STEC-HUS). **Soliris** is contraindicated in patients with unresolved *Neisseria meningitides* infection and patients who are not currently vaccinated against *N. meningitides,* unless the risks of delaying **Soliris** treatment outweigh the risks of developing meningococcal infection. Prescribers must enroll in the **Soliris** REMS Program (1-888-SOLIRIS, 1-888-765-4747), counsel patients about the risk of meningococcal infection, provide patients with **Soliris** REMS educational materials, and ensure that patients are vaccinated with meningococcal vaccine. The most frequently reported adverse reactions in the PNH randomized trial (incidence ≥10%) are headache, nasopharyngitis, back pain, and nausea. There are no adequate and well-controlled human studies of **Soliris** in pregnancy or effects on the breastfed infant. Based on animal studies, **Soliris** may cause fetal harm. It is not known whether **Soliris** is excreted in human milk. Immunoglobulin G (IgG) is excreted in human milk, so it is expected that **Soliris** will be present in human milk. However, published data suggest that antibodies in human milk do not enter the neonatal and infant circulation in substantial amounts. Caution should be exercised when **Soliris** is administered to a breastfeeding patient.

HEMOPHAGOCYTIC LYMPHOHISTIOCYTOSIS (HLH)

INTERFERON GAMMA (IFNγ)-BLOCKING ANTIBODY

▷ *emapalumab-lzsg* Starting dose: 1 mg/kg via IV infusion over 1 hour twice per week; administer concomitant *dexamethasone*

> Gamifant *Vial:* 10 mg/2 ml (5 mg/ml), 50 mg/10 ml (5 mg/ml), single dose, for dilution and IV infusion

Comment: Gamifant *(emapalumab-lzsg)* is indicated for the treatment of adult and pediatric (newborn and older) patients with primary hemophagocytic lymphohistiocytosis (HLH) with refractory, recurrent, or progressive disease or intolerance with conventional HLH therapy. The most common adverse reactions (incidence ≥20%) have been infections, hypertension, infusion-related reactions, and pyrexia. Monitor patients for signs and symptoms of infection and treat promptly. Test for latent tuberculosis. Administer prophylactic treatment against herpes zoster, *Pneumocystis jirovecii* and fungal infections. Do not administer live or live attenuated vaccines to patients receiving **Gamifant.** Monitor patients for infusion-related reactions; interrupt infusion for severe reaction and institute appropriate medical management. There are no available data on **Gamifant** use in pregnant females to inform a drug-associated risk of adverse developmental outcomes. In animal studies, no maternal toxicity occurred and there was no evidence of teratogenicity or effects on embryo/fetal survival or growth. There is no information regarding the presence of *emapalumab-lzsg* in human milk or effects on the breastfed infant. Developmental and health benefits of breastfeeding should be considered along with the mother's clinical need for **Gamifant** and any potential adverse effects on the breastfed infant from **Gamifant** or from the underlying maternal condition.

HEMOPHILIA A (CHRISTMAS DISEASE, CONGENITAL FACTOR VIII DEFICIENCY), HEMOPHILIA B (CHRISTMAS DISEASE, FACTOR IX DEFICIENCY), VON WILLEBRAND DISEASE (VWF DEFICIENCY)

BISPECIFIC FACTOR IXA- AND FACTOR X-DIRECTED ANTIBODY

▷ *emicizumab-kxwh* initially 3 mg/kg by SC injection once weekly for the first 4 weeks; followed by 1.5 mg/kg once weekly
Pediatric: same as adult

> Hemlibra *Vial:* 30 mg/ml (single-dose), 60 mg/0.4 ml (single-dose), 105 mg 0.7 ml (single-dose), 150 mg/ml (single-dose)

(continued)

Comment: Hemlibra is a bispecific factor IXa- and factor X-directed antibody indicated for routine prophylaxis to prevent or reduce the frequency of bleeding episodes in adult and pediatric patients with hemophilia A (congenital factor VIII deficiency) with factor VIII (FVIII) inhibitors. *Laboratory Coagulation Test Interference:* Hemlibra interferes with activated clotting time (ACT), activated partial thromboplastin time (aPTT), and coagulation laboratory tests based on aPTT, including one stage aPTT-based single-factor assays, aPTT-based activated protein C resistance (APC-R), and Bethesda assays (clotting-based) for FVIII inhibitor titers. Intrinsic pathway clotting-based laboratory tests should not be used. *Boxed Warning:* Cases of thrombotic microangiopathy and thrombotic events were reported when on average a cumulative amount of >100 U/kg/24 hours of activated prothrombin complex concentrate (aPCC) was administered for 24 hours or more to patients receiving Hemlibra prophylaxis. Monitor for the development of thrombotic microangiopathy and thrombotic events if aPCC is administered. Discontinue aPCC and suspend dosing of Hemlibra if symptoms occur. The most common adverse reactions have been injection site reactions, headache, and arthralgia. There are no available data on Hemlibra use in pregnant females to inform a drug-associated risk of major birth defects and miscarriage. Women of childbearing potential should use contraception while receiving Hemlibra, and Hemlibra should be used during pregnancy only if the potential benefit for the mother outweighs the risk to the fetus. There is no information regarding the presence of *emicizumab-kxwh* in human milk or effects on the breastfed infant.

COAGULATION FACTOR VIIA (RECOMBINANT)-JNCW

▷ *coagulation factor VIIa (recombinant)-jncw Mild/moderate bleed:* 75 mcg/kg; repeated every 3 hours until hemostasis is achieved or initial dose 225 mcg/kg; if hemostasis is not achieved within 9 hours, additional 75 mcg/kg doses may be administered every 3 hours as needed to achieve hemostasis; *Severe bleed:* 225 mcg/kg, followed if necessary 6 hours later with 75 mcg/kg every 2 hours
Pediatric: <12 years: safety and efficacy not established; ≥12 years: same as adult
  Sevenfact *Vial:* 1, 5 mg, 1 mg/ml (1,000 mcg/ml) after reconstitution (see mfr pkg insert), single-use, pwdr for reconstitution and IV infusion w. prefilled syringe with water for injection diluent
  Comment: Sevenfact *(coagulation factor VIIa [recombinant]-jncw)* is a recombinant analog of human factor VII (FVII) for the treatment and control of bleeding episodes in patients with hemophilia A or B with inhibitors (neutralizing antibodies). Sevenfact is not indicated for the treatment of congenital (FVII) deficiency. Sevenfact is contraindicated in patients with known allergy to rabbits or rabbit proteins. Patients with hemophilia A or B with inhibitors who have other risk factors for thrombosis may be at increased risk of serious arterial and venous thrombotic events. If a hypersensitivity reaction occurs, including anaphylaxis, discontinue Sevenfact immediately and institute appropriate medical care. Clinical experience with pharmacologic use of factor VIIa (FVIIa)-containing products indicates an elevated risk of serious thrombotic events when used simultaneously with aPCC. There are no adequate and well-controlled animal or human studies of Sevenfact use in pregnancy to determine whether there is a drug-associated embryo/fetal risk. There is no information regarding the presence of Sevenfact in human milk or effect on the breastfed infant. The developmental and health benefits of breastfeeding should be considered along with the mother's clinical need for Sevenfact and any potential adverse effects on the breastfed infant from Sevenfact or from the underlying maternal condition. The most common adverse reactions (incidence ≥1%) have been headache, dizziness, infusion site discomfort, infusion site hematoma, infusion-related reaction, and fever.

RECOMBINANT DNA-DERIVED FACTOR VIII CONCENTRATE

▷ *antihemophilic factor (recombinant), Fc-VWF-XTEN fusion protein-ehtl* for IV use only; each Altuviiio vial label states FVIII activity in international units (IU or unit); *routine prophylaxis:* 50 IU/kg once weekly; *on-demand treatment and control of bleeding episodes and perioperative management:* 50 IU/kg; estimated increment of FVIII (IU/dL or % of normal) = 50 IU/kg x 2 (IU/dL per IU/kg) To achieve a specific target FVIII activity level, use the following formula: dosage (IU) = body weight (kg) x desired FVIII increase (IU/dL or % normal) x 0.5 (IU/kg per IU/dL); *Prior to reconstitution:* store in the original package to protect the vials from light; store in powder form at 2°C to 8°C (36°F to 46°F); do not freeze to avoid damage to the prefilled diluent syringe; may be stored at room temperature, not to exceed 30°C (86°F), for a single period of up to 6 months, within the expiration date printed on the label; if stored at room temperature, record the date removed from refrigeration on the carton in the area provided; after storage at room temperature, do not return the product to the refrigerator; do not use beyond the expiration date printed on the vial or 6 months after the date that was written on the carton, whichever is earlier; *After reconstitution:* may be stored at room temperature, not to exceed 30°C (86°F), for up to 3 hours; protect from direct sunlight; if the reconstituted product is not used within 3 hours, it must be discarded; do not use if the reconstituted solution is cloudy or has particulate matter; discard any unused reconstituted product
Pediatric: same as adult (no dose adjustment is needed for this population)
  Altuviiio *Vial:* 250, 500, 750, 1,000, 2,000, 3,000, 4,000 IU of FVIII potency, single-dose, pwdr for reconstitution, dilution, and IV infusion plus *prefilled syringe* of 3 ml sterile water for injection (diluent) and a sterile vial adapter (reconstitution device) (natural rubber latex-free)

Comment: Altuviiio is a recombinant DNA-derived FVIII concentrate indicated for use in adults and children with hemophilia A (congenital factor VIII deficiency) as a once-weekly FVIII therapy for (1) routine prophylaxis to reduce the frequency of bleeding episodes, (2) on-demand treatment and control of bleeding episodes, and (3) perioperative management of bleeding. Altuviiio is not indicated for the treatment of von Willebrand disease. Do not use in patients who have had severe hypersensitivity reactions, including anaphylaxis, to Altuviiio or excipients of Altuviiio. Should symptoms of a hypersensitivity reaction occur, immediately discontinue Altuviiio and initiate appropriate treatment. Neutralizing antibodies (inhibitors) to FVIII have been reported. If expected plasma FVIII activity levels are not attained or if bleeding is not controlled with an appropriate dose, obtain an assay that measures FVIII inhibitor concentration. The most common adverse reactions (incidence >10%) have been headache and arthralgia. There are no data with Altuviiio use in human or animal pregnancy to inform a drug-associated risk of fetal harm or effect on reproductive capacity. There are no data on the presence of Altuviiio in human milk or effects on the breastfed infant. The developmental and health benefits of breastfeeding should be considered along with the mother's clinical need for Altuviiio and any potential adverse effects on the breastfed infant from Altuviiio or from the underlying maternal condition. To report suspected adverse reactions, contact Bioverativ Therapeutics at 1-800-633-1610 or FDA at 1-800-FDA-1088 or www.fda.gov/medwatch.

FACTOR VIII MOLECULE

Comment: Esperoct (*turoctocog alfa pegol, N8-GP*) is an extended half-life FVIII molecule for treatment of adults and children with hemophilia A for routine prophylaxis to reduce the frequency of bleeding episodes, on-demand treatment and control of bleeding episodes, and perioperative management of bleeding. Esperoct has been evaluated in 270 people (202 adults/adolescents and 68 children) in five prospective, multicenter clinical trials in previously treated people (PTPs) with severe hemophilia A (<1% endogenous FVIII activity) and no history of inhibitors. Total exposure to Esperoct was 80,425 exposure days corresponding to 889 patient years of treatment. Esperoct was well tolerated across all age groups and indications, and no safety concerns were identified after more than 5 years of clinical exposure.

▷ *turoctocog alfa pegol, N8-GP* dosage must be individualized according to the needs of the patient (weight, severity of hemorrhage, presence of inhibitors); the following general dosages are suggested: Number of American Hospital Formulary Service® (AHFS) IU required = (body weight [kg] x desired FVIII increase [% normal]) x 0.5 (see mfr pkg insert);
Minor hemorrhage (superficial, early hemorrhages, hemorrhages into joints): therapeutically necessary plasma level of factor VIII activity is 20-40% of normal, repeated every 12 to 24 hours as necessary until resolved (at least 1 day, depending upon the severity of the bleeding episode)
Moderate (bleeding into muscles, mild head trauma, bleeding into the oral cavity): therapeutically necessary plasma level of factor VIII activity is 30-60% of normal, repeated every 12-24 hours for 3-4 days or until adequate local hemostasis is achieved
Major (gastrointestinal bleeding, intracranial, intra-abdominal or intrathoracic bleeding, fractures): therapeutically necessary plasma level of factor VIII activity is 60-100% of normal, repeated every 8-24 hours until bleeding is resolved, or in the case of surgery until adequate local hemostasis and wound healing are achieved
Esperoct *Vial:* 500, 1,000, 1,500, 2,000, 3,000 IU, pwdr, single-dose for reconstitution and IV infusion
Pediatric: individualized, same as adult

DESMOPRESSIN (DDAVP)

Comment: Desmopressin (DDAVP) acetate 0.3 mcg/kg administered in 50 ml 0.9% saline solution via IV infusion over 15-30 minutes may enable patients with certain types of hemophilia to undergo minor procedures (e.g., tooth extraction, minor surgery) without needing replacement therapy. If a replacement product is needed, desmopressin may reduce the required dose. One dose of desmopressin is effective for about 8-10 hours. The dose required for hemostasis is approximately 15 times the dose used to treat diabetes insipidus. The regular intranasal preparation (0.1 mg/ml) used to treat diabetes insipidus is too dilute to elicit a hemostatic response. A high-concentration intranasal preparation (i.e., Stimate Nasal Spray) has been licensed and has shown a similar response as the IV form.

▷ **Stimate Nasal Spray**
Nasal spray: 1.5 mg/ml, 150 mcg/actuation 25 sprays/bottle
Pediatric: <11 months, in the treatment of hemophilia A or von Willebrand's disease: safety and efficacy not established; ≥11 months: same as adult
Stimate Nasal Spray is administered by nasal insufflation, 1 spray per nostril, to provide a total dose of 300 mcg. In patients weighing less than 50 kg, 150 mcg administered as a single spray provided the expected effect on FVIII coagulant activity, FVIII ristocetin cofactor activity, and skin bleeding time. If **Stimate Nasal Spray** is used preoperatively, it should be administered 2 hours prior to the scheduled procedure. The necessity for repeat administration of **Stimate Nasal Spray** or use of any blood products for hemostasis should be determined by laboratory response as well as the clinical condition of the patient. Fluid restriction should be observed, and fluid intake should be limited to a minimum, from 1 hour before desmopressin administration until at least

(continued)

24 hours after administration. Use of DDAVP in infants and children will require careful fluid intake restriction to prevent possible hyponatremia and water intoxication. **Stimate Nasal Spray** should not be used in infants younger than 11 months in the treatment of hemophilia A or von Willebrand disease; safety and effectiveness in children between 11 months and 12 years of age have been demonstrated. Treatment of von Willebrand disease involves control of bleeding with replacement therapy (cryoprecipitate or pasteurized intermediate-purity FVIII concentrate) or desmopressin. Desmopressin (DDAVP) is a synthetic analog of the antidiuretic hormone vasopressin; it has enhanced antidiuretic activity and no significant pressor activity related to vasopressin. DDAVP controls bleeding by stimulating the body to release more of the von Willebrand factor (VWF) into the plasma, thus increasing levels of FVIII necessary for normal platelet function. DDAVP causes a 2-fold to 5-fold increase in plasma VWF and factor VIII concentrations in individuals who are healthy and patients who are responsive. DDAVP is often considered the first treatment for managing von Willebrand disease type 1 (the most common form of VWD). Some women use the nasal spray at the beginning of their menstrual periods to control excessive bleeding. To ensure adequate response to the drug, a test dose is typically done and the response of VWF antigen is measured. DDAVP will stop bleeding in patients with mild-to-moderate von Willebrand disease and hemophilia A with episodes of spontaneous or trauma-induced injuries, such as hemarthroses, intramuscular hematomas, mucosal bleeding, or menorrhagia. In the outpatient setting during two clinical trials where patients recorded bleeding episodes, desmopressin nasal spray (i.e., **Stimate Nasal Spray**) provided effective hemostasis 100% of the time in 75% of the 106 patients (n = 16). For those patients not responding in 100% of bleeding occasions, 78% (64 of 82) of bleeding episodes were effectively controlled with **Stimate Nasal Spray**. In the outpatient setting during two clinical trials where patients recorded bleeding episodes, **Stimate Nasal Spray** provided effective hemostasis 100% of the time in two of the five patients. For those patients not responding in 100% of bleeding occasions, 45% (14 of 31) of bleeding episodes were effectively controlled with **Stimate Nasal Spray**. **Stimate Nasal Spray** is not indicated for treatment of severe classic von Willebrand disease (type I) and when there is evidence of an abnormal molecular form of FVIII antigen. **Stimate Nasal Spray** is indicated for patients with hemophilia A with FVIII coagulant activity levels greater than 5%. **Stimate Nasal Spray** is not indicated for the treatment of hemophilia A with FVIII coagulant activity levels equal to or less than 5%, or for the treatment of hemophilia B, or in patients who have FVIII antibodies. **Stimate Nasal Spray** is not appropriate for patients with changes in the nasal mucosa, such as scarring, edema, or other disease process which may cause erratic, unreliable absorption.

VON WILLEBRAND FACTOR (RECOMBINANT) (rVWF)

▶ *von Willebrand factor (recombinant) (rVWF)* physician supervision of the treatment regimen is required; administer via IV injection only at max rate 4 ml/min

Pediatric: <18 years: not established; ≥18 years: same as adult

On-demand treatment and control of bleeding episode: for each bleeding episode, administer the first dose of **Vonvendi** with an approved recombinant (non-VWF-containing) FVIII, if FVIII baseline levels are below 40% or are unknown; adjust dose based on the extent and location of bleeding

    Minor: initially 40-50 IU/kg; then 40-50 IU/kg every 8-24 hours

    Major: initially 50-80 IU/kg; then 40-60 IU/kg every 8-24 hours for approximately 2-3 days

Perioperative management of bleeding: continue to monitor the VWF:RCo and FVIII:C plasma levels after any surgical procedure

Elective surgical procedure: a single dose of **Vonvendi** may be administered 12-24 hours prior to surgery to allow the endogenous FVIII levels to increase to at least 30 IU/dl (minor surgery) or 60 IU/dl (major surgery); assess FVIII:C levels within 3 hours prior to surgery; if the FVIII:C levels are at or above the recommended minimum target levels, administer a single dose of **Vonvendi** within 1 hour prior to the procedure; if the FVIII:C levels are below the recommended minimum target levels, administer recombinant FVIII in addition to **Vonvendi** to raise VWF:RCo and FVIII:C

Emergency surgery: assess baseline VWF:RCo and FVIII:C levels within 3 hours prior to surgery; if not available, use weight-based dosing calculation; administer **Vonvendi** 1 hour before surgery with or without recombinant FVIII and adjust the dose to raise VWF:RCo and FVIII:C to adequate level

Type of Surgery	Target Peak Plasma Level		Calculation of rVWF Dose (IU VWF:RCo required)
	VWF:RCo	FVIII:C	
Minor	50-60 IU/dL	40-50 IU/dL	Δ VWF:RCo x BW (kg)/IR
Major	100 IU/dL	80-100 IU/dL	

BW, body weight; FVIII, factor VIII; rVWF, von Willebrand factor (recombinant); VWF, von Willebrand factor.

    Vonvendi Vial: 650, 1,300 IU VWF:RCo, single-use, pwdr for reconstitution with diluent supplied, and IV injection (non-pyrogenic)

    Comment: Do not use **Vonvendi** in patients who have had life-threatening hypersensitivity reactions to **Vonvendi** or its components (trisodium citrate dihydrate, glycine, mannitol, trehalose-dihydrate, polysorbate 80, and hamster or mouse proteins). The most common adverse reactions observed (incidence ≥2%) have been generalized pruritus, vomiting, nausea, dizziness, and vertigo.

Thromboembolic reactions can occur, particularly in patients with risk factors for thrombosis. Monitor for early signs of thrombosis and have prophylaxis measures against thromboembolism instituted according to current recommendations. One out of 80 von Willebrand disease subjects treated with **Vonvendi** in clinical trials developed proximal deep vein thrombosis in the perioperative period after undergoing total hip replacement surgery. In patients requiring frequent doses of **Vonvendi,** in combination with recombinant FVIII, monitor plasma levels for FVIII:C because sustained excessive FVIII plasma levels can increase the risk of thromboembolic events. Hypersensitivity reactions, including anaphylaxis, may occur. Discontinue **Vonvendi** if hypersensitivity symptoms occur and administer appropriate emergency treatment. Inhibitors to VWF <u>and/or</u> FVIII can occur. If the expected plasma levels of VWF activity (VWF:RCo) are <u>not</u> attained <u>or</u> if bleeding is <u>not</u> controlled with an appropriate dose, perform an appropriate assay to determine if an anti-VWF <u>or</u> anti-FVIII inhibitors are present.

HEMORRHOIDS

Bulk-Forming Agents, Stool Softeners, and Stimulant Laxatives *see Constipation*

RECTAL PREPARATIONS
➤ *dibucaine* (OTC)(G) 1 applicatorful <u>or</u> suppository bid and after each stool; max 6 suppositories/day
  Pediatric: <12 years: <u>not</u> recommended; ≥12 years: same as adult
    Nupercainal (OTC) *Rectal oint:* 1% (30, 60 gm); *Rectal supp:* 1% (12, 14/pck)
➤ *hydrocortisone* (OTC)(G)
  Pediatric: <12 years: <u>not</u> recommended; ≥12 years: same as adult
    Anusol-HC 1 suppository rectally bid-tid <u>or</u> 2 suppositories bid x 2 weeks
      Rectal supp: 25 mg (12, 24/pck)
    Anusol-HC Cream 2.5% apply bid-qid prn
      Rectal crm: 2.5% (30 gm)
    Anusol-HC-1 apply tid-qid prn; max 7 days
      Rectal crm: 1% (0.7 oz)
    Hydrocortisone Rectal Cream
      Rectal crm: 1, 2.5% (30 gm)
    Nupercainal apply tid-qid prn
      Rectal crm: 1% (30 gm)
    Proctocort 1 suppository rectally bid-tid prn <u>or</u> 2 suppositories bid x 2 weeks
      Rectal supp: 30 mg (12/pck)
    Proctocream HC 2.5% apply rectally bid-qid prn
      Rectal crm: 2.5% (30 gm)
    Proctofoam HC 1% apply rectally tid-qid prn
      Rectal foam: 1% (14 applications/10 gm)
➤ *hydrocortisone+pramoxine* 1 applicatorful tid-qid and after each stool; max 2 weeks
  Pediatric: <12 years: <u>not</u> recommended; ≥12 years: same as adult
    Procort *Rectal crm:* hydrocort 1.85%+pramox 1.15% (30 gm)
➤ *hydrocortisone+lidocaine* apply bid-tid prn
  Pediatric: <12 years: <u>not</u> recommended; ≥12 years: same as adult
    AnaMantle HC, LidaMantle HC *Crm/Lotn:* hydrocort 5%+lido 3% (1 oz)
➤ *petrolatum+mineral oil+shark liver oil+phenylephrine* (OTC)(G)
    Preparation H Ointment apply up to qid prn
      Rectal oint: 1, 2 oz
➤ *petrolatum+glycerin+shark liver oil+phenylephrine* (OTC)(G)
    Preparation H Cream apply up to qid prn
      Rectal crm: 0.9, 1.8 oz
➤ *phenylephrine+cocoa butter+shark liver oil* (OTC)(G)
    Preparation H Suppositories 1 suppository <u>or</u> 1 application of rectal ointment <u>or</u> cream, up to qid
      Rectal supp: phenyle 0.25%+cocoa 85.5%+shark 3% (12, 24, 45/pck); *Rectal oint:* phenyle 0.25%+petro 1.9%+mineral oil 14%+shark liv 3% (1, 2 oz); *Rectal crm:* phenyle 0.25%+petro 18%+gly 12%+shark liv 3% (0.9, 1.8 oz)

TOPICAL AND TRANSDERMAL ANALGESICS
➤ *capsaicin* 8% patch apply up to 4 patches for one 60-minute application to clean dry skin; may prep area with topical anesthetic; wear non-latex gloves; patches may be cut to size/shape; treatment may be repeated every 3 months
  Pediatric: <18 years: <u>not</u> recommended; ≥18 years: same as adult
    Qutenza *Patch:* 8% 1640 mcg/cm (179 mg) (1 <u>or</u> 2 patches w. 1-50 gm tube cleansing gel/carton)
➤ *diclofenac sodium* apply qid prn to intact skin
  Pediatric: <12 years: <u>not</u> established; ≥12 years: same as adult

(continued)

Pennsaid 1.5% in 10 drop increments, dispense and rub into front, side, and back of knee; usually 40 drops (40 mg) qid
> *Topical soln:* 1.5% (150 ml)

Pennsaid 2% apply 2 pump actuations (40 mg) and rub into front, side, and back of knee bid
> *Topical soln:* 2% (20 mg/pump actuation, 112 gm)

Solaraze Gel massage in to clean skin bid prn
> *Gel:* 3% (50 gm) (benzyl alcohol)

Voltaren Gel **(G)(OTC)** apply qid prn to intact skin
> *Gel:* 1% (100 gm)

Comment: *Diclofenac* is contraindicated with **aspirin** allergy. As with other NSAIDs, should be avoided in late pregnancy (≥30 weeks) because it may cause premature closure of the ductus arteriosus.

▷ *doxepin* **(G)** cream apply to affected area qid at intervals of at least 3-4 hours; max 8 days
Pediatric: <12 years: not recommended; >12 years: same as adult
> Prudoxin *Crm:* 5% (45 gm)
> Zonalon *Crm:* 5% (30, 45 gm)

▷ *pimecrolimus* 1% cream **(G)** <2 years: not recommended; ≥2 years: apply to affected area bid; do not apply an occlusive dressing
> Elidel *Crm:* 1% (30, 60, 100 gm)

Comment: *Pimecrolimus* is indicated for short-term and intermittent long-term use. Discontinue use when resolution occurs. Contraindicated if the patient is immunosuppressed. Change to the 0.1% preparation or if secondary bacterial infection is present.

▷ *trolamine salicylate* apply tid-qid
Pediatric: <2 years: not recommended; ≥2 years: same as adult
> Mobisyl Creme *Crm:* 10% (100 gm)

▷ *witch hazel* topical soln/gel **(OTC)**
> Tucks apply up to 6 x a day; leave on x 5-15 minutes
> *Pad:* 12, 40, 100/pck; *Gel:* 19.8 gm

TOPICAL AND TRANSDERMAL ANESTHETICS

Comment: *Lidocaine* should not be applied to non-intact skin.

▷ *lidocaine* cream apply to affected area bid prn
Pediatric: <12 years: not recommended; ≥12 years: same as adult
> LidaMantle *Crm:* 3% (1, 2 oz)
> Lidoderm *Crm:* 3% (85 gm)
> ZTlido *lidocaine* topical system 1% (30/carton)

Comment: Compared to Lidoderm (*lidocaine* patch 5%), which contains 700 mg/patch, ZTlido requires 35 mg per topical system to achieve the same therapeutic dose.

▷ *lidocaine* lotion apply to affected area bid prn
Pediatric: <12 years: not recommended; ≥12 years: same as adult
> LidaMantle *Lotn:* 3% (177 ml)

▷ *lidocaine* 5% patch **(G)** apply up to 3 patches at one time for up to 12 hours/24-hour period (12 hours on/12 hours off); patches may be cut into smaller sizes before removal of the release liner; do not reuse
Pediatric: <12 years: not recommended; ≥12 years: same as adult
> Lidoderm *Patch:* 5% (10x14 cm, 30/carton)

▷ *lidocaine+dexamethasone*
Pediatric: <12 years: not recommended; ≥12 years: same as adult
> Decadron Phosphate with Xylocaine *Lotn:* dexa 4 mg+lido 10 mg per ml (5 ml)

▷ *lidocaine+hydrocortisone* **(G)** apply to affected area bid prn
Pediatric: <12 years: not recommended; ≥12 years: same as adult
> LidaMantle HC *Crm:* lido 3%+hydro 0.5% (1, 3 oz); *Lotn:* (177 ml)

▷ *lidocaine* 2.5%+*prilocaine* 2.5% apply sparingly to the burn bid-tid prn
Pediatric: <12 years: not recommended; ≥12 years: same as adult
> Emla Cream 5, 30 gm/tube

HAEMOPHILUS INFLUENZAE B (HIB)

NOTE: Individual vaccines are located under each respective diagnosis. Hib vaccine and more combination vaccines are under development and will be posted online during the 2025 copyright year.

COMBINATION VACCINES

▷ *diphtheria, tetanus toxoid, acellular pertussis, inacivated poliovirus, Haemophilus b conjugate, and hepatitis B* Vaxelis *Vial:* 0.5 ml susp, single dose; *Prefilled syringe:* 0.5 ml susp, single-dose (preservative-free)

Comment: Vaxelis is a single, fixed-dose, combination of six vaccines; the 3-dose immunization series consists of a 0.5 ml IM injection, administered at 2, 4, and 6 months of age. See mfr pkg insert for full prescribing information, including product storage, preparation, administration, contraindications, warnings, and precautions.

HEPATIC PORPHYRIA, ACUTE (AHP)

AMINOLEVULINATE SYNTHASE 1-DIRECTED SMALL INTERFERING RNA

▷ *givosiran* 2.5 mg/kg SC once monthly; administration only by a qualified healthcare provider with access to medical support to appropriately manage anaphylactic reaction; administer injection into the back or side of the upper arm, abdomen, or thigh; rotate injection sites; avoid a 5 cm diameter circle around the navel; if more than one injection is needed for a single dose, separate injection sites at least 2 cm from previous injection sites; divide doses requiring volumes greater than 1.5 ml equally into multiple syringes

Givlaari *Vial:* 189 mg/ml (ml), single-dose

Comment: Givlaari *(givosiran)* is an aminolevulinate synthase 1-directed small interfering RNA indicated for the treatment of adults with acute hepatic porphyria (AHP). Avoid concomitant use of **Givlaari** with CYP1A2 and CYP2D6 substrates for which minimal concentration changes may lead to serious or life-threatening toxicities. The most common adverse reactions (≥20% of patients) included nausea and injection site reactions. If anaphylaxis occurs, discontinue **Givlaari** and administer appropriate medical treatment. Measure liver function at baseline and periodically during the first 6 months of treatment with **Givlaari.** Interrupt or discontinue treatment for severe or clinically significant transaminase elevations. Monitor renal function during treatment with **Givlaari** as clinically indicated. Injection site reaction may occur, including recall reaction; monitor for reactions and manage clinically as needed. Porphyria attacks during pregnancy, often triggered by hormonal changes, occur in 24-95% of AHP patients, with maternal mortality ranging from 2% to 42%. Pregnancy in AHP patients is associated with higher rates of spontaneous abortion, hypertension, and low birthweight infants. In animal reproduction studies, SC administration of *givosiran* during the period of organogenesis resulted in adverse developmental outcomes at doses that produced maternal toxicity. There are no available data with **Givlaari** use in pregnant females to evaluate a drug-associated risk of major birth defects, miscarriage, or adverse maternal or fetal outcomes. Consider benefits and risks of **Givlaari** for the mother and potential adverse embryo/fetal risk when prescribing **Givlaari** in pregnancy.

HEPATITIS A VIRUS (HAV)

Comment: Administer a 2-dose series. Schedule first immunization at least 2 weeks before expected exposure. Booster dose recommended 6-12 months later. Under 1 year of age, administer in the vastus lateralis; over 1 year of age, administer in the deltoid.

HEPATITIS A VIRUS (HAV) PROPHYLAXIS VACCINE

▷ *hepatitis A vaccine, inactivated*
Pediatric: <12 years: not approved; ≥12 years: same as adult
Havrix 1,440 El.U IM; repeat in 6-12 months
Pediatric: <2 years: not recommended; 2-18 years: 720 El.U IM; repeat in 6-12 months or 360 El.U IM; repeat in 1 month
Vaqta 25 U (1 ml) IM; repeat in 6 months
Pediatric: <2 years: not recommended; 2-18 years: 0.5 ml IM; repeat in 6-18 months
Vial: 25 U/ml single-dose (preservative-free); *Prefilled syringe:* 25 U/ml, (0.5, 1 ml, single-dose)

HAV+HEPATITIS B VIRUS (HBV) COMBINATION VACCINE

▷ *Twinrix Vial:* 1 ml soln, *single-dose (1 ml), multidose (10 ml); Prefilled syringe:* 1 ml soln, single-dose
Pediatric: <18 years: not approved; ≥18 years: same as adult
Comment: Twinrix is a fixed-dose combination of two vaccines, hepatitis A inactivated+hepatitis B surface antigen (recombinant vaccine), administered in the deltoid muscle at 0, 1, and 6 months. An alternate accelerated 4-dose schedule is approved for administration at 0, 7 days, and 21-30 days, followed by a booster dose at 12 months. See mfr pkg insert for full prescribing information, including dosing schedules, storage, preparation, administration, contraindications, warnings, and precautions.

PRE- AND POST-EXPOSURE PROPHYLAXIS
Immune Globulin (Human)

▷ *immune globulin* (human) administer via IM injection only (never IV); ensure adequate hydration prior to administration; *Household and institutional hepatitis A virus (HAV) case contacts:* 0.1 ml/kg IM as a single dose; *Planned travel to HAV endemic area:* administer as a single dose at least 2 weeks prior to travel
Pediatric: 0.25 ml/kg IM (0.5 mg/kg in immunocompromised children)

Length of Stay	Prior Dose Dose
Up to 1 month	0.1 ml/kg
Up to 2 months	0.2 ml/kg
More than 2 months	repeat 0.2 ml/kg every 2 months
Less than 3 months	0.02 ml/kg
3 months or longer	0.06 ml/kg repeat every 4-6 months

(continued)

GamaSTAN S/D *Vial:* 2, 10 ml single-dose
Comment: GamaSTAN S/D is the <u>only</u> gamma globulin product FDA-approved for measles and HAV post-exposure prophylaxis (PEP). **GamaSTAN S/D** is also FDA-approved for varicella PEP. Other **GamaSTAN S/D** indications: to prevent <u>or</u> modify measles in a susceptible person exposed fewer than 6 days previously, to modify varicella, and to modify rubella in females exposed during pregnancy. **GamaSTAN S/D** is <u>not</u> indicated for routine prophylaxis <u>or</u> treatment of viral hepatitis B, rubella, poliomyelitis, mumps, <u>or</u> varicella. Contraindications to **GamaSTAN S/D** include persons with cancer, chronic liver disease, and persons allergic to gamma globulin, the HAV vaccine, <u>or</u> a component of the HAV vaccine. Dosage is higher for HAV PEP than for measles and varicella PEP based on recently observed decreasing concentrations of HAV antibodies in **GamaSTAN S/D**, attributed to the decreasing prevalence of previous HAV infection among plasma donors; Defer live vaccines for at least 6 months.

HEPATITIS B VIRUS (HBV)

HEPATITIS B VIRUS (HBV) PROPHYLAXIS VACCINE
Comment: The Advisory Committee on Immunization Practices (ACIP) 2021 recommends vaccination for the hepatitis B virus (HBV) infection in the setting of adults who have high risk factors for HBV <u>or</u> adults requesting protection against HBV without risk factors. HBV vaccination is recommended by shared clinical decision-making for persons with diabetes age 60 years <u>or</u> older.

Comment: Administer IM. Under 1 year of age, administer in vastus lateralis. Over 1 year of age, administer in the deltoid. Administer a 3-dose series; *First dose:* newborn (<u>or</u> now); *Second dose:* 1-2 months after first dose; *Third dose:* 6 months after first dose.
▷ *hepatitis B recombinant vaccine*
    Engerix-B Adult 20 mcg (1 ml) IM; repeat in 1 and 6 months
    Pediatric: infant-19 years: 10 mcg (1/2 ml) IM; repeat in 1 and 6 months
        Vial: 20 mcg/ml single-dose (preservative-free, thimerosal); *Prefilled syringe:* 20 mcg/ml
    Engerix-B Pediatric/Adolescent
    Pediatric: infant-19 years: 10 mcg IM; repeat at 1 and 6 months
    Vial: 10 mcg/0.5 ml single-dose (preservative-free, thimerosal); *Prefilled syringe:* 10 mcg/0.5 ml
    PreHevbrio administer as a three-dose series (each dose 1 ml) via IM injection on a 0-, 1-, and 6-month schedule
    Pediatric: <18 years: <u>not</u> indicated; ≥18 years: same as adult
        Vial: 1 ml, single-dose
    Comment: PreHevbrio is indicated for the prevention of infection caused by all known subtypes of HBV in adults ≥18 years of age
    Recombivax HB Adult 10 mcg (1 ml) IM in deltoid; repeat in 1 and 6 months
        Vial: 10 mcg/ml single-dose; *Vial:* 10 mcg/3 ml multidose
    Recombivax HB Pediatric/Adolescent 5 mcg (0.5 ml) IM; repeat in 1 and 6 months
    Pediatric: birth-19 years: 5 mcg (0.5 ml) IM; repeat in 1 and 6 months; >19 years: use adult formulation <u>or</u> 10 mcg (1 ml) pediatric/adolescent formulation
        Vial: 5 mcg/0.5 ml single-dose

HEPATITIS A VIRUS (HAV)+HBV COMBINATION
▷ **Twinrix** *Vial:* 1 ml soln, single-dose (1 ml), multidose (10 ml); *Prefilled syringe:* 1 ml soln, single-dose
    Pediatric: <18 years: <u>not</u> approved; ≥18 years: same as adult
    Comment: Twinrix is a fixed-dose combination of two vaccines: hepatitis A inactivated+hepatitis B surface antigen (recombinant vaccine), administered in the deltoid muscle at 0, 1, and 6 months. An alternate accelerated 4-dose schedule is approved for administration at 0, 7 days, and 21-30 days, followed by a booster dose at 12 months. See mfr pkg insert for full prescribing information, including dosing schedules, storage, preparation, administration, contraindications, warnings, and precautions.

OTHER COMBINATION VACCINES
▷ **Vaxelis** *Vial:* 0.5 ml susp, single-dose; *Prefilled syringe:* 0.5 ml susp, single-dose (preservative-free)
    Comment: Vaxelis is a single, fixed-dose combination of six vaccines. diphtheria, tetanus toxoid, acellular pertussis, inactivated poliovirus, haemophilus b conjugate, and hepatitis b. The 3-dose immunization series consists of a 0.5 ml IM injection, administered at 2, 4, and 6 months of age. See mfr pkg insert for full prescribing information, including product storage, preparation, administration, contraindications, warnings, and precautions.
▷ **Pentacel (DTaP-IPV/Hib)** is commercially available as a kit containing single-dose vial of fixed-combination vaccine containing diphtheria, tetanus, pertussis, and poliovirus antigens (DTaP-IPV vaccine) and single-dose vial of lyophilized Hib vaccine (PRP-T; ActHIB). Prior to administration, reconstitute vial of lyophilized PRP-T (ActHIB) vaccine by adding the entire content of a vial of DTaP-IPV vaccine in the kit according to manufacturer's instructions to provide a combination vaccine containing diphtheria,

tetanus, pertussis, IPV, and Hib antigens. Gently swirl until cloudy, uniform, white to off-white (yellow tinge) suspension is obtained. Administer IM immediately after reconstitution. **Pentacel** is approved for use as a four-dose series in children 6 weeks through 4 years of age (prior to the fifth birthday). **Pentacel** is to be administered as a four-dose series at 2, 4, 6, and 15-18 months of age. The first dose may be given as early as 6 weeks of age. Four doses of **Pentacel** constitute a primary immunization course against pertussis. Three doses of **Pentacel** constitute an immunization course against diphtheria, tetanus, *Haemophilus influenzae* type b invasive disease, and poliomyelitis; the fourth dose is a booster for diphtheria, tetanus, *H. influenzae* type b invasive disease, and poliomyelitis immunizations. See mfr pkg insert for full prescribing information, including product storage, preparation, administration, contraindications, warnings, and precautions.

CHRONIC HBV INFECTION TREATMENT
Nucleoside Analogs (Reverse Transcriptase Inhibitors and HBV Polymerase Inhibitors)
Comment: Nucleoside analogs are indicated for chronic hepatitis infection with viral replication and either elevated alanine aminotransferase (ALT)/aspartate aminotransferase (AST) or histologically active disease.
▷ *adefovir dipivoxil* (G) 10 mg daily; *CrCl 20-49 ml/min:* 10 mg q 48 hours; *CrCl 10-19 ml/min:* 10 mg q 72 hours
　　Pediatric: <12 years: not recommended; ≥12 years: same as adult
　　Hepsera *Tab:* 10 mg
▷ *entecavir* (G) take on an empty stomach; *nucleoside-naïve:* 0.5 mg daily; *Nucleoside-naïve, CrCl 30-49 ml/min:* 0.25 mg daily; *Nucleoside-naïve, CrCl 10-29 ml/min:* 0.15 mg daily; *Nucleoside-naïve, CrCl <10 ml/min:* 0.05 mg daily; *lamivudine-refractory:* 1 mg daily; *lamivudine-refractory, renal impairment: see* mfr pkg insert
　　Pediatric: <18 years: not recommended; ≥18 years: same as adult
　　Baraclude *Tab:* 0.5, 1 mg; *Oral soln:* 0.05 mg/ml (orange; parabens)
▷ *lamivudine* (G) 100 mg daily; *CrCl <5 ml/min:* 35 mg for 1st dose, then 10 mg once daily; *CrCl 5-14 ml/min:* 35 mg for the 1st dose, then 15 mg once daily; *CrCl 15-29 ml/min:* 100 mg for the 1st dose, then 25 mg once daily; *CrCl 30-49 ml/min:* 100 mg for the 1st dose, then 50 mg once daily
　　Pediatric: <2 years: not recommended; 2-17 years: 3 mg/kg (max 100 mg) once daily
　　Epivir-HBV *Tab:* 100 mg
　　Epivir-HBV Oral Solution *Oral soln:* 5 mg/ml (240 ml) (strawberry-banana)
▷ *telbivudine* 600 mg daily; *CrCl <40 ml/min:* 600 mg q 72 hours; *CrCl 30-49 ml/min:* 600 mg q 48 hours
　　Pediatric: <16 years: not recommended; ≥16 years: same as adult
　　Tyzeka *Tab:* 600 mg
▷ *tenofovir alafenamide (TAF)* (G) take with food; take 1 tab once daily with concomitant *carbamazepine* 2 tablets
　　Pediatric: <18 years: not established; ≥18 years: same as adult
　　Vemlidy *Tab:* 25 mg
　　Comment: No dosage adjustment of **Vemlidy** is required for patients with mild hepatic impairment (Child-Pugh Class A) or compensated liver disease. **Vemlidy** is not recommended in patients with decompensated (Child-Pugh Class B or C) hepatic impairment. No dosage adjustment is required for patients with mild/moderate/severe renal impairment or patients with end-stage renal disease (ESRD) who are receiving chronic hemodialysis. Administer **Vemlidy** after the dialysis treatment is completed. **Vemlidy** is contraindicated in patients with ESRD who are not receiving dialysis. Healthcare providers are encouraged to register patients by calling the Antiretroviral Pregnancy Registry (APR) at 1-800-258-4263.

Interferon Alfa
▷ *interferon alfa-2b* 5 million IU SC or IM daily or 10 million IU SC or IM 3 x/week x 16 weeks; reduce dose by half or interrupt dose if white blood cells (WBCs), granulocyte count, or platelet count decreases
　　Pediatric: <1 year: not recommended; ≥1 year: 3 million IU/m², 3 x/week x 1 week; then increase to 6 million IU/m², 3 x/week up to 16-24 weeks; max 10 million IU/dose; reduce dose by half or interrupt dose if WBCs, granulocyte count, or platelet count decreases
　　Intron A *Vial (pwdr):* 5, 10, 18, 25, 50 million IU/vial (pwdr+diluent; single-dose) (benzoyl alcohol); *Vial (soln):* 3, 5, 10 million IU/vial (single-dose); *Multidose vials (soln):* 18, 25 million IU/vial soln; *Multidose pens (soln):* 3, 5, 10 million IU/0.2 ml (6 doses/pen)

Integrase Strand Transfer Inhibitor (INSTI)
▷ *tenofovir disoproxil fumarate* (G) 300 mg once daily; *CrCl 30-49 ml/min:* 300 mg q 48 hours; *CrCl 10-29 ml/min:* 300 mg q 72-96 hours; *Hemodialysis:* 300 mg once q 7 days or after a total of 12 hours of dialysis; *CrCl <10 ml/min:* not recommended
　　Pediatric: <12 years: not recommended; ≥12 years, 35 kg: 300 mg once daily; mix oral pwdr with 2-4 oz soft food
　　Viread *Tab:* 150, 200, 250, 300 mg; *Oral pwdr:* 40 mg/gm (60 gm w. dosing scoop)
　　Comment: Published studies in HBV-infected subjects do not report an increased risk of adverse pregnancy-related outcomes with the use of **Viread** during the third trimester of pregnancy.

HEPATITIS C VIRUS (HCV)

CHRONIC HEPATITIS C VIRUS (HCV) INFECTION TREATMENT
Nucleoside Analogs (Reverse Transcriptase Inhibitors)

Comment: Nucleoside analogs are indicated for patients with compensated liver disease previously untreated with *alpha interferon* or who have relapsed after *alpha interferon* therapy. Primary toxicity is hemolytic anemia. Contraindicated in male partners of pregnant females; use 2 forms of contraception during therapy and for 6 months after discontinuation.

▷ *ribavirin* (G) take with food in 2 divided doses; *Genotype 2, 3:* 800 mg/day x 24 weeks; *Genotype 1, 4, <75 kg:* 1 gm/day x 48 weeks; ≥75 kg 1.2 gm/day x 48 weeks; *HIV coinfection:* 800 mg/day x 48 weeks; *CrCl 30-50 ml/min:* alternate 200 mg and 400 mg every other day; *CrCl <30 ml/min* or *hemodialysis:* reduce dose or discontinue if hematologic abnormalities occur
   Pediatric: <5 years: not established; ≥5-<18 years: 23-33 kg: 400 mg/day; 34-46 kg: 600 mg/day; 47-59 kg: 800 mg/day; 60-75 kg: 1 gm/day; 1.2 gm/day; ≥75 kg: *Genotype 2, 3:* treat for 24 weeks; *Genotype 1, 4:* treat for 48 weeks; reduce dose or discontinue if hematologic abnormalities occur; ≥18 years: same as adult
   Copegus *Tab:* 200 mg
   Rebetol *Cap:* 200 mg
   Rebetol Oral Solution *Oral soln:* 40 mg/ml (120 ml) (bubble gum)
   Ribasphere RibaPak 600 mg *Tab:* 600 mg (14/pck)
   Virazole *Vial:* 6 gm for inhalation

Interferon Alfa

▷ *interferon alfacon-1*
   Pediatric: <18 years: not recommended; ≥18 years: same as adult
   Infergen 9 mcg SC 3 x/week x 24 weeks, then 15 mcg SC 3 x/week x 6 months; allow at least 48 hours between doses
   Vial (soln): 9, 15 mcg/vial soln (6 single-dose/pck) (preservative-free)
▷ *interferon alfa-2b*
   Intron A *Vial (pwdr):* 5, 10, 18, 25, 50 million IU/vial (pwdr w. diluent; single-dose) (benzoyl alcohol); *Vial (soln):* 3, 5, 10 million IU/vial (single-dose); *Multidose vials (soln):* 18, 25 million IU/vial; *Multidose pens (soln):* 3, 5, 10 million IU/0.2 ml (6 doses/pen)
▷ *peginterferon alfa-2a* administer 180 mcg SC once weekly (on the same day of the week); treat for 48 weeks; consider discontinuing if adequate response after 12-24 weeks
   Pediatric: <18 years: not recommended; ≥18 years: same as adult
   PEGasys *Vial:* 180 mcg/ml (single-dose); *Monthly pck (vials):* 180 mcg/ml (1 ml, 4/pck)
▷ *peginterferon alfa-2b* administer SC once weekly (on the same day of the week); treat for 1 year; consider discontinuing if inadequate response after 24 weeks; 37-45 kg: 40 mcg (100 mg/ml, 0.4 ml); 46-56 kg: 50 mcg (100 mg/ml, 0.5 ml); 57-72 kg: 64 mcg (160 mg/ml, 0.4 ml); 73-88 kg: 80 mcg (160 mg/ml, 0.5 ml); 89-106 kg: 96 mcg (240 mg/ml, 0.4 ml); 107-136 kg: 120 mcg (240 mg/ml, 0.5 ml); 137-160 kg: 150 mcg (300 mg/ml, 0.5 ml)
   Pediatric: <18 years: not recommended; ≥18 years: same as adult
   PEG-Intron *Vial:* 50, 80, 120, 150 mcg/ml (single-dose)
   PEG-Intron Redipen *Pen:* 50, 80, 120, 150 mcg/ml (disposable pens)

HCV NS5A Inhibitor

▷ *daclatasvir* 60 mg once daily for 12 weeks (with *sofosbuvir*); if *sofosbuvir* is discontinued, *daclatasvir* should also be discontinued; with concomitant CY3P inhibitors, reduce dose to 30 mg once daily; with concomitant CY3P inducers, increase dose to 90 mg once daily
   Daklinza *Tab:* 30, 60 mg
   Comment: Daklinza is indicated in combination with *sofosbuvir* with or without *ribavirin*, for the treatment of HCV genotypes 1 and 3, and in patients with comorbid HIV-1 infection, advanced cirrhosis, or post-liver transplant recurrence of HCV.

HCV NS5A Inhibitor+HCV NS3+4A Protease Inhibitor Combinations

▷ *elbasvir+grazoprevir* 1 tab as a single dose once daily; see mfr pkg insert for length of treatment
   Pediatric: <18 years: not recommended; ≥18 years: same as adult
   Zepatier *Tab:* elba 50 mg+grazo 100 mg
   Comment: Zepatier is contraindicated with moderate or severe hepatic impairment, and concomitant *atazanavir, carbamazepine, cyclosporine, darunavir, efavirenz, lopinavir, phenytoin, rifampin, saquinavir,* St. John's wort, *tipranavir.*
▷ *glecaprevir+pibrentasvir* take 3 tablets (total daily dose: *glecaprevir* 300 mg and *pibrentasvir* 120 mg) once daily with food
   Pediatric: <12 years, <45 kg: not established; ≥12 years, ≥45 kg: same as adult
   Mavyret *Tab:* gleca 100 mg+pibre 40 mg
   Comment: Mavyret is a drug for the treatment of adults who have chronic HCV genotypes 1, 2, 3, 4, 5, or 6 infection and who do not have cirrhosis or who have early-stage cirrhosis. **Mavyret** may cause serious

liver problems including liver failure and death in patients who had hepatitis b virus (HBV) infection. This is because the HBV could become active again (i.e., reactivated) during or after treatment with **Mavyret**. Test all patients for HBV infection by measuring HBsAg and anti-HBc prior to initiating therapy with **Mavyret**. The most common side effects of **Mavyret** are headache and tiredness. See mfr insert for table of recommended duration of treatment based on patient characteristics. No adequate human data are available to establish whether or not **Mavyret** poses a risk to pregnancy outcomes. It is not known whether the components of **Mavyret** are excreted in human breast milk or have effects on the breastfed infant.

HCV NS5A Inhibitor+HCV NS3/4A Protease Inhibitor+CYP3A Inhibitor Combinations

▶ *ombitasvir+paritaprevir+ritonavir* take 2 tabs once daily in the AM x 12 weeks
  Pediatric: <18 years: not established; ≥18 years: same as adult
    Technivie *Tab:* omvi 25 mg+pari 75 mg+rito 50 mg (4 x 7 daily dose pcks/carton)
    Comment: Technivie is indicated for use in chronic HCV genotype 4 without cirrhosis. **Technivie** is not for use with moderate hepatic impairment.

HCV NS3/4A Protease Inhibitor

▶ *simeprevir* 150 mg once daily; swallow whole; take with food, not for monotherapy; do not reduce dose or interrupt therapy; if discontinued, do not reinitiate; discontinue if HCV-RNA levels indicate futility; discontinue if *peginterferon, ribavirin, or sofosbuvir* is permanently discontinued; *Treatment-naïve, treatment relapses, with or without cirrhosis:* treat x 12 weeks (*simeprevir+peginterferon+ribavirin*), followed by additional 12 weeks of *peginterferon+ribavirin* (total=24 weeks); *Partial and non-responders, with or without cirrhosis:* treat x 12 weeks (*simeprevir+peginterferon+ribavirin*), followed by additional 36 weeks of *peginterferon+ribavirin* (total=48 weeks); *Treatment-naïve or treatment-experienced without cirrhosis:* treat x 12 weeks (*simeprevir+sofosbuvir*); *Treatment-naïve or treatment-experienced with cirrhosis:* treat x 24 weeks (*simeprevir+sofosbuvir*)
    Olysio *Cap:* 150 mg

HCV NS5A Inhibitor+HCV NS5B Polymerase Inhibitor Combinations

▶ *ledipasvir+sofosbuvir Treatment-naïve, without cirrhosis, with pretreatment HCV RNA <6 million IU/ml:* 1 tab daily x 8 weeks; *Treatment-naïve with or without cirrhosis or treatment-experienced without cirrhosis:* 1 tab daily x 12 weeks; *Treatment-experienced with cirrhosis:* 1 tab daily x 24 weeks; *In combination with ribavirin:* 1 tab daily x 12 weeks
  Pediatric: <18 years: not established; ≥18 years: same as adult
    Harvoni *Tab:* ledi 90 mg+sofo 400 mg
    Comment: Harvoni is indicated for patients with advanced liver disease, genotype 1, 4, 5, or 6 infection, chronic HCV genotype 1- or 4-infected liver transplant recipients with or without cirrhosis or with compensated cirrhosis (Child-Pugh Class A), and for HCV genotype 1-infected patients with decompensated cirrhosis (Child-Pugh Class B or C), including those who have undergone liver transplantation. No adequate human data are available to establish whether or not **Harvoni** poses a risk to pregnancy outcomes; the background risk of major birth defects and miscarriage for the indicated population is unknown. If **Harvoni** is administered with *ribavirin*, the combination regimen is contraindicated in pregnant females and in men whose female partners are pregnant. It is not known whether **Harvoni** and its metabolites are present in human breast milk, affect human milk production, or have effects on the breastfed infant. If **Harvoni** is administered with *ribavirin*, the nursing mother's information for *ribavirin* also applies to this combination regimen.

▶ *sofosbuvir+velpatasvir Without cirrhosis or compensated cirrhosis (Child-Pugh Class A):* 1 tablet daily x 12 weeks; *Decompensated cirrhosis (Child Pugh Class B or C):* 1 tablet daily plus *ribavirin*
  Pediatric: <18 years: not established; ≥18 years: same as adult
    Epclusa *Tab:* sofo 400 mg+velpa 100 mg
    Comment: Epclusa is indicated for patients with chronic HCV with genotype 1, 2, 3, 4, 5, or 6 infection.

HCV NS5A Inhibitor+HCV NS3/4A Protease Inhibitor+CYP3A Inhibitor Combination

▶ *sofosbuvir+velpatasvir* 1 tab daily
  Pediatric: <12 years: not established; ≥12 years: same as adult
    Viekira XR *Tab:* dasa 200 mg+omvi 8.33 mg+pari 50 mg+rito 33.33 mg ext-rel (4 weekly cartons, each containing 7 daily dose pcks/carton)
    Comment: Viekira XR is indicated for HCV genotype 1 with mild liver dysfunction (Child-Pugh Class A). **Viekira XR** is contraindicated in moderate (Child-Pugh Class B) to severe (Child-Pugh Class C) liver dysfunction. No adjustment is recommended with mild, moderate, or severe renal dysfunction.

HCV NS5A Inhibitor+HCV NS3/4A Protease Inhibitor+CYP3A Inhibitor+HCV NS5B Polymerase Inhibitor Combination

▶ *ombitasvir+paritaprevir+ritonavir* plus *dasabuvir*
  Pediatric: <12 years: not established; ≥12 years: same as adult

(continued)

Viekira Pak *ombitasvir+paritaprevir+ritonavir* fixed-dose combination tablet: 2 tablets orally once a day (in the morning); *dasabuvir*: 250 mg orally bid (morning and evening)

Tab: omvi 12.5 mg+pari 75 mg+rito 50 mg plus *Tab*: dasa 250 mg (28 day supply/pck)

Comment: Viekira Pak is indicated for mild liver dysfunction (Child-Pugh Class A). **Viekira Pak** is contraindicated in moderate (Child-Pugh Class B) to severe (Child-Pugh Class C) liver dysfunction. No adjustment is recommended with mild, moderate, or severe renal dysfunction.

HCV NS5B Polymerase Inhibitor+HCV NS5A Inhibitor+HCV NS3/4A Protease Inhibitor Combination

▷ *sofosbuvir+velpatasvir+voxilaprevir* 1 tablet once daily with food x 12 weeks; pretest for HBV infection by measuring HBsAg and anti-HBc prior to the initiation of therapy

Pediatric: <12 years: not established; ≥12 years: same as adult

Vosevi *Tab*: sofo 400 mg+velpa 100 mg+voxil 100 mg fixed-dose combination

Comment: Vosevi is not recommended in patients with moderate or severe hepatic impairment (Child-Pugh Class B or C). A dosage recommendation cannot be made for patients with severe renal impairment or end-stage renal disease. **Vosevi** is contraindicated while taking any medicines containing *rifampin* (**Rifater, Rifamate, Rimactane, Rifadin**). **Vosevi** is indicated for the treatment of adult patients with chronic HCV infection without cirrhosis or with compensated cirrhosis (Child-Pugh Class A) who have (1) genotype 1, 2, 3, 4, 5, or 6 infection and have previously been treated with an HCV regimen containing an NS5A inhibitor or (2) genotype 1a or 3 infection and have previously been treated with an HCV regimen containing *sofosbuvir* without an NS5A inhibitor. Duration of treatment is 12 weeks. Additional benefit of **Vosevi** over *sofosbuvir+velpatasvir* has not been demonstrated with genotype 1b, 2, 4, 5, or 6 infection previously treated with *sofosbuvir* without an NS5A inhibitor. Because there is risk of HBV reactivation, test all patients for evidence of current or prior HBV infection before initiation of HCV treatment. Monitor HCV/HBV coinfected patients for HBV reactivation and hepatitis flare during HCV treatment and posttreatment follow-up. Initiate appropriate patient management for HBV infection as clinically indicated. The most common adverse reactions are headache, fatigue, diarrhea, and nausea.

DUAL TREATMENT REGIMEN
Harvoni+Sovaldi

Comment: Patients who are coinfected with hepatitis B are at risk of HBV reactivation during or after treatment with HCV direct-acting retrovirals. Therefore, patients should be screened for current or past HBV infection before starting this treatment protocol.

TRIPLE TREATMENT REGIMEN
Sovaldi+Harvoni+Ribavirin

Comment: For this FDA-approved triple therapy regimen, follow the recommended regimen for each individual drug. Patients who are coinfected with hepatitis B are at risk of HBV reactivation during or after treatment with HCV direct-acting retrovirals. Therefore, patients should be screened for current or past HBV infection before starting this triple therapy regimen.

HEREDITARY ANGIOEDEMA (HAE)/C1 ESTERASE INHIBITOR DEFICIENCY

Comment: Agents administered for the treatment of hereditary angioedema (HAE) carry a risk of hypersensitivity reactions, which are similar to HAE attacks, and the patient should be monitored closely for signs and symptoms accordingly (e.g., hives, urticaria, tightness of the chest, wheezing, hypotension, and/or anaphylaxis).

HEREDITARY ANGIOEDEMA (HAE) PROPHYLAXIS
Synthetic Steroid

▷ *danazol Females:* start on 3rd or 4th day of menstrual period or after a negative pregnancy test; *Males/Females:* dosage requirements for continuous treatment of HAE should be adjusted based on individual clinical response; initially 200 mg bid-tid; after a favorable initial response is achieved (prevention of episodes of edematous attacks), continuing dosage should be determined by decreasing the dosage by 50% or less at intervals of 1 to 3 months or longer if frequency of attacks prior to treatment dictates; if an attack occurs, daily dosage may be increased by up to 200 mg; during the dose adjusting phase, close monitoring of the patient's response is indicated, particularly if the patient has a history of airway involvement.

Pediatric: <18 years: not recommended; ≥18 years: same as adult

Danocrine *Cap*: 50, 100, 200 mg

Comment: *Danazol* is a synthetic steroid derived from ethisterone. It suppresses the pituitary-ovarian axis. This suppression is probably a combination of depressed hypothalamic-pituitary response to lowered *estrogen* production, the alteration of sex steroid metabolism, and interaction of *danazol* with sex hormone receptors. The only other demonstrable hormonal effects are weak androgenic activity and depression of both follicle-stimulating hormone (FSH) and luteinizing hormone (LH) output. Recent evidence suggests a direct inhibitory effect at gonadal sites and a binding of **Danocrine** to receptors of gonadal steroids at target organs. In addition, **Danocrine** has been shown to significantly decrease immunoglobulin G (IgG), immunoglobulin M (IgM), and immunoglobulin A (IgA) levels, as well as phospholipid and IgG isotope autoantibodies, in patients with endometriosis and associated elevations of autoantibodies, suggesting this could be another mechanism by which it facilitates regression of fibrocystic breast disease. Changes in the menstrual pattern may occur. Generally, the pituitary-suppressive action of **Danocrine** is reversible. Ovulation and cyclic bleeding usually return within 60-90 days when therapy with **Danocrine** is discontinued. In the treatment of HAE, **Danocrine** at effective doses prevents attacks of the disease characterized by episodic edema of the abdominal viscera, extremities, face, and airway, which may be disabling and, if the airway is involved, fatal. In addition, **Danocrine** corrects partially or completely the primary biochemical abnormality of HAE by increasing the levels of the deficient C1 esterase inhibitor (C1EI). As a result of this action, the serum levels of the C4 component of the complement system are also increased. **Danocrine** is also used to treat endometriosis (to relieve associated abdominal pain) and fibrocystic breast disease (to reduce breast tissue nodularity and breast pain/tenderness). Contraindications include pregnancy, breastfeeding, active or history of thromboembolic disease/event, porphyria, undiagnosed abnormal genital bleeding, androgen-dependent tumor, and markedly impaired hepatic, renal, or cardiac function.

C1 Esterase Inhibitor (Human)

▶ *C1 esterase inhibitor (human)* administer 60 IU per kilogram of body weight SC in the abdomen twice weekly (every 3 or 4 days); administer at room temperature within 8 hours after reconstitution; use a silicone-free syringe for reconstitution and administration; use either the Mix2Vial transfer set provided with **Haegarda** or a commercially available 566 double-ended needle and vented filter spike
   Pediatric: <12 years: not recommended; ≥12 years: same as adult
      Haegarda *Vial:* 2,000, 3,000 IU C1 INH pwdr for reconstitution, single-use
      Comment: Haegarda is a plasma-derived concentrate of C1EI (human), a serine proteinase inhibitor. Indicated for routine prophylaxis to prevent HAE attacks in adults and adolescents. It is not indicated for treating acute attacks of HAE. **Haegarda** is the first C1EI (human) SC injection approved for self-administration by the patient or caregiver after healthcare provider instruction. An international consensus panel states that human plasma-derived C1EI is considered to be the therapy of choice for both treatment and prophylaxis of maternal HAE during lactation. There are no prospective clinical data from **Haegarda** use in pregnant females. C1-INH is a normal component of human plasma. There is no information regarding the excretion of **Haegarda** in human milk or effect on the breastfed infant. The developmental and health benefits of breastfeeding should be considered along with the mother's clinical need for **Haegarda** and any potential adverse effects on the breastfed infant from **Haegarda** or from the underlying maternal condition.

Plasma Kallikrein Inhibitor (Monoclonal Antibody)

▶ *berotralstat* take 1 capsule once daily; take with food; max 150 mg/day
   Pediatric: <12 years: not established; ≥12 years: same as adult
      Orladeyo *Cap:* 110, 150 mg
      Comment: Orladeyo (berotralstat), a plasma kallikrein inhibitor, is the first oral, once daily, prophylaxis therapy to prevent attacks of HAE. **Orladeyo** works by binding to plasma kallikrein and inhibiting its proteolytic activity. **Orladeyo** is not used to treat an acute HAE attack. The most common adverse reactions (incidence ≥10%) have been abdominal pain, vomiting, diarrhea, back pain, and gastroesophageal reflux disease. Additionally, an increase in QT prolongation can occur at dosages higher than the recommended 150 mg once daily dosage; additional doses or doses higher than 150 mg once daily are not recommended. Reduce **Orladeyo** dosage when co-administered with P-glycoprotein (P-gp) or breast cancer resistance protein (BCRP) inhibitors. Avoid P-gp inducer use with **Orladeyo**. When co-administered with **Orladeyo**, monitor or titrate dose of drugs with a narrow therapeutic index that are predominantly metabolized by CYP2D6, CYP3A4, or are P-gp substrates. There are insufficient data in pregnant females available to inform drug-related risks with **Orladeyo** use in pregnancy. There are no data on the presence of *berotralstat* in human milk or its effects on the breastfed infant.

▶ *lanadelumab-flyo* initially administer 300 mg SC q 2 weeks into the upper arm, abdomen, or thigh; dosing interval of 300 mg q 4 weeks is also effective and may be considered if the patient is well-controlled (i.e., attack-free) for more than 6 months; with appropriate healthcare provider instruction, patients may self-administer
   Pediatric: <12 years: not established; ≥12 years: same as adult
      Takhzyro *Vial:* 300 mg/2 ml (2 ml), soln, single-dose (preservative-free)
      Comment: Takhzyro (lanadelumab-flyo) is a plasma kallikrein inhibitor (monoclonal antibody) indicated for prophylaxis to prevent attacks of HAE. No dedicated drug interaction studies have been conducted. There are no available data on **Takhzyro** use in pregnant females to inform any drug-associated risks. Monoclonal antibodies such as *lanadelumab-flyo* are transported across the placenta during the 3rd trimester of pregnancy; therefore, potential effects on the fetus are likely to be greater during the 3rd trimester of pregnancy. Animal studies have revealed no evidence of harm to the developing fetus. There are no data on the presence of *lanadelumab-flyo* in human milk or effects on the breastfed infant.

(continued)

HAE ACUTE ATTACK
C1EI (Human)

▷ *C1 esterase inhibitor (human)*
Berinert reconstitute pwdr using the sterile water provided; administer 20 IU/kg body weight via intravenous push (IVP) injection at approximately 4 ml/min, at room temperature within 8 hours of reconstitution; store the vial at room temperature in the original carton to protect from light; appropriately trained patients may self-administer upon recognition of an HAE attack; hypersensitivity reactions may occur; therefore, have epinephrine immediately available for the treatment of acute severe hypersensitivity reaction
Pediatric: <12 years: not established; ≥12 years: same as adult
  Vial: 500 units/10 ml vial, single-use, pwdr for reconstitution with the 10 ml sterile water diluent (provided)
Cinryze administer 1,000 units (2 x 500 U vials) via IVP injection, after reconstitution with 5 ml sterile H₂O/vial; reconstitute 1,000 U pwdr in a 10 ml syringe with 10 ml sterile water; administer over 10 minutes (1 ml/min) at room temperature within 3 hours of reconstitution; each 1,000 unit treatment is administered every 3-4 days; hypersensitivity reactions may occur; therefore, have epinephrine immediately available for the treatment of acute severe hypersensitivity reaction
Pediatric: <16 years: not established; ≥16 years: same as adult
  Vial: 500 units/8 ml vial pwdr for reconstitution (sterile water diluent not provided)
Comment: No adequate and well-controlled studies have been conducted in pregnant women. It is not known whether **Cinryze** can cause fetal harm when administered to a pregnant female or can affect reproduction capacity. **Cinryze** should be administered to a pregnant woman only if clearly needed. It is not known whether **Cinryze** is excreted in human milk.

C1EI (Recombinant)

▷ *C1 esterase inhibitor (recombinant)* reconstitute 2.100 IU pwdr (1 vial) with 14 ml sterile H2O; administer reconstituted solution at room temperature, slow IVP injection over approximately 5 minutes; appropriately trained patients may self-administer upon recognition of HAE attack; weight-based dose: <84 kg: 50 IU /kg [wt in kg ÷ 3 = vol (ml) reconst soln for administration]; ≥84 kg: 4,200 IU (28 ml, 2 vials); if the attack symptoms persist, an additional (second) dose can be administered at the recommended dose level; do not exceed 4,200 IU per dose; max 2 doses within a 24-hour period; hypersensitivity reactions may occur; therefore, have epinephrine immediately available for the treatment of acute severe hypersensitivity reaction
Pediatric: <13 years: not established; ≥13 years: same as adult
  Ruconest *Vial:* 2,100 IU, pwdr, single-use for IVP injection after reconstitution (sterile water diluent not provided)

Bradykinin B2 Receptor Antagonist

▷ *icatibant* administer 30 mg SC injection in the abdominal area; if response is inadequate or symptoms recur, additional injections of 30 mg may be administered at intervals of at least 6 hours; max 3 injections/24 hours; patients may self-administer upon recognition of an HAE attack
Pediatric: <18 years: not established; ≥18 years: same as adult
  Firazyr *Prefilled syringe:* 10 mg/ml (3 ml), single-dose w. 25 gauge Luer lock needle (1/carton, 3 cartons/pck)
  Comment: **Firazyr**, as a bradykinin B2 receptor antagonist, may attenuate the antihypertensive effect of angiotensin-converting enzyme (ACE) inhibitors. The most commonly reported adverse reaction is injection site reaction (97% in clinical trials).

Plasma Kallikrein Inhibitor

▷ *ecallantide* administer 30 mg (3 ml) SC in three 10 mg (1 ml) injections; if an attack persists, an additional dose of 30 mg may be administered within a 24-hour period; should only be administered by a healthcare professional with appropriate medical support to manage anaphylaxis and HAE
Pediatric: <12 years: not established; ≥12 years: same as adult
  Kalbitor *Vial:* 10 mg/ml (1/carton, 3 vials/pkg), single-use
  Comment: Anaphylaxis has occurred in 3.9% of patients treated with **Kalbitor**. Therefore, **Kalbitor** should only be administered in a setting equipped to manage anaphylaxis and HAE. Given the similarity in hypersensitivity symptoms and acute HAE symptoms, monitor patients closely for hypersensitivity reactions.

HERPANGINA

Other Oral Analgesics *see Pain*

ORAL ANALGESICS
▷ *acetaminophen see Fever*

➤ *tramadol* (IV)(G)

    Rybix ODT initially 100 mg once daily; may increase by 100 mg every 5 days; max 300 mg/day; *CrCl <30 ml/min* or *severe hepatic impairment:* not recommended; *Cirrhosis:* max 50 mg q 12 hours

    Pediatric: <18 years: not recommended; ≥18 years: same as adult

        ODT: 50 mg (mint) (phenylalanine)

    Ryzolt initially 100 mg once daily; may increase by 100 mg every 5 days; max 300 mg/day; *CrCl <40 ml/min* or *severe hepatic impairment:* not recommended

    Pediatric: <18 years: not recommended; ≥18 years: same as adult

        Tab: 100, 200, 300 mg ext-rel

    Ultram 50-100 mg q 4-6 hours prn; max 400 mg/day; *CrCl <40 ml/min:* max 100 mg q 12 hours; *Cirrhosis:* max 50 mg q 12 hours

    Pediatric: <18 years: not recommended; ≥18 years: same as adult

        Tab: 50*mg

    Ultram ER initially 100 mg once daily; may increase by 100 mg every 5 days; max 300 mg/day; *CrCl <40 ml/min* or *severe hepatic impairment:* not recommended

    Pediatric: <18 years: not recommended; ≥18 years: same as adult

        Tab: 100, 200, 300 mg ext-rel

➤ *tramadol+acetaminophen* (IV)(G) 2 tabs q 4-6 hours; max 8 tabs/day; 5 days; *CrCl <40 ml/min:* max 2 tabs q 12 hours; max 4 tabs/day x 5 days

    Pediatric: <18 years: not recommended; ≥18 years: same as adult

    Ultracet *Tab:* tram 37.5+acet 325 mg

TOPICAL AND TRANSDERMAL ANESTHETICS

Comment: *Lidocaine* should not be applied to non-intact skin.

➤ *lidocaine* cream apply to affected area bid prn

    Pediatric: <12 years: not recommended; ≥12 years: same as adult

    LidaMantle *Crm:* 3% (1, 2 oz)

    Lidoderm *Crm:* 3% (85 gm)

    ZTlido *lidocaine* topical system 1% (30/carton)

    Comment: Compared to **Lidoderm** (*lidocaine* patch 5%), which contains 700 mg/patch, **ZTlido** only requires 35 mg per topical system to achieve the same therapeutic dose.

➤ *lidocaine* lotion apply to affected area bid prn

    Pediatric: <12 years: not recommended; ≥12 years: same as adult

    LidaMantle *Lotn:* 3% (177 ml)

➤ *lidocaine* 5% patch (G) apply up to 3 patches at one time for up to 12 hours/24-hour period (12 hours on/12 hours off); patches may be cut into smaller sizes before removal of the release liner; do not reuse

    Pediatric: <12 years: not recommended; ≥12 years: same as adult

    Lidoderm *Patch:* 5% (10x14 cm; 30/carton)

➤ *lidocaine+dexamethasone*

    Pediatric: <12 years: not recommended; ≥12 years: same as adult

    Decadron Phosphate with Xylocaine *Lotn:* dexa 4 mg+lido 10 mg per ml (5 ml)

➤ *lidocaine+hydrocortisone* (G) apply to affected area bid prn

    Pediatric: <12 years: not recommended; ≥12 years: same as adult

    LidaMantle HC *Crm:* lido 3%+hydro 0.5% (1, 3 oz); *Lotn:* (177 ml)

➤ *lidocaine* 2.5%+*prilocaine* 2.5% apply sparingly to the burn bid-tid prn

    Pediatric: <12 years: not recommended; ≥12 years: same as adult

    Emla Cream 5, 30 gm/tube

HERPES GENITALIS (HERPES SIMPLEX [HSV] TYPE II)

Comment: The following treatment regimens are published in the **2021 CDC Sexually Transmitted Diseases Treatment Guidelines**. Treatment regimens are for adults only; consult a specialist for the treatment of patients less than 18 years of age. Treatment regimens are presented in alphabetical order by generic drug name, followed by brands and dose forms.

RECOMMENDED REGIMENS: FIRST CLINICAL EPISODE
Regimen 1

➤ *acyclovir* 400 mg tid x 7-10 days or 200 mg 5 x/day x 10 days or until clinically resolved

Regimen 2

➤ *acyclovir* cream apply q 3 hours 6 x/day x 7 days

Regimen 3

➤ *famciclovir* 250 mg tid x 7-10 days or until clinically resolved

Regimen 4
▷ *valacyclovir* 1 gm bid x 10 days <u>or</u> until clinically resolved

RECOMMENDED RECURRENT/EPISODIC REGIMENS
Comment: Initiate treatment of recurrent episodes within 1 day of onset of lesions.

Regimen 1
▷ *acyclovir* 200 mg 5 x/day x 5 days

Regimen 2
▷ *famciclovir* 125 mg bid x 5 days

Regimen 3
▷ *valacyclovir* 500 mg bid x 3-5 days <u>or</u> until clinically resolved

SUPPRESSION THERAPY REGIMENS
Regimen 1
▷ *acyclovir* 400 mg bid x 1 year

Regimen 2
▷ *famciclovir* 250 mg bid x 1 year

Regimen 3
▷ *valacyclovir* 500 mg daily x 1 year (for ≤9 recurrences/year) <u>or</u> 1 gm daily x 1 year (for ≥10 recurrences/year)

DAILY SUPPRESSIVE REGIMENS FOR PERSONS WITH HIV
Regimen 1
▷ *acyclovir* 400-800 mg bid-tid

Regimen 2
▷ *famciclovir* 500 mg bid

Regimen 3
▷ *valacyclovir* 500 mg bid

RECURRENT/EPISODIC REGIMENS FOR PERSONS WITH HIV
Regimen 1
▷ *acyclovir* 400 mg tid x 5-10 days

Regimen 2
▷ *famciclovir* 500 mg bid x 5-10 days

Regimen 3
▷ *valacyclovir* 1 gm bid x 5-10 days

DRUG BRANDS AND DOSE FORMS
▷ *acyclovir* (G)
 Zovirax *Cap:* 200 mg; *Tab:* 400, 800 mg
 Zovirax Oral Suspension *Oral susp:* 200 mg/5 ml (banana)
 Zovirax Cream *Crm:* 5% (3, 15 gm); *Oint:* 5% (3, 15 gm)
▷ *famciclovir*
 Famvir *Tab:* 125, 250, 500 mg
▷ *valacyclovir*
 Valtrex *Cplt:* 500, 1 gm

HERPES LABIALIS/HERPES FACIALIS (HERPES SIMPLEX [HSV] TYPE I, COLD SORE, FEVER BLISTER)

PRIMARY INFECTION
▷ *acyclovir* (G) do <u>not</u> chew, crush, <u>or</u> swallow the buccal tab; apply within 1 hour of symptom onset and before appearance of lesion; apply a single buccal tab to the upper gum region on the affected side and hold in place for 30 seconds
 Pediatric: see Appendix BB.1. *acyclovir* (G) (Zovirax Suspension) *for dose by weight*
 Sitavig *Buccal tab:* 50 mg
 Comment: Sitavig is contraindicated with allergy to milk protein concentrate.

▷ *valacyclovir* 2 gm q 12 hours x 1 day
  Pediatric: <12 years: not recommended; ≥12 years: same as adult
    Valtrex *Cplt:* 500, 1,000 mg

SUPPRESSION THERAPY (≥6 OUTBREAKS/YEAR)
▷ *acyclovir* (G) 200 mg 2-5 x/day x 1 year
  Pediatric: <2 years: not recommended; ≥2 years, <40 kg: 20 mg/kg 2-5 x/day x 1 year; ≥2 years, >40 kg: 200 mg
  2-5 x/day x 1 year; *see* Appendix BB.1. *acyclovir* (G) (Zovirax Suspension) *for dose by weight*
    Zovirax *Cap:* 200 mg; *Tab:* 400, 800 mg
    Zovirax Oral Suspension *Oral susp:* 200 mg/5 ml (banana)

TOPICAL ANTIVIRAL THERAPY
▷ *acyclovir* (G) apply q 3 hours 6 x/day x 7 days
  Pediatric: <2 years: not recommended; ≥2 years: same as adult
    Zovirax Cream *Crm:* 5% (3, 15 gm); *Oint:* 5% (3, 15 gm)
▷ *docosanol* (G) apply and gently rub in 5 x daily until healed
  Pediatric: <12 years: not recommended; ≥12 years: same as adult
    Abreva (OTC) *Crm:* 10% (2 gm)
▷ *penciclovir* (G) apply q 2 hours while awake x 4 days
  Pediatric: <12 years: not recommended; ≥12 years: same as adult
    Denavir *Crm:* 1% (2 gm)

TOPICAL ANTIVIRAL+CORTICOSTEROID THERAPY
▷ *acyclovir+hydrocortisone* (G) cream apply to affected area 5 x/day x 5 days
  Pediatric: <12 years: not recommended; ≥12 years: same as adult
    Crm: 1% (2, 5 gm)

HERPES ZOSTER (HZ, SHINGLES)

See Postherpetic Neuralgia

PROPHYLAXIS VACCINES
Comment: Herpes zoster (shingles) vaccine is indicated for adults ≥50 years of age (<50 years: not recommended). The vaccine is not for preventing primary infection (chickenpox) or treatment of shingles. Contraindications to Herpes zoster vaccine are history of anaphylactic/anaphylactoid reaction to gelatin, neomycin, or any other component of the vaccine, immunosuppression or immunodeficiency, and pregnancy. Pregnancy should be avoided for 3 months following *Varicella zoster* vaccine administration.
▷ *zoster vaccine recombinant, adjuvanted* administer one 0.5 ml dose at month 0 followed by second dose
  2 and 6 months later; administer immediately upon reconstitution or store refrigerated and use within 6
  hours
  Pediatric: <18 years: not established
    Shingrix *Vial:* 0.5 ml single-dose susp for IM injection after reconstitution with diluent (10/carton)
    (preservative-free)
    Comment: Local adverse reactions to **Shingrix** include injection site pain (78%), redness (38.1%), and
    swelling (25.9%). Generalized adverse reactions include myalgia (44.7%), fatigue (44.5%), headache
    (37.7%), shivering (26.8%), fever (20.5%), and gastrointestinal symptoms (17.3%). There are no
    available human data to inform whether there is vaccine-associated risk with **Shingrix** in pregnancy. It is
    not known whether **Shingrix** is excreted in human milk or effects on the breastfed infant.

ORAL ANTIVIRALS
▷ *acyclovir* (G) 800 mg 5 x/day x 7-10 or 14 days
  Pediatric: <2 years: not recommended; ≥2 years, <40 kg: 20 mg/kg 5 x/day x 7-10 days; *see* Appendix BB.1.
  acyclovir (G) (Zovirax Suspension) *for dose by weight;* >2 years, >40 kg: 800 mg 5 x/day x 7-10 days
    Zovirax *Cap:* 200 mg; *Tab:* 400, 800 mg
    Zovirax Oral Suspension *Oral susp:* 200 mg/5 ml (banana)
▷ *famciclovir* 500 mg tid x 7-10 days
  Pediatric: <18 years: not recommended; ≥18 years: same as adult
    Famvir *Tab:* 125, 250, 500 mg
▷ *valacyclovir* 1 gm tid x 7-10 days
  Pediatric: <12 years: not recommended; ≥12 years: same as adult
    Valtrex *Cplt:* 500, 1,000 mg

PROPHYLAXIS AGAINST SECONDARY INFECTION
▷ *silver sulfadiazine* apply qid
  Pediatric: <12 years: not recommended; ≥12 years: same as adult
    Silvadene *Crm:* 1% (20, 50, 85, 400, 1,000 gm jar; 20 gm tube)

ORAL ANALGESICS
Other Oral Analgesics *see Pain*

▷ *acetaminophen see Fever*
▷ *aspirin* (G) *see Fever*
  Comment: *Aspirin*-containing medications are contraindicated with history of allergic-type reaction to *aspirin*, children and adolescents with *varicella* or other viral illness, and the 3rd trimester of pregnancy.
▷ *tramadol* (IV)(G)
  Rybix ODT initially 100 mg once daily; may increase by 100 mg q 5 days; max 300 mg/day; *CrCl <30 ml/min or severe hepatic impairment:* not recommended; *Cirrhosis:* max 50 mg q 12 hours
  Pediatric: <18 years: not recommended; ≥18 years: same as adult
    ODT: 50 mg (mint) (phenylalanine)
  Ryzolt initially 100 mg once daily; may increase by 100 mg q 5 days; max 300 mg/day; *CrCl <30 ml/min or severe hepatic impairment:* not recommended
  Pediatric: <18 years: not recommended; ≥18 years: same as adult
    Tab: 100, 200, 300 mg ext-rel
  Ultram 50-100 mg q 4-6 hours prn; max 400 mg/day; *CrCl <40 ml/min:* max 100 mg q 12 hours; *Cirrhosis:* max 50 mg q 12 hours
  Pediatric: <18 years: not recommended; ≥18 years: same as adult
    Tab: 50* mg
  Ultram ER initially 100 mg once daily; may increase by 100 mg q 5 days; max 300 mg/day; *CrCl <30 ml/min or severe hepatic impairment:* not recommended
  Pediatric: <18 years: not recommended; ≥18 years: same as adult
    Tab: 100, 200, 300 mg ext-rel
▷ *tramadol+acetaminophen* (IV)(G) 2 tabs q 4-6 hours; max 8 tabs/day x 5 days; *CrCl <40 ml/min:* max 2 tabs q 12 hours; max 4 tabs/day x 5 days
  Pediatric: <18 years: not recommended; ≥18 years: same as adult
    Ultracet *Tab:* tram 37.5+acet 325 mg

TOPICAL AND TRANSDERMAL ANESTHETICS
Comment: *Lidocaine* should not be applied to non-intact skin.
▷ *lidocaine* cream apply to affected area bid prn
  Pediatric: <12 years: not recommended; ≥12 years: same as adult
    LidaMantle *Crm:* 3% (1, 2 oz)
    Lidoderm *Crm:* 3% (85 gm)
    ZTlido *lidocaine* topical system 1% (30/carton)
    Comment: Compared to Lidoderm (*lidocaine* patch 5%) which contains 700 mg/patch, **ZTlido** only requires 35 mg per topical system to achieve the same therapeutic dose.
▷ *lidocaine* lotion apply to affected area bid prn
  Pediatric: <12 years: not recommended; ≥12 years: same as adult
    LidaMantle *Lotn:* 3% (177 ml)
▷ *lidocaine* 5% patch (G) apply up to 3 patches at one time for up to 12 hours/24-hour period (12 hours on/12 hours off); patches may be cut into smaller sizes before removal of the release liner; do not reuse
  Pediatric: <12 years: not recommended; ≥12 years: same as adult
    Lidoderm *Patch:* 5% (10x14 cm; 30/carton)
▷ *lidocaine+dexamethasone*
  Pediatric: <12 years: not recommended; ≥12 years: same as adult
    Decadron Phosphate with Xylocaine *Lotn:* dexa 4 mg+lido 10 mg per ml (5 ml)
▷ *lidocaine+hydrocortisone* (G) apply to affected area bid prn
  Pediatric: <12 years: not recommended; ≥12 years: same as adult
    LidaMantle HC *Crm:* lido 3%+hydro 0.5% (1, 3 oz); *Lotn:* (177 ml)
▷ *lidocaine 2.5%+prilocaine 2.5%* apply sparingly to the burn bid-tid prn
  Pediatric: <12 years: not recommended; ≥12 years: same as adult
    Emla Cream 5, 30 gm/tube

SECONDARY INFECTION PROPHYLAXIS
▷ *silver sulfadiazine* apply qid
  Pediatric: <12 years: not recommended; ≥12 years: same as adult
    Silvadene *Crm:* 1% (20, 50, 85, 400, 1,000 gm/jar; 20 gm tube)

HERPES ZOSTER OPHTHALMICUS (HZO, HERPETIC DENDRITIC)

Comment: Herpes zoster ophthalmicus (HZO, herpetic dendritic) is an ophthalmologic emergency. Standard therapy involves initiating systemic (oral or IV) antiviral therapy as soon as possible. Pharmacotherapy options include *acyclovir*, *valacyclovir*, and *famciclovir*. IV acyclovir is recommended for immunocompromised persons. Duration of treatment is 7-10 or 14 days, depending on severity. Ocular complications include conjunctivitis with or without superimposed bacterial infections, episcleritis, scleritis, keratitis, and uveitis, involvement of 3rd, 4th, and 5th cranial nerves III, IV, V, acute optic neuritis, and necrotizing retinopathy (which often leads to permanent vision loss). Corticosteroids reduce the duration of pain during the acute phase; however, they have <u>not</u> been shown to decrease the incidence of postherpetic neuralgia and can exacerbate some ocular complications. Ophthalmology consultation is mandatory before initiating corticosteroid therapy.

OPHTHALMIC ANTIVIRAL

➤ *acyclovir* ophthalmic ointment apply a 1 cm ribbon in the lower cul-de-sac of the affected eye 5 x/day until healed; then, 3 x a day for 7 more days
   Pediatric: <2 years: <u>not</u> established; ≥2years: same as adult
      Avaclyr *Ophth oint:* 3% (3.5 gm), single-patient, multiuse tube
      Comment: Avaclyr *(acyclovir)* is a herpes simplex virus nucleoside analog DNA polymerase inhibitor indicated for the treatment of acute herpetic keratitis (dendritic ulcers) in patients with herpes simplex (HSV-1 and HSV-2) virus. **Avaclyr** is contraindicated in patients with a known hypersensitivity to *acyclovir* <u>or</u> *valacyclovir*. The most common adverse reactions (incidence 2-10%) have been eye pain (stinging), punctate keratitis, and follicular conjunctivitis. There is no information regarding embryo/fetal effects of maternal use of ophthalmic *acyclovir* during pregnancy <u>or</u> presence of ophthalmic *acyclovir* in human milk <u>or</u> effects on the breastfed infant.

ORAL ANTIVIRALS

➤ *acyclovir* (G) 800 mg 5 x/day x 7-10 days
   Pediatric: <2 years: <u>not</u> recommended; 2 years, ≤40 kg: 20 mg/kg 5 x a day x 7-10 days; 2 years, >40 kg: 800 mg 5 x/day x 7-10 days; *see* Appendix BB.1. *acyclovir* (G) (Zovirax Suspension) *for dose by weight*
      Zovirax *Cap:* 200 mg; *Tab:* 400, 800 mg; *IVF bag:* 500 mg, 1 gm premixed in 0.9% NS
      Zovirax Oral Suspension *Oral susp:* 200 mg/5 ml (banana)
➤ *famciclovir* 500 mg tid x 7-10 days
   Pediatric: <18 years: <u>not</u> recommended; ≥18 years: same as adult
      Famvir *Tab:* 125, 250, 500 mg
➤ *valacyclovir* 1 gm tid x 7-10 days
   Pediatric: <12 years: <u>not</u> recommended; ≥12 years: same as adult
      Valtrex *Cplt:* 500, 1 gm

HICCUPS: INTRACTABLE

➤ *chlorpromazine* 25-50 mg tid-qid
   Pediatric: <6 months: <u>not</u> recommended; ≥6 months: 0.25 mg/lb orally q 4-6 hours prn <u>or</u> 0.5 mg/lb rectally q 6-8 hours prn
      Thorazine *Tab:* 10, 25, 50, 100, 200 mg; *Spansule:* 30, 75, 150 mg sust-rel; *Syr:* 10 mg/5 ml (4 oz; orange custard); *Oral conc:* 30 mg/ml (4 oz), 100 mg/ml (2, 8 oz); *Supp:* 25, 100 mg

HIDRADENITIS SUPPURATIVA

ORAL ANTI-INFECTIVES

➤ *doxycycline* (G) 100 mg bid x 7-14 days
   Pediatric: <8 years: <u>not</u> recommended; ≥8 years, <100 lb: 2 mg/lb on the first day in 2 divided doses, followed by 1 mg/lb/day in 1-2 divided doses; ≥8 years, ≥100 lb: same as adult; *see Appendix BB.19: doxycycline* (G) (Vibramycin Syrup/Suspension) *for dose by weight*
      Acticlate *Tab:* 75, 150**mg
      Adoxa *Tab:* 50, 75, 100, 150 mg ent-coat
      Doryx *Tab:* 50, 75, 100, 150, 200 mg del-rel
      Doxteric *Tab:* 50 mg del-rel
      Monodox *Cap:* 50, 75, 100 mg
      Oracea *Cap:* 40 mg del-rel
      Vibramycin *Tab:* 100 mg; *Cap:* 50, 100 mg; *Syr:* 50 mg/5 ml (raspberry-apple) (sulfites); *Oral susp:* 25 mg/5 ml (raspberry)
      Vibra-Tab *Tab:* 100 mg film-coat
➤ *erythromycin base* (G) 1-1.5 gm divided qid x 7-14 days
   Pediatric: <45 kg: 30-50 mg in 2-4 divided doses x 7-14 days; ≥45 kg: same as adult
      Ery-Tab *Tab:* 250, 333, 500 mg ent-coat
      PCE *Tab:* 333, 500 mg
➤ *erythromycin ethylsuccinate* (G) 1,200-1,600 mg divided qid x 7-14 days
   Pediatric: 30-50 mg/kg/day in 4 divided doses x 7 days; may double dose with severe infection; max 100 mg/kg/day; *see* Appendix BB.21. *erythromycin ethylsuccinate* (G) (E.E.S. Suspension, EryPed Drops/Suspension) for dose by weight

(continued)

EryPed *Oral susp:* 200 mg/5 ml (100, 200 ml) (fruit); 400 mg/5 ml (60, 100, 200 ml) (banana); *Oral drops:* 200, 400 mg/5 ml (50 ml) (fruit); *Chew tab:* 200 mg wafer (fruit)
E.E.S. *Oral susp:* 200, 400 mg/5 ml (100 ml) (fruit)
E.E.S. Granules *Oral susp:* 200 mg/5 ml (100, 200 ml) (cherry)
E.E.S. 400 Tablets *Tab:* 400 mg

▷ *minocycline* (G) 100 mg bid x 7-14 days
Pediatric: <8 years: not recommended, ≥8 years: same as adult
    Dynacin *Cap:* 50, 100 mg
    Minocin *Cap:* 50, 75, 100 mg; *Oral susp:* 50 mg/5 ml (60 ml) (custard) (sulfites, alcohol 5%)

▷ *tetracycline* (G) 250 mg qid or 500 mg tid x 7-14 days
Pediatric: <8 years: not recommended; ≥8 years, <100 lb: 25-50 mg/kg/day in 2-4 divided doses x 7-14 days; ≥8 years, ≥100 lb: same as adult; *see Appendix BB.31. tetracycline* (G) (Sumycin Suspension) *for dose by weight*
    Achromycin V *Cap:* 250, 500 mg
    Sumycin *Tab:* 250, 500 mg; *Cap:* 250, 500 mg; *Oral susp:* 125 mg/5 ml (100, 200 ml) (fruit) (sulfites)

TOPICAL ANTI-INFECTIVE

▷ *clindamycin* topical apply bid x 7-14 days
    Cleocin T *Pad:* 1% (60/pck; alcohol 50%); *Lotn:* 1% (60 ml); *Gel:* 1% (30, 60 gm); *Soln w. applicator:* 1% (30, 60 ml) (alcohol 50%)

▷ *adalimumab* 160 mg on Day 1 (administered in 1 day or split over 2 consecutive days), 80 mg on Day 15, and 40 mg every week or 80 mg every other week starting on Day 29; discontinue in patients without evidence of clinical remission by eight weeks (Day 57); administer SC in the abdomen or thigh; rotate sites
Pediatric: <12 years: safety and efficacy not established; ≥12 years: <30 kg (<60 lb) to 60 kg (132 lb): Day 1: 80 mg; Day 8 *and subsequent doses:* 40 mg every other week; >60 kg (>132 lb): same as adult; administer SC in the abdomen or thigh; rotate sites
    Humira *Prefilled pen (Humira Pen):* 40 mg/0.4 ml, 40 mg/0.8 ml, 80 mg/0.8 ml, single-dose; *Prefilled glass syringe:* 10 mg/0.1 ml, 10 mg/0.2 ml, 20 mg/0.2 ml, 20 mg/0.4 ml, 40 mg/0.4 ml. 40 mg/0.8 ml, 80 mg/0.8 ml, single-dose; *Vial:* 40 mg/0.8 ml, single dose, institutional use only (preservative-free)

HOMOCYSTINURIA

METHYLATING AGENT

▷ *betaine anhydrous* (G) *Recommended:* 6 gm/day, administered orally in divided doses of 3 gm bid; measure the prescribed amount of **Cystadane** with the measuring scoop provided and then dissolve in 4-6 oz of water, juice, or milk until completely dissolved, or mix with food for immediate ingestion
Pediatric: <3 years: *Recommended starting dose:* 100 mg/kg/day, administered orally in divided doses of 50 mg/kg bid; then increase dose weekly in 50 mg/kg increments; monitor patient response by plasma homocysteine concentrations; increase the dose gradually until the plasma total homocysteine concentration is undetectable or present only in small amounts; measure the prescribed amount of **Cystadane** with the measuring scoop provided and then dissolve in 4-6 oz of water, juice, milk, or formula until completely dissolved, or mix with food for immediate ingestion; ≥3 years: same as adult
Cystadane *Pwdr for oral soln:* 180 gm bottle w. measuring scoop (1 level scoop = 1 gm *betaine anhydrous* pwdr)
Comment: **Cystadane** is the first generic treatment for homocystinuria. **Cystadane** is a methylating agent indicated in pediatric and adult patients for the treatment of homocystinuria to decrease elevated homocysteine blood concentrations. Included within the category of homocystinuria are (1) cystathionine beta-synthase (CBS) deficiency, (2) 5,10-methylenetetrahydrofolate reductase (MTHFR) deficiency, and (3) cobalamin cofactor metabolism (cbl) defect. There is potential for hypermethioninemia in patients with CBS deficiency using **Cystadane**. Worsening elevated plasma methionine concentrations and cerebral edema have been reported. Monitor plasma methionine concentrations in patients with CBS deficiency. Keep plasma methionine concentrations below 1,000 micromol/L through dietary modification and, if necessary, a reduction of the **Cystadane** dosage. Based on physician surveys, the most common adverse reactions (>2%) have been nausea and gastrointestinal distress. Available data from a limited number of published case reports and postmarketing experience with **Cystadane** use in pregnancy have not identified any drug associated risks of major birth defects, miscarriage, or adverse maternal or fetal outcomes. Animal reproduction studies have not been conducted with *betaine*. There are no data on the presence of *betaine* in human or animal milk or effects on the breastfed infant. Developmental and health benefits of breastfeeding should be considered along with the mother's clinical need for **Cystadane** and any potential adverse effects on the breastfed infant from **Cystadane** or from the underlying maternal condition.

HOOKWORM (UNCINARIASIS, CUTANEOUS LARVAE MIGRANS)

ANTHELMINTICS

▷ *albendazole* 400 mg as a single dose; may repeat in 3 weeks
Pediatric: <2 years: 200 mg daily x 3 days, may repeat in 3 weeks; ≥2-12 years: 400 mg daily x 3 days, may repeat in 3 weeks
    Albenza *Tab:* 200 mg

▷ **ivermectin** take with water; chew or crush and mix with food; may repeat in 3 months if needed; *<15 kg:* not recommended; *≥15 kg:* 200 mcg/kg as a single dose
Pediatric: <15 kg: not recommended; ≥15 kg: same as adult
    Stromectol *Tab:* 3, 6*mg

▷ **mebendazole** (G) chew, swallow, or mix with food; 100 mg bid x 3 days; may repeat in 3 weeks if needed; take with a meal
Pediatric: <2 years: not recommended; ≥2 years: same as adult
    Emverm *Chew tab:* 100 mg
    Vermox *Chew tab:* 100 mg

▷ **pyrantel pamoate** 11 mg/kg x 1 dose; max 1 gm/dose
Pediatric: 25-37 lb: 1/2 tsp x 1 dose; 38-62 lb: 1 tsp x 1 dose; 63-87 lb: 1 tsp x 1 dose; 88-112 lb: 2 tsp x 1 dose; 113-137 lb: 2 tsp x 1 dose; 138-162 lb: 3 tsp x 1 dose; 163-187 lb: 3 tsp x 1 dose; >187 lb: 4 tsp x 1 dose
    Antiminth *Cap:* 180 mg; *Liq:* 50 mg/ml (30 ml), 144 mg/ml (30 ml); *Oral susp:* 50 mg/ml (60 ml)
    Pin-X (OTC) *Cap:* 180 mg; *Liq:* 50 mg/ml (30 ml), 144 mg/ml (30 ml); *Oral susp:* 50 mg/ml (30 ml)

▷ **thiabendazole** take with a meal; may crush and mix with food; treat x 7 days; <30 lb: consult mfr pkg insert; ≥30 lb: 25 mg/kg/dose bid with meals; 30-50 lb: 250 mg bid with meals; >50 lb: 10 mg/lb/dose bid with meals; max 1.5 gm/dose; max 3 gm/day
Pediatric: same as adult
    Mintezol *Chew tab:* 500*mg (orange); *Oral susp:* 500 mg/5 ml (120 ml) (orange)
Comment: *Thiabendazole* is not for prophylaxis. May impair mental alertness. May not be available in the United States.

HUMAN IMMUNODEFICIENCY VIRUS (HIV) INFECTION, HIV PRE-EXPOSURE PROPHYLAXIS (PrEP), HIV OCCUPATIONAL POST-EXPOSURE PROPHYLAXIS (oPEP), HIV NON-OCCUPATIONAL POST-EXPOSURE PROPHYLAXIS (nPEP)

ANTIRETROVIRAL HIV PRE-EXPOSURE PROPHYLAXIS (PrEP)
Comment: **Descovy** and **Truvada** are each individually used in the treatment of HIV-1 infection and for pre-exposure prophylaxis (PrEP) to reduce the risk of sexually acquired HIV-1 in adults and adolescents weighing ≥35 kg, at high risk for exposure, in combination with safe sex practices. HIV-1 PrEP is contraindicated in individuals with unknown or positive HIV-1 status. HIV-1 PrEP must only be prescribed to individuals confirmed to be HIV-negative immediately prior to initiating and at least every 3 months during use.

▷ **Descovy** (G) *emtricitabine+tenofovir disoproxil fumarate* take 1 tablet once daily with or without food
Pediatric: <12 years, <35 kg: not established; ≥12 years, ≥35 kg: same as adult
    Descovy *Tab:* emt 200 mg+teno ala 25 mg

▷ **Truvada** (G) *emtricitabine+tenofovir disoproxil fumarate* <17 kg: not established; *17-<22 kg:* 100/150 once daily; *22-<28 kg:* 133/200 once daily; *28-35 kg:* 167/250 once daily; *≥35 kg:* 200/300 once daily
Pediatric: same as adult
    Tab: **Truvada 100/150** emt 100 mg+teno ala 150 mg
         Truvada 133/200 emt 133 mg+teno ala 200 mg
         Truvada 167/250 emt 167 mg+teno 250 mg
         Truvada 200/300 emt 200 mg+teno 300 mg

HIV-1 INTEGRASE STRAND TRANSFER INHIBITOR (INSTI)
▷ **cabotegravir** screen the patient for HIV-1 infection immediately prior to initiating **Apretude** for HIV-1 PrEP and prior to each injection while on **Apretude** for PrEP; prior to initiating **Apretude**, oral lead-in dosing may be used for approximately 1 month with the recommended oral dose to assess the patient tolerability of **cabotegravir**; each **Apretude** dose is a single 600 mg (3 ml) IM injection in the gluteus muscle; *Recommended dosing schedule:* administer Apretude dose 1; then, dose 2: administer 1 month after Dose #1; Dose 3: administer 2 months after Dose 2; then, administer a dose once every 2 months (i.e., every other month) thereafter; *if using a 1-month oral cabotegravir lead-in:* administer **Apretude** Dose 1 on the last (or within 3 days of the last) lead-in day
Pediatric: Weight <35 kg (<77 lb): not recommended; ≥35 kg (≥77 lb): same as adult
    Apretude *Vial:* 600 mg/3 ml (200 mg/ml), single-dose (of *cabotegravir* extended-release injectable suspension) for IM injection
Comment: **Apretude** is a long-acting injectable HIV-1 integrase strand transfer inhibitor (INSTI) indicated for PrEP to reduce the risk of sexually acquired HIV-1 infection in at-risk adults and adolescents weighing ≥35 kg. Patients must have a negative HIV-1 test prior to initiating **Apretude** (with or without an oral lead-in with oral *cabotegravir*) for HIV-1 PrEP. **Apretude** is contraindicated (1) in patients with unknown HIV-1 status or with known positive HIV-1 status, (2) a previous hypersensitivity reaction to *cabotegravir*, and (3) co-administration with drugs that significantly decrease *cabotegravir* plasma concentration. Drugs that induce uridine diphosphate glucuronosyltransferase (UGT1A1) may significantly decrease plasma concentration of *cabotegravir*. See mfr pkg insert for other important drug interactions. The most common adverse reactions (all grades) observed in at least 1% of subjects receiving **Apretude** treatment were

(continued)

injection site reaction, diarrhea, headache, pyrexia, fatigue, sleep disorders, nausea, dizziness, flatulence, abdominal pain, vomiting, myalgia, rash, decreased appetite, somnolence, back pain, and upper respiratory tract infection. *Boxed Warning:* Individuals must be tested for HIV-1 infection prior to initiating **Apretude** or oral *cabotegravir*, and with each subsequent injection of **Apretude**, using a test approved or cleared by the FDA for the diagnosis of acute or primary HIV-1 infection. Drug-resistant HIV-1 variants have been identified with use of **Apretude** for HIV-1 PrEP by individuals with undiagnosed HIV-1 infection. Do not initiate **Apretude** for HIV-1 PrEP unless negative infection status is confirmed. Individuals who become infected with HIV-1 while receiving **Apretude** for PrEP must transition to a complete HIV-1 treatment regimen. Hypersensitivity reactions have been reported in association with other integrase inhibitors; discontinue **Apretude** immediately if signs or symptoms of hypersensitivity reactions develop. Hepatotoxicity has been reported in patients receiving *cabotegravir*. Clinical and laboratory monitoring should be considered to identify impaired hepatic function. Discontinue **Apretude** if hepatotoxicity is suspected. Depressive disorders have been reported with **Apretude**. Prompt evaluation is recommended for depressive symptoms. Animal studies have demonstrated that *cabotegravir* crosses the placenta and can be detected in fetal tissue. However, there are insufficient human data on the use of **Apretude** during pregnancy to adequately assess a drug-associated risk of birth defects and miscarriage. In animal studies, *cabotegravir* was administered orally to pregnant animals at 0, 30,500, or 2,000 mg/kg/day from gestation days (GDs) 7-19. No drug-related fetal toxicities were observed at 2,000 mg/kg/day (approximately 0.7 times the exposure in humans at the recommended human dose [RHD]). When *cabotegravir* was administered orally to animals at 0, 0.5, 5, or 1,000 mg/kg/day from 15 days before co-habitation, during co-habitation, and from GDs 0-17. There were no effects on fetal viability when fetuses were delivered by Cesarean, although a minor decrease in fetal body weight was observed at 1,000 mg/kg/day (>28 times the exposure in humans at the RHD). No drug-related fetal toxicities were observed at 5 mg/kg/day (approximately 13 times the exposure in humans at the RHD), and no drug-related fetal malformations were observed at any dose. While there are insufficient human data to assess the risk of neural tube defects (NTDs) with exposure to **Apretude** during pregnancy, NTDs were associated with *dolutegravir*, another integrase inhibitor. Healthcare providers should discuss the benefit/risk of using **Apretude** with individuals of childbearing potential or during pregnancy. Advise patients of reproductive potential to use effective contraception. **Apretude** for PrEP should be used during pregnancy only if the expected benefit justifies potential risks to the fetus, with knowledge of the vertical transmission of HIV-1 *in utero* and via breastfeeding, and associated potential adverse embryo/fetal and infant outcomes from *cabotegravir* exposure. Residual concentrations of *cabotegravir* may remain in the systemic circulation of patients up to 12 months or longer; therefore, consideration should be given to the potential for fetal exposure during pregnancy and breastfeeding. Assess risk/benefit to mothers and the breastfed infants prior to planned pregnancy and initiation of breastfeeding. There is a pregnancy exposure registry that monitors pregnancy outcomes in women exposed to **Apretude** during pregnancy. Healthcare providers are encouraged to register individuals by calling the Antiretroviral Pregnancy Registry (APR) at 1-800-258-4263.

ANTIRETROVIRAL HIV POST-EXPOSURE PROPHYLAXIS (OCCUPATIONAL POSTEXPOSURE PROPHYLAXIS [oPEP] AND NON-OCCUPATIONAL POSTEXPOSURE PROPHYLAXIS [nPEP])

Comment: Antiretroviral prophylactic treatment regimens for occupational HIV post-exposure prophylaxis (oPEP) and non-occupational HIV post-exposure prophylaxis (nPEP) are referenced from the **2021 CDC Sexually Transmitted Diseases Treatment Guidelines,** Morbidity and Mortality Weekly Report (MMWR), and National Institutes of Health (NIH) available at https://www.cdc.gov/hiv/pdf/programresources/cdc-hiv-npep-guidelines.pdf.

In this section, the 2021 CDC-recommended highly active antiretroviral treatment (HAART) regimens are followed by a listing of the single and combination drugs with dosing regimens and dose forms. Appendix R. is an alphabetical listing of the HIV drugs and dose forms. For more information on the management of HIV infection in adults and adolescents, see *Guidelines for the Use of Antiretroviral Agents in HIV-1-Infected Adults and Adolescents:* https://aidsinfo.nih.gov/contentfiles/lvguidelines/adultandadolescentgl.pdf.

For specific dosing information on the management of HIV infection in children, see *Guidelines for Use of Antiretroviral Agents in Pediatric HIV Infection:* www.aidsinfo.nih.gov/contentfiles/lvguidelines/pediatricguidelines.pdf. Providers should consult, and/or refer HIV-infected patients to, a specialist and/or specialty community services for age-appropriate dosing regimens and other patient-specific needs.

Initiation of oPEP/nPEP with antiretroviral therapy (ART) as soon as possible increases the likelihood of prophylactic benefit. Treatment regimens must be initiated ≥72 hours following exposure. A 28-day course of ART is recommended for persons with **substantial risk for HIV exposure** (i.e., exposure of vagina, rectum, eye, mouth, or other mucous membrane, non-intact skin, or percutaneous contact with blood, semen, vaginal secretions, breast milk, or any body fluid that is visibly contaminated with blood, when the source is known to be infected with HIV). ART is not recommended for persons with *negligible risk for HIV exposure* (i.e., exposure of vagina, rectum, eye, mouth, or other mucus membrane, intact or non-intact skin, or percutaneous contact with urine, nasal secretions, saliva, sweat, or tears, if not visibly contaminated with blood, regardless of the known or suspected HIV status of the source). There is no evidence indicating any specific antiretroviral medication or combination of medications is optimal for suppressing local viral replication. There is no evidence to indicate that a 3-drug ART regimen is any more beneficial than a 2-drug regimen. When the source person is available for interview and testing, their history of retroviral medication use and most recent/current viral load measurement should be considered when selecting an ART treatment regimen (e.g., to help avoid prescribing an antiretroviral medication to which the source virus is likely to be resistant). Register pregnant patients exposed to antiretroviral agents to the Antiretroviral Pregnancy Registry (APR) at 800-258-4263. The CDC recommends that HIV-infected mothers not breastfeed their infants to avoid risking postnatal transmission of HIV infection.

HIV-1 INFECTION ANTIRETROVIRAL TREATMENT REGIMENS

Comment: Immune reconstitution syndrome (IRS) has been reported in patients treated with combination ART. During the initial phase of combination antiretroviral treatment, patients whose immune system responds may develop an inflammatory response to indolent or residual opportunistic infections (such as *Mycobacterium avium* infection, cytomegalovirus, *Pneumocystis jirovecii* pneumonia [PCP], or tuberculosis), which may necessitate further evaluation and treatment. Autoimmune disorders (such as Graves' disease, polymyositis, and Guillain-Barré syndrome) have also been reported to occur in the setting of immune reconstitution; however, the time to onset is more variable and can occur many months after initiation of treatment. Patients with HIV-1 should be tested for the presence of chronic hepatitis B virus (HBV) before initiating ART.

NON-NUCLEOSIDE REVERSE TRANSCRIPTASE INHIBITOR (NNRTI)-BASED REGIMEN

▷ *efavirenz* plus (*lamivudine* or *emtricitabine*) plus (*zidovudine* or *tenofovir*)

PROTEASE INHIBITOR (PI)-BASED REGIMENS

▷ *lopinavir+ritonavir* (co-formulated as **Kaletra**) plus (*lamivudine* or *emtricitabine*) plus *zidovudine*
▷ *darunavir+cobicistat* (co-formulated as **Prezcobix**) plus *other retroviral agents*

ALTERNATIVE REGIMENS
NNRTI-Based Regimen

▷ *efavirenz* plus (*lamivudine* or *emtricitabine*) plus (*abacavir* or *didanosine* or *stavudine*)
Comment: *Efavirenz* should be avoided in pregnant females and females of childbearing potential.

PI-Based Regimens
Regimen 1

▷ *atazanavir* plus (*lamivudine* or *emtricitabine*) plus (*zidovudine* or *stavudine* or *abacavir* or *didanosine*) or (*tenofovir* plus *ritonavir*) (100 mg/day)

Regimen 2

▷ *fosamprenavir* plus (*lamivudine* or *emtricitabine*) plus (*zidovudine* or *stavudine*) or (*abacavir* or *tenofovir* or *didanosine*)

Regimen 3

▷ *fosamprenavir+ritonavir* plus (*lamivudine* or *emtricitabine*) plus (*zidovudine* or *stavudine* or *abacavir* or *tenofovir* or *didanosine*)

Regimen 4

▷ *indinavir+ritonavir* plus (*lamivudine* or *emtricitabine*) plus (*zidovudine* or *stavudine* or *abacavir* or *tenofovir* or *didanosine*)
Comment: Using *ritonavir* with *indinavir* may increase risk of renal adverse events.

Regimen 5

▷ *lopinavir+ritonavir* (co-formulated as **Kaletra**) plus (*lamivudine* or *emtricitabine*) plus (*stavudine* or *abacavir* or *tenofovir* or *didanosine*)

Regimen 6

▷ *nelfinavir* plus (*lamivudine* or *emtricitabine*) plus (*zidovudine* or *stavudine* or *abacavir* or *tenofovir* or *didanosine*)

Regimen 7

▷ *saquinavir+ritonavir* plus (*lamivudine* or *emtricitabine*) plus (*zidovudine* or *stavudine* or *abacavir* or *tenofovir* or *didanosine*)

Triple Nucleoside Reverse Transcriptase Inhibitor (NRTI)-Based Regimen

abacavir plus *lamivudine* plus *zidovudine*
Comment: Triple nucleoside reverse transcriptase inhibitor (NRTI) therapy should be used only when a non-nucleoside reverse transcriptase inhibitor (NNRTI)- or protease inhibitor (PI)-based regimen cannot or should not be used.

BRAND NAMES, DOSING, AND DOSE FORMS: SINGLE AGENTS
Integrase Strand Transfer Inhibitors

▶ *cabotegravir*

Vocabria *Tab:* 30 mg film-coat

Comment: Vocabria *(cabotegravir)* is indicated in combination with **Edurant** *(rilpivirine)* for short-term treatment of HIV-1 infection in adults who are virologically suppressed (HIV-1 RNA less than 50 copies/ml) on a stable antiretroviral regimen with <u>no</u> history of treatment failure and with <u>no</u> known <u>or</u> suspected resistance to either *cabotegravir* <u>or</u> *rilpivirine*, for use as (1) oral lead-in to assess the tolerability of *cabotegravir* prior to administration of **Cabenuva** *(cabotegravir+rilpivirine)* extended-release injectable suspensions and (2) oral therapy for patients who will miss planned injection dosing with **Cabenuva**.

▶ *dolutegravir Treatment-naïve <u>or</u> treatment-experienced but INSTI naïve:* 50 mg once daily; *Treatment-experienced <u>or</u> treatment naïve and co-administered with efavirenz, fosamprenavir/ritonavir* (FPV/r) <u>or</u> *tipranavir/ritonavir* (TPV/r), <u>or</u> *rifampin:* 50 mg bid; *INSTI experienced with certain INSTI-associated resistance substitutions:* 50 mg bid

Pediatric: <12 years, <40 kg: <u>not</u> established; ≥12 years, ≥40 kg: same as adult

Tivicay *Tab:* 10, 25, 50 mg

▶ *raltegravir (as potassium)* 400 mg (1 film-coat tab) bid; take with concomitant *rifampin* 800 mg bid; swallow whole; do <u>not</u> crush <u>or</u> chew

Pediatric: ≥4 weeks, 3-11 kg: (oral susp) 3 to <4 kg: 20 mg bid; 4 to <6 kg: 30 mg bid; 6 to <8 kg: 40 mg bid; 8 to <11 kg: 60 mg bid; ≥11 to <25 kg: (use oral susp/chew tab): 6 mg/kg/dose bid; see mfr pkg insert for dose by weight; ≥25 kg and unable to swallow tablet, use chew tab; 25 to <28 kg: 150 mg bid; 28 to <40 kg: 200 mg bid; ≥40 kg: 300 mg bid; 6 years, ≥25 kg, and able to swallow tablets, use film-coat tab: 400 mg bid

Isentress *Tab:* 400 mg film-coat; *Chew tab:* 25, 100*mg (orange banana) (phenylalanine)

Isentress HD *Tab:* 600 mg film-coat

Isentress Oral Suspension *Oral susp:* 100 mg/pkt pwdr for oral susp (banana)

Comment: Oral suspension, chewable tablets, and film-coat *raltegravir* tablets are <u>not</u> bioequivalent. Maximum dose for chewable tablets is 300 mg bid. Previously, the maximum dose for film-coat tablets was 400 mg bid. However, the U.S. FDA has recently approved a new 1,200 mg daily dosage of **Isentress HD** *(raltegravir)* for the treatment of HIV-1 infection in adults, and pediatric patients who weigh ≥40 kg and are treatment-naïve <u>or</u> whose virus has been suppressed on an initial regimen of 400 mg twice-daily dose of **Isentress HD**. **Isentress HD** is administered as two 600 mg film-coat oral tablets, in combination with other antiretroviral agents, and can be taken with <u>or</u> without food. Co-administration of **Isentress HD** can include a wide range of antiretroviral agents and non-antiretroviral agents; however, aluminum and/or magnesium-containing antacids, calcium carbonate antacids, *rifampin, tipranavir+ritonavir, etravirine,* and other strong inducers of drug metabolizing enzymes are <u>not</u> recommended to be combined with **Isentress HD**. Healthcare providers should consider the potential for drug-drug interactions prior to and during treatment with **Isentress HD** and any other recommended agents. Adverse effects associated with treatment included abdominal pain, diarrhea, vomiting, and decreased appetite. In addition, severe, potentially life-threatening and fatal skin reactions can occur, including Stevens-Johnson syndrome, hypersensitivity reaction, and toxic epidermal necrolysis. Treatment should be immediately discontinued if severe hypersensitivity, severe rash, <u>or</u> rash with systemic symptoms <u>or</u> liver aminotransferase elevations develop.

Nucleoside Reverse Transcriptase Inhibitors (NRTIs)

▶ *abacavir sulfate* (G) 600 mg once daily <u>or</u> 300 mg bid; *Mild hepatic impairment:* use oral solution for titration

Pediatric: 3 months-16 years: (tab/oral soln) 16 mg/kg qd <u>or</u> 8 mg/kg bid; max 300 mg bid; >14 kg: see mfr pkg insert for tablet dosing by weight band

Ziagen (as sulfate) *Tab:* 300*mg

Ziagen Oral Solution *Oral soln:* 20 mg/ml (240 ml) (strawberry-banana) (parabens, propylene glycol)

▶ *didanosine*

Videx EC take once daily on an empty stomach; swallow whole; <20 kg: use oral solution; 20 to <25 kg: 200 mg; 25 to <60 kg: 250 mg; ≥60 kg: 400 mg; *CrCl 30-59 ml/min:* <60 kg: 125 mg; ≥60 kg: 200 mg; *CrCl 10-29 ml/min:* 125 mg; *CrCl <10 ml/min <u>or</u> dialysis:* <60 kg: use oral soln: ≥60 kg: 125 mg

Pediatric: same as adult

Cap: 125, 200, 250, 400 mg ent-coat del-rel; *Chew tab:* 25, 50, 100, 150, 200 mg (mandarin orange) (buffered with calcium carbonate and magnesium hydroxide)

Videx Pediatric Pwdr for Solution <60 kg: 125 mg bid; ≥60 kg: 200 mg bid; *If once-daily dosing required:* <60 kg: 250 mg once daily; ≥60 kg: 400 mg once daily; *CrCl 30-59 ml/min:* <60 kg: 150 mg once daily <u>or</u> 75 mg bid; ≥60 kg: 200 mg once daily <u>or</u> 100 mg bid; *CrCl 10-29 ml/min:* <60 kg: 100 mg once daily; ≥60 kg: 150 mg once daily; *CrCl <10 ml/min <u>or</u> dialysis:* <60 kg: 75 mg once daily; ≥60 kg: 100 mg once daily; take on an empty stomach *Pediatric:* <2 weeks: <u>not</u> recommended; 2 weeks-8 months: 100 mg/m² bid; >8 months: 120 mg/m² bid; *Renal impairment:* consider reducing dose <u>or</u> increasing dosing interval; take on an empty stomach

Pwdr for oral soln: 2, 4 gm (120, 240 ml)

Comment: *Didanosine* is contraindicated with concomitant *allopurinol <u>or</u> ribavirin.*

▶ *emtricitabine* (G) 200 mg once daily; *CrCl 30-49 ml/min:* 200 mg q 48 hours; *CrCl 15-29 ml/min:* 200 mg q 72 hours; *CrCl <15 ml/min or dialysis:* 200 mg q 96 hours
Pediatric: <3 months: 3 mg/kg oral soln once daily; 3 months to 17 years: 6 mg/kg once daily; ≤33 kg: use oral soln, max 240 mg (24 ml); >33 kg: 200 mg cap once daily; max 240 mg/day; ≥18 years: same as adult
   Emtriva *Cap:* 200 mg
   Emtriva Oral Solution *Oral soln:* 10 mg/ml (170 ml) (cotton candy)

▶ *lamivudine* (G) *CrCl ≥50 ml/min:* 300 mg qd or 150 mg bid; *CrCl >30-50 ml/min:* 150 mg qd; *CrCl 15-29 ml/min:* first dose 150 mg, then 100 mg once daily; *CrCl 5-14 ml/min:* first dose 150 mg, then 50 mg qd; *CrCl <5 ml/min:* first dose 50 mg; then 25 mg once daily; max 8 mg/kg once daily or 150 mg bid
Pediatric: <3 months: not established; 3 months to 16 years: 4 mg/kg oral soln or tab bid; (tab) 14 to <20 kg: 150 mg once daily or 75 mg bid; ≥20 to <25 kg: 225 mg once daily or 75 mg in the AM and 150 mg in the PM; ≥25 kg: 300 mg once daily or 150 mg bid; max 8 mg/kg once daily or 150 mg bid or 300 mg once daily
   Epivir *Tab:* 150*, 300 mg
   Epivir Oral Solution *Oral soln:* 10 mg/ml (240 ml) (strawberry-banana) (sucrose 3 gm/15 ml)
   Comment: With renal impairment, reduce *lamivudine* dose or extend dosing interval.

▶ *stavudine* (G) ≥60 kg: 40 mg q 12 hours; ≤60 kg: 30 mg q 12 hours; *If peripheral neuropathy develops:* discontinue; *After resolution, ≥60 kg:* may restart at 20 mg q 12 hours; *After resolution, ≤60 kg:* may restart at 15 mg q 12 hours; *If neuropathy returns:* consider permanent discontinuation; *CrCl 10-50 ml/min, ≥60 kg:* 20 mg q 12 hours; *CrCl 10-50 ml/min, ≥60 kg:* 15 mg q 12 hours; *Hemodialysis, ≥60 kg:* 20 mg q 24 hours; *Hemodialysis, ≤60 kg:* 15 mg q 24 hours; administer at the same time of day; *Hemodialysis:* administer at the end of dialysis
Pediatric: birth-13 days: (use oral soln) 0.5 mg/kg q 12 hours; >14 days, <30 kg: (use oral soln) 1 mg/kg q 12 hours; ≥30-<60 kg: 30 mg q 12 hours; ≥60 kg: 40 mg q 12 hours
   Zerit *Cap:* 15, 20, 30, 40 mg
   Zerit for Oral Solution *Oral soln:* 1 mg/ml pwdr for reconstitution (fruit) (dye-free)
   Comment: Withdraw *stavudine* if peripheral neuropathy occurs. After complete resolution, may restart at half the recommended dose. If peripheral neuropathy recurs, consider permanent discontinuation.

▶ *tenofovir disoproxil fumarate* (G) 300 mg once daily; *CrCl 30-49 ml/min:* 300 mg q 48 hours; *CrCl 10-29 ml/min:* 300 mg q 72-96 hours; *Hemodialysis:* 300 mg once every 7 days or after a total of 12 hours of dialysis; *CrCl <10 ml/min:* not recommended
Pediatric: <2 years: not established; 2-12 years: 8 mg/kg once daily; >12 years, 35 kg: 300 mg once daily; mix oral pwdr with 2-4 oz soft food
   Viread *Tab:* 150, 200, 250, 300 mg; *Oral pwdr:* 40 mg/gm (60 gm w. dosing scoop)
   Comment: Published studies in HBV-infected subjects do not report an increased risk of adverse pregnancy-related outcomes with the use of **Viread** during the third trimester of pregnancy.

▶ *zidovudine* (G) 600 mg daily divided bid-tid; *End-stage renal disease (ESRD)/dialysis:* 100 mg q 6-8 hours; *Vertical transmission, severe anemia, or neutropenia:* see mfr pkg insert
Pediatric: Treatment of HIV-1 infection: 4-<9 kg: 24 mg/kg/day divided bid or tid; ≥9-<30 kg: 18 mg/kg/day divided bid or tid; ≥30 kg: 600 mg/day divided bid or tid; *Prevention of maternal-fetal neonatal transmission:* <12 hours after birth until 6 weeks of age: (use oral syr) 2 mg/kg q 6 hours until 6 weeks of age; (IV) 1.5 mg/kg infused over 30 minutes q 6 hours until 6 weeks of age; max 200 mg q 8 hours
   Retrovir Tablets *Tab:* 300 mg
   Retrovir Capsules *Cap:* 100 mg
   Retrovir Syrup *Syrup:* 50 mg/5 ml (strawberry)
   Retrovir IV *Vial:* 10 mg/ml after dilution (20 ml) (preservative-free)

Non-nucleoside Reverse Transcriptase Inhibitors (NNRTIs)

▶ *delavirdine mesylate* 400 mg (4 x 100 mg or 2 x 200 mg) tablets tid in combination with other antiretroviral agents
Pediatric: <16 years: not established; ≥16 years: same as adult
   Rescriptor *Tab:* 100, 200 mg
   Comment: The 100 mg **Rescriptor** tablets may be dispersed in water prior to consumption. To prepare a dispersion, add four 100 mg **Rescriptor** tablets to at least 3 oz of water, allow to stand for a few minutes, and then stir until a uniform dispersion occurs. The dispersion should be consumed promptly. The glass should be rinsed with water and the rinse swallowed to insure the entire dose is consumed. The 200 mg tablets should be taken as intact tablets because they are not readily dispersed in water.

▶ *doravirine* 100 mg once daily in combination with other antiretroviral agents; as a dosage adjustment when taking *rifabutin* with **Delstrigo** (fixed dose combination of *doravirine+lamivudine+tenofovir disoproxil fumarate),* administer 100 mg of *doravirine* (Pifeltro) approximately 12 hours after the dose of **Delstrigo**
Pediatric: <18 years: not established; ≥18 years: same as adult
   Pifeltro *Tab:* 100 mg

▶ *efavirenz* (G) 600 mg once daily
Pediatric: >3 months, 3.5 kg: (tab/cap) 3.5 to < 5 kg: 100 mg once daily; 5 to <7.5 kg: 150 mg once daily; 7.5 to <15 kg: 200 mg once daily; 15 to <20 kg: 250 mg once daily; 20 to <25 kg: 300 mg once daily; 25 to <32.5 kg: 350 once daily; 32.5 to <40 kg: 400 mg once daily; >40 kg: 600 mg once daily; max 600 mg once daily

(continued)

Comment: For children who cannot swallow capsules, the capsule contents can be administered with a small amount of food or infant formula using the capsule sprinkle method of administration. See mfr pkg insert for instructions. Tablets should not be crushed or chewed. Administer at bedtime to limit central nervous system (CNS) effects.

   Sustiva *Tab:* 75, 150, 600, 800 mg; *Cap:* 50, 200 mg

▷ *etravirine* 200 mg (1 x 200 mg tablet or 2 x 100 mg tablets) bid following a meal

   Pediatric: <3 years: not recommended; ≥3 years, >16 kg: 16-< 20 kg: 100 mg bid; 20 to <25 kg: 125 mg bid; 25 to <30 kg: 150 mg bid; ≥30 kg: 200 mg bid; max 200 mg bid; take following a meal

   Intelence *Tab:* 25*, 100, 200 mg

▷ *nevirapine* (G) initially one 200 mg tablet of immediate-release Viramune once daily for the first 14 days, in combination with other antiretroviral agents; then one 400 mg tablet of **Viramune XR** once daily

   Comment: The 14-day lead-in period has been found to lessen the frequency of rash.

   Pediatric: <6 years: not recommended; 6-<18 years: body surface area (BSA) 0.58-0.83 kg/m²: 200 mg once daily; BSA 0.84-1.16 kg/m²: 300 mg once daily; BSA ≥1.17 kg/m²: 400 mg once daily; max 400 mg once daily

   Comment: Children must initiate therapy with immediate-release **Viramune** for the first 14 days; ≥15 days: (oral susp/tab): 150 mg/m² once daily x 14 days then 150 mg/m² bid

   Viramune *Tab:* 200*mg

   Viramune Oral Suspension *Oral susp:* 50 mg/5 ml (240 ml)

   Viramune XR *Tab:* 100, 400 mg ext-rel

▷ *rilpivirine* 25 mg once daily; *If concomitant rifabutin:* 50 mg once daily: *If concomitant rifabutin stopped:* 25 mg once daily

   Pediatric: <12 years: not recommended; ≥12 years, >35 kg: same as adult

   Edurant *Tab:* 25 mg

Protease Inhibitors

▷ *atazanavir* (G) *ritonavir* is required with several **Reyataz** dosage regimens (see the *ritonavir* complete prescribing information about the safe and effective use of *ritonavir*); The use of **Reyataz** in treatment-experienced adult patients without *ritonavir* is not recommended; Once daily doses of **Reyataz** and *ritonavir* must be taken together with food; **Reyataz Oral Powder** must be mixed with food or a beverage for administration

Recommended Once Daily Dosage of **Reyataz** and *ritonavir* for Adult Patients		
	Once Daily Dose of **Reyataz**	*ritonavir* Daily Dose
Treatment-Naïve Adults		
Recommended Regimen	300 mg	100 mg
Unable to Tolerate *ritonavir*	400 mg	N/A
In Combination with *efavirenz*	400 mg	100 mg
Treatment-Experienced Adults		
Recommended Regimen	300 mg	100 mg
In Combination with an H2RA and *tenofovir*	400 mg	100 mg

See the table below for the recommended dosage of **Reyataz** and *ritonavir* in treatment-naive and treatment-experienced pregnant patients; In these patients, **Reyataz** must be administered with **ritonavir**; There are no dosage adjustments for postpartum patients

Recommended Once Daily Dosage of **Reyataz** and *ritonavir* for Pregnant Patients		
	Once Daily Dose of **Reyataz**	Once Daily Dose of *ritonavir*
Treatment-Naïve and Treatment-Experienced		
Recommended Regimen	300 mg	100 mg
Treatment-Experienced During Second or Third Trimester when Co-Administered with Either H2RA or Tenofovir DF		
Recommended Regimen	400 mg	100 mg

Pediatric: <3 months, <5 kg: not recommended; ≥3 months, ≥5 kg: see dosage tables below; Take **Reyataz** and *ritonavir* together, once daily, at the same time and with food; **Reyataz Oral Powder** must be mixed with food or a beverage for administration

Recommended Dosage of **Reyataz Oral Powder** and *ritonavir* Oral Solution for Patients ≥3 Months-of-Age and at Least 5 kg		
Body Weight	Reyataz Oral Powder Once Daily Dose	*ritonavir* Oral Solution Once Daily Dose
5 kg to <15 kg	200 mg (4 pkts)	80 mg
15 kg to <25 kg	250 mg (5 pkts)	80 mg

Recommended Dosage of **Reyataz Capsules** and *ritonavir* Oral Solution for patients ≥6 years to <18 years		
Body Weight	Reyataz Daily Dose	*ritonavir* Daily Dose
Treatment Naïve and Treatment Experienced		
<15 kg	Capsules not recommended	N/A
15 kg to <35 kg	200 mg	100 mg
≥35 mg	300 mg	100 mg
Treatment Naïve, and ≥13 Years of Age to <40 kg		
≥40 kg	400 mg	N/A

▷ *darunavir* **(G)** *Treatment-naïve and treatment-experienced with no* ***darunavir*** *resistance-associated substitutions*: 800 mg once daily with **ritonavir** 100 mg once daily; *Treatment-experienced with at least one* ***darunavir*** *resistance-associated substitution*: 600 mg bid with **ritonavir** 100 mg bid; *severe hepatic impairment*: not recommended

Pediatric: ≥3 years, 10 kg (oral soln/tab/cap); *Treatment-naïve* or *treatment-experienced without* ***darunavir*-**associated substitutions: 10-<15 kg: 35 mg/kg once daily plus **ritonavir** 7 mg/kg once daily; 15-<30 kg: 600 mg plus **ritonavir** 100 mg once daily; 30-<40 kg: 675 mg plus **ritonavir** 100 mg once daily; >40 kg: 800 mg plus **ritonavir** 100 mg once daily; *Treatment-experienced with ≥1* ***darunavir*-**associated substitution(s): 10-15 kg: 20 mg/kg bid plus **ritonavir** 3 mg/kg bid; 15-<30 kg: 375 mg plus **ritonavir** 48 mg bid; 30-<40 kg: 450 mg plus **ritonavir** 60 mg bid; >40 kg: 600 mg plus **ritonavir** 100 mg bid

    Prezista *Tab*: 75, 150, 600, 800 mg film-coat

    Prezista Oral Suspension *Susp*: 100 mg/ml (strawberry cream)

    Comment: Prezista is FDA-approved for treatment of HIV-1-infected pregnant females and for the treatment of children >3 years of age in combination with **ritonavir** and other antiretrovirals.

▷ *fosamprenavir* **(G)** *Treatment-naïve:* 1,400 mg bid or 1,400 mg once daily plus **ritonavir** 200 mg once daily or 1,400 mg once daily plus **ritonavir** 100 mg once daily or 700 mg bid plus **ritonavir** 100 mg bid; *PI-experienced:* 700 mg bid plus **ritonavir** 100 mg bid

Pediatric: <4 weeks: not recommended; *PI-naïve, ≥4 weeks* or *PI-experienced:* ≥6 months, <11 kg: 45 mg/kg plus **ritonavir** 7 mg/kg bid; 11 to <15 kg: 30 mg/kg plus **ritonavir** 3 mg/kg bid; 15 kg to <20 kg: 23 mg/kg plus **ritonavir** 3 mg/kg bid; ≥20 kg: 18 mg/kg plus **ritonavir** 3 mg/kg bid; *protease inhibitor-naive, ≥2 years:* 30 mg/kg bid without **ritonavir**, max dose 700 mg plus **ritonavir** 100 mg bid

    Lexiva: *Tab*: 700 mg film-coat

    Lexiva Oral Suspension *Oral susp*: 50 mg/ml (225 ml) (grape-bubble gum-peppermint)

    Comment: *Fosamprenavir* 1 ml is equivalent to approximately 43 mg of **amprenavir** 1 ml.

▷ *indinavir sulfate* 800 mg q 8 hours; *Concomitant* **rifabutin**: 1 gm q 8 hours and reduce **rifabutin** dose by half; *Hepatic insufficiency* or *concomitant* **ketoconazole**, **itraconazole**, *or* **delavirdine**: 600 mg q 8 hours; take with water on an empty stomach or with a light meal

Pediatric: <3 years: not established; *≥3 to 18 years:* doses of 500 mg/m² q 8 hours have been used; see mfr pkg insert

    Crixivan *Cap*: 100, 200, 333, 400 mg

▷ *nelfinavir mesylate* 1250 mg (5 x 250 mg tablets or 2 x 625 mg tablets) bid or 750 mg (3 x 250 mg tablets) tid; take with a meal; may dissolve tablets in a small amount of water; max 2,500 mg/day

Pediatric: <2 years: not established; *2-13 years:* 45-55 mg/kg bid or 25-35 mg/kg tid; take with a meal; max 2,500 mg/day; *≥13 years:* same as adult

    Viracept *Tab*: 250, 625 mg

    Viracept Oral Powder *Oral pwdr*: 50 mg/gm (144 gm) (phenylalanine)

    Comment: The 250 mg Viracept tabs are interchangeable with oral powder; the 625 mg tabs are not.

▷ *raltegravir (as potassium)* 400 mg bid

Pediatric: ≥4 weeks, 3-11 kg: (oral susp) 3 to <4 kg: 20 mg bid; 4 to <6 kg: 30 mg bid; 6 to <8 kg: 40 mg bid; 8 to <11 kg: 60 mg bid; ≥11 to <25 kg: (oral susp/chew tab) 6 mg/kg/dose bid; see mfr pkg insert for

(continued)

dosage by weight; ≥25 kg and unable to swallow tablet: (chew tab) 25-<28 kg: 150 mg bid; 28-<40 kg: 200 mg bid; ≥40 kg: 300 mg bid; ≥6 years, ≥25 kg, able to swallow tablets: 400 mg film-coat tablet bid

Comment: Oral suspension, chewable tablets, and film-coat tablets are not bioequivalent. Chewable tablet max dose is 300 mg bid. Film-coat tablets max dose is 400 mg bid. Oral suspension max dose is 100 mg bid

    Isentress *Tab:* 400 mg film-coat; *Chew tab:* 25, 100*mg (orange-banana) (phenylalanine)

    Isentress Oral Suspension *Oral susp:* 100 mg/pkt pwdr for oral susp (banana)

▷ *ritonavir* (G) initially 300 mg bid; increase at 2 to 3 day intervals by 100 mg bid; max 600 mg bid

    Pediatric: <1 month: not recommended; ≥1 month: 350-400 mg/m² bid; initiate at 250 mg/m² bid and titrate upward every 2 to 3 days by 50 mg/m² bid; max dose 600 mg bid

    Comment: Lower doses of *ritonavir* have been used to boost other PIs but the *ritonavir* doses used for boosting have not been specifically approved in children.

    Norvir *Tab:* 100 mg film-coat; *Gelcap:* 100 mg (alcohol)

    Norvir Oral Solution *Oral soln:* 80 mg/ml, 600 mg/7.5 ml (8 oz) (peppermint-caramel) (alcohol)

    Comment: **Norvir** tablets should be swallowed whole. Take **Norvir** with meals. Patients may improve the taste of **Norvir Oral Solution** by mixing with chocolate milk, **Ensure,** or **Advera** within 1 hour of dosing. Dose reduction of **Norvir** is necessary when used with other PIs (*atazanavir, darunavir, fosamprenavir, saquinavir,* and *tipranavir*). Patients who take the 600 mg gelcap bid may experience more gastrointestinal side effects such as nausea, vomiting, abdominal pain, or diarrhea when switching from the gelcap to the tablet because of greater maximum plasma concentration (Cmax) achieved with the tablet. These adverse events (gastrointestinal or paresthesias) may diminish as treatment is continued.

▷ *saquinavir mesylate*

    Pediatric: <16 years: not established; ≥16 years: same as adult

    Fortovase *Tab/Cap:* 200 mg

    Invirase *Tab:* 500 mg; *Cap:* 200 mg

▷ *tipranavir* 500 mg bid plus *ritonavir* 200 mg bid

    Pediatric: <2 years: not recommended; 2 to 18 years: (cap/oral soln) 14 mg/kg plus *ritonavir* 6 mg/kg bid or 375 mg/m² plus *ritonavir* 150 mg/m² bid; max 500 mg plus *ritonavir* 200 mg bid

    Aptivus *Gelcap:* 250 mg (alcohol)

    Aptivus Oral Solution *Oral soln:* 100 mg/ml (buttermint-butter toffee) (vit E 116 IU/ml)

FUSION INHIBITORS—CCR5 CO-RECEPTOR ANTAGONISTS

▷ *enfuvirtide* 90 mg (1 ml) SC bid; administer in upper arm, abdomen, or anterior thigh; rotate injection sites

    Pediatric: <6 years: not established; 6-16 years: administer 2 mg/kg SC bid; max 90 mg SC bid; >16 years: same as adult; rotate injection sites

    Fuzeon *Vial:* 90 mg/ml pwdr for SC inj after reconstitution (1 ml, 60 vials/kit) (preservative-free)

▷ *maraviroc* (G) must be administered concomitant with other retrovirals; *Concomitant potent CYP3A inhibitors (with or without a potent CYP3A inducer) including PIs (*except *tipranavir+ritonavir*)*, delavirdine, ketoconazole, itraconazole, clarithromycin, other potent CYP3A inhibitors (e.g., nefazodone, telithromycin): CrCl ≥30 ml/min: 150 mg bid; <30 ml/min, dialysis:* not recommended; *Potent CYP3A inducers (without a potent CYP3A inhibitor) including efavirenz, rifampin, etravirine, carbamazepine, phenobarbital, and phenytoin:* 300 mg bid; *CrCl ≥30 ml/min:* 600 mg bid; *<30 ml/min:* not recommended; *Other concomitant agents, including tipranavir+ritonavir, nevirapine, raltegravir, all NRTIs, and enfuvirtide:* 300 mg bid

    Pediatric: <16 years: not established; ≥16 years: same as adult

    Selzentry *Tab:* 150, 300 mg film-coat

CD4-DIRECTED POST-ATTACHMENT HIV-1 INHIBITOR

▷ *ibalizumab-uiyk* administer as an IV injection once q 14 days

    Pediatric: <18 years: not established; ≥18 years: same as adult

    Trogarzo *Vial:* 200 mg/1.33 ml (1.33 ml), single-dose

    Comment: **Trogarzo** *(ibalizumab)* is indicated for the treatment of patients with HIV infection who are heavily treatment-experienced (HTE) and multidrug-resistant (MDR) infection. It is intended for use in combination with other antiretroviral medications.

GP120-DIRECTED ATTACHMENT INHIBITOR

▷ *fostemsavir* take 1 tablet bid, with or without food

    Pediatric: not established

    Rukobia *Tab:* 600 mg, film-coat, ext-rel

    Comment: **Rukobia** *(fostemsavir),* an HIV-1 gp120-directed attachment inhibitor, in combination with other antiretroviral(s), is indicated for the treatment of HIV-1 infection in HTE adults with MDR HIV-1 infection failing their current antiretroviral regimen due to resistance, intolerance, or safety considerations. The most common adverse reaction (incidence 5%) has been nausea. See mfr pkg insert for complete list of significant drug interactions. Co-administration of **Rukobia** with strong cytochrome P450 (CYP)3A inducers is contraindicated as significant decreases in *temsavir* plasma concentrations may occur, which may result in loss of virologic response. IRS has been reported in patients treated with combination antiretroviral therapies. Concomitant oral contraceptive should not contain more than 30 mcg of *ethinyl estradiol* per day. Use **Rukobia** with caution in patients with a history of QTc prolongation or with relevant preexisting cardiac disease or who are taking drugs with a known risk of torsade de pointes. Elevations in hepatic transaminases have been observed in a greater proportion of subjects with HBV and/or hepatitis C virus (HCV) coinfection, compared with those with HIV mono-infection. There are insufficient human data on the use of **Rukobia** during pregnancy to adequately assess a drug-associated risk of birth defects and miscarriage. In animal reproduction studies, oral administration of *fostemsavir* during organogenesis resulted in no adverse developmental effects at clinically relevant *temsavir* exposures. There is a pregnancy exposure registry that monitors pregnancy outcomes in individuals exposed to **Rukobia** during pregnancy. Healthcare providers are encouraged to register patients by calling the Antiretroviral Pregnancy Registry (APR) at 1-800-258-4263. Breastfeeding is not recommended due to the potential for HIV-1 transmission.

CYP3A INHIBITOR

▷ *cobicistat* 150 mg once daily; must be co-administered with *atazanavir* 300 mg once daily or *darunavir* 800 mg once daily, at the same time, with food, and in combination with other HIV-1 antiretroviral agents
Pediatric: <35 kg: not established; ≥35 kg: 150 mg once daily, co-administered with *atazanavir* or ≥40 kg: 150 mg once daily, co-administered with *darunavir*; at the same time, with food, and in combination with other HIV-1 antiretroviral agents; for dosage recommendations of the coadministered PI *atazanavir* or darunavir, refer to Table 2 of the **Tybost** pkg insert
  Tybost *Tab:* 150 mg
  Comment: Tybost *(cobicistat)* is a CYP3A inhibitor indicated to increase systemic exposure of *atazanavir* or *darunavir* in combination with other antiretroviral agents in the treatment of HIV-1 infection. **Tybost**, in combination with *atazanavir* or *darunavir*, can alter the concentration of drugs metabolized by CYP3A or CYP2D6. Drugs that induce CYP3A can alter the concentrations of **Tybost**, *atazanavir* and *darunavir*. Consult the mfr pkg insert prior to and during treatment for potential drug interactions. Assess CrCl before initiating treatment. When **Tybost** is used in combination with a *tenofovir disoproxil fumarate (TDF)*-containing regimen, cases of acute renal failure (ARF) and Fanconi syndrome have been reported. Assess urine glucose and urine protein at baseline and monitor CrCl, urine glucose, and urine protein. Monitor serum phosphorus in patients with or at risk for renal impairment. **Tybost** in combination with more than one antiretroviral agent that requires pharmacokinetic enhancement (i.e., two PIs or *elvitegravir* in combination with a PI) is not recommended. Use with HIV-1 PIs other than *atazanavir* or *darunavir* administered once daily is not recommended. Co-administration with drugs or regimens containing *ritonavir* is not recommended. **Tybost** co-administered with *atazanavir* or *darunavir* is not recommended during pregnancy or lactation.

HIV-1 CAPSID INHIBITOR

▷ *lenacapavir* initiate treatment with one of two options followed by once every 6 months maintenance dosing; tablets may be taken without regard to food; 2 x 1.5 ml SC injections are required for a complete dose; see the mfr pkg insert for full prescribing information prior to and during treatment for preparation, administration, and important drug interactions

Initiation Option 1	
Day 1	927 mg via SC inj (2 x 1.5 ml) or 600 mg orally (2 x 300 mg tabs)
Day 2	600 mg orally (2 x 300 mg tabs)
Initiation Option 2	
Day 1	600 mg orally (2 x 300 mg tabs)
Day 2	600 mg orally (2 x 300 mg tabs)
Day 8	300 mg orally (1 x 300 mg tab)
Day 15	927 mg via SC inj (2 x 1.5 ml)
Maintenance	
927 mg by SC inj (2 x 1.5 ml) every 6 months (26 weeks) from the date of the last injection +/-2 weeks	
Missed Dose	
If more than 28 weeks since last injection and clinically appropriate to continue treatment with **Sunlenca**, restart initiation from Day 1, using either Option 1 or Option 2	

Pediatric: safety and efficacy not established
  Sunlenca *Tab:* 300 mg; *Vial:* 463.5 mg/1.5 ml (309 mg/ml), single-dose for SC administration
  Comment: Sunlenca is a long-acting HIV-1 capsid inhibitor for use in combination with other antiretroviral(s) for the treatment of HIV-1 infection in HTE people with MDR HIV-1 infection failing their current antiretroviral regimen due to resistance, intolerance, or safety considerations. The most common reported adverse reactions (incidence greater than or equal to 3%, all grades) have been nausea and injection site reactions. Occurrence of IRS may necessitate further evaluation and treatment. Residual

(continued)

concentrations of *lenacapavir* may remain in systemic circulation for up to 12 months or longer. Counsel patients regarding the dosing schedule; non-adherence could lead to loss of virologic response and development of resistance. Concomitant administration of **Sunlenca** is contraindicated with strong CYP3A inducers. *Lenacapavir* may increase exposure and risk of adverse reactions to drugs primarily metabolized by CYP3A initiated within 9 months after the last SC dose of **Sunlenca**. If **Sunlenca** is discontinued, initiate an alternative, fully suppressive antiretroviral regimen where possible no later than 28 weeks after the final injection of **Sunlenca**. If virologic failure occurs, switch to an alternative regimen if possible. Injection site reactions may occur, and nodules and indurations may be persistent. There is a pregnancy exposure registry that monitors pregnancy outcomes in individuals exposed to **Sunlenca** during pregnancy. Healthcare providers are encouraged to register patients by calling the Antiretroviral Pregnancy Registry (APR) at 1-800-258- 4263. Individuals infected with HIV should be instructed not to breastfeed due to the potential for HIV transmission. It is not known whether **Sunlenca** is present in human breast milk or its effects on the breastfed infant. To report suspected adverse reactions, contact Gilead Sciences at 1-800-GILEAD-5 or FDA at 1-800-FDA-1088 or www.fda.gov/medwatch.

BRAND NAMES, DOSING, AND DOSE FORMS: COMBINATION AGENTS

▷ **Atripla (G)** *efavirenz+emtricitabine+tenofovir disoproxil fumarate* 1 tablet once daily on an empty stomach; bedtime dosing may improve the tolerability of nervous system symptoms; *CrCl <50 ml/min:* not recommended
Pediatric: <12 years, <40 kg: not established; ≥12 years, ≥40 kg: same as adult
  Tab: efa 600 mg+emtri 200 mg+teno dis fum 300 mg film-coat

▷ **Biktarvy** *bictegravir+emtricitabine+tenofovir alafenamide* take 1 tablet once daily with or without food
Pediatric: <18 years: not established; ≥18 years: same as adult
  Tab: bict 50 mg+emtri 200 mg+teno alaf 25 mg
Comment: Biktarvy is a 3-drug fixed-dose combination of *bictegravir*, a human immunodeficiency virus type 1 (HIV-1) integrase strand transfer inhibitor (INSTI), and *emtricitabine* and *tenofovir alafenamide*, both HIV-1 nucleoside analog reverse transcriptase inhibitors (NRTIs), indicated as a complete regimen for the treatment of HIV-1 infection in adults who have no antiretroviral treatment history or to replace the current antiretroviral regimen in those who are virologically suppressed (HIV-1 RNA less than 50 copies per ml) on a stable antiretroviral regimen for at least 3 months with no history of treatment failure and no known substitutions associated with resistance to the individual components of **Biktarvy. Biktarvy** is not recommended in patients with estimated CrCl <30 ml/min and/or with severe hepatic impairment.

▷ **Cabenuva** *cabotegravir* and *rilpivirine*
  2 Vial kit: cabo 400 mg single-dose and rilpiv 600 mg single-dose; *2 Vial kit:* cabo 400 mg single-dose and rilpiv 900 mg single-dose
Comment: Cabenuva *(cabotegravir* and *rilpivirine)* is a 2-drug co-packaged product containing a single-dose vial of **cabotegravir** (HIV-1 integrase the strand transfer inhibitor [NSTI]) and a single-dose vial of *rilpivirine* (HIV-1 non-nucleoside reverse transcriptase inhibitor [NNRTI]). This combination provides a complete long-acting once-monthly injectable regimen (depot) option for treatment of HIV-1 infection in adults. Prior to initiation with **Cabenuva**, an oral lead-in should be used for approximately 1 month (at least 28 days) to assess the tolerability of *cabotegravir* and *rilpivirine.*

▷ **Cimduo** *lamivudine+tenofovir disoproxil fumarate* 1 tablet once daily with or without food
Pediatric: <35 kg: not recommended; ≥35 kg: same as adult
  Tab: lami 300 mg+teno diso 300 mg
Comment: Cimduo is a two-drug fixed-dose combination of *lamivudine* and *tenofovir disoproxil fumarate,* both nucleoside reverse transcriptase inhibitors (NRTIs) and indicated for the treatment of HIV-1 infection in combination with other antiretroviral agents. Prior to initiation and during treatment with **Cimduo**, patients should be tested for hepatitis b virus (HBV) infection, and estimated CrCl, serum phosphorus, urine glucose, and urine protein should be obtained. **Cimduo** is not recommended in patients with CrCl <50 ml/min or patients with ESRD requiring hemodialysis. Discontinue treatment in patients who develop symptoms or laboratory findings suggestive of lactic acidosis or pronounced hepatotoxicity.

▷ **Combivir (G)** *lamivudine+zidovudine*
Pediatric: <12 years: not recommended; ≥12 years, ≥30 kg: 1 tablet bid with food
  Tab: lami 150 mg+zido 300 mg

▷ **Complera** *emtricitabine+tenofovir disoproxil fumarate+rilpivirine* 1 tablet once daily; *CrCl <50 ml/min:* not recommended
Pediatric: <12 years, <40 kg: not recommended; ≥12 years, ≥40 kg: same as adult
  Tab: emtri 200 mg+teno dis 300 mg+rilpiv 25 mg

▷ **Delstrigo** *doravirine+lamivudine+tenofovir disoproxil fumarate* 1 tablet once daily with or without food; *CrCl <50 ml/min:* not recommended
Pediatric: <18 years: not established; ≥18 years: same as adult
  Tab: dora 100 mg+lami 300 mg+teno 300 mg
Comment: Delstrigo is approved as a complete three-drug fixed-dose once-daily regimen for patients with no prior antiretroviral treatment experience. Monitor for new-onset or worsening renal impairment. Prior to or when initiating **Delstrigo**, and during treatment on a clinically appropriate schedule, assess serum creatinine, estimated creatinine clearance, urine glucose, and urine protein in all patients. Avoid administering **Delstrigo** with concurrent or recent use of nephrotoxic drugs. In patients with chronic kidney disease (CKD), also

assess serum phosphorus. Severe acute exacerbations of hepatitis B (HBV) have been reported in patients coinfected with HIV-1 and HBV who have discontinued *lamivudine* or *TDF*, two of the components of **Delstrigo.** Closely monitor hepatic function in these patients. If appropriate, initiation of anti-hepatitis B therapy may be warranted. *Dosage Adjustment with rifabutin:* Take 1 tablet of **Delstrigo** once daily, followed by 1 tablet of *doravirine* 100 mg **(Pifeltro)** approximately 12 hours after the dose of **Delstrigo.** There is a pregnancy exposure registry that monitors pregnancy outcomes in individuals exposed to **Delstrigo** during pregnancy. Healthcare providers are encouraged to register patients by calling the Antiretroviral Pregnancy Registry (APR) at 1-800-258-4263.

▷ Descovy *emtricitabine+tenofovir alafenamide* 1 tablet once daily with or without food; *CrCl <30 ml/min:* not recommended
　　Pediatric: <12 years, <35 kg: not recommended; ≥12 years, ≥35 kg: same as adult
　　　　Tab: emtri 200 mg+teno ala 25 mg
　　Comment: Patients with HIV-1 should be tested for the presence of chronic hepatitis b virus (HBV) before initiating ART. **Descovy** is not approved for the treatment of chronic HBV infection, and the safety and efficacy of **Descovy** have not been established in patients coinfected with HIV-1 and HBV.

▷ Dovato *dolutegravir+lamivudine* 1 tab daily
　　Pediatric: safety and efficacy not established
　　　　Tab: dolu 50 mg+lami 300 mg film-coat
　　Comment: Dovato **(dolutegravir+lamivudine)** is a once-daily, single-tablet, two-drug fixed-dose combination of *dolutegravir* (Tivicay), an integrase strand transfer inhibitor (INSTI) and *lamivudine* (Epivir, a nucleoside analog reverse transcriptase inhibitor [NRTI]) indicated for the treatment of HIV-1 infection in adults with no antiretroviral treatment history and with no known resistance to either *dolutegravir* or *lamivudine.*

▷ Epzicom (G) *abacavir sulfate+lamivudine* 1 tab daily; *Mild hepatic impairment or CrCl<50 ml/min:* not recommended
　　Pediatric: <25 kg: use individual components: ≥25 kg: one tablet once daily; *Mild hepatic impairment or CrCl <50 ml/min:* not recommended
　　　　Tab: aba 600 mg/lami 300 mg

▷ Evotaz *atazanavir+cobicistat* 1 tab once daily
　　Pediatric: <12 years, <35 kg: not established; ≥12 years, ≥35 kg: same as adult
　　　　Tab: ataz 600 mg+cobi 300 mg

▷ Genvoya *elvitegravir+cobicistat+emtricitabine+tenofovir alafenamide* 1 tab once daily; *Severe hepatic impairment or CrCl <30 ml/min:* not recommended; take with food
　　Pediatric: <12 years, <35 kg: not established; ≥12 years, ≥35 kg: same as adult
　　　　Tab: elvi 150 mg+cobi 150 mg+emtri 200 mg+teno 10 mg

▷ Juluca *dolutegravir+rilpivirine* take 1 tablet once daily with or without food
　　Pediatric: <18 years: not established; ≥18 years: same as adult
　　　　Tab: dolu 50 mg+rilp 25 mg film-coat
　　Comment: Juluca is a complete two-drug fixed-dose combination of *dolutegravir,* a human immunodeficiency virus type 1 (HIV-1) integrase strand transfer inhibitor (INSTI) and *rilpivirine,* a HIV-1 non-nucleoside reverse transcriptase inhibitor (NNRTI), indicated for treatment of HIV infection to replace the current antiretroviral regimen in those who are virologically suppressed (HIV-1 RNA <50 copies per ml) on a stable antiretroviral regimen for at least 6 months, with no history of treatment failure, and no known substitutions associated with resistance to the individual components of Juluca. Pregnancy testing and contraception are recommended before initiation of Juluca in females of childbearing potential. Avoid use of Juluca at the time of conception through the first trimester due to the risk of neural tube defects.

▷ Kaletra, Kaletra Oral Solution (G) *lopinavir+ritonavir* 800+200 mg (4 tablets or 10 ml) once daily or 400/100 (2 tablets or 5 ml) bid; *May administer once daily or bid:* patients with <3 *lopinavir* resistance-associated substitutions; *May dose bid only:* patients with ≥3 resistance-associated substitutions; *Dose must be increased:* when administered in combination with *efavirenz, nevirapine,* or *nelfinavir* (500 mg/125 mg [2 x 200/50 tab plus 1 x 100/25 tab] bid or 520/130 [6.5 ml] bid); *Once-daily dosing regimen not recommended:* in combination with ≥3 *lopinavir* resistance-associated substitutions or in combination with *carbamazepine, phenobarbital,* or *phenytoin*; patients receiving *nevirapine* or *efavirenz* with Kaletra should have their Kaletra dose increased; swallow whole with or without food
　　Pediatric: dose calculation is based on the *lopinavir* component; 14 days-6 months: 16 mg/kg bid; 6 months to 12 years: (tab/cap/soln), 7 to <15 kg: 12 mg/kg bid (13 mg/kg plus *nevirapine*); 15-40 kg: 10 mg/kg bid (11 mg/kg plus *nevirapine),* ≥40 kg, >12 years: *lopinavir* 400 mg bid (533 mg plus *nevirapine*); max *lopinavir* 400 mg bid for patients who are not receiving *nevirapine* or *efavirenz*; Kaletra should not be used in combination with NNRTIs in children <6 months of age; see mfr pkg insert for BSA-based dosing
　　　　Tab: **Kaletra 100/25** lopin 100 mg+riton 25 mg
　　　　　　Kaletra 200/50 lopin 200 mg+riton 50 mg
　　　　Oral soln: lopin 80 mg+riton 20 mg per ml, lopin 400 mg+riton 500 mg per 5 ml (160 ml) (cotton candy) (alcohol 42.4%)

▷ Odefsey *emtricitabine+rilpivirine+tenofovir alafenamide* 1 tab once daily with food; *CrCl <30 ml/min:* not recommended
　　Pediatric: <12 years, <35 kg: not established; ≥12 years, >35 kg: same as adult
　　　　Tab: emtri 200 mg+rilpi 25 mg+teno alafen 25 mg

(continued)

▷ **Prezcobix** *darunavir+cobicistat* 1 tab once daily; *Treatment-naïve and treatment-experienced with no darunavir resistance-associated substitution:* 800 mg once daily plus **ritonavir** 100 mg once daily; *Treatment-experienced with at least one darunavir resistance associated substitution:* 600 mg bid plus **ritonavir** 100 mg bid; take with food; *CrCl <70 ml/min:* not recommended
Pediatric: not recommended
    Tab: darun 800 mg+cobi 150 mg

▷ **Stribild (G)** *elvitegravir+cobicistat+emtricitabine+tenofovir disoproxil fumarate* 1 tab once daily; *CrCl <70 ml/min:* not recommended; *if CrCl declines to <50 ml/min during treatment:* discontinue; *Severe hepatic impairment:* not recommended
Pediatric: <12 years: not recommended; ≥12 years: same as adult
    Tab: elvi 150 mg+cobi 150 mg+emtri 200 mg+teno dis fum 300 mg

▷ **Symfi** *efavirenz+lamivudine+tenofovir disoproxil fumarate* take 1 tablet once daily with or without food
Pediatric: <40 kg: not studied; ≥40 kg: same as adult
    Tab: efav 600 mg+lami 300 mg+teno diso fum 300 mg
Comment: Symfi is a complete 3-drug fixed-dose, regimen for the treatment of HIV-1 infection in adults and children weighing >40 kg. It contains the same triple-combination ingredients found in **Symfi Lo** but with a 600 mg dose of *efavirenz* versus the 400 mg in **Symfi Lo**. Safety and effectiveness of **Symfi** as a fixed-dose tablet in pediatric patients weighing ≥40 kg have been established based on clinical studies using the individual components.

▷ **Symfi Lo** *efavirenz+lamivudine+tenofovir disoproxil fumarate* 1 tablet once daily with or without food
Pediatric: <35 kg: not studied; ≥35 kg: same as adult
    Tab: efav 400 mg+lami 300 mg+teno diso fum 300 mg
Comment: Symfi Lo is a complete 3-drug, fixed-dose, regimen for the treatment HIV-1 infection in adults and children weighing ≥45 kg. It contains the same triple-combination ingredients found in **Symfi** but with a 400 mg dose of *efavirenz* versus the 600 mg in **Symfi Lo**. Safety and effectiveness of **Symfi** as a fixed-dose tablet in pediatric patients weighing ≥40 kg have been established based on clinical studies using the individual components.

▷ **Symtuza** *darunavir+cobicistat+emtricitabine+tenofovir alafenamide* 1 tablet once daily with food
Pediatric: <18 years: not recommended; ≥18 years: same as adult
    Tab: daru 800 mg+cobic 150 mg+emtri 200 mg+tenofo alafen 10 mg
Comment: Symtuza is indicated as a complete regimen for the treatment of HIV infection in adults who have no prior antiretroviral treatment history or who are virologically suppressed (HIV-1 RNA less than 50 copies/ml) on a stable antiretroviral regimen for at least 6 months and have no known substitutions associated with resistance to *darunavir* or *tenofovir*. Assess serum creatinine, estimated creatinine clearance, urine glucose, and urine protein on a clinically appropriate schedule. In patients with CKD, also assess serum phosphorus. **Symtuza** is not recommended in patients with estimated CrCl <30 ml/min and patients with severe hepatic impairment. **Symtuza** is not recommended during pregnancy due to substantially lower exposures of *darunavir* and *cobicistat* during pregnancy. Breastfeeding is not recommended. Co-administration of **Symtuza** with other drugs can alter the concentration of other drugs, and other drugs may alter the concentrations of **Symtuza** components. Consult the mfr pkg insert prior to and during treatment for potential drug interactions.

▷ **Temixys** *lamivudine+tenofovir disoproxil fumarate* 1 tab once daily with or without food
Pediatric: <35 kg: not recommended; ≥35 kg: same as adult
    Tab: lami 300 mg+teno diso fum 300mg
Comment: Temixys, a fixed-dose combination of two nucleoside reverse transcriptase inhibitors (NRTIs), is indicated in combination with other antiretroviral agents. Discontinue treatment in patients who develop symptoms or laboratory findings suggestive of lactic acidosis or pronounced hepatotoxicity including severe hepatomegaly with steatosis. In patients at risk for renal dysfunction, assess estimated creatinine clearance, serum phosphorus, urine glucose, and urine protein before initiating treatment with **Temixys** and periodically during treatment. Avoid administering **Temixys** with concurrent or recent use of nephrotoxic drugs. Healthcare providers are encouraged to register patients exposed to **Temixys** by calling the Antiretroviral Pregnancy Registry (APR) at 1-800-258-4263. Instruct mothers not to breastfeed if they are receiving **Temixys**.

▷ **Triumeq (G)** *abacavir sulfate+dolutegravir+lamivudine* 1 tab once daily
Pediatric: <12 years: not recommended; ≥12 years: same as adult
    Tab: aba 600 mg+dolu 50 mg+lami 300 mg

▷ **Trizivir (G)** *abacavir sulfate+lamivudine+zidovudine* 1 tab bid
Pediatric: <40 kg: not recommended; ≥40 kg: same as adult
    Tab: aba 300 mg+lami 150 mg+zido 300 mg

▷ **Truvada (G)** *emtricitabine+tenofovir disoproxil fumarate* <17 kg: not established; *17 to <22 kg:* 100/150 once daily; *22 to <28 kg:* 133/200 once daily; *28 to 35 kg:* 167/250 once daily; *≥35 kg:* 200/300 once daily
Pediatric: same as adult
    Tab: **Truvada 100/150** emt 100 mg+teno ala 150 mg
          Truvada 133/200 emt 133 mg+teno ala 200 mg
          Truvada 167/250 emt 167 mg+teno 250 mg
          Truvada 200/300 emt 200 mg+teno 300 mg

HIV INSTI AND HIV NNRTI

➤ *cabotegravir+rilpivirine* for gluteal IM injection only; prior to initiating treatment, oral lead-in dosing with **Cabenuva** may be considered to assess the tolerability of *cabotegravir* and *rilpivirine* with the recommended dosage used for approximately 1 month; *Recommended once monthly dosing schedule:* initiate **Cabenuva** (*cabotegravir* 600 mg IM and *rilpivirine* 900 mg IM) on the last day of the current antiretroviral therapy (ART) or oral lead-in and continue with injections of **Cabenuva** (*cabotegravir* 400 mg IM and *rilpivirine* 600 mg IM) every month thereafter; *Recommended Every-2-month dosing schedule:* initiate **Cabenuva** (*cabotegravir* 600 mg IM and *rilpivirine* 900 mg IM) on the last day of the current ART or oral lead-in for 2 consecutive months and continue **Cabenuva** every 2 months thereafter
Pediatric: safety and efficacy not established
Cabenuva 2-*Vial co-packaged kit (in 2 dosage strengths):* (1) 400 mg/600 mg (*cabotegravir* 400 mg/2 ml [200 mg/ml], single-dose, ext-rel susp, plus *rilpivirine* 600 mg/2 ml [300 mg/ml], single dose, ext-rel susp), (2) 600 mg/900 mg (*cabotegravir* 600 mg/3 ml [200 mg/ml], single-dose, ext-rel susp, plus *rilpivirine* 900 mg/3 ml [300 mg/ml], single-dose, ext-rel susp)
Comment: Cabenuva is a two-drug co-packaged regimen with *cabotegravir* (HIV integrase strand transfer inhibitor [ISTI]) and *rilpivirine* (HIV non-nucleoside reverse transcriptase inhibitor [NNRTI]). **Cabenuva** indicated for the treatment of on is reverse transcriptase inhibitor [NNRTI]). **Cabenuva** indicated for the treatment of HIV-1 infection in adults to replace the current antiretroviral regimen in patients who are virologically suppressed (HIV-1 RNA ≤50 copies/ml), on a stable antiretroviral treatment regimen with no history of treatment failure, and with no known or suspected resistance to either *cabotegravir* or *rilpivirine*. The contraindications to **Cabenuva** use are (1) previous hypersensitivity reaction to *cabotegravir* or *rilpivirine* and (2) co-administration with drugs where significant decreases in *cabotegravir* and/or *rilpivirine* plasma concentrations may occur, which may result in loss of virologic response. Refer to the mfr pkg insert for full prescribing information, including important drug interactions with **Cabenuva**. Hypersensitivity reactions have been reported with *rilpivirine*-containing regimens and in association with other integrase inhibitors. Discontinue **Cabenuva** immediately if signs or symptoms of hypersensitivity reaction develop. Serious postinjection reactions with *rilpivirine* have been reported. Monitor and treat as clinically indicated. Hepatotoxicity has been reported in patients receiving *cabotegravir* or *rilpivirine*. Monitoring of liver chemistries is recommended. Discontinue **Cabenuva** if hepatotoxicity is suspected. Depressive disorders have been reported with **Cabenuva**. Immediate medical evaluation is recommended for depressive symptoms. Residual concentrations of *cabotegravir* and *rilpivirine* may remain in the systemic circulation of patients up to 12 months or longer. It is essential to initiate an alternative, fully suppressive antiretroviral regimen no later than 1 month after the final injection doses of **Cabenuva**. If virologic failure is suspected, prescribe an alternative regimen as soon as possible. Because **Cabenuva** is a complete regimen, co-administration with other antiretroviral medications for the treatment of HIV-1 infection is not recommended. Drugs that induce uridine diphosphate glucuronosyltransferase (UGT1A1) or cytochrome P450 (CYP)3A4 may decrease the plasma concentrations of the components of **Cabenuva**. **Cabenuva** should be used with caution in combination with drugs with a known risk of torsade de pointes. The most common adverse reactions (grades 1-4) observed in ≥2% of subjects receiving **Cabenuva** have been injection site reactions, pyrexia, fatigue, headache, musculoskeletal pain, nausea, sleep disorders, dizziness, and rash. There are insufficient human data on the use of **Cabenuva** during pregnancy to adequately assess a drug-associated risk of birth defects and miscarriage. While there are insufficient human data to assess the risk of neural tube defects (NTDs) with exposure to **Cabenuva** during pregnancy, NTDs were associated with *dolutegravir*, another integrase inhibitor. *Cabotegravir* and *rilpivirine* are detected in systemic circulation for up to 12 months or longer after discontinuing **Cabenuva** injection; therefore, consideration should be given to the potential for fetal exposure during pregnancy. Discuss the risk/benefit of using **Cabenuva** with individuals of childbearing potential and pregnant patients. Advise patients of reproductive potential to use effective contraception throughout the period of **Cabenuva** exposure. The CDC recommends that HIV-infected mothers in the United States not breastfeed their infants to avoid risking postnatal transmission of HIV-infected. See the mfr pkg insert for animal study reports of **Cabenuva** administered in pregnancy and lactation. There is a pregnancy exposure registry that monitors pregnancy outcomes in females exposed to **Cabenuva** during pregnancy. Healthcare providers are encouraged to register patients by calling the Antiretroviral Pregnancy Registry (APR) at 1-800-258-4263. To report suspected adverse reactions, contact ViiV Healthcare at 1-877-844-8872 or FDA at 1-800-FDA-1088 or www.fda.gov/medwatch.

HUMAN PAPILLOMAVIRUS (HPV, VENEREAL WART)

Comment: Vaccination for human papillomavirus (HPV) is recommended at 11-12 years of age, but can also be started at age 9 years. Catch-up is recommended through age 26 years. Although public health benefit is generally minimal for adults aged 27 through 45 years, shared clinical decision-making is recommended because some may benefit from the HPV vaccine. Additional doses of HPV are not recommended after completing a series at the recommended dosing intervals using any HPV vaccine. The 3-dose series is recommended regardless of age of initial vaccination in immunocompromising conditions. The dose series does not need to be restarted if the vaccination schedule is interrupted (ACIP, 2021).

TREATMENT
see Wart: Venereal

PROPHYLAXIS

▷ *human papillomavirus 9-valent (types 6, 11, 16, 18, 31, 33, 45, 52, and 58) vaccine, recombinant, aluminum adsorbed* Males and females 9-45 years of age: administer IM in the deltoid or thigh; *9-14 years (2-dose regimen):* 0.5 ml IM at 0 and 6-12 months (if the second dose is administered earlier than 5 months after the first dose, administer a third dose at least 4 months after the second dose); *9-14 years (3-dose regimen):* administer 0.5 ml IM at 0, 2, and 6 months; *15-45 years (3-dose regimen):* administer 0.5 ml IM at 0, 2, and 6 months

   Gardasil 9 *Vial:* 0.5 ml (single-dose); *Prefilled syringe w. needles or tip caps:* 0.5 ml (single-dose) (preservative-free)

   Comment: Gardasil 9 is indicated for prevention of genital warts *(condyloma acuminata)* caused by HPV types 6 and11 and prevention of cervical, vulvar, vaginal, and anal cancer caused by HPV types 16, 18, 31, 33, 45, 52, and 58. There are no adequate and well-controlled studies of **Gardasil 9** in pregnancy. Available human data do not demonstrate vaccine-associated increase in risk of major birth defects and miscarriages when **Gardasil 9** is administered during pregnancy. Register pregnant patients exposed to **Gardasil 9** by calling 1-800-986-8999. Available data are not sufficient to assess the effects of **Gardasil 9** on the breastfed infant.

HUNTINGTON DISEASE-ASSOCIATED CHOREA

VESICULAR MONOAMINE TRANSPORTER 2 (VMAT2) INHIBITOR

▷ *deutetrabenazine* take with food; initially 6 mg once daily; titrate up at weekly intervals by 6 mg/day to a tolerated dose that reduces chorea; administer total daily dosages ≥12 mg in 2 divided doses; max recommended daily dose 36 mg/day divided bid (18 mg bid); swallow whole; do not chew, crush, or break; if switching from *tetrabenazine,* discontinue *tetrabenazine* and initiate **Austedo** the following day; see mfr pkg insert for full prescribing information and for a recommended conversion table
Pediatric: <12 years: not established; ≥12 years: same as adult

   Austedo *Tab:* 6, 9, 12 mg

   Comment: The most common adverse effects of *deutetrabenazine* are somnolence, diarrhea, dry mouth, fatigue, and sedation, as well as an increased risk of depression and suicidal thoughts and behaviors. **Austedo** is contraindicated in patients with untreated or inadequately treated depression, who are suicidal, have hepatic impairment, are taking monoamine oxidase inhibitors (MAOIs), *reserpine,* or *tetrabenazine.* **Austedo** may increase the risk of akathisia, agitation, and restlessness, and may cause parkinsonism in patients with Huntington disease. There are no adequate data on the developmental risk associated with the use of **Austedo** in pregnant females or lactation.

▷ *tetrabenazine* individualization of dose with careful weekly titration is required; Week 1: starting dose is 12.5 mg daily; Week 2: 25 mg (12.5 mg bid); then slowly titrate dose by 12.5 mg/day at weekly intervals as tolerated to a dose that reduces chorea; doses of 37.5 mg and up to 50 mg/day should be administered in 3 divided doses per day with a maximum recommended single dose not to exceed 25 mg; patients requiring doses above 50 mg/day should be genotyped for the drug metabolizing enzyme CYP2D6 to determine if the patient is a poor metabolizer (PM) or an extensive metabolizer (EM); max daily dose in PMs is 50 mg, with a max single dose of 25 mg
Pediatric: <12 years: not established; ≥12 years: same as adult

   Xenazine *Tab:* 12.5, 25*mg

   Comment: The most common adverse reactions are sedation/somnolence, fatigue, insomnia, depression, akathisia, anxiety/anxiety aggravated, and nausea. *Boxed Warning:* **Xenazine** increases the risk of depression and suicidal thoughts and behavior (suicidality) in patients with Huntington disease. Balance risks of depression and suicidality with the clinical need for control of chorea when considering the use of **Xenazine.** Monitor patients for the emergence or worsening of depression, suicidality, or unusual changes in behavior. Inform patients, caregivers, and families of the risk of depression and suicidality and instruct to report behaviors of concern promptly to the treating healthcare provider. Exercise caution when treating patients with a history of depression or prior suicide attempts or ideation. **Xenazine** is contraindicated in patients who are actively suicidal, and in patients with untreated or inadequately treated depression, hepatic impairment, concomitant MAOI or *reserpine,* and taking *deutetrabenazine* or *valbenazine.*

▷ *valbenazine* initially 40 mg once daily; after 1 week, increase to the recommended 80 mg once daily; take with or without food; recommended dose for patients with moderate or severe hepatic impairment is 40 mg once daily; consider dose reduction based on tolerability in known CYP2D6 poor metabolizers (PMs); concomitant use of strong CYP3A4 inducers is not recommended; avoid concomitant use of MAOIs
Pediatric: <18 years: not established; ≥18 years: same as adult

   Ingrezza *Cap:* 40 mg

   Comment: Safety and effectiveness of **Ingrezza** have not been established in pediatric patients. No dose adjustment is required for elderly patients. The limited available data on **Ingrezza** use in pregnant females are insufficient to inform a drug-associated risk. There is no information regarding the presence of **Ingrezza** or its metabolites in human milk, the effects on the breastfed infant, or the effects on milk production. However, women are advised not to breastfeed during treatment and for 5 days after the final dose.

HYPERAMMONEMIA

CARBAMOYL PHOSPHATE SYNTHETASE 1 (CPS 1) ACTIVATOR

▷ *carglumic acid* treatment should be initiated by a physician experienced in metabolic disorders; recommended initial dose range for acute hyperammonemia is 100 mg/kg/day to 250 mg/kg/day; adjust dose to maintain normal plasma ammonia levels based on age; divide the total daily dose into 2-4 doses to be administered immediately before meals or feedings; each divided dose should be rounded to the nearest 100 mg; do not swallow whole or crushed; each 200 mg tablet should be dispersed in a minimum of 2.5 ml of water and taken immediately; may be administered orally or via a nasogastric tube (NGT) or percutaneous endoscopic gastrostomy (PEG) tube

Pediatric: recommended initial dose range for acute hyperammonemia is 100-250 mg/kg/day; divide the total daily dose into 2-4 doses to be administered immediately before meals or feedings; disperse each 200 mg tablet in 2.5 ml of water to yield a concentration of 80 mg/ml; may be administered orally with an oral syringe or via an NGT or percutaneous endoscopic gastrostomy (PEG) tube

Carbaglu *Tab:* 200*mg (5, 60/bottle)

Comment: Carbaglu is a carbamoyl phosphate synthetase 1 (CPS 1) activator indicated as (1) adjunctive therapy for the treatment of acute hyperammonemia due to the deficiency of the hepatic enzyme N-acetylglutamate synthase (NAGS) and (2) maintenance therapy for the treatment of chronic hyperammonemia due to the deficiency of the hepatic enzyme NAGS. Monitor plasma ammonia levels during treatment. Prolonged exposure to elevated plasma ammonia levels can rapidly result in injury to the brain or death. Prompt use of all therapies necessary to reduce plasma ammonia levels is essential. Plasma ammonia levels should be maintained within normal range for age via individual dose adjustment. In the initial treatment of NAGS deficiency, protein restriction is recommended. When plasma ammonia level is normalized, dietary protein intake can usually be reintroduced. The most common adverse reactions (in ≥13% of patients) are infections, vomiting, abdominal pain, pyrexia, tonsillitis, anemia, ear infection, diarrhea, headache, and nasopharyngitis. There are no adequate and well-controlled studies or available human data with **Carbaglu** use in human pregnancy; however, decreased survival and impaired growth occurred in offspring born to animals that received *carglumic acid* at doses similar to the maximum recommended starting human dose during pregnancy and lactation. Further, untreated N-acetylglutamate synthase (NAGS) deficiency results in irreversible neurologic damage and death. Because females with NAGS must remain on treatment throughout pregnancy, advise females of reproductive potential of the maternal and fetal risks of pregnancy. Verify pregnancy status prior to initiating **Carbaglu** and advise females of reproductive potential to use effective contraception. It is not known whether **Carbaglu** is excreted in human milk. However, *carglumic acid* is excreted in animal milk. Increase in mortality and impaired weight gain occurred in animal neonates fed by mothers receiving *carglumic acid*. Hence, advise mothers that breastfeeding is not recommended. To report suspected adverse reactions, contact Orphan Europe at 877-894-0312 or FDA at 1-800-FDA-1088 or www.fda.gov/medwatch.

HYPERCALCEMIA

CALCIUM-SENSING RECEPTOR AGONIST

see Hyperparathyroidism (HPT) for *cinacalcet* dosing in adult patients with secondary hyperparathyroidism (HPT) due to chronic kidney disease (CKD).

▷ *cinacalcet* (G) take tabs whole, with food or shortly after a meal; *Hypercalcemia, including hypercalcemia in patients with primary HPT:* initially 30 mg 2 bid; titrate dose every 2 to 4 weeks through sequential doses of 30 mg 2 bid, 60 mg 2 bid, 90 mg 2 x a day, and 90 mg tid or qid as necessary to normalize serum calcium levels; once the maintenance dose has been established, monitor serum calcium approximately every 2 months; intact parathyroid hormone (iPTH) levels should be measured no earlier than 12 hours after most recent dose
Pediatric: <18 years: not indicated; ≥18 years: same as adult
Sensipar *Tab:* 30, 60, 90 mg
Comment: Sensipar is indicated for the treatment of hypercalcemia in adult patients with parathyroid carcinoma and patients with primary HPT for whom parathyroidectomy would be indicated on the basis of serum calcium levels, but who are unable to undergo parathyroidectomy. Co-administration with a strong CYP3A4 inhibitor may increase serum levels of *cinacalcet*; dose adjustment and monitoring of iPTH serum phosphorus and serum calcium may be required. *Cinacalcet* is a strong inhibitor of CYP2D6. Dose adjustments may be required for concomitant medications that are predominantly metabolized by CYP2D6. **Sensipar** has been shown to cross the placental barrier in animal studies. There are no adequate and well-controlled studies of Sensipar in pregnancy. **Sensipar** should be used during pregnancy only if the potential benefit justifies the potential risk to the fetus. Animal studies have shown that **Sensipar** is excreted in milk with a high milk-to-plasma ratio. It is not known whether **Sensipar** is excreted in human milk. Because of the potential for clinically significant adverse reactions in infants from **Sensipar**, risk/benefit should be discussed and a decision should be made whether to discontinue breastfeeding or to discontinue the drug. No differences in the safety and efficacy of **Sensipar** were observed in patients > or < than 65 years of age.

HYPEREMESIS GRAVIDARUM/NAUSEA AND VOMITING OF PREGNANCY

ANTIHISTAMINE+VITAMIN B ANALOG

Comment: Bonjesta and **Diclegis** are indicated for nausea/vomiting of pregnancy in women who do not respond to conservative management. Somnolence (severe drowsiness) can occur when used in combination

(continued)

with alcohol or other sedating medications. Use with caution in patients with asthma, increased intraocular pressure, narrow angle glaucoma, stenosing peptic ulcer, pyloroduodenal obstruction, and urinary bladderneck obstruction. Concomitant monoamine oxidase inhibitors (MAOIs) are contraindicated because MAOIs prolong and intensify the anticholinergic effects of antihistamines, especially long-acting formulations. *Doxylamine* is secreted in breast milk; therefore, breastfeeding is not recommended.

▶ *doxylamine succinate+pyridoxine hydrochloride* take 1 tab at HS prn; if symptoms are not adequately controlled, the dose can be increased to max 1 tablet in the AM and 1 tablet at HS
Pediatric: <18 years: not established; ≥18 years: same as adult
    Bonjesta *Tab:* doxy 20 mg+pyri 20 mg ext-rel
    Diclegis *Tab:* doxy 10 mg+pyri 10 mg ext-rel

HYPERHIDROSIS (PERSPIRATION, EXCESSIVE)

Comment: Hyperhidrosis is a common, self-limiting problem that affects 2-3% of the U.S. population. Patients may complain of localized sweating of the hands, feet, face, or underarms, or more systemic, generalized sweating in multiple locations, and report a significant impact on their quality of life.

REFERENCE
Varella, A. Y., Fukuda, J. M., Telvelis, M. P., Campos, J. R., Kauffman, P., Cucato, G. G. et al. Wolosker, N. (2016). Translation and validation of hyperhidrosis disease severity scale. *Revista da Associação Médica Brasileira, 62*(9), 843–847. doi:10.1590/1806-9282.62.09.843

▶ *aluminum chloride* 20% solution apply q HS; wash treated area the following morning; after 1-2 treatments, may reduce frequency to 1-2 x a week
    Drysol *Soln:* 35, 60 ml (alcohol 93%) cont-rel
    Comment: Apply to clean dry skin (e.g., underarms). Do not apply to broken, irritated, or recently shaved skin.

TOPICAL ANTICHOLINERGIC
▶ *glycopyrronium* unfold 1 Qbrexza cloth and apply by wiping across one entire underarm one time; using the same cloth, wipe across the other underarm one time; discard used cloth; wash hands immediately; repeat once every 24 hours
Pediatric: <9 years: not recommended; ≥9 years:
    Qbrexza Premoistened cloth (single-use pouch)
    Comment: Qbrexza (*glycopyrronium*) is the first FDA-approved, once-daily topical treatment indicated for patients ≥9 years of age with primary axillary hyperhidrosis. *Glycopyrronium* is anticholinergic; it is important to wash hands after **Qbrexza** cloths are used because it can cause blurred vision if the eyes are touched. Do not reuse **Qbrexza** cloths. **Qbrexza** is flammable. Avoid heat and flame while applying **Qbrexza**. **Qbrexza** is contraindicated in patients with medical conditions that can be exacerbated by the anticholinergic effect of *glycopyrronium* (e.g., glaucoma, paralytic ileus, unstable cardiovascular status in acute hemorrhage, severe ulcerative colitis, toxic megacolon complicating ulcerative colitis, myasthenia gravis, and Sjogren's syndrome). The most common adverse reactions (incidence ≥2%) have been dry mouth (24.2%), mydriasis (6.8%), oropharyngeal pain (5.7%), headache (5.0%), urinary hesitation (3.5%), vision blurred (3.5%), nasal dryness (2.6%), dry throat (2.6%), dry eye (2.4%), dry skin (2.2%), and constipation (2.0%). Local skin reactions include erythema (17.0%), burning/stinging (14.1%), and pruritus (8.1%). Co-administration of **Qbrexza** with anticholinergic medications may result in additive interaction; therefore, avoid co-administration of **Qbrexza** with other anticholinergic drugs. There are no available data on **Qbrexza** use in pregnancy to inform a drug-associated risk of adverse developmental outcomes. There are no data on the presence of *glycopyrrolate* or its metabolites in human milk or effects on the breastfed infant.

ORAL ANTICHOLINERGIC
Comment: *Oxybutynin*, a cholinergic antagonist commonly prescribed for overactive bladder, is the first oral agent to emerge as a treatment option for hyperhidrosis.

▶ *oxybutynin chloride* (G)
    Ditropan 5 mg bid-tid; max 20 mg/day
    Pediatric: <5 years: not recommended; 5-12 years: 5 mg bid; max 15 mg/day; ≥16 years: same as adult
      Tab: 5*mg; *Syr:* 5 mg/5 ml
    Ditropan XL initially 5 mg daily; may increase weekly in 5-mg increments as needed; max 30 mg/day
    Pediatric: <6 years: not recommended; ≥6 years: initially 5 mg once daily; may increase weekly in 5-mg increments as needed; max 20 mg/day
      Tab: 5, 10, 15 mg ext-rel
    GelniQUE 3 mg Pump apply 3 pumps (84 mg) once daily to clean dry intact skin on the abdomen, upper arm, shoulders, or thighs; rotate sites; wash hands; avoid washing application site for 1 hour after application
    Pediatric: <12 years: not recommended; ≥12 years: same as adult
      Gel: 3% (92 gm, metered pump dispenser) (alcohol)

GelniQUE 1 gm Sachet apply 1 gm gel (1 sachet) once daily to dry intact skin on the abdomen, upper arms/shoulders, <u>or</u> thighs; rotate sites; wash hands; avoid washing application site for 1 hour after application

Pediatric: <12 years: <u>not</u> recommended; ≥12 years: same as adult

Gel: 10%, 1 gm/sachet (30/carton) (alcohol)

Oxytrol Transdermal Patch (OTC) apply patch to clean dry area of the abdomen, hip, <u>or</u> buttock; one patch twice weekly; rotate sites

Pediatric: <12 years: <u>not</u> recommended; ≥12 years: same as adult

Transdermal patch: 3.9 mg/day

▷ *etelcalcetide Starting dose:* 5 mg via IV bolus 3 x/week at the end of hemodialysis treatment; *Maintenance dose:* individualized, determined by titration, based on parathyroid hormone (PTH) and corrected serum calcium response; *Dose range:* 2.5 to 15 mg 3 x/week; dose may be increased in 2.5 mg <u>or</u> 5 mg increments <u>no</u> more frequently than every 4 weeks; ensure corrected serum calcium is at <u>or</u> above the lower limit of normal prior to initiation, dose increase, <u>or</u> reinitiation; do <u>not</u> mix <u>or</u> dilute prior to administration; administer via IV bolus injection into the venous line of the dialysis circuit after hemodialysis, during rinse back <u>or</u> after rinse back; administer a sufficient volume of saline (e.g., 150 ml of rinse back) after injection into the dialysis tubing; if administered after rinse back, administer intravenously followed by at least 10 ml of saline flush

Parsabiv *Vial:* 2.5 mg/0.5 ml, 5 mg/ml, 10 mg/2 ml soln, single-dose

Comment: Parsabiv *(etelcalcetide)* is indicated for secondary hyperparathyroidism (HPT) in adult patients with chronic kidney disease (CKD) on hemodialysis. **Parsabiv** has <u>not</u> been studied in adult patients with parathyroid carcinoma, primary hyperparathyroidism, <u>or</u> with CKD who are <u>not</u> on hemodialysis and is <u>not</u> recommended for use in these populations. Measure serum calcium within 1 week after initiation <u>or</u> dose adjustment and every 4 weeks for maintenance. Measure PTH after 4 weeks from initiation <u>or</u> dose adjustment. Decrease <u>or</u> temporarily discontinue **Parsabiv** in individuals with PTH levels below the target range. Consider decreasing <u>or</u> temporarily discontinuing **Parsabiv** <u>or</u> use concomitant therapies to increase corrected serum calcium in patients with a corrected serum calcium below the lower limit of normal but at <u>or</u> above 7.5 mg/dL without symptoms of hypocalcemia. Stop **Parsabiv** and treat hypocalcemia if the corrected serum calcium falls below 7.5 mg/dL <u>or</u> patients report symptoms of hypocalcemia. The most common adverse reactions (incidence ≥5%) have been decreased serum calcium, muscle spasms, diarrhea, nausea, vomiting, headache, hypocalcemia, and paresthesia. Hypocalcemia may sometimes be severe and severe hypocalcemia can cause paresthesias, myalgias, muscle spasms, seizures, QT prolongation, and ventricular arrhythmias. Patients predisposed to QT interval prolongation, ventricular arrhythmias, and seizures may be at increased risk and require close monitoring. Educate patients on the symptoms of hypocalcemia and advise them to contact a healthcare provider if they occur. Reductions in corrected serum calcium may be associated with congestive heart failure (CHF); however, a causal relationship with **Parsabiv** could <u>not</u> be completely excluded. Closely monitor patients for worsening signs and symptoms of heart failure (HF). Patients with risk factors for upper gastrointestinal (GI) bleeding may be at increased risk. Monitor patients and promptly evaluate and treat any suspected GI bleeding. Adynamic bone may develop if PTH levels are chronically suppressed. If PTH levels decrease below the recommended target range, the dose of **Parsabiv** should be reduced <u>or</u> discontinued. **Parsabiv** is <u>not</u> recommended when breastfeeding.

HYPERHOMOCYSTEINEMIA, HOMOCYSTINURIA

Comment: Elevated homocysteine is associated with cognitive impairment, vascular dementia, and dementia of the Alzheimer's type.

HOMOCYSTEINE-LOWERING NUTRITIONAL SUPPLEMENTS

▷ *L-methylfolate calcium (as* Metafolin*)+pyridoxal 5-phosphate+methylcobalamin* take 1 cap daily

Pediatric: <12 years: <u>not</u> recommended; ≥12 years: same as adult

Metanx *Cap:* metafo 3 mg+pyrid 35 mg+methyl 2 mg (gluten-free, yeast-free, lactose-free)

Comment: Metanx is indicated as adjunct treatment for endothelial dysfunction <u>and/or</u> hyperhomocysteinemia in patients who have lower extremity ulceration.

▷ *L-methylfolate calcium (as* Metafolin*)+methylcobalamin+n-acetylcysteine* take 1 cap daily

Pediatric: <12 years: <u>not</u> recommended; ≥12 years: same as adult

Cerefolin *Cap:* metafo 5.6 mg+methyl 2 mg+n-ace 600 mg (gluten-free, yeast-free, lactose-free)

Comment: Cerefolin is indicated in the dietary management of patients treated for early memory loss, with emphasis on those at risk for neurovascular oxidative stress, hyperhomocysteinemia, mild-to-moderate cognitive impairment with <u>or</u> without vitamin B12 deficiency, vascular dementia, <u>or</u> Alzheimer's disease.

METHYLATING AGENT

▷ *betaine anhydrous for oral solution* (G) *Recommended dose:* 6 gm/day, administered orally in divided doses of 3 gm bid

Pediatric: <3 years: recommended starting dose: 100 mg/kg/day, administered orally in divided doses of 50 mg/kg bid; then increase weekly by 50 mg/kg increments; monitor patient response by plasma homocysteine concentrations; increase the dose gradually until the plasma total homocysteine concentration is undetectable <u>or</u> present only in small amounts; ≥3 years: same as adult

(continued)

Cystadane *Bottle:* 180 gm of betaine anhydrous with measuring scoop for dissolving in 4-6 oz water, juice, milk, or formula, or mixed with food

Comment: Cystadane is a methylating agent indicated in pediatric and adult patients for the treatment of homocystinuria to decrease elevated homocysteine blood concentrations. Included within the category of homocystinuria are (1) cystathionine beta-synthase (CBS) deficiency, (2) 5, 10-methylenetetrahydrofolate reductase (MTHFR) deficiency, and (3) cobalamin cofactor metabolism (cbl) defect. The prescribed amount of Cystadane should be measured with the measuring scoop provided and then dissolved in 4-6 oz of water, juice, milk, or formula until completely dissolved, or mixed with food, for immediate ingestion. Safety and efficacy of Cystadane have been established in pediatric patients. The majority of case studies of homocystinuria patients treated with Cystadane have been pediatric patients, including patients ranging in age from 24 days to 17 years. *Warning/Precaution—Hypermethioninemia in Patients with CBS Deficiency:* Cystadane may worsen elevated plasma plasma methionine concentrations and cerebral edema has been reported; monitor plasma methionine concentrations in patients with CBS deficiency. Keep plasma methionine concentrations below 1,000 micromol/L through dietary modification and, if necessary, a reduction of Cystadane dose. The most common adverse reactions (incidence >2%) have been nausea and gastrointestinal distress, based on physician survey. Available data from a limited number of published case reports and postmarketing experience with Cystadane use in pregnancy have not identified any drug-associated risks of major birth defects, miscarriage, or adverse maternal or fetal outcomes. Animal reproduction studies have not been conducted with *betaine*. There are no data on the presence of *betaine* in human or animal milk or effects on the breastfed infant. Developmental and health benefits of breastfeeding should be considered along with the mother's clinical need for Cystadane and any potential adverse effects on the breastfed infant from Cystadane or from the underlying maternal condition. To report suspected adverse reactions, contact Recordati Rare Diseases at 1-888-575-8344, or FDA at 1-800-FDA-1088 or www.fda.gov/medwatch.

HYPERKALEMIA

POTASSIUM BINDERS

Comment: Normal serum K+ range is approximately 3.5-5.5 mEq/L. Hyperkalemia is associated with cardiac dysrhythmias and metabolic acidosis. Risk factors include kidney disease, heart failure, and drugs that inhibit the renin-angiotensin-aldosterone system (RAAS), including angiotensin-converting enzyme inhibitors (ACEIs), angiotensin receptor blockers (ARBs), direct renin inhibitors, and aldosterone antagonists. Cation exchange resins are not for emergency treatment of life-threatening hyperkalemia, severe constipation, and bowel obstruction or impaction. May cause gastrointestinal (GI) irritability, ulceration, necrosis, sodium retention, hypocalcemia, hypomagnesemia, fecal impaction, and ischemic colitis. Avoid non-absorbable cation-donating antacids and laxatives (e.g., *magnesium hydroxide, aluminum hydroxide*). Concomitant sorbitol should be avoided because it may cause intestinal necrosis.

▷ *patiromer sorbitex calcium* initially 8.4 gm once daily; adjust dosage as prescribed based on potassium concentration and target range; may increase dosage at 1-week (or longer) intervals in increments of 8.4 gm; max dose 25.2 gm once daily; prepare immediately prior to administration; do not take in dry form; administer with food; measure 1/3 cup of water and pour half into a glass; then add Veltassa and stir; add the remaining water and stir well; the powder will not dissolve and the mixture will look cloudy; add more water as needed for desired consistency; take with or without food; do not heat or mix with heated food or fluids; take other oral drugs at least 6 hours before or 6 hours after taking Veltassa
Pediatric: <18 years: not recommended; ≥18 years: same as adult
   Veltassa *Pkt:* 8, 4, 16.8, 25.2 gm pwdr for oral susp, 30 single-use pkts/carton
   Comment: Store packets in the refrigerator. If stored at room temperature, product must be used within 3 months.

▷ *sodium polystyrene sulfonate* (G) *Oral:* average total daily adult dose is 15-60 gm, administered as a 15 gm dose (4 level teaspoons), 1-4 x a day; *Rectal:* average adult dose is 30-50 gm q 6 hours
Pediatrics: use 1 gm/1 mEq of K+ as basis of calculation; in pediatric patients, as in adults, Kayexalate is expected to bind potassium at the practical exchange ratio of 1 mEq potassium per 1 gm of resin; in neonates, Kayexalate should not be given by the oral route; in both children and neonates, excessive dosage or inadequate dilution could result in impaction of the resin; premature infants or low birthweight infants may have an increased risk for GI adverse effects
   Kayexalate *Jar:* 1 lb (453.6 gm) pwdr for dilution
   Comment: Kayexalate should not be used as emergency treatment for life-threatening hyperkalemia because of its delayed onset of action. Contraindications are hypersensitivity to polystyrene sulfonate resins, obstructive bowel disease, and neonates with reduced gut motility. Take other orally administered drugs at least 3 hours before or 3 hours after Kayexalate. Cation-donating antacids may reduce the resin's potassium exchange capability and increase risk of systemic alkalosis. Concomitant use of sorbitol may contribute to the risk of intestinal necrosis and is not recommended. Kayexalate is not absorbed systemically so breastfeeding is not expected to result in risk to the infant.

▷ *sodium zirconium cyclosilicate Starting dose:* 10 gm administered 3 tid for up to 48 hours; *Maintenance treatment:* 10 gm once daily; adjust dose at 1-week intervals by 5 gm daily, as needed, to obtain desired serum potassium target range; in general, other oral medications should be administered at least 2 hours before or 2 hours after a Lokelma dose

Pediatric: <18 years: <u>not</u> established; >18 years: same as adult

Lokelma for Oral Suspension *Pwdr for oral susp:* 5, 10 gm/pkt (30 pkts/box)

Comment: Lokelma (*sodium zirconium cyclosilicate*) is a potassium binder. *In vitro*, Lokelma has a high affinity for potassium ions, even in the presence of other cations such as calcium and magnesium. Lokelma increases fecal potassium excretion through binding of potassium in the lumen of the GI tract. Lokelma should <u>not</u> be used as an emergency treatment for life-threatening hyperkalemia because of its delayed onset of action. The most common adverse reaction with Lokelma is mild-to-moderate edema. Patients with motility disorders may experience GI adverse reactions. As Lokelma is <u>not</u> absorbed systemically, maternal use is <u>not</u> expected to result in fetal exposure and breastfeeding is <u>not</u> expected to result in infant exposure.

HYPERPARATHYROIDISM (HPT)

➤ *calcifediol* **(G)** 1 cap daily

Pediatric: <18 years: <u>not</u> established; ≥18 years: same as adult

Rayaldee *Cap:* 30 mcg ext-rel

Comment: Rayaldee is indicated for the prevention and treatment of secondary hyperparathyroidism associated with chronic kidney disease (CKD) stage 3 <u>or</u> 4 and serum total 25-hydroxyvitamin D levels <30 mg/ml.

➤ *paricalcitol* **(G)** administer 0.04-1 mcg/kg (2.8-7 mcg) IV bolus, during dialysis, no more than every other day; may be increased by 2-4 mcg q 2-4 weeks; monitor serum calcium and phosphorus during dose adjustment periods; if Ca x P ≥75, immediately reduce dose <u>or</u> discontinue until these levels normalize; discard unused portion of single-use vials immediately

Pediatric: <18 years: <u>not</u> established; ≥18 years: same as adult

Zemplar *Vial:* 2, 5 mcg/ml soln for inj

Comment: Zemplar is indicated for the prevention and treatment of sHPT associated with CKD stage 5.

CALCIUM-SENSING RECEPTOR AGONIST

➤ *cinacalcet* *Initial dose:* 30 mg bid; titrate every 2 to 4 weeks through sequential doses of 30 mg bid, then 60 mg bid, then 90 mg bid, then 90 mg tid-qid as needed to normalize serum calcium levels; swallow whole, do <u>not</u> break; take with food <u>or</u> shortly after a meal; *Maintenance:* serum calcium and serum phosphorus should be measured approximately monthly and parathyroid hormone (PTH) q 1-3 months

Sensipar *Tab* 30, 60, 90 mg

Comment: Sensipar (*cinacalcet*) is indicated (1) for the treatment of hypercalcemia in adult patients with primary hyperparathyroidism (pHPT) for whom parathyroidectomy would be indicated on the basis of serum calcium levels, but who are unable to undergo parathyroidectomy, (2) for the treatment of secondary hyperparathyroidism in patients with CKD on dialysis (see *Hypercalcemia*), and (3) for the treatment of hypercalcemia in patients with parathyroid carcinoma. Sensipar can be used as monotherapy <u>or</u> in combination with vitamin D sterols <u>and/or</u> phosphate binders. Secondary hyperparathyroidism (sHPT) in patients with CKD is a progressive disease associated with increases in PTH levels and derangements in calcium and phosphorus metabolism. Increased PTH stimulates osteoclastic activity resulting in cortical bone resorption and marrow fibrosis. The goal of treatment of secondary hyperparathyroidism are to lower levels of PTH, calcium, and phosphorus in the blood in order to prevent progressive bone disease and the systemic consequences of disordered mineral metabolism. In CKD patients on dialysis with uncontrolled secondary HPT, reductions in PTH are associated with a favorable impact on bone-specific alkaline phosphatase (BALP), bone turnover, and bone fibrosis. The calcium-sensing receptor on the surface of the chief cell of the parathyroid gland is the principal regulator of PTH secretion. Sensipar directly lowers PTH levels by increasing the sensitivity of the calcium-sensing receptor to extracellular calcium. The reduction in PTH is associated with a concomitant decrease in serum calcium levels. Patients should be aware of potential manifestations of hypocalcemia, including paresthesias, myalgias, cramping, tetany, and convulsions. Sensipar treatment should <u>not</u> be initiated if serum calcium is less than the lower limit of the normal range (8.4 mg/dL). Serum calcium should be measured within 1 week after any Sensipar dose adjustment. If serum calcium falls below 8.4 mg/dL but remains above 7.5 mg/dL, <u>or</u> if symptoms of hypocalcemia occur, calcium-containing phosphate binders <u>and/or</u> vitamin D sterols can be used to raise serum calcium. If serum calcium falls below 7.5 mg/dL, <u>or</u> if symptoms of hypocalcemia persist and the dose of vitamin D cannot be increased, withhold administration of Sensipar until serum calcium levels reach 8.0 mg/dL, <u>and/or</u> symptoms of hypocalcemia have resolved. Treatment should be reinitiated using the next lowest dose of Sensipar. Adynamic bone disease may develop if intact parathyroid hormone (iPTH) levels are suppressed below 100 pg/ml. Sensipar is metabolized in part by the enzyme CYP3A4. Co-administration of *ketoconazole*, a strong inhibitor of CYP3A4, can cause an approximate 2-fold increase in *cinacalcet* exposure. Dose adjustment of Sensipar may be required and PTH and serum calcium concentrations should be closely monitored if a patient initiates <u>or</u> discontinues therapy with a strong CYP3A4 inhibitor (e.g., *ketoconazole, erythromycin, itraconazole*). Patients with congenital long QT syndrome, history of QT interval prolongation, family history of long QT syndrome <u>or</u> sudden cardiac death, and other conditions that predispose to QT interval

(continued)

prolongation and ventricular arrhythmia may be at increased risk for QT interval prolongation and ventricular arrhythmias if they develop hypocalcemia due to **Sensipar**. Closely monitor corrected serum calcium and QT interval in patients at risk receiving **Sensipar**. Seizure threshold is lowered by significant reductions in serum calcium levels. Monitor patients with seizure disorders receiving **Sensipar**. Patients with risk factors for upper GI bleeding (e.g., known gastritis, esophagitis, ulcers, or severe vomiting) may be at increased risk for GI bleeding when receiving **Sensipar** treatment. In postmarketing safety surveillance, isolated, idiosyncratic cases of hypotension, worsening heart failure (HF), and/or arrhythmia have been reported in patients with impaired cardiac function.

▷ *etelcalcetide Starting dose:* 5 mg via IV bolus 3 x a week at the end of hemodialysis treatment; *Maintenance dose:* individualized, determined by titration, based on PTH and corrected serum calcium response; *Dose range:* 2.5-15 mg 3 x/week; dose may be increased in 2.5 mg or 5 mg increments no more frequently than every 4 weeks; ensure corrected serum calcium is at or above the lower limit of normal prior to initiation, dose increase, or reinitiation; do not mix or dilute prior to administration; administer via IV bolus injection into the venous line of the dialysis circuit after hemodialysis, during rinse back or after rinse back; administer a sufficient volume of saline (e.g., 150 ml of rinse back) after injection into the dialysis tubing; if administered after rinse back, administer intravenously followed by at least 10 ml of saline flush

Parsabiv *Vial:* 2.5 mg/0.5 ml, 5 mg/ml, 10 mg/2 ml soln, single-dose

Comment: Parsabiv *(etelcalcetide)* is indicated for secondary hyperparathyroidism in adult patients with CKD on hemodialysis. **Parsabiv** has not been studied in adult patients with parathyroid carcinoma, primary hyperparathyroidism, or with CKD who are not on hemodialysis, and is not recommended for use in these populations. Measure serum calcium within 1 week after initiation or dose adjustment and every 4 weeks for maintenance. Measure PTH after 4 weeks from initiation or dose adjustment. Decrease or temporarily discontinue **Parsabiv** in individuals with PTH levels below the target range. Consider decreasing or temporarily discontinuing **Parsabiv** or use concomitant therapies to increase corrected serum calcium in patients with a corrected serum calcium below the lower limit of normal but at or above 7.5 mg/dL without symptoms of hypocalcemia. Stop **Parsabiv** and treat hypocalcemia if the corrected serum calcium falls below 7.5 mg/dL or patients report symptoms of hypocalcemia. The most common adverse reactions (incidence ≥5%) have been decreased serum calcium, muscle spasms, diarrhea, nausea, vomiting, headache, hypocalcemia, and paresthesia. Hypocalcemia may sometimes be severe and severe hypocalcemia can cause paresthesias, myalgias, muscle spasms, seizures, QT prolongation, and ventricular arrhythmias. Patients predisposed to QT interval prolongation, ventricular arrhythmias, and seizures may be at increased risk and require close monitoring. Educate patients on the symptoms of hypocalcemia and advise them to contact a healthcare provider if they occur. Reductions in corrected serum calcium may be associated with congestive heart failure (CHF); however, a causal relationship with **Parsabiv** could not be completely excluded. Closely monitor patients for worsening signs and symptoms of HF. Patients with risk factors for upper GI bleeding may be at increased risk. Monitor patients and promptly evaluate and treat any suspected GI bleeding. Adynamic bone may develop if PTH levels are chronically suppressed. If PTH levels decrease below the recommended target range, the dose of **Parsabiv** should be reduced or discontinued. **Parsabiv** is not recommended when breastfeeding.

HYPERPHOSPHATEMIA

FERRIC CITRATE

▷ **ferric citrate** *Hyperphosphatemia in chronic kidney disease (CKD) on dialysis:* starting dose is 2 tabs tid with meals; adjust dose by 1 to 2 tabs as needed to maintain serum phosphorus at target levels, up to max of 12 tabs/day; dose can be titrated at 1 week or longer intervals; *Iron deficiency anemia in CKD not on dialysis:* starting dose is 1 tablet 3 tid with meals; adjust dose as needed to achieve and maintain hemoglobin goal; max max 12 tabs/day

Pediatric: <18 years: not recommended; ≥18 years: same as adult

Auryxia *Tab:* 210 mg *ferric iron* (equivalent to 1 gm *ferric citrate*)

Comment: Auryxia is a phosphate binder indicated for the control of serum phosphorus levels in patients ≥18 years of age with CKD on dialysis. Ferric iron binds dietary phosphate in the gastrointestinal (GI) tract and precipitates as ferric phosphate. This compound is insoluble and is excreted in the stool. **Auryxia** is also an iron replacement product indicated for the treatment of iron deficiency anemia in patients >18 years of age with CKD not on dialysis. Ferric iron is reduced from the ferric to the ferrous form by ferric reductase in the GI tract. After transport through the enterocytes into the blood, oxidized ferric iron circulates bound to the plasma protein transferrin, for incorporation into hemoglobin. **Auryxia** is contraindicated in iron overload syndromes (e.g., hemochromatosis). Monitor ferritin and transferrin saturation (TSAT). When clinically significant drug interactions are expected, consider separation of the timing of administration. Consider monitoring clinical responses or blood levels of the concomitant medication. The most common adverse reactions (incidence ≥5%) are discolored feces, diarrhea, constipation, nausea, vomiting, cough, abdominal pain, and hyperkalemia. There are no available data on **Auryxia** use in pregnancy to inform a drug-associated risk of major birth defects and miscarriage; however, an overdose of iron may carry a risk of spontaneous abortion, gestational diabetes, and fetal malformation. There are no human data regarding the effects of **Auryxia** on the breastfed infant. Accidental overdose of iron-containing products is a leading cause of fatal poisoning in children under 6 years of age. Keep this product out of reach of children. In case of accidental overdose, contact poison control center immediately and transfer to emergency care.

PHOSPHATE BINDERS
Comment: Monitor for development of hypercalcemia. Normal serum PO_4^- is 2.5 to 4.5 mg/dL and normal serum calcium is 8.5-10.5 mg/dL.
➤ *calcium acetate* (G) initially 2 tabs or caps with each meal; then titrate gradually to keep serum phosphate at <6 mg/dL; usual maintenance is 3-4 tabs or caps with each meal
    Pediatric: <12 years: not recommended; ≥12 years: same as adult
        PhosLo *Tab:* 667 mg; *Cap:* 667 mg
➤ *lanthanum carbonate* (G) initially 750 mg to 1.5 gm per day in divided doses; take with meals; titrate at 2 to 3-week intervals in increments of 750 mg/day based on serum phosphate; usual range 1.5-3 gm/day; usual max 3,750 mg/day
    Pediatric: <12 years: not recommended; ≥12 years: same as adult
        Fosrenol *Chew tab:* 250, 500, 750 mg; 1 gm
➤ *sevelamer* (G) for patients not taking a phosphate binder, take tid with meals; swallow whole; titrate by 1 tab per meal at 1-week intervals to keep serum phosphorus 3.5-5.5 mg/dL; switching from calcium acetate to *sevelamer*, see mfr pkg insert. *Serum phosphorus* ≥5.5 to ≤7.5 mg/dL: 800 mg tid; *Serum phosphorus 7.5-9 mg/dL:* 1.2-1.6 tid
    Pediatric: <12 years: not recommended; ≥12 years: same as adult
        Renagel *Tab:* 400, 800 mg
        Renvela *Tab:* 800 mg

HYPERPIGMENTATION

Comment: Depigmenting agents may be used for hyperpigmented skin conditions, including chloasma, melasma, freckles, and senile lentigines. Limit treatments to small areas at one time. Sunscreen ≥30 SPF recommended.
➤ *hydroquinone* (G) apply sparingly to affected area and rub in bid
        Lustra *Crm:* 4% (1, 2 oz) (sulfites)
        Lustra AF *Crm:* 4% (1, 2 oz) (sunscreen, sulfites)
➤ *monobenzone* apply sparingly to affected area and rub in bid-tid; depigmentation occurs in 1-4 months
        Benoquin *Crm:* 20% (1.25 oz)
➤ *tazarotene* (G) apply daily at HS
    Pediatric: <12 years: not recommended; ≥12 years: same as adult
        Avage Cream *Crm:* 0.1% (30 gm)
        Tazorac Cream *Crm:* 0.05, 0.1% (15, 30, 60 gm)
        Tazorac Gel *Gel:* 0.05, 0.1% (30, 100 gm)
➤ *tretinoin* (G) apply daily at HS
    Pediatric: <12 years: not recommended; ≥12 years: same as adult
        Avita *Crm/Gel:* 0.025% (20, 45 gm)
        Renova *Crm:* 0.02% (40 gm); 0.05% (40, 60 gm)
        Retin-A Cream *Crm:* 0.025, 0.05, 0.1% (20, 45 gm)
        Retin-A Gel *Gel:* 0.01, 0.025% (15, 45 gm) (alcohol 90%)
        Retin-A Liquid *Liq:* 0.05% (28 ml) (alcohol 55%)
        Retin-A Micro *Microspheres:* 0.04, 0.1% (20, 45 gm)

COMBINATION AGENTS
➤ *hydroquinone+fluocinolone+tretinoin* apply sparingly to affected area and rub in daily at HS
    Pediatric: <12 years: not recommended; ≥12 years: same as adult
        Tri-Luma *Crm:* hydroquin 4%+fluo 0.01%+tretin 0.05% (30 gm) (parabens, sulfites)
➤ *hydroquinone+padimate o+oxybenzone+octyl methoxycinnamate* apply sparingly to affected area and rub in bid
    Pediatric: <12 years: not recommended; ≥16 years: same as adult
        Glyquin *Crm:* 4% (1 oz jar)
➤ *hydroquinone+ethyl dihydroxypropyl PABA+dioxybenzone+oxybenzone* apply sparingly to affected area and rub in bid; max 2 months
    Pediatric: <12 years: not recommended; ≥12 years: same as adult
        Solaquin *Crm:* hydroquin 2%+PABA 5%+dioxy 3%+oxy 2% (1 oz) (sulfites)
➤ *hydroquinone+padimate+dioxybenzone+oxybenzone* apply sparingly to affected area and rub in bid; max 2 months
    Pediatric: <12 years: not recommended; ≥12 years: same as adult
        Solaquin Forte *Crm:* hydroquin 4%+pad 0.5%+dioxy 3%+oxy 2% (1 oz) (sunscreen, sulfites)
➤ *hydroquinone+padimate+dioxybenzone* apply sparingly to affected area and rub in bid; max 2 months
    Pediatric: <12 years: not recommended; ≥12 years: same as adult
        Solaquin Forte Gel: hydroquin 4%+pad 0.5%+dioxy 3% (1 oz) (alcohol, sulfites)

HYPERPROLACTINEMIA

DOPAMINE RECEPTOR AGONIST

▷ *cabergoline* (G) initial therapy is 0.25 mg twice a week; may increase by 0.25 mg twice weekly up to 1 mg twice a week according to the patient's serum prolactin level; dose increases should <u>not</u> occur more than every 4 weeks; after a normal serum prolactin level has been maintained for 6 months, may be discontinued, with periodic monitoring of serum prolactin level to determine if/when treatment should be reinstituted
Pediatric: <12 years: <u>not</u> established; ≥12 years: same as adult
> Dostinex *Tab:* 0.5 mg
> **Comment: Dostinex** is indicated to treat hyperprolactinemia disorders due to idiopathic <u>or</u> pituitary adenoma.

HYPERTENSION: PRIMARY, ESSENTIAL

see JNC-8 Recommendations

BETA-BLOCKERS (CARDIOSELECTIVE)

Comment: Cardioselective beta-blockers are less likely to cause bronchospasm, peripheral vasoconstriction, <u>or</u> hypoglycemia than non-cardioselective beta-blockers.

▷ *acebutolol* (G) initially 400 mg in 1-2 divided doses; usual range 200-800 mg/day; max 1.2 gm/day in 2 divided doses
Pediatric: <12 years: <u>not</u> recommended; ≥12 years: same as adult
> Sectral *Cap:* 200, 400 mg
▷ *atenolol* (G) initially 50 mg daily; may increase after 1-2 weeks to 100 mg daily; max 100 mg/day
Pediatric: <12 years: <u>not</u> recommended; ≥12 years: same as adult
> Tenormin *Tab:* 25, 50, 100 mg
▷ *betaxolol* initially 10 mg daily; may increase to 20 mg/day after 7-14 days; usual max 20 mg/day
Pediatric: <12 years: <u>not</u> recommended; ≥12 years: same as adult
> Kerlone *Tab:* 10*, 20 mg
▷ *bisoprolol* 5 mg daily; max 20 mg daily
Pediatric: <12 years: <u>not</u> recommended; ≥12 years: same as adult
> Zebeta *Tab:* 5*, 10 mg
▷ *metoprolol succinate*
Pediatric: <12 years: <u>not</u> recommended; ≥12 years: same as adult
> Toprol-XL initially 25-100 mg in a single dose once daily; increase weekly if needed; max 400 mg/day; as monotherapy <u>or</u> with a diuretic
>> *Tab:* 25*, 50*, 100*, 200*mg ext-rel
▷ *metoprolol tartrate* initially 25-50 mg bid; increase weekly if needed; max 400 mg/day; as monotherapy <u>or</u> with a diuretic
Pediatric: <12 years: <u>not</u> recommended; ≥12 years: same as adult
> Lopressor (G) *Tab:* 25, 37.5, 50, 75, 100 mg
▷ *nebivolol* (G) initially 5 mg once daily; may increase at 2-week intervals; max 40 mg/day
Pediatric: <12 years: <u>not</u> recommended; ≥12 years: same as adult
> Bystolic *Tab:* 2.5, 5, 10, 20 mg

BETA-BLOCKERS (NON-CARDIOSELECTIVE)

Comment: Non-cardioselective beta-blockers are more likely to cause bronchospasm, peripheral vasoconstriction, <u>and/or</u> hypoglycemia than cardioselective beta-blockers.

▷ *nadolol* (G) initially 40 mg daily; usual maintenance 40-80 mg daily; max 320 mg/day
Pediatric: <12 years: <u>not</u> recommended; ≥12 years: same as adult
> Corgard *Tab:* 20*, 40*, 80*, 120*, 160*mg
▷ *penbutolol* 10-20 mg once daily
Pediatric: <12 years: <u>not</u> recommended; ≥12 years: same as adult
> Levatol *Tab:* 20*mg
▷ *pindolol* (G) initially 5 mg bid; may increase after 3-4 weeks in 10 mg increments; max 60 mg/day
Pediatric: <12 years: <u>not</u> recommended; ≥12 years: same as adult
> Pindolol *Tab:* 5, 10 mg
> Visken *Tab:* 5, 10 mg
▷ *propranolol* (G)
> Inderal initially 40 mg bid; usual maintenance 120-240 mg/day; max 640 mg/day
> *Pediatric:* initially 1 mg/kg/day; usual range 2-4 mg/kg/day in 2 divided doses; max 16 mg/kg/day
>> *Tab:* 10*, 20*, 40*, 60*, 80*mg
> Inderal LA initially 80 mg daily in a single dose; increase q 3-7 days; usual range 120-160 mg/day; max 320 mg/day in a single dose
> *Pediatric:* <12 years: <u>not</u> recommended; ≥12 years: same as adult
>> *Cap:* 60, 80, 120, 160 mg sust-rel

InnoPran XL initially 80 mg q HS; max 120 mg/day
Pediatric: <12 years: <u>not</u> recommended; ≥12 years: same as adult
    Cap: 80, 120 mg ext-rel
▷ **timolol (G)** initially 10 mg bid, increase weekly if needed; usual maintenance 20-40 mg/day; max 60 mg/day in 2 divided doses
Pediatric: <12 years: <u>not</u> recommended; ≥12 years: same as adult
    Blocadren *Tab:* 5, 10*, 20*mg

BETA-BLOCKER (NON-CARDIOSELECTIVE)+ALPHA-1 BLOCKER COMBINATIONS
▷ **carvedilol (G)**
Pediatric: <12 years: <u>not</u> recommended; ≥12 years: same as adult
    Coreg initially 6.25 mg bid; may increase at 1 to 2-week intervals to 12.5 mg bid; max 25 mg bid
      Tab: 3.125, 6.25, 12.5, 25 mg
    Coreg CR initially 20 mg once daily for 2 weeks; may increase at 1 to 2-week intervals; max 80 mg once daily
      Tab: 10, 20, 40, 80 mg cont-rel
▷ **carteolol** initially 2.5 mg daily, gradually increase to 5 <u>or</u> 10 mg once daily; usual maintenance 2.5-5 mg once daily
Pediatric: <12 years: <u>not</u> recommended; ≥12 years: same as adult
    Cartrol *Tab:* 2.5, 5 mg
▷ **labetalol (G)** initially 100 mg bid; increase after 2-3 days if needed; usual maintenance 200-400 mg bid; max 2.4 gm/day
Pediatric: <12 years: <u>not</u> recommended; ≥12 years: same as adult
    Normodyne *Tab:* 100*, 200*, 300 mg
    Trandate *Tab:* 100*, 200*, 300*mg

DIURETICS
Thiazide Diuretics
▷ **chlorthalidone (G)** initially 15 mg daily; may increase to 30 mg once daily based on clinical response; max 45-60 mg/day
Pediatric: <12 years: <u>not</u> established; ≥12 years: same as adult
    Chlorthalidone *Tab:* 25, 50 mg
    Thalitone *Tab:* 15 mg
▷ **chlorothiazide (G)** 0.5-1 gm/day in a single <u>or</u> divided doses; max 2 gm/day
Pediatric: <6 months: up to 15 mg/lb/day in 2 divided doses; ≥6 months: 10 mg/lb/day in 2 divided doses
    Diuril *Tab:* 250*, 500*mg; *Oral susp:* 250 mg/5 ml (237 ml)
▷ **hydrochlorothiazide (G)**
Pediatric: <12 years: <u>not</u> recommended; ≥12 years: same as adult
    Esidrix 25-100 mg once daily
      Tab: 25, 50, 100 mg
    Hydrochlorothiazide 12.5 mg once daily; usual max 50 mg/day
      Tab: 25*, 50*mg
    Microzide 12.5 mg once daily; usual max 50 mg/day
      Cap: 12.5 mg
▷ **methyclothiazide+deserpidine** initially 5/0.25 mg once daily; titrate individual components
Pediatric: <12 years: <u>not</u> recommended; ≥12 years: same as adult
    Enduronyl *Tab:* methy 5 mg+deser 0.25 mg*
    Enduronyl Forte *Tab:* methy 5 mg+deser 0.5 mg*
▷ **polythiazide** 2-4 mg once daily
Pediatric: <12 years: <u>not</u> recommended; ≥12 years: same as adult
    Renese *Tab:* 1, 2, 4 mg

Potassium-Sparing Diuretics
▷ **amiloride** initially 5 mg; may increase to 10 mg; max 20 mg
Pediatric: <12 years: <u>not</u> recommended; ≥12 years: same as adult
    Midamor *Tab:* 5 mg
▷ **spironolactone (G)** initially 50-100 mg in a single <u>or</u> divided doses; titrate at 2-week intervals
Pediatric: <12 years: <u>not</u> established; ≥12 years: same as adult
    Aldactone *Tab:* 25, 50*, 100*mg
    CaroSpir *Oral susp:* 25 mg/5 ml (118, 473 ml) (banana)
▷ **triamterene** 100 mg bid; max 300 mg
Pediatric: <12 years: <u>not</u> recommended; ≥12 years: same as adult
    Dyrenium *Cap:* 50, 100 mg

Loop Diuretics
▷ **bumetanide (G)** 0.5-2 mg daily; may repeat at 4 to 5 hour intervals; max 10 mg/day
Pediatric: <18 years: <u>not</u> recommended; ≥18 years: same as adult

(continued)

Tab: 1*mg
Comment: *Bumetanide* is contraindicated with sulfa drug allergy.

▶ *ethacrynic acid* (G) initially 50-200 mg/day
Pediatric: <1 month: <u>not</u> recommended; ≥1 month: initially 25 mg/day; then adjust dose in 25 mg increments
   Edecrin *Tab:* 25, 50 mg

▶ *ethacrynate sodium* (G) <1 month: <u>not</u> recommended; ≥1 month-12 years: use the smallest effective dose; initially 25 mg; then careful stepwise increments in dosage of 25 mg to achieve effective maintenance; ≥12 years: administer the smallest dose required to produce gradual weight loss (about 1-2 lb/day); onset of diuresis usually occurs at 50-100 mg in children ≥12 years; after diuresis has been achieved, the minimally effective dose (usually 50-200 mg/day) may be administered on a continuous <u>or</u> intermittent dosage schedule; dose titrations are usually in 25-50 mg increments to avoid electrolyte derangement and water excretion; the patient should be weighed under standard conditions before and during administration of *ethacrynate sodium;* the following schedule may be helpful in determining the lowest effective dose; *Day 1:* 50 mg once daily after a meal; *Day 2:* 50 mg bid after meals, if necessary; *Day 3:* 100 mg in the morning and 50-100 mg following the afternoon <u>or</u> evening meal, depending on the response to the morning dose; a few patients may require initial and maintenance doses as high as 200 mg bid; these higher doses, which should be achieved gradually, are most often required in patients with severe, refractory edema
   Sodium Edecrin *Vial:* 50 mg single-dose
Comment: Sodium Edecrin is more potent than more commonly used loop and thiazide diuretics. Treatment of the edema associated with congestive heart failure, cirrhosis of the liver, and renal disease, including nephrotic syndrome; short-term management of ascites due to malignancy, idiopathic edema, and lymphedema; and short-term management of hospitalized pediatric patients, other than infants, with congenital heart disease <u>or</u> nephrotic syndrome. IV **Sodium Edecrin** is indicated when a rapid onset of diuresis is desired, for example, in acute pulmonary edema <u>or</u> when gastrointestinal absorption is impaired <u>or</u> oral medication is <u>not</u> practical.

▶ *furosemide* (G) initially 40 mg bid
Pediatric: <12 years: <u>not</u> recommended; ≥12 years: same as adult
   Lasix *Tab:* 20, 40*, 80 mg; *Oral Soln:* 10 mg/ml (2, 4 oz w. dropper)
Comment: *Furosemide* is contraindicated with sulfa drug allergy.

▶ *torsemide* 5 mg once daily; may increase to 10 mg once daily
Pediatric: <12 years: <u>not</u> recommended; ≥12 years: same as adult
   Demadex *Tab:* 5*, 10*, 20*, 100*mg

▶ *torsemide (reformulated) Recommended initial dose:* 20 mg orally once daily; titrate dose by approximately doubling until desired diuretic response is obtained; doses >200 mg have <u>not</u> been studied
Pediatric: safety and efficacy <u>not</u> established
   Soaanz *Tab:* 20, 40, 60 mg film-coat
Comment: Soaanz is a reformulated loop diuretic indicated for the treatment of edema associated with heart failure <u>or</u> renal disease in adults. **Soaanz** is contraindicated with hypersensitivity to **Soaanz**, anuria, and hepatic coma. Taking concomitant NSAIDs reduces the diuretic, natriuretic, and antihypertensive effects, and increases risk of renal impairment. Concomitant use with CYP2C9 inhibitors can decrease *torsemide* clearance. *Torsemide* may affect the efficacy and safety of sensitive CYP2C9 substrates <u>or</u> of substrates with a narrow therapeutic range, such as *warfarin* <u>or</u> *phenytoin*. Concomitant *colestyramine* decreases exposure of **Soaanz**. Co-administered organic anion drugs (e.g., *probenecid*) may decrease the diuretic activity of **Soaanz**. Like other diuretics, **torsemide** reduces the renal clearance of *lithium*, inducing a high risk of *lithium* toxicity. Monitor *lithium* levels periodically when **Soaanz** is co-administered. Renin-angiotensin inhibitors (angiotensin-converting enzyme inhibitors [ACEIs] and angiotensin II receptor blockers [ARBs]) increase risk of hypotension and renal impairment. Radiocontrast agents increased risk of renal toxicity. Corticosteroids and adrenocorticotropic hormone (ACTH) increase risk of hypokalemia.

Indoline Diuretic

▶ *indapamide* initially 1.25 mg daily; may titrate dosage upward every 4 weeks if needed; max 5 mg/day
Pediatric: <12 years: <u>not</u> recommended; ≥12 years: same as adult
   Lozol *Tab:* 1.25, 2.5 mg
Comment: *Indapamide* is contraindicated with sulfa drug allergy.

Quinazoline Diuretic

▶ *metolazone* 2.5-5 mg daily
Pediatric: <12 years: <u>not</u> recommended; ≥12 years: same as adult
   Zaroxolyn 2.5-5 mg daily
   Tab: 2.5, 5, 10 mg
Comment: *Metolazone* is contraindicated with sulfa drug allergy.

DIURETIC COMBINATIONS

▶ *amiloride+hydrochlorothiazide* (G) initially 1 tab daily; may increase to 2 tabs/day in a single <u>or</u> divided doses
Pediatric: <12 years: <u>not</u> recommended; ≥12 years: same as adult
   Moduretic *Tab:* amil 5 mg+hctz 50 mg*

▶ *methylclothiazide* +*deserpidine* initially 5/0.25 mg once daily; titrate individual components
Pediatric: safety and effectiveness in children not established; therefore, age at which this drug may be initially prescribed is not specified

> Enduronyl *Tab:* methyl 5 mg+deser 0.25 mg*
> Enduronyl Forte *Tab:* methyl 5 mg+deser 0.5 mg*
> **Comment:** Enduronyl (*methylclothiazide* and *deserpidine*) is indicated in the treatment of mild-to-moderately severe hypertension. The combined antihypertensive actions of *methyclothiazide* and *deserpidine* result in a total clinical antihypertensive effect, which is greater than can ordinarily be achieved by either drug, given individually and more potent agents can be administered at reduced dosage. *Methylclothiazide* (**Enduron**) is a thiazide (benzothiadiazine) diuretic-antihypertensive. *Deserpidine* is a purified rauwolfia alkaloid. The pharmacologic actions of *deserpidine* are essentially the same as those of other active rauwolfia alkaloids. *Deserpidine* probably produces its antihypertensive effects through depletion of tissue stores of catecholamines (epinephrine and norepinephrine) from peripheral sites. By contrast, its sedative and tranquilizing properties are thought to be related to depletion of 5-hydroxytryptamine from the brain. The antihypertensive effect is often accompanied by bradycardia. There is no significant alteration in cardiac output or renal blood flow. The carotid sinus reflex is inhibited, but postural hypotension is rarely seen with the use of conventional doses of **deserpidine** alone. *Methyclothiazide* is contraindicated in patients with anuria and in patients with a history of hypersensitivity to this or other sulfonamide-derived drugs. *Deserpidine* is contraindicated in patients with known hypersensitivity, active peptic ulcer, history of mental depression, especially with suicidal tendencies, and patients receiving electroconvulsive therapy. Animal reproduction studies have not been conducted with methyclothiazide or deserpidine. It is also not known whether **methylclothiazide** or *deserpidine* can cause fetal harm when administered to a pregnant woman. **methylclothiazide** and *deserpidine* should be given to a pregnant woman only if clearly needed. *methyclothiazide* and *deserpidine* are excreted in human milk. Effects on the breastfed infant are unknown; therefore, assess maternal need/benefit as against potential fetal risk.

▶ *spironolactone*+*hydrochlorothiazide* (G)
Pediatric: <12 years: not recommended; ≥12 years: same as adult

> Aldactazide 25 usual maintenance 1-4 tabs in a single or divided doses
> *Tab:* spiro 25 mg+hctz 25 mg
> Aldactazide 50 usual maintenance 1-2 tabs in a single or divided doses
> *Tab:* spiro 50 mg+hctz 50 mg

▶ *triamterene*+*hydrochlorothiazide* (G)
Pediatric: <12 years: not recommended; ≥12 years: same as adult

> Dyazide 1-2 caps once daily
> *Cap:* triam 37.5 mg/hctz 25 mg
> Maxzide 1 tab once daily
> *Tab:* triam 75 mg/hctz 50 mg*
> Maxzide-25 1-2 tabs once daily
> *Tab:* triam 37.5 mg/hctz 25 mg*

ANGIOTENSIN CONVERTING ENZYME INHIBITORS (ACEIs)

Comment: Black patients receiving ACEI monotherapy have been reported to have a higher incidence of angioedema as compared with non-Blacks. Non-Blacks have a greater decrease in BP when ACEIs are used as compared with Black patients.

▶ *benazepril* (G) initially 10 mg daily; usual maintenance 20-40 mg/day in 1-2 divided doses; usual max 80 mg/day
Pediatric: <12 years: not recommended; ≥12 years: same as adult

> Lotensin *Tab:* 5, 10, 20, 40 mg

▶ *captopril* (G) initially 25 mg bid-tid; after 1-2 weeks increase to 50 mg bid-tid
Pediatric: <12 years: not recommended; ≥12 years: same as adult

> Capoten *Tab:* 12.5*, 25*, 50*, 100*mg

▶ *enalapril* (G) initially 5 mg daily; usual dosage range 10-40 mg/day; max 40 mg/day
Pediatric: <12 years: not recommended; ≥12 years: same as adult

> Epaned Oral Solution *Oral soln:* 1 mg/ml (150 ml) (mixed berry)
> Vasotec (G) *Tab:* 2.5*, 5*, 10, 20 mg

▶ *fosinopril* initially 10 mg daily; usual maintenance 20-40 mg/day in a single or divided doses; max 80 mg/day
Pediatric: <6 years, <50 kg: not recommended; ≥6-12 years, ≥50 kg: 5-10 mg once daily

> Monopril *Tab:* 10*, 20, 40 mg

▶ *lisinopril*

> Prinivil initially 10 mg daily; usual range 20-40 mg/day
> *Pediatric:* <12 years: not recommended; ≥12 years: same as adult
> *Tab:* 5*, 10*, 20*, 40 mg
> Qbrelis Oral Solution administer as a single dose once daily
> *Pediatric:* <6 years, GFR <30 ml/min: not recommended; ≥6 years, GFR >30 ml/min: initially 0.07 mg/kg, max 5 mg; adjust according to BP; max 0.61 mg/kg (40 mg) once daily
> *Oral soln:* 1 mg/ml (150 ml)

(continued)

Zestril initially 10 mg daily; usual range 20-40 mg/day
  Pediatric: <12 years: not recommended; ≥12 years: same as adult
    Tab: 2.5, 5*, 10, 20, 30, 40 mg
▷ *moexipril* initially 7.5 mg daily; usual range 15-30 mg/day in 1-2 divided doses; max 30 mg/day
  Pediatric: <12 years: not recommended; ≥12 years: same as adult
    Univasc *Tab:* 7.5*, 15*mg
▷ *perindopril* initially 2-8 mg daily-bid; max 16 mg/day
  Pediatric: <12 years: not recommended; ≥12 years: same as adult
    Aceon *Tab:* 2*, 4*, 8*mg
▷ *quinapril* initially 10 mg once daily; usual maintenance 20-80 mg daily in 1-2 divided doses
  Pediatric: <12 years: not recommended; ≥12 years: same as adult
    Accupril *Tab:* 5*, 10, 20, 40 mg
▷ *ramipril* (G) initially 2.5 mg bid; usual maintenance 2.5-20 mg in 1-2 divided doses
  Pediatric: <12 years: not established; ≥12 years: same as adult
    Altace *Tab/Cap:* 1.25, 2.5, 5, 10 mg
▷ *trandolapril* initially 1-2 mg once daily; adjust at 1-week intervals; usual range 2-4 mg in 1-2 divided doses; max 8 mg/day
  Pediatric: <12 years: not recommended; ≥12 years: same as adult
    Mavik *Tab:* 1*, 2, 4 mg

ANGIOTENSIN II RECEPTOR BLOCKERS (ARBs)

▷ *azilsartan medoxomil* (G) *Monotherapy, not volume depleted:* 80 mg once daily; *Volume-depleted (concomitant high-dose diuretic):* initially 40 mg once daily
  Pediatric: <12 years: not recommended; ≥12 years: same as adult
    Edarbi *Tab:* 40, 80 mg
▷ *candesartan* (G) initially 16 mg daily; range 8-32 mg in 1-2 divided doses
  Pediatric: <12 years: not recommended; ≥12 years: same as adult
    Atacand *Tab:* 4, 8, 16, 32 mg
▷ *eprosartan* (G) initially 400 mg bid or 600 mg once daily; max 800 mg/day
  Pediatric: <12 years: not established; ≥12 years: same as adult
    Teveten *Tab:* 400, 600 mg
▷ *irbesartan* (G) initially 150 mg daily; titrate up to 300 mg
  Pediatric: <12 years: not recommended; ≥12 years: same as adult
    Avapro *Tab:* 75, 150, 300 mg
▷ *losartan* (G) initially 50 mg daily; max 100 mg/day
  Pediatric: <12 years: not recommended; ≥12 years: same as adult
    Cozaar *Tab:* 25, 50, 100 mg
▷ *olmesartan medoxomil* (G) initially 20 mg once daily; after 2 weeks, may increase to 40 mg daily
  Pediatric: <6 years: not recommended; ≥6-16 years: 20-35 kg: initially 10 mg once daily; after 2 weeks, may increase to max 20 mg once daily; ≥6-16 years: >35 kg: initially 20 mg once daily; after 2 weeks may increase to max 40 mg once daily
    Benicar *Tab:* 5, 20, 40 mg
▷ *valsartan* (G) initially 80 mg once daily; may increase to 160 or 320 mg once daily after 2-4 weeks; usual range 80-320 mg/day
  Pediatric: <12 years: not recommended; ≥12 years: same as adult
    Diovan *Tab:* 40*, 80, 160, 320 mg
    Prexxartan Oral Solution *Oral soln:* 20 mg/5 ml, 80 mg/20 ml (120, 473 ml; 20 ml unit dose cup)

CALCIUM CHANNEL BLOCKERS (CCBs)
Benzothiazepines

▷ *diltiazem* (G)
  Pediatric: <12 years: not established; ≥12 years: same as adult
    Cardizem initially 30 mg qid; may increase gradually every 1-2 days; max 360 mg/day in divided doses
      Tab: 30, 60, 90, 120 mg
    Cardizem CD initially 120-180 mg daily; adjust at 1 to 2-week intervals; max 480 mg/day
      Cap: 120, 180, 240, 300, 360 mg ext-rel
    Cardizem LA initially 180-240 mg daily; titrate at 2-week intervals; max 540 mg/day
      Tab: 120, 180, 240, 300, 360, 420 mg ext-rel
    Cardizem SR initially 60-120 mg bid; adjust at 2-week intervals; max 360 mg/day
      Cap: 60, 90, 120 mg sust-rel
    Cartia XT initially 180 or 240 mg once daily; max 540 mg once daily
      Cap: 120, 180, 240, 300 mg ext-rel
    Dilacor XR initially 180 or 240 mg in the AM; usual range 180-480 mg/day; max 540 mg/day
      Cap: 120, 180, 240 mg ext-rel
    Tiazac (G) initially 120-240 mg daily; adjust at 2-week intervals; usual max 540 mg/day
      Cap: 120, 180, 240, 300, 360, 420 mg ext-rel

▷ *diltiazem maleate* initially 120-180 mg daily; adjust at 2-week intervals; usual range 120-480 mg daily
　　Pediatric: <12 years: not recommended; ≥12 years: same as adult
　　　　Tiamate *Cap:* 120, 180, 240 mg ext-rel

Dihydropyridines

▷ *amlodipine* initially 5 mg once daily; max 10 mg/day
　　Pediatric: <12 years: not recommended; ≥12 years: same as adult
　　　　Norvasc *Tab:* 2.5, 5, 10 mg
▷ *amlodipine benzoate* (G) *Recommended starting dose:* 5 mg orally once daily; max 10 mg once daily; small
　　stature, fragile, or elderly patients, or patients with hepatic insufficiency may be started on 2.5 mg once daily
　　Pediatric: <6 years: not studied; ≥6 years: starting dose: 2.5-5 mg once daily
　　　　Katerzia *Oral susp:* 1 mg/ml (150 ml), keep refrigerated
　　Comment: Katerzia *(amlodipine benzoate)* is a calcium channel blocker (CCB) in an oral suspension
　　formulation indicated for the treatment of hypertension in adults and children ≥6 years of age, to lower
　　blood pressure. Lowering blood pressure reduces the risk of fatal and non-fatal cardiovascular events,
　　primarily strokes and myocardial infarctions. **Katerzia** is also indicated for adult patients with coronary
　　artery disease (CAD), chronic stable angina (CSA), vasospastic angina (Prinzmetal's or variant angina),
　　and angiographically documented CAD in patients without heart failure or an ejection fraction <40%, at
　　the same dose as for blood pressure management (2.5-10 mg once daily).
▷ *clevidipine butyrate* administer by IV infusion; initially 1-2 mg/hour; double dose at 90-second intervals
　　until BP approaches goal; then titrate slower; adjust at 5 to 10 minute intervals; maintenance 4-6 mg/hour;
　　usual max 16-32 mg/hour; do not exceed 1,000 ml (21 mg/hour for 24 hours) due to lipid load
　　Pediatric: <18 years: not recommended; ≥18 years: same as adult
　　　　Cleviprex *Vial:* 0.5 mg/ml soln for IV infusion (single-use, 50, 100 ml) (lipids)
　　Comment: Cleviprex is indicated to reduce blood pressure when oral therapy is not feasible or desirable.
　　Cleviprex is contraindicated with egg or soy allergy.
▷ *felodipine* (G) initially 5 mg daily; usual range 2.5-10 daily; adjust at 2-week intervals; max 10 mg/day
　　Pediatric: <12 years: not recommended; ≥12 years: same as adult
　　　　Plendil *Tab:* 2.5, 5, 10 mg ext-rel
▷ *isradipine*
　　Pediatric: <12 years: not recommended; ≥12 years: same as adult
　　　　DynaCirc initially 2.5 mg bid; adjust in increments of 5 mg/day at 2 to 4-week intervals; max 20 mg/day
　　　　　　Cap: 2.5, 5 mg
　　　　DynaCirc CR initially 5 mg daily; adjust in increments of 5 mg/day at 2 to 4-week intervals; max 20 mg/day
　　　　　　Tab: 5, 10 mg cont-rel
▷ *levamlodipine maleate* initially 2.5 mg once daily; max 5 mg/day; small, fragile, or elderly patients, or
　　patients with hepatic insufficiency may be started on 1.25 mg once daily
　　Pediatric: <6 years: not established; ≥6 years: initially 1.25-2.5 mg once daily
　　　　Conjupri *Tab:* 1.25*, 2.5*, 5*mg
▷ *nicardipine* (G)
　　Pediatric: <18 years: not recommended; ≥18 years: same as adult
　　　　Cardene initially 10-20 mg tid; adjust at intervals of at least 3 days; max 120 mg/day
　　　　　　Cap: 20, 30 mg
　　　　Cardene SR 30-60 mg bid
　　　　　　Cap: 30, 45, 60 mg sust-rel
▷ *nifedipine* (G)
　　Pediatric: <12 years: not recommended; ≥12 years: same as adult
　　　　Adalat initially 10 mg tid; usual range 10-20 mg tid; max 180 mg/day
　　　　　　Cap: 10, 20 mg
　　　　Adalat CC initially 10 mg tid; usual range 10-20 mg tid; max 180 mg/day
　　　　　　Cap: 30, 60, 90 mg ext-rel
　　　　Afeditab CR initially 30 mg once daily; titrate over 7-14 days; max 90 mg/day
　　　　　　Cap: 30, 60 mg ext-rel
　　　　Procardia initially 10 mg tid; titrate over 7-14 days: max 30 mg/dose and 180 mg/day in divided doses
　　　　　　Cap: 10, 20 mg
　　　　Procardia XL initially 30-60 mg daily; titrate over 7-14 days; max dose 90 mg/day
　　　　　　Tab: 30, 60, 90 mg ext-rel
▷ *nisoldipine* initially 20 mg daily; may increase by 10 mg weekly; usual maintenance 20-40 mg/day; max 60 mg/day
　　Pediatric: <12 years: not recommended; ≥12 years: same as adult
　　　　Sular *Tab:* 10, 20, 30, 40 mg ext-rel

Diphenylalkylamines

▷ *verapamil* (G)
　　Pediatric: <12 years: not recommended; ≥12 years: same as adult
　　　　Calan 80-120 mg tid; may titrate up; usual max 360 mg in divided doses
　　　　　　Tab: 40, 80*, 120*mg

(continued)

Calan SR initially 120 mg in the AM; may titrate up; max 480 mg/day in divided doses
Cplt: 120, 180*, 240*mg sust-rel
Covera HS initially 180 mg q HS; titrate to 240 mg; then to 360 mg; then to 480 mg if needed
Tab: 180, 240 mg ext-rel
Isoptin initially 80-120 mg tid
Tab: 40, 80, 120 mg
Isoptin SR initially 120-180 mg in the AM; may increase to 240 mg in the AM; then 180 mg q 12 hours
or 240 mg in the AM and 120 mg in the PM; then 240 mg q 12 hours
Tab: 120, 180*, 240*mg sust-rel
Verelan initially 240 mg once daily; adjust in 120 mg increments; max 480 mg/day
Cap: 120, 180, 240, 360 mg sust-rel
Verelan PM initially 200 mg q HS; may titrate upward to 300 mg; then 400 mg if needed
Cap: 100, 200, 300 mg ext-rel

ALPHA-1 ANTAGONISTS
Comment: Educate the patient regarding potential side effects of hypotension when taking an alpha-1 antagonist, especially with first dose ("first dose effect"). Start at lowest dose and titrate upward.
▷ *doxazosin* (G) initially 1 mg once daily at HS; increase dose slowly every 2 weeks if needed; max 16 mg/day
Pediatric: <12 years: not recommended; ≥12 years: same as adult
Cardura *Tab:* 1*, 2*, 4*, 8*mg
Cardura XL *Tab:* 4, 8 mg
▷ *prazosin* (G) first dose at HS, 1 mg bid-tid; increase dose slowly; usual range 6-15 mg/day in divided doses; max 20-40 mg/day
Pediatric: <12 years: not recommended; ≥12 years: same as adult
Minipress *Cap:* 1, 2, 5 mg
▷ *terazosin* 1 mg at bedtime, then increase dose slowly; usual range 1-5 mg at bedtime; max 20 mg/day
Pediatric: <12 years: not recommended; ≥12 years: same as adult
Hytrin *Cap:* 1, 2, 5, 10 mg

CENTRAL ALPHA-AGONISTS
▷ *clonidine*
Pediatric: <12 years: not recommended; ≥12 years: same as adult
Catapres initially 0.1 mg bid; usual range 0.2-0.6 mg/day in divided doses; max 2.4 mg/day
Tab: 0.1*, 0.2*, 0.3*mg
Catapres-TTS initially 0.1 mg patch weekly; increase after 1-2 weeks if needed; max 0.6 mg/day
Patch: 0.1, 0.2 mg/day (12/carton), 0.3 mg/day (4/carton)
Kapvay (G) initially 0.1 mg bid; usual range 0.2-0.6 mg/day in divided doses; max 2.4 mg/day
Tab: 0.1, 0.2 mg
Nexiclon XR initially 0.18 mg (2 ml) suspension or 0.17 mg tab once daily; usual max 0.52 mg (6 ml suspension) once daily
Tab: 0.17, 0.26 mg ext-rel; *Oral susp:* 0.09 mg/ml ext-rel (4 oz)
▷ *guanabenz* (G) initially 4 mg bid; may increase by 4-8 mg/day every 1-2 weeks; max 32 mg/day
Pediatric: <12 years: not recommended; ≥12 years: same as adult
Tab: 4, 8 mg
▷ *guanfacine* (G) initially 1 mg/day q HS; may increase to 2 mg/day q HS; usual max 3 mg/day
Pediatric: <12 years: not recommended; ≥12 years: same as adult
Tenex *Tab:* 1, 2 mg
▷ *methyldopa* (G) initially 250 mg bid-tid; titrate at 2-day intervals; usual maintenance 500 mg/day to 2 gm/day; max 3 gm/day
Pediatric: initially 10 mg/kg/day in 2-4 divided doses; max 65 mg/kg/day or 3 gm/day, whichever is less
Aldomet *Tab:* 125, 250, 500 mg; *Oral susp:* 250 mg/5 ml (473 ml)

ALDOSTERONE RECEPTOR BLOCKER
▷ *eplerenone* initially 25-50 mg daily; may increase to 50 mg bid; max 100 mg/day
Pediatric: <12 years: not recommended; ≥12 years: same as adult
Inspra *Tab:* 25, 50 mg
Comment: Contraindicated with concomitant potent CYP3A4 inhibitors. Risk of hyperkalemia with concomitant ACEI or ARB. Monitor serum potassium at baseline, 1 week, and 1 month. Caution with serum creatinine (sCr)>2 mg/dL (male) or >1.8 mg/dL (female) and/or CrCl <50 ml/min, and diabetes mellitus (DM) with proteinuria.

PERIPHERAL ADRENERGIC BLOCKER
▷ *guanethidine* initially 10 mg daily; may adjust dose at 5 to 7 day intervals; usual range 25-50 mg/day
Pediatric: <12 years: not recommended; ≥12 years: same as adult
Ismelin *Tab:* 10, 25 mg

DIRECT RENIN INHIBITOR
▷ *aliskiren* (G) initially 150 mg once daily; max 300 mg/day
Pediatric: <18 years: not recommended; ≥18 years: same as adult
Tekturna *Tab:* 150, 300 mg

PERIPHERAL VASODILATORS

▶ *hydralazine* (G) initially 10 mg qid x 2-4 days; then increase to 25 mg 4 x/day for remainder of the 1st week; then increase to 50 mg qid; max 300 mg/day
  Pediatric: initially 0.75 mg/kg/day in 4 divided doses; increase gradually over 3-4 weeks; max 7.5 mg/kg/day or 2,000 mg/day
  Tab: 10, 25, 50, 100 mg

▶ *minoxidil* initially 5 mg daily; may increase at 3-day intervals to 10 mg/day, then 20 mg/day, then 40 mg/day; usual range 10-40 mg/day; max 100 mg/day
  Pediatric: initially 0.2 mg/kg daily; may increase in 50%-100% increments every 3 days; usual range 0.25-1 gm/kg/day; max 50 mg/day
    Loniten *Tab:* 2.5*, 10*mg

ACEI+DIURETIC COMBINATIONS

▶ *benazepril+hydrochlorothiazide*
  Pediatric: <12 years: not recommended; ≥12 years: same as adult
    Lotensin HCT
    Tab: Lotensin HCT 5/6.25 benaz 5 mg+hctz 6.25 mg*
       Lotensin HCT 10/12.5 benaz 10 mg+hctz 12.5 mg*
       Lotensin HCT 20/12.5 benaz 20 mg+hctz 12.5 mg*
       Lotensin HCT 20/25 benaz 20 mg+hctz 25 mg*

▶ *captopril+hydrochlorothiazide* (G)
  Pediatric: <12 years: not recommended; ≥12 years: same as adult
    Capozide 1 tab once daily; titrate individual components
    Tab: Capozide 25/15 capt 25 mg+hctz 15 mg*
       Capozide 25/25 capt 25 mg+hctz 25 mg*
       Capozide 50/15 capt 50 mg+hctz 15 mg*
       Capozide 50/25 capt 50 mg+hctz 25 mg*

▶ *enalapril+hydrochlorothiazide*
  Pediatric: <12 years: not recommended; ≥12 years: same as adult
    Vaseretic 1 tab once daily; titrate individual components
    Tab: Vaseretic 5/12.5 enal 5 mg+hctz 12.5 mg
       Vaseretic 10/25 enal 10 mg+hctz 25 mg

▶ *lisinopril+hydrochlorothiazide*
  Pediatric: <12 years: not recommended; ≥12 years: same as adult
    Prinzide 1 tab once daily; titrate individual components
    Tab: Prinzide 10/12.5 lis 10 mg+hctz 12.5 mg
       Prinzide 20/12.5 lis 20 mg+hctz 12.5 mg
       Prinzide 20/25 lis 20 mg+hctz 25 mg
    Zestoretic 1 tab once daily; titrate individual components; *CrCl <40 ml/min:* not recommended
    Tab: Zestoretic 10/12.5 lis 10 mg+hctz 12.5 mg
       Zestoretic 20/12.5 lis 20 mg+hctz 12.5 mg*
       Zestoretic 20/25 lis 20 mg+hctz 25 mg

▶ *moexipril+hydrochlorothiazide*
  Pediatric: <12 years: not recommended; ≥12 years: same as adult
    Uniretic 1 tab once daily; titrate individual components
    Tab: Uniretic 7.5/12.5 moex 7.5 mg+hctz 12.5 mg*
       Uniretic 15/12.5 moex 15 mg+hctz 12.5 mg*
       Uniretic 15/25 moex 15 mg+hctz 25 mg*

▶ *quinapril+hydrochlorothiazide*
  Pediatric: <12 years: not recommended; ≥12 years: same as adult
    Accuretic 1 tab once daily; titrate individual components
    Tab: Accuretic 10/12.5 quin 10 mg+hctz 12.5 mg*
       Accuretic 20/12.5 quin 20 mg+hctz 12.5 mg*
       Accuretic 20/25 quin 20 mg+hctz 25 mg*

ARB+DIURETIC COMBINATIONS

▶ *azilsartan+chlorthalidone*
  Pediatric: <18 years: not recommended; ≥18 years: same as adult
    Edarbyclor 1 tab once daily; titrate individual components
    Tab: Edarbyclor 40/12.5 azil 40 mg+chlor 12.5 mg
       Edarbyclor 40/25 azil 40 mg+chlor 25 mg

▶ *candesartan+hydrochlorothiazide*
  Pediatric: <12 years: not recommended; ≥12 years: same as adult
    Atacand HCT
    Tab: Atacand HCT 16/12.5 cande 16 mg+hctz 12.5 mg
       Atacand HCT 32/12.5 cande 32 mg+hctz 12.5 mg

(continued)

▷ *eprosartan+hydrochlorothiazide*
  Pediatric: <12 years: <u>not</u> recommended; ≥12 years: same as adult
    Teveten HCT 1 tab once daily; titrate individual components
      Tab: Teveten HCT **600/12.5** epro 600 mg+hctz 12.5 mg
        Teveten HCT **600/25** epro 600 mg+hctz 25 mg
▷ *irbesartan+hydrochlorothiazide*
  Pediatric: <12 years: <u>not</u> recommended; ≥12 years: same as adult
    Avalide 1 tab once daily; titrate individual components
      Tab: Avalide **150/12.5** irbes 150 mg+hctz 12.5 mg
        Avalide **300/12.5** irbes 300 mg+hctz 12.5 mg
▷ *losartan+hydrochlorothiazide* (G)
  Pediatric: <12 years: <u>not</u> recommended; ≥12 years: same as adult
    Hyzaar 1 tab once daily; titrate individual components
      Tab: Hyzaar **50/12.5** losar 50 mg+hctz 12.5 mg
        Hyzaar **100/12.5** losar 100 mg+hctz 12.5 mg
        Hyzaar **100/25** losar 100 mg+hctz 25 mg
▷ *olmesartan medoxomil+hydrochlorothiazide* (G)
  Pediatric: <12 years: <u>not</u> recommended; ≥12 years: same as adult
    Benicar HCT 1 tab once daily; titrate individual components
      Tab: Benicar HCT **20/12.5** olmi 20 mg+hctz 12.5 mg
        Benicar HCT **40/12.5** olmi 40 mg+hctz 12.5 mg
        Benicar HCT **40/25** olmi 40 mg+hctz 25 mg
▷ *telmisartan+hydrochlorothiazide* (G)
  Pediatric: <12 years: <u>not</u> recommended; ≥12 years: same as adult
    Micardis HCT 1 tab once daily; titrate individual components
      Tab: Micardis HCT **40/12.5** telmi 40 mg+hctz 12.5 mg
        Micardis HCT **80/12.5** telmi 80 mg+hctz 12.5 mg
        Micardis HCT **80/25** telmi 80 mg+hctz 25 mg
▷ *valsartan+hydrochlorothiazide* (G)
  Pediatric: <12 years: <u>not</u> recommended; ≥12 years: same as adult
    Diovan HCT 1 tab once daily; titrate individual components
      Tab: Diovan HCT **80/12.5** vals 80 mg+hctz 12.5 mg
        Diovan HCT **160/12.5** vals 160 mg+hctz 12.5 mg
        Diovan HCT **160/25** vals 160 mg+hctz 25 mg
        Diovan HCT **320/12.5** vals 320 mg+hctz 12.5 mg
        Diovan HCT **320/25** vals 320 mg+hctz 25 mg

CENTRAL ALPHA-AGONIST+DIURETIC COMBINATIONS
▷ *clonidine+chlorthalidone*
  Pediatric: <12 years: <u>not</u> recommended; ≥12 years: same as adult
    Combipres 1 tab daily-bid
      Tab: Combipres **0.1** clon 0.1 mg+chlor 15 mg*
        Combipres **0.2** clon 0.2 mg+chlor 15 mg*
        Combipres **0.3** clon 0.3 mg+chlor 15 mg*
▷ *methyldopa+hydrochlorothiazide* (G)
  Pediatric: <12 years: <u>not</u> recommended; ≥12 years: same as adult
    Aldoril initially **Aldoril 15** bid-tid <u>or</u> **Aldoril 25** bid; titrate individual components
      Tab: Aldoril **15** meth 250 mg+hctz 15 mg
        Aldoril **25** meth 250 mg+hctz 25 mg
        Aldoril **D30** meth 500 mg+hctz 30 mg
        Aldoril **D50** meth 500 mg+hctz 50 mg

BETA-BLOCKER (CARDIOSELECTIVE)+DIURETIC COMBINATIONS
▷ *atenolol+chlorthalidone* (G)
  Pediatric: <12 years: <u>not</u> recommended; ≥12 years: same as adult
    Tenoretic initially **Tenoretic 50** mg once daily; may increase to **Tenoretic** 100 mg once daily
      Tab: Tenoretic **50/25** aten 50 mg+chlor 25 mg*
        Tenoretic **100/25** aten 100 mg+chlor 25 mg
▷ *bisoprolol+hydrochlorothiazide*
  Pediatric: <12 years: <u>not</u> recommended; ≥12 years: same as adult
    Ziac initially one 2.5/6.25 mg tab daily; adjust at 2-week intervals; max two 10/6.25 mg tabs daily
      Tab: Ziac **2.5** biso 2.5 mg+hctz 6.25 mg
        Ziac **5** biso 5 mg+hctz 6.25 mg
        Ziac **10** biso 10 mg+hctz 6.25 mg
▷ *metoprolol succinate+hydrochlorothiazide*
  Pediatric: <12 years: <u>not</u> recommended; ≥12 years: same as adult
    Lopressor HCT titrate individual components

   Tab: **Lopressor HCT 50/25** meto succ 50 mg+hctz 25 mg*
     Lopressor HCT 100/25 meto succ 100 mg+hctz 25 mg*
     Lopressor HCT 100/50 meto succ 100 mg+hctz 50 mg*
▷ *metoprolol succinate+ext-rel hydrochlorothiazide*
 Pediatric: <12 years: <u>not</u> established; ≥12 years: same as adult
  Dutoprol titrate individual components; may titrate to max 200/25 mg once daily
   Tab: **Dutoprol 25/12.5** meto succ 25 mg+hctz 12.5 mg ext-rel
    Dutoprol 50/12.5 meto succ 50 mg+hctz 12.5 mg ext-rel
    Dutoprol 100/12.5 meto succ 100 mg+hctz 12.5 mg ext-rel

BETA-BLOCKER (NON-CARDIOSELECTIVE)+DIURETIC COMBINATIONS
▷ *nadolol+bendroflumethiazide*
 Pediatric: <12 years: <u>not</u> recommended; ≥12 years: same as adult
  Corzide titrate individual components
   Tab: **Corzide 40/5** nado 40 mg+bend 5 mg*
    Corzide 80/5 nado 80 mg+bend 5 mg*
▷ *propranolol+hydrochlorothiazide* (G)
 Pediatric: <12 years: <u>not</u> recommended; ≥12 years: same as adult
  Inderide titrate individual components
   Tab: **Inderide 40/25** prop 40 mg+hctz 25 mg*
    Inderide 80/25 prop 80 mg+hctz 25 mg*
  Inderide LA titrate individual components
   Cap: **Inderide LA 80/50** prop 80 mg+hctz 50 mg sust-rel
    Inderide LA 120/50 prop 120 mg+hctz 50 mg sust-rel
    Inderide LA 160/50 prop 160 mg+hctz 50 mg sust-rel
▷ *timolol+hydrochlorothiazide*
 Pediatric: <12 years: <u>not</u> recommended; ≥12 years: same as adult
  Timolide usual maintenance 2 tabs/day in a single <u>or</u> 2 divided doses
   Tab: timo 10 mg+hctz 25 mg

BETA-BLOCKER (CARDIOSELECTIVE)+ARB COMBINATION
▷ *nebivolol+valsartan* (G) 1 tab daily; may initiate when inadequately controlled on *nebivolol* 10 mg <u>or</u>
 valsartan 80 mg
 Pediatric: <12 years: <u>not</u> established; ≥12 years: same as adult
  Byvalson *Tab:* nebi 5 mg+val 80 mg

ALPHA-1 ANTAGONIST+DIURETIC COMBINATIONS
▷ *prazosin+polythiazide*
 Pediatric: <12 years: <u>not</u> recommended; ≥12 years: same as adult
  Minizide titrate individual components
   Cap: **Minizide 1** praz 1 mg+poly 0.5 mg
    Minizide 2 praz 2 mg+poly 0.5 mg
    Minizide 5 praz 5 mg+poly 0.5 mg

PERIPHERAL ADRENERGIC BLOCKER+HYDROCHLOROTHIAZIDE (HCTZ) COMBINATION
▷ *guanethidine+hydrochlorothiazide*
 Pediatric: <12 years: <u>not</u> recommended; ≥12 years: same as adult
  Esimil titrate individual components
   Tab: **Esimil 10/25** guan 10 mg+hctz 25 mg

ACEI+CCB COMBINATIONS
▷ *amlodipine+benazepril*
 Pediatric: <12 years: <u>not</u> recommended; ≥12 years: same as adult
  Lotrel titrate individual components
   Cap: **Lotrel 2.5/10** amlo 2.5 mg+benaz 10 mg
    Lotrel 5/10 amlo 5 mg+benaz 10 mg
    Lotrel 5/20 amlo 5 mg+benaz 20 mg
    Lotrel 10/20 amlo 10 mg+benaz 20 mg
    Lotrel 5/40 amlo 5 mg+benaz 40 mg
    Lotrel 10/40 amlo 10 mg+benaz 40 mg
▷ *amlodipine+perindopril*
 Pediatric: <12 years: <u>not</u> recommended; ≥12 years: same as adult
  Prestalia titrate individual components
   Cap: **Prestalia 2.5/3.5** amlo 2.5 mg+peri 3.5 mg
    Prestalia 5/7 amlo 5 mg+peri 7 mg
    Prestalia 5/14 amlo 5 mg+peri 14 mg

(continued)

▷ *enalapril+diltiazem*
   Pediatric: <12 years: <u>not</u> recommended; ≥12 years: same as adult
      Teczem titrate individual components
        Tab: enal 5 mg+dil 180 mg ext-rel
▷ *enalapril+felodipine*
   Pediatric: <18 years: <u>not</u> recommended; ≥18 years: same as adult
      Lexxel titrate individual components
        Tab: **Lexxel 5/2.5** enal 5 mg+felo 2.5 mg ext-rel
           Lexxel 5/5 enal 5 mg+felo 5 mg ext-rel
▷ *perindopril+amlodipine*
   Pediatric: <12 years: <u>not</u> established; ≥12 years: same as adult
      Prestalia titrate individual components; max 14/10 once daily
        Tab: **Prestalia 3.5/2.5** peri 3.5 mg+amlo 2.5 mg
           Prestalia 7/5 peri 7 mg+amlo 5 mg
           Prestalia 14/10 peri 14 mg+amlo 10 mg
▷ *trandolapril+verapamil*
   Pediatric: <12 years: <u>not</u> established; ≥12 years: same as adult
      Tarka titrate individual components
        Tab: **Tarka 1/240** tran 1 mg+ver 240 mg ext-rel
           Tarka 2/180 tran 2 mg+ver 180 mg ext-rel
           Tarka 2/240 tran 2 mg+ver 240 mg ext-rel
           Tarka 4/240 tran 4 mg+ver 240 mg ext-rel

DIRECT RENIN INHIBITOR (DRI)+HCTZ COMBINATIONS

▷ *aliskiren+hydrochlorothiazide*
   Pediatric: <18 years: <u>not</u> recommended; ≥18 years: same as adult
      Tekturna HCT initially *aliskiren* 150 mg once daily; max *aliskiren* 300 mg/day
        Tab: **Tekturna HCT 150/12.5** alisk 150 mg+hctz 12.5 mg
           Tekturna HCT 150/25 alisk 150 mg+hctz 25 mg
           Tekturna HCT 300/12.5 alisk 300 mg+hctz 12.5 mg
           Tekturna HCT 300/25 alisk 300 mg+hctz 25 mg

DRI+ARB COMBINATION

▷ *aliskiren+valsartan*
   Pediatric: <12 years: <u>not</u> recommended; ≥12 years: same as adult
      Valturna initially 150/160 once daily; may increase to max 300/320 once daily
        Tab: **Valturna 150/160** alisk 150 mg+vals 160 mg
           Valturna 300/320 alisk 300 mg+vals 320 mg

DRI+CCB COMBINATION

▷ *aliskiren+amlodipine*
   Pediatric: <12 years: <u>not</u> recommended; ≥12 years: same as adult
      Tekamlo initially 150/5 once daily; may increase to max 300/10 once daily
        Tab: **Tekamlo 150/5** alisk 150 mg+amlo 5 mg
           Tekamlo 150/10 alisk 150 mg+amlo 10 mg
           Tekamlo 300/5 alisk 300 mg+amlo 5 mg
           Tekamlo 300/10 alisk 300 mg+amlo 10 mg

DRI+CCB+HCTZ COMBINATIONS

▷ *aliskiren+amlodipine+hydrochlorothiazide*
   Pediatric: <12 years: <u>not</u> established; ≥12 years: same as adult
      Amturnide initially 150/5/12.5 once daily; may increase to max 300/10/25 once daily
        Tab: **Amturnide 150/5/12.5** alisk 150 mg+amlo 5 mg+hctz 12.5 mg
           Amturnide 300/5/12.5 alisk 300 mg+amlo 5 mg+hctz 12.5 mg
           Amturnide 300/5/25 alisk 300 mg+amlo 5 mg+hctz 25 mg

ARB+CCB COMBINATIONS

▷ *amlodipine+valsartan medoxomil* (G)
   Pediatric: <12 years: <u>not</u> recommended; ≥12 years: same as adult
      Exforge 1 tab daily; titrate individual components at 1-week intervals; max 10/320 once daily
        Tab: **Exforge 5/160** amlo 5 mg+vals 160 mg
           Exforge 5/320 amlo 5 mg+vals 320 mg
           Exforge 10/160 amlo 10 mg+vals 160 mg
           Exforge 10/320 amlo 10 mg+vals 320 mg
▷ *amlodipine+olmesartan medoxomil* (G)
   Pediatric: <12 years: <u>not</u> established; ≥12 years: same as adult
      Azor titrate individual components
        Tab: **Azor 5/20** amlo 5 mg+olme 20 mg
           Azor 10/20 amlo 10 mg+olme 20 mg

Azor 5/40 amlo 5 mg+olme 40 mg
Azor 10/40 amlo 10 mg+olme 40 mg
▷ *telmisartan+amlodipine* (G)
Pediatric: <12 years: <u>not</u> established; ≥12 years: same as adult
Twynsta initially 40/5 once daily; titrate at 1 week intervals; max 80/10 once daily
Tab: Twynsta 40/5 telmi 40 mg+amlo 5 mg
Twynsta 40/10 telmi 40 mg+amlo 10 mg
Twynsta 80/5 telmi 80 mg+amlo 5 mg
Twynsta 80/10 telmi 80 mg+amlo 10 mg

ARB+CCB+HCTZ COMBINATIONS
▷ *amlodipine+valsartan medoxomil+hydrochlorothiazide* (G)
Pediatric: <12 years: <u>not</u> recommended; ≥12 years: same as adult
Exforge HCT: initially 5/160/12.5 once daily; may titrate at 1-week intervals to max 10/320/25 once daily
Tab: Exforge HCT 5/160/12.5 amlo 5 mg+vals 160 mg+hctz 12.5 mg
Exforge HCT 5/160/25 amlo 5 mg+vals 160 mg+hctz 25 mg
Exforge HCT 10/160/12.5 amlo 10 mg+vals 160 mg+hctz 12.5 mg
Exforge HCT 10/160/25 amlo 10 mg+vals 160 mg+hctz 25 mg
Exforge HCT 10/320/25 amlo 10 mg+vals 320 mg+hctz 25 mg
▷ *olmesartan medoxomil+amlodipine+hydrochlorothiazide* (G)
Pediatric: <12 years: <u>not</u> recommended; ≥12 years: same as adult
Tribenzor: initially 20/5/12.5 once daily; may titrate at 1-week intervals to max 40/10/25 daily
Tab: Tribenzor 20/5/12.5 olme 20 mg+amlo 5 mg+hctz 12.5 mg
Tribenzor 40/5/12.5 olme 40 mg+amlo 5 mg+hctz 12.5 mg
Tribenzor 40/5/25 olme 40 mg+amlo 5 mg+hctz 25 mg
Tribenzor 40/10/12.5 olme 40 mg+amlo 10 mg+hctz 12.5 mg
Tribenzor 40/10/25 olme 40 mg+amlo 10 mg+hctz 25 mg

OTHER COMBINATION AGENTS
▷ *clonidine+chlorthalidone*
Pediatric: <12 years: <u>not</u> recommended; ≥12 years: same as adult
Clorpres initially 0.1/15 once daily; may titrate to max 0.3/15 bid
Tab: Clorpres 0.1/15 clon 0.1 mg+chlor 15 mg
Clorpres 0.2/15 clon 0.2 mg+chlor 15 mg
Clorpres 0.3/15 clon 0.3 mg+chlor 15 mg
▷ *reserpine+hydroflumethiazide*
Pediatric: <12 years: <u>not</u> recommended; ≥12 years: same as adult
Salutensin initially 1.25/25 once daily; may titrate to 1.25/25 bid <u>or</u> 1.25/50 once daily
Tab: Salutensin 1.25/25 enal 1.25 mg+hydro 25 mg
Salutensin 1.25/50: enal 1.25 mg+hydro 50 mg

ANTIHYPERTENSION+ANTILIPID COMBINATIONS
CCB+Statin Combinations
▷ *amlodipine+atorvastatin*
Pediatric: <10 years: <u>not</u> established; ≥10 years (female postmenarche): same as adult
Caduet select dose according to blood pressure and lipid values; titrate *amlodipine* over 7-14 days; titrate *atorvastatin* according to monitored lipid values; max *amlodipine* 10 mg/day and max *atorvastatin* 80 mg/day; see mfr pkg insert for contraindications and precautions for CCB and statin therapy
Tab: Caduet 2.5/10 amlo 2.5 mg+ator 10 mg
Caduet 2.5/20 amlo 2.5 mg+ator 20 mg
Caduet 5/10 amlo 5 mg+ator 10 mg
Caduet 5/20 amlo 5 mg+ator 20 mg
Caduet 5/40 amlo 5 mg+ator 40 mg
Caduet 5/80 amlo 5 mg+ator 80 mg
Caduet 10/10 amlo 10 mg+ator 10 mg
Caduet 10/20 amlo 10 mg+ator 20 mg
Caduet 10/40 amlo 10 mg+ator 40 mg
Caduet 10/80 amlo 10 mg+ator 80 mg

HYPERTHYROIDISM

▷ **methimazole** initially 15-60 mg/day in 3 divided doses; maintenance 5-15 mg/day
Pediatric: initially 0.4 mg/kg/day in 3 divided doses; maintenance 0.2 mg/kg/day <u>or</u> 1/2 initial dose
Tapazole *Tab:* 5*, 10*mg
Comment: *Methimazole* potentiates anticoagulants. Contraindicated in nursing mothers.

(continued)

▷ *propylthiouracil (ptu) (G)*
　　Propyl-Thyracil initially 100-900 mg/day in 3 divided doses; maintenance usually 50-600 mg/day in 2
　　divided doses
　　　　Pediatric: <6 years: <u>not</u> recommended; ≥6-10 years: initially 50-150 mg/day <u>or</u> 5-7 mg/kg/day in 3
　　　　divided doses; ≥10 years: initially 150-300 mg/day <u>or</u> 5-7 mg/kg/day in 3 divided doses; *maintenance:*
　　　　0.2 mg/kg/day <u>or</u> 1/2 to 2/3 of initial dose
　　　　　　Tab: 50*mg
　　Comment: Preferred agent in pregnancy. Side effects include dermatitis, nausea, agranulocytosis, and
　　hypothyroidism. Should be taken regularly for 2 years. Do <u>not</u> discontinue abruptly.

BETA-ADRENERGIC BLOCKER
▷ *propranolol* (G) 40-240 mg daily
　　Pediatric: <12 years: <u>not</u> recommended; ≥12 years: same as adult
　　　　Inderal *Tab:* 10*, 20*, 40*, 60*, 80*mg
　　　　Inderal LA initially 80 mg daily in a single dose; increase q 3-7 days; usual range 120-160 mg/day; max
　　　　320 mg/day in a single dose
　　　　　　Cap: 60, 80, 120, 160 mg sust-rel
　　　　InnoPran XL initially 80 mg q HS; max 120 mg/day
　　　　　　Cap: 80, 120 mg ext-rel

HYPERTRIGLYCERIDEMIA

OMEGA-3 FATTY ACID ETHYL ESTERS
Comment: Vascepa, Lovaza, and Epanova are indicated for the treatment of triglyceride (TG) ≥500 mg/dL.
▷ *icosapent ethyl (omega-3 fatty acid ethyl ester of EPA)* (G) 2 caps bid with food; max 4 gm/day; swallow
　　whole, do <u>not</u> crush <u>or</u> chew
　　Pediatric: <18 years: <u>not</u> recommended; ≥18 years: same as adult
　　　　Vascepa sgc: 0.5, 1 gm (alpha-tocopherol 4 mg/cap)
▷ *omega 3-fatty acid ethyl esters* (G) 2 gm bid <u>or</u> 4 gm daily; swallow whole, do <u>not</u> crush <u>or</u> chew
　　Pediatric: <18 years: <u>not</u> recommended; ≥18 years: same as adult
　　　　Lovaza *Gelcap:* 1 gm (alpha-tocopherol 4 mg/cap) *omega 3-carcartonyl acids* take 2-4 gelcaps (2-4 gm)
　　　　daily without regard to meals
　　　　Epanova *Gelcap:* 1 gm

ISOBUTYRIC ACID DERIVATIVE
▷ *gemfibrozil* (G)
　　Pediatric: <12 years: <u>not</u> recommended; ≥12 years: same as adult
　　　　Lopid 600 mg bid 30 minutes before AM and PM meals
　　　　　　Tab: 600*mg

FIBRATES (FIBRIC ACID DERIVATIVES)
▷ *fenofibrate* take with meals; adjust at 4 to 8-week intervals; discontinue if inadequate response after 2
　　months; lowest dose <u>or</u> contraindicated with renal impairment and the elderly
　　Pediatric: <12 years: <u>not</u> recommended; ≥12 years: same as adult
　　　　Antara 43-130 mg once daily; max 130 mg/day
　　　　　　Cap: 43, 87, 130 mg
　　　　FibriCor 30-105 mg once daily; max 105 mg/day
　　　　　　Tab: 30, 105 mg
　　　　TriCor (G) 48-145 mg once daily; max 145 mg/day
　　　　　　Tab: 48, 145 mg
　　　　TriLipix (G) 45-135 mg once daily; max 135 mg/day
　　　　　　Cap: 45, 135 mg del-rel
　　　　Lipofen (G) 50-150 mg once daily; max 150 mg/day
　　　　　　Cap: 50, 150 mg
　　　　Lofibra 67-200 mg daily; max 200 mg/day
　　　　　　Tab: 67, 134, 200 mg

NICOTINIC ACID DERIVATIVES
Comment: Contraindicated in liver disease. decrease total cholesterol, LDL-C, and TG and increase high-
density lipoprotein cholesterol (HDL-C). Before initiating and at 4-6 weeks, 3 months, and 6 months of
therapy, check fasting lipid profile, liver function tests (LFTs) glucose, and uric acid. A common side effect of
NADs is transient skin flushing. It is recommend to take a single dose of aspirin 325 mg 30 minutes before a
meal, and then take the NAD dose with the meal, to reduce flushing.
▷ *niacin*
　　Niaspan 375 mg daily for the 1st week; then 500 mg daily for the 2nd week; then 750 mg daily for 3rd
　　week; then 1 gm daily for weeks 4-7; then may increase by 500 mg q 4 weeks if needed; usual range 1-3
　　gm/day

    Pediatric: <12 years: not recommended; ≥12 years: same as adult
      Tab: 500, 750, 1,000 mg ext-rel
Slo-Niacin 250 mg or 500 mg or 750 mg q AM or HS
    Pediatric: <12 years: not recommended; ≥12 years: same as adult
      Tab: 250, 500, 750 mg cont-rel

HMG-COA REDUCTASE INHIBITORS (STATINS)

▷ *atorvastatin* (G) initially 10 mg daily; usual range 10-80 mg daily
    Pediatric: <10 years: not recommended; ≥10 years (female postmenarche): same as adult
      Lipitor *Tab:* 10, 20, 40, 80 mg
▷ *fluvastatin* (G) initially 20-40 mg q HS; usual range 20-80 mg/day
    Pediatric: <18 years: not established; ≥18 years: same as adult
      Lescol *Cap:* 20, 40 mg
      Lescol XL *Tab:* 80 mg ext-rel
▷ *lovastatin* initially 20 mg daily at evening meal; may increase at 4-week intervals; max 80 mg/day in a single or divided doses; *Concomitant fibrates, niacin,* or *CrCl <40 ml/min:* usual max 20 mg/day
    Pediatric: <10 years: not recommended; 10-17 years: initially 10-20 mg daily at evening meal; may increase at 4-week intervals; max 40 mg daily; *Concomitant fibrates, niacin,* or *CrCl <40 ml/min:* usual max 20 mg/day
      Mevacor *Tab:* 10, 20, 40 mg
▷ *pravastatin* (G) initially 10-20 mg q HS; usual range 10-80 mg/day; may start at 40 mg/day
    Pediatric: <8 years: not recommended; 8-13 years: 20 mg q HS; 14-17 years: 40 mg q HS; >17 years: same as adult
      Pravachol *Tab:* 10, 20, 40, 80 mg
▷ *rosuvastatin* initially 20 mg q HS; usual range 5-40 mg/day; adjust at 4-week intervals
    Pediatric: <10 years: not recommended; 10-17 years: 5-20 mg q HS; max 20 mg q HS; >17 years: same as adult
      Crestor *Tab:* 5, 10, 20, 40 mg
▷ *simvastatin* (G) initially 20 mg q HS; usual range 5-80 mg/day; adjust at 4-week intervals
    Pediatric: <10 years: not recommended; 10-17 years: initially 10 mg q HS; may increase at 4-week intervals; max 40 mg q HS; >17 years: same as adult
      Zocor *Tab:* 5, 10, 20, 40, 80 mg

NICOTINIC ACID DERIVATIVE+HMG-COA REDUCTASE INHIBITOR COMBINATION

Comment: Nicotinic acid derivatives decrease total cholesterol, LDL-C, and TG, and increase HDL-C. Before initiating and at 4-6 weeks, 3 months, and 6 months of therapy, check fasting lipid profile, liver function tests (LFTs), glucose, and uric acid. Side effects *Relative contraindications:* diabetes, hyperuricemia (gout), and peptic ulcer disease (PUD). *Absolute contraindications:* severe gout and chronic liver disease. It is recommend to take a single dose of aspirin 325 mg 30 minutes before a meal, and then take the NAD dose with the meal, to reduce flushing.

▷ *niacin+lovastatin*
    Pediatric: <18 years: not recommended; ≥18 years: same as adult
      Advicor monitor lab values; may titrate up to max 1,000/20 once daily
        Tab: **Advicor 500/20** niac 500 mg ext-rel+lova 20 mg
          Advicor 750/20 niac 750 mg ext-rel+lova 20 mg
          Advicor 1000/20 niac 1,000 mg ext-rel+lova 20 mg

HYPOCALCEMIA

Comment: Hypocalcemia resulting in metabolic bone disease may be secondary to hyperparathyroidism, pseudohypoparathyroidism, and chronic renal disease (CRD). Normal serum Ca^{++} range is approximately 8.5-12 mg/dL. Signs and symptoms of hypocalcemia include confusion, increased neuromuscular excitability, muscle spasms, paresthesias, hyperphosphatemia, positive Chvostek's sign, and positive Trousseau's sign. Signs and symptoms of hypercalcemia include fatigue, lethargy, decreased concentration and attention span, frank psychosis, anorexia, nausea, vomiting, constipation, bradycardia, heart block, and shortened QT interval. Foods high in calcium include almonds, broccoli, baked beans, salmon, sardines, buttermilk, turnip greens, collard greens, spinach, pumpkin, rhubarb, and bran. *Recommended daily calcium intake:* 1-3 years: 700 mg; 4-8 years: 1,000 mg; 9-18 years: 1,300 mg; 19-50 years: 1,000 mg; 51-70 years (males): 1,000 mg; ≥51 years (females): 1,200 mg; pregnancy or nursing: 1,000-1,300 mg. *Recommended daily vitamin D intake:* >1 year: 600 IU; 50+ years: 800-1,000 IU. The American Academy of Rheumatology (AAR) recommends the following daily doses for anyone on a chronic oral corticosteroid regimen: calcium 1,200-1,500 mg/day and vitamin D 800-1,000 IU/day.

CALCIUM SUPPLEMENTS

Comment: Take *calcium* supplements after meals to avoid gastric upset. Dosages of *calcium* over 2,000 mg/day have not been shown to have any additional benefit. *Calcium* decreases *tetracycline* absorption. *Calcium* absorption is decreased by corticosteroids.

(continued)

▷ *calcitonin-salmon*
    Miacalcin 200 units (1 spray intranasally) once daily; alternate nostrils each day
      Nasal spray: 14 dose (2 ml)
    Miacalcin injection 100 units/day SC <u>or</u> IM
      Vial: 2 ml
▷ *calcium carbonate* (OTC)(G)
    Rolaids chew 2 tabs bid; max 14 tabs/day
      Tab: calcium carbonate: 550 mg
    Rolaids Extra Strength chew 2 tabs bid; max 8 tabs/day
      Tab: 1,000 mg
    Tums chew 2 tabs bid; max 16 tabs/day
      Tab: 500 mg
    Tums Extra Strength chew 2 tabs bid; max 10 tabs/day
      Tab: 750 mg
    Tums Ultra chew 2 tabs bid; max 8 tabs/day
      Tab: 1,000 mg
    Os-Cal 500 (OTC) 1-2 tab bid-tid
      Tab: elemental calcium carbonate 500 mg
▷ *calcium carbonate+vitamin D* (G)
    Os-Cal 250+D (OTC) 1-2 tabs tid
      Tab: elemental calcium carbonate 250 mg+vit d 125 IU
    Os-Cal 500+D (OTC) 1-2 tabs bid-tid
      Tab: elemental calcium carbonate 500 mg+vit d 125 IU
    Viactiv (OTC) 1 tab tid
      Chew tab: elemental calcium 500 mg+vit d and vit a 100 IU+vit k 40 mEq
▷ *calcium citrate*
    Citracal (OTC) 1-2 tabs bid
      Tab: elemental calcium citrate 200 mg
▷ *calcium citrate+vitamin D* (G)
    Citracal+D (OTC) 1-2 cplts bid
      Cplt: elemental calcium citrate 315 mg+vit d 200 IU
    Citracal 250+D (OTC) 1-2 tabs bid
      Tab: elemental calcium citrate 250 mg+vit d 62.3 IU

VITAMIN D ANALOGS

Comment: Concurrent *vitamin D* supplementation is contraindicated in patients taking *calcitriol* <u>or</u> *doxercalciferol* due to the risk of *vitamin D* toxicity. Symptoms of hypervitaminosis D include hypercalcemia, hypercalciuria, elevated creatinine, erythema multiforme, and hyperphosphatemia. Maintain adequate daily calcium and fluid intake. Keep serum calcium times phosphate (Ca x P) product below 70. Monitor serum calcium (especially during dose titration), phosphorus, and other lab values (see literature for frequency).

▷ *calcitriol* (G) *Predialysis:* initially 0.25 mcg daily; may increase to 0.5 mcg daily; *Dialysis:* initially 0.25 mcg daily; may increase by 0.25 mcg/day at 4 to 8-week intervals; usual maintenance 0.5-1 mcg/day; *Hypoparathyroidism:* initially 0.25 mcg q AM; may increase by 0.25 mcg/day at 4 to 8-week intervals; usual maintenance 0.5-2 mcg/day
Pediatric: <12 years: *Predialysis:* <3 years: 10-15 ng/kg per day; ≥3 years: initially 0.25 mcg once daily; may increase to 0.5 mcg daily; *Dialysis:* <u>not</u> recommended; *Hypoparathyroidism:* initially 0.25 mcg daily in the AM; may increase by 0.25 mcg/day at 2 to 4-week intervals; usual maintenance: 1-5 years: 0.25-0.75 mcg daily; ≥6 years: 0.5-2 mcg daily; *Pseudohypoparathyroidism:* <6 years: insufficient data, see mfr pkg insert; ≥12 years: *Predialysis:* initially 0.25 mcg daily, may increase to 0.5 mcg daily; *Dialysis:* initially 0.25 mcg daily; may increase by 0.25 mcg daily at 4 to 8-week intervals; usual maintenance: 0.5-1 mcg daily
    Rocaltrol *Cap:* 0.25, 0.5 mcg
    Rocaltrol Solution *Soln:* 1 mcg/ml (15 ml, single-use dispensers)
Comment: *Calcitriol* is indicated for the treatment of secondary hyperparathyroidism and resultant metabolic bone disease in predialysis patients (CrCl 15-55 ml/min), hypocalcemia and resultant metabolic bone disease in patients on chronic renal dialysis, hypocalcemia in hypoparathyroidism, and pseudohypoparathyroidism.

▷ *doxercalciferol* (G) *Dialysis:* initially 10 mcg 3 x/week at dialysis; adjust to maintain intact parathyroid hormone (iPTH) level at 150-300 pg/ml; if iPTH is <u>not</u> lowered by 50% and fails to reach target range, may increase by 2.5 mcg at 8-week intervals; max 20 mcg 3 x/week; if iPTH <100 pg/ml, suspend for 1 week, then resume at a dose that is at least 2.5 mcg lower; *Predialysis:* initially 1 mcg once daily; may increase by 0.5 mcg at 2-week intervals to target iPTH level; max 3.5 mcg/day
Pediatric: <12 years: <u>not</u> established; ≥12 years: same as adult
    Hectorol *Cap:* 0.25, 0.5, 1, 2.5 mcg
    Comment: Oral **Hectorol** is indicated for the treatment of secondary hyperparathyroidism in patients with chronic kidney disease (CKD) on dialysis; *Predialysis stage 3 or 4 CKD:* use oral form <u>only</u>.

Hectorol Injection <12 years: <u>not</u> recommended; ≥12 years: 4 mcg 3 x weekly after dialysis; adjust dose to maintain intact parathyroid hormone (iPTH) 150-300 pg/ml; if iPTH is <u>not</u> lowered by 50% and fails to reach target range, may increase by 1-2 mcg at 8- week intervals; max 18 mcg/week; if iPTH <100 pg/ml, suspend for 1 week, then resume at a dose that is at least 1 mcg lower

   Vial: 2 mcg/ml (1, 2 ml single-dose; 2 ml multi-dose)

   Comment: *Hectorol Injection* is indicated for the treatment of secondary hyperparathyroidism in patients with CKD on dialysis.

➤ *paricalcitol* (G) administer 0.04-1 mcg/kg (2.8-7 mcg) IV bolus, during dialysis, no more than every other day; may be increased by 2-4 mcg/dose q 2-4 weeks; monitor serum calcium and phosphorus during dose adjustment periods; if Ca x P >75, immediately reduce dose <u>or</u> discontinue until these levels normalize; discard unused portion of single-use vials immediately

Pediatric: <18 years: <u>not</u> established; ≥18 years: same as adult

   Zemplar *Vial:* 2, 5 mcg/ml soln for inj

   Comment: *Paricalcitol* is indicated for the prevention and treatment of secondary hyperparathyroidism associated with CKD stage 5.

BIOENGINEERED REPLICA OF HUMAN PARATHYROID HORMONE

➤ *bioengineered replica of human parathyroid hormone* before starting, confirm 25-hydroxyvitamin D stores are sufficient; if insufficient, replace to sufficient levels per standard of care; confirm serum calcium is above 7.5 mg/dL; the goal of treatment is to achieve serum calcium within the lower half of the normal range; administer SC into the thigh once daily; alternate thighs; initially 50 mcg/day; when initiating, decrease dose of active vitamin D by 50%, if serum calcium is above 7.5 mg/dL; monitor serum calcium levels every 3 to 7 days after starting <u>or</u> adjusting dose and when adjusting either active vitamin D <u>or</u> calcium supplements dose; abrupt interruption <u>or</u> discontinuation of **Natpara** can result in severe hypocalcemia; resume treatment with, <u>or</u> increase the dose of, an active form of vitamin D and calcium supplements; monitor for signs and symptoms of hypocalcemia and monitor serum calcium levels; in the case of a missed dose, the next **Natpara** dose should be administered as soon as reasonably feasible and additional exogenous calcium should be taken in the event of hypocalcemia

   Natpara *Soln for inj:* 25, 50, 75, 100 mcg (2/pkg), multi-dose, dual-chamber glass cartridge containing a sterile powder and diluent

   Comment: Natpara is indicated as an adjunct to calcium and vitamin D in patients with hypoparathyroidism. Because of a potential risk of osteosarcoma, use **Natpara** <u>only</u> in patients who cannot be well-controlled on calcium and active forms of vitamin D alone and for whom the potential benefits are considered to outweigh the potential risk. Avoid use of **Natpara** in patients who are at increased baseline risk for osteosarcoma, such as patients with Paget's disease of bone <u>or</u> unexplained elevations of alkaline phosphatase, pediatric and young adult patients with open epiphyses, patients with hereditary disorders predisposing to osteosarcoma, <u>or</u> patients with a history of external beam <u>or</u> implant radiation therapy involving the skeleton. Because of the risk of osteosarcoma, **Natpara** is available <u>only</u> through a restricted program under the Risk Evaluation and Mitigation Strategy (REMS) (www.natparaREMS.com).

HYPOGLYCEMIA: ACUTE

GLUCAGON/GLUCAGON ANALOG

Comment: Necrolytic migratory erythema (NME), a skin rash, has been reported postmarketing following continuous *glucagon* infusion and resolved with discontinuation of the *glucagon*. The following are alternative treatments for the treatment of acute hypoglycemia: *glucagon* (Gvoke) injection for SC administration; *glucagon* nasal powder (Baqsimi) for nasal administration; *glucagon analog (dasiglucagon,* Zegalogue*)* for SC administration; orally administered glucose <u>or</u> a parenteral form of glucose for IV administration; orally administered non-diuretic benzothiadiazine derivative *diazoxide* (**Proglycem**) for patients with pheochromocytoma <u>or</u> insulinoma.

➤ *glucagon injection*

   Gvoke 1 mg SC; administer via SC injection <u>only</u> in the upper outer arm, lower abdomen, <u>or</u> outer thigh; call for emergency assistance immediately after administration of the dose; if there has been no response after 15 minutes, an additional weight-appropriate dose may be administered while waiting for emergency assistance; do <u>not</u> reuse an injection device; when the patient has responded to treatment, administer oral carbohydrates

Pediatric: <2 years: <u>not</u> established; 2-12 years: <45 kg: 0.5 mg SC; ≥45 kg: same as adult

   HypoPen *autoinjector:* 0.5 mg/0.1 ml, 1 mg/0.2 ml, single-use; *Prefilled syringe:* 0.5 mg/0.1 ml, 1 mg/0.2 ml, single-use

   Comment: Gvoke *(glucagon injection)* is a ready-to-use, room-temperature stable, liquid *glucagon* for the treatment of severe hypoglycemia in adult and pediatric patients ≥2 years of age with diabetes. Patients taking a beta-blocker may have a transient increase in pulse and BP. In patients taking *indomethacin*, **Gvoke** may lose its ability to raise glucose <u>or</u> may produce hypoglycemia. **Gvoke** may increase the anticoagulant effect of *warfarin*. **Gvoke** is contraindicated in patients with pheochromocytoma because

(continued)

Gvoke may stimulate the release of catecholamines from the tumor. In patients with insulinoma, Gvoke administration may produce an initial increase in blood glucose; however, Gvoke may stimulate exaggerated insulin release from an insulinoma and cause hypoglycemia; if a patient develops symptoms of hypoglycemia after a dose of Gvoke, administer glucose orally or intravenously. Allergic reactions have been reported and include generalized rash, anaphylactic shock with breathing difficulties, and hypotension. Gvoke is effective in treating hypoglycemia only if sufficient hepatic glycogen is present; patients in states of starvation with adrenal insufficiency or chronic hypoglycemia may not have adequate levels of hepatic glycogen for Gvoke to be effective (use glucose instead). *Glucagon* administered to patients with glucagonoma may cause secondary hypoglycemia. Test patients suspected of having glucagonoma for blood levels of glucagon prior to treatment, and monitor blood glucose levels during treatment; if hypoglycemia develops, administer glucose orally or intravenously. The most common adverse reactions to Gvoke (incidence ≥2%) reported have been the following: *Adult:* nausea, vomiting, injection site edema raised ≥1 mm, and headache; *Pediatric:* nausea, hypoglycemia, vomiting, headache, abdominal pain, hyperglycemia, injection site discomfort and reaction, and urticaria. Available data from case reports and a small number of observational studies with *glucagon* use in pregnant females over decades of use have not identified a drug-associated risk of major birth defects, miscarriage, or adverse maternal or embryo/fetal outcomes. There is no information available on the presence of *glucagon* in human or animal milk or effects on the breastfed infant. However, *glucagon* is a peptide and would be expected to be broken down to its constituent amino acids in the infant's digestive tract and is therefore unlikely to cause harm to an exposed infant.

▶ *glucagon nasal powder* 3 mg administered as 1 actuation of the intranasal device into one nostril; administer the dose by inserting the tip into one nostril and pressing the device plunger all the way in until the green line is no longer showing; the dose does not need to be inhaled; call for emergency assistance immediately after administering the dose; when the patient responds to treatment, administer oral carbohydrates; do not attempt to reuse the device (each device contains only 1 dose of *glucagon*); if there has been no response after 15 minutes, administer an additional 3 mg using an unused device
Pediatric: <4 years: not approved; ≥4 years: same as adult
  Baqsimi *Intranasal device:* 3 mg pwdr, single-dose
  Comment: Baqsimi is a nasally administered antihypoglycemic agent indicated for the treatment of severe hypoglycemia in diabetes patients ≥4 years of age. Pheochromocytoma (Baqsimi may stimulate the release of catecholamines from the tumor) and insulinoma (Baqsimi may stimulate exaggerated insulin release from an insulinoma) are contraindications to Baqsimi use. Patients taking a beta-blocker may experience a transient increase in HR and BP. For patients taking *indomethacin*, Baqsimi may lose its ability to raise glucose or may produce hypoglycemia. Baqsimi may increase the anticoagulant effect of *warfarin*. Baqsimi is effective in treating hypoglycemia only if sufficient hepatic glycogen is present. Patients in states of starvation, with adrenal insufficiency, or chronic hypoglycemia may not have adequate levels of hepatic glycogen for Baqsimi to be effective; therefore, patients with any of these conditions should be treated with glucose. The most common (incidence ≥10%) adverse reactions associated with Baqsimi are nausea, vomiting, headache, upper respiratory tract irritation (i.e., rhinorrhea, nasal discomfort, nasal congestion, cough, and epistaxis), watery eyes, redness of eyes, and itchy nose, throat, and eyes.

GLUCAGON ANALOG
▶ *dasiglucagon* 0.6 mg SC into the outer upper arm, lower abdomen, thigh, or buttocks; if there has been no response after 15 minutes, an additional dose from a new device may be administered while waiting for emergency assistance; when the patient has responded to treatment, give oral carbohydrates
Pediatric: <6 years: safety and efficacy not established; ≥6 years: same as adult
  Zegalogue *Prefilled syringe:* 0.6 mg/0.6 ml, single-dose; *Autoinjector:* 0.6 mg/0.6 ml, single-dose
  Comment: Zegalogue is a glucagon analog for the treatment of severe hypoglycemia in patients with diabetes. Contraindications to Zegalogue include pheochromocytoma and insulinoma. In patients with pheochromocytoma, Zegalogue may stimulate the release of catecholamines from the tumor. In patients with insulinoma, Zegalogue may produce an initial increase in blood glucose, but then stimulate exaggerated insulin release from an insulinoma, causing subsequent hypoglycemia. If the patient develops symptoms of hypoglycemia after a dose of Zegalogue, administer glucose orally or intravenously. Zegalogue is effective in treating hypoglycemia only if sufficient hepatic glycogen is present. Patients in states of starvation or with adrenal insufficiency or chronic hypoglycemia may not have adequate levels of hepatic glycogen for Zegalogue to be effective and patients with these conditions should be treated with glucose. Drug interactions with Zegalogue include beta-blockers, *indomethacin*, and *warfarin*. Patients taking a beta-blocker may have a transient increase in HR and BP. With patients taking *indomethacin*, Zegalogue may lose its ability to raise serum glucose or may produce hypoglycemia. Co-administration of Zegalogue with *warfarin* may increase *warfarin's* anticoagulant effect. The most common adverse reactions (incidence ≥2%) associated with Zegalogue have been the following: *Adult:* nausea, vomiting, headache, diarrhea, and injection site pain; *Pediatric:* nausea, vomiting, headache, and injection site pain. Allergic reactions have been reported with glucagon products. These reactions may include generalized rash, and in some cases anaphylactic shock with breathing difficulties and hypotension. There are no available data on *dasiglucagon* use in pregnant women to evaluate for a drug-associated risk of major birth defects, miscarriage, or adverse maternal or

embryo/fetal outcomes. In animal reproduction studies, daily SC administration of *dasiglucagon* during the period of organogenesis did not cause adverse developmental effects at exposures 7 and 709 times the human dose of 0.6 mg based on area under the curve (AUC), respectively. There is no information on the presence of *dasiglucagon* in either human or animal milk or effects on the breastfed infant. *Dasiglucagon* is a peptide and would be expected to be broken down to its constituent amino acids in the infant's digestive tract and is therefore unlikely to cause harm to the exposed infant.

NONDIURETIC BENZOTHIADIAZINE DERIVATIVE
➤ *diazoxide* (G)

Proglycem *Cap:* 50 mg; *Oral susp:* 50 mg/ml (chocolate mint) (sodium benzoate) (alcohol 7.25%)
Comment: Proglycem is useful in the management of hypoglycemia due to hyperinsulinism associated with the following conditions: *Adults:* inoperable islet cell adenoma or carcinoma, or extrapancreatic malignancy; *Infants and children:* leucine sensitivity, islet cell hyperplasia, nesidioblastosis, extrapancreatic malignancy, islet cell adenoma, or adenomatosis. Proglycem may be used preoperatively as a temporary measure and postoperatively if hypoglycemia persists. Treatment with Proglycem should be initiated under close clinical supervision, with careful monitoring of blood glucose and clinical response until the patient's condition has stabilized. This usually requires several days. If not effective in 2 to 3 weeks, Proglycem should be discontinued. Proglycem-induced hyperglycemia is reversed by the administration of insulin or *tolbutamide*. The inhibition of insulin release by Proglycem is antagonized by alpha-adrenergic blocking agents. The antidiuretic property of *diazoxide* may lead to significant fluid retention, which in patients with compromised cardiac reserve may precipitate congestive heart failure (CHF). The fluid retention will respond to conventional therapy with diuretics. There have been postmarketing reports of pulmonary hypertension occurring in infants and neonates treated with *diazoxide*. The cases were reversible upon discontinuation of the drug. Monitor patients, especially those with risk factors for pulmonary hypertension, for respiratory distress and discontinue *diazoxide* if pulmonary hypertension is suspected. Development of abnormal facial features in four children treated chronically (>4 years) with Proglycem for hypoglycemia hyperinsulinism has been reported. *Diazoxide* is highly bound to serum proteins (>90%) and therefore may displace other substances which are also protein-bound, such as bilirubin or *coumarin* and its derivatives, resulting in higher blood levels of these substances. Concomitant administration of oral *diazoxide* and *diphenylhydantoin* may result in a loss of seizure control. IV administration of Proglycem during labor may cause cessation of uterine contractions, and administration of oxytocic agents may be required to reinstate labor; caution is advised in administering Proglycem at that time. *Diazoxide* crosses the placental barrier and appears in cord blood. When given to the mother prior to delivery of the infant, the drug may produce fetal or neonatal hyperbilirubinemia, thrombocytopenia, altered carbohydrate metabolism, and possibly other side effects that have occurred in adults. Alopecia and hypertrichosis lanuginosa have occurred in infants whose mothers received oral *diazoxide* during the last 19-60 days of pregnancy. Reproduction animal studies using the oral preparation have revealed increased fetal resorptions and delayed parturition, as well as fetal skeletal anomalies; evidence of skeletal and cardiac teratogenic effects have also been noted with IV administration. Proglycem has also been demonstrated to cross the placental barrier in animals and to cause degeneration of the fetal pancreatic beta cells. When use of Proglycem is considered, potential benefits to the mother must be weighed against possible harmful effects to the fetus. Information is not available concerning the passage of diazoxide in breast milk. Because many drugs are excreted in human milk and because of the potential for adverse reactions from *diazoxide* in nursing infants, a decision should be made whether to discontinue nursing or to discontinue the drug, taking into account the importance of the drug to the mother.

HYPOKALEMIA

Comment: Normal serum K+ range is approximately 3.5-5.5 mEq/L. Signs and symptoms of hypokalemia include neuromuscular weakness, muscle twitching and cramping, hyporeflexia, postural hypotension, anorexia, nausea and vomiting, depressed ST segments, flattened T waves, and cardiac tachyarrhythmias. Signs and symptoms of hyperkalemia include peaked T waves, elevated ST segment, and widened QRS complexes.

PROPHYLAXIS
Comment: Usual dose range is 8-10 mEq/day.

TREATMENT OF HYPOKALEMIA: NON-EMERGENCY (K+ <3.5 mEq/L)
Comment: Usual dose range 40-120 mEq/day in divided doses. Solutions are preferred; potentially serious GI side effects may occur with tablet formulations or when taken on an empty stomach.

POTASSIUM SUPPLEMENTS
Comment: Potassium supplements should be taken with food. Solutions are the preferred form. Extended-release and sustained-release forms should be swallowed whole; do not crush or chew. Potassium supplementation is indicated for hypokalemia, including that caused by diuretic use, and digitalis intoxication without atrioventricular (AV) block.

(continued)

▷ *potassium* (G)
  Pediatric: <12 years: not established; ≥12 years: same as adult
    KCL Solution *Oral soln:* 10% (30 ml unit dose, 50/case)
    K-Dur (as chloride) *Tab:* 10, 20* mEq sust-rel
    K-Lor for Oral Solution (as chloride) *Pkts for reconstitution:* 20 mEq/pkt (fruit)
    Klor-Con/25 (as chloride) *Pkts for reconstitution:* 25 mEq/pkt
    Klor-Con/EF 25 (as bicarbonate) *Pkts for reconstitution:* 25 mEq/pkt (effervescent) (fruit)
    Klor-Con Extended-Release (as chloride) *Tab:* 8, 10 mEq ext-rel
    Klor-Con M (as chloride) *Tab:* 10, 15*, 20* mEq ext-rel
    Klor-Con Powder (as chloride) 20, 25 mEq *Pkts for reconstitution:* (30/carton) (fruit)
    Klorvess (as bicarbonate and citrate) *Tab:* 20 mEq effervescent for solution; *Granules:* 20 mEq/pkt
      effervescent for solution; *Oral liq:* 20 mEq/15 ml (16 oz)
    Klotrix (as chloride) *Tab:* 10 mEq sust-rel
    K-Lyte (as bicarbonate and citrate) *Tab:* 25 mEq effervescent for solution (lime, orange)
    K-Lyte/CL (as chloride) *Tab:* 25 mEq effervescent for solution (citrus, fruit)
    K-Lyte/CL 50 (as chloride) *Tab:* 50 mEq effervescent for solution (citrus, fruit)
    K-Lyte/DS (as bicarbonate and citrate) *Tab:* 50 mEq effervescent for solution (lime, orange)
    K-Tab (as chloride) *Tab:* 10 mEq sust-rel
    Micro-K (as chloride) *Cap:* 8, 10 mEq sust-rel
    Potassium Chloride Extended Release Caps *Cap:* 8, 10 mEq ext-rel
    Potassium Chloride Sust-Rel Tabs *Tab/Cap:* 10 mEq sust-rel
    Potassium Chloride ER *Tab:* 8 mEq (600 mg), 10 mEq (750 mg)

HYPOMAGNESEMIA

Comment: Normal serum Mg^{++} range is approximately 1.2-2.6 mEq/L. Signs and symptoms of hypomagnesemia include confusion, disorientation, hallucinations, hyperreflexia, tetany, convulsions, tachyarrhythmia, positive Chvostek's sign, and positive Trousseau's sign. Signs and symptoms of hypermagnesemia include drowsiness, lethargy, muscle weakness, hypoactive reflexes, slurred speech, bradycardia, hypotension, convulsions, and cardiac arrhythmias.

MAGNESIUM SUPPLEMENTS
▷ *magnesium* 2 tabs daily
  Slow-Mag
    Tab: 64 mg (as chloride)+110 mg (as carbonate)
▷ *magnesium oxide* 1-2 tabs daily
  Mag-Ox 400
    Tab: 400 mg

HYPOPARATHYROIDISM

VITAMIN D ANALOGS
Comment: Concurrent vitamin D supplementation is contraindicated in patients taking *calcitriol* or *doxercalciferol* owing to the risk of vitamin D toxicity.
▷ *calcitriol* initially 0.25 mcg q AM; may increase by 0.25 mcg/day at 4 to 8-week intervals; usual maintenance
  0.5-2 mcg/day
  Pediatric: initially 0.25 mcg daily; may increase by 0.25 mcg/day at 2 to 4-week intervals; usual maintenance:
  1-5 years: 0.25-0.75 mcg/day; ≥6 years: 0.5-2 mcg/day
    Rocaltrol *Cap:* 0.25, 0.5 mcg
    Rocaltrol Solution *Soln:* 1 mcg/ml (15 ml, single-use dispensers)
▷ *doxercalciferol* initially 0.25 mcg q AM; may increase by 0.25 mcg/day at 4 to 8-week intervals; usual
  maintenance 0.5-2 mcg/day
  Pediatric: initially 0.25 mcg daily; may increase by 0.25 mcg/day at 2 to 4-week intervals; usual maintenance:
  1-5 years: 0.25-0.75 mcg/day; ≥6 years: 0.5-2 mcg/day
    Hectorol *Cap:* 0.25, 0.5 mcg

HUMAN PARATHYROID HORMONE
▷ *teriparatide* 20 mcg SC daily in the thigh or abdomen; may treat for up to 2 years
    Forteo *Multidose pen:* 250 mcg/ml (3 ml)
    Comment: Forteo is indicated for the treatment of postmenopausal osteoporosis in women who are at high
    risk for fracture and to increase bone mass in men with primary or hypogonadal osteoporosis who are at
    high risk for fracture.

HUMAN PARATHYROID HORMONE-RELATED PEPTIDE (PTHrP) ANALOG
▷ *abaloparatide* administer 80 mcg SC once daily into the periumbilical region of the abdomen; sit or lie
  down in case of orthostatic hypotension, especially for first dose; patients should receive supplemental
  calcium and vitamin D if dietary intake is inadequate

Tymlos *Multidose pen:* 3,120 mcg/1.56 ml (2,000 mcg/ml, 30 daily doses) disposable

Comment: **Tymlos** is indicated to increase bone density in adult men and menopausal women who are at high risk for fracture (defined as a history of osteoporotic fracture, or multiple risk factors for fracture, or patients who have failed or are intolerant to other available osteoporosis therapy). **Tymlos** is not indicated for use in females of reproductive potential. There are no human data with use in pregnant females to inform any drug-associated risks, and animal reproduction studies with *abaloparatide* have not been conducted. There is no information on the presence of *abaloparatide* in human milk or effects on the breastfed infant; however, breastfeeding is not recommended while using **Tymlos**. **Tymlos** is not recommended in patients who are at risk for osteosarcoma (boxed warning). Cumulative use of **Tymlos** or other parathyroid analogs (e.g., *teriparatide*) for >2 years during a patient's lifetime is not recommended (boxed warning). Avoid use in patients with preexisting hypercalcemia and those known to have an underlying hypercalcemic disorder, such as primary hyperparathyroidism. Monitor urine calcium if preexisting hypercalciuria or active urolithiasis is suspected.

BIOENGINEERED REPLICA OF HUMAN PARATHYROID HORMONE

➤ *bioengineered replica of human parathyroid hormone* initially inject mg IM into the thigh once daily; when initiating, decrease dose of active vitamin D by 50% if serum calcium is above 7.5 mg/day; monitor serum calcium levels every 3-7 days after starting or adjusting dose and when adjusting either active vitamin D or calcium supplement dose

Natpara *Soln for inj:* 25, 50, 75, 100 mcg (2/pkg), multi-dose, dual-chamber glass cartridge containing a sterile powder and diluent

Comment: **Natpara** is indicated as an adjunct to calcium and vitamin D in patients with parathyroidism.

HYPOPHOSPHATASIA (OSTEOMALACIA, RICKETS)

Comment: Hypophosphatasia (HPP) is an inborn error of metabolism marked by abnormally low serum alkaline phosphatase activity and phosphoethanolamine in the urine. It is manifested by osteomalacia in adults and rickets in infants and children. It is most severe in infants under 6 months of age. With congenital absence of alkaline phosphatase, an enzyme essential to the calcification of bone tissue, complications include vomiting, growth retardation, and often death in infancy. Surviving children have numerous skeletal abnormalities and dwarfism.

➤ *asfotase alfa* 6 mg/kg/week SC, administered as 2 mg/kg or 1 mg/kg 6 x/week; max 9 mg/kg/week SC administered as 3 mg/kg 3 x/week

Pediatric: same as adult

Strensiq *Vial:* 18 mg/0.45 ml, 28 mg/0.7 ml, 40 mg/ml, 80 mg/0.8 ml for SC inj, single-use (1, 12/carton) (preservative-free)

Comment: **Strensiq** is the first FDA-approved (2015) treatment for perinatal, infantile, and juvenile onset HPP. Prior to the availability of **Strensiq**, there was no effective treatment and patient prognosis was very poor.

HYPOPHOSPHATEMIA, X-LINKED (XLH)

FIBROBLAST GROWTH FACTOR (FGF23)-BLOCKING ANTIBODY

➤ *burosumab-twza* 1 mg/kg body weight rounded to the nearest 10 mg up to max dose of 90 mg administered q 4 weeks

Pediatric: <1 year: not recommended; ≥1-17 years: starting dose 0.8 mg/kg rounded to the nearest 10 mg; min starting dose 10 mg; max dose 90 mg; administer SC q 2 weeks; dose may be increased up to approximately 2 mg/kg (max 90 mg), administered q 2 weeks to achieve normal serum phosphorus; ≥18 years: same as adult

Crysvita *Vial:* 10, 20, 30 mg/ml (1 ml), single-dose

Comment: The most common adverse side effects associated with **Crysvita** in pediatric X-linked hypophosphatemia (XLH) patients are headache, injection site reaction, vomiting, pyrexia, pain in extremity, and decreased serum vitamin D. The most common adverse side effects associated with **Crysvita** in patients with XLH ≥18 years of age are back pain, headache, tooth infection, restless leg syndrome, dizziness, constipation, decreased serum vitamin D, and increased serum phosphorus. There are no available data on *burosumab-twza* use to inform a drug-associated risk of adverse developmental outcomes in pregnancy. There are no data to inform the presence of *burosumab-twza* in human milk or effects on the breastfed infant.

HYPOTENSION: NEUROGENIC, ORTHOSTATIC

ALPHA-1 AGONIST

➤ *midodrine* (G) 10 mg tid at 3 to 4 hour intervals; take while upright; take last dose at least 4 hours before bedtime

Pediatric: <12 years: not recommended; ≥12 years: same as adult

ProAmatine *Tab:* 2.5*, 5*, 10*mg

SYNTHETIC AMINO ACID PRECURSOR OF NOREPINEPHRINE

▷ *droxidopa* (G) initially 100 mg, taken 3 tid (upon arising in the morning, at midday, and in the late afternoon at least 3 hours prior to bedtime to reduce the potential for supine hypertension during sleep); administer with or without; swallow whole; titrate to symptomatic response in increments of 100 mg tid every 24-48 hours; max 600 mg tid (max total 1,800 mg/day)
Pediatric: <12 years: not recommended; ≥12 years: same as adult
  Northera *Cap:* 100, 200, 300 mg
  Comment: Northera is indicated for the treatment of orthostatic dizziness, lightheadedness, or feeling about to black out in adult patients with symptomatic neurogenic orthostatic hypotension (NOH) caused by primary autonomic failure (Parkinson's disease [PD], multiple system atrophy [MSA], and pure autonomic failure), dopamine beta-hydroxylase deficiency, and non-diabetic autonomic neuropathy. Effectiveness beyond 2 weeks of treatment has not been established. The continued effectiveness of **Northera** should be assessed. Administering **Northera** in combination with other agents that increase blood pressure (e.g., norepinephrine, ephedrine, midodrine, triptans) would be expected to increase the risk for supine hypertension.

HYPOTHYROIDISM

Comment: Take thyroid replacement hormone in the morning on an empty stomach. For the elderly, start thyroid hormone replacement at 25 mcg/day. Target thyroid-stimulating hormone (TSH) is 0.4-5.5 mIU/L; target T4 is 4.5-12.5 ng/L. Signs and symptoms of thyroid toxicity include tachycardia, palpitations, nervousness, chest pain, heat intolerance, and weight loss.

ORAL THYROID HORMONE SUPPLEMENTS
T3
▷ *liothyronine* initially 25 mcg daily; may increase by 25 mcg every 1-2 weeks as needed; usual maintenance 25-75 mcg/day
Pediatric: initially 5 mcg/day; may increase by 5 mcg/day every 3-4 days; *Cretinism:* maintenance dose: <1 year: 20 mcg/day; 1-3 years: 50 mcg/day; >3 years: same as adult
  Cytomel *Tab:* 5, 25, 50 mcg

T4
▷ *levothyroxine* (G)
  Levoxyl initially 25-100 mcg/day; increase by 25 mcg/day q 2-3 weeks as needed; maintenance 100-200 mcg/day
  Pediatric: <6 months: 8-10 mcg/kg/day; 6-12 months: 6-8 mcg/kg/day; >1-5 years: 5-6 mcg/kg/day; 6-12 years: 4-5 mcg/kg/day; >12 years: same as adult
    Tab: 25*, 50* (dye-free), 75*, 88*, 100*, 112*, 125*, 137*, 150*, 175*, 200*, 300*mcg
  Synthroid initially 50 mcg/day; increase by 25 mcg/day q 2-3 weeks as needed; max 300 mcg/day
  Pediatric: <6 months: 8-10 mcg/kg/day; 6-12 months: 6-8 mcg/kg/day; >1-5 years: 5-6 mcg/kg/day; 6-12 years: 4-5 mcg/kg/day; >12 years: same as adult
    Tab: 25*, 50* (dye-free), 75*, 88*, 100*, 112*, 125*, 137*, 150*, 175*, 200*, 300*mcg
  Tirosint/Tirosint-Sol starting dose depends on a variety of factors, including age, body weight, cardiovascular status, concomitant medical conditions (including pregnancy), concomitant medications, co-administered food, and specific nature of the condition being treated; peak therapeutic effect may not be attained for 4-6 weeks
  Pediatric: 0-3 months: 10-15 mcg/kg/day; 3-6 months: 8-10 mcg/kg/day; 6-12 months: 6-8 mcg/kg/day; 1-5 years: 5-6 mcg/kg/day; 6-12 years: 4-5 mcg/kg/day; >12 years, growth and puberty incomplete: 12-3 mcg/kg/day; growth and puberty complete: 1.7 mcg/kg/day
    Tirosint *Cap:* 0.013, 0.025, 0.0375, 0.044, 0.05, 0.0625, 0.075, 0.088, 0.1, 0.112, 0.125, 0.137, 0.15, 0.175, 0.2 mg
    Tirosint-Sol *Oral sol:* 12, 25, 37.5, 44, 50, 62.5, 75, 88, 100, 112, 125, 137, 150, 175, 200 ml
  Unithroid initially 50 mcg/day; increase by 25 mcg/day every 2-3 weeks as needed; max 300 mcg/day
  Pediatric: 0-3 months: 10-15 mcg/kg/day; 3-6 months: 8-10 mcg/kg/day; 6-12 months: 6-8 mcg/kg/day; 1-5 years: 5-6 mcg/kg/day; 6-12 years: 4-5 mcg/kg/day; >12 years: 2-3 mcg/kg/day; growth and puberty complete: same as adult
    Tab: 25*, 50* (dye-free), 75*, 88*, 100*, 112*, 125*, 150*, 175*, 200*, 300*mcg

T3+T4 Combination
▷ *liothyronine+levothyroxine* initially 15-30 mg/day; increase by 15 mg/day q 2-3 weeks to target goal; usual maintenance 60-120 mg/day
Pediatric: <6 months: 4.6-6 mcg/kg/day; 6-12 months: 3.6-4.8 mcg/kg/day; >1-5 years: 3-3.6 mcg/kg/day; 6-12 years: 2.4-3 mcg/kg/day; >12 years: 1.2-1.8 mcg/kg/day; growth and puberty complete: same as adult
  Armour Thyroid Tab *Tab:* per grain: T3 9 mcg+T4 38 mcg: ¼, ½, 1, 1, 2, 3*, 4*, 5* gr; 15, 30, 60, 90, 120, 180*, 240*, 300*mg
  Thyrolar *Tab:* per grain: T3 12.5 mcg+T4 50 mcg: 1/4, 1/5, 1, 2, 3 gr

PARENTERAL THYROID HORMONE SUPPLEMENT

➤ *levothyroxine sodium* (G) 1/2 oral dose by IV or IM and titrate; *Myxedema Coma:* 200-500 mcg IV x 1 dose; may administer 100-300 mcg (or more) IV on the second day if needed; then 50-100 mcg IV daily; switch to oral form as soon as possible
Pediatric: <12 years: not recommended; ≥12 years: same as adult
T4 *Vial:* 100, 200, 500 mcg (pwdr for IM or IV administration after reconstitution)

HYPOTRICHOSIS (THIN/SPARSE EYELASHES)

PROSTAGLANDIN ANALOG

➤ *bimatoprost* ophthalmic solution (G) apply 1 drop nightly directly to the skin of the upper eyelid margin at the base of the eyelashes using the accompanying applicators; blot any excess solution beyond the eyelid margin; dispose of the applicator after one use; repeat for the opposite eyelid margin using a new sterile applicator; repeat treatment of the opposite eye using a new applicator
Pediatric: <16 years: not recommended; ≥16 years: same as adult
Latisse *Ophth soln:* 0.03% (3 ml in 5 ml bottle w. 70 disposable sterile applicators; 5 ml in 5 ml bottle w. 140 disposable sterile applicators)
Comment: Latisse is indicated for treatment of hypotrichosis of the eyelashes by increasing their growth, including length, thickness, and darkness. Ensure the face is clean, all makeup is removed, and contact lenses removed. Place 1 drop of **Latisse** on the disposable sterile applicator and brush cautiously along the skin of the upper eyelid margin at the base of the eyelashes. Do not to apply to the lower eyelash line. If eyelid skin darkening occurs, it may be reversible after discontinuation of **Latisse**. If any **Latisse** solution gets into the eye proper, it will not cause harm; the eye should not be rinsed. Any excess solution outside the upper eyelid margin should be blotted with a tissue or other absorbent material. Onset of effect is gradual but is not significant in the majority of patients until 2 months. The effect is not permanent and can be expected to gradually return to previous. Additional applications of **Latisse** will not increase the growth of eyelashes.

IDIOPATHIC (IMMUNE) THROMBOCYTOPENIA PURPURA (ITP)

IMMUNOGLOBULIN INTRAVENOUS (IGIV), HUMAN

➤ *immune globulin intravenous (human) Dose:* 2 g/kg divided in equal doses administered over 2 consecutive days; *Initial infusion rate:* 1 mg/kg/min (0.01 ml/kg/min); *Maintenance infusion rate:* up to 12 mg/kg/min (up to 0.12 ml/kg/min); in patients >65 years or in any person at risk of developing renal insufficiency, do not exceed the recommended dose and infuse **Octagam** 10% at the minimum infusion rate practical
Pediatric: safety and efficacy not established
Octagam 10% IgG 100 mg/ml, soln for IV infusion (vol: 20, 50, 100, 200, 300 ml) (protein: 2, 5, 10, 20, 30 gm, respectively)
Comment: **Octagam** is a ready-to-use immunoglobulin intravenous (IGIV) product indicated for the treatment of primary humoral immunodeficiency, chronic immune thrombocytopenic purpura (ITP), and dermatomyositis. The most common adverse reactions reported (>5% of subjects during a clinical trial) in patients treated for chronic ITP have been headache, fever, and increased heart rate. *Boxed Warning: thrombosis, renal dysfunction, acute renal failure (ARF).* Thrombosis may occur with IGIV products, including **Octagam 10%**. Risk factors may include advanced age, prolonged immobilization, hypercoagulable conditions, history of venous or arterial thrombosis, use of estrogens, indwelling vascular catheters, hyperviscosity, and cardiovascular risk factors. Renal dysfunction, ARF, osmotic nephropathy, and death may occur with the administration of IGIV products in predisposed patients. Renal dysfunction and ARF occur more commonly in patients receiving IGIV products containing sucrose. **Octagam 10%** does not contain sucrose. For patients at risk of thrombosis, renal dysfunction, or renal failure, administer **Octagam 10%** at the minimum practical infusion rate. Ensure adequate hydration in patients before administration. Monitor for signs and symptoms of thrombosis and assess blood viscosity in patients at risk for hyperviscosity. **Octagam 10%** is contraindicated with patient history of anaphylactic or severe systemic reactions to human immunoglobulin, immunoglobulin A (IgA)-deficient patients with antibodies against IgA, and a history of hypersensitivity. IgA-deficient patients with antibodies against IgA are at greater risk of developing severe hypersensitivity and anaphylactic reactions to **Octagam 10%**; epinephrine should be available immediately to treat any severe acute hypersensitivity reaction. Monitor renal function, including blood urea nitrogen (BUN) and serum creatinine (sCr), and urine output in patients at risk of developing ARF. Falsely elevated blood glucose readings may occur during and after the infusion of **Octagam 10%**. Hyperproteinemia, increased serum osmolarity, and hyponatremia may occur in patients receiving **Octagam 10%**. Hemolysis that is either intravascular or due to enhanced red blood cell sequestration can develop subsequent to **Octagam 10%** treatments. Risk factors for hemolysis include high doses and non-O-blood group; closely monitor patients for hemolysis and hemolytic anemia. Aseptic meningitis

(continued)

syndrome (AMS) may occur, especially with high doses or rapid infusion. Monitor patients for pulmonary adverse reactions (transfusion-related acute lung injury [TRALI]). **Octagam 10%** is made from human plasma and may contain infectious agents (e.g., viruses and theoretically the Creutzfeldt-Jakob disease [CJD] agent). The passive transfer of antibodies may confound the results of serologic testing and interfere with the immune response to live viral vaccines (such as measles, mumps, and rubella). There are no human or animal data; use only if clearly needed. It is not known whether **Octagam 10%** can cause fetal harm when administered to a pregnant patient or can affect reproduction capacity. Immune globulins cross the placenta from maternal circulation increasingly after 30 weeks of gestation. **Octagam 10%** should be administered to pregnant women only if clearly needed. No human data are available to assess the presence or absence of **Octagam 10%** in human milk or effects of **Octagam 10%** on the breastfed infant. Developmental and health benefits of breastfeeding should be considered along with the mother's clinical need for **Octagam 10%** and any potential adverse effects on the breastfed infant from **Octagam 10%** or from the underlying maternal condition. Immunoglobulins are excreted into the milk and may contribute to the transfer of protective antibodies to the neonate.

SPLEEN TYROSINE KINASE (SYK) INHIBITOR

▷ *fostamatinib disodium hexahydrate* initially 100 mg bid; increase to 150 mg bid if platelet count not at ≥50 x 10^9/L after 4 weeks; discontinue if insufficient increase in platelet count after 12 weeks; for dose modifications, see mfr pkg insert

Pediatric: <18 years: not recommended; ≥18 years: same as adult

Tavalisse *Tab:* 100, 150 mg

Comment: Tavalisse (*fostamatinib*) is an oral spleen tyrosine kinase (SYK) inhibitor for the treatment of patients with chronic immune thrombocytopenia (ITP). Monitor complete blood counts (CBCs), including platelets, monthly until stable count (≥50 x 10^9/L) achieved, then periodically thereafter. Monitor liver function tests (LFTs) monthly. Discontinue if AST/ALT >5 x ULN for ≥2 weeks or >3 x ULN7 and total bilirubin >2 x ULN. Monitor blood pressure (BP) every 2 weeks until stable dose established, then monthly thereafter. Interrupt or discontinue dose if hypertensive crisis (>180/120 mm Hg) occurs; discontinue if repeat BP >160/100 mm Hg for >4 weeks. Temporarily interrupt if severe diarrhea (grade ≥3) occurs; resume at next lower daily dose if improved to grade 1. Monitor absolute neutrophil count (ANC) monthly and for signs/symptoms of infection. Temporarily interrupt if ANC <1 x 10^9/L occurs and remains low after 72 hours until resolved; resume at next lower daily dose. Use lowest effective dose. Due to potential for embryo/fetal toxicity, use effective contraception during and for ≥1 month after last dose. Confirm negative pregnancy status prior to initiation. Breastfeeding not recommended (during and for ≥1 month after last dose). Concomitant strong CYP3A4 inducers not recommended. Concomitant strong CYP3A4 inhibitors or substrates, monitor for toxicity. May potentiate concomitant breast cancer resistance protein (BCRP) (e.g., *rosuvastatin*) or P-glycoprotein (P-gp) (e.g., *digoxin*) substrates, monitor for toxicity. Adverse reactions include diarrhea, hypertension, nausea, respiratory infection, dizziness, ALT/AST increase, rash, abdominal pain, fatigue, chest pain, and neutropenia.

IMMUNODEFICIENCY: PRIMARY HUMORAL (PHI), CONGENITAL AGAMMAGLOBULINEMIA, COMMON VARIABLE IMMUNODEFICIENCY, X-LINKED AGAMMAGLOBULINEMIA, WISKOTT-ALDRICH SYNDROME, CHRONIC IMMUNE THROMBOCYTOPENIA PURPURA (ITP), DERMATOMYOSITIS

IMMUNOGLOBULIN INTRAVENOUS (IGIV), HUMAN

▷ *immune globulin intravenous (human) Dose:* 2 gm/kg divided in equal doses administered over 2 consecutive days; *Initial infusion rate:* 1 mg/kg/min (0.01 ml/kg/min); *Maintenance infusion rate:* up to 12 mg/kg/min (up to 0.12 ml/kg/min); in patients >65 years or in any person at risk of developing renal insufficiency, do not exceed the recommended dose and infuse **Octagam 10%** at the minimum infusion rate practical

Pediatric: safety and efficacy not established

Octagam 10% IgG 100 mg/ml, soln for IV infusion (vol: 20, 50, 100, 200, 300 ml) (protein: 2, 5, 10, 20, 30 gm, respectively)

Comment: Octagam is a ready-to-use immunoglobulin intravenous (IGIV) (human) 5% liquid indicated for treatment of PHI, such as congenital agammaglobulinemia, CVID, X-linked agammaglobulinemia, Wiskott-Aldrich syndrome and severe combined immunodeficiencies, chronic immune thrombocytopenic purpura (ITP), and dermatomyositis. The most common adverse reactions reported (>5% of subjects during a clinical trial) in patients treated for dermatomyositis were headache, fever, nausea, vomiting, increased blood pressure, chills, musculoskeletal pain, increased heart rate, dyspnea, and infusions site reactions. *Boxed Warning: thrombosis, renal dysfunction, acute renal failure (ARF).* Thrombosis may occur with immune globulin intravenous (IGIV) products, including **Octagam 10%**. Risk factors may include advanced age, prolonged immobilization, hypercoagulable conditions, history of venous or arterial thrombosis, use of estrogens, indwelling vascular catheters, hyperviscosity, and cardiovascular risk factors. Renal dysfunction, ARF, osmotic nephropathy, and death may occur with the administration of IGIV products in predisposed patients. Renal dysfunction and ARF occur more commonly in patients receiving IGIV products containing sucrose. **Octagam 10%** does not contain sucrose. For patients at risk of thrombosis, renal dysfunction, or renal failure, administer **Octagam 10%** at the minimum practical infusion rate. Ensure adequate hydration in patients before administration. Monitor for signs and symptoms of thrombosis and assess blood viscosity in patients at risk for hyperviscosity. **Octagam 10%** is contraindicated with patient history of anaphylactic or severe systemic reactions to human immunoglobulin, immunoglobulin A (IgA)-deficient patients with antibodies against IgA, and a history of hypersensitivity. IgA-deficient patients with antibodies against IgA are at greater risk of developing severe hypersensitivity and anaphylactic reactions to **Octagam 10%**; epinephrine should be available immediately to treat any severe acute hypersensitivity reaction. Monitor renal function, including blood urea nitrogen (BUN) and serum creatinine (sCr), and urine output in patients at risk of developing ARF; falsely elevated blood glucose readings may occur during and after the infusion of **Octagam 10%**. Hyperproteinemia, increased serum osmolarity, and hyponatremia may occur in patients receiving **Octagam 10%**. Hemolysis that is either intravascular or due to enhanced red blood cell (RBC) sequestration can develop subsequent to **Octagam 10%** treatments. Risk factors for hemolysis include high doses and non-O-blood group; closely monitor patients for hemolysis and hemolytic anemia. Aseptic meningitis syndrome (AMS) may occur, especially with high doses or rapid infusion. Monitor patients for pulmonary adverse reactions (transfusion-related acute lung injury [TRALI]). **Octagam 10%** is made from human plasma and may contain infectious agents (e.g. viruses and theoretically the Creutzfeldt-Jakob disease [CJD] agent). The passive transfer of antibodies may confound the results of serologic testing and interfere with the immune response to live viral vaccines (such as measles, mumps, and rubella). There are no human or animal data; use only if clearly needed. It is not known whether **Octagam 10%** can cause fetal harm when administered to a pregnant patient or can affect reproduction capacity. Immune globulins cross the placenta from maternal circulation increasingly after 30 weeks of gestation. **Octagam 10%** should be administered to pregnant women only if clearly needed. No human data are available to assess the presence or absence of **Octagam 10%** in human milk or effects of **Octagam 10%** on the breastfed infant. Developmental and health benefits of breastfeeding should be considered along with the mother's clinical need for **Octagam 10%** and any potential adverse effects on the breastfed infant from **Octagam 10%** or from the underlying maternal condition. Immunoglobulins are excreted into the milk and may contribute to the transfer of protective antibodies to the neonate.

IMMUNE GLOBULIN, HUMAN

▶ *immune globulin intravenous, human–slra* 300-800 mg/kg via IV infusion q 3-4 weeks; rate 0.5 mg/kg/min (0.005 ml/kg/min) for the first 15 minutes; then increase rate gradually q 5 minutes as tolerated; max 8 mg/kg/min (0.08 ml/kg/min); ≥65 years of age: infuse **Asceniv** at the minimum infusion rate practicable; monitor renal function, including BUN, sCr, and urine output; ensure that patients with preexisting renal insufficiency are not volume-depleted; discontinue **Asceniv** if renal function deteriorates; for patients at risk of renal dysfunction or thrombotic events, administer **Asceniv** at the minimum infusion rate practicable; IgA-deficient patients with antibodies against IgA are at greater risk of developing severe hypersensitivity and anaphylactic reactions; have epinephrine available to treat any acute severe hypersensitivity reaction

Pediatric: **Asceniv** was evaluated in 11 pediatric subjects (6 children [age 12 years] and 5 adolescents [ages 12-16 years]) with PHI. The pharmacokinetic (PK), safety, and effectiveness profile of **Asceniv** in adolescent subjects appeared to be comparable to that demonstrated in adult subjects. There are insufficient PK, safety, and effectiveness data from pediatric subjects <12 years of age and safety and effectiveness have not been studied in pediatric patients with PHI who are <3 years of age.

Asceniv *Vial:* 5 gm/50 ml (100 mg/ml), single use, liquid solution containing 10% immunoglobulin G (IgG) for IV infusion (preservative-free)

Comment: Asceniv *(immune globulin intravenous, human–slra)* is a 10% immune globulin liquid for IV infusion, indicated for the treatment of PHI in adults and adolescents (12-17 years of age). Clinical studies of **Asceniv** have not included sufficient numbers of subjects ≥65 years of age to determine whether they respond differently from younger subjects. Hyperproteinemia, increased serum viscosity, and hyponatremia or pseudohyponatremia can occur in patients receiving IGIV treatment. AMS has been reported with IGIV treatment, especially with high doses or rapid infusion. Hemolytic anemia can develop subsequent to IGIV treatment; monitor patients for hemolysis and hemolytic anemia. Monitor patients for pulmonary adverse reactions (transfusion-related acute lung injury [TRALI]). If TRALI is suspected, test the product and the patient for antineutrophil antibodies. Because this product is made from human blood, it may carry a risk of transmitting infectious agents, for example, viruses and theoretically the CJD agent. There are no controlled data in human pregnancy. Intact immune globulins cross the placenta increasingly after 30 weeks gestation. Clinical experience with immunoglobulins does not suggest a harmful effect on pregnancy or the fetus. When administered prior to delivery in mothers with immune thrombocytopenic purpura (I~TP), the platelet response and clinical effect were similar in the mother and the neonate.

▶ *immune globulin subcutaneous (human) 20% liquid* administer via SC infusion only; up to 8 infusion sites are allowed simultaneously, with at least 2 inches between sites; *Infusion volume:* for the first infusion, up to 15 ml per injection site; may increase to 20 ml per site after the fourth infusion; max 25 ml per

(continued)

site as tolerated; *Infusion rate:* first infusion, up to 15 ml/hour per site; may increase to max of 25 ml/hour per site as tolerated; however, maximum flow rate is not to exceed a total of 50 ml/hour for all sites combined; before switching to **Hizentra**, obtain the patient's serum IgG trough level to guide subsequent dose adjustments; adjust the dose based on clinical response and serum IgG trough levels; administer at regular intervals from daily up to q 2 week; *Weekly dosing:* start **Hizentra** 1 week after last IGIV human infusion; initial weekly dose: (previous IGIV dose [in grams] x 1.37) divided by number of weeks between IGIV doses; *Biweekly dosing (every 2 weeks):* start **Hizentra** 1 or 2 weeks after the last IGIV infusion or 1 week after the last weekly immune globulin subcutaneous [human] (IGSC) infusion; administer twice the calculated weekly dose; *Frequent dosing (2-7 times per week):* start **Hizentra** 1 week after the last IGIV or IGSC infusion; divide the calculated weekly dose by the desired number of times per week

Pediatric: <12 years: not established; ≥12 years: same as adult

Hizentra *Vial:* 0.2 mg/ml (20%; 5, 10, 20, 50 ml)

Comment: IgA-deficient patients with anti-IgA antibodies are at greater risk of severe hypersensitivity and anaphylactic reactions. Thrombosis may occur following treatment with immune globulin products, including **Hizentra**. AMS has been reported with IGIV and IGSC, including **Hizentra**. Monitor renal function in patients at risk of ARF. Monitor for clinical signs and symptoms of hemolysis. Monitor for pulmonary adverse reactions (TRALI). **Hizentra** is made from human blood and may contain infectious agents (e.g., viruses, the variant Creutzfeldt-Jakob disease [vCJD] agent, and theoretically the Creutzfeldt-Jakob disease [CJD] agent). Monitor for clinical signs and symptoms of hemolysis. The most common adverse reactions observed in ≥5% of study subjects were local infusion site reactions, headache, diarrhea, fatigue, back pain, nausea, pain in extremity, cough, upper respiratory tract infection, rash, pruritus, vomiting, abdominal pain (upper), migraine, arthralgia, pain, fall, and nasopharyngitis. No human or animal reproduction studies have been conducted with **Hizentra**. It is not known whether **Hizentra** can cause fetal harm when administered during pregnancy. No human data are available to inform maternal use of **Hizentra** on the breastfed infant.

IMMUNE GLOBULIN WITH A RECOMBINANT HUMAN HYALURONIDASE

▷ *immune globulin* and *hyaluronidase* Hyqvia should be administered by a qualified healthcare professional or caregiver or self-administered by the patient after appropriate training; suggested site(s) for the SC infusions are the abdomen and thighs; if two sites are used, the two infusion sites should be on opposite sides of the body; avoid bony prominences, or areas that are scarred, inflamed, or infected; administer up to 600 ml per site for patients whose body weight is ≥40 kg and up to 300 ml per site for patients whose body weight is <40 kg; a second site can be used at the discretion of the physician and the patient based on tolerability and total volume; if a second site is used, administer half the total volume of *recombinant human hyaluronidase* of Hyqvia in each site; administer the *recombinant human hyaluronidase* of Hyqvia at an initial rate per site of approximately 1-2 ml per minute or as tolerated; see mfr pkg insert for scheduling infusions (spacing intervals) and for ramping up of successive infusions, product storage, preparation, warnings, precautions, and adverse reactions

Pediatric: <2 years: safety and efficacy not established; ≥2 years: same as adult

Hyqvia *Dual vial unit:* consisting of 1 vial of a liquid solution containing *immune globulin infusion 10% (human)* and 1 vial of a liquid solution containing 160 U/ml *recombinant human hyaluronidase* soln for SC infusion (preservative-free) (natural rubber latex-free)

Comment: Hyqvia is an immune globulin with a *recombinant human hyaluronidase* indicated for the treatment of primary immunodeficiency (PI) in adults and pediatric patients ≥2 years of age. This includes, but is not limited to, CVID, X-linked agammaglobulinemia, congenital agammaglobulinemia, Wiskott-Aldrich syndrome, and severe combined immunodeficiencies. Safety and efficacy of chronic use of *recombinant human hyaluronidase* in Hyqvia have not been established in conditions other than PI or in patients <2 years of age. Hyqvia is contraindicated in (1) patients who have had a history of anaphylactic or severe systemic reactions to the administration of IgG, (2) IgA-deficient patients with antibodies to IgA and a history of hypersensitivity, (3) patients with known systemic hypersensitivity to hyaluronidase including *recombinant human hyaluronidase* of Hyqvia, and (4) patients with known systemic hypersensitivity to human albumin (in the hyaluronidase solution). Thrombosis may occur following treatment with immune globulin products, including Hyqvia. Risk factors may include advanced age, prolonged immobilization, hypercoagulable conditions, history of venous or arterial thrombosis, use of estrogens, indwelling central vascular catheters, hyperviscosity, and cardiovascular risk factors. Thrombosis may occur in the absence of known risk factors. For patients at risk of thrombosis, administer Hyqvia at the minimum dose and infusion rate practicable. Ensure adequate hydration in patients before administration. Monitor for signs and symptoms of thrombosis and assess blood viscosity in patients at risk for hyperviscosity. AMS has been reported to occur with IgG products, including *immune globulin infusion 10% (human)*, administered intravenously and subcutaneously. AMS may occur more frequently in female patients. Discontinuation of IgG treatment has resulted in remission of AMS within several days without sequelae. The syndrome usually begins within several hours to 2 days following intravenously administered IgG. AMS is characterized by the following signs and symptoms: severe headache, nuchal rigidity, drowsiness, fever, photophobia, painful eye movements, nausea, and vomiting. Cerebrospinal fluid (CSF) studies frequently reveal pleocytosis up to several thousand cells per mm³, predominantly from the granulocytic series, and elevated protein levels up to several hundred mg/dl, but negative culture results. Conduct a thorough neurologic examination on patients exhibiting such symptoms and signs, including CSF studies, to rule out other causes of meningitis. IgG products, including **Hyqvia**, contain blood group antibodies which may act as hemolysins and induce *in vivo* coating of RBCs with IgG. These antibodies may cause a positive direct antiglobulin reaction and hemolysis. Acute intravascular hemolysis has been reported following intravenously administered IgG, including *immune globulin infusion 10% (human),* administered intravenously, and delayed hemolytic anemia can develop due to enhanced RBC sequestration. Acute renal dysfunction/failure, acute tubular necrosis (ATN), proximal tubular nephropathy, osmotic nephrosis, and death may occur upon use of IgG products administered intravenously, especially those containing sucrose. **Hyqvia** does not contain sucrose. Acute renal dysfunction/failure has been reported in association with *immune globulin infusion 10% (human)* administered intravenously. Ensure that patients are not volume-depleted prior to the initiation of infusion of **Hyqvia**. Patients at risk of developing renal dysfunction due to preexisting renal insufficiency or predisposition to ARF include patients with diabetes mellitus, age ≥65 years, volume depletion, sepsis, paraproteinemia, or patients receiving known nephrotoxic drugs. Periodic monitoring of renal function and urine output is particularly important in patients judged to be at increased risk for developing ARF. Assess renal function, including measurement of BUN and sCr, before the initial infusion of **Hyqvia** and again at appropriate intervals thereafter. If renal function deteriorates, consider discontinuation of **Hyqvia**. TRALI (i.e., non-cardiogenic pulmonary edema) may occur with intravenously administered IgG and has been reported to occur *with immune globulin infusion 10% (human)* administered intravenously. TRALI is characterized by severe respiratory distress, pulmonary edema, hypoxemia, normal left ventricular function, and fever. Symptoms typically occur within 1-6 hours after treatment. Monitor patients for pulmonary adverse reactions. If TRALI is suspected, conduct an evaluation, including appropriate tests for the presence of antineutrophil and anti-HLA antibodies in both the product and patient serum. TRALI may be managed using oxygen therapy with adequate ventilatory support. No human data are available to indicate the presence or absence of drug-associated risk in human pregnancy. Animal reproduction studies have not been conducted with the *immune globulin infusion 10% (human)* component of **Hyqvia**. It is not known whether **Hyqvia** can cause fetal harm when administered to a pregnant female or can affect reproduction capacity. Immune globulins cross the placenta from maternal circulation increasingly after 30 weeks of gestation. Effects of the *recombinant human hyaluronidase* component of **Hyqvia** on the human embryo or on human fetal development are unknown. **Hyqvia** should be administered to a pregnant female only if clearly indicated. No human data are available to indicate the presence or absence of drug-associated risk. In animal studies, maternal antibodies binding to *recombinant human hyaluronidase* were transferred to offspring during lactation. Effects of antibodies that bind to *recombinant human hyaluronidase* of **Hyqvia** transferred during human lactation are unknown. Developmental and health benefits of breastfeeding should be considered along with the mother's clinical need for **Hyqvia** and any potential adverse effects on the breastfed infant from **Hyqvia** or from the underlying maternal condition.

IMPETIGO CONTAGIOSA (INDIAN FIRE)

Comment: The most common infectious organisms are *Staphylococcus aureus* and *Streptococcus pyogenes.*

TOPICAL ANTI-INFECTIVES
➤ *mupirocin* (G) apply to lesions bid; apply to walls of nares bid
  Pediatric: same as adult
    Bactroban *Oint:* 2% (22 gm); *Crm:* 2% (15, 30 gm)
    Centany *Oint:* 2% (15, 30 gm)

ORAL ANTI-INFECTIVES
➤ *amoxicillin* (G) 500-875 mg bid or 250-500 mg tid x 10 days
  Pediatric: <40 kg (88 lb): 20-40 mg/kg/day in 3 divided doses x 10 days or 25-45 mg/kg/day in 2 divided doses x 10 days; ≥40 kg: same as adult; *see Appendix BB.3. amoxicillin* (G) (Amoxil Suspension, Trimox Suspension) *for dose by weight*
    Amoxil *Cap:* 250, 500 mg; *Tab:* 875*mg; *Chew tab:* 125, 200, 250, 400 mg (cherry-banana-peppermint) (phenylalanine); *Oral susp:* 125, 250 mg/5 ml (80, 100, 150 ml) (strawberry); 200, 400 mg/5 ml (50, 75, 100 ml) (bubble gum); *Oral drops:* 50 mg/ml (30 ml) (bubble gum)
    Moxatag *Tab:* 775 mg ext-rel
    Trimox *Tab:* 125, 250 mg; *Cap:* 250, 500 mg; *Oral susp:* 125, 250 mg/5 ml (80, 100, 150 ml) (raspberry-strawberry)
➤ *amoxicillin+clavulanate* (G)
    Augmentin 500 mg tid or 875 mg bid x 7-10 days
    Pediatric: 40-45 mg/kg/day divided tid x 10 days or 90 mg/kg/day divided bid x 10 days; *see Appendix BB.4. amoxicillin+clavulanate* (G) (Augmentin Suspension) *for dose by weight*
      Tab: 250, 500, 875 mg; *Chew tab:* 125, 250 mg (lemon-lime); 200, 400 mg (cherry-banana) (phenylalanine); *Oral susp:* 125 mg/5 ml (banana), 250 mg/5 ml (75, 100, 150 ml) (orange); 200, 400 mg/5 ml (50, 75, 100 ml) (orange) (phenylalanine)
    Augmentin ES-600 not recommended for adults

(continued)

Pediatric: <3 months: <u>not</u> recommended; ≥3 months, <40 kg: 90 mg/kg/day in 2 divided doses x 7-10 days; ≥40 kg: <u>not</u> recommended

    Oral susp: 42.9 mg/5 ml (50, 75, 100, 125, 150, 200 ml) (strawberry cream) (phenylalanine)

Augmentin XR 2 tabs q 12 hours x 7-10 days

Pediatric: <16 years: use other forms; ≥16 years: same as adult

    Tab: 1,000*mg ext-rel

▸ *azithromycin* **(G)** 500 mg x 1 dose on day 1, then 250 mg daily on days 2-5 <u>or</u> 500 mg daily x 3 days <u>or</u> 2 gm in a single dose

    Zithromax *Tab:* 250, 500, 600 mg; *Oral susp:* 100 mg/5 ml (15 ml), 200 mg/5 ml (15, 22.5, 30 ml) (cherry); *Pkt:* 1 gm for reconstitution (cherry-banana)

    Zithromax Tri-Pak *Tab:* 3 x 500 mg tabs/pck

    Zithromax Z-Pak *Tab:* 6 x 250 mg tabs/pck

    Zmax *Oral susp:* 2 gm ext-rel for reconstitution (cherry-banana) (148 mg Na$^+$)

▸ *cefaclor* **(G)**

    Ceclor 250 mg tid <u>or</u> 375 mg bid 3-10 days

    Pediatric: <1 month: <u>not</u> recommended; 1 month-12 years: 20-40 mg/kg divided bid <u>or</u> q 12 hours x 3-10 days; max 1 gm/day; *see Appendix BB.8. cefaclor (G) (Ceclor Suspension) for dose by weight;* >12 years: same as adult

    Tab: 500 mg; *Cap:* 250, 500 mg; *Susp:* 125 mg/5 ml (75, 150 ml) (strawberry), 187 mg/5 ml (50, 100 ml) (strawberry), 250 mg/5 ml (75, 150 ml) (strawberry), 375 mg/5 ml (50, 100 ml) (strawberry)

    Ceclor Extended Release 375-500 mg bid x 3-10 days

    Pediatric: <16 years: ext-rel <u>not</u> recommended; ≥16 years: same as adult

    Tab: 375, 500 mg ext-rel

▸ *cefadroxil* 1-2 gm in 1-2 divided doses x 10 days

    Pediatric: 30 mg/kg/day in 2 divided doses x 10 days; *see Appendix BB.9. cefadroxil (Duricef Suspension) for dose by weight*

    Duricef *Cap:* 500 mg; *Tab:* 1 gm; *Oral susp:* 250 mg/5 ml (100 ml), 500 mg/5 ml (75, 100 ml) (orange-pineapple)

▸ *cefpodoxime proxetil* 200 mg bid x 10 days

    Pediatric: <2 months: <u>not</u> recommended; 2 months-12 years: 10 mg/kg/day (max 400 mg/dose) <u>or</u> 5 mg/kg/day bid (max 200 mg/dose) x 10 days; *see Appendix BB.12. cefpodoxime proxetil (G) (Vantin Suspension) for dose by weight*

    Vantin *Tab:* 100, 200 mg; *Oral susp:* 50, 100 mg/5 ml (50, 75, 100 mg) (lemon creme)

▸ *cefprozil* 500 mg bid x 10 days

    Pediatric: ≤6 months: <u>not</u> recommended; 6 months-12 years: *see Appendix BB.13. cefprozil (G) (Cefzil Suspension) for dose by weight*

    Cefzil *Tab:* 250, 500 mg; *Oral susp:* 125, 250 mg/5 ml (50, 75, 100 ml) (bubble gum) (phenylalanine)

▸ *ceftaroline fosamil* administer by IV infusion after reconstitution q 12 hours x 5-14 days; *CrCl >50 ml/min:* 600 mg; *CrCl >30 to <50 ml/min:* 400 mg; *CrCl >15 to <30 ml/min:* 300 mg; *ESRD:* 200 mg

    Teflaro *Vial:* 400, 600 mg

▸ *cephalexin* **(G)** 250-500 mg qid <u>or</u> 500 mg bid x 10 days

    Pediatric: 25-50 mg/kg/day in 4 divided doses x 10 days; *see Appendix BB.15. cephalexin (G) (Keflex Suspension) for dose by weight*

    Keflex *Cap:* 250, 333, 500, 750 mg; *Oral susp:* 125, 250 mg/5 ml (100, 200 ml) (strawberry)

▸ *clarithromycin* **(G)** 500 mg bid <u>or</u> 500 mg ext-rel once daily x 7 days

    Pediatric: <6 months: <u>not</u> recommended; ≥6 months: 7.5 mg/kg bid x 7 days; *see Appendix BB.16. clarithromycin (G) (Biaxin Suspension) for dose by weight*

    Biaxin *Tab:* 250, 500 mg

    Biaxin Oral Suspension *Oral susp:* 125, 250 mg/5 ml (50, 100 ml) (fruit punch)

    Biaxin XL *Tab:* 500 mg ext-rel

▸ *dicloxacillin* **(G)** 500 mg q 6 hours x 10 days

    Pediatric: 12.5-25 mg/kg/day in 4 divided doses x 10 days; *see Appendix BB.18. dicloxacillin (G) (Dynapen Suspension) for dose by weight*

    Dynapen *Cap:* 125, 250, 500 mg; *Oral susp:* 62.5 mg/5 ml (80, 100, 200 ml)

▸ *erythromycin base* **(G)** 250 mg qid, <u>or</u> 333 mg tid, <u>or</u> 500 mg bid x 7-10 days

    Pediatric: ≤45 kg: 30-50 mg in 2-4 divided doses x 7-10 days; ≥45 kg: same as adult

    Ery-Tab *Tab:* 250, 333, 500 mg ent-coat

    PCE *Tab:* 333, 500 mg

▸ *erythromycin ethylsuccinate* **(G)** 400 mg tid x 7-10 days

    Pediatric: 30-50 mg/kg/day in 4 divided doses x 7-10 days; may double dose with severe infection; max 100 mg/kg/day; *see Appendix BB.21. erythromycin ethylsuccinate (G) (E.E.S. Suspension, EryPed Drops/ Suspension) for dose by weight*

    EryPed *Oral susp:* 200 mg/5 ml (100, 200 ml) (fruit), 400 mg/5 ml (60, 100, 200 ml) (banana); *Oral drops:* 200, 400 mg/5 ml (50 ml) (fruit); *Chew tab:* 200 mg wafer (fruit)

    E.E.S. *Oral susp:* 200, 400 mg/5 ml (100 ml) (fruit)

E.E.S. Granules *Oral susp:* 200 mg/5 ml (100, 200 ml) (cherry)
E.E.S. 400 Tablets *Tab:* 400 mg
➤ *loracarbef* 200 mg bid x 10 days
Pediatric: 15 mg/kg/day in 2 divided doses x 10 days; *see* Appendix BB.27. *loracarbef* (G) (Lorabid Suspension) *for dose by weight*
Pediatric: 30 mg/kg/day in 2 divided doses x 7 days
Lorabid *Pulvule:* 200, 400 mg; *Oral susp:* 100 mg/5 ml (50, 100 ml), 200 mg/5 ml (50, 75, 100 ml) (strawberry bubble gum)
➤ *ozenoxacin* <2 months: not recommended; ≥2 months: apply a thin layer topically to the affected area bid x 5 days; affected area may be up to 100 cm² in patients ≥12 years of age or 2% of the total body surface area (BSA) and not exceeding 100 cm² in patients <12 years of age
Xepi *Crm:* 1% 10 mg/gm (45 gm)
Comment: Xepi is indicated for the topical treatment of impetigo due to *Staphylococcus aureus* or *Streptococcus pyogenes*. There are no available data on the use of **Xepi** in pregnancy to inform a drug-associated risk; however, systemic absorption of *ozenoxacin* in humans is negligible following topical administration. No data are available regarding the presence of *ozenoxacin* in human milk or effects on the breastfed infant; however, breastfeeding is not expected to result in infant exposure due to the negligible systemic absorption.
➤ *penicillin g (benzathine)* (G) 1.2 million units IM x 1 dose
Pediatric: <60 lb: 300,000-600,000 units IM x 1 dose; ≥60 lb: 900,000 units x 1 dose
Bicillin L-A *Cartridge-needle unit:* 600,000 units (1 ml), 1.2 million units (2 ml)
➤ *penicillin g (benzathine procaine)* (G) 2.4 million units IM x 1 dose
Pediatric: <30 lb: 600,000 units IM x 1 dose; 30-60 lb: 900,000-1.2 million units IM x 1 dose
Bicillin C-R *Cartridge-needle unit:* 600,000 units (1 ml), 1.2 million units (2 ml), 2.4 million units (4 ml)
➤ *penicillin v potassium* 250-500 mg q 6 hours x 10 days
Pediatric: 50 mg/kg/day in 4 divided doses x 3 days; ≥12 years: same as adult; *see* Appendix BB.29. *penicillin v potassium* (G) (Pen-Vee K Solution, Veetids Solution) *for dose by weight*
Pen-Vee K *Tab:* 250, 500 mg; *Oral soln:* 125 mg/5 ml (100, 200 ml), 250 mg/5 ml (100, 150, 200 ml)

INCONTINENCE: FECAL

Comment: Treatment of fecal incontinence in patients who have failed conservative therapy (e.g., diet, fiber therapy, antimotility agents).
➤ *dextranomer microspheres+sodium hyaluronate*
Pediatric: <18 years: not recommended; ≥18 years: same as adult
Pretreatment: bowel preparation using enema (required) and prophylactic antibiotics (recommended) prior to injection;
Treatment: inject slowly into the deep submucosal layer in the proximal part of the high pressure zone of the anal canal about 5 mm above the dentate line; four 1ml injections in the following order: posterior, left lateral, anterior, right lateral; keep needle in place 15-30 seconds to minimize leakage; use a new needle for each syringe and injection site;
Posttreatment: avoid hot baths and physical activity during the first 24 hours; avoid antidiarrheal drugs, sexual intercourse, and strenuous activity for 1 week; avoid anal manipulation for 1 month;
Retreatment: may repeat if needed with max 4 ml, no sooner than 4 weeks after the first injection; point of injection should be made in between initial injection sites (i.e., shifted 1/8 of a turn)
Solesta dex micro 50 mg+sod hyal 15 mg per ml
Syringe: 1 ml (4 w. needles)

INCONTINENCE: URINARY OVERACTIVE BLADDER, STRESS INCONTINENCE, URGE INCONTINENCE, NEUROGENIC DETRUSOR OVERACTIVITY (NDO)

see Enuresis
➤ *estrogen* replacement *see Menopause*
➤ *pseudoephedrine* (G) 30-60 mg tid
Sudafed (OTC) *Tab:* 30 mg; *Liq:* 15 mg/5 ml (1, 4 oz)

VASOPRESSIN
➤ *desmopressin acetate (DDAVP)* (G)
DDAVP usual dosage 0.1-1.2 mg/day in 2-3 divided doses; 0.2 mg q HS prn for nocturnal enuresis
Pediatric: <6 years: not recommended; ≥6 years: 0.5 mg daily or q HS prn
Tab: 0.1*, 0.2*mg
DDAVP Rhinal Tube

(continued)

Pediatric: <6 years: <u>not</u> recommended; ≥6 years: 10 mcg <u>or</u> 0.1 ml of soln each nostril (20 mcg total dose) q HS prn; max 40 mcg total dose
  Rhinal tube: 0.1 mg/ml (2.5 ml)

BETA-3 ADRENERGIC AGONIST
▷ **mirabegron** initially 25 mg once daily; max 50 mg once daily; *Severe renal impairment:* 25 mg once daily
  Myrbetriq *Tab:* 25, 50 mg ext-rel
  Comment: Myrbetriq *(mirabegron)* is FDA-approved to be taken in combination with **VESIcare** *(solifenacin succinate)* for the treatment of overactive bladder (OAB) with symptoms of frequency, urgency, and urge urinary incontinence.

MUSCARINIC RECEPTOR ANTAGONISTS
▷ **vibegron** take one 75 mg tablet once daily; swallow tablet whole with water; may be crushed and mixed with applesauce
  Pediatric: safety and efficacy <u>not</u> established
    Gemtesa *Tab:* 75 mg
    Comment: Gemtesa is a beta-3 adrenergic agonist indicated for the treatment of overactive bladder (OAB) with symptoms of urge urinary incontinence, urgency, and urinary frequency in adults. The most common adverse reactions (incidence ≥2%) have been headache, urinary tract infection (UTI), nasopharyngitis, diarrhea, nausea, and upper respiratory infection (URI). Measure serum *digoxin* concentrations before initiating **Gemtesa**; monitor serum *digoxin* concentrations to titrate *digoxin* dose to desired clinical effect. Monitor for urinary retention, especially in patients with bladder outlet obstruction and patients taking muscarinic antagonist medications for OAB, in whom the risk of urinary retention may be greater. If urinary retention develops, discontinue **Gemtesa**. *End-Stage Renal Disease (ESRD) With or Without hemodialysis:* <u>Not</u> recommended. *Severe hepatic impairment:* <u>Not</u> recommended. There are <u>no</u> available data on **Gemtesa** use in pregnant females to evaluate for a drug-associated risk of major birth defects, miscarriage, <u>or</u> adverse maternal <u>or</u> fetal outcomes. In animal studies, <u>no</u> effects on embryo/fetal development were observed following administration of *vibegron* during organogenesis at exposures approximately 275-fold and 285-fold greater than clinical exposure at the recommended daily dose. There are <u>no</u> data on the presence of *vibegron* in human milk <u>or</u> effects on the breastfed infant. Developmental and health benefits of breastfeeding should be considered along with the mother's clinical need for **Gemtesa** and any potential adverse effects on the breastfed infant from **Gemtesa** <u>or</u> from the underlying maternal condition.
▷ **fesoterodine** (G) *OAB:* 4-8 mg once daily
  Pediatric: Neurogenic detrusor overactivity (NDO): <6 years, <25 kg: safety and efficacy <u>not</u> established; ≥6 years, 25-35 kg: 4 mg orally once daily; if needed, dosage may be increased to 8 mg orally once daily; ≥6 years, >35 kg: recommended starting dose: is 4 mg orally once daily; after 1 week, increase to 8 mg orally once daily
    Toviaz *Tab:* 4, 8 mg ext-rel
▷ **tolterodine tartrate** (G) **Detrol** 1-2 mg bid <u>or</u> **Detrol LA** 2-4 mg once daily <u>or</u> **Detrol XL** 1 tab daily
  Pediatric: <12 years: <u>not</u> recommended; ≥12 years: same as adult
    Detrol *Tab:* 1, 2 mg
    Detrol *Cap:* 2, 4 mg ext-rel
    Detrol XL *Tab:* 5, 10, 15 mg ext-rel

ANTISPASMODIC/ANTICHOLINERGICS AGENTS
▷ **darifenacin** 7.5-15 mg daily with liquid; max 15 mg/day
  Pediatric: <12 years: <u>not</u> recommended; ≥12 years: same as adult
    Enablex 7.5-15 mg daily with liquid; max 15 mg/day
      Tab: 7.5, 15 mg ext-rel
▷ **dicyclomine** (G) 10-20 mg qid
  Pediatric: <12 years: <u>not</u> recommended; ≥12 years: same as adult
    Bentyl *Tab:* 20 mg; *Cap:* 10 mg; *Syr:* 10 mg/5 ml (16 oz)
▷ **flavoxate** 100-200 mg tid-qid
  Pediatric: <12 years: <u>not</u> recommended; ≥12 years: same as adult
    Urispas *Tab:* 100 mg
▷ **hyoscyamine** (G)
    Anaspaz 1-2 tabs q 4 hours prn; max 12 tabs/day
    Pediatric: <2 years: <u>not</u> recommended; 2-12 years: 0.0625-0.125 mg q 4 hours prn; max 0.75 mg/day
      Tab: 0.125*mg
    Levbid 1-2 tabs q 12 hours prn; max 4 tabs/day
    Pediatric: <12 years: <u>not</u> recommended; ≥12 years: same as adult
      Tab: 0.375*mg ext-rel
    Levsin 1-2 tabs q 4 hours prn; max 12 tabs/day
    Pediatric: <6 years: <u>not</u> recommended; 6-12 years: 1 tab q 4 hours prn
      Tab: 0.125*mg

Levsin Drops 1-2 ml q 4 hours prn; max 60 ml/day
Pediatric: 3.4 kg: 4 drops q 4 hours prn, max 24 drops/day; 5 kg: 5 drops q 4 hours prn; max 30 drops/day; 7 kg: 6 drops q 4 hours prn; max 36 drops/day; 10 kg: 8 drops q 4 hours prn; max 40 drops/day; 2-12 years: 0.25-1 ml; max 6 ml/day
    Oral drops: 0.125 mg/ml (15 ml) (orange) (alcohol 5%)
Levsin Elixir 5-10 ml q 4 hours prn
Pediatric: <10 kg: use drops; 10-19 kg: 1.25 ml q 4 hours prn; 20-39 kg: 2.5 ml q 4 hours prn; 40-49 kg: 3.75 ml q 4 hours prn; ≥50 kg: 5 ml q 4 hours prn
    Elix: 0.125 mg/5 ml (16 oz) (orange) (alcohol 20%)
Levsinex SL 1-2 tabs q 4 hours SL <u>or</u> PO; max 12 tabs/day
Pediatric: <2 years: <u>not</u> recommended; 2-12 years: 1 tab q 4 hours; max 6 tabs/day; >12 years: same as adult
    Tab: 0.125 mg sublingual
Levsinex Timecaps 1-2 caps q 12 hours; may adjust to 1 cap q 8 hours
Pediatric: 2-12 years: 1 cap q 12 hours; max 2 caps/day; >12 years: same as adult
    Cap: 0.375 mg time-rel
NuLev dissolve 1-2 tabs on tongue, with <u>or</u> without water, q 4 hours prn; max 12 tabs/day
Pediatric: <2 years: <u>not</u> recommended; 2-12 years: dissolve 1 tab on tongue, with <u>or</u> without water, q 4 hours prn; max 6 tabs/day; ≥12 years: same as adult
    ODT: 0.125 mg (mint) (phenylalanine)
➤ *oxybutynin chloride*
Ditropan 5 mg bid-tid; max 20 mg/day
Pediatric: <5 years: <u>not</u> recommended; 5-12 years: 5 mg bid; max 15 mg/day; ≥16 years: same as adult
    Tab: 5*mg; *Syr:* 5 mg/5 ml
Ditropan XL initially 5 mg daily; may increase weekly in 5 mg increments as needed; max 30 mg/day
Pediatric: <6 years: <u>not</u> recommended; ≥6 years: initially 5 mg once daily; may increase weekly in 5 mg increments as needed; max 20 mg/day
    Tab: 5, 10, 15 mg ext-rel
GelniQUE 3 mg Pump apply 3 pumps (84 mg) once daily to clean dry intact skin on the abdomen, upper arm, shoulders, <u>or</u> thighs; rotate sites; wash hands; avoid washing application site for 1 hour after application
Pediatric: <12 years: <u>not</u> recommended; ≥12 years: same as adult
    Gel: 3% (92 gm, metered pump dispenser) (alcohol)
GelniQUE 1 gm Sachet apply 1 gm gel (1 sachet) once daily to dry intact skin on the abdomen, upper arms/shoulders, <u>or</u> thighs; rotate sites; wash hands; avoid washing application site for 1 hour after application
Pediatric: <12 years: <u>not</u> recommended; ≥12 years: same as adult
    Gel: 10%, 1 gm/sachet (30/carton) (alcohol)
Oxytrol Transdermal Patch (OTC) apply patch to clean dry area of the abdomen, hip, <u>or</u> buttock; one patch twice weekly; rotate sites
Pediatric: <12 years: <u>not</u> recommended; ≥12 years: same as adult
    Transdermal patch: 3.9 mg/day
➤ *propantheline* 15-30 mg tid
Pediatric: <12 years: <u>not</u> recommended; ≥12 years: same as adult
    Pro-Banthine *Tab:* 7.5, 15 mg
➤ *solifenacin* (G) 5-10 mg daily
Pediatric: <12 years: <u>not</u> recommended; ≥12 years: same as adult
    VESIcare *Tab:* 5, 10 mg
    Comment: VESIcare *(solifenacin succinate)* is FDA-approved to be taken in combination with **Myrbetriq** *(mirabegron)* for the treatment of overactive bladder (OAB) with symptoms of frequency, urgency, and urge urinary incontinence.
➤ *trospium chloride* (G)
Pediatric: <12 years: <u>not</u> recommended; ≥12 years: same as adult
    Sanctura 20 mg bid; ≥75 years: *CrCl ≤30 ml/min:* 20 mg once daily
    Tab: 20 mg
    Sanctura XR 60 mg daily in the morning
    Cap: 60 mg ext-rel
Comment: Take *trospium chloride* on an empty stomach.

OVERFLOW INCONTINENCE: ATONIC BLADDER
➤ *bethanechol* 10-30 mg tid
    Urecholine *Tab:* 5, 10, 25, 50 mg

OVERFLOW INCONTINENCE: PROSTATIC ENLARGEMENT
Alpha-1 Blockers
Comment: Educate the patient regarding the potential side effect of hypotension when taking an alpha-1 blocker, especially with first dose. Start at the lowest dose and titrate upward.

(continued)

▷ **terazosin** initially 1 mg q HS; titrate to 10 mg q HS; max 20 mg/day
    Hytrin *Cap:* 1, 2, 5, 10 mg
▷ **doxazosin** initially 1 mg q HS; may double dose every 1-2 weeks; max 8 mg/day
    Cardura *Tab:* 1*, 2*, 4*, 8*mg
    Cardura XL *Tab:* 4, 8 mg
▷ **prazosin** (G) 1-15 mg q HS; max 15 mg/day
    Minipress *Tab:* 1, 2, 5 mg
▷ **tamsulosin** initially 0.4 mg daily q HS; may increase to 0.8 mg once daily after 2-4 weeks if needed
    Flomax *Cap:* 0.4 mg

5-ALPHA REDUCTASE INHIBITOR
▷ **finasteride** (G) 5 mg daily
    Proscar *Tab:* 5 mg

ALPHA 1A-BLOCKER
▷ **silodosin** (G) take 8 mg with food once daily; *CrCl 30-50 ml/min:* take 4 mg
    Rapaflo *Cap:* 4, 8 mg

INFLUENZA, SEASONAL (FLU)

Comment: Routine annual influenza vaccination is recommended for all persons aged 6 months and older without contraindications for the 2020-2021 flu season. The Advisory Committee on Immunization Practices (ACIP) does <u>not</u> prefer one vaccine over another for persons in which more than one influenza vaccine product is applicable based on age and health status.

The live attenuated influenza vaccine (LAIV4) is an option for adults through age 49 years, except with immunocompromising conditions. According to the LAIV4 mfr pkg insert, antiviral agents may reduce the effectiveness of LAIV4 if it is given within the interval from 48 hours before to 14 days after vaccination. Considering the longer half-lives of newer antiviral agents, ACIP recommends that LAIV4 should <u>not</u> be used if a person received either **oseltamivir** <u>or</u> **zanamivir** within the previous 48 hours, **peramivir** within the previous 5 days, <u>or</u> **baloxavir** within the previous 17 days.

Regarding persons with egg allergy with symptoms other than hives, if an influenza vaccine other than **Flublok** <u>or</u> **Flucelvax** is used, the vaccine should be administered in a medical setting under supervision of a healthcare provider who can recognize and manage severe allergic reactions.

The influenza vaccine is contraindicated in persons with a previous severe allergic reaction to the vaccine. Adults who have received a previous influenza dose and developed Guillain-Barre syndrome within 6 weeks of vaccination should <u>not</u> be vaccinated again unless benefits outweigh the risks.

PROPHYLAXIS (NASAL SPRAY)
▷ **trivalent, live attenuated influenza vaccine, types A and B** 1 spray each nostril; ≥50 years; <u>not</u> recommended
    Pediatric: ≤5 years: <u>not</u> recommended; ≥5 years: same as adult
    Never vaccinated with FluMist: 5-8 years: 2 doses spaced 46-74 days apart; *Previously vaccinated*
    with FluMist: 5-8 years: same as adult
    FluMist Nasal Spray 0.5 ml spray annually
      Nasal spray: 0.5 ml (0.25 ml/spray) (10/carton) (preservative-free)

PROPHYLAXIS (INJECTABLE)
▷ **quadrivalent inactivated influenza subvirion vaccine, types a and b**
    Afluria Quadrivalent <6 months: <u>not</u> recommended; 6 months-18 years: 1-2 doses/season at least 4 weeks apart; >9 years: 1 dose/season
    Vial/Prefilled pen/PharmaJet Stratis Needle-Free Injection System: 0.5 ml single-dose (preservative-free);
    Vial: 5 ml multidose (thimerosal)
    Comment: Contraindicated with allergy to egg <u>or</u> chicken protein, neomycin, polymyxin, <u>or</u> history of life-threatening reaction to any previous flu vaccine. PharmaJet Stratis Needle-Free Injection System is <u>only</u> approved as a method of administration for patients 18-64 years of age.
      Fluad 0.5 ml IM annually
      Comment: Fluad is the first seasonal influenza vaccine with adjuvant indicated for persons ≥65 years of age. Adjuvants are incorporated into some vaccine formulations to enhance <u>or</u> direct the immune response.
      Fluarix Quadrivalent 0.5 ml IM annually
      Pediatric: <3 years: <u>not</u> recommended; ≥3 years: same as adult
        Prefilled syringe: 0.5 ml (10/carton) (preservative-free, latex-free)
▷ **trivalent inactivated influenza subvirion vaccine, types a and b**
    Fluarix 0.5 ml IM annually

Pediatric: <3 years: <u>not</u> recommended; 3-9 years (previously unvaccinated <u>or</u> vaccinated for the first time last season with 1 dose of flu vaccine): 2 doses per season spaced at least 1 month apart; 3-9 years (previously vaccinated with 2 doses of flu vaccine); >9 years: 1 dose per season
> *Prefilled syringe:* 0.5 ml single-dose (5/carton) (may contain trace amounts of hydrocortisone, gentamicin; preservative-free)

Flublok 0.5 ml IM annually; ≥49 years: <u>not</u> recommended
Pediatric: <18 years: <u>not</u> recommended; ≥18 years: same as adult
> *Vial:* 0.5 ml single-dose (10/carton) (preservative-free, egg protein-free, antibiotic-free, latex-free)

Comment: Flublok is a cell culture-derived vaccine and therefore is an alternative to the traditional egg-based vaccines. Contains 3 times the amount of active ingredient in traditional flu vaccines

Flucelvax 0.5 ml IM annually
Pediatric: <18 years: <u>not</u> recommended; ≥18 years: same as adult
> *Prefilled syringes:* 0.5 ml (10/carton; preservative-free, latex-free)

Comment: Flucelvax is a cell culture-derived vaccine and therefore is an alternative to the traditional egg-based vaccines.

FluLaval 0.5 ml IM annually
Pediatric: <6 months: <u>not</u> recommended; ≥6 years: same as adult
> *Vial:* 5 ml

FluShield 0.5 ml IM annually
Pediatric: <6 months: <u>not</u> recommended; *Never vaccinated:* <9 years: 2 doses at least 4 weeks apart; 9-12 years: same as adult; *Previously vaccinated:* 6-35 months: 0.25 ml IM x 1 dose; 3-8 years: same as adult

Fluzone 0.5 ml IM annually
> *Vial:* 5 ml (thimerosal)

Fluzone High-Dose Quadrivalent 0.5 ml IM annually
> *Vial:* 5 ml (thimerosal)

Fluzone Preservative-Free: Adult Dose 0.5 ml IM annually
Pediatric: <6 months: <u>not</u> recommended; <u>not</u> *previously vaccinated:* 6 months to 8 years: 0.25 ml IM, repeat in 1 month; *Previously vaccinated:* 6-35 months: 0.25 ml IM x 1 dose; ≥3 years: same as adult
> *Prefilled syringe:* 0.5 ml (10/carton) (preservative-free, trace thimerosal)

Fluzone Preservative-Free: Pediatric Dose
Pediatric: <6 months: <u>not</u> recommended; <u>Not</u> *previously vaccinated:* 6 months to 8 years: 0.25 ml IM; repeat in 1 month; *Previously vaccinated:* 6-35 months: 0.25 ml IM x 1 dose; ≥3 years: 0.5 ml IM (use **Fluzone for Adult**)
> *Prefilled syringe:* 0.5 ml (10/carton; preservative-free; trace thimerosal)

Comment: Contraindicated with allergy to egg protein <u>or</u> history of life-threatening reaction to any previous flu vaccine.

PROPHYLAXIS AND TREATMENTS
Neuraminidase Inhibitors
Comment: Effective for influenza type A and B. Indicated for treatment of uncomplicated acute illness in patients who have been symptomatic for no more than 2 days; therefore, start within 2 days of symptom onset <u>or</u> exposure. Indicated for influenza prophylaxis in patients ≥3 months of age.

▷ *oseltamivir* phosphate (G)
Prophylaxis: 75 mg daily for at least 7 days and up to 6 weeks for community outbreak
> *Pediatric:* <1 year: <u>not</u> recommended; 1-12 years: <15 kg: 30 mg once daily x 10 days; 16-23 kg: 45 mg once daily x 10 days; 24-40 kg: 60 mg once daily x 10 days; >40 kg: same as adult

Treatment: 75 mg bid x 5 days; initiate treatment <u>only</u> if symptomatic <2 days
> *Pediatric:* <1 year: <u>not</u> recommended; 1-12 years: <15 kg: 30 mg bid x 5 days; 16-23 kg: 45 mg bid x 5 days; 24-40 kg: 60 mg bid x 5 days; >40 kg: same as adult
> **Tamiflu** *Cap:* 30, 45, 75 mg; *Oral susp:* 6 mg/ml pwdr for reconstitution (60 ml w. oral dispenser) (tutti-frutti)
> **Comment:** Tamiflu is effective for influenza type A and B.

▷ *peramivir* start within 2 days of symptom onset; administer via IV infusion over 15-30 minutes; 600 mg as a single dose; *CrCl 30-49 ml/min:* 200 mg; *CrCl 10-29 ml/min:* 100 mg; *Hemodialysis:* administer after dialysis
Pediatric: start within 2 days of symptom onset; administer via IV infusion over 15-30 minutes; <2 years: safety and efficacy <u>not</u> established; 2-12 years: 12 mg/kg as a single dose; max 600 mg; ≥13 years: same as adult; *CrCl 30-49 ml/min:* 4 mg/kg; *CrCl 10-29 ml/min:* 2 mg/kg; *Hemodialysis:* administer after dialysis
> **Rapivab** *Vial:* 10 mg/ml (20 ml), single-use, soln for IV administration after dilution (preservative-free)
> **Comment:** Avoid live attenuated influenza vaccine (LAIV) 2 weeks prior to, and 48 hours after, treatment with **Rapivab** *(peramivir).*

▷ *zanamivir* 2 inhalations (10 mg) bid x 5 days
Pediatric: <7 years: <u>not</u> recommended; ≥7 years: same as adult
> **Relenza Inhaler** *Inhaler:* 5 mg/inh blister; 4 blisters/Rotadisk (5 Rotadisks/carton w. 1 inhaler)
> **Comment:** Relenza Inhaler is effective for influenza type A and B. Use caution with asthma and chronic obstructive pulmonary disease (COPD).

Polymerase Acidic (PA) Endonuclease Inhibitor

▷ *baloxavir marboxil* take as a single dose within 48 hours of symptom onset; *40-<80 kg*: 40 mg; *≥80 kg*: 80 mg; take with or without food; do not take with dairy products, calcium-fortified beverages, laxatives, antacids, or oral supplements containing iron, zinc, selenium, calcium, or magnesium (polyvalent cations)

Pediatric: <12 years, <88 lb (40 kg): not established; ≥12 years, ≥88 lb (40 kg): same as adult

    Xofluza *Tab*: 20, 40 mg

    Comment: Xofluza *(baloxavir marboxil)* is a first-in-class, single-dose, oral antiviral drug with a novel mechanism of action designed to target the influenza A and B viruses, including *oseltamivir-*resistant strains and avian strains (e.g., H7N9, H5N1). Unlike other currently available antiviral treatments, *baloxavir marboxil* is the first polymerase acidic (PA) endonuclease inhibitor designed to inhibit the cap-dependent endonuclease protein within the flu virus, which is essential for viral replication, thereby reducing symptoms and duration of the illness. This is the first new antiviral flu treatment with a novel mechanism of action approved by the FDA in nearly 20 years. Safety and efficacy of **Xofluza** were demonstrated in two randomized controlled clinical trials of 1,832 patients where participants were randomly assigned to receive a single dose of 40 mg or 80 mg of *baloxavir marboxil* (according to body weight), placebo, or 75 mg of *oseltamivir* twice a day for 5 days within 48 hours of experiencing flu symptoms. **Xofluza** was granted priority review (FDA action on an application within an expedited time frame where the agency determines that the drug, if approved, would significantly improve the safety or effectiveness of treating, diagnosing, or preventing a serious condition). Co-administration with polyvalent cation-containing products may decrease plasma concentrations of *baloxavir,* which may reduce **Xofluza** efficacy. Therefore, avoid co-administration of **Xofluza** with polyvalent cation-containing laxatives, antacids, or oral supplements (e.g., calcium, iron, magnesium, selenium, or zinc). The concurrent use of **Xofluza** with intranasal LAIV has not been evaluated. Concurrent administration of antiviral drugs may inhibit viral replication of LAIV and thereby decrease the effectiveness of LAIV vaccination. Interactions between inactivated influenza vaccines and **Xofluza** have not been evaluated. It is not known if **Xofluza** is safe and effective in children younger than 12 years of age or weighing less than 88 lb (40 kg). Safety in pregnancy is unknown. It is not known whether **Xofluza** is present in breast milk or effects on the breastfed infant.

INSECT BITE/STING

Topical Corticosteroids *see* Appendix J. Topical Corticosteroids by Potency
Parenteral Corticosteroids *see* Appendix L. Parenteral Corticosteroids
Oral Corticosteroids *see* Appendix K. Oral Corticosteroids

TOPICAL AND TRANSDERMAL ANESTHETICS

Comment: *Lidocaine* should not be applied to non-intact skin.

▷ *lidocaine* cream apply to affected area bid prn
Pediatric: <12 years: not recommended; ≥12 years: same as adult
    LidaMantle *Crm*: 3% (1, 2 oz)
    Lidoderm *Crm*: 3% (85 gm)
    ZTlido *lidocaine* topical system 1% (30/carton)
    Comment: Compared to Lidoderm (*lidocaine* patch 5%), which contains 700 mg/patch, ZTlido only requires 35 mg per topical system to achieve the same therapeutic dose.

▷ *lidocaine* lotion apply to affected area bid prn
Pediatric: <12 years: not recommended; ≥12 years: same as adult
    LidaMantle *Lotn*: 3% (177 ml)

▷ *lidocaine* 5% patch **(G)** apply up to 3 patches at one time for up to 12 hours/24-hour period (12 hours on/12 hours off); patches may be cut into smaller sizes before removal of the release liner; do not reuse
Pediatric: <12 years: not recommended; ≥12 years: same as adult
    Lidoderm *Patch*: 5% (10 x 14 cm; 30/carton)

▷ *lidocaine+dexamethasone*
Pediatric: <12 years: not recommended; ≥12 years: same as adult
    Decadron Phosphate with Xylocaine *Lotn*: dexa 4 mg+lido 10 mg per ml (5 ml)

▷ *lidocaine+hydrocortisone* **(G)** apply to affected area bid prn
Pediatric: <12 years: not recommended; ≥12 years: same as adult
    LidaMantle HC *Crm*: lido 3%+hydro 0.5% (1, 3 oz); *Lotn*: (177 ml)

▷ *lidocaine* 2.5%+*prilocaine* 2.5% apply sparingly to the burn bid-tid prn
Pediatric: <12 years: not recommended; ≥12 years: same as adult
    Emla Cream 5, 30 gm/tube

EPINEPHRINE

▷ *epinephrine* **(G)** 1:1,000 0.3-0.5 ml SC
Pediatric: 0.01 ml/kg SC

TETANUS PROPHYLAXIS
▷ **tetanus toxoid** vaccine **(G)** 0.5 ml IM x 1 dose if previously immunized
Vial: 5 Lf units/0.5 ml (0.5, 5 ml); *Prefilled syringe:* 5 Lf units/0.5 ml (0.5 ml) (for patients not previously immunized, *see* Tetanus)

INSOMNIA

Tricyclic Antidepressants *see* Depression

MELATONIN RECEPTOR AGONIST
▷ **ramelteon (IV)** 8 mg within 30 minutes of bedtime; delayed effect if taken with a meal
Pediatric: <12 years: not recommended; ≥12 years: same as adult
  Rozerem *Tab:* 8 mg

NON-BENZODIAZEPINES
▷ **eszopiclone (IV)(G)** (pyrrolopyrazine) 1-3 mg; max 3 mg/day x 1 month; do not take if unable to sleep for at least 8 hours before required to be active again; delayed effect if taken with a meal
Pediatric: <18 years: not recommended; ≥18 years: same as adult
  Lunesta *Tab:* 1, 2, 3 mg
▷ **zaleplon (IV)** (imidazopyridine) 5-10 mg at HS or after going to bed if unable to sleep; do not take if unable to sleep for at least 4 hours before required to be active again; max 20 mg/day x 1 month; delayed effect if taken with a meal
Pediatric: <12 years: not recommended; ≥12 years: same as adult
  Sonata *Cap:* 5, 10 mg (tartrazine)
  Comment: Sonata is indicated for the treatment of insomnia when a middle-of-the-night awakening is followed by difficulty returning to sleep.
▷ **zolpidem** oral solution spray **(IV)** (imidazopyridine hypnotic) 2 actuations (10 mg) immediately before bedtime; *Elderly, debilitated, or hepatic impairment:* 2 actuations (5 mg); max 2 actuations (10 mg)
Pediatric: <18 years: not recommended; ≥18 years: same as adult
  ZolpiMist *Oral soln spray:* 5 mg/actuation (60 metered actuations) (cherry)
  Comment: The lowest dose of *zolpidem* in all forms is recommended for persons >50 years of age and women as drug elimination is slower than in men.
▷ **zolpidem** tabs **(IV)(G)** (pyrazolopyrimidine hypnotic) 5-10 mg or 6.25-12.5 ext-rel q HS prn; max 12.5 mg/day x 1 month; do not take if unable to sleep for at least 8 hours before required to be active again; delayed effect if taken with a meal
Pediatric: <18 years: not recommended; ≥18 years: same as adult
  Ambien *Tab:* 5, 10 mg
  Ambien CR *Tab:* 6.25, 12.5 mg ext-rel
  Comment: The lowest dose of *zolpidem* in all forms is recommended for persons >50 years of age and women as drug elimination is slower than in men.
▷ **zolpidem** sublingual tabs **(IV)(G)** (imidazopyridine hypnotic) dissolve 1 tab under the tongue; allow to disintegrate completely before swallowing; take only once per night and only if at least 4 hours of bedtime remain before planned time for awakening
Pediatric: <18 years: not recommended; ≥18 years: same as adult
  Edluar *SL Tab:* 5, 10 mg
  Intermezzo *SL Tab:* 1.75, 3.5 mg
  Comment: Intermezzo is indicated for the treatment of insomnia when a middle-of-the-night awakening is followed by difficulty returning to sleep. The lowest dose of *zolpidem* in all forms is recommended for persons >50 years of age and women as drug elimination is slower than in men.

OREXIN RECEPTOR ANTAGONIST
▷ **suvorexant (IV)** use lowest effective dose; take 30 minutes before bedtime; do not take if unable to sleep for ≥7 hours, max 20 mg
Pediatric: <12 years: not recommended; ≥12 years: same as adult
  Belsomra *Tab:* 5, 10, 15, 20 mg (30/blister pck)

BENZODIAZEPINES
▷ **estazolam (IV)(G)** initially 1 mg q HS prn; may increase to 2 mg q HS
Pediatric: <18 years: not recommended; ≥18 years: same as adult
  ProSom *Tab:* 1*, 2*mg
▷ **flurazepam (IV)(G)** 30 mg q HS prn; Elderly or debilitated: 15 mg
Pediatric: <15 years: not recommended; ≥15 years: same as adult
  Dalmane *Cap:* 15, 30 mg
▷ **temazepam (IV)(G)** 7.5-30 mg q HS prn; short term, 7-10 days; max 30 mg; max 1 month
Pediatric: <18 years: not recommended; ≥18 years: same as adult
  Restoril *Cap:* 7.5, 15, 22.5, 30 mg

(continued)

▷ *triazolam* (IV) 0.125-0.25 mg q HS prn; short term, 7-10 days; max 0.5 mg; max 1 month
  Pediatric: <18 years: <u>not</u> recommended; ≥18 years: same as adult
    Halcion *Tab:* 0.125, 0.25*mg
    Barbiturates
▷ *pentobarbital* (II)(G)
    Nembutal 100 mg q HS prn
      Cap: 50, 100 mg
    Nembutal Suppository 120 <u>or</u> 200 mg suppository rectally q HS prn
    Pediatric: 2-12 months (10-20 lb): 30 mg supp; 1-4 years (21-40 lb): 30 <u>or</u> 60 mg supp; 5-12 years (41-80 lb):
    60 mg supp; 12-14 years (81-110 lb): 60 <u>or</u> 120 mg sup
      Rectal supp: 30, 60, 120, 200 mg

ORAL H1 RECEPTOR AGONIST (FIRST-GENERATION ANTIHISTAMINE)

▷ *doxepin*
    Silenor 3-6 mg q HS prn; *Elderly, hepatic impairment, tendency to urinary retention:* initially 3 mg
      Tab: 3, 6 mg

Other Oral 1st Generation Antihistamines *see* Appendix Z. Drugs for the Management of Allergy, Cough,
and Cold Symptoms online at https://connect.springerpub.com/content/reference-book/978-0-8261-7935-7/
back-matter/part02/back-matter/bmatter27

DUAL OREXIN RECEPTOR ANTAGONIST (DORA)

▷ *lemborexant* (controlled substance schedule pending) *Recommended dose:* 5 mg once nightly, immediately before
  going to bed, with at least 7 hours remaining before the planned time of awakening; time to sleep onset may be
  delayed if taken with <u>or</u> soon after a meal; may increase to max 10 mg based on clinical response and tolerability;
  Moderate hepatic impairment: max 5 mg once nightly; *Severe hepatic impairment:* <u>not</u> recommended
  Pediatric: safety and efficacy <u>not</u> established
    Dayvigo *Tab:* 5, 10 mg
    Comment: Dayvigo *(lemborexant)* is dual orexin receptor antagonist (DORA) for the treatment of adult
    patients with insomnia, characterized by difficulties with sleep onset and/or sleep maintenance. The central
    nervous system (CNS) depressant effects of **Dayvigo** impair alertness and motor coordination, including
    morning impairment. Risk increases with dose and concomitant use with other CNS depressants. **Dayvigo**
    is contraindicated in patients with narcolepsy. Sleep paralysis, hypnogogic/hypnopompic hallucinations,
    and cataplexy-like symptoms may be experienced. Complex sleep behaviors (CSB) including sleepwalking,
    sleepdriving, and engaging in other activities while <u>not</u> fully awake may occur; if this happens, discontinue
    Dayvigo immediately. Patients should be cautioned regarding potential worsening of depression <u>or</u>
    suicidal ideation. The most common adverse reaction reported (incidence ≥5% and at least twice the rate
    of placebo) has been somnolence. Avoid concomitant use of strong <u>or</u> moderate CYP3A inhibitors, weak
    CYP3A inhibitors, and strong <u>or</u> moderate CYP3A inducers. There are no available data on **Dayvigo** use
    in pregnant women to assess drug-associated risk of major birth defects, miscarriage, <u>or</u> adverse maternal
    <u>or</u> fetal outcomes. There are no data on the presence of *lemborexant* in human milk <u>or</u> effects on the
    breastfed infant. There is a pregnancy exposure registry that monitors pregnancy outcomes in women who
    are exposed to **Dayvigo** during pregnancy. Healthcare providers are encouraged to register patients in the
    Dayvigo pregnancy registry by calling 1-888-274-2378.

ANALGESIC+FIRST-GENERATION ANTIHISTAMINE COMBINATIONS

▷ *acetaminophen+diphenhydramine*
    Excedrin PM (OTC) 2 tabs q HS prn
      Pediatric: <12 years: <u>not</u> recommended; ≥12 years: same as adult
      Tab/Geltab: acet 500 mg+diphen 38 mg
    Tylenol PM (OTC) 2 caps q HS prn
      Pediatric: <12 years: <u>not</u> recommended; ≥12 years: same as adult
      Tab/Cap/Gelcap: acet 500 mg+diphen 25 mg

DUAL OREXIN RECEPTOR ANTAGONIST (DORA)

▷ *daridorexant* *Recommended dose:* 25-50 mg once per night, within 30 minutes before bedtime, with at
  least 7 hours remaining prior to planned awakening; time to sleep onset may be delayed if taken with <u>or</u>
  soon after a meal; *Child-Pugh Class B:* max 25 mg once per night; *Child-Pugh Class C:* <u>not</u> recommended;
  Concomitant strong CYP3A4 inhibitors and/or *moderate* <u>or</u> *strong CYP3A4 inducers:* avoid use; *Concomitant*
  CYP3A4 inhibitors: max 25 mg once per night
  Pediatric: safety and efficacy <u>not</u> established
    Quviviq *Tab:* 25, 50 mg
    Comment: Quviviq is a dual orexin receptor antagonist (DORA) for the treatment of adult patients with
    insomnia. The most common adverse reactions (reported in ≥5% of patients treated with **Quviviq** and at
    an incidence ≥than placebo) have been headache and somnolence <u>or</u> fatigue. The only contraindication
    to **Quviviq** is narcolepsy. **Quviviq**'s CNS depressant effects impair alertness and motor coordination
    including morning impairment. Risk increases when **Quviviq** is used with other CNS depressants.

Caution against next-day driving and other activities requiring complete mental alertness. Worsening of depression or suicidal ideation may occur. Sleep paralysis, hypnagogic hallucinations (occur falling asleep), hypnopompic hallucinations (occur when waking up), or cataplexy-like symptoms may occur with use of **Quviviq**. CSBs, including sleepwalking, sleepdriving, and engaging in other activities while not fully awake may occur. Discontinue **Quviviq** immediately if any CSBs occur. Monitor patients for compromised respiratory function (e.g., hypopnea, hypoxia, obstructive sleep apnea [OSA]). Evaluate patients for comorbid diagnoses and re-evaluate if insomnia persists after 7-10 days of using **Quviviq**. There are no available data on **Quviviq** use in human pregnancy to evaluate for drug-associated risks of major birth defects, miscarriage, or other adverse maternal or fetal outcomes. In animal reproduction studies, oral administration of ***daridorexant*** during the period of organogenesis did not cause fetal toxicity or malformation. There is a pregnancy exposure registry that monitors pregnancy outcomes in females exposed to **Quviviq** during pregnancy. Pregnant patients exposed to **Quviviq** and healthcare providers are encouraged to call Idorsia Pharmaceuticals Ltd at 1-833-400-9611. Infants exposed to **Quviviq** through breast milk should be monitored for excessive sedation. Developmental and health benefits of breastfeeding should be considered along with the mother's clinical need for **Quviviq** and any potential adverse effects on the breastfed infant from **Quviviq** or from the underlying maternal condition.

INTERSTITIAL CYSTITIS

Acetaminophen for IV Infusion *see Pain*
Oral Prescription NSAIDs *see* Appendix I. NSAIDs online at https://connect.springerpub.com/content/reference-book/978-0-8261-7935-7/back-matter/part02/back-matter/bmatter10
Comment: Avoid peppers and spicy food, citrus, vinegar, caffeine (e.g., coffee, tea, colas), alcohol, carbonated beverages, and other genitourinary (GU) tract irritants.

MANAGEMENT OF PAIN AND URINARY URGENCY
➤ **phenazopyridine** (G) 95-200 mg q 6 hours prn; max 2 days
Pediatric: <12 years: not recommended; ≥12 years: same as adult
   AZO Standard, Prodium, Uristat (OTC) *Tab:* 95 mg
   AZO Standard Maximum Strength (OTC) *Tab:* 97.5 mg
   Azo Standard (OTC) *Tab:* 95 mg
   Azo Standard Maximum Strength (OTC) *Tab:* 97.5 mg
   Pyridium *Tab:* 100, 200 mg ent-coat
   Uristat (OTC) *Tab:* 95 mg
   Urogesic *Tab:* 100, 200 mg
➤ **hyoscyamine** (G)
   Anaspaz 1-2 tabs q 4 hours prn; max 12 tabs/day
   Pediatric: <2 years: not recommended; 2-12 years: 0.0625-0.125 mg q 4 hours prn; max 0.75 mg/day; ≥12 years: same as adult
      Tab: 0.125*mg
   Levbid 1-2 tabs q 12 hours prn; max 4 tabs/day
   Pediatric: <12 years: not recommended; ≥12 years: same as adult
      Tab: 0.375*mg ext-rel
   Levsin 1-2 tabs q 4 hours prn; max 12 tabs/day
   Pediatric: <6 years: not recommended; 6-12 years: 1 tab q 4 hours prn; ≥12 years: same as adult
      Tab: 0.125*mg
   Levsin Drops 1-2 ml q 4 hours prn; max 60 ml/day
   Pediatric: 3.4 kg: 4 drops q 4 hours prn; max 24 drops/day; 5 kg: 5 drops q 4 hours prn; max 30 drops/day; 7 kg: 6 drops q 4 hours prn; max 36 drops/day; 10 kg: 8 drops q 4 hours prn; max 40 drops/day
      Oral drops: 0.125 mg/ml (15 ml) (orange) (alcohol 5%)
   Levsin Elixir 5-10 ml q 4 hours prn
   Pediatric: <10 kg: use drops; 10-19 kg: 1.25 ml q 4 hours prn; 20-39 kg: 2.5 ml q 4 hours prn; 40-49 kg: 3.75 ml q 4 hours prn; ≥50 kg: 5 ml q 4 hours prn
      Elix: 0.125 mg/5 ml (16 oz) (orange) (alcohol 20%)
   Levsinex SL 1-2 tabs q 4 hours SL or PO; max 12 tabs/day
   Pediatric: <2 years: not recommended; 2-12 years: 1 tab q 4 hours; max 6 tabs/day; ≥12 years: same as adult
      SL tab: 0.125 mg
   Levsinex Timecaps 1-2 caps q 12 hours; may adjust to 1 cap q 8 hours
   Pediatric: <2 years: not recommended; 2-12 years: 1 cap q 12 hours; max 2 caps/day; ≥12 years: same as adult
      Cap: 0.375 mg time-rel
   NuLev dissolve 1-2 tabs on tongue, with or without water, q 4 hours prn; max 12 tabs/day
   Pediatric: <2 years: not recommended; 2-12 years: dissolve 1 tab on tongue, with or without water, q 4 hours prn; max 6 tabs/day; ≥12 years: same as adult
      ODT: 0.125 mg (mint) (phenylalanine)

(continued)

▷ *methenamine+sod phosphate monobasic+phenyl salicylate+methylene blue+hyoscyamine sulfate* 1 cap qid
    Pediatric: <6 years: <u>not</u> recommended; ≥6 years: individualize dose
        Uribel *Cap*: meth 118 mg+sod phos 40.8 mg+phenyl sal 36 mg+meth blue 10 mg+hyoscy 0.12 mg
▷ *methenamine+phenyl salicylate+methylene blue+benzoic acid+atropine sulfate+hyoscyamine sulfate* (G) 2 tabs qid
    Pediatric: <6 years: <u>not</u> recommended; ≥6 years: same as adult
        Urised *Tab*: meth 40.8 mg+phenyl sal 18.1 mg+meth blue 5.4 mg+benz acid 4.5 mg+atro sul 0.03 mg+hyoscy 0.03 mg
        Comment: Urised imparts a blue-green color to urine which may stain fabrics.
▷ *oxybutynin chloride*
    Ditropan 5 mg bid-tid; max 20 mg/day
        Pediatric: <5 years: <u>not</u> recommended; 5-12 years: 5 mg bid; max 15 mg/day; ≥12 years: same as adult
        Tab: 5*mg; Syr: 5 mg/5 ml
    Ditropan XL initially 5 mg daily; may increase weekly in 5 mg increments as needed; max 30 mg/day
        Pediatric: <5 years: <u>not</u> recommended; ≥5 years: same as adult
        Tab: 5, 10, 15 mg ext-rel
▷ *pentosan* 100 mg tid; re-evaluate at 3 and 6 months
    Pediatric: <16 years: <u>not</u> recommended; ≥16 years: same as adult
        Elmiron *Cap*: 100 mg

URINARY TRACT ANALGESIA

▷ *phenazopyridine* (G) 95-200 mg q 6 hours prn; max 2 days
    Pediatric: <12 years: <u>not</u> recommended; ≥12 years: same as adult
        AZO Standard, Prodium, Uristat (OTC) *Tab*: 95 mg
        AZO Standard Maximum Strength (OTC) *Tab*: 97.5 mg
        Pyridium, Urogesic *Tab*: 100, 200 mg
        Azo Standard (OTC) *Tab*: 95 mg
        Azo Standard Maximum Strength (OTC) *Tab*: 97.5 mg
        Pyridium *Tab*: 100, 200 mg ent-coat
        Uristat (OTC) *Tab*: 95 mg
        Urogesic *Tab*: 100, 200 mg
    Comment: *Phenazopyridine* imparts an orange-red color to urine which may stain fabrics.
▷ *propantheline* 15-30 mg tid
        Pro-Banthine *Tab*: 7.5, 15 mg
▷ *tolterodine tartrate* (G) Detrol 1-2 mg bid <u>or</u> Detrol LA 2-4 mg once daily <u>or</u> Detrol XL 1 tab daily
    Pediatric: <12 years: <u>not</u> recommended; ≥12 years: same as adult
        Detrol *Tab*: 1, 2 mg
        Detrol *Cap*: 2, 4 mg ext-rel
        Detrol XL *Tab*: 5, 10, 15 mg ext-rel

ANTICHOLINERGIC+SEDATIVE COMBINATION

▷ *chlordiazepoxide+clidinium* (IV) 1-2 caps ac and HS; max 8 caps/day
    Pediatric: <12 years: <u>not</u> recommended; ≥12 years: same as adult
        Librax *Cap*: chlor 5 mg+clid 2.5 mg

TRICYCLIC ANTIDEPRESSANTS (TCAs)

▷ *amitriptyline* (G) 25-50 mg q HS
    Pediatric: <12 years: <u>not</u> recommended; ≥12 years: same as adult
        Tab: 10, 25, 50, 75, 100, 150 mg
▷ *imipramine* (G)
    Pediatric: <12 years: <u>not</u> recommended; ≥12 years: same as adult
        Tofranil initially 75 mg daily (max 200 mg); adolescents initially 30-40 mg daily (max 100 mg/day); if maintenance dose exceeds 75 mg daily, may switch to Tofranil PM for divided <u>or</u> bedtime dose
        Tab: 10, 25, 50 mg
        Tofranil PM initially 75 mg daily 1 hour before HS; max 200 mg
        Cap: 75, 100, 125, 150

INTERTRIGO

see **Candidiasis: Skin**
Topical Antifungals *see* **Tinea Corporis**
Topical Anti-Infectives *see* **Skin Infection: Bacterial**
Topical Corticosteroids *see* Appendix J. Topical Corticosteroids by Potency
OTC Hydrocortisone 1% Paste <u>or</u> Ointment
OTC Zinc Oxide Paste <u>or</u> Ointment
OTC A&D Ointment

Comment: Intertrigo is an irritant dermatitis in the intertriginous zones (skin creases and folds) characterized by inflammation and excoriation caused by skin-to-skin friction, moisture, and heat, and may be itching, stinging, and burning with a musty odor. Common areas at risk include breast folds, axillae, groin folds, buttocks folds, and the abdominal panniculus in obese persons, finger, and toe webs. Treatment includes keeping the areas clean, moisture-free, application of a steroid cream, and a protective lubricant barrier. Intertrigo may be complicated by a superimposed infection such as yeast (*Candida albicans*), dermatophytic fungi, or bacteria. Oral agents may be required based on severity of the skin breakdown and invasive infectious process. Apply appropriate topical anti-infective first and barrier product last. Non-medicated powders (e.g., cornstarch) are contraindicated in the affected areas as they trap moisture. Exposure to light and air when possible and as appropriate facilitates integumentary healing.

INTRA-ABDOMINAL INFECTION: COMPLICATED (cIAI)

PARENTERAL CEPHALOSPORIN ANTIBACTERIAL+BETA-LACTAMASE INHIBITOR

➤ *ceftazidime+avibactam* infuse dose over 2 hours; *Recommended duration of treatment*: 5-14 days; *CrCl 31-50 ml/min*: 1.25 gm q 8 hours; *CrCl 16-30 ml/min*: 0.94 gm q 12 hours; *CrCl 6-15 ml/min*: 0.94 gm q 24 hours; *CrCl ≤5 ml/min*: 0.94 gm q 48 hours; both *ceftazidime* and *avibactam* are hemodialyzable; thus, administer **Avycaz** after hemodialysis on hemodialysis days

Pediatric: <18 years: not recommended; ≥18 years: same as adult

    Avycaz *Vial:* 2.5 gm, single-dose, pwdr for reconstitution and IV infusion

    Comment: Avycaz 2.5 gm contains *ceftazidime* (a cephalosporin) 2 gm (equivalent to 2.635 gm of *ceftazidime pentahydrate/sodium carbonate powder*) and *avibactam* (a beta-lactamase inhibitor) 0.5 gm (equivalent to 0.551 gm of *avibactam sodium*). As only limited clinical safety and efficacy data for **Avycaz** are currently available, reserve **Avycaz** for use in patients who have limited or no alternative treatment options. To reduce the development of drug-resistant bacteria and maintain the effectiveness of **Avycaz** and other antibacterial drugs, **Avycaz** should be used only to treat infections that are proven or strongly suspected to be caused by susceptible bacteria. Seizures and other neurologic events may occur, especially in patients with renal impairment. Adjust dose in patients with renal impairment. Decreased efficacy in patients with baseline CrCl 30 ≤50 ml/min. Monitor CrCl at least daily in patients with changing renal function and adjust the dose of **Avycaz** accordingly. Monitor for hypersensitivity reactions, including anaphylaxis and serious skin reactions. Cross-hypersensitivity may occur in patients with a history of penicillin allergy. If an allergic reaction occurs, discontinue **Avycaz**. *Clostridioides difficile*-associated diarrhea (CDAD) has been reported with nearly all systemic antibacterial agents, including **Avycaz**. There are no adequate and well-controlled studies of **Avycaz**, *ceftazidime*, or *avibactam* in pregnant females. *Ceftazidime* is excreted in human milk in low concentrations. It is not known whether *avibactam* is excreted into human milk. There are no studies to inform effects on the breastfed infant.

➤ *ceftolozane+tazobactam* administer 1.5 gm q 8 hours via IV infusion over 1 hour x 4-14 days; *CrCl 30-50 ml/min*: 750 mg via IV infusion q 8 hours; *CrCl 15-29 ml/min*: 375 mg via IV infusion q 8 hours; *End-stage renal disease (ESRD):* a single loading dose of 750 mg via IV infusion, followed by 150 mg via IV infusion q 8 hours for the remainder of the treatment period (on hemodialysis days, administer the dose at the earliest possible time following completion of dialysis)

Pediatric: <18: not established; ≥18 years: same as adult

    Zerbaxa *Vial:* 1.5 gm (*ceftolozane* 1 gm+*tazobactam* 0.5 gm), single-dose, pwdr for reconstitution and IV infusion

    Comment: For doses >1.5 gm, reconstitute a second vial in the same manner as the first one, withdraw an appropriate volume (see Table 3 in the mfr pkg insert) and add to the same infusion bag. The most common adverse reactions in patients with complicated intra-abdominal infection (cIAI) (incidence ≥5%) have been nausea, diarrhea, headache, and pyrexia.

PARENTERAL PENEM ANTIBACTERIAL+RENAL DEHYDROPEPTIDASE INHIBITOR+BETA-LACTAMASE INHIBITOR

➤ *imipenem+cilastatin+relebactam* administer dose via IV infusion over 30 minutes every 6 hours; *CrCl ≥90 ml/min*: 1.25 gm/dose (*imipenem* 500 mg, *cilastatin* 500 mg, *relebactam* 250 mg); *CrCl 60-89 ml/min*: 1 gm/dose (*imipenem* 400 mg, *cilastatin* 400 mg, *relebactam* 200 mg); *CrCl 30-59 ml/min*: 0.75 gm/dose (*imipenem* 300 mg, *cilastatin* 300 mg, *relebactam* 150 mg); *CrCl 15-29 ml/min*: 0.5 gm/dose (*imipenem* 200 mg, *cilastatin* 200 mg, *relebactam* 100 mg); *ESRD/Dialysis:* 0.5 gm/dose (*imipenem* 200 mg, *cilastatin* 200 mg, *relebactam* 100 mg)

Pediatric: <18 years: not established; ≥18 years: same as adult

    Recarbrio *Vial:* imipen 500 mg+cilast 500 mg+relebac 250 mg, single-dose, pwdr for reconstitution, dilution, and IV infusion

    Comment: Recarbrio (*imipenem+cilastatin+relebactam*) is a fixed-dose triple combination of *imipenem* (a penem antibacterial), *cilastatin* (a renal dehydropeptidase inhibitor), and *relebactam* (a beta-lactamase inhibitor) indicated for the treatment of complicated urinary tract infection (cUTI), including pyelonephritis, and cIAI caused by susceptible gram-negative bacteria in patients who have limited or no alternative treatment options, hospital-acquired bacterial pneumonia (HABP), and ventilator-associated bacterial pneumonia (VABP) in adults. Avoid concomitant use of **Recarbrio** with *ganciclovir*, *valproic*

(continued)

acid, or *divalproex sodium.* Based on clinical reports on patients treated with *imipenem/cilastatin* plus *relebactam* 250 mg, the most frequent adverse reactions (incidence ≥2 %) have been diarrhea, nausea, headache, vomiting, increased alanine aminotransferase (ALT), increased aspartate aminotransferase (AST), phlebitis/infusion site reactions, pyrexia, and hypertension. There are insufficient human data to establish whether there is a drug-associated risk of major birth defects, miscarriage, or adverse maternal or fetal outcomes with *imipenem, cilastatin,* or *relebactam* in pregnancy. However, embryonic loss has been observed in monkeys treated with *imipenem/cilastatin,* and fetal abnormalities have been observed in *relebactam*-treated mice; therefore, advise pregnant females of the potential risks to pregnancy and the fetus. There are insufficient data on the presence of *imipenem/cilastatin* and *relebactam* in human milk and no data on the effects on the breastfed infant; however, *relebactam* is present in the milk of lactating rats and therefore developmental and health benefits of breastfeeding should be considered along with the mother's clinical need for **Recarbrio** and any potential adverse effects on the breastfed child from **Recarbrio** or from the underlying maternal condition.

PARENTERAL TETRACYCLINE-CLASS (FLUOROCYCLINE) ANTIBACTERIAL

▶ *eravacycline* 1 mg/kg by IV infusion over approximately 60 minutes q 12 hours x 4-14 days; *severe hepatic impairment (Child-Pugh Class C):* 1 mg/kg q 12 hours on Day 1, then 1 mg/kg q 24 hours starting on Day 2 for a total duration of 4-14 days; *Concomitant use of a strong cytochrome P450 isoenzyme (CYP)3A inducer:* 1.5 mg/kg q 12 hours x 4-14 days
Pediatric: <18 years: not established; ≥18 years: same as adult
   Xerava *Vial:* 50 mg pwdr for IV reconstitution and further dilution for IV infusion, single-use
   Comment: Xerava *(eravacycline)* is a tetracycline-class (fluorocycline) antibacterial indicated for the treatment of complicated intra-abdominal infections in patients ≥18 years of age. **Xerava** is not indicated for the treatment of complicated urinary tract infections (cUTI). Patients who are on anticoagulant therapy may require downward adjustment of their anticoagulant dosage. The most common adverse reactions (incidence ≥3%) have been infusion site reactions, nausea, and vomiting. The use of **Xerava** during tooth development (last half of pregnancy, infancy, and childhood up to 8 years of age) may cause permanent discoloration of the teeth (yellow-gray-brown) and enamel hypoplasia. The use of **Xerava** during the 2nd and 3rd trimesters of pregnancy, infancy, and childhood up to 8 years of age may cause reversible inhibition of bone growth. *Eravacycline* and its metabolites are excreted in breast milk. Breastfeeding is not recommended; consider fetal risk and maternal benefit.

IRITIS: ACUTE

▶ *loteprednol etabonate* **(G)** 1-2 drops qid; may increase to 1 drop hourly as needed
Pediatric: <12 years: not recommended; ≥12 years: same as adult
   Lotemax Ophthalmic Gel *Ophth gel:* 0.5% (5 gm)
   Lotemax Ophthalmic Ointment *Oint:* 0.5% (3.5 gm)
   Lotemax Ophthalmic Solution *Ophth soln:* 0.3% (2.5, 5, 10, 15 ml)
   Lotemax SM *Ophth gel:* 0.38% (5 gm)
▶ *prednisone acetate* **(G)** 1 drop q 1 hour x 24-48 hours, then 1 drop q 2 hours while awake x 24-48 hours, then 1 drop bid-qid until resolved
Pediatric: <12 years: not recommended; ≥12 years: same as adult
   Pred Forte *Ophth soln:* 1% (1, 5, 10, 15 ml)

IRON OVERLOAD

IRON CHELATING AGENTS

▶ *deferiprone* 25-33 mg/kg 3 tid (total daily dose 75-99 mg/kg)
Pediatric: <3 years: safety and efficacy not established; ≥3-8 years: same as adult (use oral soln); ≥8 years: same as adult (use tablet form)
   Ferriprox *Tab:* 500, 1,000 mg film-coat (5 x 10-count blister packs/carton), adults and patients ≥8 years of age; *Oral soln:* 80, 100 mg/ml (20 gm/250 ml, 40 gm/500 ml w. graduated measuring cup)
   Comment: Ferriprox is an iron chelator agent indicated for the treatment of transfusional iron overload in patients with thalassemia syndromes and patients with sickle cell disease or other anemias. Safety and efficacy have not been established for the treatment of transfusional iron overload in patients with myelodysplastic syndrome or in patients with Diamond-Blackfan anemia. The most common adverse reactions in patients with thalassemia (incidence ≥6%) have been nausea, vomiting, abdominal pain, arthralgia, increased alanine aminotransferase (ALT), and neutropenia. The most common adverse reactions in patients with sickle cell disease or other anemias (incidence ≥6%) have been pyrexia, abdominal pain, bone pain, headache, vomiting, pain in extremity, sickle cell anemia with crisis, back pain, increased ALT, increased aspartate aminotransferase (AST), arthralgia, oropharyngeal pain,

nasopharyngitis, decreased neutrophil count, cough, and nausea. Monitor liver enzymes monthly and discontinue for persistent elevations. Monitor for zinc deficiency and supplement as indicated. *Boxed Warning:* **Ferriprox** can cause agranulocytosis that can lead to serious infections and death. Neutropenia may precede the development of agranulocytosis. Measure the absolute neutrophil count (ANC) before starting **Ferriprox** and monitor weekly while on therapy. Interrupt **Ferriprox** if infection develops and monitor the ANC more frequently. Advise patients to immediately report any symptoms indicative of infection. Avoid co-administration of drugs associated with neutropenia or agranulocytosis. If co-administration is unavoidable, closely monitor the absolute neutrophil count (ANC). Avoid co-administration with UGT1A6 inhibitors. Allow at least a 4-hour interval between administration of **Ferriprox** and drugs or supplements containing polyvalent cations (e.g., iron, aluminum, or zinc). Limited available data from *deferiprone* use in pregnant females are insufficient to inform a drug-associated risk of major birth defects and miscarriage. Based on animal studies, **Ferriprox** can cause embryo/fetal harm. Advise pregnant females and males and females of reproductive potential of the potential risk and advise to use effective contraception. Advise not to breastfeed.

▷ *deferasirox (tridentate ligand)* (G) initially 20 mg/kg/day; titrate; may increase 5-10 mg/kg q 3-6 months based on serum ferritin trends; max 30 mg/kg/day
  Pediatric: <2 years: not recommended; ≥2 years: same as adult
    Exjade *Tab for oral soln:* 125, 250, 500 mg
    Jadenu *Tab:* 90, 180, 360 mg film-coat
    Jadenu Sprinkle *Sachet:* 90, 180, 360 mg (30/carton)
  Comment: *Deferasirox* is an orally active chelator selective for iron. It is indicated for the treatment of chronic iron overload due to blood transfusions (transfusional hemosiderosis). Monitor serum ferritin monthly. Consider interrupting therapy if serum ferritin falls below 500 mcg/L. Take *deferasirox* (**Exjade, Jadenu, Jadenu Sprinkle**) on an empty stomach. Completely disperse tablet(s) or granules in 3.5 oz liquid if dose is ≤1 gm or 7 oz liquid if dose is ≥1 gm.

▷ *Succimer* initially 10 mg/kg q 8 hours x 5 days; then reduce frequency to q 12 hours x 14 more days; allow at least 14 days between courses unless blood lead levels indicate need for prompt treatment
  Pediatric: <12 months: not recommended; ≥12 months: same as adult
    Chemet *Cap:* 100 mg
  Comment: Chemet is indicated for the treatment of lead poisoning when blood lead level is 45 mcg/dL. Treatment for more than 3 consecutive weeks is not recommended. Monitor hydration, renal, and hepatic function.

IRRITABLE BOWEL SYNDROME WITH CONSTIPATION (IBS-C)

Bulk-Producing Agents, Laxatives, Stool Softeners *see Constipation*

GUANYLATE CYCLASE-C AGONIST
Comment: Guanylate cyclase-c agonists increase intestinal fluid and intestinal transit time may induce diarrhea and bloating and, therefore are contraindicated with known or suspected mechanical GI obstruction.
▷ *linaclotide* (G) 290 mcg once daily; take on an empty stomach at least 30 minutes before the first meal of the day; swallow whole or may open cap and sprinkle on applesauce or in water for administration
  Pediatric: <6 years: not recommended; 6-17 years: avoid; >17 years: same as adult
    Linzess *Cap:* 145, 290 mcg
  Comment: *Linaclotide* and its active metabolite are negligibly absorbed systemically following oral administration and maternal use is not expected to result in fetal exposure to the drug. There is no information regarding the presence of *plecanatide* in human milk or its effects on the breastfed infant.

CHLORIDE CHANNEL ACTIVATOR
▷ *lubiprostone* 8 mcg bid; *Severe hepatic impairment (Child-Pugh Class C):* 8 mcg once daily; take with food and water; do not break apart or chew
  Pediatric: <18 years: not recommended; ≥18 years: same as adult
    Amitiza *Cap:* 8, 24 mcg
  Comment: Amitiza increases intestinal fluid and intestinal transit time. Suspend dosing and rehydrate if severe diarrhea occurs. **Amitiza** is contraindicated with known or suspected mechanical GI obstruction. The most common adverse reactions in chronic idiopathic constipation (CIC) are nausea, diarrhea, headache, abdominal pain, abdominal distension, and flatulence.

SODIUM/HYDROGEN EXCHANGER 3 (NHE3) INHIBITOR
▷ *tenapanor* 50 mg bid; administer immediately prior to breakfast or the first meal of the day and immediately prior to dinner; if a dose is missed, skip the missed dose and take the next dose at the regular time; do not take 2 doses at the same time

(continued)

Pediatric: <6 years: contraindicated; 6-<12 years: avoid use; <18 years: safety not established; ≥18 years: same as adult

Ibsrela *Tab:* 50 mg

Comment: Ibsrela *(tenapanor)* is a first-in-class, sodium/hydrogen exchanger 3 (NHE3) inhibitor indicated for the treatment of adults with irritable bowel syndrome with constipation (IBS-C). Ibsrela is contraindicated in pediatric patients <6 years of age and patients with known or suspected mechanical GI obstruction. The most common adverse reactions (incidence ≥2%) have been diarrhea, abdominal distension, flatulence, and dizziness. If severe diarrhea occurs, suspend dosing and rehydrate the patient. *Tenapanor* is minimally absorbed systemically, with plasma concentrations below the limit of quantification (<0.5 ng/ml) following oral administration. Therefore, maternal use is not expected to result in embryo/fetal exposure to the drug. Animal studies and available data on Ibsrela exposure from a small number of pregnant females have not identified any drug-associated risk of major birth defects, miscarriage, or adverse maternal or embryo/fetal outcomes. The minimal systemic absorption of *tenapanor* will not result in a clinically relevant exposure to breastfed infants.

GUANYLATE CYCLASE-C AGONIST

▷ *plecanatide* 3 mg once daily; take with or without food; swallow whole; for patients who have difficulty swallowing tablets whole or those with a nasogastric or gastric feeding tube, see mfr pkg insert for full prescribing information with instructions for crushing the tablet and administering with applesauce or water; if serious dehydration occurs, suspend dosing and institute rehydration measures
Pediatric: <6 years: contraindicated; 6-<18 years: avoid use, safety and efficacy not established; ≥18 years: same as adult

Trulance *Tab:* 3 mg

Comment: Trulance *(plecanatide)* is a guanylate cyclase-C agonist indicated for adults for treatment of chronic idiopathic constipation (CIC) and irritable bowel syndrome with constipation (IBS-C). Trulance is contraindicated children <6 years of age (due to risk of serious dehydration) and patients with known or suspected GI obstruction. *Plecanatide* and its active metabolite are negligibly absorbed systemically following oral administration and maternal use is not expected to result in fetal exposure. No lactation studies in animals have been conducted and there is no information regarding the presence of *plecanatide* in human milk or effects on the breastfed infant.

IRRITABLE BOWEL SYNDROME WITH DIARRHEA (IBS-D)

Bulk-Producing Agents *see Constipation*

CONSTIPATING AGENTS

▷ *difenoxin+atropine* 2 tabs, then 1 tab after each loose stool or 1 tab q 3-4 hours as needed; max 8 tab/day x 2 days
Pediatric: <12 years: not recommended; ≥12 years: same as adult

Motofen *Tab:* difen 1 mg+atro 0.025 mg
▷ *diphenoxylate+atropine* (G) 2 tabs or 10 ml qid
Pediatric: <2 years: not recommended; 2-12 years: initially 0.3-0.4 mg/kg/day in 4 divided doses; ≥12 years: same as adult

Lomotil *Tab:* difen 2.5 mg+atro 0.025 mg; *Liq:* difen 2.5 mg+atro 0.025 mg per 5 ml (2 oz)
▷ *eluxadoline* (IV) 100 mg bid; 75 mg bid if unable to tolerate 100 mg, or without a gall bladder, or mild-to-moderate hepatic impairment, or receiving concomitant OATP1B1 inhibitors
Pediatric: <12 years: not established; ≥12 years: same as adult

Viberzi 4 mg initially, then 2 mg after each loose stool; max 16 mg/day

Tab: 75, 100 mg film-coat

Comment: *Eluxadoline* is a mu-opioid receptor agonist. It is contraindicated with biliary obstruction, Sphincter of Oddi disease or dysfunction, alcohol abuse or addiction, pancreatitis, pancreatic duct obstruction, severe hepatic impairment, and mechanical GI obstruction.
▷ *loperamide* (G)

Imodium (OTC) 4 mg initially, then 2 mg after each loose stool; max 16 mg/day
Pediatric: <5 years: not recommended; ≥5 years: same as adult

Cap: 2 mg

Imodium A-D (OTC) 4 mg initially, then 2 mg after each loose stool; usual max 8 mg/day x 2 days
Pediatric: <2 years: not recommended; 2-5 years (24-47 lb): 1 mg up to tid x 2 days; 6-8 years (48-59 lb): 2 mg initially, then 1 mg after each loose stool; max 4 mg/day x 2 days; 9-11 years (60-95 lb): 2 mg initially, then 1 mg after each loose stool; max 6 mg/day x 2 days; ≥12 years: same as adult

Cplt: 2 mg; *Liq:* 1 mg/5 ml (2, 4 oz)
▷ *loperamide+simethicone* (G)

Imodium Advanced (OTC) 2 tabs chewed after loose stool, then 1 after the next loose stool; max 4 tabs/day

Pediatric: <6 years: not recommended; 6-8 years: 1 tab chewed after loose stool, then 1/2 after next loose stool; max 2 tabs/day; 9-11 years: 1 tab chewed after loose stool, then 1/2 after next loose stool; max 3 tabs/day; ≥12 years: same as adult
Chew tab: lop 2 mg+sim 125 mg

SEROTONIN (5-HT3) RECEPTOR ANTAGONIST

▷ *alosetron* (G) initially 0.5 mg bid; may increase to 1 mg bid after 4 weeks if starting dose is tolerated but inadequate
Pediatric: <12 years: not recommended; ≥12 years: same as adult
  Lotronex *Tab:* 0.5, 1 mg

ANTISPASMODIC+ANTICHOLINERGIC COMBINATIONS

▷ *dicyclomine* (G) initially 20 mg bid-qid; may increase to 40 mg qid PO; usual IM dose 80 mg/day divided qid; do not use IM route for more than 1-2 days
Pediatric: <12 years: not recommended; ≥12 years: same as adult
  Bentyl *Tab:* 20 mg; *Cap:* 10 mg; *Syr:* 10 mg/5 ml (16 oz); *Vial:* 10 mg/ml (10 ml); *Amp:* 10 mg/ml (2 ml)
▷ *methscopolamine bromide* 1 tab q 6 hours prn
Pediatric: <12 years: not recommended; ≥12 years: same as adult
  Pamine *Tab:* 2.5 mg
  Pamine Forte *Tab:* 5 mg

ANTICHOLINERGICS

▷ *hyoscyamine* (G)
  Anaspaz 1-2 tabs q 4 hours prn; max 12 tabs/day
  Pediatric: <2 years: not recommended; 2-12 years: 0.0625-0.125 mg q 4 hours prn; max 0.75 mg/day; ≥12 years: same as adult
    Tab: 0.125*mg
  Levbid 1-2 tabs q 12 hours prn; max 4 tabs/day
  Pediatric: <12 years: not recommended; ≥12 years: same as adult
    Tab: 0.375*mg ext-rel
  Levsin 1-2 tabs q 4 hours prn; max 12 tabs/day
  Pediatric: <6 years: not recommended; 6-12 years: 1 tab q 4 hours prn; >12 years: same as adult
    Tab: 0.125*mg
  Levsinex SL 1-2 tabs q 4 hours SL or PO; max 12 tabs/day
  Pediatric: <2 years: not recommended; 2-12 years: 1 tab q 4 hours; max 6 tabs/day; >12 years: same as adult
    Tab: 0.125 mg sublingual
  Levsinex Timecaps 1-2 caps q 12 hours; may adjust to 1 cap q 8 hours
  Pediatric: <2 years: not recommended; 2-12 years: 1 cap q 12 hours; max 2 caps/day; >12 years: same as adult
    Cap: 0.375 mg time-rel
  NuLev dissolve 1-2 tabs on tongue, with or without water, q 4 hours prn; max 12 tabs/day
  Pediatric: <2 years: not recommended; 2-12 years: dissolve 1 tab on tongue, with or without water, q 4 hours prn; max 6 tabs/day; >12 years: same as adult
    ODT: 0.125 mg (mint; phenylalanine)
▷ *simethicone* (G) 0.3 ml qid pc and HS
  Mylicon Drops (OTC) *Oral drops:* 40 mg/0.6 ml (30 ml)
▷ *phenobarbital+hyoscyamine+atropine+scopolamine* (IV)(G)
  Donnatal 1-2 tabs ac and HS
  Pediatric: <12 years: not recommended; ≥12 years: same as adult
    Tab: pheno 16.2 mg+hyo 0.1037 mg+atro 0.0194 mg+scop 0.0065 mg
  Donnatal Elixir 1-2 tsp ac and HS
  Pediatric: 20 lb: 1 ml q 4 hours or 1.5 ml q 6 hours; 30 lb: 1.5 ml q 4 hours or 2 ml q 6 hours; 50 lb: 1/2 tsp q 4 hours or 3/4 tsp q 6 hours; 75 lb: 3/4 tsp q 4 hours or 1 tsp q 6 hours; 100 lb: 1 tsp q 4 hours or 1 tsp q 6 hours
    Elix: pheno 16.2 mg+hyo 0.1037 mg+atro 0.0194 mg+scop 0.0065 mg per 5 ml (4, 16 oz)
  Donnatal Extentabs 1 tab q 12 hours
  Pediatric: <12 years: not recommended; ≥12 years: same as adult
    Tab: pheno 48.6 mg+hyo 0.3111 mg+atro 0.0582 mg+scop 0.0195 mg ext-rel

ANTICHOLINERGIC+SEDATIVE COMBINATION

▷ *chlordiazepoxide+clidinium* (IV) 1-2 caps ac and HS: max 8 caps/day
  Pediatric: <12 years: not recommended; ≥12 years: same as adult
    Librax *Cap:* chlor 5 mg+clid 2.5 mg

TRICYCLIC ANTIDEPRESSANTS (TCAs)

▷ *amitriptyline* (G) 25-50 mg q HS
  Pediatric: <12 years: <u>not</u> recommended; ≥12 years: same as adult
    Tab: 10, 25, 50, 75, 100, 150 mg
▷ *imipramine* (G) 25-50 mg tid
  Pediatric: <12 years: <u>not</u> recommended; ≥12 years: same as adult
    Tofranil initially 75 mg daily (max 200 mg); adolescents initially 30-40 mg daily (max 100 mg/day); if
    maintenance dose exceeds 75 mg daily, may switch to **Tofranil PM** for divided <u>or</u> bedtime dose
      Tab: 10, 25, 50 mg
    Tofranil PM initially 75 mg daily 1 hour before HS; max 200 mg
      Cap: 75, 100, 125, 150
    Tofranil Injection 50 mg IM; lower dose for adolescents; switch to oral form as soon as possible
      Amp: 25 mg/2 ml (2 ml)
▷ *nortriptyline* (G) initially 25 mg tid-qid; max 150 mg/day
  Pediatric: <12 years: <u>not</u> recommended; ≥12 years: same as adult
    Pamelor *Cap:* 10, 25, 50, 75 mg; *Oral soln:* 10 mg/5 ml (16 oz)
▷ *protriptyline* initially 5 mg tid; usual dose 15-40 mg/day in 3-4 divided doses; max 60 mg/day
  Pediatric: <12 years: <u>not</u> recommended; ≥12 years: same as adult
    Vivactil *Tab:* 5, 10 mg
▷ *trimipramine* initially 75 mg/day in divided doses; max 200 mg/day
  Pediatric: <12 years: <u>not</u> recommended; ≥12 years: same as adult
    Surmontil *Cap:* 25, 50, 100 mg

JAPANESE ENCEPHALITIS VIRUS (JEV)

Comment: Japanese encephalitis is a viral disease spread by the bite of an infected mosquito. It is <u>not</u> spread
from person-to-person. Currently there is no cure. A person with encephalitis can experience fever, neck
stiffness, seizures, and coma. About 1 person in 4 with encephalitis die. Up to half of those who do <u>not</u> die
have permanent disability. There is one vaccine for Japanese encephalitis, currently licensed in the UK, for
use in adults and children >2 months of age. The live attenuated vaccine is administered in 2 doses for full
protection, with the second dose administered 28 days after the first. The second dose should be given at least
a week before travel. Children younger than 3 years of age get a smaller dose than patients who are 3 <u>or</u> older.
A booster dose might be recommended for anyone 17 <u>or</u> older who was vaccinated more than a year ago
and is still at risk of exposure. There is no information yet on the need for a booster dose for children. The
Japanese encephalitis virus (JEV) vaccine is usually available through the local health department.

▷ *Japanese encephalitis vaccine (JEV), inactivated, adsorbed* shake the prefilled syringe containing 0.5 ml to
  obtain a homogeneous suspension; *18-65 years:* 0.5 ml IM x 2 doses 7-28 days apart; *>65 years:* 0.5 ml IM x
  2 doses 28 days apart
  Pediatric: shake the prefilled syringe containing 0.5 ml to obtain a homogeneous suspension; <2 months:
  <u>not</u> recommended; 2 months to <3 years: 0.25 ml IM x 2 doses 28 days apart; 3 to <18 years: 0.5 ml IM x 2
  doses 28 days apart
    Ixiaro *Prefilled syringe:* 0.5 ml (protamine sulfate)
    Comment: Administer **Ixiaro** intramuscularly <u>only</u>. Preferred injection sites are the anterolateral aspect
    of the thigh (LAT) in infants 2 to 11 months of age, the LAT <u>or</u> the deltoid muscle if muscle mass
    is adequate in children 1 to <3 years of age, and the deltoid muscle in patients ≥3 years of age. To
    administer a 0.25 ml JEV dose, expel and discard half of the volume from the 0.5 ml prefilled syringe
    by pushing the plunger stopper up to the edge of the red line on the syringe barrel prior to injection.
    Complete the primary immunization series at least 1 week prior to potential exposure to JEV. A
    booster dose (third dose) may be administered at least 11 months after completion of the primary
    immunization series if ongoing exposure <u>or</u> re-exposure to JEV is expected. Embryo/fetal effects of
    JEV exposure in pregnancy and effects on the breastfed infant have <u>not</u> been studied.

JUVENILE IDIOPATHIC ARTHRITIS (JIA), POLYARTICULAR JUVENILE IDIOPATHIC ARTHRITIS (PJIA), SYSTEMIC JUVENILE IDIOPATHIC ARTHRITIS (SJIA)

Acetaminophen for IV Infusion *see Pain*
NSAIDs *see* Appendix I. NSAIDs online at https://connect.springerpub.com/content/reference-book/978-0-8261-7935-7/back-matter/part02/back-matter/bmatter10
Opioid Analgesics *see Pain*
Topical and Transdermal Analgesics *see Pain*
Parenteral Corticosteroids *see* Appendix L. Parenteral Corticosteroids
Oral Corticosteroids *see* Appendix K. Oral Corticosteroids
Topical Analgesic and Anesthetic Agents *see* Appendix H. Anesthetic Agents for Local Infiltration and
Dermal/Mucosal Membrane Application online at https://connect.springerpub.com/content/reference-book/978-0-8261-7935-7/back-matter/part02/back-matter9

TOPICAL AND TRANSDERMAL ANALGESICS

▷ *capsaicin* (G) apply tid <u>or</u> qid prn to intact skin
  Pediatric: <2 years: <u>not</u> recommended; ≥2 years: same as adult
      Axsain *Crm:* 0.075% (1, 2 oz)
      Capsin *Lotn:* 0.025, 0.075% (59 ml)
      Capzasin-HP (OTC) *Crm:* 0.075% (1.5 oz), 0.025% (45, 90 gm); *Lotn:* 0.075% (2 oz); 0.025% (45, 90 gm)
      Capzasin-P (OTC) *Crm:* 0.025% (1.5 oz); *Lotn:* 0.025% (2 oz)
      Dolorac *Crm:* 0.025% (28 gm)
      Double Cap (OTC) *Crm:* 0.05% (2 oz)
      R-Gel *Gel:* 0.025% (15, 30 gm)
      Zostrix (OTC) *Crm:* 0.025% (0.7, 1.5, 3 oz)
      Zostrix HP (OTC) *Emol crm:* 0.075% (1, 2 oz)
▷ *capsaicin* 8% patch apply up to 4 patches for one 60-minute application to clean dry skin; may prep area
  with topical anesthetic; wear non-latex gloves; patches may be cut to size/shape; treatment may be repeated
  every 3 months
  Pediatric: <18 years: <u>not</u> recommended; ≥18 years: same as adult
      Qutenza *Patch:* 8% 1640 mcg/cm (179 mg) (1 <u>or</u> 2 patches w. 1-50 gm tube cleansing gel/carton)
▷ *diclofenac sodium* apply qid prn to intact skin
  Pediatric: <12 years: <u>not</u> established; ≥12 years: same as adult
      Pennsaid 1.5% in 10 drop increments, dispense and rub into front, side, and back of the knee: usually;
      40 drops (40 mg) qid
          Topical soln: 1.5% (150 ml)
      Pennsaid 2% apply 2 pump actuations (40 mg) and rub into front, side, and back of the knee bid
          Topical soln: 2% (20 mg/pump actuation, 112 gm)
      Solaraze Gel massage in to clean skin bid prn
          Gel: 3% (50 gm) (benzyl alcohol)
      Voltaren Gel (OTC)(G) apply qid prn to intact skin
          Gel: 1% (100 gm)
  Comment: *Diclofenac* is contraindicated with *aspirin* allergy. As with other NSAIDs, should be avoided in
  late pregnancy (≥30 weeks) because it may cause premature closure of the ductus arteriosus.
▷ *doxepin* (G) cream apply to affected area qid at intervals of at least 3-4 hours; max 8 days
  Pediatric: <12 years: <u>not</u> recommended; >12 years: same as adult
      Prudoxin *Crm:* 5% (45 gm)
      Zonalon *Crm:* 5% (30, 45 gm)
▷ *pimecrolimus* 1% cream (G) <2 years: <u>not</u> recommended; ≥2 years: apply to affected area bid; do <u>not</u> apply
  an occlusive dressing
      Elidel *Crm:* 1% (30, 60, 100 gm)
  Comment: *Pimecrolimus* is indicated for short-term and intermittent long-term use. Discontinue use when
  resolution occurs. Contraindicated if the patient is immunosuppressed. Change to the 0.1% preparation <u>or</u>
  if secondary bacterial infection is present.
▷ *trolamine salicylate* apply tid-qid
  Pediatric: <2 years: <u>not</u> recommended; ≥2 years: same as adult
      Mobisyl Creme *Crm:* 10% (100 gm)

TOPICAL AND TRANSDERMAL ANESTHETICS

Comment: *Lidocaine* should <u>not</u> be applied to non-intact skin.
▷ *lidocaine* cream apply to affected area bid prn
  Pediatric: <12 years: <u>not</u> recommended; ≥12 years: same as adult
      LidaMantle *Crm:* 3% (1, 2 oz)
      Lidoderm *Crm:* 3% (85 gm)
      ZTlido *lidocaine* topical system 1% (30/carton)
      Comment: Compared to Lidoderm (*lidocaine* patch 5%), which contains 700 mg/patch, **ZTlido** requires
      35 mg per topical system to achieve the same therapeutic dose.
▷ *lidocaine* lotion apply to affected area bid prn
  Pediatric: <12 years: <u>not</u> recommended; ≥12 years: same as adult
      LidaMantle *Lotn:* 3% (177 ml)
▷ *lidocaine* 5% patch (G) apply up to 3 patches at one time for up to 12 hours/24-hour period (12 hours on/12
  hours off); patches may be cut into smaller sizes before removal of the release liner; do <u>not</u> reuse
  Pediatric: <12 years: <u>not</u> recommended; ≥12 years: same as adult
      Lidoderm *Patch:* 5% (10 x 14 cm; 30/carton)
▷ *lidocaine+dexamethasone*
  Pediatric: <12 years: <u>not</u> recommended; ≥12 years: same as adult
      Decadron Phosphate with Xylocaine *Lotn:* dexa 4 mg+lido 10 mg per ml (5 ml)
▷ *lidocaine+hydrocortisone* (G) apply to affected area bid prn
  Pediatric: <12 years: <u>not</u> recommended; ≥12 years: same as adult
      LidaMantle HC *Crm:* lido 3%+hydro 0.5% (1, 3 oz); *Lotn:* (177 ml)

(continued)

▷ *lidocaine* 2.5%+prilocaine 2.5% apply sparingly to the burn bid-tid prn
  Pediatric: <12 years: <u>not</u> recommended; ≥12 years: same as adult
      Emla Cream 5, 30 gm/tube

ORAL SALICYLATES

▷ *indomethacin* initially 25 mg bid <u>or</u> tid, increase as needed at weekly intervals by 25-50 mg/day; max 200
  mg/day
  Pediatric: <14 years: usually <u>not</u> recommended; >2 years, if risk warranted: 1-2 mg/kg/day in divided doses,
  max 3-4 mg/kg/day (<u>or</u> 150-200 mg/day, whichever is less); <14 years: ER cap <u>not</u> recommended
  Cap: 25, 50 mg; *Susp:* 25 mg/5 ml (pineapple-coconut, mint) (alcohol 1%); *Supp:* 50 mg; *ER Cap:* 75 mg ext-rel
  Comment: *Indomethacin* is indicated <u>only</u> for acute painful flares. Administer with food <u>and/or</u> antacids. Use
  lowest effective dose for shortest duration.

METHOTREXATE (MTX)

▷ *methotrexate* (MTX) 7.5 mg x 1 dose per week <u>or</u> 2.5 mg x 3 at 12 hour intervals once a week; max 20 mg/
  week; therapeutic response begins in 3-6 weeks; administer *MTX* injection SC <u>only</u> into the abdomen <u>or</u>
  thigh
  Pediatric: <2 years: <u>not</u> recommended; ≥2 years: 10 mg/m² once weekly; max 20 mg/m²
      Rasuvo *Autoinjector:* 7.5 mg/0.15 ml, 10 mg/0.20 ml, 12.5 mg/0.25 ml, 15 mg/0.30 ml, 17.5 mg/0.35 ml, 20
      mg/0.40 ml, 22.5 mg/0.45 ml, 25 mg/0.50 ml, 27.5 mg/0.55 ml, 30 mg/0.60 ml (solution concentration for
      SC injection is 50 mg/ml)
      RediTrex *Prefilled syringe (in needle safety device):* 7.5, 10, 12.5, 15, 17.5, 20, 22.5, 25 mg, single-dose
      Rheumatrex *Tab:* 2.5*mg (5, 7.5, 10, 12.5, 15 mg/week, 4/card unit dose pack)
      Trexall *Tab:* 5*, 7.5*, 10*, 15*mg (5, 7.5, 10, 12.5, 15 mg/week, 4/card unit dose pack)
  Comment: *Methotrexate* (MTX) is contraindicated with immunodeficiency, blood dyscrasias, alcoholism, and
  chronic liver disease.

INTERLEUKIN-6 RECEPTOR ANTAGONIST

▷ *tocilizumab* IV infusion: administer over 1 hour; do <u>not</u> administer as bolus <u>or</u> IV push; *Adults, polyarticular
  juvenile idiopathic arthritis (PJIA), and systemic juvenile idiopathic arthritis (SJIA),* ≥30 kg: dilute to 100 ml
  in 0.9% <u>or</u> 0.45% NaCl; *PJIA and SJIA,* <30 kg: dilute to 50 ml in 0.9% <u>or</u> 0.45% NaCl.
  Pediatric: <2 years: <u>not</u> recommended; ≥2 years: same as adult
      Adults: IV infusion: whether used in combination with disease-modifying antirheumatic drugs
      (DMARDs) <u>or</u> as monotherapy, the recommended IV infusion starting dose is 4 mg/kg IV q 4 weeks
      followed by an increase to 8 mg/kg IV q 4 weeks based on clinical response; max 800 mg per infusion
      in rheumatoid arthritis (RA) patients; *SC administration:* ≥100 kg: 162 mg SC once weekly on the same
      day; <100 kg: 162 mg SC every other week on the same day followed by an increase according to clinical
      response
      Pediatric: <2 years: <u>not</u> recommended; ≥2 years: weight-based dosing according to diagnosis: *PJIA:* ≥30
      kg: 8 mg/kg SC q 4 weeks; <30 kg: 10 mg/kg SC q 4 weeks; *SJIA:* ≥30 kg: 8 mg/kg SC q 2 weeks; <30 kg:
      12 mg/kg SC q 2 weeks
          Actemra *Vial:* 80 mg/4 ml, 200 mg/10 ml, 400 mg/20 ml, single-use, for IV infusion after dilution;
          Prefilled syringe: 162 mg (0.9 ml, single-dose); *Prefilled ACTPen autoinjector:* 162 mg/0.9 ml, single-
          dose, for SC administration
  Comment: *Tocilizumab* is an interleukin-6 receptor-alpha inhibitor indicated for use in moderate-to-severe
  RA that has <u>not</u> responded to conventional therapy and also for some subtypes of juvenile idiopathic arthritis
  (JIA). **Actemra** may be used alone <u>or</u> in combination with *methotrexate* (MTX) and in RA other DMARDs
  may be used. Monitor patients for dose-related laboratory changes, including elevated liver function tests
  (LFTs), neutropenia, and thrombocytopenia. **Actemra** should <u>not</u> be initiated in patients with an absolute
  neutrophil count (ANC) below 2,000 per mm³, platelet count below 100,000 per mm³, <u>or</u> who have alanine
  aminotransferase (ALT) <u>or</u> aspartate aminotransferase (AST) above 1.5 times the upper limit of normal
  (ULN). Registration in the Pregnancy Exposure Registry (1-877-311-8972) is encouraged for monitoring
  pregnancy outcomes in women exposed to **Actemra** during pregnancy. The limited available data with
  Actemra in pregnant females are <u>not</u> sufficient to determine whether there is a drug-associated risk of
  major birth defects and miscarriage. Monoclonal antibodies, such as *tocilizumab*, are actively transported
  across the placenta during the third trimester of pregnancy and may affect immune response in the infant
  exposed *in utero*. It is <u>not</u> known whether *tocilizumab* passes into breast milk; therefore, breastfeeding is <u>not</u>
  recommended while using **Actemra**.

Selective Co-Stimulation Modulator

▷ *abatacept* <2 years: <u>not</u> recommended; 2-17 years: administer as an IV infusion over 30 minutes at weeks 0,
  2, and 4; then q 4 weeks thereafter; <75 kg: administer 10 mg/kg; same as adult (max 1 gm); administer as
  an IV infusion over 30 minutes at weeks 0, 2, and 4; then q 4 weeks thereafter; <60 kg: administer 500 mg/
  dose; 60-100 kg: administer 750 mg/dose; >100 kg: administer 1 gm/dose
      Orencia *Vial:* 250 mg pwdr for IV infusion after reconstitution (silicone-free) (preservative-free);
      Prefilled syringe: 125 mg/ml soln for SC injection (preservative-free); *ClickJect autoinjector:* 125 mg/ml
      soln for SC injection

Comment: Orencia is indicated to reduce signs/symptoms of moderate-to-severe active polyarticular juvenile idiopathic arthritis (PJIA) in patients >2 years of age as monotherapy or with *methotrexate* (MTX). **Orencia** is also indicated to reduce signs/symptoms, induce major clinical response, inhibit progression of structural damage, and improve physical function in adult patients with moderate-to-severe active RA. **Orencia** may be used as monotherapy or with DMARDs, other than tumor necrosis factor (TNF) antagonists.

TUMOR NECROSIS FACTOR (TNF) BLOCKER

▷ *adalimumab* <10 kg (<22 lb): safety and efficacy not established; 10 kg (22 lb) to <15 kg (<33 lb): 10 mg every other week; 15 kg (33 lb) to <30 kg (<66 lb): 20 mg every other week; ≥30 kg (66 lb): 40 mg every other week; administer SC in the abdomen or thigh; rotate sites

Humira *Prefilled pen (Humira Pen):* 40 mg/0.4 ml, 40 mg/0.8 ml, 80 mg/0.8 ml, single-dose; *Prefilled glass syringe:* 10 mg/0.1 ml, 10 mg/0.2 ml, 20 mg/0.2 ml, 20 mg/0.4 ml, 40 mg/0.4 ml, 40 mg/0.8 ml, 80 mg/0.8 ml, single-dose; *Vial:* 40 mg/0.8 ml, single-dose, institutional use only (preservative-free)

Comment: May use with *MTX*, DMARDs, corticosteroids, salicylates, NSAIDs, or analgesics.

▷ *adalimumab-aacf*
Pediatric: <2 years: not recommended; ≥2 years, ≥30 kg (≥ 66 lb): 40 mg SC every other week

Idacio *Prefilled pen (Idacio Pen):* 40 mg/0.8 ml, single-dose; *Prefilled glass syringe:* 40 mg/0.8 ml, single-dose

Comment: Idacio is biosimilar to **Humira**.

▷ *adalimumab-adaz* <4 years, <30 kg (<66 lb): not recommended; ≥4 years, ≥30 kg (≥66 lb): 40 mg every other week; inject into thigh or abdomen; rotate sites

Hyrimoz *Prefilled syringe:* 40 mg/0.8 ml, single-dose (preservative-free)

Comment: Hyrimoz is biosimilar to **Humira** *(adalimumab)*.

▷ *adalimumab-adbm* <30 kg, <66 lb: not recommended; ≥30 kg, ≥66 lb: 40 mg every other week; inject into thigh or abdomen; rotate sites

Cyltezo *Prefilled syringe:* 40 mg/0.8 ml, single-dose (preservative-free)

Comment: Cyltezo is biosimilar to **Humira** *(adalimumab)*.

▷ *adalimumab-afzb* 40 mg SC every other week; some patients with RA not receiving *MTX* may benefit from increasing the frequency to 40 mg SC every week

Abrilada *Prefilled pen:* 40 mg/0.8 ml, single-dose; *Prefilled syringe:* 40 mg/0.8 ml, 20 mg/0.4 ml, 10 mg/0.2 ml, single-dose; *Vial:* 40 mg/0.8 ml, single-use (for institutional use only) (preservative-free)

Comment: Abrilada is biosimilar to **Humira** *(adalimumab)*.

▷ *adalimumab-bwwd* Initial dose (Day 1): 160 mg SC; *Second dose:* 2 weeks later (Day 15): 80 mg SC; *2 weeks later* (Day 29): begin maintenance dose: 40 mg every other week

Hadlima *Prefilled autoinjector:* 40 mg/0.8 ml, single-dose (Hadlima PushTouch); *Prefilled syringe:* 40 mg/0.8 ml, single-dose

Comment: Hadlima is biosimilar to **Humira** *(adalimumab)*.

▷ *etanercept* inject SC into thigh, abdomen, or upper arm; rotate sites; initially 50 mg twice weekly (3-4 days apart) for 3 months; then 50 mg/week maintenance or 25 mg or 50 mg per week for 3 months; then 50 mg/week maintenance

Pediatric: <4 years: not recommended; 4-17 years: chronic moderate-to-severe plaque psoriasis; >17 years: same as adult

Enbrel *Vial:* 25 mg pwdr for SC injection after reconstitution (4/carton w. supplies) (preservative-free, diluent contains benzyl alcohol); *Prefilled syringe:* 25, 50 mg/ml (preservative-free); *SureClick autoinjector:* 50 mg/ml (preservative-free)

▷ *etanercept-ykro* 50 mg SC once weekly
Pediatric: <4 years: not established; ≥4 years, ≥63 kg, 138 lb: same as adult

Eticovo *Prefilled syringe:* 25 mg/0.5 ml, 50 mg/ml solution, single-dose

Comment: Eticovo *(etanercept-ykro)* is a TNF blocker biosimilar to **Enbrel** *(etanercept)*.

▷ *golimumab* administer SC or IV infusion
Simponi 50 mg SC once monthly; rotate sites
Pediatric: <18 years: not recommended; ≥18 years: same as adult

Prefilled syringe, SmartJect autoinjector: 50 mg/0.5 ml, single-use (preservative-free)

Simponi Aria 2 mg/kg IV infusion weeks 0 and 4; then q 8 weeks thereafter
Pediatric: <2 years: not recommended; ≥2 years, with active (pJIA): 80 mg/m² via IV infusion over 30 minutes at weeks 0 and 4 and q 8 weeks thereafter

Vial: 50 mg/4 ml, single-use, soln for IV infusion after dilution (latex-free, preservative-free)

JUVENILE RHEUMATOID ARTHRITIS (JRA)

see Juvenile Idiopathic Arthritis (JIA), Polyarticular Juvenile Idiopathic Arthritis (PJIA), Systemic Juvenile Idiopathic Arthritis (SJIA)

Acetaminophen for IV Infusion *see* Pain

NSAIDs *see* Appendix I. NSAIDs online at https://connect.springerpub.com/content/reference-book/978-0-8261-7935-7/back-matter/part02/back-matter/bmatter10

(continued)

Opioid Analgesics *see Pain*
Topical and Transdermal Analgesics *see Pain*
Parenteral Corticosteroids *see* Appendix L. Parenteral Corticosteroids
Oral Corticosteroids *see* Appendix K. Oral Corticosteroids

TOPICAL AND TRANSDERMAL ANALGESICS

▷ *capsaicin* (G) apply tid-qid prn to intact skin
  Pediatric: <2 years: <u>not</u> recommended; ≥2 years: same as adult
    Axsain *Crm:* 0.075% (1, 2 oz)
    Capsin *Lotn:* 0.025, 0.075% (59 ml)
    Capzasin-HP (OTC) *Crm:* 0.075% (1.5 oz), 0.025% (45, 90 gm); *Lotn:* 0.075% (2 oz), 0.025% (45, 90 gm)
    Capzasin-P (OTC) *Crm:* 0.025% (1.5 oz); *Lotn:* 0.025% (2 oz)
    Dolorac *Crm:* 0.025% (28 gm)
    Double Cap (OTC) *Crm:* 0.05% (2 oz)
    R-Gel *Gel:* 0.025% (15, 30 gm)
    Zostrix (OTC) *Crm:* 0.025% (0.7, 1.5, 3 oz)
    Zostrix HP (OTC) *Emol crm:* 0.075% (1, 2 oz)
▷ *capsaicin* 8% patch apply up to 4 patches for one 60-minute application to clean dry skin; may prep area
  with topical anesthetic; wear non-latex gloves; patches may be cut to size/shape; treatment may be repeated
  q 3 months
  Pediatric: <18 years: <u>not</u> recommended; ≥18 years: same as adult
    Qutenza *Patch:* 8% 1,640 mcg/cm (179 mg) (1 <u>or</u> 2 patches w. 1-50 gm tube cleansing gel/carton)
▷ *diclofenac sodium* (C; D ≥30 weeks) apply qid prn to intact skin
  Pediatric: <12 years: <u>not</u> established; ≥12 years: same as adult
    Pennsaid 1.5% in 10 drop increments, dispense and rub into front, side, and back of knee: usually
    40 drops (40 mg) qid
      Topical soln: 1.5% (150 ml)
    Pennsaid 2% apply 2 pump actuations (40 mg) and rub into front, side, and back of knee bid
      Topical soln: 2% (20 mg/pump actuation, 112 gm)
    Solaraze Gel massage into clean skin bid prn
      Gel: 3% (50 gm) (benzyl alcohol)
    Voltaren Gel (OTC)(G) apply qid prn to intact skin
      Gel: 1% (100 gm)
  Comment: *Diclofenac* is contraindicated with **aspirin** allergy. As with other non-steroidal anti-inflammatory
  drugs (NSAIDs), should be avoided in late pregnancy (≥30 weeks) because it may cause premature closure
  of the ductus arteriosus.
▷ *doxepin* (G) cream apply to affected area qid at intervals of at least 3-4 hours; max 8 days
  Pediatric: <12 years: <u>not</u> recommended; >12 years: same as adult
    Prudoxin *Crm:* 5% (45 gm)
    Zonalon *Crm:* 5% (30, 45 gm)
▷ *pimecrolimus* 1% cream (G) <2 years: <u>not</u> recommended; ≥2 years: apply to affected area bid; do <u>not</u> apply
  an occlusive dressing
    Elidel *Crm:* 1% (30, 60, 100 gm)
  Comment: *Pimecrolimus* is indicated for short-term and intermittent long-term use. Discontinue use when
  resolution occurs. Contraindicated if the patient is immunosuppressed. Change to the 0.1% preparation <u>or</u>
  if secondary bacterial infection is present.
▷ *trolamine salicylate* apply tid-qid
  Pediatric: <2 years: <u>not</u> recommended; ≥2 years: same as adult
    Mobisyl Creme *Crm:* 10% (100 gm)

TOPICAL AND TRANSDERMAL ANESTHETICS

Comment: *Lidocaine* should <u>not</u> be applied to non-intact skin.
▷ *lidocaine* cream apply to affected area bid prn
  Pediatric: <12 years: <u>not</u> recommended; ≥12 years: same as adult
    LidaMantle *Crm:* 3% (1, 2 oz)
    Lidoderm *Crm:* 3% (85 gm)
    ZTlido *lidocaine* topical system 1% (30/carton)
    Comment: Compared to Lidoderm (*lidocaine* patch 5%), which contains 700 mg/patch, ZTlido requires
    35 mg per topical system to achieve the same therapeutic dose.
▷ *lidocaine* lotion apply to affected area bid prn
  Pediatric: <12 years: <u>not</u> recommended; ≥12 years: same as adult
    LidaMantle *Lotn:* 3% (177 ml)
▷ *lidocaine* 5% patch (G) apply up to 3 patches at one time for up to 12 hours/24-hour period (12 hours on/12
  hours off); patches may be cut into smaller sizes before removal of the release liner; do <u>not</u> reuse
  Pediatric: <12 years: <u>not</u> recommended; ≥12 years: same as adult
    Lidoderm *Patch:* 5% (10 x 14 cm; 30/carton)

▷ *lidocaine+dexamethasone*
  Pediatric: <12 years: <u>not</u> recommended; ≥12 years: same as adult
    Decadron Phosphate with Xylocaine *Lotn:* dexa 4 mg+lido 10 mg per ml (5 ml)
▷ *lidocaine+hydrocortisone* **(G)** apply to affected area bid prn
  Pediatric: <12 years: <u>not</u> recommended; ≥12 years: same as adult
    LidaMantle HC *Crm:* lido 3%+hydro 0.5% (1, 3 oz); *Lotn:* (177 ml)
  lidocaine 2.5%+prilocaine 2.5% apply sparingly to the burn bid-tid prn
  Pediatric: <12 years: <u>not</u> recommended; ≥12 years: same as adult
    Emla Cream 5, 30 gm/tube

ORAL SALICYLATE

▷ *indomethacin* initially 25 mg bid-tid, increase as needed at weekly intervals by 25-50 mg/day; max 200 mg/day
  Pediatric: <14 years: usually <u>not</u> recommended; ≥2 years, if risk warranted: 1-2 mg/kg/day in divided doses, max 3-4 mg/kg/day (<u>or</u> total 150-200 mg/day, whichever is less); ≤14 years: ER cap <u>not</u> recommended
  Cap: 25, 50 mg; *Susp:* 25 mg/5 ml (pineapple-coconut, mint)(alcohol 1%); *Supp:* 50 mg; *ER cap:* 75 mg ext-rel
  Comment: *Indomethacin* is indicated <u>only</u> for acute painful flares. Administer with food <u>and/or</u> antacids. Use lowest effective dose for shortest duration.

METHOTREXATE (MTX)

▷ *methotrexate (MTX)* 7.5 mg x 1 dose per week <u>or</u> 2.5 mg x 3 at 12-hour intervals once a week; max 20 mg/week; therapeutic response begins in 3-6 weeks; administer MTX injection SC <u>only</u> into the abdomen <u>or</u> thigh
  Pediatric: <2 years: <u>not</u> recommended; ≥2 years: 10 mg/m^2 once weekly; max 20 mg/m^2
    Rasuvo *Autoinjector:* 7.5 mg/0.15 ml, 10 mg/0.20 ml, 12.5 mg/0.25 ml, 15 mg/0.30 ml, 17.5 mg/0.35 ml, 20 mg/0.40 ml, 22.5 mg/0.45 ml, 25 mg/0.50 ml, 27.5 mg/0.55 ml, 30 mg/0.60 ml (solution concentration for SC injection is 50 mg/ml)
    Rheumatrex *Tab:* 2.5*mg (5, 7.5, 10, 12.5, 15 mg/week, 4/card unit-of-use dose pack)
    Trexall *Tab:* 5*, 7.5*, 10*, 15*mg (5, 7.5, 10, 12.5, 15 mg/week, 4/card unit-of-use dose pack)
  Comment: *Methotrexate* (MTX) is contraindicated with immunodeficiency, blood dyscrasias, alcoholism, and chronic liver disease.

INTERLEUKIN-6 RECEPTOR ANTAGONIST

▷ *tocilizumab* <2 years: <u>not</u> recommended; ≥2 years: weight-based dosing: ≥30 kg: 8 mg/kg SC q 2 weeks; *<30 kg:* 12 mg/kg SC q 2 weeks; *IV infusion:* administer over 1 hour; do <u>not</u> administer as a bolus <u>or</u> IV push; ≥30 kg: dilute to 100 ml in 0.9% <u>or</u> 0.45% NaCl; <30 kg: dilute to 50 ml in 0.9% <u>or</u> 0.45% NaCl; *≥18 years:* whether used in combination with disease-modifying antirheumatic drugs (DMARDs) <u>or</u> as monotherapy, the recommended IV infusion starting dose is 4 mg/kg IV q 4 weeks followed by an increase to 8 mg/kg IV q 4 weeks based on clinical response; max 800 mg per infusion in rheumatoid arthritis (RA) patients; *SC administration:* ≥100 kg: 162 mg SC once weekly on the same day; *<100 kg:* 162 mg SC every other week on the same day followed by an increase according to clinical response
    Actemra *Vial:* 80 mg/4 ml, 200 mg/10 ml, 400 mg/20 ml, single-use, for IV infusion after dilution; *Prefilled syringe:* 162 mg (0.9 ml, single-dose); *Prefilled ACTPen autoinjector:* 162 mg/0.9 ml, single-dose, for SC administration
  Comment: *Tocilizumab* is an interleukin-6 receptor-alpha inhibitor indicated for use in moderate-to-severe rheumatoid arthritis (RA) that has <u>not</u> responded to conventional therapy, and also for some subtypes of juvenile rheumatoid arthritis (JRA). **Actemra** may be used alone <u>or</u> in combination with MTX, and in RA other DMARDs may be used. Monitor patient for dose-related laboratory changes, including elevated liver function tests (LFTs), neutropenia, and thrombocytopenia. **Actemra** should <u>not</u> be initiated in patients with an absolute neutrophil count (ANC) below 2,000 per mm^3, platelet count below 100,000 per mm^3, <u>or</u> who have alanine aminotransferase (ALT) <u>or</u> aspartate aminotransferase (AST) above 1.5 times the upper limit of normal (ULN). Registration in the Pregnancy Exposure Registry (1-877-311-8972) is encouraged for monitoring pregnancy outcomes in women exposed to **Actemra** during pregnancy. Monoclonal antibodies, such as *tocilizumab*, are actively transported across the placenta during the third trimester of pregnancy and may affect immune response in the infant exposed *in utero*. It is <u>not</u> known whether *tocilizumab* passes into breast milk; therefore, breastfeeding is <u>not</u> recommended while using **Actemra**.

Selective Co-Stimulation Modulator

▷ *abatacept* <2 years: <u>not</u> recommended; 2-17 years: administer as an IV infusion over 30 minutes at weeks 0, 2, and 4; then every 4 weeks thereafter; <75 kg: administer 10 mg/kg; same as adult (max 1 gm); administer as an IV infusion over 30 minutes at weeks 0, 2, and 4; then every 4 weeks thereafter; <60 kg: administer 500 mg/dose; 60-100 kg: administer 750 mg/dose; >100 kg: administer 1 gm/dose
    Orencia *Vial:* 250 mg pwdr for IV infusion after reconstitution (silicone-free) (preservative-free); *Prefilled syringe:* 125 mg/ml soln for SC injection (preservative-free); *ClickJect autoinjector:* 125 mg/ml soln for SC injection

(continued)

Comment: Orencia is also indicated to reduce signs/symptoms, induce major clinical response, inhibit progression of structural damage, and improve physical function in adult patients with moderate-to-severe active RA. **Orencia** may be used as monotherapy or with DMARDs other than tumor necrosis factor (TNF) antagonists. **Orencia** is also indicated to reduce signs/symptoms of moderate-to-severe active polyarticular juvenile idiopathic arthritis (PJIA) in patients >2 years of age as monotherapy or with MTX.

KERATITIS/KERATOCONJUNCTIVITIS SICCA/DRY EYE SYNDROME

▷ *cyclosporine* using 1 single-use disposable vial, instill 1 drop in each eye bid q 12 hours
Pediatric: <16 years: not recommended; ≥16 years: same as adult
   Cequa *Ophth soln:* 0.09% single-use vials (0.25 ml, 6 pouches, 10 vials/pouch per carton) (preservative-free)
   Comment: Cequa ophthalmic solution is a calcineurin inhibitor immune-suppressant indicated to increase tear production in patients with keratoconjunctivitis sicca. It is the first *cyclosporine* product to utilize nanomicellar technology, facilitating the drug molecule to penetrate the eye's aqueous layer and preventing the release of active lipophilic molecule prior to penetration.
   Restasis (G) *Ophth emul:* 0.05% (0.4 ml) (preservative-free)

KERATITIS/KERATOCONJUNCTIVITIS: HERPES SIMPLEX

▷ *acyclovir* ophthalmic ointment apply a 1 cm ribbon in the lower cul-de-sac of the affected eye 5x a day until healed; then, 3 tid for 7 more days
Pediatric: <2 years: not established; ≥2 years: same as adult
   Avaclyr *Ophth oint:* 3% (3.5 gm), single-patient multiuse tube
   Comment: Avaclyr *(acyclovir)* is a herpes simplex virus nucleoside analog DNA polymerase inhibitor indicated for the treatment of acute herpetic keratitis (dendritic ulcers) in patients with herpes simplex (HSV-1 and HSV-2) virus. **Avaclyr** is contraindicated in patients with a known hypersensitivity to *acyclovir* or *valacyclovir*. The most common adverse reactions (incidence 2%-10%) have been eye pain (stinging), punctate keratitis, and follicular conjunctivitis. There is no information regarding embryo/fetal effects of maternal use of ophthalmic *acyclovir* during pregnancy or presence of ophthalmic *acyclovir* in human milk or effects on the breastfed infant.
▷ *ganciclovir* instill 1 drop 5 x/day (every 3 hours) while awake until corneal ulcer heals; then 1 drop tid x 7 days
Pediatric: <2 years: not recommended; ≥2 years: same as adult
   Zirgan *Ophth gel:* 0.15% (5 gm) (benzalkonium chloride)
▷ *idoxuridine* instill 1 drop q 1 hour during the day and every other hour at night or 1 drop every minute for 5 minutes and repeat q 4 hours during day and night
   Herplex *Ophth soln:* 0.1% (15 ml)
▷ *trifluridine* instill 1 drop q 2 hours while awake (max 9 drops/day until re-epithelialization; then 1 drop q 4 hours x 7 more days; at least 5 drops/day); max 21 days
Pediatric: <6 years: not recommended; ≥6 years: same as adult
   Viroptic *Ophth soln:* 1% (7.5 ml) (thimerosal)
▷ *vidarabine* apply 1/2 inch in lower conjunctival sac 5 x/day q 3 hours until re-epithelialization occurs, then bid x 7 more days
Pediatric: <2 years: not recommended; ≥2 years: same as adult
   Vira-A *Ophth oint:* 3% (3.5 gm)

KERATITIS: NEUROTROPHIC

Comment: Oxervate is a recombinant form of human nerve growth factor (hNGF) structurally similar to endogenous NGF protein. NGF is an endogenous protein involved in the differentiation and maintenance of neurons, which acts through specific high-affinity (i.e., TrkA) and low-affinity (i.e., p75NTR) nerve growth factor receptors in the anterior segment of the eye to support corneal innervation and integrity. Prior to FDA approval of **Oxervate**, treatment was limited to symptomatic relief such as artificial tears, antibiotics, autologous serum-derived eye drops, tarsorrhaphy, and botulinum-induced ptosis, or surgical intervention.

▷ *cenegermin-bkbj* 1 drop in affected eye(s) 6 x/ day at 2-hour intervals x 8 weeks; pharmacy storage of the weekly carton in the freezer at or below −4°F (−20°C) until dispensed in the insulated pack in the Delivery System Kit; within 5 hours of leaving the pharmacy, store the weekly carton in the refrigerator between 36°F to 46°F (2°C to 8°C) for up to 14 days; opened vials may be stored in the original weekly carton in the refrigerator between 36°F to 46°F (2°C to 8°C) or at room temperature up to 77°F (25°C) for up to 12 hours; do not refreeze; do not shake the vial; discard any unused portion after 12 hours

Pediatric: <2 years: not recommended; ≥2 years: same as adult
    Oxervate *Vial:* 0.002% multidose (7/carton; Delivery System Kit contains insulated pack, 8 vial adapters, 45 pipettes, 45 sterile disinfectant wipes, dose card) (preservative-free)

KERATITIS/KERATOCONJUNCTIVITIS: VERNAL

OPHTHALMIC MAST CELL STABILIZERS

Comment: Contact lens wear is contraindicated.

▷ *cromolyn sodium* 1-2 drops 4-6 x/day
  Pediatric: <4 years: not recommended; ≥4 years: same as adult
    Crolom, Opticrom *Ophth soln:* 4% (10 ml) (benzalkonium chloride)
▷ *lodoxamide tromethamine* 1-2 drops qid; max 3 months
  Pediatric: <2 years: not recommended; ≥2 years: same as adult
    Alomide *Ophth susp:* 0.1% (10 ml)

LABYRINTHITIS

▷ *meclizine* 25 mg tid
  Pediatric: <12 years: not recommended; ≥12 years: same as adult
    Antivert *Tab:* 12.5, 25, 50*mg
    Bonine (OTC) *Cap:* 15, 25, 30 mg; *Tab:* 12.5, 25, 50 mg; *Chew tab/Film-coat tab:* 25 mg
    Dramamine II (OTC) *Tab:* 25*mg
    Zentrip *Strip:* 25 mg orally disintegrating
▷ *promethazine* (G) 25 mg tid
  Pediatric: <2 years: not recommended; ≥2 years: 0.5 mg/lb or 6.25-25 mg tid
    Phenergan *Tab:* 12.5*, 25*, 50 mg; *Plain syr:* 6.25 mg/5 ml; *Fortis syr:* 25 mg/5 ml; *Rectal supp:* 12.5, 25, 50 mg
Comment: *Promethazine* is contraindicated in children with uncomplicated nausea, dehydration, Reye's syndrome, history of sleep apnea, asthma, and lower respiratory disorders. *Promethazine* lowers the seizure threshold in children and may cause cholestatic jaundice, anticholinergic effects, extrapyramidal effects, and potentially fatal respiratory depression.
▷ *scopolamine*
    Transderm Scop 1 patch behind the ear at least 4 hours before travel; each patch is effective for 3 days
      Transdermal patch: 1.5 mg (4/carton)

LACTOSE INTOLERANCE

▷ *lactase* enzyme 9,000 FCC units taken with dairy food; adjust based on abatement of symptoms; usual max 18,000 units/dose
  Pediatric: same as adult
    Lactaid Drops (OTC) 5-7 drops to each quart of milk and shake gently; may increase to 10-15 drops if needed; hydrolyzes 70%-99% of lactose at refrigerator temperature in 24 hours
      Oral drops: 1,250 units/5 gtts (7 ml w. dropper)
    Lactaid Extra (OTC) *Cplt:* 4,500 FCC units
    Lactaid Fast ACT (OTC) *Cplt:* 9,000 FCC units; *Chew tab:* 9,000 FCC units (vanilla twist)
    Lactaid Original (OTC) *Cplt:* 3,000 FCC units
    Lactaid Ultra (OTC) *Cplt:* 9,000 FCC units; *Chew tab:* 9,000 FCC units (vanilla twist)

LAMBERT-EATON MYASTHENIC SYNDROME (LEMS)

BROAD-SPECTRUM POTASSIUM CHANNEL BLOCKER

▷ *amifampridine*
  Pediatric: <6 years: not established; 6-<17 years, <45 kg: initially 7.5-15 mg daily in divided doses; then increase daily in 2.5-5 mg increments, divided in up to 5 doses daily; max single dose is 15 mg; max total 50 mg/day; 6-<17 years, ≥45 kg: initially 15-30 mg daily in divided doses; then increase daily in 5-10 mg increments, divided in up to 5 doses daily; max single dose is 30 mg; max total 100 mg/day; if the patient requires doses in less than 5 mg increments, has difficulty swallowing, or requires a feeding tube, a 1 mg/ml suspension can be prepared; for patients with renal or hepatic impairment or are poor N-acetyltransferase 2 metabolizers, use the lowest recommended initial dose of **Rusurgi**.
    Ruzurgi *Tab:* 10*mg
  Comment: **Ruzurgi** *(amifampridine)* is a broad-spectrum potassium channel blocker. **Ruzurgi** is contraindicated in patients with a history of seizures or hypersensitivity to *amifampridine* or other *aminopyridine*. **Ruzurgi** can cause seizures. Consider discontinuation or dose reduction of **Ruzurgi**

(continued)

in patients who have a seizure while on treatment. If a hypersensitivity reaction such as anaphylaxis occurs, **Ruzurgi** should be discontinued and appropriate therapy initiated. Concomitant use of **Ruzurgi** and drugs known to lower seizure threshold may lead to an increased risk of seizures. Concomitant use of **Ruzurgi** and drugs with cholinergic effects (e.g., direct or indirect cholinesterase inhibitors) may increase the cholinergic effects of **Ruzurgi** and of those drugs and increase the risk of adverse reaction. The most common adverse reactions (incidence 10% and 2% greater than placebo) are paresthesia/dysesthesia, abdominal pain, dyspepsia, dizziness, and nausea. There are no human or animal data on the developmental risk associated with the use of **Ruzurgi** in pregnancy. There are no data on the presence of *amifampridine* or the 3-N-acetyl-amifampridine metabolite in human milk or effects on the breastfed infant.

LARVA MIGRANS: CUTANEOUS, VISCERAL

▷ *thiabendazole* adult and pediatric dosing schedules are the same; dosing is bid, is based on weight in pounds, and must be taken with meals
  Cutaneous larva migrans: treat bid x 2 days
  Visceral larva migrans: treat bid x 7 days
    <30 lb: consult mfr pkg insert; *30 lb*: 250 mg bid; *50 lb*: 500 mg bid; *75 lb*: 750 mg bid; *100 lb*: 1,000 mg bid; *125 lb*: 1,250 mg bid; ≥*150 lb*: 1,500 mg bid; max 3,000 mg/day
    Mintezol *Chew tab*: 500*mg (orange); *Oral susp*: 500 mg/5 ml (120 ml) (orange)
  Comment: *Thiabendazole* is not for prophylaxis. May impair mental alertness. May not be available in the United States.

LEAD POISONING

Comment: Chelation therapy for lead poisoning requires maintenance of adequate hydration, close monitoring of renal and hepatic function, and monitoring for neutropenia; discontinue therapy at first sign of toxicity. Contraindicated with severe renal disease or anuria.

CHELATING AGENTS
▷ *deferoxamine mesylate* initially 1 gm IM, followed by 500 mg IM q 4 hours x 2 doses; then repeat q 4-12 hours if needed; max 6 gm/day
  Pediatric: <3 months: not recommended; ≥3 months: same as adult
    Desferal *Vial*: 250 mg/ml after reconstitution (500 mg)
▷ *edetate calcium disodium (EDTA)* administer IM or IV; use IM route of administration for children and overt lead encephalopathy
  Pediatric: same as adult; *Serum lead level: 20-70 mcg/dL*: 1 gm/m² per day; *IV*: infuse over 8-12 hours; *IM*: divided doses q 8-12 hours; treat for 5 days; then stop for 2-4 days; may repeat if serum lead level is ≥70 mcg/dL
    Calcium Disodium Versenate *Amp*: 200 mg/ml (5 ml)
▷ *succimer* may swallow caps whole or put contents onto a small amount of soft food or a spoon and swallow, followed by a fruit drink
  Pediatric: <12 months: not recommended; ≥12 months: same as adult; *Serum lead level: >45 mcg/dL*: initially 10 mg/kg (or 350 mg/m²) q 8 hours for 5 days; then reduce frequency to q 12 hours for 14 more days; allow at least 14 days between courses unless serum lead levels indicate a need for more prompt treatment; for more than 3 consecutive weeks not recommended
    Chemet *Cap*: 100 mg

LEG CRAMPS: NOCTURNAL, RECUMBENCY

▷ *quinine sulfate* (G) 1 tab or cap q HS
  Pediatric: <16 years: not recommended; ≥16 years: same as adult
    Qualaquin *Tab*: 260 mg; *Cap*: 260, 300, 325 mg
  Comment: If hypokalemia is the cause of leg cramps, treat with potassium supplementation (*see Hypokalemia*).

LEISHMANIASIS: CUTANEOUS, MUCOSAL, VISCERAL

Comment: The leishmanial parasite species addressed in this section are **cutaneous leishmaniasis** (due to *Leishmania braziliensis, L. guyanensis, L. panamensis*), **mucosal leishmaniasis** (due to *L. braziliensis*), and **visceral leishmaniasis** (due to *L. donovani*). The weight-based treatment for adults and adolescents is the same for each of the species, the anti-leishmanial drug *miltefosone* (Impavido). Contraindications to this drug include pregnancy, lactation, and Sjogren-Larsson syndrome. The contraindication in pregnancy is due to embryo/fetal toxicity, teratogenicity, and fetal death. Obtain a serum or urine pregnancy test for females of reproductive potential and advise females to use effective contraception during therapy and for 5 months following treatment. Breastfeeding is contraindicated while taking this drug and for 5 months following termination of breastfeeding. Potential adverse side effects (ASEs) include loss of appetite, abdominal pain, nausea, vomiting, diarrhea, headache, dizziness, pruritis, somnolence, elevated liver transaminases, bilirubin, and serum creatinine and thrombocytopenia. *Miltefosine* is associated with impaired fertility in females and males in animal studies.

▶ *miltefosine* (G) 30-44 kg: 1 cap bid x 28 consecutive days; ≥45 kg: 1 cap tid x 28 consecutive days; take with a full meal
    Pediatric: <12 years, <30 kg (60 lb): not established; ≥12 years, ≥30 kg (≥60 lb): same as adult
      Impavido *Cap:* 50 mg

LENNOX-GASTAUT SYNDROME (LGS)/DRAVET SYNDROME

CANNABINOID-DERIVED TREATMENT
Comment: The FDA Peripheral and Central Nervous System Drugs Advisory Committee's **Epidiolex** (*cannabidiol*) recommendation was based on three randomized, double-blind, placebo-controlled clinical trials. These trials showed a 50% reduction in drop seizure frequency in 40%-44% of patients with Lennox-Gastaut syndrome (LGS) and a 39% decrease in convulsive seizure frequency for trial participants with Dravet syndrome. A total of 516 patients with one of the two seizure disorders participated in the clinical trials. The FDA Advisory Committee judged that CBD-OS, derived from a non-psychoactive chemical found in marijuana, was very unlikely to have potential for abuse.

▶ *cannabidiol* initially 2.5 mg/kg 2 bid (5 mg/kg/day); after 1 week, may be increased to a maintenance dose of 5 mg/kg 2 bid (10 mg/kg/day); max 10 mg/kg 2 bid (20 mg/kg/day); titration based on effectiveness and tolerability; dose adjustment is recommended for patients with moderate or severe hepatic impairment.
    Pediatric: <1 years: not established; ≥1 year: weight-based dosing as above
      Epidiolex *Oral soln:* 100 mg/ml (100 ml) (strawberry)
      Comment: Epidiolex (*cannabidiol*) is a prescription pharmaceutical formulation of highly purified, marijuana plant-derived cannabidiol (CBD) indicated for the treatment of seizures associated with Lennox-Gastaut syndrome, Dravet syndrome, and tuberous sclerosis complex in patients ≥2 years of age. Obtain serum transaminases (ALT and AST) and total bilirubin levels in all patients prior to starting treatment. Concomitant use of *valproate* and higher doses of **Epidiolex** increase the risk of transaminase elevations. Consider dose reduction of **Epidiolex** with concomitant moderate or strong inhibitors of CYP3A4 or CYP2C19. Consider dose increase of **Epidiolex** with strong inducers of CYP3A4 or CYP2C19. Consider dose reduction of substrates of UGT1A9, UGT2B7, CYP2C8, CYP2C9, and CYP2C19 (e.g., *clobazam*). Substrates of CYP1A2 and CYP2B6 may also require dose adjustment. Monitor for somnolence and sedation and advise patients not to drive or operate machinery until they have gained sufficient experience on **Epidiolex**. Monitor patients for suicidal behavior and thoughts. Advise patients to seek immediate medical care for any hypersensitivity reaction. Discontinue and do not restart **Epidiolex** if hypersensitivity occurs. **Epidiolex** should be gradually withdrawn to minimize the risk of increased seizure frequency and status epilepticus. The most common adverse reactions (incidence ≥10%) include somnolence; decreased appetite; diarrhea; transaminase elevations; fatigue, malaise, and asthenia; rash; insomnia, sleep disorder, and poor quality sleep; and infections. There are no adequate data on the developmental risks associated with the use of **Epidiolex** in pregnant females. However, animal studies have demonstrated **Epidiolex** may cause fetal harm. There are no data on the presence of *cannabidiol* or its metabolites in human milk or effects on the breastfed infant. Encourage females who take **Epidiolex** during pregnancy to enroll in the North American Antiepileptic Drug (NAAED) Pregnancy Registry by calling 1-888-233-2334 or www.aedpregnancyregistry.org/.

OTHER ANTICONVULSANTS
▶ *clobazam* (IV) (G) take with or without food; for doses above 5 mg/day, administer in 2 divided doses; ≤30 *kg body weight:* initiate at 5 mg daily and titrate as tolerated up to 20 mg daily; *>30 kg body weight:* initiate at 10 mg daily and titrate as tolerated up to 40 mg daily; *Tablets:* administer whole, broken in half along the score line, or crushed and mixed in applesauce; *Suspension:* measure prescribed amount using provided adapter and dosing syringe; *Mild-to-moderate hepatic impairment:* reduce dose or discontinue gradually; *Severe hepatic impairment:* no information; *Geriatric patients and CYP2C19 poor metabolizers:* adjust dose
    Pediatric: <2 years: not recommended; ≥2 years: same as adult
      Onfi *Tab:* 10*, 20*mg
      Onfi Oral Suspension *Oral susp:* 2.5 mg/ml (120 ml w. adapter and 2 dosing syringes) (berry)
      Sympazan Oral Film *Oral film:* 5, 10, 20 mg, single-dose (60/pkg) (berry)
    Comment: *Clobazam* is a benzodiazepine indicated for adjunctive treatment of seizures associated with Lennox-Gastaut syndrome (LGS) in patients ≥2 years of age. Monitor for central nervous system (CNS) depression (somnolence, sedation), caution with concomitant CNS depressants, and avoid rapid dose reduction or discontinuation. Monitor for potential Stevens-Johnson syndrome and toxic epidermal necrolysis. Discontinue *clobazam* at first sign of rash unless the rash is clearly not drug-related. Monitor patients with a history of substance abuse for signs of habituation and dependence. Monitor for suicidal thoughts or behaviors. Adverse reactions which have occurred (incidence ≥10%) with any *clobazam*

(continued)

dose included constipation, somnolence or sedation, pyrexia, lethargy, and drooling. *Clobazam* is excreted in human milk. Breastfed infants of mothers taking benzodiazepines, such as *clobazam*, may have effects of lethargy, somnolence, and poor sucking. There is insufficient evidence to assess the effect of benzodiazepine pregnancy exposure on neurodevelopment. Prescribers are advised to recommend pregnant patients taking **Onfi** or **Sympazan** self-enroll in the North American Antiepileptic Drug (NAAED) Pregnancy Registry by calling 1-888-233-2334 or www.aedpregnancyregistry.org

▶ *stiripentol* 50 mg/kg/day in 2 or 3 divided doses; reduce dose or discontinue dose gradually; capsules must be swallowed whole with a glass of water during a meal; do not break or open capsules; mix contents of 1 packet in a glass of water and take immediately after mixing during a meal
Pediatric: <2 years: not recommended; ≥2 years: same as adult
    Diacomit *Cap:* 250, 500 mg; *Pwdr for oral susp:* 250, 500 mg (60 pkts/carton)(fruit)
    Comment: Diacomit is indicated for the treatment of seizures associated with Dravet syndrome in patients ≥2 years of age taking *clobazam*. There are no clinical data to support the use of **Diacomit** as monotherapy in Dravet syndrome.

▶ *topiramate* initial dose, titration, and recommended maintenance dose vary by indication and age group; see mfr pkg insert for full prescribing information for recommended dosage, and dosing considerations in patients with renal impairment, geriatric patients, and patients undergoing hemodialysis
Pediatric: <2 years: safety and efficacy not established; >2 years: see adult comment above
    Eprontia *Oral soln:* 25 mg/ml (473 ml)
    Comment: Eprontia is an anticonvulsant indicated (1) for initial monotherapy for the treatment of partial-onset or primary generalized tonic-clonic seizures in patients ≥2 years of age and (2) as adjunctive therapy for the treatment of partial-onset seizures, primary generalized tonic-clonic seizures, or seizures associated with (LGS) in patients ≥2 years of age and older. The most common (incidence ≥10% more frequent than placebo or low-dose *topiramate*) adverse reactions in adult and pediatric patients have been paresthesia, anorexia, weight loss, speech disorders/related speech problems, fatigue, dizziness, somnolence, nervousness, psychomotor slowing, abnormal vision, and fever. There are no contraindications. However, patients must be monitored for the following conditions. If acute myopia or secondary angle closure glaucoma (which can lead to permanent visual loss) occurs, discontinue **Eprontia** as soon as possible. If visual field defects occur, consider discontinuation of **Eprontia**. Oligohidrosis and hyperthermia may occur; monitor decreased sweating and increased body temperature, especially in pediatric patients. Metabolic acidosis can occur; baseline and periodic measurement of serum bicarbonate is recommended and consider dose reduction or discontinuation of **Eprontia** as clinically appropriate. Antiepileptic drugs (AEDs) increase the risk of suicidal behavior or ideation; monitor for depression and mood problems. Cognitive/neuropsychiatric adverse reactions may occur; advise caution when operating machinery, including motor vehicles. Hyperammonemia/ encephalopathy may occur; measure ammonia if encephalopathy symptoms occur; kidney stones can develop; avoid use with other carbonic anhydrase inhibitors, drugs causing metabolic acidosis, and patients on a ketogenic diet. Hypothermia has been reported with and without hyperammonemia during *topiramate* treatment with concomitant *valproic acid* use. Concomitant oral contraceptives with **Eprontia** can result in decreased contraceptive efficacy and increased breakthrough bleeding, especially at doses greater than 200 mg/day. Monitor *lithium* levels if *lithium* is used with high-dose **Eprontia**. Withdrawal of AEDs, including **Eprontia**, should be gradual. Use during pregnancy can cause cleft lip and/or palate and fetal size small for gestational age (SGA). In multiple animal species, *topiramate* produced developmental toxicity, including increased incidences of fetal malformations, in the absence of maternal toxicity at clinically relevant doses. *Topiramate* can cause fetal harm when administered in human pregnancy. Data from pregnancy registries indicate that infants exposed to *topiramate in utero* have an increased risk for cleft lip and/or cleft palate (oral clefts) and for being SGA. SGA has been observed at all doses and appears to be dose-dependent. The prevalence of SGA is greater in infants of females who received higher doses of *topiramate* during pregnancy. In addition, the prevalence of SGA in infants of females who continued *topiramate* use until later in pregnancy is higher compared to the prevalence in infants of women who stopped *topiramate* use before the third trimester. The development of *topiramate*-induced metabolic acidosis in the mother and/or in the fetus can affect the fetus' ability to tolerate labor. Females who are planning a pregnancy should be counseled regarding the relative risks and benefits of *topiramate* use during pregnancy and alternative therapeutic options should be considered for these patients. Advise patients of reproductive potential to use an effective non-hormonal contraceptive. *Topiramate* is excreted in human milk. Diarrhea and somnolence have been reported in breastfed infants whose mothers receive *topiramate* treatment. Developmental and health benefits of breastfeeding should be considered along with the mother's clinical need for *topiramate* and any potential adverse effects on the breastfed infant from *topiramate* or from the underlying maternal condition. There is a pregnancy exposure registry that monitors pregnancy outcomes in women exposed to *topiramate* during pregnancy. Patients should be encouraged to enroll in the North American Antiepileptic Drug (NAAED) Pregnancy Registry if they become pregnant. This registry is collecting information about the safety of antiepileptic drugs (AEDs) during pregnancy. To enroll, patients can call the toll-free number at 888-233-2334. Information about the North American Drug Pregnancy Registry can be found at http://www.aedpregnancyregistry.org/. To report suspected adverse reactions, contact Azurity Pharmaceuticals at 855-379-0383 or FDA at 1-800-FDA-1088 or www.fda.gov/medwatch.

LENTIGINES: BENIGN, SENILE

Comment: Wash affected area with a soap-free cleanser; pat dry and wait 20-30 minutes; then apply agent sparingly to affected area; use <u>only</u> once daily in the PM. Avoid eyes, ears, nostrils, mouth, and healthy skin. Avoid sun exposure. Cautious use of concomitant astringents, alcohol-based products, sulfur-containing products, salicylic acid-containing products, soap, and other topical agents.

TOPICAL RETINOIDS
▷ *tazarotene* (G) apply daily at HS
   Pediatric: <12 years: <u>not</u> recommended; ≥12 years: same as adult
      Avage Cream *Crm:* 0.1% (30 gm)
      Tazorac Cream *Crm:* 0.05, 0.1% (15, 30, 60 gm)
      Tazorac Gel *Gel:* 0.05, 0.1% (30, 100 gm)
▷ *tretinoin* (G) apply daily at HS
   Pediatric: <12 years: <u>not</u> recommended; ≥12 years: same as adult
      Avita *Crm:* 0.025% (20, 45 gm); *Gel:* 0.025% (20, 45 gm)
      Renova *Crm:* 0.02% (40 gm); 0.05% (40, 60 gm)
      Retin-A Cream *Crm:* 0.025, 0.05, 0.1% (20, 45 gm)
      Retin-A Gel *Gel:* 0.01, 0.025% (15, 45 gm) (alcohol 90%)
      Retin-A Liquid *Liq:* 0.05% (28 ml; alcohol 55%)
      Retin-A Micro *Microspheres:* 0.04, 0.1% (20, 45 gm)
      Retin-A Micro Gel *Gel:* 0.04, 0.1% (20, 45 gm)

LISTERIOSIS (*LISTERIA MONOCYTOGENES*)

Comment: *Listeria monocytogenes* is a potentially lethal foodborne pathogen that is a common contaminant of food and food preparation equipment, and has been isolated in soil, farm environments, produce, raw foods, dairy products, and the feces of asymptomatic people. IV *ampicillin* is the mainstay of treatment, but penicillin may be as effective. Some experts recommend combination antibiotic therapy for neuroinvasive *L. monocytogenes*. The most common antimicrobial combination is IV *ampicillin* and IV *gentamycin* (which is usually discontinued when the patient shows signs of improvement to limit the potential for toxicity). If the patient is penicillin-allergic, IV *trimethoprim-sulfamethoxazole* (TMP-SMX) as monotherapy x 28 days. Patients with bacteremia but without central nervous system (CNS) involvement may be treated with combination (*ampicillin+gentamycin*) therapy for 14 days, but patients with meningitis require a full 21-day combination course of antibiotics. Endocarditis, encephalitis, and brain abscesses may require a longer duration of high-dose antimicrobials. Cephalosporins are ineffective. Supportive care and standard isolation precautions are required.

▷ *ampicillin* (G) 2 gm IV infusion q 4 hours (in combination with IV gentamycin q 8 hours)
   Pediatric: 50-100 mg/kg (max 3 gm) IV infusion q 6 hours
      Unasyn *Vial:* 1.5, 3 gm
▷ *gentamicin* (G) 1-2 mg/kg q 8 hours (in combination with IV ampicillin q 4 hours; monitor plasma levels; dilution <u>not</u> less than 1 mg/ml in D5W <u>or</u> NS; administer dose over 30 minutes-2 hours
   Pediatric: 2 mg/kg/dose q 8 hours; monitor plasma levels; dilution <u>not</u> less than 1 mg/ml in D5W <u>or</u> NS; administer dose over 30 minutes-2 hours
      Garamycin *Vial:* 20, 80 mg/2 ml (2 ml) for dilution (<u>not</u> less than 1 mg/ml) and IV infusion (over 30 minutes-2 hours
▷ *penicillin g potassium* (G) 4 million units via IV infusion q 4 hours
   Pediatric: 65,000 units/kg/dose via IV infusion q 4 hours; max 4 million units/dose; infuse dose over 1-2 hours
      Vial: 5, 20 MU pwdr for reconstitution (in D5W <u>or</u> NS) and IV infusion; *Premixed bag:* 1, 2, 3 MU (50 ml); infuse dose over 1-2 hours
▷ *trimethoprim-sulfamethoxazole (TMP-SMX)* (G) TMP 5 mg/kg IV infusion q 6 hours; max TMP 160 mg/dose
   Pediatric: <2 months: contraindicated: ≥2 months: 2-5 mg/kg/dose q 8 hours; max TMP 160 mg/dose

LIVER FLUKES: FASCIOLIASIS (*FASCIOLA GIGANTICA, FASCIOLA HEPATICA*)

BENZIMIDAZOLE ANTHELMINTIC
▷ *triclabendazole* recommended dose is 2 doses of 10 mg/kg administered 12 hours apart; take with food; swallow dose with waters; swallow whole <u>or</u> divide tablet in half; may crush and administer with applesauce; if the dose cannot be adjusted exactly, round dose upwards
   Pediatric: <6 years: <u>not</u> established; ≥6 years: same as adult
      Egaten *Tab:* 250*mg

(continued)

Comment: *Triclabendazole* is indicated for the treatment of fascioliasis, a neglected tropical disease (NTD) caused by liver flukes *Fasciola hepatica* and *F. gigantica*. It is contraindicated in patients with known hypersensitivity to *triclabendazole* or other *benzimidazole* derivatives. *Triclabendazole* may prolong QT interval; therefore, monitor ECG in patients with a history of QT prolongation or who are taking medications which prolong the QT interval. The most common adverse reactions (incidence >2%) with *triclabendazole* ≥20 mg/kg dose are abdominal pain, hyperhidrosis, nausea, decreased appetite, headache, urticaria, diarrhea, vomiting, musculoskeletal chest pain, and pruritus. There are no available data on **Egaten** use in pregnant females to inform a drug-associated risk of major birth defects, miscarriage, or adverse maternal or fetal outcomes. There are no data on the presence of *triclabendazole* in human milk or effects on the breastfed infant. Clinical studies of **Egaten** have not included sufficient numbers of patients ≥65 to inform whether the elderly respond differently from younger patients.

TREMATODICIDE

Comment: *Praziquantel* is a trematodicide indicated for the treatment of infections due to all species of *Schistosoma* (e.g., *Schistosoma mekongi, S. japonicum, S. mansoni,* and *S. haematobium*) and infections due to liver flukes (i.e., *Clonorchis sinensis, Opisthorchis viverrini*). *Praziquantel* induces a rapid contraction of schistosomes by a specific effect on the permeability of the cell membrane. The drug further causes vacuolization and disintegration of the schistosome tegument.

▷ *praziquantel* 25 mg/kg tid as a 1-day treatment; take the 3 doses at intervals of not less than 4 hours and not more than 6 hours; swallow whole with water during meals; holding the tablets in the mouth leaves a bitter taste which can trigger gagging or vomiting
  Pediatric: <4 years: not established; >4 years: same as adult
    Biltricide *Tab:* 600 mg*** film-coat (3 scores, 4 segments, 150 mg/segment)
  Comment: Concomitant administration with strong cytochrome P450 (P450) inducers, such as *rifampin*, is contraindicated since therapeutically effective blood levels of *praziquantel* may not be achieved. In patients receiving *rifampin* who need immediate treatment for schistosomiasis, alternative agents for schistosomiasis should be considered. However, if treatment with *praziquantel* is necessary, *rifampin* should be discontinued 4 weeks before administration of *praziquantel*. Treatment with *rifampin* can then be restarted 1 day after completion of *praziquantel* treatment. Concomitant administration of other P450 inducers (e.g., antiepileptic drugs such as *phenytoin, phenobarbital, carbamazepine*) and *dexamethasone* may also reduce plasma levels of *praziquantel*. Concomitant administration of P450 inhibitors (e.g., *cimetidine, ketoconazole, itraconazole, erythromycin*) may increase plasma levels of *praziquantel*. Patients should be warned not to drive a car or operate machinery on the day of **Biltricide** treatment and the following day. There are no adequate or well-controlled studies in pregnant females. This drug should be used during pregnancy only if clearly needed. *Praziquantel* appears in the milk of nursing women at a concentration of about 1/4 that of maternal serum. It is not known whether a pharmacologic effect is likely to occur in children. Women should not nurse on the day of **Biltricide** treatment and during the subsequent 72 hours.

LOW BACK STRAIN (LBS)

Acetaminophen for IV Infusion *see Pain*
NSAIDs *see* Appendix I. NSAIDs online at https://connect.springerpub.com/content/reference-book/978-0-8261-7935-7/back-matter/part02/back-matter/bmatter10
Opioid Analgesics *see Pain*
Topical and Transdermal Analgesics *see Pain*
Muscle Relaxants *see Muscle Strain*
Parenteral Corticosteroids *see* Appendix L. Parenteral Corticosteroids
Oral Corticosteroids *see* Appendix K. Oral Corticosteroids
Topical Analgesic and Anesthetic Agents *see* Appendix H. Anesthetic Agents for Local Infiltration and Dermal/Mucosal Membrane Application online at https://connect.springerpub.com/content/reference-book/978-0-8261-7935-7/back-matter/part02/back-matter/bmatter9

LOW LIBIDO, HYPOACTIVE SEXUAL DESIRE DISORDER (HSDD)

5-HT1A AGONIST/5-HT2A
▷ *flibanserin* 1 tab once daily at bedtime; discontinue if no improvement in 8 weeks
  Pediatric: <18 years: not recommended; ≥18 years: same as adult
    Addyi *Tab:* 100 mg
    Comment: **Addyi** is for use in premenopausal women. **Addyi** is not for use in men, postmenopausal women, and is not recommended in pregnancy or lactation. Potential adverse side effects (ASEs) include dry mouth, nausea, hypotension, dizziness, syncope, fatigue, somnolence, and insomnia.

MELANOCORTIN RECEPTOR AGONIST (MRA)

▷ *bremelanotide* inject 1.75 mg SC via the autoinjector to the abdomen or thigh, as needed, at least 45 minutes before anticipated sexual activity; do not administer more than 1 dose within 24 hours; more than 8 doses per month is not recommended

Pediatric: <18 years: not established; ≥18 years: same as adult

Vyleesi *Prefilled autoinjector:* 1.75 mg (0.3 ml) solution, single-dose (4/carton)

Comment: Vyleesi *(bremelanotide)* is a melanocortin receptor agonist for the treatment of acquired, generalized, and hypoactive sexual desire disorder (HSDD) in premenopausal women as characterized by low sexual desire that causes marked distress or interpersonal difficulty and is not due to a coexisting medical or psychiatric condition, problems with the relationship, or effects of a medication or drug. Vyleesi is not indicated for treatment of HSDD in postmenopausal women or in men to enhance sexual performance. Vyleesi is contraindicated in patients with uncontrolled hypertension or known cardiovascular disease. Transient increase in blood pressure (BP) and decrease in heart rate occur after each dose and usually resolve within 12 hours. Consider the patient's cardiovascular risk before initiating Vyleesi and periodically. Focal hyperpigmentation has been reported by 1% of patients who received up to 8 doses per month, including involvement of the face, gingiva, and breasts, with higher risk in patients with darker skin and with daily dosing. Resolution was not confirmed in some patients. Consider discontinuing Vyleesi if hyperpigmentation develops. Nausea has been reported by 40% of patients receiving up to 8 monthly doses, requiring antiemetic therapy in 13% of patients and leading to premature discontinuation for 8% of patients. Improvement has been reported for most patients with the second dose. Consider discontinuing Vyleesi or initiating antiemetic therapy for persistent or severe nausea. Vyleesi may slow gastric emptying and impact absorption of concomitantly administered oral medications. Avoid use of Vyleesi with orally administered *naltrexone*-containing products intended to treat alcohol or opioid addiction as Vyleesi may significantly decrease the systemic exposure of orallyadministered *naltrexone.* Use of Vyleesi during pregnancy is not recommended. Advise females of reproductive potential to use effective contraception while taking Vyleesi and to discontinue Vyleesi if pregnancy is suspected. Pregnant females exposed to Vyleesi and healthcare providers are encouraged to call the Vyleesi Pregnancy Exposure Registry at 877-411-2510. There is no information on the presence of *bremelanotide* or its metabolites in human milk or effects on the breastfed infant.

▷ *selpercatinib* <50 kg: 120 mg bid; ≥50 kg: 160 mg bid; reduce dose in patients with severe hepatic impairment

Pediatric: <12 years: not established; ≥12 years: same as adult

Retevmo *Cap:* 40, 80 mg

Comment: Retevmo *(selpercatinib)* is a kinase inhibitor indicated for adult patients with metastatic RET (rearranged during transfection) fusion-positive non-small cell lung cancer, adult and pediatric patients ≥12 years of age with advanced or metastatic RET-mutant medullary thyroid cancer (MTC) who require systemic therapy, and adult and pediatric patients ≥12 years of age with advanced or metastatic RET fusion-positive thyroid cancer who require systemic therapy and who are radioactive iodine-refractory (if radioactive iodine is appropriate). The most common adverse reactions (incidence ≥25%), including laboratory abnormalities, (incidence ≥25%) have been increased aspartate aminotransferase (AST), increased alanine aminotransferase (ALT), increased glucose, decreased leukocytes, decreased albumin, decreased calcium, dry mouth, diarrhea, increased creatinine, increased alkaline phosphatase, hypertension, fatigue, edema, decreased platelets, increased total cholesterol, rash, decreased sodium, and constipation. Monitor ALT and AST prior to initiating Retevmo every 2 weeks during the first 3 months, then monthly thereafter and as clinically indicated. Do not initiate Retevmo in patients with uncontrolled hypertension; optimize BP prior to initiating Retevmo and monitor BP after 1 week, at least monthly thereafter and as clinically indicated. Monitor patients who are at significant risk of developing QTc prolongation. Assess QT interval, electrolytes, and thyroid-stimulating hormone (TSH) at baseline and periodically during treatment. Monitor QT interval more frequently when Retevmo is concomitantly administered with strong and moderate CYP3A inhibitors or drugs known to prolong QTc interval. Permanently discontinue Retevmo in patients with severe or life-threatening hemorrhage. Withhold Retevmo and initiate corticosteroids in the occurrence of any hypersensitivity reaction and, upon resolution, resume at a reduced dose and increase dose by 1 dose level each week until reaching the dose taken prior to onset of hypersensitivity. Continue steroids until the patient reaches target dose of Retevmo and then taper. Withhold Retevmo for at least 7 days prior to elective surgery. Do not administer for at least 2 weeks following major surgery and until adequate wound healing. The safety of resumption of Retevmo after resolution of wound healing complications has not been established. Avoid co-administration with proton pump inhibitors (PPIs); if co-administration cannot be avoided, take Retevmo with food (with PPI) or modify its administration time (with H2 receptor antagonist or locally acting antacid). Avoid co-administration with strong and moderate CYP3A inhibitors; if co-administration cannot be avoided, reduce the Retevmo dose. Avoid co-administration with strong and moderate CYP3A inducers. Avoid co-administration with CYP2C8 and CYP3A substrates; if co-administration cannot be avoided, modify the substrate dosage as recommended in its product labeling. Based on findings

(continued)

from animal studies and its mechanism of action, **Retevmo** can cause fetal harm. There are <u>no</u> available data on **Retevmo** use in pregnant females to inform drug-associated risk. Therefore, verify pregnancy status in females of reproductive potential prior to initiating **Retevmo** and advise females of reproductive potential of the possible risk to the fetus and to use effective contraception. There are <u>no</u> data on the presence of *selpercatinib* <u>or</u> its metabolites in human milk <u>or</u> effects on the breastfed infant. Because of the potential for serious adverse embryo/fetal effects, advise women <u>not</u> to breastfeed during treatment with **Retevmo** and for 1 week after the final dose.

LUPUS NEPHRITIS

CALCINEURIN INHIBITOR IMMUNOSUPPRESSANT

▶ *voclosporin Recommended starting dose:* 23.7 mg bid; *Severe renal impairment:* 15.8 mg bid; *Mild/Moderate hepatic impairment:* 15.8 mg bid; *Severe hepatic impairment:* avoid use with administer consistently as close to an every 12hour schedule as possible and with at least 8 hours between doses; if a dose is missed, take it as soon as possible within 4 hours after the missed dose; beyond the 4-hour time frame, wait until the usual scheduled time to take the next regular dose; do <u>not</u> double the next dose; must be swallowed whole on an empty stomach; do <u>not</u> break, crush, chew or dissolve **Lupkynis** capsules before swallowing; avoid eating grapefruit <u>or</u> drinking grapefruit juice while taking **Lupkynis** it is <u>not</u> known if taking Lupkynis is safe <u>or</u> effective beyond a year.

    Lupkynis *Cap:* 7.9 mg
    Comment: **Lupkynis** is indicated in combination with a background immunosuppressive therapy regimen. Use **Lupkynis** in combination with *mycophenolate mofetil* (*MMF*) and corticosteroids. Before initiating **Lupkynis**, establish an accurate baseline estimated glomerular filtration rate (eGFR) and blood pressure.

    Baseline eGFR ≤45 ml/min: <u>not</u> recommended unless the benefit exceeds the risk (these patients may be at increased risk for acute and/<u>or</u> chronic nephrotoxicity). Assess eGFR every 2 weeks for the first month and every 4 weeks thereafter. If eGFR <60 ml/min and reduced from baseline by >20% and <30%, reduce the dose by 7.9 mg bid; then reassess within 2 weeks; if eGFR is still reduced from baseline by >20%, reduce the dose again by 7.9 mg bid.

    If eGFR <60 ml/min and reduced from baseline by ≥30%, discontinue **Lupkynis**; then reassess eGFR within 2 weeks; consider reinitiating **Lupkynis** at a lower dose (7.9 mg bid) <u>only</u> if eGFR has returned to ≥80% of baseline.

    For patients who had a decrease in dose due to eGFR, consider increasing the dose by 7.9 mg bid for each eGFR measurement that is ≥80% of baseline; do <u>not</u> exceed the starting dose. Do <u>not</u> initiate **Lupkynis** in patients with baseline BP >165/105 <u>or</u> with hypertensive emergency. Monitor BP every 2 weeks for the first month and as clinically indicated thereafter. If BP >165/105 <u>or</u> with hypertensive emergency, discontinue **Lupkynis** and initiate antihypertensive therapy.

    Concomitant use of strong CYP3A4 inhibitors (e.g., *ketoconazole, itraconazole, clarithromycin*) with **Lupkynis** is contraindicated. The most commonly reported adverse reactions (incidence ≥3%) have been decreased eGFR, hypertension, diarrhea, headache, anemia, cough, urinary tract infection, abdominal pain upper, dyspepsia, alopecia, renal impairment, abdominal pain, mouth ulceration, fatigue, tremor, acute kidney injury, and decreased appetite. When **Lupkynis** is co-administered with moderate CYP3A4 inhibitors, reduce the **Lupkynis** daily dose to 15.8 mg in the morning and 7.9 mg in the evening. Avoid co-administration of **Lupkynis** with strong and moderate CYP3A4 inducers. Reduce dosage of certain P-glycoprotein (P-gp) substrates with a narrow therapeutic window when co-administered with **Lupkynis**. Avoid live vaccines. **Lupkynis** may cause embryo/fetal harm. Advise <u>not</u> to breastfeed.

LYME DISEASE (*ERYTHEMA CHRONICUM MIGRANS*)

Comment: The bite of the deer tick (*Ixodes scapularis*) carries the *Borrelia burgdorferi* organism causing Lyme disease. Proper removal of the tick and early diagnosis and treatment are essential to effective management of this disease.

STAGE 1

▶ *amoxicillin* (G) 500-875 mg bid <u>or</u> 250-500 mg tid x 10 days
    Pediatric: <40 kg (88 lb): 20-40 mg/kg/day in 3 divided doses x 10 days <u>or</u> 25-45 mg/kg/day in 2 divided doses x 10 days; ≥40 kg: same as adult; *see* Appendix BB.3. *amoxicillin* (G) (Amoxil Suspension, Trimox Suspension) *for dose by weight*
        Amoxil *Cap:* 250, 500 mg; *Tab:* 875*mg; *Chew tab:* 125, 200, 250, 400 mg (cherry-banana-peppermint) (phenylalanine); *Oral susp:* 125, 250 mg/5 ml (80, 100, 150 ml) (strawberry); 200, 400 mg/5 ml (50, 75, 100 ml) (bubble gum); *Oral drops:* 50 mg/ml (30 ml) (bubble gum)
        Moxatag *Tab:* 775 mg ext-rel
        Trimox *Tab:* 125, 250 mg; *Cap:* 250, 500 mg; *Oral susp:* 125, 250 mg/5 ml (80, 100, 150 ml) (raspberry-strawberry)

▷ **clarithromycin (G)** 500 mg bid or 500 mg ext-rel once daily x 14-21 days
Pediatric: <6 months: not recommended; ≥6 months: 7.5 mg/kg bid x 7 days; *see* Appendix BB.16.
clarithromycin (G) (Biaxin Suspension) *for dose by weight*
   Biaxin *Tab:* 250, 500 mg
   Biaxin Oral Suspension *Oral susp:* 125, 250 mg/5 ml (50, 100 ml)
   Biaxin XL *Tab:* 500 mg ext-rel
▷ **doxycycline (G)** 100 mg bid x 14-21 days
Pediatric: <8 years: not recommended; ≥8 years, ≤100 lb: 2 mg/lb on first day in 2 divided doses, followed
by 1 mg/lb/day in 1-2 divided doses; ≥8 years, >100 lb: same as adult; *see* Appendix BB.19. doxycycline (G)
(Vibramycin Syrup/Suspension) *for dose by weight*
   Acticlate *Tab:* 75, 150**mg
   Adoxa *Tab:* 50, 75, 100, 150 mg ent-coat
   Doryx *Tab:* 50, 75, 100, 150, 200 mg del-rel
   Doxteric *Tab:* 50 mg del-rel
   Monodox *Cap:* 50, 75, 100 mg
   Oracea *Cap:* 40 mg del-rel
   Vibramycin *Tab:* 100 mg; *Cap:* 50, 100 mg; *Syr:* 50 mg/5 ml (raspberry-apple) (sulfites); *Oral susp:* 25
   mg/5 ml (raspberry)
   Vibra-Tab *Tab:* 100 mg film-coat
▷ **minocycline (G)** 200 mg on first day; then 100 mg q 12 hours x 9 more days
Pediatric: ≤8 years: not recommended; ≥8 years, <100 lb: 2 mg/lb on first day in 2 divided doses, followed by
1 mg/lb q 12 hours x 9 more days; ≥8 years, >100 lb: same as adult
   Dynacin *Cap:* 50, 100 mg
   Minocin *Cap:* 50, 75, 100 mg; *Oral susp:* 50 mg/5 ml (60 ml) (custard) (sulfites, alcohol 5%)
▷ **tetracycline (G)** 250-500 mg qid ac x 21 days
Pediatric: <8 years: not recommended; ≥8 years, ≤100 lb: 25-50 mg/kg/day in 2-4 divided doses x 7 days; ≥8
years, >100 lb: same as adult; *see* Appendix BB.31. tetracycline (G) (Sumycin Suspension) *for dose by weight*
   Achromycin V *Cap:* 250, 500 mg
   Sumycin *Tab:* 250, 500 mg; *Cap:* 250, 500 mg; *Oral susp:* 125 mg/5 ml (100, 200 ml) (fruit) (sulfites)

LYMPHADENITIS

Comment: Therapy should continue for no less than 5 days after resolution of symptoms.

▷ **amoxicillin+clavulanate (G)**
   Augmentin 500 mg tid or 875 mg bid x 7-10 days
   Pediatric: 40-45 mg/kg/day divided tid x 10 days or 90 mg/kg/day divided bid x 10 days; *see* Appendix
   BB.4. amoxicillin+clavulanate (G) (Augmentin Suspension) *for dose by weight*
      Tab: 250, 500, 875 mg; *Chew tab:* 125, 250 mg (lemon-lime); 200, 400 mg (cherry-banana) (phenylal-
      anine); *Oral susp:* 125 mg/5 ml (banana), 250 mg/5 ml (75, 100, 150 ml) (orange); 200, 400 mg/5 ml
      (50, 75, 100 ml) (orange) (phenylalanine)
   Augmentin ES-600 not recommended for adults
   Pediatric: <3 months: not recommended; ≥3 months, <40 kg: 90 mg/kg/day in 2 divided doses x 7-10
   days; ≥40 kg: not recommended
      Oral susp: 42.9 mg/5 ml (50, 75, 100, 125, 150, 200 ml) (strawberry cream) (phenylalanine)
   Augmentin XR 2 tabs q 12 hours x 7-10 days
   Pediatric: <16 years: use other forms; ≥16 years: same as adult
      Tab: 1,000*mg ext-rel
▷ **cephalexin (G)** 500 mg bid x 10 days
Pediatric: 25-50 mg/kg/day in 4 divided doses x 10 days; *see* Appendix BB.15. cephalexin (G) (Keflex
Suspension) *for dose by weight*
   Keflex *Cap:* 250, 333, 500, 750 mg; *Oral susp:* 125, 250 mg/5 ml (100, 200 ml) (strawberry)
▷ **dicloxacillin** 500 mg qid x 10 days
Pediatric: 12.5-25 mg/kg/day in 4 divided doses x 10 days; *see* Appendix BB.18. dicloxacillin (G) (Dynapen
Suspension) *for dose by weight*
   Dynapen *Cap:* 125, 250, 500 mg; *Oral susp:* 62.5 mg/5 ml (80, 100, 200 ml)

LYMPHOGRANULOMA VENEREUM

Comment: The following treatment regimens are published in the **2021 CDC Sexually Transmitted Diseases
Treatment Guidelines.** This section contains treatment regimens for adults only; consult a specialist for treatment
of patients less than 18 years of age. Treatment regimens are presented in alphabetical order by generic drug name,
followed by brands and dose forms. Treat all sexual contacts. Persons with both lymphogranuloma venereum
(LGV) and HIV infection should receive the same treatment regimens as those who are HIV-negative; however,
prolonged treatment may be required and delay in resolution of symptoms may occur.

RECOMMENDED REGIMEN
Regimen 1
▷ *doxycycline* 100 mg bid x 21 days

ALTERNATIVE REGIMEN
Regimen 1
▷ *erythromycin base* 500 mg qid x 21 days or *erythromycin ethylsuccinate* 400 mg qid x 21 days

RECOMMENDED REGIMENS FOR THE MANAGEMENT OF SEXUAL CONTACTS
Comment: LGV is caused by *Chlamydia trachomatis* serovars L1, L2, or L3. Persons who have had sexual contact with a patient who has LGV within 60 days before onset of the patient's symptoms should be examined, tested for urethral or cervical chlamydial infection, and treated with a chlamydia regimen.

Regimen 1
▷ *azithromycin* 1 gm in a single dose

Regimen 2
▷ *doxycycline* 100 mg bid x 7 days

DRUG BRANDS AND DOSE FORMS
▷ *azithromycin* (G)
    Zithromax *Tab:* 250, 500, 600 mg; *Oral susp:* 100 mg/5 ml (15 ml), 200 mg/5 ml (15, 22.5, 30 ml) (cherry); *Pkt:* 1 gm for reconstitution (cherry-banana)
    Zithromax Tri-Pak *Tab:* 3 x 500 mg tabs/pck
    Zithromax Z-Pak *Tab:* 6 x 250 mg tabs/pck
    Zmax *Oral susp:* 2 gm ext-rel for reconstitution (cherry-banana) (148 mg Na$^+$)
▷ *doxycycline* (G)
    Acticlate *Tab:* 75, 150**mg
    Adoxa *Tab:* 50, 75, 100, 150 mg ent-coat
    Doryx *Tab:* 50, 75, 100, 150, 200 mg del-rel
    Doxteric *Tab:* 50 mg del-rel
    Monodox *Cap:* 50, 75, 100 mg
    Oracea *Cap:* 40 mg del-rel
    Vibramycin *Tab:* 100 mg; *Cap:* 50, 100 mg; *Syr:* 50 mg/5 ml (raspberry-apple) (sulfites); *Oral susp:* 25 mg/5 ml (raspberry)
    Vibra-Tab *Tab:* 100 mg film-coat
▷ *erythromycin base* (G)
    Ery-Tab *Tab:* 250, 333, 500 mg ent-coat
    PCE *Tab:* 333, 500 mg
▷ *erythromycin ethylsuccinate* (G)
    EryPed *Oral susp:* 200 mg/5 ml (100, 200 ml) (fruit), 400 mg/5 ml (60, 100, 200 ml) (banana); *Oral drops:* 200, 400 mg/5 ml (50 ml) (fruit); *Chew tab:* 200 mg wafer (fruit)
    E.E.S. *Oral susp:* 200, 400 mg/5 ml (100 ml) (fruit)
    E.E.S. Granules *Oral susp:* 200 mg/5 ml (100, 200 ml) (cherry)
    E.E.S. 400 Tablets *Tab:* 400 mg

MALARIA (*PLASMODIUM FALCIPARUM, PLASMODIUM VIVAX*)

▷ *doxycycline* (G) 100 mg daily; initiate 1-2 days prior to travel; take during travel; continue for 4 weeks after leaving the endemic area
    Pediatric: ≤8 years: not recommended; ≥8 years, ≤100 lb: 1 mg/lb/day prior to travel; take during travel; continue for 4 weeks after leaving the endemic area; ≥8 years, ≥100 lb: same as adult; *see* Appendix BB.19.
    doxycycline (G) (Vibramycin Syrup/Suspension) *for dose by weight*
    Acticlate *Tab:* 75, 150**mg
    Adoxa *Tab:* 50, 75, 100, 150 mg ent-coat
    Doryx *Tab:* 50, 75, 100, 150, 200 mg del-rel
    Doxteric *Tab:* 50 mg del-rel
    Monodox *Cap:* 50, 75, 100 mg
    Oracea *Cap:* 40 mg del-rel
    Vibramycin *Tab:* 100 mg; *Cap:* 50, 100 mg; *Syr:* 50 mg/5 ml (raspberry-apple) (sulfites); *Oral susp:* 25 mg/5 ml (raspberry)
    Vibra-Tab *Tab:* 100 mg film-coat
▷ *minocycline* (G) 100 mg daily; initiate 1-2 days prior to travel; take during travel; continue for 4 weeks after leaving the endemic area
    Pediatric: <8 years: not recommended; ≥8 years, ≤100 lb: 2 mg/lb on first day in 2 divided doses, followed by 1 mg/lb q 12 hours x 9 more days; ≥8 years, >100 lb: same as adult

Dynacin *Cap:* 50, 100 mg

Minocin *Cap:* 50, 75, 100 mg; *Oral susp:* 50 mg/5 ml (60 ml) (custard) (sulfites, alcohol 5%)

▷ *tetracycline* 250 mg daily; initiate 1-2 days prior to travel; take during travel; continue for 4 weeks after leaving the endemic area

Pediatric: <8 years: not recommended; ≥8 years, ≤100 lb: 25-50 mg/kg/day in 4 divided doses x 10 days; ≥8 years, >100 lb: same as adult; *see* Appendix BB.31. *tetracycline* (G) (Sumycin Suspension) *for dose by weight*

Achromycin V *Cap:* 250, 500 mg

Sumycin *Tab:* 250, 500 mg; *Cap:* 250, 500 mg; *Oral susp:* 125 mg/5 ml (100, 200 ml) (fruit) (sulfites)

INITIAL BOLUS TREATMENT FOR SEVERE MALARIA

▷ *artesunate for injection* 2.4 mg/kg administered IV at 0 hours, 12 hours, and 24 hours; thereafter, administer once daily until the patient is able to tolerate oral antimalarial therapy; using only the sterile diluent supplied, swirl gently (do not shake) for up to 5-6 minutes until the powder is fully dissolved; administer as a slow IV bolus over 1-2 minutes within 1.5 hours after reconstitution; do not administer via continuous IV infusion; see mfr pkg insert for instructions on preparation

Pediatric: for patients <6 months, a pharmacokinetic (PK) extrapolation approach using modeling and simulation indicated comparable or higher predicted PK steady-state area under the curve (AUC) of dihydroartemisinin (DHA) between this age group and older children or adults at the recommended 2.4 mg/kg dose regimen; no notable safety issues have been identified in limited published safety and outcome data in patients <6 months with severe malaria; no dose adjustment is necessary for pediatric patients regardless of age or body weight; based on animal data, **Artesunate** may cause fetal harm. However, administration of **Artesunate** for Injection for the treatment of severe malaria. Treatment should not be delayed due to pregnancy. Delaying treatment of severe malaria in pregnancy may result in serious morbidity and mortality to the mother and fetus. DHA, a metabolite of artesunate, is present in human milk. DHA is present in breast milk and effects on the breastfed infant are unknown. The developmental and health benefits of breastfeeding should be considered along with the mother's clinical need for **Artesunate for Injection** and any potential adverse effects on the breastfed infant from **Artesunate for Injection** or from the underlying maternal condition.

Artesunate for Injection *Vial:* 110 mg, single-dose, pwdr for reconstitution w. supplied sterile diluent (12 ml) (natural rubber latex-free)

Comment: Artesunate for Injection is an antimalarial indicated for the initial treatment of severe malaria in adult and pediatric patients. Treatment of severe malaria with **Artesunate for Injection** should always be followed by a complete treatment course of an appropriate oral antimalarial regimen. **Artesunate for Injection** does not treat the hypnozoite liver stage forms of *Plasmodium* and will, therefore, not prevent relapses of malaria due to *Plasmodium vivax* or *P. ovale*. Concomitant therapy with an antimalarial agent, such as an 8-aminoquinoline drug, is necessary for the treatment of severe malaria due to *P. vivax* or *P. ovale*. Cases of posttreatment hemolytic anemia severe enough to require transfusion have been reported; monitor patients for 4 weeks after treatment for evidence of hemolytic anemia. Serious hypersensitivity reactions, including anaphylaxis, have been reported; discontinue if signs of serious hypersensitivity occur. The most common adverse reactions (incidence ≥2%) reported in clinical trials of severe malaria include acute renal failure requiring dialysis, hemoglobinuria, and jaundice. Monitor for possible reduced antimalarial efficacy if **Artesunate for Injection** is used concomitantly with *nevirapine* or *ritonavir* antiretrovirals or strong UGT inducers (e.g., *rifampin, carbamazepine, phenytoin*). Delaying treatment of severe malaria in pregnancy may result in serious morbidity and mortality to the mother and the fetus. Based on animal data, **Artesunate for Injection** may cause fetal harm. However, administration for the treatment of severe malaria may be lifesaving for the pregnant female and the fetus; therefore, treatment should not be delayed due to pregnancy.

ANTIMALARIALS

▷ *atovaquone* (G) take as a single dose with food or a milky drink at the same time each day; repeat dose if vomited within 1 hour; *Prophylaxis:* 1,500 mg once daily; *Treatment:* 750 mg bid x 21 days

Mepron *Susp:* 750 mg/5 ml

▷ *atovaquone+proguanil* (G) take as a single dose with food or a milky drink at the same time each day; repeat dose if vomited within 1 hour; *Prophylaxis:* 1 tab daily starting 1-2 days before entering endemic area, during stay, and for 7 days after return; *Treatment (acute, uncomplicated):* 4 tabs daily x 3 days

Pediatric: <5 kg: not recommended; 5-40 kg: *Prophylaxis:* daily dose starting 1-2 days before entering endemic area, during stay, and for 7 days after return; 5-20 kg: 1 ped tab; 21-30 kg: 2 ped tabs; 31-40 kg: 3 ped tabs; ≥40 kg: same as adult; *Treatment (acute, uncomplicated):* daily dose x 3 days; 5-8 kg: 2 ped tabs; 9-10 kg: 3 ped tabs; 11-20 kg: 1 adult tab; 21-30 kg: 2 adult tabs; 31-40 kg: 3 adult tabs; >40 kg: same as adult

Malarone *Tab:* atov 250 mg+prog 100 mg

Malarone Pediatric *Tab:* atov 62.5 mg+prog 25 mg

Comment: *Atovaquone* is antagonized by *tetracycline* and *metoclopramide*. Concomitant *rifampin* is not recommended (may elevate liver function tests [LFTs]).

▷ *chloroquine* (G) *Prophylaxis:* 500 mg once weekly (on the same day of each week); start 2 weeks prior to exposure, continue while in the endemic area, and continue 4 weeks after departure; *Treatment:* initially 1

(continued)

gm; then 500 mg 6 hours, 24 hours, and 48 hours after initial dose or initially 200-250 mg IM; may repeat in 6 hours; max 1 gm in the first 24 hours; continue to 1.875 gm in 3 days
Pediatric: Suppression: 8.35 mg/kg (max 500 mg) weekly (on the same day of each week); *Treatment:* initially 16.7 mg/kg (max 1 gm); then 8.35 mg/kg (max 500 mg) 6 hours, 24 hours, and 48 hours after initial dose, or initially 6.25 mg/kg IM; may repeat in 6 hours; max 12.5 mg/kg/day
    Aralen *Tab:* 500 mg; *Amp:* 50 mg/ml (5 ml)

▶ *hydroxychloroquine* (G) *Prophylaxis:* 400 mg once weekly (on the same day of each week); start 2 weeks prior to exposure, continue while in the endemic area, and continue 8 weeks after departure; *Treatment:* initially 800 mg; then 400 mg 6 hours, 24 hours, and 48 hours after initial dose
Pediatric: Suppression: 6.45 mg/kg (max 400 mg) weekly (on the same day of each week) beginning 2 weeks prior to arrival, continuing while in endemic area, and continuing 4 weeks after departure; *Treatment:* initially 12.9 mg/kg (max 800 mg); then 6.45 mg/kg (max 400 mg) 6 hours, 24 hours, and 48 hours after initial dose hours after initial dose
    Plaquenil *Tab:* 200 mg

▶ *mefloquine Prophylaxis:* 250 mg once weekly (on the same day of each week); start 1 week prior to exposure, continue while in the endemic area, and continue for 4 weeks after departure; *Treatment:* 1,250 mg as a single dose
Pediatric: <6 months: not recommended; *Prophylaxis:* ≥6 months: 3-5 mg/kg (max 250 mg) weekly (on the same day of each week); start 1 week prior to exposure, continue while in the endemic area, and continue for 4 weeks after departure; *Treatment:* ≥6 months: 25-50 mg/kg as a single dose; max 250 mg
    Lariam *Tab:* 250*mg
    Comment: *Mefloquine* is contraindicated with active or recent history of depression, generalized anxiety disorder, psychosis, schizophrenia or any other psychiatric disorder, or history of convulsions.

▶ *quinine sulfate* (G) 1 tab or cap q 8 hours x 7 days
Pediatric: <16 years: not recommended; ≥16 years: same as adult
    Tab: 260 mg; *Cap:* 260, 300, 325 mg
    Qualaquin *Cap:* 324 mg
    Comment: *Qualaquin* is indicated in the treatment of uncomplicated *P. falciparum* malaria (including *chloroquine*-resistant strains).

▶ *tafenoquine* (G) *Loading regimen:* take 200 mg (2 x 100 mg tabs) once daily x 3 days before travel to endemic area; *Maintenance:* take 200 mg (2 x 100 mg tabs) once weekly beginning 7 days after the last loading regimen dose; maintenance dose may be continued for up to 6 months; take with food
Pediatric: <18 years: not recommended; ≥18 years: same as adult
    Arakoda *Tab:* 100 mg
    Comment: **Arakoda** *(tafenoquine)* is an 8-aminoquinoline antimalarial drug indicated for the prophylaxis of malaria. **Arakoda** provides effective protection against both of the major types of malaria (*P. vivax* and *P. falciparum*), killing the parasites in both the blood and liver. **Arakoda** is not recommended with a history of psychosis or current psychotic symptoms. **Arakoda** is not recommended for patients with glucose-6-phosphate dehydrogenase (G6PD) deficiency or unknown G6PD status. Because **Arakoda** may cause fetal harm when administered to a pregnant female with a G6PD-deficient fetus, **Arakoda** is not recommended during pregnancy, breastfeeding when the infant is found to be G6PD-deficient or if G6PD status is unknown, and during treatment and for 3 months after the last dose of **Arakoda**. All patients must be G6PD deficiency prior to prescribing **Arakoda** and pregnancy testing is recommended for females of reproductive potential prior to initiating treatment. Due to the long half-life of **Arakoda** (approximately 17 days), psychiatric effects, hemolytic anemia, methemoglobinemia, and hypersensitivity reactions may be delayed in onset and/or duration. Avoid co-administration with drugs that are substrates of organic cation transporter-2 (OCT2) or multidrug and toxin extrusion (MATE) transporters. The most common adverse reactions (incidence ≥1%) have been headache, dizziness, back pain, diarrhea, nausea, vomiting, increased alanine aminotransferase (ALT), motion sickness, insomnia, depression, abnormal dreams, and anxiety.

RADICAL CURE (PREVENTION OF RELAPSE)
8-AMINOQUINOLINE DERIVATIVE

▶ *tafenoquine* take 300 mg (2 x 150 mg tabs) as a single dose with food; co-administer on the first or second day of the appropriate antimalarial therapy for acute *P. vivax* malaria
Pediatric: <16 years: not recommended; ≥16 years: same as adult
    Krintafel *Tab:* 150 mg
    Comment: **Krintafel** *(tafenoquine)* is an 8-aminoquinoline derivative antimalarial for the radical cure (prevention of relapse) of *P. vivax* malaria in patients who are receiving appropriate antimalarial therapy for acute *P. vivax* infection. **Krintafel** is not indicated for the treatment of acute *P. vivax* malaria. Contraindications are G6PD deficiency or unknown G6PD status and breastfeeding by a lactating woman when the infant is found to be G6PD-deficient or if G6PD status is unknown (due to the risk of hemolytic anemia in patients with G6PD deficiency). All patients must be tested for G6PD deficiency prior to prescribing **Krintafel** and pregnancy testing is recommended for females of reproductive potential prior to initiating treatment with **Krintafel**. Also, the G6PD-deficient infant may be at risk for hemolytic anemia from exposure to **Krintafel** through breast milk; check the infant's G6PD status before breastfeeding begins.

Asymptomatic elevations in blood methemoglobin have been observed; initiate appropriate therapy if signs or symptoms of methemoglobinemia occur. Serious psychiatric adverse reactions have been observed in patients with a history of psychiatric conditions at doses higher than the approved dose. Therefore, benefit of treatment with **Krintafel** must be weighed against the potential risk for psychiatric adverse reactions in patients with a history of psychiatric illness. Due to the long half-life of **Krintafel** (15 days), psychiatric effects and hypersensitivity reactions may be delayed in onset and/or duration. Common adverse reactions (incidence ≥5%) have been dizziness, nausea, vomiting, headache, and decreased hemoglobin.

MASTITIS (BREAST ABSCESS)

ANTI-INFECTIVES
▷ *amoxicillin+clavulanate* (G)
    Augmentin 500 mg tid or 875 mg bid x 7-10 days
    Pediatric: 40-45 mg/kg/day divided tid x 10 days or 90 mg/kg/day divided bid x 10 days; *see* Appendix BB.4. *amoxicillin+clavulanate* (G) (Augmentin Suspension) *for dose by weight*
        Tab: 250, 500, 875 mg; *Chew tab:* 125, 250 mg (lemon-lime); 200, 400 mg (cherry-banana) (phenylalanine); *Oral susp:* 125 mg/5 ml (banana), 250 mg/5 ml (75, 100, 150 ml) (orange); 200, 400 mg/5 ml (50, 75, 100 ml) (orange) (phenylalanine)
    Augmentin ES-600 not recommended for adults
    Pediatric: <3 months: not recommended; ≥3 months, <40 kg: 90 mg/kg/day in 2 divided doses x 7-10 days; ≥40 kg: not recommended
        Oral susp: 42.9 mg/5 ml (50, 75, 100, 125, 150, 200 ml) (strawberry cream) (phenylalanine)
    Augmentin XR 2 tabs q 12 hours x 7-10 days
    Pediatric: <16 years: use other forms; ≥16 years: same as adult
        Tab: 1,000*mg ext-rel
▷ *cefaclor* (G)
    Ceclor 250 mg tid or 375 mg bid 3-10 days
    Pediatric: <1 month: not recommended; 1 month-12 years: 20-40 mg/kg divided bid or q 12 hours x 3-10 days; max 1 gm/day; *see* Appendix BB.8. *cefaclor* (G) (Ceclor Suspension) for *dose by weight*; >12 years: same as adult
        Tab: 500 mg; *Cap:* 250, 500 mg; *Susp:* 125 mg/5 ml (75, 150 ml) (strawberry), 187 mg/5 ml (50, 100 ml) (strawberry), 250 mg/5 ml (75, 150 ml) (strawberry), 375 mg/5 ml (50, 100 ml) (strawberry)
    Ceclor Extended Release 375-500 mg bid x 3-10 days
    Pediatric: <16 years: ext-rel not recommended; ≥16 years: same as adult
        Tab: 375, 500 mg ext-rel
▷ *ceftriaxone* (G) 1-2 gm IM daily continued 2 days after signs of infection have disappeared; max 4 gm/day
    Pediatric: 50 mg/kg IM daily continued 2 days after signs of infection have disappeared
        Rocephin *Vial:* 250, 500 mg; 1, 2 gm
▷ *cephalexin* (G) 500 mg bid x 10 days
    Pediatric: 25-50 mg/kg/day in 4 divided doses x 10 days; *see* Appendix BB.15. *cephalexin* (G) (Keflex Suspension) *for dose by weight*
        Keflex *Cap:* 250, 333, 500, 750 mg; *Oral susp:* 125, 250 mg/5 ml (100, 200 ml) (strawberry)
▷ *clindamycin* (G) 300 mg tid x 10 days
    Pediatric: <12 years: not recommended; ≥12 years: same as adult
        Cleocin *Cap:* 75 (tartrazine), 150 (tartrazine), 300 mg
        Cleocin Pediatric Granules *Oral susp:* 75 mg/5 ml (100 ml) (cherry)
▷ *erythromycin base* (G) 250-500 mg qid x 10 days
    Pediatric: <45 kg: 30-40 mg/kg/day in 4 divided doses x 10 days; ≥45 kg: same as adult
        Ery-Tab *Tab:* 250, 333, 500 mg ent-coat
        PCE *Tab:* 333, 500 mg

MELASMA/CHLOASMA

SKIN DEPIGMENTING AGENTS
▷ *hydroquinone* apply a thin film to clean dry affected areas bid; discontinue if lightening does not occur after 2 months
    Pediatric: <12 years: not recommended; ≥12 years: same as adult
        Lustra *Crm:* hydro 4% (1, 2 oz) (sulfites)
        Lustra AF *Crm:* hydro 4% (1, 2 oz) (sunscreens, sulfites)
▷ *hydroquinone+fluocinolone acetonide+tretinoin* apply a thin film to clean dry affected areas once daily at least 30 minutes before bedtime
    Pediatric: <12 years: not recommended; ≥12 years: same as adult
        Tri-Luma *Crm:* hydro 4%+fluo acet 0.01%+tret 0.05% (30 gm) (sulfites, parabens)

MÉNIÈRE'S DISEASE

▷ *diazepam* (IV) (G) initially 1-2.5 mg tid-qid; may increase gradually
  Pediatric: <6 months: not recommended; ≥6 months: same as adult
    Diastat *Rectal gel delivery system* 2.5 mg
    Diastat AcuDial *Rectal gel delivery system* 10, 20 mg
    Valium *Tab:* 2*, 5*, 10*mg
    Valium Intensol Oral Solution *Conc oral soln:* 5 mg/ml (30 ml w. dropper) (alcohol 19%)
    Valium Oral Solution *Oral soln:* 5 mg/5 ml (500 ml) (wintergreen-spice)
▷ *dimenhydrinate* (OTC) (G) 50 mg q 4-6 hours
  Pediatric: <2 years: not recommended; 2-6 years: 12.5-25 mg q 6-8 hours, max 75 mg/day; >6-11 years:
  25-50 mg q 6-8 hours, max 150 mg/day; >11 years: same as adult
    Dramamine (OTC) *Tab:* 50*mg; *Chew tab:* 50 mg (phenylalanine, tartrazine); *Liq:* 12.5 mg/5 ml (4 oz)
▷ *diphenhydramine* (OTC) (G) 25-50 mg q 6-8 hours; max 100 mg/day
  Pediatric: <2 years: not recommended; 2-6 years: 6.25 mg q 4-6 hours, max 37.5 mg/day; >6-12 years:
  12.5-25 mg q 4-6 hours, max 150 mg/day; >12 years: same as adult
    Benadryl (OTC) *Chew tab:* 12.5 mg (grape; phenylalanine); *Liq:* 12.5 mg/5 ml (4, 8 oz); *Cap:* 25 mg; *Tab:*
    25 mg; *Dye-free softgel:* 25 mg; *Dye-free liq:* 12.5 mg/5 ml (4, 8 oz)
▷ *meclizine* (G) 25-100 mg/day in divided doses
  Pediatric: <12 years: not recommended; ≥12 years: same as adult
    Antivert *Tab:* 12.5, 25, 50*mg; *Amp:* 50 mg/ml (1 ml); *Vial:* 50 mg/ml (1 ml single-use), 50 mg/ml (10
    ml multidose)
    Bonine (OTC) *Cap:* 15, 25, 30 mg; *Tab:* 12.5, 25, 50 mg; *Chew tab/Film-coat tab:* 25 mg
    Dramamine II 25 mg bid; max 50 mg/day
      Tab: 25*mg
    Zentrip *Strip:* 25 mg orally disintegrating
▷ *promethazine* 12.5-25 q 4-6 hours PO or rectally
  Pediatric: <2 years: not recommended; ≥2 years: 0.5 mg/lb or 6.25-25 mg q 4-6 hours PO or rectally
    Phenergan *Tab:* 12.5*, 25*, 50 mg; *Plain syr:* 6.25 mg/5 ml; *Fortis syr:* 25 mg/5 ml; *Rectal supp:* 12.5, 25,
    50 mg
  Comment: *Promethazine* is contraindicated in children with uncomplicated nausea, dehydration, Reye's
  syndrome, history of sleep apnea, asthma, and lower respiratory disorders. *Promethazine* lowers the seizure
  threshold in children and may cause cholestatic jaundice, anticholinergic effects, extrapyramidal effects, and
  potentially fatal respiratory depression.
▷ *scopolamine* transdermal patch 1 patch behind the ear; each patch is effective for 3 days; change patch every
  4th day; alternate sites
  Pediatric: <12 years: not recommended; ≥12 years: same as adult
    Transderm Scop *Patch:* 1.5 mg (4/carton)

MENINGITIS (*NEISSERIA MENINGITIDIS*)

PROPHYLAXIS
Comment: Meningitis vaccine is a 3-dose series (0, 2, 6-month schedule) indicated for persons ≥10-25 years of
age. Have epinephrine 1:1,000 readily available and monitor for 15 minutes post-dose of meningitis vaccine.
  Meningococcal A, C, W, Y Vaccination
  The Advisory Committee on Immunization Practices (ACIP) recommends routine vaccination with a
  quadrivalent meningococcal conjugate vaccine (**MenACWY**) for persons at risk for meningococcal disease
  caused by serogroups A, C, W, or Y and booster doses for those who were previously vaccinated who
  become or remain at risk. **MenACWY-TT** was first licensed in 2020 for the prevention of meningococcal
  disease caused by serogroups A, C, W, and Y in persons ≥2 years of age.
  Meningococcal B Vaccination
  ACIP recommends routine vaccination with serogroup B meningococcal (**MenB**) vaccine in persons >10
  years of age who are at risk for serogroup B meningococcal disease and **MenB** boosters are recommended
  for those who were previously vaccinated who become or remain at risk. ACIP recommends a **MenB** series
  for adolescents and young adults 16-23 years of age by shared clinical decision-making to provide short-
  term protection against most strains of the serogroup B meningococcal disease.

▷ *meningococcal group b vaccine (recombinant, absorbed)* administer first dose IM in the deltoid; administer
  second dose 2 months later; administer the third dose 6 months from the first dose
  Pediatric: <10 years: not established; ≥10 years: same as adult
    Bexsero *Susp for IM inj:* 0.5 ml single-dose prefilled syringes (1, 10/carton)
    Trumenba *Susp for IM inj:* 0.5 ml single-dose prefilled syringes (5, 10/carton)
▷ *Neisseria meningitides oligosaccharide conjugate* quadrivalent meningococcal vaccine contains
  Corynebacterium diphtheria CRM197 protein; 10 mcg of Group A + 5 mcg each of Group C, Y, and W-135
  + 32.7-64.1 mcg of diphtheria CRM197 protein per 0.5 ml.
  Pediatric: <11 years: not recommended; ≥11-55 years: 0.5 ml IM x 1 dose in the deltoid

Menveo *Vial multidose:* 5 doses/vial (MenA conjugate component pwdr for reconstitution + 1 vial liquid MenCWY conjugate component for reconstitution) (preservative-free)

▷ *Neisseria meningitidis polysaccharides* vaccine 0.5 ml SC x 1 dose; if at high risk, may revaccinate after 3-5 years; age ≥55 years: contact mfr

Menactra (Group A/C/Y/W-135)

Pediatric: <2 years: see mfr pkg insert; ≥2 years: same as adult; if at high risk, may revaccinate children first vaccinated ≤4 years of age after 2-3 years

Vial (single-dose): 4 mcg each of Groups A, C, Y, and W-135 per 0.5 ml (pwdr for SC inj after reconstitution) (preservative-free diluent); *Vial (multidose):* 4 mcg each of Group A, C, Y, and W-130 per 0.5 ml pwdr for SC inj after reconstitution (5 doses/vial) (preservative-free)

Comment: Latex allergy is a contraindication to **Menactra**.

Menomune-(Group A/C/Y/W-135)

Pediatric: <2 years: <u>not</u> recommended (except ≥3 months of age as short-term protection against group A); ≥2 years: same as adult; if at high risk, may revaccinate children first vaccinated ≤4 years of age after 2-3 years (older children after 3-5 years)

Vial (single-dose): 50 mcg each of Group A, C, Y, and W-135 per 0.5 ml (pwdr for SC inj after reconstitution; preservative-free diluent); *Vial (multidose):* 50 mcg each of Group A, C, Y, and W-130 per 0.5 ml pwdr for SC inj after reconstitution (10 doses/vial) (thimerosal-preserved diluent)

Comment: Use precaution with latex allergy.

▷ *meningococcal (groups A, C, W, Y) conjugate vaccine* *Primary vaccination:* 0.5 ml IM as a single one-time dose; *Booster vaccination:* a single 0.5 ml IM dose may be administered to individuals ≥15 years of age and older who are at continued risk for meningococcal disease if at least 4 years have elapsed since a prior dose of meningococcal (Groups A, C, W, Y) conjugate vaccine

Pediatric: <2 years: <u>not</u> established; ≥2 years: same as adult

MenQuadfi *Vial:* 0.5 ml, single-dose

Comment: MenQuadfi is a quadrivalent (MenACWY) vaccine indicated for active immunization for the prevention of invasive meningococcal disease caused by *Neisseria meningitidis* serogroups A, C, W, and Y. MenQuadfi is contraindicated with patient history of severe allergic reaction to any component of the vaccine, <u>or</u> after a previous dose of **MenQuadfi** <u>or</u> any other tetanus toxoid-containing vaccine. The most commonly reported adverse reactions following a primary dose in Study 2 and Study 3 were as follows: *2-9 years:* injection site pain (38.6%, 42.4%), injection site erythema (22.6%, 31.5%), injection site swelling (13.8%, 21.5%), malaise (21.1%, 21.4%), myalgia (20.1%, 23.0), headache (12.5%, 11.5%) and fever (1.9%, 2.7%); *10-17 years:* injection site pain (45.2%, 34.%), injection site erythema (4.5%, 5%), injection site swelling (4.1%, 5.4%) myalgia (35,3%, 27.4%), headache (30.2%, 26.5%), myalgia (27.4%-35.3), fever (0.7%-1.4) malaise (26.0%, 19.4%), and fever (0.2%, 1.4%); *18-55 years:* injection site pain (41.9%, 35.0%), injection site erythema (5.1%, 3.7%), injection site swelling (4.3%, 3.4%), myalgia (35.6%, 51.2%), headache (29.0%, 27.6%), malaise (22.9%, 18.9%), and fever (1.4%, 1.7%). In Study 4, the most commonly reported adverse reactions in patients who had received a prior dose were as follows: injection site pain (16.7%), injection site erythema (3.7%), injection site swelling (3.7%), myalgia (21.6%), headache 18.5%), malaise (13.6%), and fever (0.6%.) ≥56 *years:* injection site pain (25.5%), injection site erythema (5.2%), injection site swelling (4.5%), myalgia (21.9%), malaise (14.5%), headache (14.5%), and fever (2.1).

MENOMETRORRHAGIA: IRREGULAR HEAVY MENSTRUAL BLEEDING, MENORRHAGIA: HEAVY CYCLICAL MENSTRUAL BLEEDING

Combined Oral Contraceptives *see* Appendix G.3. 28-Day Oral Contraceptives with Estrogen and Progesterone Content

Intrauterine Contraceptives *see* Appendix G.10. Intrauterine Contraceptives

ANTIFIBRINOLYTIC AGENT

▷ *tranexamic acid* (G) 1,300 mg tid; treat for up to 5 days during menses; *Normal renal function (serum creatinine (sCr) ≤1.4 mg/dL):* 1,300 mg tid; *sCr ≥1.4-2.8 mg/dL:* 1,300 mg bid; *SCr ≥2.8-5.7 mg/dL:* 1,300 mg once daily; *sCr ≥5.7 mg/dL:* 650 mg once daily

Pediatric: <18 years: <u>not</u> recommended; ≥18 years: same as adult

Lysteda *Tab:* 650 mg

Injectable Progesterone-Only Contraceptives

▷ *medroxyprogesterone* (G)

Depo-Provera 150 mg deep IM q 3 months

Vial: 150 mg/ml (1 ml)

Prefilled syringe: 150 mg/ml

Depo-SubQ 104 mg SC q 3 months

Prefilled syringe: 104 mg/ml (0.65 ml) (parabens)

Comment: Administer first dose within 5 days of onset of normal menses, within 5 days postpartum if <u>not</u> breastfeeding, <u>or</u> at 6 weeks postpartum if breastfeeding exclusively. Do <u>not</u> use for >2 years unless other methods are inadequate.

MENOPAUSE

Comment:
Adverse Side Effects of Estrogen Supplementation: Inform patients of possible less serious but common adverse reactions that may occur with estrogen-alone therapy: headaches, breast/nipple tenderness/pain, and nausea/vomiting. Estrogen-alone therapy increases the risk of gallbladder disease; discontinue estrogen if severe hypercalcemia, loss of vision, severe hypertriglyceridemia, or cholestatic jaundice occurs.

Estrogen Therapy: should be used with caution in women with hypoparathyroidism as estrogen-induced hypocalcemia may occur. Monitor thyroid function in women on thyroid replacement therapy. Retinal vascular thrombosis has been reported in women receiving estrogen; discontinue medication pending examination if there is sudden partial or complete loss of vision, or a sudden onset of proptosis, diplopia, or migraine. If examination reveals papilledema or retinal vascular lesions, estrogens should be permanently discontinued. In a small number of case reports, substantial increases in blood pressure have been attributed to idiosyncratic reactions to estrogens. In a large, randomized, placebo-controlled clinical trial, a generalized effect of estrogens on blood pressure was not seen. Exogenous estrogen may exacerbate symptoms of angioedema in women with hereditary angioedema. Estrogen therapy may cause exacerbation of asthma, diabetes mellitus, epilepsy, migraine, porphyria, systemic lupus erythematosus, and hepatic hemangiomas; use with caution in women with any of these conditions. Inducers and inhibitors of CYP3A4 may alter estrogen drug metabolism and decrease or increase the estrogen plasma concentration.

Contraindications to Estrogen-Replacement Therapy (ERT): known or suspected pregnancy, undiagnosed abnormal genital bleeding, breast cancer or a history of breast cancer, estrogen-dependent neoplasia, active DVT, PE or history of these conditions, active arterial thromboembolic disease (e.g., stroke, MI) or history of these conditions, known anaphylactic reaction, angioedema, or hypersensitivity to exogenous estrogen, hepatic impairment/disease, protein C, protein S, or antithrombin deficiency or other known thrombophilic disorder. A woman who takes estrogen but does not have a uterus generally does not need a progestin. In some cases, however, hysterectomized women who have a history of endometriosis may need a progestin. Use estrogen-alone (recommended) or in combination with a progestin, at the lowest effective dose and for the shortest duration consistent with treatment goals and risks for the individual woman. Re-evaluate postmenopausal women periodically as clinically appropriate to determine if treatment is still necessary.

Estrogen-Alone Therapy: There is increased risk of endometrial cancer in a woman with a uterus who uses unopposed estrogens. Estrogen-alone therapy should not be used for the prevention of cardiovascular disease or dementia. The Women's Health Initiative (WHI) estrogen-alone substudy reported increased risks of stroke and deep vein thrombosis (DVT). The WHI Memory Study (WHIMS), estrogen-alone ancillary study of WHI, reported an increased risk of probable dementia in postmenopausal women ≥65 years of age.

Estrogen plus Progestin Therapy: Estrogen plus progestin therapy should not be used for the prevention of cardiovascular disease or dementia. The Womens Health Initiative Hormone Therapy Trials (WHIHTT) estrogen plus progestin substudy reported increased risks of stroke, DVT, pulmonary embolism (PE), and myocardial infarction (MI). The WHIHTT substudy also reported estrogen plus progestin study also reported increased risks of invasive breast cancer. The WHIMS estrogen plus progestin ancillary study of WHIHTT further reported an increased risk of probable dementia in post-menopausal women ≥65 years of age.

VAGINAL RINGS
▷ *estradiol, acetate*
 Femring Vaginal Ring insert high into the vagina; replace every 90 days
▷ *estradiol, micronized*
 Estring Vaginal Ring insert high into the vagina; replace every 90 days
 Vag ring: 7.5 mcg/24 hours (1/pck)

REGIMENS FOR PATIENTS WITH INTACT UTERUS
Vaginal Preparations (With Uterus)
Comment: Vaginal preparations provide relief from vaginal and urinary symptoms only (i.e., atrophic vaginitis, dyspareunia, dysuria, and urinary frequency).
▷ *estradiol (G)*
 Vagifem Tabs insert one 10 mcg or 25 mcg vaginal tablet once daily x 2 weeks; then twice weekly for 2 weeks (e.g., Tuesday/Friday); consider the addition of a progestin
 Vag tab: 10, 25 mcg (8, 18/blister pck with applicator)
 Yuvafem Vaginal Tablet 1 tab intravaginally daily x 2 weeks; then 1 tab intravaginally twice weekly
 Vag tab: 10 mcg (15 tabs w. applicators)
▷ *estradiol, micronized (G)*
 Estrace Vaginal Cream 2-4 gm daily x 1-2 weeks, then gradually reduced to 1/2 initial dose x 1-2 weeks, then maintenance dose of 1 gm 1-3 x/week
 Vag crm: 0.01% (12, 42.5 gm w. calib applicator)
▷ *estrogen, conjugated equine*
 Premarin Vaginal Cream 0.5-2 gm/day intravaginally; cyclically (3 weeks on, 1 week off)
 Vag crm: 1.5 oz w. applicator marked in 1/2 gm increments to max of 2 gm

Transdermal Systems (With Uterus)

Comment: Alternate sites. Do <u>not</u> apply patches on <u>or</u> near breasts.

➤ *estradiol* (G)

    Climara initially apply 1 0.025 mg/day patch to the trunk once weekly x 3 weeks, changing the patch on the same day of the week (3 weeks on and 1 week off)

        Transdermal patch: 0.025, 0.0375, 0.05, 0.075, 0.1 mg/day (4/pck)

    Esclim apply twice weekly x 3 weeks, then 1 week off; use with an oral progestin to prevent endometrial hyperplasia

        Transdermal patch: 0.025, 0.0375, 0.05, 0.075, 0.1 mg/day (8, 48/pck)

    Vivelle initially apply 1 0.0375 mg/day patch twice weekly to trunk area; use with an oral progestin to prevent endometrial hyperplasia

        Transdermal patch: 0.025, 0.0375, 0.05, 0.075, 0.1 mg/day (8, 48/pck)

    Vivelle-Dot initially apply 0.05 mg/day patch twice weekly to lower-abdomen, below the waist; use with an oral progestin to prevent endometrialhyperplasia

        Transdermal patch: 0.025, 0.0375, 0.05, 0.075, 0.1 mg/day (8, 24/pck)

➤ *estradiol+levonorgestrel* apply 1 patch weekly to lower abdomen; avoid waistline; alternate sites

    Climara Pro *Transdermal patch:* estra 0.045 mg+levo 0.015 mg per day (4/pck)

➤ *estradiol+norethindrone*

    CombiPatch apply 1 patch twice weekly <u>or</u> q 3-4 days

        Transdermal patch: 9 cm^2: estra 0.05 mg+noreth 0.14 mg; 16 cm^2: estra 0.05 mg+noreth 0.25 mg

Comment: May cause irregular bleeding in the first 6 months of therapy, but usually decreases over time (often to amenorrhea).

ORAL AGENTS (WITH UTERUS)

➤ *estradiol* (G)

    Estrace 1-2 mg daily cyclically (3 weeks on and 1 week off)

        Tab: 0.5, 1, 2*mg (tartrazine)

➤ *estradiol+drospirenone*

    Angeliq 1 tab daily

        Tab: **Angeliq 0.5/0.25** estra 0.5 mg+dros 0.25 mg

            Angeliq 1/0.5 estra 1 mg+dros 0.5 mg

➤ *estradiol+norethindrone* 1 tab daily

    Activella (G) *Tab:* estra 1 mg+noreth 0.5 mg

    FemHRT (G) **1/5** *Tab:* estra 5 mcg+noreth 1 mg

    Fyavolv (G) *Tab:* estra 0.25 mg+noreth 1 mg; *Tab:* estra 0.5 mg+noreth 1 mg

    Mimvey LO *Tab:* estra 0.5 mg+noreth 0.1 mg

➤ *estradiol+norgestimate* 1 x estradiol 1 mg tab once daily x 3 days, then 1 x estradiol 1 mg+norgestimate 0.09 mg tab daily x 3 days; repeat this pattern continuously

    Ortho-Prefest *Tab:* estra 1 mg+norgest 0.09 mg (30/blister pck)

➤ *estradiol+progesterone* (G) 1 cap each evening with food

    Bijuva *Cap:* estradiol 1 mg+progesterone 100 mg

➤ *estrogen, conjugated+medroxyprogesterone*

    Prempro 1 tab daily

        Tab: **Prempro 0.3/1.5** estro, conj 0.3 mg+medroxy 1.5 mg

            Prempro 0.45/1.5 estro, conj 0.45 mg+medroxy 1.5 mg

            Prempro 0.625/2.5 estro, conj 0.625 mg+medroxy 2.5 mg

            Prempro 0.625/5 estro, conj 0.625 mg+medroxy 5 mg

    Premphase 0.625 *estrogen* on days 1-14, then 0.625 mg *estrogen*+5 mg *medroxyprogesterone* on days 15-28

        Tab (in dial dispenser): estro, conj 0.625 mg (14 maroon tabs)+medroxy 5 mg (14 blue tabs)

➤ *estrogen, esterified (plant-derived)*

    Menest 0.3-2.5 mg daily cyclically, 3 weeks on and 1 week off (with progestins in the latter part of the cycle to prevent endometrial hyperplasia)

        Tab: 0.3, 0.625, 1.25, 2.5 mg

➤ *estrogen, esterified+methyltestosterone*

    Estratest 1 tab daily cyclically, 3 weeks on and 1 week off

        Tab: estro ester 1.25 mg+meth 2.5 mg

    Estratest HS 1-2 tabs daily cyclically, 3 weeks on and 1 week off

        Tab: estro ester 0.625 mg+meth 1.25 mg

➤ *ethinyl estradiol* 0.02-0.05 mg q 1-2 days cyclically, 3 weeks on and 1 week off (with progestins in the latter part of the cycle to prevent endometrial hyperplasia)

    Estinyl *Tab:* 0.02 (tartrazine), 0.05 mg

➤ *estropipate, piperazine estrone sulfate* (G)

    Ogen 0.625-1.25 mg daily cyclically (3 weeks on and 1 week off)

        Tab: 0.625, 1.25, 2.5 mg

(continued)

Ortho-Est 0.75-6 mg daily cyclically (3 weeks on and 1 week off)
Tab: 0.625, 1.25 mg
▷ *medroxyprogesterone* 5-10 mg daily for 12 sequential days of each 28-day cycle to prevent endometrial hyperplasia in the postmenopausal women with an intact uterus receiving conjugated estrogens
Provera *Tab:* 2.5, 5, 10 mg
▷ *norethindrone acetate* 2.5-10 mg daily x 5-10 days during the second half of menstrual cycle
Aygestin *Tab:* 5*mg
▷ *progesterone, micronized* (G)
Prometrium 200 mg daily in the PM for 12 sequential days of each 28-day cycle to prevent endometrial hyperplasia in the postmenopausal woman with an intact uterus receiving conjugated estrogens
Cap: 100, 200 mg (peanut oil)

BIOIDENTICAL ESTRADIOL+PROGESTERONE
▷ *estradiol+progesterone (bioidentical)* take 1 gelcap once daily
Bijuva *Gelcap:* estro 1 mg+progest 100 mg
Comment: Bijuva is the first and only bioidentical estradiol and bioidentical progesterone product offering women an alternative to the available FDA-approved synthetic (non-bioidentical) hormones, the separate FDA-approved bioidentical estrogen and progesterone products that are used together but are not approved for combination use, and the unapproved compounded bioidentical hormone products.

ESTROGENS, CONJUGATED+ESTROGEN AGONIST-ANTAGONIST
▷ *estrogen, conjugated+bazedoxifene*
Duavee 1 tab daily
Tab: conj estra 0.45 mg+baze 20 mg

REGIMENS FOR PATIENTS WITHOUT UTERUS
Oral Agents (Without Uterus)
▷ *estradiol* (G)
Estrace 1-2 mg daily
Tab: 0.5*, 1*, 2*mg (tartrazine)
▷ *estrogen, conjugated (equine)*
Premarin 1 tab daily
Tab: 0.3, 0.45, 0.625, 0.9, 1.25, 2.5 mg
▷ *estrogen, conjugated (synthetic)* 1 tab daily; may titrate up to max 1.25 mg/day
Cenestin *Tab:* 0.3, 0.625, 0.9, 1.25 mg
Enjuvia *Tab:* 0.3, 0.45, 0.625 mg
▷ *estrogen, esterified (plant derived)* 1 tab daily
Estratab *Tab:* 0.3, 0.625, 2.5 mg
Menest *Tab:* 0.3, 0.625, 1.25, 2.5 mg
▷ *ethinyl estradiol* 0.02-0.05 mg q 1-2 days
Estinyl *Tab:* 0.02 (tartrazine), 0.05 mg

Vaginal Preparations (Without Uterus)
Comment: Vaginal preparations provide relief from vaginal and urinary symptoms only (i.e., atrophic vaginitis, dyspareunia, dysuria, and urinary frequency).
▷ *estradiol* (G)
Vagifem Tabs insert one 10 mcg or 25 mcg vaginal tablet once daily x 2 weeks; then twice weekly for 2 weeks (e.g., Tuesday/Friday); consider the addition of a progestin
Vag tab: 10, 25 mcg (8, 18/blister pck with applicator)
Yuvafem Vaginal Tablet 1 tab intravaginally daily x 2 weeks; then 1 tab intravaginally twice weekly
Vag tab: 10 mcg (15 tabs w. applicators)

Topical Agents (Without Uterus)
▷ *estradiol*
Divigel apply 0.25-1.25 gm of **Divigel** to the right or left upper thigh once daily; alternate thighs every other day; start with the lowest effective dose and re-evaluate periodically; max 1.25 mg (1.25 gm/pkt) once daily
Gel: 0.25 mg (0.25 gm/pkt), 0.5 mg (0.5 gm/pkt), 0.75 mg (0.75 gm/pkt), 1.0 mg (1.0 gm/pkt), 1.25 mg (1.25 gm/pkt), single-dose, foil packets (30 pkts/carton) (alcohol)
Elestrin once daily, apply 1 pump actuation (0.87 gm of gel, 0.52 mg *estradiol*) or 2 pump actuations (1.7 gm of gel, 1.04 *mg estradiol*) to the upper arm; alternate arms every other day
Metered dose pump: 0.52 mg of *estradiol* in 0.87 gm of gel per non-aerosol pump actuation (30 metered doses/container) (hydroalcohol)
Estrasorb apply 3.48 gm (2 pouches) every morning; apply 1 pouch to each leg from the upper thigh to the calf; rub in for 3 minutes; rub excess on hands onto buttocks
Emul: 0.025 mg/day/pouch (2.5 mg/gm; 1.74 gm/pouch) (56 pouches/carton)

EstroGel apply 1.25 gm (one compression) to one arm from wrist to shoulder once daily at the same time each day
> *Gel:* (32 metered 1.25 gm doses/pump container) (50 gm)

Evamist apply 1 spray once daily each morning to forearm; may increase to 2 or 3 sprays once daily to forearm based on clinical response
> *Spray:* 1.53 mg (90 mcl) per metered spray actuation (56 sprays) (alcohol)

Transdermal Systems (Without Uterus)

Comment: Do not apply patches on or near breasts. Alternate sites.
▷ *estradiol*

Alora initially 0.05 mg/day apply patch twice weekly to lower abdomen, upper quadrant of buttocks, or outer aspect of hip
> *Transdermal patch:* 0.025, 0.05, 0.075, 0.1 mg/day (8, 24/pck)

Climara initially 0.025 mg/day patch once weekly to trunk
> *Transdermal patch:* 0.025, 0.0375, 0.05, 0.075, 0.1 mg/day (4, 8, 24/pck)

Esclim initially 0.025 mg/day apply patch twice weekly to buttocks, femoral triangle, or upper arm
> *Transdermal patch:* 0.025, 0.0375, 0.05, 0.075, 0.1 mg/day (8/pck)

Estraderm initially apply one 0.05 mg/day patch twice weekly to trunk
> *Transdermal patch:* 0.05, 0.1 mg/day (8, 24/pck)

Menostar apply 1 patch weekly to lower abdomen, below the waist; avoid the breasts; alternate sites
> *Transdermal patch:* 14 mcg/day (4/pck)

Minivelle initially one 0.0375 mg/day patch twice weekly to trunk area; adjust after 1 month of therapy
> *Transdermal patch:* 0.025, 0.0375, 0.05, 0.075, 0.1 mg/day (8/pck)

Vivelle initially one 0.0375 mg/day patch twice weekly to trunk area; adjust after 1 month of therapy
> *Transdermal patch:* 0.025, 0.0375, 0.05, 0.075, 0.1 mg/day (8, 48/pck)

Vivelle-Dot initially apply one 0.05 mg/day patch twice weekly to lower abdomen, below the waist; adjust after 1 month of therapy
> *Transdermal patch:* 0.025, 0.0375, 0.05, 0.075, 0.1 mg/day (8, 24/pck)

Comment: The estrogens in **Alora, Climara, Estraderm,** and **Vivelle-Dot** are plant-derived.

MESOTHELIOMA

KINASE INHIBITOR
▷ *capmatinib* 400 mg bid with or without food

Tabrecta *Tab:* 150, 200 mg

Comment: Tabrecta *(capmatinib)* is a kinase inhibitor indicated for the treatment of adult patients with metastatic non-small cell lung cancer (NSCLC) whose tumors have a mutation that leads to mesenchymal-epithelial transition (MET) exon 14 skipping as detected by an FDA-approved test. The most common adverse reactions (incidence ≥20%) have been peripheral edema, nausea, fatigue, vomiting, dyspnea, and decreased appetite. Monitor for new or worsening pulmonary symptoms indicative of interstitial lung disease (ILD)/pneumonitis. Permanently discontinue **Tabrecta** in patients with ILD/pneumonitis. Monitor liver function tests. In the event of hepatotoxicity, withhold, reduce dose, or permanently discontinue **Tabrecta** based on severity. **Tabrecta** may cause photosensitivity reactions. Advise patients to limit direct (UV) exposure. **Tabrecta** can cause embryo/fetal harm. Advise patients of reproductive potential to use effective contraception. Advise not to breastfeed.

FOLATE ANALOG METABOLIC INHIBITOR
▷ *pemetrexed* (G) for injection *Recommended dose, administered as a single agent or with* **cisplatin,** *in patients with CrCl ≥45 ml/min:* 500 mg/m² via IV infusion over 10 minutes on Day 1 of each 21-day cycle; *Initiate folic acid:* 400-1,000 mcg orally once daily beginning 7 days prior to the first dose and continue until 21 days after the last dose; *Administer vitamin B12:* 1 mg IM 1 week prior to the first dose and every 3 cycles thereafter; *Administer* **dexamethasone:** 4 mg orally bid the day before, the day of, and the day after **Pemfexy** administration
Pediatric: safety and efficacy not established

Pemfexy *Vial:* 500 mg/20 ml (25 mg/ml), single dose, for dilution and IV infusion

Comment: Pemfexy is a branded alternative to **Alimta** for the treatment of non-squamous non-small cell lung cancer (NSCLC) and malignant pleural mesothelioma. **Pemfexy** is indicated (1) in combination with **cisplatin** for the initial treatment of patients with locally advanced or metastatic non-squamous NSCLC, (2) as a single agent for the maintenance treatment of patients with locally advanced or metastatic non-squamous NSCLC whose disease has not progressed after 4 cycles of *platinum-based first-line chemotherapy,* and (3) as a single agent for the treatment of patients with recurrent, metastatic non-squamous NSCLC after prior chemotherapy. **Pemfexy** is not indicated for the treatment of patients with squamous cell NSCLC. **Pemfexy** can cause severe bone marrow suppression resulting in cytopenia and an increased risk of infection. Do not administer **Pemfexy** when the absolute neutrophil count is less than 1,500 cells/mm³ and platelets are <100,000 cells/mm³. Initiate supplementation with oral folic

(continued)

acid and vitamin B12 IM to reduce the severity of hematologic and gastrointestinal toxicity. **Pemfexy** can cause severe, and sometimes fatal, renal failure. Do not administer when CrCl <45 ml/min. Permanently discontinue for severe and life-threatening bullous, blistering, or exfoliating skin toxicity. Withhold for acute onset of new or progressive unexplained pulmonary symptoms and permanently discontinue if interstitial pneumonitis is confirmed. Radiation recall can occur in patients who received radiation weeks to years previously; permanently discontinue for signs of radiation recall. The most common adverse reactions (incidence ≥20%) of *pemetrexed* when administered as a single agent have been fatigue, nausea, and anorexia. The most common adverse reactions (incidence ≥20%) of *pemetrexed* when administered with *cisplatin* have been vomiting, neutropenia, anemia, stomatitis/pharyngitis, thrombocytopenia, and constipation. **Pemfexy** is embryo/fetal toxic. Advise males and females of reproductive potential of the potential risk and to use effective contraception. Advise not to breastfeed.

METHAMPHETAMINE-INDUCED PSYCHOSIS

ANTIPSYCHOSIS AGENTS
For more antipsychotics, see Appendix P. Antipsychosis Drugs
see Tardive Dyskinesia

Comment: First-generation antipsychotics (e.g., *haloperidol* or *fluphenazine*) should be used sparingly and cautiously in patients with methamphetamine-induced psychosis because of the risk of developing extrapyramidal symptoms (EPS) and because these patients are prone to develop motor complications as a result of methamphetamine abuse. Second-generation antipsychotics (e.g., *risperidone* and *olanzapine*) may be more appropriate because of the lower risks of EPS. The presence of high norepinephrine levels in some patients with recurrent methamphetamine psychosis suggests that drugs that block norepinephrine receptors (e.g., *prazosin* or *propranolol*) might be of therapeutic benefit, although they have not been studied in controlled trials.

▷ *aripiprazole* (G) initially 15 mg once daily; may increase to max 30 mg/day
  Pediatric: <10 years: not recommended; ≥10-17 years: initially 2 mg/day in a single dose for 2 days; then increase to 5 mg/day in a single dose for 2 days; then increase to target dose of 10 mg/day in a single dose; may increase by 5 mg/day at weekly intervals as needed to max 30 mg/day
  Abilify *Tab:* 2, 5, 10, 15, 20, 30 mg
  Abilify Discmelt *Tab:* 15 mg orally-disint (vanilla) (phenylalanine)
  Abilify Maintena *Vial:* 300, 400 mg ext-rel pwdr for IM injection after reconstitution; 300, 400 mg single-dose prefilled dual-chamber syringes w. supplies
▷ *aripiprazole lauroxil* administer by IM injection in the deltoid (441 mg dose only) or gluteal (441 mg, 662 mg, 882 mg, or 1,064 mg) muscle; initiate at a dose of 441 mg, 662 mg, or 882 mg administered monthly, or 882 mg every 6 weeks, or 1,064 mg every 2 months
  Pediatric: <18 years: not recommended; ≥18 years: same as adult
  Aristada *Prefilled syringe:* 441, 662, 882, 1,064 mg single-use, ext-rel susp
  Comment: Aristada *(aripiprazole)* is an atypical antipsychotic available in 4 doses with 3 dosing duration options for flexible dosing. For patients naïve to *aripiprazole*, establish tolerability with oral *aripiprazole* prior to initiating treatment with **Aristada**. **Aristada** can be initiated at any of the 4 doses at the appropriate dosing duration option. In conjunction with the first injection, administer treatment with oral *aripiprazole* for 21 consecutive days for all 4 dose sizes. The most common adverse event associated with **Aristada** is akathisia. Patients are also at increased risk for developing neuroleptic malignant syndrome (NMS), tardive dyskinesia, pathologic gambling or other compulsive behaviors, orthostatic hypotension, hyperglycemia, dyslipidemia, and weight gain. Hypersensitive reactions can occur and range from pruritus or urticaria to anaphylaxis. Stroke, transient ischemic attacks, and falls have been reported in elderly patients with dementia-related psychosis who were treated with *aripiprazole*. **Aristada** is not for treatment of people who have lost touch with reality (psychosis) due to confusion and memory loss (dementia). May cause extrapyramidal and/or withdrawal symptoms in neonates exposed *in utero* in the third trimester of pregnancy. *Aripiprazole* is present in human breast milk; however, there are insufficient data to assess the amount in human milk or the effects on the breastfed infant. The development and health benefits of breastfeeding should be considered along with the mother's clinical need for **Aristada** and any potential adverse effects on the breastfed infant from **Aristada** or from the underlying maternal condition. For more information or to report adverse side effects (ASEs), contact the National Pregnancy Registry for Atypical Antipsychotics at 1-866-961-2388 or http://womensmentalhealth.org/clinical-and-research-programs/pregnancyregistry. Limited published data on *aripiprazole* use in pregnant females are not sufficient to inform any drug-associated risks of birth defects or miscarriage.
  Aristada Initio administer a single 675 mg **Aristada Initio** injection plus a single 30 mg dose of oral *aripiprazole*; administer the IM injection into the deltoid or gluteal muscle; must be administered only by a qualified healthcare professional; **Aristada Initio** is only to be used as a single dose and is not for repeated dosing
  Prefilled pen: 675 mg/2.4 ml ext-rel single-dose

Comment: Aristada Initio (*aripiprazole lauroxil*) is a smaller particle-size version of extended-release injectable (*aripiprazole*) for adults with schizophrenia. It is the first and only long-acting atypical antipsychotic that can be initiated on day 1. Combining **Aristada Initio** with a single 30 mg dose of oral *aripiprazole* provides an alternative regimen to initiate patients onto any dose of **Aristada** on day 1. Previously, the initiation process for the older *aripiprazole* product was to give the first dose and to then give oral *aripiprazole* for 21 consecutive days. **Aristada Initio** releases relevant levels of *aripiprazole* within 4 days of initiation. **Aristada Initio** carries a warning that it is not approved for use by older patients with dementia-related psychosis, as this patient population is at risk for increased mortality when treated with antipsychotics. For patients naïve to *aripiprazole*, establish tolerability with oral *aripiprazole* prior to initiating treatment with **Aristada Initio**. Avoid use in known CYP2D6 poor metabolizers. Avoid use with strong CYP2D6 or CYP 3A4 inhibitors and strong CYP3A4 inducers. **Aristada Initio** is not interchangeable with **Aristada**. The most commonly observed adverse reaction (incidence ≥5%) has been akathisia. May cause extrapyramidal and/or withdrawal symptoms in neonates in females exposed during the third trimester of pregnancy. There is a pregnancy exposure registry that monitors pregnancy outcomes in women exposed to **Aristada Initio** during pregnancy. *Aripiprazole* is present in human breast milk; however, there are insufficient data to assess the amount in human milk and the effects on the breastfed infant. For more information, contact the National Pregnancy Registry for Atypical Antipsychotics at 1-866-961-2388 or http://womensmentalhealth.org/clinical-and-research-programs/pregnancyregistry

▶ *fluphenazine hcl* (Prolixin) (G)
    Pediatric: <18 years: not studied
        Tab: 1, 2.5, 5, 10 mg; *Elixir:* 2.5 mg/5 ml; *Conc:* 5 mg/ml; *Vial:* 2.5 mg/ml for injection
▶ *fluphenazine decanoate* (Prolixin Decanoate) (G)
    Pediatric: <18 years: not studied
        Vial: 2.5 mg/ml (5 ml)
Comment: Previously, *fluphenazine* was marketed as **Prolixin**, but is currently only available in generic form. Optimal dose and frequency of administration of *fluphenazine* must be determined for each patient since dosage requirements have been found to vary with clinical circumstances as well as with individual response; dosage should not exceed 100 mg; if doses >50 mg are deemed necessary, the next dose and succeeding doses should be increased cautiously in increments of 12.5 mg. *Fluphenazine decanoate injection* and *fluphenazine enanthate injection* are long-acting parenteral antipsychotic forms intended for use in the management of patients requiring prolonged parenteral neuroleptic therapy. *Fluphenazine* has activity at all levels of the central nervous system (CNS) as well as on multiple organ systems. The mechanism whereby its therapeutic action is exerted is unknown. *Fluphenazine* differs from other phenothiazine derivatives in several respects: It is more potent on a milligram basis, it has less potentiating effect on CNS depressants and anesthetics than do some of the phenothiazines and appears to be less sedating, and it is less likely than some of the older phenothiazines to produce hypotension (nevertheless, appropriate cautions should be observed). Neuroleptic malignant syndrome (NMS), a potentially fatal symptom complex, is associated with all antipsychotic drugs. Clinical manifestations of NMS are hyperpyrexia, muscle rigidity, altered mental status, and evidence of autonomic instability (irregular pulse or blood pressure, tachycardia, diaphoresis, and cardiac dysrhythmias). Anticholinergic effects may be potentiated with concomitant *atropine* and *fluphenazine*. Safety and efficacy in children have not been established. Safety during pregnancy has not been established; therefore, the possible hazards should be weighed against the potential benefits when administering this drug to pregnant patients.

▶ *haloperidol* (G) *Oral route of administration: Moderate symptomology:* 0.5-2 mg orally bid-tid; *Severe symptomology:* 3-5 mg orally 2-3 x a day; initial doses of up to 100 mg/day have been necessary in some severely resistant cases; *Maintenance:* after achieving a satisfactory response, the dose should be adjusted as practical to achieve optimum control; *Parenteral route of administration: Prompt control of acute agitation:* 2-5 mg IM q 4-8 hours; *Maintenance:* frequency of IM administration should be determined by patient response and may be given as often as every hour; max: 20 mg/day
    Haldol *Tab:* 0.5*, 1*, 2*, 5*, 10*, 20*mg
    Haldol Lactate *Vial:* 5 mg for IM injection, single-dose
▶ *mesoridazine* initially 25 mg tid; max 300 mg/day
    Serentil *Tab:* 10, 25, 50, 100 mg; *Conc:* 25 mg/ml (118 ml)
▶ *olanzapine* initially 2.5-10 mg daily; increase to 10 mg/day within a few days; then by 5 mg/day at weekly intervals; max 20 mg/day
    Zyprexa *Tab:* 2.5, 5, 7.5, 10 mg
    Zyprexa Zydis *ODT:* 5, 10, 15, 20 mg (phenylalanine)
▶ *quetiapine fumarate* (G)
    Seroquel initially 25 mg bid, titrate q 2nd or 3rd day in increments of 25-50 mg bid-tid; usual maintenance 400-600 mg/day in 2-3 divided doses
        Tab: 25, 50, 100, 200, 300, 400 mg
    Seroquel XR administer once daily in the PM; *Day 1:* 50 mg; *Day 2:* 100 mg; *Day 3:* 200 mg; *Day 4:* 300 mg; usual range 400-600 mg/day
        Tab: 50, 150, 200, 300, 400 mg ext-rel

(continued)

▷ *risperidone* 0.5 mg bid x 1 day; adjust in increments of 0.5 mg bid; usual range 0.5-5 mg/day
    Risperdal *Tab:* 1, 2, 3, 4 mg; *Oral soln:* 1 mg/ml (100 ml)
    Risperdal M-Tab *Tab:* 0.5, 1, 2 mg
▷ *thioridazine* (G) 10-25 mg bid
    Mellaril *Tab:* 10, 15, 25, 50, 100, 150, 200 mg; *Oral susp:* 25 mg/5 ml, 100 mg/5 ml; *Oral conc:* 30 mg/ml,
    100 mg/ml (4 oz)

MITRAL VALVE PROLAPSE (MVP)

▷ *propranolol* (G)
    Inderal 10-30 mg tid-qid
      Tab: 10*, 20*, 40*, 60*, 80*mg
    Inderal LA initially 80 mg daily in a single dose; increase q 3-7 days; usual range 120-160 mg/day; max
    320 mg/day in a single dose
      Cap: 60, 80, 120, 160 mg sust-rel
    InnoPran XL initially 80 mg q HS; max 120 mg/day
      Cap: 80, 120 mg ext-rel

MONONUCLEOSIS (MONO)

    Opioid Analgesics *see* **Pain**
    Parenteral Corticosteroids *see* Appendix L. Parenteral Corticosteroids
    Oral Corticosteroids *see* Appendix K. Oral Corticosteroids

▷ *prednisone* initially 40-80 mg/day, then taper off over 5-7 days
Comment: Corticosteroids are recommended in patients with significant pharyngeal edema.

MOTION SICKNESS

▷ *dimenhydrinate* (OTC) 50-100 mg q 4-6 hours; start 1 hour before travel; max 400 mg/day
Pediatric: <2 years: <u>not</u> recommended; 2-6 years: 12.5-25 mg, max 75 mg/day, start 1 hour before travel, may
repeat q 6-8 hours; 6-11 years: 25-50 mg, max 150 mg/day, start 1 hour before travel, may repeat q 6-8 hours;
≥12 years: same as adult
    Dramamine *Tab:* 50*mg; *Chew tab:* 50 mg (phenylalanine, tartrazine); *Liq:* 12.5 mg/5 ml (4 oz)
▷ *meclizine* (G) 25-50 mg 1 hour before travel; may repeat q 24 hours as needed; max 50 mg/day
Pediatric: <12 years: <u>not</u> recommended; ≥12 years: same as adult
    Antivert *Tab:* 12.5, 25, 50*mg
    Bonine (OTC) *Cap:* 15, 25, 50 mg; *Tab:* 12.5, 25, 50 mg; *Chew tab/Film-coat tab:* 25 mg
    Dramamine II (OTC) *Tab:* 25 mg
    Zentrip *Strip:* 25 mg orally disint
▷ *prochlorperazine* (G)
Pediatric: <12 years: <u>not</u> recommended; ≥12 years: same as adult
    Compazine 5-10 mg q 4 hours as needed
      Tab: 5 mg; *Syr:* 5 mg/5 ml (4 oz; fruit); *Rectal supp:* 2.5, 5, 25 mg
    Compazine Spansule 15 mg q AM <u>or</u> 10 mg q 12 hours
      Spansules: 10, 15 mg sust-rel
▷ *promethazine* (G) 25 mg 30-60 minutes before travel; may repeat in 8-12 hours
Pediatric: <2 years: <u>not</u> recommended; ≥2 years: 12.5-25 mg 30-60 minutes before travel; may repeat in 8-12
hours
    Phenergan *Tab:* 12.5*, 25*, 50 mg; *Plain syr:* 6.25 mg/5 ml; *Fortis syr:* 25 mg/5 ml; *Rectal supp:* 12.5, 25,
    50 mg
Comment: *Promethazine* is contraindicated in children with uncomplicated nausea, dehydration, Reye's
syndrome, history of sleep apnea, asthma, and lower respiratory disorders. *Promethazine* lowers the seizure
threshold in children and may cause cholestatic jaundice, anticholinergic effects, extrapyramidal effects, and
potentially fatal respiratory depression.
▷ *scopolamine*
Pediatric: <12 years: <u>not</u> recommended; ≥12 years: same as adult
    Scopace 0.4-0.8 mg 1 hour before travel; may repeat in 8 hours
      Tab: 0.4 mg
    Transderm Scop 1 patch behind the ear at least 4 hours before travel; each patch is effective for 3 days
      Transdermal patch: 1.5 mg (4/carton)

MULTIPLE SCLEROSIS (MS)

NICOTINIC ACID RECEPTOR AGONIST

▷ *dimethyl fumarate* initially 120 mg bid x 7 days; then maintenance 240 mg bid
   Pediatric: <18 years: not recommended; ≥18 years: same as adult
      Tecfidera *Cap:* 120, 240 mg del-rel; *Starter pack:* 14 x 120 mg, 46 x 240 mg
   Comment: The mechanism by which *dimethyl fumarate* (DMF) exerts its therapeutic effect in multiple sclerosis (MS) is unknown. DMF and the metabolite *monomethyl fumarate* (MMF) have been shown to activate the nuclear factor (erythroid-derived 2)-like 2 (Nrf2) pathway *in vitro* and *in vivo* in animals and humans. The Nrf2 pathway is involved in the cellular response to oxidative stress. MMF has been identified as a nicotinic acid receptor agonist *in vitro*.

POTASSIUM CHANNEL BLOCKER

▷ *dalfampridine* (G) 10 mg q 12 hours
   Pediatric: <18 years: not recommended; ≥18 years: same as adult
      Ampyra *Tab:* 10 mg ext-rel
   Comment: *Dalfampridine* is indicated to improve walking speed.

PURINE ANTIMETABOLITE

▷ *cladribine* swallow whole with water; do not chew; may take with or without food; separate administration from any other oral drug by at least 3 hours; swallow immediately following removal; **Mavenclad** is an uncoated oral cytotoxic tablet and therefore requires special handling and disposal (see comment); avoid contact with skin; wash hands thoroughly after touching; cumulative dosage of **Mavenclad** is 3.5 mg/kg divided into 2 yearly treatment courses (1.75 mg/kg per treatment course); each treatment course is divided into 2 treatment cycles; see mfr pkg insert for kilogram weight-based # of tablets per dose; administer the cycle dosage as 1 or 2 tablets once daily over 4 or 5 consecutive days; do not administer more than 2 tablets daily; if a dose is missed, do not take double or extra doses; if a dose is not taken on the scheduled day, take the missed dose on the following day and extend the number of days in that treatment cycle; if 2 consecutive doses are missed, extend the treatment cycle by 2 days
   First course/first cycle: start any time
   First course/second cycle: administer 23 to 27 days after the last dose of the first course/first cycle
   Second course/first cycle: administer at least 43 weeks after the last dose of the first course/second cycle
   Second course/second cycle: administer 23-27 days after the last dose of the second course/first cycle
   Following the 2 treatment courses, do not administer additional **Mavenclad** during the next 2 years; treatment during these 2 years may further increase the risk of malignancy; safety and efficacy of reinitiating **Mavenclad** more than 2 years after completing 2 treatment courses have not been studied
   Pediatric: <18 years: safety and efficacy not studied; >18 years, <40 kg: safety and efficacy not studied; >18 years, >40 kg: same as adult
      Mavenclad Tab: 10 mg
   Comment: Mavenclad *(cladribine)* is a purine antimetabolite indicated for the treatment of highly active relapsing forms of MS, to include relapsing-remitting disease and active secondary progressive disease, in adults. Because of its safety profile, use of **Mavenclad** is generally recommended for patients who have had an inadequate response to, or are unable to tolerate, an alternate drug indicated for the treatment of MS. **Mavenclad** is not recommended for use in patients with clinically isolated syndrome (CIS) because of its safety profile. Hands must be dry when handling the tablets and washed thoroughly afterwards. Avoid prolonged contact with skin. If a tablet is left on a surface or if a broken or fragmented tablet is released from the blister, the area must be thoroughly washed with water. Follow applicable special handling and disposal procedures. Contraindications to **Mavenclad** use include current malignancy, HIV infection, active chronic infection (e.g., hepatitis, tuberculosis), history of hypersensitivity to *cladribine*, pregnancy (embryo/fetal teratogenic), failure to use effective contraception during **Mavenclad** dosing and for 6 months after the last dose in each treatment course, breastfeeding on a **Mavenclad** treatment day, and for 10 days after the last dose. *Warnings and Precautions:* Monitor lymphocyte counts before, during, and after treatment; screen patients for latent infections, consider delaying treatment until infection is fully controlled, and monitor for signs of developing infection; vaccinate patients antibody-negative to varicella zoster virus (VZV) prior to treatment; administer anti-herpes prophylaxis in patients with lymphocyte counts less than 200 cells per microliter; measure complete blood count (CBC) annually if clinically indicated after treatment; monitor for graft versus host disease (GVHD) with blood transfusion (irradiation of cellular blood components is recommended); obtain liver function tests (LFTs) prior to treatment and discontinue treatment if clinically significant hepatic injury is suspected. Concomitant use of immunosuppressive drugs is not recommended. Monitor patients for additive effects of hematotoxic drugs on the hematologic profile. Avoid concomitant use of antiviral and antiretroviral drugs. Avoid concomitant use of breast cancer resistance protein (BCRP) or quilibrative nucleoside transporter (ENT)/concentratice nucleoside transpoeter (CNT) inhibitors as these may alter the bioavailability of *cladribine*. The most common adverse reactions (incidence >20%) have been upper respiratory tract infection, headache, and lymphopenia.

PYRIMIDINE SYNTHESIS INHIBITOR (DISEASE-MODIFYING ANTIRHEUMATIC DRUG [DMARD])

▷ *teriflunomide* 7 mg or 14 mg once daily

Pediatric: <12 years: not recommended; ≥12 years: same as adult

Aubagio *Tab:* 7, 14 mg

Comment: Contraindicated with severe hepatic impairment and women of childbearing potential not using reliable contraception. Co-administer *teriflunomide* with the disease-modifying antirheumatic drugs (DMARD) *leflunomide* (**Arava**).

IMMUNOMODULATORS

Comment: The role of immunomodulators in the treatment of MS is to slow the progression of physical disability and to decrease frequency of clinical exacerbations.

▷ *alemtuzumab* administer two treatment courses: *First treatment course:* 12 mg/day x 5 days (total 60 mg); *Second treatment course:* 12 months later, administer 12 mg/day x 3 days (total 36 mg); complete all immunizations 6 weeks prior to the first treatment; premedicate with 1,000 mg methylprednisolone or equivalent immediately prior to the first 3 treatment days in each treatment course

Pediatric: <18 years: not recommended; ≥18 years: same as adult

Lemtrada *Vial:* 12 mg/1.2 ml soln for IV infusion, single-use vial

Comment: Lemtrada is indicated for the treatment of patients with relapsing forms of MS. Because of its safety profile, the use of **Lemtrada** should generally be reserved for patients who have had an inadequate response to two or more drugs indicated for the treatment of MS. **Lemtrada REMS** is a restricted distribution program which allows early detection and management of some of the serious risks associated with its use.

▷ *fingolimod* 0.5 mg once daily

Pediatric: <10 years: not recommended; ≥10 years: same as adult

Gilenya *Cap:* 0.5 mg

Comment: First-dose monitoring for bradycardia. In the first 2 weeks, first-dose monitoring is recommended after an interruption of 1 day or more. During weeks 3 and 4, first-dose monitoring is recommended after an interruption of more than 7 days. *FDA Warning:* When **Gilenya** *(fingolimod)* is stopped, the MS disability can become much worse than before the medicine was started or while it was being taken. This MS worsening is rare but can result in permanent disability. Before starting treatment with **Gilenya**, patient should be warned about the potential risk of severe increase in disability after stopping **Gilenya**.

▷ *glatiramer acetate* (G)

Copaxone 20-40 mg SC once daily

Pediatric: <18 years: not recommended; ≥18 years: same as adult

Prefilled syringe: 20, 40 mg/ml (1 ml), single-dose (mannitol 40 mg; preservative-free)

Glatopa 20 mg SC once daily or 40 mg SC 3 x weekly at least 48 hours apart

Pediatric: <18 years: not recommended; ≥18 years: same as adult

Prefilled syringe: 20, 40 mg/ml (1 ml), single-dose (mannitol 40 mg; preservative-free)

Comment: *Glatiramer acetate* injection (**Copaxone**, **Glatopa**) is indicated for the treatment of patients with relapsing forms of MS. Mechanisms by which *glatiramer acetate* exerts its effects in patients with MS are not fully understood. However, *glatiramer acetate* is thought to act by modifying immune processes that are believed to be responsible for the pathogenesis of MS. The biological activity of *glatiramer acetate* is informed by its ability to block the induction of experimental autoimmune encephalomyelitis (EAE) in animal studies. Further, studies in animals and *in vitro* systems suggest that upon its administration, *glatiramer acetate*-specific suppressor T-cells are induced and activated in the periphery. **Glatopa** is a fully substitutable, AP-rated generic version of **Copaxone**.

▷ *interferon beta-1a*

Pediatric: <18 years: not recommended; ≥18 years: same as adult

Avonex 30 mcg IM weekly; rotate sites; may titrate to reduce flu-like symptoms; may use concurrent analgesics/antipyretics on treatment days; *Titration schedule:* 7.5 mcg week 1, 15 mcg week 2, 22.5 mcg week 3, 30 mcg week 4 and ongoing

Vial: 30 mcg/vial pwdr for reconstitution (single-dose w. diluent, 4 vials/kit) (albumin [human], preservative-free); *Prefilled syringe:* 30 mcg, single-dose (0.5 ml) (4/pck)

▷ *peginterferon beta-1a* *Recommended therapeutic dose:* 125 mcg SC or IM once every 14 days; dose should be titrated—Day 1: 63 mcg SC or IM; Day 15: 94 mcg SC or IM; Day 29: 125 mcg SC or IM; a qualified healthcare professional should train patients and/or caregivers in the proper technique for self-administering SC injections using the prefilled pen or syringe or SC injections using the prefilled syringe; analgesics and/or antipyretics on treatment days may help ameliorate flu-like symptoms

Pediatric: safety and efficacy not established

Plegridy *Prefilled pen/Prefilled syringe:* 63, 94, 125 mcg/0.5 ml, single-dose, for SC injection; *Prefilled syringe:* 125 mcg/0.5 ml, single-dose, with a 23 g, 1.25 inch staked needle, for IM injection (starter packs available for prefilled pens and prefilled syringes) (preservative-free)

Comment: **Plegridy** is an interferon beta-1a indicated for the treatment of relapsing forms of MS, to include clinically isolated syndrome (CIS), relapsing-remitting disease, and active secondary progressive disease, in adults. The most common adverse reactions in clinical trials of subcutaneous **Plegridy** (incidence ≥10% and at least 2% more frequent with **Plegridy** than with placebo) have been injection site erythema, influenza-like illness, pyrexia, headache, myalgia, chills, injection site pain, asthenia, injection site pruritus, and arthralgia. Monitor liver function tests and patients for signs and symptoms of hepatic injury; consider discontinuation of **Plegridy** if hepatic injury occurs. Advise patients to report immediately any symptom of depression or suicidal ideation to their healthcare provider and consider discontinuation of **Plegridy** if depression occurs. Discontinue **Plegridy** if a serious allergic reaction occurs. Do not administer **Plegridy** into affected area until fully healed; if multiple lesions occur, change injection site or discontinue **Plegridy** until skin lesions fully healed. Monitor patients with preexisting significant cardiac disease for worsening of cardiac symptoms. Monitor labs for decreased peripheral blood count (e.g., CBC). Cases of thrombotic microangiopathy (TMA) have been reported with interferon beta products. Discontinue if **Plegridy** clinical symptoms and laboratory findings consistent with TMA occur. Consider discontinuation of **Plegridy** if a new autoimmune disorder occurs. Epidemiologic data do not suggest a clear relationship between interferon beta use and major congenital malformations; however, based on animal data, interferon beta may cause fetal harm. Limited published literature has described the presence of interferon beta-1a products in human milk at low levels. Therefore, the developmental and health benefits of breastfeeding should be considered along with the mother's clinical need for **Plegridy** and any potential adverse effects on the breastfed infant from **Plegridy** or from the underlying maternal condition.

Rebif, administer SC 3x/week (at least 48 hours apart and preferably in the late afternoon or evening); increase over 4 weeks to prescribed usual dose of 22-44 mcg 3x/week; *Titration schedule (22 mcg prescribed dose):* 4.4 mcg week 1 and 2; 11 mcg week 3 and 4; 22 mcg week 5 and ongoing; *Titration schedule (44 mcg prescribed dose):* 8.8 mcg week 1 and 2; 22 mcg week 3 and 4; 44 mcg week 5 and ongoing

Prefilled syringe: 22, 44 mcg/0.5 ml w. needle (12/carton) (albumin [human], preservative-free); (titration pack, 6 doses of 8.8 mcg [0.2 ml] w. needle per carton) (albumin [human], preservative-free)

Comment: Only prefilled syringes (**Rebif**) can be used to titrate to the 22 mcg prescribed dose. Prefilled syringes or autoinjectors (**Rebif Rebidose**) can be used to titrate to the 44 mcg prescribed dose.

Rebif Rebidose administer SC 3x/week (at least 48 hours apart and preferably in the late afternoon or evening) after titration to 22 mcg or 44 mcg; *Titration schedule:* see the **Rebif** mfr pkg insert
Prefilled autoinjector: 22, 44 mcg/0.5 ml (0.5 ml, 12/carton) (titration pack, 6 doses of 8.8 mcg [0.2 ml] per carton) (albumin [human], preservative-free)

Comment: Only prefilled syringes (**Rebif**) can be used to titrate to the 22 mcg prescribed dose. Prefilled syringes or autoinjectors (**Rebif Rebidose**) can be used to titrate to the 44 mcg prescribed dose.

▷ *interferon beta-1b*
Pediatric: <18 years: not recommended; ≥18 years: same as adult
Actimmune *BSA* ≤0.5m²: 1.5 mcg/kg SC in a single dose 3 x weekly; *BSA* ≥0.5m²: 50 mcg/m² SC in a single dose 3 x weekly; do not shake; store vials in the refrigerator at 2 to 8°C (36°F to 46°F); do not freeze; an unused vial can be stored at room temperature up to 12 hours prior to use; discard vials if not used within the 12 hour period; do not return vials to the refrigerator
Vial: 100 mcg/0.5 ml, single-dose for SC injection (12 vials/carton)
Betaseron, Extavia 0.0625 mg (0.25 ml) SC every other day; increase over 6 weeks to 0.25 mg (1 ml) SC every other day; Before reconstitution with diluent, store **Extavia** at room temperature 25°C (77°F). Excursions of 15° to 30°C (59° to 86°F) are permitted; after reconstitution, if not used immediately, the product should be refrigerated and used within three hours; do not freeze
Vial: 0.3 mg/vial pwdr for reconstitution (single-dose w. prefilled diluents syringes) (albumin [human], mannitol, preservative-free)

▷ *natalizumab* administer 300 mg by IV infusion over 1 hour q 4 weeks; monitor during infusion and for 1 hour postinfusion
Pediatric: <18 years: not recommended; ≥18 years: same as adult
Tysabri *Vial:* 300 mg/15 ml (15 ml)

CD20-DIRECTED CYTOLYTIC ANTIBODY
▷ *ocrelizumab* premedicate with corticosteroid and antihistamine, and consider antipyretic, prior to each infusion; initially administer 300 mg via IV infusion followed by another 300 mg via IV infusion 2 weeks later; then administer 600 mg every 6 months; see mfr pkg insert for infusion rates and dose modifications
Pediatric: <18 years: not recommended; ≥18 years: same as adult
Ocrevus *Vial:* 30 mg/ml (10 ml, single-dose) for dilution (preservative-free)
Comment: **Ocrevus** is a CD20-directed cytolytic antibody indicated for the treatment of patients with relapsing or primary progressive forms of MS. The precise mechanism of action is unknown; however, it is thought to involve binding to CD20, a cell surface antigen present on pre-B and mature B lymphocytes which results

(continued)

in antibody-dependent cellular cytolysis and complement-mediated lysis. **Ocrevus** is contraindicated with active hepatitis b virus (HBV) infection. Screen for HBV infection (HBsAg/anti-HB) prior to initiation. Concomitant live or attenuated vaccine not recommended during treatment and until B-cell repletion. Administer these at least 6 weeks prior to initiation of treatment. Additive immunosuppressive effects with other immunosuppressants. Monitor for infusion reaction (pruritis, rash, urticaria, erythema, throat irritation, bronchospasm). Delay treatment with active infection. Withhold at first sign/symptom of progressive multifocal leukoencephalopathy (PML) or HBV reactivation. Females of reproductive potential should use effective contraception during treatment and for 6 months after the last dose of **Ocrevus**. It is not known whether *ocrelizumab* is excreted in human breast milk or has any effect on the breastfed infant.

▷ *ofatumumab* initially 20 mg SC at Week 0, 1, and 2; then 20 mg SC monthly starting at Week 4
Pediatric: <18 years: not recommended; ≥18 years: same as adult

> **Kesimpta** *Prefilled sensoready:* 20 mg/0.4 ml, single-dose; *Prefilled syringe:* 20 mg/0.4 ml, single-dose (preservative-free)
> **Comment:** Kesimpta *(ofatumumab)* is indicated for the treatment of relapsing forms of MS, to include clinically isolated syndrome (CIS), relapsing-remitting disease, and active secondary progressive disease, in adults. **Kesimpta** is contraindicated with active HBV infection; HBV and quantitative serum immunoglobulins screening required before the first dose. The most common adverse reactions (incidence >10%) are upper respiratory tract infection, headache, injection-related reactions, and local injection site reactions. Delay **Kesimpta** administration in patients with an active infection until the infection is resolved. Vaccination with live attenuated or live vaccines is not recommended during treatment and after discontinuation until B-cell repletion. Management for injection-related reactions depends on the type and severity of the reaction. Monitor the level of immunoglobulins at the beginning, during, and after discontinuation of treatment until B-cell repletion. Consider discontinuing **Kesimpta** if the patient develops a serious opportunistic infection or recurrent infections if immunoglobulin levels indicate immune compromise. **Kesimpta** may cause fetal harm based on animal data. Advise females of reproductive potential of potential embryo/fetal risk and to use an effective method of contraception during treatment and for 6 months after stopping **Kesimpta**.

▷ *ublituximab-xiiy* HBV screening and quantitative serum immunoglobulin screening are required before the first dose; premedicate with *methylprednisolone* (or an equivalent corticosteroid) and an antihistamine (e.g., *diphenhydramine*) prior to each infusion; administer **Briumvi** via IV infusion; *First infusion:* 150 mg via IV infusion; *Second infusion:* 450 mg via IV infusion 2 weeks after the first infusion; *Subsequent infusions:* 450 mg via IV infusion 24 weeks after the first infusion and every 24 weeks thereafter; **Briumvi** must be diluted in 0.9% NaCl inj prior to administration; monitor patients closely during and for at least 1 hour after the completion of the first two infusions; postinfusion monitoring of subsequent infusions is at physician discretion unless infusion reaction and/or hypersensitivity has been observed
Pediatric: safety and efficacy not established

> **Briumvi** *Vial:* 150 mg/6 ml (25 mg/ml), single-dose, soln for dilution in 0.09% NaCl and IV infusion
> **Comment:** Briumvi *(ublituximab-xiiy)* is a CD20-directed cytolytic antibody indicated for the treatment of relapsing forms of MS, to include CIS, relapsing remitting disease, and active secondary progressive disease, in adults. Contraindications include active HBV infection and history of life-threatening infusion reaction to **Briumvi**. The most common adverse reactions (≥10%) have been infusion reactions and upper respiratory tract infections. Management recommendations for infusion reactions depend on the type and severity of the reaction; permanently discontinue **Briumvi** if a life-threatening or disabling infusion reaction occurs. Serious infections, including life-threatening and fatal infections, have occurred; delay **Briumvi** administration in patients with an active infection until the infection is resolved. Consider discontinuing **Briumvi** in patients with serious opportunistic or recurrent serious infections, and if prolonged hypogammaglobulinemia requires treatment with IV immunoglobulins. Vaccination with live attenuated or live vaccines is not recommended during treatment with **Briumvi** and after discontinuation until B-cell repletion. Monitor the level of immunoglobulins at the beginning, during, and after discontinuation of treatment with **Briumvi**. Although there are no data on *ublituximab-xiiy*, monoclonal antibodies can be actively transported across the placenta and therefore **Briumvi** may cause immunosuppression in the *in utero* exposed infant. Advise females and males of reproductive potential of the potential risk to the fetus and to use effective contraception during treatment and for at least 6 months after stopping treatment. There are no data on the presence of *ublituximab-xiiy* in human milk or effects on the breastfed infant. However, human immunoglobulin G (IgG) is excreted in human milk, and the potential for absorption of *ublituximab-xiiy* to lead to B-cell depletion in the infant is unknown. The developmental and health benefits of breastfeeding should be considered along with the mother's clinical need for **Briumvi** and any potential adverse effects on the breastfed infant from **Briumvi** or from the underlying maternal condition.

SPHINGOSINE 1-PHOSPHATE RECEPTOR MODULATOR

Comment: Sphingosine 1-phosphate receptor modulators are indicated for the treatment of relapsing forms of MS, to include CIS, relapsing-remitting disease, and active secondary progressive disease, in adults. This drug class is contraindicated in patients who have experienced myocardial infarction, unstable angina, stroke, transient ischemic attack, decompensated heart failure requiring hospitalization, or Class III/IV heart failure in the preceding 6 months. The presence of Mobitz type II second-degree and third-degree atrioventricular (AV) block or sick sinus syndrome (SSS), are contraindications unless the patient has a functioning pacemaker.

Obtain a CBC, transaminase, and bilirubin before initiating treatment. Monitor for infection during treatment; do not initiate treatment in patients with active infection. Avoid live attenuated vaccines during and for up to 4 weeks after treatment. Test patients for antibodies to varicella zoster virus (VZV) before initiating treatment. VZV vaccination of antibody-negative patients is recommended prior to commencing treatment. CYP2C9 and CYP3A4 inhibitors increase in exposure to this class; therefore, concomitant use with moderate CYP2C9 and moderate or strong CYP3A4 inhibitors is not recommended. CYP2C9 and CYP3A4 inducers decrease exposure; therefore, concomitant use with moderate CYP2C9 or strong CYP3A4 inducers is not recommended. There are no adequate data on the developmental risk associated with the use in pregnant females. However, reproductive and developmental data in animal studies have demonstrated embryo/fetal toxicity. Before initiation of treatment, females of childbearing potential should be counseled on the potential for serious risk to the fetus and the need for contraception during treatment. Because of the time it takes to eliminate the drug from the body after stopping treatment, the potential risk to the fetus may persist and females of childbearing age should also use effective contraception for 3 months after stopping. There are no data on the presence in human milk or effects on the breastfed infant.

▷ **ozanimod** assessments are required prior to initiating **Zeposia**; titration is required for treatment initiation; recommended maintenance dose is 0.92 mg once daily; if a dose is missed within the first 2 weeks of treatment, reinitiate with the titration regimen
Pediatric: safety and efficacy not established
  Zeposia *Caps:* 0.23, 0.46, 0.92 mg
  Comment: Zeposia is a sphingosine 1-phosphate receptor modulator indicated for the treatment of relapsing forms of MS, to include CIS, relapsing-remitting disease, and active secondary progressive disease, in adults. **Zeposia** is contraindicated (1) if in the last 6 months the patient has experienced myocardial infarction, unstable angina, stroke, transient ischemic attack, decompensated heart failure requiring hospitalization, or class III or IV heart failure; (2) there is presence of Mobitz type II second-degree or third-degree AV block, SSS, or sinoatrial block (unless the patient has a functioning pacemaker); (3) the patient has severe untreated sleep apnea; and (4) the patient would have concomitant use of a monoamine oxidase inhibitor (MAOI). The most common adverse reactions (incidence ≥4%) have been upper respiratory infection, hepatic transaminase elevation, orthostatic hypotension, urinary tract infection, back pain, and hypertension. **Zeposia** may increase the risk of infections. Obtain a CBC before initiation of treatment. Monitor for infection during treatment and for 3 months after **Zeposia** discontinuation. Do not start **Zeposia** in patients with active infection. Bradyarrhythmias and AV conduction delays may result in transient decrease in heart rate; titration is required for treatment initiation. Check an ECG to assess for preexisting cardiac conduction abnormalities before starting **Zeposia**. Consider cardiology consultation for conduction abnormalities or concomitant use with other drugs that decrease heart rate. Obtain liver function tests before initiating **Zeposia**. Discontinue **Zeposia** if significant liver injury is confirmed. Monitor BP during treatment. **Zeposia** may cause a decline in pulmonary function. Assess pulmonary function (e.g., spirometry) if clinically indicated. Macular edema can occur. A prompt ophthalmic evaluation is recommended if there is any change in vision while taking **Zeposia**. Diabetes mellitus and uveitis increase the risk of macular edema; patients with a history of these conditions should have an ophthalmic evaluation of the fundus, including the macula, prior to treatment initiation. Avoid use of live attenuated vaccines during and for up to 3 months after stopping treatment with **Zeposia**. Co-administration of strong CYP2C8 inhibitors with **Zeposia** is not recommended. Co-administration of BCRP inhibitors with **Zeposia** is not recommended. Co-administration of strong CYP2C8 inducers with **Zeposia** should be avoided. **Zeposia** can cause fetal harm. Advise females of the risk to the fetus and exclude pregnancy prior to initiating **Zeposia**. Advise females of reproductive use to use effective contraception during treatment and for 3 months after stopping **Zeposia**. There are no data on the presence of *ozanimod* in human milk or effects on the breastfed infant. However, following oral administration of *ozanimod*, *ozanimod* and/or metabolites were detected in the milk of lactating animals at levels higher than those in maternal plasma. Therefore, the developmental and health benefits of breastfeeding should be considered along with the mother's clinical need for **Zeposia** and any potential adverse effects on the breastfed infant from **Zeposia** or from the underlying maternal condition.

▷ **siponimod** initiate treatment with a 5-day titration regimen (starter pack); Day 1: 0.25 mg (1 x 0.25 mg); Day 2: 0.25 mg (1 x 0.25 mg); Day 3: 0.50 mg (2 x 0.25 mg); Day 4: 0.75 mg (3 x 0.25 mg); Day 5: 1.25 mg (5 x 0.25 mg); Day 6 and thereafter: 2 mg once daily; if one titration dose is missed for more than 24 hours, reinitiate using day 1 of the initial titration regimen; see mfr pkg insert for titration and maintenance doses for patients with CYP2C9 genotypes *1/*3 or *2/*3
Pediatric: safety and efficacy not established
  Mayzent *Tab:* 0.25, 2 mg film-coat; titration pck

Nrf2 PATHWAY ACTIVATOR

▷ **monomethyl fumarate** *Starting dose:* 95 mg bid x 7 days; *Maintenance:* 190 mg (2 x 95 mg) bid; swallow whole and intact; do not crush, chew, or mix contents with food; take with or without food
Pediatric: not established
  Bafiertam *Cap:* 95 mg del-rel

(continued)

Comment: Bafiertam is indicated for the treatment of relapsing forms of MS, to include CIS, relapsing-remitting disease, and active secondary progressive disease, in adults. The most common adverse reactions (incidence for *dimethyl fumarate* [the prodrug of Bafiertam] ≥10% and ≥2% more than placebo) have been flushing, abdominal pain, diarrhea, and nausea. Co-administration of Bafiertam with *(DMF)* or *diroximel fumarate* is contraindicated. Blood tests are required prior to initiation of Bafiertam. Obtain a CBC including lymphocyte count before initiating Bafiertam, after 6 months, and every 6-12 months thereafter. Consider interruption of Bafiertam if lymphocyte counts <0.5 x 10⁹/L persist for more than 6 months. Obtain serum aminotransferase, alkaline phosphatase, and total bilirubin levels before initiating Bafiertam and during treatment, as clinically indicated. Discontinue Bafiertam if clinically significant liver injury induced by Bafiertam is suspected. Discontinue and do not restart Bafiertam if anaphylaxis or angioedema occurs. Withhold Bafiertam at the first sign or symptom suggestive of PML. Consider withholding Bafiertam in cases of serious infection (e.g., herpes zoster and other serious opportunistic infections) until the infection has resolved. There are no adequate data on the developmental risk associated with the use of Bafiertam or *DMF* (the prodrug of Bafiertam) in pregnant females. In animals, adverse effects on offspring survival, growth, sexual maturation, and neurobehavioral function were observed when *DMF* was administered during pregnancy and lactation at clinically relevant doses. There are no data on the presence of DMF or MMF in human milk or effects on the breastfed infant. Developmental and health benefits of breastfeeding should be considered along with the mother's clinical need for Bafiertam and any potential adverse effects on the breastfed infant from the drug or from the underlying maternal condition.

PSEUDOBULBAR AFFECT (PBA)
Comment: Pseudobulbar affect (PBA), emotional lability, labile affect, or emotional incontinence refers to a neurologic disorder characterized by involuntary crying or uncontrollable episodes of crying and/or laughing or other emotional outbursts. PBA occurs secondary to a neurologic disease or brain injury, such as traumatic brain injury (TBI), stroke, Parkinson's disease, MS, and amyotrophic lateral sclerosis (ALS, or Lou Gehrig's disease).

▷ **dextromethorphan+quinidine** (G) 1 cap once daily x 7 days; then starting on day 8, 1 cap bid
Pediatric: <12 years: not recommended; ≥12 years: same as adult
   Nuedexta *Cap:* dextro 20 mg+quini 10 mg
   Comment: *Dextromethorphan hydrobromide* is an uncompetitive N-methyl D-aspartate (NMDA) receptor antagonist and sigma-1 agonist. *Quinidine sulfate* is a CYP450 2D6 inhibitor. Nuedexta is contraindicated with an MAOI or within 14 days of stopping an MAOI, with prolonged QT interval, congenital long QT syndrome, history suggestive of torsades de pointes, or heart failure, complete AV block without implanted pacemaker or patients at high risk of complete AV block, and concomitant drugs that both prolong QT interval and are metabolized by CYP2D6 (e.g., *thioridazine* or *pimozide*). Discontinue Nuedexta if the following occurs: hepatitis or thrombocytopenia or any other hypersensitivity reaction. Monitor ECG in patients with left ventricular hypertrophy (LVH) or left ventricular dysfunction (LVD). *Desipramine* exposure increases Nuedexta 8-fold; reduce *desipramine* dose and adjust based on clinical response. Use of Nuedexta with selective serotonin reuptake inhibitors (SSRIs) or tricyclic antidepressants (TCAs) increases the risk of *serotonin syndrome*. *Paroxetine* exposure increases Nuedexta 2-fold; therefore, reduce *paroxetine* dose and adjust based on clinical response (*digoxin* exposure may increase *digoxin* substrate plasma concentration). Nuedexta is not recommended in pregnancy or breastfeeding. Safety and effectiveness of Nuedexta in children have not been established.

ORAL FUMARATE
▷ **diroximel fumarate** *Starting dose:* 231 mg bid x 7 days; *Maintenance dose:* 462 mg (2 x 231 mg capsules) bid; swallow whole, do not crush, chew, or open capsules, and do not sprinkle contents onto food; avoid administration with a high-fat, high-calorie meal/snack; avoid co-administration with alcohol
Pediatric: safety and efficacy not established
   Vumerity *Cap:* 231 mg del-rel
   Comment: Vumerity (*diroximel fumarate*) is a novel oral fumarate for the treatment of relapsing forms of MS, to include CIS, relapsing-remitting disease, and active secondary progressive disease, in adults. *Contraindications:* Known hypersensitivity to *diroximel fumarate*, *DMF*, or to any of the excipients of Vumerity, and co-administration with *DMF*. Vumerity is not recommended in patients with moderate or severe renal impairment. The most common adverse reactions have been flushing, nausea, abdominal pain, and diarrhea. Based on animal studies, discontinue and do not restart Vumerity if anaphylaxis or angioedema occurs. Withhold Vumerity at the first sign or symptom suggestive of lymphopenia or PML. Obtain a CBC including lymphocyte count before initiating Vumerity, after 6 months, and every 6-12 months thereafter. Consider interruption of Vumerity if lymphocyte counts <0.5 × 10⁹/L persist for more than 6 months. Obtain serum aminotransferase, alkaline phosphatase, and total bilirubin levels before initiating Vumerity and during treatment, as clinically indicated. Discontinue Vumerity if clinically significant liver injury induced by Vumerity is suspected. There are no adequate human data on the developmental risk associated with the use of Vumerity or *DMF* (which has the same

active metabolite as **Vumerity**) in pregnancy. Animal studies have demonstrated the administration of *diroximel fumarate* during pregnancy or throughout pregnancy and lactation resulted in adverse effects on embryo/fetal and offspring development (increased incidences of skeletal abnormalities, increased mortality, decreased body weight, neurobehavioral impairment) at clinically relevant drug exposure. There are no data on the presence of *diroximel fumarate* or metabolites (MMF, HES) in human milk or effects on the breastfed infant. The developmental and health benefits of breastfeeding should be considered along with the mother's clinical need for **Vumerity** and any potential adverse effects on the breastfed infant from the drug or from the underlying maternal condition.

MUMPS (INFECTIOUS PAROTITIS, *PARAMYXOVIRUS*)

see Childhood Immunizations
Parenteral Corticosteroids *see* Appendix L. Parenteral Corticosteroids
Oral Corticosteroids *see* Appendix K. Oral Corticosteroids
Antipyretics *see Fever*

PROPHYLAXIS VACCINE
▷ *measles, mumps, rubella, live, attenuated, neomycin vaccine*
  MMR II 25 mcg SC (preservative-free)
Comment: Contraindications include hypersensitivity to *neomycin* or eggs, primary or acquired immune deficiency, immunosuppressant therapy, bone marrow or lymphatic malignancy, and pregnancy (within 3 months after vaccination).

MUSCLE STRAIN

Acetaminophen for IV Infusion *see Pain*
Parenteral Corticosteroids *see* Appendix L. Parenteral Corticosteroids
Oral Corticosteroids *see* Appendix K. Oral Corticosteroids
Opioid Analgesics *see Pain*

Comment: Usual length of treatment for acute injury is approximately 5 days.

SKELETAL MUSCLE RELAXANTS
▷ *baclofen* (G) 5 mg tid; titrate up by 5 mg q 3 days to 20 mg tid; max 80 mg/day
  Pediatric: <12 years: <u>not</u> recommended; ≥12 years: same as adult
    Lioresal *Tab:* 10*, 20*mg
  Comment: *Baclofen* is indicated for muscle spasm pain and chronic spasticity associated with multiple sclerosis and spinal cord injury or disease. Potential for seizures or hallucinations on abrupt withdrawal.
▷ *carisoprodol* (G) 1 tab tid or qid
  Pediatric: <12 years: <u>not</u> recommended; ≥12 years: same as adult
    Soma *Tab:* 350 mg
▷ *chlorzoxazone* (G) 1 caplet qid; max 750 mg qid
  Pediatric: <12 years: <u>not</u> recommended; ≥12 years: same as adult
    Parafon Forte DSC *Cplt:* 500*mg
▷ *cyclobenzaprine* (G) 10 mg tid; usual range 20-40 mg/day in divided doses; max 60 mg/day x 2-3 weeks or 15 mg ext-rel once daily; max 30 mg ext-rel/day x 2-3 weeks
  Pediatric: <15 years: <u>not</u> recommended; ≥15 years: same as adult
    Amrix *Cap:* 15, 30 mg ext-rel
    Fexmid *Tab:* 7.5 mg
    Flexeril *Tab:* 5, 10 mg
▷ *dantrolene* 25 mg daily x 7 days; then 25 mg tid x 7 days; then 50 mg tid x 7 days; max 100 mg qid
  Pediatric: 0.5 mg/kg daily x 7 days; then 0.5 mg/kg tid x 7 days; then 1 mg/kg tid x 7 days; then 2 mg/kg tid; max 100 mg qid
    Dantrium *Tab:* 25, 50, 100 mg
  Comment: *Dantrolene* is indicated for chronic spasticity associated with multiple sclerosis and spinal cord injury or disease.
▷ *diazepam* (IV) 2-10 mg bid-qid; may increase gradually
  Pediatric: <6 months: <u>not</u> recommended; ≥6 months: initially 1-2.5 mg bid-qid; may increase gradually
    Diastat *Rectal gel delivery system:* 2.5 mg
    Diastat AcuDial *Rectal gel delivery system:* 10, 20 mg
    Valium *Tab:* 2, 5, 10 mg
    Valium Intensol Oral Solution *Conc oral soln:* 5 mg/ml (30 ml w. dropper)(alcohol 19%)
    Valium Oral Solution *Oral soln:* 5 mg/5 ml (500 ml) (wintergreen spice)

(continued)

▷ **metaxalone** 1 tab tid-qid
    Pediatric: <12 years: <u>not</u> recommended; ≥12 years: same as adult
        Skelaxin *Tab:* 800*mg
▷ **methocarbamol** (G) initially 1.5 gm qid x 2-3 days; maintenance, 750 mg every 4 hours <u>or</u> 1.5 gm 3x daily;
    max 8 gm/day
    Pediatric: <16 years: <u>not</u> recommended; ≥16 years: same as adult
        Robaxin *Tab:* 500 mg
        Robaxin 750 *Tab:* 750 mg
        Robaxin Injection 10 ml IM <u>or</u> IV; max 30 ml/day; max 3 days; max 5 ml/gluteal injection q 8 hours;
        max IV rate 3 ml/min
          Vial: 100 mg/ml (10 ml)
▷ **nabumetone**
    Pediatric: <12 years: <u>not</u> recommended; ≥12 years: same as adult
        Relafen *Tab:* 500, 750 mg
        Relafen 500 *Tab:* 500 mg
▷ **orphenadrine citrate** (G) 1 tab bid
    Pediatric: <12 years: <u>not</u> recommended; ≥12 years: same as adult
        Norflex *Tab:* 100 mg sust-rel
▷ **tizanidine** 1-4 mg q 6-8 hours; max 36 mg/day
    Pediatric: <12 years: <u>not</u> recommended; ≥12 years: same as adult
        Zanaflex *Tab:* 2*, 4**mg; *Cap:* 2, 4, 6 mg

SKELETAL MUSCLE RELAXANT+NON-STEROIDAL ANTI-INFLAMMATORY DRUG (NSAID) COMBINATIONS

▷ **carisoprodol+aspirin** (III)(G) 1-2 tabs qid
    Pediatric: <12 years: <u>not</u> recommended; ≥12 years: same as adult
        Soma Compound *Tab:* caris 200 mg+asp 325 mg (sulfites)
▷ **meprobamate+aspirin** (IV) 1-2 tabs tid <u>or</u> qid
    Pediatric: <12 years: <u>not</u> recommended; ≥12 years: same as adult
        Equagesic *Tab:* mepro 200 mg+asp 325*mg

SKELETAL MUSCLE RELAXANT+NSAID+CAFFEINE COMBINATIONS

▷ **orphenadrine+aspirin+caffeine** (G)
    Pediatric: <12 years: <u>not</u> recommended; ≥12 years: same as adult
        Norgesic 1-2 tabs tid-qid
          Tab: orphen 25 mg+asp 385 mg+caf 30 mg
        Norgesic Forte 1 tab tid <u>or</u> qid; max 4 tabs/day
          Tab: orphen 50 mg+asp 770 mg+caf 60 mg*

SKELETAL MUSCLE RELAXANT+NSAID+CODEINE COMBINATIONS

▷ **carisoprodol+aspirin+codeine** (III)(G) 1-2 tabs qid prn
    Pediatric: <12 years: contraindicated; 12-<18: use extreme caution; <u>not</u> recommended for children and
    adolescents with obesity, asthma, obstructive sleep apnea, <u>or</u> other chronic breathing problem, <u>or</u> for post-
    tonsillectomy/adenoidectomy pain; ≥18 years: same as adult
        Soma Compound w. Codeine
        Tab: caris 200 mg+asp 325 mg+cod 16 mg (sulfites)

TOPICAL AND TRANSDERMAL ANALGESICS

▷ **capsaicin** (G) apply tid-qid prn to intact skin
    Pediatric: <2 years: <u>not</u> recommended; ≥2 years: apply sparingly tid-qid prn
        Axsain *Crm:* 0.075% (1, 2 oz)
        Capsin *Lotn:* 0.025, 0.075% (59 ml)
        Capzasin-HP (OTC) *Crm:* 0.075% (1.5 oz), 0.025% (45, 90 gm); *Lotn:* 0.075% (2 oz); 0.025% (45, 90 gm)
        Capzasin-P (OTC) *Crm:* 0.025% (1.5 oz); *Lotn:* 0.025% (2 oz)
        Dolorac *Crm:* 0.025% (28 gm)
        Double Cap (OTC) *Crm:* 0.05% (2 oz)
        R-Gel *Gel:* 0.025% (15, 30 gm)
        Zostrix (OTC) *Crm:* 0.025% (0.7, 1.5, 3 oz)
        Zostrix HP (OTC) *Emol crm:* 0.075% (1, 2 oz)
▷ **capsaicin** 8% patch apply up to 4 patches for one 60-minute application to clean dry skin; may prep area
    with topical anesthetic; wear non-latex gloves; patches may be cut to size/shape; treatment may be repeated
    q 3 months
    Pediatric: <18 years: <u>not</u> recommended; ≥18 years: same as adult
        Qutenza *Patch:* 8% 1640 mcg/cm (179 mg) (1 <u>or</u> 2 patches w. 1-50 gm tube cleansing gel/carton)
▷ **diclofenac sodium** apply qid prn to intact skin; not for use in pregnancy after 30 weeks gestation
    Pediatric: <12 years: <u>not</u> established; ≥12 years: same as adult

Pennsaid 1.5% in 10 drop increments, dispense and rub into front, side, and back of knee; usually 40 drops (40 mg) qid
　Topical soln: 1.5% (150 ml)
Pennsaid 2% apply 2 pump actuations (40 mg) and rub into front, side, and back of knee bid
　Topical soln: 2% (20 mg/pump actuation, 112 gm)
Solaraze Gel massage into clean skin bid prn
　Gel: 3% (50 gm) (benzyl alcohol)
Voltaren Gel (OTC) (G) apply qid prn to intact skin
　Gel: 1% (100 gm)
Comment: *Diclofenac* is contraindicated with *aspirin* allergy. As with other NSAIDs, should be avoided in late pregnancy (≥30 weeks) because it may cause premature closure of the ductus arteriosus.
▷ *doxepin* **(G)** cream apply to affected area qid at intervals of at least 3-4 hours; max 8 days
　Pediatric: <12 years: not recommended; >12 years: same as adult
　　Prudoxin *Crm:* 5% (45 gm)
　　Zonalon *Crm:* 5% (30, 45 gm)
▷ *pimecrolimus* **1% cream (G)** <2 years: not recommended; ≥2 years: apply to affected area bid; do not apply an occlusive dressing
　　Elidel *Crm:* 1% (30, 60, 100 gm)
Comment: *Pimecrolimus* is indicated for short-term and intermittent long-term use. Discontinue use when resolution occurs. Contraindicated if the patient is immunosuppressed. Change to the 0.1% preparation or if secondary bacterial infection is present.
▷ *trolamine salicylate* apply tid-qid
　Pediatric: <2 years: not recommended; ≥2 years: same as adult
　　Mobisyl Creme *Crm:* 10% (100 gm)

TOPICAL AND TRANSDERMAL ANESTHETICS

Comment: *Lidocaine* should not be applied to non-intact skin.
▷ *lidocaine* cream apply to affected area bid prn
　Pediatric: <12 years: not recommended; ≥12 years: same as adult
　　LidaMantle *Crm:* 3% (1, 2 oz)
　　Lidoderm *Crm:* 3% (85 gm)
　　ZTlido *lidocaine* topical system 1% (30/carton)
　　Comment: Compared to **Lidoderm** (*lidocaine* patch 5%), which contains 700 mg/patch, **ZTlido** only requires 35 mg per topical system to achieve the same therapeutic dose.
▷ *lidocaine* lotion apply to affected area bid prn
　Pediatric: <12 years: not recommended; ≥12 years: same as adult
　　LidaMantle *Lotn:* 3% (177 ml)
▷ *lidocaine* **5% patch (G)** apply up to 3 patches at one time for up to 12 hours/24-hour period (12 hours on/12 hours off); patches may be cut into smaller sizes before removal of the release liner; do not reuse
　Pediatric: <12 years: not recommended; ≥12 years: same as adult
　　Lidoderm *Patch:* 5% (10 x 14 cm; 30/carton)
▷ *lidocaine+dexamethasone*
　Pediatric: <12 years: not recommended; ≥12 years: same as adult
　　Decadron Phosphate with Xylocaine *Lotn:* dexa 4 mg+lido 10 mg per ml (5 ml)
▷ *lidocaine+hydrocortisone* **(G)** apply to affected area bid prn
　Pediatric: <12 years: not recommended; ≥12 years: same as adult
　　LidaMantle HC *Crm:* lido 3%+hydro 0.5% (1, 3 oz); *Lotn:* (177 ml)
▷ *lidocaine* **2.5%+prilocaine 2.5%** apply sparingly to the burn bid-tid prn
　Pediatric: <12 years: not recommended; ≥12 years: same as adult
　　Emla Cream 5, 30 gm/tube

ORAL NSAIDs

For an expanded list of NSAIDs *see* Appendix I. NSAIDs online at https://connect.springerpub.com/content/reference-book/978-0-8261-7935-7/back-matter/part02/back-matter/bmatter10
▷ *diclofenac* **(C; D ≥30 wks)** take on empty stomach; 35 mg tid; *Hepatic impairment:* use lowest dose
　Pediatric: <18 years: not recommended; ≥18 years: same as adult
　　Zorvolex *Gelcap:* 18, 35 mg
▷ *diclofenac sodium*
　Pediatric: <18 years: not recommended; ≥18 years: same as adult
　　Voltaren 50 mg bid-qid or 75 mg bid or 25 mg qid with an additional 25 mg at HS if necessary
　　　Tab: 25, 50, 75 mg ent-coat
　　Voltaren XR 100 mg once daily; rarely, 100 mg bid may be used
　　　Tab: 100 mg ext-rel
Comment: *Diclofenac* is contraindicated with *aspirin* allergy. As with other NSAIDs, should be avoided in late premature closure of the ductus arteriosus.

ORAL NSAIDs+PROTON PUMP INHIBITOR (PPI) COMBINATIONS

▷ *esomeprazole+naproxen* (G) 1 tab bid; use lowest effective dose for the shortest duration; swallow whole; take at least 30 minutes before a meal

Pediatric: <18 years: not recommended; ≥18 years: same as adult

Vimovo *Tab:* nap 375 mg+eso 20 mg ext-rel; nap 500 mg+eso 20 mg ext-rel

Comment: Vimovo is indicated to improve signs/symptoms, and risk of gastric ulcer in patients at risk of developing NSAID-associated gastric ulcer.

COX-2 INHIBITORS

Comment: Cox-2 inhibitors are contraindicated with history of asthma, urticaria, and allergic-type reactions to *aspirin*, other NSAIDs, and sulfonamides, 3rd trimester of pregnancy, and coronary artery bypass graft (CABG) surgery.

▷ *celecoxib* (G) 100-400 mg daily bid; max 800 mg/day

Pediatric: <18 years: not recommended; ≥18 years: same as adult

Celebrex *Cap:* 50, 100, 200, 400 mg

▷ *meloxicam* (G)

Mobic <2 years, <60 kg: not recommended; ≥2 years, >60 kg: 0.125 mg/kg; max 7.5 mg once daily; ≥18 years: initially 7.5 mg once daily, max 15 mg once daily; *Hemodialysis:* max 7.5 mg/day

Tab: 7.5, 15 mg; *Oral susp:* 7.5 mg/5 ml (100 ml) (raspberry)

Vivlodex <18 years: not established; ≥18 years: initially 5 mg once daily, may increase to max 10 mg/day; *Hemodialysis:* max 5 mg/day

Cap: 5, 10 mg

▷ *meloxicam injection* administer 30 mg via IV bolus once daily; administer dose over 15 seconds; monitor analgesic response and administer a short-acting, non-NSAID, immediate-release analgesic if response is inadequate; patients must be well hydrated before **Anjeso** administration; use **Anjeso** for the shortest duration consistent with individual patient treatment goals

Pediatric: safety and efficacy not established

Anjeso *Vial:* 30 mg/ml (1 ml), single dose

Comment: Anjeso *(meloxicam)* is an NSAID injection indicated for use in adults for the management of moderate-to-severe pain, alone or in combination with non-NSAID analgesics. Because of delayed onset of analgesia, **Anjeso** as monotherapy is not recommended for use when rapid onset of analgesia is required. The most common adverse reactions (incidence ≥2%) in controlled clinical trials have included constipation, increased gamma-glutamyltransferase (GGT), and anemia. Use of NSAIDs during the third trimester of pregnancy increases the risk of premature closure of the fetal ductus arteriosus; therefore, avoid **Anjeso** use after 30 weeks gestation. There are no human data available on whether *meloxicam* is present in human milk or on the effects on breastfed infants. NSAIDs are associated with reversible infertility. Consider withdrawal of **Anjeso** in women who have difficulties conceiving. **Anjeso** may also compromise fertility in males of reproductive potential; it is not known if this effect on male fertility is reversible.

TOPICAL AND TRANSDERMAL LIDOCAINE

▷ *lidocaine* transdermal patch (G) apply 1 patch to affected area for 12 hours (then off for 12 hours); remove during bathing; avoid non-intact skin

Pediatric: <12 years: not recommended; ≥12 years: same as adult

Lidoderm *Patch:* 5% (10 cm x 14 cm; 30/carton)

MYASTHENIA GRAVIS (MG)

COMPLEMENT INHIBITORS

▷ *eculizumab* dilute to a final admixture concentration of 5 mg/ml using the following steps: (1) withdraw the required amount of **Soliris** from the vial into a sterile syringe; (2) transfer the dose to an infusion bag; (3) add IV fluid equal to the drug volume (0.9% NaCl or 0.45% NaCl or D5W or Ringer's lactate); the final admixed **Soliris** 5 mg/ml infusion volume is 300 mg dose (60 ml), 600 mg dose (120 ml), 900 mg dose (180 ml), and 1,200 mg dose (240 ml); administer 900 mg IV infusion once weekly for the first 4 weeks; then 1,200 mg IV infusion for the 5th dose 1 week after the 4th dose; then 1,200 mg IV infusion once every 2 weeks thereafter

Pediatric: <18 years: safety and efficacy not established; ≥18 years: same as adult

Soliris *Vial:* 300 mg (10 mg/ml, 30 ml), single-use, concentrated solution for IV infusion (preservative-free)

Comment: Soliris *(eculizumab)* is a complement inhibitor indicated for the treatment of patients with paroxysmal nocturnal hemoglobinuria (PNH) to reduce hemolysis, patients with atypical hemolytic uremic syndrome (aHUS) to inhibit complement-mediated thrombotic microangiopathy (TMA), and adult patients with generalized myasthenia gravis (gMG) who are anti-acetylcholine receptor (AchR) antibody-positive. **Soliris** should be administered for gMG at the above recommended dosage regimen time points or within 2 days of each time point. Supplemental dosing of **Soliris** is required in the setting of concomitant support with plasmapheresis (PI) or plasma exchange (PE) or fresh frozen plasma (FFP) infusion (see mfr pkg insert for supplemental dosing). **Soliris** is not indicated for the treatment of patients with Shiga toxin *Escherichia coli*-related hemolytic uremic syndrome (STEC-HUS). **Soliris** is contraindicated in patients with unresolved *Neisseria meningitides* infection and patients who are not currently vaccinated against *N. meningitides,* unless the risks of delaying **Soliris** treatment outweigh the risks of developing meningococcal infection. Prescribers must enroll in the **Soliris** REMS Program (888-SOLIRIS, 1-888-765-4747), counsel patients about the risk of meningococcal infection, provide patients with **Soliris** REMS educational materials, and ensure that patients are vaccinated with a meningococcal vaccine. There are no adequate and well-controlled human studies of **Soliris** in pregnancy or effects on the breastfed infant. Based on animal studies, **Soliris** may cause fetal harm. It is not known whether **Soliris** is excreted in human milk. Immunoglobulin G (IgG) is excreted in human milk so it is expected that **Soliris** will be present in human milk. However, published data suggest that antibodies in human milk do not enter the neonatal and infant circulation in substantial amounts. Caution should be exercised when **Soliris** is administered to a breastfeeding patient.

NEONATAL Fc RECEPTOR BLOCKER
▷ *efgartigimod alfa-fcab* **Vyvgart** must be diluted with 0.9% NaCl Injection, USP prior to administration; *Recommended dose:*10 mg/kg, via IV infusion with a 0.2 micron in-line filter, over 1 hour, once weekly for 4 weeks; *Patient weight ≥120 kg:*1,200 mg per infusion; administer subsequent treatment cycles based on clinical evaluation; the safety of initiating subsequent cycles sooner than 50 days from the start of the previous treatment cycle has not been established
Pediatric: safety and efficacy not established
> **Vyvgart** *Vial:* 400 mg/20 ml (20 mg/ml), single-dose, soln for dilution and IV infusion (preservative-free)
> **Comment:** **Vyvgart** is a neonatal Fc receptor blocker indicated for the treatment of gMG in adult patients who are anti-acetylcholine receptor (AchR) antibody positive. Store vials refrigerated at 2°C to 8°C (36°F to 46°F) in the original carton to protect from light until time of use; do not freeze; do not shake. The most common adverse reactions (≥10%) in patients treated with **Vyvgart** have been respiratory tract infections, headache, and urinary tract infection. Hypersensitivity reactions, including angioedema, dyspnea, and rash, have occurred. If a hypersensitivity reaction occurs, discontinue the infusion and institute appropriate therapy. Monitor for signs and symptoms of infection in patients treated with **Vyvgart.** If serious infection occurs, administer appropriate treatment and consider withholding **Vyvgart** until the infection has resolved. Evaluate the need to administer age-appropriate vaccines according to immunization guidelines before initiation of a new treatment cycle. Closely monitor for reduced effectiveness of medications that bind to the human neonatal Fc receptor. When concomitant long-term use of such medications is essential for patient care, consider discontinuing **Vyvgart** and using alternative therapies. There are no available data on the use of **Vyvgart** during human pregnancy. There is no evidence of adverse developmental outcomes following the administration of **Vyvgart** at up to 100 mg/kg/day in animal studies. Monoclonal antibodies are increasingly transported across the placenta as pregnancy progresses, with the largest amount transferred during the third semester. Therefore, *efgartigimod alfa-fcab* may be transmitted from the mother to the developing fetus. As **Vyvgart** is expected to reduce maternal IgG antibody levels, reduction in passive protection to the newborn is anticipated. Risk and benefits should be considered prior to administering live or live attenuated vaccines to infants exposed to **Vyvgart** *in utero.* IV administration of *efgartigimod alfa-fcab* (0, 30, or 100 mg/kg/day) in animal studies throughout organogenesis resulted in no adverse effects on embryo/fetal development. The doses tested were 3 and 10 times the recommended human dose (RHD) of 10 mg/kg, on a body weight (mg/kg) basis. There is no information regarding the presence of *efgartigimod alfa-fcab* in human milk or effects on the breastfed infant. Maternal IgG is known to be present in human milk. Developmental and health benefits of breastfeeding should be considered along with the mother's clinical need for **Vyvgart** and any potential adverse effects on the breastfed infant from **Vyvgart** or from the underlying maternal condition.

MYELODYSPLASTIC SYNDROMES (MDS)

NUCLEOSIDE METABOLIC INHIBITOR+CYTIDINE DEAMINASE INHIBITOR
▷ *decitabine+cedazuridine* take 1 tablet once daily on Days 1 through 5 of each 28-day cycle; take on an empty stomach
Pediatric: not established
> **Inqovi** *Tab:* deci 35 mg+cedaz 100 mg film-coat
> **Comment:** **Inqovi** *(decitabine+cedazuridine)* is a nucleoside metabolic inhibitor *(decitabine)* and cytidine deaminase inhibitor *(cedazuridine)* combination indicated for the treatment of adults with intermediate and high-risk myelodysplastic syndromes (MDS), including chronic myelomonocytic leukemia (CMML). The most common adverse reactions (incidence ≥20%) have been fatigue, constipation, hemorrhage, myalgia, mucositis, arthralgia, nausea, dyspnea, diarrhea, rash, dizziness, febrile neutropenia, edema, headache, cough, decreased appetite, upper respiratory infection,

(continued)

pneumonia, and increased transaminase. The most common grade 3 or 4 laboratory abnormalities (≥50%) have been decreased leukocytes, platelet count, neutrophil count, and hemoglobin. Fatal and serious myelosuppression and infectious complications can occur. Obtain CBC prior to initiation of **Inqovi**, prior to each cycle, and as clinically indicated to monitor for response and toxicity (sCr ≥2 mg/dL, serum bilirubin ≥2 x ULN), AST or ALT ≥2 x ULN, active or uncontrolled infection). Manage persistent severe neutropenia and febrile neutropenia with supportive treatment. Following resolution, delay the next cycle and resume at the same or reduced dose as indicated. See mfr pkg insert for recommended dose reductions for myelosuppression. **Inqovi** can cause fetal harm. Avoid co-administration of **Inqovi** with other drugs metabolized by cytidine deaminase. **Inqovi** can impair fertility. Advise patients of reproductive potential of potential embryo/fetal risk and to use effective contraception for 6 months (females) or 3 months (males) after the last dose. Based on animal studies of *decitabine* and *cedazuridine*, **Inqovi** may impair male fertility. Reversibility of the effect on fertility is unknown. Advise females not to breastfeed.

MYELOFIBROSIS

KINASE INHIBITORS

▶ *fedratinib* 400 mg once daily with or without food for patients with a baseline platelet count of greater than or equal to 50 x 10⁹/L (2.1); reduce dose for patients taking strong CYP3A inhibitors or with severe renal impairment; avoid use in patients with severe hepatic impairment

Inrebic *Cap:* 100 mg

Comment: Inrebic *(fedratinib)* is a highly selective Janus kinase 2 (JAK2) inhibitor indicated for the treatment of adult patients with intermediate- or high-risk primary or secondary (post-polycythemia vera or post-essential thrombocythemia) myelofibrosis. Reduce **Inrebic** dose as recommended with concomitant use of strong CYP3A4 inhibitors. Avoid use of **Inrebic** with concomitant use of strong and moderate CYP3A4 inducers and dual CYP3A4 and CYP2C19 inhibitors. *Boxed Warning*; Serious and fatal encephalopathy, including Wernicke's, has occurred in patients treated with **Inrebic**. Wernicke's encephalopathy is a neurologic emergency; therefore, assess thiamine levels in all patients prior to starting **Inrebic**, periodically during treatment, and as clinically indicated. Do not start **Inrebic** in patients with thiamine deficiency. Replete thiamine prior to treatment initiation. If encephalopathy is suspected, immediately discontinue **Inrebic** and initiate parenteral thiamine. Monitor until symptoms resolve or improve and thiamine levels normalize. Warnings and precautions with use of **Inrebic** include anemia and thrombocytopenia (manage by dose reduction, interruption, or transfusion); gastrointestinal toxicity (manage by dose reduction or interruption if the patient develops severe diarrhea, nausea, or vomiting—prophylaxis with antiemetics and treatment with antidiarrheal medications are recommended and hepatic toxicity (manage amylase and lipase elevation by dose reduction or interruption). There are no available data on **Inrebic** use in pregnant females to evaluate for a drug-associated risk of major birth defects, miscarriage, or adverse maternal or fetal outcomes. However, in animal reproduction studies, oral administration of *fedratinib* during organogenesis at doses considerably lower than the recommended human daily dose of 400 mg/day resulted in adverse developmental outcomes. Consider the benefits and risks of **Inrebic** to the mother and possible embryo/fetal risk when prescribing during pregnancy. There are no data on the presence of *fedratinib* or its metabolites in human milk or effects on the breastfed infant and patients should be advised not to breastfeed during treatment with **Inrebic** and for at least 1 month after the last dose.

▶ *pacritinib* *Recommended dose:* 200 mg bid; take with or without food; avoid use in patients with eGFR <30 ml/min; avoid use in Child-Pugh Class B or C
Pediatric: safety and efficacy not established

Vonjo *Cap:* 100 mg

Comment: Vonjo is a kinase inhibitor indicated for the treatment of adults with intermediate- or high-risk primary or secondary (post-polycythemia vera or post-essential thrombocythemia) myelofibrosis with a platelet count <50 × 10⁹/L. This indication is approved under accelerated approval based on spleen volume reduction. Continued approval for this indication may be contingent upon verification and description of clinical benefit in a confirmatory trial(s). Concomitant use of **Vonjo** with strong CYP3A4 inhibitors or inducers is contraindicated. Avoid use in patients with active bleeding and hold **Vonjo** prior to any planned surgical procedures. May require dose interruption, dose reduction, or permanent discontinuation depending on severity. Manage significant diarrhea with antidiarrheals, dose reduction, or dose interruption. Manage thrombocytopenia by dose reduction or interruption. Avoid use of **Vonjo** in patients with baseline QTc >480 msec. Interrupt and reduce **Vonjo** dose in patients who have a QTcF >500 msec. Correct hypokalemia prior to and during **Vonjo** administration. Risk of major adverse cardiac events (MACE) may be increased in current/past smokers and patients with other cardiovascular risk factors; monitor for signs, evaluate, and treat promptly. Thrombosis, including deep venous thrombosis (DVT), pulmonary embolism (PE), and arterial thrombosis may occur. Monitor for signs, evaluate, and treat promptly. Secondary malignancies (e.g., lymphoma) and other malignancies may occur; past/current smokers may be at increased risk. Delay starting **Vonjo** until active serious infections have resolved. Observe for signs and symptoms of infection and manage promptly. Avoid use of **Vonjo** concomitant with moderate CYP3A4 inhibitors or inducers. Co-administration of **Vonjo** can alter the concentration of drugs that are P-glycoprotein (P-gp), breast cancer resistance protein (BCRP), or organic cation transporter 1 (OCT1) substrates. Avoid **Vonjo** use with sensitive substrates. The most common (≥20% of patients) adverse reactions have been diarrhea, thrombocytopenia, nausea, anemia, and peripheral edema. There are no available data on **Vonjo** use in human pregnancy to evaluate a drug-associated risk of major birth defects, miscarriage, or adverse maternal or fetal outcomes. In animal reproduction studies, administration of *pacritinib* at exposures that were considerably lower than those observed at the recommended human dose was associated with maternal toxicity and embryonic and fetal loss. *Pacritinib* was administered orally at doses of 30, 100, or 250 mg/kg/day from gestation day 6 to gestation day 15. *Pacritinib* was also administered orally at doses of 15, 30, or 60 mg/kg/day from gestation day 7 until gestation day 20. *Pacritinib* was associated with maternal toxicity, which resulted in postimplantation loss, abortions, and reduced fetal body weights at exposures 0.1 and 0.3 times the exposure at the recommended human dose (area under the curve [AUC]-based). The high dose was associated with an increased incidence of an external malformation (cleft palate) in the presence of maternal toxicity. In a pre- and postnatal development study, pregnant animals were dosed with *pacritinib* from implantation through lactation at 30, 100, or 250 mg/kg/day. Maternal toxicity was noted at 250 mg/kg and associated with increased gestation length and dystocia, lowered mean birth weights and neonatal survival, and transiently delayed startle response, learning, and memory development at weaning. Advise pregnant women of the potential risk to the fetus. Consider the benefits and risks of **Vonjo** for the mother and possible risks to the fetus when prescribing **Vonjo** to a pregnant female. Advise females of reproductive potential to use effective contraception. There are no data on the presence of *pacritinib* in either human or animal milk or effects on the breastfed infant. It is not known whether **Vonjo** is excreted in human milk. Because of the potential for serious adverse reactions in the breastfed infant, advise mothers that breastfeeding is not recommended during treatment with **Vonjo** and for 2 weeks after the last dose. *Pacritinib* reduced male mating and fertility indices in animal studies. *Pacritinib* may impair male fertility in humans. Advise male patients of this risk and to consider risk/benefit. To report suspected adverse reactions, contact CTI BioPharma at 844-428-4246 (844-4CTIBIO) or FDA at 1-800-FDA-1088 or www.VONJO.com or www.fda.gov/medwatch.

▶ *ruxolitinib* Starting dose: based on baseline platelet count: >200 x 10⁹/L: 20 mg bid; 100 x 10⁹/L to 200 x 10⁹/L: 15 mg bid; 50 x 10⁹/L to <100 x 10⁹/L: 5 mg bid; therapeutic dose should be individualized based on safety and efficacy; monitor CBC every 2 to 4 weeks until doses are stabilized and then as clinically indicated; modify or interrupt dosing for thrombocytopenia; *Renal impairment:* reduce starting dose or avoid use; *Hepatic impairment:* reduce starting dose or avoid use
Pediatric: <12 years: not established; ≥12 years: same as adult
Jakafi *Tab:* 5, 10, 15, 20, 25 mg
Comment: Jakafi *(ruxolitinib)* is a kinase inhibitor indicated for treatment of adults with intermediate- and high-risk myelofibrosis, including primary myelofibrosis, polycythemia vera with inadequate response to, or intolerance to, hydroxyurea, post-polycythemia vera myelofibrosis, and post-essential thrombocythemia myelofibrosis. Manage thrombocytopenia, anemia, and neutropenia with dose reduction, or treatment interruption, or transfusion. Serious infections should be resolved before starting therapy with **Jakafi**. Assess patients for signs and symptoms of infection during **Jakafi** therapy and initiate appropriate treatment promptly. Manage symptom exacerbation following interruption or discontinuation of **Jakafi** with supportive care and then consider resuming treatment with **Jakafi**. There is risk of non-melanoma skin cancer (NMSC) with **Jakafi** use; perform periodic skin examinations. Assess lipid levels 8-12 weeks from start of **Jakafi** therapy and treat as appropriate. Avoid use of **Jakafi** with *fluconazole* doses greater than 200 mg except in patients with acute graft versus host disease (GVHD). With myelofibrosis and polycythemia vera, the most common hematologic adverse reactions (incidence >20%) have been thrombocytopenia and anemia. The most common non-hematologic adverse reactions (incidence >10%) have been bruising, dizziness, and headache. There are no studies with the use of **Jakafi** in pregnant females to inform drug-associated risks. No data are available regarding the presence of *ruxolitinib* in human milk or the effects on the breastfed infant. Patients should be advised to discontinue breastfeeding during treatment with **Jakafi** and for 2 weeks after the final dose.

NARCOLEPSY, CATAPLEXY, EXCESSIVE DAYTIME SLEEPINESS (EDS)

STIMULANTS

▶ *amphetamine sulfate* (II) administer first dose on awakening and additional doses at 4- to 6-hour intervals; usual range 5-60 mg/day
Pediatric: <6 years: not recommended; 6-12 years: 5 mg daily in the AM; may increase by 5 mg/day at weekly intervals; ≥12-18 years: initially 10 mg in the AM; may increase by 10 mg daily at weekly intervals; >18 years: same as adult
Evekeo initially 10 mg once or twice daily at the same time(s) each day; may increase by 10 mg/day at weekly intervals; max 40 mg/day
Tab: 5, 10 mg

(continued)

▷ *armodafinil (IV)(G) Obstructive sleep apnea hypopnea syndrome (OSAHS)* 50-250 mg once daily in the AM; *Shift work sleep disorder (SWSD)* 150 mg 1 hour before starting shift; reduce dose with severe hepatic impairment
Pediatric: <17 years: not recommended; ≥17 years: same as adult
    Nuvigil *Tab:* 50, 150, 200, 250 mg
▷ *modafinil (IV)(G)* 100-200 mg q AM; max 400 mg/day
Pediatric: <17 years: not recommended; ≥17 years: same as adult
    Provigil *Tab:* 100, 200*mg
    Comment: Provigil also promotes wakefulness in patients with shift work sleep disorder (SWSD) and excessive sleepiness due to obstructive sleep apnea (OSA)/hypopnea syndrome.
▷ *sodium oxybate (III)(G)* initiate dosage at 4.5 gm per night orally divided into 2 doses; titrate to effect in increments of 1.5 gm per night at weekly intervals (0.75 gm at bedtime and 0.75 gm taken 2½ to 4 hours later)

Total Nightly Dose (gm)	4.5 gm	6 gm	7.5 gm	9 gm
Bedtime (gm)	2.25 gm	3 gm	3.75 gm	4.5 gm
2½ to 4 hours later (gm)	2.25 gm	3 gm	3.75 gm	4.5 gm

Pediatric: <7 years: not recommended; ≥7-17 years: see mfr pkg insert for weight-based (in kilograms) dosing table; ≥18 years: same as adult
    Xyrem *Oral soln:* 500 mg/ml
    Comment: Xyrem is used to reduce the number of cataplexy attacks (sudden and transient episode of muscle weakness coupled with full conscious awareness, typically triggered by emotions such as laughing, crying, or terror) and reduce daytime sleepiness in patients with narcolepsy. The rapid onset of sedation coupled with amnesia, particularly when combined with alcohol, has posed risks for voluntary and involuntary users (e.g., assault victims). Contraindicated with *alcohol* and central nervous system (CNS) depressants (may impair consciousness; may lead to respiratory depression, coma, or death) and in patients with succinic semialdehyde dehydrogenase deficiency (SSDD) (an inborn error of metabolism). Prepare both doses prior to bedtime and do not attempt to get out of bed after taking the first dose. Place both doses within reach at the bedside. Set the bedside clock to awaken for the second dose. Dilute each dose in 60 ml (1/4 cup, 4 tbsp) water in child-resistant dosing containers. Food significantly reduces the bioavailability of *sodium oxybate*; take at least 2 hours after ingesting food. There are no adequate data on the fetal developmental risk associated with the use of *sodium oxybate* in pregnant females. Gamma-hydroxybutyrate (GHB) is excreted in human milk. There is insufficient information on risk to the breastfed infant.
    Comment: Xyrem is a schedule III controlled substance. The active ingredient of **Xyrem**, sodium oxybate or GHB, is a schedule I controlled substance. **Xyrem** is available only through a restricted distribution with the **Xyrem** Risk Evaluation and Mitigation Strategy (REMS) Program because of the risks of CNS depression and abuse and misuse. Healthcare providers who prescribe **Xyrem** are specially certified. **Xyrem** is dispensed only by the central pharmacy that is specially certified and **Xyrem** is dispensed and shipped only to patients who are enrolled in the **Xyrem** REMS Program with documentation of safe use (www.XYREMREMS.com or 1-866-XYREM88 [1-866-997-3688]).
▷ *sodium oxybate, extended-release (III)* take dose at least 2 hours after eating; *Prepare the dose:* prior to bedtime by suspending the dose in approximately 1/3 cup of water in the mixing cup provided; take a single dose once at bedtime after getting into bed; usual time to sleep onset is 5 to 15 minutes after ingesting the dose; *Initial dose:* 4.5 gm orally once per night; *Titrate to effect:* at weekly intervals in increments of 1.5 gm per night; *Recommended dose range:* 6-9 gm orally once per night
Pediatric: <18 years: safety and efficacy not established; ≥18 years: same as adult
    Lumryz *Pkts:* 4.5, 6. 7.5, 9 grams/pkt, single-dose, ext-rel granules for oral suspension (7, 30 pkts/carton w. mixing cup)
    Comment: Lumryz is a CNS depressant indicated for the treatment of cataplexy or excessive daytime sleepiness (EDS) in adults with narcolepsy. **Lumryz** is the first and only FDA-approved once-at-bedtime *sodium oxybate* therapy for people with narcolepsy. The approval is based on data from the phase 3 REST-ON study. As reported in *Medscape Medical News*, compared with placebo, extended-release *sodium oxybate* demonstrated statistically significant (P <.001) and clinically meaningful improvement at all three doses assessed (6 g, 7.5 g, and 9 g) across all three co-primary endpoints: (1) the Maintenance of Wakefulness Test (MWT), (2) Clinical Global Impression-Improvement (CGII), and (3) mean weekly attacks of cataplexy. "**Lumryz** fills an unmet need by avoiding the burden of a second middle-of-the-night dose that immediate-release *oxybate* products require," principal investigator Michael J. Thorpy, MD, Director at the Sleep-Wake Disorders Center at Montefiore Medical Center, New York City, said in a news release. "The once-at-bedtime dosing regimen of **Lumryz** may help restore a more natural sleep-wake cycle," noted Thorpy, Professor of Neurology, Albert Einstein College of Medicine. **Lumryz** is available only through the Lumryz Risk Evaluation and Mitigation Strategy (REMS) program. The most common adverse reactions (incidence >5% than with placebo) reported for all doses of **Lumryz** combined were nausea, dizziness, enuresis, headache, and vomiting. Inform patients that **Lumryz** may impair respiratory drive, especially in patients with compromised respiratory function, and may

cause apnea. Contraindications to **Lumryz** use are concurrent use of sedative hypnotics or alcohol and succinic semialdehyde dehydrogenase deficiency (SSDD). Monitor for impaired motor/cognitive function. Caution patients against hazardous activities requiring complete mental alertness or motor coordination within the first 6 hours of dosing or after first initiating treatment until certain that **Lumryz** does not affect them adversely. Monitor patients for emergent or increased depression and suicidality. **Lumryz** has a high sodium content; monitor patients with heart failure, hypertension, or impaired renal function. Parasomnias may occur; evaluate episodes of sleepwalking. **Lumryz** is the sodium salt of GHB. Abuse or misuse of illicit GHB is associated with CNS adverse reactions, including seizure, respiratory depression, decreased consciousness, coma, and death. Because of an increase in exposure, **Lumryz** should not be initiated in patients with hepatic impairment because appropriate dosage adjustments for initiation of **Lumryz** cannot be made. Based on animal data, **Lumryz** may cause fetal harm. Advise females of reproductive potential of the potential risk to the fetus and to use effective contraception during treatment with **Lumryz**. GHB is excreted in human milk after oral administration of *sodium oxybate*. There is insufficient information on the risk to the breastfed infant. Developmental and health benefits of breastfeeding should be considered along with the mother's clinical need for **Lumryz** and any adverse effects on the breastfed infant from **Lumryz** or from the underlying maternal condition. To report suspected adverse reactions, contact Avadel CNS Pharmaceuticals at 888-828-2335 or FDA at 800-FDA-1088 or www.fda.gov/medwatch.

SELECTIVE DOPAMINE AND NOREPINEPHRINE REUPTAKE INHIBITOR (DNRI)

▷ *solriamfetol* administer once daily upon awakening; avoid administration within 9 hours of planned bedtime because of the potential to interfere with sleep; *Starting dose for patients with narcolepsy:* 75 mg once daily; *Starting dose for patients with OSA:* 37.5 mg once daily; dose may be increased at intervals of at least 3 days; max 150 mg once daily; *Moderate renal impairment:* starting dose is 37.5 mg once daily; may increase to 75 mg once daily after at least 7 days; *Severe renal impairment:* starting dose and max dose is 37.5 mg once daily; *end-stage renal disease (ESRD):* not recommended.
Pediatric: safety and efficacy not established
    Sunosi *Tab:* 75*, 150 mg film-coat
Comment: Sunosi *(solriamfetol)* is a dopamine and norepinephrine reuptake inhibitor (DNRI) indicated to improve wakefulness in adult patients with excessive daytime sleepiness associated with narcolepsy or OSA. **Sunosi** is not indicated to treat the underlying airway obstruction in OSA. Ensure that the underlying airway obstruction is treated (e.g., with continuous positive airway pressure [CPAP]) for at least 1 month prior to initiating **Sunosi** for excessive daytime sleepiness. Modalities to treat the underlying airway obstruction should be continued during treatment with **Sunosi**. **Sunosi** is not a substitute for these modalities. Use caution when co-administering **Sunosi** with drugs that increase BP and/or HR and dopaminergic drugs. Measure HR and BP prior to initiating and periodically throughout treatment. Control hypertension before and during therapy. Avoid use in patients with unstable cardiovascular disease, serious heart arrhythmias, or other serious heart problems. Use caution in treating patients with a history of psychosis or bipolar disorder. Consider **Sunosi** dose reduction or discontinuation if psychiatric symptoms develop. **Sunosi** is contraindicated in patients receiving treatment with a monoamine oxidase inhibitor (MAOI) and within 14 days following discontinuation of an MAOI. Available data from case reports are not sufficient to determine drug-associated risks of major birth defects, miscarriage, or adverse maternal or fetal outcomes. There are no data available on the presence of *solriamfetol* or its metabolites in human milk or effects on the breastfed infant. The developmental and health benefits of breastfeeding should be considered along with the mother's clinical need for **Sunosi** and any potential adverse effects on the breastfed infant from **Sunosi** or from the underlying maternal condition. Healthcare providers are encouraged to register pregnant patients, or pregnant females may enroll themselves, in the Sunosi Pregnancy Exposure Registry by calling 877-283-6220 or www.SunosiPregnancyRegistry.com

AMPHETAMINES

▷ *dextroamphetamine sulfate* (II)(G) initially start with 10 mg daily; increase by 10 mg at weekly intervals if needed; may switch to daily dose with sust-rel spansules when titrated
Pediatric: <3 years: not recommended; 3-5 years: 2.5 mg daily; may increase by 2.5 mg daily at weekly intervals if needed; 6-12 years: initially 5 mg daily-bid; may increase by 5 mg/day at weekly intervals; usual max 40 mg/day; >12 years: initially 10 mg daily; may increase by mg/day at weekly intervals; max 40 mg/day 10
    Dexedrine *Tab:* 5*mg (tartrazine)
    Dexedrine Spansule *Cap:* 5, 10, 15 mg sust-rel
    Dextrostat *Tab:* 5, 10 mg (tartrazine)
▷ *dextroamphetamine saccharate+dextroamphetamine sulfate+amphetamine aspartate+amphetamine sulfate* (II)(G)
    Adderall initially 10 mg daily; may increase weekly by 10 mg/day; usual max 60 mg/day in 2-3 divided doses; first dose on awakening and then q 4-6 hours prn
    Pediatric: <6 years: not indicated; 6-12 years: initially 5 mg daily; may increase weekly by 5 mg/day; usual max 40 mg/day in 2-3 divided doses; >12 years: same as adult
    Tab: 5**, 7.5**, 10**, 12.5**, 15**, 20**, 30**mg

(continued)

Adderall XR
Pediatric: <6 years: not recommended; 6-12 years: initially 10 mg daily in the AM, may increase by 10 mg weekly; max 30 mg/day; 13-17 years: initially 10 mg daily; may increase to 20 mg/day after 1 week, max 30 mg/day; Do not crush or chew; may sprinkle on apple sauce
    Cap: 5, 10, 15, 20, 25, 30 mg ext-rel
Comment: Adderall is also indicated to improve wakefulness in patients with shift-work sleep disorder and excessive sleepiness due to OSA/hypopnea syndrome.

▷ *dexmethylphenidate* (II)(G) take once daily in the AM
Pediatric: <6 years: not recommended; ≥6 years: same as adult
    Focalin initially 2.5 mg bid; allow at least 4 hours between doses; may increase at 1-week intervals; max 40 mg/day
      Tab: 2.5, 5, 10*mg (dye-free)
    Focalin XR 20-40 mg q AM; max 40 mg/day
      Tab: 5, 10, 15, 20, 30, 40 mg ext-rel (dye-free)

▷ *methylphenidate (regular-acting)* (II)(G)
Pediatric: <6 years: not recommended; ≥6 years: initially 5 mg bid ac (before breakfast and lunch); may gradually increase by 5-10 mg at weekly intervals as needed; max 60 mg/day
    Methylin, Methylin Chewable, Methylin Oral Solution usual dose 20-30 mg/day in 2-3 divided doses 30-45 minutes before a meal; may increase to 60 mg/day
    Ritalin 10-60 mg/day in 2-3 divided doses 30-45 minutes ac; max 60 mg/day
      Tab: 5, 10*, 20*mg

▷ *methylphenidate (long-acting)* (II)
    Adhansia XR recommended starting dose is 25 mg once daily in the morning; may be increased in increments of 10-15 mg at intervals of at least 5 days; dosage ≥85 mg daily (adults) and ≥70 mg daily (children) are associated with disproportionate increases in the incidence of certain adverse reactions; administer with or without food; may be swallowed whole or opened and the capsule contents sprinkled onto a tablespoon of applesauce or yogurt; do not crush or chew capsule contents
      Cap: 25, 35, 45, 55, 70, 85 mg ext-rel
    Concerta (G) initially 18 mg q AM; may increase in 18 mg increments as needed; max 54 mg/day; do not crush or chew
      Tab: 18, 27, 36, 54 mg sust-rel
    Metadate CD (G) 1 cap daily in the AM; may sprinkle on food; do not crush or chew
Pediatric: <6 years: not recommended; ≥6 years: initially 20 mg daily; may gradually increase by 20 mg/day at weekly intervals as needed; max 60 mg/day
      Cap: 10, 20, 30, 40, 50, 60 mg immed- and ext-rel beads
    Metadate ER 1 tab daily in the AM; do not crush or chew
Pediatric: <6 years: not recommended; ≥6 years: use in place of regular-acting *methylphenidate* when the 8-hour dose of **Metadate-ER** corresponds to the titrated 8-hour dose of regular-acting *methylphenidate*
      Tab: 10, 20 mg ext-rel (dye-free)
    Ritalin LA 1 cap daily in the AM
Pediatric: <6 years: not recommended; ≥6 years: use in place of regular-acting *methylphenidate* when the 8-hour dose of **Ritalin LA** corresponds to the titrated 8-hour dose of regular-acting *methylphenidate*; max 60 mg/day
      Cap: 10, 20, 30, 40 mg ext-rel (immed- and ext-rel beads)
    Ritalin SR 1 cap daily in the AM
Pediatric: <6 years: not recommended; ≥6 years: use in place of regular-acting *methylphenidate* when the 8-hour dose of **Ritalin SR** corresponds to the titrated 8-hour dose of regular-acting *methylphenidate*; max 60 mg/day
      Tab: 20 mg sust-rel (dye-free)

▷ *methylphenidate (transdermal patch)* (II)(G) 1 patch daily in the AM
Pediatric: <6 years: not recommended; ≥6 years: initially 10 mg patch daily in the AM; may increase by 5-10 mg/week; max 60 mg/day
    Transdermal patch: 10, 15, 20, 30 mg

HISTAMINE-3 (H3) RECEPTOR ANTAGONIST/INVERSE AGONIST

▷ *pitolisant* administer once daily in the morning upon wakening; recommended range is 17.8 mg to 35.6 mg once daily; titrate dose as follows: Week 1: initially 8.9 mg once daily; Week 2: increase to 17.8 mg once daily; Week 3: may increase to max 35.6 mg once daily
Moderate hepatic impairment: initially 8.9 mg once daily; titrate to max 17.8 mg once daily after 14 days
Severe hepatic impairment: contraindicated;
Moderate/Severe renal impairment: initially 8.9 mg once daily; titrate to max 17.8 mg once daily after 7 days;
ESRD: not recommended; *Poor metabolizers of CYP2D6:* max 17.8 mg once daily; *Strong CYP2D6 inhibitors:* max 17.8 mg once daily; *Strong CYP3A4 inducers:* decrease exposure to **Wakix**; consider dose adjustment; *Sensitive CYP3A4 substrates* (including hormonal contraceptives): **Wakix** may reduce effectiveness of sensitive CYP3A4 substrates; recommend using an alternative non-hormonal contraceptive method during treatment with **Wakix** and for at least 21 days after discontinuation of treatment

Wakix *Tab*: 4.45, 17.8 mg

Comment: Wakix (*pitolisant*) is a first-in-class drug, a histamine-3 (H$_3$) receptor antagonist/inverse agonist, for the treatment of EDS in adult patients with narcolepsy. The most common adverse reactions (incidence ≥5%) have been insomnia, nausea, and anxiety. Avoid use of **Wakix** with drugs that also increase the QT interval and in patients with risk factors for prolonged QT interval, and monitor patients with hepatic or renal impairment for increased QTc. There is a pregnancy exposure registry that monitors pregnancy outcomes in women who are exposed to **Wakix** during pregnancy. Patients should be encouraged to enroll in the **Wakix** pregnancy registry if they become pregnant. To enroll or obtain information from the registry, patients can call 1-800-833-7460. There are no data on the presence of *pitolisant* in human milk or effects on the breastfed infant; however, *pitolisant* is present in the milk of lactating rats. The developmental and health benefits of breastfeeding should be considered along with the mother's clinical need for treatment with **Wakix**.

CENTRAL NERVOUS SYSTEM (CNS) DEPRESSANT

▷ *calcium, magnesium, potassium, and sodium oxybate oral solution (CIII)* prepare 2 doses prior to bedtime; dilute each dose with approximately ¼ cup of water in pharmacy-provided containers; take the first nightly dose at least 2 hours after eating; take each dose while in bed and lie down after dosing; see mfr pkg insert for adult dosing

Pediatric: <7 years: not established; ≥7 years: recommended starting dose, titration regimen, and maximum total nightly dose is based on body weight (see mfr pkg insert for dosing by weight table)

Xywav *Oral soln*: 0.5 gm/ml total salts (equivalent to 0.413 gm/ml of oxybate)

Comment: Xywav is a CNS depressant indicated for the treatment of cataplexy or EDS in patients ≥7 years of age with narcolepsy. The most common adverse reactions in adults (incidence ≥5%) have been headache, nausea, dizziness, decreased appetite, parasomnia, diarrhea, hyperhidrosis, anxiety, and vomiting. In a pediatric study with sodium oxybate (same active moiety as **Xywav**), the most common adverse reactions (incidence ≥5%) were enuresis, nausea, headache, vomiting, decreased weight, decreased appetite, and dizziness. **Xywav** is contraindicated in combination with sedative hypnotics or alcohol or when the patient has succinic semialdehyde dehydrogenase deficiency (SSDD). When used with concomitant *divalproex sodium*, an initial reduction in **Xywav** dose of at least 20% is recommended. If transitioning from **Xyrem** to **Xywav**, initiate **Xywav** at the same dose and regimen as **Xyrem** (gram for gram) and titrate as needed based on efficacy and tolerability. If the patient has hepatic impairment, the recommended starting dosage of **Xywav** is one-half of the original dosage per night administered orally, divided into 2 doses. Use caution when considering the concurrent use of **Xywav** with other CNS depressants, and caution patients against hazardous activity requiring complete mental alertness or motor coordination within the first 6 hours of dosing or after first initiating treatment until certain that **Xywav** does not affect them adversely. Monitor patients for emergent or increased depression and suicidality. Monitor for impaired motor/cognitive function. Evaluate episodes of sleepwalking (parasomnia). Based on animal data, **Xywav** may cause embryo/fetal harm. Advise females of reproductive potential of the potential embryo/fetal risk and to use an effective method of contraception during treatment. GHB is excreted in human milk after oral administration of *sodium oxybate*. There is insufficient information on risk to a breastfed infant. Developmental and health benefits of breastfeeding should be considered along with the mother's clinical need for **Xywav**, and any potential adverse effects on the breastfed infant from **Xywav** or from the underlying maternal condition.

NAUSEA/VOMITING: CHEMOTHERAPY-INDUCED (CINV)

SUBSTANCE P/NEUROKININ-1 (NK-1) RECEPTOR ANTAGONIST AND SEROTONIN-3 (5-HT3) RECEPTOR ANTAGONIST COMBINATION

▷ *fosnetupitant+palonosetron*

Akynzeo 1 capsule cap administered approximately 1 hour prior to the start of chemotherapy, with or without food

Akynzeo for Injection: 1 vial reconstituted in 50 ml of D5W or 0.9% NS administered as a 30-minute IV infusion; start the infusion approximately 30 minutes prior to the start of chemotherapy

Pediatric: <18 years: not established; ≥18 years: same as adult

Akynzeo *Cap*: 300 mg netu+palo 0.5 mg

Akynzeo for Injection *Vial*: fosnetu 235 mg+palo 0.25 mg, single-dose, pwdr for reconstitution and IV infusion

Comment: Akynzeo for Injection is indicated in combination with *dexamethasone* for the prevention of acute and delayed nausea and vomiting associated with initial and repeat courses of highly emetogenic cancer chemotherapy. **Akynzeo for Injection** has not been studied for the prevention of nausea and vomiting associated with *anthracycline* plus *cyclophosphamide* chemotherapy. **Akynzeo** capsules are indicated in combination with *dexamethasone* for prevention of acute and delayed nausea and vomiting associated with initial and repeat courses of cancer chemotherapy, including, but not limited to, highly emetogenic chemotherapy. Avoid in patients with severe hepatic impairment and patients with severe renal disease and end-stage renal disease (ESRD). May cause fetal harm.

NAUSEA/VOMITING: POSTANESTHESIA

Rx ANTIEMETICS
DOPAMINE-2 (D2) ANTAGONIST

▷ **amisulpride** *Prevention of PONV (either alone or in combination with another antiemetic):* 5 mg as a single IV dose infused over 1-2 minutes at the time of induction of anesthesia; *Treatment of PONV:* 10 mg as a single IV dose infused over 1-2 minutes in the event of nausea and/or vomiting after a surgical procedure; dilution is not required prior to administration
Pediatric: safety and efficacy not established
  Barhemsys *Vial:* 5 mg/2 ml (2 ml), single-dose
  Comment: **Barhemsys** *(amisulpride)* is a dopamine-2 (D2) antagonist for the management of postoperative nausea/vomiting (PONV). The most common adverse reactions (incidence ≥2%) have been the following: *prevention of PONV:* increased blood prolactin concentrations, chills, hypokalemia, procedural hypotension, and abdominal distension; *treatment of PONV:* infusion site pain. QT prolongation occurs in a dose- and concentration-dependent manner. Avoid use in patients with congenital long QT syndrome and in patients taking **droperidol**. ECG monitoring is recommended in patients with preexisting arrhythmias/cardiac conduction disorders, electrolyte abnormalities (e.g., hypokalemia or hypomagnesemia), congestive heart failure, and in patients taking other medicinal products (e.g., **ondansetron**) or with other medical conditions known to prolong the QT interval. There are no reports of adverse effects on the breastfed infant. A lactating woman may pump and discard breast milk for 48 hours after **Barhemsys** administration to reduce infant exposure.

5-HT3 RECEPTOR ANTAGONIST

▷ **ondansetron** (G) 8 mg q 8 hours x 2 doses; then 8 mg q 12 hours
Pediatric: <4 years: not recommended; 4-11 years: 4 mg q 4 hours x 3 doses; then 4 mg q 8 hours
  Zofran *Tab:* 4, 8, 24 mg
  Zofran ODT *ODT:* 4, 8 mg (strawberry) (phenylalanine)
  Zofran Oral Solution *Oral soln:* 4 mg/5 ml (50 ml) (strawberry) (phenyl-alanine); *Parenteral form:* see mfr pkg insert
  Zofran Injection *Vial:* 2 mg/ml (2 ml single-dose); 2 mg/ml (20 ml multidose); 32 mg/50 ml (50 ml multidose); *Prefilled syringe:* 4 mg/2 ml, single-use (24/carton)
  Zuplenz Oral Soluble Film: 4, 8 mg oral-dis (10/carton) (peppermint)
  Comment: The FDA has issued a warning against **ondansetron** use in pregnancy. **Ondansetron** is a 5-HT3 receptor antagonist approved by the FDA for preventing nausea and vomiting related to cancer chemotherapy and surgery. However, it has been used "off label" to treat the nausea and vomiting of pregnancy. The FDA has cautioned against the use of **ondansetron** in pregnancy in light of studies of **ondansetron** in early pregnancy associated with congenital cardiac malformations and oral clefts (i.e., cleft lip and cleft palate). Further, there are potential maternal risks in pregnancy with electrolyte imbalance caused by severe nausea and vomiting (as with hyperemesis gravidarum). These risks include *serotonin syndrome* (a triad of cognitive and behavioral changes including confusion, agitation, autonomic instability, and neuromuscular changes). Therefore, **ondansetron** should not be taken during pregnancy.

▷ **palonosetron** (G) administer 0.25 mg IV over 30 seconds; max 1 dose/week
Pediatric: <1 month: not recommended; 1 month to 17 years: 20 mcg/kg; max 1.5 mg/single dose; infuse over 15 minutes beginning 30 minutes
  Aloxi *Vial (single-use):* 0.075 mg/1.5 ml; 0.25 mg/5 ml (mannitol)

RECEPTOR-BLOCKING AGENT

▷ **promethazine** (G) 25 mg PO or rectally q 4-6 hours prn
Pediatric: <2 years: not recommended; ≥2 years: 0.5 mg/lb or 6.25-25 mg q 4-6 hours prn
  Phenergan *Tab:* 12.5*, 25*, 50 mg; *Plain syr:* 6.25 mg/5 ml; *Fortis syr:* 25 mg/5 ml; *Rectal supp:* 12.5, 25, 50 mg
  Comment: *Promethazine* is contraindicated in children with uncomplicated nausea, dehydration, Reye's syndrome, history of sleep apnea, asthma, and lower respiratory disorders. *Promethazine* lowers the seizure threshold in children and may cause cholestatic jaundice, anticholinergic effects, extrapyramidal effects, and potentially fatal respiratory depression.

NEPHROPATHY: PRIMARY, IMMUNOGLOBULIN A (IGAN)

▷ **budesonide** swallow whole, in the morning, at least 1 hour before a meal
Pediatric: safety and efficacy not established
  Tarpeyo *Cap:* 4 mg del-rel (120/bottle)
  Comment: **Tarpeyo** is indicated to reduce proteinuria in adults with primary immunoglobulin A nephropathy (IgAN) at risk of rapid disease progression, generally a urine protein-to-creatinine ratio (UPCR) of at least 1.5 gm/gm. Grapefruit juice should be avoided for the duration of **Tarpeyo** therapy; it can increase systemic exposure of **budesonide**. It has not been established whether **Tarpeyo** slows kidney function decline in patients with IgAN. Continued approval for the proteinuria indication may be contingent upon verification and description of clinical benefit in a confirmatory clinical trial.

SUBSTANCE P/NEUROKININ-1 (NK1) RECEPTOR ANTAGONIST

▷ *omidenepag isopropyl Recommended* dose: 32 mg administered as a 30-second IV infusion prior to induction of anesthesia; flush the infusion line with normal saline before and after administration of **Aponvie. Aponvie** is compatible with 0.9% Sodium Chloride Injection, USP or 5% Dextrose Injection, USP, and solutions containing divalent cations (e.g., calcium, magnesium), including lactated Ringer's solution
Pediatric: safety and efficacy not established

    Aponvie *Vial:* 32 mg/4.4 ml (7.2 mg/ml), single-dose, emulsion

    Comment: Aponvie is an IV formulation of the approved antiemetic *aprepitant* indicated for the prevention of postoperative nausea and vomiting (PONV). Contraindications are known hypersensitivity to any component of this product and concurrent use with *pimozide*. Inhibition of CYP3A4 by *aprepitant* could result in elevated plasma concentrations of *pimozide*, which is a CYP3A4 substrate, potentially causing serious or life-threatening reactions, such as QT prolongation, a known adverse reaction of *pimozide*.

NERVE AGENT POISONING

▷ *atropine sulfate* (G) 2 mg IM
    Pediatric: <15 lb: not recommended; ≥15-40 lb: 0.5 mg IM; ≥40-90 lb: 1 mg IM; >90 lb: same as adult
    AtroPen *Pen (single-use):* 0.5, 1, 2 mg (0.5 ml)

NEUROGENIC DETRUSOR OVERACTIVITY (NDO)

Comment: *Solifenacin* is a muscarinic receptor antagonist. **VESIcare** *(solifenacin)* and **VESIcare LS** *(solifenacin succinate)* are FDA-approved to be taken in combination with **Myrbetriq** *(mirabegron)* for the treatment of overactive bladder (OAB) with symptoms of frequency, urgency, and urge urinary incontinence.

▷ *solifenacin* initially 25 mg once daily; max 50 mg once daily; *Severe renal impairment:* 25 mg once daily
    VESIcare *Tab:* 5, 10 mg 5-10 mg once daily
▷ *solifenacin succinate* see weight-based chart for once daily dosing; follow with a liquid drink (e.g., water or milk); initiate at recommended starting dose; titrate to the lowest effective dose; do not exceed max recommended dose
    Pediatric: <2 years: not established; ≥2 years: see mfr pkg insert for weight-based once-daily dosing; follow with a liquid drink (e.g., water or milk); initiate at recommended starting dose; titrate to the lowest effective dose; do not exceed max recommended dose
    VESIcare LS *Oral susp:* 5 mg/5 ml (1 mg/ml, 150 ml) (orange)
    Comment: Do not exceed the recommended starting dose of **VESIcare LS** in patients with severe renal impairment (CrCl <30 ml/min), moderate hepatic impairment (Child-Pugh Class B), or concomitant use of strong CYP3A4 inhibitors. **VESIcare LS** is contraindicated in patients with severe hepatic impairment (Child-Pugh Class C), gastric retention, and uncontrolled narrow-angle glaucoma. The most common adverse reactions (incidence >2%) have been constipation, dry mouth, and urinary tract infection. Somnolence has been reported. **VESIcare LS** is not recommended for use in patients at high risk of QT prolongation, including patients with a known history of QT prolongation and patients taking medications known to prolong the QT interval.

NEUROFIBROMATOSIS TYPE 1

MITOGEN-ACTIVATED PROTEIN KINASE 1 AND 2 (MEK1/2) INHIBITOR

▷ *selumetinib* 25 mg/m² bid; do not consume food 2 hours before each dose or 1 hour after each dose; *Moderate hepatic impairment (Child-Pugh Class B):* 20 mg/m² bid; *Severe hepatic impairment (Child-Pugh Class C):* not established
    Pediatric: <2 years: safety and efficacy not established; ≥2 years: same as adult
    Koselugo *Cap:* 10, 25 mg
    Comment: Koselugo *(selumetinib)* is a kinase inhibitor (inhibitor of mitogen-activated protein kinase 1 and 2 [MEK1/2]) indicated for the treatment of pediatric patients 2 years of age and older with neurofibromatosis type 1 (NF1) who have symptomatic, inoperable plexiform neurofibromas (PN). Withhold, reduce dose, or permanently discontinue **Koselugo** based on severity of any adverse reaction. Assess ejection fraction prior to initiating treatment, every 3 months during the first year, then every 6 months thereafter and as clinically indicated. Conduct ophthalmic assessments prior to initiating **Koselugo**, at regular intervals during treatment and for new or worsening visual changes. Permanently discontinue **Koselugo** for retinal vein occlusion (RVO). Withhold **Koselugo** for retinal pigment epithelial detachment (RPED), monitor with optical coherence tomography assessments until resolution, and resume at reduced dose. Advise patients to start an antidiarrheal agent immediately after the first episode of loose stool and to increase fluid intake. Monitor for severe skin rashes. Increased creatinine phosphokinase (CPK) and rhabdomyolysis can occur. Obtain serum CPK prior to initiating **Koselugo**, periodically during treatment and as clinically indicated. If increased CPK occurs, evaluate for rhabdomyolysis or other causes. **Koselugo** capsules contain vitamin E, and daily intake of vitamin

(continued)

E that exceeds the recommended or safe limits may increase the risk of bleeding. An increased risk of bleeding may occur in patients co-administered vitamin K antagonists or antiplatelet agents. Avoid co-administration of strong or moderate CYP3A4 inhibitors or *fluconazole* with **Koselugo**. If co-administration with strong or moderate CYP3A4 inhibitors or *fluconazole* cannot be avoided, reduce the dose of **Koselugo**. Avoid concomitant use of strong and moderate CYP3A4 inducers. The most common adverse reactions (incidence ≥40%) are vomiting, rash (all), abdominal pain, diarrhea, nausea, dry skin, fatigue, musculoskeletal pain, pyrexia, acneiform rash, stomatitis, headache, paronychia, and pruritus. Based on findings from animal studies and its mechanism of action, **Koselugo** can cause fetal harm when administered to a pregnant woman. There are no available data on the use of **Koselugo** in pregnant females to evaluate drug-associated risk. There are no data on the presence of *selumetinib* or its active metabolite in human milk or effects on the breastfed infant. Due to potential for adverse reactions, advise women not to breastfeed during treatment with **Koselugo** and for 1 week after the last dose. To report suspected adverse reactions, contact AstraZeneca at 1-800-236-9933 or FDA at 1-800-FDA-1088 or www.fda.gov/medwatch.

NEUROMYELITIS OPTICA SPECTRUM DISORDER (NMOSD)

COMPLEMENT INHIBITOR

▷ *eculizumab* administer 900 mg via IV infusion once weekly for the first 4 weeks; followed by a single 1,200 mg dose via IV infusion 1 week later (the fifth week); then 1,200 mg via IV infusion once every 2 weeks thereafter; administer at the recommended dosage regimen time points or within 2 days of these time points; see mfr pkg insert for dose preparation instructions

Pediatric: safety and efficacy not established

Soliris *Vial:* 10 mg/ml (30 ml), single-dose (preservative-free) solution for dilution and IV infusion

Comment: Soliris *(eculizumab)* is indicated for the treatment of neuromyelitis optica spectrum disorder (NMOSD) in adult patients who are anti-aquaporin-4 (AQP4) antibody-positive. **Soliris** is available only through a restricted program under a Risk Evaluation and Mitigation Strategy (REMS). Under the Soliris REMS, prescribers must enroll in the program.

NEUTROPENIA: CHEMOTHERAPY-ASSOCIATED, NEUTROPENIA: FEBRILE, NEUTROPENIA: MYELOSUPPRESSION-ASSOCIATED

LEUKOCYTE GROWTH FACTOR

▷ *pegfilgrastim* <45 kg: see mfr pkg insert for a weight-based dosing table; ≥45 kg: *Patients with cancer receiving myelosuppressive chemotherapy:* 6 mg SC once per chemotherapy cycle; do not administer between 14 days before and 24 hours after administration of cytotoxic chemotherapy; *Patients acutely exposed to myelosuppressive doses of radiation,* <45 kg: see mfr pkg insert for a weight-based dosing table; ≥45 kg: 6 mg SC x 2 doses 1 week apart; administer the first dose as soon as possible after suspected or confirmed exposure to myelosuppressive doses of radiation

Neulasta *Prefilled syringe:* 6 mg/0.6 ml, single-dose, for manual use only; 6 mg/0.6 ml, single-dose, co-packaged with the on-body **Neulasta** autoinjector

Comment: *Pegfilgrastim* is a leukocyte growth factor that helps reduce the risk/incidence of infection, as manifested by febrile neutropenia, in patients with non-myeloid malignancies receiving myelosuppressive anticancer drugs and to increase survival in patients acutely exposed to myelosuppressive doses of radiation (i.e., hematopoietic subsyndrome of acute radiation syndrome [HSARS]). **Neulasta** is not indicated for the mobilization of peripheral blood progenitor cells for hematopoietic stem cell transplantation. Warnings and precautions associated with **Neulasta** include fatal splenic rupture, acute respiratory distress syndrome (ARDS), serious allergic reaction/anaphylaxis, allergic reaction to acrylic adhesive (used to attach the autoinjector), fatal sickle cell crisis, glomerulonephritis, and on-body injector failure. There are no adequate or well-controlled studies of **Neulasta** use in pregnancy. Based on animal data, may cause fetal harm. It is not known whether *pegfilgrastim* is secreted in human milk. Other recombinant granulocyte colony-stimulating factor (G-CSF) products are poorly secreted in breast milk and G-CSF is not orally absorbed by neonates. Caution should be exercised when administered to a nursing female.

▷ *pegfilgrastim-bmez* <45 kg: see mfr pkg insert for a weight-based dosing table; ≥45 kg: administer 6 mg SC once per chemotherapy cycle; do not administer between 14 days before and 24 hours after administration of cytotoxic chemotherapy

Ziextenzo *Prefilled pen:* 6 mg/0.6 ml, single-dose

Comment: Ziextenzo is biosimilar to **Neulasta** *(pegfilgrastim)*.

▷ *pegfilgrastim-cbqv*

Udenyca *Prefilled autoinjector:* 6 mg/0.6 ml, single-dose

Comment: Udenyca is biosimilar to **Neulasta** *(pegfilgrastim)*.

▷ *pegfilgrastim-jmdb*

Fulphila *Prefilled syringe:* 6 mg/0.6 ml, single-dose, for manual use only

Comment: Fulphila is biosimilar to **Neulasta** *(pegfilgrastim)*.

FILGRASTIM PRODUCTS

Comment: *Filgrastim* (**Neupogen**) and *filgrastim* biosimilar products (**Nivestym, Releuko, Zarxio, Granix**) are contraindicated in patients with a history of serious allergic reactions to human granulocyte colony-stimulating factors (e.g., *filgrastim, pegfilgrastim*). Administration to patients <18 years is not recommended. Direct administration of less than 0.3 ml is not recommended due to potential for dosing errors. Use during pregnancy only if the potential benefit justifies the potential risk to the fetus. It is not known whether *filgrastim* or biosimilar products are excreted in human milk or effects on the breastfed infant. Prior to using *filgrastim* or a *filgrastim* biosimilar product, remove the vial or prefilled syringe from the refrigerator and allow to reach room temperature for a minimum of 30 minutes and a maximum of 24 hours. Discard any vial or prefilled syringe left at room temperature for greater than 24 hours. Visually inspect for particulate matter and discoloration prior to administration (the solution is clear and colorless). Do not administer if particulates or discoloration is observed. Discard any unused portion. Do not re-enter a vial. Inject subcutaneously in the outer area of upper arms, abdomen, thighs, or upper outer areas of the buttock. Patients or caregivers may administer the SC dose after appropriate education and supervised training by a qualified healthcare provider. For IV infusion, may be diluted in D5%W USP from a concentration of 300 mcg/ml to 5 mcg/ml (do not dilute to a final concentration <5 mcg/ml). Dilution to concentrations from 5 mcg/ml to 15 mcg/ml should be protected from adsorption to plastic materials by the addition of albumin (human) to a final concentration of 2 mg/ml. When diluted in D5%W USP or D5%W plus albumin (human), *filgrastim* and *filgrastim* biosimilar products are compatible with glass bottles, polyvinyl chloride (PVC) and polyolefin IV bags, and polypropylene syringes. Do not dilute with saline at any time because the product may precipitate. Warnings and precautions include splenic rupture, acute respiratory distress syndrome (ARDS), serious allergic reaction, sickle cell disorders, glomerulonephritis, alveolar hemorrhage and hemoptysis, capillary leak syndrome (CLS), thrombocytopenia, leukocytosis, and cutaneous vasculitis (see mfr pkg insert for detailed discussion of potential adverse side effects (ASEs) and complications).

▷ *filgrastim*

Patients with cancer receiving myelosuppressive chemotherapy or induction and/or consolidation chemotherapy for acute myeloid leukemia (AML): recommended starting dose is 5 mcg/kg/day via SC injection, short IV infusion (over 15-30 minutes), or continuous IV infusion; see mfr pkg insert for recommended dosage adjustments and timing of administration; obtain a complete blood count (CBC) and platelet count before instituting *filgrastim* therapy and monitor twice weekly during therapy; consider dose escalation in increments of 5 mcg/kg for each chemotherapy cycle, according to the duration and severity of the absolute neutrophil count (ANC) nadir; recommend stopping *filgrastim* if the ANC increases beyond 10,000/mm^3

Patients with cancer undergoing bone marrow transplantation: 10 mcg/kg/day via IV infusion over ≤24 hour; see mfr pkg insert for recommended dosage adjustments and timing of administration based on ANC

Patients undergoing autologous peripheral blood progenitor cell collection and therapy: 10 mcg/kg/day via SC injection; administer for at least 4 days before first leukapheresis procedure and continue until last leukapheresis

Patients with severe chronic congenital neutropenia: recommended starting dose is 6 mcg/kg via SC injection bid

Patients with cyclic or idiopathic neutropenia: recommended starting dose is 5 mcg/kg via SC injection once daily

Patients acutely exposed to myelosuppressive doses of radiation (i.e., hematopoietic syndrome of acute radiation syndrome [HSARS]): recommended dose is 10 mcg/kg via SC injection once daily for patients exposed to myelosuppressive doses of radiation; administer as soon as possible after suspected or confirmed exposure to radiation doses greater than 2 gray (Gy); estimate the patient's absorbed radiation dose (i.e., level of radiation exposure) based on information from public health authorities, biodosimetry if available, or clinical findings such as time to onset of vomiting or lymphocyte depletion kinetics; obtain a baseline CBC and then serial CBCs approximately every 3rd day until the ANC remains >1,000/mm^3 for 3 consecutive CBCs; do not delay administration of *filgrastim* if a CBC is not readily available; continue administration until the ANC remains >1,000/mm^3 for 3 consecutive CBCs or exceeds 10,000/mm^3 after a radiation-induced nadir

Neupogen *Vial:* 300 mcg/ml (1 ml), 480 mcg/1.6 ml (1.6 ml), single-dose (preservative-free); *Prefilled syringe:* 300 mcg/0.5 ml (0.5 ml), 480 mcg/0.8 ml (0.8 ml), single-dose (preservative-free)

▷ *filgrastim-aafi* see *filgrastim* (**Neupogen**) above for prescribing information

Nivestym *Vial:* 300 mcg/ml (1 ml), 480 mcg/1.6 ml (1.6 ml), single-dose (preservative-free); *Prefilled syringe:* 300 mcg/0.5 ml (0.5 ml), 480 mcg/0.8 ml (0.8 ml), single-dose (preservative-free)

▷ *filgrastim-ayow* see *filgrastim* (**Neupogen**) above for prescribing information

Releuko *Vial:* 300 mcg/ml (1 ml), 480 mcg/1.6 ml (1.6 ml), single-dose vial (3); *Prefilled syringe:* 300 mcg/0.5 ml (0.5 ml), 480 mcg/0.8ml (0.8 ml), single-dose

▷ *filgrastim-cbqv* see *filgrastim* (**Neupogen**) above for prescribing information

Udenyca *Prefilled syringe:* 6 mg/0.6 ml (0.6 ml), single-dose; the needle cap on the prefilled syringe is not made with natural rubber latex (preservative-free)

(continued)

➤ **filgrastim-sndz** *see* **filgrastim** (Neupogen) above for prescribing information
  Zarxio *Vial:* 300 mcg/ml (1 ml), 480 mcg/1.6 ml (1.6 ml), single-dose (preservative-free); *Prefilled syringe:* 300 mcg/0.5 ml (0.5 ml), 480 mcg/0.8 ml (0.8 ml), single-dose (preservative-free)

➤ **tbo-filgrastim** *Recommended dose:* 5 mcg/kg/day via SC injection; administer the first dose no earlier than 24 hours following myelosuppressive chemotherapy; do not administer within 24 hours prior to chemotherapy
  Granix *Prefilled syringe:* 300 mcg/0.5 ml (0.5 ml), 480 mcg/0.8 ml (0.8 ml), single-dose (preservative-free)
  Comment: Granix *(tbo-filgrastim)* is a leukocyte growth factor indicated for reduction in the duration of severe neutropenia in patients with non-myeloid malignancies receiving myelosuppressive anticancer drugs associated with a clinically significant incidence of febrile neutropenia. **Granix** should be used during pregnancy only if the potential benefit justifies the potential risk to the fetus. It is not known if *tbo-filgrastim* is excreted in human milk or effects on the breastfed infant.

NON-24 SLEEP-WAKE DISORDER

Comment: For other drug options (stimulants, sedative hypnotics), *see* **Insomnia** or *see* **Sleepiness: Excessive, Shift Work Sleep Disorder**

MELATONIN RECEPTOR AGONIST
➤ **tasimelteon** (G) take 1 gelcap before bedtime at the same time every night; do not take with food
  Pediatric: <12 years: not established; ≥12 years: same as adult
    Hetlioz *Gelcap:* 20 mg

OREXIN RECEPTOR ANTAGONIST
➤ **suvorexant** (IV) use lowest effective dose; take 30 minutes before bedtime; do not take if unable to sleep for ≥7 hours; max 20 mg
  Pediatric: <12 years: not recommended; ≥12 years: same as adult
    Belsomra *Tab:* 5, 10, 15, 20 mg (30/blister pck)

OBESITY

Comment: Target body mass index (BMI) is 25-30 (≤27 preferred). Approximately 17% of children and adolescents in the United States aged 2-19 years are obese. Almost 32% of children and adolescents are either overweight or obese, and the proportion of children with severe obesity continues to rise. Obesity in childhood increases the risk of having obesity as an adult and children with obesity are about 5 times more likely to have obesity as adults than children without obesity. The immediate consequences of childhood obesity include increased incidence of psychological issues, asthma, obstructive sleep apnea, orthopedic problems, high blood pressure, elevated lipid levels, and insulin resistance. The U.S. Preventive Services Task Force (USPSTF) recommends that clinicians screen for obesity in children and adolescents 6 years and older and offer or refer them to comprehensive, intensive behavioral interventions (at least 26 hours of contact) to promote improvements in weight status.

STIMULANTS
➤ **amphetamine sulfate** (II)
  Pediatric: <12 years: not recommended; ≥12 years: same as adult
    Evekeo initially 5 mg 30-60 minutes before meals; usually up to 30 mg/day
      Tab: 5, 10 mg

LIPASE INHIBITOR
➤ **orlistat** (G) 1 cap tid 1 hour before or during each main meal containing fat
  Pediatric: <12 years: not recommended; ≥12 years: same as adult
    Alli (OTC) *Cap:* 60 mg
    Xenical *Cap:* 120 mg
  Comment: For use when BMI >30 kg/m^2 or BMI >27 kg/m^2 in the presence of other risk factors (i.e., hypertension, diabetes mellitus, dyslipidemia).

ANOREXIGENICS
Sympathomimetics
Comment: Adverse side effects (ASEs) of sympathomimetics include hypertension, tachycardia, restlessness, insomnia, and dry mouth.

➤ **benzphetamine** (III) initially 25-50 mg daily in the mid-morning or mid-afternoon; may increase to bid-tid as needed
  Pediatric: <12 years: not recommended; ≥12 years: same as adult
    Didrex *Tab:* 50*mg

▷ *naltrexone+bupropion* (G) swallow whole; avoid high-fat meals; initially 10 mg bid; evaluate weight loss after 12 weeks; discontinue if less than 5% weight loss
Pediatric: <18 years: <u>not</u> recommended; ≥18 years: same as adult
    Contrave *Tab:* nal 8 mg+bup 900 mg ext-rel
▷ *methamphetamine* (II) 10-15 mg q AM
Pediatric: <12 years: <u>not</u> recommended; ≥12 years: same as adult
    Desoxyn *Tab:* 5, 10, 15 mg sust-rel
▷ *phendimetrazine* (III)
Pediatric: <12 years: <u>not</u> recommended; ≥12 years: same as adult
    Bontril PDM 35 mg bid-tid 1 hour ac; may reduce to 17.5 mg (1/2 tab)/dose; max 210 mg/day in 3 divided doses
        Tab: 35*mg
    Bontril Slow-Release 105 mg in the AM 30-60 minutes before breakfast
        Cap: 105 mg slow-rel
▷ *phentermine* (IV)(G)
Pediatric: <16 years: <u>not</u> recommended; ≥16 years: same as adult
    Adipex-P 1 cap <u>or</u> tab before breakfast <u>or</u> 1/2 tab bid ac
        Cap: 37.5 mg; *Tab:* 37.5*mg
    Fastin 1 cap before breakfast
        Cap: 30 mg
    Ionamin 1 cap before breakfast <u>or</u> 10-14 hours prior to HS
        Cap: 15, 30 mg
    Suprenza ODT (IV) dissolve 1 tab on top of tongue once daily in the morning, with <u>or</u> without food; use lowest effective dose
        Tab: 15, 30, 37.5 mg orally-disint
Comment: Contraindicated with history of cardiovascular disease (e.g., coronary artery disease, stroke, arrhythmias, congestive heart failure, uncontrolled hypertension, during <u>or</u> within 14 days following the administration of a monoamine oxidase inhibitor (MAOI), hyperthyroidism, glaucoma, agitated states, history of drug abuse, pregnancy, and nursing).

Sympathomimetic+Antiepileptic Combination

▷ *phentermine+topiramate ext-rel* (IV)(G) initially 3.75/23 daily in the AM x 14 days; then increase to 7.5/46 and evaluate weight loss on this dose after 12 weeks; if ≤3% weight loss from baseline, discontinue <u>or</u> increase dose to 11.25/69 x 14 days; then increase to 15/92 and evaluate weight loss on this dose after 12 weeks; if ≤5% weight loss from baseline, discontinue by taking a dose every other day for at least 1 week prior to stopping; max 7.5/46 for moderate-to-severe renal impairment <u>or</u> moderate hepatic impairment.
Pediatric: <12 years: <u>not</u> recommended; ≥12 years with BMI in the ≥95th percentile standardized for age and sex: same as adult
    Qsymia
      Cap: **Qsymia 3.75/23** phen 3.75 mg+topir 23 mg ext-rel
           Qsymia 7.5/46 phen 7.5 mg+topir 46 mg ext-rel
           Qsymia 11.25/69 phen 11.25 mg+topir 69 mg ext-rel
           Qsymia 15/92 phen 15 mg+topir 92 mg ext-rel
Comment: Qsymia is a combination of *phentermine*, a sympathomimetic amine anorectic, and *topiramate*, indicated as an adjunct to a reduced-calorie diet and increased physical activity for chronic weight management in (1) adults with an initial body mass index (BMI) of ≥30 kg/m^2 (obese) <u>or</u> 27 kg/m^2 (overweight) in the presence of at least one weight-related comorbidity, such as hypertension, type 2 diabetes mellitus (T2DM), <u>or</u> dyslipidemia; <u>and</u> (2) pediatric patients ≥12 years of age with an initial BMI in the ≥95th percentile standardized for age and sex (obese). The most common adverse reactions in adults (incidence ≥5% and at least 1.5 times placebo) have been paresthesia, dizziness, dysgeusia, insomnia, constipation, and dry mouth. The most common adverse reactions in patients ≥12 years (incidence ≥4% and greater than placebo) have been depression, dizziness, arthralgia, pyrexia, influenza, and ligament sprain. Contraindications to **Qsymia** include pregnancy, glaucoma, hyperthyroidism, either taking <u>or</u> within 14 days of stopping MAOIs, known hypersensitivity to any component of **Qsymia,** <u>or</u> idiosyncrasy to sympathomimetic amines. CNS depressants, including alcohol, may potentiate CNS depressant effects of **Qsymia.** Non-potassium-sparing diuretics may potentiate hypokalemia; monitor potassium before and during treatment. The effect of **Qsymia** on cardiovascular morbidity and mortality has <u>not</u> been established. Safety and effectiveness of **Qsymia** in combination with other products intended for weight loss, including prescription and OTC drugs, and herbal preparations, have <u>not</u> been established. Monitor heart rate, especially in those with cardiac <u>or</u> cerebrovascular disease. Monitor for depression <u>or</u> suicidal thoughts <u>or</u> suicidal behavior; discontinue **Qsymia** if symptoms develop. Acute myopia and secondary angle closure glaucoma have been reported; immediately discontinue **Qsymia** if symptoms develop (e.g., if visual field defects occur). Consider dosage reduction <u>or</u> discontinuation for clinically significant <u>or</u> persistent mood <u>or</u> sleep disorder symptoms. **Qsymia** may cause disturbances in attention <u>or</u> memory, <u>or</u> speech/language problems. Caution patients about driving a motor vehicle <u>or</u> other operating hazardous

(continued)

machinery. **Qsymia** may slow linear growth; consider dose reduction or discontinuation if pediatric patients are not growing or gaining height as expected. Monitor electrolytes before and during treatment. If persistent metabolic acidosis develops, reduce dose or discontinue **Qsymia**. Measure creatinine before and during treatment. For persistent creatinine elevations, reduce dosage or discontinue **Qsymia**. **Qsymia** should be discontinued at the first sign of a rash, unless the rash is clearly not drug-related. **Qsymia** is embryo/fetal toxic. Animal reproduction studies have not been conducted with *phentermine*. Limited data from studies conducted with the *phentermine/topiramate* combination indicate that *phentermine* alone was not teratogenic but resulted in lower body weight and reduced survival of offspring. Developmental toxicity, including teratogenicity, has occurred at clinically relevant doses in multiple animal species in which *topiramate* was administered during the period of organogenesis. Therefore, a negative pregnancy test is recommended before initiating **Qsymia** and monthly during therapy; advise the use of effective contraception. Diarrhea and somnolence have been reported in breastfed infants with maternal use of *topiramate*. There are no data on the effects of *phentermine* in breastfed infants. Because of the potential for serious adverse reactions, including changes in sleep, irritability, hypertension, vomiting, tremor, and weight loss in breastfed infants with maternal use of *phentermine*, advise patients that breastfeeding is not recommended. **Qsymia** is available through a limited program under a Risk Evaluation and Mitigation Strategy (REMS).

Serotonin 2C Receptor Agonist
▶ *lorcaserin* (G) 10 mg bid; discontinue if 5% weight loss is not achieved by week 12
  Pediatric: <18 years: not recommended; ≥18 years: same as adult
    Belviq *Tab:* 10 mg film-coat
    Comment: **Belviq** is indicated as an adjunct to a reduced-calorie diet and increased physical activity for chronic weight management in adults with an initial BMI of 30 kg/m² or greater (obese) or 27 kg/m² or greater (overweight) in the presence of at least one weight-related comorbid condition (e.g., hypertension, dyslipidemia, T2DM). Serotonin 2C receptor agonists interact with serotonergic drugs (selective serotonin reuptake inhibitors [SSRIs], serotonin norepinephrine reuptake inhibitors [SNRIs], MAOIs, triptans, *bupropion, dextromethorphan, St. John's wort*); therefore, use with extreme caution due to the risk of *serotonin syndrome*.

GLUCAGON-LIKE PEPTIDE-1 (GLP-1) RECEPTOR AGONIST
▶ *liraglutide* administer SC in the upper arm, abdomen, or thigh once daily; escalate dose gradually over 5 weeks to 3 mg SC daily; *Week 1:* 0.6 mg SC daily; *Week 2:* 1.2 mg SC daily; *Week 3:* 1.8 mg SC daily; *Week 4:* 2.4 mg SC daily; *Week 5:* 3 mg SC daily
  Pediatric: <12 years: not recommended; ≥12 years, >60 kg, initial BMI ≥30 kg/m²: same as adult
    Saxenda *Soln for SC inj:* 6 mg/ml multidose prefilled pen (3 ml; 3, 5 pens/carton)
    Comment: **Saxenda** is indicated as an adjunct to a reduced-calorie diet and increased physical activity for chronic weight management in adults with an initial BMI of 30 kg/m² or greater (obese) or 27 kg/m² or greater (overweight) in the presence of at least one weight-related comorbid condition (e.g., hypertension, dyslipidemia, T2DM). Not indicated for treatment of T2DM. Do not use with **Victoza**, other glucagon-like peptide-1 (GLP-1) receptor agonists, or insulin. Contraindicated with personal or family history of medullary thyroid carcinoma (MTC) and multiple endocrine neoplasia syndrome (MENS) type 2. Monitor for signs/symptoms of pancreatitis. Discontinue if gastroparesis or renal or hepatic impairment occurs.
▶ *semaglutide* Administer once weekly, on the same day each week, at any time of day, with or without meals; inject SC in the upper arm, abdomen, or thigh or upper arm; in patients with T2DM, monitor blood glucose prior to starting and during treatment; *Starting dose:* 0.25 mg once weekly x 4 weeks; *Step up the dose:* at 4-week intervals until a dose of 2.4 mg is reached; *Maintenance and max:* 2.4 mg SC once weekly; rotate sites
  Pediatric: <12 years: not recommended; ≥12 years with an initial BMI in the ≥95th percentile standardized for age and sex: same as adult
    Wegovy *Pre-filled pen:* 0.25, 0.5, 1, 1.7, 2.4 mg, single-dose
    Comment: **Wegovy** is a GLP-1 receptor agonist indicated as an adjunct to diet and exercise for chronic weight management in (1) adult patients with an initial BMI of ≥30 kg/m² (obese) or 27 kg/m² (overweight) in the presence of at least one weight-related comorbidity, such as hypertension, T2DM, or dyslipidemia; and (2) pediatric patients ≥12 years of age with an initial BMI in the ≥95th percentile standardized for age and sex (obesity). The most common adverse reactions (incidence ≥5%) in adults and pediatric patients ≥12 years of age have been nausea, diarrhea, vomiting, constipation, abdominal pain, headache, fatigue, dyspepsia, dizziness, abdominal distension, eructation, hypoglycemia in patients with T2DM, flatulence, gastroenteritis, gastroesophageal reflux disease, and nasopharyngitis. *Boxed Warning:* In rodents, *semaglutide* causes thyroid C-cell tumors at clinically relevant exposures. It is unknown whether **Wegovy** causes thyroid C-cell tumors, including medullary thyroid carcinoma (MTC), in humans as the human relevance of *semaglutide*-induced rodent thyroid C-cell tumors has not been determined. **Wegovy** is contraindicated in patients with a personal or family history of MTC or in patients with multiple endocrine neoplasia syndrome (MENS) type 2. Counsel patients regarding the potential risk of MTC and symptoms of thyroid tumors. **Wegovy** is also contraindicated in patients

with known hypersensitivity to *semaglutide* or any of the excipients in **Wegovy**. **Wegovy** should not be used in combination with other *semaglutide*-containing products or any other GLP-1 receptor agonist. Safety and efficacy of co-administration with other products for weight loss have not been established. **Wegovy** has not been studied in patients with a history of pancreatitis. Acute pancreatitis has occurred in clinical trials; discontinue **Wegovy** promptly if pancreatitis is suspected and do not restart if pancreatitis is confirmed. Acute gallbladder disease has occurred in clinical trials; if cholelithiasis is suspected, gallbladder studies and clinical follow-up are indicated. Concomitant use of **Wegovy** with an insulin secretagogue or insulin may increase the risk of hypoglycemia, including severe hypoglycemia. Reducing the dose of insulin secretagogue or insulin may be necessary. Inform all patients of the risk of hypoglycemia and signs and symptoms of hypoglycemia. Acute kidney injury (AKI) has occurred; monitor renal function when initiating or escalating doses of **Wegovy** in patients reporting severe adverse gastrointestinal reactions as well as those with renal impairment who report severe adverse gastrointestinal reactions. Anaphylactic reactions and angioedema have been reported postmarketing; discontinue **Wegovy** if suspected and promptly seek medical advice. Diabetic retinopathy complications in patients with T2DM have been reported in trials with *semaglutide*; monitor patients with a history of diabetic retinopathy. Monitor heart rate at regular intervals. *Suicidal behavior and ideation:* Monitor for depression or suicidal thoughts or behavior; discontinue **Wegovy** if symptoms develop. **Wegovy** delays gastric emptying, which may impact absorption of concomitantly administered oral medications. **Wegovy** may cause fetal harm. Advise females and males of reproductive potential to use effective contraception during treatment with **Wegovy** and to discontinue **Wegovy** at least 2 months before a planned pregnancy because of the long half-life of *semaglutide*. If pregnancy is recognized, discontinue **Wegovy**. In animal studies, *semaglutide* was present in the milk of lactating rats. There are no data on the presence of *semaglutide* or its metabolites in human milk or effects on the breastfed infant. Advise females that when a drug is present in animal milk, it is likely that the drug will be present in human milk, and the developmental and health benefits of breastfeeding should be considered along with the mother's clinical need for **Wegovy** and any potential adverse effects on the breastfed infant from **Wegovy** or from the underlying maternal condition.

OBSESSIVE-COMPULSIVE DISORDER (OCD)

SELECTIVE SEROTONIN REUPTAKE INHIBITORS (SSRIs)
Comment: Co-administration of SSRIs with tricyclic antidepressants (TCAs) requires extreme caution. Concomitant use of monoamine oxidase inhibitors (MAOIs) and SSRIs is absolutely contraindicated. Avoid other serotonergic drugs. A potentially fatal adverse event is *serotonin syndrome*, caused by serotonin excess. Milder symptoms require healthcare provider intervention to avert severe symptoms which can be rapidly fatal without urgent/emergent medical care. Symptoms include restlessness, agitation, confusion, hallucinations, tachycardia, hypertension, dilated pupils, muscle twitching, muscle rigidity, loss of muscle coordination, diaphoresis, diarrhea, headache, shivering, piloerection, hyperpyrexia, cardiac arrhythmias, seizures, loss of consciousness, coma, and death. Abrupt withdrawal or interruption of treatment with an antidepressant medication is sometimes associated with an *antidepressant discontinuation syndrome (ADS)*, which may be mediated by gradually tapering the drug over a period of 2 weeks or longer, depending on the dose strength and length of treatment. Common symptoms of the *serotonin discontinuation syndrome* include flu-like symptoms (nausea, vomiting, diarrhea, headaches, sweating), sleep disturbances (insomnia, nightmares, constant sleepiness), mood disturbances (dysphoria, anxiety, agitation), cognitive disturbances (mental confusion, hyperarousal), and sensory and movement disturbances (imbalance, tremors, vertigo, dizziness, and electric-shock-like sensations in the brain, often described by sufferers as "brain zaps").

▷ *fluoxetine* (G)
   Prozac initially 20 mg daily; may increase after 1 week; doses >20 mg/day may be divided into AM and noon doses; max 80 mg/day
   Pediatric: <8 years: not recommended; 8-17 years: initially 10 mg/day; may increase after 2 weeks to 20 mg/day, range 20-60 mg/day; range for lower weight children 20-30 mg/day; >17 years: same as adult
      Cap: 10, 20, 40 mg; *Tab:* 30*, 60*mg; *Oral soln:* 20 mg/5 ml (4 oz) (mint)
   Prozac Weekly following daily *fluoxetine* therapy at 20 mg/day for 13 weeks; may initiate **Prozac Weekly** 7 days after the last 20 mg *fluoxetine* dose
   Pediatric: <12 years: not recommended; ≥12 years: same as adult
      Cap: 90 mg ent-coat del-rel pellets
▷ *fluvoxamine* (G)
   Luvox initially 50 mg q HS; adjust in 50 mg increments at 4 to 7-day intervals; range 100-300 mg/day; over 100 mg/day, divide into 2 doses giving the larger dose at HS
   Pediatric: <8 years: not recommended; 8-17 years: initially 25 mg q HS; adjust in 25 mg increments q 4-7 days; usual range 50-200 mg/day; over 50 mg/day, divide into 2 doses giving the larger dose at HS
      Tab: 25, 50*, 100*mg
   Luvox CR initially 100 mg once daily at HS; may increase by 50 mg increments at 1-week intervals; max 300 mg/day; swallow whole; do not crush or chew
   Pediatric: <18 years: not recommended; ≥18 years: same as adult
      Cap: 100, 150 mg ext-rel

(continued)

▷ **paroxetine maleate (G)**
  Pediatric: <12 years: <u>not</u> recommended; ≥12 years: same as adult
    Paxil initially 20 mg daily in the AM; may increase by 10 mg/day at weekly intervals as needed; max 60 mg/day
      Tab: 10*, 20*, 30, 40 mg
    Paxil CR initially 25 mg daily in the AM; may increase by 12.5 mg at weekly intervals as needed; max 62.5 mg/day
      Tab: 12.5, 25, 37.5 mg cont-rel ent-coat
    Paxil Oral Suspension initially 20 mg daily in AM; may increase by 10 mg/day at weekly intervals as needed; max 60 mg/day
      Oral susp: 10 mg/5 ml (250 ml) (orange)
▷ **paroxetine mesylate (G)** initially 7.5 mg daily in AM; may increase by 10 mg/day at weekly intervals as needed; max 60 mg/day
  Pediatric: <12 years: <u>not</u> recommended; ≥12 years: same as adult
    Brisdelle *Cap:* 7.5 mg
▷ **sertraline** initially 50 mg daily; increase at 1 week intervals if needed; max 200 mg daily
  Pediatric: <6 years: <u>not</u> recommended; 6-12 years: initially 25 mg daily; max 200 mg/day; 13-17 years: initially 50 mg daily; max 200 mg/day; >17 years: same as adult
    Zoloft *Tab:* 15*, 50*, 100*mg; *Oral conc:* 20 mg/ml (60 ml [dilute just before administering in 4 oz water, ginger ale, lemon-lime soda, lemonade, <u>or</u> orange juice]) (alcohol 12%)

TRICYCLIC ANTIDEPRESSANTS (TCAs)

▷ **clomipramine (G)** initially 25 mg daily in divided doses; gradually increase to 100 mg during first 2 weeks; max 250 mg/day; total maintenance dose may be given at HS
  Pediatric: <10 years: <u>not</u> recommended; ≥10 years: initially 25 mg daily in divided doses; gradually increase; max 3 mg/kg <u>or</u> 100 mg, whichever is smaller
    Anafranil *Cap:* 25, 50, 75 mg
▷ **imipramine (G)**
    Tofranil initially 75 mg/day; max 200 mg/day
    Pediatric: adolescents initially 30-40 mg/day; max 100 mg/day
      Tab: 10, 25, 50 mg
    Tofranil PM initially 75 mg/day; max 200 mg/day
    Pediatric: <12 years: <u>not</u> recommended; ≥12 years: same as adult
      Cap: 75, 100, 125, 150 mg

ONYCHOMYCOSIS (FUNGAL NAIL)

ORAL AGENTS

▷ **griseofulvin, microsize (G)** 1 gm daily for at least 4 months for fingernails and at least 6 months for toenails
  Pediatric: 5 mg/lb/day; *see* Appendix BB.25. griseofulvin, microsize (G) (Grifulvin V Suspension) *for dose by weight*
    Grifulvin V *Tab:* 250, 500 mg; *Oral susp:* 125 mg/5 ml (120 ml; alcohol 0.02%)
▷ **griseofulvin, ultramicrosize** 750 mg in a single <u>or</u> divided doses for at least 4 months for fingernails and at least 6 months for toenails
  Pediatric: <2 years: <u>not</u> recommended; ≥2 years: 3.3 mg/lb in a single <u>or</u> divided doses
    Gris-PEG *Tab:* 125, 250 mg
▷ **itraconazole (G)** 200 mg daily x 12 consecutive weeks for toenails; 200 mg bid x 1 week, off 3 weeks, then 200 mg bid x 1 additional week for fingernails
  Pediatric: <12 years: <u>not</u> recommended; ≥12 years: same as adult
    Sporanox *Cap:* 100 mg; *Soln:* 10 mg/ml (150 ml) (cherry-caramel)
    Pulse Pack: 100 mg caps (7/pck)
▷ **terbinafine (G)** 250 mg daily x 6 weeks for fingernails; 250 mg daily x 12 weeks for toenails
  Pediatric: <12 years: <u>not</u> recommended; ≥12 years: same as adult
    Lamisil *Tab:* 250 mg

TOPICAL AGENTS

Comment: File and trim nail while nail is free from drug. Remove unattached infected nail as frequently as monthly. For use with mild-to-moderate onychomycosis of the fingernails and toenails without lunula involvement due to *Trichophyton rubrum* immunocompetent patients as part of a comprehensive treatment program. For use on nails and adjacent skin <u>only</u>. Apply evenly to entire onycholytic nail and surrounding 5 mm of skin daily, preferably at HS <u>or</u> 8 hours before washing; apply to nail bed, hyponychium, and under surface of nail plate when it is free of the nail bed; apply over previous coats, then remove with alcohol once per week; treat for up to 48 weeks.

▷ **ciclopirox**
  Pediatric: <12 years: <u>not</u> established; ≥12 years: same as adult
    Penlac Nail Lacquer *Topical soln (lacquer):* 8% (6.6 ml w. applicator)
▷ **efinaconazole (G)**
  Pediatric: <12 years: <u>not</u> established; ≥12 years: same as adult
    Jublia *Topical soln:* 5% (10 ml w. brush applicator)

▷ *tavaborole* (G)
  Pediatric: <12 years: <u>not</u> established; ≥12 years: same as adult
    Kerydin *Topical soln:* 10% (10 ml w. dropper)

OPHTHALMIA NEONATORUM: CHLAMYDIAL

PROPHYLAXIS
▷ *erythromycin* ophthalmic ointment 0.5-1 cm ribbon into lower conjunctival sac of each eye x 1 application
    Ilotycin Ophthalmic Ointment *Ophth oint:* 5 mg/gm (1/8 oz)
    Comment: The following treatment regimens are published in the **2021 CDC Sexually Transmitted Diseases Treatment Guidelines.** Treatment regimens are presented by generic drug name first, followed by information about brands and dose forms.

RECOMMENDED TREATMENT REGIMENS
Regimen 1
▷ *erythromycin base* 50 mg/kg/day in 4 doses x 14 days

Regimen 2
▷ *erythromycin ethylsuccinate* 50 mg/kg/day in 4 doses x 14 days; *see* Appendix BB.21: *erythromycin ethylsuccinate* (E.E.S. Suspension, EryPed Drops/Suspension) *for dose by weight*

DRUG BRANDS AND DOSE FORMS
▷ *erythromycin base* (G)
    Ery-Tab *Tab:* 250, 333, 500 mg ent-coat
    PCE *Tab:* 333, 500 mg
▷ *erythromycin ethylsuccinate* (G)
    EryPed *Oral susp:* 200 mg/5 ml (100, 200 ml) (fruit), 400 mg/5 ml (60, 100, 200 ml) (banana); *Oral drops:* 200, 400 mg/5 ml (50 ml) (fruit); *Chew tab:* 200 mg wafer (fruit)
    E.E.S. *Oral susp:* 200, 400 mg/5 ml (100 ml) (fruit)
    E.E.S. Granules *Oral susp:* 200 mg/5 ml (100, 200 ml) (cherry)

OPHTHALMIA NEONATORUM: GONOCOCCAL

Comment: The following prophylaxis and treatment regimens for gonococcal conjunctivitis are published in the **2021 CDC Sexually Transmitted Diseases Treatment Guidelines.**

PROPHYLAXIS
▷ *erythromycin 0.5%* ophthalmic ointment 0.5-1 cm ribbon into lower conjunctival sac of each eye x 1 application
    Ilotycin Ophthalmic Ointment *Ophth oint:* 5 mg/gm (1/8 oz)

TREATMENT
▷ *ceftriaxone* (G) 25-50 mg/kg IV <u>or</u> IM in a single dose, <u>not</u> to exceed 125 mg
    Rocephin *Vial:* 250, 500 mg; 1, 2 gm

OPIOID DEPENDENCE, OPIOID USE DISORDER (OUD), OPIOID WITHDRAWAL SYNDROME

Comment: Safety labeling for all immediate-release (IR) opioids has been issued by the FDA. The *Boxed Warning* includes serious risks of misuse, abuse, addiction, overdose, and death. The dosing section offers clear steps regarding administration and patient monitoring, including initial dose, dose changes, and the abrupt cessation of treatment in physical dependence. Chronic maternal use of opioids during pregnancy can lead to potentially life-threatening neonatal opioid withdrawal. The American Pain Society (APS) has released new evidence-based clinical practice guidelines that include 32 recommendations related to postop pain management in adults and children. The Transmucosal Immediate Release Fentanyl (TIRF) Risk Evaluation and Mitigation Strategy (REMS) Program is an FDA-required program designed to ensure informed risk-benefit decisions before initiating treatment and while patients are treated to ensure appropriate use of TIRF medicines. The purpose of the TIRF REMS Access Program is to mitigate the risk of misuse, abuse, addiction, overdose and serious complications due to medication errors with the use of TIRF medicines. You must enroll in the TIRF REMS Access Program to prescribe, dispense, <u>or</u> distribute TIRF medicines. To register, call the TIRF REMS Access Program at 1-866-822-1483 <u>or</u> register online at https://www.tirfremsaccess.com/TirfUI/rems/home.action.

SELECTIVE ALPHA 2-ADRENERGIC RECEPTOR AGONIST
Comment: Lucemyra *(lofexidine)* is the first FDA-approved non-opioid treatment for the management of opioid withdrawal symptoms, for the mitigation of withdrawal symptoms to facilitate abrupt discontinuation of opioids in adults. While **Lucemyra** may lessen the severity of withdrawal symptoms, it may <u>not</u> completely prevent them. This oral selective alpha 2-adrenergic receptor agonist reduces the release of norepinephrine. The actions of norepinephrine in the autonomic nervous system are believed to play a role in many of the symptoms of opioid withdrawal and is <u>only</u> approved for treatment for up to 14 days.

(continued)

▷ *lofexidine* 0.18 mg x 3 tabs taken orally 4 qid at 5 to 6-hour intervals; max 14 days with dosing guided by symptoms; discontinue with a gradual dose reduction over 2 to 4 days
Pediatric: <17 years: not established; ≥17 years: same as adult
    Lucemyra *Tab:* 0.18 mg
Comment: Lucemyra is not a treatment for opioid use disorder (OUD), per se, but can be used as part of a broader, long-term treatment plan for managing OUD. The most common side effects from treatment with **Lucemyra** include hypotension, bradycardia, somnolence, sedation, and dizziness. **Lucemyra** has also been associated with a few cases of syncope. *Methadone* and **Lucemyra** both prolong the QT interval. Therefore, ECG monitoring is recommended when used concomitantly. Concomitant use of oral *naltrexone* with **Lucemyra** may reduce efficacy of oral *naltrexone*. Concomitant use of *paroxetine* has resulted in increased plasma levels of **Lucemyra**. Monitor for symptoms of orthostasis and bradycardia with concomitant use of CYP2D6 inhibitors. The safety of **Lucemyra** in pregnant females has not been established. There is no information regarding the presence of **Lucemyra** or its metabolites in human milk or effects on the breastfed infant.

OPIOID AGONISTS
Methadone Detoxification and Methadone Maintenance
Comment: *Methadone* is not indicated as an as-needed (prn) analgesic. For use in chronic moderately severe-to-severe pain management (e.g., hospice care).

▷ *methadone* (II)(G) a single dose of 20 to 30 mg may be sufficient to suppress withdrawal syndrome; *Narcotic detoxification:* 15-40 mg daily in decreasing doses, not to exceed 21 days; *Narcotic maintenance:* >21 days; see mfr pkg insert; clinical stability is most commonly achieved at doses between 80 to 120 mg/day; monitor patients with periodic ECGs (e.g., risk of lethal QT interval prolongation, *torsades de pointes*)
Pediatric: <12 years: not recommended; ≥12 years: same as adult
    Dolophine *Tab:* 5, 10 mg; *Dispersible tab:* 40 mg (dissolve in 120 ml orange juice or other citrus drink); *Oral soln:* 5, 10 mg/ml; *Oral conc:* 10 mg/ml; *Syr:* 10 mg/30 ml; *Vial:* 10 mg/ml (200 mg/20 ml multidose) for injection
Comment: *Methadone* administration is allowed only by approved providers with strict state and federal regulations (as stipulated in 42 CFR 8.12). *Boxed Warning: Dolophine* exposes users to risks of addiction, abuse, and misuse, which can lead to overdose and death. Assess each patient's risk and monitor regularly for development of these behaviors and conditions. Serious, life-threatening, or fatal respiratory depression may occur. The peak respiratory depressant effect of *methadone* occurs later and persists longer than the peak analgesic effect. Accidental ingestion, especially by children, can result in fatal overdose. QT interval prolongation and serious arrhythmia (torsades de pointes) have occurred during treatment with *methadone*. Closely monitor patients with risk factors for development of prolonged QT interval, a history of cardiac conduction abnormalities, and those taking medications affecting cardiac conduction. Neonatal opioid withdrawal syndrome (NOWS) is an expected and treatable outcome of use of *methadone* during pregnancy. NOWS may be life-threatening if not recognized and treated in the neonate. The balance between the risks of NOWS and the benefits of maternal *methadone* use should be considered and the patient advised of the risk of NOWS so that appropriate planning for management of the neonate can occur. *Methadone* has been detected in human milk. Concomitant use with CYP3A4, 2B6, 2C19, 2C9, or 2D6 inhibitors or discontinuation of concomitantly used CYP3A4 2B6, 2C19, or 2C9 inducers can result in a fatal overdose of *methadone*. Concomitant use of opioids with benzodiazepines or other central nervous system (CNS) depressants, including alcohol, may result in profound sedation, respiratory depression, coma, and death.

OPIOID ANTAGONIST
▷ *naltrexone*
Pediatric: <12 years: not established; ≥12 years: same as adult
    ReVia 50 mg daily
      Tab: 50 mg
    Vivitrol (G) 380 mg IM once monthly; alternate buttocks
      Vial: 380 mg

PARTIAL OPIOID AGONIST
▷ *buprenorphine extended-release for subcutaneous injection* preparation and administration are required by an authorized qualified healthcare provider; administer slowly into the subcutaneous tissue of the upper arm, abdomen, buttock, or thigh; serious harm or death could result if administered IV; **Brixadi (weekly)** and **Brixadi (monthly)** are different formulations; therefore, doses of **Brixadi (weekly)** cannot be combined to yield an equivalent **Brixadi (monthly)** dose; strongly consider prescribing *naloxone* at the time **Brixadi** is initiated or renewed because patients being treated for OUD have the potential for relapse, putting them at risk for opioid overdose; injection sites for **Brixadi (weekly)** should be alternated/rotated for each SC injection; see mfr pkg insert for full prescribing information for preparation and administration
Pediatric: safety and efficacy not established
    Brixadi (monthly) *Prefilled syringe:* 64 mg/0.18 ml, 96 mg/0.27 ml, 128 mg/0.36 ml, single-dose, ext-rel soln w. 23 g, 1/2 inch needle, for once-monthly SC administration (natural rubber latex)

Brixadi (weekly) *Prefilled syringe*: 8 mg/0.16 ml, 16 mg/0.32 ml, 24 mg/0.48 ml, 32 mg/0.64 ml, single-dose, ext-rel soln w. 23 g, 1/2 inch needle, for once-weekly SC administration (natural rubber latex)
Comment: **Brixadi** is an injectable extended-release form of *buprenorphine*, a partial opioid agonist, indicated for the treatment of moderate-to-severe OUD in patients who have initiated treatment with a single dose of a transmucosal *buprenorphine* product or who are already being treated with *buprenorphine*. **Brixadi** should be used as part of a complete treatment plan that includes counseling and psychosocial support. **Brixadi** is only available through a restricted program called the Brixadi Risk Evaluation and Mitigation Strategy (REMS) program. Healthcare settings and pharmacies that order and dispense **Brixadi** must be certified in the Brixadi REMS program and comply with the REMS requirements. Adverse reactions commonly associated with **Brixadi** administration (incidence >5%) were injection site pain, headache, constipation, nausea, injection site erythema, injection site pruritus, insomnia, and urinary tract infection. *Buprenorphine* can be abused in a manner similar to other opioids; monitor patients for conditions indicative of diversion or progression of opioid dependence and addictive behaviors. Life-threatening respiratory depression and death have occurred in association with *buprenorphine*. Monitor geriatric patients for sedation and respiratory depression and treat as appropriate. Warn patients of the potential danger of self-administration of *benzodiazepines* or other CNS depressants while under treatment with **Brixadi**. Neonatal opioid withdrawal syndrome (NOWS) is an expected and treatable outcome of prolonged use of opioids during pregnancy. If adrenal insufficiency is diagnosed, treat with physiologic replacement of corticosteroids, and wean the patient off **Brixadi**. There is risk of opioid withdrawal syndrome (OWS) with abrupt discontinuation of *buprenorphine*: If treatment with **Brixadi** is discontinued, monitor patients for withdrawal and treat as appropriate. There is risk of hepatitis and other hepatic events; monitor liver function tests prior to and during treatment and treat as appropriate. **Brixadi** is not recommended for patients with moderate-to-severe hepatic impairment. The packaging of this product contains natural rubber latex which may cause allergic reactions; assess for latex allergy prior to initiation of treatment with **Brixadi**; if latex allergy develops, initiate appropriate treatment to wean from **Brixadi**. There is risk of OWS in patients dependent on full agonist opioids; administer a test dose of transmucosal *buprenorphine* and monitor for precipitated withdrawal before initiating **Brixadi**. Treat acute pain with a non-opioid analgesic whenever possible. If opioid therapy is required, monitor patients closely because higher doses may be required for analgesic effect. Monitor patients starting or ending CYP3A4 inhibitors or inducers for potential over- or underdosing. If concomitant use of a serotonergic drug is warranted, monitor for serotonin syndrome, particularly during treatment initiation and during dose adjustment of the serotonergic drug. Studies have been conducted to evaluate neonatal outcomes in women exposed to *buprenorphine* during pregnancy. Limited data from trials, observational studies, case series, and case reports on *buprenorphine* use in pregnancy do not indicate an increased risk of major malformations specifically due to *buprenorphine*. Several factors may complicate the interpretation of investigations of the children of females who take *buprenorphine* during pregnancy, including maternal use of illicit drugs, late presentation for prenatal care, infection, poor compliance, poor nutrition, and psychosocial circumstances. Interpretation of data is complicated further by the lack of information on untreated opioid-dependent pregnant women, who would be the most appropriate group for comparison. Rather, women on another form of opioid medication-assisted treatment, or women in the general population are generally used as the comparison group. However, women in these comparison groups may be different from women prescribed *buprenorphine*-containing products with respect to maternal factors that may lead to poor pregnancy outcomes. In a multicenter, double-blind, randomized, controlled trial (Maternal Opioid Treatment: Human Experimental Research [MOTHER]) designed primarily to assess neonatal opioid withdrawal effects, opioid-dependent pregnant women were randomized to *buprenorphine* (n = 86) or *methadone* (n = 89) treatment, with enrollment at an average gestational age of 18.7 weeks in both groups. A total of 28 of the 86 women in the *buprenorphine* group (33%) and 16 of the 89 women in the *methadone* group (18%) discontinued treatment before the end of pregnancy. Among women who remained in treatment until delivery, there was no difference between *buprenorphine*-treated and *methadone*-treated groups in the number of neonates requiring NOWS treatment or in the peak severity of NOWS. *Buprenorphine*-exposed neonates required less *morphine* (mean total dose, 1.1 mg vs 10.4 mg), had shorter hospital stays (10.0 days vs 17.5 days), and shorter duration of treatment for NOWS (4.1 days vs 9.9 days) compared to the *methadone*-exposed group. There were no differences between groups in other primary outcomes (neonatal head circumference) or secondary outcomes (weight and length at birth, preterm birth, gestational age at delivery, and 1-minute and 5-minute Apgar scores), or in the rates of maternal or neonatal adverse events. Advise mothers that *buprenorphine* passes into the mother's milk. Based on two studies in 13 lactating women maintained on sublingual *buprenorphine* treatment, *buprenorphine* and its metabolite *norbuprenorphine* were present in low levels in human milk. Available data have not shown adverse reactions in breastfed infants. Development and health benefits of breastfeeding should be considered along with the mother's clinical need for *buprenorphine* treatment and any potential adverse effects on the breastfed infant from the drug or from the underlying maternal condition. See the mfr pkg insert for more in-depth discussion of human and animal studies of opioid use in the setting of pregnancy and lactation. To report suspected adverse reactions, contact Braeburn at 833-274-9234 or FDA at 800-FDA-1088 or www.fda.gov/medwatch.

OPIOID PARTIAL AGONIST-ANTAGONIST

Comment: Belbuca, Butrans, Probuphine, Sublocade, and Subutex maintenance are allowed only by approved providers with strict state and federal regulations. These drugs are potentiated by CYP3A4 inhibitors (e.g., azole antifungals, macrolides, HIV protease inhibitors) and antagonized by CYP3A4 inducers (monitor for opioid withdrawal). Concomitant non-nucleoside reverse transcriptase inhibitors (NNRTIs) (e.g., *efavirenz, nevirapine, etravirine, delavirdine*) or protease inhibitors (e.g., *atazanavir* with or without *ritonavir*): monitor. There is risk of respiratory or CNS depression with concomitant opioid analgesics, general anesthetics, benzodiazepines, phenothiazines, other tranquilizers, sedative/hypnotics, alcohol, or other CNS depressants. There is risk of *serotonin syndrome* with concomitant selective serotonin reuptake inhibitors (SSRI), serotonin norepinephrine reuptake inhibitor (SNRI), and tricyclic antidepressants (TCAs), 5-HT3 receptor antagonists, *mirtazapine, trazodone, tramadol*, and monoamine oxidase inhibitors (MAOIs).

▷ *buprenorphine* (III)

Belbuca apply buccal film to inside of cheek; do not chew or swallow; *Opioid-naïve:* initially 75 mcg once daily-q 12 hours x at least 4 days; then, increase to 150 mcg q 12 hours; may increase in increments of 150 mcg q 12 hours no sooner than every 4 days; max 900 mcg q 12 hours; see mfr pkg insert for conversion from other opioids; *Severe hepatic impairment or oral mucositis:* reduce initial and titration doses by half
Pediatric: <12 years: not established; ≥12 years: same as adult
  Buccal film: 75, 150, 300, 450, 600, 750, 900 mcg (60/pck) (peppermint)
Butrans Transdermal System apply 1 patch to clean, dry, hairless, intact skin on the upper outer arm, upper chest, upper back, or side of chest every 7 days; rotate sites and do not re-use a site for at least 21 days; *Opioid-naïve or oral morphine <30 mg/day or equivalent:* one 5 mcg/hour patch; *Converting from oral morphine equivalents 30-80 mg/day:* taper current opioids for up to 7 days to ≤30 mg/day oral morphine equivalents before starting; then initiate with 10 mcg/hour patch; may use a short-acting analgesic until efficacy is attained; increase dose only after exposure to previous dose x at least 72 hours; max one 20 mcg/hour patch/week; *Conversion from higher opioid doses:* not recommended
Pediatric: <12 years: not established; ≥12 years: same as adult
  Transdermal patch: 5, 7.5, 10, 15, 20 mcg/hour (4/pck)
Probuphine initiate when stable on *buprenorphine* ≤8 mg/day; insertion site is the inner side of the upper arm; 4 implants are intended to be in place for 6 months; remove the implants by the end of the 6th month and insert 4 new implants on the same day in the contralateral arm; if a new implant is not inserted on the same day as removal of a previous implant, maintain the patient on the previous dose of transmucosal *buprenorphine* (i.e., the dose from which the patient was transferred to **Probuphine** treatment).
Pediatric: <16 years: not established; ≥16 years: same as adult
  Subdermal implant: 74.2 mg of *buprenorphine* (equivalent to 80 mg of *buprenorphine hydrochloride*)
Comment: Healthcare providers who prescribe, perform insertions and/or perform removals of **Probuphine** must successfully complete a live training program and demonstrate procedural competency prior to inserting or removing the implants. For further information, visit www.ProbuphineREMS.com or call 1-844-859-6341
Subutex (G) 8 mg in a single dose on day 1; then 16 mg in a single dose on day 2; target dose is 16 mg/day in a single dose; dissolve under tongue; do not chew or swallow whole
Pediatric: <12 years: not established; ≥12 years: same as adult
  SL tab (lemon-lime) or SL film (lime): 2, 8 mg (30/pck)
Sublocade verify that the patient is clinically stable on transmucosal *buprenorphine* before initiating **Sublocade**; doses must be prepared by an authorized healthcare provider and administered once monthly only by SC injection in the abdominal region; initially 300 mg SC once monthly x the first 2 months, followed by 100 mg SC once monthly maintenance dose; increasing the maintenance dose to 300 mg once monthly may be considered for patients in which the benefits outweigh the risks
Pediatric: <12 years: not established; ≥12 years: same as adult
  Prefilled syringe: 100 mg/0.5 ml, 300 mg/1.5 ml, single-dose w. 19 gauge 5/8-inch needle
Comment: Serious harm or death could result if **Sublocade** is administered IV. NOWS is an expected and treatable outcome of prolonged use of opioids during pregnancy. (**Sublocade** is not recommended with moderate-to-severe hepatic impairment. Monitor liver function tests prior to and during treatment. If diagnosed with adrenal insufficiency, treat with physiologic replacement of corticosteroids and wean patient off of the opioid. **Sublocade** is only available through the restricted Sublocade REMS program. Healthcare settings and pharmacies that order and dispense **Sublocade** must be certified in this program.

▷ *buprenorphine hcl* (III) *Initial Dose:* 0.3 mg (1 ml) deep IM or slow IV (over at least 2 minutes); may repeat once (up to 0.3 mg) if required, 30-60 minutes after initial dose; usual frequency every 6 hours prn; fixed interval or "round-the-clock" dosing should not be undertaken until the appropriate interdose interval has been established by clinical observation
Pediatric: <2 years: not recommended; 2-12 years: 2-6 mcg/kg deep IM or slow IV every 4-6 hours or q 6-8 hours prn; >12 years: same as adult; fixed interval or "round-the-clock" dosing should not be undertaken until the appropriate interdose interval has been established by clinical observation
  Buprenex *Amp:* 0.3 mg/ml (1 ml) (5 ampules/carton)

OPIOID PARTIAL AGONIST-ANTAGONIST+OPIOID ANTAGONIST

Comment: Bunavail, Cassipa, Suboxone, Sucartonone, Troxyca ER, and Zubsolv maintenance may be prescribed only by Drug Addiction Treatment Act (DATA) certified providers with strict state and federal regulations. These drugs are potentiated by CYP3A4 inhibitors (e.g., azole antifungals, macrolides, HIV protease inhibitors) and antagonized by CYP3A4 inducers (monitor for opioid withdrawal). Concomitant NNRTIs (e.g., *efavirenz, nevirapine, etravirine, delavirdine*) or protease inhibitors (e.g., *atazanavir* with or without *ritonavir*): monitor. There is risk of respiratory or CNS depression with concomitant opioid analgesics, general anesthetics, benzodiazepines phenothiazines, other tranquilizers, sedative/ hypnotics, alcohol, or other CNS depressants. There is risk of serotonin syndrome with concomitant SSRIs, SNRIs, TCAs, 5-HT3 receptor antagonists, *mirtazapine, trazodone, tramadol*, MAO inhibitors. *Buprenorphine/ naloxone* products are not recommended in patients with severe hepatic impairment and may not be appropriate for patients with moderate hepatic impairment. *Buprenorphine* passes into human breast milk. NOWS may occur in newborn infants of mothers who are receiving treatment with *buprenorphine*.

▷ *buprenorphine+naloxone* (III) (G)
    Bunavail administer 1 buccal film once daily at the same time each day; target dose is 8.4/1.4 once daily; place the side of the **Bunavail** film with the text (BN2, BN4, or BN6) against the inside of the cheek; press and hold the film in place for 5 seconds; maintenance is usually 2.1/0.3 to 12.6/2.1 once daily
    Pediatric: <16 years: not recommended; ≥16 years: same as adult
      SL film:
        Bunavail 2.1/0.3 bup 2.1 mg+nal 0.3 mg (30/carton)
        Bunavail 4.2/0.7 bup 4.2 mg+nal 0.7 mg (30/carton)
        Bunavail 6.3/1 bup 6.3 mg+nal 1 mg (30/carton)
    Comment: One Bunavail 4.2/0.7 mg buccal film provides equivalent *buprenorphine* exposure to a Sucartonone 8/2 mg sublingual tablet.
    Cassipa place 1 film under the tongue, close to the base on the left or right side, and allow to completely dissolve as a single daily dose; initiate only after induction and stabilization of the patient, and the patient has been titrated to a dose of 16 mg *buprenorphine* using another marketed product; do not cut, chew, or swallow whole
    Pediatric: <12 years: not recommended; ≥12 years: adjust in 2-4 mg of
    buprenorphine SL film
      Cassipa 16/4 *SL film:* bupre 16 mg+nalox 4 mg
    Suboxone (G) adjust dose in increments/decrements of 2/0.5 or 4/1 once daily *buprenorphine+naloxone*, based on the patient's daily dose of *buprenorphine*, to a level that suppresses opioid withdrawal signs and symptoms; *Recommended target dosage:* 16/4 as a single daily dose; *Maintenance dose:* generally in the range of 4/1 to 24/6 per day; higher once-daily doses have not been demonstrated to provide any clinical advantage
    Pediatric: <12 years: not established; ≥12 years: same as adult
    Suboxone
      SL tab, SL film: **Suboxone 2/0.5** bup 2 mg+nal 0.5 mg (30/bottle) (lime)
        Suboxone 4/1 bup 4 mg+nal 1 mg (30/bottle) (lime)
        Suboxone 8/2 bup 8 mg+nal 2 mg (30/bottle) (lime)
        Suboxone 12/3 bup 12 mg+nal 3 mg (30/bottle) (lime)
    Sucartonone adjust in 2-4 mg of *buprenorphine* per day in a single dose; usual range is 4-24 mg/day in a single dose; target dose is 6 mg/day in a single dose; dissolve under tongue; do not chew or swallow whole
    Pediatric: <16 years: not recommended; ≥16 years: same as adult
    Sucartonone
      SL film: **Sucartonone 2/0.5** bup 2 mg+nal 0.5 mg (30/pck) (lime)
        Sucartonone 4/1 bup 4 mg+nal 1 mg (30/pck) (lime)
        Sucartonone 8/2 bup 8 mg+nal 2 mg (30/pck) (lime)
        Sucartonone 12/3 bup 12 mg+nal 3 mg (30/pck) (lime)
    Zubsolv initial induction with *buprenorphine* sublingual tabs; administer as a single dose once daily; titrate dose in increments of 1.4/0.36 or 2.9/0.72 per day; recommended target dose is 11.4/2.9 per day; usual max 17.2/4.2 per day
    Pediatric: <16 years: not recommended; ≥16 years: same as adult
    Zubsolv
    SL tab: **Zubsolv 1.4/0.36** bup 1.4 mg+nal 0.36 mg
        Zubsolv 2.9/0.72 bup 2.9 mg+nal 0.72 mg
        Zubsolv 5.7/1.4 bup 5.7 mg+nal 1.4 mg
        Zubsolv 8.6/2.1 bup 8.6 mg+nal 2.1 mg
        Zubsolv 11.4/2.9 bup 11.4 mg+nal 2.9 mg
    Comment: One Subutex 5.7/1.4 SL tab is bioequivalent to one Sucartonone 8/2 SL film.
▷ *oxycodone+naloxone* (II) *Opioid-naïve and opioid non-tolerant:* initially 10/1.2 q 12 hours; *Opioid-tolerant:* single dose >40/4.8 or a total daily dose >80/9.6 is only for use in patients for whom tolerance to an opioid of comparable potency has been established; swallow whole, or sprinkle contents on applesauce and swallow immediately without chewing
    Pediatric: <18 years: not recommended; ≥18 years: same as adult
    Troxyca ER
      Cap: **Troxyca ER 10/1.2** oxy 10 mg+nalox 1.2 mg ext-rel
        Troxyca ER 20/2.4 oxy 20 mg+nalox 2.4 mg ext-rel
        Troxyca ER 30/3.6 oxy 30 mg+nalox 3.6 mg ext-rel

(continued)

> Troxyca ER 40/4.8 oxy 40 mg+nalox 4.8 mg ext-rel
> Troxyca ER 60/7.2 oxy 60 mg+nalox 7.2 mg ext-rel
> Troxyca ER 80/9.6 oxy 80 mg+nalox 9.6 mg ext-rel

Comment: Opioid-tolerant patients are those taking, for 1 week or longer, at least 60 mg oral *morphine* per day, 25 mcg transdermal *fentanyl* per hour, 30 mg oral *oxycodone* per day, 8 mg oral *hydromorphone* per day, 25 mg oral *oxymorphone* per day, 60 mg oral *hydrocodone* per day, or an equianalgesic dose of another opioid.

SELECTIVE ALPHA 2-ADRENERGIC RECEPTOR AGONIST

Comment: Lucemyra *(lofexidine)* is the first FDA-approved non-opioid treatment for the management of opioid withdrawal symptoms, for the mitigation of withdrawal symptoms to facilitate abrupt discontinuation of opioids in adults. While **Lucemyra** may lessen the severity of withdrawal symptoms, it may not completely prevent them. This oral selective alpha 2-adrenergic receptor agonist reduces the release of norepinephrine. The actions of norepinephrine in the autonomic nervous system are believed to play a role in many of the symptoms of opioid withdrawal and is only approved for treatment for up to 14 days.

> *lofexidine* 0.18 mg x 3 tabs taken orally 4 qid at 5 to 6-hour intervals; max 14 days with dosing guided by symptoms; discontinue with a gradual dose reduction over 2 to 4 days
> *Pediatric:* <17 years: not recommended; ≥17 years: same as adult
> Lucemyra *Tab:* 0.18 mg
> **Comment:** Lucemyra is not a treatment for OUD, per se, but can be used as part of a broader, long-term treatment plan for managing OUD. The most common side effects from treatment with **Lucemyra** include hypotension, bradycardia, somnolence, sedation, and dizziness. **Lucemyra** has also been associated with a few cases of syncope. *Methadone* and **Lucemyra** both prolong the QT interval. Therefore, ECG monitoring is recommended when used concomitantly. Concomitant use of oral *naltrexone* with **Lucemyra** may reduce efficacy of oral *naltrexone*. Concomitant use of *paroxetine* has resulted in increased plasma levels of **Lucemyra**. Monitor for symptoms of orthostasis and bradycardia with concomitant use of CYP2D6 inhibitors. The safety of **Lucemyra** in pregnant females has not been established. There is no information regarding the presence of **Lucemyra** or its metabolites in human milk or effects on the breastfed infant.

OPIOID-INDUCED CONSTIPATION (OIC)

> *lubiprostone* (G) swallow whole; take with food and water; initially 24 mcg bid; *Moderate hepatic impairment (Child-Pugh Class B):* 16 mg bid; *Severe hepatic impairment (Child-Pugh Class C):* 8 mg bid
> Amitiza *Cap:* 8, 24 mg
> **Comment:** Amitiza increases intestinal fluid and intestinal transit time. Suspend dosing and rehydrate if severe diarrhea occurs. **Amitiza** is contraindicated with known or suspected mechanical GI obstruction. The most common adverse reactions in OIC are nausea, diarrhea, headache, abdominal pain, abdominal distension, and flatulence .

> *methylnaltrexone bromide* 1 oral dose or 1 weight-based SC dose every other day as needed; max 1 dose per 24 hours; administer SC; inject into the upper arm, abdomen, or thigh; rotate sites; *Chronic non-cancer pain:* 450 mg once daily in the morning (take with water on an empty stomach at least 30 minutes before the first meal of the day) or 12 mg SC once daily in the morning; *Severe hepatic impairment:* <38 kg: 0.075 mg/kg; 38-<62 kg: 4 mg (0.2 ml); 62-114 kg: 6 mg (0.3 ml); >114 kg: 0.075 mg/kg
> *Advanced illness, receiving palliative care:* <38 kg: 0.15 mg/kg; 38-<62 kg: 8 mg (0.4 ml); 62-114 kg: 12 mg (0.6 ml); >114 kg: 0.15 mg/kg; *Moderate and severe renal impairment (CrCl <60 ml/min):* <38 kg: 0.075 mg/kg; 38 to <62 kg: 4 mg (0.2 ml); 62 to 114 kg: 6 mg (0.3 ml); >114 kg: 0.075 mg/kg
> *Pediatric:* <18 years: not established; ≥18 years: same as adult
> Relistor *Tab:* 150 mg film-coat; *Vial:* 12 mg, single-dose (0.6 ml, 7/carton)
> Relistor Injection: *Prefilled syringe:* 8 mg (0.4 ml), 12 mg (0.6 ml) (7/carton)
> **Comment:** Relistor injection is indicated for patients with advanced illness or pain caused by active cancer who require opioid dosage escalation for palliative care. **Relistor** is an opioid antagonist indicated for the treatment of opioid-induced constipation (OIC) in adult patients with chronic non-cancer pain, including patients with chronic pain related to prior cancer or its treatment who do not require frequent (e.g., weekly) opioid dosage escalation. *Methylnaltrexone* is a selective antagonist of opioid binding at the mu-opioid receptor in the gut. As a quaternary amine, the ability of *methylnaltrexone* to cross the blood-brain barrier is restricted. This allows *methylnaltrexone* to function as a peripherally acting mu-opioid receptor antagonist in tissues such as the GI tract, thereby decreasing the constipating effects of opioids without impacting opioid-mediated analgesic effects on the central nervous system. The prefilled syringe is only for patients who require a **Relistor** injection dose of 8 mg or 12 mg. Use the vial for patients who require other doses. **Relistor** is contraindicated with known or suspected GI obstruction and patients at increased risk of recurrent obstruction due to the potential for GI perforation. Be within close proximity to toilet facilities once **Relistor** is administered. Discontinue all maintenance laxative therapy prior to initiation. Laxative(s) can be used as needed if there is a suboptimal response after 3 days. Discontinue if treatment with the opioid pain medication is also discontinued. Safety and effectiveness of **Relistor** have not been established in pediatric patients. Avoid concomitant use with other opioid antagonists because of the potential for additive effects of opioid receptor antagonism and increased risk of opioid withdrawal symptoms (sweating, chills, diarrhea, abdominal pain,

anxiety, and yawning). Advise females of reproductive potential, who become pregnant or are planning to become pregnant, that the use of **Relistor** during pregnancy may precipitate opioid withdrawal in the fetus due to the undeveloped blood-brain barrier. Breastfeeding is not recommended during treatment.

➤ *naldemedine* <12 years: not established; ≥12 years: take 1 tab once daily; take with or without food; discontinue if opioid pain therapy discontinued
Pediatric: <12 years: not established; ≥12 years: same as adult

Symproic *Tab:* 0.2 mg

Comment: **Symproic** is contraindicated with known or suspected GI obstruction and patients at increased risk for recurrent obstruction. Avoid with severe hepatic impairment (Child-Pugh Class C). Not recommended in pregnancy and breastfeeding (during and 3 days after final dose). There is risk of perforation in persons with conditions associated with reduction in structural integrity of the GI tract wall (e.g., peptic ulcer disease [PUD], Ogilvie's syndrome, diverticulitis disease, infiltrative GI tract malignancies, or peritoneal metastases).

➤ *naloxegol* swallow whole; take on an empty stomach; initially 25 mg once daily in the AM; discontinue other laxatives; *CrCl <60 ml/min:* 12.5 mg
Pediatric: <12 years: not established; ≥12 years: same as adult

Movantik *Tab:* 12.5, 25 mg

Comment: **Movantik** is an opioid antagonist indicated for the treatment of OIC in adult patients with chronic non-cancer pain, including patients with chronic pain related to prior cancer or treatment who do not require frequent (e.g., weekly) opioid dosage escalation. Alteration in analgesic dosing regimen prior to starting **Movantik** is not required. Patients receiving opioids for less than 4 weeks may be less responsive to **Movantik**. Take on an empty stomach at least 1 hour prior to the first meal of the day or 2 hours after the meal. For patients who are unable to swallow the **Movantik** tablet whole, the tablet can be crushed and given orally or administered via nasogastric tube. Avoid consumption of grapefruit or grapefruit juice. Discontinue if treatment with the opioid pain medication is also discontinued.

OPIOID-INDUCED NAUSEA/VOMITING (OINV)

Comment: Opioid analgesics bind to μ (mu), κ (kappa), or δ (delta) opioid receptors in the brain, spinal cord, and digestive tract. However, opioids cause adverse effects that may interfere with their therapeutic use. Opioid-induced nausea/vomiting (OINV) treatment options include serotonin receptor antagonists, dopamine receptor antagonists, and neurokinin-1 receptor antagonists.

SEROTONIN RECEPTOR ANTAGONISTS

➤ *dolasetron* administer 100 mg IV over 30 seconds; max 100 mg/dose
Pediatric: <2 years: not recommended; 2-16 years: 1.8 mg/kg; >16 years: same as adult

Anzemet *Tab:* 50, 100 mg; *Amp:* 12.5 mg/0.625 ml; *Prefilled carpuject syringe:* 12.5 mg (0.625 ml); *Vial:* 100 mg/5 ml (single-use); *Vial:* 500 mg/25 ml (multidose)

➤ *granisetron*

Kytril administer IV over 30 seconds, 30 min; max 1 dose/week
Pediatric: <2 years: not recommended; ≥2 years: 10 mcg/kg

Tab: 1 mg; *Oral soln:* 2 mg/10 ml (30 ml; orange); *Vial:* 1 mg/ml (1 ml single-dose) (preservative-free); 1 mg/ml (4 ml multidose) (benzyl alcohol)

Sancuso apply 1 patch 24-48 hours before chemo; remove 24 hours (minimum) to 7 days (maximum) after completion of treatment
Pediatric: <12 years: not recommended; ≥12 years: same as adult

Transdermal patch: 3.1 mg/day

➤ *ondansetron* (G) 8 mg q 8 hours x 2 doses; then 8 mg q 12 hours
Pediatric: <4 years: not recommended; 4-11 years: 4 mg q 4 hours x 3 doses; then 4 mg q 8 hours

Zofran *Tab:* 4, 8, 24 mg
Zofran ODT *ODT:* 4, 8 mg (strawberry) (phenylalanine)
Zofran Oral Solution *Oral soln:* 4 mg/5 ml (50 ml) (strawberry) (phenylalanine); *Parenteral form:* see mfr pkg insert
Zofran Injection *Vial:* 2 mg/ml (2 ml single-dose), 2 mg/ml (20 ml multi-dose), 32 mg/50 ml (50 ml multidose); *Prefilled syringe:* 4 mg/2 ml, single-use (24/carton)
Zuplenz Oral Soluble Film *Oral-dis:* 4, 8 mg oral-dis (10/carton) (peppermint)

Comment: The FDA has issued a warning against **ondansetron** use in pregnancy. **Ondansetron** is a 5-HT3 receptor antagonist approved by the FDA for preventing nausea and vomiting related to cancer chemotherapy and surgery. However, it has been used "off label" to treat the nausea and vomiting of pregnancy. The FDA has cautioned against the use of **ondansetron** in pregnancy in light of studies of **ondansetron** in early pregnancy and associated with congenital cardiac malformations and oral clefts (i.e., cleft lip and cleft palate). Further, there are potential maternal risks in pregnancy with electrolyte imbalance caused by severe nausea and vomiting (as with hyperemesis gravidarum). These risks include *serotonin syndrome* (a triad of cognitive and behavioral changes including confusion, agitation, autonomic instability, and neuromuscular changes). Therefore, **ondansetron** should not be taken during pregnancy.

(continued)

▷ *palonosetron* (G) administer 0.25 mg IV over 30 seconds; max 1 dose/week
Pediatric: <1 month: not recommended; 1 month to 17 years: 20 mcg/kg; max 1.5 mg/single dose; infuse over 15 minutes
    Aloxi *Vial (single-use):* 0.075 mg/1.5 ml, 0.25 mg/5 ml (mannitol)

DOPAMINE RECEPTOR ANTAGONISTS
▷ *prochlorperazine* (G)
    Compazine 5-10 mg tid-qid prn; usual max 40 mg/day
    Pediatric: <2 years or <20 lb: not recommended; 20-29 lb: 2.5 mg daily bid prn; max 7.5 mg/day; 30-39 lb: 2.5 mg bid-tid prn; max 10 mg/day; 40-85 lb: 2.5 mg tid or 5 mg bid prn; max 15 mg/day
        Tab: 5, 10 mg; *Syr:* 5 mg/5 ml (4 oz) (fruit)
    Compazine Suppository 25 mg rectally bid prn; usual max 50 mg/day
    Pediatric: <2 years or <20 lb: not recommended; 20-29 lb: 2.5 mg daily-bid prn; max 7.5; mg/day; 30-39 lb: 2.5 mg bid-tid prn; max 10 mg/day; 40-85 lb: 2.5 mg tid or 5 mg bid prn; max 15 mg/day
        Rectal supp: 2.5, 5, 25 mg
    Compazine Injectable 5-10 mg tid or qid prn
    Pediatric: <2 years or <20 lb: not recommended; ≥2 years or ≥20 lb: 0.06 mg/kg x 1 dose
        Vial: 5 mg/ml (2, 10 ml)
    Compazine Spansule 15 mg q AM prn or 10 mg q 12 hours prn; usual max 40 mg/day
    Pediatric: <12 years: not recommended; ≥12 years: same as adult
        Spansule: 10, 15 mg sust-rel

NEUROKININ-1 RECEPTOR ANTAGONISTS
▷ *aprepitant* (G) administer with 5HT-3 receptor antagonist; *Day 1:* 125 mg; Days 2 and 3: 80 mg in the morning
    Pediatric: <6 months: not recommended; ≥6 months: use oral suspension (see mfr pkg insert for dose by weight
        Emend *Cap:* 40, 80, 125 mg (2 x 80 mg bifold pck; 1 x 25 mg/2 x 80 mg trifold pck); *Oral susp:* 125 mg pwdr for oral suspension, single-dose pouch w. dispenser; *Vial:* 150 mg pwdr for reconstitution and IV infusion

OPIOID OVERDOSE/OPIOID REVERSAL

Comment: Patients should be transported to an emergency care facility. Seek emergency medical support (activate EMS) immediately.
Opioid Reversal Risks:
(1) *Risk of recurrent respiratory and central nervous system (CNS) depression:* Due to the duration of action of **naloxone** relative to the opioid, keep the patient under continued surveillance and administer repeat doses of **naloxone** using a new administration device as necessary, while awaiting emergency medical assistance.
(2) *Risk of limited efficacy with partial agonists or mixed agonist/antagonists:* Reversal of respiratory depression caused by partial agonists or mixed agonist/antagonists, such as **buprenorphine** and **pentazocine**, may be incomplete. Larger or repeat doses may be necessary.
(3) *Precipitation of severe opioid withdrawal:* Use of **naloxone** in patients who are opioid-dependent may precipitate opioid withdrawal. In neonates, opioid withdrawal may be life-threatening if not recognized and properly treated. Monitor for the development of opioid withdrawal.
(4) *Risk of cardiovascular (CV) effects:* Abrupt postoperative reversal of opioid depression may result in adverse CV effects. These events have primarily occurred in patients who had preexisting CV disorders or received other drugs that may have similar adverse CV effects. Monitor these patients closely in an appropriate healthcare setting after use of **naloxone** hydrochloride.

OPIOID ANTAGONISTS
▷ *nalmefene* Recommended initial dose (for non-opioid dependent patients): 0.5 mg/70 kg; If needed, may be followed, 2 to 5 minutes later, by a second dose of 1 mg/70 kg; If a total dose of 1.5 mg/70 kg has been administered without clinical response, additional **nalmefene** is not likely to have an effect; Patients should not be administered more **nalmefene** injection than is required to restore the respiratory rate to normal, thus minimizing the likelihood of cardiovascular stress and precipitated withdrawal syndrome; If IV access is lost or not readily obtainable: **nalmefene** injection should be effective within 5 to 15 minutes after IM or SC doses of 1 mg
    Pediatric: Safety and efficacy not established
        Nalmefene *Vial:* 2 mg/2 ml (1 mg/ml) soln, single-dose (10 vials/carton)
    Comment: *Nalmefene* was developed as an alternative to **naloxone** for complete or partial reversal of the effects of opioids including respiratory depression, sedation, and hypotension, induced by either natural or synthetic opioids, and in the management of known or suspected opioid overdose. *Nalmefene* was previously marketed under the brand name **Revex** (which has since been discontinued). Pharmacodynamic studies have shown that **nalmefene** has a longer duration of action than **naloxone**. *Nalmefene* can be administered via the IV, IM, or SC route. The most common adverse reactions reported in clinical trials have been nausea (18%), vomiting (9%), tachycardia (5%), hypertension (5%), postoperative pain (4%), fever (3%), and dizziness (3%). The duration of action of **nalmefene** injection is as long as most opioid analgesics. The apparent duration of action of **nalmefene** injection will vary, however, depending on the half-life and plasma concentration of the narcotic being reversed, the presence

or absence of other drugs affecting the brain or muscles of respiration, and the dose of *nalmefene* injection administered. Partially reversing doses of *nalmefene* injection (1 mcg/kg) lose their effect as the drug is redistributed through the body, and the effects of these low doses may not last more than 30 to 60 minutes in the presence of persistent opioid effects. Fully reversing doses (1 mg/70 kg) have been shown to last many hours in both experimental and clinical studies, but may complicate the management of patients who are in pain, at high cardiovascular risk, or who are physically dependent on opioids. The recommended doses represent a compromise between a desirable controlled reversal and the need for prompt response and adequate duration of action. Using higher dosages or shorter intervals between incremental doses is likely to increase the incidence and severity of symptoms related to acute withdrawal such as nausea, vomiting, elevated blood pressure, and anxiety. *Nalmefene* injection may cause acute withdrawal symptoms in individuals who have some degree of tolerance to, and dependence on, opioids. These patients should be closely observed for symptoms of withdrawal following administration of the initial and subsequent injections of *nalmefene* injection. Subsequent doses should be administered with intervals of at least 2 to 5 minutes between doses to allow the full effect of each incremental dose of *nalmefene* injection to be reached. The recommended initial dose of *nalmefene* injection for non-opioid dependent patients is 0.5 mg/70 kg. If needed, this may be followed by a second dose of 1 mg/70 kg, 2 to 5 minutes later. If a total dose of 1.5 mg/70 kg has been administered without clinical response, additional *nalmefene* injection is unlikely to have an effect. Patients should not be given more *nalmefene* injection than is required to restore the respiratory rate to normal, thus minimizing the likelihood of cardiovascular stress and precipitated withdrawal syndrome. *Nalmefene* has been administered after benzodiazepines, inhalational anesthetics, muscle relaxants, and muscle relaxant antagonists administered in conjunction with general anesthesia. It also has been administered in outpatient settings, both in trials in conscious sedation and in the emergency management of overdose following a wide variety of agents. No deleterious interactions have been observed. The following side effects of *nalmefene* are very common (≥10% incidence): insomnia, dizziness, headache, and nausea. **Nalmefene** is extensively metabolized in the liver, mainly by conjugation with glucuronic acid and also by *N*-dealkylation. Less than 5% of the dose is excreted unchanged.

➤ *naloxone* (G) 0.4-2 mg; repeat in 2-3 minutes if no response
  Pediatric: 0.01 mg/kg initially, repeat in 2-3 minutes at 0.1 mg/kg if response inadequate
    Evzio *Prefilled autoinjector:* 0.4 mg/0.4, 2 mg/0.4 ml IM/SC only
    Comment: **Evzio** 2 mg/0.4 ml comes with two autoinjectors and one trainer. This strength is indicated for the emergency treatment of known or suspected opioid overdose manifested by CNS depression. If the electronic voice instruction system does not operate properly, **Evzio** will still deliver the intended dose of *naloxone* when used according to the printed instructions on the flat surface of the autoinjector label. **Evzio** cannot be administered IV. Due to the short duration of action of naloxone, as compared to opioids which are longer acting, monitoring of the patient is critical as the opioid reversal effects of *naloxone* may wear off before the effects of the opioid.
    Kloxxado administer 1 spray in one nostril; if an additional dose is needed, spray into the opposite nostril using a new **Kloxxado** nasal spray device with each dose; if the patient does not respond or responds and then relapses into respiratory depression, additional doses may be administered every 2-3 minutes until emergency medical assistance arrives
    Pediatric: same as adult
      Nasal spray: 8 mg/0.1 ml, single-dose (2 blisters, each containing a single dose of *naloxone* and 2 nasal spray devices and /carton)
    Narcan *Vial/Amp:* 0.4 mg/ml (1 ml), 1 mg/ml (2 ml); *Prefilled syringe:* 0.4 mg/ml (1 ml), 1 mg/ml (2 ml) IV, IM, or SC (parabens-free)
    Narcan Nasal Spray position supine with head tilted back; 1 spray in one nostril; if an additional dose is needed, spray into the opposite nostril
      Nasal spray: 4 mg/0.1 ml, single-dose (2 blister pcks, each w. a single nasal spray/carton)
➤ **RiVive Nasal Spray (OTC)**
  Nasal spray: 3 mg, single-dose, disposable delivery unit
  Comment: **RiVive** may be purchased and used by anyone of any age without a prescription. There are no contraindications. **RiVive** is intended for urgent/emergent use immediately, on site, by professional healthcare providers, first-responders, and lay persons, when opioid overdose is suspected (independent of whether the potential overdose is witnessed or unwitnessed, confirmed or unconfirmed). Animal studies have not demonstrated terogenicity or other embryo/fetal harm. Because **RiVive** is not orally bioavailable, it is unlikely to affect the breastfed infant. Studies in nursing mothers have shown that **RiVive** does not affect prolactin or oxytocin hormone levels.

ORGAN TRANSPLANT REJECTION PROPHYLAXIS (OTRP)

SELECTIVE IMMUNOMODULATORY AGENTS
Comment: Selective immunosuppressive agents are drugs that suppress the immune system due to a selective point of action. They are used to reduce the risk of rejection in organ transplants, in autoimmune diseases, and can be used as cancer chemotherapy. As immunosuppressive agents lower the immunity, there is increased risk of infection.

CHIMERIC (MURINE/HUMAN) MONOCLONAL ANTIBODY

▶ *basiliximab* recommended regimen is 2 doses of 20 mg each; the first 20 mg dose should be administered within 2 hours prior to transplantation surgery; the second dose should be administered 4 days after transplantation; the second dose should be withheld if complications such as severe hypersensitivity reactions to **Simulect** or graft loss occur

Pediatric: <35 kg: 2 doses of 10 mg each; ≥35 kg: 2 doses of 20 mg each; the first dose should be administered within 2 hours prior to transplantation surgery; the second dose should be administered 4 days after transplantation; the second dose should be withheld if complications such as severe hypersensitivity reactions to **Simulect** or graft loss occur

    Simulect *Vial:* 10, 20 mg (6 ml) for reconstitution and IV infusion (preservative-free); 10 mg vial: contains 10 mg *basiliximab*, 3.61 mg monobasic potassium phosphate, 0.50 mg disodium hydrogen phosphate (anhydrous), 0.80 mg sodium chloride, 10 mg sucrose, 40 mg mannitol, and 20 mg glycine, to be reconstituted in 2.5 ml of Sterile Water for Injection, USP; 20 mg vial: contains 20 mg *basiliximab*, 7.21 mg monobasic potassium phosphate, 0.99 mg disodium hydrogen phosphate (anhydrous), 1.61 mg sodium chloride, 20 mg sucrose, 80 mg mannitol, and 40 mg glycine, to be reconstituted in 5 ml of Sterile Water for Injection

INOSINE MONOPHOSPHATE DEHYDROGENASE (IMPDH) INHIBITOR)

▶ *mycophenolate mofetil (MMF)* <3 years: not recommended; 3 months to 18 years: recommended dose of **CellCept** oral suspension is 600 mg/m² administered bid (up to total max 2 gm daily); patients with body surface area (BSA) 1.25 m² to 1.5 m² may be dosed with **CellCept** capsules at 750 mg bid (total 1.5 gm daily); patients with BSA >1.5 m² may be dosed with **CellCept** capsules or tablets at 1 gm bid (total 2 gm daily); >18 years: 1.5 gm bid orally (total 3 gm daily) or via IV infusion (infuse over no less than 2 hours; do not administer by bolus or rapid infusion)

    CellCept *Cap:* 250, 500 mg; *Oral susp:* 200 mg/ml (225 ml) after reconstitution w. bottle adapter and 2 oral dispensers; *Vial:* 500 mg MMF hcl for IV infusion after reconstitution and dilution in D5W

    Comment: CellCept (*MMF*) is the 2-morpholinoethyl ester of mycophenolic acid (MPA), an inosine monophosphate dehydrogenase (IMPDH) inhibitor. MMF has been demonstrated in experimental animal models to prolong the survival of allogeneic transplants (kidney, heart, liver, intestine, limb, small bowel, pancreatic islets, and bone marrow). MMF has demonstrated teratogenic effects in humans; however, there are no adequate and well-controlled studies in pregnancy. Females of reproductive potential must be made aware of the increased risk of 1st trimester pregnancy loss and congenital malformations and must be counseled regarding pregnancy prevention and planning. To prevent unplanned exposure during pregnancy, females of reproductive potential should have a serum or urine pregnancy test with a sensitivity of at least 25 mIU/ml immediately before starting **CellCept**, repeated testing 8-10 days later and during routine follow-up visits. In the event of a positive pregnancy test, females should be counseled with regard to maternal-fetal risk/benefit. Animal studies have shown MPA to be excreted in milk. It is not known whether MMF is excreted in human milk. Because of the potential for serious adverse reactions in breastfed infants from MMF exposure, risk/benefit of breastfeeding should be discussed with the patient.

Mammalian Target of Rapamycin (mTOR) Inhibitors (mTORi)

Comment: The most frequently occurring adverse events associated with mammalian target of rapamycin (mTOR) inhibitors (≥30%) include aphthous stomatitis, rash, anemia, fatigue, hyperglycemia, hypertriglyceridemia, hypercholesterolemia, decreased appetite, nausea, diarrhea, abdominal pain, headache, peripheral edema, hypertension, increased serum creatinine, fever, urinary tract infection (UTI), arthralgia, pain, thrombocytopenia, and interstitial lung disease. There are no adequate and well-controlled studies in pregnant females. Effective contraception must be initiated before mTOR inhibitor (mTORi) therapy, continued during therapy, and for 12 weeks after therapy has been stopped. It is not known whether *sirolimus*-based drugs are excreted in human milk. The pharmacokinetic and safety profiles in breastfed infants are not known; therefore, a decision should be made whether to discontinue nursing or to discontinue the drug, taking into account the importance of the drug to the mother.

▶ *everolimus* (G) administer consistently with or without food at the same time as *cyclosporine (CsA)* or *tacrolimus;* monitor *everolimus* concentrations; adjust maintenance dose to achieve trough concentrations within the 3-8 ng/ml target range (using the liquid chromatography-tandem mass spectrometry [LC-MS/MS] assay method); *Mild hepatic impairment:* reduce initial daily dose by one-third; *Moderate or severe hepatic impairment:* reduce initial daily dose by one-half *Kidney transplant:* indicated for patients at low-moderate immunologic risk; use in combination with *basiliximab*, *CsA* (reduced doses), and *corticosteroids*; starting dose is 0.75 mg bid; initiate as soon as possible after transplantation; *Liver transplant:* use in combination with *tacrolimus* (reduced doses) and *corticosteroids*; starting dose is 1.0 mg bid; initiate 30 days after transplantation

    Pediatric: <18 years: not established/not recommended; ≥18 years: same as adult

    Zortress *Tab:* 0.25, 0.5, 0.75 mg

▶ *sirolimus* (G)

    Tab: 1, 2 mg

    Rapamune administer consistently with or without food at the same time as *CsA; Low- to moderate-immunologic risk:* Day 1: 6 mg as a single loading dose; Day 2: initiate 2 mg once-daily maintenance; use initially with CsA and *corticosteroids*; initiate CsA withdrawal over 4-8 weeks beginning 2-4 months posttransplantation; *High-immunologic risk:* Day 1: up to 15 mg as a single loading dose; Day 2: initiate 5 mg once-daily maintenance; use with CsA for the first 12 months posttransplantation

Pediatric: <13 years: <u>not</u> established/not recommended; ≥13 years: same as adult

Tab: 0.5, 1, 2, mg; *Oral soln:* 60 mg/60 ml in amber glass bottle, 1 oral syringe adapter for fitting into the neck of the bottle, sufficient disposable amber oral syringes and caps for daily dosing, and a carrying case; bottles should be stored protected from light and refrigerated at 2°C to 8°C (36°F to 46°F); once the bottle is opened, the contents should be used within 1 month; if necessary, bottles may be stored the bottles at room temperatures up to 25°C (77°F) for a short period of time (<u>not</u> more than 15 days)

CALCINEURIN-INHIBITOR IMMUNOSUPPRESSANTS

Comment: *Tacrolimus* products are available in immediate-release (capsule, granules, parenteral form for IV administration) and extended-release tablet form. The forms are <u>not</u> interchangeable. Consider dose reduction <u>or</u> discontinuation in the event of myocardial hypertrophy and discontinue in the event of pure red cell aplasia. Avoid live vaccines during treatment with *tacrolimus*. Monitor for new-onset diabetes after transplant. Monitor for acute <u>and/or</u> chronic nephrotoxicity and consider dosage reduction with concomitant nephrotoxic drugs <u>and/or</u> neurotoxic drugs. The most common adverse reactions (incidence 10%-15%) have included diarrhea, constipation, anemia, UTI, hypertension, tremor, peripheral edema, hyperkalemia, diabetes mellitus, and headache. Monitor for hypertension, hyperkalemia, other abnormal electrolytes, and QT prolongation. Data from postmarketing surveillance and the Transplant Pregnancy Registry International (TPRI) suggests that infants exposed to *tacrolimus in utero* are at risk for prematurity, birth defects/congenital anomalies, low birth weight, and fetal distress. Risk/benefit to the mother and the infant should be considered. Adult organ recipients and parents of pediatric organ recipients should be encouraged to enroll in The Transplant Pregnancy Registry International (TPRI) by calling 1-877-955-6877 <u>or</u> www.transplantpregnancyregistry.org. Controlled lactation studies have <u>not</u> been conducted in humans; however, *tacrolimus* has been reported in human breast milk and effects on the breastfed infant are unknown. Risk/benefit of maternal health and infant health should be discussed.

➤ *tacrolimus* see mfr pkg insert for dosing table; dosing is based on patient age (<18 years <u>or</u> ≥18 years), organ transplanted, whether concomitant with *azathioprine* <u>or</u> MMF/interleukin 2 receptor antagonist, dosage formulation, whole blood trough concentration range in ng/ml, and specific months in the treatment schedule; see the mfr pkg insert also for dosage adjustments for African-American patients and patients with hepatic <u>and/or</u> renal impairment

Envarsus XR take once daily on an empty stomach at the same time of day, preferably in the morning

	Initial Oral Dose	Whole Blood Trough Concentration Range
De novo kidney transplantation with antibody induction	0.14 mg/kg/day	Month 1: 6-11 ng/ml >Month 1: 4-11 ng/ml
Conversion from *tacrolimus* immediate-release formulation	80% of the precon-version dose of *tacrolimus* immediate-release	Titrate to 4-11 ng/ml

Tab: 0.75, 1, 4 mg ext-rel

Comment: Envarsus XR (*tacrolimus* extended-release) is indicated to prevent organ rejection in *de novo* kidney transplant patients in combination with other immunosuppressants. Envarsus XR was initially approved for the prophylaxis of organ rejection in kidney transplant patients converted from *tacrolimus* immediate-release formulations. Envarsus XR is <u>not</u> interchangeable with other *tacrolimus* products. Prograf *Cap:* 0.5, 1, 5 mg; *Granules:* 0.2, 1 mg unit-dose pkts for oral suspension (50 pkts/carton); *Amp:* 5 mg/ml solution for dilution and IV infusion (1 ml, 10/box)

Comment: Prograf *(tacrolimus)* is indicated for the prophylaxis of organ rejection in patients receiving an allogenic liver, kidney, <u>or</u> heart transplant with other immunosuppressants. Frequent monitoring of trough concentration is recommended. Capsules and suspension should be consistently administered either with <u>or</u> without food. IV administration is intended for patients who are unable to swallow capsules <u>or</u> tablets. Prograf is <u>not</u> interchangeable with other extended-release *tacrolimus* products. Monitor for and implement appropriate management for new-onset diabetes, nephrotoxicity, neurotoxicity, hyperkalemia, hypertension, and anaphylaxis. Prograf is <u>not</u> recommended with concomitant use of *sirolimus* with liver and heart transplantation due to increased risk of adverse reactions.

OSGOOD-SCHLATTER DISEASE

Acetaminophen for IV Infusion *see Pain*

NSAIDs *see* Appendix I. NSAIDs online at https://connect.springerpub.com/content/reference-book/978-0-8261-7935-7/back-matter/part02/back-matter/bmatter10

Opioid Analgesics *see Pain*

Topical and Transdermal Analgesics *see Pain*

(continued)

Parenteral Corticosteroids *see* Appendix L. Parenteral Corticosteroids
Oral Corticosteroids *see* Appendix K. Oral Corticosteroids
Topical Analgesic and Anesthetic Agents *see* Appendix H. Anesthetic Agents for Local Infiltration and Dermal/Mucosal Membrane Application online at https://connect.springerpub.com/content/reference-book/978-0-8261-7935-7/back-matter/part02/back-matter/bmatter9

OSTEOARTHRITIS (OA), ANKYLOSING SPONDYLITIS

Acetaminophen for IV Infusion *see Pain*
NSAIDs *see* Appendix I. NSAIDs online at https://connect.springerpub.com/content/reference-book/978-0-8261-7935-7/back-matter/part02/back-matter/bmatter10
Opioid Analgesics *see Pain*
Topical and Transdermal Analgesics *see Pain*
Parenteral Corticosteroids *see* Appendix L. Parenteral Corticosteroids
Oral Corticosteroids *see* Appendix K. Oral Corticosteroids
Topical Analgesic and Anesthetic Agents *see* Appendix H. Anesthetic Agents for Local Infiltration and Dermal/Mucosal Membrane Application online at https://connect.springerpub.com/content/reference-book/978-0-8261-7935-7/back-matter/part02/back-matter/bmatter9

TOPICAL AND TRANSDERMAL ANALGESICS

➤ *capsaicin* (G) apply tid-qid prn to intact skin
 Pediatric: <2 years: not recommended; ≥2 years: same as adult
   Axsain *Crm:* 0.075% (1, 2 oz)
   Capsin *Lotn:* 0.025, 0.075% (59 ml)
   Capsaicin-HP (OTC) *Crm:* 0.075% (1.5 oz), 0.025% (45, 90 gm); *Lotn:* 0.075% (2 oz), 0.025% (45, 90 gm)
   Capzasin-P (OTC) *Crm:* 0.025% (1.5 oz); *Lotn:* 0.025% (2 oz)
   Dolorac *Crm:* 0.025% (28 gm)
   Double Cap (OTC) *Crm:* 0.05% (2 oz)
   R-Gel *Gel:* 0.025% (15, 30 gm)
   Zostrix (OTC) *Crm:* 0.025% (0.7, 1.5, 3 oz)
   Zostrix HP (OTC) *Emol crm:* 0.075% (1, 2 oz)
➤ *capsaicin* 8% patch apply up to 4 patches for one 60-minute application to clean dry skin; may prep area with topical anesthetic; wear non-latex gloves; patches may be cut to size/shape; treatment may be repeated every 3 months
 Pediatric: <18 years: not recommended; ≥18 years: same as adult
   Qutenza *Patch:* 8% 1,640 mcg/cm (179 mg) (1 or 2 patches w. 1-50 gm tube cleansing gel/carton)
➤ *diclofenac sodium* apply qid prn to intact skin
 Pediatric: <12 years: not established; ≥12 years: same as adult
   Pennsaid 1.5% in 10 drop increments, dispense and rub into front, side, and back of knee; usually 40 drops (40 mg) qid
    Topical soln: 1.5% (150 ml)
   Pennsaid 2% apply 2 pump actuations (40 mg) and rub into front, side, and back of knee bid
    Topical soln: 2% (20 mg/pump actuation, 112 gm)
   Solaraze Gel massage into clean skin bid prn
    Gel: 3% (50 gm) (benzyl alcohol)
   Voltaren Gel (G)(OTC) apply qid prn to intact skin
    Gel: 1% (100 gm)
   Comment: *Diclofenac* is contraindicated with **aspirin** allergy. As with other NSAIDs, should be avoided in late pregnancy (≥30 weeks) because it may cause premature closure of the ductus arteriosus (PCDA).
➤ *doxepin* (G) cream apply to affected area qid at intervals of at least 3-4 hours; max 8 days
 Pediatric: <12 years: not recommended; >12 years: same as adult
   Prudoxin *Crm:* 5% (45 gm)
   Zonalon *Crm:* 5% (30, 45 gm)
➤ *pimecrolimus* 1% cream (G) <2 years: not recommended; ≥2 years: apply to affected area bid; do not apply an occlusive dressing
   Elidel *Crm:* 1% (30, 60, 100 gm)
   Comment: *Pimecrolimus* is indicated for short-term and intermittent long-term use. Discontinue use when resolution occurs. Contraindicated if the patient is immunosuppressed. Change to the 0.1% preparation or if secondary bacterial infection is present.
➤ *trolamine salicylate* apply tid-qid
 Pediatric: <2 years: not recommended; ≥2 years: same as adult
   Mobisyl Creme *Crm:* 10% (100 gm)

ORAL SALICYLATE

➤ *indomethacin* initially 25 mg bid-tid, increase as needed at weekly intervals by 25-50 mg/day; max 200 mg/day
 Pediatric: <14 years: usually not recommended; >2 years, if risk warranted: 1-2 mg/kg/day in divided doses, max 3-4 mg/kg/day (or 150-200 mg/day, whichever is less); <14 years: ER cap not recommended
   Cap: 25, 50 mg; *Susp:* 25 mg/5 ml (pineapple-coconut, mint) (alcohol 1%); *Supp:* 50 mg; *ER Cap:* 75 mg ext-rel

Comment: *Indomethacin* is indicated only for acute painful flares. Administer with food and/or antacids. Use lowest effective dose for shortest duration.

ORAL NON-STEROIDAL ANTI-INFLAMMATORY DRUGS (NSAIDs)

See more oral NSAIDs at https://connect.springerpub.com/content/reference-book/978-0-8261-7935-7/back-matter/part02/back-matter/bmatter10

▷ **diclofenac** take on empty stomach; 35 mg tid; *Hepatic impairment:* use lowest dose
  Pediatric: <18 years: not recommended; ≥18 years: same as adult
    Zorvolex *Gelcap:* 18, 35 mg
▷ **diclofenac sodium**
  Pediatric: <18 years: not recommended; ≥18 years: same as adult
    Voltaren 50 mg bid-qid or 75 mg bid or 25 mg qid with an additional 25 mg at HS if necessary
      Tab: 25, 50, 75 mg ent-coat
    Voltaren XR 100 mg once daily; rarely, 100 mg bid may be used
      Tab: 100 mg ext-rel
  Comment: *Diclofenac* is contraindicated with *aspirin* allergy. As with other NSAIDs, should be avoided in late pregnancy (≥30 weeks) because it may cause premature closure of the ductus arteriosus (PCDA).

IBUPROFEN+ESOMEPRAZOLE COMBINATION

▷ **naproxen+esomeprazole magnesium** (G) take 1 tablet bid; use the lowest effective dose; not recommended in moderate/severe renal insufficiency or in severe hepatic insufficiency (Child-Pugh Class C); consider dose reduction in mild/moderate hepatic insufficiency (Child-Pugh Class A or B)
  Pediatric: <18 years: safety and efficacy not established; ≥18 years: same as adult
    Vimovo *Tab:* nap 375 mg+eso 20 mg, nap 500 mg+eso mg, del-rel, film-coat
  Comment: **Vimovo** is a fixed-dose combination of the NSAID *naproxen* (375 mg or 500 mg) and proton pump inhibitor (PPI) 20 mg indicated for relief of signs and symptoms of rheumatoid arthritis (RA), osteoarthritis (OA), and ankylosing spondylitis and to decrease the risk of developing gastric ulcers in patients at risk of developing NSAID-associated gastric ulcers. The most common adverse reactions (incidence ≥5% have been erosive gastritis, dyspepsia, gastritis, diarrhea, gastric ulcer, upper abdominal pain, and nausea. Contraindications to **Vimovo** use are (1) known hypersensitivity to any component of **Vimovo** or substituted benzimidazoles; (2) history of asthma, urticaria, or other allergic-type reactions after taking *aspirin* or other NSAIDs; (3) use during the perioperative period in the setting of coronary artery bypass graft (CABG) surgery; and (4) late pregnancy. Starting at 30 weeks' gestation, **Vimovo** should not be used by pregnant females as premature closure of the ductus arteriosus (PCDA) in the fetus may occur. *Boxed Warnings: Naproxen,* a component of **Vimovo,** may cause an increased risk of serious cardiovascular (CV) thrombotic events, myocardial infarction, and stroke, which can be fatal. This risk may increase with duration of use. Patients with cardiovascular disease (CVD) or risk factors for CVD may be at greater risk. **Vimovo** is contraindicated for the treatment of perioperative pain in the setting of CABG surgery. NSAIDs, including *naproxen,* can cause an increased risk of serious gastrointestinal (GI) adverse events including bleeding, ulceration, and perforation of the stomach or intestines, which can be fatal. These events can occur at any time during use and without warning symptoms. Elderly patients are at greater risk for serious GI events. *Other Warnings and Precautions:* Monitor patients for elevated liver enzymes and, rarely occurring, severe hepatic reactions; discontinue use immediately if abnormal liver enzymes persist or worsen. New onset or worsening of preexisting hypertension may occur; Monitor BP during treatment with **Vimovo.** Congestive heart failure (CHF) and edema can occur; **Vimovo** should be used with caution in patients with fluid retention or heart failure (HF). Renal papillary necrosis and other renal injury may occur with long-term use. Use **Vimovo** with caution in the elderly, those with impaired renal function, hypovolemia, salt depletion, HF, and liver dysfunction, and those taking diuretics or angiotensin-converting enzyme (ACE) inhibitors. Do not use **Vimovo** in patients with the *aspirin* triad. Serious skin adverse reactions such as exfoliative dermatitis, Steven-Johnson syndrome (SJS), and toxic epidermal necrolysis (TEN) can be fatal and can occur without warning. Discontinue **Vimovo** at first appearance of skin rash or any other sign of hypersensitivity. Long-term PPI therapy is associated with an increased risk for osteoporosis-related fractures of the hip, wrist, or spine. Symptomatic response to *esomeprazole* does not preclude the presence of gastric malignancy. Atrophic gastritis has been noted on biopsy with long-term *omeprazole* therapy. *Drug-drug interactions:* Concomitant use of NSAIDs may reduce the antihypertensive effect of ACE inhibitors, diuretics, and beta-blockers. Concomitant use of NSAIDs increases *lithium* plasma levels. Concomitant use of **Vimovo** with *methotrexate* may increase the toxicity of *methotrexate.* Concomitant use of **Vimovo** and *warfarin* may result in increased risk of bleeding complications; monitor for increases in international normalized ratio (INR) and PT/PTT. *Esomeprazole* inhibits gastric acid secretion and may interfere with the absorption of drugs where gastric pH is an important determinant of bioavailability (e.g., *ketoconazole,* iron salts, and *digoxin*). **Vimovo** is contraindicated in pregnancy starting at 30 weeks gestation; may cause fetal harm (premature closure of the ductus arteriosus (PCDA). The *naproxen* anion has been found in the milk of lactating females. Because of the possible adverse effects of prostaglandin-inhibiting drugs on neonates and potential for tumorigenicity shown for *esomeprazole* in animal carcinogenicity studies, a decision should be made whether to discontinue breastfeeding or discontinue the **Vimovo,** taking into account the importance of the drug to the mother.

IBUPROFEN+FAMOTIDINE COMBINATION

▷ *ibuprofen+famotidine* take 1 tablet tid or take 1 tablet q 8 hours; max 3 tabs/24 hours
  Pediatric: safety and efficacy not established
    Duexis *Tab:* ibu 800 mg+famo 26.6 mg, film-coat, single-dose
    Comment: Duexis is a fixed-dose combination of the NSAID *ibuprofen* (800 mg) and the histamine H2 receptor antagonist *famotidine* (26.6 mg) indicated for relief of signs and symptoms of rheumatoid arthritis (RA) and osteoarthritis and to decrease the risk of developing upper GI ulcers, which in clinical trials was defined as a gastric and/or duodenal ulcer in patients who are taking **ibuprofen** for those indications. The clinical trials primarily enrolled patients less than 65 years of age without a history of GI ulcer. The most common adverse reactions (incidence ≥1% and greater than *ibuprofen* alone) have been nausea, diarrhea, constipation, upper abdominal pain, and headache. Contraindications to **Duexis** use are (1) preexisting asthma, urticaria, or allergic reactions after taking *aspirin* or other NSAIDs; (2) use during the perioperative period in the setting of CABG surgery; (3) starting at 30 weeks gestation (**Duexis** should not be used by pregnant females as premature closure of the ductus arteriosus (PCDA) in the fetus may occur); and (4) known hypersensitivity to other H2 receptor antagonists. *Boxed Warnings: Ibuprofen,* a component of **Duexis,** may increase the risk of serious CV thrombotic events, myocardial infarction, and stroke, which can be fatal. Risk may increase with duration of use. Patients with CVD or risk factors for CVD may be at greater risk. NSAIDs, including *ibuprofen,* a component of **Duexis,** increase the risk of serious GI adverse reactions including bleeding, ulceration, and perforation of the stomach or intestines, which can be fatal. Reactions can occur at any time without warning symptoms. Elderly patients are at greater risk. *Other Warnings and Precautions with Duexis Use:* Hypertension can occur with NSAID treatment; BP closely during treatment with **Duexis.** Congestive heart failure (CHF) and edema can occur with NSAID treatment; use **Duexis** with caution in patients with fluid retention or heart failure (HF). Active and clinically significant bleeding from any source can occur; discontinue **Duexis** if active bleeding occurs. Long-term administration of NSAIDs can result in renal papillary necrosis and other renal injury; use **Duexis** with caution in patients at risk (e.g., the elderly, those with renal impairment, HF, liver impairment, and those taking diuretics or ACE inhibitors). Anaphylaxis may occur in patients with the *aspirin* triad or in patients without prior exposure to **Duexis;** discontinue **Duexis** immediately if an anaphylactoid reaction occurs. Serious skin reactions including exfoliative dermatitis, SJS, and TEN can occur and can be fatal; discontinue **Duexis** if rash or other signs of local skin reaction occur. Hepatic injury ranging from transaminase elevations to liver failure can occur; discontinue **Duexis** immediately if abnormal liver tests persist or worsen, if clinical signs and symptoms of liver disease develop, or if systemic manifestations occur. *Drug Interactions:* Concomitant use of NSAIDs and anticoagulants (e.g., *warfarin*) increases the risk of serious GI bleeding. Concomitant administration with other NSAIDs, including *aspirin,* may increase the risk of adverse reactions, including GI bleeding. *Ibuprofen,* a component of **Duexis,** may reduce the effectiveness of ACE inhibitors and diuretics. *Ibuprofen,* a component of **Duexis,** may increase **lithium** levels. **Duexis** is contraindicated in pregnancy starting at 30 weeks gestation; may cause fetal harm. Mothers' use of **Duexis** when lactating has not been studied; effects on the breastfed infant are unknown.

COX-2 INHIBITORS

Comment: Cox-2 inhibitors are contraindicated with history of asthma, urticaria, and allergic-type reactions to *aspirin,* other NSAIDs, and sulfonamides, 3rd trimester of pregnancy, and coronary artery bypass graft (CABG) surgery.
▷ *celecoxib* (G) 100-400 mg daily bid; max 800 mg/day
  Pediatric: <18 years: not recommended; ≥18 years: same as adult
    Celebrex *Cap:* 50, 100, 200, 400 mg
▷ *meloxicam* (G)
    Mobic <2 years, <60 kg: not recommended; ≥2 years, >60 kg: 0.125 mg/kg; max 7.5 mg once daily; ≥18 years: initially 7.5 mg once daily; max 15 mg once daily; *Hemodialysis:* max 7.5 mg/day
      Tab: 7.5, 15 mg; *Oral susp:* 7.5 mg/5 ml (100 ml) (raspberry)
    Vivlodex <18 years: not established; ≥18 years: initially 5 mg once daily; may increase to max 10 mg/day; *Hemodialysis:* max 5 mg/day
      Cap: 5, 10 mg

INTRA-ARTICULAR STEROID INJECTIONS

▷ *triamcinolone acetonide* ext-rel injectable synthetic corticosteroid indicated as an intra-articular injection for the management of osteoarthritic knee pain
    Zilretta *Vial:* 32 mg single-dose microsphere pwdr for injection + 5 ml diluent and vial adapter/single-use kit
    Comment: Zilretta is not intended for repeat administration. Zilretta is not interchangeable with other formulations of injectable *triamcinolone acetonide.*

INTRA-ARTICULAR SODIUM HYALURONATE INJECTIONS

Comment: *Sodium hyaluronate* intra-articular injection is indicated for the treatment of pain in osteoarthritis (OA) of the knee in patients who have failed to respond adequately to conservative non-pharmacologic therapy and simple analgesics (e.g., *acetaminophen*); alternative practices and procedures include NSAIDs, intra-articular injection of corticosteroid, unmodified hyaluronan injections, avoidance of activities that cause joint pain, exercise, weight loss, physical therapy, and removal of excess fluid from the knee. For patients who have failed the above treatments, surgical interventions such as arthroscopic surgery and total knee replacement surgery are also alternative treatments. Do not inject this product in the knees of patients with infections or skin diseases in the area of the injection site. Potential adverse effects occur in association with intra-articular injections: arthralgia, joint stiffness, joint effusion, joint swelling, joint warmth, injection site pain, arthritis, allergic reaction, and bleeding at the injection site. *Sodium hyaluronate* has not been formally assigned to a pregnancy category by the FDA. Animal studies have failed to reveal evidence of fertility impairment or teratogenicity. There are no controlled data in human pregnancy.

▷ *sodium hyaluronate* using strict aseptic technique, administer by intra-articular injection into the synovial space of the affected knee(s) for the prescribed number of weeks (see mfr pkg insert); after preparing the injection site and attaining local analgesia, remove joint synovial fluid or effusion prior to injection; do not inject intravascularly, extra-articularly, or in the synovial tissues or capsule; for at least 48 hours following an injection, avoid jogging, strenuous activity, or high-impact sports such as soccer or tennis, weight-bearing activity, or standing for longer than 1 hour at a time

Pediatric: <12 years: not recommended; ≥12 years: same as adult

  Durolane administer a single intra-articular knee injection
  Pediatric: <21 years: not recommended
    Prefilled syringe: 60 mg (20 mg/ml, 3 ml), single-use
  Euflexxa administer 3-5 intra-articular knee injections 1 week apart
  Pediatric: <21 years: not recommended
    Prefilled syringe: 20 mg (10 mg/ml, 2.0 ml), single-use
  Gel-One administer a single intra-articular knee injection
  Pediatric: <21 years: not recommended
    Prefilled syringe: 30 mg (10 mg/ml, 3 ml), single-use
  GelSyn-3 administer 3-5 intra-articular injections 1 week apart
  Pediatric: <21 years: not recommended
    Prefilled syringe: 16.5 mg (8.4 mg/ml, 2 ml), single-use
  GenVisc 850 administer 3-5 intra-articular knee injections 1 week apart
  Pediatric: <21 years: not recommended
    Prefilled syringe: 25 mg (10 mg/ml, 2.5 ml), single-use
  Hyalgan administer 3 to 5 intra-articular injections 1 week apart
  Pediatric: <21 years: not recommended
    Prefilled syringe: 10 mg/ml (20 mg, 2 ml), single-use
  Monovisc administer a single intra-articular knee injection
  Pediatric: <21 years: not recommended
    Prefilled syringe: 88 mg (22 mg/ml, 4 ml), single-use
  Orthovisc administer 3 to 4 intra-articular knee injections 1 week apart
  Pediatric: <21 years: not recommended
    Prefilled syringe: 30 mg (15 mg/ml, 2 ml), single-use
  Supartz, Supartz FX administer 3- to 5 intra-articular knee injections 1 week apart
  Pediatric: <21 years: not recommended
    Prefilled syringe: 25 mg (10 mg/ml, 2.5 ml), single-use
  Synvisc administer 3 intra-articular knee injections 1 week apart
  Pediatric: <21 years: not recommended
    Prefilled syringe: 16 mg (8 mg/ml, 2 ml), juvenile idiopathic arthritis single-use
  Synvisc-One administer a single intra-articular knee injection
  Pediatric: <21 years: not recommended
    Prefilled syringe: 48 mg (8 mg/ml, 6 ml), single-use
  Triluron administer 3 intra-articular knee injections 1 week apart
  Pediatric: <21 years: not established
    Vial: 20 mg/2 ml (2 ml); *Prefilled syringe:* 20 mg/2 ml (2 ml), single-use
  TriVisc administer 3 intra-articular knee injections 1 week apart
  Pediatric: <21 years: not recommended
    Prefilled syringe: 30 mg (10 mg/ml, 3 ml), single-use
  Visco-3 administer 3 intra-articular knee injections 1 week apart
  Pediatric: <21 years: not recommended
    Prefilled syringe: 25 mg (10 mg/ml, 2.5 ml), single-use

TUMOR NECROSIS FACTOR (TNF) ALPHA BLOCKERS FOR ANKYLOSING SPONDYLITIS

▷ *adalimumab* 40 mg SC once every other week; may increase to once weekly; administer SC in abdomen or thigh; rotate sites
  Pediatric: NA
    Humira *Prefilled pen* (Humira Pen): 40 mg/0.4 ml, 40 mg/0.8 ml, 80 mg/0.8 ml, single-dose;
    Prefilled glass syringe: 10 mg/0.1 ml, 10 mg/0.2 ml, 20 mg/0.2 ml, 20 mg/0.4 ml, 40 mg/0.4 ml,

(continued)

40 mg/0.8 ml, 80 mg/0.8 ml, single-dose; *Vial:* 40 mg/0.8 ml, single-dose, institutional use only (preservative-free)

Comment: Humira may be used with *methotrexate* (MTX), disease-modifying antirheumatic drugs (DMARDs), corticosteroids, salicylates, NSAIDs, or analgesics.

▷ *adalimumab-aacf* 40 mg SC every other week; if not receiving *methotrexate* may benefit from increasing the dose to 40 mg SC every week or 80 mg SC every other week

Idacio *Prefilled pen* (Idacio Pen): 40 mg/0.8 ml, single-dose; *Prefilled glass syringe:* 40 mg/0.8 ml, single-dose

Comment: Idacio is biosimilar to Humira (*Iadalimumab*).

▷ *adalimumab-adaz* 40 mg SC every other week; some patients with RA not receiving *methotrexate* (MTX) may benefit from increasing the frequency to 40 mg SC every week

Pediatric: <18 years: not recommended; ≥18 years: same as adult

Hyrimoz *Prefilled syringe:* 40 mg/0.8 ml, single-dose (preservative-free)

Comment: Hyrimoz is biosimilar to Humira (*adalimumab*).

▷ *adalimumab-adbm* initially 80 SC; then 40 mg SC every other week starting 1 week after initial dose; inject into thigh or abdomen; rotate sites

Pediatric: <18 years: not recommended; ≥18 years: same as adult

Cyltezo *Prefilled syringe:* 40 mg/0.8 ml, single-dose (preservative-free)

Comment: Cyltezo is biosimilar to Humira (*adalimumab*).

▷ *adalimumab-afzb* 40 mg SC every other week; some patients with RA not receiving *methotrexate* may benefit from increasing the frequency to 40 mg SC every week

Abrilada *Prefilled pen:* 40 mg/0.8 ml, single-dose; *Prefilled syringe:* 40 mg/0.8 ml, 20 mg/0.4 ml, 10 mg/0.2 ml, single-dose (for institutional use only) (preservative-free)

Comment: Abrilada is biosimilar to Humira (*adalimumab*).

▷ *adalimumab-bwwd Initial dose* (Day 1): 160 mg SC; *Second dose, two weeks later* (Day 15): 80 mg SC; *2 weeks later* (Day 29): begin maintenance dose of 40 mg every other week

Hadlima *Prefilled autoinjector:* 40 mg/0.8 ml, single-dose (Hadlima PushTouch); *Prefilled syringe:* 40 mg/0.8 ml, single-dose

Comment: Hadlima is biosimilar to Humira (*adalimumab*).

▷ *etanercept* inject SC into thigh, abdomen, or upper arm; rotate sites; initially 50 mg twice weekly (3-4 days apart) for 3 months; then 50 mg/week maintenance or 25 mg or 50 mg per week for 3 months; then 50 mg/week maintenance

Pediatric: <4 years: not recommended; 4-17 years: chronic moderate-to-severe plaque psoriasis; >17 years: same as adult

Enbrel *Vial:* 25 mg pwdr for SC injection after reconstitution (4/carton w. supplies) (preservative-free, diluent contains benzyl alcohol); *Prefilled syringe:* 25, 50 mg/ml (preservative-free); *SureClick autoinjector:* 50 mg/ml (preservative-free)

▷ *etanercept-ykro* 50 mg SC once weekly

Pediatric: <4 years: not established; ≥4 years, ≥63 kg, 138 lb: same as adult

Eticovo *Prefilled syringe:* 25 mg/0.5 ml, 50 mg/ml solution, single-dose

Comment: Eticovo is biosimilar to Enbrel (*etanercept*).

▷ *infliximab* must be refrigerated at 2°C to 8°C (36°F to 46°F); administer dose intravenously over a period of not less than 2 hours; do not use beyond the expiration date as this product contains no preservative; 5 mg/kg at 0, 2, and 6 weeks, then every 8 weeks

Pediatric: safety and efficacy not established

Remicade *Vial:* 100 mg pwdr for reconstitution to 10 ml administration volume, single-dose (preservative-free)

Comment: Remicade is indicated to reduce signs and symptoms and induce and maintain clinical remission in adults and children ≥6 years of age with moderately to severely active disease who have had an inadequate response to conventional therapy, and reduce the number of draining enterocutaneous and rectovaginal fistulas and maintain fistula closure in adults with fistulizing disease. Common adverse effects associated with **Remicade** included abdominal pain, headache, pharyngitis, sinusitis, and upper respiratory infections. In addition, **Remicade** might increase the risk for serious infections, including tuberculosis, bacterial sepsis, and invasive fungal infections. Available data from published literature on the use of *infliximab* products during pregnancy have not reported a clear association with *infliximab* products and adverse pregnancy outcomes. *Infliximab* products cross the placenta and infants exposed *in utero* should not be administered live vaccines for at least 6 months after birth. Otherwise, the infant may be at increased risk of infection, including disseminated infection, which can become fatal. Available information is insufficient to inform the amount of *infliximab* products present in human milk or effects on the breastfed infant.

▷ *infliximab-abda*

Renflexis *Vial:* 100 mg pwdr for reconstitution to 10 ml administration volume, single-dose

Comment: Renflexis is biosimilar to Remicade (*infliximab*).

▷ *infliximab-dyyb*

Inflectra *Vial:* 100 mg pwdr for reconstitution to 10 ml administration volume, single-dose

Comment: Inflectra is biosimilar to Remicade (*infliximab*).

➤ *infliximab-axxq*

Avsola *Vial*: 100 mg pwdr in a 20 ml single-dose vial, for reconstitution, dilution, and IV infusion

Comment: Avsola is biosimilar to **Remicade** *(infliximab).*

➤ *infliximab-qbtx*

Ixifi *Vial*: 100 mg pwdr for reconstitution to 10 ml administration volume, single-dose

Comment: Ixifi is biosimilar to **Remicade** *(infliximab).*

SELECTIVE INTERLEUKIN 17A (IL-17A) INHIBITOR

➤ *secukinumab Recommended dose:* 300 mg via SC injection at Weeks 0, 1, 2, 3, and 4 followed by 300 mg every 4 weeks; for some patients, a dose of 150 mg may be acceptable; see mfr pkg insert for full prescribing information for preparation of the Sensoready pen and prefilled syringe; reconstitute lyophilized powder in a vial with Sterile Water for Injection; reconstitution and administration should be performed by a qualified healthcare provider. *Pediatric:* safety and efficacy not established

Cosentyx *Prefilled syringe/Sensoready pen:* 150 mg/ml soln, single-use; *Vial:* 150 mg, pwdr, single-use; Cosentyx is for use only by a qualified healthcare professional

Comment: **Cosentyx** is a selective interleukin-17A (IL-17A) inhibitor for the treatment of adult patients with moderate-to-severe plaque psoriasis who are candidates for systemic therapy or phototherapy, psoriatic arthritis, ankylosing spondylitis, and psoriatic arthritis, and non-radiographic axial spondyloarthritis. **Cosentyx** may be used as monotherapy or in combination with *methotrexate* (MTX). The most common adverse reactions (incidence >1%) have been nasopharyngitis, diarrhea, and upper respiratory tract infection. Doses up to 30 mg/kg (i.e., approximately 2,000-3,000 mg) have been administered IV in clinical trials without dose-limiting toxicity. In the event of overdosage, it is recommended that the patient be monitored for any signs or symptoms of adverse reactions and appropriate symptomatic treatment be instituted immediately. Caution should be exercised when considering the use of **Cosentyx** in patients with a chronic infection or a history of recurrent infection. If a serious infection develops, discontinue **Cosentyx** until the infection resolves. Prior to initiating treatment with **Cosentyx**, evaluate the patient for tuberculosis. Exacerbations of Crohn's disease have been observed in clinical trials; therefore, caution should be exercised when prescribing **Cosentyx** to patients with active Crohn's disease. History of a serious hypersensitivity reaction to *secukinumab* or to any of the **Cosentyx** excipients is a contraindication to **Cosentyx** administration. If an anaphylactic reaction or other serious allergic reaction occurs, discontinue **Cosentyx** immediately and initiate appropriate therapy. Prior to initiating treatment with **Cosentyx**, consider completion of all age-appropriate immunizations according to current immunization guidelines. Patients treated with **Cosentyx** should not receive live vaccines. Non-live vaccinations received during a course of **Cosentyx** may not elicit an immune response sufficient to prevent disease. There are no adequate and well-controlled trials of **Cosentyx** in human pregnancy. Animal studies found no evidence of fetal harm. However, **Cosentyx** should be used during pregnancy only if the potential benefit justifies the potential risk to the fetus. It is not known whether *secukinumab* is excreted in human milk or absorbed systemically after ingestion. Because many drugs are excreted in human milk, caution should be exercised when **Cosentyx** is administered to a breastfeeding mother. To report suspected adverse reactions, contact Novartis Pharmaceuticals at 1-888-669-6682 or FDA at 1-800-FDA-1088 or www.fda.gov/medwatch.

OSTEOPOROSIS

Comment: Indications for bone density screening include postmenopausal women not receiving hormone replacement therapy (HRT), maternal history of hip fracture, personal history of fragility fracture, presence of high serum markers of bone resorption, smoker, height >67 inches, weight <125 lb, taking a steroid, gonadotropin-releasing hormone (GnRH) agonist or antiseizure drug, immobilization, hyperthyroidism, posttransplantation, malabsorption syndrome, hyperparathyroidism. The mnemonic **ABONE** (**A**ge >65, **B**ulk [weight <140 lb at menopause], and **N**ever **E**strogens [for more than 6 months]) represents other indications for bone density screening. Foods high in calcium include almonds, broccoli, baked beans, salmon, sardines, buttermilk, turnip greens, collard greens, spinach, pumpkin, rhubarb, and bran. *Recommended daily calcium intake:* 1-3 years: 700 mg; 4-8 years: 1,000 mg; 9-18 years: 1,300 mg; 19-50 years: 1,000 mg: 51-70 years (males): 1,000 mg; ≥51 years (females): 1,200 mg; pregnancy or nursing: 1,000-1,300 mg; *Recommended daily vitamin D intake:* >1 year: 600 IU; 50+ years: 800-1,000 IU. Prior to initiating, or concomitant prescribing, corticosteroids in patients at risk for, or diagnosed with, osteoporosis, referral to the following American College of Rheumatology (ACR) guidelines is recommended: ACR Guidelines on Prevention & Treatment of Glucocorticoid-Induced Osteoporosis (press release, June 7, 2017). Atlanta, Georgia. American College of Rheumatology, www.rheumatology.org/About-Us/Newsroom/Press-Releases/ID/812/ACR-Releases-Guideline-on-Prevention-Treatment-of-Glucocorticoid-Induced-Osteoporosis.

ESTROGEN REPLACEMENT THERAPY

Comment: Estrogen plus progesterone is indicated for postmenopausal women with an intact uterus. *Estrogen* monotherapy is indicated in women without a uterus. The following list is not inclusive; for more estrogen replacement therapies, *see Menopause.*

(continued)

▷ *estradiol*
    Alora initially 0.05 mg/day apply patch twice weekly to lower abdomen, upper quadrant of buttocks, <u>or</u> outer aspect of hip
      Transdermal patch: 0.025, 0.05, 0.075, 0.1 mg/day (8, 24/pck)
    Climara initially 0.025 mg/day patch once a week to trunk
      Transdermal patch: 0.025, 0.0375, 0.05, 0.075, 0.1 mg/day (4, 8, 24/pck)
    Estrace 1-2 mg daily cyclically (3 weeks on and 1 week off)
      Tab: 0.5, 1, 2*mg (tartrazine)
    Estraderm initially apply one 0.05 mg/day patch twice weekly to trunk
      Transdermal patch: 0.05, 0.1 mg/day (8, 24/pck)
    Menostar apply 1 patch weekly to lower abdomen, below the waist; avoid the breasts; alternate sites;
    Transdermal patch: 14 mcg/day (4/pck)
    Minivelle initially one 0.0375 mg/day patch twice weekly to trunk area; adjust after 1 month of therapy
      Transdermal patch: 0.025, 0.0375, 0.05, 0.075, 0.1 mg/day (8/pck)
    Vivelle initially one 0.0375 mg/day patch twice weekly to trunk area; use with an oral progestin to prevent endometrial hyperplasia
      Transdermal patch: 0.025, 0.0375, 0.05, 0.075, 0.1 mg/day (8, 48/pck)
    Vivelle-Dot initially one 0.05 mg/day patch twice weekly to lower abdomen, below the waist; use with an oral progestin to prevent endometrial hyperplasia
      Transdermal patch: 0.025, 0.0375, 0.05, 0.075, 0.1 mg/day (8, 24/pck)
▷ *estradiol+levonorgestrel* apply 1 patch weekly to lower abdomen; avoid waistline; alternate sites
    Climara Pro *Transdermal patch:* estra 0.045 mg+levo 0.015 mg per day (4/pck)
▷ *estradiol+norethindrone* 1 tab daily
    Activella (G) *Tab:* estra 1 mg+noreth 0.5 mg
    FemHRT 1/5 *Tab:* estra 5 mcg+noreth 1 mg
▷ *estradiol+norgestimate* one x 1 mg *estradiol* tab daily x 3 days, then 1 x *estradiol* 1 mg+*norgestimate* 0.09 mg tab once daily x 3 days; repeat this pattern continuously
    Ortho-Prefest *Tab:* estra 1 mg+norgest 0.09 mg (30/blister pck)
▷ *estrogen, conjugated (equine)*
    Premarin 1 tab daily
      Tab: 0.3, 0.45, 0.625, 0.9, 1.25, 2.5 mg
▷ *estropipate, piperazine estrone sulfate (G)*
    Ogen 0.625-1.25 mg daily cyclically (3 weeks on and 1 week off)
      Tab: 0.625, 1.25, 2.5 mg
    Ortho-Est 0.75-6 mg daily cyclically (3 weeks on and 1 week off)
      Tab: 0.625, 1.25 mg

ESTROGENS, CONJUGATED+ESTROGEN AGONIST-ANTAGONIST COMBINATION
▷ *estrogen, conjugated+bazedoxifene*
    Duavee 1 tab daily
      Tab: estra, conj 0.45 mg+baze 20 mg

CALCIUM SUPPLEMENTS
Comment: Take calcium supplements after meals to avoid gastric upset. Dosages of calcium over 2,000 mg/day have <u>not</u> been shown to have any additional benefit. Calcium decreases *tetracycline* absorption. Calcium absorption is decreased by corticosteroids.
▷ *calcitonin-salmon*
    Fortical 200 IU intranasally daily; alternate nostrils each day
    Nasal spray: 200 IU/actuation (30 doses, 3.7 ml)
    Miacalcin Nasal spray 200 IU spray in one nostril once daily; alternate nostrils each day
      Nasal spray: 200 IU/actuation (30 doses, 3.7 ml)
    Miacalcin Injection 100 units SC <u>or</u> IM every other day
      Vial: 200 units/ml (2 ml)
    Comment: Supplement diet with calcium (1 gm/day) and vitamin D (400 IU/day).
▷ *calcium carbonate (OTC)(G)*
    Rolaids chew 2 tabs bid; max 14 tabs/day
      Chew tab: 550 mg
    Rolaids Extra Strength chew 2 tabs bid; max 8 tabs/day
      Chew tab: 1,000 mg
    Tums chew 2 tabs bid; max 16 tabs/day
      Chew tab: 500 mg
    Tums Extra Strength chew 2 tabs bid; max 10 tabs/day
      Chew tab: 750 mg
    Tum Sultra chew 2 tabs bid; max 8 tabs/day
      Chew tab: 1,000 mg
    Os-Cal 500 1-2 tab bid-tid
      Chew tab: elemental calcium carbonate 500 mg

▷ *calcium carbonate+vitamin D* (G)
    Os-Cal 250+D 1-2 tab tid
      Tab: calc carb 250 mg+vit d 125 IU
    Os-Cal 500+D 1-2 tab bid-tid
      Tab: calc carb 500 mg+vit d 125 IU
    Viactiv 1 tab tid
      Chew tab: calc carb 500 mg+vit d 100 IU+vit k 40 mcg
▷ *calcium citrate* (OTC) (G)
    Citracal 1-2 tabs bid
      Tab: 200 mg
▷ *calcium citrate+vitamin D* (OTC) (G)
    Citracal+D 1-2 cplts bid
      Cplt: calc cit 315 mg+vit d 200 IU
    Citracal 250+D 1-2 tabs bid
      Tab: calc cit 250 mg+vit d 62.3 IU

VITAMIN D ANALOGS

Comment: Concurrent vitamin D supplementation is contraindicated in patients taking *calcitriol* or *doxercalciferol* due to the risk of vitamin D toxicity.

▷ *calcitriol Predialysis:* initially 0.25 mcg daily; may increase to 0.5 mcg daily; *Dialysis:* initially 0.25 mcg daily; may increase by 0.25 mcg/day at 4-8 week intervals; usual maintenance 0.5-1 mcg/day; *Hypoparathyroidism:* initially 0.25 mcg q AM; may increase by 0.25 mcg/day at 4- to 8-week intervals; usual maintenance 0.5-2 mcg/day
  Pediatric: Predialysis: <3 years: 10-15 ng/kg/day; ≥3 years: initially 0.25 mcg daily; may increase to 0.5 mcg/day; *Dialysis:* not recommended; *Hypoparathyroidism:* initially 0.25 mcg daily; may increase by 0.25 mcg/day at 2 to 4-week intervals; usual maintenance: 1-5 years: 0.25-0.75 mcg/day: ≥6 years: 0.5-2 mcg/day
    Rocaltrol *Cap:* 0.25, 0.5 mcg
    Rocaltrol Solution *Soln:* 1 mcg/ml (15 ml, single-use dispensers)
▷ *doxercalciferol* initially 0.25 mcg q AM; may increase by 0.25 mcg/day at 4 to 8-week intervals; usual maintenance 0.5-2 mcg/day
  Pediatric: initially 0.25 mcg daily; may increase by 0.25 mcg; 0.25 mcg/day at 2 to 4-week intervals; usual maintenance: -1-5 years) 0.25-0.75 mcg/day: ≥6 years 0.5-2 mcg/day
    Hectorol *Cap:* 0.25, 0.5 mcg

BISPHOSPHONATES (CALCIUM MODIFIERS)

Comment: Bisphosphonates should be swallowed whole in the AM with 6-8 oz of plain water 30 minutes before first meal, beverage, or other medications of the day. Monitor serum alkaline phosphatase. Contraindications include abnormalities of the esophagus which delay esophageal emptying such as stricture or achalasia, inability to stand or sit upright for at least 30 minutes post-dose, patients at risk of aspiration, and hypocalcemia. Co-administration of bisphosphonates and *calcium*, antacids, or oral medications containing multivalent cations will interfere with absorption of the bisphosphonate. Therefore, instruct patients to wait at least half hour after taking the bisphosphonate before taking any other oral medications.

▷ *alendronate (as sodium)* (G) take once weekly, in the AM, 30 minutes before the first food, beverage, or medication of the day; do not lie down (remain upright) for at least 30 minutes and after the first food of the day; *CrCl <35 ml/min:* not recommended
  Pediatric: <12 years: not recommended; ≥12 years: same as adult
    Binosto dissolve the effervescent tab in 4 oz (120 ml) of plain, room temperature, water (not mineral or flavored); wait 5 minutes after the effervescence has subsided, then stir for 10 seconds, then drink
      Tab: 70 mg effervescent for buffered solution (4, 12/carton) (strawberry)
    Fosamax (G) swallow tab whole; dosing regimens are the same for men and postmenopausal women; *Prevention:* 5 mg once daily or 35 mg once weekly; *Treatment:* 10 mg once daily or 70 mg once weekly
      Tab: 5, 10, 35, 40, 70 mg
▷ *alendronate+cholecalciferol (vit d3)* (G) take 1 tab once weekly, in the AM, with plain water (not mineral) 30 minutes before the first food, beverage, or medication of the day; do not lie down (remain upright) for at least 30 minutes and after the first food of the day
  Pediatric: <12 years: not recommended; ≥12 years: same as adult
    Fosamax Plus D
      Tab: **Fosamax Plus D 70/2800** alen 70 mg+chole 2,800 IU
    Fosamax Plus D 70/5600 alen 70 mg+chole 5,600 IU
▷ *ibandronate (as monosodium monohydrate)* (G)
  Pediatric: <12 years: not recommended; ≥12 years: same as adult
    Boniva take 2.5 mg once daily or 150 mg once monthly on the same day; take in the AM, with plain water (not mineral) 60 minutes before the first food, beverage, or medication of the day; do not lie down (remain upright) for at least 30 minutes and after the first food of the day
      Tab: 2.5, 150 mg

(continued)

Boniva Injection administer 3 mg every 3 months by IV bolus over 15-30 seconds; if dose is missed, administer as soon as possible; then every 3 months from the date of the last dose

Prefilled syringe: 3 mg/3 ml (5 ml)

Comment: Boniva Injection must be administered by a healthcare professional.

▷ *risedronate (as sodium)* (G) take in the AM; swallow whole with a full glass of plain water (not mineral); do not lie down (remain upright) for 30 minutes afterward

Pediatric: <12 years: not recommended; ≥12 years: same as adult

Actonel take at least 30 minutes before any food or drink; *Women:* 5 mg once daily or 35 mg once weekly or 75 mg on 2 consecutive days monthly or 150 mg once monthly; *Men:* 35 mg once weekly

Tab: 5, 30, 35, 75, 150 mg

Atelvia 35 mg once weekly immediately after breakfast

Tab: 35 mg del-rel

▷ *risedronate+calcium* 1 x 5 mg *risedronate* tab weekly plus 1 x 500 mg calcium tab on days 2-7 weekly

Actonel with Calcium *Tab: risedronate* 5 mg and *Tab:* calcium 500 mg (4 *risedronate* tabs + 30 calcium tabs/pck)

▷ *zoledronic acid* (G)

Pediatric: <12 years: not recommended; ≥12 years: same as adult

Reclast administer 5 mg via IV infusion over at least 15 minutes mg once a year (for osteoporosis) or once every 2 years (for osteopenia or prophylaxis)

Bottle: 5 mg/100 ml (single-dose)

Comment: Reclast is indicated for the treatment of postmenopausal osteoporosis in women who are at high risk for fracture and to increase bone mass in men with primary or hypogonadal osteoporosis who are at high risk for fracture. Administered by a healthcare professional. Contraindicated in hypocalcemia.

Zometa *Bottle:* 4 mg/5 ml administer 4 mg via IV infusion over at least 15 minutes every 3-4 weeks; optimal duration of treatment not known

Vial: 4 mg/5 ml (single-dose)

Comment: Zometa is indicated for the treatment of hypercalcemia of malignancy. The safety and efficacy of Zometa in the treatment of hypercalcemia associated with hyperparathyroidism or with other non-tumor-related conditions have not been established.

SELECTIVE ESTROGEN RECEPTOR MODULATOR (SERMs)

▷ *raloxifene* (G) 60 mg once daily

Evista *Tab:* 60 mg

Comment: Contraindicated in women who have history of, or current, venous thrombotic event.

HUMAN PARATHYROID HORMONE RELATED PEPTIDE (PTHrP[1-34]) ANALOG

▷ *abaloparatide* 80 mcg (40 mcl) SC once daily

Tymlos *Pen:* 80 mcg/40 mcl (1.56 ml, 2,000 mcg/ml) (30 doses) preassembled, single-patient use, disposable w. glass cartridge

Comment: Tymlos is indicated for increasing bone density in adult men and postmenopausal women with osteoporosis at high risk for fracture (defined as a history of osteoporotic fracture, or multiple risk factors for fracture, or patients who have failed or are intolerant to other available osteoporosis therapy). Tymlos is not indicated for use in females of reproductive potential. There are no human data with use in pregnant females to inform any drug-associated risks, and animal reproduction studies with *abaloparatide* have not been conducted. There is no information on the presence of *abaloparatide* in human milk or effects on the breastfed infant; however, breastfeeding is not recommended while using Tymlos. Tymlos is not recommended for use in pediatric patients with open epiphyses or hereditary disorders predisposing to osteosarcoma because of an increased baseline risk of osteosarcoma. Tymlos may cause hypercalciuria. It is unknown whether Tymlos may exacerbate urolithiasis in patients with active or a history of urolithiasis. If active urolithiasis or preexisting hypercalciuria is suspected, measurement of urinary calcium excretion should be considered. No dosage adjustment is required for patients with any degree of renal impairment. Currently, there are no specific drug-drug interaction studies.

▷ *teriparatide*

Forteo Multidose Pen 20 mcg SC daily in the thigh or abdomen; may treat for up to 2 years

Pediatric: <12 years: not recommended; ≥12 years: same as adult

Multidose pen: 250 mcg/ml (3 ml)

Comment: Forteo is indicated for the treatment of postmenopausal osteoporosis in women who are at high risk for fracture and to increase bone mass in men with primary or hypogonadal osteoporosis who are at high risk for fracture. **Bonsity** 20 mcg SC once daily; administer via SC injection only into the abdominal wall or thigh; initial administration under circumstances in which the patient can sit or lie down if symptoms of orthostatic hypotension occur; during the use period, time out of the refrigerator should be minimized; the dose may be delivered immediately following removal from the refrigerator

Pediatric: not recommended

Prefilled pen: 620 mcg/2.48 ml (250 mcg/ml), single-patientuse, containing 28 daily SC doses of 20 mcg

Comment: Bonsity *(teriparatide)* is a parathyroid hormone analog (PTH 1-34) indicated for the treatment of osteoporosis in certain patients at high risk for fracture, increase bone mass in men with primary or hypogonadal osteoporosis at high risk for fracture, and treatment of men and women with osteoporosis associated with sustained systemic glucocorticoid therapy at high risk for fracture. Use of **Bonsity** *(teriparatide)* more than 2 years during a patient's lifetime is not recommended. Patients with Paget's disease of bone, pediatric and young adult patients with open epiphyses, and patients with prior external beam or implant radiation involving the skeleton should not be treated with **Bonsity**. Use of **Bonsity** for more than 2 years during a patient's lifetime is not recommended. Patients with bone metastases, history of skeletal malignancies, metabolic bone diseases other than osteoporosis, or hypercalcemic disorders should not be treated with **Bonsity**. **Bonsity** may *increase* serum calcium, urinary calcium, and serum uric acid. Use with caution in patients with active or recent urolithiasis due to risk of exacerbation. Transient orthostatic hypotension may occur with initial doses of **Bonsity**; therefore, administer under circumstances in which the patient can sit or lie down. Use **Bonsity** with caution in patients receiving *digoxin* as transient hypercalcemia may predispose the patient to digitalis toxicity. Consider discontinuing **Bonsity** when pregnancy is recognized. Breastfeeding is not recommended during treatment with **Bonsity**. The most common adverse reactions (incidence >10%) reported have been arthralgia, pain, and nausea.

BIOENGINEERED REPLICA OF HUMAN PARATHYROID HORMONE

▶ *bioengineered replica of human parathyroid hormone* initially inject mg IM into the thigh once daily; when initiating, decrease dose of active vitamin D by 50% if serum calcium is above 7.5 mg/dL; monitor serum calcium levels every 3-7 days; after starting or adjusting dose; and when adjusting either active vitamin D or calcium supplements dose

Pediatric: <18 years: not recommended; ≥18 years: same as adult

Natpara *Soln for inj:* 25, 50, 75, 100 mcg (2/pkg), multidose, dual-chamber glass cartridge containing a sterile powder and diluent

Comment: **Natpara** is indicated as adjunct to calcium and vitamin D in patients with parathyroidism.

OSTEOCLAST INHIBITOR (RANK LIGAND [RANKL] INHIBITOR)

▶ *denosumab*

Pediatric: <18 years: not established; treatment with **Prolia** may impair bone growth in children with open growth plates and may inhibit eruption of dentition; ≥18 years: same as adult

Prolia for SC route only; should not be administered intravenously, intramuscularly, or intradermally; 60 mcg SC once every 6 months in the upper arm, abdomen, or upper thigh

Vial/Pen: 60 mg/ml (1 ml), single-dose

Comment: **Prolia** is indicated for the treatment of postmenopausal osteoporosis in females who are at high risk for fracture, defined as a history of osteoporotic fracture or multiple risk factors for fracture or patients who have failed or are intolerant to other therapy, and treatment to increase bone mass in women at high risk for fracture receiving adjuvant aromatase inhibitor therapy for breast cancer. **Prolia** is also indicated for treatment to increase bone mass in men at high risk for fracture receiving androgen deprivation therapy for non-metastatic prostate cancer. **Prolia** must be administered by a healthcare professional. *Denosumab* is contraindicated with hypocalcemia. Instruct patients to take calcium 1,000 mg daily and at least 400 IU vitamin D daily. There is no information regarding the presence of *denosumab* in human milk or effects on the breastfed infant.

Xgeva *Multiple myeloma and bone metastasis from solid tumors:* administer 120 mg administer SC in the upper arm, abdomen, or upper thigh; SC every 4 weeks; *Giant cell tumor of bone:* administer 120 mg SC q 4 weeks with additional 120 mg doses on days 8 and 15 of the first month of therapy and administer calcium and vitamin D as necessary to treat or prevent hypocalcemia; *Hypercalcemia of malignancy:* administer 120 mg every 4 weeks with additional 120 mg doses on Days 8 and 15 of the first month of therapy

Pediatric: recommended only for treatment of skeletally mature adolescents with giant cell tumor of bone; treatment with **Xgeva** may impair bone growth in children with open growth plates and may inhibit eruption of dentition

Vial: 120 mg/1.7 ml (70 mg/ml) solution in a single-dose

Comment: **Xgeva** is indicated for prevention of skeletal-related events in patients with multiple myeloma and in patients with bone metastases from solid tumors, treatment of adults and skeletally mature adolescents with giant cell tumor of bone that is unresectable or where surgical resection is likely to result in severe morbidity, and treatment of hypercalcemia of malignancy refractory to bisphosphonate therapy. CrCl <30 ml/min or receiving dialysis are at risk for hypocalcemia. Adequately supplement with calcium and vitamin D. There is no information regarding the presence of *denosumab* in human milk or effects on the breastfed invent.

ANTI-SCLEROSTIN MONOCLONAL ANTIBODY

▶ *romosozumab-aqqg* a full dose of **Evenity** requires two single-use prefilled syringes (2 x 105 mg = 210 mg) administered SC (administered one after the other) in the upper arm, abdomen, or thigh once each month for 12 full doses (12 months) along with adequately supplemented calcium and vitamin D during treatment; **Evenity** should be administered by a qualified healthcare provider; limit duration of use to 12 monthly treatments

Evenity *Prefilled syringe:* 105 mg/1.17 ml, single-use (2/carton) (no natural rubber latex)

Comment: **Evenity** *(romosozumab-aqqg)* is an anti-sclerostin monoclonal antibody for the treatment of osteoporosis in postmenopausal women at increased risk of fracture, defined as a history of osteoporotic fracture or multiple risk factors for fracture or patients who have failed or are intolerant to other available

(continued)

osteoporosis therapy. If after the 12 monthly treatments osteoporosis therapy remains warranted, continued therapy with an antiresorptive agent should be considered. Monitor serum calcium; patients with severe renal impairment or receiving dialysis are at greater risk of developing hypocalcemia. **Evenity** should be <u>not</u> be initiated in patients who have had a myocardial infarction or stroke within the preceding year. Consider whether the benefits outweigh the risks in patients with other cardiovascular risk factors. If a patient experiences a myocardial infarction or stroke during therapy, **Evenity** should be discontinued. **Evenity** is <u>not</u> indicated for use in women of reproductive potential or in pediatric patients.

OTITIS EXTERNA

OTIC ANALGESIC
▷ *antipyrine+benzocaine+zinc acetate dihydrate* fill ear canal with solution; then insert a cotton plug into meatus; may repeat every 1-2 hours prn
   Pediatric: same as adult
   Otozin *Otic soln:* antipyr 5.4%+benz 1%+zinc 1% per ml (10 ml w. dropper)

OTIC ANTI-INFECTIVE
▷ *chloroxylenol+pramoxine* 4-5 drops tid x 5-10 days
   Pediatric: <1 year: <u>not</u> recommended; 1-12 years: 5 drops bid x 10 days; ≥12 years: same as adult
   PramOtic *Otic drops:* chlorox+pramox (5 ml w. dropper)
▷ *finafloxacin* otic 4-5 drops tid x 5-10 days
   Pediatric: <1 year: <u>not</u> recommended; ≥1 year: same as adult
   Xtoro *Otic soln:* 0.3% (5, 8 ml)
▷ *ofloxacin* (G) 10 drops bid x 10 days
   Pediatric: <1 year: <u>not</u> recommended; 1-12 years: 5 drops bid x 10 days; ≥12 years: same as adult
   Floxin *Otic Otic soln:* 0.3% (5, 10 ml w. dropper; 0.25 ml, 5 drop singles, 20/carton)
   Comment: Floxin Otic is indicated for adult patients with perforated tympanic membranes and pediatric patients with percutaneous ear tubes (i.e., PE tubes, tympanostomy tubes) PE tubes.

OTIC ANTI-INFECTIVE+CORTICOSTEROID COMBINATIONS
▷ *chloroxylenol+pramoxine+hydrocortisone* (G) drops 4 drops tid-qid x 5-10 days
   Pediatric: 3 drops tid-qid x 5-10 days
   Cortane B, Cortane B Aqueous *Otic soln:* chlo 1 mg+pram 10 mg+hydro 10 mg per ml (10 ml w. dropper)
   Comment: Cortane B Aqueous may be used to saturate a cotton wick.
▷ *ciprofloxacin+hydrocortisone* susp 3 drops bid x 7 days
   Pediatric: <1 year: <u>not</u> recommended; ≥1 year: same as adult
   Cipro HC *Otic Otic susp:* cipro 0.2%+hydro 1% (10 ml w. dropper)
▷ *ciprofloxacin+dexamethasone* (G) 4 drops bid x 7 days
   Pediatric: <6 months: <u>not</u> recommended; ≥6 months: same as adult
   Ciprodex *Otic susp:* cipro 0.3%+dexa 1% (7.5 ml)
   Comment: Ciprodex is indicated for the treatment of otitis media in pediatric patients with tympanostomy tubes.
▷ *colistin+neomycin+hydrocortisone+thonzonium* (G) 5 drops tid or qid x 5-10 days
   Pediatric: 4 drops tid-qid x 5-10 days
   Coly-Mycin S *Otic susp:* 5, 10 ml
   Cortisporin-TC *Otic Otic susp:* colis 3 mg+neo 3.3 mg+hydro 10 mg+thon 0.5 mg per ml (10 ml w. dropper) (thimerosal)
▷ *polymyxin b+neomycin+hydrocortisone* (G) 4 drops tid-qid; max 10 days
   Pediatric: 3 drops tid-qid; max 10 days
   Cortisporin Otic Suspension *Otic susp:* poly b 10,000 u+neo 3.5 mg+hydro 10 mg per 5 ml (10 ml w. dropper)
   Cortisporin Otic Solution *Otic soln:* poly b 10,000 u+neo 3.5 mg+hydro 10 mg per 5 ml (10 ml w. dropper)

OTIC ASTRINGENTS
▷ *acetic acid 2% in aluminum sulfate* (G) 4-6 drops q 2-3 hours
   Pediatric: same as adult
   Domeboro *Otic Otic soln:* 60 ml w. dropper
▷ *acetic acid+propylene glycol+benzethonium chloride+sodium acetate* (G) 3-5 drops q 4-6 hours
   Pediatric: same as adult
   VoSol *Otic soln:* acet 2% (15, 30 ml)
▷ *acetic acid+propylene glycol+hydrocortisone+benzethonium chloride+sodium acetate* (G) 3-5 drops q 4-6 hours
   Pediatric: same as adult
   VoSol HC *Otic soln:* acet 2%+hydro 1% (10 ml)

OTIC ANESTHETIC+ANALGESIC COMBINATIONS

➤ *antipyrine+benzocaine+glycerine* (G) fill ear canal and insert cotton plug; may repeat q 1-2 hours as needed
  Pediatric: same as adult
    A/B Otic *Otic soln:* 15 ml w. dropper
➤ *benzocaine* (G) 4-5 drops q 1-2 hours
  Pediatric: <1 year: <u>not</u> recommended; ≥1 year: same as adult
    Americaine Otic *Otic soln:* 20% (15 ml w. dropper)
    Benzotic *Otic soln:* 20% (15 ml w. dropper)

SYSTEMIC ANTI-INFECTIVES

Comment: Used for severe disease <u>or</u> with culture.
➤ *amoxicillin+clavulanate* (G)
    Augmentin 500 mg tid <u>or</u> 875 mg bid x 7-10 days
    Pediatric: 40-45 mg/kg/day divided tid x 10 days <u>or</u> 90 mg/kg/day divided bid x 10 days; *see* Appendix
    BB.4. *amoxicillin+clavulanate* (G) (Augmentin Suspension) *for dose by weight*
      Tab: 250, 500, 875 mg; *Chew tab:* 125, 250 mg (lemon-lime); 200, 400 mg (cherry-banana) (phenylal-
      anine); *Oral susp:* 125 mg/5 ml (banana), 250 mg/5 ml (75, 100, 150 ml) (orange); 200, 400 mg/5 ml
      (50, 75, 100 ml) (orange) (phenylalanine)
    Augmentin ES-600 <u>not</u> recommended for adults
    Pediatric: <3 months: <u>not</u> recommended; ≥3 months, <40 kg: 90 mg/kg/day in 2 divided doses x 7-10
    days; ≥40 kg: <u>not</u> recommended
      Oral susp: 42.9 mg/5 ml (50, 75, 100, 125, 150, 200 ml) (strawberry cream) (phenylalanine)
    Augmentin XR 2 tabs q 12 hours x 7-10 days
    Pediatric: <16 years: use other forms; ≥16 years: same as adult
      Tab: 1,000*mg ext-rel
➤ *cefaclor* (G)
    Ceclor 250 mg tid <u>or</u> 375 mg bid 3-10 days
    Pediatric: <1 month: <u>not</u> recommended; 1 month-12 years: 20-40 mg/kg divided bid <u>or</u> q 12 hours x
    3-10 days; max 1 gm/day; see Appendix BB.8. *cefaclor* (G) (Ceclor Suspension) for *dose by weight*; >12
    years: same as adult
      Tab: 500 mg; *Cap:* 250, 500 mg; *Susp:* 125 mg/5 ml (75, 150 ml) (strawberry), 187 mg/5 ml (50, 100 ml)
      (strawberry), 250 mg/5 ml (75, 150 ml) (strawberry), 375 mg/5 ml (50, 100 ml) (strawberry)
    Ceclor Extended Release 375-500 mg bid x 3-10 days
    Pediatric: <16 years: ext-rel <u>not</u> recommended; ≥16 years: same as adult
      Tab: 375, 500 mg ext-rel
➤ *dicloxacillin* 500 mg qid x 7-10 days
  Pediatric: 12.5-25 mg/kg/day in 4 divided doses x 7-10 days; *see* Appendix BB.18. *dicloxacillin* (G) (Dynapen
  Suspension) *for dose by weight*
    Dynapen *Cap:* 125, 250, 500 mg; *Oral susp:* 62.5 mg/5 ml (80, 100, 200 ml)
➤ *trimethoprim+sulfamethoxazole (TMP-SMX)* (G)
  Pediatric: <2 months: <u>not</u> recommended; ≥2 months: 40 mg/kg/day of *sulfamethoxazole* in 2 doses bid x 10
  days; *see* Appendix BB.33: *trimethoprim+sulfamethoxazole* (G) (Bactrim Suspension, Septra Suspension) *for
  dose by weight*
    Bactrim, Septra 2 tabs bid x 10 days
      Tab: trim 80 mg+sulfa 400 mg*
    Bactrim DS, Septra DS 1 tab bid x 10 days
      Tab: trim 160 mg+sulfa 800 mg*
    Bactrim Pediatric Suspension, Septra Pediatric Suspension
      Oral susp: trim 40 mg+sulfa 200 mg per 5 ml (100 ml) (cherry) (alcohol 0.3%)

OTITIS MEDIA: ACUTE

OTIC ANALGESIC

➤ *antipyrine+benzocaine+zinc acetate dihydrate* otic fill ear canal with solution; then insert cotton plug into
  meatus; may repeat every 1-2 hours prn
  Pediatric: same as adult
    Otozin *Otic soln:* antipyr 5.4%+benz 1%+zinc 1% per ml (10 ml w. dropper)

SYSTEMIC ANTI-INFECTIVES

➤ *amoxicillin* (G) 500-875 mg bid <u>or</u> 250-500 mg tid x 10 days
  Pediatric: <40 kg (88 lb): 20-40 mg/kg/day in 3 divided doses x 10 days <u>or</u> 25-45 mg/kg/day in 2 divided
  doses x 10 days; *see* Appendix BB.3. *amoxicillin* (G) (Amoxil Suspension, Trimox Suspension) *for dose by
  weight*
    Amoxil *Cap:* 250, 500 mg; *Tab:* 875*mg; *Chew tab:* 125, 200, 250, 400 mg (cherry-banana-peppermint)
    (phenylalanine); *Oral susp:* 125, 250 mg/5 ml (80, 100, 150 ml) (strawberry); 200, 400 mg/5 ml (50, 75,
    100 ml) (bubble gum); *Oral drops:* 50 mg/ml (30 ml) (bubble gum)

(continued)

Moxatag *Tab:* 775 mg ext-rel
Trimox *Tab:* 125, 250 mg; *Cap:* 250, 500 mg; *Oral susp:* 125, 250 mg/5 ml (80, 100, 150 ml) (raspberry-strawberry)
Comment: Consider 80-90 mg/kg/day in 3 divided doses for resistant cases

▷ *amoxicillin+clavulanate* (G)
Augmentin 500 mg tid <u>or</u> 875 mg bid x 7-10 days
Pediatric: 40-45 mg/kg/day divided tid x 10 days <u>or</u> 90 mg/kg/day divided bid x 10 days; *see* Appendix BB.4. *amoxicillin+clavulanate* (G) (Augmentin Suspension) *for dose by weight*
Tab: 250, 500, 875 mg; *Chew tab:* 125, 250 mg (lemon-lime); 200, 400 mg (cherry-banana) (phenylalanine); *Oral susp:* 125 mg/5 ml (banana), 250 mg/5 ml (75, 100, 150 ml) (orange); 200, 400 mg/5 ml (50, 75, 100 ml) (orange) (phenylalanine)
Augmentin ES-600 <u>not</u> recommended for adults
Pediatric: <3 months: <u>not</u> recommended; ≥3 months, <40 kg: 90 mg/kg/day in 2 divided doses x 7-10 days; ≥40 kg: <u>not</u> recommended
Oral susp: 42.9 mg/5 ml (50, 75, 100, 125, 150, 200 ml) (strawberry cream) (phenylalanine)
Augmentin XR 2 tabs q 12 hours x 7-10 days
Pediatric: <16 years: use other forms; ≥16 years: same as adult
Tab: 1,000*mg ext-rel

▷ *ampicillin* 250-500 mg qid x 10 days
Pediatric: 50-100 mg/kg/day in 4 divided doses x 10 days; *see* Appendix BB.6. *ampicillin* (Omnipen Suspension, Principen Suspension) *for dose by weight*
Omnipen, Principen *Cap:* 250, 500 mg; *Oral susp:* 125, 250 mg/5 ml (100, 150, 200 ml) (fruit)

▷ *azithromycin* (G) 500 mg x 1 dose on day 1, then 250 mg daily on days 2-5 <u>or</u> 500 mg daily x 3 days <u>or</u>
Zmax 2 gm in a single dose
Pediatric: 12 mg/kg/day x 5 days; max 500 mg/day; *see* Appendix BB.7. *azithromycin* (G) (Zithromax Suspension, Zmax Suspension) *for dose by weight*
Zithromax *Tab:* 250, 500, 600 mg; *Oral susp:* 100 mg/5 ml (15 ml), 200 mg/5 ml (15, 22.5, 30 ml) (cherry); *Pkt:* 1 gm for reconstitution (cherry-banana)
Zithromax Tri-Pak *Tab:* 3 x 500 mg tabs/pck
Zithromax Z-Pak *Tab:* 6 x 250 mg tabs/pck
Zmax *Oral susp:* 2 gm ext-rel for reconstitution (cherry-banana) (148 mg Na$^+$)

▷ *cefaclor* (G)
Ceclor 250 mg tid <u>or</u> 375 mg bid 3-10 days
Pediatric: <1 month: <u>not</u> recommended; 1 month-12 years: 20-40 mg/kg divided bid <u>or</u> q 12 hours x 3-10 days; max 1 gm/day; *see* Appendix BB.8. *cefaclor* (G) (Ceclor Suspension) for *dose by weight;* >12 years: same as adult
Tab: 500 mg; *Cap:* 250, 500 mg; *Susp:* 125 mg/5 ml (75, 150 ml) (strawberry), 187 mg/5 ml (50, 100 ml) (strawberry), 250 mg/5 ml (75, 150 ml) (strawberry), 375 mg/5 ml (50, 100 ml) (strawberry)
Ceclor Extended Release 375-500 mg bid x 3-10 days
Pediatric: <16 years: ext-rel <u>not</u> recommended; ≥16 years: same as adult
Tab: 375, 500 mg ext-rel

▷ *cefdinir* 300 mg bid <u>or</u> 600 mg daily x 5-10 days
Pediatric: <6 months: <u>not</u> recommended; 6 months-12 years: 14 mg/kg/day in 1-2 divided doses x 10 days; >12 years: same as adult; *see* Appendix BB.10. *cefdinir* (G) (Omnicef Suspension) *for dose by weight*
Omnicef *Cap:* 300 mg; *Oral susp:* 125 mg/5 ml (60, 100 ml) (strawberry)

▷ *cefixime* (G)
Pediatric: <6 months: <u>not</u> recommended; 6 months-12 years, <50 kg: 8 mg/kg/day in 1-2 divided doses x 10 days; >12 years, ≥50 kg: same as adult; *see* Appendix BB.11. *cefixime* (G) (Suprax Oral Suspension) *for dose by weight*
Suprax *Tab:* 400 mg; *Cap:* 400 mg; *Oral susp:* 100, 200, 500 mg/5 ml (50, 75, 100 ml) (strawberry)

▷ *cefpodoxime proxetil* 100 mg bid x 5 days
Pediatric: <2 months: <u>not</u> recommended; 2 months-12 years: 10 mg/kg/day (max 400 mg/dose) <u>or</u> 5 mg/kg/day bid (max 200 mg/dose) x 5 days; >12 years: same as adult; *see* Appendix BB.12. *cefpodoxime proxetil* (G) (Vantin Suspension) *for dose by weight*
Vantin *Tab:* 100, 200 mg; *Oral susp:* 50, 100 mg/5 ml (50, 75, 100 ml) (lemon creme)

▷ *cefprozil* 250-500 mg bid <u>or</u> 500 mg daily x 10 days
Pediatric: <2 years: same as adult; 2-12 years: 7.5 mg/kg bid x 10 days; *see* Appendix BB.13. *cefprozil* (G) (Cefzil Suspension) *for dose by weight;* >12 years: same as adult
Cefzil *Tab:* 250, 500 mg; *Oral susp:* 125, 250 mg/5 ml (50, 75, 100 ml) (bubble gum) (phenylalanine)

▷ *ceftibuten* 400 mg daily x 10 days
Pediatric: 9 mg/kg daily x 10 days; max 400 mg/day; *see* Appendix BB.14. *ceftibuten* (G) (Cedax Suspension) *for dose by weight*
Cedax *Cap:* 400 mg; *Oral susp:* 90 mg/5 ml (30, 60, 90, 120 ml), 180 mg/5 ml (30, 60, 120 ml) (cherry)

▷ *ceftriaxone* (G) 1-2 gm IM x 1 dose; max 4 gm
Pediatric: 50 mg/kg IM x 1 dose
Rocephin *Vial:* 250, 500 mg; 1, 2 gm

▷ *cephalexin* (G) 250 mg qid x 10 days
  Pediatric: 25-50 mg/kg/day in 4 doses x 10 days; *see Appendix BB.15. cephalexin* (G) (Keflex Suspension) *for dose by weight*
    Keflex *Cap:* 250, 333, 500, 750 mg; *Oral susp:* 125, 250 mg/5 ml (100, 200 ml) (strawberry)
▷ *clarithromycin* (G) 500 mg bid or 500 mg ext-rel once daily x 10 days
  Pediatric: <6 months: not recommended; ≥6 months: 7.5 mg/kg divided bid x 7 days; *see Appendix BB.16. clarithromycin* (G) (Biaxin Suspension) *for dose by weight*
    Biaxin *Tab:* 250, 500 mg
    Biaxin Oral Suspension *Oral susp:* 125, 250 mg/5 ml (50, 100 ml) (fruit punch)
    Biaxin XL *Tab:* 500 mg ext-rel
▷ *erythromycin+sulfisoxazole* (G)
  Pediatric: <2 months: not recommended; ≥2 months: 50 mg/kg/day in 3 divided doses x 10 days; *see Appendix BB.22. erythromycin+sulfamethoxazole* (G) (Eryzole, Pediazole) *for dose by weight*
    Eryzole *Oral susp:* eryth 200 mg+sulfa 600 mg per 5 ml (100, 150, 200, 250 ml)
    Pediazole *Oral susp:* eryth 200 mg+sulfa 600 mg per 5 ml (100, 150, 200 ml) (strawberry-banana)
▷ *loracarbef* 400 mg bid x 10 days
  Pediatric: 30 mg/kg/day in divided bid x 7 days; *see Appendix BB.27. loracarbef* (G) (Lorabid Suspension) *for dose by weight*
    Lorabid *Pulvule:* 200, 400 mg; *Oral susp:* 100 mg/5 ml (50, 100 ml), 200 mg/5 ml (50, 75, 100 ml) (strawberry bubble gum)
▷ *trimethoprim+sulfamethoxazole (TMP-SMX)* (G)
  Pediatric: <2 months: not recommended; >2 months: 40 mg/kg/day of *sulfamethoxazole* in divided doses bid x 10 days; *see Appendix BB.33. trimethoprim+sulfamethoxazole* (G) (Bactrim Suspension, Septra Suspension) *for dose by weight*
    Bactrim, Septra 2 tabs bid x 10 days
      Tab: trim 80 mg+sulfa 400 mg*
    Bactrim DS, Septra DS 1 tab bid x 10 days
      Tab: trim 160 mg+sulfa 800 mg*
    Bactrim Pediatric Suspension, Septra Pediatric Suspension
      Oral susp: trim 40 mg+sulfa 200 mg per 5 ml (100 ml) (cherry) (alcohol 0.3%)

OTIC ANTI-INFECTIVE

▷ *ofloxacin* (G) 10 drops bid x 14 days
  Pediatric: <6 months: not recommended; 6 months-12 years: 5 drops bid x 14 days; >12 years: same as adult
    Floxin Otic *Otic soln:* 0.3% (5, 10 ml w. dropper)

OTIC ANTI-INFECTIVE+CORTICOSTEROID COMBINATIONS

Comment: *Neomycin* may cause ototoxicity. Do not use with known or suspected tympanic membrane rupture.

▷ *chloroxylenol+pramoxine+hydrocortisone* 4 drops tid-qid x 5-10 days
  Pediatric: 3 drops tid-qid x 5-10 days
    Cortane Ear Drops, *Otic drops:* 10 ml
▷ *ciprofloxacin+hydrocortisone* otic susp 3 drops bid x 7 days
  Pediatric: <1 year: not recommended; ≥1 year: same as adult
    Cipro HC *Otic susp:* cipro 0.3%+dexa 0.1% (10 ml)
▷ *ciprofloxacin+dexamethasone* (G) otic susp 4 drops bid x 7 days
  Pediatric: <6 months: not recommended; ≥6 months: same as adult
    Ciprodex *Otic susp:* cipro 0.3%+dexa 1% (7.5 ml)
    Comment: Ciprodex is indicated for the treatment of otitis media in pediatric patients with tympanostomy tubes (PE tubes).
▷ *colistin+neomycin+hydrocortisone+thonzonium* 5 drops tid-qid x 5-10 days
  Pediatric: 4 drops tid-qid x 5-10 days
    Coly-Mycin S *Otic susp:* 5, 10 ml
▷ *polymyxin b+neomycin+hydrocortisone* (G) 4 drops tid-qid; max 10 days
  Pediatric: 3 drops tid-qid; max 10 days
    Cortisporin *Otic susp:* 10 ml w. dropper; *Otic soln:* 10 ml w. dropper
    PediOtic *Otic susp:* 7.5 ml w. dropper
▷ *polymyxin b+neomycin+hydrocortisone+surfactant* 4 drops tid-qid
  Pediatric: 3 drops tid-qid; max 10 days
    Cortisporin-TC *Otic susp:* 10 ml w. dropper

OTIC ANESTHETIC+ANALGESIC COMBINATIONS

▷ *antipyrine+benzocaine+glycerine* fill ear canal and insert cotton plug; may repeat q 1-2 hours as needed
  Pediatric: same as adult
    A/B Otic *Otic soln:* antipy 5.4%+benzo 1.4% 15 ml w. dropper

(continued)

▷ *benzocaine* (OTC) 4-5 drops q 1-2 hours
   Pediatric: <1 year: <u>not</u> recommended; ≥1 year: same as adult
   benzocaine *Otic drops*: 20% (15 ml dropper-top bottle)
      Americaine Otic *Otic soln*: 15 ml w. dropper
      Benzotic *Otic soln*: 20% (15 ml w. dropper)

OTITIS MEDIA: SEROUS (SOM), OTITIS MEDIA WITH EFFUSION

Anti-Infectives *see Otitis Media: Acute*
Antihistamines and Decongestants *see* Appendix Z. Drugs for the Management of Allergy, Cough, and Cold
Symptoms online at https://connect.springerpub.com/content/reference-book/978-0-8261-7935-7/back-matter/
part02/back-matter/bmatter27
Oral Corticosteroids *see* Appendix K. Oral Corticosteroids

INTRATYMPANIC AGENT

▷ *ciprofloxacin otic suspension* <6 months: <u>not</u> recommended; ≥6 months: instill 0.1 ml in each ear, via
   intratympanic administration <u>only</u> by a qualified healthcare professional, following suctioning of the middle
   ear effusion
      Otiprio *Vial*: 6% otic suspension (6 mg/ml, 1 ml) single-patient use with two 0.1 ml doses in each vial
      (preservative-free)
      Comment: Otiprio is *ciprofloxacin,* a synthetic fluoroquinolone antibacterial, indicated for the
      treatment of acute otitis media (AOM) due to *Pseudomonas aeruginosa* and *Staphylococcus aureus*
      and for intratympanic administration in pediatric patients ≥6 months of age with bilateral AOM
      with effusion undergoing tympanostomy tube placement. The bactericidal action of *ciprofloxacin*
      results from interference with the enzyme DNA gyrase, which is needed for the synthesis of bacterial
      DNA. *Ciprofloxacin* has been shown to be active against most isolates of the following bacteria:
      gram-positive bacteria (i.e., *Staphylococcus aureus, Streptococcus pneumoniae*) and gram-negative
      bacteria (*Haemophilus influenzae, Moraxella catarrhalis, Pseudomonas aeruginosa*). **Otiprio** is for
      intratympanic administration <u>only</u>. The most frequently occurring adverse reactions (incidence >
      3 %) were nasopharyngitis and irritability. Because of the negligible systemic exposure associated
      with clinical administration of **Otiprio,** this product is expected to be of minimal risk for maternal
      and fetal toxicity during pregnancy and nursing infants of mothers receiving **Otiprio** should <u>not</u> be
      affected.

OVULATION INDUCTION

Comment: Fertility treatments are prescribed by physicians who are trained and experienced in this specialty
field. Pregnancy must be excluded prior to initiating any fertility treatment.

SYNTHETIC OVULATION STIMULANTS

▷ *clomiphene citrate* (G) take 50 mg once daily x 5 days, starting on the 5th day of the menstrual period;
   impediments to achieving pregnancy must be excluded <u>or</u> adequately treated before beginning **Clomid**
   therapy; using **Clomid** for longer than 3 treatment cycles may increase the risk of developing an ovarian
   tumor; patients should be evaluated carefully to exclude pregnancy, ovarian enlargement, <u>or</u> ovarian cyst
   formation between each treatment cycle; store **Clomid** at room temperature away from moisture, heat, and
   light.
      Clomid *Tab*: 50*mg
      Comment: Clomid is a non-steroidal fertility medicine indicated for anovulatory patients (e.g.,
      polycystic ovary syndrome, POS) desiring pregnancy. It causes the pituitary gland to release
      hormones needed to stimulate ovulation. *Clomiphene citrate* is capable of interacting with
      estrogen receptor-containing tissues, including the hypothalamus, pituitary, ovary, endometrium,
      vagina, and cervix. It may compete with estrogen for estrogen receptor-binding sites and may
      delay replenishment of intracellular estrogen receptors. *Clomiphene citrate* initiates a series of
      endocrine events culminating in a preovulatory gonadotropin surge and subsequent follicular
      rupture. The first endocrine event in response to a course of *clomiphene* therapy is an increase in
      the release of pituitary gonadotropins. This initiates steroidogenesis and folliculogenesis, resulting
      in growth of the ovarian follicle and an increase in the circulating level of estradiol. Following
      ovulation, plasma progesterone and estradiol rise and fall as they would in a normal ovulatory cycle.
      Clomiphene citrate has <u>no</u> apparent progestational, androgenic, <u>or</u> antiandrogenic effects and does
      <u>not</u> appear to interfere with pituitary-adrenal <u>or</u> pituitary-thyroid function. Although there is no
      evidence of a "carryover effect" of **Clomid,** spontaneous ovulatory menses have been noted in some
      patients after **Clomid** therapy. **Clomid** should <u>not</u> be used in patients with liver disease, abnormal
      vaginal bleeding, an uncontrolled adrenal gland <u>or</u> thyroid disorder, an ovarian cyst (unrelated to
      POS), <u>or</u> patients who are pregnant. Fertility treatment may increase the patient's chance of having
      multiple births (twins, triplets). These are high-risk pregnancies both for the mother and the

babies. Ovulation usually occurs within 5 to 10 days after taking the **Clomid**. Advise patients that sexual intercourse while ovulating improves the chance of becoming pregnant. Common **Clomid** side effects may include flushing (warmth, redness, or tingly feeling), breast pain or tenderness, headache, or breakthrough bleeding or spotting. **Clovid** may cause blurred vision. Advise patients to be careful when driving or doing anything that requires alertness and clear vision. *Clomiphene* can pass into breast milk and may harm the breastfeeding infant.

SYNTHETIC DECAPEPTIDE WITH GONADOTROPIN-RELEASING HORMONE (GNRH) ANTAGONISTIC ACTIVITY

▷ *cetrorelix acetate* (G) administer doses via SC injection in the lower abdominal region; before starting treatment with **Cetrotide**, pregnancy must be excluded; ovarian stimulation therapy with gonadotropins (follicle-stimulating hormone [FSH], human menopausal gonadotropin [HMG]) is started on cycle Day 2 or 3; the dose of gonadotropins should be adjusted according to individual response; **Cetrotide** is administered SC either once daily (0.25 mg dose) or a one-time single dose (3 mg dose) during the early- to mid-follicular phase

Single dose regimen: 3 mg of **Cetrotide** is administered when the serum estradiol level is indicative of an appropriate stimulation response, usually on stimulation day 7 (range day 5-9); if human chorionic gonadotropin (hCG) has not been administered within 4 days after injection of **Cetrotide** 3 mg, **Cetrotide** 0.25 mg should be administered once daily until the day of hCG administration

Multiple-dose regimen: 0.25 mg of **Cetrotide** is administered on either stimulation day 5 (morning or evening) or day 6 (morning) and continued daily until the day of hCG administration; when assessment by ultrasound shows a sufficient number of follicles of adequate size, hCG is administered to induce ovulation and final maturation of the oocytes; no hCG should be administered if the ovaries show an excessive response to the treatment with gonadotropins to reduce the chance of developing ovarian hyperstimulation syndrome (OHSS)

Cetrotide *Vial:* 0.25 mg w. 1 ml diluent, 3 mg w. 3 ml diluent, pwdr for reconstitution co-packaged w. supplied diluent in prefilled syringe, and SC injection; each vial of **Cetrotide** 0.25 mg (multiple-dose regimen) contains 0.26-0.27 mg *cetrorelix acetate* equivalent to 0.25 mg *cetrorelix* and 54.80 mg mannitol; each vial of **Cetrotide** 3 mg (single-dose regimen) contains 3.12-3.24 mg *cetrorelix acetate*, equivalent to 3 mg *cetrorelix* and 164.40 mg mannitol

Comment: **Cetrotide** is indicated for the inhibition of premature luteinizing hormone (LH) surges in women undergoing controlled ovarian stimulation. **Cetrotide** is a synthetic decapeptide with gonadotropin-releasing hormone (GnRH) antagonistic activity. GnRH induces the production and release of LH and FSH from the gonadotrophic cells of the anterior pituitary. Due to a positive estradiol (E2) feedback at midcycle, GnRH liberation is enhanced, resulting in an LH surge. This LH surge induces the ovulation of the dominant follicle, resumption of oocyte meiosis, and subsequently luteinization as indicated by rising progesterone levels. **Cetrotide** competes with natural GnRH for binding to membrane receptors on pituitary cells and thus controls the release of LH and FSH in a dose-dependent manner. The onset of LH suppression is approximately 1 hour with the 3 mg dose and 2 hours with the 0.25 mg dose. This suppression is maintained by continuous treatment and there is a more pronounced effect on LH than on FSH. An initial release of endogenous gonadotropins has not been detected with **Cetrotide**, which is consistent with an antagonist effect. The effects of **Cetrotide** on LH and FSH are reversible after discontinuation of treatment. In women, **Cetrotide** delays the LH surge, and consequently ovulation, in a dose-dependent fashion. FSH levels are not affected at the doses used during controlled ovarian stimulation. Following a single 3 mg dose of **Cetrotide**, duration of action of at least 4 days has been established. A 0.25 mg dose of **Cetrotide** every 24 hours has been shown to maintain the effect. **Cetrotide** is contraindicated under the following conditions: (1) hypersensitivity to *cetrorelix acetate*, extrinsic peptide hormones, or mannitol; (2) known hypersensitivity to GnRH or any other GnRH analogs; and (3) known or suspected pregnancy and lactation. Patients may self-administer **Cetrotide** injections as prescribed with appropriate education and training and approval of the prescribing physician. It is not known whether **Cetrotide** is excreted in human milk. Because the effects of **Cetrotide** on the breastfed infant have not been determined, **Cetrotide** should not be used by breastfeeding mothers.

PAGET'S DISEASE: BONE

Comment: Calcium decreases *tetracycline* absorption. Calcium absorption is decreased by corticosteroids. Calcium absorption is decreased by foods such as rhubarb, spinach, and bran.

BISPHOSPHONATES (CALCIUM MODIFIERS)

Comment: Bisphosphonates should be swallowed whole in the AM with 6-8 oz of plain water 30 minutes before first meal, beverage, or other medications of the day. Monitor serum alkaline phosphatase. Contraindications include abnormalities of the esophagus which delay esophageal emptying, such as stricture or achalasia, inability to stand or sit upright for at least 30 minutes post-dose, patients at risk of aspiration, and hypocalcemia. Co-administration of bisphosphonates and calcium, antacids, or oral medications containing multivalent cations will interfere with absorption of the bisphosphonate. Therefore, instruct patients to wait at least half hour after taking the bisphosphonate before taking any other oral medications.

(continued)

▷ *alendronate (as sodium)* (G) take once weekly, in the AM, 30 minutes before the first food, beverage, or medication of the day; do not lie down (remain upright) for at least 30 minutes and after the first food of the day; not recommended with *CrCl <35 ml/min*
Pediatric: <12 years: not recommended; ≥12 years: same as adult
  Binosto dissolve the effervescent tab in 4 oz (120 ml) of plain, room temperature, water (not mineral or flavored); wait 5 minutes after the effervescence has subsided, then stir for 10 seconds, then drink
    Tab: 70 mg effervescent for buffered solution (4, 12/carton) (strawberry)
  Fosamax (G) swallow tab whole; dosing regimens are the same for men and postmenopausal women; *Prevention:* 5 mg once daily or 35 mg once weekly; *Treatment:* 10 mg once daily or 70 mg once weekly
    Tab: 5, 10, 35, 40, 70 mg
▷ *alendronate+cholecalciferol (vit d3)* (G) take 1 tab once weekly, in the AM, with plain water (not mineral) 30 minutes before the first food, beverage, or medication of the day; do not lie down (remain upright) for at least 30 minutes and after the first food of the day
Pediatric: <12 years: not recommended; ≥12 years: same as adult
  Fosamax Plus D
    Tab: Fosamax Plus D 70/2800 alen 70 mg+chole 2,800 IU
    Fosamax Plus D 70/5600 alen 70 mg+chole 5,600 IU
▷ *ibandronate (as monosodium monohydrate)* (G)
Pediatric: <12 years: not recommended; ≥12 years: same as adult
  Boniva take 2.5 mg once daily or 150 mg once monthly on the same day; take in the AM, with plain water (not mineral) 60 minutes before the first food, beverage, or medication of the day; do not lie down (remain upright) for at least 30 minutes and after the first food of the day
    Tab: 2.5, 150 mg
  Boniva Injection administer 3 mg every 3 months by IV bolus over 15-30 seconds; if dose is missed, administer as soon as possible, then every 3 months from the date of the last dose
    Prefilled syringe: 3 mg/3 ml (5 ml)
    Comment: Boniva Injection must be administered by a qualified healthcare professional.
▷ *risedronate (as sodium)* (G) take in the AM; swallow whole with a full glass of plain water (not mineral); do not lie down (remain upright) for 30 minutes afterward
Pediatric: <12 years: not recommended; ≥12 years: same as adult
  Actonel take at least 30 minutes before any food or drink; *Women:* 5 mg once daily or 35 mg once weekly or 75 mg on 2 consecutive days monthly or 150 mg once monthly; *Men:* 35 mg once weekly
    Tab: 5, 30, 35, 75, 150 mg
  Atelvia 35 mg once weekly immediately after breakfast
    Tab: 35 mg del-rel
▷ *risedronate+calcium* 1 x 5 mg *risedronate* tab weekly and 1 x 500 mg *calcium* tab on days 2-7 weekly
  Actonel with Calcium *Tab: risedronate* 5 mg and *Tab: calcium* 500 mg (4 *risedronate* tabs + 30 *calcium* tabs/pck)
▷ *zoledronic acid* (G)
Pediatric: <12 years: not recommended; ≥12 years: same as adult
  Reclast administer 5 mg via IV infusion over at least 15 minutes mg once a year (for osteoporosis) or once q 2 years (for osteopenia or prophylaxis)
    Bottle: 5 mg/100 ml (single-dose)
    Comment: Reclast is indicated for the treatment of postmenopausal osteoporosis in women who are at high risk for fracture and to increase bone mass in men with primary or hypogonadal osteoporosis who are at high risk for fracture. Administered by a qualified healthcare professional. Contraindicated in hypocalcemia.
  Zometa administer 4 mg via IV infusion over at least 15 minutes q 3-4 weeks; optimal duration of treatment not known
    Bottle: 4 mg/5 ml; *Vial:* 4 mg/5 ml (single-dose)
    Comment: Zometa is indicated for the treatment of hypercalcemia of malignancy. The safety and efficacy of Zometa in the treatment of hypercalcemia associated with hyperparathyroidism or with other non-tumor-related conditions have not been established.

PAIN

Antidepressants *see Depression*
Skeletal Muscle Relaxants *see Muscle Strain*

ACETAMINOPHEN FOR IV INFUSION

▷ *acetaminophen* injectable administer by IV infusion over 15 minutes; 1,000 mg q 6 hours prn or 650 mg q 4 hours prn; max 4,000 mg/day
Pediatric: <2 years: not recommended; 2-13 years, <50 kg: 15 mg/kg q 6 hours prn or 2.5 mg/kg q 4 hours prn; max 750 mg/single-dose; max 75 mg/kg per day; >13 years: same as adult
  Ofirmev *Vial:* 10 mg/ml (100 ml) (preservative-free)

Comment: The **Ofirmev** vial is intended for single-use. If any portion is withdrawn from the vial, use within 6 hours. Discard the unused portion. For pediatric patients, withdraw the intended dose and administer via syringe pump. Do not admix **Ofirmev** with any other drugs. **Ofirmev** is physically incompatible with *diazepam* and *chlorpromazine hydrochloride*.

IBUPROFEN FOR IV INFUSION

▷ *ibuprofen* dilute dose in 0.9% NS, D5W, or lactated Ringers (LR) solution; administer by IV infusion over at least 10 minutes; do not administer via IV bolus or IM; 400-800 mg q 6 hours prn; maximum 3,200 mg/day
Pediatric: <6 months; not recommended; 6 months-<12 years: 10 mg/kg q 4-6 hours prn; max 400 mg/dose; max 40 mg/kg or 2,400 mg/24 hours, whichever is less; 12-17 years: 400 mg q 4-6 hours prn; max 2,400 mg/24 hours

   Caldolor *Vial:* 800 mg/8 ml, single-dose
   Comment: Prepare **Caldolor** solution for IV administration as follows: 100 mg dose: dilute 1 ml of **Caldolor** in at least 100 ml of diluent (intravenous infusion [IVF]); 200 mg dose: dilute 2 ml of **Caldolor** in at least 100 ml of diluent; 400 mg dose: dilute 4 ml of **Caldolor** in at least 100 ml of diluent; 800 mg dose: dilute 8 ml of **Caldolor** in at least 200 ml of diluent. **Caldolor** is also indicated for management of fever. For adults with fever, 400 mg via IV infusion, followed by 400 mg q 4-6 hours or 100-200 mg q 4 hours prn.

MELOXICAM FOR IV INFUSION

▷ *meloxicam injection* administer 30 mg via IV bolus once daily; administer dose over 15 seconds; monitor analgesic response and administer a short-acting, non-NSAID, immediate-release analgesic if response is inadequate; patients must be well hydrated before **Anjeso** administration; use **Anjeso** for the shortest duration consistent with individual patient treatment goals
Pediatric: not established

   Anjeso *Vial:* 30 mg/ml (1 ml), single-dose
   Comment: Anjeso *(meloxicam)* is an NSAID injection indicated for use in adults for the management of moderate-to-severe pain, alone or in combination with non-NSAID analgesics. Because of delayed onset of analgesia, **Anjeso** as monotherapy is not recommended for use when rapid onset of analgesia is required. The most common adverse reactions (incidence ≥2%) in controlled clinical trials have included constipation, increased gamma-glutamyltransferase (GGT), and anemia. Use of NSAIDs during the third trimester of pregnancy increases the risk of premature closure of the fetal ductus arteriosus (PCDA); therefore, avoid **Anjeso** use after 30 weeks gestation. There are no human data available on whether *meloxicam* is present in human milk or on the effects on breastfed infants. NSAIDs are associated with reversible infertility. Consider withdrawal of **Anjeso** in women who have difficulties conceiving. **Anjeso** may also compromise fertility in males of reproductive potential; it is not known if this effect on male fertility is reversible.

ACETAMINOPHEN+IBUPROFEN COMBINATION

▷ *ibuprofen+acetaminophen* (G)
   Advil Dual Action with Acetaminophen (OTC) take 2 caplets every 8 hours prn pain; max 6 caplets/24 hours
   Pediatric: <12 years: safety and efficacy not established; ≥12 years: 1-2 caplets every 8 hours prn pain; max 6 caplets/24 hours
   Cplt: fixed-dose combination of *ibuprofen* 125 mg (NSAID, antipyretic, analgesic) and *acetaminophen* 250 mg (antipyretic, analgesic)

IBUPROFEN+FAMOTIDINE COMBINATION

▷ *ibuprofen+famotidine* take 1 tablet 3 x/day or take 1 tablet every 8 hours; max 3 tabs/24 hours
   Pediatric: safety and efficacy not established
   Duexis *Tab:* ibu 800 mg+famo 26.6 mg, film-coat, single-dose
   Comment: Duexis is a fixed-dose combination of the NSAID *ibuprofen* (800 mg) and the histamine H2 receptor antagonist *famotidine* (26.6 mg) indicated for relief of signs and symptoms of rheumatoid arthritis and osteoarthritis and to decrease the risk of developing upper gastrointestinal (GI) ulcers, which in clinical trials was defined as a gastric and/or duodenal ulcer in patients who are taking *ibuprofen* for those indications. The clinical trials primarily enrolled patients less than 65 years of age without a history of GI ulcer. The most common adverse reactions (incidence ≥1% and greater than *ibuprofen* alone) have been nausea, diarrhea, constipation, upper abdominal pain, and headache. Contraindications to Duexis use are (1) pre-existing asthma, urticaria, or allergic reactions after taking *aspirin* or other NSAIDs; (2) use during the perioperative period in the setting of coronary artery bypass graft (CABG) surgery; (3) starting at 30 weeks' gestation (**Duexis** should not be used by pregnant females as PCDA in the fetus may occur); and (4) known hypersensitivity to other H2 receptor antagonists. *Boxed Warnings:* *Ibuprofen*, a component of **Duexis**, may increase the risk of serious cardiovascular (CV) thrombotic events, myocardial infarction, and stroke, which can be fatal.

(continued)

Risk may increase with duration of use. Patients with cardiovascular disease (CVD) or risk factors for CVD may be at greater risk. NSAIDs, including *ibuprofen*, a component of **Duexis**, increase the risk of serious GI adverse reactions, including bleeding, ulceration, and perforation of the stomach or intestines, which can be fatal. Reactions can occur at any time without warning symptoms. Elderly patients are at greater risk. *Other Warnings and Precautions with Duexis Use:* Hypertension can occur with NSAID treatment; monitor blood pressure closely during treatment with **Duexis**. Congestive heart failure (CHF) and edema can occur with NSAID treatment; use **Duexis** with caution in patients with fluid retention or heart failure (HF). Active and clinically significant bleeding from any source can occur; discontinue **Duexis** if active bleeding occurs. Long-term administration of NSAIDs can result in renal papillary necrosis and other renal injury; use **Duexis** with caution in patients at risk (e.g., the elderly, those with renal impairment, HF, liver impairment, and those taking diuretics or angiotensin-converting enzyme [ACE] inhibitors). Anaphylaxis may occur in patients with the *aspirin* triad or in patients without prior exposure to **Duexis**; discontinue **Duexis** immediately if an anaphylactoid reaction occurs. Serious skin reactions, including exfoliative dermatitis, Stevens-Johnson Syndrome (SJS), and toxic epidermal necrolysis (TEN), can occur and can be fatal; discontinue **Duexis** if rash or other signs of local skin reaction occur. Hepatic injury ranging from transaminase elevations to liver failure can occur; discontinue **Duexis** immediately if abnormal liver tests persist or worsen, if clinical signs and symptoms of liver disease develop, or if systemic manifestations occur. *Drug Interactions:* Concomitant use of NSAIDs and anticoagulants (e.g., *warfarin*) increases the risk of serious GI bleeding. Concomitant administration with other NSAIDs, including *aspirin*, may increase the risk of adverse reactions, including GI bleeding. *Ibuprofen*, a component of **Duexis**, may reduce the effectiveness of ACE inhibitors and diuretics. *Ibuprofen*, a component of **Duexis**, may increase *lithium* levels. **Duexis** is contraindicated in pregnancy starting at 30 weeks' gestation; may cause fetal harm. Mothers' use of **Duexis** when lactating has not been studied; effects on the breastfed infant are unknown.

IBUPROFEN+ESOMEPRAZOLE COMBINATION

▶ *naproxen+esomeprazole magnesium* (G) take 1 tablet bid; use the lowest effective dose; not recommended in moderate/severe renal insufficiency or in severe hepatic insufficiency (Child-Pugh Class C); consider dose reduction in mild/moderate hepatic insufficiency (Child-Pugh Class A or B)
Pediatric: <18 years: safety and efficacy not established; ≥18 years: same as adult

Vimovo *Tab:* nap 375 mg+eso 20 mg, nap 500 mg +eso mg, del-rel, film-coat
Comment: **Vimovo** is a fixed-dose combination of the NSAID *naproxen* (375 mg or 500 mg) and the proton pump inhibitor (PPI) 20 mg indicated for relief of signs and symptoms of rheumatoid arthritis, osteoarthritis, and ankylosing spondylitis and to decrease the risk of developing gastric ulcers in patients at risk of developing NSAID-associated gastric ulcers. The most common adverse reactions (incidence ≥5%) have been erosive gastritis, dyspepsia, gastritis, diarrhea, gastric ulcer, upper abdominal pain, and nausea. *Contraindications to Vimovo use are* (1) known hypersensitivity to any component of **Vimovo** or substituted benzimidazoles; (2) history of asthma, urticaria, or other allergic-type reactions after taking *aspirin* or other NSAIDs; (3) use during the perioperative period in the setting of CABG surgery; and (4) late pregnancy. Starting at 30 weeks' gestation, **Vimovo** should not be used by pregnant females as PCDA in the fetus may occur. *Boxed Warnings:* *Naproxen*, a component of **Vimovo**, may cause an increased risk of serious CV thrombotic events, myocardial infarction, and stroke, which can be fatal. This risk may increase with duration of use. Patients with CVD or risk factors for CVD may be at greater risk. **Vimovo** is contraindicated in the treatment of perioperative pain in the setting of CABG surgery. NSAIDs, including *naproxen,* can cause an increased risk of serious GI adverse events, including bleeding, ulceration, and perforation of the stomach or intestines, which can be fatal. These events can occur at any time during use and without warning symptoms. Elderly patients are at greater risk for serious GI events. *Other Warnings and Precautions:* Monitor patients for elevated liver enzymes and, rarely occurring, severe hepatic reactions; discontinue use immediately if abnormal liver enzymes persist or worsen. New onset or worsening of preexisting hypertension may occur; monitor blood pressure during treatment with **Vimovo**. CHF and edema can occur; **Vimovo** should be used with caution in patients with fluid retention or HF. Renal papillary necrosis and other renal injury may occur with long-term use. Use **Vimovo** with caution in the elderly, those with impaired renal function, hypovolemia, salt depletion, HF, and liver dysfunction, and those taking diuretics or ACE inhibitors. Do not use **Vimovo** in patients with the *aspirin* triad. Serious skin adverse reactions such as exfoliative dermatitis, SJS, and TEN can be fatal and can occur without warning. Discontinue **Vimovo** at first appearance of skin rash or any other sign of hypersensitivity. Long-term PPI therapy is associated with an increased risk for osteoporosis-related fractures of the hip, wrist, or spine. Symptomatic response to *esomeprazole* does not preclude the presence of gastric malignancy. Atrophic gastritis has been noted on biopsy with long-term *omeprazole* therapy. *Drug-Drug Interactions:* Concomitant use of NSAIDs may reduce the antihypertensive effect of ACE inhibitors, diuretics, and beta-blockers. Concomitant use of NSAIDs increases *lithium* plasma levels. Concomitant use of **Vimovo** with *methotrexate* may increase the toxicity of *methotrexate*. Concomitant use of **Vimovo** and *warfarin* may result in increased risk of

bleeding complications; monitor for increases in international normalized ratio (INR) and PT/PTT. *Esomeprazole* inhibits gastric acid secretion and may interfere with the absorption of drugs where gastric pH is an important determinant of bioavailability (e.g., *ketoconazole*, iron salts, and *digoxin*). Vimovo is contraindicated in pregnancy starting at 30 weeks' gestation; may cause fetal harm PCDA. The *naproxen* anion has been found in the milk of lactating females. Because of the possible adverse effects of prostaglandin-inhibiting drugs on neonates and potential for tumorigenicity shown for *esomeprazole* in animal carcinogenicity studies, a decision should be made whether to discontinue breastfeeding or discontinue the **Vimovo**, taking into account the importance of the drug to the mother.

OCULAR PAIN

▷ *dexamethasone ophthalmic insert* postsurgical insertion in the lower lacrimal punctum and into the canaliculus by a qualified healthcare provider; insert is resorbable (does not require removal); saline irrigation or manual expression can be performed if removal is necessary; a single insert provides sustained delivery of *dexamethasone* up to 30 days
Pediatric: safety and efficacy not established
   Dextenza 0.4 mg single-dose in a foam carrier within a foil laminate pouch (preservative-free)
   Comment: Dextenza is the first FDA-approved intracanalicular insert delivering *dexamethasone* to treat postsurgical ocular pain for up to 30 days with a single administration.
▷ *difluprednate* (G) apply 1 drop to affected eye qid; for postop ocular pain, begin treatment 24 hours postop and continue x 2 weeks; then bid daily x 1 week; then taper
Pediatric: <12 years: not recommended; ≥12 years: same as adult
   Durezol *Ophth emul:* 0.05% (5 ml)
   Comment: Durezol is an ophthalmic steroid.
▷ *nepafenac* apply 1 drop to affected eye tid; for postop ocular pain, begin treatment 24 hours before surgery and continue day of surgery and for 2 weeks postop
Pediatric: <10 years: not recommended; ≥10 years: same as adult
   Nevanac *Ophth susp:* 0.1% (3 ml) (benzalkonium chloride)
   Comment: Nevanac is an ophthalmic NSAID.

TOPICAL AND TRANSDERMAL ANALGESICS

▷ *capsaicin* (G) apply tid-qid prn to intact skin
Pediatric: <2 years: not recommended; ≥2 years: apply sparingly tid-qid prn
   Axsain *Crm:* 0.075% (1, 2 oz)
   Capsin (OTC) *Lotn:* 0.025, 0.075% (59 ml)
   Capzasin-HP (OTC) *Crm:* 0.075% (1.5 oz), 0.025% (45, 90 gm); *Lotn:* 0.075% (2 oz), 0.025% (45, 90 gm)
   Capzasin-P (OTC) *Crm:* 0.025% (1.5 oz); *Lotn:* 0.025% (2 oz)
   Dolorac *Crm:* 0.025% (28 gm)
   Double Cap (OTC) *Crm:* 0.05% (2 oz)
   R-Gel *Gel:* 0.025% (15, 30 gm)
   Zostrix (OTC) *Crm:* 0.025% (0.7, 1.5, 3 oz)
   Zostrix HP (OTC) *Emol crm:* 0.075% (1, 2 oz)
▷ *capsaicin* 8% patch apply up to 4 patches for one 60-minute application to clean dry skin; may prep area with topical anesthetic; wear non-latex gloves; patches may be cut to size/shape; treatment may be repeated every 3 months
Pediatric: <18 years: not recommended; ≥18 years: same as adult
   Qutenza *Patch:* 8% 1,640 mcg/cm (179 mg) (1 or 2 patches w. 1-50 gm tube cleansing gel/carton)
▷ *diclofenac sodium* apply qid prn to intact skin
Pediatric: <12 years: not established; ≥12 years: same as adult
   Pennsaid 1.5% in 10 drop increments, dispense and rub into front, side, and back of knee: usually 40 drops (40 mg) qid
      Topical soln: 1.5% (150 ml)
   Pennsaid 2% apply 2 pump actuations (40 mg) and rub into front, side, and back of knee bid
      Topical soln: 2% (20 mg/pump actuation, 112 gm)
   Solaraze Gel massage into clean skin bid prn
      Gel: 3% (50 gm) (benzyl alcohol)
   Voltaren Gel (OTC) (G) apply qid prn to intact skin
      Gel: 1% (100 gm)
   Comment: *Diclofenac* is contraindicated with *aspirin* allergy. As with other NSAIDs, should be avoided in late pregnancy (≥30 weeks) because it may cause premature closure of the ductus arteriosus (PCDA).
▷ *doxepin* (G) cream apply to affected area qid at intervals of at least 3-4 hours; max 8 days
Pediatric: <12 years: not recommended; >12 years: same as adult
   Prudoxin *Crm:* 5% (45 gm)
   Zonalon *Crm:* 5% (30, 45 gm)

(continued)

➤ *pimecrolimus* 1% cream (G) <2 years: <u>not</u> recommended; ≥2 years: apply to affected area bid; do <u>not</u> apply an occlusive dressing

  Elidel *Crm:* 1% (30, 60, 100 gm)

  Comment: *Pimecrolimus* is indicated for short-term and intermittent long-term use. Discontinue use when resolution occurs. Contraindicated if the patient is immunosuppressed. Change to the 0.1% preparation <u>or</u> if secondary bacterial infection is present.

➤ *trolamine salicylate* apply tid-qid

  Pediatric: <2 years: <u>not</u> recommended; ≥2 years: same as adult

  Mobisyl Creme *Crm:* 10% (100 gm)

TOPICAL AND TRANSDERMAL ANESTHETICS

Comment: *Lidocaine* should <u>not</u> be applied to non-intact skin.

➤ *lidocaine* cream apply to affected area bid prn

  Pediatric: <12 years: <u>not</u> recommended; ≥12 years: same as adult

  LidaMantle *Crm:* 3% (1, 2 oz)

  Lidoderm *Crm:* 3% (85 gm)

  ZTlido *lidocaine* topical system 1% (30/carton)

  Comment: Compared to Lidoderm (*lidocaine* patch 5%), which contains 700 mg/patch, ZTlido <u>only</u> requires 35 mg per topical system to achieve the same therapeutic dose.

➤ *lidocaine* lotion apply to affected area bid prn

  Pediatric: <12 years: <u>not</u> recommended; ≥12 years: same as adult

  LidaMantle *Lotn:* 3% (177 ml)

➤ *lidocaine* 5% patch (G) apply up to 3 patches at one time for up to 12 hours/24-hour period (12 hours on/12 hours off); patches may be cut into smaller sizes before removal of the release liner; do <u>not</u> reuse

  Pediatric: <12 years: <u>not</u> recommended; ≥12 years: same as adult

  Lidoderm *Patch:* 5% (10 x 14 cm; 30/carton)

➤ *lidocaine+dexamethasone*

  Pediatric: <12 years: <u>not</u> recommended; ≥12 years: same as adult

  Decadron Phosphate with Xylocaine *Lotn:* dexa 4 mg+lido 10 mg per ml (5 ml)

➤ *lidocaine+hydrocortisone* (G) apply to affected area bid prn

  Pediatric: <12 years: <u>not</u> recommended; ≥12 years: same as adult

  LidaMantle HC *Crm:* lido 3%+hydro 0.5% (1, 3 oz); *Lotn:* (177 ml)

➤ *lidocaine* 2.5%+*prilocaine* 2.5% apply sparingly to the burn bid-tid prn

  Pediatric: <12 years: <u>not</u> recommended; ≥12 years: same as adult

  Emla Cream 5, 30 gm/tube

OPIOID ANALGESICS

Comment: According to the American Society of Interventional Pain Physicians (ASIPP), presumptive urine drug testing (UDT) should be performed when opioid therapy for chronic pain is initiated, along with subsequent use as adherence monitoring, using in-office point-of-service testing, to identify patients who are non-compliant <u>or</u> abusing prescription drugs <u>or</u> illicit drugs. Opiate agonists may produce significant central nervous system (CNS) and respiratory depression of varying duration, particularly when given in high dosages <u>and/or</u> by rapid IV administration. Apnea may result from decreased respiratory drive as well as increased airway resistance, and rigidity of respiratory muscles may occur during rapid IV administration <u>or</u> when these agents are used in the induction of anesthesia. At therapeutic analgesic dosages, the respiratory effects are usually <u>not</u> clinically important except in patients with preexisting pulmonary impairment. Therapy with opiate agonists should be avoided <u>or</u> administered with extreme caution and initiated at reduced dosages in patients with severe CNS depression (e.g., sleep apnea, hypoxia, anoxia, <u>or</u> hypercapnia, upper airway obstruction, chronic pulmonary insufficiency, limited ventilatory reserve, and other respiratory disorders). In the presence of excessive respiratory secretions, the use of opiate agonists may also be problematic because they decrease ciliary activity and reduce the cough reflex. Caution is also advised in patients who may be at increased risk for respiratory depression, such as comatose patients <u>or</u> those with head injury, intracranial lesions, <u>or</u> intracranial hypertension. Clinical monitoring of pulmonary function is recommended, and equipment for resuscitation should be immediately available if parenteral <u>or</u> neuraxial routes are used. *Naloxone* may be administered to reverse clinically significant respiratory depression, which may be prolonged depending on the opioid agent, cumulative dose, and route of administration.

➤ *benzhydrocodone+acetaminophen* (II) <18 years: <u>not</u> recommended; ≥18 years: initiate treatment with 1-2 tabs q 4-6 hours prn; max 12 tabs/24 hours; max 14 days

  Apadaz *Tab:* benz 6.12 mg+acet 325 mg

  Comment: *Benzhydrocodone* 6.12 mg is equivalent to 4.54 mg *hydrocodone* <u>or</u> 7.5 mg *hydrocodone bitartrate*. If switching from immediate-release *hydrocodone bitartrate+acetaminophen*, substitute Apadaz 6.12 mg/325 mg for 7.5 mg/325 mg *hydrocodone bitartrate+acetaminophen*. Dosage of Apadaz should be adjusted according to the severity of the pain and the response of the patient. Do <u>not</u> stop Apadaz abruptly in the physically-dependent patient.

➤ *butalbital+acetaminophen* (G) 1 tab q 4 hours prn; max 6 tabs/day
    Pediatric: <12 years: <u>not</u> recommended; ≥12 years: same as adult
        Tab: but 50 mg+acet 325 mg
      Phrenilin 1-2 tabs q 4 hours prn; max 6 tabs/day
        Tab: but 50 mg+acet 325 mg
      Phrenilin Forte 1 tab <u>or</u> cap q 4 hours prn; max 6 caps/day
        Cap: but 50 mg+acet 325 mg; *Tab:* but 50 mg+acet 325 mg
➤ *butalbital+acetaminophen+caffeine* (G)
    Pediatric: <12 years <u>not</u> recommended; ≥12 years: same as adult
      Fioricet 1-2 tabs q 4 hours prn; max 6/day
        Tab: but 50 mg+acet 325 mg+caf 40 mg
      Zebutal 1 cap q 4 hours prn; max 5/day
        Cap: but 50 mg+acet 325 mg+caf 40 mg
➤ *butalbital+aspirin+caffeine* (III) (G)
    Pediatric: <12 years: <u>not</u> recommended; ≥12 years: same as adult
      Fiorinal 1-2 tabs <u>or</u> caps q 4 hours prn; max 6 caps/day
        Tab/Cap: but 50 mg+asp 325 mg+caf 40 mg
➤ *butalbital+aspirin+codeine+caffeine* (III)(G)
    Pediatric: <18 years: <u>not</u> recommended; ≥18 years: same as adult
      Fiorinal with Codeine 1-2 caps q 4 hours prn; max 6 caps/day
        Cap: but 50 mg+asp 325 mg+cod 30 mg+caf 40 mg
➤ *codeine sulfate* (III)(G) 15-60 q 4-6 hours prn; max 60 mg/day
    Pediatric: <18 years: <u>not</u> recommended; ≥18 years: same as adult
        Tab: 15, 30, 60 mg
➤ *codeine+acetaminophen* (III)(G) 15-60 mg of *codeine* q 4 hours prn; max 360 mg of *codeine* per day
    Pediatric: <18 years: <u>not</u> recommended; ≥18 years: same as adult
        Tab: **Tylenol #1** cod 7.5 mg+acet 300 mg (sulfites)
            Tylenol #2 cod 15 mg+acet 300 mg (sulfites)
            Tylenol #3 cod 30 mg+acet 300 mg (sulfites)
            Tylenol #4 cod 60 mg+acet 300 mg (sulfites)
            Tylenol with Codeine Elixir (III)
        Elix: cod 12 mg+acet 120 mg per 5 ml (cherry) (alcohol)
➤ *dihydrocodeine+acetaminophen+caffeine* (III)(G)
    Pediatric: <18 years: <u>not</u> recommended; ≥18 years: same as adult
      Panlor DC 1-2 caps q 4-6 hours prn; max 10 caps/day
        Cap: dihydro 16 mg+acet 325 mg+caf 30 mg
      Panlor SS 1 tab q 4 hours prn; max 5 tabs/day
        Tab: dihydro 32 mg+acet 325 mg+caf 60*mg
➤ *dihydrocodeine+aspirin+caffeine* (III)(G) 1-2 caps q 4 hours prn
    Pediatric: <18 years: <u>not</u> recommended; ≥18 years: same as adult
      Synalgos-DC
        Cap: dihydro 16 mg+asp 356.4 mg+caf 30 mg
➤ *hydrocodone bitartrate* (G)(II)
    Pediatric: <18 years: <u>not</u> recommended; ≥18 years: same as adult
      Hysingla ER swallow whole; 1 tab once daily at the same time each day
        Tab: 20, 30, 40, 60, 80, 100, 120 mg ext-rel
      Vantrela ER swallow whole; 1 tab once daily at the same time each day
        Tab: 15, 30, 45, 60, 90 mg ext-rel
      Zohydro ER swallow whole; *Opioid-naïve:* 10 mg q 12 hours; may increase by 10 mg q 12 hours every 3-7 days; when discontinuing, titrate downward every 2-4 days
        Cap: 10, 15, 20, 30, 40, 50 mg ext-rel
➤ *hydrocodone bitartrate+acetaminophen* (II)(G)
    Pediatric: <18: <u>not</u> recommended; ≥18 years: same as adult
      Hycet 5/325 1-2 tabs q 4-6 hours prn; max 8 tabs/day
        Tab: hydro 5 mg+acet 325 mg*
      Hycet 7.5/325 1 tab q 4-6 hours prn; max 6 tabs/day
        Tab: hydro 7.5 mg+acet 325 mg*
      Hycet 10/325 1 tab q 4-6 hours prn; max 6 tab/day
        Tab: hydro 10 mg+acet 325 mg*
      Hycet Oral Solution 2.5/325 3 tsp (15 ml) q 4-6 hours prn; max 24 tsp (90 ml)/day (alcohol 7%)
        Liq: hydro 2.5 mg+acet 108 mg per 15 ml (alcohol 7%)
      Hycet Oral Solution 7.5/325 1 tsp (5 ml) q 4-6 hours prn; max 8 tsp (90 ml)/day (alcohol 7%)
        Liq: hydro 7.5 mg+acet 325 mg per 15 ml (alcohol 7%)
      Lorcet 1-2 tabs q 4-6 hours prn; max 8 caps/day*
        Tab: hydro 5 mg+acet 325 mg

(continued)

Lorcet Plus 1 tab q 4-6 hours prn; max 6 tabs/day*
Tab: hydro 7.5 mg+acet 325 mg
Lorcet-HD 1 cap q 4-6 hours prn; max 6 tabs/day*
Tab: hydro 10 mg+acet 325 mg
Lortab 5/325 1-2 tabs q 4-6 hours prn; max 8 tabs/day
Tab: hydro 5 mg+acet 325 mg*
Lortab 7.5/325 1 tab q 4-6 hours prn; max 6 tabs/day
Tab: hydro 7.5 mg+acet 325 mg*
Lortab 10/500 1 tab q 4-6 hours prn; max 6 tabs/day
Tab: hydro 10 mg+acet 500 mg*
Maxidone 1 tab q 4-6 hours prn; max 5 tabs/day
Tab: hydro 10 mg+acet 750 mg*
Norco 5/325 1-2 tab2 q 4-6 hours prn; max 8 tabs/day
Tab: hydro 5 mg+acet 325 mg*
Norco 7.5/325 1 tab q 4-6 hours prn; max 6 tabs/day
Tab: hydro 7.5 mg+acet 325 mg*
Norco 10/325 1 tab q 4-6 hours prn; max 6 tabs/day
Tab: hydro 10 mg+acet 325 mg*
Vicodin 1-2 tabs q 4-6 hours prn; max 8 tabs/day
Tab: hydro 5 mg+acet 300 mg*
Vicodin ES 1 tab q 4-6 hours prn; max 6 tabs/day
Tab: hydro 7.5 mg+acet 300 mg*
Vicodin HP 1 tab q 4-6 hours prn; max 6 tabs/day
Tab: hydro 10 mg+acet 300 mg*
Xodol 5/300 1-2 tabs q 4-6 hours prn; max 8 tabs/day
Tab: hydro 5 mg+acet 300 mg*
Xodol 7.5/300 1 tab q 4-6 hours prn; max 6 tabs/day
Tab: hydro 7.5 mg+acet 300 mg*
Xodol 10/300 1 tab q 4-6 hours prn; max 6 tabs/day
Tab: hydro 10 mg+acet 300 mg*
Zamicet Oral Solution 5/163 3 tsp (15 ml) q 4-6 hours prn; max 24 tsp (90 ml)/day (alcohol 7.7%)
Liq: hydro 5 mg+acet 325 mg per 163 ml (alcohol 7%)
Zamicet Oral Solution 10/325 3 tsp (15 ml) q 4-6 hours prn; max 24 tsp (90 ml)/day (alcohol 7.7%)
Liq: hydro 10 mg+acet 325 mg per 15 ml (alcohol 7%)
Zydone 5/400 1-2 tabs q 4-6 hours prn; max 8 tabs/day
Tab: hydro 5 mg+acet 400 mg
Zydone 7.5/400 1 tab q 4-6 hours prn; max 6 tabs/day
Tab: hydro 7.5 mg+acet 400 mg
Zydone 10/400 1 tab q 4-6 hours prn; max 6 tabs/day
Tab: hydro 10 mg+acet 400 mg
▷ *hydrocodone+ibuprofen* (II)(G)
Pediatric: <18: <u>not</u> recommended; ≥18 years: same as adult
Ibudone 5/200 1 tab q 4-6 hours prn; max 5 tabs/day
Tab: hydro 5 mg+ibup 200 mg
Ibudone 10/200 1 tab q 4-6 hours prn; max 5 tabs/day
Tab: hydro 10 mg+ibup 200 mg
Reprexain 1 tab q 4-6 hours prn; max 5 tabs/day
Tab: hydro 5 mg+ibup 200 mg
Vicoprofen 1 tab q 4-6 hours prn; max 5 tabs/day
Tab: hydro 7.5 mg+ibup 200 mg
Comment: *Ibuprofen is contraindicated for use in the 3rd trimester of pregnancy.*
▷ *hydromorphone* (II)(G)
Pediatric: <18: <u>not</u> recommended; ≥18 years: same as adult
Dilaudid initially 2-4 mg q 4-6 hours prn
Tab: 2, 4, 8 mg (sulfites)
Dilaudid Oral Liquid 2.5-10 mg q 3-6 hours prn
Liq: 5 mg/5 ml (sulfites)
Dilaudid Rectal Suppository 2.5-10 mg q 6-8 hours prn
Rectal supp: 3 mg
Dilaudid Injection initially 1-2 mg SC <u>or</u> IM q 4-6 hours prn
Amp: 1, 2, 4 mg/ml (1 ml)
Dilaudid-HP Injection initially 1-2 mg SC <u>or</u> IM q 4-6 hours prn
Amp: 10 mg/ml (1 ml)
Exalgo initially 8-64 mg once daily
Tab: 8, 12, 16, 32 mg ext-rel (sulfites)

▷ *meperidine* (II)(G) 50-150 mg q 3-4 hours prn
  Pediatric: 0.5-0.8 mg/lb q 3-4 hours prn; max adult dose
    Demerol *Tab:* 50, 100 mg; *Syr:* 50 mg/5 ml (banana) (alcohol-free)
▷ *meperidine+promethazine* (II)(G)
  Pediatric: <18: not recommended; ≥18 years: same as adult
    Mepergan 1-2 tsp q 3-4 hours prn
      Syr: mep 25 mg+prom 25 mg per ml
    Mepergan Fortis 1-2 tsp q 4-6 hours prn
      Tab: mep 50 mg+prom 25 mg
▷ *methadone* (II)(G) 2.5-10 mg PO, SC, or IM q 3-4 hours; for use only in chronic moderately severe-to-severe pain management (e.g., hospice care). For opioid-naïve patients, initiate **Dolophine** tablets with 2.5 mg every 8-12 hours; unlike other opioid analgesics, *methadone* is not indicated as an as-needed (prn) analgesic, per se; titrate slowly with dose increases no more frequent than every 3 to 5 days; to convert to **Dolophine** tablets from another opioid, use available conversion factors to obtain estimated dose (see mfr pkg insert); do not abruptly discontinue **Dolophine** in a physically dependent patient
  Pediatric: <18: not recommended; ≥18 years: same as adult
    Dolophine *Tab:* 5, 10 mg; *Dispersible tab:* 40 mg (dissolve in 120 ml orange juice or other citrus drink); *Oral soln:* 5, 10 mg/ml; *Oral conc:* 10 mg/ml; *Syr:* 10 mg/30 ml; *Vial:* 10 mg/ml (200 mg/20 ml multidose) for injection
Comment: *Methadone* administration is allowed only by approved providers with strict state and federal regulations (as stipulated in 42 CFR 8.12). *Boxed Warning: Dolophine* exposes users to risks of addiction, abuse, and misuse, which can lead to overdose and death. Assess each patient's risk and monitor regularly for development of these behaviors and conditions. Serious, life-threatening, or fatal respiratory depression may occur. The peak respiratory depressant effect of *methadone* occurs later and persists longer than the peak analgesic effect. Accidental ingestion, especially by children, can result in fatal overdose. QT interval prolongation and serious arrhythmias (torsades de pointes) have occurred during treatment with *methadone*. Closely monitor patients with risk factors for development of prolonged QT interval, a history of cardiac conduction abnormalities, and those taking medications affecting cardiac conduction. Neonatal opioid withdrawal syndrome (NOWS) is an expected and treatable outcome of use of *methadone* use during pregnancy. NOWS may be life-threatening if not recognized and treated in the neonate. The balance between the risks of NOWS and the benefits of maternal *methadone* use should be considered and the patient advised of the risk of NOWS so that appropriate planning for management of the neonate can occur. *Methadone* has been detected in human milk. Concomitant use with CYP3A4, 2B6, 2C19, 2C9, or 2D6 inhibitors or discontinuation of concomitantly used CYP3A4 2B6, 2C19, or 2C9 inducers can result in a fatal overdose of *methadone*. Concomitant use of opioids with benzodiazepines or other CNS depressants, including alcohol, may result in profound sedation, respiratory depression, coma, and death.
▷ *morphine sulfate (immed-release)* (II)(G) usually 15-30 mg q 4 hours prn; solution, usually 10-20 mg q 4 hours prn
  Pediatric: <18 years: not recommended; ≥18 years: same as adult
    Tab: 15*, 30*mg; *Oral soln:* 10 mg/5 ml, 20 mg/5 ml (100, 500 ml), 100 mg/5 ml (30, 120 ml)
▷ *morphine sulfate (immed- and sust-rel)* (II)
  Comment: Dosage dependent upon previous opioid dosage; see mfr pkg insert for conversion guidelines; not for prn use; swallow whole or sprinkle contents of caps on applesauce (do not crush, chew, or dissolve). Generic *morphine sulfate* is available in the following forms: *Tab:* 15*, 30*mg; *Oral soln:* 10, 20 mg/5 ml (100 ml), 100 mg/5 ml (30, 120 ml w. oral syringe)
  Pediatric: <18 years: not recommended; ≥18 years: same as adult
    Arymo ER swallow whole; 1 tab once daily at the same time each day
      Tab: 15, 30, 60 mg ext-rel
    Duramorph administer per anesthesia
      IV/Intrathecal/Epidural: 0.5, 1 mg/ml
    Infumorph administer per anesthesia
      Intrathecal/Epidural: 10, 20 mg/ml
    Kadian (G) 1 cap every 12-24 hours
      Cap: 10, 20, 30, 50, 60, 80, 100, 200 mg sust-rel
    MS Contin (G) 1 tab every 24 hours
      Tab: 15, 30, 60, 100, 200 mg sust-rel
    MSIR 5-30 mg q 4 hours prn
      Tab: 15*, 30*mg; *Cap:* 15, 30 mg
    MSIR Oral Solution 5-30 mg q 4 hours prn
      Oral soln: 10, 20 mg/5 ml (120 ml)
    MSIR Oral Solution Concentrate 5-30 mg q 4 hours prn
      Oral conc: 20 mg/ml (30, 120 ml w. dropper)
    Oramorph SR 1 cap q 12-24 hours
      Tab: 15, 30, 60, 100 mg sust-rel

(continued)

Roxanol Oral Solution 10-30 mg q 4 hours prn
Oral soln: 20 mg/ml (1, 4, 8 oz)
Roxanol Rescudose
Oral soln: 10 mg/2.5 ml (25 single-dose)

▷ *morphine sulfate (ext-rel)* (II)
Pediatric: <18 years: not recommended; ≥18 years: same as adult
MorphaBond ER *Tab:* 15, 30, 60, 100 mg ext-rel
Comment: MorphaBond may be prescribed only by a qualified healthcare provider knowledgeable in use of potent opioids for management of chronic pain. Do not abruptly discontinue in a physically dependent patient. Instruct patients to swallow **MorphaBond ER** tablets intact and not to cut, break, crush, chew, or dissolve **MorphaBond ER** to avoid the risk of release and absorption of potentially fatal dose of *morphine*. **MorphaBond ER** 100 mg tablets, a single dose greater than 60 mg, or a total daily dose >120 mg, are only for use in patients in whom tolerance to an opioid of comparable potency has been established. Patients considered opioid-tolerant are those taking, for 1 week or longer, at least 60 mg oral *morphine* per day, 25 mcg transdermal *fentanyl* per hour, 30 mg oral *oxycodone* per day, 8 mg oral *hydromorphone* per day, 25 mg oral *oxymorphone* per day, 60 mg oral *hydrocodone* per day, or an equianalgesic dose of another opioid. Use the lowest effective dosage for the shortest duration consistent with individual patient treatment goals. Individualize dosing based on the severity of pain, patient response, prior analgesic experience, and risk factors for addiction, abuse, and misuse.

▷ *morphine sulfate+naltrexone* (II)
Pediatric: <18 years: not recommended; ≥18 years: same as adult
Embeda 1 cap q 12-24 hours
Cap: **Embeda 20/0.8** morph 20 mg+nal 0.8 mg ext-rel
Embeda 30/1.2 morph 30 mg+nal 1.2 mg ext-rel
Embeda 50/2 morph 50 mg+nal 2 mg ext-rel
Embeda 60/2.4 morph 60 mg+nal 2.4 mg ext-rel
Embeda 80/3.2 morph 80 mg+nal 3.2 mg ext-rel
Embeda 100/4 morph 100 mg+nal 4 mg ext-rel
Comment: Embeda is not for prn use; for use in opioid-tolerant patients only; swallow whole or sprinkle contents of caps on applesauce (do not crush, chew, or dissolve); do not administer via nasogastric tube (NG tube) or gastric tube (percutaneous endoscopic gastrostomy [PEG] tube).

▷ *oxycodone* (II) 5-15 mg q 4-6 hours prn
Comment: Concomitant use of CYP3A4 inhibitors may increase opioid effects and CYP3A4 inducers may decrease effects or possibly cause the development of an abstinence syndrome (withdrawal symptoms) in patients who are physically *oxycodone*-dependent/addicted.
Pediatric: <18 years: not recommended; ≥18 years: same as adult
Oxaydo *Tab:* 5, 7.5 mg
Comment: Oxaydo is the first and only immediate-release oral *oxycodone* that discourages intranasal abuse. **Oxaydo** is formulated with sodium lauryl sulfate, an inactive ingredient that may cause nasal burning and throat irritation when snorted and thus potentially reducing abuse liability. There is no generic equivalent.
Oxecta *Tab:* 5, 7.5 mg
Oxycodone Oral Solution (G) *Oral soln:* 5 mg/5 ml (15, 30 ml)
OxyIR (G) *Cap:* 5 mg
RoxyBond *Tab:* 5, 15, 30 mg
Comment: The FDA recently approved **RoxyBond** immediate-release tablets for the management of severe pain that does not respond to alternative treatment and requires an opioid analgesic. **RoxyBond** is the first immediate-release opioid analgesic to receive FDA approval, with a label describing its abuse-deterrent properties under the FDA 2015 Guidance for Industry: Abuse-Deterrent Opioids Evaluation and Labeling. The drug is formulated with inactive ingredients, making it more difficult to misuse and abuse. When compared with another approved immediate-release tablet, **RoxyBond** was shown to be more resistant to cutting, crushing, grinding, or breaking, and more resistant to extraction. Adverse events associated with **RoxyBond** include nausea, constipation, vomiting, headache, pruritus, insomnia, dizziness, asthenia, somnolence, and addiction.
Roxycodone *Tab:* 5, 15*, 30*mg; *Oral soln:* 5 mg/ml
Roxycodone Intensol *Oral soln:* 20 mg/ml

▷ *oxycodone cont-rel* (II)(G) dosage dependent upon previous opioid dosages; see mfr pkg insert: <11 years: not recommended; 11-16 years: the child's pain must be severe enough to require around-the-clock, long-term treatment not managed well by other treatments; must already be taking and tolerating minimum opium dose equal to *oxycodone* 20 mg/day x 5 consecutive days; >16 year: same as adult; no previous treatment with *oxycodone* required
OxyContin dose q 12 hours
Tab: 10, 15, 20, 30, 40, 60, 80 mg cont-rel
OxyFast dose q 6 hours
Oral conc: 20 mg/ml (30 ml w. dropper)

Xtampza ER dose q 12 hours
Cap: 10, 15, 20, 30, 40 mg ext-rel
Comment: May open the **Xtampza ER** capsule and sprinkle in water or on soft food.

➤ *oxycodone+acetaminophen* (II)(G)
Comment: Maximum 4 gm acetaminophen per day.
Pediatric: not recommended
    Magnacet **2.5/400** 1 tab q 6 hours prn; max 10 tabs/day
      Tab: oxy 2.5 mg+acet 325 mg
    Magnacet **5/400** 1 tab q 6 hours prn; max 10 tabs/day
      Tab: oxy 5 mg+acet 325 mg
    Magnacet **7.5/400** 1 tab q 6 hours prn; max 8 tabs/day
      Tab: oxy 7.5 mg+acet 325 mg
    Magnacet **10/400** 1 tab q 6 hours prn; max 6 tabs/day
      Tab: oxy 10 mg+acet 325 mg
    Percocet **2.5/325** 1 tab q 6 hours prn; max 4 gm acet/day
      Tab: oxy 2.5 mg+acet 325 mg
    Percocet **5/325** 1 tab q 6 hours prn; max 4 gm acet/day
      Tab: oxy 5 mg+acet 325*mg
    Percocet **7.5/325** 1 tab q 6 hours prn; max 4 gm acet/day
      Tab: oxy 7.5 mg+acet 325 mg
    Percocet **7.5/500** 1 tab q 6 hours prn; max 4 gm acet/day
      Tab: oxy 7.5 mg+acet 325 mg
    Percocet **10/325** 1 tab q 6 hours prn; max 4 gm acet/day
      Tab: oxy 10 mg+acet 325 mg
    Percocet **10/650** 1 tab q 6 hours prn; max 4 gm acet/day
      Tab: oxy 10 mg+acet 325 mg
    Roxicet **5/325** 1 tab/tsp q 6 hours prn
      Tab: oxy 5 mg+acet 325 mg; *Oral soln:* oxy 5 mg+acet 325 mg per 5 ml
    Roxicet **5/500** 1 caplet q 6 hours prn
      Cplt: oxy 5 mg+acet 325 mg
    Roxicet **Oral Solution** 1 tsp q 6 hours prn
      Oral soln: oxy 5 mg+acet 325 mg per 5 ml (alcohol 0.4%)
    Tylox 1 cap q 6 hours prn
      Cap: oxy 5 mg+acet 325 mg
    Xartemis XR 2 tabs q 12 hours prn
      Tab: oxy 7.5 mg+acet 325 mg

➤ *oxycodone+aspirin* (II)(G)
    Percodan 1 tab q 6 hours prn
      Pediatric: not recommended
      Tab: oxy 4.8355 mg+asp 325*mg
    Percodan-Demi 1-2 tabs q 6 hours prn
      Pediatric: 6-12 years: 1/4 tab q 6 hours prn; >12-18 years: 1/2 tab q 6 hours prn
      Tab: oxy 2.25 mg+asp 325 mg

➤ *oxycodone+ibuprofen* (II)(G)
Pediatric: <14 years: not recommended; ≥14 years: same as adult
    Combunox 1 tab q 6 hours prn
      Tab: oxy 5 mg+ibu 400*mg

➤ *oxycodone+naloxone* (II) 1 tab q 3-4 hours prn
Pediatric: <12 years: not recommended; ≥12 years: same as adult
    Targiniq
      Tab: **Targiniq 10/5** oxy 10 mg+nal 5 mg
        Targiniq 20/10 oxy 20 mg+nal 10 mg
        Targiniq 40/20 oxy 40 mg+nal 20 mg

➤ *oxymorphone* (II)(G)
Pediatric: <18 years: not recommended; ≥18 years: same as adult
    Numorphan 1 supp q 4-6 hours prn
    Rectal supp: 5 mg; *Vial:* 1 mg/ml (1 ml); *Amp:* 1.5 mg/ml (10 ml);
    Comment: Store in refrigerator in original package. 1 mg of **Numorphan** is approximately equivalent in analgesic activity to 10 mg of *morphine sulfate.*
    Opana 1-1 tab q 4-6 hours prn
      Tab: 5, 10 mg
    Opana ER 1 tab q 12 hours prn
      Tab: 5, 7.5, 10, 15, 20, 30, 40 mg ext-rel, crush-resist
    Opana Injection initially 0.5 mg IV or IM; 1 x 1 mg IM or IV q 4-6 hours prn
      Amp: 1 mg/ml (1 ml) (paraben/sodium dithionite-free)

(continued)

▷ *pentazocine+aspirin* **(IV)** 2 cplts tid or qid prn
    Pediatric: <12 years: not recommended; ≥12 years: same as adult
      Talwin Compound *Cplt:* pent 12.5 mg+asp 325 mg
▷ *pentazocine+naloxone* **(IV)** 1 tab q 3-4 hours prn
    Pediatric: <12 years: not recommended; ≥12 years: same as adult
      Talwin NX *Tab:* pent 50 mg+nal 0.5*mg
▷ *pentazocine lactate* **(IV)** 30 mg IM, SC, or IV q 3-4 hours; max 360 mg/day
    Pediatric: <1 year: not recommended; ≥1 year: 0.5 mg/kg IM
      Talwin Injectable *Amp:* pent 30 mg/ml (1, 1.5, 2 ml)
▷ *propoxyphene napsylate+acetaminophen* **(IV) (G)**
    Comment: Maximum 4 gm acetaminophen per day.
    Pediatric: <12 years: not recommended; ≥12 years: same as adult
      Balacet 325 1 tab q 4 hours prn; max 6 tabs/day
      Tab: prop 100 mg+acet 325 mg
▷ *tramadol* **(IV)(G)**
    Conzip initially 100 mg once daily; may titrate up by 100 mg increments every 5 days according to need and tolerance; max 300 mg once daily
    Cap: 100, 150, 200, 300 mg ext-rel
    Comment: Conzip is an opioid agonist indicated for the management of pain severe enough to require daily, around-the-clock, long-term opioid treatment and for which alternative treatment options are inadequate. **Conzip** is not indicated as an as-needed (prn) analgesic. **Conzip** is contraindicated in children <12 years of age, postoperative pain management of patients <18 years of age following tonsillectomy and/or adenoidectomy, acute or severe bronchial asthma in an unmonitored setting or in the absence of resuscitative equipment, known or suspected GI obstruction, including paralytic ileus, and concurrent use of monoamine oxidase inhibitors (MAOIs) or use within the previous 14 days. Potentially life-threatening *serotonin syndrome* can result from concomitant serotonergic drug administration. Risk of seizure is present within the recommended dose range; risk is increased with higher than recommended doses and concomitant use of selective serotonin reuptake inhibitors (SSRIs), serotonin norepinephrine reuptake inhibitors (SNRIs), anorectics, tricyclic antidepressants (TCAs) and other tricyclic compounds, other opioids, MAOIs, neuroleptics, other drugs that reduce seizure threshold, and patients with epilepsy or at risk for seizures. Do not use **Conzip** in suicidal or addiction-prone patients. If adrenal insufficiency is diagnosed, treat with physiologic replacement of corticosteroids and wean off of the opioid. Life-threatening respiratory depression can occur with chronic obstructive pulmonary disease (COPD) or patients who are elderly, cachectic, or debilitated; monitor closely, particularly during initiation and titration. Use caution in patients with increased intracranial pressure (ICP) brain tumor, head injury, or impaired consciousness. Prolonged use of opioid analgesics during pregnancy may cause neonatal opioid withdrawal syndrome (NOWS). Available data within pregnant females are insufficient to inform a drug-associated risk of major birth defects and miscarriage. Based on animal data, advise pregnant females of the potential embryo/fetal risk. *Tramadol* and its metabolite, O-desmethyltramadol (M1), are present in human milk. **Conzip** is not recommended for obstetrical preoperative medication or for postdelivery analgesia in nursing mothers because its safety in infants and newborns has not been studied.
    Rybix ODT initially 100 mg once daily; may increase by 100 mg every 5 days; max 300 mg/day; *CrCl <30 ml/min or severe hepatic impairment:* not recommended; *Cirrhosis:* max 50 mg q 12 hours
  Pediatric: <12 years: contraindicated; 12-<18 years: use extreme caution; not recommended for children and adolescents with obesity, asthma, obstructive sleep apnea, or other chronic breathing problem, or for posttonsillectomy/adenoidectomy pain; ≥18 years: same as adult
      ODT: 50 mg (mint) (phenylalanine)
    Ryzolt initially 100 mg once daily; may increase by 100 mg every 5 days; max 300 mg/day; *CrCl <30 ml/min or severe hepatic impairment:* not recommended
  Pediatric: <12 years: contraindicated; 12-<18 years: use extreme caution; not recommended for children and adolescents with obesity, asthma, obstructive sleep apnea, or other chronic breathing problem, or for posttonsillectomy/adenoidectomy pain; ≥18 years: same as adult
      Tab: 100, 200, 300 mg ext-rel
    Ultram 50-100 mg q 4-6 hours prn; max 400 mg/day; *CrCl <30 ml/min:* max 100 mg q 12 hours; *Cirrhosis:* max 50 mg q 12 hours
  Pediatric: <12 years: contraindicated; 12-<18 years: use extreme caution; not recommended for children and adolescents with obesity, asthma, obstructive sleep apnea, or other chronic breathing problem, or for posttonsillectomy/adenoidectomy pain; ≥18 years: same as adult
      Tab: 50*mg
    Ultram ER initially 100 mg once daily; may increase by 100 mg every 5 days; max 300 mg/day; *CrCl <30 ml/min or severe hepatic impairment:* not recommended
  Pediatric: <12 years: contraindicated; 12-<18 years: use extreme caution; not recommended for children and adolescents with obesity, asthma, obstructive sleep apnea, or other chronic breathing problem, or for posttonsillectomy/adenoidectomy pain; ≥18 years: same as adult
      Tab: 100, 200, 300 mg ext-rel

▷ *tramadol+acetaminophen* (IV)(G) 2 tabs q 4-6 hours; max 8 tabs/day; 5 days; *CrCl <30 ml/min:* max 2 tabs q 12 hours; max 4 tabs/day x 5 days
  Pediatric: <12 years: contraindicated; 12-<18 years: use extreme caution; not recommended for children and adolescents with obesity, asthma, obstructive sleep apnea, or other chronic breathing problem, or for posttonsillectomy/adenoidectomy pain; ≥18 years: same as adult
    Ultracet *Tab:* tram 37.5+acet 325 mg
▷ *buprenorphine* (III) change patch every 7 days; do not increase the dose until previous dose has been worn for at least 72 hours; after removal, do not reuse the site for at least 3 weeks; do not expose the patch to heat
  Pediatric: <16 years: not recommended; ≥16 years: same as adult
    Butrans Transdermal System *Transdermal patch:* 5, 10, 20 mcg/hour (4/pck)
▷ *fentanyl* transdermal system (II) apply to clean, dry, non-irritated, intact, skin; hold in place for 30 seconds; start at lowest dose and titrate upward; *Opioid-naïve:* change patch every 3 days (72 hours)
  Pediatric: <18 years or <110 lb: not recommended; ≥18 years or ≥110 lb: same as adult
    Duragesic *Transdermal patch:* 12, 25, 37.5, 50, 62.5, 75, 87.5, 100 mcg/hour (5/pck)
▷ *fentanyl iontophoretic transdermal system*
    Ionsys is a transdermal patient-controlled device that sticks to the arm or chest; it is activated when the patient pushes the button
    Comment: Ionsys is for in-hospital use only and should be discontinued prior to hospital discharge. It is indicated for postop pain relief.

TRANSMUCOSAL (SUBLINGUAL, BUCCAL) OPIOIDS
Comment: For chronic severe pain. For management of breakthrough pain in patients with cancer who are already receiving and who are tolerant to opioid therapy. Opioid-tolerant patients are those taking oral *morphine* ≥60 mg/day, transdermal *fentanyl* ≥25 mcg/hour, *oxycodone* ≥30 mg/day, oral *hydromorphone* ≥8 mg/day, or an equianalgesic dose of another opioid, for ≥1 week

ORAL OPIOID PARTIAL AGONIST-ANTAGONIST
▷ *buprenorphine*
  Pediatric: <16 years: not recommended; ≥16 years: same as adult
    Subutex 8 mg in a single dose on day 1; then 16 mg in a single dose on day 2; target dose is 16 mg/day in a single dose; dissolve under tongue; do not chew or swallow whole
    SL tab (lemon-lime) or *SL film (lime):* 2, 8 mg (30/pck)
▷ *fentanyl* buccal soluble film (II) dissolve 1 film on moistened area inside cheek; initially 200 mcg; no more than 4 doses/day at least 2 hours apart; max 1,200 mcg/dose; do not cut film
  Pediatric: <18 years: not recommended; ≥18 years: same as adult
    Onsolis *Buccal film:* 200, 400, 600, 800, 1,200 mcg (30 films/pck)
▷ *fentanyl citrate* transmucosal unit (II)(G) initially one 200 mcg unit placed between cheek and lower gum; move from side to side; suck (not chew); use 6 units before titrating; titrate dose as needed; max 4 units/day
  Pediatric: <18 years: not recommended; ≥18 years: same as adult
    Actiq *Unit:* 200, 400, 600, 800, 1,200, 1,600 mcg (24 units/pck)
    Fentora *Unit:* 100, 200, 400, 600, 800 mcg (24 units/pck)
▷ *fentanyl* sublingual tab (II) initially one 100 mcg dose; if inadequate after 30 minutes, may repeat; titrate in increments of 100 mcg; max 2 doses per episode, up to 4 episodes per day; wait at least 2 hours before treating another episode; *Maintenance:* use only 1 tablet of appropriate strength; do not chew, suck, or swallow tablets; do not convert from other *fentanyl* products on a mcg-per-mcg basis or interchange with other *fentanyl* products
  Pediatric: <18 years: not recommended; ≥18 years: same as adult
    Abstral *SL tab:* 100, 200, 300, 400, 600, 800 mcg (32 tabs/pck)
▷ *fentanyl sublingual spray* (II)
  Pediatric: <18 years: not recommended; ≥18 years: same as adult
    Subsys 100, 200, 400, 600, 800 mcg/SL spray
    Comment: Subsys is not bioequivalent with other *fentanyl* products. Do not convert patients from other *fentanyl* products to Subsys on a mcg-per-mcg basis. There are no conversion directions available for patients on any other *fentanyl* products other than Actiq. (NOTE: This includes oral, transdermal, or parenteral formulations of *fentanyl*.)
▷ *sufentanil* 30 mcg sublingually prn; minimum 1 hour between doses; max 12 tablets/24 hours; max 72 hours
  Pediatric: <18 years: not established; ≥18 years: same as adult
    Dsuvia *SL tab:* 30 mcg in a single use applicator (SDA)
    Comment: Dsuvia *(sufentanil)* is a synthetic opioid analgesic formulation for the management of acute severe pain that is severe enough to require an opioid analgesic and for which alternative treatments are inadequate. Dsuvia is indicated for use only in adults in a certified medically supervised healthcare settings, such as hospitals, surgical centers, and emergency departments. Dsuvia is only available through the Dsuvia REMS Program; Dsuvia is not for home use or for use in children; discontinue treatment with Dsuvia before patients leave the certified medically supervised healthcare setting. Do not discontinue Dsuvia abruptly in the physically dependent patient. Concomitant use with CYP3A4

(continued)

inhibitors (or discontinuation of CYP3A4 inducers) can result in a fatal overdose of *sufentanil*. The most commonly reported adverse reactions (incidence ≥2%) have been nausea, headache, vomiting, dizziness, and hypotension.

PARENTERAL OPIOID AGONIST-ANTAGONISTS

▷ *buprenorphine hcl Initial dose:* 0.3 mg (1 ml) deep IM or slow IV (over at least 2 minutes); may repeat once (up to 0.3 mg) if required, 30-60 minutes after initial dose; usual frequency every 6 hours prn; fixed interval or "round-the-clock" dosing should not be undertaken until the appropriate interdose interval has been established by clinical observation
Pediatric: <2 years: not recommended; 2-12 years: 2-6 mcg/kg deep IM or slow IV every 4-6 hours or every 6-8 hours prn; >12 years: same as adult; fixed interval or "round-the-clock" dosing should not be undertaken until the appropriate interdose interval has been established by clinical observation
Buprenex *Amp:* 0.3 mg/ml (1 ml) (5 ampules/carton)
▷ *nalbuphine* (G) 10 mg/70 kg IM, SC, or IV q 3-6 hours prn
Pediatric: <18 years: not recommended; ≥18 years: same as adult
Nubain *Amp:* 10, 20 mg/ml (1 ml) (sulfite-free, parabens-free)
▷ *pentazocine+naloxone* (IV) 1-2 tabs q 3-4 hours prn; max 12 tabs/day
Pediatric: <12 years: not recommended; ≥12 years: same as adult
Talwin-NX *Tab:* pent 50 mg+nal 0.5*mg

TRANSMUCOSAL (INTRANASAL) OPIOIDS

▷ *butorphanol tartrate* nasal spray (IV) initially 1 spray (1 mg) in one nostril and may repeat after 60-90 minutes (*Elderly:* 90-120 minutes) in opposite nostril if needed or 1 spray in each nostril and may repeat q 3-4 hours prn
Pediatric: <18 years: not recommended; ≥18 years: same as adult
Butorphanol Nasal Spray *Nasal spray:* 1 mg/actuation (10 mg/ml, 2.5 ml)
Stadol Nasal Spray *Nasal spray:* 1 mg/actuation (10 mg/ml, 2.5 ml)
▷ *fentanyl* nasal spray (II) initially 1 spray (100 mcg) in one nostril and may repeat after 2 hours; when adequate analgesia is achieved, use that dose for subsequent breakthrough episodes
Titration steps: 100 mcg using 1 x 100 mcg spray; 200 mcg using 2 x 100 mcg spray (1 in each nostril); 400 mcg using 1 x 400 mcg spray; 800 mcg using 2 x 400 mcg (1 in each nostril); max 800 mcg; limit to ≤4 doses per day
Pediatric: <18 years: not recommended; ≥18 years: same as adult
Lazanda Nasal Spray *Nasal spray:* 100, 400 mcg/100 mcl (8 sprays/bottle)
Comment: **Lazanda Nasal Spray** is available by restricted distribution program. To enroll, call 855-841-4234 or https://www.fda.gov/downloads/drugs/drugsafety/postmarketdrugsafetyinformationforpatientsandproviders/ucm261983.pdf. **Lazanda Nasal Spray** is indicated for the management of breakthrough pain in cancer patients who are already receiving and who are tolerant to opioid therapy for their underlying persistent cancer pain. Patients considered opioid-tolerant are those who are taking at least 60 mg of oral morphine/day, 25 mcg of transdermal *fentanyl*/hour, 30 mg oral *oxycodone*/day, 8 mg oral *hydromorphone*/day, 25 mg oral *oxymorphone*/day, or an equianalgesic dose of another opioid for a week or longer. Patients must remain on around-the-clock opioids when using **Lazanda Nasal Spray**. As such, it is contraindicated in the management of acute or postop pain, including headache/migraine or dental pain.

INTRATHECAL OPIOID

▷ *ziconotide* intrathecal (IT) infusion initially no more than 2.4 mcg/day (0.1 mcg/hour) and titrate to upward by up to 2.4 mcg/day (0.1 mcg/day at intervals of no more than 2-3 times per week), up to a recommended maximum of 19.2 mcg/day (0.8 mcg/hour) by Day 21; dose increases in increments of less than 2.4 mcg/day (0.1 mcg/hour) and increases in dose less frequently than 2-3 times per week may be used
Pediatric: <12 years: not recommended; ≥12 years: same as adult
Prialt *Vial:* 25 mcg/ml (20 ml), 100 mcg/ml (1, 2, 5 ml)
Comment: Patients with a preexisting history of psychosis should not be treated with *ziconotide*. Contraindications to the use of IT analgesia include conditions such as the presence of infection at the microinfusion injection site, uncontrolled bleeding diathesis, and spinal canal obstruction that impairs circulation of cerebrospinal fluid (CSF).

PANCREATIC ENZYME INSUFFICIENCY

Comment: Seen in chronic pancreatitis, postpancreatectomy, cystic fibrosis, steatorrhea, post-gastrointestinal (GI) tract bypass surgery, and ductal obstruction from neoplasia. May sprinkle cap; however, do not crush or chew cap or tab. May mix with applesauce or other acidic food; follow with water or juice. Do not let any drug remain in the mouth. Take dose just prior to each meal or snack. Base dose on lipase units; adjust per diet and clinical response (i.e., steatorrhea). Pancrelipase products are interchangeable. Contraindicated with pork protein hypersensitivity.

PANCRELIPASE PRODUCTS
▷ *pancreatic enzymes*

Creon 500 units/kg per meal; max 2,500 units/kg per meal or <10,000 units/kg per day or <4,000 units/gm fat ingested per day
Pediatric: <12 months: 2,000-4,000 units per 120 ml formula or per breastfeeding (do not mix directly into formula or breast milk; 12 months to 4 years: 1,000 units/kg per meal; max 2,500 units/kg per meal <10,000 units/kg per day; >4 years: same as adult
> *Cap:* **Creon 3000** lip 3,000 units+pro 9,500 units+amyl 15,000 units del-rel
> **Creon 6000** lip 6,000 units+pro 19,000 units+amyl 30,000 units del-rel
> **Creon 12000** lip 12,000 units+pro 38,000 units+amyl 60,000 units del-rel
> **Creon 24000** lip 24,000 units+pro 76,000 units+amyl 120,000 units del-rel
> **Creon 36000** lip 36,000 units+pro 114,000 units+amyl 180,000 units del-rel

Cotazym 1-3 tabs just prior to each meal or snack
Pediatric: <12 years: not recommended; ≥12 years: same as adult
> *Tab:* **Cotazym** lip 1,000 units+pro 12,500 units+amyl 12,500 units del-rel
> **Cotazym-S** lip 5,000 units+pro 20,000 units+amyl 20,000 units del-rel

Donnazyme 1-3 caps just prior to each meal or snack
Pediatric: <12 years: not recommended; ≥12 years: same as adult
> *Cap:* **Donnazyme** lip 5,000 units+pro 20,000 units+amyl 20,000 units del-rel

Ku-Zyme 1-2 caps just prior to each meal or snack
Pediatric: <12 years: not recommended; ≥12 years: same as adult
> *Cap:* **Ku-Zyme:** lip 12,000 units+pro 15,000 units+amyl 15,000 units del-rel

Kutrase 1-2 caps just prior to each meal or snack
Pediatric: <12 years: not recommended; ≥12 years: same as adult
> *Cap:* **Kutrase:** lip 12,000 units+pro 30,000 units+amyl 30,000 units del-rel

Pancreaze 2,500 lipase units/kg per meal or <10,000 lipase units/kg per day or <4,000 lipase units/gm fat ingested per day
Pediatric: <12 months: 2,000-4,000 lipase units per 120 ml formula or per breastfeeding; >12 months-<4 years 1,000 lipase units/kg per meal; >4 years: 500 lipase units/kg per meal; max: adult dose
> *Cap:* **Pancreaze 4200** lip 4,200 units+pro 10,000 units+amyl 17,500 units ec-microtabs
> **Pancreaze 10500** lip 10,500 units+pro 25,000 units+amyl 43,750 units ec-microtabs
> **Pancreaze 16800** lip 16,800 units+pro 40,000 units+amyl 70,000 units ec-microtabs
> **Pancreaze 21000** lip 21,000 units+pro 37,000 units+amyl 61,000 units ec-microtabs

Pertzye 12 months to 4 years, ≥8 kg: initially 1,000 lipase units/kg per meal; ≥4 years, ≥16 kg: initially 500 lipase units/kg per meal; *Both:* 2,500 lipase units/kg per meal or <10,000 units/kg per day or <4,000 lipase units/gm fat ingested per day
> *Cap:* **Pertzye 8000** lip 8,000 units+pro 28,750 units+amyl 30,250 units del-rel

Pertzye 16000 lip 16,000 units+pro 57,500 units+amyl 65,000 units del-rel
Ultrase 1-3 tabs just prior to each meal or snack
Pediatric: same as adult
> *Cap:* **Ultrase** lip 4,500 units+pro 20,000 units+amyl 25,000 units del-rel
> **Ultrase MT** lip 12,000 units+pro 39,000 units+amyl 39,000 units del-rel
> **Ultrase MT 18** lip 18,000 units+pro 58,500 units+amyl 58,500 units del-rel
> **Ultrase MT 20** lip 20,000 units+pro 65,000 units+amyl 65,000 units del-rel

Viokace initially 500 lip units/kg per meal; max 2,500 lipase units/kg per meal, or <10,000 lipase units/kg per meal, or <4,000 units/gm fat ingested per day
Pediatric: same as adult
> *Tab:* **Viokace 8** lip 8,000 units+pro 30,000 units+amyl 30,000 units
> **Viokace 16** lip 16,000 units+pro 60,000 units+amyl 60,000 units

Viokace 0440 lip 10,440 units+pro 39,150 units+amyl 39,150 units
Viokace 20880 lip 20,880 units+pro 78,300 units+amyl 78,300 units
Comment: Viokace 10440 and Viokace 20880 should be taken with a daily proton pump inhibitor (PPI).
Viokace Powder 1/4 tsp (0.7 gm) with meals
Viokace Powder lip 16,800 units+pro 70,000 units+amyl 70,000 units per 1/4 tsp (8 oz)

Zenpep initially 500 lipase units/kg per meal; max 2,500 lipase units/kg per meal or <10,000 units/kg per day or <4,000 units/gm fat ingested per day
Pediatric: Infant-12 months: infants may be given 3,000 lipase units (1 capsule) per 120 ml of formula or per breastfeeding; do not mix capsule contents directly into formula or breast milk prior to administration; Children >12 months to <4 years: enzyme dosing should begin with 1,000 lipase units/kg of body weight per meal to a maximum of 2,500 lipase units/kg of body weight per meal (or ≤10,000 lipase units/kg/day), or <4,000 lipase units/gm fat ingested per day; Children ≥4 years: same as adult
> *Cap:* **Zenpep 3000** lip 3,000 units+pro 10,000 units+amyl 14,000 units del-rel
> **Zenpep 5000** lip 5,000 units+pro 17,000 units+amyl 24,000 units

(continued)

Zenpep 10000 lip 10,000 units+pro 32,000 units+amyl 42,000 units del-rel
Zenpep 15000 lip 15,000 units+pro 47,000 units+amyl 63,000 units del-rel
Zenpep 20000 lip 20,000 units+pro 63,000 units+amyl 84,000 units del-rel
Zenpep 25000 lip 25,000 units+pro 79,000 units+amyl 105,000 units del-rel
Zenpep 40000 lip 40,000 units+pro 126,000 units+amyl 168,000 units del-rel
Comment: Zenpep is not interchangeable with any other pancrelipase product. Dosing should not exceed the recommended maximum dosage set forth by the Cystic Fibrosis Foundation Consensus Conferences Guidelines. **Zenpep** should be swallowed whole. For infants or patients unable to swallow intact capsules, the contents may be sprinkled on soft acidic food (e.g., applesauce).
Zymase 1-3 caps just prior to each meal or snack
Pediatric: <12 years: not recommended; ≥12 years: same as adult
Cap: **Zymase** lip 12,000 units+prot 24,000 units+amyl 24,000 units del-rel

PANIC DISORDER

Comment: If possible when considering a benzodiazepine to treat anxiety, a short-acting benzodiazepine should be used only prn to avert intense anxiety and panic for the least time necessary while a different non-addictive antianxiety regimen (e.g., selective serotonin reuptake inhibitor [SSRI], serotonin norepinephrine reuptake inhibitor [SNRI], tricyclic antidepressant [TCA], *buspirone*, beta-blocker) is established and effective treatment goals achieved. Co-administration of SSRIs with TCAs requires extreme caution. Concomitant use of monoamine oxidase inhibitors (MAOIs) and SSRIs is absolutely contraindicated. Avoid other serotonergic drugs. A potentially fatal adverse event is *serotonin syndrome*, caused by serotonin excess. Milder symptoms require healthcare provider intervention to avert severe symptoms which can be rapidly fatal without urgent/emergent medical care. Symptoms include restlessness, agitation, confusion, hallucinations, tachycardia, hypertension, dilated pupils, muscle twitching, muscle rigidity, loss of muscle coordination, diaphoresis, diarrhea, headache, shivering, piloerection, hyperpyrexia, cardiac arrhythmias, seizures, loss of consciousness, coma, and death. Abrupt withdrawal or interruption of treatment with an antidepressant medication is sometimes associated with an *antidepressant discontinuation syndrome*, which may be mediated by gradually tapering the drug over a period of 2 weeks or longer, depending on the dose strength and length of treatment. Common symptoms of the *serotonin discontinuation syndrome* include flu-like symptoms (nausea, vomiting, diarrhea, headaches, sweating), sleep disturbances (insomnia, nightmares, constant sleepiness), mood disturbances (dysphoria, anxiety, agitation), cognitive disturbances (mental confusion, hyperarousal), and sensory and movement disturbances (imbalance, tremors, vertigo, dizziness, electric-shock-like sensations in the brain, often described by sufferers as "brain zaps").

SELECTIVE SEROTONIN REUPTAKE INHIBITORS (SSRIs)

▷ *escitalopram* (G) initially 10 mg daily; may increase to 20 mg daily after 1 week; *Elderly or hepatic impairment:* 10 mg once daily
Pediatric: <12 years: not recommended; ≥12 years: same as adult; 12-17 years: initially 10 mg once daily; may increase to 20 mg once daily after 3 weeks
Lexapro *Tab:* 5, 10*, 20*mg
Lexapro Oral Solution *Oral soln:* 1 mg/ml (240 ml) (peppermint) (parabens)
▷ *fluoxetine* (G)
Prozac initially 20 mg daily; may increase after 1 week; doses >20 mg/day should be divided into AM and noon doses; max 80 mg/day
Pediatric: <8 years: not recommended; 8-17 years: initially 10 mg/day, may increase after 2 weeks to 20 mg/day, range 20-60 mg/day, range for lower weight children 20-30 mg/day; >17 years: same as adult
Cap: 10, 20, 40 mg; *Tab:* 30*, 60*mg; *Oral soln:* 20 mg/5 ml (4 oz) (mint)
Prozac Weekly following daily *fluoxetine* therapy at 20 mg/day for 13 weeks, may initiate **Prozac Weekly** 7 days after the last 20 mg *fluoxetine* dose
Pediatric: <12 years: not recommended; ≥12 years: same as adult
Cap: 90 mg ent-coat del-rel pellets
▷ *paroxetine maleate* (G)
Pediatric: <12 years: not recommended; ≥12 years: same as adult
Paxil initially 20 mg daily in the AM; may increase by 10 mg/day at weekly intervals as needed; max 60 mg/day
Tab: 10*, 20*, 30, 40 mg
Paxil CR initially 25 mg daily in the AM; may increase by 12.5 mg at weekly intervals as needed; max 62.5 mg/day
Tab: 12.5, 25, 37.5 mg cont-rel ent-coat
Paxil Oral Suspension initially 20 mg daily in the AM; may increase by 10 mg/day at weekly intervals as needed; max 60 mg/day
Oral susp: 10 mg/5 ml (250 ml) (orange)

▷ *paroxetine mesylate* (G) initially 7.5 mg daily in the AM; may increase by 10 mg/day at weekly intervals as needed; max 60 mg/day
    Pediatric: <12 years: <u>not</u> recommended; ≥12 years: same as adult
        Brisdelle *Cap:* 7.5 mg
▷ *sertraline* initially 50 mg daily; increase at 1-week intervals if needed; max 200 mg daily
    Pediatric: <6 years: <u>not</u> recommended; 6-12 years: initially 25 mg daily; max 200 mg/day; 13-17 years: initially 50 mg daily; max 200 mg/day; ≥17 years: same as adult
        Zoloft *Tab:* 15*, 50*, 100*mg; *Oral conc:* 20 mg per ml (60 ml, dilute just before administering in 4 oz water, ginger ale, lemon-lime soda, lemonade, <u>or</u> orange juice) (alcohol 12%)

SEROTONIN NOREPINEPHRINE REUPTAKE INHIBITORS (SNRIs)
▷ *desvenlafaxine* (G) swallow whole; initially 50 mg once daily; max 120 mg/day
    Pediatric: <12 years: <u>not</u> recommended; ≥12 years: same as adult
        Pristiq *Tab:* 50, 100 mg ext-rel
▷ *venlafaxine* (G)
        Effexor initially 75 mg/day in 2-3 doses; may increase at 4-day intervals in 75 mg increments to 150 mg/day; max 375 mg/day
    Pediatric: <18 years: <u>not</u> recommended; ≥18 years: same as adult
        Tab: 25, 37.5, 50, 75, 100 mg
        Effexor XR initially 75 mg q AM; may start at 37.5 mg daily x 4-7 days, then increase by increments of up to 75 mg/day at intervals of at least 4 days; usual max 375 mg/day
    Pediatric: <18 years: <u>not</u> recommended; ≥18 years: same as adult
        Cap: 37.5, 75, 150 mg ext-rel

TRICYCLIC ANTIDEPRESSANTS (TCAs)
▷ *doxepin* (G)
    Pediatric: <12 years: <u>not</u> recommended; ≥12 years: same as adult
        Cap: 10, 25, 50, 75, 100, 150 mg; *Oral conc:* 10 mg/ml (4 oz w. dropper)
▷ *imipramine* (G)
    Pediatric: <12 years: <u>not</u> recommended; ≥12 years: same as adult
        Tofranil initially 75 mg daily, max 200 mg; *Adolescents:* initially 30-40 mg daily, max 100 mg/day; if maintenance dose exceeds 75 mg daily, may switch to **Tofranil PM** for divided <u>or</u> bedtime dose
        Tab: 10, 25, 50 mg
        Tofranil PM initially 75 mg daily 1 hour before HS; max 200 mg
            Cap: 75, 100, 125, 150
        Tofranil Injection 50 mg IM; lower dose for adolescents; switch to oral form as soon as possible
            Amp: 25 mg/2 ml (2 ml)

FIRST-GENERATION ANTIHISTAMINE
▷ *hydroxyzine* (G) 50-100 mg qid; max 600 mg/day
    Pediatric: <6 years: 50 mg/day divided qid; ≥6 years: 50-100 mg/day divided qid
        Atarax *Tab:* 10, 25, 50, 100 mg; *Syr:* 10 mg/5 ml (alcohol 0.5%)
        Vistaril *Cap:* 25, 50, 100 mg; *Oral susp:* 25 mg/5 ml (4 oz) (lemon)
Comment: *Hydroxyzine* is contraindicated in early pregnancy and in patients with a prolonged QT interval. It is <u>not</u> known whether this drug is excreted in human milk; therefore, *hydroxyzine* should <u>not</u> be given to nursing mothers.

AZAPIRONES
▷ *buspirone* initially 7.5 mg bid; may increase by 5 mg/day q 2-3 days; max 60 mg/day
    Pediatric: <6 years: <u>not</u> recommended; 6-17 years: same as adult
        BuSpar *Tab:* 5, 10, 15*, 30*mg

BENZODIAZEPINES
Short-Acting
▷ *alprazolam* (IV)(G)
    Pediatric: <18 years: <u>not</u> recommended; ≥18 years: same as adult
        Niravam initially 0.25-0.5 mg tid; may titrate every 3-4 days; max 4 mg/day
          Tab: 0.25*, 0.5*, 1*, 2*mg orally-disint
        Xanax initially 0.25-0.5 mg tid; may titrate every 3-4 days; max 4 mg/day
          Tab: 0.25*, 0.5*, 1*, 2*mg
        Xanax XR initially 0.5-1 mg once daily, preferably in the AM; increase at intervals of at least 3-4 days by up to 1 mg/day; taper no faster than 0.5 mg every 3 days; max 10 mg/day; when switching from immediate-release *alprazolam*, give total daily dose of immediate-release once daily
          Tab: 0.5, 1, 2, 3 mg ext-rel
▷ *oxazepam* (IV)(G) 10-15 mg tid-qid for moderate symptoms; 15-30 mg tid-qid for severe symptoms
    Pediatric: <12 years: <u>not</u> recommended; ≥12 years: same as adult
        oxazepam Tab: 15 mg; *Cap:* 10, 15, 30 mg

Intermediate-Acting

▷ *lorazepam* (IV)(G) 1-10 mg/day in 2-3 divided doses
  Pediatric: <12 years: <u>not</u> recommended; ≥12 years: same as adult
    Ativan *Tab:* 0.5, 1*, 2*mg
    Lorazepam Intensol *Oral conc:* 2 mg/ml (30 ml w. graduated dropper)

Long-Acting

▷ *chlordiazepoxide* (IV)(G)
  Pediatric: <6 years: <u>not</u> recommended; ≥6 years: 5 mg bid-qid; increase to 10 mg bid-tid
    Librium 5-10 mg tid-qid for moderate symptoms; 20-25 mg tid-qid for severe symptoms
      Cap: 5, 10, 25 mg
    Librium Injectable 50-100 mg IM or IV; then 25-50 mg IM tid-qid prn; max 300 mg/day
      Inj: 100 mg
▷ *chlordiazepoxide+clidinium* (IV) 1-2 caps tid-qid; max 8 caps/day
  Pediatric: <12 years: <u>not</u> recommended; ≥12 years: same as adult
    Librax *Cap:* chlor 5 mg+clid 2.5 mg
▷ *clonazepam* (IV)(G) initially 0.25 mg bid; increase to 1 mg/day after 3 days
  Pediatric: <18 years: <u>not</u> recommended; ≥18 years: same as adult
    Klonopin *Tab:* 0.5*, 1, 2 mg
    Klonopin Wafers dissolve in mouth with or without water
      Wafer: 0.125, 0.25, 0.5, 1, 2 mg orally-disint
▷ *clorazepate* (IV)(G) 30 mg/day in divided doses; max 60 mg/day
  Pediatric: <9 years: <u>not</u> recommended; ≥9 years: same as adult
    Tranxene *Tab:* 3.75, 7.5, 15 mg
    Tranxene SD do <u>not</u> use for initial therapy
      Tab: 22.5 mg ext-rel
    Tranxene SD Half Strength do <u>not</u> use for initial therapy
      Tab: 11.25 mg ext-rel
    Tranxene T-Tab *Tab:* 3.75*, 7.5*, 15*mg
▷ *diazepam* (IV)(G) 2-10 mg bid-qid
  Pediatric: <12 years: <u>not</u> recommended; ≥12 years: same as adult
    Diastat *Rectal gel delivery system:* 2.5 mg
    Diastat AcuDial *Rectal gel delivery system:* 10, 20 mg
    Valium *Tab:* 2*, 5*, 10*mg
    Valium Injectable *Vial:* 5 mg/ml (10 ml); *Amp:* 5 mg/ml (2 ml); *Prefilled syringe:* 5 mg/ml (5 ml)
    Valium Intensol Oral Solution *Conc oral soln:* 5 mg/ml (30 ml w. dropper) (alcohol 19%)
    Valium Oral Solution *Oral soln:* 5 mg/5 ml (500 ml) (wintergreen spice)

PHENOTHIAZINES

▷ *prochlorperazine* (G)
  Pediatric: <12 years: <u>not</u> recommended; ≥12 years: same as adult
    Compazine 5 mg tid-qid
      Tab: 5 mg; *Syr:* 5 mg/5 ml (4 oz) (fruit); *Rectal supp:* 2.5, 5, 25 mg
    Compazine Spansule 15 mg q AM or 10 mg q 12 hours
      Spansule: 10, 15 mg sust-rel
▷ *trifluoperazine* (G) 1-2 mg bid; max 6 mg/day; max 12 weeks
  Pediatric: <12 years: <u>not</u> recommended; ≥12 years: same as adult
    Stelazine *Tab:* 1, 2, 5, 10 mg

PARKINSON'S DISEASE (PD)

Parkinson's Disease-Associated Dementia *see Dementia*
Comment: When administering *carbidopa* and *levodopa* separately, administer each at the same time. Titrate daily dose ratio of 1:10 *carbidopa* to *levodopa*. Max daily *carbidopa* is 200 mg. Most patients will require *levodopa* 400-1600 mg/day in divided doses every 4-8 hours. After titrating both drugs to the desired effects without intolerable side effects, switch to a *carbidopa+levodopa* combination form.

DOPAMINE PRECURSOR (LEVODOPA)

▷ *levodopa* (G)
    Tab: 125, 150, 200 mg

DECARBOXYLASE INHIBITOR (CARBIDOPA)

▷ *carbidopa* (G)
    Lodosyn *Tab:* 25 mg

TREATMENT OF DOPAMINE OFF EPISODES

▶ *levodopa inhalation powder* for oral inhalation only; do not swallow capsules; administer capsules only with the Inbrija inhaler; max 1 dose (2 capsules) for any *Off* period; max 5 doses (10 capsules), 420 mg/day

Inbrija *Inhal cap:* 42 mg inhal pwdr (60 caps; 4 caps/foil blister card, 15 cards/carton) w. Inbrija inhaler

Comment: Inbrija is an aromatic amino acid oral inhalation powder for the intermittent (on-demand) treatment of *Off* episodes in people with Parkinson's disease (PD) treated with ***carbidopa/levodopa***. *Off* episodes, also known as *Off* periods, are defined as the return of Parkinson's symptoms that result from low levels of dopamine between doses of oral carbidopa/levodopa, the standard oral baseline Parkinson's treatment. **Inbrija** is not recommended for patients with asthma, chronic obstructive pulmonary disease (COPD), or other chronic underlying lung disease. **Inbrija** is contraindicated within 14 days before and 7 days after taking a non-selective monoamine oxidase inhibitor (MAOI). Monitor patients on MAO-B inhibitors for orthostatic hypotension. Concomitant dopamine D2 antagonists, respiratory tract infection, and discolored sputum.

NON-ERGOLINE DOPAMINE AGONIST

▶ *apomorphine hcl* (G) *Injection;* for SC administration only; rotate sites; therapeutic dosing is based on effectiveness and tolerance; *Start:* at 0.2 ml (2 mg) SC; may titrate up to a maximum recommended dose of 0.6 ml (6 mg) SC; *Patients in an "Off" State:* administer a 0.2 ml (2 mg) SC test dose in a setting where BP can be closely monitored by medical personnel; supine and standing BP should be checked pre-dose and at 20, 40, and 60 minutes post-dose; patients who develop clinically significant orthostatic hypotension in response to this test dose should not be considered candidates for treatment with **Apokyn**; if the patient tolerates the 0.2 ml (2 mg) SC dose and responds, the starting dose should be 0.2 ml (2 mg) SC on an "as needed" basis to treat existing *Off* episodes; do not exceed max 0.6 ml (6 mg) SC

Apokyn (G) *Amp:* 20 mg/2 ml (10 mg/ml), single-use, soln (metabisulfite); *Cartridge:* 30 mg/3 ml (10 mg/ml), multi-dose, soln (metabisulfite) (benzyl alcohol)

Comment: Apokyn is indicated for the acute, intermittent treatment of hypomobility, "off" episodes ("end-of-dose wearing off" and unpredictable "on/off" episodes) associated with advanced Parkinson's disease. **Apokyn** is contraindicated in patients who have demonstrated hypersensitivity to the drug or its ingredients (notably, sodium metabisulfite). Based on reports of profound hypotension and loss of consciousness when *apomorphine* was administered with *ondansetron*, the concomitant use of *apomorphine* with drugs of the 5-HT3 antagonist class (including, for example, *ondansetron*, *granisetron*, *dolasetron*, *palonosetron*, and *alosetron*) is contraindicated. Serious adverse events (such as IV crystallization of *apomorphine*, leading to thrombus formation and pulmonary embolism), have followed the IV administration of *apomorphine*. Consequently, *apomorphine* should not be administered intravenously. Adverse side effects have included nausea and vomiting, syncope, QT prolongation and potential for proarrhythmic effects, symptomatic hypotension, falls, hallucinations, sedation, somnolence, and falling asleep during activities of daily living (ADLs). Alcohol, antihypertensive medications, and vasodilating medications may potentiate the hypotensive effect of *apomorphine*. Because *apomorphine* has been shown to reduce resting systolic and diastolic BP, it has the potential to exacerbate coronary (and cerebral) ischemia. During clinical development, 4% of patients treated with *apomorphine* experienced angina, myocardial infarction, cardiac arrest, and/or sudden death. Extra caution should be used in prescribing *apomorphine* for patients with known cardiovascular and cerebrovascular disease. If patients develop signs and symptoms of coronary or cerebral ischemia, the continued use of *apomorphine* should be carefully re-evaluated. **Apokyn** contains sodium metabisulfite, a sulfite that may cause allergic-type reactions, including anaphylactic symptoms and life-threatening or less severe asthmatic episodes in certain susceptible people. Sulfite sensitivity is seen more frequently in asthmatic than in non-asthmatic people. Among the 550 patients treated with *apomorphine* SC injections during development, 26% of patients complained of injection site reactions, including bruising (16%), granuloma (4%), and pruritus (2%). There was a limited experience (both for overall numbers of patients as well as the total number of injections per patient) with *apomorphine* injections in controlled trials. In this limited controlled experience, the number of injection site reactions reported by patients receiving *apomorphine* was similar to that reported by patients receiving placebo. *Apomorphine* may cause dyskinesia or exacerbate preexisting dyskinesia. During clinical development, dyskinesia or worsening of dyskinesia was reported in 24% of patients, and 2% of patients withdrew from studies due to dyskinesias. During clinical development, painful erection (priapism) was reported by 3 of 361 males (<1%). Caution should be exercised when administrating *apomorphine* to patients with mild and moderate hepatic impairment (Child-Pugh Class A or B) due to the increased maximum plasma concentration (Cmax) and area under the curve (AUC) in these patients. Studies of subjects with severe hepatic impairment (Child-Pugh Class C) have not been conducted. The starting dose should be reduced to 1 mg when administering *apomorphine* to patients with mild or moderate renal impairment because the Cmax and AUC are increased in these patients. Studies in subjects with severe renal impairment have not been conducted. Patients and caregivers should be urged to read the attached Patient Package Insert and Directions for Use of the ampule and dosing pen. Patients should be instructed to use **Apokyn** only as prescribed. Patients and/or caregivers who are advised to administer **Apokyn** in medically unsupervised situations should receive instruction on the proper use

(continued)

of the product from the physician **Apokyn** and other suitably qualified healthcare professional and then observed during the initial dosing. Particular attention paid to two issues: (1) Patients need to be aware that the drug is dosed in milliliters, not milligrams and (2) a dose of 1 mg is represented on the dosing pen as 0.1 ml, and not as 1.0 ml (the latter representing a dose of 10 mg). Reproduction studies have not been conducted with *apomorphine*; it is not known whether apomorphine can cause fetal harm when administered to a pregnant woman or can affect reproductive capacity. It is not known whether *apomorphine* is excreted in human milk. Because many drugs are excreted in human milk and because of the potential for serious adverse reactions in nursing infants from *apomorphine*, a decision should be made as to whether to discontinue nursing or to discontinue the drug, taking into account the importance of the drug to the mother.

▷ *apomorphine sublingual film* 10-30 mg SL as a single dose prn; do not cut, chew, or swallow; separate doses by at least 2 hours; max single dose 30 mg; max 5 doses per day; initiation and titration should be supervised by an appropriate healthcare provider; a concomitant antiemetic (e.g., *trimethobenzamide*) is recommended beginning 3 days prior to initial dose

Kynmobi *SL film:* 10, 15, 20, 25, 30 mg, single-dose in an individual foil pouch

Comment: Kynmobi *(apomorphine sublingual film)* is a novel formulation of the approved dopamine agonist *apomorphine* for the on-demand management of *Off* episodes associated with PD. Contraindications include concomitant use with 5-HT3 antagonists and hypersensitivity to *apomorphine* or any of its ingredients (including sodium metabisulfite). The most common adverse reactions (incidence ≥10%) have been nausea, oral/pharyngeal soft tissue swelling, oral/pharyngeal soft tissue pain and paresthesia, dizziness, and somnolence. Discontinue if falling asleep during ADLs and daytime somnolence occurs at lowest dose. Syncope and hypotension/orthostatic hypotension may occur; monitor BP. Oral mucosal irritation may require a drug pause or discontinuation. Falls may occur or increase. If hallucinations and psychotic-like behavior, loss of impulse control, or impulsive behaviors occur, consider dose reduction or discontinuation. Withdrawal-emergent hyperpyrexia and confusion may occur with rapid dose reduction or withdrawal. May prolong QTc and cause torsades de pointes or sudden death; consider risk factors prior to initiation. Concomitant use of antihypertensive medications and vasodilators may increase risk for hypotension, myocardial infarction, falls, and injuries. Avoid use of **Kynmobi** in patients with severe hepatic impairment (Child-Pugh Class C). No dosage adjustment is required for patients with mild or moderate hepatic impairment (Child-Pugh Class A or B). Avoid use of **Kynmobi** in patients with severe and end-stage renal disease (ESRD; CrCl <30 ml/min). No dosage adjustment is required for patients with mild or moderate renal impairment. Concomitant dopamine antagonists may diminish effectiveness of **Kynmobi.** *Apomorphine* is not a controlled substance. In premarketing clinical experience, **Kynmobi** did not reveal any tendency for a withdrawal syndrome or any drug-seeking behavior. However, there are rare postmarketing reports of abuse of medications containing *apomorphine*. Advise patients that **Kynmobi** may cause prolonged painful erections (priapism) and if this occurs to seek immediate medical attention. Based on animal data, **Kynmobi** may cause fetal harm. There are no data on the presence of *apomorphine* in human milk or effects on the breastfed infant.

DOPAMINE RECEPTOR AGONISTS

▷ *amantadine*

Gocovri take once daily at bedtime; initially 137 mg; after 1 week, increase to the recommended daily dosage of 274 mg; swallow whole; may sprinkle contents on soft food; take with or without food; avoid use with alcohol; a lower dosage is recommended for patients with moderate or severe renal impairment; contraindicated in patients with ESRD

Cap: 68.5, 137 mg ext-rel

Comment: Gocovri is a chronosynchronous *amantadine* therapy indicated for the treatment of dyskinesia in patients with Parkinson's disease (PD) receiving *levodopa*-based therapy, with or without concomitant dopaminergic medications, and as adjunctive treatment to *levodopa/carbidopa* in patients with PD experiencing "*off*" episodes. The most commonly observed adverse reactions (incidence ≥10%) have been hallucination, dizziness, dry mouth, peripheral edema, constipation, fall, and orthostatic hypotension. Advise patients prior to treatment about the potential to fall asleep during ADLs; discontinue if this occurs. Monitor patients for depressed mood, depression, or suicidal ideation or behavior. Patients with major psychotic disorder should ordinarily not be treated with **Gocovri**; observe patients for the occurrence of hallucinations throughout treatment, especially at initiation and after dose increases. Monitor patients for dizziness and orthostatic hypotension, especially after starting **Gocovri** and after dose increases. Avoid sudden discontinuation, which can result in withdrawal-emergent hyperpyrexia and confusion. Impulse control and compulsive behaviors may occur, such as gambling urges, sexual urges, and uncontrolled spending; consider dose reduction or discontinuation if any occur. Increased risk of anticholinergic effects may require reduction of **Gocovri** or dose of the anticholinergic drug(s). Excretion of *amantadine* increases with acidic urine, resulting in possible accumulation with urine change toward alkaline. Live attenuated vaccines (LAVs) are not recommended during treatment with **Gocovri**. Concomitant use of alcohol is not recommended due to increased potential for central nervous system (CNS) effects. There are no adequate data on embryo/fetal risk associated with use of *amantadine* in pregnant females. Animal studies suggest a potential risk for fetal harm with *amantadine*. *Amantadine* is excreted in human milk, but amounts have <u>not</u> been quantified. There is <u>no</u> information on the risk to the breastfed infant.

Osmolex ER initial dose 129 mg orally once daily in the morning; may increase dose in weekly intervals; max daily dose 322 mg in the morning; dose frequency reduction and monitoring required for renal impairment; swallow whole; do <u>not</u> chew, crush, <u>or</u> divide

    Tab: 129, 193, 258 mg ext-rel

Comment: **Osmolex ER** is <u>not</u> interchangeable with other *amantadine* immediate- <u>or</u> extended-release products. The most common adverse reactions (incidence ≥5%) are nausea, dizziness/lightheadedness, and insomnia. **Osmolex ER** is contraindicated in patients with ESRD. Advise patients prior to treatment about potential for falling asleep during ADLs and somnolence and discontinue **Osmolex ER** if occurs. Monitor patients for depressed mood, depression, <u>and</u> suicidal ideation <u>or</u> behavior. Patients with major psychotic disorder should ordinarily <u>not</u> be treated with **Osmolex ER**; observe patients throughout treatment for the occurrence of hallucinations, especially at initiation and after dose increases. Monitor patients for dizziness and orthostatic hypotension, especially after starting **Osmolex ER** <u>or</u> increasing the dose. Avoid sudden withdrawal/discontinuation due to risk of withdrawal-emergent hyperpyrexia and confusion. Monitor patient for development of impulse control/compulsive behaviors. Ask patients about increased gambling urges, sexual urges, uncontrolled spending, <u>or</u> other urges, and consider dose reduction <u>or</u> discontinuation if any occur. Increased risk of anticholinergic effects may require reduction of **Osmolex ER** <u>or</u> dose of the anticholinergic drug(s). Excretion of *amantadine* increases with acidic urine, resulting in possible accumulation with urine change toward alkaline. Live attenuated vaccines (LAVs) are <u>not</u> recommended during treatment with **Osmolex ER**. Concomitant use of alcohol is <u>not</u> recommended due to increased potential for CNS effects. There are <u>no</u> adequate data on the developmental risk associated with use of *amantadine* in pregnant females. Animal studies suggest a potential risk for fetal harm with *amantadine*. *Amantadine* is excreted in human milk, but amounts have <u>not</u> been quantified. There is <u>no</u> information on the risk to the breastfed infant.

Symadine (G) initially 100 mg bid; may increase after 1-2 weeks by 100 mg/day; max 400 mg/day in divided doses; for extrapyramidal effects, 100 mg bid; max 300 mg/day in divided doses

    Cap: 100 mg

Symmetrel (G) initially 100 mg bid; may increase after 1-2 weeks by 100 mg/day; max 400 mg/day in divided doses; for extrapyramidal effects, 100 mg bid; max 300 mg/day in divided doses

    Cap: 100 mg; *Syr:* 50 mg/5 ml (16 oz) (raspberry)

➤ *bromocriptine* **(G)** initially 1.25 mg bid to 2.5 mg tid with meals; increase as needed every 2-4 weeks by 2.5 mg/day; max 100 mg/day

    Parlodel *Tab:* 2.5*mg; *Cap:* 5 mg

➤ *pramipexole* **(G)** initially 0.125 mg tid; increase at intervals q 5-7 days; max 1.5 mg tid

    Mirapex *Tab:* 0.125, 0.25*, 0.5*, 1*, 1.5*mg

➤ *ropinirole* initially 0.25 mg tid for the first week; then 0.5 mg tid for the second week; then 0.75 mg tid for the third week; then 1 mg tid for the fourth week; may increase by 1.5 mg/day at 1-week intervals to 9 mg/day; then increase up to 3 mg/day at 1-week intervals; max 24 mg/day

    Requip *Tab:* 0.25, 0.5, 1, 2, 4, 5 mg

➤ *rotigotine* transdermal patch apply to clean, dry, intact skin on abdomen, thigh, hip, flank, shoulder, <u>or</u> upper arm; rotate sites and allow 14 days before reusing site; if hairy, shave site at least 3 days before application to site; avoid abrupt cessation; taper by 2 mg/24 hours every other day; *Early stage:* initially 2 mg/24 hr patch once daily; may increase weekly by 2 mg/24 hours if needed; max 6 mg/24 hours once daily; *Advanced stage:* initially a 4 mg/24 hours patch once daily; may increase weekly by 2 mg/24 hours if needed; max 8 mg/24 hours once daily

    Neupro *Trans patch:* 1 mg/24 hours, 2 mg/24 hours, 3 mg/24 hours, 4 mg/24 hours, 6 mg/24 hours, 8 mg/24 hours (30/carton) (sulfites)

DOPA-DECARBOXYLASE INHIBITORS

Comment: Contraindicated in narrow-angle glaucoma. Use with caution with sympathomimetics and antihypertensive agents.

➤ *carbidopa+levodopa* **(G)** usually 400-1,600 mg *levodopa* per day

    Duopa *Ent susp:* carb 4.63 mg+levo 20 mg single-use cassettes for use w. CADD Legacy 1400 Pump

    Sinemet 10/100 initially 1 tab tid-qid; increase if needed daily <u>or</u> every other day up to qid

        Tab: carb 10 mg+levo 100 mg*

    Sinemet 25/100 initially 1 tab bid-tid; increase if needed daily <u>or</u> every other day up to qid

        Tab: carb 25 mg+levo 100 mg*

    Sinemet 25/250 1 tab tid-qid

        Tab: carb 25 mg+levo 250 mg*

    Sinemet CR 25/100 initially one 25/100 tab bid; allow 3 days between dosage adjustments

        Tab: carb 25 mg+levo 100 mg cont-rel

    Sinemet CR 50/200 initially one 50/200 tab bid; allow 3 days between dosage adjustments

        Tab: carb 50 mg+levo 200 mg cont-rel*

(continued)

DOPA-DECARBOXYLASE INHIBITOR+DOPAMINE PRECURSOR+CATECHOL-O-METHYLTRANSFERASE (COMT) INHIBITOR COMBINATION

▷ *carbidopa+levodopa+entacapone* titrate individually with separate components; then switch to corresponding strength *levodopa* and *carbidopa*; max 8 tabs/day

Tab: **Stalevo 50** carb 12.5 mg+levo 50 mg+enta 200 mg
Stalevo 75 carb 12.5 mg+levo 75 mg+enta 200 mg
Stalevo 100 carb 12.5 mg+levo 100 mg+enta 200 mg
Stalevo 125 carb 12.5 mg+levo 125 mg+enta 200 mg
Stalevo 150 carb 12.5 mg+levo 150 mg+enta 200 mg
Stalevo 200 carb 12.5 mg+levo 200 mg+enta 200 mg

MONOAMINE OXIDASE INHIBITORS (MAOIs)

▷ *rasagiline* (G) *Usual maintenance:* 0.5-1 mg/day; max 1 mg/day; initial dose for patients on concomitant *levodopa* 0.5 mg daily; initial dose for patients not on concomitant *levodopa* 1 mg daily
Azilect *Tab:* 0.5, 1 mg
Comment: Azilect is indicated as monotherapy or as adjunct to *levodopa*. With mild hepatic dysfunction (Child-Pugh 5-6), limit **Azilect** dose to 0.5 mg daily. With moderate-to-severe hepatic dysfunction (Child-Pugh 7-15), **Azilect** is not recommended. Contraindications include co-administration with *meperidine, methadone, mirtazapine, propoxyphene, tramadol, dextromethorphan, St. John's wort, cyclobenzaprine, methylphenidate, dexmethylphenidate,* or other MAOIs.

▷ *selegiline* (G) 5 mg at breakfast and at lunch; max 10 mg/day
Tab/Cap: 5 mg

▷ *selegiline* (G) 1.25 mg daily; max 2.5 mg/day
Zelapar *ODT:* 1.25 mg orally-disint (phenylalanine)

MONOAMINE OXIDASE TYPE B (MOA-B) INHIBITOR

▷ *safinamide* (G) initially 50 mg once daily at the same time each day; after 2 weeks, dose may be increased to 100 mg once daily based on individual need and tolerability; *Moderate hepatic impairment:* do not exceed 50 mg once daily; *Severe hepatic impairment:* contraindicated
Xadago *Tab:* 50, 100 mg
Comment: Xadago *(safinamide)* has not been shown to be effective as monotherapy; it is adjunctive treatment to *levodopa/carbidopa* in patients experiencing *Off* episodes. **Xadago** *drug interactions:* selective serotonin reuptake inhibitors (SSRIs) (monitor for *serotonin syndrome*); sympathomimetics (monitor for hypertension); tyramine (monitor for severe hypertension); substrates of breast cancer resistance protein [BCRP] as there us potential for increase plasma concentration of BRCP substrates). **Xadago** is contraindicated with concomitant use of other MAOIs or other drugs that are potent inhibitors of monoamine oxidase (e.g., *linezolid; isoniazid* has some monoamine oxidase-inhibiting activity), opioids and their derivatives, serotonin-norepinephrine reuptake inhibitors (SNRIs), tri- or tetracyclic or triazolopyridine antidepressants, *cyclobenzaprine, methylphenidate,* and *amphetamine* and their derivatives, *dextromethorphan,* St. John's Wort, and severe hepatic impairment (Child-Pugh Class C). The most common adverse effects (incidence ≥2%) are dyskinesia, fall, nausea, and insomnia. Other adverse side effects include falling asleep during activities of daily living (ADLs), hallucinations, psychotic behavior, compulsive and impulsive behaviors, and withdrawal-emergent hyperpyrexia and confusion. Dopaminergic antagonists (e.g., antipsychotics, *metoclopramide*) may decrease the effectiveness of **Xadago** and exacerbate symptoms of PD. There are no adequate and well-controlled human studies of **Xadago** use in pregnancy. Based on animal studies, **Xadago** may cause fetal harm. It is not known whether **Xadago** is present in human milk or effects on the breastfed infant. Mothers should be advised regarding the risk/benefit to the mother and the infant, and decide whether or not to discontinue the **Xadago** or breastfeeding.

ADENOSINE A$_{2A}$ RECEPTOR ANTAGONIST

▷ *istradefylline* 20 mg once daily; may increase to max 40 mg once daily; may take with or without food; *Moderate hepatic impairment:* max 20 mg once daily; *Severe hepatic impairment:* avoid; *Smokers (≥20 cigarettes/day or the equivalent of another tobacco product):* recommend 40 mg once daily
Nourianz *Tab:* 20, 40 mg
Comment: Nourianz *(istradefylline)* is an adenosine A$_{2A}$ receptor antagonist intended for use as adjunctive treatment to *levodopa/carbidopa* in adult patients with PD experiencing "*Off*" episodes. Recommended maximum dosage with concomitant use of strong CYP 3A4 inhibitors is 20 mg once daily. Avoid use of **Nourianz** with strong CYP 3A4 inducers. Monitor patients for dyskinesia or exacerbation of existing dyskinesia. Consider dosage reduction or stopping **Nourianz** if hallucinations or other signs/symptoms of psychosis occur, or loss of impulse control or compulsive behaviors occur. The most common adverse reactions (incidence ≥5%) have been dyskinesia, dizziness, constipation, nausea, hallucination, and insomnia. Based on data from animal studies, **Nourianz** may cause embryo/fetal harm in pregnancy. There are no data on the presence of *istradefylline* in human milk or effects on the breastfed infant.

COMT INHIBITORS
▷ *entacapone* 1 tab with each dose of *levodopa* or *carbidopa*; max 8 tabs/day
　　Comtan *Tab:* 200 mg
　　Comment: Comtan is an adjunct to *levodopa+carbidopa* in patients with end-of-dose wearing off.
▷ *opicapone* 50 mg once daily at bedtime; *Moderate hepatic impairment:* 25 mg once daily at bedtime; *Severe hepatic impairment:* avoid use; do not eat food for 1 hour before and for at least 1 hour after taking dose
　　Ongentys *Cap:* 25, 50mg
　　Comment: Ongentys *(opicapone)* is an adjunctive treatment to *levodopa/carbidopa* in patients experiencing "*Off*" episodes.
▷ *tolcapone* **(G)** 100-200 mg tid; max 600 mg/day
　　Tasmar *Tab:* 100, 200 mg
　　Comment: Monitor liver function tests (LFTs) every 2 weeks. Withdraw **Tasmar** if no substantial improvement in the first 3 weeks of treatment.

CENTRALLY ACTING ANTICHOLINERGICS
▷ *benztropine mesylate* initially 0.5-1 mg q HS, increase if needed; for extrapyramidal disorders 1-4 mg once daily-bid; max 6 mg/day
　　Cogentin *Tab:* 0.5*, 1*, 2*mg
▷ *biperiden hydrochloride* initially 1 tab tid or qid, then increase as needed; max 8 tabs/day
　　Akineton *Tab:* 2 mg
▷ *procyclidine* initially 2.5 mg tid; may increase as needed to 5 mg tid-qid every 3-5 days; max 15 mg/day
　　Kemadrin *Tab:* 5 mg
▷ *trihexyphenidyl* **(G)** initially 1 mg; increase as needed by 2 mg every 3-5 days; max 15 mg/day
　　Artane *Tab:* 2*, 5*mg

PSEUDOBULBAR AFFECT (PBA)
Comment: Pseudobulbar affect (PBA), emotional lability, labile affect, or emotional incontinence refers to a neurologic disorder characterized by involuntary crying or uncontrollable episodes of crying and/or laughing, or other emotional outbursts. PBA occurs secondary to a neurologic disease or brain injury, such as traumatic brain injury (TBI), stroke, Parkinson's disease (PD), multiple sclerosis, and amyotrophic lateral sclerosis (ALS, or Lou Gehrig's disease).
▷ *dextromethorphan+quinidine* **(G)** 1 cap once daily x 7 days; then starting on day 8, 1 cap bid
　Pediatric: <12 years: not recommended; ≥12 years: same as adult
　　Nuedexta *Cap:* dextro 20 mg+quini 10 mg
　　Comment: *Dextromethorphan hydrobromide* is an uncompetitive N-methyl D-aspartate (NMDA) receptor antagonist and sigma-1 agonist. *Quinidine sulfate* is a CYP450 2D6 inhibitor. **Nuedexta** is contraindicated with an MAOI or within 14 days of stopping an MAOI, with prolonged QT interval, congenital long QT syndrome, history suggestive of torsades de pointes, or heart failure, complete atrioventricular (AV) block without implanted pacemaker or patients at high risk of complete AV block, and concomitant drugs that both prolong QT interval and are metabolized by CYP2D6 (e.g., *thioridazine* or *pimozide*). Discontinue **Nuedexta** if the following occurs: hepatitis or thrombocytopenia or any other hypersensitivity reaction. Monitor ECG in patients with left ventricular hypertrophy (LVH) or left ventricular dysfunction (LVD). *Desipramine* exposure increases **Nuedexta** 8-fold; reduce *desipramine* dose and adjust based on clinical response. Use of **Nuedexta** with SSRIs or tricyclic antidepressants (TCAs) increases the risk of *serotonin syndrome*. *Paroxetine* exposure increases **Nuedexta** 2-fold; therefore, reduce *paroxetine* dose and adjust based on clinical response (*digoxin* exposure may increase *digoxin* substrate plasma concentration). **Nuedexta** is not recommended in pregnancy or breastfeeding. Safety and effectiveness of **Nuedexta** in children have not been established.

PARKINSON'S PSYCHOSIS
Atypical Antipsychotic
▷ *pimavanserin* take 34 mg once daily with or without food; no titration needed
　　Nuplazid *Tab:* 10 (2 x 17 mg tabs); *Cap:* 34 mg
　　Comment: Nuplazid *(pimavanserin)* is an atypical antipsychotic indicated for the treatment of hallucinations and delusions associated with (PD) psychosis. **Nuplazid** is not indicated for dementia-related psychosis unrelated to PD as elderly patients with dementia-related psychosis treated with antipsychotic drugs are at increased risk of death. There is risk of QT interval prolongation with **Nuplazid**; therefore, avoid use in patients with risk factors for prolonged QT interval and concomitant use of other drugs that also increase the QT interval. **Nuplazid** does not affect motor function. Reduce **Nuplazid** dose by one-half with strong CYP3A4 inhibitors (e.g., *ketoconazole*). Strong CYP3A4 inducers may reduce efficacy of **Nuplazid**; increase in **Nuplazid** dosage may be needed. No **Nuplazid** dose adjustment is needed in patients with mild-to-moderate renal impairment. **Nuplazid** is not recommended for use in patients with severe renal impairment or hepatic impairment. There are no data on **Nuplazid** use in pregnancy that would allow assessment of the drug-associated risk of major congenital malformations or miscarriage, presence of *pimavanserin* in human milk, or effects on the breastfed infant. The most common adverse reactions (incidence ≥5%) are peripheral edema and confusional state.

PARKINSONISM; PARKINSONISM FOLLOWING CARBON MONOXIDE INTOXICATION; PARKINSONISM FOLLOWING MANGANESE INTOXICATION; PARKINSONISM: POST-ENCEPHALITIC

DOPA-DECARBOXYLASE INHIBITORS

Comment: This drug class is contraindicated in narrow-angle glaucoma and non-selective MAOIs. Use with caution with sympathomimetics and antihypertensive agents. The most common adverse reactions reported with *carbidopa/levodopa* tablets have included dyskinesias, such as choreiform, dystonic, and other involuntary movements, and nausea. Warnings and Precautions: (1) May cause falling asleep during activities of daily living; (2) Avoid sudden discontinuation or rapid dose reduction to reduce the risk of withdrawal-emergent hyperpyrexia and confusion; (3) Monitor patients with a history of cardiovascular disease for potential cardiovascular ischemic events; (4) Hallucinations/Psychosis may occur; (5) Consider dose reduction or discontinuation if disordered impulse control occurs; (6) May cause or exacerbate dyskinesia—consider dose reduction.

▷ *carbidopa+levodopa*
   Dhivy initially 1 tab tid; may increase dose by up to one whole tablet every day or every other day, as needed, until max total daily dose is 8 whole tabs (i.e., total 50 mg/200 mg/day)
      Tab: carb 25 mg+levo 100 mg*** (each tablet has 3 functional scores with each of the four segments containing 6.25 mg of *carbidopa* and 25 mg of *levodopa*)
   Comment: *Dhivy* is a fixed combination of *carbidopa* (an aromatic amino acid decarboxylation inhibitor) and *levodopa* (an aromatic amino acid) indicated for the treatment of Parkinson's disease, post-encephalitic parkinsonism, and symptomatic parkinsonism that may follow carbon monoxide intoxication or manganese intoxication.

PARONYCHIA (PERIUNGUAL ABSCESS)

▷ *cephalexin* (**G**) 500 mg bid x 10 days
   Pediatric: 25-50 mg/day in 2 divided doses x 10 days
      Keflex *Cap:* 250, 333, 500, 750 mg; *Oral susp:* 125, 250 mg/5 ml (100, 200 ml) (strawberry)
▷ *clindamycin* (**G**) 150-300 mg q 6 hours x 10 days
   Pediatric: 8-16 mg/kg/day in 3-4 divided doses x 10 days
      Cleocin *Cap:* 75 (tartrazine), 150 (tartrazine), 300 mg
      Cleocin Pediatric Granules *Oral susp:* 75 mg/5 ml (100 ml) (cherry)
▷ *dicloxacillin* (**G**) 500 mg q 6 hours x 10 days
   Pediatric: 12.5-25 mg/kg/day in 4 divided doses x 10 days; *see* Appendix BB.18. *dicloxacillin* (**G**) (Dynapen Suspension) *for dose by weight*
      Dynapen *Cap:* 125, 250, 500 mg; *Oral susp:* 62.5 mg/5 ml (80, 100, 200 ml)
▷ *erythromycin base* (**G**) 500 mg q 6 hours x 10 days
   Pediatric: <45 kg: 30-50 mg in 2-4 doses x 10 days; ≥45 kg: same as adult
      Ery-Tab *Tab:* 250, 333, 500 mg ent-coat
      PCE *Tab:* 333, 500 mg
▷ *erythromycin ethylsuccinate* (**G**) 400 mg q 6 hours x 10 days
   Pediatric: 30-50 mg/kg/day in 4 divided doses q 6 hours x 10 days; may double dose with severe infection; max 100 mg/kg/day; *see* Appendix BB.21. *erythromycin ethylsuccinate* (**G**) (E.E.S. Supension, EryPed Drops/ Suspension) *for dose by weight*
      EryPed *Oral susp:* 200 mg/5 ml (100, 200 ml) (fruit), 400 mg/5 ml (60, 100, 200 ml) (banana); *Oral drops:* 200, 400 mg/5 ml (50 ml) (fruit); *Chew tab:* 200 mg wafer (fruit)
      E.E.S. *Oral susp:* 200, 400 mg/5 ml (100 ml) (fruit)
      E.E.S. Granules *Oral susp:* 200 mg/5 ml (100, 200 ml) (cherry)
      E.E.S. 400 Tablets *Tab:* 400 mg

PAROXYSMAL NOCTURNAL HEMOGLOBINURIA (PNH)

COMPLEMENT INHIBITOR

▷ *eculizumab* dilute to a final admixture concentration of 5 mg/ml using the following steps: (1) withdraw the required amount of **Soliris** from the vial into a sterile syringe; (2) transfer the dose to an infusion bag; (3) add IV fluid equal to the drug volume (0.9% NaCl or 0.45% NaCl or D5W or Ringer's lactate); the final admixed **Soliris** 5 mg/ml infusion volume is 300 mg dose (60 ml), 600 mg dose (120 ml), 900 mg dose (180 ml), and 1,200 mg dose (240 ml)
   Pediatric: <18 years: safety and efficacy not established
      Soliris *Vial:* 300 mg (10 mg/ml, 30 ml), single-use, concentrated solution for IV infusion (preservative-free)

Comment: Soliris *(eculizumab)* is a complement inhibitor indicated for the treatment of patients with paroxysmal nocturnal hemoglobinuria (PNH) to reduce hemolysis, patients with atypical hemolytic uremia syndrome (aHUS) to inhibit complement-mediated thrombotic microangiopathy (TMA), and adult patients with generalized myasthenia gravis (gMG) who are anti-acetylcholine receptor (AchR) antibody-positive. **Soliris** *(eculizumab)* should be administered at the above recommended dosage regimen time points or within 2 days of each time point. Supplemental dosing of **Soliris** is required in the setting of concomitant support with plasmapheresis (PI) or plasma exchange (PE) or fresh frozen plasma (FFP) infusion. See mfr pkg insert for supplemental dosing. **Soliris** is not indicated for the treatment of patients with Shiga toxin *Escherichia coli*-related hemolytic uremic syndrome (STEC-HUS). **Soliris** is contraindicated in patients with unresolved *Neisseria meningitides* infection and patients who are not currently vaccinated against *N. meningitides,* unless the risks of delaying **Soliris** treatment outweigh the risks of developing meningococcal infection. Prescribers must enroll in the **Soliris** Risk Evaluation and Mitigation Strategy (REMS) Program (1-888-SOLIRIS, 1-888-765-4747), counsel patients about the risk of meningococcal infection, provide patients with **Soliris** REMS educational materials, and ensure that patients are vaccinated with a meningococcal vaccine. The most frequently reported adverse reactions in the PNH randomized trial (incidence ≥10%) are headache, nasopharyngitis, back pain, and nausea. The most frequently reported adverse reactions in aHUS single-arm prospective trials (incidence ≥15%) are hypertension, upper respiratory infection (URI), diarrhea, headache, anemia, vomiting, nausea, urinary tract infection (UTI), and leukopenia. There are no adequate and well-controlled human studies of **Soliris** in pregnancy or effects on the breastfed infant. Based on animal studies, **Soliris** may cause fetal harm. It is not known whether **Soliris** is excreted in human milk. Immunoglobulin G (IgG) is excreted in human milk so it is expected that **Soliris** will be present in human milk. However, published data suggest that antibodies in human milk do not enter the neonatal and infant circulation in substantial amounts. Caution should be exercised when **Soliris** is administered to the breastfeeding patient.

▶ *pegcetacoplan* administer 1,080 mg via SC infusion twice weekly using a commercially available infusion pump; see mfr pkg insert for instructions on preparation and administration
Pediatric: safety and efficacy not established

Empaveli *Vial:* 1,080 mg/20 ml (54 mg/ml), single-dose

Comment: Empaveli is available only through the restricted **Empaveli** REMS Program. Prescribers must enroll in the program. The most common adverse reactions in patients with PNH (incidence ≥10%) have been injection site reactions, infections, diarrhea, abdominal pain, respiratory tract infection, viral infection, and fatigue. **Empaveli** is contraindicated in (1) patients with hypersensitivity to *pegcetacoplan* or any of the excipients; (2) patients who are not currently vaccinated against certain encapsulated bacteria unless the risks of delaying **Empaveli** treatment outweigh the risks of developing a serious bacterial infection with an encapsulated organism; and (3) patients with unresolved serious infection caused by encapsulated bacteria. Use caution when administering **Empaveli** to patients with serious infections caused by encapsulated bacteria. *Boxed Warning:* Meningococcal infections may occur in patients treated with **Empaveli** and may become rapidly life-threatening or fatal if not recognized and treated early. Use of **Empaveli** may predispose individuals to serious infections, especially those caused by encapsulated bacteria, such as *Streptococcus pneumoniae, N. meningitidis, types A, C, W, Y, and B,* and *Haemophilus influenzae, type B.* Comply with the most current Advisory Committee on Immunization Practices (ACIP) recommendations for vaccinations against encapsulated bacteria. Vaccinate patients against encapsulated bacteria as recommended at least 2 weeks prior to administering the first dose of **Empaveli** unless the risks of delaying **Empaveli** therapy outweigh the risks of developing a serious infection. See the mfr pkg insert for additional guidance on managing the risk of serious infections. Vaccination reduces, but does not eliminate, the risk of serious infections. Monitor patients for early signs of serious infections and evaluate immediately if infection is suspected. Monitor patients for infusion-related reactions and institute appropriate medical management as needed. Use of silica reagents in coagulation panels may result in artificially prolonged activated partial thromboplastin time (aPTT). The use of **Empaveli** may be considered following a risk/benefit assessment. Clinical considerations include disease-associated maternal risk/benefit and embryo/fetal/neonatal risks. There are insufficient data on **Empaveli** use in pregnant females to inform a drug-associated risk of major birth defects, miscarriage, or adverse maternal or fetal outcomes, and there are risks to the mother and the fetus associated with untreated PNH in pregnancy. In animal studies, treatment of pregnant cynomolgus monkeys with *pegcetacoplan* at SC dose of 28 mg/kg/day (2.9 times human exposure based on area under the curve [AUC]) from the gestation period through parturition resulted in a statistically significant increase in abortions or stillbirths compared to controls. PNH in pregnancy is associated with adverse maternal outcomes, including worsening cytopenias, thrombotic events, infections, bleeding, miscarriages, and increased maternal mortality, as well as adverse fetal outcomes, including premature delivery and fetal death. Because it is not known whether *pegcetacoplan* is secreted in human milk or whether there is potential for absorption and harm to the infant, breastfeeding should be discontinued during treatment and for 40 days after the last dose.

(continued)

➤ *ravulizumab-cwvz* withdraw the calculated volume of **Ultomiris** from the appropriate number of vials (according to the weight-based reference table) and dilute in an infusion bag using 0.9% NS to a final concentration of 5 mg/ml; administer all doses via IV infusion only; starting 2 weeks after administration of the loading dose, begin maintenance doses at once every 8-week intervals; the dosing schedule is allowed to occasionally vary within 7 days of the scheduled infusion day (except for the first maintenance dose of **Ultomiris**) but the subsequent dose should be administered according to the original schedule; for patients switching from *eculizumab* (Soliris) to **Ultomiris**, administer the loading dose of **Ultomiris** 2 weeks after the last *eculizumab* (Soliris) infusion, and then administer maintenance doses once every 8 weeks, starting 2 weeks after loading dose administration; dilute the appropriate number of vials to a final concentration of 5 mg/ml prior to administration

Weight-Based Dosing Regimen		
	Loading	Maintenance
≥40-<60 mg/kg	2,400 mg	3,000 mg
≥60-<100 mg/kg	2,700 mg	3,300 mg
≥100 mg/kg	3,000 mg	3,600 mg

Pediatric: <18 years: not recommended; ≥18 years: same as adult

Ultomiris *Vial:* 300 mg/30 ml (10 mg/ml) in a single-dose

Comment: Ultomiris *(ravulizumab-cwvz)* is a long-acting C5 complement inhibitor for the treatment of paroxysmal nocturnal hemoglobinuria (PNH). Vaccinate patients for meningococcal disease according to current ACIP guidelines to reduce the risk of serious infection. Provide 2 weeks of antibacterial drug prophylaxis to patients if **Ultomiris** must be initiated immediately and vaccines are administered less than 2 weeks before starting **Ultomiris** therapy. There are no available data on **Ultomiris** use in pregnant females to inform a drug-associated risk of major birth defects, miscarriage, or adverse maternal or fetal outcomes (PNH in pregnancy is associated with adverse maternal outcomes, including worsening cytopenias, thrombotic events, infections, bleeding, miscarriages, and increased maternal mortality, and adverse fetal outcomes, including fetal death and premature delivery). There are no data on the presence of *ravulizumab-cwvz* in human milk or effect on the breastfed infant. However, breastfeeding should be discontinued during treatment and for 8 months after the final dose. Healthcare professionals who prescribe **Ultomiris** must enroll in the **Ultomiris REMS** program by telephone at 1-888-765-4747 or by www.ultomirisrems.com.

PEANUT (ARACHIS HYPOGAEA) ALLERGY

ORAL IMMUNOTHERAPY

➤ *arachis hypogaea allergen powder-dnfp* open capsule(s) or sachet and empty the entire dose onto refrigerated or room temperature semi solid food; mix well; consume the entire volume; do not swallow capsule(s); do not inhale powder

Initial dose escalation, Day 1: the first 5 doses, and all new dose escalations, must be administered by a qualified healthcare provider, on a single day, under continuous observation by qualified healthcare staff, in an appropriate healthcare setting, with epinephrine and other emergency support readily available to treat anaphylaxis

Up-dosing phase (begins on day 2): 11 up-dosing levels starting with *Level 1* (3 mg) and finishing with *Level 11* (300 mg); see mfr pkg insert for level dosing regimen; remain at each dose level for a period of at least 2 weeks; a dose level cannot be skipped

Maintenance therapy: 300 mg/day; all doses must be taken daily, at the same time each day, to maintain treatment effect; patients must be co-prescribed injectable epinephrine for home use, provided with instruction and training on appropriate use, and instruction to seek immediate medical care upon its use

Pediatric: <4 years: not established; ≥4 years: same as adult

Palforzia *Cap:* 0.5 ,1, 10, 20, 100 mg; *Sachet:* 300 mg

Comment: Palforzia is an oral immunotherapy indicated to help reduce the severity of allergic reactions, including anaphylaxis, that may occur with accidental exposure to peanut. **Palforzia** does not treat allergic reactions and should not be taken during an allergic reaction. Patients must maintain a strict peanut-free diet while taking **Palforzia**. The first dose, and all dose increases, must be administered in a healthcare setting under the observation of trained healthcare staff for at least 1 hour. The most common adverse reactions reported in subjects treated with **Palforzia** (incidence ≥5%) have been abdominal pain, vomiting, nausea, oral pruritus, oral paresthesia, throat irritation, cough, rhinorrhea, sneezing, throat tightness, wheezing, dyspnea, pruritus, urticaria, anaphylactic reaction, and ear pruritus. Patients should be advised to stop taking **Palforzia** and seek emergency medical treatment right away if they have any of the following symptoms after taking **Palforzia**: trouble breathing or wheezing, chest discomfort or tightness, throat tightness, difficulty swallowing or speaking, swelling of the face, lips, eyes, or tongue, dizziness or fainting, severe stomach cramps or pain, vomiting, or diarrhea, hives, and severe flushing of the skin. Contraindications to **Palforzia** are uncontrolled asthma, history of eosinophilic esophagitis (EoE) or other eosinophilic gastrointestinal disease. No human or animal data are available to establish the presence or absence of the risks due to **Palforzia** in pregnancy. Anaphylaxis can cause a dangerous decrease in blood pressure, which could result in compromised placental perfusion and significant risk to the fetus. There is a pregnancy exposure registry that monitors pregnancy outcomes in women exposed to **Palforzia** during pregnancy. Women exposed to **Palforzia** during pregnancy or their healthcare professionals are encouraged to contact Aimmune by calling 1-833-246-2566. There are no data available on the presence of **Palforzia** in human milk or effects on the breastfed infant. The developmental and health benefits of breastfeeding should be considered, along with the mother's clinical need for **Palforzia** and any other potential adverse effects on the breastfed infant from **Palforzia** or from the underlying maternal condition. **Palforzia** is available only through a restricted program under a Risk Evaluation and Mitigation Strategy (REMS) called the Palforzia REMS. **Palforzia** is only dispensed and distributed to certified healthcare settings and only administered to patients in certified healthcare settings.

PEDICULOSIS HUMANUS CAPITIS (HEAD LICE), PEDICULOSIS PHTHIRUS (PUBIC LICE)

▶ *abametapir* shake well before use; apply to dry hair in an amount sufficient (up to the full content of one bottle) to thoroughly coat the hair and scalp; avoid contact with eyes; massage into scalp and throughout the hair; leave on the hair and scalp for 10 minutes and then rinse off with warm water
Pediatric: <6 months: not established; ≥6 months: same as adult
   Xeglyze Lotion *Lotn:* 0.74% (approx 7 oz or 210 ml), single-use, amber glass bottle
   Comment: **Xeglyze** is a pediculicide indicated for the topical treatment of head lice infestation. Systemic exposure to benzyl alcohol has been associated with serious adverse reactions and death in neonates and low birthweight infants. **Xeglyze** use is not recommended in pediatric patients under <6 months of age because of the potential for increased systemic absorption. Direct supervision of children by an adult is required due to the risk of accidental ingestion. Treatment involves a single application. Discard any unused product. Do not flush contents down the sink or toilet. The most common adverse reactions (incidence of ≥1%) have been erythema, rash, skin burning sensation, contact dermatitis, vomiting, eye irritation, pruritus, and hair color changes. Other than age, there are no contraindications to **Xeglyze** use. For 2 weeks after a **Xeglyze** application, avoid taking drugs that are substrates of CYP3A4, CYP2B6, or CYP1A2. There are no available data on **Xeglyze** use in pregnancy to evaluate for a drug-associated risk of major birth defects, miscarriage, or adverse maternal or fetal outcomes. In animal embryo/fetal development studies conducted with oral administration of *abametapir* during organogenesis, there was no evidence of fetal harm or malformations. No data are available regarding the presence of *abametapir* in human milk or effects on the breastfed infant.
▶ *ivermectin* (G) thoroughly wet hair; leave on for 10 minutes; then rinse off with water; do not re-treat
Pediatric: <6 months, <33 lb: not recommended; ≥6 months, ≥33 lb: same as adult
   Sklice *Lotn:* 0.5% (4 oz, 117 gm, laminate tube)
▶ *lindane* (G) apply, leave on for 4 minutes, then thoroughly wash off
Pediatric: <2 years: not recommended; ≥2 years: same as adult
   Kwell Shampoo *Shampoo:* 1% (60 ml)
▶ *malathion* (G) thoroughly wet hair; allow to dry naturally; shampoo and rinse after 8-12 hours; use a fine-tooth comb to remove lice and nits; if lice persist after 7-9 days, may repeat treatment
Pediatric: same as adult
   Ovide (OTC) *Lotn:* 59% (2 oz)
▶ *permethrin* (G) apply to washed and towel-dried hair; allow to remain on for 10 minutes, then rinse off; repeat after 7 days if needed
Pediatric: <2 months: not recommended; ≥2 months: same as adult
   Nix (OTC) *Crm rinse:* 1% (2 oz w. comb)
▶ *pyrethrins with piperonyl butoxide* (G) apply and leave on for 10 minutes, then wash off
   A-200 *Shampoo:* pyr 0.33%+pip but 3%
   Rid Mousse *Shampoo:* pyr 0.33%+pip but 4%
   Rid Shampoo *Shampoo:* pyr 0.33%+pip but 3%
   Comment: To remove nits, soak hair in equal parts of white vinegar and water for 15-20 minutes.
▶ *spinosad* shake bottle well; apply a sufficient amount to cover dry scalp, then apply to dry hair; rinse off with warm water after 10 minutes; repeat treatment only if live lice are seen 7 days after the first treatment
Pediatric: <6 months: safety and efficacy not established; >6 months: same as adult
   Natroba *Topical susp:* 0.9% (9 mg/gm; 120ml)
   Comment: **Natroba** is a pediculicide/scabicide indicated for the topical treatment of head lice infestation in patients ≥6 months and scabies infestation in patients ≥4 years. The most common adverse reactions (incidence >1%) have been application site erythema and ocular erythema. *Spinosad*, the active ingredient in **Natroba**, is not absorbed systemically following topical application, and maternal use is not expected to result in embryo/fetal exposure to the drug. **Natroba** contains benzyl alcohol. Topical benzyl alcohol is unlikely to be absorbed through the skin in clinically relevant amounts; therefore, maternal use is not expected to result in embryo/fetal exposure to the drug. Breastfeeding is not expected to result in the exposure of the infant to *spinosad*.

PELVIC INFLAMMATORY DISEASE (PID)

Comment: The following treatment regimens are published in the **2021 CDC Sexually Transmitted Diseases Treatment Guidelines.** Treatment regimens are presented by generic drug name first, followed by information about brands and dose forms. Treat all sexual partners. Because of the high risk for maternal morbidity and preterm delivery, pregnant females who have suspected pelvic inflammatory disease (PID) should be hospitalized and treated with parenteral antibiotics. HIV-infected women with PID respond equally well to standard parenteral and antibiotic regimens as HIV-negative females.

OUTPATIENT REGIMENS
Regimen 1
➤ *ceftriaxone* 250 mg IM in a single dose plus *doxycycline*
➤ *doxycycline* 100 mg bid x 14 days with or without *metronidazole*
➤ *metronidazole* 500 mg PO bid x 14 days

Regimen 2
➤ *cefoxitin* 2 gm IM in a single dose plus *probenecid*
➤ *probenecid* 1 gm PO in a single dose administered concurrently plus *doxycycline* 100 mg bid x 14 days with or without *metronidazole*
➤ *metronidazole* 500 mg PO bid x 14 days

Regimen 3
➤ Other parenteral third-generation cephalosporin (e.g., *ceftizoxime* or *cefotaxime*) in a single dose plus *doxycycline*
➤ *doxycycline* 100 mg bid x 14 days with or without *metronidazole*
➤ *metronidazole* 500 mg PO bid x 14 days

DRUG BRANDS AND DOSE FORMS
➤ *cefoxitin* (G)
　　Mefoxin *Vial:* 1, 2 g
➤ *ceftriaxone* (G)
　　Rocephin *Vial:* 250, 500 mg; 1, 2 gm
➤ *doxycycline* (G)
　　Acticlate *Tab:* 75, 150**mg
　　Adoxa *Tab:* 50, 75, 100, 150 mg ent-coat
　　Doryx *Tab:* 50, 75, 100, 150, 200 mg del-rel
　　Doxteric *Tab:* 50 mg del-rel
　　Monodox *Cap:* 50, 75, 100 mg
　　Oracea *Cap:* 40 mg del-rel
　　Vibramycin *Tab:* 100 mg; *Cap:* 50, 100 mg; *Syr:* 50 mg/5 ml (raspberry-apple) (sulfites); *Oral susp:* 25 mg/5 ml (raspberry)
　　Vibra-Tab *Tab:* 100 mg film-coat
➤ *metronidazole* (G)
　　Flagyl *Tab:* 250*, 500*mg
　　Flagyl 375 *Cap:* 375 mg
　　Flagyl ER *Tab:* 750 mg ext-rel
➤ *probenecid* (G)
　　Benemid *Tab:* 500*mg; *Cap:* 500 mg

PEMPHIGUS VULGARIS (PV), PEMPHIGUS FOLIACEUS (PF)

Comment: Pemphigus is a rare bullous autoimmune disorder that has no cure and is fatal if left untreated. It is characterized by autoantibody-mediated blistering of the skin (primarily affecting the chest and back; usually sparing the palms and soles of the feet) and oral mucosa. There are two histologic subtypes. Pemphigus vulgaris (PV), accounting for 70% of pemphigus cases, affects the mid-to-deep layers of the epidermis. The hallmark of PV is involvement of the oral mucosa. Pemphigus foliaceus (PF) affects the superficial skin layers and does not affect the oral mucosa. Systemic administration of corticosteroids is the standard first-line treatment to suppress the immune response. Adjuvant non-steroidal immunosuppressants may be used (e.g., *azathioprine, cyclophosphamide, mycophenolate mofetil* [MMF], *dapsone*).

GLUCOCORTICOSTEROID
➤ *prednisone* 1.0-1.5 mg/kg (oral or parenteral) daily with slow tapering and discontinuation after lesions have resolved

MYCOPHENOLIC ACID
➤ *azathioprine* 1 mg/kg/day in a single or divided doses; may increase by 0.5 mg/kg/day q 4 weeks; max 2.5 mg/kg/day; minimum trial to ascertain effectiveness is 12 weeks; administer IV doses over no less than 2 hours

Pediatric: <12 years: <u>not</u> recommended; >12 years: same as adult
    Azasan *Tab* 75*, 100*mg
    Imuran *Tab* 50*mg

▷ *cyclophosphamide* **(G)** *Oral:* Usually 1 mg per kg per day to 5 mg per kg per day for both initial and maintenance dosing the IV form has been discontinued
    Cytoxan *Tab:* 25, 50 mg;

SULFONE

▷ *dapsone* topical **(G)** apply to affected area bid
Pediatric: <12 years: <u>not</u> recommended; ≥12 years: same as adult
    Aczone *Gel:* 5, 7.5% (30, 60, 90 gm pump)

CD20-DIRECTED CYTOLYTIC MONOCLONAL ANTIBODY

▷ *rituximab* *Month* 0: 1,000 mg x 2 IV infusions separated by 2 weeks in combination with a tapering course of glucocorticoids; then a 500 mg IV infusion at *Month* 12 and every 6 months thereafter <u>or</u> based on clinical evaluation; *Relapse:* 1,000 mg IV infusion with considerations to resume <u>or</u> increase the glucocorticoid dose based on clinical evaluation; subsequent infusions may be no sooner than 16 weeks after the previous infusion; methylprednisolone 100 mg IV <u>or</u> equivalent glucocorticoid recommended 30 minutes prior to each infusion
Pediatric: <6 years: <u>not</u> recommended; ≥6 years: same as adult
    Rituxan *Vial:* 100 mg/10 ml (10 mg/ml), 500 mg/50 ml (10 mg/ml), single-use (preservative-free)
    Comment: Rituxan *(rituximab)* is a CD20-targeting cytolytic monoclonal antibody that received FDA Breakthrough Therapy Designation for treatment of PV in 2017. Safety and efficacy in recalcitrant PV have been demonstrated in approximately 500 patients across several small trials and case studies, with clinical remission occurring within six weeks in up to 95% of cases. In a recent phase 2 trial comparing *rituximab* <u>plus</u> *prednisone* with *prednisone* alone in patients with newly diagnosed PV, a 55% increase in 2-year remission rate (89% vs 34%) was observed in those receiving *rituximab* <u>plus</u> *prednisone*. Consider intravenous immunoglobulin (IVIG).

INTERLEUKIN-6 (IL-6) RECEPTOR ANTAGONIST

▷ *tocilizumab* *<100 kg:* 162 mg SC every other week on the same day followed by an increase according to clinical response; *≥100 kg:* 162 mg SC once weekly on the same day; SC injections may be self-administered after being trained and supervised by a qualified healthcare provider
    Actemra *Vial:* 80 mg/4 ml, 200 mg/10 ml, 400 mg/20 ml, single-use, for IV infusion after dilution; *Prefilled syringe:* 162 mg (0.9 ml, single-dose); *Prefilled ACTPen autoinjector:* 162 mg/0.9 ml, single-dose, for SC administration
    Comment: Actemra *(tocilizumab)* has received FDA Orphan Drug Designation in PV and is currently being investigated in a phase 2 trial. It is indicated for active recalcitrant PV that has failed 2 lines of prior treatment comprising *prednisone, mycophenolate mofetil (MMF),* and IV immunoglobulin (IVIG).

B-LYMPHOCYTE STIMULATOR (BLYS)-SPECIFIC INHIBITOR

▷ *belimumab* *SC administration:* 200 mg SC once weekly; may be self-administered by the patient in the home setting; *IV infusion:* 10 mg/kg at 2-week intervals by a qualified healthcare provider
Pediatric: <5 years: <u>not</u> established; ≥5 years: same as adult
    Benlysta *Prefilled syringe:* 200 mg/ml (1 ml), single-dose (4/carton); *Autoinjector:* 200 mg (1 ml), single-dose (4/carton); *Vial:* 120 mg/5 ml, 400 mg/20 ml, single-dose, pwdr for reconstitution and IV infusion (4/carton)
    Comment: Benlysta *(belimumab)* is an immunoglobulin G1 (IgG1)-lambda monoclonal antibody that prevents the survival of B-lymphocytes by blocking the binding of soluble human B-lymphocyte stimulator protein (BLyS) to receptors on B-lymphocytes. This reduces the activity of B-cell-mediated immunity and the autoimmune response. Benlysta was initially approved as an IV formulation administered in a hospital <u>or</u> clinic setting as a weight-dosed IV infusion every 4 weeks. Patients can now self-administer **Benlysta** as a once-weekly SC injection after being trained and supervised by a qualified healthcare provider.

PEPTIC ULCER DISEASE (PUD)

Helicobacter pylori Eradication Regimens *see Helicobacter Pylori (H. Pylori)* Infection
Antacids *see* Gastroesophageal Reflux Disease (GERD)

H2 ANTAGONISTS

▷ *cimetidine* **(G)**
Pediatric: <16 years: <u>not</u> recommended; ≥16 years: same as adult
    Tagamet 800 mg bid <u>or</u> 400 mg qid; max 2.4 gm/day
    Tab: 300, 400*, 800*mg

(continued)

Tagamet HB (OTC) *Prophylaxis:* 1 tab ac; *Treatment:* 1 tab bid
    Tab: 200 mg
Tagamet HB Oral Suspension (OTC) *Prophylaxis:* 1 tsp ac; *Treatment:* 1 tsp bid
    Oral susp: 200 mg/20 ml (12 oz)
Tagamet Liquid *Liq:* 300 mg/5 ml (mint-peach) (alcohol 2.8%)

➤ *famotidine* **(G)** 20 mg bid or 40 mg q HS; max 6 weeks
  Pediatric: 0.5 mg/kg/day q HS or in 2 divided doses; max 40 mg/day
    Pepcid *Tab:* 20, 40 mg; *Oral susp:* 40 mg/5 ml (50 ml)
    Pepcid AC (OTC) 1 tab ac; max 2 doses/day
      Tab/Rapid dissolv tab: 10 mg
    Pepcid Complete (OTC) 1 tab ac; max 2 doses/day
      Tab: fam 10 mg+CaCO2 800 mg+mag hydrox 165 mg
    Pepcid RPD
      Tab: 20, 40 mg rapid-dissolv

➤ *nizatidine* **(G)** 150 mg bid; max 12 weeks
  Pediatric: <12 years: <u>not</u> recommended; ≥12 years: same as adult
    Axid *Cap:* 150, 300 mg
    Axid AR (OTC) 1 tab ac; max 150 mg/day
      Tab: 75 mg

➤ *ranitidine* **(G)**
  Pediatric: <1 month: <u>not</u> recommended; 1 month-16 years: 2-4 mg/kg/day in 2 divided doses, max 300 mg/
  day; *Duodenal/gastric ulcer:* 2-4 mg/kg/day divided bid, max 300 mg/day; *Erosive esophagitis:* 5-10 mg/kg/
  day divided bid; max 300 mg/day; >16 years: same as adult
    Zantac 150 mg bid or 300 mg q HS
      Tab: 150, 300 mg
    Zantac 75 (OTC) 1 tab ac
      Tab: 75 mg
    Zantac EFFERdose dissolve 25 mg tab in 5 ml water; dissolve 150 mg tab in 6-8 oz water
      Efferdose: 25, 150 mg effervescent (phenylalanine)
    Zantac Syrup *Syr:* 15 mg/ml (peppermint) (alcohol 7.5%)

➤ *ranitidine bismuth citrate* 400 mg bid
  Pediatric: <12 years: <u>not</u> recommended; ≥12 years: same as adult
    Tritec *Tab:* 400 mg

PROTON PUMP INHIBITORS (PPIs)

Comment: If hepatic impairment, or if patient is Asian, consider reducing the proton pump inhibitor (PPI) dosage. Research has demonstrated associations between PPI use and fractures of the hip, wrist, and spine, hypomagnesemia, kidney injuries and chronic kidney disease, possible cardiovascular drug interactions, and infections (e.g., *Clostridioides difficile* and pneumonia). Reducing the acidity of the stomach allows bacteria to thrive and spread to other organs like the lungs and intestines. This risk is increased with high dose and chronic use and greatest in the elderly. The most recent class-wide FDA warning cites reports of cutaneous and systemic lupus erythematosus (CLS/SLE) associated with PPIs in patients with both new onset and exacerbation of existing autoimmune disease. PPI treatment should be discontinued and the patient should be referred to a specialist (http://www.fda.gov/Drugs/DrugSafety/InformationbyDrugClass/ucm213259.htm).

➤ *dexlansoprazole* **(G)** 30-60 mg daily for up to 4 weeks
  Pediatric: <18 years: <u>not</u> recommended; ≥18 years: same as adult
    Dexilant *Cap:* 30, 60 mg ent-coat, del-rel granules; may open and sprinkle on applesauce; do <u>not</u> crush
    or chew granules
    Dexilant SoluTab *Tab:* 30 mg del-rel, orally-disint

➤ *esomeprazole* **(OTC)(G)** 20-40 mg daily; max 8 weeks; take 1 hour before food; swallow whole or mix granules with food or juice and take immediately; do <u>not</u> crush or chew granules
  Pediatric: <1 year: <u>not</u> recommended; 1-11 years, <20 kg: 10 mg; ≥20 kg: 10-20 mg once daily; 12-17 years: 20-40 mg once daily; max 8 weeks; >17 years: same as adult
    Nexium *Cap:* 20, 40 mg ent-coat, del-rel pellets
    Nexium for Oral Suspension *Oral susp:* 10, 20, 40 mg ent-coat, del-rel granules/pkt (30 pkt/carton); mix
    in 2 tbsp water and drink immediately

➤ *lansoprazole* **(OTC)(G)** 15-30 mg daily for up to 8 weeks; may repeat course; take before eating
  Pediatric: <1 year: <u>not</u> recommended; 1-11 years, <30 kg: 15 mg once daily; ≥12 years: same as adult
    Prevacid *Cap:* 15, 30 mg ent-coat, del-rel granules; swallow whole or mix granules with food or juice and
    take immediately; do <u>not</u> crush or chew granules; follow with water
    Prevacid for Oral Suspension *Oral susp:* 15, 30 mg ent-coat, del-rel granules/pkt (30 pkt/carton); mix in
    2 tbsp water and drink immediately (strawberry)
    Prevacid SoluTab *ODT:* 15, 30 mg (strawberry) (phenylalanine)
    Prevacid 24HR 15 mg ent-coat, del-rel granules; swallow whole or mix granules with food or juice and
    take immediately; do <u>not</u> crush or chew granules; follow with water

➤ *omeprazole* **(OTC)(G)** 20-40 mg daily; take before eating; swallow whole or mix granules with applesauce
  and take immediately; do <u>not</u> crush or chew; follow with water

Pediatric: <1 year: <u>not</u> recommended; 5-<10 kg: 5 mg daily; 10-<20 kg: 10 mg daily; ≥20 kg: same as adult
  Prilosec *Cap:* 10, 20, 40 mg ent-coat, del-rel granules
  Prilosec OTC *Tab:* 20 mg del-rel (regular, wild berry)
▷ *pantoprazole* (G) initially 40 mg bid
  Pediatric: <12 years: <u>not</u> recommended; ≥12 years: same as adult
    Protonix *Tab:* 40 mg ent-coat, del-rel
    Protonix for Oral Suspension *Oral susp:* 40 mg ent-coat, del-rel granules/pkt; mix in 1 tsp apple juice for 5 seconds <u>or</u> sprinkle on 1 tsp apple sauce, and swallow immediately; do <u>not</u> mix in water <u>or</u> any other liquid <u>or</u> food; take approximately 30 minutes prior to a meal; 30 pkt/carton
▷ *rabeprazole* (OTC)(G) initially 20 mg daily; then titrate; may take 100 mg daily in divided doses <u>or</u> 60 mg bid
  Pediatric: <12 years: <u>not</u> recommended; ≥12 years: 20 mg once daily; max 8 weeks
    AcipHex *Tab:* 20 mg ent-coat, del-rel
    AcipHex Sprinkle *Cap:* 5, 10 mg del-rel

ANTICHOLINERGICS

▷ *glycopyrrolate Recommended dose:* 1.7 mg (1 ODT) administered 2 <u>or</u> 3 times daily on top of the tongue; allow to disintegrate and swallow without water; max 6.8 mg/day; administer at least 1 hour before <u>or</u> 2 hours after food; use the lowest effective dose to control symptoms; switch patients who are titrated to a lower dose to another oral tablet dose form of *glycopyrrolate*; patients receiving the 2 mg dose strength of another oral tablet dose form of *glycopyrrolate* may be switched to **Dartisla ODT**; <u>not</u> recommended for patients initiating treatment <u>or</u> receiving maintenance treatment with a lower dosage strength of another oral *glycopyrrolate* product (e.g., 1 mg tablet)
  Pediatric: safety and efficacy <u>not</u> established
    Dartisla ODT *ODT:* 1.7 mg (10 orally-disintegrating tablets per blister card, 3 blister cards per carton)
    Comment: Dartisla ODT is an anticholinergic indicated in adults to reduce symptoms of a peptic ulcer as an adjunct to treatment of peptic ulcer. **Dartisla ODT** is <u>not</u> indicated as monotherapy for treatment of peptic ulcer because effectiveness in peptic ulcer healing has <u>not</u> been established. Adverse reactions include blurred vision, drowsiness, decreased sweating, flushing, vomiting, constipation, dry mouth, tachycardia, and urinary retention. **Dartisla ODT** may impair mental and/or physical function. Inform patients <u>not</u> to operate motor vehicles <u>or</u> perform other hazardous tasks until reasonably certain they are <u>not</u> adversely affected; discontinue use if signs <u>or</u> symptoms develop. Heat prostration resulting in fever and heat stroke can occur, especially in geriatric patients; avoid exposure to hot <u>or</u> very warm environmental temperatures. Use of **Dartisla ODT** is <u>not</u> recommended in patients with autonomic neuropathy, hyperthyroidism, cardiac disease, hiatal hernia, etc., as these conditions are exacerbated by anticholinergic adverse reactions. Anticholinergic adverse reactions in geriatric patients can cause <u>or</u> exacerbate complications such as urinary retention, bowel obstruction, heat prostration, arrythmias, delirium, and falls <u>or</u> fractures; therefore, **Dartisla ODT** may <u>not</u> be recommended for geriatric patients and may be contraindicated in some patients with underlying medical conditions. **Dartisla ODT** is contraindicated in patients at risk for anticholinergic toxicity due to underlying medical condition(s) and patients with hypersensitivity to *glycopyrrolate* <u>or</u> the inactive ingredients in the product. Concomitant use of *glycopyrrolate* with other anticholinergic drugs is <u>not</u> recommended. Concomitant use of **Dartisla ODT** with drugs with altered absorption due to decreased gastrointestinal (GI) motility is <u>not</u> recommended. Delayed gastric emptying, constipation, and intestinal pseudo-obstruction may occur and precipitate <u>or</u> aggravate paralytic ileus and toxic megacolon. Concomitant use of **Dartisla ODT** with solid oral dose forms of potassium chloride (KCl) is <u>not</u> recommended. Monitor patients with renal impairment; if anticholinergic adverse reactions occur, discontinue **Dartisla ODT**. Over decades of *glycopyrrolate* use, there is an absence of published data on orally administered *glycopyrrolate* in pregnant women, including an absence of any reports of a drug-associated risk of major birth defects, miscarriage, <u>or</u> other adverse human maternal <u>or</u> fetal outcomes. In animal studies, at non-maternally toxic doses of oral *glycopyrrolate*, there were <u>no</u> adverse developmental effects. An animal pre- and postnatal developmental study of oral *glycopyrrolate* showed a decrease in pup mean body weight that recovered post nursing, with <u>no</u> other developmental effects observed. In a published reproductive and developmental study, male and female rats were administered *glycopyrrolate* in the diet at 0, 32.5, 63, and 130 mg/kg/day for 3 to 5 weeks and through up to three consecutive litters. There was <u>no</u> indication of abnormalities in the pups of treated dams. There was a decreased rate of conception and in survival rate at weaning for all treated animals in a dose-related manner. There are <u>no</u> data on the presence of *glycopyrrolate* in either human <u>or</u> animal milk <u>or</u> effects on the breastfed infant. As with other anticholinergic drugs, *glycopyrrolate* may cause suppression of lactation. Developmental and health benefits of breastfeeding should be considered along with the mother's clinical need for **Dartisla ODT** and any potential adverse effects on the breastfed infant from **Dartisla ODT**.
▷ **Robinul** (G) initially 1-2 mg bid-tid; *Maintenance:* 1 mg bid; max 8 mg/day
  Pediatric: <12 years: <u>not</u> recommended; ≥12 years: same as adult
    Tab: 1 mg (dye-free)
▷ **Robinul Forte** (G) initially 1-2 mg bid-tid; *Maintenance:* 1 mg bid; max 8 mg/day
  Pediatric: <12 years: <u>not</u> recommended; ≥12 years: same as adult
    Tab: 2 mg (dye-free)
    Comment: Robinul/Robinul Forte is an anticholinergic adjunct to peptic ulcer disease (PUD) treatment.

OTHER AGENTS

▷ *mepenzolate* (G) 25-50 mg divided qid, with meals and at HS
    Cantil *Tab:* 25 mg
▷ *sucralfate* (G) Active ulcer: 1 gm qid; *Maintenance:* 1 gm bid
    Carafate *Tab:* 1*gm; *Oral susp:* 1 gm/10 ml (14 oz)

PROPHYLAXIS

▷ *misoprostol* 200 mg qid with food for prevention of non-steroidal anti-inflammatory drug (NSAID)-induced gastric ulcers
    Cytotec *Tab:* 100, 200 mg
    Comment: *Misoprostol* is a prostaglandin E1 analog indicated for the prevention of NSAID-induced gastric ulcers. Females of childbearing potential should have a negative serum pregnancy test within 2 weeks before starting the first dose on the second or third day of the next menstrual period. A contraceptive method should be maintained during therapy. Risks to pregnant females include: spontaneous abortion, premature birth, fetal anomalies, and uterine rupture.

PERIPHERAL NEURITIS, DIABETIC NEUROPATHIC PAIN, PERIPHERAL NEUROPATHIC PAIN

▷ Acetaminophen for IV Infusion *see Pain*
▷ Ibuprofen for IV Infusion *see Pain*
▷ *Acetaminophen* (G) *see Fever*
▷ *Aspirin* (G) *see Fever*

ALPHA-2 DELTA LIGAND

▷ *pregabalin (GABA analog)* (G)(V) initially 150 mg daily divided bid-tid; may titrate within 1 week; max 600 mg divided bid-tid; discontinue over 1 week
    Pediatric: <18 years: not recommended; ≥18 years: same as adult
        Lyrica *Cap:* 25, 50, 75, 100, 150, 200, 225, 300 mg; *Oral soln:* 20 mg/ml

SEROTONIN NOREPINEPHRINE REUPTAKE INHIBITOR (SNRI)

▷ *duloxetine* swallow whole; 30-60 mg once daily; may increase by 30 mg at 1-week intervals; usual target 60 mg daily; max 120 mg/day
    Pediatric: <12 years: not recommended; ≥12 years: same as adult
        Cymbalta *Cap:* 20, 30, 60 mg ent-coat pellets
        Comment: Cymbalta is indicated for chronic pain syndromes (e.g., arthritis, fibromyalgia, low back pain).

TOPICAL AND TRANSDERMAL ANALGESICS

▷ *capsaicin* (G) apply tid-qid prn to intact skin
    Pediatric: <2 years: not recommended; ≥2 years: apply sparingly tid-qid prn
        Axsain *Crm:* 0.075% (1, 2 oz)
        Capsin *Lotn:* 0.025, 0.075% (59 ml)
        Capzasin-HP (OTC) *Crm:* 0.075% (1.5 oz), 0.025% (45, 90 gm); *Lotn:* 0.075% (2 oz); 0.025% (45, 90 gm)
        Capzasin-P (OTC) *Crm:* 0.025% (1.5 oz); *Lotn:* 0.025% (2 oz)
        Dolorac *Crm:* 0.025% (28 gm)
        Double Cap (OTC) *Crm:* 0.05% (2 oz)
        R-Gel *Gel:* 0.025% (15, 30 gm)
        Zostrix (OTC) *Crm:* 0.025% (0.7, 1.5, 3 oz)
        Zostrix HP (OTC) *Emol crm:* 0.075% (1, 2 oz)
▷ *capsaicin* 8% patch apply up to 4 patches for one 60-minute application to clean dry skin; may prep area with topical anesthetic; wear non-latex gloves; patches may be cut to size/shape; treatment may be repeated every 3 months
    Pediatric: <18 years: not recommended; ≥18 years: same as adult
        Qutenza *Patch:* 8% 1640 mcg/cm (179 mg) (1 or 2 patches w. 1-50 gm tube cleansing gel/carton)
▷ *diclofenac sodium* apply qid prn to intact skin
    Pediatric: <12 years: not established; ≥12 years: same as adult
        Pennsaid 1.5% in 10 drop increments, dispense and rub into front, side, and back of knee; usually 40 drops (40 mg) qid
            Topical soln: 1.5% (150 ml)
        Pennsaid 2% apply 2 pump actuations (40 mg) and rub into front, side, and back of knee bid
            Topical soln: 2% (20 mg/pump actuation, 112 gm)
        Solaraze Gel massage into clean skin bid prn
            Gel: 3% (50 gm) (benzyl alcohol)
        Voltaren Gel (G)(OTC) apply qid prn to intact skin
            Gel: 1% (100 gm)
    Comment: *Diclofenac* is contraindicated with *aspirin* allergy. As with other NSAIDs, should be avoided in late pregnancy (≥30 weeks) because it may cause premature closure of the ductus arteriosus.
▷ *doxepin* (G) cream apply to affected area qid at intervals of at least 3-4 hours; max 8 days
    Pediatric: <12 years: not recommended; >12 years: same as adult

Prudoxin *Crm:* 5% (45 gm)
Zonalon *Crm:* 5% (30, 45 gm)
▷ *pimecrolimus* 1% cream (G) <2 years: <u>not</u> recommended; ≥2 years: apply to affected area bid; do <u>not</u> apply an occlusive dressing
Elidel *Crm:* 1% (30, 60, 100 gm)
Comment: *Pimecrolimus* is indicated for short-term and intermittent long-term use. Discontinue use when resolution occurs. Contraindicated if the patient is immunosuppressed. Change to the 0.1% preparation <u>or</u> if secondary bacterial infection is present.
▷ *trolamine salicylate* apply tid-qid
Pediatric: <2 years: <u>not</u> recommended; ≥2 years: same as adult
Mobisyl Creme *Crm:* 10% (100 gm)

TOPICAL AND TRANSDERMAL ANESTHETICS
Comment: *Lidocaine* should <u>not</u> be applied to non-intact skin.
▷ *lidocaine* cream apply to affected area bid prn
Pediatric: <12 years: <u>not</u> recommended; ≥12 years: same as adult
LidaMantle *Crm:* 3% (1, 2 oz)
Lidoderm *Crm:* 3% (85 gm)
ZTlido *lidocaine* topical system 1% (30/carton)
Comment: Compared to Lidoderm (*lidocaine* patch 5%), which contains 700 mg/patch, ZTlido requires 35 mg per topical system to achieve the same therapeutic dose.
▷ *lidocaine* lotion apply to affected area bid prn
Pediatric: <12 years: <u>not</u> recommended; ≥12 years: same as adult
LidaMantle *Lotn:* 3% (177 ml)
▷ *lidocaine* 5% patch (G) apply up to 3 patches at one time for up to 12 hours/24-hour period (12 hours on/12 hours off); patches may be cut into smaller sizes before removal of the release liner; do <u>not</u> reuse
Pediatric: <12 years: <u>not</u> recommended; ≥12 years: same as adult
Lidoderm *Patch:* 5% (10 x 14 cm; 30/carton)
▷ *lidocaine+dexamethasone*
Pediatric: <12 years: <u>not</u> recommended; ≥12 years: same as adult
Decadron Phosphate with Xylocaine *Lotn:* dexa 4 mg+lido 10 mg per ml (5 ml)
▷ *lidocaine+hydrocortisone* (G) apply to affected area bid prn
Pediatric: <12 years: <u>not</u> recommended; ≥12 years: same as adult
LidaMantle HC *Crm:* lido 3%+hydro 0.5% (1, 3 oz); *Lotn:* (177 ml)
▷ *lidocaine* 2.5%+*prilocaine* 2.5% apply sparingly to the burn bid-tid prn
Pediatric: <12 years: <u>not</u> recommended; ≥12 years: same as adult
Emla Cream 5, 30 gm/tube

ORAL ANALGESICS
▷ *tramadol* (IV)(G)
Rybix ODT initially 100 mg once daily; may increase by 100 mg every 5 days; max 300 mg/day; *CrCl <30 ml/min* <u>or</u> *severe hepatic impairment:* <u>not</u> recommended; *Cirrhosis:* max 50 mg q 12 hours
Pediatric: <12 years: contraindicated; 12 to <18 years: use extreme caution; <u>not</u> recommended for children and adolescents with obesity, asthma, obstructive sleep apnea, <u>or</u> other chronic breathing problem, <u>or</u> for posttonsillectomy/adenoidectomy pain; ≥18 years: same as adult
ODT: 50 mg (mint) (phenylalanine)
Ryzolt initially 100 mg once daily; may increase by 100 mg every; 5 days; max 300 mg/day; *CrCl <30 ml/min* <u>or</u> *severe hepatic impairment:* <u>not</u> recommended
Pediatric: <18 years: <u>not</u> recommended; ≥18 years: same as adult
Tab: 100, 200, 300 mg ext-rel
Ultram 50-100 mg q 4-6 hours prn; max 400 mg/day; *CrCl <30 ml/min:* max 100 mg q 12 hours; *Cirrhosis:* max 50 mg q 12 hours
Pediatric: <18 years: <u>not</u> recommended; ≥18 years: same as adult
Tab: 50 mg
Ultram ER initially 100 mg once daily; may increase by 100 mg every 5 days; max 300 mg/day; *CrCl <30 ml/min* <u>or</u> *severe hepatic impairment:* <u>not</u> recommended
Pediatric: <18 years: <u>not</u> recommended; ≥18 years: same as adult
Tab: 100, 200, 300 mg ext-rel
▷ *tramadol+acetaminophen* (IV)(G) 2 tabs q 4-6 hours; max 8 tabs/day; 5 days; *CrCl <30 ml/min:* max 2 tabs q 12 hours; max 4 tabs/day x 5 days
Pediatric: <18 years: <u>not</u> recommended; ≥18 years: same as adult
Ultracet *Tab:* tram 37.5+acet 325 mg

OPIOID AGONIST
▷ *tapentadol* (II)
Pediatric: <18 years: <u>not</u> recommended; ≥18 years: same as adult
Nucynta 50-100 mg q 4-6 hours prn; max 700 mg/day on the first day; 600 mg/day on subsequent days

(continued)

Tab: 50, 75, 100 mg

Nucynta ER *Opioid-naïve:* initially 50 mg q 12 hours, then titrate to optimal dose within therapeutic range; usual therapeutic range 100-250 mg q 12 hours; doses >500 mg <u>not</u> recommended; *Converting from Nucynta:* divide total **Nucynta** daily dose into 2 **Nucynta ER** doses and administer q 12 hours; *Converting from oxycodone CR and other opioids:* see mfr recommendations

Tab: 50, 100, 150, 200, 250 mg ext-rel

PERIPHERAL VASCULAR DISEASE (PVD, ARTERIAL INSUFFICIENCY, INTERMITTENT CLAUDICATION)

ANTIPLATELET THERAPY

▷ *aspirin* (OTC) usually 81 mg once daily; range 75-325 mg once daily
  Ecotrin *Tab/Cap:* 81, 325, 500 mg ent-coat
▷ *cilostazol* 100 mg bid ½ hour before <u>or</u> 2 hours after breakfast <u>or</u> dinner; may reduce to 50 mg bid if used with CYP3A4 (e.g., azole antifungals, macrolides, *diltiazem, fluvoxamine, fluoxetine, nefazodone, sertraline*) <u>or</u> CYP2C19 (e.g., *omeprazole*) inhibitors
  Tab: 50, 100 mg
  Comment: *Cilostazol* may be used with *aspirin.* Cautious use with other antiplatelet agents and anticoagulants.
  clopidogrel 75 mg daily
  Plavix *Tab:* 75 mg
▷ *dipyridamole* (G) 25-100 mg tid-qid
  Persantine *Tab:* 25, 50, 75 mg
  Comment: *Dipyridamole* does <u>not</u> potentiate *warfarin* and may be taken concomitantly. Do <u>not</u> administer *dipyridamole* concomitantly with *aspirin.*
▷ *pentoxifylline* 400 mg tid with food
  PentoPak *Tab:* 400 mg ext-rel
  Trental *Tab:* 400 mg sust-rel
▷ *ticlopidine* 250 mg bid with food
  Ticlid *Tab:* 250 mg
  Comment: Monitor for neutropenia; resolves after discontinuation.
▷ *warfarin* adjust dose to maintain international normalized ratio (INR) in recommended range; For *Anticoagulation Therapy Appendix S. Anticoagulants*
  Coumadin *Tab:* 1*, 2*, 2.5*, 5*, 7.5*, 10*mg
  Coumadin for Injection *Vial:* 2 mg/ml (5 mg) pwdr for reconstitution
  Comment: Treatment for overanticoagulation with *warfarin* is *vitamin K.*

PERLECHE (ANGULAR STOMATITIS)

Comment: Perleche is a form of intertrigo. This localized tissue inflammation and maceration is characterized by constant exposure to saliva, which normally contains bacteria, yeast, and other organisms, in the natural anatomical furrow at the corners of the mouth. Perleche is often misdiagnosed as yeast infection, but almost never responds to antiyeast agents. Patients with severe vitamin deficiencies (e.g., chronic alcoholism, malnutrition) are often at increased risk. Sensitivities <u>or</u> allergies to toothpaste may be contributing irritants.

Treatment: apply a small amount of a combination of 2.5% *hydrocortisone* cream and *miconazole* cream (which kills yeast, fungi, and many bacteria) to the affected area bid; once the area is clear, recurrence can be prevented with local application of petroleum jelly.

PERTUSSIS (WHOOPING COUGH)

Prophylaxis *see Childhood Immunizations*

COMBINATION VACCINES

▷ **Pentacel** (DTaP-IPV/Hib) is commercially available as a kit containing single-dose vial of fixed-combination vaccine containing diphtheria, tetanus, pertussis, and poliovirus antigens (DTaP-IPV vaccine) and single-dose vial of lyophilized Hib vaccine (PRP-T; ActHIB). Prior to administration, reconstitute vial of lyophilized PRP-T (ActHIB) vaccine by adding the entire content of the vial of DTaP-IPV vaccine in the kit according to manufacturer's instructions to provide a combination vaccine containing diphtheria, tetanus, pertussis, IPV, and Hib antigens. Gently swirl until cloudy, uniform, white to off-white (yellow tinge) suspension is obtained. Administer IM immediately after reconstitution. **Pentacel** is approved for use as a four-dose series in children 6 weeks through 4 years of age (prior to ghe 5th birthday). **Pentacel** is to be administered as a 4-dose series at 2, 4, 6, and 15-18 months of age. The first dose may be given as early as 6 weeks of age. Four doses of **Pentacel** constitute a primary immunization course against pertussis. Three doses of **Pentacel** constitute an immunization course against diphtheria, tetanus, *Haemophilus influenzae, type b* invasive disease, and poliomyelitis; the fourth dose is a booster for diphtheria, tetanus, *Haemophilus influenzae, type b* invasive disease, and poliomyelitis immunizations. See mfr pkg insert for full prescribing information, including product storage, preparation, administration, contraindications, warnings, and precautions.

▷ **Vaxelis** *Vial:* 0.5 ml susp, single-dose; *Prefilled syringe:* 0.5 ml susp, single-dose (preservative-free)
Comment: Vaxelis is a single fixed-dose combination of six vaccines: diphtheria, tetanus toxoid, acellular pertussis, inactivated poliovirus, *Haemophilus* b conjugate, and hepatitis b (HBV). The 3-dose immunization series consists of a 0.5 ml IM injection, administered at 2, 4, and 6 months of age. See mfr pkg insert for full prescribing information, including product storage, preparation, administration, contraindications, warnings, and precautions.

POST-EXPOSURE PROPHYLAXIS AND TREATMENT

Comment: Antibiotics do not alter the course of illness, but they do prevent transmission. Infected persons should be isolated until after the fifth day of antibiotic treatment.

▷ *azithromycin* (G) 500 mg x 1 dose on day 1, then 250 mg daily on days 2-5 or 500 mg daily x 3 days
Pediatric: 12 mg/kg/day x 5 days; max 500 mg/day; *see* Appendix BB.7. *azithromycin* (Zithromax Suspension, Zmax Suspension) *for dose by weight*
    Zithromax *Tab:* 250, 500, 600 mg; *Oral susp:* 100 mg/5 ml (15 ml), 200 mg/5 ml (15, 22.5, 30 ml) (cherry); *Pkt:* 1 gm for reconstitution (cherry-banana)
    Zithromax Tri-Pak *Tab:* 3 x 500 mg tabs/pck
    Zithromax Z-Pak *Tab:* 6 x 250 mg tabs/pck
    Zmax *Oral susp:* 2 gm ext-rel for reconstitution (cherry-banana) (148 mg Na$^+$)
    Comment: *Azithromycin* is the drug of choice for infants <1 month of age.

▷ *clarithromycin* (G) 250 mg bid or 500 mg ext-rel once daily x 10 days
Pediatric: <6 months: not recommended; ≥6 months: 7.5 mg/kg divided bid x 10 days; *see* Appendix BB.16. *clarithromycin* (G) (Biaxin Suspension) *for dose by weight*
    Biaxin *Tab:* 250, 500 mg
    Biaxin Oral Suspension *Oral susp:* 125, 250 mg/5 ml (50, 100 ml) (fruit punch)
    Biaxin XL *Tab:* 500 mg ext-rel

▷ *erythromycin base* (G) 1 gm/day divided qid x 14 days
Pediatric: 40 mg/kg/day in divided doses x 14 days
    Ery-Tab *Tab:* 250, 333, 500 mg ent-coat
    PCE *Tab:* 333, 500 mg

▷ *erythromycin ethylsuccinate* (G) 1 gm/day in 4 divided doses x 14 days
Pediatric: 40-50 mg/kg/day in 4 divided doses x 7 days; may double dose with severe infection; max 100 mg/kg/day; *see* Appendix BB.21. *erythromycin ethylsuccinate* (G) (E.E.S. Suspension, EryPed Drops/Suspension) *for dose by weight*
    EryPed *Oral susp:* 200 mg/5 ml (100, 200 ml) (fruit), 400 mg/5 ml (60, 100, 200 ml) (banana); *Oral drops:* 200, 400 mg/5 ml (50 ml) (fruit); *Chew tab:* 200 mg wafer (fruit)
    E.E.S. *Oral susp:* 200, 400 mg/5 ml (100 ml) (fruit)
    E.E.S. Granules *Oral susp:* 200 mg/5 ml (100, 200 ml) (cherry)
    E.E.S. 400 Tablets *Tab:* 400 mg

▷ *trimethoprim+sulfamethoxazole (TMP-SMX)* (G)
Pediatric: <2 months: not recommended; ≥2 months: 40 mg/kg/day of *sulfamethoxazole* in 2 doses bid x 10 days; *see* Appendix BB.33. *trimethoprim+ sulfamethoxazole* (G) (Bactrim Suspension, Septra Suspension) *for dose by weight*
    Bactrim, Septra 2 tabs bid x 10 days
      Tab: trim 80 mg+sulfa 400 mg*
    Bactrim DS, Septra DS 1 tab bid x 10 days
      Tab: trim 160 mg+sulfa 800 mg
    Bactrim Pediatric Suspension, Septra Pediatric Suspension
      Oral susp: trim 40 mg+sulfa 200 mg per 5 ml (100 ml) (cherry) (alcohol 0.3%)

PHARYNGITIS: GONOCOCCAL

Comment: Treat all sexual contacts. Empiric therapy requires concomitant treatment for chlamydia. Posttreatment culture recommended with history of rheumatic fever.

PRIMARY THERAPY

▷ *azithromycin* (G) 1 gm x 1 dose
Pediatric: 12 mg/kg/day x 5 days; max 500 mg/day; *see* Appendix BB.7. *Azithromycin* (G) (Zithromax Suspension, Zmax Suspension) *for dose by weight*
    Zithromax *Tab:* 250, 500, 600 mg; *Oral susp:* 100 mg/5 ml (15 ml), 200 mg/5 ml (15, 22.5, 30 ml) (cherry); *Pkt:* 1 gm for reconstitution (cherry-banana)
    Zithromax Tri-Pak *Tab:* 3 x 500 mg tabs/pck
    Zithromax Z-Pak *Tab:* 6 x 250 mg tabs/pck
    Zmax *Oral susp:* 2 gm ext-rel for reconstitution (cherry-banana) (148 mg Na$^+$)
    Comment: Per the CDC 2015 STD Treatment Guidelines, *azithromycin* should be used with *ceftriaxone* 250 mg.

▷ *ceftriaxone* (G) 250 mg IM x 1 dose
Pediatric: <45 kg: 125 mg IM x 1 dose; ≥45 kg: same as adult
    Rocephin *Vial:* 250, 500 mg; 1, 2 gm

PHARYNGITIS: STREPTOCOCCAL (STREP THROAT)

Comment: Acute rheumatic fever is a rare but serious autoimmune disease that may occur following a group A streptococcal throat infection. It causes inflammatory lesions in connective tissue, especially that of the heart, kidneys, joints, blood vessels, and subcutaneous tissue. Prior to the broad availability of penicillin, rheumatic fever was a leading cause of death in children and one of the leading causes of acquired heart disease in adults. Strep throat is highly responsive to the penicillins and cephalosporins.

▷ *amoxicillin* (G) 500-875 mg bid or 250-500 mg tid x 10 days
  Pediatric: <40 kg (88 lb): 20-40 mg/kg/day in 3 divided doses x 10 days or 25-45 mg/kg/day in 2 divided doses x 10 days; ≥40 kg: same as adult; *see Appendix BB.3. amoxicillin (G) (Amoxil Suspension, Trimox Suspension) for dose by weight*
    Amoxil *Cap:* 250, 500 mg; *Tab:* 875*mg; *Chew tab:* 125, 200, 250, 400 mg (cherry-banana-peppermint) (phenylalanine); *Oral susp:* 125, 250 mg/5 ml (80, 100, 150 ml) (strawberry); 200, 400 mg/5 ml (50, 75, 100 ml) (bubble gum); *Oral drops:* 50 mg/ml (30 ml) (bubble gum)
    Moxatag *Tab:* 775 mg ext-rel
    Trimox *Tab:* 125, 250 mg; *Cap:* 250, 500 mg; *Oral susp:* 125, 250 mg/5 ml (80, 100, 150 ml) (raspberry-strawberry)

▷ *amoxicillin+clavulanate* (G)
    Augmentin 500 mg tid or 875 mg bid x 7-10 days
    Pediatric: 40-45 mg/kg/day divided tid x 10 days or 90 mg/kg/day divided bid x 10 days; *see Appendix BB.4. amoxicillin+clavulanate (G) (Augmentin Suspension) for dose by weight*
      Tab: 250, 500, 875 mg; *Chew tab:* 125, 250 mg (lemon-lime); 200, 400 mg (cherry-banana) (phenylalanine); *Oral susp:* 125 mg/5 ml (banana), 250 mg/5 ml (75, 100, 150 ml) (orange); 200, 400 mg/5 ml (50, 75, 100 ml) (orange) (phenylalanine)
    Augmentin ES-600 not recommended for adults
    Pediatric: <3 months: not recommended; ≥3 months, <40 kg: 90 mg/kg/day in 2 divided doses x 7-10 days; ≥40 kg: not recommended
      Oral susp: 42.9 mg/5 ml (50, 75, 100, 125, 150, 200 ml) (strawberry cream) (phenylalanine)
    Augmentin XR 2 tabs q 12 hours x 7-10 days
    Pediatric: <16 years: use other forms; ≥16 years: same as adult
      Tab: 1,000*mg ext-rel

▷ *azithromycin* (G) 500 mg x 1 dose on day 1, then 250 mg daily on days 2-5 or 500 mg daily x 3 days
    Pediatric: 12 mg/kg/day x 5 days; max 500 mg/day; *see Appendix BB.7. azithromycin (G) (Zithromax Suspension, Zmax Suspension) for dose by weight*
      Zithromax *Tab:* 250, 500, 600 mg; *Oral susp:* 100 mg/5 ml (15 ml), 200 mg/5 ml (15, 22.5, 30 ml) (cherry); *Pkt:* 1 gm for reconstitution (cherry-banana)
      Zithromax Tri-Pak *Tab:* 3 x 500 mg tabs/pck
      Zithromax Z-Pak *Tab:* 6 x 250 mg tabs/pck
      Zmax *Oral susp:* 2 gm ext-rel for reconstitution (cherry-banana) (148 mg Na$^+$)

▷ *cefaclor* (G)
    Ceclor 250 mg tid or 375 mg bid 3-10 days
    Pediatric: <1 month: not recommended; 1 month-12 years: 20-40 mg/kg divided bid or q 12 hours x 3-10 days; max 1 gm/day; *see Appendix BB.8. cefaclor (G) (Ceclor Suspension) for dose by weight;* >12 years: same as adult
      Tab: 500 mg; *Cap:* 250, 500 mg; *Susp:* 125 mg/5 ml (75, 150 ml) (strawberry), 187 mg/5 ml (50, 100 ml) (strawberry), 250 mg/5 ml (75, 150 ml) (strawberry), 375 mg/5 ml (50, 100 ml) (strawberry)
    Cefaclor Extended Release 375-500 mg bid x 3-10 days
    Pediatric: <16 years: ext-rel not recommended; ≥16 years: same as adult
      Tab: 375, 500 mg ext-rel

▷ *cefadroxil* 1 gm in 1-2 doses x 10 days
    Pediatric: 30 mg/kg/day in 2 divided doses x 10 days; *see Appendix BB.9. cefadroxil (G) (Duricef Suspension) for dose by weight*
      Duricef *Cap:* 500 mg; *Tab:* 1 gm; *Oral susp:* 250 mg/5 ml (100 ml), 500 mg/5 ml (75, 100 ml) (orange-pineapple)

▷ *cefdinir* 300 mg bid x 10 days
    Pediatric: <6 months: not recommended; 6 months-12 years: 14 mg/kg/day in 1-2 doses x 10 days; *see Appendix BB.10. cefdinir (G) (Omnicef Suspension) for dose by weight;* >12 years: same as adult
      Omnicef *Cap:* 300 mg; *Oral susp:* 125 mg/5 ml (60, 100 ml) (strawberry)

▷ *cefditoren pivoxil* 200 mg bid x 10 days
    Pediatric: <12 years: not recommended; ≥12 years: same as adult
      Spectracef *Tab:* 200 mg
      Comment: Spectracef is contraindicated with milk protein allergy or carnitine deficiency.

▷ *cefixime* (G) 400 mg daily x 5 days
    Pediatric: <6 months: not recommended; 6 months-12 years, <50 kg: 8 mg/kg/day in 1-2 divided doses x 10 days; *see Appendix BB.11. cefixime (G) (Suprax Oral Suspension) for dose by weight;* >12 years, ≥50 kg: same as adult
      Suprax *Tab:* 400 mg; *Cap:* 400 mg; *Oral susp:* 100, 200, 500 mg/5 ml (50, 75, 100 ml) (strawberry)

▷ **cefpodoxime proxetil** 100 mg bid x 5-7 days
Pediatric: <2 months: <u>not</u> recommended; 2 months-12 years: 10 mg/kg/day in 2 divided doses x 5-7 days; *see* Appendix BB.12. *cefpodoxime proxetil* (G) (Vantin Suspension) *for dose by weight;* >12 years: same as adult
  Vantin *Tab:* 100, 200 mg; *Oral susp:* 50, 100 mg/5 ml (50, 75, 100 ml) (lemon creme)
▷ **cefprozil** 500 mg daily x 10 days
Pediatric: <2 years: <u>not</u> recommended; 2-12 years: 7.5 mg/kg divided bid x 10 days; *see* Appendix BB.13. *cefprozil* (G) (Cefzil Suspension) *for dose by weight;* >12 years: same as adult
  Cefzil *Tab:* 250, 500 mg; *Oral susp:* 125, 250 mg/5 ml (50, 75, 100 ml) (bubble gum) (phenylalanine)
▷ **ceftibuten** 400 mg daily x 5 days
Pediatric: 9 mg/kg daily x 5 days; *see* Appendix BB.14. *ceftibuten* (G) (Cedax Suspension) *for dose by weight*
  Cedax *Cap:* 400 mg; *Oral susp:* 90 mg/5 ml (30, 60, 90, 120 ml), 180 mg/5 ml (30, 60, 120 ml) (cherry)
▷ **cephalexin** (G) 500 mg bid x 10 days
Pediatric: 25-50 mg/kg/day in 2 divided doses x 10 days; *see* Appendix BB.15. *cephalexin* (G) (Keflex Suspension) *for dose by weight*
  Keflex *Cap:* 250, 333, 500, 750 mg; *Oral susp:* 125, 250 mg/5 ml (100, 200 ml) (strawberry)
▷ **clarithromycin** (G) 250 mg bid <u>or</u> 500 mg ext-rel once daily x 10 days
Pediatric: <6 months: <u>not</u> recommended; ≥6 months: 7.5 mg/kg divided bid x 10 days; *see* Appendix BB.16. *clarithromycin* (G) (Biaxin Suspension) *for dose by weight*
  Biaxin *Tab:* 250, 500 mg
  Biaxin Oral Suspension *Oral susp:* 125, 250 mg/5 ml (50, 100 ml) (fruit punch)
  Biaxin XL *Tab:* 500 mg ext-rel
▷ **dirithromycin** (G) 500 mg daily x 10 days
Pediatric: <12 years: <u>not</u> recommended; ≥12 years: same as adult
  Dynabac *Tab:* 250 mg
▷ **erythromycin base** (G) 500 mg qid x 10 days
Pediatric: <45 kg: 30-50 mg divided bid-qid x 10 days; ≥45 kg: same as adult
  Ery-Tab *Tab:* 250, 333, 500 mg ent-coat
  PCE *Tab:* 333, 500 mg
▷ **erythromycin estolate** (G) 250-500 mg qid x 10 days
Pediatric: 20-50 mg/kg divided q 6 hours x 10 days; *see* Appendix BB.20. *erythromycin* estolate (G) (Ilosone Suspension) *for dose by weight*
  Ilosone *Pulvule:* 250 mg; *Tab:* 500 mg; *Liq:* 125, 250 mg/5 ml (100 ml)
▷ **erythromycin ethylsuccinate** (G) 400 mg <u>or</u> 800 mg bid x 10 days
Pediatric: 30-50 mg/kg/day in 4 divided doses x 7 days; may double dose with severe infection; max 100 mg/kg/day; *see* Appendix BB.21: *erythromycin ethylsuccinate* (G) (E.E.S. Suspension, EryPed Drops/Suspension) *for dose by weight*
  EryPed *Oral susp:* 200 mg/5 ml (100, 200 ml) (fruit), 400 mg/5 ml (60, 100, 200 ml) (banana); *Oral drops:* 200, 400 mg/5 ml (50 ml) (fruit); *Chew tab:* 200 mg wafer (fruit)
  E.E.S. *Oral susp:* 200, 400 mg/5 ml (100 ml) (fruit)
  E.E.S. Granules *Oral susp:* 200 mg/5 ml (100, 200 ml) (cherry)
  E.E.S. 400 Tablets *Tab:* 400 mg
▷ **loracarbef** 200 mg bid x 5 days
Pediatric: 15 mg/kg/day in 2 divided doses x 5 days; *see* Appendix BB.27. *loracarbef* (G) (Lorabid Suspension) *for dose by weight*
  Lorabid *Pulvule:* 200, 400 mg; *Oral susp:* 100 mg/5 ml (50, 100 ml), 200 mg/5 ml (50, 75, 100 ml) (strawberry bubble gum)
▷ **penicillin g (benzathine)** (G) 1.2 million units IM x 1 dose
Pediatric: <60 lb: 300,000-600,000 units IM x 1 dose; ≥60 lb: 900,000 units x 1 dose
  Bicillin L-A *Cartridge-needle unit:* 600,000 units (1 ml), 1.2 million units (2 ml)
▷ **penicillin g (benzathine and procaine)** (G) 2.4 million units IM x 1 dose
Pediatric: <30 lb: 600,000 units IM x 1 dose; 30-60 lb: 900,000-1.2 million units IM x 1 dose; >60 lb: same as adult
  Bicillin C-R *Cartridge-needle unit:* 600,000 units (1 ml), 1.2 million units, (2 ml), 2.4 million units (4 ml)
▷ **penicillin v potassium** (G) 500 mg bid <u>or</u> 250 mg qid x 10 days
Pediatric: <12 years: 25-50 mg/kg day in 4 divided doses x 10 days; *see* Appendix BB.29. *penicillin v potassium* (G) (Pen-Vee K Solution, Veetids Solution) *for dose by weight;* >12 years: same as adult
  Pen-Vee K *Tab:* 250, 500 mg; *Oral soln:* 125 mg/5 ml (100, 200 ml), 250 mg/5 ml (100, 150, 200 ml)
  Veetids *Tab:* 250, 500 mg; *Oral soln:* 125, 250 mg/5 ml (100, 200 ml)

PHENYLKETONURIA (PKU)

PHENYLALANINE-METABOLIZING ENZYME

Comment: Palynziq (**pegvaliase-pqpz**) is a phenylalanine-metabolizing enzyme indicated to reduce serum phenylalanine (Phe) concentrations in adult patients with phenylketonuria (PKU) who have uncontrolled

(continued)

serum phenylalanine concentrations >600 micromol/L on existing management. **Palynziq** is to be used in conjunction with a Pha-restricted diet.

▷ *pegvaliase-pqpz* recommended initial dosage is 2.5 mg SC once weekly x 4 weeks; titrate dosage in a step-wise manner over at least 5 weeks based on tolerability to achieve a dosage of 20 mg SC once daily; see mfr pkg insert for titration regimen; consider increasing the dosage to max 40 mg SC once daily in patients who have been on 20 mg once daily continuously for at least 24 weeks and who have <u>not</u> achieved either a 20% reduction in blood phenylalanine concentration from pretreatment baseline <u>or</u> a blood phenylalanine concentration ≤600 micromol/L; discontinue **Palynziq** in patients who have <u>not</u> achieved at least a 20% reduction in blood phenylalanine concentration from pretreatment baseline <u>or</u> a blood phenylalanine concentration ≤600 micromol/L after 16 weeks of continuous treatment with the maximum dosage of 40 mg once daily; reduce the dosage <u>and/or</u> modify dietary protein and phenylalanine intake, as needed, to maintain blood phenylalanine concentrations within a clinically acceptable range and >30 micromol/L *ALWAYS co-prescribe autoinjectable epinephrine*
Pediatric: <18 years: <u>not</u> recommended; ≥18 years: same as adult
   Palynziq *Prefilled syringe:* 2.5, 10 mg/0.5 ml; 20 mg/ml, single-dose (preservative-free)
Comment: Obtain serum phenylalanine (Phe) concentrations every 4 weeks until a maintenance dosage is established. After a maintenance dosage is established, periodically monitor blood phenylalanine concentrations. Counsel patients to monitor dietary protein and phenylalanine intake, and adjust as directed by their healthcare provider. Anaphylaxis has been reported after administration of **Palynziq** and may occur at any time during treatment. Administer the initial dose under the supervision of a healthcare provider equipped to manage anaphylaxis and closely observe patients for at least 60 minutes following injection. Prior to self-injection, confirm patient competency with self-administration, and the patient's and observer's (if applicable) ability to recognize signs and symptoms of anaphylaxis and to administer autoinjectable epinephrine, if needed. *Prescribe autoinjectable epinephrine.* Prior to first dose, instruct the patient and the observer (if applicable) on its appropriate use. Instruct the patient to seek immediate medical care upon its use. Instruct patients to carry autoinjectable epinephrine with them at all times during **Palynziq** treatment. **Palynziq** is available <u>only</u> through the restricted **Palynziq** Risk Evaluation and Mitigation Strategy (REMS) pogram. **Palynziq** may cause fetal harm when administered to a pregnant woman. Limited available data with *pegvaliase-pqpz* use in pregnant females are insufficient to inform a drug-associated risk of adverse developmental outcomes. There are risks to the fetus associated with poorly controlled phenylalanine concentrations in women with PKU during pregnancy, including increased risk of miscarriage, major birth defects (including microcephaly, major cardiac malformations), intrauterine fetal growth retardation, and future intellectual disability with low IQ; therefore, phenylalanine concentrations should be closely monitored in women with PKU during pregnancy. There are no data on the presence of *pegvaliase-pqpz* in human milk <u>or</u> the effects on the breastfed infant.

PHENYLALANINE HYDROXYLASE ACTIVATOR (PHA)
Comment: Kuvan *(sapropterin)* is a phenylalanine hydroxylase activator (PHA) indicated to reduce serum phenylalanine (Phe) levels in patients with hyperphenylalaninemia (HPA) due to tetrahydrobiopterin- (BH4-) responsive phenylketonuria (PKU). **Kuvan** is to be used in conjunction with a Phe-restricted diet.

▷ *sapropterin* (G) recommended starting dose is 10 mg/kg/day taken once daily; doses may be adjusted in the range of 5-20 mg/kg taken once daily. Serum phenylalanine (Phe) must be monitored regularly; take with food to increase absorption; tabs may be swallowed whole <u>or</u> dissolved in 4-8 oz (120-240 ml) of water <u>or</u> apple juice; once dissolved, dose should be taken within 15 minutes; pwdr for oral soln should be dissolved in 4-8 oz (120-240 ml) of water <u>or</u> apple juice and consumed within 30 minutes of preparation
Pediatric: <18 years: <u>not</u> recommended; ≥18 years: same as adult
   Kuvan *Tab:* 100 mg; *Pwdr for oral soln:* 100 mg/unit dose pkt

PHEOCHROMOCYTOMA (ADRENAL GLAND TUMOR)

▷ *metyrosine* (G) initially 250 mg 4 x/day; may increase by 250 mg to 500 mg every day; max 4 g/day in divided doses; *Preoperative preparation:* the optimally effective dose should be administered for at least 5-7 days prior to surgery
Pediatric: <12 years: <u>not</u> established; ≥12 years: same as adult
   Demser Capsules *Cap:* 250 mg
   Comment: Demser is indicated in the treatment of patients with pheochromocytoma for preoperative preparation of patients for surgery, management of patients when surgery is contraindicated, and chronic treatment of patients with malignant pheochromocytoma. **Demser** is <u>not</u> recommended for the control of essential hypertension. When **Demser** is used preoperatively, alone <u>or</u> especially in combination with alpha-adrenergic blocking drugs, adequate intravascular volume must be maintained intraoperatively (especially after tumor removal) and postoperatively to avoid hypotension and decreased perfusion of vital organs resulting from vasodilatation and expanded volume capacity. Following tumor removal, large volumes of plasma may be needed to maintain BP and central venous pressure within the normal range. In addition, life-threatening arrhythmias may

occur during anesthesia and surgery and may require treatment with a beta-blocker or lidocaine. During surgery, patients should have continuous BP and ECG monitoring. While the preoperative use of **Demser** in patients with pheochromocytoma is thought to decrease intraoperative problems with BP control, **Demser** does not eliminate the danger of hypertensive crises or arrhythmias during manipulation of the tumor, and the alpha-adrenergic blocking drug, *phentolamine*, may be needed. **Demser** may add to the sedative effects of alcohol and other central nervous system (CNS) depressants (e.g., hypnotics, sedatives, and tranquilizers). *Metyrosine* crystalluria and urolithiasis have been found in animal studies with **Demser** at doses similar to those used in humans, and crystalluria has also been observed in a few patients. To minimize the risk of crystalluria, patients should be urged to maintain water intake sufficient to achieve a daily urine volume of 2,000 ml or more, particularly with doses greater than 2 g/day. Routinely monitor urine clarity. *Metyrosine* will crystallize as needles or rods, causing the urine to appear cloudy. If *metyrosine* crystalluria occurs, fluid intake should be increased further. If crystalluria persists, the dose regimen should be reduced or the drug discontinued. Caution should be observed when administering **Demser** to patients receiving phenothiazines or *haloperidol* because the extrapyramidal effects of these drugs can be expected to be potentiated by inhibition of catecholamine synthesis. Common side effects of **Demser** may include drowsiness or involuntary muscle movement. Adverse side effects requiring urgent/emergent medical intervention include drooling, trouble speaking, confusion, hallucinations, tremors, muscle spasms, painful or difficult urination, cloudy urine, and severe or ongoing diarrhea. If patients are not adequately controlled by the use of **Demser**, an alpha-adrenergic blocking agent *(phenoxybenzamine)* should be added. It is not known whether **Demser** can cause embryo/fetal harm when administered in pregnancy or can affect reproduction capacity. **Demser** should be used in pregnancy only if clearly needed after a risk/benefit assessment. It is not known whether **Demser** is excreted in human milk or if it may have effect on the breastfed infant.

ALPHA-BLOCKER
➤ *phenoxybenzamine* initially 10 mg bid; increase every other day as needed; usually 20-40 mg bid-tid
  Pediatric: <18 years: not established; ≥18 years: same as adult
    Dibenzyline *Cap:* 10 mg
    Comment: Dibenzyline *(phenoxybenzamine hydrochloride)* is a long-acting, adrenergic, alpha-receptor blocking agent which can produce and maintain "chemical sympathectomy" by oral administration. It increases blood flow to the skin, mucosa, and abdominal viscera, and lowers both supine and erect BPs. It has no effect on the parasympathetic system. **Dibenzyline** is indicated in the treatment of pheochromocytoma, to control episodes of hypertension and sweating. If tachycardia is excessive, it may be necessary to use a beta-blocking agent concomitantly. **Dibenzyline**-induced alpha-adrenergic blockade leaves beta-adrenergic receptors unopposed. Compounds that stimulate both types of receptors may, therefore, produce an exaggerated hypotensive response and tachycardia.

PHEOCHROMOCYTOMA: UNRESECTABLE, LOCALLY ADVANCED, OR METASTATIC

ALPHA-BLOCKER
➤ *phenoxybenzamine* initially 10 mg bid; increase every other day as needed; usually 20-40 mg bid-tid
  Pediatric: <18 years: not established; ≥18 years: same as adult
    Dibenzyline *Cap:* 10 mg
  (see **Pheochromocytoma** for comment)

ANTINEOPLASIA AGENT
➤ *iobenguane I 131* to be administered only by a qualified healthcare professional; verify pregnancy status in females of reproductive potential prior to administration; initiate thyroid-blocking medication prior to **Azedra** administration and continue after each dose; do not administer if platelet count <80,000/mcL or absolute neutrophil count <1,200/mcL; administer IV as a dosimetric dose followed by two therapeutic doses administered 90 days apart
  Recommended Dosimetric dose:
    >50 kg: 185-222 MBq (5-6 mCi)
    ≤50 kg: 3.7 MBq/kg (0.1 mCi/kg)
  Recommended Therapeutic dose for each of the 2 doses:
    > 62.5 kg: 18,500 MBq (500 mCi)
    ≤62.5 kg: 296 MBq/kg (8 mCi/kg)
  Adjust therapeutic doses based on radiation dose estimate results from dosimetry, if needed
  Pediatric: <12 years: not established; ≥12 years: same as adult
    Azedra *Vial:* 555 MBq/ml (15 mCi/ml), single-dose for IV infusion
    Comment: Azedra *(iobenguane I 131)* is a radioactive therapeutic agent indicated for the treatment of patients with iobenguane scan-positive, unresectable, locally advanced, or metastatic pheochromocytoma or paraganglioma who require systemic anticancer therapy. Monitor for

(continued)

hypothyroidism and thyroid-stimulating hormone (TSH) before starting **Azedra** and annually thereafter. Monitor blood pressure frequently during the first 24 hours after each dose. **Azedra** can cause fetal harm; advise females and males of reproductive potential of the potential risk to the fetus and to use effective contraception. **Azedra** may cause infertility. Advise women not to breastfeed.

PINWORM (*ENTEROBIUS VERMICULARIS*)

Comment: Treatment of all family members is recommended.

ANTHELMINTICS
Comment: Oral bioavailability of anthelmintics is enhanced when administered with a fatty meal (estimated fat content 40 gm). Treatment of all family members is recommended. Some clinicians recommend all household contacts of infected patients receive treatment, especially when multiple or repeated symptomatic infections occur, since such contacts commonly also are infected; retreatment after 14-21 days may be needed.

▷ *albendazole* 400 mg x 1 dose; may repeat in 2-3 weeks if needed; take with a meal
 Pediatric: <20 kg: 200 mg as a single dose; ≥20 kg: same as adult
   Albenza *Tab:* 200 mg
▷ *mebendazole* chew, swallow, or mix with food; 100 mg x 1 dose; may repeat in 3 weeks if needed; take with a meal
 Pediatric: <2 years: not recommended; ≥2 years: same as adult
   Emverm *Chew tab:* 100 mg
   Vermox (G) *Chew tab:* 100 mg
▷ *pyrantel pamoate* 11 mg/kg x 1 dose; max 1 gm/dose; may repeat in 2-3 weeks if needed; take with a meal
 Pediatric: 25-37 lb: 1/2 tsp x 1 dose; 38-62 lb: 1 tsp x 1 dose; 63-87 lb: 1 tsp x 1 dose; 88-112 lb: 2 tsp x 1 dose; 113-137 lb: 2 tsp x 1 dose; 138-162 lb: 3 tsp x 1 dose; 163-187 lb: 3 tsp x 1 dose; >187 lb: 4 tsp x 1 dose
   Pin-X (OTC); *Cap:* 180 mg; *Liq:* 50 mg/ml (30 ml), 144 mg/ml (30 ml); *Oral susp:* 50 mg/ml (30 ml)
▷ *thiabendazole* 50 mg/kg x 1 dose after a meal; max 3 gm; may repeat in 2-3 weeks if needed; take with a meal
 Pediatric: same as adult
   Mintezol *Chew tab:* 500*mg (orange); *Oral susp:* 500 mg/5 ml (120 ml) (orange)
   Comment: *Thiabendazole* is not for prophylaxis and should not be used as first-line therapy for pinworms. May impair mental alertness. May not be available in the United States.

PITYRIASIS ALBA

Topical Corticosteroids *see* Appendix J. Topical Corticosteroids by Potency

Comment: Pityriasis alba is a chronic skin disorder seen in children with a genetic predisposition to atopic disease. Treatment is directed toward controlling roughness and pruritus. There is no known treatment for the associated skin pigment changes. Pityriasis alba resolves spontaneously and permanently in the 2nd or 3rd decade of life.

COAL TAR PREPARATIONS
▷ *coal tar*
 Pediatric: same as adult
   Scytera (OTC) apply qd-qid; use lowest effective dose
     Foam: 2%
   T/Gel Shampoo Extra Strength (OTC) use every other day; max 4 x/week; massage into affected area for 5 minutes; rinse; repeat
     Shampoo: 1%
   T/Gel Shampoo Original Formula (OTC) use every other day; max 7 x/week; massage into affected area for 5 minutes; rinse; repeat
     Shampoo: 0.5%
   T/Gel Shampoo Stubborn Itch Control (OTC) use every other day; max 7 x/week; massage into affected area for 5 minutes; rinse; repeat
     Shampoo: 0.5%

EMOLLIENTS AND OTHER MOISTURIZING AGENTS
see *Dermatitis: Atopic*

PITYRIASIS ROSEA

Topical Corticosteroids *see* Appendix J. Topical Corticosteroids by Potency
Antihistamines *see* Appendix Z. Drugs for the Management of Allergy, Cough, and Cold Symptoms online at https://connect.springerpub.com/content/reference-book/978-0-8261-7935-7/back-matter/part02/back-matter/bmatter27

PLAGUE (*YERSINIA PESTIS*)

Comment: *Yersinia pestis* is transmitted via the bite of a flea from an infected rodent or the bite, lick, or scratch of an infected cat. Untreated bubonic plague may progress to secondary pneumonic plague, which may be transmitted via contaminated respiratory droplet spread.

➤ *streptomycin* (G) 15 mg/kg IM bid x 10 days
  Pediatric: same as adult
  Amp: 1 gm/2.5 ml or 400 mg/ml (2.5 ml)
  Comment: For patients with renal impairment, reduce dose of *streptomycin* to 20 mg/kg/day if mild and 8 mg/kg/day q 3 days if advanced. For patients who are pregnant or who have hearing impairment, shorten the course of treatment to 3 days after fever has resolved.

➤ *moxifloxacin* (G) 400 mg daily x 10 days
  Pediatric: <18 years: not recommended; ≥18 years: same as adult
    Avelox *Tab:* 400 mg; *IV soln:* 400 mg/250 mg (latex-free, preservative-free)

➤ *tetracycline* (G) 500 mg qid or 25-50 mg/kg/day divided q 6 hours x 10 days
  Pediatric: <8 years: not recommended; ≥8 years: same as adult

PNEUMONIA: BACTERIAL, HOSPITAL-ACQUIRED (HABP)

PARENTERAL CEPHALOSPORIN ANTIBACTERIAL+BETA-LACTAMASE INHIBITOR

➤ *ceftazidime+avibactam* infuse dose over 2 hours; recommended duration of treatment is 4-5 days; *CrCl 31-50 ml/min:* 1.25 gm every 8 hours; *CrCl 16-30 ml/min:* 0.94 gm every 12 hours; *CrCl 6-15 ml/min:* 0.94 gm every 24 hours; *CrCl ≤5 ml/min:* 0.94 gm every 48 hours; both *ceftazidime* and *avibactam* are hemodialyzable; thus, administer **Avycaz** after hemodialysis on hemodialysis days
  Pediatric: <18 years: not recommended; ≥18 years: same as adult
    Avycaz *Vial:* 2.5 gm, single-dose, pwdr for reconstitution and IV infusion
    Comment: Avycaz 2.5 gm contains *ceftazidime* (a cephalosporin) 2 gm (equivalent to 2.635 gm of *ceftazidime pentahydrate/sodium carbonate powder*) and *avibactam* (a beta-lactam inhibitor) 0.5 gm (equivalent to 0.551 gm of *avibactam sodium*). As only limited clinical safety and efficacy data for **Avycaz** are currently available, reserve **Avycaz** for use in patients who have limited or no alternative treatment options. To reduce the development of drug-resistant bacteria and maintain the effectiveness of **Avycaz** and other antibacterial drugs, **Avycaz** should be used only to treat infections that are proven or strongly suspected to be caused by susceptible bacteria. Seizures and other neurologic events may occur, especially in patients with renal impairment. Adjust dose in patients with renal impairment. Decreased efficacy in patients with baseline CrCl 30 ≤50 ml/min. Monitor CrCl at least daily in patients with changing renal function and adjust the dose of **Avycaz** accordingly. Monitor for hypersensitivity reactions, including anaphylaxis and serious skin reactions. Cross-hypersensitivity may occur in patients with a history of penicillin allergy. If an allergic reaction occurs, discontinue **Avycaz**. *Clostridioides difficile*-associated diarrhea (CDAD) has been reported with nearly all systemic antibacterial agents, including **Avycaz**. There are no adequate and well-controlled studies of **Avycaz**, *ceftazidime*, or *avibactam* in pregnant females. *Ceftazidime* is excreted in human milk in low concentrations. It is not known whether *avibactam* is excreted into human milk. There are no studies to inform effects on the breastfed infant.

➤ *ceftolozane+tazobactam* administer 3 gm every 8 hours via IV infusion over 1 hour x 8-14 days; *CrCl 30-50 ml/min:* 1.5 gm via IV infusion every 8 hours; *CrCl 15-29 ml/min:* 750 mg via IV infusion q 8 hours; *end-stage renal disease (ESRD):* a single loading dose of 2.25 gm via IV infusion, followed by 450 mg via IV infusion q 8 hours for the remainder of the treatment period (on hemodialysis days, administer the dose at the earliest possible time following completion of dialysis)
  Pediatric: <18 years: not established; ≥18 years: same as adult
    Zerbaxa *Vial:* 1.5 gm (*ceftolozane* 1 gm+*tazobactam* 0.5 gm), single-dose, pwdr for reconstitution and IV infusion
  Comment: For doses >1.5 gm, reconstitute a second vial in the same manner as the first one, withdraw an appropriate volume and add to the same infusion bag. The most common adverse reactions in patients with hospital-acquired bacterial pneumonia (HABP) (incidence ≥5%) have been increase in hepatic transaminases, renal impairment/renal failure, and diarrhea.

PARENTERAL PENEM ANTIBACTERIAL+RENAL DEHYDROPEPTIDASE INHIBITOR+BETA-LACTAMASE INHIBITOR

➤ *imipenem+cilastatin+relebactam* administer dose via IV infusion over 30 minutes every 6 hours; *CrCl ≥90 ml/min:* 1.25 gm/dose (*imipenem* 500 mg, *cilastatin* 500 mg, *relebactam* 250 mg); *CrCl 60-89 ml/min:* 1 gm/dose (*imipenem* 400 mg, *cilastatin* 400 mg, *relebactam* 200 mg); *CrCl 30-59 ml/min:* 0.75 gm/dose (*imipenem* 300 mg, *cilastatin* 300 mg, *relebactam* 150 mg); *CrCl 15-29 ml/min:* 0.5 gm/dose (*imipenem* 200 mg, *cilastatin* 200 mg, *relebactam* 100 mg); *ESRD/Dialysis:* 0.5 gm/dose (*imipenem* 200 mg, *cilastatin* 200 mg, *relebactam* 100 mg)

(continued)

Pediatric: <18 years: not established; ≥18 years: same as adult

> **Recarbrio** *Vial:* imipen 500 mg+cilast 500 mg+relebac 250 mg, single-dose, pwdr for reconstitution, dilution, and IV infusion

Comment: Recarbrio *(imipenem+cilastatin+relebactam)* is a fixed-dose triple combination of *imipenem* (a penem antibacterial), *cilastatin* (a renal dehydropeptidase inhibitor), and *relebactam* (a beta-lactamase inhibitor) indicated for the treatment of complicated urinary tract infection (cUTI), including pyelonephritis, complicated intra-abdominal infection (cIAI) caused by susceptible gram-negative bacteria in patients who have limited or no alternative treatment options, HABP, and ventilator-associated bacterial pneumonia (VABP) in adults. Avoid concomitant use of **Recarbrio** with *ganciclovir, valproic acid,* or *divalproex sodium.* Based on clinical reports on patients treated with imipenem/cilastatin plus relebactam 250 mg, the most frequent adverse reactions (incidence ≥2%) have been diarrhea, nausea, headache, vomiting, increased alanine aminotransferase, increased aspartate aminotransferase, phlebitis/infusion site reactions, pyrexia, and hypertension. There are insufficient human data to establish whether there is a drug-associated risk of major birth defects, miscarriage, or adverse maternal or fetal outcomes with *imipenem, cilastatin,* or *relebactam* in pregnancy. However, embryonic loss has been observed in monkeys treated with *imipenem/cilastatin,* and fetal abnormalities have been observed in *relebactam*-treated mice; therefore, advise pregnant females of the potential risks to pregnancy and the fetus. There are insufficient data on the presence of *imipenem/cilastatin* and *relebactam* in human milk and no data on the effects on the breastfed infant; however, *relebactam* is present in the milk of lactating rats and therefore developmental and health benefits of breastfeeding should be considered along with the mother's clinical need for **Recarbrio** and any potential adverse effects on the breastfed infant from **Recarbrio** or from the underlying maternal condition.

SIDEROPHORE CEPHALOSPORIN

> *cefiderocol* administer 2 gm via IV infusion every 8 hours; infuse dose over 3 hours in patients with CrCl 60-119 ml/min; see mfr pkg insert for dose adjustments required in patients with CrCl <60 ml/min and CrCl ≥120 ml/min; see mfr pkg insert for dose preparation

> **Fetroja** *Vial:* 1 gm pwdr for reconstitution and IV infusion, single-dose

Comment: Fetroja *(cefiderocol)* is a siderophore cephalosporin for the treatment of complicated urinary tract infection (cUTI), including pyelonephritis, caused by susceptible gram-negative microorganisms, in patients ≥18 years of age with limited or no alternative treatment options. Approval of this indication is based on limited clinical safety and efficacy data. An increase in all-cause mortality was observed in Fetroja-treated patients compared to those treated with best available therapy (BAT). Closely monitor the clinical response to therapy in patients with cUTI. Serious and occasionally fatal hypersensitivity (anaphylactic) reactions have been reported in patients receiving beta-lactam antibacterial drugs. Hypersensitivity was observed with **Fetroja.** Cross-hypersensitivity may occur in patients with a history of penicillin allergy. If an allergic reaction occurs, discontinue **Fetroja.** *Clostridioides difficile*-associated diarrhea (CDAD) has been reported with nearly all systemic antibacterial agents, including **Fetroja.** Seizures and other central nervous system (CNS) adverse reactions have been reported with **Fetroja.** If focal tremors, myoclonus, or seizures occur, evaluate patients to determine whether **Fetroja** should be discontinued. The most frequently occurring adverse reactions (incidence ≥2%) of patients treated with **Fetroja** have been diarrhea, infusion site reactions, constipation, rash, candidiasis, cough, elevations in liver tests, headache, hypokalemia, nausea, and vomiting. There are no available data on **Fetroja** use in pregnant females to evaluate for a drug-associated risk of major birth defects, miscarriage, or adverse maternal or fetal outcomes. Available data from published prospective cohort studies, case series, and case reports over several decades with *cephalosporin* use in pregnant females have not established drug-associated risks of major birth defects, miscarriage, or adverse maternal or fetal outcomes. Developmental toxicity studies with *cefiderocol* administered during organogenesis in animal studies showed no evidence of embryo/fetal toxicity, including drug-induced fetal malformations. It is not known whether *cefiderocol* is excreted into human milk. No information is available on the effects of **Fetroja** on the breastfed infant. Developmental and health benefits of breastfeeding should be considered along with the mother's clinical need for **Fetroja** and any potential adverse effects on the breastfed infant or from the underlying maternal condition.

PNEUMONIA: BACTERIAL, VENTILATOR-ASSOCIATED (VABP)

PARENTERAL CEPHALOSPORIN ANTIBACTERIAL+BETA-LACTAMASE INHIBITOR

> *ceftazidime+avibactam* infuse dose over 2 hours; recommended duration of treatment is 4-5 days; *CrCl 31-50 ml/min:* 1.25 gm every 8 hours; *CrCl 16-30 ml/min:* 0.94 gm every 12 hours; *CrCl 6-15 ml/min:* 0.94 gm every 24 hours; *CrCl ≤5 ml/min:* 0.94 gm every 48 hours; both *ceftazidime* and *avibactam* are hemodializable; thus, administer **Avycaz** after hemodialysis on hemodialysis days

Pediatric: <18 years: not recommended; ≥18 years: same as adult

> **Avycaz** *Vial:* 2.5 gm, single-dose, pwdr for reconstitution and IV infusion

Comment: Avycaz 2.5 gm contains *ceftazidime* (a cephalosporin) 2 gm (equivalent to 2.635 gm of *ceftazidime pentahydrate/sodium carbonate powder*) and *avibactam* (a beta-lactam inhibitor) 0.5 gm (equivalent to 0.551 gm of *avibactam sodium*). As only limited clinical safety and efficacy data for

Avycaz are currently available, reserve **Avycaz** for use in patients who have limited or no alternative treatment options. To reduce the development of drug-resistant bacteria and maintain the effectiveness of **Avycaz** and other antibacterial drugs, **Avycaz** should be used only to treat infections that are proven or strongly suspected to be caused by susceptible bacteria. Seizures and other neurologic events may occur, especially in patients with renal impairment. Adjust dose in patients with renal impairment. Decreased efficacy in patients with baseline CrCl 30 ≤50 ml/min. Monitor CrCl at least daily in patients with changing renal function and adjust the dose of **Avycaz** accordingly. Monitor for hypersensitivity reactions, including anaphylaxis and serious skin reactions. Cross-hypersensitivity may occur in patients with a history of penicillin allergy. If an allergic reaction occurs, discontinue **Avycaz**. *Clostridioides difficile*-associated diarrhea (CDAD) has been reported with nearly all systemic antibacterial agents, including **Avycaz**. There are no adequate and well-controlled studies of **Avycaz**, *ceftazidime*, or *avibactam* in pregnant females. *Ceftazidime* is excreted in human milk in low concentrations. It is not known whether *avibactam* is excreted into human milk. There are no studies to inform effects on the breastfed infant.

▶ *ceftolozane+tazobactam* administer 3 gm every 8 hours via IV infusion over 1 hour x 8-14 days; *CrCl 30-50 ml/min:* 1.5 gm via IV infusion q 8 hours; *CrCl 15-29 ml/min:* 750 mg via IV infusion q 8 hours; *end-stage renal disease (ESRD):* a single loading dose of 2.25 gm via IV infusion, followed by 450 mg via IV infusion q 8 hours for the remainder of the treatment period (on hemodialysis days, administer the dose at the earliest possible time following completion of dialysis)
Pediatric: <18 years: not established; ≥18 years: same as adult
    Zerbaxa *Vial:* 1.5 gm (*ceftolozane* 1 gm+*tazobactam* 0.5 gm), single-dose, pwdr for reconstitution and IV infusion
Comment: For doses >1.5 gm, reconstitute a second vial in the same manner as the first one, withdraw an appropriate volume and add to the same infusion bag. The most common adverse reactions in patients with ventilator-associated bacterial pneumonia (VABP) (incidence ≥5%) have been increase in hepatic transaminases, renal impairment/renal failure, and diarrhea.

PARENTERAL PENEM ANTIBACTERIAL+RENAL DEHYDROPEPTIDASE INHIBITOR+BETA-LACTAMASE INHIBITOR

▶ *imipenem+cilastatin+relebactam* administer dose via IV infusion over 30 minutes q 6 hours; *CrCl ≥90 ml/min:* 1.25 gm/dose (*imipenem* 500 mg, *cilastatin* 500 mg, *relebactam* 250 mg); *CrCl 60-89 ml/min:* 1 gm/dose (*imipenem* 400 mg, *cilastatin* 400 mg, *relebactam* 200 mg); *CrCl 30-59 ml/min:* 0.75 gm/dose (*imipenem* 300 mg, *cilastatin* 300 mg, *relebactam* 150 mg); *CrCl 15-29 ml/min:* 0.5 gm/dose (*imipenem* 200 mg, *cilastatin* 200 mg, *relebactam* 100 mg); *ESRD/Dialysis:* 0.5 gm/dose (*imipenem* 200 mg, *cilastatin* 200 mg, *relebactam* 100 mg)
Pediatric: <18 years: not established; ≥18 years: same as adult
    Recarbrio *Vial:* imipen 500 mg+cilast 500 mg+relebac 250 mg, single-dose, pwdr for reconstitution, dilution, and IV infusion
Comment: Recarbrio (*imipenem+cilastatin+relebactam*) is a fixed-dose triple combination of *imipenem* (a penem antibacterial), *cilastatin* (a renal dehydropeptidase inhibitor), and *relebactam* (a beta-lactamase inhibitor) indicated for the treatment of complicated urinary tract infection (cUTI), including pyelonephritis, complicated intra-abdominal infection (cIAI) caused by susceptible gram-negative bacteria in patients who have limited or no alternative treatment options, hospital-acquired bacterial pneumonia (HABP), and ventilator-associated bacterial pneumonia (VABP) in adults. Avoid concomitant use of **Recarbrio** with *ganciclovir, valproic acid,* or *divalproex sodium.* Based on clinical reports on patients treated with *imipenem/cilastatin* plus *relebactam* 250 mg, the most frequent adverse reactions (incidence ≥2%) have been diarrhea, nausea, headache, vomiting, increased alanine aminotransferase, increased aspartate aminotransferase, phlebitis/infusion site reactions, pyrexia, and hypertension. There are insufficient human data to establish whether there is a drug-associated risk of major birth defects, miscarriage, or adverse maternal or fetal outcomes with *imipenem, cilastatin,* or *relebactam* in pregnancy. However, embryonic loss has been observed in monkeys treated with *imipenem/cilastatin,* and fetal abnormalities have been observed in *relebactam*-treated mice; therefore, advise pregnant females of the potential risks to pregnancy and the fetus. There are insufficient data on the presence of *imipenem/cilastatin* and *relebactam* in human milk and no data on the effects on the breastfed infant; However, *relebactam* is present in the milk of lactating rats and therefore developmental and health benefits of breastfeeding should be considered along with the mother's clinical need for **Recarbrio** and any potential adverse effects on the breastfed infant from **Recarbrio** or from the underlying maternal condition.

SIDEROPHORE CEPHALOSPORIN

▶ *cefiderocol* administer 2 gm via IV infusion q 8 hours; infuse dose over 3 hours in patients with CrCl 60-119 ml/min; see mfr pkg insert for dose adjustments required in patients with CrCl <60 ml/min and CrCl ≥120 ml/min; see mfr pkg insert for dose preparation
    Fetroja *Vial:* 1 gm, pwdr for reconstitution and IV infusion, single-dose
Comment: Fetroja (*cefiderocol*) is a siderophore cephalosporin for the treatment of cUTI, including pyelonephritis, caused by susceptible gram-negative microorganisms, in patients ≥18 years of age with

(continued)

limited or no alternative treatment options. Approval of this indication is based on limited clinical safety and efficacy data. An increase in all-cause mortality was observed in **Fetroja**-treated patients compared to those treated with best available therapy (BAT). Closely monitor the clinical response to therapy in patients with cUTI. Serious and occasionally fatal hypersensitivity (anaphylactic) reactions have been reported in patients receiving beta-lactam antibacterial drugs. Hypersensitivity was observed with **Fetroja**. Cross-hypersensitivity may occur in patients with a history of penicillin allergy. If an allergic reaction occurs, discontinue **Fetroja**. *Clostridioides difficile*-associated diarrhea (CDAD) has been reported with nearly all systemic antibacterial agents, including **Fetroja**. Seizures and other central nervous system (CNS) adverse reactions have been reported with **Fetroja**. If focal tremors, myoclonus, or seizures occur, evaluate patients to determine whether **Fetroja** should be discontinued. The most frequently occurring adverse reactions (incidence ≥2%) of patients treated with **Fetroja** have been diarrhea, infusion site reactions, constipation, rash, candidiasis, cough, elevations in liver tests, headache, hypokalemia, nausea, and vomiting. There are no available data on **Fetroja** use in pregnant females to evaluate for a drug-associated risk of major birth defects, miscarriage, or adverse maternal or fetal outcomes. Available data from published prospective cohort studies, case series, and case reports over several decades with cephalosporin use in pregnant women have not established drug-associated risks of major birth defects, miscarriage, or adverse maternal or fetal outcomes. Developmental toxicity studies with *cefiderocol* administered during organogenesis in animal studies showed no evidence of embryo/fetal toxicity, including drug-induced fetal malformations. It is not known whether *cefiderocol* is excreted into human milk. No information is available on the effects of **Fetroja** on the breastfed infant. Developmental and health benefits of breastfeeding should be considered along with the mother's clinical need for **Fetroja** and any potential adverse effects on the breastfed infant or from the underlying maternal condition.

PNEUMONIA: CHLAMYDIAL

RECOMMENDED REGIMEN
▷ *erythromycin base* (G) 500 mg qid hours x 10-14 days
 Pediatric: <45 kg: 50 mg in 4 divided doses x 10-14 days; ≥45 kg: same as adult
  Ery-Tab *Tab:* 250, 333, 500 mg ent-coat
  PCE *Tab:* 333, 500 mg
▷ *erythromycin ethylsuccinate* (G) 400 mg qid x 10-14 days
 Pediatric: <45 kg: 50 mg/kg/day in 4 divided doses x 10-14 days; ≥45 kg: same as adult; *see* Appendix BB.21.
 erythromycin ethylsuccinate (G) (E.E.S. Suspension, EryPed Drops/Suspension) *for dose by weight*
  EryPed *Oral susp:* 200 mg/5 ml (100, 200 ml) (fruit), 400 mg/5 ml (60, 100, 200 ml) (banana); *Oral drops:* 200, 400 mg/5 ml (50 ml) (fruit); *Chew tab:* 200 mg wafer (fruit)
  E.E.S. *Oral susp:* 200, 400 mg/5 ml (100 ml) (fruit)
  E.E.S. Granules *Oral susp:* 200 mg/5 ml (100, 200 ml) (cherry)
  E.E.S. 400 Tablets *Tab:* 400 mg

ALTERNATE REGIMENS
▷ *azithromycin* (G) 500 mg once daily x 10 days
 Pediatric: 20 mg/kg per dose once daily x 3 days; max 500 mg/day; *see* Appendix BB.7. *azithromycin* (G) (Zithromax Suspension, Zmax Suspension) *for dose by weight*
  Zithromax *Tab:* 250, 500, 600 mg; *Oral susp:* 100 mg/5 ml (15 ml), 200 mg/5 ml (15, 22.5, 30 ml) (cherry); *Pkt:* 1 gm for reconstitution (cherry-banana)
  Zithromax Tri-Pak *Tab:* 3 x 500 mg tabs/pck
  Zithromax Z-Pak *Tab:* 6 x 250 mg tabs/pck
  Zmax *Oral susp:* 2 gm ext-rel for reconstitution (cherry-banana) (148 mg Na+)
▷ *levofloxacin* Uncomplicated: 500 mg daily x 7 days; *Complicated:* 750 mg daily x 7 days
 Pediatric: <18 years: not recommended; ≥18 years: same as adult
  Levaquin *Tab:* 250, 500, 750 mg; *Oral soln:* 25 mg/ml (480 ml) (benzyl alcohol); *Inj conc:* 25 mg/ml for IV infusion after dilution (20, 30 ml single-use vial) (preservative-free); *Premix soln:* 5 mg/ml for IV infusion (50, 100, 150 ml) (preservative-free)

PNEUMONIA: COMMUNITY-ACQUIRED PNEUMONIA (CAP) AND COMMUNITY-ACQUIRED BACTERIAL PNEUMONIA (CABP)

Comment: Over 70% of patients with uncomplicated community-acquired pneumonia (CAP) received prescriptions for antibiotics that exceeded national duration recommendations, according to a retrospective study that included 22,128 patients from 18 to 64 years of age with private insurance and 130,746 patients aged >65 years with Medicare who were hospitalized with uncomplicated CAP. Length of antibiotic therapy (LOT) during hospital stay was estimated using the MarketScan Hospital Drug Database and outpatient LOT was determined using prescriptions filled at discharge. The researchers defined excessive duration as a LOT of more than 3 days.

▷ *pneumococcal 15-valent conjugate vaccine*
  Pediatric: <18 years: not indicated; ≥18 years: same as adult
  Comment: *Pneumococcal 15-valent conjugate vaccine* is indicated for active immunization for the prevention of invasive disease caused by *Streptococcus pneumoniae* serotypes 1, 3, 4, 5, 6A, 6B, 7F, 9V, 14, 18C, 19A, 19F, 22F, 23F, and 33F in patients ≥18 years of age and older.

ANTI-INFECTIVES

▷ *amoxicillin* (G) 500-875 mg bid or 250-500 mg tid x 3-10 days
  Pediatric: <40 kg (88 lb): 20-40 mg/kg/day in 3 divided doses x 3-10 days or 25-45 mg/kg/day in 2 divided doses x 3-10 days; ≥40 kg: same as adult
    Amoxil *Cap:* 250, 500 mg; *Tab:* 875 mg; *Chew tab:* 125, 200, 250, 400 mg (cherry-banana-peppermint) (phenylalanine); *Oral susp:* 125, 250 mg/5 ml (80, 100, 150 ml) (strawberry); 200, 400 mg/5 ml (50, 75, 100 ml) (bubble gum); *Oral drops:* 50 mg/ml (30 ml) (bubble gum)
    Moxatag *Tab:* 775 mg ext-rel
    Trimox *Tab:* 125, 250 mg; *Cap:* 250, 500 mg; *Oral susp:* 125, 250 mg/5 ml (80, 100, 150 ml) (raspberry-strawberry)
▷ *amoxicillin+clavulanate* (G) 500 mg tid or 875 mg bid x 3-10 days
    Augmentin 500 mg tid or 875 mg bid x 3-10 days
    Pediatric: 40-45 mg/kg/day divided tid x 10 days or 90 mg/kg/day divided bid x 10 days; *see* Appendix BB.4. *amoxicillin+clavulanate* (G) (Augmentin Suspension) *for dose by weight*
    Tab: 250, 500, 875 mg; *Chew tab:* 125, 250 mg (lemon-lime); 200, 400 mg (cherry-banana) (phenylalanine); *Oral susp:* 125 mg/5 ml (banana), 250 mg/5 ml (75, 100, 150 ml) (orange); 200, 400 mg/5 ml (50, 75, 100 ml) (orange) (phenylalanine)
    Augmentin ES-600 not recommended for adults
    Pediatric: <3 months: not recommended; ≥3 months, <40 kg: 90 mg/kg/day in 2 divided doses x 3-10 days; ≥40 kg: not recommended
    Oral susp: 42.9 mg/5 ml (50, 75, 100, 125, 150, 200 ml) (strawberry cream) (phenylalanine)
    Augmentin XR 2 tabs q 12 hours x 3-10 days
    Pediatric: <16 years: use other forms; ≥16 years: same as adult
    Tab: 1,000*mg ext-rel
▷ *azithromycin* (G) *Day 1,* 500 mg as a single dose and *Days 2-5,* 250 mg once daily or 500 mg once daily x 3 days
  Pediatric: <6 months: not recommended; ≥6 months: 10 mg/kg x 1 dose on day 1; then 5 mg/kg/day on days 2-5; max 500 mg/day; *see* Appendix BB.7. *azithromycin* (G) (Zithromax Suspension, Zmax Suspension) *for dose by weight*
    Zithromax *Tab:* 250, 500, 600 mg; *Oral susp:* 100 mg/5 ml (15 ml), 200 mg/5 ml (15, 22.5, 30 ml) (cherry); *Pkt:* 1 gm for reconstitution (cherry-banana)
    Zithromax Tri-Pak *Tab:* 3 x 500 mg tabs/pck
    Zithromax Z-Pak *Tab:* 6 x 250 mg tabs/pck
    Zmax *Oral susp:* 2 gm ext-rel for reconstitution (cherry-banana) (148 mg Na$^+$)
▷ *cefaclor* (G)
  Ceclor 250 mg tid or 375 mg bid 3-10 days
  Pediatric: <1 month: not recommended; 1 month-12 years: 20-40 mg/kg divided bid or q 12 hours x 3-10 days; max 1 gm/day; *see* Appendix BB.8. *cefaclor* (G) (Ceclor Suspension) *for dose by weight*; >12 years: same as adult
    Tab: 500 mg; *Cap:* 250, 500 mg; *Susp:* 125 mg/5 ml (75, 150 ml) (strawberry), 187 mg/5 ml (50, 100 ml) (strawberry), 250 mg/5 ml (75, 150 ml) (strawberry), 375 mg/5 ml (50, 100 ml) (strawberry)
  Cefaclor Extended Release 375-500 mg bid x 3-10 days
  Pediatric: <16 years: ext-rel not recommended; ≥16 years: same as adult
    Tab: 375, 500 mg ext-rel
▷ *cefdinir* 300 mg bid or 600 mg daily x 3-10 days
  Pediatric: <6 months: not recommended; 6 months-12 years: 14 mg/kg/day in a single or 2 divided doses x 3-10 days; *see* Appendix BB.10. *cefdinir* (G) (Omnicef Suspension) *for dose by weight*; >12 years: same as adult
    Omnicef *Cap:* 300 mg; *Oral susp:* 125 mg/5 ml (60, 100 ml) (strawberry)
▷ *cefpodoxime proxetil* 200 mg bid x 3-10 days
  Pediatric: 2 months-12 years: 10 mg/kg/day in 2 divided doses x 3-5 days; *see* Appendix BB.12. *cefpodoxime proxetil* (G) (Vantin Suspension) *for dose by weight*; >12 years: same as adult
    Vantin *Tab:* 100, 200 mg; *Oral susp:* 50, 100 mg/5 ml (50, 75, 100 ml) (lemon creme)
▷ *ceftaroline fosamil* administer by IV infusion after reconstitution q 12 hours x 3-10 days; *CrCl ≥50 ml/min:* 600 mg; *CrCl >30-<50 ml/min:* 400 mg; *CrCl: >15-<30 ml/min:* 300 mg; *End-stage renal disease (ESRD):* 200 mg
  Pediatric: <18 years: not recommended; ≥18 years: same as adult
    Teflaro *Vial:* 400, 600 mg
▷ *ceftriaxone* (G) 1-2 gm IM daily x 1-3 days
  Pediatric: 50-75 mg/kg IM in 2 divided doses; max 2 gm/day x 1-3 days
    Rocephin *Vial:* 250, 500 mg; 1, 2 gm

(continued)

▷ **clarithromycin (G)** 500 mg bid or 500 mg ext-rel once daily x 3-10 days
  Pediatric: <6 months: not recommended; ≥6 months: 7.5 mg/kg bid x 3-10 days
    Biaxin *Tab:* 250, 500 mg
    Biaxin Oral Suspension *Oral susp:* 125, 250 mg/5 ml (50, 100 ml) (fruit punch)
    Biaxin XL *Tab:* 500 mg ext-rel
▷ **dirithromycin (G)** 500 mg daily x 3-10 days
  Pediatric: <12 years: not recommended; ≥12 years: same as adult
    Dynabac *Tab:* 250 mg
▷ **doxycycline (G)** 100 mg bid x 3-10 days
  Pediatric: <8 years: not recommended; ≥8 years, ≤100 lb: 2 mg/lb on first day in 2 divided doses, followed
  by 1 mg/lb/day in 1-2 divided doses; ≥8 years, >100 lb: same as adult; *see Appendix BB.19. doxycycline (G)*
  (Vibramycin Syrup/Suspension) for dose by weight
    Acticlate *Tab:* 75, 150**mg
    Adoxa *Tab:* 50, 75, 100, 150 mg ent-coat
    Doryx *Tab:* 50, 75, 100, 150, 200 mg del-rel
    Doxteric *Tab:* 50 mg del-rel
    Monodox *Cap:* 50, 75, 100 mg
    Oracea *Cap:* 40 mg del-rel
    Vibramycin **Tab: 100 mg;** *Cap:* 50, 100 mg; *Syr:* 50 mg/5 ml (raspberry-apple) (sulfites); *Oral susp:* 25
    mg/5 ml (raspberry)
    Vibra-Tab *Tab:* 100 mg film-coat
▷ **ertapenem (G)** 1 gm daily; *CrCl <30 ml/min:* 500 mg daily x 3-10 days; may switch to an oral antibiotic after 3
  days if warranted; *IV infusion:* administer over 30 minutes; *IM injection:* reconstitute with **lidocaine** only
    Invanz *Vial:* 1 gm pwdr for reconstitution
▷ **erythromycin base (G)** 500 mg q 6 hours x 14-21 days; <45 kg: 30-50 mg in 2-4 doses x 3-10 days; ≥45 kg:
  same as adult
    Ery-Tab *Tab:* 250, 333, 500 mg ent-coat
    PCE *Tab:* 333, 500 mg
▷ **erythromycin estolate** 500 mg q 6 hours x 3-10 days
    Ilosone *Pulvule:* 250 mg; *Tab:* 500 mg; *Liq:* 125, 250 mg/5 ml (100 ml)
▷ **gemifloxacin (G)** 320 mg daily x 3-10 days
  Pediatric: <18 years: not recommended; ≥18 years: same as adult
    Factive *Tab:* 320*mg
▷ **levofloxacin** 250 mg once daily x 3-10 days
  Pediatric: <18 years: not recommended; ≥18 years: same as adult
    Levaquin *Tab:* 250, 500, 750 mg; *Oral soln:* 25 mg/ml (480 ml) (benzyl alcohol); *Inj conc:* 25 mg/ml for
    IV infusion after dilution (20, 30 ml single-use vial) (preservative-free); *Premix soln:* 5 mg/ml for IV
    infusion (50, 100, 150 ml) (preservative-free)
▷ **linezolid (G)** 400-600 mg q 12 hours x 10-14 days
  Pediatric: <5 years: 10 mg/kg q 8 hours x 10-14 days; 5-11 years: 10 mg/kg q 12 hours x 10-14 days; >11
  years: same as adult
    Zyvox *Tab:* 400, 600 mg; *Oral susp:* 100 mg/5 ml (150 ml) (orange) (phenylalanine)
  Comment: *Linezolid* is indicated to treat susceptible vancomycin-resistant *Enterococcus faecium* infections.
▷ **loracarbef** 400 mg bid x 3-10 days
  Pediatric: <12 years: 15 mg/kg/day in 2 divided doses x 7 days; *see Appendix BB.27. loracarbef (G)*
  (Lorabid Suspension) for dose by weight table; ≥12 years: 200 mg bid x 7 days
    Lorabid *Pulvule:* 200, 400 mg; *Oral susp:* 100 mg/5 ml (50, 100 ml), 200 mg/5 ml (50, 75, 100 ml)
    (strawberry bubble gum)
▷ **moxifloxacin (G)** 400 mg daily x 3-10 days
  Pediatric: <18 years: not recommended; ≥18 years: same as adult
    Avelox *Tab:* 400 mg; *IV soln:* 400 mg/250 mg (latex-free, preservative-free)
▷ **ofloxacin (G)** 400 mg bid x 3-10 days
  Pediatric: <18 years: not recommended; ≥18 years: same as adult
    Floxin *Tab:* 200, 300, 400 mg
▷ **penicillin v potassium (G)** 250-500 mg q 6 hours x 3-10 days
  Pediatric: <12 years: 25-75 mg/kg day divided q 6-8 hours x 5-7 days; *see Appendix BB.29. penicillin v*
  potassium (G) (Pen-Vee K Solution, Veetids Solution) for dose by weight table; ≥12 years: same as adult
    Pen-VK *Tab:* 250, 500 mg; *Oral soln:* 125 mg/5 ml (100, 200 ml), 250 mg/5 ml (100, 150, 200 ml)
▷ **tedizolid phosphate** administer 200 mg once daily x 6 days, via PO or IV infusion over 1 hour
    Sivextro *Tab:* 200 mg (6/blister pck)
  Comment: Sivextro is indicated for the treatment of community-acquired bacterial pneumonia (CABP).
▷ **telithromycin** 2 x 400 mg tabs in a single dose once daily x 3-5 days
  Pediatric: <8 years: not recommended; ≥8 years: same as adult
    Ketek *Tab:* 300, 400 mg
  Comment: *Telithromycin* is contraindicated with a history of hepatitis or jaundice associated with macrolide
  use.

▶ *tigecycline* (G) 100 mg once; then 50 mg q 12 hours x 3-5 days; *Severe hepatic impairment (Child-Pugh Class C):* 100 mg once; then 25 mg q 12 hours x 3-5 days
Pediatric: <18 years: not recommended; ≥18 years: same as adult
   Tygacil *Vial:* 50 mg pwdr for reconstitution and IV infusion (preservative-free)
   Comment: Tygacil is indicated only for the treatment of adults (≥18 years of age) with community-acquired bacterial pneumonia (CABP). *tigecycline* is contraindicated in pregnancy and lactation (discolors developing tooth enamel). A side effect may be photosensitivity (photophobia). Do not give with antacids, calcium supplements, milk or other dairy, or within 2 hours of taking another drug.
▶ *trimethoprim+sulfamethoxazole (TMP-SMX)* (G)
Pediatric: <2 months: not recommended; ≥2 months: 40 mg/kg/day of *sulfamethoxazole* in 2 doses bid x 3-10 days; *see* Appendix BB.33. *trimethoprim+ sulfamethoxazole* (Bactrim Suspension, Septra Suspension) *for dose by weight*
   Bactrim, Septra 2 tabs bid x 3-10 days
      Tab: trim 80 mg+sulfa 400 mg*
   Bactrim DS, Septra DS 1 tab bid x 3-10 days
      Tab: trim 160 mg+sulfa 800 mg*
   Bactrim Pediatric Suspension, Septra Pediatric Suspension 160/800 bid x 3-10 days
      Oral susp: trim 40 mg+sulfa 200 mg per 5 ml (100 ml) (cherry) (alcohol 0.3%)

AMINOMETHYLCYCLINE TETRACYCLINE

▶ *omadacycline Loading Dose* Day 1: 200 mg via IV infusion over 60 minutes or 100 mg via IV infusion over 30 minutes twice; *Maintenance:* 100 mg via IV infusion over 30 minutes once daily or 300 mg orally once daily; total treatment duration 7-14 days; before oral dosing, fast x at least 4 hours and then take tablets with water; after oral dosing, no food or drink (except water) x 2 hours and no dairy products, antacids, or multivitamins x 4 hours
Pediatric: <18 years: not recommended; ≥18 years: same as adult
   Nuzyra *Tab:* 150 mg; *Vial:* 100 mg, single-dose for reconstitution, dilution, and IV infusion
   Comment: Nuzyra *(omadacycline)* is an aminomethylcycline tetracycline antibiotic for the treatment of community-acquired bacterial pneumonia (CABP) and acute bacterial skin and skin structure infection (ABSSSI). The most common adverse reactions (incidence ≥2%) are nausea, vomiting, infusion site reactions, increased alanine aminotransferase (ALT), increased aspartate aminotransferase (AST), increased gamma-glutamyltransferase (GGT), hypertension, headache, diarrhea, insomnia, and constipation. Like other tetracycline-class antibacterial drugs, **Nuzyra** may cause discoloration of deciduous teeth and reversible inhibition of bone growth when administered during the 2nd and third trimesters of pregnancy. The limited available data of **Nuzyra** use in pregnancy are insufficient to inform drug-associated risk of major birth defects and miscarriages. There is no information on the presence of *omadacycline* in human milk or effects on the breastfed infant.

SEMISYNTHETIC PLEUROMUTILIN ANTIBIOTIC

▶ *lefamulin Tab:* 600 mg q 12 hours x 5 days; take at least 1 hour before or 2 hours after a meal; swallow whole with 6-8 oz of water; *Moderate-to-severe hepatic impairment (Child-Pugh Class B or C):* tablets have not been studied in and are not recommended; *IV infusion:* 150 mg q 12 hours x 5-7 days; infuse over 60 minutes; *Severe hepatic impairment (Child-Pugh Class C):* reduce the IV infusion dose to 150 mg q 24 hours
Pediatric: <18 years: not established; ≥18 years: same as adult
   Xenleta *Tab:* 600 mg; *Vial:* 150 mg/15 ml 0.9% NS, single-dose, for dilution and IV infusion
   Comment: Xenleta *(lefamulin)* is a first-in-class, semisynthetic pleuromutilin antibiotic for the treatment of community-acquired bacterial pneumonia (CABP). To reduce the development of drug-resistant bacteria and maintain effectiveness of **Xenleta** and other antibacterial drugs, **Xenleta** should be used only to treat or prevent infections that are proven or strongly suspected to be caused by bacteria. *IV Infusion:* Avoid use of **Xenleta** via IV infusion with concomitant strong or moderate CYP3A inducers or P-glycoprotein (P-gp) inducers, unless benefit outweighs risk, and monitor for reduced **Xenleta** efficacy. *Tablet:* Concomitant use of **Xenleta** tablets with CYP3A substrates that prolong the QT interval is contraindicated. Avoid use of **Xenleta** tablet in patients with known QT prolongation, ventricular arrhythmias including torsades de pointes, and patients receiving drugs that prolong the QT interval such as antiarrhythmic agents. Avoid **Xenleta** tablet with strong CYP3A inhibitors or P-gp inhibitors; monitor for adverse reactions with concomitant CYP3A inhibitors or P-gp inhibitors, **midazolam** (Versed), and other sensitive CYP3A substrates. The most common adverse reactions (incidence ≥2%) have been diarrhea, nausea, vomiting, and hepatic enzyme elevation for tab, and administration site reactions, hepatic enzyme elevation, nausea, hypokalemia, insomnia, and headache for IV infusion. Evaluate patients who develop diarrhea for *Clostridium difficile*-associated diarrhea (CDAD). **Xenleta** may cause embryo/fetal toxicity. Verify pregnancy status prior to initiation of treatment and advise females of reproductive potential of the potential risk and to use effective contraception for the duration of treatment and for 2 days after the final dose. There is a pregnancy pharmacovigilance program. If **Xenleta** is inadvertently administered during pregnancy or if the patient becomes pregnant while receiving **Xenleta**, healthcare providers should report **Xenleta** exposure by calling 1-855-5NABRIVA to enroll. Lactating females should pump and discard breast milk for the duration of treatment with **Xenleta** and for 2 days after the final dose.

PNEUMONIA: LEGIONELLA

ANTI-INFECTIVES

▷ *ciprofloxacin* 500 mg bid x 14-21 days
   Pediatric: <18 years: not recommended; ≥18 years: same as adult
      Cipro (G) *Tab:* 250, 500, 750 mg; *Oral susp:* 250, 500 mg/5 ml (100 ml) (strawberry)
      Cipro XR *Tab:* 500, 1,000 mg ext-rel
      ProQuin XR *Tab:* 500 mg ext-rel
▷ *clarithromycin* (G) 500 mg bid or 500 mg ext-rel once daily x 14-21 days
      Biaxin *Tab:* 250, 500 mg
      Biaxin Oral Suspension *Oral susp:* 125, 250 mg/5 ml (50, 100 ml) (fruit punch)
      Biaxin XL *Tab:* 500 mg ext-rel
▷ *dirithromycin* (G) 500 mg once daily x 14-21 days
      Dynabac *Tab:* 250 mg
▷ *erythromycin base* (G) 500 mg qid x 14-21 days
   Pediatric: <45 kg: 30-50 mg in 2-4 divided doses x 14-21 days; ≥45 kg: same as adult
      Ery-Tab *Tab:* 250, 333, 500 mg ent-coat
      PCE *Tab:* 333, 500 mg
▷ *erythromycin estolate* (G) 1-2 gm daily in divided doses x 14-21 days
   Pediatric: 30-50 mg/kg/day in divided doses x 14-21 days; *see Appendix BB.20. erythromycin* estolate (G)
   (Ilosone Suspension) *for dose by weight*
      Ilosone *Pulvule:* 250 mg; *Tab:* 500 mg; *Liq:* 125, 250 mg/5 ml (100 ml)
▷ *trimethoprim+sulfamethoxazole (TMP-SMX)* (G)
   Pediatric: <2 months: not recommended; ≥2 months: 40 mg/kg/day of *sulfamethoxazole* in 2 doses bid x 10
   days
      Bactrim, Septra 2 tabs bid x 10 days
         Tab: trim 80 mg+sulfa 400 mg*
      Bactrim DS, Septra DS 1 tab bid x 10 days
         Tab: trim 160 mg+sulfa 800 mg*
      Bactrim Pediatric Suspension, Septra Pediatric Suspension
         Oral susp: trim 40 mg+sulfa 200 mg per 5 ml (100 ml) (cherry) (alcohol 0.3%)

PNEUMONIA: MYCOPLASMA

ANTI-INFECTIVES

▷ *azithromycin* (G) 500 mg x 1 dose on day 1, then 250 mg daily on days 2-5 or 500 mg daily x 3 days or
   Zmax 2 gm in a single dose
   Pediatric: 12 mg/kg/day x 5 days; max 500 mg/day; *see Appendix BB.7. azithromycin* (G) (Zithromax
   Suspension, Zmax Suspension) *for dose by weight*
      Zithromax *Tab:* 250, 500, 600 mg; *Oral susp:* 100 mg/5 ml (15 ml), 200 mg/5 ml (15, 22.5, 30 ml)
      (cherry); *Pkt:* 1 gm for reconstitution (cherry-banana)
      Zithromax Tri-Pak *Tab:* 3 x 500 mg tabs/pck
      Zithromax Z-Pak *Tab:* 6 x 250 mg tabs/pck
      Zmax *Oral susp:* 2 gm ext-rel for reconstitution (cherry-banana) (148 mg Na$^+$)
▷ *clarithromycin* (G) 500 mg bid or 500 mg ext-rel once daily x 14-21 days
   Pediatric: <6 months: not recommended; ≥6 months: 7.5 mg/kg bid x 7 days; *see* Appendix BB.16.
   clarithromycin (G) (Biaxin Suspension) *for dose by weight*
      Biaxin *Tab:* 250, 500 mg
      Biaxin Oral Suspension *Oral susp:* 125, 250 mg/5 ml (50, 100 ml) (fruit-punch)
      Biaxin XL *Tab:* 500 mg ext-rel
▷ *erythromycin base* (G) 500 mg q 6 hours x 14-21 days
   Pediatric: <45 kg: 30-50 mg in 2-4 doses x 14-21 days; ≥45 kg: same as adult
      Ery-Tab *Tab:* 250, 333, 500 mg ent-coat
      PCE *Tab:* 333, 500 mg
▷ *erythromycin ethylsuccinate* (G) 400 mg qid x 14-21 days
   Pediatric: 30-50 mg/kg/day in 4 divided doses x 14-21 days; may double dose with severe infection; max
   100 mg/kg/day; *see* Appendix BB.21. *erythromycin ethylsuccinate* (G) (E.E.S. Suspension, EryPed Drops/
   Suspension) *for dose by weight*
      EryPed *Oral susp:* 200 mg/5 ml (100, 200 ml) (fruit), 400 mg/5 ml (60, 100, 200 ml) (banana); *Oral
      drops:* 200, 400 mg/5 ml (50 ml) (fruit); *Chew tab:* 200 mg wafer (fruit)
      E.E.S. *Oral susp:* 200, 400 mg/5 ml (100 ml) (fruit)
      E.E.S. Granules *Oral susp:* 200 mg/5 ml (100, 200 ml) (cherry)
      E.E.S. 400 Tablets *Tab:* 400 mg
▷ *tetracycline* (G) 500 mg qid
   Pediatric: <8 years: not recommended; ≥8 years, <100 lb: 25-50 mg/kg/day in 2-4 divided doses; ≥8 years,
   ≥100 lb: same as adult; *see* Appendix BB.31. *tetracycline* (G) (Sumycin Suspension) *for dose by weight*

Achromycin V *Cap:* 250, 500 mg
Sumycin *Tab:* 250, 500 mg; *Cap:* 250, 500 mg; *Oral susp:* 125 mg/5 ml (100, 200 ml) (fruit) (sulfites)

PNEUMONIA: PNEUMOCOCCAL

PNEUMOCOCCAL VACCINATION

The Advisory Committee on Immunization Practices (ACIP) recommends a routine single dose of PPSV23 (pneumococcal 23-valent polysaccharide vaccine) in adults age ≥65 years. If not previously administered PCV13, PCV13 is recommended by shared clinical decision-making in persons age ≥65 years who do not have an immunocompromising condition, cerebrospinal fluid leak, or cochlear implant. If PCV13 is to be administered, it should be administered first, followed by PPSV23 at least 1 year later.

TREATMENT

See Pneumonia: Community-Acquired (CAP) and Community-Acquired Bacterial Pneumonia (CABP)

PROPHYLAXIS

➤ *pneumococcal* vaccine 0.5 ml IM or SC in deltoid x 1 dose
  Pneumovax
  Pediatric: <2 years: not recommended; ≥2 years: same as adult
    Vial: 25 mcg/0.5 ml (single-dose, 10/pck; multidose, 2.5 ml, 10/pck)
  Pnu-Imune 23
  Pediatric: <2 years: not recommended; ≥2 years: same as adult
    Vial: 25 mcg/0.5 ml (0.5 ml single-dose, 5/pck; 2.5 ml)
  Prevnar 13 for adults ≥50 years of age
  Pediatric: total 4 doses: 2, 4, 6, and 12-15 months of age; may start at 6 weeks of age; administer first 3 doses 4-8 weeks apart and the 4th dose at least 2 months after the 3rd dose
    Vial: 25 mcg/0.5 ml (single-dose, 10/pck); *Prefilled syringe:* 0.5 ml (single-dose, 10/pck; 2.5 ml, multidose)
➤ *pneumococcal 20-valent conjugate vaccine* injection 0.5 ml IM as a one-time single dose in the deltoid muscle; ≥60 years: 0.5 ml IM as a one-time single dose (if not previously immunized with **Prevnar 20**)
  Pediatric: Infants: administer 0.5 ml IM in the anterolateral thigh; *Toddlers and young children:* administer 0.5 ml IM in the deltoid muscle; *Ages 6 weeks through 2 months, 4 months, 6 months, and 12 through 15 months:* administer 0.5 ml IM (total 4 doses according to age [the four-dose schedule]); *Age 15 months through 17 years:* administer 0.5 ml IM as a one-time single dose (if not previously immunized with **Prevnar 20**); *Age ≥18 years:* same as adult (if not previously immunized with the 4-dose series
  Prevnar 20 *Susp for IM injection: Prefilled syringe:* 0.5 ml, single-dose (1, 10/carton)
  Comment: Prevnar 20 *(pneumococcal 20-valent conjugate vaccine)* is a vaccine indicated for (1) patients 6 weeks of age and older for prevention of pneumonia and invasive disease caused by *Streptococcus pneumoniae* serotypes 1, 3, 4, 5, 6A, 6B, 7F, 8, 9V, 10A, 11A, 12F, 14, 15B, 18C, 19A, 19F, 22F, 23F, and 33F and (2) patients 6 weeks through 5 years of age for the prevention of otitis media (middle ear infection) caused by 7 of the 20 pneumococcal strains. **Prevnar 20** is approved under accelerated approval based on immune responses as measured by opsonophagocytic activity (OPA) assay; continued approval for this indication may be contingent upon verification and description of clinical benefit in a confirmatory trial. Do not freeze (discard if frozen). Administer as soon as possible after removal from refrigeration. Vaccine can be used as long as total time out of refrigeration (cumulative multiple excursions) does not exceed 96 hours. Store syringes in refrigerator horizontally to minimize resuspension time. Resuspend product by shaking vigorously until product is a homogenous white suspension; do not use if vaccine cannot be resuspended. Attach a sterile needle after resuspension. **Prevnar 20** is contraindicated in patients with a history of severe allergic reaction (e.g., anaphylaxis) to any component of **Prevnar 20** or to diphtheria toxoid. *Common Adverse Side Effects in Adults >60 years:* (incidence >10%) pain at the injection site (>50%), muscle pain and fatigue (>30%), headache (>20%), and arthralgia (>10%). *Common Adverse Side Effects in Adults 18-59 years:* (incidence >10%), pain at the injection site (>70%), muscle pain (>50%), fatigue (>40%), headache (>30%), and arthralgia and injection site swelling (>10%). *Common Adverse Side Effects in Pediatric Patients 5 Months Through 17 Years of age Vaccinated with A Single Dose:* (incidence >10%), irritability (<2 years of age, 60%), pain at the injection site (>50%), drowsiness (<2 years of age, >40%), fatigue and muscle pain (≥2 years of age, >20%), decreased appetite (<2 years of age, <20%), injection site swelling and injection site redness (>10%), headache (≥5 years of age, >10%), and fever (<2 years of age, >10%). *Common side effects in pediatric patients 2, 4, 6, and 12 through 15 months of age, vaccinated with a 4-dose schedule:* (incidence >10%), irritability (>60%), pain at the injection site (>30%), drowsiness (>30%), decreased appetite and injection site redness (>20%), injection site swelling (>10%), and fever (>10%). There are no data available on use of **Prevnar 20** in human pregnancy to inform a drug-related risk. An animal developmental toxicity study of administration of a single human dose prior to mating and during gestation revealed no evidence of harm to the fetus. There is no information regarding this drug on the presence in human milk or effects on the breastfed infant. Consider the developmental and health benefits of breastfeeding along with the mother's clinical need for this medication as well as any potential

(continued)

adverse effects from this drug or the underlying maternal condition. To report suspected adverse reactions, contact the Vaccine Adverse Event Reporting System (VAERS) at https://vaers.hhs.gov.

Effective April 2023—The U.S. FDA has approved **Prevnar 20** (*20-valent pneumococcal conjugate vaccine*) for the prevention of invasive pneumococcal disease (IPD) caused by the 20 *Streptococcus pneumoniae* (pneumococcal) serotypes contained in the vaccine in infants and children 6 weeks through 17 years of age, and for the prevention of otitis media in infants 6 weeks through 5 years of age caused by the original seven serotypes contained in **Prevnar**. The FDA's decision is based on results from the phase 2 and phase 3 clinical trial programs for the pediatric indication for **Prevnar 20**. Three core phase 3 pediatric studies contributed to data on the safety, tolerability, and immunogenicity of **Prevnar 20**, including previously announced positive, top-line results of the pivotal U.S. phase 3 study (NCT04382326). Further positive data from a proof-of-concept phase 2 study (NCT03512288) that assessed the safety and immunogenicity of **Prevnar 20** also supported the FDA's decision. —From www.Drugs.com

PNEUMONIA (*PNEUMOCYSTIS JIROVECII*)

QUINONE ANTIMICROBIAL

▷ *atovaquone* (G) take as a single dose with food or a milky drink at the same time each day; repeat dose if vomited within 1 hour; *Prophylaxis:* 1,500 mg once daily; *Treatment:* 750 mg bid x 21 days
Pediatric: <12 years: not recommended; ≥12 years: same as adult
Mepron *Susp:* 750 mg/5 ml (210 ml; 5 ml pouches) (citrus)
Comment: Mepron (*atovaquone*) suspension is a quinone antimicrobial drug indicated for the prevention of *Pneumocystis jirovecii* pneumonia (PCP) and treatment of mild-to-moderate PCP in adults and adolescents ≥13 years of age who cannot tolerate *trimethoprim+sulfamethoxazole (TMP-SMX)*. Treatment of severe PCP (alveolar arterial oxygen diffusion gradient [(A-a)DO2] >45 mm Hg) with **Mepron** and the efficacy of **Mepron** in subjects who are failing therapy with TMP-SMX have not been studied. Elevated liver chemistry tests and cases of hepatitis and fatal liver failure have been reported. Failure to administer **Mepron** suspension with food may result in lower plasma *atovaquone* concentrations and may limit response to therapy. Patients with gastrointestinal disorders may have limited absorption resulting in suboptimal *atovaquone* concentrations. Concomitant administration of the following drugs reduce *atovaquone* concentrations: *rifampin* and *rifabutin, tetracyclines,* and *metoclopramide*. Concomitant administration of *indinavir* reduces *indinavir* trough concentrations. The most frequent adverse reactions (≥25% that required discontinuation) attributed to **Mepron** taken for prophylaxis have been diarrhea, rash, headache, nausea, and fever. The most frequent adverse reactions (≥14% that required discontinuation) attributed to **Mepron** taken for prophylaxis have been rash (including maculopapular), nausea, diarrhea, headache, vomiting, and fever. There are no adequate and well-controlled studies of **Mepron** use in pregnancy. *Atovaquone* was not teratogenic and did not cause reproductive toxicity in animal studies at plasma concentrations up to 2 to 3 times the estimated human exposure (dose of 1,000 mg/kg/day). However, **Mepron** should be used during pregnancy only if the potential benefit justifies the potential risk to the fetus. It is not known whether *atovaquone* is excreted into human milk or the effects on the breastfed infant. In an animal study (with doses of 10 and 250 mg/kg), *atovaquone* concentrations in milk were 30% of the concurrent *atovaquone* concentrations in maternal plasma at both doses; therefore, caution should be exercised when **Mepron** is administered to patients who are breastfeeding.
▷ *trimethoprim+sulfamethoxazole (TMP-SMX)* (G) *Prophylaxis:* 1 tab 3 x/week; *Treatment:* 1 tab daily x 3 weeks; *Septra* can be given if intolerable to *Bactrim*
Pediatric: <2 months: not recommended; ≥2 months: 40 mg/kg/day of *sulfamethoxazole* in 2 doses bid x 10 days
Bactrim, Septra 2 tabs bid x 10 days
Tab: trim 80 mg+sulfa 400 mg*
Bactrim DS, Septra DS 1 tab bid x 10 days
Tab: trim 160 mg+sulfa 800 mg*
Bactrim Pediatric Suspension, Septra Pediatric Suspension
Oral susp: trim 40 mg+sulfa 200 mg per 5 ml (100 ml) (cherry) (alcohol 0.3%)

POLIOMYELITIS (POLIOVIRUS)

PROPHYLAXIS

▷ *trivalent poliovirus vaccine, inactivated (type 1, 2, and 3)*
Pediatric: <6 weeks: not recommended; ≥6 weeks: 1 dose at 2, 4, 6-18 months, and 1 dose at 4-6 years of age
Ipol 0.5 ml SC or IM in deltoid area

COMBINATION VACCINES

▷ **Pentacel** (DTaP-IPV/Hib) is commercially available as a kit containing single-dose vial of fixed-combination vaccine containing diphtheria, tetanus, pertussis, and poliovirus antigens (DTaP-IPV vaccine) and single-dose vial of lyophilized Hib vaccine (PRP-T; ActHIB). Prior to administration, reconstitute vial of lyophilized PRP-T (ActHIB) vaccine by adding the entire content of the vial of DTaP-IPV vaccine in the kit according to manufacturer's instructions to provide a combination vaccine containing diphtheria, tetanus, pertussis, IPV, and Hib antigens. Gently swirl until cloudy, uniform, white to off-white (yellow tinge) suspension is obtained. Administer IM immediately after reconstitution. **Pentacel** is approved for use as a four-dose series in children 6 weeks through 4 years of age (prior to the 5th birthday). **Pentacel** is to be administered as a 4-dose series at 2, 4, 6, and 15-18 months of age. The first dose may be given as early as 6 weeks of age. Four doses of **Pentacel** constitute a primary immunization course against pertussis. Three doses of **Pentacel** constitute an immunization course against diphtheria, tetanus, *Haemophilus influenzae*, type b invasive disease, and poliomyelitis; the fourth dose is a booster for diphtheria, tetanus, *H. influenzae*, type b invasive disease, and poliomyelitis immunizations. See mfr pkg insert for full prescribing information, including product storage, preparation, administration, contraindications, warnings, and precautions.

▷ **Vaxelis** *Vial:* 0.5 ml susp, single-dose; *Prefilled syringe:* 0.5 ml susp, single-dose (preservative-free)
Comment: **Vaxelis** is a single fixed-dose combination of six vaccines: diphtheria, tetanus toxoid, acellular pertussis, inactivated poliovirus, *Haemophilus* b conjugate, and hepatitis b (HBV). The 3-dose immunization series consists of a 0.5 ml IM injection, administered at 2, 4, and 6 months of age. See mfr pkg insert for full prescribing information, including product storage, preparation, administration, contraindications, warnings, and precautions.

POLYANGIITIS

CD20-DIRECTED CYTOLYTIC ANTIBODY

▷ *rituximab* *Induction:* 375 mg/m² via IV infusion once weekly x 4 weeks, in combination with glucocorticoids; *Follow up, patients who have achieved disease control with induction treatment, in combination with glucocorticoids:* two 500 mg IV infusions separated by 2 weeks, followed by one 500 mg IV infusion every 6 months thereafter, based on clinical evaluation; **Rituxan** should <u>only</u> be administered by a qualified healthcare professional with appropriate medical support to manage severe infusion-related reactions that can be fatal if they occur
Pediatric: <2 years: safety and efficacy <u>not</u> established; ≥2 years: *Induction:* 375 mg/m² via IV infusion once weekly x 4 weeks, in combination with glucocorticoids; *Follow up, patients who have achieved disease control with induction treatment, in combination with glucocorticoids:* two 250 mg/m² via IV infusions separated by 2 weeks, followed by one 250 mg/m² via IV infusion every 6 months thereafter, based on clinical evaluation; **Rituxan** should <u>only</u> be administered by a qualified healthcare professional with appropriate medical support to manage severe infusion-related reactions that can be fatal if they occur
    Rituxan *Vial:* 100 mg/10 ml (10 mg/ml), 500 mg/50 ml (10 mg/ml), single-dose, soln for dilution and IV infusion (preservative-free)
    Comment: **Rituxan** is indicated for the treatment of Wegener's granulomatosis, in combination with glucocorticoids, for adults and pediatric patients ≥2 years of age. The most adverse common reactions (incidence ≥15%) in clinical trials have been infections, nausea, diarrhea, headache, muscle spasms, anemia, peripheral edema, and infusion-related reactions. For tumor lysis syndrome (TLS), administer aggressive IV hydration and antihyperuricemic agents, and monitor renal function. Monitor for infections; withhold **Rituxan** and institute appropriate anti-infective therapy. For cardiac adverse reactions, discontinue infusions in case of serious <u>or</u> life-threatening events. Discontinue **Rituxan** in patients with rising serum creatinine <u>or</u> oliguria. Bowel obstruction and perforation can occur; consider and evaluate for abdominal pain, vomiting, <u>or</u> related symptoms. Live virus vaccinations prior to <u>or</u> during **Rituxan** treatment is <u>not</u> recommended. **Rituxan** is embryo/fetal toxic. Advise males and females of reproductive potential of the potential risk and to use effective contraception. Advise women <u>not</u> to breastfeed during treatment and for at least 6 months after the last dose.

▷ *rituximab-arrx* *Induction:* 375 mg/m² once weekly x 4 weeks; then if disease control is achieved, 500 mg via IV infusion x 2 doses separated by 2 weeks; then 500 mg via IV infusion once every 6 months based on clinical evaluation; administer <u>all</u> doses of **Riabni** in combination with glucocorticoids; **Riabni** should <u>only</u> be administered by a qualified healthcare professional with appropriate medical support to manage severe infusion-related reactions that can be fatal
Pediatric: safety and efficacy <u>not</u> established
    Riabni *Vial:* 100 mg/10 ml (10 mg/ml), 500 mg/50 ml (10 mg/ml) soln, single-dose
    Comment: **Riabni** *(rituximab-arrx)* is a biosimilar to **Rituxan** indicated for the treatment of adult patients with microscopic polyangiitis (MPA) in combination with glucocorticoids. The most common adverse reactions in clinical trials with MPA (incidence ≥15%) have been infections, nausea, diarrhea, headache, muscle spasms, anemia, peripheral edema, and infusion-related reactions. Monitor renal function. Discontinue **Riabni** in patients with rising serum creatinine <u>or</u> oliguria. If tumor lysis syndrome (TLS) is suspected, administer aggressive IV hydration and antihyperuricemic agents. If infection occurs, withhold **Riabni** and institute appropriate anti-infective therapy. Bowel obstruction and perforation can occur; evaluate for abdominal pain, vomiting, and related symptoms. Live virus vaccine administration

(continued)

prior to or during treatment with **Riabni** is not recommended. **Riabni** is embryo/fetal toxic. Advise females of reproductive potential of embryo/fetal risk and to use effective contraception. Advise not to breastfeed.

POLYCYSTIC KIDNEY DISEASE, AUTOSOMAL DOMINANT (ADPKD)

SELECTIVE VASOPRESSIN V2 RECEPTOR ANTAGONIST

➤ *tolvaptan* usual starting dose is 15 mg once daily with or without food; may titrate the dose once daily after at least 24 hours to 30 mg; then may titrate once daily dose to 60 mg as needed to achieve the desired level of serum sodium; do not administer for more than 30 days to minimize the risk of liver injury; initiation and reinitiation of therapy too should occur in a hospital environment to evaluate the therapeutic response and because too rapid correction of hyponatremia can cause osmotic demyelination resulting in dysarthria, mutism, dysphagia, lethargy, affective changes, spastic quadriparesis, seizures, coma, and death; avoid fluid restriction during the first 24 hours of therapy; patients receiving *tolvaptan* should be advised that they can continue ingestion of fluid in response to thirst; following discontinuation from *tolvaptan*, patients should be advised to resume fluid restriction and should be monitored for changes in serum sodium and volume status

Pediatric: <18 years: not established; ≥18 years: same as adult

    Jynarque *Tab:* 15, 30, 45, 60, 90 mg (7, 28/pck)

    Samsca *Tab:* 15, 30 mg

Comment: *Tolvaptan* is indicated to slow kidney function decline patients at risk of rapidly progressing autosomal dominant polycystic kidney disease (ADPKD). Further, *tolvaptan* is indicated for the treatment of clinically significant hypervolemic and euvolemic hyponatremia (serum sodium <125 mEq/L or less marked hyponatremia that is symptomatic and has resisted correction with fluid restriction), including patients with heart failure (HF) and syndrome of inappropriate antidiuretic hormone (SIAD). Contraindications to *tolvaptan* include use in patients with ADPKD outside of FDA-approved Risk Evaluation and Mitigation Strategy (REMS), patients requiring intervention to raise serum sodium urgently to prevent or to treat serious neurologic symptoms, patients unable to respond appropriately to thirst, hypovolemic hyponatremia, concomitant use of strong CYP 3A inhibitors, anuria, and hypersensitivity to the drug. Avoid use in patients with underlying liver disease; if hepatic injury is suspected, discontinue. Avoid use with CYP 3A inducers and moderate CYP 3A inhibitors. Dehydration and hypovolemia may require intervention. Avoid use with hypertonic saline. Consider dose reduction if co-administered with P-glycoprotein (P-gp) inhibitors. Monitor serum K^+ in patients with potassium >5 mEq/L or on drugs known to increase potassium. Based on animal data, *tolvaptan* may cause fetal harm. Discontinue *tolvaptan* or breastfeeding taking into consideration the importance of the drug to mother.

POLYCYSTIC OVARIAN SYNDROME (PCOS, STEIN-LEVENTHAL DISEASE)

See **Contraceptives**
See **Type 2 Diabetes Mellitus**

POLYCYTHEMIA VERA

INTERFERON ALFA-2b

➤ *ropeginterferon-alfa-2b-njft Recommended starting dose:* 100 mcg SC q 2 weeks (50 mcg if receiving hydroxyurea); increase by 50 mcg SC q 2 weeks; max 500 mcg/dose) until hematologic parameters are stabilized; interrupt or discontinue if certain adverse reactions occur

Pediatric: safety and efficacy not established

    Besremi *Prefilled syringe:* 500 mcg/ml, single-dose, solution for SC administration

Comment: **Besremi** is an interferon alfa-2b indicated for the treatment of adults with polycythemia vera (PV). **Besremi** received FDA orphan drug designation for this indication. Orphan drug designation provides incentives to assist and encourage drug development for rare diseases. **Besremi** is the first FDA-approved medication for polycythemia vera (PV) that patients can take regardless of their treatment history and the first interferon therapy specifically approved for PV. Untreated PV during pregnancy is associated with adverse maternal outcomes such as thrombosis and hemorrhage. Adverse pregnancy outcomes associated with PV include increased risk for miscarriage. *Boxed Warning:* Risk of serious disorders: Interferon alfa products may cause or aggravate fatal or life-threatening neuropsychiatric, autoimmune, ischemic, and infectious disorders. Monitor closely and withdraw therapy with persistently severe or worsening signs or symptoms of the above disorders. See mfr pkg insert for full prescribing information and complete boxed warning. **Besremi** is contraindicated with (1) existence of or history of severe psychiatric disorders, particularly severe depression, suicidal ideation, or suicide attempt; (2) hypersensitivity to interferon or to any component of **Besremi;** (3) hepatic impairment (Child-Pugh Class B or C); (4) history or presence of active serious or untreated autoimmune disease; and (5) immunosuppressed transplant recipients. Monitor for signs and symptoms of depression and suicideal ideation. Monitor for endocrine toxicity; discontinue **Besremi** if endocrine disorders occur that cannot be medically managed. Monitor for signs and symptoms of cardiovascular toxicity; avoid **Besremi** in patients with severe, acute, or unstable cardiovascular disease. Monitor patients with history of cardiovascular disorders more frequently. Obtain blood counts at baseline, every 2 weeks during titration, and at least every 3-6 months during maintenance treatment. For any hypersensitivity reactions, stop treatment and immediately manage the reaction. Consider discontinuation of **Besremi** if pancreatitis is confirmed. Discontinue **Besremi** for indications of colitis. Monitor for pulmonary toxicity and discontinue **Besremi** if pulmonary infiltrates develop or pulmonary function declines. Monitor for ophthalmologic toxicity; advise patients to have eye examinations before and during treatment. Evaluate eye symptoms promptly and discontinue **Besremi** if new or worsening eye disorder develops. Monitor serum triglycerides before **Besremi** treatment and intermittently during therapy and manage elevations. Monitor liver enzymes and hepatic function at baseline and during treatment; reduce dose or discontinue depending on severity. Monitor serum creatinine at baseline and during therapy and discontinue **Besremi** if severe renal impairment develops. Advise patients to maintain good oral hygiene and to have regular dental examinations as prophylaxis against dental and periodontal toxicity. Consider discontinuing if clinically significant dermatologic toxicity develop. Advise patients to avoid driving or using machinery if experience dizziness, somnolence, or hallucinations. Monitor patients taking CYP450 substrates with a narrow therapeutic index for adverse reactions to inform dose adjustment of the concomitant drug. Avoid use of **Besremi** with myelosuppressive agents and monitor patients receiving the combination for effects of excessive myelosuppression. Avoid use of **Besremi** with narcotics, hypnotics, or sedatives; monitor patients receiving the combination for excessive CNS toxicity. The most common adverse reactions reported in ≥40% of patients were influenza-like illness, arthralgia, fatigue, pruritus, nasopharyngitis, and musculoskeletal pain. Monitor patients taking CYP450 substrates with a narrow therapeutic index for adverse reactions to inform dose adjustment of the concomitant drug. Avoid use of **Besremi** with myelosuppressive agents and monitor patients receiving the combination for effects of excessive myelosuppression. Available data with **Besremi** use in human pregnancy are insufficient to identify a drug-associated risk of major birth defects, miscarriage, or adverse maternal or fetal outcomes. Animal studies assessing reproductive toxicity of **Besremi** have not been conducted. Based on mechanism of action and role of interferon alfa in pregnancy and fetal development, **Besremi** may cause fetal harm and should be assumed to have abortifacient potential when administered to a pregnant patient. Confirm pregnancy status prior to initiating **Besremi**. Advise females/males of reproductive potential to use effective contraception. There are no data on presence of **Besremi** in human or animal milk or effects on the breastfed infant. Because of potential for serious adverse reactions in breastfed infants from **Besremi**, advise mothers not to breastfeed during treatment and for 8 weeks after final dose. To report suspected adverse reactions, contact PharmaEssentia at 1-800-999-2449 or FDA at 1-800-FDA-1088 or www.fda.gov/medwatch.

▷ *ruxolitinib* initially 10 mg bid; therapeutic dose should be individualized based on safety and efficacy; *Renal impairment:* reduce starting dose or avoid use; *Hepatic impairment:* reduce starting dose or avoid use
Pediatric: safety and efficacy not established
Jakafi *Tab:* 5, 10, 15, 20, 25 mg
Comment: Jakafi *(ruxolitinib)* is a kinase inhibitor indicated for treatment of adults with intermediate- and high-risk myelofibrosis, including primary myelofibrosis, polycythemia vera (PV) with inadequate response to, or intolerance to, hydroxyurea, post-PV myelofibrosis, and postessential thrombocythemia myelofibrosis. Manage thrombocytopenia, anemia, and neutropenia with dose reduction, or treatment interruption, or transfusion. Serious infections should be resolved before starting therapy with Jakafi. Assess patients for signs and symptoms of infection during Jakafi therapy and initiate appropriate treatment promptly. Manage symptom exacerbation following interruption or discontinuation of Jakafi with supportive care and then consider resuming treatment with Jakafi. There is risk of non-melanoma skin cancer (NMSC) with Jakafi use; perform periodic skin examinations. Assess lipid levels 8-12 weeks from start of Jakafi therapy and treat as appropriate. Avoid use of Jakafi with *fluconazole* doses greater than 200 mg except in patients with acute graft versus host disease (GVHD). With myelofibrosis and PV, the most common hematologic adverse reactions (incidence >20%) have been thrombocytopenia and anemia, and the most common non-hematologic adverse reactions (incidence >10%) have been bruising, dizziness, and headache. There are no studies with the use of Jakafi in pregnant females to inform drug-associated risks. No data are available regarding the presence of *ruxolitinib* in human milk or the effects on the breastfed infant. Patients should be advised to discontinue breastfeeding during treatment with Jakafi and for 2 weeks after the final dose.

POLYMYALGIA RHEUMATICA

Oral Corticosteroids *see* Appendix K. Oral Corticosteroids
Calcium and Vitamin D Supplementation *see* Hypocalcemia

Comment: Initial treatment is low-dose prednisone at 12-25 mg/day. May attempt a very slow tapering regimen after 2-4 weeks. If relapse occurs, increase the daily dose of corticosteroid to the previous effective dose. Most people with polymyalgia rheumatica need to continue corticosteroid treatment for at least a year. Approximately 30%-60% of people will have at least one relapse during corticosteroid tapering. Joint guidelines from the American Academy of Rheumatology (AAR) and the European League Against Rheumatism (EULAR) suggest using concomitant *methotrexate* (MTX) along with corticosteroids in some patients. It may be useful early in the course of treatment or later, if the patient relapses or does not respond to corticosteroids. The AAR recommends the following daily doses for anyone on a chronic oral corticosteroid regimen: calcium 1,200-1,500 mg/day and vitamin D 800-1,000 IU/day.

METHOTREXATE

➤ *methotrexate* (MTX) 7.5 mg x 1 dose per week or 2.5 mg x 3 at 12-hour intervals once a week; max 20 mg/week; therapeutic response begins in 3-6 weeks; administer *MTX* injection SC only into the abdomen or thigh
Pediatric: <2 years: not recommended; ≥2 years: 10 mg/m² once weekly; max 20 mg/m²
   Rasuvo Autoinjector: 7.5 mg/0.15 ml, 10 mg/0.20 ml, 12.5 mg/0.25 ml, 15 mg/0.30 ml, 17.5 mg/0.35 ml, 20 mg/0.40 ml, 22.5 mg/0.45 ml, 25 mg/0.50 ml, 27.5 mg/0.55 ml, 30 mg/0.60 ml (solution concentration for SC injection is 50 mg/ml)
   Rheumatrex Tab: 2.5*mg (5, 7.5, 10, 12.5, 15 mg/week, 4/card unit dose pack)
   Trexall Tab: 5*, 7.5*, 10*, 15*mg (5, 7.5, 10, 12.5, 15 mg/week, 4/card unit dose pack)
Comment: *MTX* is contraindicated with immunodeficiency, blood dyscrasias, alcoholism, and chronic liver disease.

INTERLEUKIN-6 (IL-6) RECEPTOR ANTAGONIST

➤ *sarilumab* 200 mg SC q 2 weeks on the same day; if necessary, the dosage can be reduced 150 mg q 2 weeks to manage potential laboratory abnormalities, such as neutropenia, thrombocytopenia, and liver enzyme elevations; SC injections may be self-administered
Pediatric: safety and efficacy not established
   Kevzara Prefilled syringe: 150, 200 mg (1.4 ml, single-use)
   Comment: *Sarilumab* is a human monoclonal antibody that binds to the interleukin-6 receptor (IL-6R) and has been shown to inhibit IL-6R-mediated signaling. IL-6 is a cytokine in the body that, in excess and over time, can contribute to the inflammation associated with rheumatoid arthritis (RA). **Kevzara** is indicated for the treatment of adult patients with polymyalgia rheumatica and patients with active moderate-to-severe RA in adults who have had an inadequate response or intolerance to one or more disease-modifying antirheumatic drugs (DMARDs). **Kevzara** may be used as monotherapy or in combination with *MTX* or other conventional DMARDs. Monitor the patient for dose-related laboratory changes including elevated liver function tests (LFTs), neutropenia, and thrombocytopenia. **Kevzara** should not be initiated in patients with an absolute neutrophil count (ANC) <2,000/mm³, platelet count <150,000/mm³, or liver transaminases above 1.5 times the upper limit of normal (ULN). Registration in the Pregnancy Exposure Registry (1-877-311-8972) is encouraged for monitoring pregnancy outcomes in women exposed to **Kevzara** during pregnancy. Negative side effects of **Kevzara** should be reported to the FDA at www.fda.gov/medwatch or call 1-800-FDA-1088 or call Sanofi-Aventis at 1-800-633-1610. The limited available data with **Kevzara** in pregnant females are not sufficient to determine whether there is a drug-associated risk of major birth defects and miscarriage. Monoclonal antibodies, such as *sarilumab*, are actively transported across the placenta during the third trimester of pregnancy and may affect immune response in the infant exposed *in utero*. It is not known whether *sarilumab* passes into breast milk; therefore, breastfeeding is not recommended while using **Kevzara**.

POLYMYOSITIS, DERMATOMYOSITIS

➤ *immune globulin intravenous (human)* Dose: 2 g/kg divided in equal doses administered over 2-5 consecutive days q 4 weeks; *Initial infusion rate:* mg/kg/min (0.01 ml/kg/min); *Maintenance infusion rate:* up to 4 mg/kg/min (up to 0.04 ml/kg/min); patients >65 years or in any person at risk of developing renal insufficiency, do not exceed the recommended dose and infuse **Octagam** 10% at the minimum infusion rate practical
Pediatric: safety and efficacy not established
   Octagam 10% IgG (100 mg/ml), soln for IV infusion (vol: 20, 50, 100, 200, 300 ml) (protein: 2, 5, 10, 20, 30 gm, respectively)
   Comment: *Octagam* is a ready-to-use immunoglobulin intravenous (IGIV) product indicated for the treatment of primary humoral immunodeficiency, chronic immune thrombocytopenic purpura (ITP) and dermatomyositis. The most common adverse reactions reported (>5% of subjects during a clinical trial) in patients treated for dermatomyositis were headache, fever, nausea, vomiting, increased blood pressure, chills, musculoskeletal pain, increased heart rate, dyspnea, and infusions site reactions. *Boxed Warning:* thrombosis, renal dysfunction, and acute renal failure (ARF). See mfr pkg insert for full prescribing information and full boxed warning. Thrombosis may occur with IGIV products, including **Octagam** 10%. Risk factors may include advanced age, prolonged immobilization, hypercoagulable conditions, history of venous or arterial thrombosis, use of estrogens, indwelling vascular catheters, hyperviscosity, and cardiovascular risk factors. Renal dysfunction, acute renal failure (ARF), osmotic

nephropathy, and death may occur with the administration of IGIV products in predisposed patients. Renal dysfunction and ARF occur more commonly in patients receiving IGIV products containing sucrose. **Octagam 10%** does not contain sucrose. For patients at risk of thrombosis, renal dysfunction, or renal failure, administer **Octagam 10%** at the minimum practical infusion rate. Ensure adequate hydration in patients before administration. Monitor for signs and symptoms of thrombosis and assess blood viscosity in patients at risk for hyperviscosity. **Octagam 10%** is contraindicated with patient history of anaphylactic or severe systemic reactions to human immunoglobulin, immunoglobulin A (IgA)-deficient patients with antibodies against IgA, and a history of hypersensitivity. IgA-deficient patients with antibodies against IgA are at greater risk of developing severe hypersensitivity and anaphylactic reactions to **Octagam 10%**; epinephrine should be available immediately to treat any severe acute hypersensitivity reactions. Monitor renal function, including blood urea nitrogen (BUN) and serum creatinine (sCr), and urine output in patients at risk of developing ARF. Falsely elevated blood glucose readings may occur during and after the infusion of **Octagam 10%**. Hyperproteinemia, increased serum osmolarity, and hyponatremia may occur in patients receiving **Octagam 10%**. Hemolysis that is either intravascular or due to enhanced red blood cell sequestration can develop subsequent to **Octagam 10%** treatments. Risk factors for hemolysis include high doses and non-O-blood group; closely monitor patients for hemolysis and hemolytic anemia. Aseptic meningitis syndrome (AMS) may occur, especially with high doses or rapid infusion. Monitor patients for pulmonary adverse reactions (transfusion-related acute lung injury [TRALI]). **Octagam 10%** is made from human plasma and may contain infectious agents (e.g., viruses and theoretically the Creutzfeldt-Jakob disease agent). The passive transfer of antibodies may confound the results of sero logic testing and interfere with the immune response to live viral vaccines (such as measles, mumps, and rubella). There are no human or animal data; use only if clearly needed. It is not known whether **Octagam 10%** can cause fetal harm when administered to a pregnant patient or can affect reproduction capacity. Immune globulins cross the placenta from maternal circulation increasingly after 30 weeks of gestation. **Octagam 10%** should be administered to pregnant women only if clearly needed. No human data are available to assess the presence or absence of **Octagam 10%** in human milk or effects of **Octagam 10%** on the breastfed infant. Developmental and health benefits of breastfeeding should be considered along with the mother's clinical need for **Octagam 10%** and any potential adverse effects on the breastfed infant from **Octagam 10%** or from the underlying maternal condition. Immunoglobulins are excreted into the milk and may contribute to the transfer of protective antibodies to the neonate.

POLYNEUROPATHY, CHRONIC INFLAMMATORY DEMYELINATING (CIDP)

IMMUNE GLOBULIN, HUMAN

▷ *immune globulin subcutaneous (human) 20% liquid* initiate therapy with **Hizentra** 1 week after the last immunoglobulin intravenous (IGIV) infusion; recommended SC dose is 0.2 gm/kg (1 ml/kg) body weight per week, administered in 1 or 2 sessions over 1 or 2 consecutive days; in the clinical study after transitioning from IGIV to **Hizentra** treatment, a dose of 0.4 gm/kg (2 ml/kg) body weight per week was also safe and effective in preventing chronic inflammatory demyelinating polyneuropathy (CIDP) relapse; if CIDP symptoms worsen on 0.2 g/kg (1 ml/kg) body weight per week, consider increasing the **Hizentra** dose from 0.2 gm/kg (1 ml/kg) to 0.4 gm/kg (2 ml/kg) body weight per week, administered in 2 sessions per week over 1 or 2 consecutive days; if CIDP symptoms worsen on the 0.4 gm/kg body weight per week dose, consider reinitiating therapy with an IGIV product approved for treatment of CIDP, while discontinuing **Hizentra**; monitor the patient's clinical response and adjust the duration of therapy based on patient need; **Hizentra** is intended for SC administration using an infusion pump; infuse **Hizentra** in the upper arm, abdomen, thigh, and/or lateral hip; use up to eight infusion sites in parallel; using aseptic technique, pinch up the injection site with 2 fingers, clean the site, insert the needle straight into the site, and secure with sterile gauze and tape or transparent dressing to secure the needle in place; more than one infusion device can be used simultaneously; infusion sites should be at least 2 inches apart; change the actual site of infusion with each administration; inspect each prefilled syringe or vial of **Hizentra**; do not use the prefilled syringe or vial if the liquid looks cloudy, contains particles, has changed color, the protective cap of the prefilled syringe or the vial is missing or defective, or the expiration date on the label has passed; Do not use the prefilled syringe or vial if the liquid looks cloudy, contains particles, has changed color, the protective cap of the prefilled syringe or the vial is missing or defective, or the expiration date on the label has passed. Do not mix **Hizentra** with other products; do not shake the prefilled syringe or vial; use aseptic technique when preparing and administering this product; both the **Hizentra** prefilled syringe and vial are single-dose containers; multiple **Hizentra** prefilled syringes or vials can be administered to achieve the prescribed dose; discard all used administration supplies and any unused product immediately after each infusion in accordance with local requirements; *Volume:* for the first infusion of **Hizentra**, do not exceed a volume of 20 ml per infusion site in patients with CIDP; for subsequent infusions, the volume may be increased up to 50 ml per site for patients with CIDP; *Rate:* for the first infusion of **Hizentra**, the recommended flow rate is 20 ml per hour per site in patients with CIDP; for subsequent infusions, the flow rate may be increased up to 50 ml per hour per site in patients with CIDP
Pediatric: <18 years: safety and efficacy not established; ≥18 years: same as adult

(continued)

Hizentra *Vial:* 0.2 gm/ml (20%) (5, 10, 20, 50 ml); *Prefilled syringe:* 0.2 gm/ml (20%) (5, 10, 20 ml), single-dose, protein solution for SC infusion

Comment: Hizentra is indicated for the treatment of patients with primary humoral immunodeficiency (PI) and chronic inflammatory demyelinating polyneuropathy (CIDP). Patients with CIDP require maintenance therapy to prevent relapse of neuromuscular disability and impairment. The most common adverse reactions (ARs) observed in ≥5% of study subjects receiving **Hizentra** were local reactions (e.g., swelling, redness, heat, pain, hematoma, and itching at the infusion site), headache, diarrhea, fatigue, back pain, nausea, pain in extremity, cough, upper respiratory tract infection, rash, pruritus, vomiting, abdominal pain (upper), migraine, arthralgia, pain, fall, and nasopharyngitis. **Hizentra** is contraindicated in patients with (1) history of anaphylactic or severe systemic reaction to human immune globulin or inactive ingredients of **Hizentra**, such as polysorbate 80; (2) hyperprolinemia type I or II because it contains L-proline as a stabilizer; and (3) immunoglobulin A (IgA) deficiency with antibodies against IgA and a history of hypersensitivity. Acute renal dysfunction/failure, acute tubular necrosis, proximal tubular nephropathy, osmotic nephrosis, and death may occur with use of human immune globulin products, especially those containing sucrose. (NOTE: **Hizentra** does not contain sucrose.) Ensure that patients are not volume depleted before administering **Hizentra**. For patients judged to be at risk for developing renal dysfunction, including patients with any degree of preexisting renal insufficiency, diabetes mellitus, age >65 years, volume-depletion, sepsis, paraproteinemia, or patients receiving known nephrotoxic drugs, monitor renal function and consider lower, more frequent dosing. Periodic monitoring of renal function and urine output is particularly important in patients judged to have a potential increased risk of developing acute renal failure. Assess renal function, including measurement of blood urea nitrogen (BUN) and serum creatinine, before the initial infusion of **Hizentra** and at appropriate intervals thereafter. If renal function deteriorates, consider discontinuing **Hizentra**. Non-cardiogenic pulmonary edema may occur in patients administered human immune globulin products. *Transfusion-related acute lung injury* (TRALI) is characterized by severe respiratory distress, pulmonary edema, hypoxemia, normal left ventricular, function, and fever. If TRALI is suspected, perform appropriate tests for the presence of antineutrophil antibodies in both the product and the patient's serum. Typically, it occurs within 1 to 6 hours following transfusion. Patients with TRALI may be managed using oxygen therapy with adequate ventilatory support. Thrombosis may occur with immune globulin products1-3, including **Hizentra**. Risk factors may include advanced age, prolonged immobilization, hypercoagulable conditions, history of venous or arterial thrombosis, use of estrogens, indwelling central vascular catheters, hyperviscosity, and cardiovascular risk factors. Thrombosis may occur in the absence of known risk factors. For patients at risk of thrombosis, administer **Hizentra** at the minimum dose and infusion rate practicable. Ensure adequate hydration in patients before administration. Monitor for signs and symptoms of thrombosis and assess blood viscosity in patients at risk for hyperviscosity. **Hizentra** can contain blood group antibodies that may act as hemolysins and induce *in vivo* coating of red blood cells (RBCs) with immunoglobulin, causing a positive direct antiglobulin (Coombs') test result and hemolysis. Delayed hemolytic anemia can develop subsequent to immune globulin therapy due to enhanced RBC sequestration, and acute hemolysis, consistent with intravascular hemolysis, has been reported. Aseptic meningitis syndrome (AMS) has been reported with use of immune globulin intravenous (IGIV) or immune globulin subcutaneous (IGSC), including **Hizentra**. The syndrome usually begins within several hours to 2 days following immune globulin treatment. AMS is characterized by the following signs and symptoms: severe headache, nuchal rigidity, drowsiness, fever, photophobia, painful eye movements, nausea, and vomiting. Cerebrospinal fluid (CSF) studies frequently show pleocytosis up to several thousand cells per cubic millimeter, predominantly from the granulocytic series, and elevated protein levels up to several hundred mg/dL. AMS may occur more frequently in association with high doses (≥2 gm/kg) and/or rapid infusion of immune globulin product. Patients exhibiting such signs and symptoms should receive a thorough neurologic examination, including CSF studies, to rule out other causes of meningitis. Discontinuation of immune globulin treatment has resulted in remission of AMS within several days without sequelae. *Switching to* **Hizentra** *From IGIV*: Establish the initial weekly dose of **Hizentra** by converting the monthly IGIV dose into a weekly equivalent and increasing it using the dose adjustment factor. The goal is to achieve a systemic serum immunoglobulin G (IgG) exposure (area under the concentration-time curve [AUC]) not inferior to that of the previous IGIV treatment. To calculate the initial weekly dose of **Hizentra**, divide the previous IGIV dose in grams by the number of weeks between doses during the patient's IGIV treatment (e.g., 3 or 4); then multiply this by the dose adjustment factor of 1.37. *Switching to* **Hizentra** *From IGSC*: The previous weekly IGSC dose should be maintained. For biweekly dosing, multiply the previous weekly dose by 2. For frequent dosing (2 to 7 times per week), divide the previous weekly dose by the desired number of times per week (e.g., for 3 times per week dosing, divide weekly dose by 3). *Measles Exposure:* Administer a minimum total weekly **Hizentra** dose of 0.2 gm/kg body weight for 2 consecutive weeks if a patient is *at risk* of measles exposure (i.e., due to an outbreak in the United States or travel to endemic areas outside of the United States). For biweekly dosing, one infusion of a minimum at 400 mg/kg is recommended. If a patient has *been exposed* to measles, ensure this minimum dose is administered as soon as possible after exposure. No human data are available to indicate the presence or absence of drug-associated fetal risk. Animal reproduction studies have not been conducted with **Hizentra**. It is not known whether **Hizentra** can cause fetal harm when administered to a pregnant female. However, it is known that immune globulins cross the placenta from maternal circulation increasingly after 30 weeks gestation. Therefore, **Hizentra** should be administered in pregnancy only if clearly needed. No human data are available to indicate the presence or absence of drug-associated risk to the breastfeeding infant. Developmental and health benefits of breastfeeding should be considered along with the mother's clinical need for **Hizentra** and any potential adverse effects on the breastfed infant from **Hizentra** or from the underlying maternal condition.

POLYPS: NASAL

LONG-ACTING CORTICOSTEROID SINUS IMPLANT

▶ *mometasone furoate* the **Sinuva Sinus Implant** must be inserted by a physician trained in otolaryngology; the implant is loaded into a sterile delivery system supplied with the implant and placed in the ethmoid sinus under endoscopic visualization; the implant is left in the sinus to gradually release the corticosteroid over 90 days; the implant is removed at Day 90 or earlier at the physician's discretion using standard surgical instruments; repeat administration has not been studied
Pediatric: <18 years: not established: ≥18 years: same as adult
  Sinuva Sinus Implant *Sinus implant:* 1,350 mcg w. sterile delivery system
  Comment: Sinuva is a corticosteroid-eluting sinus implant indicated for the treatment of recurrent nasal polyp disease in patients who have ethmoid sinus surgery. Monitor nasal mucosa adjacent to the **Sinuva Sinus Implant** for any signs of bleeding (epistaxis), irritation, infection, or perforation. Avoid use in patients with nasal ulcers or trauma. Monitor patients with a change in vision or with a history of increased intraocular pressure, glaucoma, and/or cataracts closely. Potential worsening of existing tuberculosis; fungal, bacterial, viral, parasitic infection, or ocular herpes simplex. More serious or even fatal course of chickenpox or measles in susceptible patients. If corticosteroid effects such as hypercorticism and adrenal suppression appear in patients, consider sinus implant removal.

NASAL SPRAY CORTICOSTEROIDS

▶ *beclomethasone dipropionate*
  Beconase 1 spray in each nostril bid-qid
  Pediatric: <6 years: not recommended; 6-12 years: 1 spray in each nostril tid; >12 years: same as adult
    Nasal spray: 42 mcg/actuation (6.7 gm, 80 sprays; 16.8 gm, 200 sprays)
  Beconase AQ 1-2 sprays in each nostril bid
  Pediatric: <6 years: not recommended; ≥6 years: same as adult
    Nasal spray: 42 mcg/actuation (25 gm, 180 sprays)
  Beconase Inhalation Aerosol 1-2 sprays in each nostril bid-qid
  Pediatric: <6 years: not recommended; 6-12 years: 1 spray in each nostril tid; >12 years: same as adult
    Nasal spray: 42 mcg/actuation (6.7 gm, 80 sprays; 16.8 gm, 200 sprays)
  Vancenase AQ 1-2 sprays in each nostril bid
  Pediatric: <6 years: not recommended; ≥6 years: same as adult
    Nasal spray: 84 mcg/actuation (25 gm, 200 sprays)
  Vancenase AQ DS 1-2 sprays in each nostril once daily
  Pediatric: <6 years: not recommended; ≥6 years: same as adult
    Nasal spray: 84, 168 mcg/actuation (19 gm, 120 sprays)
  Vancenase Pockethaler 1 spray in each nostril bid or qid
  Pediatric: <6 years: not recommended; ≥6 years: 1 spray in each nostril tid
    Pockethaler: 42 mcg/actuation (7 gm, 200 sprays)
  QNASL Nasal Aerosol 2 sprays, 80 mcg/spray, in each nostril once daily
  Pediatric: <12 years: 2 sprays, 40 mcg/spray, in each nostril once daily; ≥12 years: same as adult
    Nasal spray: 40 mcg/actuation (4.9 gm, 60 sprays), 80 mcg/actuation (8.7 gm, 120 sprays)
▶ *budesonide*
  Rhinocort initially 2 sprays in each nostril bid in the AM and PM, or 4 sprays in each nostril in the AM; max 4 sprays each nostril/day; use lowest effective dose
  Pediatric: <6 years: not recommended; ≥6 years: same as adult
    Nasal spray: 32 mcg/actuation (7 gm, 200 sprays)
  Rhinocort Aqua Nasal Spray initially 1 spray in each nostril once daily; max 4 sprays in each nostril once daily
  Pediatric: <6 years: not recommended; ≥6-12 years: initially 1 spray in each nostril once daily; max 2 sprays in each nostril once daily
    Nasal spray: 32 mcg/actuation (10 ml, 60 sprays)
▶ *ciclesonide*
  Pediatric: <6 years: not recommended; ≥6 years: same as adult
  Omnaris 2 sprays in each nostril once daily
    Nasal spray: 50 mcg/actuation (12.5 gm, 120 sprays)
  Zetonna 1-2 sprays in each nostril once daily
    Nasal spray: 37 mcg/actuation (6.1 gm, 60 sprays) (HFA)

(continued)

▷ *dexamethasone* 2 sprays in each nostril bid-tid; max 12 sprays/day; maintain at lowest effective dose
  Pediatric: <6 years: not recommended; ≥6-12 years: 1-2 sprays in each nostril bid; max 8 sprays/day; maintain at lowest effective dose; >12 years: same as adult
      Dexacort Turbinaire *Nasal spray:* 84 mcg/actuation (12.6 gm, 170 sprays)

▷ *flunisolide* 2 sprays in each nostril bid; may increase to 2 sprays in each nostril tid; max 8 sprays/nostril/day
  Pediatric: <6 years: not recommended; 6-14 years: initially 1 spray in each nostril tid or 2 sprays in each nostril bid; max 4 sprays/nostril/day; >14 years: same as adult
      Nasalide *Nasal spray:* 25 mcg/actuation (25 ml, 200 sprays)
      Nasarel *Nasal spray:* 25 mcg/actuation (25 ml, 200 sprays)

▷ *fluticasone furoate* 2 sprays in each nostril once daily; may reduce to 1 spray each nostril once daily
  Pediatric: <2 years: not recommended; ≥2-11 years: 1 spray in each nostril once daily; ≥12 years: same as adult
      Veramyst *Nasal spray:* 27.5 mcg/actuation (10 gm, 120 sprays) (alcohol-free)

▷ *fluticasone propionate*
      Flonase (OTC) (G) initially 2 sprays in each nostril once daily or 1 spray bid; maintenance 1 spray once daily
      Pediatric: <4 years: not recommended; ≥4 years: initially 1 spray in each nostril once daily; may increase to 2 sprays in each nostril once daily; maintenance 1 spray in each nostril once daily; max 2 sprays in each nostril/day
        Nasal spray: 50 mcg/actuation (16 gm, 120 sprays)
      Xhance 1 spray per nostril bid (total daily dose 372 mcg); 2 sprays per nostril bid may also be effective in some patients (total daily dose 744 mcg)
      Pediatric: <12 years: not established; ≥12 years: same as adult
        Nasal spray: 93 mcg/actuation (16 ml, 120 metered sprays)
  Comment: Available data from published literature on the use of inhaled or intranasal *fluticasone propionate* in pregnant females have not reported a clear association with adverse developmental outcomes. There are no available data on the presence of *fluticasone propionate* in human milk or effects on the breastfed infant. The safety and efficacy of **Xhance** in pediatric patients have not been established.

▷ *mometasone furoate* **(G)** 2 sprays in each nostril once daily
  Pediatric: <2 years: not recommended; 2-11 years: 1 spray in each nostril once daily; >11 years: same as adult
      Nasonex *Nasal spray:* 50 mcg/actuation (17 gm, 120 sprays)

▷ *mometasone furoate monohydrate* **(OTC) (G)** 1-2 sprays in each nostril once daily
  Pediatric: <2 years: not recommended; 2-11 years: 1 spray in each nostril once daily; ≥11 years: same as adult
      Nasonex 24HR Allergy
      Comment: Nasonex 24HR Allergy is a corticosteroid nasal spray for the temporary relief of the symptoms of hayfever or other upper respiratory allergies.

▷ *olopatadine* 2 sprays in each nostril bid
  Pediatric: <6 years: not recommended; 6-11 years: 1 spray each nostril bid; >11 years: same as adult
      Patanase *Nasal spray:* 0.6%; 665 mcg/actuation (30.5 gm, 240 sprays) (benzalkonium chloride)

▷ *triamcinolone acetonide* **(G)** initially 2 sprays in each nostril once daily; max 4 sprays in each nostril once daily or 2 sprays in each nostril bid or 1 spray in each nostril qid; maintain at lowest effective dose
  Pediatric: <6 years: not recommended; ≥6 years: 1 spray in each nostril once daily; max 2 sprays in each nostril once daily
      Nasacort Allergy 24HR (OTC) *Nasal spray:* 55 mcg/actuation (10 gm, 120 sprays)
      Tri-Nasal *Nasal spray:* 50 mcg/actuation (15 ml, 120 sprays)

POLYURIA: NOCTURNAL

VASOPRESSIN ANALOG

▷ *desmopressin acetate* administer a single sublingual dose 1 hour prior to bedtime; *Females:* 27.7 mcg; *Males:* 55.3 mcg
      Nocdurna *SL tab:* 27.7, 55.3 mcg
      Comment: Nocdurna is a vasopressin analog and the first sublingual tab indicated for the treatment of nocturia due to nocturnal polyuria in adults. **Nocdurna** is indicated for patients ≥18 years of age with nocturnal polyuria who awaken at least 2 x/night to void. **Nocdurna** is available in two strengths: 27.7 mcg of *desmopressin acetate* (equivalent to 25 mcg of *desmopressin*) and 55.3 mcg of *desmopressin acetate* and dose is gender-based. **Nocdurna** is contraindicated with the following conditions: hyponatremia or a history of hyponatremia, polydipsia, concomitant use with loop diuretics or systemic or inhaled glucocorticoids, estimated glomerular filtration rate (eGFR) <50 ml/min/1.73 m^2, syndrome of inappropriate antidiuretic hormone secretion (SIADH), during illnesses that can cause fluid or electrolyte imbalance, heart failure (HF), and uncontrolled hypertension. **Nocdurna** can cause hyponatremia, which may be life-threatening if severe. Ensure serum sodium concentration is normal before starting or resuming **Nocdurna**. Measure serum sodium within 1 week and approximately 1 month after initiating therapy and periodically during treatment. Monitor serum sodium more

frequently in patients ≥65 years of age and in patients at increased risk of hyponatremia. Monitor serum sodium more frequently when **Nocdurna** is concomitantly used with drugs that may increase the risk of hyponatremia (e.g., tricyclic antidepressants [TCAs], selective serotonin reuptake inhibitors [SSRIs], *chlorpromazine*, opiate analgesics, thiazide diuretics, NSAIDs, *lamotrigine*, *chlorpropamide*, and *carbamazepine*). Nocdurna is not recommended in patients at risk of increased intracranial pressure or history of urinary retention. Limit fluid intake to a minimum from 1 hour before until 8 hours after administration; treatment without concomitant reduction of fluid intake may lead to fluid retention and hyponatremia. If hyponatremia occurs, **Nocdurna** may need to be temporarily or permanently discontinued. Use of **Nocdurna** is not recommended for the treatment of nocturia in pregnancy (nocturia is usually related to normal, physiologic changes during pregnancy that do not require treatment). There are no data with **Nocdurna** use in pregnancy to inform any drug-associated risks. *Desmopressin* is present in small amounts in human milk; however, there is no information on the effects of *desmopressin* on the breastfed infant.

POSTHERPETIC NEURALGIA (PHN)

Acetaminophen for IV Infusion *see Pain*
Oral Analgesics *see Pain*

GAMMA AMINOBUTYRIC ACID ANALOGS

Comment: The gabapentinoids (*gabapentin* [Gralise, Neurontin, Horizant] and *pregabalin* [Lyrica]) have respiratory depression risk potential. Therefore, when co-prescribed with other central nervous system (CNS) depressant agents, initiate the gabapentinoid at the lowest possible dose and monitor the patient for respiratory depression (especially elders and patients with compromised pulmonary function). Side effects include fatigue, somnolence/sedation, dizziness, vertigo, feeling drunk, headache, nausea, and dry mouth. To discontinue a gabapentinoid, withdraw gradually over 1 week or longer.

► *gabapentin* CrCl 30-60 ml/min: 600-1,800 mg; CrCl <30 ml/min or on hemodialysis: not recommended
 Gralise initially 300 mg on Day 1; then 600 mg on Day 2; then 900 mg on Days 3-6; then 1,200 mg on Days 7-10; then 1,500 mg on Days 11-14; titrate up to 1,800 mg on Day 15; take entire dose once daily with the evening meal; do not crush, split, or chew
 Pediatric: <18 years: not recommended; ≥18 years: same as adult
 Tab: 300, 600 mg
 Neurontin (G) 300 mg daily x 1 day, then 300 mg bid x 1 day, then 300 mg tid continuously; max 1,800 mg/day in 3 divided doses; taper over 7 days
 Pediatric: <3 years: not recommended; 3-12 years: initially 10-15 mg/kg/day in 3 divided doses; max 12 hours between doses, titrate over 3 days; 3-4 years: titrate to 40 mg/kg/day; 5-12 years: titrate to 25-35 mg/kg/day, max 50 mg/kg/day
 Tab: 600*, 800*mg; *Cap:* 100, 300, 400 mg
 Neurontin Oral Solution (G) *Oral soln:* 250 mg/5 ml (480 ml) (strawberry-anise)
► *gabapentin enacarbil* 600 mg once daily at about 5:00 PM; if dose not taken at recommended time, next dose should be taken the following day; swallow whole; take with food; CrCl 30-59 ml/min: 600 mg on Day 1, Day 3, and every day thereafter; CrCl <30 ml/min or on hemodialysis: not recommended
 Pediatric: <18 years: not recommended; ≥18 years: same as adult
 Horizant *Tab:* 300, 600 mg ext-rel
► *pregabalin (GABA analog)* (V)
 Pediatric: <12 years: not recommended; ≥12 years: same as adult
 Lyrica initially 50 mg tid; may titrate to 100 mg tid within 1 week; max 600 mg divided tid; discontinue over 1 week
 Cap: 25, 50, 75, 100, 150, 200, 225, 300 mg; *Oral soln:* 20 mg/ml
 Lyrica CR *Tab:* usual dose: 165 mg once daily; may increase to 330 mg/day within 1 week; max 660 mg/day
 Tab: 82.5, 165, 330 mg ext-rel

Tricyclic Antidepressants (TCAs)

Comment: Co-administration of selective serotonin reuptake inhibitors (SSRIs) and tricyclic antidepressants (TCAs) requires extreme caution.

► *amitriptyline* (G) initially 75 mg/day in divided doses of 50-100 mg/day q HS; max 300 mg/day
 Pediatric: <12 years: not recommended; ≥12 years: same as adult
 Tab: 10, 25, 50, 75, 100, 150 mg
► *amoxapine* initially 50 mg bid-tid; after 1 week may increase to 100 mg bid-tid; usual effective dose 200-300 mg/day; if total dose exceeds 300 mg/day, give in divided doses (max 400 mg/day); may give as a single bedtime dose (max 300 mg q HS)
 Pediatric: <12 years: not recommended; ≥12 years: same as adult
 Tab: 25, 50, 100, 150 mg

(continued)

▷ *desipramine* **(G)** 100-200 mg/day in single or divided doses; max 300 mg/day
  Pediatric: <12 years: not recommended; ≥12 years: same as adult
    Norpramin *Tab:* 10, 25, 50, 75, 100, 150 mg
▷ *doxepin* **(G)** 75 mg/day; max 150 mg/day
  Pediatric: <12 years: not recommended; ≥12 years: same as adult
    Cap: 10, 25, 50, 75, 100, 150 mg; *Oral conc:* 10 mg/ml (4 oz w. dropper)
▷ *imipramine* **(G)**
  Pediatric: <12 years: not recommended; ≥12 years: same as adult
    Tofranil initially 75 mg daily (max 200 mg); adolescents initially 30-40 mg daily (max 100 mg/day); if
    maintenance dose exceeds 75 mg daily, may switch to **Tofranil PM** for divided or bedtime dose
      Tab: 10, 25, 50 mg
    Tofranil PM initially 75 mg daily 1 hour before HS; max 200 mg
      Cap: 75, 100, 125, 150 mg
    Tofranil Injection 50 mg IM; lower dose for adolescents; switch to oral form as soon as possible
      Amp: 25 mg/2 ml (2 ml)
▷ *nortriptyline* **(G)** initially 25 mg tid-qid; max 150 mg/day
  Pediatric: <12 years: not recommended; ≥12 years: same as adult
    Pamelor *Cap:* 10, 25, 50, 75 mg; *Oral soln:* 10 mg/5 ml (16 oz)
▷ *protriptyline* initially 5 mg tid; usual dose 15-40 mg/day in 3-4 divided doses; max 60 mg/day
  Pediatric: <12 years: not recommended; ≥12 years: same as adult
    Vivactil *Tab:* 5, 10 mg
▷ *trimipramine* initially 75 mg/day in divided doses; max 200 mg/day
  Pediatric: <12 years: not recommended; ≥12 years: same as adult
    Surmontil *Cap:* 25, 50, 100 mg

ALPHA-2 DELTA LIGAND
▷ *pregabalin* **(GABA analog) (V) (G)** initially 150 mg daily divided bid-tid and may titrate within 1 week; max
  600 mg divided bid-tid; discontinue over 1 week
  Pediatric: <18 years: not recommended; ≥18 years: same as adult
    Lyrica *Cap:* 25, 50, 75, 100, 150, 200, 225, 300 mg; *Oral soln:* 20 mg/ml

TOPICAL AND TRANSDERMAL ANALGESICS
▷ *capsaicin* 8% patch apply up to 4 patches for one 60-minute application to clean dry skin; may prep area
  with topical anesthetic; wear non-latex gloves; patches may be cut to size/shape; treatment may be repeated
  every 3 months
  Pediatric: <18 years: not recommended; ≥18 years: same as adult
    Qutenza *Patch:* 8% 1,640 mcg/cm (179 mg) (1 or 2 patches w. 1-50 gm tube cleansing gel/carton)
▷ *diclofenac sodium* apply qid prn to intact skin
  Pediatric: <12 years: not established; ≥12 years: same as adult
    Pennsaid 1.5% in 10 drop increments, dispense and rub into front, side, and back of knee: usually 40
    drops (40 mg) qid
      Topical soln: 1.5% (150 ml)
    Pennsaid 2% apply 2 pump actuations (40 mg) and rub into front, side, and back of knee bid
      Topical soln: 2% (20 mg/pump actuation, 112 gm)
    Solaraze Gel massage into clean skin bid prn
      Gel: 3% (50 gm) (benzyl alcohol)
    Voltaren Gel (G)(OTC) apply qid prn to intact skin
      Gel: 1% (100 gm)
  Comment: *Diclofenac* is contraindicated with *aspirin* allergy. As with other NSAIDs, should be avoided in
  late pregnancy (≥30 weeks) because it may cause premature closure of the ductus arteriosus.
▷ *doxepin* **(G)** cream apply to affected area qid at intervals of at least 3-4 hours; max 8 days
  Pediatric: <12 years: not recommended; >12 years: same as adult
    Prudoxin *Crm:* 5% (45 gm)
    Zonalon *Crm:* 5% (30, 45 gm)
▷ *pimecrolimus* 1% cream **(G)** <2 years: not recommended; ≥2 years: apply to affected area bid; do not apply
  an occlusive dressing
    Elidel *Crm:* 1% (30, 60, 100 gm)
  Comment: *Pimecrolimus* is indicated for short-term and intermittent long-term use. Discontinue use when
  resolution occurs. Contraindicated if the patient is immunosuppressed. Change to the 0.1% preparation or
  if secondary bacterial infection is present.
▷ *trolamine salicylate* apply tid-qid
  Pediatric: <2 years: not recommended; ≥2 years: same as adult
    Mobisyl Creme *Crm:* 10% (100 gm)

TOPICAL AND TRANSDERMAL ANESTHETICS

Comment: *Lidocaine* should <u>not</u> be applied to non-intact skin.

▷ *lidocaine* cream apply to affected area bid prn
  Pediatric: <12 years: <u>not</u> recommended; ≥12 years: same as adult
    LidaMantle *Crm:* 3% (1, 2 oz)
    Lidoderm *Crm:* 3% (85 gm)
    ZTlido *lidocaine* topical system 1% (30/carton)
    Comment: Compared to **Lidoderm** (*lidocaine* patch 5%), which contains 700 mg/patch, **ZTlido** requires 35 mg per topical system to achieve the same therapeutic dose.

▷ *lidocaine* lotion apply to affected area bid prn
  Pediatric: <12 years: <u>not</u> recommended; ≥12 years: same as adult
    LidaMantle *Lotn:* 3% (177 ml)

▷ *lidocaine* 5% patch **(G)** apply up to 3 patches at one time for up to 12 hours/24-hour period (12 hours on/12 hours off); patches may be cut into smaller sizes before removal of the release liner; do <u>not</u> reuse
  Pediatric: <12 years: <u>not</u> recommended; ≥12 years: same as adult
    Lidoderm *Patch:* 5% (10 x 14 cm; 30/carton)

lidocaine+dexamethasone
  Pediatric: <12 years: <u>not</u> recommended; ≥12 years: same as adult
    Decadron Phosphate with Xylocaine *Lotn:* dexa 4 mg+lido 10 mg per ml (5 ml)

▷ *lidocaine+hydrocortisone* **(G)** apply to affected area bid prn
  Pediatric: <12 years: <u>not</u> recommended; ≥12 years: same as adult
    LidaMantle HC *Crm:* lido 3%+hydro 0.5% (1, 3 oz); *Lotn:* (177 ml)

▷ *lidocaine* 2.5%+*prilocaine* 2.5% apply sparingly to the burn bid-tid prn
  Pediatric: <12 years: <u>not</u> recommended; ≥12 years: same as adult
    Emla Cream 5, 30 gm/tube

ORAL ANALGESICS

▷ *acetaminophen* **(G)** *see Fever*
▷ *aspirin* **(G)** *see Fever*
▷ *tramadol* **(IV)(G)**
    Rybix ODT initially 100 mg once daily; may increase by 100 mg every 5 days; max 300 mg/day; *CrCl <30 ml/min* <u>or</u> *severe hepatic impairment:* <u>not</u> recommended; *Cirrhosis:* max 50 mg q 12 hours
    Pediatric: <18 years: <u>not</u> recommended; ≥18 years: same as adult
      ODT: 50 mg (mint) (phenylalanine)
    Ryzolt initially 100 mg once daily; may increase by 100 mg every 5 days; max 300 mg/day; *CrCl <30 ml/min* <u>or</u> *severe hepatic impairment:* <u>not</u> recommended
    Pediatric: <18 years: <u>not</u> recommended; ≥18 years: same as adult
      Tab: 100, 200, 300 mg ext-rel
    Ultram 50-100 mg q 4-6 hours prn; max 400 mg/day; *CrCl <30 ml/min:* max 100 mg q 12 hours; *Cirrhosis:* max 50 mg q 12 hours
    Pediatric: <18 years: <u>not</u> recommended; ≥18 years: same as adult
      Tab: 50*mg
    Ultram ER initially 100 mg once daily; may increase by 100 mg every 5 days; max 300 mg/day; *CrCl <30 ml/min* <u>or</u> *severe hepatic impairment:* <u>not</u> recommended
    Pediatric: <18 years: <u>not</u> recommended; ≥18 years: same as adult
      Tab: 100, 200, 300 mg ext-rel

▷ *tramadol+acetaminophen* **(IV)(G)** 2 tabs q 4-6 hours; max 8 tabs/day; 5 days; *CrCl <30 ml/min:* max 2 tabs q 12 hours; max 4 tabs/day x 5 days
  Pediatric: <18 years: <u>not</u> recommended; ≥18 years: same as adult
    Ultracet *Tab:* tram 37.5+acet 325 mg

TRICYCLIC ANTIDEPRESSANTS (TCAs)

Comment: Co-administration of TCAs with SSRIs requires extreme caution.

▷ *amitriptyline* **(G)** titrate to achieve pain relief; max 300 mg/day
  Pediatric: <12 years: <u>not</u> recommended; ≥12 years: same as adult
    Tab: 10, 25, 50, 75, 100, 150 mg

▷ *amoxapine* titrate to achieve pain relief; if total dose exceeds 300 mg/day, give in divided doses; max 400 mg/day
  Pediatric: <12 years: <u>not</u> recommended; ≥12 years: same as adult
    Tab: 25, 50, 100, 150 mg

▷ *desipramine* **(G)** titrate to achieve pain relief; max 300 mg/day
  Pediatric: <12 years: <u>not</u> recommended; ≥12 years: same as adult
    Norpramin *Tab:* 10, 25, 50, 75, 100, 150 mg

(continued)

▷ **doxepin (G)** titrate to achieve pain relief; max 150 mg/day
  Pediatric: <12 years: <u>not</u> recommended; ≥12 years: same as adult
    Cap: 10, 25, 50, 75, 100, 150 mg; *Oral conc:* 10 mg/ml (4 oz w. dropper)
▷ **imipramine (G)**
  Pediatric: <12 years: <u>not</u> recommended; ≥12 years: same as adult
    Tofranil titrate to achieve pain relief; max 200 mg/day; adolescents max 100 mg/day; if maintenance dose
    exceeds 75 mg/day, may switch to **Tofranil PM** at bedtime
    Tab: 10, 25, 50 mg
    Tofranil PM titrate to achieve pain relief; initially 75 mg at HS; max 200 mg at HS
    Cap: 75, 100, 125, 150 mg
    Tofranil Injection 50 mg IM; lower dose for adolescents; switch to oral form as soon as possible
    Amp: 25 mg/2 ml (2 ml)
▷ **nortriptyline (G)** titrate to achieve pain relief; initially 10-25 mg tid-qid; max 150 mg/day; lower doses for
  elderly and adolescents
  Pediatric: <12 years: <u>not</u> recommended; ≥12 years: same as adult
    Pamelor titrate to achieve pain relief; max 150 mg/day
    Cap: 10, 25, 50, 75 mg; *Oral soln:* 10 mg/5 ml (16 oz)
▷ **protriptyline** titrate to achieve pain relief; initially 5 mg tid; max 60 mg/day
  Pediatric: <12 years: <u>not</u> recommended; ≥12 years: same as adult
    Vivactil *Tab:* 5, 10 mg
▷ **trimipramine** titrate to achieve pain relief; max 200 mg/day
  Pediatric: <12 years: <u>not</u> recommended; ≥12 years: same as adult
    Surmontil *Cap:* 25, 50, 100 mg

POSTTRAUMATIC STRESS DISORDER (PTSD)

Comment: No one pharmacologic agent has emerged as the best treatment for PTSD. A combination of pharmacological agents (e.g., antidepressants, non-adrenergic agents, antipsychosis drugs) may comprise an individualized treatment plan to successfully manage core symptoms of PTSD, as well as associated anxiety, depression, sleep disturbances, and co-occurring psychiatric disorders.

SELECTIVE SEROTONIN REUPTAKE INHIBITORS (SSRIs)
Comment: The FDA has approved two selective serotonin reuptake inhibitors (SSRIs) for the treatment of PTSD: *paroxetine* and *sertraline*. However, the safety and efficacy of other SSRIs (*fluoxetine, citalopram, escitalopram, fluvoxamine*) have been tested in clinical practice. Co-administration of SSRIs with tricyclic antidepressants (TCAs) requires extreme caution. Concomitant use of monoamine oxidase inhibitors (MAOIs) and SSRIs is absolutely contraindicated. Avoid St. John's wort and other serotonergic agents. A potentially fatal adverse event is *serotonin syndrome,* caused by serotonin excess. Milder symptoms require healthcare provider intervention to avert severe symptoms which can be rapidly fatal without urgent/emergent medical care. Symptoms include restlessness, agitation, confusion, hallucinations, tachycardia, hypertension, dilated pupils, muscle twitching, muscle rigidity, loss of muscle coordination, diaphoresis, diarrhea, headache, shivering, piloerection, hyperpyrexia, cardiac arrhythmias, seizures, loss of consciousness, coma, and death. Abrupt withdrawal <u>or</u> interruption of treatment with an antidepressant medication is sometimes associated with an *antidepressant discontinuation syndrome* (ADS) which may be mediated by gradually tapering the drug over a period of 2 weeks <u>or</u> longer, depending on the dose strength and length of treatment. Common symptoms of the *serotonin discontinuation syndrome* include flu-like symptoms (nausea, vomiting, diarrhea, headaches, sweating), sleep disturbances (insomnia, nightmares, constant sleepiness), mood disturbances (dysphoria, anxiety, agitation), cognitive disturbances (mental confusion, hyperarousal), and sensory and movement disturbances (imbalance, tremors, vertigo, dizziness, electric-shock-like sensations in the brain, often described by sufferers as "brain zaps").
▷ **paroxetine maleate (G)**
  Pediatric: <12 years: <u>not</u> recommended; ≥12 years: same as adult
    Paxil initially 20 mg daily in the AM; may increase by 10 mg/day at 1-week intervals as needed; max 60
    mg/day
      Tab: 10*, 20*, 30, 40 mg
    Paxil CR initially 25 mg daily in the AM; may increase by 12.5 mg at 1-week intervals as needed; max
    62.5 mg/day
      Oral Tab: 12.5, 25, 37.5 mg cont-rel ent-coat
    Paxil Suspension initially 20 mg daily in the AM; may increase by 10 mg/day at 1-week intervals as
    needed; max 60 mg/day
      Oral susp: 10 mg/5 ml (250 ml; orange)
▷ **paroxetine mesylate (G)** initially 7.5 mg daily in the AM; may increase by 10 mg/day at 1-week intervals as
  needed; max 60 mg/day
  Pediatric: <12 years: <u>not</u> recommended; ≥12 years: same as adult
    Brisdelle *Cap:* 7.5 mg

➤ *sertraline* initially 50 mg daily; increase at 1-week intervals if needed; max 200 mg daily
    Pediatric: <6 years: not recommended; 6-12 years: initially 25 mg daily; max 200 mg/day; 13-17 years: initially 50 mg daily; max 200 mg/day; ≥17 years: same as adult
        Zoloft *Tab:* 15*, 50*, 100*mg; *Oral conc:* 20 mg per ml (60 ml [dilute just before administering in 4 oz water, ginger ale, lemon-lime soda, lemonade, or orange juice]) (alcohol 12%)

ATYPICAL ANTIPSYCHOSIS DRUGS

➤ *olanzapine* (G) initially 2.5-5 mg once daily at HS; increase by 5 mg every week to 20 mg at HS; usual maintenance 10-20 mg/day
        Zyprexa *Tab:* 2.5, 5, 7.5, 10, 15, 20 mg
        Zyprexa Zydis *ODT:* 5, 10, 15, 20 mg (phenylalanine)
➤ *quetiapine* (G) initially 25 mg bid; increase total daily dose by 50 mg, as needed and tolerated, to max 300-600 mg/day
        Seroquel *Tab:* 25, 100, 200, 300 mg
        Seroquel XR *Tab:* 50, 150, 200, 300, 400 mg ext-rel
➤ *risperidone* (G) initially 0.5-1 mg bid; titrate to 3 mg bid by the end of the first week; usual maintenance 4-6 mg/day
        Risperdal *Tab:* 0.25, 0.5, 1, 2, 3, 4 mg; *Soln:* 1 mg/ml (30 ml w. pipette); *Consta (Inj):* 25, 37.5, 50 mg
        Risperdal M-Tabs *M-tab:* 0.5, 1, 2, 3, 4 mg orally-disint (phenylalanine)

NON-ADRENERGIC AGENTS
ALPHA-1 ANTAGONISTS

Comment: *Prazosin* is useful in reducing combat-trauma nightmares, normalizing dreams for combat veterans, and mediating other sleep disturbances.
➤ *prazosin* (G) first dose at HS, 1 mg bid-tid; increase dose slowly; usual range 6-15 mg/day in divided doses; max 20-40 mg/day
    Pediatric: <12 years: not recommended; ≥12 years: same as adult
        Minipress *Cap:* 1, 2, 5 mg

CENTRAL ALPHA-2 AGONISTS

Comment: *Clonidine* is useful in reducing nightmares, hypervigilance, startle reactions, and outbursts of rage.
➤ *clonidine*
    Pediatric: <12 years: not recommended; ≥12 years: same as adult
        Catapres initially 0.1 mg bid; usual range 0.2-0.6 mg/day in divided doses; max 2.4 mg/day
           Tab: 0.1*, 0.2*, 0.3*mg
        Catapres-TTS initially 0.1 mg patch weekly; increase after 1-2 weeks if needed; max 0.6 mg/day
           Patch: 0.1, 0.2 mg/day (12/carton); 0.3 mg/day (4/carton)
        Kapvay (G) initially 0.1 mg bid; usual range 0.2-0.6 mg/day in divided doses; max 2.4 mg/day
           Tab: 0.1, 0.2 mg
        Nexiclon XR initially 0.18 mg (2 ml) suspension or 0.17 mg tab once daily; usual max 0.52 mg (6 ml suspension) once daily
           Tab: 0.17, 0.26 mg ext-rel; *Oral susp:* 0.09 mg/ml ext-rel (4 oz)

BETA-ADRENERGIC BLOCKER (NON-CARDIOSELECTIVE)

Comment: *Propranolol* is useful in mediating hyperarousal. For other non-cardioselective beta-adrenergic blockers, see **Hypertension**
➤ *propranolol* (G) 40-240 mg daily
    Pediatric: <12 years: not recommended; ≥12 years: same as adult
        Inderal *Tab:* 10*, 20*, 40*, 60*, 80*mg
        Inderal LA initially 80 mg daily in a single dose; increase q 3-7 days; usual range 120-160 mg/day; max 320 mg/day in a single dose

SEROTONIN NOREPINEPHRINE REUPTAKE INHIBITORS (SNRIs)

➤ *desvenlafaxine* (G) swallow whole; initially 50 mg once daily; max 120 mg/day
    Pediatric: <12 years: not recommended; ≥12 years: same as adult
        Pristiq *Tab:* 50, 100 mg ext-rel
➤ *duloxetine* (G) swallow whole; initially 30 mg once daily x 1 week; then increase to 60 mg once daily; max 120 mg/day
    Pediatric: <12 years: not recommended; ≥12 years: same as adult
        Cymbalta *Cap:* 20, 30, 40, 60 mg del-rel
➤ *venlafaxine* (G)
        Effexor initially 75 mg/day in 2-3 divided doses; may increase at 4-day intervals in 75 mg increments to 150 mg/day; max 225 mg/day
    Pediatric: <18 years: not recommended; ≥18 years: same as adult
        Tab: 37.5, 75, 150, 225 mg

(continued)

Effexor XR initially 75 mg q AM; may start at 37.5 mg daily x 4-7 days, then increase by increments of up to 75 mg/day at intervals of at least 4 days; usual max 375 mg/day
Pediatric: <18 years: not recommended; ≥18 years: same as adult
Tab/Cap: 37.5, 75, 150 mg ext-rel

5HT2/3 RECEPTOR BLOCKERS

▷ *mirtazapine* initially 15 mg q HS; increase at intervals of 1-2 weeks; 1-2 weeks; usual range 15-60 mg/day; max 60 mg/day
Pediatric: <12 years: not recommended; ≥12 years: same as adult
Remeron *Tab:* 15*, 30*, 45*mg
Remeron SolTab *ODT:* 15, 30, 45 mg (orange) (phenylalanine)

SEROTONIN+ACETYLCHOLINE+NOREPINEPHRINE+DOPAMINE BLOCKER

▷ *trazodone* (G) initially 150 mg/day in divided doses with food; increase by 50 mg/day q 3-4 days; max 400 mg/day in divided doses or 50-400 mg at HS
Pediatric: <18 years: not recommended; ≥18 years: same as adult
Oleptro *Tab:* 50, 100*, 150*, 200, 250, 300 mg

TRICYCLIC ANTIDEPRESSANTS (TCAs)

▷ *amitriptyline* (G) 10-20 mg at HS
Pediatric: <12 years: not recommended; ≥12 years: same as adult
Tab: 10, 25, 50, 75, 100, 150 mg
▷ *doxepin* (G) 10-200 mg at HS
Pediatric: <12 years: not recommended; ≥12 years: same as adult
Cap: 10, 25, 50, 75, 100, 150 mg; *Oral conc:* 10 mg/ml (4 oz w. dropper)
▷ *imipramine* (G) 10-200 mg q HS
Tofranil 100-300 mg at HS or divided bid or tid
Pediatric: <6 years: not recommended; 6-12 years: initially 25 mg; >12 years: 50 mg; max 2.5 mg/kg/day
Tab: 10, 25, 50 mg
Tofranil PM initially 75 mg daily 1 hour before HS; max 200 mg
Pediatric: <12 years: not recommended; ≥12 years: same as adult
Cap: 75, 100, 125, 150 mg
Tofranil Injection 50 mg IM; lower dose for adolescents; switch to oral form as soon as possible
Amp: 25 mg/2 ml (2 ml)
▷ *nortriptyline* (G) 10-150 mg q HS
Pediatric: <12 years: not recommended; ≥12 years: same as adult
Pamelor *Cap:* 10, 25, 50, 75 mg; *Oral soln:* 10 mg/5 ml

MONOAMINE OXIDASE INHIBITORS (MAOIs)

Comment: Many drug and food interactions with this class of drugs, use cautiously. MAOIs should be reserved for refractory depression that has not responded to other classes of antidepressants. Concomitant use of MAOIs and SSRIs is contraindicated. See mfr pkg insert for drug and food interactions. MAOIs have been used to reduce recurrent recollections of the trauma, nightmares, flashbacks, numbing, sleep disturbances, and social withdrawal in PTSD.
▷ *phenelzine* (G) initially 15 mg tid; max 90 mg/day
Pediatric: <16 years: not recommended; ≥16 years: same as adult
Nardil *Tab:* 15 mg
▷ *selegiline* initially 10 mg tid; max 60 mg/day
Pediatric: <12 years: not recommended; ≥12 years: same as adult
Emsam *Transdermal patch:* 6 mg/24 hours, 9 mg/24 hours, 12 mg/24 hours
Comment: At the Emsam transdermal patch 6 mg/24 hours dose, the dietary restrictions commonly required when using non-selective MAOIs are not necessary.

PRECOCIOUS PUBERTY, CENTRAL (CPP)

Comment: Gonadotropin-releasing hormone (GnRH)-dependent central precocious puberty (CPP) is defined by pubertal development occurring before the age of 8 years in girls and 9 years in boys. It is characterized by early pubertal changes such as breast development and start of menses in girls and increased testicular and penile growth in boys, appearance of pubic hair, as well as acceleration of growth velocity and bone maturation and tall stature during childhood, which often results in reduced adult height due to premature fusion of the growth plates.

GONADOTROPIN RELEASING HORMONE (GnRH) AGONIST

▷ *leuprolide acetate*
Pediatric: <2 years: safety and efficacy not established; ≥2 years: 45 mg SC once every 6 months in the abdomen, upper buttocks, or another location with adequate amounts of subcutaneous tissue that does not

have excessive pigment, nodules, lesions, or hair; avoid areas with brawny or fibrous subcutaneous tissue or locations that could be rubbed or compressed (e.g., by a belt or clothing waistband); rotate sites; refrigerate the kit; if the kit remains sealed, may remain at room temperature for up to 8 weeks; allow to reach room temperature before reconstitution; administer within 30 minutes of reconstitution or discard; must be administered by a qualified healthcare professional

Fensolvi *Administration kit:* 45 mg/pwdr (prefilled syringe) for reconstitution w. diluent (prefilled syringe), single-dose

Comment: Fensolvi *(leuprolide acetate)* is a gonadotropin releasing hormone (GnRH) agonist indicated for the treatment of pediatric patients 2 years of age and older with central precocious puberty (CPP). Monitor response to **Fensolvi** with a GnRH agonist stimulation test, basal serum luteinizing hormone (LH) levels, or serum concentration of sex steroid levels at 1 to 2 months following initiation of therapy and as needed to confirm adequate suppression of pituitary gonadotropins, sex steroids, and progression of secondary sexual characteristics. Measure height every 3-6 months and monitor bone age periodically. The most common adverse reactions (incidence ≥5%) have been injection site pain, nasopharyngitis, pyrexia, headache, cough, abdominal pain, injection site erythema, nausea, constipation, vomiting, upper respiratory tract infection, bronchospasm, productive cough, and hot flush. Initial rise in gonadotropins and sex steroid levels are expected during the early phase of therapy because of the initial stimulatory effect of the drug. Therefore, an increase in clinical signs and symptoms of puberty, including vaginal bleeding, may be observed during the first weeks of therapy or after subsequent doses. Instruct patients and caregivers to notify the healthcare provider if these symptoms continue beyond the second month after **Fensolvi** administration. Psychiatric events have been reported in patients taking GnRH agonists, including emotional lability, such as crying, irritability, impatience, anger, and aggression. Monitor for development or worsening of psychiatric symptoms. Convulsions have been observed in patients with or without a history of seizures, epilepsy, cerebrovascular disorder, central nervous system anomalies or tumors, and in patients on concomitant medications that have been associated with convulsions. Non-compliance with drug regimen or inadequate dosing may lead to gonadotropins and/or sex steroids increasing above prepubertal levels, resulting in inadequate control of the pubertal process. If the dose of **Fensolvi** is not adequate, switching to an alternative GnRH agonist for the treatment of CPP with the ability for dose adjustment may be necessary. Discontinue **Fensolvi** treatment at the appropriate age of onset of puberty. Anaphylactic reactions to synthetic GnRH or GnRH agonists have been reported. **Fensolvi** is contraindicated in pregnancy; may cause embryo/fetal harm. Exclude pregnancy in females of reproductive potential prior to initiating **Fensolvi** if clinically indicated. **Fensolvi** is not a contraceptive. If contraception is indicated, advise females of reproductive potential to use a non-hormonal method of contraception during treatment. Based on its pharmacodynamic effects of decreasing secretion of gonadal steroids, fertility is expected to be decreased while on treatment with **Fensolvi**. Clinical and pharmacologic studies in adults (>18 years) with *leuprolide acetate* and similar analogs have shown reversibility of fertility suppression when the drug is discontinued after continuous administration for periods of up to 24 weeks. There are no data on the presence of *leuprolide acetate* in either animal or human milk or effects on the breastfed infant. Developmental and health benefits of breastfeeding should be considered along with the mother's clinical need for **Fensolvi** and any potential adverse effects on the breastfed infant from **Fensolvi** or from the underlying maternal condition.

▶ **triptorelin**

Pediatric: <2 years: not recommended; ≥2 years: administer as a single 22.5 mg IM injection once q 24 weeks; must be administered under the supervision of a physician; monitor response with LH levels after a GnRH or GnRH agonist stimulation test, basal LH, or serum concentration of sex steroid levels beginning 1-2 months following initiation of therapy, during therapy as necessary to confirm maintenance of efficacy, and with each subsequent dose; measure height every 3-6 months and monitor bone age periodically; see mfr pkg insert for reconstitution and administration instructions

Triptodur *Single-use kit:* 1 single-dose vial of **triptorelin** 22.5 mg w. Flip-Off seal containing sterile lyophilized white to slightly yellow powder cake, 1 sterile, glass syringe prefilled with 2 ml of sterile water for injection, 2 sterile 21 gauge, 1½ inch needles (thin-wall) with safety cover

Comment: Triptodur is contraindicated in females who are pregnant since expected hormonal changes that occur with *triptorelin* treatment increase the risk for pregnancy loss. Available data with *triptorelin* use in pregnant females are insufficient to determine a drug-associated risk of adverse developmental outcomes. Based on mechanism of action in humans and findings of increased pregnancy loss in animal studies, *triptorelin* may cause fetal harm when administered to pregnant females. Advise pregnant females of the potential risk to the fetus. The estimated background risk of major birth defects and miscarriage is unknown. There are no data on the presence of *triptorelin* in human milk or the effects of the drug on the breastfed infant. The developmental and health benefits of breastfeeding should be considered along with the mother's clinical need for *triptorelin* and any potential adverse effects on the breastfed infant from *triptorelin* or from the underlying maternal condition. During the early phase of therapy, gonadotropins and sex steroids rise above baseline because of the initial stimulatory effect of the drug. Therefore, a transient increase in clinical signs and symptoms of puberty, including vaginal bleeding, may be observed during the first weeks of therapy. Postmarketing reports with this class of drugs include symptoms of emotional lability, such as crying, irritability, impatience, anger,

(continued)

and aggression. Monitor for development or worsening of psychiatric symptoms during treatment with **Triptodur**. Postmarketing reports of convulsions have been observed in patients receiving GnRH agonists, including *triptorelin*. These included patients with a history of seizures, epilepsy, cerebrovascular disorders, central nervous system anomalies or tumors, and patients on concomitant medications that have been associated with convulsions such as bupropion and selective serotonin reuptake inhibitors (SSRIs). Convulsions have also been reported in patients in the absence of any of the conditions mentioned above.

PREGNANCY

See **Prescription Prenatal Vitamins**
Comment: Prenatal vitamins should have at least 400 mcg of folic acid content. Take 1 dose once daily. It is recommended that prenatal vitamins be started at least 3 months prior to conception to improve preconception nutritional status, and continued throughout pregnancy and the postnatal period, in lactating and non-lactating women, and throughout the childbearing years.

NAUSEA/VOMITING
➤ *doxylamine succinate+pyridoxine* (G) do not crush or chew; take on an empty stomach with water; initially 2 tabs at HS on day 1; may increase to 1 tab in the AM and 2 tabs at HS day 2; may increase to 1 tab in the AM, 1 tab mid-afternoon, 2 tabs at HS; max 4 tabs/day
    Diclegis *Tab:* doxyl 10 mg+pyri 10 mg del-rel
    Comment: Diclegis is the only FDA-approved drug for the treatment of morning sickness. It has not been studied in women with hyperemesis gravidarum.
➤ *promethazine* (G) 12.5-50 mg PO/IM/rectally q 4-6 hours prn
    Phenergan *Tab:* 12.5*, 25*, 50 mg; *Plain syr:* 6.25 mg/5 ml; *Fortis syr:* 25 mg/5 ml; *Rectal supp:* 12.5, 25, 50 mg; *Amp:* 25, 50 mg/ml (1 ml)
    Comment: *Promethazine* is contraindicated in children with uncomplicated nausea, dehydration, Reye's syndrome, history of sleep apnea, asthma, and lower respiratory disorders. *Promethazine* lowers the seizure threshold in children and may cause cholestatic jaundice, anticholinergic effects, extrapyramidal effects, and potentially fatal respiratory depression.

PREMENSTRUAL DYSPHORIC DISORDER (PMDD)

NSAIDs *see* Appendix I. NSAIDs online at https://connect.springerpub.com/content/reference-book/978-0-8261-7935-7/back-matter/part02/back-matter/bmatter10
Opioid Analgesics *see* **Pain**
Oral Contraceptives *see* Appendix G. Contraceptives

ORAL ESTROGEN+PROGESTERONE COMBINATIONS
Comment: Rajani (a generic form of **Beyaz**) and Yaz, also available in generic forms (**Gianvi, Ocella, Syeda, Vestura, Yasmin, Zarah**), have an FDA indication for treatment of premenstrual dysphoric disorder (PMDD) in females who choose to use oral contraceptive pill (OCP). Contraindicated with renal and adrenal insufficiency. Monitor K+ level during the first cycle if the patient is at risk for hyperkalemia for any reason. If the patient is taking a drug that increases serum potassium (e.g., angiotensin-converting enzyme inhibitors [ACEIs], angiotensin II receptor blockers [ARBs], non-steroidal anti-inflammatory drugs [NSAIDs], K+-sparing diuretics), the patient is at risk for hyperkalemia.
➤ *ethinyl estradiol+drospirenone* (G) *Premenarchal:* not indicated; *Postmenarchal:* 1 tab once daily x 28 days; repeat cycle; start on first Sunday after menses begins or on first day of next menses
    Yaz *Tab:* ethin estra 20 mcg+drospir 3 mg
➤ *ethinyl+estradiol+drospirenone+levomefolate calcium* (G) *Premenarchal:* not indicated; *Postmenarchal:* 1 tab once daily x 28 days; repeat cycle; start on first Sunday after menses begins or on first day of next menses preceded by a negative pregnancy test
    Beyaz *Tab:* ethin estra 20 mcg+drospir 3 mg+levo 0.451 mg
    Rajani *Tab:* ethin estra 20 mcg+drospir 3 mg+levo 0.451 mg

DIURETICS
➤ *spironolactone* (G) initially 50-100 mg once daily or in divided doses; titrate at 2-week intervals
    Pediatric: <12 years: not recommended; ≥12 years: same as adult
    Aldactone *Tab:* 25, 50*, 100*mg

ANTIDEPRESSANTS
➤ *fluoxetine* (G)
    Prozac initially 20 mg daily; may increase after 1 week; doses >20 mg/day should be divided into AM and noon doses; max 80 mg/day

Pediatric: <8 years: <u>not</u> recommended; 8-17 years: initially 10 <u>or</u> 20 mg/day; start lower weight children at 10 mg/day; if starting at 10 mg/day, may increase after 1 week to 20 mg/day; ≥17 years: same as adult

    Tab: 10*mg; *Cap:* 10, 20, 40 mg; *Oral soln:* 20 mg/5 ml (4 oz) (mint)

Prozac Weekly following daily *fluoxetine* therapy at 20 mg/day for 13 weeks, may initiate **Prozac Weekly** 7 days after the last 20 mg *fluoxetine* dose

Pediatric: <12 years: <u>not</u> recommended; ≥12 years: same as adult

    Cap: 90 mg ent-coat del-rel pellets

Sarafem administer daily <u>or</u> 14 days before expected menses and through first full day of menses; initially 20 mg/day; max 80 mg/day

Pediatric: <8 years: <u>not</u> recommended; 8-17 years: initially 10 <u>or</u> 20 mg/day; start lower weight children at 10 mg/day; if starting at 10 mg/day, may increase after 1 week to 20 mg/day

    Tab: 10, 15, 20 mg; *Cap:* 20 mg

▷ *paroxetine maleate* **(G)**

Pediatric: <12 years: <u>not</u> recommended; ≥12 years: same as adult

    Paxil initially 20 mg daily in the AM; may increase by 10 mg/day at weekly intervals as needed; max 60 mg/day

    Tab: 10*, 20*, 30, 40 mg

    Paxil CR initially 25 mg daily in the AM; may increase by 12.5 mg at weekly intervals as needed; max 62.5 mg/day; may start 14 days before and continue through day 1 of menses

    Tab: 12.5, 25, 37.5 mg cont-rel ent-coat

    Paxil Oral Suspension initially 20 mg daily in the AM; may increase by 10 mg/day at weekly intervals as needed; max 60 mg/day

    Oral susp: 10 mg/5 ml (250 ml) (orange)

▷ *paroxetine mesylate* **(G)** initially 7.5 mg daily in the AM; may increase by 10 mg/day at weekly intervals as needed; max 60 mg/day

Pediatric: <12 years: <u>not</u> recommended; ≥12 years: same as adult

    Brisdelle *Cap:* 7.5 mg

▷ *sertraline for 2 weeks prior to onset of menses:* initially 50 mg daily x 3; then increase to 100 mg daily for remainder of the cycle; *For full cycle:* initially 50 mg daily; then may increase by 50 mg/day each cycle to max 150 mg/day

Pediatric: <12 years: <u>not</u> recommended; ≥12 years: same as adult

    Zoloft *Tab:* 25*, 50*, 100*mg; *Oral conc:* 20 mg per ml (60 ml) (alcohol 12%); dilute just before administering in 4 oz water, ginger ale, lemon-lime soda, lemonade, <u>or</u> orange juice

▷ *nortriptyline* **(G)** initially 25 mg tid-qid; max 150 mg/day

Pediatric: <12 years: <u>not</u> recommended; ≥12 years: same as adult

    Pamelor *Cap:* 10, 25, 50, 75 mg; *Oral soln:* 10 mg/5 ml

CALCIUM SUPPLEMENTS

▷ *calcium* 1,200 mg/day

see **Osteoporosis**

PRESBYOPIA

CHOLINERGIC MUSCARINIC RECEPTOR AGONIST

▷ *pilocarpine hydrochloride* 1 drop in each eye once daily; if more than one topical ophthalmic product is being used, the products should be administered at least 5 minutes apart

Pediatric: <u>not</u> indicated; presbyopia does <u>not</u> occur in the pediatric population

    Vuity *Ophth Soln* 1.25% solution (12.5 mg/ml, 5 ml), 1, 3/carton

    Comment: **Vuity** is an optimized ophthalmic solution formulation of the approved cholinergic muscarinic receptor agonist *pilocarpine* indicated for the treatment of presbyopia (age-related blurry near vision) in adults. **Vuity** is contraindicated in patients with known hypersensitivity to the active ingredient <u>or</u> to any of the excipients. Miotics, including **Vuity**, may cause accommodative spasm. Patients should be advised <u>not</u> to drive <u>or</u> operate machinery if vision is <u>not</u> clear (e.g., blurred vision). In addition, patients may experience temporary dim <u>or</u> dark vision with miotics, including **Vuity**. Patients should be advised to exercise caution in night driving and other hazardous activities in poor illumination. Individuals with preexisting retinal disease are at increased risk. Therefore, examination of the retina is advised in all patients prior to the initiation of therapy. Patients should be advised to seek immediate medical care with sudden onset of flashing lights, floaters, <u>or</u> vision loss. **Vuity** is <u>not</u> recommended to be used when iritis is present because synechiae (adhesions) may form between the iris and the lens. Contact lens wearers should be advised to remove their lenses prior to the instillation of **Vuity** and to wait 10 minutes after dosing before reinserting their contact lenses. The most common adverse reactions reported in >5% of patients were headache and conjunctival hyperemia. Ocular adverse reactions reported in 1%-5% of patients were blurred vision, eye pain, visual impairment, eye irritation, and increased lacrimation. Adverse reactions have been identified during postapproval use of **Vuity**.

(continued)

Because these reactions are reported voluntarily from a population of uncertain size, it is <u>not</u> always possible to reliably estimate their frequency <u>or</u> establish a causal relationship to **Vuity** exposure: vitreous detachment, vitreomacular traction, retinal tear, and retinal detachment. There are no adequate and well-controlled studies of **Vuity** administration in pregnant patients to inform a drug-associated risk. In animal studies, oral administration of *pilocarpine* throughout organogenesis and lactation did <u>not</u> produce adverse effects at clinically relevant doses. There is no information regarding the presence of *pilocarpine* in human milk, the effects on the breastfed infants, <u>or</u> the effects on milk production to inform risk of **Vuity** to an infant during lactation. *Pilocarpine* <u>and/or</u> its metabolites are excreted in animal milk. Systemic levels of *pilocarpine* following topical ocular administration are low and it is <u>not</u> known whether measurable levels of *pilocarpine* would be present in maternal human milk following topical ocular administration. Developmental and health benefits of breastfeeding should be considered along with the mother's clinical need for **Vuity** and any potential adverse effects on the breastfed infant from **Vuity**. To report suspected adverse reactions, contact Allergan at 1-800-678-1605 <u>or</u> FDA at 1-800-FDA-1088 <u>or</u> www.fda.gov/medwatch.

PROCTITIS: ACUTE (PROCTOCOLITIS, ENTERITIS)

Comment: The following regimen for the treatment of proctitis, proctocolitis, and enteritis is published in the 2021 CDC Sexually Transmitted Diseases Treatment Guidelines.

RECOMMENDED REGIMEN
▷ *ceftriaxone* (G) 250 mg IM in a single dose
      Rocephin *Vial:* 250, 500 mg; 1, 2 gm
         plus
▷ *doxycycline* 100 mg bid x 7 days
      Acticlate *Tab:* 75, 150**mg
      Adoxa *Tab:* 50, 75, 100, 150 mg ent-coat
      Doryx *Tab:* 50, 75, 100, 150, 200 mg del-rel
      Doxteric *Tab:* 50 mg del-rel
      Monodox *Cap:* 50, 75, 100 mg
      Oracea *Cap:* 40 mg del-rel
      Vibramycin *Tab:* 100 mg; *Cap:* 50, 100 mg; *Syr:* 50 mg/5 ml (raspberry-apple) (sulfites); *Oral susp:* 25 mg/5 ml (raspberry)
      Vibra-Tab *Tab:* 100 mg film-coat

PROSTATITIS: ACUTE

ANTI-INFECTIVES
▷ *ciprofloxacin* 500 mg bid x 4-6 weeks
  Pediatric: <18 years: <u>not</u> recommended; ≥18 years: same as adult
      Cipro (G) *Tab:* 250, 500, 750 mg; *Oral susp:* 250, 500 mg/5 ml (100 ml) (strawberry)
      Cipro XR *Tab:* 500, 1,000 mg ext-rel
      ProQuin XR *Tab:* 500 mg ext-rel
▷ *norfloxacin* 400 mg bid x 28 days
  Pediatric: <18 years: <u>not</u> recommended; ≥18 years: same as adult
      Noroxin *Tab:* 400 mg
▷ *ofloxacin* (G) 300 mg x bid x 6 weeks
  Pediatric: <18 years: <u>not</u> recommended; ≥18 years: same as adult
      Floxin *Tab:* 200, 300, 400 mg
▷ *trimethoprim+sulfamethoxazole (TMP-SMX)* (G)
  Pediatric: <12 years: <u>not</u> recommended; ≥12 years: same as adult
      Bactrim, Septra 2 tabs bid x 10 days
        Tab: trim 80 mg+sulfa 400 mg*
      Bactrim DS, Septra DS 1 tab bid x 10 days
        Tab: trim 160 mg+sulfa 800 mg*
      Bactrim Pediatric Suspension, Septra Pediatric Suspension
        Oral susp: trim 40 mg+sulfa 200 mg per 5 ml (100 ml) (cherry) (alcohol 0.3%)

PROSTATITIS: CHRONIC

ANTI-INFECTIVES
▷ *carbenicillin* 2 tabs qid x 4-12 weeks
      Geocillin *Tab:* 382 mg
▷ *ciprofloxacin* 500 mg bid x 3 <u>or</u> more months
  Pediatric: <18 years: <u>not</u> recommended; ≥18 years: same as adult
      Cipro (G) *Tab:* 250, 500, 750 mg; *Oral susp:* 250, 500 mg/5 ml (100 ml) (strawberry)

Cipro XR *Tab:* 500, 1,000 mg ext-rel
ProQuin XR *Tab:* 500 mg ext-rel
➤ *norfloxacin* 400 mg bid x 4-12 weeks
   Pediatric: <18 years: <u>not</u> recommended; ≥18 years: same as adult
   Noroxin *Tab:* 400 mg
➤ *ofloxacin* (G) 300 mg bid x 4-12 weeks
   Pediatric: <18 years: <u>not</u> recommended; ≥18 years: same as adult
   Floxin *Tab:* 200, 300, 400 mg
➤ *trimethoprim+sulfamethoxazole* (G)
   Pediatric: <18 years: *see* Appendix N.33. *trimethoprim+sulfamethoxazole* (Bactrim Suspension, Septra
   Suspension) for dose by weight; ≥18 years: same as adult
      Bactrim, Septra 2 tabs bid x 10 days
         Tab: trim 80 mg+sulfa 400 mg*
      Bactrim DS, Septra DS 1 tab bid x 10 days
         Tab: trim 160 mg+sulfa 800 mg
      Bactrim Pediatric Suspension, Septra Pediatric Suspension 20 ml bid x 10 days
         Oral susp: trim 40 mg+sulfa 200 mg per 5 ml (100 ml) (cherry) (alcohol 0.3%)

SUPPRESSION THERAPY

➤ *trimethoprim+sulfamethoxazole (TMP-SMX)* (G)
   Pediatric: <18 years: <u>not</u> recommended; ≥18 years: same as adult
      Bactrim, Septra 2 tabs bid x 10 days
         Tab: trim 80 mg+sulfa 400 mg*
      Bactrim DS, Septra DS 1 tab bid x 10 days
         Tab: trim 160 mg+sulfa 800 mg*
      Bactrim Pediatric Suspension, Septra Pediatric Suspension 20 ml bid x 10 days
         Oral susp: trim 40 mg+sulfa 200 mg per 5 ml (100 ml) (cherry) (alcohol 0.3%)

PRURITUS

Antihistamines *see* Drugs for the Management of Allergy, Cough, and Cold Symptoms online at https://connect.springerpub.com/content/reference-book/ 978-0-8261-7935-7/back-matter/part02/back-matter/bmatter27
Topical Corticosteroids *see* Appendix J. Topical Corticosteroids by Potency
Parenteral Corticosteroids *see* Appendix L. Parenteral Corticosteroids
Oral Corticosteroids *see* Appendix K. Oral Corticosteroids
OTC Antihistamines
OTC Eucerin Products
OTC Lac-Hydrin Products
OTC Lubriderm Products
OTC Aveeno Products

TOPICAL OIL

➤ *fluocinolone acetonide* 0.01% topical oil
   Pediatric: <6 years: <u>not</u> recommended; ≥6 years: apply sparingly bid for up to 4 weeks
      Derma-Smoothe/FS Topical Oil apply sparingly tid
         Topical oil: 0.01% (4 oz) (peanut oil)

TOPICAL AND TRANSDERMAL ANALGESICS

➤ *capsaicin* (G) apply tid-qid prn to intact skin
   Pediatric: <2 years: <u>not</u> recommended; ≥2 years: same as adult
      Axsain *Crm:* 0.075% (1, 2 oz)
      Capsin (OTC) *Lotn:* 0.025, 0, 075% (59 ml)
      Capzasin-HP (OTC) *Crm:* 0.075% (1.5 oz); *Lotn:* 0.075% (2 oz)
      Capzasin-P (OTC) *Crm:* 0.025% (1.5 oz); *Lotn:* 0.025% (2 oz)
      Dolorac *Crm:* 0.025% (28 gm)
      Double Cap (OTC) *Crm:* 0.05% (2 oz)
      R-Gel *Gel:* 0.025% (15, 30 gm)
      Zostrix (OTC) *Crm:* 0.025% (0.7, 1.5, 3 oz)
      Zostrix HP (OTC) *Emol crm:* 0.075% (1, 2 oz)
➤ *capsaicin* 8% patch apply up to 4 patches for one 60-minute application to clean dry skin; may prep area
   with topical anesthetic; wear non-latex gloves; patches may be cut to size/shape; treatment may be repeated
   every 3 months
   Pediatric: <18 years: <u>not</u> recommended; ≥18 years: same as adult
      Qutenza *Patch:* 8% 1,640 mcg/cm (179 mg) (1 <u>or</u> 2 patches w. 1-50 gm tube cleansing gel/carton)

(continued)

▷ **diclofenac sodium** apply qid prn to intact skin
    Pediatric: <12 years: <u>not</u> established; ≥12 years: same as adult
        Pennsaid 1.5% in 10 drop increments, dispense and rub into front, side, and back of knee; usually 40
        drops (40 mg) qid
            Topical soln: 1.5% (150 ml)
        Pennsaid 2% apply 2 pump actuations (40 mg) and rub into front, side, and back of knee bid
            Topical soln: 2% (20 mg/pump actuation, 112 gm)
        Solaraze Gel massage into clean skin bid prn
            Gel: 3% (50 gm) (benzyl alcohol)
        Voltaren Gel (OTC) (G) apply qid prn to intact skin
            Gel: 1% (100 gm)
    Comment: *Diclofenac* is contraindicated with **aspirin** allergy. As with other NSAIDs, should be avoided in
    late pregnancy (≥30 weeks) because it may cause premature closure of the ductus arteriosus.
▷ **doxepin** cream apply to affected area qid at intervals of at least 3-4 hours; max 8 days
    Pediatric: <12 years: <u>not</u> recommended; >12 years: same as adult
        Prudoxin *Crm:* 5% (45 gm)
        Zonalon *Crm:* 5% (30, 45 gm)
▷ **pimecrolimus** 1% cream **(G)** <2 years: <u>not</u> recommended; ≥2 years: apply to affected area bid; do <u>not</u> apply
    an occlusive dressing
        Elidel *Crm:* 1% (30, 60, 100 gm)
    Comment: *Pimecrolimus* is indicated for short-term and intermittent long-term use. Discontinue use when
    resolution occurs. Contraindicated if the patient is immunosuppressed. Change to the 0.1% preparation <u>or</u>
    if secondary bacterial infection is present.
▷ **trolamine salicylate** apply tid-qid
    Pediatric: <2 years: <u>not</u> recommended; ≥2 years: same as adult
        Mobisyl Creme *Crm:* 10% (100 gm)

PSEUDOBULBAR AFFECT (PBA) DISORDER

Comment: Pseudobulbar affect (PBA), emotional lability, labile affect, <u>or</u> emotional incontinence refers to a
neurologic disorder characterized by involuntary crying <u>or</u> uncontrollable episodes of crying and/or laughing,
<u>or</u> other emotional outbursts. PBA occurs secondary to a neurologic disease <u>or</u> brain injury such as traumatic
brain injury (TBI), stroke, Parkinson's disease, multiple sclerosis, amyotrophic lateral sclerosis (ALS, Lou
Gehrig's disease).

▷ **dextromethorphan+quinidine (G)** 1 cap once daily x 7 days; then starting on day 8, 1 cap bid
    Pediatric: <12 years: <u>not</u> recommended; ≥12 years: same as adult
        Nuedexta *Cap:* dextro 20 mg+quini 10 mg
    Comment: *dextromethorphan hydrobromide* is an uncompetitive N-methyl D-aspartate (NMDA) receptor
    antagonist and sigma-1 agonist. *Quinidine sulfate* is a CYP450 2D6 inhibitor. **Nuedexta** is contraindicated
    with a monoamine oxidase inhibitor (MAOI) <u>or</u> within 14 days of stopping an MAOI, with prolonged QT
    interval, congenital long QT syndrome, history suggestive of torsades de pointes, <u>or</u> heart failure, complete
    atrioventricular (AV) block without implanted pacemaker <u>or</u> patients at high risk of complete AV block,
    and concomitant drugs that both prolong QT interval and are metabolized by CYP2D6 (e.g., *thioridazine*
    <u>or</u> *pimozide*). Discontinue **Nuedexta** if the following occurs: hepatitis <u>or</u> thrombocytopenia <u>or</u> any other
    hypersensitivity reaction. Monitor ECG in patients with left ventricular hypertrophy (LVH) <u>or</u> left ventricular
    dysfunction (LVD). *Desipramine* exposure increases **Nuedexta** 8-fold; reduce *desipramine* dose and adjust
    based on clinical response. Use of **Nuedexta** with selective serotonin reuptake inhibitors (SSRIs) <u>or</u> tricyclic
    antidepressants (TCAs) increases the risk of *serotonin syndrome*. *Paroxetine* exposure increases **Nuedexta**
    two-fold; therefore, reduce **paroxetine** dose and adjust based on clinical response (*digoxin* exposure
    may increase *digoxin* substrate plasma concentration). **Nuedexta** is <u>not</u> recommended in pregnancy <u>or</u>
    breastfeeding. Safety and effectiveness of **Nuedexta** in children have <u>not</u> been established.

PSEUDOGOUT

Injectable Acetaminophen *see* **Pain**
NSAIDs *see* Appendix I. NSAIDs online at https://connect.springerpub.com/content/reference-
book/978-0-8261-7935-7/back-matter/part02/back-matter/bmatter10
Opioid Analgesics *see* **Pain**
Topical and Transdermal Analgesics *see* **Pain**
Parenteral Corticosteroids *see* Appendix L. Parenteral Corticosteroids
Oral Corticosteroids *see* Appendix K. Oral Corticosteroids
Topical Analgesic and Anesthetic Agents *see* Appendix H. Anesthetic Agents for Local Infiltration and
Dermal/Mucosal Membrane Application online at https://connect.springerpub.com/content/reference-
book/978-0-8261-7935-7/back-matter/part02/back-matter/bmatter9

PSEUDOMEMBRANOUS COLITIS

Comment: Staphylococcal enterocolitis and antibiotic-associated pseudomembranous colitis caused by *Clostridioides difficile*.

ANTI-INFECTIVES
➤ *metronidazole* (G) 500 mg tid x 14 days; not for use in the first trimester of pregnancy)
    Flagyl *Tab:* 250*, 500*mg
    Flagyl 375 *Cap:* 375 mg
    Flagyl ER *Tab:* 750 mg ext-rel
➤ *vancomycin hcl capsule* (G) 500 mg to 2 gm in 3-4 doses x 7-10 days; max 2 gm/day
    Pediatric: 40 mg/kg/day in 3-4 doses x 7-10 days; max 2 gm/day; use caps or oral solution as appropriate
        Vancocin *Cap:* 125, 250 mg

GLYCOPEPTIDE ANTIBACTERIAL AGENT
Comment: Firvanq *(vancomycin hcl oral solution)* is a glycopeptide antibacterial agent FDA-approved to treat *C. difficile*-associated diarrhea (CDAD) and enterocolitis caused by *Staphylococcus aureus*, including methicillin-resistant strains (MRSA). **Firvanq** should be used only to treat or prevent infections that are proven or strongly suspected to be caused by susceptible bacteria. Orally administered *vancomycin hcl* is not effective for treatment of other types of infections. Prescribing **Firvanq** in the absence of a proven or strongly suspected bacterial infection is unlikely to provide benefit to the patient and increases the risk of the development of drug-resistant bacteria.

➤ *vancomycin hcl oral solution* (G) see mfr pkg insert for preparation and important administration information; *CDAD* 125 mg orally qid x 10 days; *Staphylococcal enterocolitis:* 500 mg to 2 gm orally in 3 or 4 divided doses x 7-10 days
    Pediatric: <18 years: *CDAD and staphylococcal enterocolitis:* 40 mg/kg orally in 3 or 4 divided doses x 7-10 days; total daily dosage max 2 gm; ≥18 years: same as adult
        Firvanq *Kit w. pwdr for oral soln:* 25, 50 mg/ml (150, 300 ml) equivalent to 3.75, 7.5, 10.5, or 15 gm *vancomycin hcl,* and grape-flavored diluent
Comment: Nephrotoxicity has occurred following oral *vancomycin hcl* therapy and can occur either during or after completion of therapy. The risk is increased in geriatric patients. Monitor renal function. Ototoxicity has occurred in patients receiving *vancomycin hcl.* Assessment of auditory function may be appropriate in some instances. The most common adverse reactions (≥10%) have been nausea (17%), abdominal pain (15%), and hypokalemia (13%). There are no available data on **Firvanq** use in pregnant females to inform a drug-associated risk of major birth defects or miscarriage. Available published data on *vancomycin hcl* use in pregnancy during the second and third trimesters have not shown an association with adverse pregnancy-related outcomes. There are insufficient data to inform the levels of *vancomycin hcl* in human milk. However, systemic absorption of *vancomycin hcl* following oral administration is expected to be minimal. There are no data on the effects of **Firvanq** on the breastfed infant.

PSITTACOSIS

ANTI-INFECTIVES
➤ *tetracycline* (G) 250 mg qid or 500 mg tid x 7-14 days
    Pediatric: <8 years: not recommended; ≥8 years, <100 lb: 25-50 mg/kg/day in 4 doses x 7-14 days; ≥8 years, ≥100 lb: same as adult
        Achromycin V *Cap:* 250, 500 mg
        Sumycin *Tab:* 250, 500 mg; *Cap:* 250, 500 mg; *Oral susp:* 125 mg/5 ml (100, 200 ml) (fruit) (sulfites)

PSORIASIS, PLAQUE PSORIASIS

Emollients *see Dermatitis: Atopic*
Topical Corticosteroids *see Appendix J. Topical Corticosteroids by Potency*

VITAMIN D-3 DERIVATIVES
➤ *calcipotriene*
    Pediatric: <12 years: not recommended; ≥12 years: same as adult
        Dovonex apply bid to lesions and gently rub in completely
            Crm: 0.005% (30, 120 gm)
        Sorilux Foam *Foam:* 0.005% (60, 120 gm)

VITAMIN D3 DERIVATIVE+CORTICOSTEROID COMBINATIONS
➤ *anhydrous calcipotriene+betamethasone dipropionate* apply to affected areas once daily for up to 8 weeks; do not use more than 100 gm per week; do not use with occlusive dressings; avoid use on the face, groin,

(continued)

or axillae, or if skin atrophy is present at the treatment site; not for oral, ophthalmic, or intravaginal use; discontinue therapy when control is achieved

Pediatric: <18 years: safety and efficacy not established; ≥18 years: same as adult

Wynzora *Crm:* 0.005%/0.064% (calci 50 mcg and beta 0.064% per gram) (60 gm)

Comment: Wynzora cream is a combination of *anhydrous calcipotriene* (a vitamin D analog) and *betamethasone dipropionate* (a corticosteroid) indicated for the topical treatment of plaque psoriasis. Hypercalcemia and hypercalciuria have been observed with use of topical *calcipotriene*. If either condition occurs, discontinue until parameters of calcium metabolism normalize. **Wynzora** can cause reversible hypothalamic-pituitary-adrenal (HPA) axis. Because of a higher ratio of skin surface area to body mass, pediatric patients are at a greater risk than adults of systemic toxicity when treated with topical corticosteroids. Pediatric patients are, therefore, at greater risk of HPA axis suppression and adrenal insufficiency with the use of topical corticosteroids, including **Wynzora** cream. Systemic toxicities such as Cushing's syndrome, linear growth retardation, delayed weight gain, and intracranial hypertension have been reported in pediatric patients, especially those with prolonged exposure to large doses of high-potency topical corticosteroids. **Wynzora** can cause reversible hypothalamicpituitary-adrenal (HPA) axis suppression with the potential for glucocorticosteroid insufficiency during and after withdrawal of treatment. Risk factors include the use of high-potency topical corticosteroid, use over a large surface area, or to areas under occlusion, prolonged use, altered skin barrier, liver failure, or young age. Modify **Wynzora** use if HPA axis suppression develops. **Wynzora** may increase the risk of cataracts and glaucoma. If visual symptoms occur, consider referral to an ophthalmologist. The most common adverse reactions reported (by more than 1% of subjects) have been upper respiratory infection (URI), headache, and application site irritation. Available data with **Wynzora** cream are not sufficient to evaluate a drug-associated risk of major birth defects, miscarriages, or adverse maternal or fetal outcomes. Although there are no available data on use of the *calcipotriene* component in pregnant women, systemic exposure to *calcipotriene* after topical administration of **Wynzora** cream is likely to be low. Observational studies suggest an increased risk of having low birthweight infants with the maternal use of potent or very potent topical corticosteroids. Advise pregnant women that **Wynzora** may increase the potential risk of having a low birthweight infant and to use **Wynzora** cream on the smallest area of skin and for the shortest duration possible. It is not known whether topically administered *calcipotriene* or corticosteroids could result in sufficient systemic absorption to produce detectable quantities in human milk. The developmental and health benefits of breastfeeding should be considered along with the mother's clinical need for **Wynzora** cream and any potential adverse effects on the breastfed child from **Wynzora** or from the underlying maternal condition.

▷ *calcipotriene+betamethasone dipropionate* (G)

Pediatric: <18 years: not recommended; ≥18 years: same as adult

Enstilar apply to affected area and gently rub in once daily x up to 4 weeks; limit treatment area to 30% of body surface area; do not cover with occlusive dressing; do not use on face, axillae, groin, or atrophic skin; max 100 gm/week

Foam: calci 0.005%+beta 0.064% (60 gm spray can)

Taclonex apply to affected area and gently rub in once daily as needed, up to 4 weeks

Taclonex Ointment apply bid to lesions and gently rub in completely; limit treatment area to 30% of body surface area; do not cover with occlusive dressing; do not use on face, axillae, groin, or atrophic skin; max 100 gm/week

Oint: calci 0.005%+beta 0.064% (60, 100 gm)

Taclonex Scalp Topical Suspension apply to affected area and gently rub in once daily x 2 weeks or until cleared; max 8 weeks; limit treatment area to 30% of body surface area; do not cover with occlusive dressing; do not use on face, axillae, groin, or atrophic skin; max 100 gm/week

Bottle: (30, 60 gm; 120 gm [2 x 60 gm])

Wynzora Cream apply to affected areas once daily for up to 8 weeks; discontinue when control is achieved; max 100 gm/week; do not cover with occlusive dressing; do not use on face, axillae, groin, or atrophic skin; max 100 gm/week

Cream: calci 0.005%+beta 0.064% (60 gm)

▷ *calcitriol* apply bid to lesions and gently rub in completely; do not cover with occlusive dressing; do not use on face, axillae, groin, or atrophic skin; max weekly dose should not exceed 200 gm

Pediatric: <18 years: not recommended; ≥18 years: same as adult

Vectical *Oint:* 3 mcg/gm (100 gm)

HIGH-POTENCY TOPICAL STEROID

Other High-Potency Topical Corticosteroids *see* Appendix J. Topical Corticosteroids by Potency

▷ *clobetasol propionate* apply a thin layer to the affected skin areas bid; rub in gently and completely; wash hands after each application; discontinue when control is achieved; max 50 gm/week; max 2 consecutive weeks per treatment course; do not use if atrophy is present at the treatment site; do not bandage, cover, or wrap the treated skin area; avoid use on the face, scalp, axilla, groin, or other intertriginous areas; topical use only; not for oral, ophthalmic, or intravaginal use

Pediatric: <18 years: not recommended; ≥18 years: same as adult

Impoyz *Crm:* 0.025% (60, 112 gm)

Comment: Impoyz *(clobetasol propionate 0.025%)* cream is a high-potency corticosteroid specifically indicated for the treatment of moderate-to-severe plaque psoriasis.

▷ *halobetasol propionate* **(G)**
Pediatric: <18 years: not recommended; ≥18 years: same as adult
Bryhali apply a thin layer to the affected skin areas bid; rub in gently and completely; wash hands after each application; discontinue when control is achieved; max 50 gm/week; max 2 consecutive weeks per treatment course; do not use if atrophy is present at the treatment site; do not bandage, cover, or wrap the treated skin area; avoid use on the face, scalp, axilla, groin, or other intertriginous areas; topical use only; not for oral, ophthalmic, or intravaginal use
Lotn: 0.01% (60, 112 gm)
Comment: Bryhali *(halobetasol propionate 0.01%)* cream is a high-potency corticosteroid specifically indicated for the treatment of moderate-to-severe plaque psoriasis.
Lexette Foam **(G)** apply a thin layer of foam to affected areas once daily
Can: 0.05% (50 gm)
Comment: Lexette Foam *(halobetasol propionate)* is a potent corticosteroid specifically indicated for the topical treatment of plaque psoriasis in adult patients.

HIGH-POTENCY TOPICAL STEROID+RETINOID PRODRUG

▷ *halobetasol propionate+tazarotene*
Pediatric: safety and efficacy not established
Duobrii *Lotn:* halo prop 0.01%+tara 0.045% per gm (100 gm tube)

IMMUNOSUPPRESSANTS

▷ *alefacept* 7.5 mg IV bolus or 15 mg IM once weekly x 12 weeks; may re-treat x 12 weeks
Pediatric: <12 years: not recommended; ≥12 years: same as adult
Amevive *IV dose pack:* 7.5 mg single-use (w. 10 ml sterile water diluents [use 0.6 ml]; 1, 4/pck); *IM dose pack:* 15 mg single-use (w. 10 ml sterile water diluent [use 0.6 ml]; 1, 4/pck
Comment: CD4+ and T-lymphocyte count should be checked prior to initiating treatment with *alefacept* and then monitored. Treatment should be withheld if CD4+ T-lymphocyte counts are below 250 cells/mcl.
▷ *cyclosporine* 1.25 mg/kg bid; may increase after 4 weeks by 0.5 mg/kg/day; then adjust at 2-week intervals; max 4 mg/kg/day; administer with meals
Pediatric: <18 years: not recommended; ≥18 years: same as adult
Neoral *Cap:* 25, 100 mg (alcohol)
Neoral Oral Solution *Oral soln:* 100 mg/ml (50 ml); may dilute in room temperature apple juice or orange juice (alcohol)

ANTIMITOTICS

▷ *anthralin* apply once daily
Pediatric: <12 years: not recommended; ≥12 years: same as adult
Zithranol-RR *Crm:* 1.2% (15, 45 gm)

RETINOIDS

▷ *acitretin* **(G)** 25-50 mg once daily with main meal
Pediatric: <12 years: not recommended; ≥12 years: same as adult
Soriatane *Cap:* 10, 25 mg
▷ *tazarotene* **(G)** apply once daily at HS
Pediatric: <12 years: not recommended; ≥12 years: same as adult
Avage Cream *Crm:* 0.1% (30 gm)
Tazorac Cream *Crm:* 0.05, 0.1% (15, 30, 60 gm)
Tazorac Gel *Gel:* 0.05, 0.1% (30, 100 gm)

COAL TAR PREPARATIONS

▷ *coal tar* **(G)**
Pediatric: same as adult
Scytera **(OTC)** apply qd-qid; use lowest effective dose
Foam: 2%
T/Gel Shampoo Extra Strength **(OTC)** use every other day; max 4 x/week; massage into affected areas for 5 minutes; rinse; repeat
Shampoo: 1%
T/Gel Shampoo Original Formula **(OTC)** use every other day; max 7 x/week; massage into affected areas for 5 minutes; rinse; repeat
Shampoo: 0.5%
T/Gel Shampoo Stubborn Itch Control **(OTC)** use every other day; max 7 x/week; massage into affected areas for 5 minutes; rinse; repeat
Shampoo: 0.5%

PHOSPHODIESTERASE 4 (PDE4) INHIBITOR

▶ *roflumilast* apply to affected area, including intertriginous areas, once daily
  Pediatric: <12 years: safety and efficacy not established; ≥12 years: same as adult

  Zoryve *Crm:* 0.3% (3 mg/gm, 60 gm tube)
  Comment: **Zoryve** is a topical phosphodiesterase 4 (PDE4) inhibitor indicated for the topical treatment of plaque psoriasis. *Child-Pugh Class B or C:* **Zoryve** use is contraindicated. Co-administration of *roflumilast* with systemic CYP3A4 inhibitors, or dual inhibitors that inhibit both CYP3A4 and CYP1A2 simultaneously, may increase *roflumilast* systemic exposure and may result in increased adverse reactions. The risk of such concurrent use should be weighed carefully against benefit. Co-administration of *roflumilast* with oral contraceptives containing *gestodene* and *ethinyl estradiol* may increase *roflumilast* systemic exposure and may result in increased side effects. The risk of such concurrent use should be weighed carefully against benefit. The most common adverse reactions (reported in ≥1% of patients) have been diarrhea, headache, insomnia, application site pain, URIs, and urinary tract infections (UTIs). **Zoryve** should not be used during labor and delivery. There are no human studies that have investigated effects of the **Zoryve** on preterm labor or labor at term; however, animal studies showed that oral *roflumilast* disrupted the labor and delivery process. To minimize potential exposure to the breastfed infant via breast milk, use **Zoryve** on the smallest area of skin and for the shortest duration possible while breastfeeding. Advise mothers not to apply **Zoryve** directly to the nipple and areola to avoid direct infant exposure. There is no information regarding the presence of **Zoryve** in human milk or effects on the breastfed infant. *Roflumilast* and/or its metabolites are excreted into animal milk in animal studies. When a drug is present in animal milk, it is likely that the drug will be present in human milk. Developmental and health benefits of breastfeeding should be considered along with the mother's clinical need for **Zoryve** and any potential adverse effects on the breastfed infant from **Zoryve** or from the underlying maternal condition.

HUMANIZED INTERLEUKIN-17A ANTAGONIST

▶ *brodalumab* inject SC into the upper arm, abdomen, or thigh; rotate sites; administer 210 mg SC (as two separate 150 mg SC injections) at weeks 0, 1, and 2; then 210 mg every 2 weeks
  Pediatric: <18 years: not recommended; ≥18 years: same as adult

  Siliq *Prefilled pen:* 210 mg/1.5 ml solution, single-use (2/carton) (preservative-free)
  Comment: **Siliq** is currently indicated for plaque psoriasis only. **Siliq** is contraindicated with Crohn's disease. *Boxed Warning:* Suicidal ideation and behavior, including completed suicides, have occurred in patients treated with **Siliq**. Prior to prescribing, weigh potential risks and benefits in patients with a history of depression and/or suicidal ideation or behavior. Patients with new or worsening suicidal thoughts and behavior should be referred to a mental health professional, as appropriate. Advise patients and caregivers to seek medical attention for manifestations of suicidal ideation or behavior, new onset or worsening depression, anxiety, or other mood changes. Avoid using live vaccines concurrently with **Siliq** therapy. There are no human data on **Siliq** use in pregnant females to inform a drug-associated risk. Human immunoglobulin G (IgG) antibodies are known to cross the placental barrier; therefore, **Siliq** may be transmitted from the mother to the developing fetus. There are no data on the presence of *brodalumab* in human milk or effects on the breastfed infant. **Siliq** is available only through the restricted **Siliq** Risk Evaluation and Mitigation Strategy (REMS) program.

▶ *ixekizumab* <18 years: not recommended; ≥18 years: recommended dose is 160 mg (2 x 80 mg injections) SC at Week 0, followed by 80 mg at Weeks 2, 4, 6, 8, 10, and 12, then 80 mg SC every 4 weeks thereafter
  Pediatric: <18 years: not recommended; ≥18 years: same as adult

  Taltz *Prefilled pen/Prefilled autoinjector:* 80 mg/ml (1 ml), single-dose
  Comment: **Taltz** injection is the first and only treatment approved by the FDA for moderate-to-severe plaque psoriasis involving the genital area. This indication is based upon positive results from a randomized, double-blind, placebo-controlled study in moderate-to-severe psoriasis involving the genital area which involved 149 patients with plaque psoriasis who were candidates for phototherapy or systemic therapy but failed to respond to or were intolerant to at least one topical therapy. There are no available data on **Taltz** use in pregnancy to inform any drug-associated risks. Human IgG is known to cross the placental barrier; therefore, **Taltz** may be transmitted from the mother to the developing fetus. There are no data on the presence of *ixekizumab* in human milk or effects on the breastfed infant.

▶ *secukinumab* inject SC into the upper arm, abdomen, or thigh; rotate sites; administer 300 mg SC (as two separate 150 mg SC injections) at weeks 0, 1, 2, 3, and 4; then 300 mg every 4 weeks; for some patients, 150 mg/dose may be sufficient
  Pediatric: safety and efficacy not established

  Cosentyx *Prefilled syringe/Sensoready pen:* 150 mg/ml soln, single-use; *Vial:* 150 mg/ml pwdr for SC inj after reconstitution, single-use (preservative-free)
  Comment: **Cosentyx** is a selective interleukin-17A (IL-17A) inhibitor for the treatment of adult patients with moderate-to-severe plaque psoriasis who are candidates for systemic therapy or phototherapy, psoriatic arthritis, ankylosing spondylitis, and psoriatic arthritis, and non-radiographic axial spondyloarthritis. **Cosentyx** may be used as monotherapy or in combination with *methotrexate* (MTX). The most common adverse reactions (incidence >1%) have been nasopharyngitis, diarrhea, and upper respiratory tract infection. Doses up to 30 mg/kg (i.e., approximately 2,000-3,000 mg)

have been administered IV in clinical trials without dose-limiting toxicity. In the event of overdosage, it is recommended that the patient be monitored for any signs or symptoms of adverse reactions and appropriate symptomatic treatment be instituted immediately. Caution should be exercised when considering the use of **Cosentyx** in patients with a chronic infection or a history of recurrent infection. If a serious infection develops, discontinue **Cosentyx** until the infection resolves. Prior to initiating treatment with **Cosentyx**, evaluate the patient for tuberculosis (TB). Exacerbations of Crohn's disease have been observed in clinical trials; therefore, caution should be exercised when prescribing **Cosentyx** to patients with active Crohn's disease. History of a serious hypersensitivity reaction to *secukinumab* or to any of the **Cosentyx** excipients is a contraindication to **Cosentyx** administration. If an anaphylactic reaction or other serious allergic reaction occurs, discontinue **Cosentyx** immediately and initiate appropriate therapy. Prior to initiating treatment with **Cosentyx**, consider completion of all age-appropriate immunizations according to current immunization guidelines. Patients treated with **Cosentyx** should not receive live vaccines. Non-live vaccinations received during a course of **Cosentyx** may not elicit an immune response sufficient to prevent disease. There are no adequate and well-controlled trials of **Cosentyx** in human pregnancy. Animal studies found no evidence of fetal harm. However, **Cosentyx** should be used during pregnancy only if the potential benefit justifies the potential risk to the fetus. It is not known whether *secukinumab* is excreted in human milk or absorbed systemically after ingestion. Because many drugs are excreted in human milk, caution should be exercised when **Cosentyx** is administered to a breastfeeding mother. To report suspected adverse reactions, contact Novartis Pharmaceuticals at 1-888-669-6682 or FDA at 1-800-FDA-1088 or www.fda.gov/medwatch.

INTERLEUKIN-23 ANTAGONIST

▶ *guselkumab* injection administer 100 mg SC at Week 0, Week 4, and every 8 weeks thereafter
Tremfya *Prefilled syringe:* 100 mg/ml (1 ml), single-dose; *OnePress:* 100 mg/ml (1 ml), single-use, patient-controlled injector
Comment: Tremfya is indicated for the treatment of patients >18 years of age with moderate-to-severe plaque psoriasis who are candidates for systemic therapy or phototherapy. Evaluate for TB prior to initiating treatment with **Tremfya**. **Tremfya** may increase the risk of infection. Instruct patients to seek medical advice if signs or symptoms of clinically important chronic or acute infection occur. If a serious infection develops, discontinue **Tremfya** until the infection resolves. Avoid use of live vaccines in patients treated with **Tremfya**. The most common (≥1%) adverse reactions associated with **Tremfya** include URIs, headache, injection site reactions, arthralgia, diarrhea, gastroenteritis, tinea infections, and herpes simplex infections. The safety and efficacy of **Tremfya** in pediatric patients (<18 years of age) have not been established. There are no available data on **Tremfya** use in pregnancy to inform a drug-associated risk of adverse developmental outcomes, presence of *guselkumab* in human milk, or effects on the breastfed infant.

▶ *risankizumab-rzaa* administer 150 mg via SC injection at Week 0, Week 4, and every 12 weeks thereafter
Pediatric: safety and efficacy not established
Skyrizi *single-dose soln for IV infusion:* Vial: 600 mg/10 ml (60 mg/ml) (preservative-free); *single-dose soln for SC injection: Prefilled pen:* 150 mg/ml (1 ml); *Prefilled syringe:* 75 mg/0.83 ml (150 mg/ml), 180 mg/1.2 ml (150 mg/ml) (NOTE: prefilled pen and prefilled syringe have a fixed 27-gauge 1/2 inch needle with needle guard); *Prefilled cartridge:* 360 mg/2.4 ml (150 mg/ml) (NOTE: Prefilled cartridge is supplied with an on-body injector device) (preservative-free)
Comment: Skyrizi is an interleukin-23 antagonist indicated for the treatment of moderate-to-severe plaque psoriasis in adults who are candidates for systemic therapy or phototherapy, active psoriatic arthritis in adults, and moderately to severely active Crohn's disease in adults. **Skyrizi** can be administered as monotherapy or in combination with non-biologic disease-modifying antirheumatic drugs (DMARDs). **Skyrizi** is contraindicated in patients with a history of serious hypersensitivity reaction to *risankizumab-rzaa* or any of the excipients. Serious hypersensitivity reactions, including anaphylaxis, may occur. **Skyrizi** may increase the risk of infection; instruct patients to seek medical advice if signs or symptoms of clinically important infection occur, and if such an infection develops, do not administer **Skyrizi** until the infection resolves. Evaluate for TB prior to initiating treatment. Drug-induced liver injury during induction has been reported. Monitor liver enzymes and bilirubin levels at baseline and, during induction, up to at least 12 weeks of treatment; thereafter, monitor according to routine patient management. Avoid use of live vaccines. Available pharmacovigilance and clinical trial data with *risankizumab-rzaa* use in pregnancy are insufficient to establish a drug-associated risk of major birth defects, miscarriage, or other adverse maternal or fetal outcomes. Although there are no data on *risankizumab-rzaa*, monoclonal antibodies can be actively transported across the placenta, and **Skyrizi** may cause immunosuppression in the infant exposed *in utero*. Transport of endogenous IgG antibodies across the placenta increases as pregnancy progresses and peaks during the third trimester. Because *risankizumab-rzaa* may interfere with immune response to infection, risks and benefits should be considered prior to administering live vaccines to infants exposed to **Skyrizi** *in utero*. There are insufficient data regarding infant serum levels of *risankizumab-rzaa* at birth and the duration of persistence of *risankizumab-rzaa* in infant serum after birth. Although a specific time frame to delay

(continued)

live virus immunizations in infants exposed *in utero* is unknown, a minimum of 5 months after birth should be considered because of the half-life of **Skyrizi**. (NOTE: Published data suggest that the risk of adverse pregnancy outcomes in females with inflammatory bowel disease [IBD] is associated with increased disease activity with adverse pregnancy outcomes including preterm delivery [<37 weeks gestation], low birthweight [<2,500 gm] infants, and small for gestational age [SGA] at birth). Advise females of reproductive potential of potential fetal risk and recommend effective contraception during treatment. There is a pregnancy exposure registry that monitors outcomes in women who become pregnant while treated with **Skyrizi**. Patients should be encouraged to enroll by calling 1-877-302-2161 or http://glowpregnancyregistry.com. There are no data on the presence of *risankizumab-rzaa* in human milk or effects on the breastfed infant. However, endogenous maternal IgG and monoclonal antibodies are transferred in human milk. The effects of local gastrointestinal exposure and limited systemic exposure in the breastfed infant to *risankizumab-rzaa* are unknown. Developmental and health benefits of breastfeeding should be considered along with the mother's clinical need for **Skyrizi** and any potential adverse effects on the breastfed infant from **Skyrizi** or from the underlying maternal condition.

▷ *tildrakizumab-asmn* inject SC; rotate sites; recommended dose is 100 mg at Weeks 0, 4, and every 12 weeks thereafter
    Pediatric: <18 years: not recommended; ≥18 years: same as adult
    Ilumya *Prefilled syringe:* 100 mg/ml (1 ml), single-use (preservative-free)
    Comment: **Ilumya** is an interleukin-23 (IL-23) antagonist indicated for the treatment of adults with moderate-to-severe plaque psoriasis who are candidates for systemic therapy or phototherapy. **Ilumya** acts by selectively binding to the p19 subunit of IL-23 and inhibiting its interaction with the IL-23 receptor, blocking the release of proinflammatory cytokines and chemokines. The most common adverse reactions associated with **Ilumya** treatment are upper respiratory infections (URIs), injection site reactions, and diarrhea. Avoid use of live vaccines in patients treated with **Ilumya**. If a serious allergic reaction occurs, discontinue **Ilumya** immediately and initiate appropriate therapy. **Ilumya** may increase the risk of infection. Evaluate for TB prior to initiating **Ilumya**. Instruct patients to seek medical advice if signs or symptoms of clinically important chronic or acute infection occur. If a serious infection develops, consider discontinuing females until the infection resolves. Limited available data with **Ilumya** use in pregnant women are insufficient to inform a drug-associated risk of adverse developmental outcomes. Human IgG is known to cross the placental barrier; therefore, **Ilumya** may be transferred from the mother to the fetus. There are no data on the presence of *tildrakizumab-asmn* in human milk or effects on the breastfed infant.

INTERLEUKIN-12+INTERLEUKIN-23 ANTAGONIST
▷ *ustekinumab* rotate sites; ≤100 kg: 45 mg SC once; then 45 mg SC once 4 weeks later; then 45 mg SC once every 12 weeks thereafter; >100 kg: 90 mg SC once; then 90 mg SC once 4 weeks later; then 90 mg SC once every 12 weeks thereafter
Pediatric: <12 years: not recommended; ≥12 years: same as adult
    Stelara *Prefilled syringe:* 45 mg/0.5 ml, single dose; *Vial:* 45 mg/0.5 ml, 90 mg/ml, single-dose; 130 mg/26 ml, single-dose (preservative-free)
    Comment: **Stelara** is indicated for patients with moderate-to-severe psoriatic arthritis and may be used as monotherapy or with *methotrexate* (*MTX*).

INTERLEUKIN-36 RECEPTOR ANTAGONIST
▷ *spesolimab-sbzo* (G) administer as a single 900 mg dose via IV infusion over 90 minutes; if flare symptoms persist, may administer an additional IV 900 mg dose 1 week after the initial dose; must be diluted before use; see mfr pkg insert for full prescribing information for preparation, administration instructions, and storage of the diluted solution
Pediatric: safety and efficacy not established
    Spevigo *Vial:* 450 mg/7.5 ml (60 mg/ml), single-dose, soln for dilution and IV infusion (2 vials/carton) (preservative-free); store in carton to protect from light
    Comment: **Spevigo** is an interleukin-36 receptor antagonist indicated for the treatment of generalized pustular psoriasis flares in adults. The most common adverse reactions (incidence ≥5%) have been asthenia and fatigue, nausea and vomiting, headache, pruritus and prurigo, infusion site hematoma and bruising, and urinary tract infection (UTI). **Spevigo** is contraindicated for severe or life-threatening hypersensitivity to *spesolimab-sbzo* or to any of the excipients in **Spevigo**. **Spevigo** may increase the risk of infections. Do not initiate **Spevigo** during any clinically important active infection. Instruct patients to seek medical advice if signs or symptoms of clinically important infection occur after treatment with **Spevigo**. Evaluate patients for TB prior to initiating treatment with **Spevigo**. Hypersensitivity and infusion-related reactions, including drug reaction with eosinophilia and systemic symptoms (DRESS), may occur. If a serious hypersensitivity reaction occurs, discontinue **Spevigo** immediately and initiate appropriate treatment. Do not administer live vaccines concurrently with **Spevigo**. The limited data on the use of **Spevigo** in human pregnancy are insufficient to inform a drug-associated risk of adverse pregnancy-related outcomes. However, human IgG is known to cross the placental barrier; therefore, **Spevigo** may be transmitted from the mother to the developing fetus. In an animal reproduction study, IV administration of a surrogate antibody against IL-36R during the period of organogenesis did not elicit any reproductive toxicity. Embryo/fetal development and pre-and postnatal development toxicity

studies were performed using a surrogate mouse-specific IL-36R antagonist monoclonal antibody. In the embryo/fetal development study, the surrogate was administered intravenously at doses up to 50 mg/kg to pregnant females twice weekly during the period of organogenesis. The surrogate was not associated with embryo/fetal lethality or fetal malformations. In the pre-and postnatal development toxicity study, the surrogate was administered intravenously at doses up to 50 mg/kg to pregnant females twice weekly from gestation day 6 through lactation day 18. There were no maternal effects and there were no treatment-related effects observed on postnatal developmental, neurobehavioral, or reproductive performance of offspring. There are no data on the presence of *spesolimab-sbzo* in human milk or effects on the breastfed infant. *Spesolimab-sbzo* is a monoclonal antibody and is expected to be present in human milk. The developmental and health benefits of breastfeeding should be considered along with the mother's clinical need for **Spevigo** and any potential adverse effects on the breastfed infant from **Spevigo** or from the underlying maternal condition. To report suspected adverse reactions, contact Boehringer Ingelheim Pharmaceuticals at (800) 542-6257 or FDA at 800-FDA-1088 or www.fda.gov/medwatch.

TUMOR NECROSIS FACTOR (TNF) BLOCKERS

▷ *adalimumab* initially 80 mg SC once followed by 40 mg once every other week starting 1 week after initial dose; inject into thigh or abdomen; rotate sites
  Pediatric: <18 years: not recommended; ≥18 years: same as adult
    Humira *Prefilled syringe:* 20 mg/0.4 ml; 40 mg/0.8 ml, single-dose (2/pck; 2, 6/starter pck) (preservative-free)
▷ *adalimumab-aacf administer:* 160 mg SC on Day 1 (may split dose over 2 consecutive days); then 80 mg SC on Day 15; then 40 mg SC every other week starting on Day 29; discontinue in patients without evidence of clinical remission by 8 weeks (Day 57)
    Idacio *Prefilled pen (Idacio Pen):* 40 mg/0.8 ml, single-dose; *Prefilled glass syringe:* 40 mg/0.8 ml, single dose
    Comment: Idacio is biosimilar to Humira *(adalimumab)*.
▷ *adalimumab-adaz* initially 80 SC; then 40 mg SC every other week starting 1 week after initial dose; inject into thigh or abdomen; rotate sites
  Pediatric: <18 years: not recommended; ≥18 years: same as adult
    Hyrimoz *Prefilled syringe/Prefilled pen:* 40 mg/0.8 ml, single-dose (preservative-free)
    Comment: Hyrimoz is biosimilar to Humira *(adalimumab)*.
▷ *adalimumab-adbm* initially 80 SC; then 40 mg SC every other week starting 1 week after initial dose; inject into thigh or abdomen; rotate sites
  Pediatric: <18 years: not recommended; ≥18 years: same as adult
    Cyltezo *Prefilled syringe:* 40 mg/0.8 ml, single-dose (preservative-free)
    Comment: Cyltezo is biosimilar to Humira *(adalimumab)*.
▷ *adalimumab-afzb* 40 mg SC every other week; some patients with rheumatoid arthritis (RA) not receiving *methotrexate* (MTX) may benefit from increasing the frequency to 40 mg SC every week
    Abrilada *Prefilled pen:* 40 mg/0.8 ml, single-dose; *Prefilled syringe:* 40 mg/0.8 ml, 20 mg/0.4 ml, 10 mg/0.2 ml, single-dose (for institutional use only) (preservative-free)
    Comment: Abrilada is biosimilar to Humira *(adalimumab)*.
▷ *adalimumab-bwwd Initial dose (Day 1):* 160 mg SC; *Second dose, 2 weeks later (Day 15):* 80 mg SC; *2 weeks later (Day 29):* begin maintenance dose of 40 mg every other week
    Hadlima *Prefilled autoinjector:* 40 mg/0.8 ml, single-dose (Hadlima PushTouch); *Prefilled syringe:* 40 mg/0.8 ml, single-dose
    Comment: Hadlima is biosimilar to Humira *(adalimumab)*.
▷ *etanercept* inject SC into thigh, abdomen, or upper arm; rotate sites; initially 50 mg twice weekly (3-4 days apart) for 3 months; then 50 mg/week maintenance or 25 mg or 50 mg per week for 3 months; then 50 mg/week maintenance
  Pediatric: <4 years: not recommended; 4-17 years: chronic moderate-to-severe plaque psoriasis; >17 years: same as adult
    Enbrel *Vial:* 25 mg pwdr for SC injection after reconstitution (4/carton w. supplies) (preservative-free, diluent contains benzyl alcohol); *Prefilled syringe:* 25, 50 mg/ml (preservative-free); *SureClick autoinjector:* 50 mg/ml (preservative-free)
▷ *etanercept-ykro* 50 mg SC once weekly
  Pediatric: <4 years: not established; ≥4 years, ≥63 kg, 138 lb: same as adult
    Eticovo *Prefilled syringe:* 25 mg/0.5 ml, 50 mg/ml solution, single-dose
    Comment: Eticovo is biosimilar to Enbrel *(etanercept)*.
▷ *golimumab* administer SC or IV infusion
  Pediatric: <18 years: not recommended; ≥18 years: same as adult
    Simponi 50 mg SC once monthly; rotate sites
      Prefilled syringe, SmartJect autoinjector: 50 mg/0.5 ml, single-use (preservative-free)
    Simponi Aria 2 mg/kg IV infusion week 0 and week 4; then every 8 weeks thereafter
      Vial: 50 mg/4 ml, single-use, soln for IV infusion after dilution (latex-free, preservative-free)

(continued)

▷ *infliximab* must be refrigerated at 2°C to 8°C (36°F to 46°F); administer dose IV over a period of not less than 2 hours; do not use beyond the expiration date as this product contains no preservative; administer in conjunction with **methotrexate (MTX)**, infuse 3 mg/kg at 0, 2, and 6 weeks, then every 8 weeks; some patients may benefit from increasing the dose up to 10 mg/kg or treatment as often as every 4 weeks

Pediatric: safety and efficacy not established

    Remicade *Vial:* 100 mg for reconstitution to 10 ml administration volume, single-dose pwdr (preservative-free)

    Comment: Remicade is indicated to reduce signs and symptoms, and induce and maintain clinical remission, in adults and children ≥6 years of age with moderately to severely active disease who have had an inadequate response to conventional therapy, and reduce the number of draining enterocutaneous and rectovaginal fistulas, and maintain fistula closure, in adults with fistulizing disease. Common adverse effects associated with **Remicade** included abdominal pain, headache, pharyngitis, sinusitis, and upper respiratory infections (URIs). In addition, **Remicade** might increase the risk for serious infections, including tuberculosis (TB), bacterial sepsis, and invasive fungal infections. Available data from published literature on the use of *infliximab* products during pregnancy have not reported a clear association with *infliximab* products and adverse pregnancy outcomes. *Infliximab* products cross the placenta and infants exposed *in utero* should not be administered live vaccines for at least 6 months after birth. Otherwise, the infant may be at increased risk of infection, including disseminated infection, which can become fatal. Available information is insufficient to inform the amount of *infliximab* products present in human milk or effects on the breastfed infant.

▷ *infliximab-abda*
    Renflexis *Vial:* 100 mg pwdr for reconstitution to 10 ml administration volume, single-dose
    Comment: Renflexis is biosimilar to **Remicade** (*infliximab*).

▷ *infliximab-dyyb*
    Inflectra *Vial:* 100 mg pwdr for reconstitution to 10 ml administration volume, single-dose
    Comment: Inflectra is biosimilar to **Remicade** (*infliximab*).

▷ *infliximab-axxq*
    Avsola *Vial:* 100 mg pwdr in a 20 ml single-dose vial, for reconstitution, dilution, and IV infusion
    Comment: Avsola is biosimilar to **Remicade** (*infliximab*).

▷ *infliximab-qbtx*
    Ixifi *Vial:* 100 mg pwdr for reconstitution to 10 ml administration volume, single-dose
    Comment: Ixifi is biosimilar to **Remicade** (*infliximab*).

MOISTURIZING AGENTS

Aquaphor Healing Ointment (OTC) *Oint:* (1.75, 3.5, 14 oz) (alcohol)
Eucerin Daily Sun Defense (OTC) *Lotn:* 6 oz (fragrance-free)
Comment: Eucerin Daily Sun Defense is a moisturizer with SPF-15.
Eucerin Facial Lotion (OTC) *Lotn:* 4 oz
Eucerin Light Lotion (OTC) *Lotn:* 8 oz
Eucerin Lotion (OTC) *Lotn:* 8, 16 oz
Eucerin Original Creme (OTC) *Crm:* 2, 4, 16 oz (alcohol)
Eucerin Plus Creme *Crm:* 4 oz
Eucerin Plus Lotion (OTC) *Lotn:* 6, 12 oz
Eucerin Protective Lotion (OTC) *Lotn:* 4 oz (alcohol)
Comment: Eucerin Protective Lotion is a moisturizer with SPF-25.
Lac-Hydrin Cream (OTC) *Crm:* 280, 385 gm
Lac-Hydrin Lotion (OTC) *Lotn:* 225, 400 gm
Lubriderm Dry Skin Scented (OTC) *Lotn:* 6, 10, 16, 32 oz
Lubriderm Dry Skin Unscented (OTC) *Lotn:* 3.3, 6, 10, 16 oz (fragrance-free)
Lubriderm Sensitive Skin Lotion (OTC) *Lotn:* 3.3, 6, 10, 16 oz (lanolin-free)
Lubriderm Dry Skin (OTC) *Lotn (scented):* 2.5, 6, 10, 16 oz; *Lotn (fragrance-free):* 1, 2.5, 6, 10, 16 oz
Lubriderm Bath 1-2 capfuls in bath or rub onto wet skin as needed; then rinse (8 oz)

PSORIATIC ARTHRITIS

Injectable Acetaminophen *see Pain*
NSAIDs *see* Appendix I. NSAIDs online at https://connect.springerpub.com/content/reference-book/978-0-8261-7935-7/back-matter/part02/back-matter/bmatter10
Opioid Analgesics *see Pain*
Topical and Transdermal Analgesics *see Pain*
Parenteral Corticosteroids *see* Appendix L. Parenteral Corticosteroids
Oral Corticosteroids *see* Appendix K. Oral Corticosteroids
Topical Analgesic and Anesthetic Agents *see* Appendix H. Anesthetic Agents for Local Infiltration and Dermal/Mucosal Membrane Application online at https://connect.springerpub.com/content/reference-book/978-0-8261-7935-7/back-matter/part02/back-matter/bmatter9

TOPICAL AND TRANSDERMAL ANALGESICS

▷ **capsaicin** (G) apply tid-qid prn to intact skin
Pediatric: <2 years: not recommended; ≥2 years: same as adult
  Axsain *Crm:* 0.075% (1, 2 oz)
  Capsin *Lotn:* 0.025, 0.075% (59 ml)
  Capzasin-HP (OTC) *Crm:* 0.075% (1.5 oz), 0.025% (45, 90 gm); *Lotn:* 0.075% (2 oz); 0.025% (45, 90 gm)
  Capzasin-P (OTC) *Crm:* 0.025% (1.5 oz); *Lotn:* 0.025% (2 oz)
  Dolorac *Crm:* 0.025% (28 gm)
  Double Cap (OTC) *Crm:* 0.05% (2 oz)
  R-Gel *Gel:* 0.025% (15, 30 gm)
  Zostrix (OTC) *Crm:* 0.025% (0.7, 1.5, 3 oz)
  Zostrix HP (OTC) *Emol crm:* 0.075% (1, 2 oz)
▷ **capsaicin** 8% patch apply up to 4 patches for one 60-minute application to clean dry skin; may prep
area with topical anesthetic; wear non-latex gloves; patches may be cut to size/shape; treatment may be
repeated every 3 months
Pediatric: <18 years: not recommended; ≥18 years: same as adult
  Qutenza *Patch:* 8% 1,640 mcg/cm (179 mg) (1 or 2 patches w. 1-50 gm tube cleansing gel/carton)
▷ **diclofenac sodium** apply qid prn to intact skin
Pediatric: <12 years: not established; ≥12 years: same as adult
  Pennsaid 1.5% in 10 drop increments, dispense and rub into front, side, and back of knee; usually 40
  drops (40 mg) qid
    Topical soln: 1.5% (150 ml)
  Pennsaid 2% apply 2 pump actuations (40 mg) and rub into front, side, and back of knee bid
    Topical soln: 2% (20 mg/pump actuation, 112 gm)
  Solaraze Gel massage into clean skin bid prn
    Gel: 3% (50 gm) (benzyl alcohol)
  Voltaren Gel (OTC) (G) apply qid prn to intact skin
    Gel: 1% (100 gm)
Comment: *Diclofenac* is contraindicated with **aspirin** allergy. As with other NSAIDs, should be avoided in
late pregnancy (≥30 weeks) because it may cause premature closure of the ductus arteriosus.
▷ **doxepin** cream apply to affected area qid at intervals of at least 3-4 hours; max 8 days
Pediatric: <12 years: not recommended; >12 years: same as adult
  Prudoxin *Crm:* 5% (45 gm)
  Zonalon *Crm:* 5% (30, 45 gm)
▷ **pimecrolimus** 1% cream (G) <2 years: not recommended; ≥2 years: apply to affected area bid; do not apply
an occlusive dressing
  Elidel *Crm:* 1% (30, 60, 100 gm)
Comment: *Pimecrolimus* is indicated for short-term and intermittent long-term use. Discontinue use when
resolution occurs. Contraindicated if the patient is immunosuppressed. Change to the 0.1% preparation or
if secondary bacterial infection is present.
▷ **trolamine salicylate** apply tid-qid
Pediatric: <2 years: not recommended; ≥2 years: same as adult
  Mobisyl Creme *Crm:* 10% (100 gm)

ORAL SALICYLATE

▷ **indomethacin** initially 25 mg bid-tid; increase as needed at weekly intervals by 25-50 mg/day; max 200 mg/day
Pediatric: <14 years: usually not recommended; >2 years, if risk warranted: 1-2 mg/kg/day in divided doses;
max 3-4 mg/kg/day or 150-200 mg/day, whichever is less; <14 years: ER cap not recommended
  Cap: 25, 50 mg; *Susp;* 25 mg/5 ml (pineapple-coconut, mint) (alcohol 1%); *Supp:* 50 mg; *ER Cap:* 75 mg ext-rel
Comment: *Indomethacin* is indicated only for acute painful flares. Administer with food and/or antacids. Use
lowest effective dose for shortest duration.

ORAL NON-STEROIDAL ANTI-INFLAMMATORY DRUGS (NSAIDs)

see more **Oral NSAIDs** NSAIDs online at https://connect.springerpub.com/content/reference-
book/978-0-8261-7935-7/back-matter/part02/back-matter/bmatter10

▷ **diclofenac** take on empty stomach; 35 mg tid; *Hepatic impairment:* use lowest dose
Pediatric: <18 years: not recommended; ≥18 years: same as adult
  Zorvolex *Gelcap:* 18, 35 mg
▷ **diclofenac sodium**
Pediatric: <18 years: not recommended; ≥18 years: same as adult
  Voltaren 50 mg bid to qid or 75 mg bid or 25 mg qid with an additional 25 mg at HS if necessary
    Tab: 25, 50, 75 mg ent-coat
  Voltaren XR 100 mg once daily; rarely, 100 mg bid may be used
    Tab: 100 mg ext-rel
Comment: *Diclofenac* is contraindicated with **aspirin** allergy. As with other NSAIDs, should be avoided in
late pregnancy (≥30 weeks) because it may cause premature closure of the ductus arteriosus.

NON-STEROIDAL ANTI-INFLAMMATORY DRUGS (NSAIDS)+PROTON PUMP INHIBITOR (PPI)

▷ *esomeprazole+naproxen* (G) 1 tab bid; use lowest effective dose for the shortest duration; swallow whole; take at least 30 minutes before a meal
Pediatric: <18 years: not recommended; ≥18 years: same as adult
  Vimovo *Tab:* nap 375 mg+eso 20 mg ext-rel; nap 500 mg+eso 20 mg ext-rel
  Comment: Vimovo is indicated to improve signs/symptoms and risk of gastric ulcer in patients at risk of developing NSAID-associated gastric ulcer.

COX-2 INHIBITORS

Comment: Cox-2 inhibitors are contraindicated with history of asthma, urticaria, and allergic-type reactions to *aspirin*, other NSAIDs, and sulfonamides, 3rd trimester of pregnancy, and coronary artery bypass graft (CABG) surgery.
▷ *celecoxib* (G) 50-400 mg once daily-bid; max 800 mg/day
Pediatric: <18 years: not recommended; ≥18 years: same as adult
  Celebrex *Cap:* 50, 100, 200, 400 mg
▷ *meloxicam* (G)
Pediatric: <18 years: not recommended; ≥18 years: same as adult
  Mobic <2 years, <60 kg: not recommended; ≥2, ≥60 kg: 0.125 mg/kg, max 7.5 mg once daily; ≥18 years: initially 7.5 mg once daily; max 15 mg once daily; *Hemodialysis:* max 7.5 mg/day
  Tab: 7.5, 15 mg; *Oral susp:* 7.5 mg/5 ml (100 ml) (raspberry)
  Vivlodex <18 years: not established; ≥18 years: initially 5 mg once daily; may increase to max 10 mg/day; *Hemodialysis:* max 5 mg/day
  Cap: 5, 10 mg

PHOSPHODIESTERASE 4 (PDE4) INHIBITOR

▷ *apremilast* (G) swallow whole; initial titration over 5 days; maintenance 30 mg bid; *Day 1:* 10 mg in AM; *Day 2:* 10 mg AM and 10 mg PM; *Day 3:* 10 mg AM and 20 mg PM; *Day 4:* 20 mg AM and 20 mg PM; *Day 5:* 20 mg AM and 30 mg PM; *Day 6 and ongoing:* 30 mg AM and 30 mg PM
Pediatric: <12 years: not recommended; ≥12 years: same as adult
  Otezla *Tab:* 10, 20, 30 mg; 2-week starter pack
  Comment: Register pregnant patients exposed to Otezla by calling 877-311-8972.

INTERLEUKIN-23 ANTAGONIST

▷ *guselkumab* 100 mg SC at Week 0, Week 4, and every 8 weeks thereafter; can be used alone or in combination with a conventional DMARD (e.g. *methotrexate* [MTX])
Pediatric: <18 years: not established; ≥18 years: same as adult
  Tremfya *Prefilled syringe:* 100 mg/ml (1 ml), single-dose; *OnePress:* 100 mg/ml (1 ml), single-use, patient-controlled injector
  Comment: Tremfya is an interleukin-23 blocker indicated for active psoriatic arthritis. Evaluate for tuberculosis (TB) prior to initiating treatment. Tremfya may increase the risk of infection. Instruct patients to seek medical advice if signs or symptoms of clinically important chronic or acute infection occur. If a serious infection develops, discontinue Tremfya until the infection resolves. Avoid use of live vaccines in patients treated with Tremfya. The most common (incidence ≥1%) adverse reactions have been upper respiratory infection (URI), headache, injection site reaction, arthralgia, diarrhea, gastroenteritis, tinea infection, and herpes simplex infection. There are no available data on Tremfya use in pregnancy to inform a drug-associated risk of adverse developmental outcomes, presence of *guselkumab* in human milk, or effects on the breastfed infant.
▷ *risankizumab-rzaa Recommended dose:* 150 mg via SC injection at Week 0, Week 4, and every 12 weeks thereafter; do not freeze; do not shake; keep in the original cartons to protect from light; no natural rubber latex
Pediatric: safety and efficacy not established
  Skyrizi *Single-dose preservative-free soln for IV infusion: Vial:* 600 mg/10 ml (60 mg/ml); *Single-dose preservative-free soln for SC injection: Prefilled pen:* 150 mg/ml (1 ml); *Prefilled syringe:* 75 mg/0.83 ml (150 mg/ml), 180 mg/1.2 ml (150 mg/ml) (NOTE: Prefilled pen and prefilled syringe have a fixed 27-gauge ½ inch needle with needle guard); *Prefilled cartridge:* 360 mg/2.4 ml (150 mg/ml) (NOTE: Prefilled cartridge is supplied with an on-body injector device)
  Comment: Skyrizi is an interleukin-23 antagonist indicated for the treatment of moderate-to-severe plaque psoriasis in adults who are candidates for systemic therapy or phototherapy, active psoriatic arthritis in adults, and moderately to severely active Crohn's disease in adults. Skyrizi can be administered as monotherapy or in combination with non-biologic disease-modifying antirheumatic drugs (DMARDs). Skyrizi is contraindicated in patients with a history of serious hypersensitivity reaction to *risankizumab-rzaa* or any of the excipients. Serious hypersensitivity reactions, including anaphylaxis, may occur. Skyrizi may increase the risk of infection; instruct patients to seek medical advice if signs or symptoms of clinically important infection occur, and if such an infection develops, do not administer Skyrizi until the infection resolves. Evaluate for TB prior to initiating treatment. Drug-induced liver injury during induction has been reported. Monitor liver enzymes and bilirubin levels

at baseline and, during induction, up to at least 12 weeks of treatment; thereafter, monitor according to routine patient management. Avoid use of live vaccines. Available pharmacovigilance and clinical trial data with *risankizumab-rzaa* use in pregnancy are insufficient to establish a drug-associated risk of major birth defects, miscarriage, or other adverse maternal or fetal outcomes. Although there are no data on *risankizumab-rzaa*, monoclonal antibodies can be actively transported across the placenta, and **Skyrizi** may cause immunosuppression in the infant exposed *in utero*. Transport of endogenous immunoglobulin G (IgG) antibodies across the placenta increases as pregnancy progresses and peaks during the third trimester. Because *risankizumab-rzaa* may interfere with immune response to infection, risks and benefits should be considered prior to administering live vaccines to infants exposed to **Skyrizi** *in utero*. There are insufficient data regarding infant serum levels of *risankizumab-rzaa* at birth and the duration of persistence of *risankizumab-rzaa* in infant serum after birth. Although a specific time frame to delay live virus immunizations in infants exposed *in utero* is unknown, a minimum of 5 months after birth should be considered because of the half-life of **Skyrizi**. (NOTE: Published data suggest that the risk of adverse pregnancy outcomes in females with inflammatory bowel disease [IBD] is associated with increased disease activity with adverse pregnancy outcomes including preterm delivery [<37 weeks gestation], low birthweight [<2,500 gm] infants, and small for gestational age [SGA] at birth). Advise females of reproductive potential of potential fetal risk and recommend effective contraception during treatment. There is a pregnancy exposure registry that monitors outcomes in women who become pregnant while treated with **Skyrizi**. Patients should be encouraged to enroll by calling 1-877-302-2161 or http://glowpregnancyregistry.com. There are no data on the presence of *risankizumab-rzaa* in human milk or effects on the breastfed infant. However, endogenous maternal IgG and monoclonal antibodies are transferred in human milk. The effects of local gastrointestinal exposure and limited systemic exposure in the breastfed infant to *risankizumab-rzaa* are unknown. Developmental and health benefits of breastfeeding should be considered along with the mother's clinical need for **Skyrizi** and any potential adverse effects on the breastfed infant from **Skyrizi** or from the underlying maternal condition.

INTERLEUKIN-12 AND INTERLEUKIN-23 ANTAGONIST

▷ *ustekinumab* inject SC; rotate sites; ≤100 kg: 45 mg SC once; then 45 mg SC once 4 weeks later; then 45 mg SC once every 12 weeks thereafter; >100 kg: 90 mg SC once; then 90 mg SC once 4 weeks later; then 90 mg SC once every 12 weeks thereafter
Pediatric: <18 years: <u>not</u> recommended; ≥18 years: same as adult
    Stelara *Prefilled syringe:* 45 mg/0.5 ml, single dose; *Vial:* 45 mg/0.5 ml, 90 mg/ml, single-dose; 130 mg/26 ml, single-dose (preservative-free)
    Comment: Stelara may be used as monotherapy or in combination with *methotrexate (MTX)*.

TUMOR NECROSIS FACTOR (TNF) BLOCKERS

▷ *adalimumab* 40 mg SC once every other week; may increase to once weekly without *methotrexate (MTX)*; administer in abdomen or thigh; rotate sites; 2-17 years, supervise first dose
Pediatric: <5 years, <20 kg: <u>not</u> recommended; 5-18 years, living with moderate-to-severe UC, weight-based: 20 kg (44 lb) to <40 kg (<88 lb): *Day 1:* 80 mg; *Day 8:* 40 mg; *Day 15:* 20 mg; *Starting on Day 29:* 20 mg every week or 40 mg every other week; >40 kg (>88 lb): *Day 1:* 160 mg (as a single dose or split over 2 consecutive days); *Day 8:* 80 mg; *Day 15:* 80 mg; *Starting on Day 29:* 40 mg every week or 80 mg every other week; it is recommended to continue the recommended pediatric dosage in patients who turn 18 years of age and who are well-controlled on their **Humira** regimen
    Humira *Prefilled syringe:* 20 mg/0.4 ml, 40 mg/0.8 ml, single-dose (2/pck; 2, 6/starter pck) (preservative-free)
    Comment: Humira may use with *methotrexate (MTX)*, DMARDS, corticoids, salicylates, NSAIDs, or analgesics.
▷ *adalimumab-aacf* 40 mg SC every other week; if <u>not</u> receiving *methotrexate (MTX)* may benefit from increasing the dose to 40 mg SC every week or 80 mg SC every other week
    Idacio *Prefilled pen* (Idacio Pen): 40 mg/0.8 ml, single-dose; *Prefilled glass syringe:* 40 mg/0.8 ml, single-dose
    Comment: Idacio is biosimilar to Humira *(adalimumab)*.
▷ *adalimumab-adaz* 40 mg SC every other week; some patients with rheumatoid arthritis (RA) <u>not</u> receiving *methotrexate (MTX)* may benefit from increasing the frequency to 40 mg SC every week
Pediatric: <18 years: <u>not</u> recommended; ≥18 years: same as adult
    Hyrimoz *Prefilled syringe/Prefilled pen:* 40 mg/0.8 ml, single-dose (preservative-free)
    Comment: Hyrimoz is biosimilar to Humira *(adalimumab)*.
▷ *adalimumab-adbm* initially 80 SC; then 40 mg SC every other week starting 1 week after initial dose; inject into thigh or abdomen; rotate sites
Pediatric: <18 years: <u>not</u> recommended; ≥18 years: same as adult
    Cyltezo *Prefilled syringe:* 40 mg/0.8 ml, single-dose (preservative-free)
    Comment: Cyltezo is biosimilar to Humira *(adalimumab)*.

(continued)

▷ *adalimumab-afzb* 40 mg SC every other week; some patients with RA <u>not</u> receiving *methotrexate (MTX)* may benefit from increasing the frequency to 40 mg SC every week
    Abrilada *Prefilled pen:* 40 mg/0.8 ml, single-dose; *Prefilled syringe:* 40 mg/0.8 ml, 20 mg/0.4 ml, 10 mg/0.2 ml, single-dose (for institutional use only) (preservative-free)
    Comment: Abrilada is biosimilar to Humira *(adalimumab)*.
▷ *adalimumab-bwwd* Initial dose (Day 1): 160 mg SC; *Second dose, 2 weeks later* (Day 15): 80 mg SC; *2 weeks later* (Day 29): begin maintenance dose of 40 mg every other week
    Hadlima *Prefilled autoinjector:* 40 mg/0.8 ml, single-dose (Hadlima PushTouch); *Prefilled syringe:* 40 mg/0.8 ml, single-dose
    Comment: Hadlima is biosimilar to Humira *(adalimumab)*.
▷ *etanercept* 25 mg SC twice weekly (72-96 hours apart) <u>or</u> 50 mg SC weekly; rotate sites
Pediatric: <4 years: not recommended; 4-17 years: 0.4 mg/kg SC twice weekly, 72-96 hours apart (max 25 mg/dose) <u>or</u> 0.8 mg/kg SC weekly (max 50 mg/dose); >17 years: same as adult
    Enbrel *Vial:* 25 mg pwdr for SC injection after reconstitution (4/carton w. supplies) (preservative-free; diluent contains benzyl alcohol); *Prefilled syringe:* 25, 50 mg/ml (preservative-free); *SureClick Autoinjector:* 50 mg/ml (preservative-free)
Comment: *Etanercept* reduces pain, morning stiffness, and swelling. May be administered in combination with *methotrexate (MTX)*. Live vaccines should <u>not</u> be administered concurrently. Do <u>not</u> administer with active infection.
▷ *etanercept-ykro* 50 mg SC once weekly
Pediatric: <4 years: <u>not</u> established; ≥4 years, ≥63 kg, 138 lb: same as adult
    Eticovo *Prefilled syringe:* 25 mg/0.5 ml, 50 mg/ml solution, single-dose
    Comment: Eticovo *(etanercept-ykro)* is biosimilar to **Enbrel.**
▷ *golimumab* administer SC <u>or</u> IV infusion
    Simponi 50 mg SC once monthly; rotate sites
    Pediatric: <18 years: <u>not</u> recommended; ≥18 years: same as adult
    Prefilled syringe, SmartJect autoinjector: 50 mg/0.5 ml, single-use (preservative-free)
    Simponi Aria 2 mg/kg IV infusion week 0 and week 4; then every 8 weeks thereafter
    Pediatric: <2 years: <u>not</u> recommended; ≥2 years, with active psoriatic arthritis (PsA): 80 mg/m² via IV infusion over 30 minutes at Week 0 and Week 4, and every 8 weeks thereafter
    Vial: 50 mg/4 ml, single-use, soln for IV infusion after dilution (latex-free, preservative-free)
    Comment: Corticosteroids, non-biologic DMARDs, <u>and/or</u> NSAIDs may be continued during treatment with *golimumab*.
▷ *infliximab* must be refrigerated at 2°C to 8°C (36°F to 46°F); administer dose intravenously over a period of <u>not</u> less than 2 hours; do <u>not</u> use beyond the expiration date as this product contains no preservative; 5 mg/kg at 0, 2, and 6 weeks, then every 8 weeks; some adult patients who initially respond to treatment may benefit from increasing the dose to 10 mg/kg if response is lost later
Pediatric: safety and efficacy <u>not</u> established
    Remicade *Vial:* 100 mg pwdr for reconstitution to 10 ml administration volume, single-dose (preservative-free)
    Comment: Remicade is indicated to reduce signs and symptoms, and induce and maintain clinical remission, in adults and children ≥6 years of age with moderately to severely active disease who have had an inadequate response to conventional therapy, <u>and</u> reduce the number of draining enterocutaneous and rectovaginal fistulas, and maintain fistula closure, in adults with fistulizing disease. Common adverse effects associated with **Remicade** included abdominal pain, headache, pharyngitis, sinusitis, and URIs. In addition, **Remicade** might increase the risk for serious infections, including TB, bacterial sepsis, and invasive fungal infections. Available data from published literature on the use of *infliximab* products during pregnancy have <u>not</u> reported a clear association with *infliximab* products and adverse pregnancy outcomes. *Infliximab* products cross the placenta and infants exposed *in utero* should <u>not</u> be administered live vaccines for at least 6 months after birth. Otherwise, the infant may be at increased risk of infection, including disseminated infection, which can become fatal. Available information is insufficient to inform the amount of *infliximab* products present in human milk <u>or</u> effects on the breastfed infant.
▷ *infliximab-abda*
    Renflexis *Vial:* 100 mg pwdr for reconstitution to 10 ml administration volume, single-dose
    Comment: Renflexis is biosimilar to Remicade *(infliximab)*.
▷ *infliximab-dyyb*
    Inflectra *Vial:* 100 mg pwdr for reconstitution to 10 ml administration volume, single-dose
    Comment: Inflectra is biosimilar to Remicade *(infliximab)*.
▷ *infliximab-axxq*
    Avsola *Vial:* 100 mg pwdr in a 20 ml single-dose vial, for reconstitution, dilution, and IV infusion
    Comment: Avsola is biosimilar to Remicade *(infliximab)*.
▷ *infliximab-qbtx*
    Ixifi *Vial:* 100 mg pwdr for reconstitution to 10 ml administration volume, single-dose
    Comment: Ixifi is biosimilar to Remicade. *(infliximab)*.

Selective Costimulation Modulator

▷ *abatacept* administer as an IV infusion over 30 minutes at weeks 0, 2, and 4; then every 4 weeks thereafter; <60 kg: administer 500 mg/dose; 60-100 kg: administer 750 mg/dose; >100 kg: administer 1 gm/dose
Pediatric: <6 years: <u>not</u> recommended; 6-17 years: administer as an IV infusion over 30 minutes at Weeks 0, 2, and 4; then every 4 weeks thereafter; <75 kg, administer 10 mg/kg; same as adult (max 1 gm); >17 years: same as adult

    Orencia *Vial:* 250 mg pwdr for IV infusion after reconstitution (silicone-free) (preservative-free); *Prefilled syringe:* 125 mg/ml soln for SC injection (preservative-free); *ClickJect Autoinjector:* 125 mg/ml soln for SC injection

CD20-DIRECTED CYTOLYTIC MONOCLONAL ANTIBODY

▷ *rituximab* administer corticosteroid 30 minutes prior to each infusion; concomitant **methotrexate** (**MTX**) therapy, administer a 1,000 mg IV infusion at 0 and 2 weeks; then every 24 weeks <u>or</u> based on response, but <u>not</u> sooner than every 16 weeks
Pediatric: <6 years: <u>not</u> recommended; ≥6 years: same as adult

    Rituxan *Vial:* 100 mg/10 ml (10 mg/ml), 500 mg/50 ml (10 mg/ml), single-use (preservative-free)
Comment: *Rituximab* is a B-cell targeting chimeric monoclonal antibody that acts against CD20 and reduces antibody titers. B-cell depletion by *rituximab* may also set the stage for production of interleukin 10-secreting B-cells that do <u>not</u> interact with T-cells, which further reduces production of antidesmoglein antibodies. *Rituximab* carries a black box warning regarding fatal infusion reactions, severe mucocutaneous reactions, hepatitis B virus reactivation, and progressive multifocal leukoencephalopathy. However, serious adverse events are rare. There was no evidence of increased mortality with longer exposure to *rituximab* <u>or</u> to multiple courses of therapy.

PUPILLARY DILATION (MYDRIASIS): SHORT-TERM

TOPICAL ANTICHOLINERGIC+ALPHA-1 ADRENERGIC AGONIST COMBINATION

▷ *tropicamide+phenylephrine hydrochloride* administer 1 metered spray to the cornea of each eye to be dilated; repeat after 5 minutes; Mydcombi acts in 15-30 minutes with maximal mydriasis occurring in 20-90 minutes; darker irides tend to dilate slower than lightly pigmented irides (and to achieve maximal effect may require more doses than lighter irides)
Pediatric: <1 year: administer 1 metered spray to the cornea of each eye to be dilated, up to a max of 3 sprays per eye per day; >1 year: same as adult

    Mydcombi *Ophth spray:* 1%/2.5% (tropi 1%+phenyle hcl 2.5%), multi-dose, metered, fixed-dose soln; each metered spray delivers 0.008 ml, which contains 0.08 mg tropicamide and 0.2 mg phenylephrine hcl; Mydcombi solution is packaged in a 2 ml vial enclosed in a dispenser cartridge; each Mydcombi cartridge holds approximately 180 sprays
Comment: Mydcombi *(phenylephrine hydrochloride and tropicamide)* is an alpha-1 adrenergic receptor agonist and anticholinergic fixed-combination ophthalmic spray indicated to induce mydriasis for diagnostic procedures and in conditions where short-term pupil dilation is desired. *Tropicamide*, the anticholinergic component of Mydcombi, blocks the responses of the sphincter muscle of the iris, dilating the pupil (mydriasis). *Phenylephrine hydrochloride*, the alpha-1 adrenergic agonist component of Mydcombi, acts as a mydriatic agent by contracting the dilator muscle of the iris. Mydcombi can cause significant elevation in blood pressure; use caution in pediatric patients <5 years of age, and in patients with cardiovascular disease (CVD) <u>or</u> hyperthyroidism. In patients at high risk, monitor blood pressure posttreatment. Atropine-like drugs may exaggerate the adrenergic pressor response. Cholinergic agonists and ophthalmic cholinesterase inhibitors may interfere with the antihypertensive action of *carbachol*, *pilocarpine,* <u>or</u> *ophthalmic cholinesterase inhibitors*. Mydcombi may potentiate the cardiovascular depressant effects of potent inhalation anesthetic agents. Mydcombi may produce a transient elevation in intraocular pressure. Rebound miosis has been reported 1 day after administration of Mydcombi. Mydcombi may rarely cause central nervous system (CNS) disturbances, which may be dangerous in pediatric patients. Systemic adverse reactions include dryness of the mouth, tachycardia, headache, allergic reaction, nausea, vomiting, and pallor. CNS disturbances and muscle rigidity have been reported with the use of *tropicamide*. The most common ocular adverse reactions to Mydcombi include transient blurred vision, reduced visual acuity, photophobia, superficial punctate keratitis, and mild eye discomfort. Increased intraocular pressure has been reported following the use of mydriatics. Mydriasis will reverse spontaneously with time, with expected recovery after 3 to 8 hours. Complete recovery from mydriasis in some individuals may require 24 hours. Advise patients that they will likely experience sensitivity to light and blurred vision while their pupils are dilated. Advise patients <u>not</u> to drive, use machinery, <u>or</u> do any activity that requires clear vision until they are sure they can perform such activities safely. There are <u>no</u> available data on Mydcombi use in human <u>or</u> animal pregnancy to inform any drug-associated risks. It is also <u>not</u> known whether *tropicamide* <u>or</u> *phenylephrine* can cause fetal harm when administered in human <u>or</u> animal pregnancy <u>or</u> can affect reproduction capacity. Mydcombi should be administered to a pregnant female only if clearly needed. There are <u>no</u> data on the presence of *tropicamide* <u>or</u> *phenylephrine* in human milk from the administration of Mydcombi <u>or</u> effects on the breastfed infant. Developmental and health benefits of breastfeeding should be considered along with the mother's clinical need for Mydcombi and any potential adverse effects on the breastfed infant from Mydcombi.

PULMONARY ARTERIAL HYPERTENSION (PAH) (WHO GROUP I)

ENDOTHELIAL RECEPTOR ANTAGONIST (ERA)

▶ *bosentan* (G) initiate at 62.5 mg orally bid; for patients weighing greater than 40 kg, increase to 125 mg orally bid after 4 weeks
Pediatric: <3 years: not established; 3-12: initiate at 62.5 mg orally bid; for patients weighing >40 kg, increase to 125 mg orally bid after 4 weeks; >12 years: same as adult
    Tracleer *Tab:* 62.5, 125 mg film-coat; *Tab for oral suspension:* 32 mg
Comment: Bosentan is an endothelin receptor antagonist (ERA) indicated for the treatment of pulmonary arterial hypertension (PAH) (WHO Group 1). **Tracleer** is the first ERA indicated for the treatment of PAH in patients aged 3 years and older with idiopathic or congenital PAH to improve pulmonary vascular resistance (PVR), which is expected to result in an improvement in exercise ability. The most common adverse events associated with **Tracleer** in clinical trials include respiratory tract infections, headache, edema, chest pain, syncope, flushing, hypotension, sinusitis, arthralgia, abnormal serum aminotransferases, palpitations, and anemia. Monitor hemoglobin levels after 1 and 3 months of treatment, then every 3 months thereafter. If signs of pulmonary edema occur, consider the diagnosis of associated pulmonary veno-occlusive disease (PVOD) and consider discontinuing **Tracleer**. Measure liver aminotransferases prior to initiation of treatment and then monthly. Reduce the dose and closely monitor patients developing aminotransferase elevations >3 x the upper limit of normal (ULN). Co-administration of **Tracleer** with drugs metabolized by CYP2C9 and CYP3A can increase exposure to **Tracleer** and/or the co-administered drug. **Tracleer** use decreases contraceptive exposure and reduces effectiveness. There are no data on the presence of *bosentan* in human milk or the effects on the breastfed infant. However, because of the potential for serious adverse reactions, such as fluid retention and hepatotoxicity in breastfed infants, advise women not to breastfeed during treatment with **Tracleer** and pregnancy is contraindicated while taking **Tracleer**. To prevent pregnancy, females of reproductive potential must use two reliable forms of contraception during treatment and for 1 month after stopping **Tracleer**. Due to the risks of hepatotoxicity and birth defects, **Tracleer** includes a boxed warning and is only available through the restricted **Tracleer** Risk Evaluation and Mitigation Strategy (REMS) program, a restricted distribution program. Patients, prescribers, and pharmacies must enroll in the program to receive and administer **Tracleer**: www.tracleerrems.com/prescribers.aspx.

▶ *macitentan* 10 mg once daily; doses >10 mg once daily have not been studied in patients with PAH and are not recommended
Pediatric: safety and efficacy not established
    Opsumit *Tab:* 10 mg film-coat (film-coat, 2 x 15/aluminum foil blisters/carton, 30 count/ bottle)
    Comment: Opsumit is an endothelin receptor antagonist (ERA) indicated for the treatment of pulmonary arterial hypertension (PAH, WHO Group 1) to delay disease progression (disease progression included death, initiation of IV or SC prostanoids, or clinical worsening of PAH [i.e., decreased 6-minute walk distance], worsened PAH symptoms, and need for additional PAH treatment). **Opsumit** also reduced hospitalization for PAH. The most common adverse reactions (more frequent than placebo by ≥3%) have been anemia, nasopharyngitis/pharyngitis, bronchitis, headache, influenza, and urinary tract infection (UTI). Because ERAs can cause hepatotoxicity and liver failure, obtain baseline liver enzymes and monitor as clinically indicated. Monitor for decreases in hemoglobin. Pulmonary edema can occur in patients with pulmonary veno-occlusive disease (PVOD). *Macitentan* was teratogenic in animal studies at all doses tested. Therefore, **Opsumit** is contraindicated in human pregnancy. Advise females of reproductive potential of the risk to the fetus and to use effective contraception during **Opsumit** treatment and for 1 month after the last **Opsumit** dose. Exclude pregnancy prior to initiating treatment with **Opsumit**, monthly during treatment, and for 1 month after the last **Opsumit** dose. If pregnancy is confirmed, discontinue **Opsumit** treatment. Advise mothers of the potential for serious adverse reactions from *macitentan* in breastfed infants and to either not breastfeed or discontinue **Opsumit**. For all female patients, **Opsumit** is available only through the Opsumit Risk Evaluation and Mitigation Strategy (REMS) program. Further information is available at www.OPSUMITREMS.com or 866-228-3546. Information on **Opsumit**-certified pharmacies or wholesale distributors is available through Actelion Pathways at 866-228-3546. Decreases in sperm count have been observed in male patients taking ERAs. To report suspected adverse reactions, contact Actelion at 866-228-3546 or FDA at 800-FDA-1088 or www.fda.gov/medwatch.

PROSTACYCLIN RECEPTOR AGONIST

▶ *macitentan* (G) 10 mg once daily; doses higher than 10 mg once daily have not been studied in patients with PAH and are not recommended
Pediatric: safety and efficacy not established
    Opsumit *Tab:* 10 mg film-coat
    Comment: Opsumit is an endothelin receptor antagonist (ERA) indicated for the treatment of pulmonary arterial hypertension (PAH, WHO Group 1) to reduce the risks of disease progression and hospitalization. The most common adverse reactions (more frequent than placebo by ≥3%) have been anemia, nasopharyngitis/pharyngitis, bronchitis, headache, influenza, and UTI. ERAs cause hepatotoxicity and liver failure. Obtain baseline liver enzymes and monitor as clinically indicated. Fluid retention may require intervention. Pulmonary edema in patients with (PVOD); if confirmed, discontinue treatment. Decreases in sperm count have been observed in patients taking ERAs. Monitor for decreases in hemoglobin. Strong CYP3A4 inducers (e.g., *rifampin*) reduce exposure to *macitentan*; avoid co-administration with

Opsumit. Strong CYP3A4 inhibitors (e.g., *ketoconazole, ritonavir*) increase exposure to *macitentan*; avoid co-administration with **Opsumit.** *Boxed Warning:* embryo/fetal toxicity; therefore, do not administer **Opsumit** to a pregnant female. For females of reproductive potential, exclude pregnancy before start of treatment, monthly during treatment, and 1 month after stopping treatment. Advise males and females of reproductive potential regarding contraception. Advise not to breastfeed. For all female patients, **Opsumit** is available only through the **Opsumit** Risk Evaluation and Mitigation Strategy (REMS) program. Further information is available at www.OPSUMITREMS.com or 1-866-228-3546. Information on **Opsumit**-certified pharmacies or wholesale distributors is available through Actelion Pathways at 1-866-228-3546.

▶ *selexipag* (G) *Starting dose:* 200 mcg bid; increase the dose by 200 mcg bid at weekly intervals to the highest tolerated dose; max 1,600 mcg bid; *Maintenance dose:* determined by tolerability; *Child-Pugh Class B: Starting dose:* 200 mcg once daily; increase the dose by 200 mcg once daily at weekly intervals to the highest tolerated dose up to 1,600 mcg once daily; *Child-Pugh Class C:* avoid use; do not, break, cut, crush, or chew; *IV infusion:* administer bid; dose is determined by the patient's current (max tolerated) dose of **Uptravi** in tablet form

Pediatric: safety and efficacy not established

    Uptravi *Tab:* 200, 400, 600, 800, 1,000, 1,200, 1,400, 1,600 mcg film-coat; *Vial:* 1,800 mcg (10 ml), single-dose, pwdr, for reconstitution, dilution, and IV infusion

    Comment: Uptravi is a prostacyclin receptor agonist indicated for the treatment of pulmonary arterial hypertension (PAH, WHO Group 1) to delay disease progression and reduce the risk of hospitalization. Adverse reactions occurring more frequently (≥5%, on **Uptravi** compared to placebo) have been headache, diarrhea, jaw pain, nausea, myalgia, vomiting, pain in extremity, and flushing. When co-administered with moderate CYP2C8 inhibitors (e.g., *clopidogrel, deferasirox,* and *teriflunomide*), reduce the dosing of **Uptravi** to once daily. Concomitant use of strong CYP2C8 inhibitors (e.g., *gemfibrozil*) is contraindicated. CYP2C8 inducers (e.g., *rifampin*) decrease exposure to the active metabolite; increase up to twice the dose of **Uptravi.** Should signs of pulmonary edema occur, consider the possibility of associated PVOD. If confirmed, discontinue **Uptravi.** There are no adequate and well-controlled studies with **Uptravi** in pregnant females. Animal reproduction studies performed with *selexipag* showed no clinically relevant effects on embryo/fetal development or survival. Because of the potential for serious adverse reactions in breastfeeding infants, discontinue breastfeeding or discontinue **Uptravi.**

ENDOTHELIN RECEPTOR ANTAGONIST, SELECTIVE FOR THE ENDOTHELIN TYPE-A (ETA) RECEPTOR

▶ *ambrisentan* (G) initiate treatment at 5 mg once daily, with or without *tadalafil* 20 mg once daily; at 4-week intervals, either the dose of **Letairis** or *tadalafil* can be increased, as needed and tolerated, to **Letairis** 10 mg or *tadalafil* 40 mg; do not split, crush, or chew

Pediatric: <12 years: not recommended; ≥12 years: same as adult

    Letairis *Tab:* 5, 10 mg film-coat

    Comment: In patients with PAH, plasma ET-1 concentrations are increased as much as 10-fold and correlate with increased mean right atrial pressure and disease severity. ET-1 and ET-1 mRNA concentrations are increased as much as 9-fold in the lung tissue of patients with PAH, primarily in the endothelium of pulmonary arteries. These findings suggest that ET-1 may play a critical role in the pathogenesis and progression of PAH. When taken with *tadalafil,* **Letairis** is indicated to reduce the risk of disease progression and hospitalization, to reduce the risk of hospitalization due to worsening PAH, and to improve exercise tolerance. **Letairis** is contraindicated in idiopathic pulmonary fibrosis (IPF). Exclude pregnancy before the initiation of treatment with **Letairis.** Females of reproductive potential must use acceptable methods of contraception during treatment with **Letairis** and for 1 month after treatment. Obtain monthly pregnancy tests during treatment and 1 month after discontinuation of treatment. Females can only receive **Letairis** through the **Letairis** Risk Evaluation and Mitigation Strategy (REMS) program, a restricted distribution program, because of the risk of embryo/fetal toxicity: www.Letairisrems.com or 1-866-664-5327.

Guanylate Cyclase Stimulator

▶ *riociguat* (G) initially 0.5-1 mg tid; titrate every 2 weeks as tolerated (SBP ≥95 and absence of hypotensive symptoms) to highest tolerated dose; max 2.5 mg tid

Pediatric: <12 years: not recommended; ≥12 years: same as adult

    Adempas *Tab:* 0.5, 1, 1.5, 2, 2.5 mg

    Comment: If **Adempas** is interrupted for ≥3 days, retitrate. Consider titrating to dosage higher than 2.5 mg tid, if tolerated, in patients who smoke. Consider a starting dose of 0.5 mg tid when initiating **Adempas** in patients receiving strong cytochrome P450 (CYP) and P-glycoprotein/breast cancer resistance protein (P-gp/BCRP) inhibitors such as azole antimycotics (e.g., *ketoconazole, itraconazole*) or HIV protease inhibitors (e.g., *ritonavir*). Monitor for signs and symptoms of hypotension with strong CYP and P-gp/BCRP inhibitors. Obtain pregnancy tests prior to initiation and monthly during treatment. **Adempas** has consistently shown to have teratogenic effects when administered to animals. Females can only receive **Adempas** through the Adempas Risk Evaluation and Mitigation Strategy (REMS) program, a restricted distribution program: www.AdempasREMS.com or 855-4 ADEMPAS. It is not known if **Adempas** is present in human milk; however, *riociguat* or its metabolites were present in the milk of rats. Because of the potential for serious adverse reactions in nursing infants from *riociguat,* discontinue nursing or **Adempas.**

(continued)

In placebo-controlled clinical trials, serious bleeding has occurred including hemoptysis, hematemesis, vaginal hemorrhage, catheter site hemorrhage, subdural hematoma, and intra-abdominal hemorrhage. Safety and efficacy have not been demonstrated in patients with creatinine clearance <15 ml/min or on dialysis or severe hepatic impairment (Child-Pugh Class C).

PHOSPHODIESTERASE TYPE 5 (PDE5) INHIBITORS AND CGMP-SPECIFIC DRUGS

➤ *sildenafil citrate* (G) *Orally:* initially 5 or 20 mg tid, 4-6 hours apart; max 20 mg tid; *IV bolus:* 2.5 mg or 10 mg bolus injection tid, 4-6 hours apart; max 10 mg tid; the dose does not need to be adjusted for body weight
Pediatric: <12 years: not recommended; ≥12 years: same as adult
    Revatio *Tab:* 20 mg film-coat; *Oral susp:* 10 mg/ml pwdr for reconstitution (1.12 gm, 112 ml) (grape) (sorbitol); *Vial:* 10 mg/12.5 ml (0.8 mg/ml)
    Comment: A 10 mg IV dose is predicted to provide pharmacologic effect equivalent to the 20 mg oral dose. Revatio is contraindicated with concomitant nitrate drugs, including *nitroglycerin, isosorbide dinitrate,* isosorbide mononitrate, and some recreational drugs such as "poppers." Taking **Revatio** with a nitrate can cause a sudden and serious decrease in blood pressure. **Revatio** is contraindicated with concomitant guanylate cyclase stimulator drugs such as *riociguat* (**Adempas**). Avoid the use of grapefruit products while taking **Revatio**. Stop **Revatio** and get emergency medical help if sudden vision loss. **Revatio** is contraindicated with other phosphodiesterase type 5 (PDE5) inhibitors and cGMP-specific drugs such as *avanafil* (**Stendra**), *tadalafil* (**Cialis**), or *vardenafil* (**Levitra**). Caution with history of recent myocardial infarction (MI), stroke, life-threatening arrhythmia, hypotension, hypertension, cardiac failure, unstable angina, retinitis pigmentosa, CYP3A4 inhibitors (e.g., *cimetidine,* the azoles, *erythromycin,* protease inhibitors) (e.g., *ritonavir*), CYP3A4 inducers (e.g., *rifampin, carbamazepine, phenytoin, phenobarbital*), alcohol, and antihypertensive agents. Side effects include headache, flushing, nasal congestion, rhinitis, dyspepsia, and diarrhea. Use **Revatio** with caution in patients with anatomical deformation of the penis (e.g., angulation, cavernosal fibrosis, or Peyronie's disease) or in patients who have conditions which may predispose them to priapism (e.g., sickle cell anemia, multiple myeloma, or leukemia). In the event of an erection that persists longer than 4 hours, the patient should seek immediate medical assistance. If priapism (painful erection greater than 6 hours in duration) is not treated immediately, penile tissue damage and permanent loss of potency could result.

➤ *tadalafil* (G) 40 mg once daily; *CrCl 31-80 ml/min:* initially 20 mg once daily; increase to 40 mg once daily if tolerated; *CrCl <30 ml/min:* not recommended; *Mild or moderate hepatic cirrhosis (Child-Pugh Class A or B):* initially 20 mg once daily; *Severe hepatic cirrhosis (Child-Pugh Class C):* not recommended; *Use with* **ritonavir**; *Receiving* **ritonavir** *for at least 1 week:* initiate *tadalafil* at 20 mg once daily; may increase to 40 mg once daily if tolerated; *Already on* **tadalafil**: stop *tadalafil* at least 24 hours prior to initiating *ritonavir*; resume *tadalafil* at 20 mg once daily after at least 1 week; may increase to 40 mg once daily if tolerated
Pediatric: <12 years: not recommended; ≥12 years: same as adult
    Adcirca *Tab:* 20 mg
    Comment: Contraindicated with concomitant organic nitrates and guanylate cyclase stimulators (e.g., *riociguat*).

➤ *treprostinil* swallow whole; take with food
    Orenitram *Tab:* 0.125, 0.25, 1, 2.5 mg ext-rel
    Comment: Orenitram is indicated to improve exercise capacity. It is contraindicated with severe hepatic impairment (Child-Pugh Class C). **Orenitram** inhibits platelet aggregation and increases the risk of bleeding. Concomitant administration of **Orenitram** with diuretics, antihypertensive agents, or other vasodilators increases the risk of symptomatic hypotension.

PULMONARY FIBROSIS, IDIOPATHIC (IPF)/INTERSTITIAL LUNG DISEASE (ILD)

Parenteral Corticosteroids *see* Appendix L. Parenteral Corticosteroids
Oral Corticosteroids *see* Appendix K. Oral Corticosteroids

Comment: Idiopathic pulmonary fibrosis (IPF) is a chronic, progressive, interstitial lung disease (ILD) of unknown etiology. There are few effective therapies and the mortality rate is high. New treatments for IPF are urgently needed. Anti-inflammatory therapy with corticosteroids or immunosuppressants fails to significantly improve the survival time of patients with IPF. Other pharmacologic interventions, including *nintedanib* (**Ofev**), *etanercept* (**Enbrel**), *warfarin, imatinib mesylate* (**Gleevec**), and *bosentan* (**Tracleer**), remain controversial. *Pirfenidone* was approved by the European Medicines Agency in 2011. In a 2016 study, *N-acetylcysteine* was found to have a significant effect only on decreases in percentage of predicted vital capacity and 6 minutes walking test distance. *N-acetylcysteine* showed no beneficial effect on changes in forced vital capacity, changes in predicted carbon monoxide diffusing capacity, rates of adverse events, or death rates.

➤ *azathioprine* 1 mg/kg/day in a single or divided doses; may increase by 0.5 mg/kg/day q 4 weeks; max 2.5 mg/kg/day; minimum trial to ascertain effectiveness is 12 weeks
Pediatric: <12 years: not recommended; ≥12 years: same as adult
    Azasan *Tab* 75*, 100*mg
    Imuran *Tab* 50*mg

▶ *nintedanib* recommended dose is 150 mg bid, approximately 12 hours apart, with food; *Mild hepatic impairment (Child-Pugh Class A):* 100 mg bid, approximately 12 hours apart, with food; *Moderate or severe hepatic impairment (Child-Pugh Class B or C):* not recommended; consider temporary dose reduction to 100 mg, treatment interruption, or discontinuation for management of adverse reactions; prior to initiation of treatment, perform a pregnancy test; monitor liver function tests (LFTs) and bilirubin before and during treatment

Pediatric: <12 years: not established; ≥12 years: same as adult

    Ofev *Cap:* 100, 150 mg

    Comment: Monitor liver enzymes. If elevated LFTs without severe liver damage, interrupt therapy or reduce dose to 100 mg bid. When liver enzymes return to baseline, restart at 100 mg bid and titrate up. Diarrhea, nausea, and vomiting have occurred with **Ofev.** Treat patients at first signs with adequate hydration and antidiarrheal medicine (e.g., *loperamide*) or antiemetics. Discontinue **Ofev** if severe diarrhea, nausea, or vomiting persists despite symptomatic treatment. Gastrointestinal perforation has been reported. Use **Ofev** with caution when treating patients with recent abdominal surgery. Discontinue **Ofev** in patients who develop gastrointestinal perforation. Only use **Ofev** in patients with known risk of gastrointestinal perforation if the anticipated benefit outweighs the potential risk. Arterial thromboembolic events have been reported. Use caution when treating patients at higher cardiovascular risk, including known coronary artery disease (CAD). Bleeding events have been reported. Use **Ofev** in patients with known bleeding risk only if anticipated benefit outweighs the potential risk. There are no human data to inform safety on the use of **Ofev** in pregnancy; however, based on animal studies and the mechanism of action, the use of **Ofev** in pregnancy can cause fetal harm (structural damage during organogenesis and embryo/fetal death). Advise patients of the potential risks to the developing fetus versus patient need/benefit and advise females of reproductive potential to use effective contraception. There is no information on the presence of *nintedanib* in human milk or effects on the breastfed infant; breastfeeding is not recommended. Safety and efficacy of **Ofev** have not been studied in patients with severe renal impairment and end-stage renal disease (ESRD). Decreased exposure has been noted in smokers, which may alter the efficacy profile of **Ofev.** The most common adverse reactions (≥5%) are diarrhea, nausea, abdominal pain, vomiting, liver enzyme elevation, decreased appetite, headache, decreased weight, and hypertension.

▶ *pirfenidone* (G) take with food at the same time each day; Days 1-7: 267 mg 3 x/day (801 mg/day); Days 8-14: 534 mg 3 x/day (1,602 mg/day); Days 15 and ongoing: 801 mg 3 x/day (2,403 mg/day)

Pediatric: <12 years: not established; ≥12 years: same as adult

    Esbriet *Gelcap:* 267, 801 mg

    Comment: Esbriet (*pirfenidone*) is a pyridone. In the postmarketing setting, non-serious and serious cases of drug-induced liver injury, including severe liver injury with fatal outcomes, have been reported. Monitor alanine aminotransferase (ALT), aspartate aminotransferase (AST), and bilirubin before and during treatment. Photosensitivity and rash have been noted with **Esbriet.** Avoid exposure to sunlight and sunlamps. **Esbriet** is not recommended for use in patients with severe hepatic impairment or patients with ESRD on dialysis. Advise patients to wear sunscreen and protective clothing. Nausea, vomiting, diarrhea, dyspepsia, gastroesophageal reflux disease, and abdominal pain have occurred with **Esbriet.** Temporary dosage reductions or discontinuations may be required for any of these adverse side effects (ASEs). The most common adverse reactions (incidence ≥10%) have been, anorexia, gastroesophageal reflux disease, abdominal pain, dyspepsia, nausea, vomiting, diarrhea, weight loss, upper respiratory infection (URI), sinusitis, fatigue, headache, dizziness, insomnia, rash, and arthralgia. Moderate (e.g., *ciprofloxacin*) and strong (e.g., *fluvoxamine*) inhibitors of CYP1A2 increase systemic exposure of **Esbriet** and may alter the adverse reaction profile of **Esbriet.** Discontinue *fluvoxamine* prior to administration of **Esbriet** or reduce **Esbriet** dose to 267 mg 3 x/day (801 mg/day). Consider dosage reduction with use of *ciprofloxacin.* Decreased exposure has been noted in smokers, which may alter the efficacy profile of **Esbriet.**

▶ *tocilizumab administer:* 8 mg/kg via a 60-minute IV infusion; do not administer as a bolus or IV push; see mfr pkg insert for instructions on preparation and administration

Pediatric: safety and efficacy not established

    Actemra *Vial:* 80 mg/4 ml (20 mg/ml), 200 mg/10 ml (20 mg/ml), 400 mg/20 ml (20 mg/ml), single-dose, for further dilution and IV infusion; *Prefilled ACTPen autoinjector:* 162 mg/0.9 ml, single-dose, for SC administration

    Comment: Actemra is a humanized interleukin-6 (IL-6) receptor-inhibiting monoclonal antibody for the treatment of rheumatoid arthritis (RA), systemic juvenile idiopathic arthritis (SJIA), polyarticular juvenile idiopathic arthritis (PJIA), giant cell arteritis (GCA), CAR T-cell-induced severe or life-threatening cytokine release syndrome (CRS), systemic sclerosis-associated ILD, and for hospitalized adult patients with COVID-19. Monitor patients for dose-related laboratory changes, including elevated LFTs, neutropenia, and thrombocytopenia. **Actemra** should not be initiated in patients with an absolute neutrophil count (ANC) below 2,000 per mm³, platelet count below 100,000 per mm³, or who have ALT or AST above 1.5 times the ULN. Registration in the Pregnancy Exposure Registry (1-877-311-8972) is encouraged for monitoring pregnancy outcomes in women exposed to **Actemra** during pregnancy. The limited available data with **Actemra** in pregnant females are not sufficient to determine whether there is a drug-associated risk of major birth defects and miscarriage. Monoclonal antibodies, such as *tocilizumab,* are actively transported

(continued)

across the placenta during the third trimester of pregnancy and may affect immune response in the infant exposed *in utero*. It is not known whether *tocilizumab* passes into breast milk; therefore, breastfeeding is not recommended while using **Actemra**.

PUPILLARY DILATION: SHORT-TERM

ANTICHOLINERGIC+ALPHA-1 ADRENERGIC RECEPTOR AGONIST
▶ *tropicamide+phenylephrine hydrochloride* ophthalmic spray administer 1 metered spray to the cornea of each eye to be dilated; repeat after 5 minutes
Pediatric: <1 year: administer 1 metered spray to the cornea of each eye to be dilated, up to max 3 sprays per eye per day
> **Mydcombi** *Ophth spray:* trop 1%+phenyle 2.5% (each metered spray delivers 0.008 ml, which contains 0.08 mg *tropicamide* and 0.2 mg *phenylephrine hcl*)
> **Comment:** Mydcombi is a fixed-combination of tropicamide, an anticholinergic, and phenylephrine hydrochloride, an alpha-1 adrenergic receptor agonist, indicated to induce mydriasis for diagnostic procedures and in conditions where short-term pupil dilation is desired.

PYELONEPHRITIS: ACUTE

URINARY TRACT ANALGESIA
▶ *phenazopyridine* (G) 95-200 mg q 6 hours prn; max 2 days
Pediatric: <12 years: not recommended; ≥12 years: same as adult
> **AZO Standard, Prodium, Uristat (OTC)** *Tab:* 95 mg
> **AZO Standard Maximum Strength (OTC)** *Tab:* 97.5 mg
> **Pyridium, Urogesic** *Tab:* 100, 200 mg
> **Urogesic** *Tab:* 100, 200 mg

OUTPATIENT ANTI-INFECTIVE TREATMENT
Comment: Acute pyelonephritis can be treated with a single IM antibiotic administration followed by a PO antibiotic regimen and close follow-up. Example: **Rocephin** 1 gm IM followed by **Bactrim DS,** *cephalexin, ciprofloxacin, levofloxacin,* or *loracarbef.*

▶ *cephalexin* (G) 1-4 gm/day in 4 divided doses x 10-14 days
Pediatric: 25-50 mg/kg/day in 4 divided doses x 10-14 days; *see* Appendix BB.15. *Cephalexin* (G) (Keflex Suspension) *for dose by weight*
> **Keflex** *Cap:* 250, 333, 500, 750 mg; *Oral susp:* 125, 250 mg/5 ml (100, 200 ml) (strawberry)
▶ *ciprofloxacin* 500 mg bid or 1,000 mg XR once daily x 3-14 days
Pediatric: <18 years: not recommended; ≥18 years: same as adult
> **Cipro** (G) *Tab:* 250, 500, 750 mg; *Oral susp:* 250, 500 mg/5 ml (100 ml) (strawberry)
> **Cipro XR** *Tab:* 500, 1,000 mg ext-rel
> **ProQuin XR** *Tab:* 500 mg ext-rel
▶ *levofloxacin Uncomplicated:* 500 mg once daily x 10 days; *Complicated:* 750 mg once daily x 10 days
Pediatric: <18 years: not recommended; ≥18 years: same as adult
> **Levaquin** *Tab:* 250, 500, 750 mg; *Oral soln:* 25 mg/ml (480 ml) (benzyl alcohol); *Inj conc:* 25 mg/ml for IV infusion after dilution for IV infusion (50, 100, 150 ml) (preservative-free)
▶ *loracarbef* 400 mg bid x 14 days
Pediatric: 15 mg/kg/day in 2 divided doses x 14 days; *see* Appendix BB.27. *Loracarbef* (G) (Lorabid Suspension) *for dose by weight*
> **Lorabid** *Pulvule:* 200, 400 mg; *Oral susp:* 100 mg/5 ml (50, 100 ml); 200 mg/5 ml (50, 75, 100 ml) (strawberry bubble gum)
▶ *trimethoprim+sulfamethoxazole* **(TMP-SMX)** (G) bid x 10 days
Pediatric: <2 months: not recommended; ≥2 months: 40 mg/kg/day of *sulfamethoxazole* in 2 divided doses x 10 days; *see Appendix BB.33.* Trimethoprim+Sulfamethoxazole (G) (Bactrim Suspension, Septra Suspension) *for dose by weight*
> **Bactrim, Septra** 2 tabs bid x 10 days
>   *Tab:* trim 80 mg+sulfa 400 mg*
> **Bactrim DS, Septra DS** 1 tab bid x 10 days
>   *Tab:* trim 160 mg+sulfa 800 mg*
> **Bactrim Pediatric Suspension, Septra Pediatric Suspension**
>   *Oral susp:* trim 40 mg+sulfa 200 mg per 5 ml (100 ml) (cherry) (alcohol 0.3%)

PYELONEPHRITIS: ACUTE, COMPLICATED (ACP)

PARENTERAL CEPHALOSPORIN ANTIBACTERIAL+BETA-LACTAMASE INHIBITOR
▶ *ceftazidime+avibactam* infuse dose over 2 hours; recommended duration of treatment is 7-14; *CrCl 31-50 ml/min:* 1.25 gm every 8 hours; *CrCl 16-30 ml/min:* 0.94 gm q 12 hours; *CrCl 6-15 ml/min:* 0.94 gm q 24

hours; *CrCl ≤5 ml/min*: 0.94 gm every 48 hours; both *ceftazidime* and *avibactam* are hemodialyzable; thus, administer **Avycaz** after hemodialysis on hemodialysis days

Pediatric: <18 years: not recommended; ≥18 years: same as adult

    Avycaz *Vial*: 2.5 gm, single-dose, pwdr for reconstitution, dilution, and IV infusion

    Comment: **Avycaz** 2.5 gm contains *ceftazidime* (a cephalosporin) 2 gm (equivalent to 2.635 gm of *ceftazidime pentahydrate/sodium carbonate powder*) and *avibactam* (a beta-lactam inhibitor) 0.5 gm (equivalent to 0.551 gm of *avibactam sodium*). As only limited clinical safety and efficacy data for **Avycaz** are currently available, reserve **Avycaz** for use in patients who have limited or no alternative treatment options. To reduce the development of drug-resistant bacteria and maintain the effectiveness of **Avycaz** and other antibacterial drugs, **Avycaz** should be used only to treat infections that are proven or strongly suspected to be caused by susceptible bacteria. Seizures and other neurologic events may occur, especially in patients with renal impairment. Adjust dose in patients with renal impairment. Decreased efficacy in patients with baseline CrCl 30-≤50 ml/min. Monitor CrCl at least daily in patients with changing renal function and adjust the dose of **Avycaz** accordingly. Monitor for hypersensitivity reactions, including anaphylaxis and serious skin reactions. Cross-hypersensitivity may occur in patients with a history of penicillin allergy. If an allergic reaction occurs, discontinue **Avycaz**. *Clostridioides difficile*-associated diarrhea (CDAD) has been reported with nearly all systemic antibacterial agents, including **Avycaz**. There are no adequate and well-controlled studies of **Avycaz**, *ceftazidime*, or *avibactam* in pregnant females. *Ceftazidime* is excreted in human milk in low concentrations. It is not known whether *avibactam* is excreted into human milk. There are no studies to inform effects on the breastfed infant.

PARENTERAL PENEM ANTIBACTERIAL+RENAL DEHYDROPEPTIDASE INHIBITOR+BETA-LACTAMASE INHIBITOR

▷ *imipenem+cilastatin+relebactam* administer dose via IV infusion over 30 minutes q 6 hours; *CrCl ≥90 ml/min*: 1.25 gm/dose (*imipenem* 500 mg, *cilastatin* 500 mg, *relebactam* 250 mg); *CrCl 60-89 ml/min*: 1 gm/dose (*imipenem* 400 mg, *cilastatin* 400 mg, *relebactam* 200 mg); *CrCl 30-59 ml/min*: 0.75 gm/dose (*imipenem* 300 mg, *cilastatin* 300 mg, *relebactam* 150 mg); *CrCl 15-29 ml/min*: 0.5 gm/dose (*imipenem* 200 mg, *cilastatin* 200 mg, *relebactam* 100 mg); *End-stage renal disease (ESRD)/Dialysis*: 0.5 gm/dose (*imipenem* 200 mg, *cilastatin* 200 mg, *relebactam* 100 mg)

Pediatric: <18 years: not established; ≥18 years: same as adult

    Recarbrio *Vial*: imipen 500 mg+cilast 500 mg+relebac 250 mg, single-dose, pwdr for reconstitution, dilution, and IV infusion

    Comment: **Recarbrio** (*imipenem+cilastatin+relebactam*) is a fixed-dose triple combination of *imipenem* (a penem antibacterial), *cilastatin* (a renal dehydropeptidase inhibitor), and *relebactam* (a beta-lactamase inhibitor) indicated for the treatment of complicated urinary tract infection (cUTI), including pyelonephritis, and complicated intra-abdominal infection (cIAI) caused by susceptible gram-negative bacteria in patients who have limited or no alternative treatment options, hospital-acquired bacterial pneumonia (HABP), and ventilator-associated bacterial pneumonia (VABP) in adults. Avoid concomitant use of **Recarbrio** with *ganciclovir, valproic acid*, or *divalproex sodium*. Based on clinical reports on patients treated with *imipenem/cilastatin* plus *relebactam* 250 mg, the most frequent adverse reactions (incidence ≥2%) have been diarrhea, nausea, headache, vomiting, increased alanine aminotransferase, increased aspartate aminotransferase, phlebitis/infusion site reactions, pyrexia, and hypertension. There are insufficient human data to establish whether there is a drug-associated risk of major birth defects, miscarriage, or adverse maternal or fetal outcomes with *imipenem, cilastatin*, or *relebactam* in pregnancy. However, embryonic loss has been observed in monkeys treated with *imipenem/cilastatin*, and fetal abnormalities have been observed in *relebactam*-treated mice; therefore, advise pregnant females of the potential risks to pregnancy and the fetus. There are insufficient data on the presence of *imipenem/cilastatin* and *relebactam* in human milk and no data on the effects on the breastfed infant; However, *relebactam* is present in the milk of lactating rats and, therefore, developmental and health benefits of breastfeeding should be considered along with the mother's clinical need for **Recarbrio** and any potential adverse effects on the breastfed infant from **Recarbrio** or from the underlying maternal condition.

PARENTERAL AMINOGLYCOSIDE ANTIBACTERIAL

▷ *plazomicin* recommended dose is 15 mg/kg once q 24 hours by IV infusion over 30 minutes x 4-7 days in patients with CrCl ≥90 ml/min; CrCl ≥60 to <90 ml/min: 15 mg/kg q 24 hours; CrCl ≥30 to <60 ml/min:10 mg/kg q 24 hours; CrCl ≥15 to <30 ml/min: 10 mg/kg q 48 hours

Pediatric: <18 years: not recommended; ≥18 years: same as adult

    Zemdri *Injection Vial*: 500 mg/10 ml (50 mg/ml), single-dose

    Comment: **Zemdri** (*plazomicin*) is an aminoglycoside antibacterial for the treatment of cUTI, including pyelonephritis. As only limited clinical safety and efficacy data are available, reserve **Zemdri** for use in patients who have limited or no alternative treatment options. Assess creatinine clearance in all patients prior to initiating therapy and daily during therapy. Adjustment of initial dose and therapeutic drug monitoring (TDM) is recommended in patients with renal impairment. There is insufficient information to recommend a dosing regimen in patients with CrCl <15 ml/min or on hemodialysis or continuous renal replacement therapy. For patients with CrCl ≥15 ml/min and <90 ml/min, TDM is recommended in order to avoid *plazomicin*-induced nephrotoxicity. Monitor *plazomicin* trough concentrations and adjust **Zemdri** as described in the mfr pkg insert. *Boxed Warning*: Aminoglycosides are associated with

(continued)

nephrotoxicity, ototoxicity, and neuromuscular blockade; therefore, administer **Zemdri** no faster than 30 minutes, monitor for adverse reactions, and stop the infusion if any of these adverse events occur. Aminoglycosides can cause fetal harm in pregnancy. There are no available data on the use of **Zemdri** in pregnancy to inform a drug-related risk of adverse developmental outcomes. *Streptomycin*, an aminoglycoside, can cause total and irreversible bilateral congenital deafness in children whose mothers received *streptomycin* in pregnancy. There are no data on the presence of **Zemdri** in human milk or effects on the breastfed infant; therefore, potential risk/benefit should be discussed with the mother. The most common adverse reactions (incidence ≥1%) are decreased renal function, diarrhea, hypertension, headache, nausea, vomiting, and hypotension.

RABIES (LYSSAVIRUS)

PRE-EXPOSURE PROPHYLAXIS (PrEP) AND POST-EXPOSURE PROPHYLAXIS (PEP)

Comment: Have *epinephrine* 1:1,000 readily available. Every exposure to possible rabies infection must be individually evaluated. Rabies vaccine and *rabies immune globulin (human) (HRIG)* should be given to all persons suspected of exposure to rabies with one exception: Persons who have been previously immunized with rabies vaccine and have a confirmed adequate rabies antibody titer should receive only vaccine. Recommendations for use of passive and active immunization after exposure to an animal suspected of having rabies have been detailed by the Health Canada National Advisory Committee on Immunization and the U.S. Public Health Service Advisory Committee on Immunization Practices (ACIP). HRIG should be used in conjunction with rabies vaccine and can be administered through the seventh day after the first dose of vaccine is administered. Beyond the seventh day, HRIG is not indicated since an antibody response to cell culture vaccine is presumed to have occurred. If the patient has previously received *HRIG*, and has a confirmed adequate rabies antibody titer, administer only the vaccine. *HRIG* should be administered as promptly as possible after exposure, but can be administered up to the eighth day after the first dose of vaccine is administered. Repeated doses of rabies immune globulin should not be administered once vaccine treatment has been initiated as this could prevent the full expression of active immunity expected from the rabies vaccine. Administer *HRIG* via IM injection only. Do not give IV. The recommended *HRIG* dose 20 IU/kg (0.133 ml/kg) of body weight administered at the time of the first vaccine dose. It may also be given through the seventh day after the first dose of vaccine is given. If anatomically feasible, up to one-half the *HRIG* dose should be thoroughly infiltrated in the area around the wound and the rest should be administered intramuscularly in the gluteal area or lateral thigh muscle using a separate syringe and needle. Because of risk of injury to the sciatic nerve, only the upper, outer quadrant should be used. *HRIG* should never be administered in the same syringe or needle or in the same anatomical site as vaccine. Because of interference with active antibody production, the recommended dose should not be exceeded. It is not known whether rabies immune globulin can cause fetal harm when administered to a pregnant female or can affect reproduction capacity. It should be administered in pregnancy only if clearly needed. Safety and effectiveness in the pediatric population have not been established.

PRE-EXPOSURE PROPHYLAXIS (PrEP)

Comment: Postpone pre-exposure prophylaxis during acute febrile illness or infection. Have *epinephrine* 1:1,000 readily available.

▷ *rabies vaccine, human diploid cell (HDVC) Infants and young children:* administer IM in the vastus lateralis; *All others:* administer IM in the deltoid; do not inject the vaccine into the gluteal area as administration in this area may result in lower neutralizing antibody titers; *not previously immunized:* Day 0, administer 1 ml IM as soon as possible after exposure; then repeat on days 7 and 21 or 28; administer the first dose with rabies immune globulin, human (HRIG); *Previously immunized:* only 2 doses are administered; Day 0: administer 1 ml IM immediately after exposure, and again 3 days later; no HRIG is needed

    Imovax, RabAvert *Vial:* 2.5 IU/ml (1 ml) (2.5 IU of freeze-dried vaccine w. diluent) for IM injection after reconstitution (preservative-free)

Comment: Administer vaccine immediately after reconstitution. If not used, discard. It is also not known whether rabies vaccine can cause fetal harm when administered to a pregnant female or can affect reproductive capacity. Rabies vaccine should be given to a pregnant female only if potential benefits outweigh potential risks. All serious systemic neuroparalytic or anaphylactic reactions to a rabies vaccine should be immediately reported to the Vaccine Adverse Event Reporting System (VAERS) at 1-800-822-7967 (http://vaers.hhs.gov) or Sanofi Pasteur at 1-800-VACCINE (1-800-822-2463).

POST-EXPOSURE PROPHYLAXIS (PEP)
Rabies Immune Globulin, Human (HRIG)

▷ *rabies immune globulin, human (HRIG)* administer 20 IU/kg infiltrated into wound area as much as feasible, then remaining dose administered IM at site remote from vaccine administration

    BayRab, KamRAB, Imogam Rabies HT *Vial:* 150 IU/ml (2, 10 ml)

Comment: Administer *rabies immune globulin, human (HRIG)* concurrently with a full course of rabies vaccine if the patient has not previously received the rabies vaccine and has confirmed adequate antibodies, administer only the vaccine.

    HyperRAB S/D *Vial:* 300 IU/2 ml (2 ml), 1,500 IU/10 ml (10 ml), single-dose

Comment: HyperRAB S/D is a high-potency rabies immunoglobulin.

Comment: If the patient has previously received rabies vaccine and has a confirmed adequate rabies antibody titer, administer <u>only</u> the vaccine. Repeated dosing of *immune globulin, human (HRIG)* after administration of rabies vaccine may suppress the immune response to the vaccine. If the patient has <u>not</u> previously received rabies vaccine, administer *HRIG* concurrently with a full course of rabies vaccine. Defer live vaccine (measles, mumps, rubella) administration for 4 months. There are <u>no</u> data with *HRIG* use in pregnant females to inform a drug-associated risk. There is <u>no</u> information regarding the presence of HRIG in human milk <u>or</u> effect on the breastfed infant.

TETANUS PROPHYLAXIS VACCINE

See *Tetanus* for patients <u>not</u> vaccinated within the past 5 years.

RESPIRATORY SYNCYTIAL VIRUS (RSV)

PROPHYLAXIS

▷ *MVA-BN RSV vaccine*

Comment: FDA has granted breakthrough therapy designation to the **MVA-BN RSV** vaccine candidate for active immunization for the prevention of lower respiratory tract disease (LRTD) caused by respiratory syncytial virus (RSV) in adults ≥60 years of age

▷ *palivizumab* 15 mg/kg IM administered monthly throughout the RSV season

Synagis *Vial:* 100 mg/ml

▷ *respiratory syncytial virus vaccine* administer as a single approximately 0.5 ml dose IM in the deltoid muscle; *Prior to reconstitution:* store refrigerated at 2°C to 8°C (36°F to 46°F) in the original carton; do <u>not</u> freeze; discard if the carton has been frozen; *After reconstitution:* administer immediately <u>or</u> store at room temperature (15°C to 30°C [59°F to 86°F]) and use within 4 hours; do <u>not</u> store reconstituted vaccine under refrigerated conditions (2°C to 8°C [36°F to 46°F]); do <u>not</u> freeze reconstituted vaccine

Pediatric: <u>not</u> approved for patients <60 years of age

Abrysvo *Vial:* 0.5 ml after reconstitution, single-dose, for IM administration (single-dose vial of lyophilized antigen component to be reconstituted with the accompanying vial of the diluent component yielding a 0.5 ml single-dose solution after reconstitution) (preservative-free) (natural rubber, latex-free) (5, 10 vials w. diluent/carton)

Comment: Abrysvo *(respiratory syncytial virus vaccine)* is a vaccine indicated for active immunization for LRTD caused by RSV in individuals ≥60 years of age. The most commonly reported solicited local and systemic adverse reactions (incidence ≥10%) were fatigue (15.5%), headache (12.8%), pain at the injection site (10.5%), and muscle pain (10.1%). To report suspected adverse reactions, contact Pfizer at 800-438-1985 <u>or</u> Vaccine Adverse Event Reporting System (VAERS) at 800-822-7967 <u>or</u> http://vaers. hhs.gov.

May 2023—The approval was based on data from the pivotal phase 3 clinical trial (NCT05035212) RENOIR (RSV vaccine Efficacy study iNOlder adults Immunized against RSV disease). RENOIR is a global, randomized, double-blind, placebo-controlled study designed to assess the efficacy, immunogenicity, and safety of a single dose of the vaccine in adults 60 years of age and older. RENOIR has enrolled approximately 37,000 participants, randomized (1:1) to receive **Abrysvo** (n = 17,197) <u>or</u> placebo (n = 17,186). Randomization was stratified by age, 60-69 years (n = 21,499, 63%), 70-79 years (n = 10,948, 32%), and ≥80 years (n = 1,934, 6%). Healthy adults and adults with stable chronic diseases were included. Among enrolled participants, 15% had stable chronic cardiopulmonary conditions such as chronic obstructive pulmonary disease (COPD), asthma, <u>or</u> congestive heart failure (CHF). The results were recently published in *The New England Journal of Medicine*. RENOIR is ongoing, with efficacy data being collected in the second RSV season in the study. —From www.empr.com; www. pfizer.com; www.drugs.com

▷ *respiratory syncytial virus vaccine, adjuvanted* administer a single 0.5 ml dose IM in the deltoid muscle; administer immediately <u>or</u> store in the refrigerator between 2°C and 8°C (36°F to 46°F) <u>or</u> at room temperature (up to 25°C [77°F]) for up to 4 hours prior to use; protect vials from light; discard reconstituted vaccine if <u>not</u> used within 4 hours; do <u>not</u> freeze; discard if the vaccine has been frozen

Pediatric: <u>not</u> approved for patients <60 years of age

Arexvy *Vial:* 0.5 ml after reconstitution, single-dose, for IM administration (single-dose vial of lyophilized antigen component to be reconstituted with the accompanying vial of adjuvant suspension component yielding a 0.5 ml single-dose suspension after reconstitution) (preservative-free) (natural rubber, latex-free) (10 vials w. diluent/carton)

Comment: Arexvy is a vaccine indicated for active immunization for the prevention of lower respiratory tract disease (LRTD) caused by the respiratory syncytial virus (RSV) in individuals ≥60 years of age. The most commonly reported solicited local adverse reaction (incidence ≥10%) was injection site pain (60.9%). The most commonly reported solicited systemic adverse reactions (incidence ≥10%) were fatigue (33.6%), myalgia (28.9%), headache (27.2%), and arthralgia (18.1%). To report suspected adverse reactions, contact GlaxoSmithKline at 888-825-5249 <u>or</u> VAERS at 800-822-7967 <u>or</u> www.vaers. hhs.gov.

(continued)

May 2023—The approval was based on data from the ongoing randomized, placebo-controlled, observer-blind phase 3 AReSVi 006 trial (ClinicalTrials.gov Identifier: NCT04886596), which included approximately 25,000 adults 60 years of age and older. The efficacy of **Arexvy** in the prevention of a first episode of confirmed RSV-A and/or B-associated LRTD during the first season was the study's primary endpoint. Vaccine efficacy was reported to be 82.6% (96.95% CI, 57.9-94.1), with 7 cases in the vaccine arm compared with 40 cases in the placebo arm. The median follow-up time was 6.7 months for both study groups. Vaccine efficacy against RSV A-associated LRTD cases and RSV B-associated LRTD cases was 84.6% (95% CI, 32.1-98.3) and 80.9% (95% CI, 49.4-94.3), respectively. Compared with placebo, **Arexvy** significantly reduced the risk of developing severe RSV-associated LRTD by 94.1% (95% CI, 62.4-99.9). —From www.empr.com; www.gsk.com; www.drugs.com

TREATMENT
*See **Bronchiolitis***

RESTLESS LEGS SYNDROME (RLS)

GAMMA AMINOBUTYRIC ACID ANALOGS

Comment: The gabapentinoids (*gabapentin* [Gralise, Neurontin, Horizant] and *pregabalin* [Lyrica]) have respiratory depression risk potential. Therefore, when co-prescribed with other central nervous system (CNS) depressant agents, initiate the gabapentinoid at the lowest possible dose and monitor the patient for respiratory depression (especially elders and patients with compromised pulmonary function). Side effects include fatigue, somnolence/sedation, dizziness, vertigo, feeling drunk, headache, nausea, and dry mouth. To discontinue a gabapentinoid, withdraw gradually over 1 week or longer.

▷ *gabapentin* 100 mg once daily x 1 day; then 100 mg bid x 1 day; then 100 mg tid thereafter; max 900 mg tid
    Gralise initially 300 mg on Day 1; then 600 mg on Day 2; then 900 mg on Days 3-6; then 1,200 mg on Days 7-10; then 1,500 mg on Days 11-14; titrate up to 1,800 mg on Day 15; take entire dose once daily with the evening meal; do not crush, split, or chew
    Pediatric: <12 years: not recommended; ≥12 years: same as adult
      Tab: 300, 600 mg
    Neurontin (OTC)(G) 100 mg daily x 1 day, then 100 mg bid x 1 day, then 100 mg tid continuously; max 900 mg tid
    Pediatric: <3 years: not recommended; 3-12 years: initially 10-15 mg/kg/day in 3 divided doses; max 12 hours between doses; titrate over 3 days; 3-4 years: titrate to 40 mg/kg/day; 5-12 years: titrate to 25-35 mg/kg/day; max 50 mg/kg/day
▷ *gabapentin enacarbil* 600 mg once daily at about 5:00 PM; if dose not taken at recommended time, next dose should be taken the following day; swallow whole; take with food; *CrCl 30-59 ml/min:* 600 mg on Day 1, Day 3, and every day thereafter; *CrCl <30 ml/min* or on hemodialysis: not recommended
    Pediatric: <12 years: not recommended; ≥12 years: same as adult
    Horizant *Tab:* 300, 600 mg ext-rel
▷ *pregabalin (GABA analog)* **(V)**
    Pediatric: <12 years: not recommended; ≥12 years: same as adult
    Lyrica initially 50 mg tid; may titrate to 100 mg tid within 1 week; max 600 mg divided tid; discontinue over 1 week
    Cap: 25, 50, 75, 100, 150, 200, 225, 300 mg; *Oral soln:* 20 mg/ml
    Lyrica CR *Tab:* usual dose: 165 mg once daily; may increase to 330 mg/day within 1 week; max 660 mg/day
    Tab: 82.5, 165, 330 mg ext-rel

DOPAMINE RECEPTOR AGONISTS

▷ *pramipexole dihydrochloride* **(G)** initially 0.125 mg once daily 2-3 hours before bedtime; may double dose every 4-7 days; max 0.75 mg/day
    Pediatric: <12 years: not recommended; ≥12 years: same as adult
    Mirapex *Tab:* 0.125, 0.25*, 0.5*, 0.75*, 1*, 1.5*mg
▷ *ropinirole* take once daily 1-3 hours prior to bedtime; initially 0.25 mg on days 1 and 2; then 0.5 mg on days 3-7; increase by 0.5 mg/day at 1-week intervals to 3 mg; max 4 mg/day
    Pediatric: <12 years: not recommended; ≥12 years: same as adult
    Requip *Tab:* 0.25, 0.5, 1, 2, 3, 4, 5 mg
▷ *rotigotine* transdermal patch apply to clean, dry, intact skin on abdomen, thigh, hip, flank, shoulder, or upper arm; initially 1 mg/24 hours patch once daily; may increase weekly by 1 mg/24 hours if needed; max 3 mg/24 hours once daily; rotate sites and allow 14 days before reusing site; if hairy, shave site at least 3 days before application to site; avoid abrupt cessation; reduce by 1 mg/24 hours every other day
    Pediatric: <12 years: not recommended; ≥12 years: same as adult
    Neupro *Trans patch:* 1 mg/24 Hrs, 2 mg/24 Hrs, 3 mg/24 Hrs, 4 mg/24 Hrs, 6 mg/24 Hrs, 8 mg/24 Hrs (30/carton) (sulfites)

RETT SYNDROME

AMINO-TERMINAL TRIPEPTIDE OF INSULIN-LIKE GROWTH FACTOR 1 (IGF-1) SYNTHETIC ANALOG

▶ *trofinetide* Recommended dosing: bid (morning and evening) according to patient weight; see dosing table below; may be administered with or without food; may be administered orally or via gastrostomy (G) tube; doses administered via gastrojejunal (GJ) tubes must be administered through the G-port; discard any unused portion 14 days after the bottle is first opened

Patient Weight	Daybue Dosage	Daybue Volume
9 kg to <12 kg	5,000 mg bid	25 ml bid
12 kg to <20 kg	6,000 mg bid	30 ml bid
20 kg to <35 kg	8,000 mg bid	40 ml bid
35 kg <50 kg	10,000 mg bid	50 ml bid
≥50 kg	12,000 mg bid	60 ml bid

Pediatric: <2 years: safety and efficacy not established; ≥2 years: see weight-based dosing table
  Daybue *Oral soln:* 200 mg/ml (450 ml) (strawberry)
  Comment: **Daybue** is a synthetic analog of the amino-terminal tripeptide of insulin-like growth factor 1 (IGF-1) indicated for the treatment of Rett syndrome (a rare *genetic neurologic disorder that* leads to severe impairments, including the ability to speak, walk, eat, and breathe easily, and requiring significant medical support and total care support) in adult and pediatric patients ≥2 years of age. The hallmark of Rett syndrome is near-constant repetitive hand movements while awake. Cognitive assessment in patients with Rett syndrome is complicated, but it is known these patients understand far more than they can communicate verbally, as evidenced by their bright and attentive eyes, and their ability to express a wide spectrum of moods and emotions. The most common adverse reactions to **Daybue** (incidence at least 10% of **Daybue**-treated patients and at least 2% greater than placebo) have been diarrhea and vomiting. Advise patients to stop laxatives before starting **Daybue**. If diarrhea occurs, patients should start antidiarrheal treatment, increase oral fluids, and notify their healthcare provider. Interrupt, reduce dose, or discontinue **Daybue** if severe diarrhea occurs or if dehydration is suspected. Weight loss may occur in patients treated with **Daybue**. Monitor weight and interrupt, reduce dose, or discontinue **Daybue** if significant weight loss occurs. Closely monitor for adverse reactions with concomitant use of orally administered (1) CYP3A4 sensitive substrates for which a small change in substrate plasma concentration may lead to serious toxicities and (2) OATP1B1 and OATP1B3 substrates for which a small change in substrate plasma concentration may lead to serious toxicities. **Daybue** is not recommended for use in patients with moderate-to-severe renal impairment. To report suspected adverse reactions, contact Acadia Pharmaceuticals at 1-844-422-2342 or FDA at 1-800-FDA-1088 or www.fda.gov/medwatch.

RHEUMATOID ARTHRITIS (RA)

Injectable Acetaminophen *see Pain*
NSAIDs *see* Appendix I. NSAIDs online at https://connect.springerpub.com/content/reference-book/978-0-8261-7935-7/back-matter/part02/back-matter/bmatter10
Opioid Analgesics *see Pain*
Topical and Transdermal Analgesics *see Pain*
Parenteral Corticosteroids *see* Appendix L. Parenteral Corticosteroids
Oral Corticosteroids *see* Appendix K. Oral Corticosteroids
Topical Analgesic and Anesthetic Agents *see* Appendix H. Anesthetic Agents for Local Infiltration and Dermal/Mucosal Membrane Application online at https://connect.springerpub.com/content/reference-book/978-0-8261-7935-7/back-matter/part02/back-matter/bmatter9

TOPICAL AND TRANSDERMAL ANALGESICS

▶ *capsaicin* cream (G) apply tid-qid prn to intact skin
  Pediatric: <2 years: not recommended; ≥2 years: same as adult
        Axsain *Crm:* 0.075% (1, 2 oz)
        Capsin *Lotn:* 0.025, 0.075% (59 ml)
        Capzasin-HP (OTC) *Crm:* 0.075% (1.5 oz), 0.025% (45, 90 gm); *Lotn:* 0.075% (2 oz)
        Capzasin-P (OTC) *Crm:* 0.025% (1.5 oz); *Lotn:* 0.025% (2 oz)
        Dolorac *Crm:* 0.025% (28 gm)
        Double Cap (OTC) *Crm:* 0.05% (2 oz)
        R-Gel *Gel:* 0.025% (15, 30 gm)
        Zostrix (OTC) *Crm:* 0.025% (0.7, 1.5, 3 oz)
        Zostrix HP (OTC) *Emol crm:* 0.075% (1, 2 oz)

(continued)

▷ *capsaicin* 8% patch apply up to 4 patches for one 60-minute application to clean dry skin; may prep area with topical anesthetic; wear non-latex gloves; patches may be cut to size/shape; treatment may be repeated every 3 months
Pediatric: <18 years: not recommended; ≥18 years: same as adult
    Qutenza *Patch:* 8% 1,640 mcg/cm (179 mg) (1 or 2 patches w. 1-50 gm tube cleansing gel/carton)
▷ *diclofenac sodium* apply qid prn to intact skin
Pediatric: <12 years: not established; ≥12 years: same as adult
    Pennsaid 1.5% in 10 drop increments, dispense and rub into front, side, and back of knee; usually 40 drops (40 mg) qid
      Topical soln: 1.5% (150 ml)
    Pennsaid 2% apply 2 pump actuations (40 mg) and rub into front, side, and back of knee bid
      Topical soln: 2% (20 mg/pump actuation, 112 gm)
    Solaraze Gel massage into clean skin bid prn
      Gel: 3% (50 gm) (benzyl alcohol)
    Voltaren Gel (OTC) (G) apply qid prn to intact skin
      Gel: 1% (100 gm)
Comment: *Diclofenac* is contraindicated with *aspirin* allergy. As with other NSAIDs, should be avoided in late pregnancy (≥30 weeks) because it may cause premature closure of the ductus arteriosus (PCDA).
▷ *doxepin* cream apply to affected area qid at intervals of at least 3-4 hours; max 8 days
Pediatric: <12 years: not recommended; >12 years: same as adult
    Prudoxin *Crm:* 5% (45 gm)
    Zonalon *Crm:* 5% (30, 45 gm)
▷ *pimecrolimus* 1% cream **(G)** <2 years: not recommended; ≥2 years: apply to affected area bid; do not apply an occlusive dressing
    Elidel *Crm:* 1% (30, 60, 100 gm)
Comment: *Pimecrolimus* is indicated for short-term and intermittent long-term use. Discontinue use when resolution occurs. Contraindicated if the patient is immunosuppressed. Change to the 0.1% preparation or if secondary bacterial infection is present.
▷ *trolamine salicylate* apply tid-qid
Pediatric: <2 years: not recommended; ≥2 years: same as adult
    Mobisyl Creme *Crm:* 10% (100 gm)

ORAL SALICYLATE

▷ *indomethacin* initially 25 mg bid-tid, increase as needed at weekly intervals by 25-50 mg/day; max 200 mg/day
Pediatric: <14 years: usually not recommended; >2 years, if risk warranted: 1-2 mg/kg/day in divided doses; max 3-4 mg/kg/day (or 150-200 mg/day, whichever is less); <14 years: ER cap not recommended
Cap: 25, 50 mg; *Susp:* 25 mg/5 ml (pineapple-coconut, mint) (alcohol 1%); *Supp:* 50 mg; *ER Cap:* 75 mg ext-rel
Comment: *Indomethacin* is indicated only for acute painful flares. Administer with food and/or antacids. Use lowest effective dose for shortest duration.

ORAL NSAID

see more **Oral NSAIDs** NSAIDs online at https://connect.springerpub.com/content/reference-book/978-0-8261-7935-7/back-matter/part02/back-matter/bmatter10

▷ *diclofenac* take on empty stomach; 35 mg tid; *Hepatic impairment:* use lowest dose
Pediatric: <18 years: not recommended; ≥18 years: same as adult
    Zorvolex *Gelcap:* 18, 35 mg
▷ *diclofenac sodium* **(G)**
Pediatric: <18 years: not recommended; ≥18 years: same as adult
    Voltaren 50 mg bid-qid or 75 mg bid or 25 mg qid with an additional 25 mg at HS if necessary
    Tab: 25, 50, 75 mg ent-coat
    Voltaren XR 100 mg once daily; rarely, 100 mg bid may be used
    Tab: 100 mg ext-rel
Comment: *Diclofenac* is contraindicated with *aspirin* allergy. As with other NSAIDs, should be avoided in late pregnancy (≥30 weeks) because it may cause premature closure of the ductus arteriosus (PCDA).

ORAL NSAID+PPI
Ibuprofen+Esomeprazole Combination

▷ *naproxen+esomeprazole magnesium* **(G)** take 1 tablet bid; use the lowest effective dose; not recommended in moderate/severe renal insufficiency or in severe hepatic insufficiency (Child-Pugh Class C); consider dose reduction in mild/moderate hepatic insufficiency (Child-Pugh Class A or B)
Pediatric: <18 years: safety and efficacy not established; ≥18 years: same as adult
    Vimovo *Tab:* nap 375 mg+eso 20 mg, nap 500 mg +eso mg, del-rel, film-coat
Comment: *Vimovo* is a fixed-dose combination of the NSAID *naproxen* (375 mg or 500 mg) and the proton pump inhibitor (PPI) 20 mg indicated for relief of signs and symptoms of rheumatoid arthritis (RA), osteoarthritis, and ankylosing spondylitis and to decrease the risk of developing gastric ulcers in patients at risk of developing NSAID-associated gastric ulcers. The most common adverse reactions (incidence

≥5%) have been erosive gastritis, dyspepsia, gastritis, diarrhea, gastric ulcer, upper abdominal pain, and nausea. *Contraindications to Vimovo use are* (1) known hypersensitivity to any component of **Vimovo** or substituted benzimidazoles; (2) history of asthma, urticaria, or other allergic-type reactions after taking *aspirin* or other NSAIDs; (3) use during the perioperative period in the setting of coronary artery bypass graft (CABG) surgery; and (4) late pregnancy. Starting at 30 weeks gestation, **Vimovo** should not be used by pregnant females as PCDA in the fetus may occur. *Boxed Warnings: Naproxen,* a component of **Vimovo**, may cause an increased risk of serious cardiovascular (CV) thrombotic events, myocardial infarction, and stroke, which can be fatal. This risk may increase with duration of use. Patients with cardiovascular disease (CVD) or risk factors for CVD may be at greater risk. **Vimovo** is contraindicated for the treatment of perioperative pain in the setting of CABG surgery. NSAIDs, including *naproxen,* can cause an increased risk of serious gastrointestinal (GI) adverse events, including bleeding, ulceration, and perforation of the stomach or intestines, which can be fatal. These events can occur at any time during use and without warning symptoms. Elderly patients are at greater risk for serious GI events. *Other Warnings and Precautions:* Monitor patients for elevated liver enzymes and, rarely occurring, severe hepatic reactions; discontinue use immediately if abnormal liver enzymes persist or worsen. New onset or worsening of preexisting hypertension may occur; monitor blood pressure during treatment with **Vimovo**. Congestive heart failure (CHF) and edema can occur; **Vimovo** should be used with caution in patients with fluid retention or heart failure (HF). Renal papillary necrosis and other renal injury may occur with long-term use. Use **Vimovo** with caution in the elderly, those with impaired renal function, hypovolemia, salt depletion, HF, and liver dysfunction, and those taking diuretics or angiotensin-converting enzyme (ACE) inhibitors. Do not use **Vimovo** in patients with the *aspirin* triad. Serious skin adverse reactions, such as exfoliative dermatitis, Steven-Johnson syndrome (SJS), and toxic epidermal necrolysis (TEN), can be fatal and can occur without warning. Discontinue **Vimovo** at first appearance of skin rash or any other sign of hypersensitivity. Long-term PPI therapy is associated with an increased risk for osteoporosis-related fractures of the hip, wrist, or spine. Symptomatic response to *esomeprazole* does not preclude the presence of gastric malignancy. Atrophic gastritis has been noted on biopsy with long-term *omeprazole* therapy. *Drug-Drug Interactions:* Concomitant use of NSAIDs may reduce the antihypertensive effect of ACE inhibitors, diuretics, and beta-blockers. Concomitant use of NSAIDs increases *lithium* plasma levels. Concomitant use of **Vimovo** with *methotrexate* (MTX) may increase the toxicity of *MTX.* Concomitant use of **Vimovo** and *warfarin* may result in increased risk of bleeding complications; monitor for increases in international normalized ratio (INR) and prothrombin time (PT). *Esomeprazole* inhibits gastric acid secretion and may interfere with the absorption of drugs where gastric pH is an important determinant of bioavailability (e.g., *ketoconazole,* iron salts, and *digoxin*). **Vimovo** is contraindicated in pregnancy starting at 30 weeks gestation; may cause fetal harm (premature closure of the ductus arteriosus (PCDA). The *naproxen* anion has been found in the milk of lactating females. Because of the possible adverse effects of prostaglandin-inhibiting drugs on neonates and potential for tumorigenicity shown for *esomeprazole* in animal carcinogenicity studies, a decision should be made whether to discontinue breastfeeding or discontinue the **Vimovo**, taking into account the importance of the drug to the mother.

Ibuprofen+Famotidine Combination

▷ *ibuprofen+famotidine* take 1 tablet 3 tid or take 1 tablet q 8 hours; max 3 tabs/24 hours
  Pediatric: safety and efficacy not established
    Duexis *Tab:* ibu 800 mg+famo 26.6 mg, film-coat, single-dose
    Comment: Duexis is a fixed-dose combination of the NSAID *ibuprofen* (800 mg) and the histamine H2 receptor antagonist *famotidine* (26.6 mg) indicated for relief of signs and symptoms of RA and osteoarthritis and to decrease the risk of developing upper gastrointestinal ulcers (which in clinical trials was defined as a gastric and/or duodenal ulcer) in patients who are taking *ibuprofen* for those indications. The clinical trials primarily enrolled patients less than 65 years of age without a history of GI ulcer. The most common adverse reactions (incidence ≥1% and greater than *ibuprofen* alone) have been nausea, diarrhea, constipation, upper abdominal pain, and headache. *Contraindications to Duexis use are* (1) preexisting asthma, urticaria, or allergic reactions after taking *aspirin* or other NSAIDs; (2) use during the perioperative period in the setting of coronary artery bypass graft (CABG) surgery; (3) starting at 30 weeks gestation (**Duexis** should not be used by pregnant females as premature closure of the ductus arteriosus (PCDA) in the fetus may occur); and (4) known hypersensitivity to other H2 receptor antagonists. *Boxed Warnings: Ibuprofen,* a component of **Duexis**, may increase the risk of serious cardiovascular (CV) thrombotic events, myocardial infarction, and stroke, which can be fatal. Risk may increase with duration of use. Patients with cardiovascular disease (CVD) or risk factors for CVD may be at greater risk. NSAIDs, including *ibuprofen,* a component of **Duexis**, increase the risk of serious GI adverse reactions, including bleeding, ulceration, and perforation of the stomach or intestines, which can be fatal. Reactions can occur at any time without warning symptoms. Elderly patients are at greater risk. *Other warnings and precautions with Duexis use:* Hypertension can occur with NSAID treatment; monitor blood pressure closely during treatment with **Duexis**. Congestive heart failure (CHF) and edema can occur with NSAID treatment; use **Duexis** with caution in patients with fluid retention or heart failure (HF). Active and clinically significant bleeding from any source can occur; discontinue **Duexis** if active bleeding occurs. Long-term administration of NSAIDs can result in renal papillary necrosis and other renal injury; use **Duexis** with caution in patients at risk (e.g., the

(continued)

elderly, those with renal impairment, HF, liver impairment, and those taking diuretics or ACE inhibitors). Anaphylaxis may occur in patients with the *aspirin* triad or in patients without prior exposure to **Duexis**; discontinue **Duexis** immediately if an anaphylactoid reaction occurs. Serious skin reactions, including exfoliative dermatitis, SJS, and TEN, can occur and can be fatal; discontinue **Duexis** if rash or other signs of local skin reaction occur. Hepatic injury ranging from transaminase elevations to liver failure can occur; discontinue **Duexis** immediately if abnormal liver tests persist or worsen, if clinical signs and symptoms of liver disease develop, or if systemic manifestations occur. *Drug Interactions:* Concomitant use of NSAIDs and anticoagulants (e.g., **warfarin**) increases the risk of serious GI bleeding. Concomitant administration with other NSAIDs, including *aspirin*, may increase the risk of adverse reactions, including GI bleeding. *Ibuprofen*, a component of **Duexis**, may reduce the effectiveness of ACE inhibitors and diuretics. *Ibuprofen*, a component of **Duexis**, may increase lithium levels. **Duexis** is contraindicated in pregnancy starting at 30 weeks' gestation; may cause fetal harm. Mothers' use of **Duexis** when lactating has not been studied; effects on the breastfed infant are unknown.

COX-2 Inhibitors

Comment: Cox-2 inhibitors are contraindicated with history of asthma, urticaria, and allergic-type reactions to *aspirin*, other NSAIDs, and sulfonamides, 3rd trimester of pregnancy, and coronary artery bypass graft (CABG) surgery.

➤ *celecoxib* (G) 50-400 mg once daily-bid; max 800 mg/day
  Pediatric: <18 years: not recommended; ≥18 years: same as adult
    Celebrex *Cap:* 50, 100, 200, 400 mg
➤ *meloxicam* (G)
    Mobic <2 years, <60 kg: not recommended; ≥2 years, ≥60 kg: 0.125 mg/kg; max 7.5 mg once daily; ≥18 years: initially 7.5 mg once daily, max 15 mg once daily; *Hemodialysis:* max 7.5 mg/day
      Tab: 7.5, 15 mg; *Oral susp:* 7.5 mg/5 ml (100 ml) (raspberry)
    Vivlodex <18 years: not established; ≥18 years: initially 5 mg once daily; may increase to max 10 mg/day; *Hemodialysis:* max 5 mg/day
      Cap: 5, 10 mg

Janus Kinase (JAK) Inhibitor (JAKI)

➤ *baricitinib Recommended dose:* 2 mg once daily; take with or without food; an alternative method of oral administration may be used for patients unable to swallow tablets; **Olumiant** may be used as monotherapy or in combination with (MTX) or other non-biologic disease-modifying antirheumatic drugs (DMARDs). *Pediatric:* safety and efficacy not established
    Olumiant *Tab:* 1, 2, 4 mg film-coat
    Comment: Olumiant is a Janus kinase (JAK) inhibitor indicated for the treatment of adult patients with moderately to severely active RA who have had an inadequate response to one or more tumor necrosis factor (TNF) blockers. **Olumiant** is not recommended for use in combination with other JAK inhibitors, biologic DMARDs, or with potent immunosuppressants such as *azathioprine* and *cyclosporine*. **Olumiant** may be used as monotherapy or in combination with *methotrexate* (MTX) or other non-biologic DMARDs. The most common adverse reactions (incidence >1%) have included upper respiratory infection (URI), nausea, herpes simplex, and herpes zoster. See the mfr pkg insert for full prescribing information, including a boxed warning regarding serious infections, mortality, malignancy, major adverse cardiovascular events (MACE), and thrombosis. See mfr pkg insert for other warnings, precautions, adverse reactions, dose modifications, drug interactions, laboratory abnormalities (cytopenias), hepatic and renal impairment, carcinogenesis, mutagenesis, and fertility impairment. Advise patients of the potential benefits and risks of **Olumiant** and advise patients to read the FDA-approved patient labeling (Medication Guide). Increased disease activity is associated with the risk of developing adverse pregnancy outcomes in females with rheumatoid arthritis (RA); adverse pregnancy outcomes include preterm delivery, low birthweight (<2,500 gm) infants, and small for gestational age (SGA) at birth. The limited data on **Olumiant** use in human pregnancy are not sufficient to inform a drug-associated risk of major birth defects or miscarriage. Pregnancy status should be determined prior to initiating treatment with **Olumiant**. Females of reproductive potential should be informed of the risks to the fetus and advised to use effective contraception during treatment. Because of the potential for serious adverse reactions in breastfed infants, advise **Olumiant**-treated mothers not to breastfeed. Report pregnancies to Eli Lilly at 1-800-LillyRx (1-800-545-5979). To report suspected adverse reactions, contact Eli Lilly at 1-800-LillyRx (1-800-545-5979) or FDA at 1-800-FDA-1088 or www.fda.gov/medwatch.
➤ *tofacitinib* 5 mg bid or 11 mg once daily; discontinue after 16 weeks if adequate therapeutic benefit is not achieved; use the lowest effective dose to maintain response; see mfr pkg insert for dosage adjustments for patients receiving CYP2C19 and/or CYP3A4 inhibitors; in patients with moderate or severe renal impairment or moderate hepatic impairment, and patients with lymphopenia, neutropenia, or anemia, use of **Xeljanz/Xeljanz XR** in patients with severe hepatic impairment is not recommended in any patient population
    Comment: FDA has issued a MedWatch Alert to the public that a recent safety clinical trial found an increased risk of blood clots in the lungs and death when a 10 mg bid dose of *tofacitinib* (**Xeljanz, Xeljanz XR**) was administered to patients with rheumatoid arthritis (RA). FDA has not approved the 10 mg bid dosing regimen for RA; this dosing regimen is only approved for patients with ulcerative colitis (UC).

Pediatric: safety and efficacy of **Xeljanz** tabs and **Xeljanz Oral Solution** in pediatric patients for indications other than juvenile idiopathic arthritis (JIA) not established

Xeljanz *Tab:* 5, 10 mg film-coat
Xeljanz Oral Solution *Oral soln:* 1 mg/ml (240 ml) with press-in bottle adapter and oral dosing syringe (no latex)
Xeljanz XR *Tab:* 11, 22 mg film-coat
Comment: Xeljanz/Xeljanz XR is indicated for moderate-to-severe RA as monotherapy in patients who have inadequate response or intolerance to *methotrexate (MTX)* and/or in combination with other non-biologic DMARDs. Use **Xeljanz/Xeljanz XR** with caution in patients who may be at increased risk for gastrointestinal perforation. The most common adverse events associated with **Xeljanz,** treatment are diarrhea, elevated cholesterol level, headache, herpes zoster (shingles), increased blood creatine phosphokinase, nasopharyngitis, rash, and upper respiratory tract infection (URI). Avoid use of **Xeljanz/Xeljanz XR** during an active serious infection, including localized infection. Patients treated with **Xeljanz/Xeljanz XR** are at increased risk for developing serious infections that may lead to hospitalization or death. **Xeljanz/Xeljanz XR** has a *Boxed Warning* for serious infections (e.g., opportunistic infections) and malignancy (e.g., lymphoma). Use of **Xeljanz/Xeljanz XR** in combination with biological therapies or with potent immunosuppressants, such as *azathioprine* and *cyclosporine,* is not recommended. Avoid live vaccine administration during treatment with **Xeljanz.** Prior to starting **Xeljanz/Xeljanz XR,** perform a test for latent tuberculosis; if it is positive, start treatment for tuberculosis prior to starting **Xeljanz/Xeljanz XR.** Recommend lab monitoring due to potential for changes in lymphocytes, neutrophils, hemoglobin, liver enzymes, and lipids. Do not initiate **Xeljanz** if absolute lymphocyte count <500 cells/mm^3, an absolute neutrophil count (ANC) <1,000 cells/mm^3 or Hgb <9 gm/dL. The safety and effectiveness of **Xeljanz/Xeljanz XR** in pediatric patients have not been established. Available data with **Xeljanz/Xeljanz XR** use in pregnancy are insufficient to establish a drug-associated risk of major birth defects, miscarriage, or adverse maternal or fetal outcomes. In animal reproduction studies, fetocidal, and teratogenic effects were noted. There is a pregnancy exposure registry that monitors pregnancy outcomes in females exposed to **Xeljanz/Xeljanz XR** during pregnancy. Consider pregnancy planning and prevention for females of reproductive potential. Patients should be encouraged to enroll in the **Xeljanz/Xeljanz XR** pregnancy registry if they become pregnant. To enroll or obtain information from the registry, patients can call the toll free number at 1-877-311-8972. There are no data on the presence of *tofacitinib* in human milk or the effects on the breastfed infant; however, mothers should be advised not to breastfeed.

▶ *upadacitinib* 15 mg once daily; may be used as monotherapy or in combination with *methotrexate (MTX)* or other non-biologic DMARDs; avoid initiation or interrupt **Rinvoq** if absolute lymphocyte count is <500 cells/mm^3, absolute neutrophil count (ANC) <1,000 cells/mm^3, or hemoglobin <8 gm/dL.
Pediatric: <18 years: not established; ≥18 years: same as adult
Rinvoq Extended-Release Tablets *Tab:* 15 mg ext-rel
Comment: Rinvoq (*upadacitinib*) is a JAK inhibitor for the treatment of adult patients with moderate-to-severe active RA who have had an inadequate response or intolerance to *methotrexate (MTX).* Use of **Rinvoq** in combination with other JAK inhibitors, biologic DMARDs, or with potent immunosuppressants such as *azathioprine* and *cyclosporine* is not recommended. Use of **Rinvoq** in patients with severe hepatic impairment (Child-Pugh Class C) is not recommended. Co-administration of **Rinvoq** with strong CYP3A4 inducers (e.g., *rifampin*) is not recommended. Use with caution in patients receiving chronic treatment with strong CYP3A4 inhibitors (e.g., *ketoconazole*). Avoid use of **Rinvoq** with live vaccines. Serious infections leading to hospitalization or death, including tuberculosis and bacterial, invasive fungal, viral, and other opportunistic infections, have occurred in patients receiving **Rinvoq.** Avoid use of **Rinvoq** in patients with active, serious infection, including localized infection. If a serious infection develops, interrupt **Rinvoq** until the infection is controlled. Prior to starting **Rinvoq,** test for latent tuberculosis; if the test is positive, start treatment for tuberculosis. Monitor all patients for active tuberculosis during treatment, even if the initial latent tuberculosis test is negative. Lymphoma and other malignancies have been observed in patients treated with **Rinvoq.** Thrombosis, including deep vein thrombosis, pulmonary embolism, and arterial thrombosis, has occurred in patients treated with Janus kinase (JAK) inhibitors used to treat inflammatory conditions. Consider risk/benefit prior to initiating **Rinvoq** in patients with a known malignancy and patients who may be at increased risk of thrombosis or gastrointestinal perforation. Monitor for potential changes in lymphocytes, neutrophils, Hgb, liver enzymes, and lipids. **Rinvoq** may cause embryo/fetal toxicity; therefore, advise females of reproductive potential to use effective contraception during treatment and for 4 weeks following the final dose. Advise lactating women that breastfeeding is not recommended during treatment with *upadacitinib* and for 6 days (approximately 10 half-lives) after the last dose.

Disease Modifying Antirheumatic Drugs (DMARDs)

Comment: DMARDs are first-line treatment options for RA. DMARDs include penicillamine, gold salts (*auranofin, aurothioglucose*), immunosuppressants, and *hydroxychloroquine.* The DMARDs reduce erythrocyte sedimentation rate (ESR), reduce rheumatoid factor (RF), and favorably affect the outcome of RA. Immunosuppressants may require 6 weeks to begin to improve and 6 months for full improvement.

(continued)

▷ *auranofin (gold salt)* 3 mg bid or 6 mg once daily; if inadequate response after 6 months, increase to 3 mg tid
    Pediatric: <12 years: not recommended; ≥12 years: same as adult
      Ridaura *Vial:* 100 mg/20 ml
▷ *azathioprine* 1 mg/kg/day in a single or divided doses; may increase by 0.5 mg/kg/day q 4 weeks; max 2.5 mg/kg/day; minimum trial to ascertain effectiveness is 12 weeks
    Pediatric: <12 years: not recommended; ≥12 years: same as adult
      Azasan *Tab* 75*, 100*mg
      Imuran *Tab* 50*mg
▷ *cyclosporine (immunosuppressant)* 1.25 mg/kg bid; may increase after 4 weeks by 0.5 mg/kg/day; then adjust at 2-week intervals; max 4 mg/kg/day; administer with meals
    Pediatric: <12 years: not recommended; ≥12 years: same as adult
      Neoral *Cap:* 25, 100 mg (alcohol)
      Neoral Oral Solution *Oral soln:* 100 mg/ml (50 ml); may dilute in room temperature apple juice or orange juice (alcohol)
      Comment: Neoral is indicated for RA unresponsive to *methotrexate (MTX).*
▷ *hydroxychloroquine* 400-600 mg/day
    Pediatric: <12 years: not recommended; ≥12 years: same as adult
      Plaquenil *Tab:* 200 mg
      Comment: May require several weeks to achieve beneficial effects. If no improvement in 6 months, discontinue.
▷ *leflunomide (G)* initially 100 mg once daily x 3 days; maintenance dose 20 mg once daily; max 20 mg daily
    Pediatric: <18 years: not recommended; ≥18 years: same as adult
      Arava *Tab:* 10, 20, 100 mg
      Comment: Arava is contraindicated with breastfeeding.
▷ *methotrexate (MTX)* 7.5 mg x 1 dose per week or 2.5 mg x 3 at 12-hour intervals once a week; max 20 mg/week; therapeutic response begins in 3-6 weeks; administer *methotrexate (MTX)* injection SC only into the abdomen or thigh
    Pediatric: <2 years: not recommended; ≥2 years: 10 mg/m² once weekly; max 20 mg/m²
      Rasuvo *Autoinjector:* 7.5 mg/0.15 ml, 10 mg/0.20 ml, 12.5 mg/0.25 ml, 15 mg/0.30 ml, 17.5 mg/0.35 ml, 20 mg/0.40 ml, 22.5 mg/0.45 ml, 25 mg/0.50 ml, 27.5 mg/0.55 ml, 30 mg/0.60 ml (solution concentration for SC injection is 50 mg/ml)
      Rheumatrex *Tab:* 2.5*mg (5, 7.5, 10, 12.5, 15 mg/week, 4/card unit-of-use dose pack)
      Trexall *Tab:* 5*, 7.5*, 10*, 15*mg (5, 7.5, 10, 12.5, 15 mg/week, 4/card unit-of-use dose pack)
      Comment: *methotrexate (MTX)* is contraindicated with immunodeficiency, blood dyscrasias, alcoholism, and chronic liver disease.
▷ *penicillamine* administer on an empty stomach, at least 1 hour before meals or 2 hours after meals, and at least 1 hour apart from any other drug, food, milk, antacid, and zinc- or iron-containing preparation; maintenance dosage must be individualized and may require adjustment during the course of treatment; *initially* a single daily dose of 125-250 mg; then increase at 1 to 3-month intervals by 125-250 mg/day, as patient response and tolerance indicate; if a satisfactory remission of symptoms is achieved, the dose associated with the remission should be continued as the patient's maintenance therapy; if there is no improvement and there are no signs of potentially serious toxicity after 2-3 months of treatment with doses of 500-750 mg/day, increase by 250 mg/day at 2 to 3-month intervals until a satisfactory remission occurs or signs of toxicity develop; if there is no discernible improvement after 3-4 months of treatment with 1,000-1,500 mg/day, discontinue **Cuprimine**; changes in maintenance dosage levels may not be reflected clinically or in the erythrocyte sedimentation rate (ESR) for 2-3 months after each dosage adjustment
      Cuprimine *Cap:* 125, 250 mg
      Depen *Tab:* 250 mg
      Comment: The use of *penicillamine* has been associated with fatalities due to certain diseases such as aplastic anemia, agranulocytosis, thrombocytopenia, Goodpasture's syndrome, and myasthenia gravis. Because of the potential for serious hematologic and renal adverse reactions to occur at any time, routine urinalysis, white and differential blood cell count, hemoglobin, and direct platelet count must be checked twice weekly, together with monitoring of the patient's skin, lymph nodes, and body temperature, during the first month of therapy, every 2 weeks for the next 5 months, and monthly thereafter. Patients should be instructed to report promptly the development of signs and symptoms of granulocytopenia and/or thrombocytopenia, such as fever, sore throat, chills, bruising, or bleeding; the above laboratory studies should then be promptly repeated.
▷ *sulfasalazine (G)* initially 0.5 gm once daily bid; gradually increase every 4 days; usual maintenance 2-3 gm/day in equally divided doses at regular intervals; max 4 gm/day
    Pediatric: <6 years: not recommended; 6-16 years: initially 1/4 to 1/3 of maintenance dose, increase weekly, maintenance 30-50 mg/kg/day in 2 divided doses at regular intervals; max 2 gm/day; >16 years: same as adult
      Azulfidine *Tab:* 500 mg
      Azulfidine EN *Tab:* 500 mg ent-coat

Tumor Necrosis Factor (TNF) Blockers

▷ *adalimumab* 40 mg SC once every other week; may increase to once weekly without *methotrexate (MTX)*; administer in abdomen or thigh; rotate sites; 2-17 years, supervise first dose

Pediatric: <2 years, <10 kg: not recommended; 10-<15 kg: 10 mg every other week; 15-<30 kg: 20 mg every other week; ≥30 kg: 40 mg every other week

Humira *Prefilled pen (Humira Pen):* 40 mg/0.4 ml, 40 mg/0.8 ml, 80 mg/0.8 ml, single-dose; *Prefilled glass syringe:* 10 mg/0.1 ml, 10 mg/0.2 ml, 20 mg/0.2 ml, 20 mg/0.4 ml, 40 mg/0.4 ml, 40 mg/0.8 ml, 80 mg/0.8 ml, single-dose; *Vial:* 40 mg/0.8 ml, single-dose, institutional use only (preservative-free)

Comment: Humira may be used with *methotrexate (MTX)*, DMARDs, corticosteroids, salicylates, NSAIDs, or analgesics.

▷ *adalimumab-aacf* 40 mg SC every other week; if not receiving *methotrexate* may benefit from increasing the dose to 40 mg SC every week or 80 mg SC every other week

Idacio *Prefilled pen (Idacio Pen):* 40 mg/0.8 ml, single-dose; *Prefilled glass syringe:* 40 mg/0.8 ml, single-dose

Comment: Idacio is biosimilar to Humira *(adalimumab).*

▷ *adalimumab-adbm* initially 80 SC; then 40 mg SC every other week starting 1 week after initial dose; inject into thigh or abdomen; rotate sites

Pediatric: <18 years: not recommended; ≥18 years: same as adult

Cyltezo *Prefilled syringe:* 40 mg/0.8 ml, single-dose (preservative-free)

Comment: Cyltezo is biosimilar to Humira *(adalimumab).*

▷ *adalimumab-afzb* 40 mg SC every other week; some patients with RA not receiving *methotrexate (MTX)* may benefit from increasing the frequency to 40 mg SC every week

Abrilada *Prefilled pen:* 40 mg/0.8 ml, single-dose; *Prefilled syringe:* 40 mg/0.8 ml, 20 mg/0.4 ml, 10 mg/0.2 ml, single-dose (for institutional use only) (preservative-free)

Comment: Abrilada is biosimilar to Humira *(adalimumab).*

▷ *adalimumab-bwwd Initial dose* (Day 1): 160 mg SC; *Second dose 2 weeks later* (Day 15): 80 mg SC; *Third dose, weeks later* (Day 29): begin maintenance dose of 40 mg every other week

Hadlima *Prefilled autoinjector:* 40 mg/0.8 ml, single-dose (Hadlima PushTouch); *Prefilled syringe:* 40 mg/0.8 ml, single-dose

Comment: Hadlima is biosimilar to Humira *(adalimumab).*

▷ *certolizumab pegol* 400 mg SC on day 1, at week 2, and at week 4; then 200 mg every other week; rotate sites

Pediatric: <12 years: not recommended; ≥12 years: same as adult

Cimzia *Vial:* 200 mg single-dose w. supplies (2/pck, 2, 6/starter pck); *Prefilled syringe:* 200 mg single-dose w. supplies (2/pck, 2, 6/starter pck) (preservative-free)

▷ *etanercept* 25 mg SC twice weekly, 72-96 hours apart or 50 mg SC weekly; rotate sites

Pediatric: <4 years: not recommended; 4-17 years: 0.4 mg/kg SC twice weekly, 72-96 hours apart (max 25 mg/dose) or 0.8 mg/kg SC weekly (max 50 mg/dose)

Enbrel *Vial:* 25 mg pwdr for SC injection after reconstitution (4/carton w. supplies) (preservative-free; diluent contains benzyl alcohol); *Prefilled syringe:* 50 mg/ml (preservative-free); *SureClick autoinjector:* 50 mg/ml (preservative-free)

Comment: *Etanercept* reduces pain, morning stiffness, and swelling. May be administered in combination with *methotrexate (MTX)*. Live vaccines should not be administered concurrently. Do not administer with active infection.

▷ *etanercept-ykro* 50 mg SC once weekly

Pediatric: <4 years: not established; ≥4 years, ≥63 kg, 138 lb: same as adult

Eticovo *Prefilled syringe:* 25 mg/0.5 ml, 50 mg/ml solution, single-dose

Comment: Eticovo is biosimilar to Enbrel *(etanercept).*

▷ *golimumab* administer SC or IV infusion (in combination with *methotrexate* [MTX])

Pediatric: <18 years: not recommended; ≥18 years: same as adult

Simponi 50 mg SC once monthly; rotate sites

Prefilled syringe, SmartJect autoinjector: 50 mg/0.5 ml, single-use (preservative-free)

Simponi Aria 2 mg/kg via IV infusion Week 0 and Week 4; then every 8 weeks thereafter

Vial: 50 mg/4 ml, single-use, soln for IV infusion after dilution (latex-free, preservative-free)

Comment: Corticosteroids, non-biologic DMARDs, and/or NSAIDs may be continued during treatment with *golimumab.*

▷ *infliximab* must be refrigerated at 2°C to 8°C (36°F to 46°F); administer dose via IV infusion over a period of not less than 2 hours; do not use beyond the expiration date as this product contains no preservative; 5 mg/kg at 0, 2, and 6 weeks, then every 8 weeks

Pediatric: <6 years: safety and efficacy not established; ≥6-17 years: 3 mg/kg at 0, 2, and 6 weeks, then every 8 weeks; ≥18 years: same as adult

Remicade *Vial:* 100 mg pwdr for reconstitution to 10 ml administration volume, single-dose (preservative-free)

Comment: Use *infliximab* concomitantly with *methotrexate (MTX)* when there has been insufficient response to *methotrexate (MTX)* alone. **Remicade** is indicated to reduce signs and symptoms, and induce and maintain clinical remission, in adults and children ≥6 years of age with moderately to severely active disease who have had an inadequate response to conventional therapy, and reduce the number of draining enterocutaneous and rectovaginal fistulas, and maintain fistula closure, in adults with fistulizing disease. Common adverse effects associated with **Remicade** included abdominal pain, headache, pharyngitis, sinusitis, and upper

(continued)

respiratory infections (URIs). In addition, **Remicade** might increase the risk for serious infections, including tuberculosis, bacterial sepsis, and invasive fungal infections. Available data from published literature on the use of *infliximab* products during pregnancy have <u>not</u> reported a clear association with *infliximab* products and adverse pregnancy outcomes. *Infliximab* products cross the placenta and infants exposed *in utero* should <u>not</u> be administered live vaccines for at least 6 months after birth. Otherwise, the infant may be at increased risk of infection, including disseminated infection, which can become fatal. Available information is insufficient to inform the amount of *infliximab* products present in human milk <u>or</u> effects on the breastfed infant.

▷ *infliximab-abda*
   Renflexis *Vial:* 100 mg pwdr for reconstitution to 10 ml administration volume, single-dose
   Comment: Renflexis is biosimilar to **Remicade** (*infliximab*).

▷ *infliximab-dyyb*
   Inflectra *Vial:* 100 mg pwdr for reconstitution to 10 ml administration volume, single-dose
   Comment: Inflectra is biosimilar to **Remicade** (*infliximab*).

▷ *infliximab-axxq*
   Avsola *Vial:* 100 mg pwdr in a 20 ml single-dose vial, for reconstitution, dilution, and IV infusion
   Comment: Avsola is biosimilar to **Remicade** *(infliximab)*. Avsola is indicated for the treatment of RA, in combination with *methotrexate*, for reducing signs and symptoms, inhibiting the progression of structural damage, and improving physical function in patients with moderate-to-severe active disease. See *infliximab* (Remicade) above for prescribing information.

▷ *infliximab-qbtx*
   Ixifi *Vial:* 100 mg pwdr for reconstitution to 10 ml administration volume, single-dose
   Comment: Ixifi is biosimilar to **Remicade** (*infliximab*).

Interleukin-1 Receptor Antagonist

▷ *anakinra (interleukin-1 receptor antagonist)* 100 mg SC once daily; discard any unused portion
   Pediatric: <12 years: <u>not</u> recommended; ≥12 years: same as adult
   Kineret *Prefilled syringe:* 100 mg/single-dose syringe (7, 28/pck) (preservative-free)

Interleukin-6 Receptor Antagonists

▷ *sarilumab* 200 mg SC every 2 weeks on the same day; if necessary, the dosage can be reduced 150 mg every 2 weeks to manage potential laboratory abnormalities, such as neutropenia, thrombocytopenia, and liver enzyme elevations; SC injections may be self-administered
   Pediatric: <18 years: <u>not</u> recommended; ≥18 years: same as adult
   Kevzara *Prefilled syringe:* 150, 200 mg (1.4 ml, single-use)
   Comment: *Sarilumab* is a human monoclonal antibody that binds to the interleukin-6 receptor (IL-6R) and has been shown to inhibit IL-6R-mediated signaling. IL-6 is a cytokine in the body that, in excess and over time, can contribute to the inflammation associated with RA. **Kevzara** is indicated for the treatment of patients with polymyalgia rheumatica and patients with active moderate-to-severe rheumatoid arthritis (RA) in adults who have had an inadequate response <u>or</u> intolerance to one <u>or</u> more disease modifying antirheumatic drugs (DMARDs). **Kevzara** may be used as monotherapy <u>or</u> in combination with *methotrexate (MTX)* <u>or</u> other conventional DMARDs. Monitor the patient for dose-related laboratory changes including elevated liver function tests (LFTs), neutropenia, and thrombocytopenia. **Kevzara** should <u>not</u> be initiated in patients with an absolute neutrophil count (ANC) <2,000/mm³, platelet count <150,000/mm³, <u>or</u> liver transaminases above 1.5 times the upper limit of normal (ULN). Registration in the Pregnancy Exposure Registry (1-877-311-8972) is encouraged for monitoring pregnancy outcomes in women exposed to **Kevzara** during pregnancy. Negative side effects of **Kevzara** should be reported to the FDA at www.fda.gov/medwatch <u>or</u> call 1-800-FDA-1088 <u>or</u> call Sanofi-Aventis at 1-800-633-1610. The limited available data with **Kevzara** in pregnant females are <u>not</u> sufficient to determine whether there is a drug-associated risk of major birth defects and miscarriage. Monoclonal antibodies, such as *sarilumab*, are actively transported across the placenta during the third trimester of pregnancy and may affect immune response in the infant exposed *in utero*. It is <u>not</u> known whether *sarilumab* passes into breast milk; therefore, breastfeeding is <u>not</u> recommended while using **Kevzara**.

▷ *tocilizumab IV Infusion:* administer IV infusion over 1 hour; do <u>not</u> administer as bolus <u>or</u> IV push; *Adults, polyarticular juvenile idiopathic arthritis (PJIA), and systemic juvenile idiopathic arthritis (SJIA),* ≥30 kg: dilute to 100 ml in 0.9% <u>or</u> 0.45% NaCl. *PJIA and SJIA; <30 kg:* dilute to 50 ml in 0.9% <u>or</u> 0.45% NaCl
   Adults: IV infusion: Whether used in combination with DMARDs <u>or</u> as monotherapy, the recommended starting dose is 4 mg/kg every 4 weeks followed by an increase to 8 mg/kg every 4 weeks based on clinical response; max 800 mg per infusion in RA patients; *SC administration:* ≥*100 kg:* 162 mg SC once weekly on the same day; *<100 kg:* 162 mg SC every other week on the same day followed by an increase according to clinical response; SC injections may be self-administered
   Pediatric: <2 years: <u>not</u> recommended; ≥2 years: weight-based dosing according to diagnosis: *PJIA:* ≥*30 kg:* 8 mg/kg SC every 4 weeks; *<30 kg:* 10 mg/kg SC every 4 weeks; *SJIA:* ≥*30 kg:* 8 mg/kg SC every 2 weeks; *<30 kg:* 12 mg/kg SC every 2 weeks
      Actemra *Vial:* 80 mg/4 ml, 200 mg/10 ml, 400 mg/20 ml, single-use, for IV infusion after dilution; *Prefilled syringe:* 162 mg (0.9 ml, single-dose); *Prefilled ACTPen autoinjector:* 162 mg/0.9 ml, single-dose, for SC administration

Comment: *Tocilizumab* is an interleukin-6 receptor-alpha inhibitor indicated for use in moderate-to-severe rheumatoid arthritis (RA) that has not responded to conventional therapy and also for some subtypes of juvenile idiopathic arthritis (JIA). **Actemra** may be used alone or in combination with *methotrexate (MTX)*, and in RA other DMARDs may be used. Monitor the patient for dose-related laboratory changes including elevated LFTs, neutropenia, and thrombocytopenia. **Actemra** should not be initiated in patients with an absolute neutrophil count (ANC) below 2,000 per mm³, platelet count below 100,000 per mm³, or who have alanine aminotransferase (ALT) or aspartate aminotransferase (AST) above 1.5 times the upper limit of normal (ULN). Registration in the Pregnancy Exposure Registry (1-877-311-8972) is encouraged for monitoring pregnancy outcomes in women exposed to **Actemra** during pregnancy. The limited available data with **Actemra** in pregnant females are not sufficient to determine whether there is a drug-associated risk of major birth defects and miscarriage. Monoclonal antibodies, such as *tocilizumab*, are actively transported across the placenta during the third trimester of pregnancy and may affect immune response in the infant exposed *in utero*. It is not known whether *tocilizumab* passes into breast milk; therefore, breastfeeding is not recommended while using **Actemra**.

Selective Co-Stimulation Modulator

➤ *abatacept* administer as an IV infusion over 30 minutes at Weeks 0, 2, and 4; then every 4 weeks thereafter; <60 kg: administer 500 mg/dose; 60-100 kg: administer 750 mg/dose; >100 kg: administer 1 gm/dose
Pediatric: <6 years: not recommended; 6-17 years: administer as an IV infusion over 30 minutes at weeks 0, 2, and 4, then every 4 weeks thereafter; <75 kg, administer 10 mg/kg; same as adult (max 1 gm)
   Orencia *Vial:* 250 mg pwdr for IV infusion after reconstitution (silicone-free) (preservative-free); *Prefilled syringe:* 125 mg/ml soln for SC injection (preservative-free); *ClickJect Autoinjector:* 125 mg/ml soln for SC injection

CD20 ANTIBODY

➤ *rituximab* administer corticosteroid 30 minutes prior to each infusion; concomitant *methotrexate* (MTX) therapy, administer a 1,000 mg IV infusion at 0 and 2 weeks; then every 24 weeks or based on response, but not sooner than every 16 weeks
Pediatric: <6 years: not recommended; ≥6 years: same as adult
   Rituxan *Vial:* 100 mg/10 ml (10 mg/ml), 50 mg/50 ml (10 mg/ml), single-use (preservative-free)

INTRA-ARTICULAR INJECTION

➤ *sodium hyaluronate* 20 mg as intra-articular injection weekly x 5 weeks
Pediatric: <12 years: not recommended; ≥12 years: same as adult
   Hyalgan *Prefilled syringe:* 20 mg/2 ml
   Comment: Remove joint effusion and inject with *lidocaine* if possible before injecting **Hyalgan**.

RHINITIS/SINUSITIS: ALLERGIC

See Appendix Z. Drugs for the Management of Allergy, Cough, and Cold Symptoms online at https://connect.springerpub.com/content/reference-book/978-0-8261-7935-7/back-matter/part02/back-matter/bmatter27
Parenteral Corticosteroids *see* Appendix L. Parenteral Corticosteroids
Oral Corticosteroids *see* Appendix K. Oral Corticosteroids

Comment: The Joint Task Force on Practice Parameters, which comprises representatives of the American Academy of Allergy, Asthma and Immunology (AAAAI) and the American College of Allergy, Asthma and Immunology (ACAAI), has provided guidance to healthcare providers on the initial pharmacologic treatment of seasonal allergic rhinitis in patients aged ≥12 years. For initial treatment of seasonal allergic rhinitis in persons aged ≥12 years, routinely prescribe monotherapy with an intranasal corticosteroid rather than an intranasal corticosteroid in combination with an oral antihistamine. For initial treatment of seasonal allergic rhinitis in persons aged ≥15 years, recommend an intranasal corticosteroid over a leukotriene. For initial treatment of seasonal allergic rhinitis in persons aged ≥15 years, recommend an intranasal corticosteroid over a leukotriene receptor antagonist. For initial treatment of moderate-to-severe seasonal allergic rhinitis in persons aged ≥12 years, recommend a combination of an intranasal corticosteroid and an intranasal antihistamine.

SECOND-GENERATION ANTIHISTAMINES

Comment: The following drugs are second-generation antihistamines. As such they are minimally sedating, much less so than the first-generation antihistamines. All antihistamines are excreted into breast milk.
➤ *cetirizine* (OTC)(G) initially 5-10 mg once daily; 5 mg once daily; ≥65 years: use with caution
Pediatric: <6 years: not recommended; ≥6 years: same as adult
   cetirizine Cap: 10 mg
   Children's Zyrtec Chewable *Chew tab:* 5, 10 mg (grape)
   Children's Zyrtec Allergy Syrup *Syr:* 1 mg/ml (4 oz) (grape, bubble gum) (sugar-free, dye-free)
   Zyrtec *Tab:* 10 mg
   Zyrtec Hives Relief *Tab:* 10 mg
   Zyrtec Liquid Gels *Liq gel:* 10 mg

(continued)

▷ **desloratadine**
    Clarinex 1/2-1 tab once daily
    Pediatric: <6 years: <u>not</u> recommended; ≥6 years: same as adult
    Tab: 5 mg
    Clarinex RediTabs 5 mg once daily
    Pediatric: <6 years: <u>not</u> recommended; 6-12 years: 2.5 mg once daily; ≥12 years: same as adult
    ODT: 2.5, 5 mg (tutti-frutti) (phenylalanine)
    Clarinex Syrup 5 mg (10 ml) once daily
    Pediatric: <6 months: <u>not</u> recommended; 6-11 months: 1 mg (2 ml) once daily; 1-5 years: 1.25 mg (2.5 ml) once daily; 6-11 years: 2.5 mg (5 ml) once daily; ≥12 years: same as adult
    Syr: 0.5 mg per ml (4 oz) (tutti-frutti) (phenylalanine)
    Desloratadine ODT 1 tab once daily
    Pediatric: <6 years: <u>not</u> recommended; 6-11 years: 1/2 tab once daily; ≥12 years: same as adult
    ODT: 5 mg
▷ **fexofenadine** (OTC)(G) 60 mg once daily-bid <u>or</u> 180 mg once daily; *CrCl <90 ml/min:* 60 mg once daily
    Pediatric: <6 months: <u>not</u> recommended; 6 months-2 years: 15 mg bid; *CrCl ≤90 ml/min:* 15 mg once daily; 2-11 years: 30 mg bid; *CrCl ≤90 ml/min:* 30 mg once daily; ≥12 years: same as adult
    Allegra *Tab:* 30, 60, 180 mg film-coat
    Allegra Allergy *Tab:* 60, 180 mg film-coat
    Allegra ODT *ODT:* 30 mg (phenylalanine)
    Allegra Oral Suspension *Oral susp:* 30 mg/5 ml (6 mg/ml) (4 oz)
▷ **levocetirizine** (OTC)(G) administer dose in the PM; *Seasonal allergic rhinitis:* <2 years: <u>not</u> recommended; may start at ≥2 years; *Chronic idiopathic urticaria (CIU), perennial allergic rhinitis:* <6 months: <u>not</u> recommended; may start at ≥ 6 months; *Dosing by age:* 6 months to 5 years: max 1.25 mg once daily; 6-11 years: max 2.5 mg once daily; ≥12 years: 2.5-5 mg once daily; *Renal dysfunction <12 years:* contraindicated; *Renal dysfunction ≥12 years:* CrCl 50-80 ml/min: 2.5 mg once daily; CrCl 30-50 ml/min: 2.5 mg every other day; CrCl 10-30 ml/min: 2.5 mg twice weekly (every 3-4 days); CrCl <10 ml/min, end-stage renal disease (ESRD), <u>or</u> hemodialysis: contraindicated
    Children's Xyzal Allergy 24HR *Oral soln:* 0.5 mg/ml (150 ml)
    Xyzal Allergy 24HR *Tab:* 5*mg
▷ **loratadine** (OTC)(G) 5 mg bid <u>or</u> 10 mg once daily; *Hepatic <u>or</u> renal insufficiency:* see mfr pkg insert
    Pediatric: <2 years: <u>not</u> recommended; 2-5 years: 5 mg once daily; ≥6 years: same as adult
    Children's Claritin Chewables *Chew tab:* 5 mg (grape) (phenylalanine)
    Children's Claritin Syrup 1 mg/ml (4 oz) (fruit) (sugar-free, alcohol-free, dye-free; sodium 6 mg/5 ml)
    Claritin *Tab:* 10 mg
    Claritin Hives Relief *Tab:* 10 mg
    Claritin Liqui-Gels *Liq gel:* 10 mg
    Claritin RediTabs 12 Hours *ODT:* 5 mg (mint)
    Claritin RediTabs 24 Hours *ODT:* 10 mg (mint)

FIRST-GENERATION ANTIHISTAMINES

▷ **diphenhydramine** (G) 25-50 mg q 6-8 hours; max 100 mg/day
    Pediatric: <2 years: <u>not</u> recommended; 2-6 years: 6.25 mg q 4-6 hours; max 37.5 mg/day; >6-12 years: 12.5-25 mg q 4-6 hours, max 150 mg/day; >12 years: same as adult
    Benadryl (OTC) *Chew tab:* 12.5 mg (grape) (phenylalanine); *Liq:* 12.5 mg/5 ml (4, 8 oz); *Cap:* 25 mg; *Tab:* 25 mg; *Dye-free soft gel:* 25 mg; *Dye-free liq:* 12.5 mg/5 ml (4, 8 oz)
▷ **diphenhydramine injectable** (G) 25-50 mg IM immediately; then q 6 hours prn
    Pediatric: <12 years: see mfr pkg insert: 1.25 mg/kg up to 25 mg IM x 1 dose; then q 6 hours prn; ≥12 years: same as adult
    Benadryl Injectable *Vial:* 50 mg/ml (1 ml single-use); 50 mg/ml (10 ml multi-dose); *Amp:* 10 mg/ml (1 ml); *Prefilled syringe:* 50 mg/ml (1 ml)
▷ **hydroxyzine** (G) 50-100 mg/day divided qid prn
    Pediatric: <6 years: 50 mg/day divided qid prn; ≥6 years to 12 years: 50 mg/day divided qid prn; >12 years: same as adult
    Atarax *Tab:* 10, 25, 50, 100 mg; *Syr:* 10 mg/5 ml (alcohol 0.5%)
    Vistaril *Cap:* 25, 50, 100 mg; *Oral susp:* 25 mg/5 ml (4 oz) (lemon)
    Comment: *Hydroxyzine* is contraindicated in early pregnancy and in patients with a prolonged QT interval. It is <u>not</u> known whether this drug is excreted in human milk; therefore, *hydroxyzine* should <u>not</u> be given to nursing mothers.

ALLERGEN EXTRACTS
Comment: Allergen extracts (**Grastek, Oralair, Ragwitek**) are <u>not</u> for immediate relief of allergic symptoms. Contraindicated with severe, unstable, and uncontrolled asthma, history of eosinophilic esophagitis, and severe local <u>or</u> systemic reaction. First dose under supervision of a qualified healthcare provider and observe ≥30 minutes. Subsequent doses may be taken at home.

▷ *short ragweed pollen allergen extract* 1 SL tab once daily
  Pediatric: <18 years: <u>not</u> established; ≥18 years: same as adult
      Ragwitek *SL tab:* Ambrosia artemisiifolia 12 amb a 1-unit (30, 90/blister pck)
      Comment: Initiate **Ragwitek** at least 12 weeks before onset of ragweed pollen season and continue throughout season.
▷ *sweet vernal, orchard, perennial rye, timothy, Kentucky blue grass mixed pollen allergen extract* 300 IR once daily
  Pediatric: <10 years: <u>not</u> established; 10-17 years: Day 1: 100 IR; Day 2: 200 IR; Day 3 and thereafter: 300 IR once daily
      Oralair *SL tab:* 100, 300 IR (index of reactivity) (30/blister pck)
      Comment: **Oralair** is indicated for grass pollen-induced allergic rhinitis with <u>or</u> without conjunctivitis confirmed by positive skin test. Initiate **Oralair** at least 4 months before onset of grass pollen season and continue throughout season.
▷ *Timothy grass pollen allergen extract* 1 SL tab once daily
  Pediatric: <5 years: <u>not</u> established; ≥5 years: same as adult
      Grastek *SL tab:* 2,800 bioequivalent allergy units (BAUS) (30/blister pck)
      Comment: **Grastek** is indicated for grass pollen-induced allergic rhinitis with <u>or</u> without conjunctivitis confirmed by positive skin test. Initiate **Grastek** at least 12 weeks before onset of grass pollen season and continue throughout season.

NASAL DECONGESTANT
▷ *tetrahydrozoline*
      Tyzine 2-4 drops <u>or</u> 3-4 sprays in each nostril q 3-8 hours prn
      Pediatric: <6 years: <u>not</u> recommended; ≥6 years: same as adult
        Nasal spray: 0.1% (15 ml); *Nasal drops:* 0.1% (30 ml)
      Tyzine Pediatric Nasal Drops 2-3 sprays <u>or</u> drops in each nostril q 3-6 hours prn
        Nasal drops: 0.05% (15 ml)

LEUKOTRIENE RECEPTOR ANTAGONISTS (LRAs)
Comment: For prophylaxis and chronic treatment <u>only</u>. <u>Not</u> for primary (rescue) treatment of acute asthma attack.
▷ *montelukast* (G) 10 mg once daily in the PM; for exercise induced bronchospasm (EIB), take at least 2 hours before exercise; max 1 dose/day
  Pediatric: <12 months: <u>not</u> recommended; 12-23 months: one 4 mg granule pkt daily; 2-5 years: one 4 mg chew tab <u>or</u> granule pkt daily; 6-14 years: one 5 mg chew tab daily; ≥15 years: same as adult
      Singulair *Tab:* 10 mg
      Singulair Chewable *Chew tab:* 4, 5 mg (cherry, phenylalanine)
      Singulair Oral Granules: 4 mg/pkt; take within 15 minutes of opening pkt; may mix with applesauce, carrots, rice, <u>or</u> ice cream
▷ *zafirlukast* (G) 20 mg bid, 1 hour ac <u>or</u> 2 hours pc
  Pediatric: <7 years: <u>not</u> recommended; 7-11 years: 10 mg bid 1 hour ac <u>or</u> 2 hours pc; >11 years: same as adult
      Accolate *Tab:* 10, 20 mg
▷ *zileuton* (G)
  Pediatric: <12 years: <u>not</u> recommended; ≥12 years: same as adult
      Zyflo 1 tab qid (total 2400 mg/day)
        Tab: 600 mg
      Zyflo CR 2 tab bid (total 2400 mg/day)
        Tab: 600 mg ext-rel

NASAL CORTICOSTEROIDS
▷ *beclomethasone dipropionate*
      Beconase 1 spray in each nostril bid-qid
        Pediatric: <6 years: <u>not</u> recommended; 6-12 years: 1 spray in each nostril tid; >12 years: same as adult
        Nasal spray: 42 mcg/actuation (6.7 gm, 80 sprays; 16.8 gm, 200 sprays)
      Beconase AQ 1-2 sprays in each nostril bid
        Pediatric: <6: <u>not</u> recommended; ≥6 years: same as adult
        Nasal spray: 42 mcg/actuation (25 gm, 180 sprays)
      Beconase Inhalation Aerosol 1-2 sprays in each nostril bid-qid
        Pediatric: <6: <u>not</u> recommended; 6-12 years: 1 spray in each nostril tid; >12 years: same as adult
        Nasal spray: 42 mcg/actuation (6.7 gm, 80 sprays; 16.8 gm, 200 sprays)
      Vancenase AQ 1-2 sprays in each nostril bid
        Pediatric: <6 years: <u>not</u> recommended; ≥6 years: same as adult
        Nasal spray: 84 mcg/actuation (25 gm, 200 sprays)
      Vancenase AQ DS 1-2 sprays in each nostril once daily
        Pediatric: <6 years: <u>not</u> recommended; ≥6 years: same as adult
        Nasal spray: 84, 168 mcg/actuation (19 gm, 120 sprays)
      Vancenase Pockethaler 1 spray in each nostril bid <u>or</u> qid
        Pediatric: <6: <u>not</u> recommended; ≥6 years: 1 spray in each nostril tid

(continued)

Pockethaler: 42 mcg/actuation (7 gm, 200 sprays)
QNASL Nasal Aerosol 2 sprays, 80 mcg/spray, in each nostril once daily
Pediatric: <12 years: 2 sprays, 40 mcg/spray, in each nostril once daily; ≥12 years: same as adult
Nasal spray: 40 mcg/actuation (4.9 gm, 60 sprays); 80 mcg/actuation (8.7 gm, 120 sprays)

▷ *budesonide*
Rhinocort initially 2 sprays in each nostril bid in the AM and PM, or 4 sprays in each nostril in the AM; max 4 sprays each nostril/day; use lowest effective dose
Pediatric: <6 years: <u>not</u> recommended; ≥6 years: same as adult
Nasal spray: 32 mcg/actuation (7 gm, 200 sprays)
Rhinocort Aqua Nasal Spray initially 1 spray in each nostril once daily; max 4 sprays in each nostril once daily
Pediatric: <6 years: <u>not</u> recommended; ≥6-12 years: initially 1 spray in each nostril once daily; max 2 sprays in each nostril once daily
Nasal spray: 32 mcg/actuation (10 ml, 60 sprays)

▷ *ciclesonide*
Pediatric: <6 years: <u>not</u> recommended; ≥6 years: same as adult
Omnaris 2 sprays in each nostril once daily
Nasal spray: 50 mcg/actuation (12.5 gm, 120 sprays)
Zetonna 1-2 sprays in each nostril once daily
Nasal spray: 37 mcg/actuation (6.1 gm, 60 sprays) (HFA)

▷ *dexamethasone* 2 sprays in each nostril bid-tid; max 12 sprays/day; maintain at lowest effective dose
Pediatric: <6 years: <u>not</u> recommended; ≥6-12 years: 1-2 sprays in each nostril bid; max 8 sprays/day; maintain at lowest effective dose; >12 years: same as adult
Dexacort Turbinaire *Nasal spray:* 84 mcg/actuation (12.6 gm, 170 sprays)

▷ *fluticasone furoate* 2 sprays in each nostril once daily; may reduce to 1 spray each nostril once daily
Pediatric: <2 years: <u>not</u> recommended; ≥2-11 years: 1 spray in each nostril once daily; ≥12 years: same as adult
Veramyst *Nasal spray:* 27.5 mcg/actuation (10 gm, 120 sprays) (alcohol-free)

▷ *fluticasone propionate* (OTC)(G) initially 2 sprays in each nostril once daily or 1 spray bid; maintenance 1 spray once daily
Pediatric: <4 years: <u>not</u> recommended; ≥4 years: initially 1 spray in each nostril once daily; may increase to 2 sprays in each nostril once daily; maintenance 1 spray in each nostril once daily; max 2 sprays in each nostril/day
Flonase *Nasal spray:* 50 mcg/actuation (16 gm, 120 sprays)

▷ *flunisolide* 2 sprays in each nostril bid; may increase to 2 sprays in each nostril tid; max 8 sprays/nostril/day
Pediatric: <6 years: <u>not</u> recommended; 6-14 years: initially 1 spray in each nostril tid or 2 sprays in each nostril bid; max 4 sprays/nostril/day; >14 years: same as adult
Nasalide *Nasal spray:* 25 mcg/actuation (25 ml, 200 sprays)
Nasarel *Nasal spray:* 25 mcg/actuation (25 ml, 200 sprays)

▷ *mometasone furoate* (G) 2 sprays in each nostril once daily
Pediatric: <2 years: <u>not</u> recommended; 2-11 years: 1 spray in each nostril once daily; max 2 sprays in each nostril once daily; >11 years: same as adult
Nasonex *Nasal spray:* 50 mcg/actuation (17 gm, 120 sprays)

▷ *olopatadine* 2 sprays in each nostril bid
Pediatric: <6 years: <u>not</u> recommended; 6-11 years: 1 spray each nostril bid; >11 years: same as adult
Patanase *Nasal spray:* 0.6%; 665 mcg/actuation (30.5 gm, 240 sprays) (benzalkonium chloride)

▷ *triamcinolone acetonide* (G) initially 2 sprays in each nostril once daily; max 4 sprays in each nostril once daily or 2 sprays in each nostril bid or 1 spray in each nostril qid; maintain at lowest effective dose
Pediatric: <6 years: <u>not</u> recommended; ≥6 years: 1 spray in each nostril once daily; max 2 sprays in each nostril once daily
Nasacort Allergy 24HR (OTC) *Nasal spray:* 55 mcg/actuation (10 gm, 120 sprays)
Tri-Nasal *Nasal spray:* 50 mcg/actuation (15 ml, 120 sprays)

NASAL MAST CELL STABILIZERS
▷ *cromolyn sodium* (OTC) 1 spray in each nostril tid-qid; max 6 sprays in each nostril/day
Pediatric: <2 years: <u>not</u> recommended; ≥2 years: same as adult
Children's NasalCrom, NasalCrom *Nasal spray:* 5.2 mg/spray (13 ml, 100 sprays; 26 ml, 200 sprays)
Comment: Begin 1-2 weeks before exposure to known allergen. May take 2-4 weeks to achieve maximum effect.

NASAL ANTIHISTAMINES
▷ *azelastine*
Astelin Ready Spray 2 sprays in each nostril bid
Pediatric: <5 years: <u>not</u> recommended; ≥5-12 years: 1 spray in each nostril once daily bid; >12 years: same as adult
Nasal spray: 137 mcg/actuation (30 ml, 200 sprays) (benzalkonium chloride)
Astepro 0.15% Nasal Spray (OTC) 1 or 2 sprays each nostril once daily bid
Pediatric: <12 years: <u>not</u> recommended; ≥12 years: same as adult
Nasal spray: 205.5 mcg/actuation (17 ml, 106 sprays; 30 ml, 200 sprays) (benzalkonium chloride)

NASAL ANTIHISTAMINE+CORTICOSTEROID COMBINATION

▷ *azelastine+fluticasone* (G) 1 spray in each nostril bid
  Pediatric: <6 years: not recommended; ≥6 years: same as adult
    Dymista *Nasal spray:* azel 137 mcg/flutic 50 mcg per actuation (23 gm, 120 sprays) (benzalkonium chloride)
▷ *olopatadine hydrochloride+mometasone furoate* 2 sprays in each nostril bid; prime before initial use by
  releasing 6 sprays; when it has not been used for 14 or more days, reprime by releasing 2 sprays or until a
  fine mist appears
  Pediatric: <12 years: safety and efficacy not established; ≥12 years: same as adult
    Ryaltris *Nasal spray: olopatadine hydrochloride* 665 mcg (histamine-1[H1]-receptor
    inhibitor)+*mometasone furoate* 25 mcg (corticosteroid), metered, fixed-dose combination (240 metered
    sprays plus 6 initial priming sprays)
    Comment: Ryaltris is a fixed-dose combination of an antihistamine and corticosteroid for adults and
    pediatrics ≥12 years of age indicated for the treatment of symptoms of seasonal allergic rhinitis. **Ryaltris** is
    contraindicated for patients with known hypersensitivity to any **Ryaltris** ingredients, including *mometasone
    furoate.* The most common adverse reactions (≥1% incidence) are dysgeusia, epistaxis, and nasal discomfort.
    Monitor patients periodically for signs of adverse reactions on the nasal mucosa: epistaxis, nasal ulcerations,
    nasal septal perforations, impaired wound healing, and *Candida albicans* infection. Avoid engaging in
    hazardous occupations requiring complete mental alertness and motor coordination. Avoid concurrent use
    of alcohol or other central nervous system (CNS) depressants with **Ryaltris** because additional reductions
    in alertness (somnolence) and additional impairment of CNS performance may occur. Monitor patients
    with a change in vision or with a history of increased intraocular pressure, glaucoma, and/or cataracts.
    Hypersensitivity reactions, including wheezing, have occurred after the nasal administration of *mometasone
    furoate.* Discontinue **Ryaltris** if such reactions occur. Immunosuppression and infections are potential
    complications of **Ryaltris** use, such as worsening of existing tuberculosis, fungal, bacterial, viral, or parasitic
    infections, ocular herpes simplex, or serious, even fatal, course of chickenpox or measles in susceptible
    patients. Hypercorticism and adrenal suppression may potentially develop with misuse or use of higher-
    than-recommended dosage or at the regular dosage in susceptible patients at risk for such effects. Routinely
    monitor the growth in pediatric patients for potential reduction in growth velocity. There are no available
    data on **Ryaltris** or *mometasone furoate* use in human pregnancy to evaluate for a drug-associated risk of
    major birth defects, miscarriage, or other adverse maternal or fetal outcomes. Postmarketing experience
    with antihistamines with similar mechanism of action to *olopatadine,* has not identified a drug-associated
    risk of major birth defects, miscarriage, or adverse maternal or fetal outcomes. However, there are no
    published human data specific to *olopatadine.* See the mfr pkg insert for a review of reproductive toxicity
    and embryo/fetal development animal studies. Risk/benefit should be considered by informed pregnant
    patients and females of reproductive potential in terms of fetal risk and the patient's condition. There are
    no available data on the presence of *olopatadine* or *mometasone furoate* or its metabolites in human milk
    or effects on the breastfed infant. Other corticosteroids similar to *mometasone furoate* are excreted in
    human milk. However, *mometasone furoate* concentrations in plasma after therapeutic nasal doses are low
    and therefore concentrations in human breast milk are likely to be correspondingly low. It is not known
    whether topical nasal administration of *olopatadine* could result in sufficient systemic absorption to produce
    detectable quantities in human breast milk. The developmental and health benefits of breastfeeding should be
    considered along with the mother's clinical need for **Ryaltris** and any potential adverse effects on the breastfed
    infant from **Ryaltris** or from the underlying maternal condition. To report suspected adverse reactions,
    contact Hikma Specialty USA at 1-800-962-8364 or FDA at 1-800-FDA-1088 or www.fda.gov/medwatch.

NASAL ANTICHOLINERGICS

▷ *ipratropium bromide* (G)
    Atrovent Nasal Spray 0.03% 2 sprays in each nostril bid-tid
    Pediatric: <6 years: not recommended; ≥6 years: same as adult
      Nasal spray: 21 mcg/actuation (30 ml, 345 sprays)
    Atrovent Nasal Spray 0.06% 2 sprays in each nostril tid-qid; max 5-7 days
    Pediatric: <5 years: not recommended; ≥5-11 years: 2 sprays in each nostril tid; >11 years: same as adult
      Nasal spray: 42 mcg/actuation (15 ml, 165 sprays)
    Comment: Avoid *ipratropium bromide* use with narrow-angle glaucoma, prostate hyperplasia, and bladder
    neck obstruction.

CHRONIC RHINOSINUSITIS WITH NASAL POLYPS (CRSwNP)
Interleukin-4 Receptor Alpha Antagonist

▷ *dupilumab* administer SC into the upper arm, abdomen, or thigh; rotate sites; 300 mg SC once every other
  week; may use with or without nasal corticosteroids
  Pediatric: safety and efficacy not established
    Dupixent *Prefilled syringe:* 200 mg/1.14 ml, 300 mg/2 ml, single-dose (2/pck without needle)
    (preservative-free)
    Comment: *Dupilumab* is a human monoclonal immunoglobulin G4 (IgG4) antibody that inhibits
    interleukin-4 (IL-4) and interleukin-13 (IL-13) signaling by specifically binding to the IL-4Ra subunit
    shared by the IL-4 and IL-13 receptor complexes, thereby inhibiting the release of proinflammatory

(continued)

cytokines, chemokines, and immunoglobulin E (IgE). *Dupilumab* is also indicated as an add-on maintenance therapy for patients ≥12 years of age with moderate-to-severe asthma with an eosinophilic subtype or with oral corticosteroid-dependent asthma and to treat moderate-to-severe atopic dermatitis. Avoid live vaccines.

INTERLEUKIN-5 ANTAGONIST MONOCLONAL ANTIBODY (IMMUNOGLOBULIN G1 (IGG1) KAPPA)

▷ *mepolizumab* Adult: *Severe asthma*: 100 mg SC once q 4 weeks; *Chronic rhinosinusitis with nasal polyps (CRSwNP)*: 100 mg SC once every 4 weeks; *eosinophilic granulomatosis with polyangiitis (EGPA) and hypereosinophilia syndromes (HES)*: 300 mg as 3 separate 100 mg SC injections once q 4 weeks
Pediatric: <6 years: safety and efficacy not established; severe asthma and with an eosinophilic phenotype in patients aged 6-11 years: 40 mg SC once every 4 weeks as an add-on maintenance treatment; may self-administer or caregiver may administer (with healthcare provider approval); severe asthma in patients aged ≥12 years: 100 mg SC once every 4 weeks
   Nucala *Vial*: 100 mg/ml, pwdr for reconstitution, single-dose; *Prefilled syringe*: 40 mg/0.4ml, 100 mg/ml, single-dose; *Prefilled autoinjector*: 100 mg/ml, single-dose
   Comment: Nucala is an interleukin-5 antagonist monoclonal antibody (immunoglobulin G1 [IgG1] kappa) indicated for the treatment of severe eosinophilic asthma, eosinophilic granulomatosis with polyangiitis (Churg-Strauss syndrome), hypereosinophilic syndrome (HES), and chronic rhinosinusitis with nasal polyps (CRSwNP). Nucala is not indicated for relief of acute bronchospasm or status asthmaticus. Hypersensitivity reactions (e.g., anaphylaxis, angioedema, bronchospasm, hypotension, urticaria, rash) have occurred after administration of Nucala; discontinue Nucala in the event of a hypersensitivity reaction. Herpes zoster (HZ) infections have occurred in patients receiving Nucala; consider vaccination if medically appropriate. Do not discontinue systemic or inhaled corticosteroids abruptly upon initiation of therapy with Nucala; decrease corticosteroids gradually, if appropriate. Treat patients with preexisting helminth infections before therapy with Nucala. If patients become infected while receiving treatment with Nucala and do not respond to antihelminth treatment, discontinue Nucala until the parasitic infection resolves. The most common adverse reactions (incidence ≥5%) are the following: *asthma*: headache, injection site reaction, back pain, and fatigue; *CRSwNP*: oropharyngeal pain and arthralgia; *EGPA and HES*: similar to asthma. In pregnant females with poorly or moderately controlled asthma, evidence demonstrates that there is an increased risk of preeclampsia in the mother, and prematurity, low birth weight (LBW), and small for gestational age (SGA) in the neonate. The level of asthma control should be closely monitored in pregnant women and treatment adjusted as necessary to maintain optimal control. Data on pregnancy exposure are insufficient to inform on Nucala-associated risk. Monoclonal antibodies, such as *mepolizumab*, are transported across the placenta in a linear fashion as pregnancy progresses; therefore, potential effects on the fetus are likely to be greater during the 2nd and 3rd trimesters of pregnancy. There is a pregnancy exposure registry that monitors pregnancy outcomes in women with asthma exposed to Nucala during pregnancy. Healthcare providers can enroll patients or encourage patients to enroll themselves by calling 1-877-311-8972 or www.mothertobaby.org/asthma. *Mepolizumab* is a humanized monoclonal antibody (IgG1 kappa), and immunoglobulin G (IgG) is present in human milk in small amounts. Developmental and health benefits of breastfeeding should be considered along with the mother's clinical need for Nucala and any potential adverse effects on the breastfed infant from *mepolizumab* or from the underlying maternal condition.

RHINITIS MEDICAMENTOSA

Comment: The nasal/oral regimen selected should be instituted with concurrent weaning from the nasal decongestant.

Nasal Corticosteroids *see Rhinitis/Sinusitis: Allergic*
Oral Corticosteroids *see Appendix K. Oral Corticosteroids*
Parenteral Corticosteroids *see Appendix L. Parenteral Corticosteroids*
OTC Decongestants
OTC Antihistamine+Decongestant Combinations

NASAL ANTICHOLINERGICS

▷ *ipratropium bromide* (G)
   Atrovent Nasal Spray 0.03% stop nasal decongestant; 2 sprays in each nostril bid-tid with progressive weaning as tolerated
   Pediatric: <6 years: not recommended; ≥6 years: same as adult
      Nasal spray: 21 mcg/actuation (30 ml, 345 sprays)
   Atrovent Nasal Spray 0.06% stop nasal decongestant; 2 sprays in each nostril tid-qid with progressive weaning as tolerated
   Pediatric: <5 years: not recommended; ≥5-11 years: 2 sprays in each nostril tid; ≥11 years: same as adult
      Nasal spray: 42 mcg/actuation (15 ml, 165 sprays)
   Comment: Avoid *ipratropium bromide* use with narrow-angle glaucoma, prostate hyperplasia, and bladder neck obstruction.

NASAL ANTIHISTAMINE

▶ *azelastine* 2 sprays in each nostril bid
  Pediatric: <5 years: not recommended; ≥5-12 years: 1 spray in each nostril bid
    Astelin Ready Spray *Nasal spray:* 137 mcg/actuation (30 ml, 200 sprays)

FIRST GENERATION ANTIHISTAMINES

▶ *diphenhydramine* (G) 25-50 mg q 6-8 hours; max 100 mg/day
  Pediatric: <2 years: not recommended; 2-6 years: 6.25 mg q 4-6 hours, max 37.5 mg/day; >6-12 years: 12.5-
  25 mg q 4-6 hours; max 150 mg/day; >12 years: same as adult
    Benadryl (OTC) *Chew tab:* 12.5 mg (grape) (phenylalanine); *Liq:* 12.5 mg/5 ml (4, 8 oz); *Cap:* 25 mg;
    Tab: 25 mg; *Dye-free soft gel:* 25 mg; *Dye-free liq:* 12.5 mg/5 ml (4, 8 oz)
▶ *diphenhydramine* injectable (G) 25-50 mg IM immediately; then q 6 hours prn
  Pediatric: <12 years: see mfr pkg insert: 1.25 mg/kg up to 25 mg IM x 1 dose; then q 6 hours prn; ≥12 years:
    Benadryl Injectable *Vial:* 50 mg/ml (1 ml single-use); 50 mg/ml (10 ml multi-dose); *Amp:* 10 mg/ml
    (1 ml); *Prefilled syringe:* 50 mg/ml (1 ml)
▶ *hydroxyzine* (G) 25 mg tid prn; max 600 mg/day
  Pediatric: <6 years: 50 mg/day divided qid prn; ≥6 years: 50-100 mg/day divided qid prn; max 600 mg/day
    Atarax *Tab:* 10, 25, 50, 100 mg; *Syr:* 10 mg/5 ml (alcohol 0.5%)
    Vistaril *Cap:* 25, 50, 100 mg; *Oral susp:* 25 mg/5 ml (4 oz) (lemon)

SECOND-GENERATION ANTIHISTAMINES

Comment: Second-generation antihistamines are sedating, but much less so than the first-generation
antihistamines. All antihistamines are excreted into breast milk.
▶ *cetirizine* (OTC)(G) <6 years: not recommended; ≥6-<65 years: initially 5-10 mg once daily; ≥65 years: 5
  mg once daily
    cetirizine Cap: 10 mg
    Children's Zyrtec Chewable *Chew tab:* 5, 10 mg (grape)
    Children's Zyrtec Allergy Syrup *Syr:* 1 mg/ml (4 oz) (grape, bubble gum) (sugar-free, dye-free)
    Zyrtec *Tab:* 10 mg
    Zyrtec Hives Relief *Tab:* 10 mg
    Zyrtec Liquid Gels *Liq gel:* 10 mg
▶ *desloratadine*
    Clarinex <6 years: not recommended; ≥6 years: 1/2-1 tab once daily
      Tab: 5 mg
    Clarinex RediTabs <6 years: not recommended; 6-12 years: 2.5 mg once daily; ≥12 years: 5 mg once daily
      ODT: 2.5, 5 mg (tutti-frutti) (phenylalanine)
    Clarinex Syrup <6 months: not recommended; 6-11 months: 1 mg (2 ml) once daily; 1-5 years: 1.25 mg
      (2.5 ml) once daily; 6-11 years: 2.5 mg (5 ml) once daily; ≥12 years: 5 mg (10 ml) once daily
      Tab: 0.5 mg per ml (4 oz) (tutti-frutti) (phenylalanine)
    Desloratadine ODT
▶ *fexofenadine* (OTC)(G) 6 months to 2 years: 15 mg bid; *CrCl ≤90 ml/min:* 15 mg once daily; 2-11 years: 30
  mg bid; *CrCl ≤90 ml/min:* 30 mg once daily; ≥12 years and older: ≥12 years: 60 mg once daily-bid or 180 mg
  once daily; *CrCl <90 ml/min:* 60 mg once daily
    Allegra *Tab:* 30, 60, 180 mg film-coat
    Allegra Allergy *Tab:* 60, 180 mg film-coat
    Allegra ODT *ODT:* 30 mg (phenylalanine)
    Allegra Oral Suspension *Oral susp:* 30 mg/5 ml (6 mg/ml) (4 oz)
▶ *levocetirizine* (OTC)(G) administer dose in the PM; *Seasonal allergic rhinitis:* <2 years: not recommended;
  may start at ≥2 years; *Chronic idiopathic urticaria (CIU), perennial allergic rhinitis:* <6 months: not
  recommended; may start at ≥ 6 months; *Dosing by age:* 6 months to 5 years: max 1.25 mg once daily; 6-11
  years: max 2.5 mg once daily; ≥12 years: 2.5-5 mg once daily; *Renal dysfunction <12 years:* contraindicated;
  Renal dysfunction ≥12 years: CrCl 50-80 ml/min: 2.5 mg once daily; CrCl 30-50 ml/min: 2.5 mg every other
  day; *CrCl 10-30 ml/min:* 2.5 mg twice weekly (every 3-4 days); *CrCl <10 ml/min, end-stage renal disease
  (ESRD), or hemodialysis:* contraindicated
    Children's Xyzal Allergy 24HR *Oral soln:* 0.5 mg/ml (150 ml)
    Xyzal Allergy 24HR *Tab:* 5*mg
▶ *loratadine* (OTC)(G) 5 mg bid or 10 mg once daily; *Hepatic or renal insufficiency:* see mfr pkg insert
  Pediatric: <2 years: not recommended; 2-5 years: 5 mg once daily; ≥6 years: same as adult
    Children's Claritin Chewables *Chew tab:* 5 mg (grape) (phenylalanine)
    Children's Claritin Syrup 1 mg/ml (4 oz) (fruit) (sugar-free, alcohol-free, dye-free, sodium 6 mg/5 ml)
    Claritin *Tab:* 10 mg
    Claritin Hives Relief *Tab:* 10 mg
    Claritin Liqui-Gels *Liq gel:* 10 mg
    Claritin RediTabs 12 Hours *ODT:* 5 mg (mint)
    Claritin RediTabs 24 Hours *ODT:* 10 mg (mint)

RHINITIS: VASOMOTOR

NASAL ANTICHOLINERGICS
Comment: Avoid use with narrow-angle glaucoma, prostate hyperplasia, and bladder neck obstruction
▷ *ipratropium bromide* (G)
> **Atrovent Nasal Spray 0.03%** stop nasal decongestant; 2 sprays in each nostril bid-tid with progressive weaning as tolerated
> *Pediatric:* <6 years: <u>not</u> recommended; ≥6 years: same as adult
> > *Nasal spray:* 21 mcg/actuation (30 ml, 345 sprays)
> **Atrovent Nasal Spray 0.06%** stop nasal decongestant; 2 sprays in each nostril tid-qid with progressive weaning as tolerated
> *Pediatric:* <5 years: <u>not</u> recommended; ≥5-11 years: 2 sprays in each nostril tid; >11 years: same as adult
> > *Nasal spray:* 42 mcg/actuation (15 ml, 165 sprays)

RIVER BLINDNESS (ONCHOCERCIASIS)

ANTHELMINTIC
▷ *moxidectin* (G) take 8 mg (4 x 2 mg tablets) as a single dose, with <u>or</u> without food
Pediatric: <12 years: <u>not</u> recommended; ≥12 years: same as adult
> *Tab:* 2 mg
Comment: *Moxidectin* is a macrocyclic lactone anthelmintic medicine indicated for the treatment of river blindness (onchocerciasis) due to *Onchocerca volvulus* in patients ≥12 years of age. *Moxidectin* does <u>not</u> kill adult *O. volvulus* parasites. Follow-up is advised. The safety and efficacy of repeat administration of *moxidectin* tablets in patients with *O. volvulus* have <u>not</u> been studied. Cutaneous, ophthalmologic, and/or systemic adverse reactions of varying severity (Mazzotti reaction) have occurred in patients with onchocerciasis following treatment. Episodes of symptomatic orthostatic hypotension, including inability to stand without support, may occur in patients following treatment. Serious <u>or</u> even fatal encephalopathy following treatment may occur in patients coinfected with *Loa loa* (assess patients for loiasis in *L. loa* endemic areas prior to treatment. Patients with hyperreactive onchodermatitis (sowda) may be more likely than others to experience severe edema and aggravation of onchodermatitis. Limited available data on the use of *moxidectin* in pregnant patients are insufficient to establish whether there is a *moxidectin*-associated risk of major birth defects and miscarriage. *Moxidectin* has been detected in human milk following a single 8 mg dose. There are no data on the effects of *moxidectin* on breastfed infants. Risk/benefit of the developmental and health benefits of breastfeeding should be considered along with the mother's clinical need for *moxidectin*. The most common adverse reactions (incidence > 10%) have been eosinophilia, pruritus, musculoskeletal pain, headache, lymphopenia, tachycardia, rash, abdominal pain, hypotension, pyrexia, leukocytosis, influenza-like illness, neutropenia, cough, lymph node pain, dizziness, diarrhea, hyponatremia, and peripheral swelling.

ROCKY MOUNTAIN SPOTTED FEVER (RMSF, *RICKETTSIA RICKETTSII*)

ANTI-INFECTIVES
▷ *doxycycline* (G) 200 mg on first day; then 100 mg bid x 7-10 days
Pediatric: <8 years: <u>not</u> recommended; ≥8 years, <100 lb: 2-2.5 mg/kg q 12 hours x 7-10 days; ≥8 years, ≥100 lb: same as adult
> **Acticlate** *Tab:* 75, 150**mg
> **Adoxa** *Tab:* 50, 75, 100, 150 mg ent-coat
> **Doryx** *Tab:* 50, 75, 100, 150, 200 mg del-rel
> **Doxteric** *Tab:* 50 mg del-rel
> **Monodox** *Cap:* 50, 75, 100 mg
> **Oracea** *Cap:* 40 mg del-rel
> **Vibramycin** *Tab:* 100 mg; *Cap:* 50, 100 mg; *Syr:* 50 mg/5 ml (raspberry-apple) (sulfites); *Oral susp:* 25 mg/5 ml (raspberry)
> **Vibra-Tab** *Tab:* 100 mg film-coat
Comment: IV therapy might be indicated for more severely ill patients who require hospitalization, particularly in patients who are vomiting <u>or</u> obtunded. Recommended duration of therapy is at least 3 days after subsidence of fever and until evidence of clinical improvement is noted. Typically, the minimum total course of treatment is 5-7 days. Severe <u>or</u> complicated disease could require a longer treatment course. Diagnostic tests for rickettsial diseases, particularly for Rocky Mountain spotted fever (RMSF), are usually <u>not</u> helpful in making a timely diagnosis during the initial stages of illness, and treatment decisions for rickettsial pathogens should <u>never</u> be delayed while awaiting laboratory confirmation. Delay in treatment can lead to severe disease and long-term sequelae <u>or</u> death. The American Academy of Pediatrics and CDC recommend *doxycycline* as the treatment of choice for children of all ages with suspected tickborne rickettsial disease. Previous concerns about tooth staining in children aged <8 years stem from experience with older tetracycline-class drugs that bind more readily to calcium than newer members of the drug class, such as *doxycycline*. *Doxycycline* used at the dose and duration recommended for treatment of RMSF in

children aged <8 years, even after multiple courses, did not result in tooth staining or enamel hypoplasia in a 2013 retrospective cohort study of 58 children. These results support the findings of a study published in 2007 reporting no evidence of tooth staining among 31 children with asthma exacerbation who were treated with *doxycycline.*

➤ *tetracycline* (G) 500 mg q 6 hours x 7-10 days
   Pediatric: <8 years: not recommended; ≥8 years, <100 lb: 10 mg/kg/day q 6 hours x 7-10 days; ≥8 years, ≥100 lb: same as adult
      Achromycin V *Cap:* 250, 500 mg
      Sumycin *Tab:* 250, 500 mg; *Cap:* 250, 500 mg; *Oral susp:* 125 mg/5 ml (100, 200 ml) (fruit) (sulfites)

ROSEOLA INFANTUM (EXANTHEM SUBITUM)

Antipyretics *see Fever*

Comment: Roseola infantum (also known as exanthem subitum, sixth disease, pseudorubella, exanthem criticum, and three-day fever) is a generally mild clinical syndrome, commonly occurring in children <3 years of age, characterized by sudden onset of high fever (may exceed 40°C [104°F]) that lasts 3 days and resolves abruptly, and is followed by development of a rash lasting ≤3 days. Roseola usually is caused by human herpesvirus 6 (HHV-6). Treatment is antipyretics (aspirin is contraindicated) and adequate hydration. Monitor for febrile seizures. As with the common cold, roseola spreads from person to person through contact with an infected person's respiratory secretions or saliva. The disease can occur at any time of year.

ROTAVIRUS GASTROENTERITIS

PROPHYLAXIS
Comment: Rotavirus is a leading cause of severe acute gastroenteritis in infants and young children, with over 95% of these children infected by the time they are 5 years old. The most severe cases occur among infants and young children between 6 and 24 months of age.

➤ *rotavirus vaccine, live*
   Pediatric:
      Rotarix *6 weeks and up to 24 weeks of age*
      Oral susp: 1.5 ml in a single-use squeezable tube for ready-to-use oral administration; 1 vial (containing lyophilized vaccine component) and 1 oral dosing applicator (containing diluent), single-use for reconstitution and oral administration
      Comment: Rotarix is indicated for the prevention of rotavirus gastroenteritis caused by G1 and non-G1 types (G3, G4, and G9) when administered as a 2-dose series. **Rotarix** vaccination is a 2-dose series. The first dose should be administered to infants beginning at 6 weeks of age. There should be an interval of at least 4 weeks between the first and second dose. The 2-dose series should be completed by 24 weeks of age.
      RotaTeq: *6 weeks and up to 32 weeks of age*
      Oral soln: 2 ml in a single-use squeezable tube for oral administration
      Comment: RotaTeq is indicated for the prevention of rotavirus gastroenteritis in infants and young children caused by types G1, G2, G3, G4, and G9 when administered as a 3-dose series to infants age 6-32 weeks of age. The first dose of **RotaTeq** should be administered between 6 and 12 weeks of age with the subsequent doses administered at 4 to 10-week intervals. The 3-dose series should be completed by 32 weeks of age.

ROUNDWORM (*ASCARIASIS*)

ANTHELMINTICS
Comment: Oral bioavailability of anthelmintics is enhanced when administered with a fatty meal (estimated fat content 40 gm).

➤ *albendazole* take with a meal; swallow, chew, crush, or mix with food; 400 mg once daily x 7 days
   Pediatric: <2 years: 200 mg once daily x 3 days; may repeat in 3 weeks if needed; 2-12 years: 400 mg once daily x 3 days; may repeat in 3 weeks if needed; >12 years: same as adult
      Albenza *Tab:* 200 mg
➤ *mebendazole* take with a meal; swallow, chew, crush, or mix with food; 100 mg bid x 3 days; may repeat in 3 weeks if needed
   Pediatric: <2 years: not recommended; ≥2 years: same as adult
      Emverm *Chew tab:* 100 mg
      Vermox (G) *Chew tab:* 100 mg
➤ *pyrantel pamoate* take with a meal; may open capsule and sprinkle or mix with food; treat x 3 days; may repeat in 2-3 weeks if needed; 11 mg/kg once daily x 3 days; max 1 gm/dose
   Pediatric: 25-37 lb: 1/2 tsp x 1 dose; 38-62 lb: 1 tsp x 1 dose; 63-87 lb: 1 tsp x 1 dose; 88-112 lb: 2 tsp x 1 dose; 113-137 lb: 2 tsp x 1 dose; 138-162 lb: 3 tsp x 1 dose; 163-187 lb: 3 tsp x 1 dose; >187 lb: 4 tsp x 1 dose
      Antiminth (OTC) *Cap:* 180 mg; *Liq:* 50 mg/ml (30 ml); 144 mg/ml (30 ml); *Oral susp:* 50 mg/ml (60 ml)
      Pin-X (OTC) *Cap:* 180 mg; *Liq:* 50 mg/ml (30 ml); 144 mg/ml (30 ml); *Oral susp:* 50 mg/ml (30 ml)

(continued)

▷ *thiabendazole* 25 mg/kg bid x 7 days; max 1.5 gm/dose; max 3000 mg/day; take with a meal
   Pediatric: same as adult
      Mintezol *Chew tab:* 500*mg (orange); *Oral susp:* 500 mg/5 ml (120 ml) (orange)
   Comment: *Thiabendazole* is <u>not</u> for prophylaxis. May impair mental alertness.
   May <u>not</u> be available in the United States.

RUBELLA (GERMAN MEASLES)

Antipyretics *see* Fever
see Childhood Immunizations

Comment: Rubella is highly contagious and highly teratogenic. Quarantine is mandatory to prevent a community outbreak. Herd immunity is the best prevention.

PROPHYLAXIS VACCINE
Comment: <12 months: <u>not</u> recommended; ≥12 months: 25 mcg SC; if vaccinated <12 months, revaccinate at 12 months; administer in the upper posterior arm.

▷ *rubella virus, live, attenuated+neomycin* vaccine
   Pediatric: <12 months: <u>not</u> recommended (if vaccinated <12 months, revaccinate at 12 months); ≥12 months: 25 mcg SC
      Meruvax II 25 mcg SC
▷ *measles, mumps, rubella, live, attenuated, neomycin vaccine*
      MMR II 25 mcg SC (preservative-free)
   Comment: Contraindications: hypersensitivity to *neomycin* <u>or</u> eggs, primary <u>or</u> acquired immune deficiency, immunosuppressant therapy, bone marrow <u>or</u> lymphatic malignancy, and pregnancy (within 3 months following vaccination).
   See Childhood Immunizations

PRE- AND POST-EXPOSURE PROPHYLAXIS
Immune Globulin

▷ *immune globulin (human)* administer via IM injection <u>only</u> (<u>never</u> IV); ensure adequate hydration prior to administration; *Household and institutional rubella case contacts:* promptly administer 0.55 ml/kg IM as a single dose; *Planned travel to rubella endemic area:* administer 0.55 ml/kg as a single dose at least 6 days prior to travel
   Pediatric: 0.25 ml/kg IM (0.5 mg/kg in immunocompromised children)
      GamaSTAN S/D *Vial:* 2, 10 ml single-dose
   Comment: GamaSTAN S/D is the <u>only</u> *gamma globulin* product FDA-approved for measles and hepatitis A virus (HAV) post-exposure prophylaxis (PEP). **GamaSTAN S/D** is also FDA-approved for varicella post-exposure prophylaxis (PEP). *Other GamaSTAN S/D Indications:* To prevent <u>or</u> modify measles in a susceptible person exposed fewer than 6 days previously; to modify varicella; to modify rubella in exposed women who will <u>not</u> consider a therapeutic abortion. **GamaSTAN S/D** is <u>not</u> indicated for routine prophylaxis <u>or</u> treatment of viral hepatitis B, rubella, poliomyelitis, mumps, <u>or</u> varicella. Contraindications to **GamaSTAN S/D** include persons with cancer, chronic liver disease, and persons allergic to *gamma globulin*, the HAV vaccine, <u>or</u> a component of the HAV vaccine. Dosage is higher for HAV PEP than for measles and varicella PEP based on recently observed decreasing concentrations of HAV antibodies in **GamaSTAN S/D**, attributed to the decreasing prevalence of previous HAV infection among plasma donors.

RUBEOLA (RED MEASLES)

Antipyretics *see* Fever
see Childhood Immunizations

PROPHYLAXIS VACCINE
▷ *measles, mumps, rubella, live, attenuated, neomycin vaccine*
      MMR II 25 mcg SC (preservative-free)
   Comment: Contraindications: hypersensitivity to *neomycin* <u>or</u> eggs, primary <u>or</u> acquired immune deficiency, immunosuppressant therapy, bone marrow <u>or</u> lymphatic malignancy, and pregnancy (within 3 months following vaccination).

PRE- AND POST-EXPOSURE PROPHYLAXIS
Immune Globulin (Human)

▷ *immune globulin (human)* administer via IM injection <u>only</u> (<u>never</u> IV); ensure adequate hydration prior to administration; *Household and institutional measles case contacts:* promptly administer 0.025 ml/kg IM as a single dose; *Planned travel to measles endemic area:* administer 0.025 ml/kg IM as a single dose at least 6 days prior to travel

Pediatric: 0.25 ml/kg IM (0.5 mg/kg in immunocompromised children)
> GamaSTAN S/D *Vial:* 2, 10 ml single-dose
> **Comment:** GamaSTAN S/D is the <u>only</u> *gamma globulin* product FDA-approved for measles and hepatitis A virus (HAV) post-exposure prophylaxis (PEP). **GamaSTAN S/D** is also FDA-approved for varicella PEP. Other **GamaSTAN S/D** Indications: To prevent <u>or</u> modify measles in a susceptible person exposed fewer than 6 days previously; to modify varicella; to modify rubella in exposed women who will <u>not</u> consider a therapeutic abortion. **GamaSTAN S/D** is <u>not</u> indicated for routine prophylaxis <u>or</u> treatment of viral hepatitis B, rubella, poliomyelitis, mumps, <u>or</u> varicella. Contraindications to **GamaSTAN S/D** include persons with cancer, chronic liver disease, and persons allergic to *gamma globulin*, the HAV vaccine, <u>or</u> a component of the HAV vaccine. Dosage is higher for HAV PEP than for measles and varicella PEP based on recently observed decreasing concentrations of HAV antibodies in **GamaSTAN S/D**, attributed to the decreasing prevalence of previous HAV infection among plasma donors.

SALMONELLOSIS

ANTI-INFECTIVES

▷ *ciprofloxacin* 500 mg bid x 3-5 days
  Pediatric: <18 years: <u>not</u> recommended; ≥18 years: same as adult
    Cipro (G) *Tab:* 250, 500, 750 mg; *Oral susp:* 250, 500 mg/5 ml (100 ml) (strawberry)
    Cipro XR *Tab:* 500, 1,000 mg ext-rel
    ProQuin XR *Tab:* 500 mg ext-rel
▷ *trimethoprim+sulfamethoxazole (TMP-SMX)* **(G)**
  Pediatric: <2 months: <u>not</u> recommended; ≥2 months: 40 mg/kg/day of *sulfamethoxazole* in 2 divided doses bid x 10 days; *see* Appendix BB.33. *trimethoprim+sulfamethoxazole* (Bactrim Suspension, Septra Suspension) *for dose by weight*
    Bactrim, Septra 2 tabs bid x 10 days
      Tab: trim 80 mg+sulfa 400 mg*
    Bactrim DS, Septra DS 1 tab bid x 10 days
      Tab: trim 160 mg+sulfa 800 mg*
    Bactrim Pediatric Suspension, Septra Pediatric Suspension
      Oral susp: trim 40 mg+sulfa 200 mg per 5 ml (100 ml) (cherry) (alcohol 0.3%)

SCABIES (*SARCOPTES SCABIEI*)

Comment: This section presents treatment regimens for scabies infestation published in the **2021 CDC Sexually Transmitted Diseases Treatment Guidelines**, as well as other available treatments.
▷ *spinosad* shake bottle well; apply product to skin by rubbing it in to completely cover the body from the neck down to the soles of the feet; patients with balding scalp should also apply product to the scalp, hairline, temples, and forehead; allow to absorb in the skin and dry for 10 minutes before getting dressed; leave on the skin for at least 6 hours before showering <u>or</u> bathing
  Pediatric: <4 years: safety and efficacy <u>not</u> established; ≥4 years: same as adult
    Natroba *Topical susp:* 0.9% (9 mg/gm; 120ml)
    Comment: **Natroba** is a pediculocide/scabicide indicated for the topical treatment of scabies infestation in patients ≥4 years. The most common adverse reactions (incidence >1%) have been application site irritation (pain and burning) and dry skin. *Spinosad*, the active ingredient in **Natroba**, is <u>not</u> absorbed systemically following topical application, and maternal use is <u>not</u> expected to result in embryo/fetal exposure to the drug. **Natroba** contains benzyl alcohol. Topical benzyl alcohol is unlikely to be absorbed through the skin in clinically relevant amounts; therefore, maternal use is <u>not</u> expected to result in embryo/fetal exposure to the drug. Breastfeeding is <u>not</u> expected to result in the exposure of the infant to *spinosad*. Advise breastfeeding females to remove **Natroba** from the breast with soap and water before breastfeeding to avoid direct infant exposure to **Natroba**.

RECOMMENDED REGIMEN

▷ *permethrin* **(G)** massage into skin from head to soles of feet; leave on x 8-14 hours, then rinse off
  Pediatric: <2 months: <u>not</u> recommended; ≥2 months: same as adult
    Acticin, Elimite *Crm:* 5% (60 gm)

ALTERNATIVE REGIMEN

▷ *lindane* **(G)** 1 oz of lotion <u>or</u> 30 gm of cream apply to all skin surfaces from neck down to the soles of the feet; leave on x 8 hours, then wash off thoroughly; may repeat if needed in 14 days
  Pediatric: <2 months: <u>not</u> recommended; ≥2 months: same as adult
    Kwell *Lotn:* 1% (60, 473 ml); *Crm:* 1% (60 gm); *Shampoo:* 1% (60, 473 ml)

OTHER TOPICAL TREATMENTS

▷ *crotamiton* massage into skin from chin down; repeat in 24 hours
  Pediatric: <12 years: <u>not</u> recommended; ≥12 years: same as adult
    Eurax *Lotn:* 10% (60 gm); *Crm:* 10% (60 gm)

SCARLET FEVER (SCARLATINA)

Comment: Microorganism responsible for scarlet fever is group A beta-hemolytic *Streptococcus* (GABHS). Strep cultures and screens will be positive.

▷ *azithromycin* (G) 500 mg x 1 dose on day 1, then 250 mg once daily on days 2-5 or 500 mg once daily x 3 days
  Pediatric: 12 mg/kg/day x 5 days; max 500 mg/day; *see* Appendix BB.7. *azithromycin* (G) (Zithromax Suspension, Zmax Suspension) *for dose by weight*
    Zithromax *Tab:* 250, 500, 600 mg; *Oral susp:* 100 mg/5 ml (15 ml); 200 mg/5 ml (15, 22.5, 30 ml) (cherry); *Pkt:* 1 gm for reconstitution (cherry-banana)
    Zithromax Tri-Pak *Tab:* 3 x 500 mg tabs/pck
    Zithromax Z-Pak *Tab:* 6 x 250 mg tabs/pck
    Zmax *Oral susp:* 2 gm ext-rel for reconstitution (cherry-banana) (148 mg Na⁺)

▷ *cefadroxil*
  Pediatric: 15-30 mg/kg/day in 2 divided doses x 10 days; *see* Appendix BB.9. *cefadroxil* (G) (Duricef Suspension) *for dose by weight*
    Duricef *Cap:* 500 mg; *Tab:* 1 gm; *Oral susp:* 250 mg/5 ml (100 ml); 500 mg/5 ml (75, 100 ml) (orange-pineapple)

▷ *cephalexin* (G)
  Pediatric: 25-50 mg/kg/day in 2 divided doses x 10 days; *see* Appendix BB.15. *cephalexin* (G) (Keflex Suspension) *for dose by weight*
    Keflex *Cap:* 250, 333, 500, 750 mg; *Oral susp:* 125, 250 mg/5 ml (100, 200 ml) (strawberry)

▷ *clarithromycin* (G) 250 mg bid or 500 mg ext-rel once daily x 10 days
  Pediatric: <6 months: not recommended; ≥6 months: 7.5 mg/kg bid x 10 days; *see* Appendix BB.16. Clarithromycin (G) (Biaxin Suspension) *for dose by weight*
    Biaxin *Tab:* 250, 500 mg
    Biaxin Oral Suspension *Oral susp:* 125, 250 mg/5 ml (50, 100 ml) (fruit punch)
    Biaxin XL *Tab:* 500 mg ext-rel

▷ *clindamycin* (G) 150-300 mg q 6 hours x 10 days
  Pediatric: 8-16 mg/kg/day in 3-4 divided doses x 10 days
    Cleocin *Cap:* 75 (tartrazine), 150 (tartrazine), 300 mg
    Cleocin Pediatric Granules *Oral susp:* 75 mg/5 ml (100 ml) (cherry)

▷ *erythromycin estolate* (G) 250 mg q 6 hours x 10 days
  Pediatric: 20-50 mg/kg q 6 hours x 10 days; *see* Appendix BB.20. *erythromycin* estolate (G) (Ilosone Suspension) *for dose by weight*
    Ilosone *Pulvule:* 250 mg; *Tab:* 500 mg; *Liq:* 125, 250 mg/5 ml (100 ml)

▷ *erythromycin ethylsuccinate* (G) 400 mg qid or 800 mg bid x 10 days
  Pediatric: 30-50 mg/kg/day in 4 divided doses x 10 days; may double dose with severe infection; max 100 mg/kg/day; *see* Appendix BB.21. *erythromycin ethylsuccinate* (G) (E.E.S. Suspension, EryPed Drops/Suspension) *for dose by weight*
    EryPed *Oral susp:* 200 mg/5 ml (100, 200 ml) (fruit); 400 mg/5 ml (60, 100, 200 ml) (banana); *Oral drops:* 200, 400 mg/5 ml (50 ml) (fruit); *Chew tab:* 200 mg wafer (fruit)
    E.E.S. *Oral susp:* 200, 400 mg/5 ml (100 ml) (fruit)
    E.E.S. Granules *Oral susp:* 200 mg/5 ml (100, 200 ml) (cherry)
    E.E.S. 400 Tablets *Tab:* 400 mg

▷ *penicillin g (benzathine and procaine)* (G) 2.4 million units IM x 1 dose
  Pediatric: <30 lb: 600,000 units IM x 1 dose; 30-60 lb: 900,000-1.2 million units IM x 1 dose
    Bicillin C-R *Cartridge-needle unit:* 600,000 units (1 ml); 1.2 million units; (2 ml); 2.4 million units (4 ml)

▷ *penicillin v potassium* 250 mg tid x 10 days
  Pediatric: 25-50 mg/kg day in 4 divided doses x 10 days; ≥12 years: same as adult; *see* Appendix BB.29. *penicillin v potassium* (G) (Pen-Vee K Solution, Veetids Solution) *for dose by weight*
    Pen-Vee K *Tab:* 250, 500 mg; *Oral soln:* 125 mg/5 ml (100, 200 ml); 250 mg/5 ml (100, 150, 200 ml)

SCHISTOSOMIASIS

TREMATODICIDE

Comment: *Praziquantel* is a trematodicide indicated for the treatment of infections due to all species of genus *Schistosoma* (e.g., *Schistosoma mekongi, S. japonicum, S. mansoni,* and *S. haematobium*) and infections due to liver flukes (i.e., *Clonorchis sinensis, Opisthorchis viverrini*). *Praziquantel* induces a rapid contraction of schistosomes by a specific effect on the permeability of the cell membrane. The drug further causes vacuolization and disintegration of the schistosome tegument.

▷ *praziquantel* 20 mg/kg tid as a 1-day treatment; take the 3 doses at intervals of not less than 4 hours and not more than 6 hours; swallow whole with water during meals; holding the tablets in the mouth leaves a bitter taste which can trigger gagging or vomiting
  Pediatric: <4 years: not established; ≥4 years: same as adult
    Biltricide *Tab:* 600 mg film-coat

Comment: Concomitant administration with strong cytochrome P450 (CYP450) inducers, such as *rifampin*, is contraindicated since therapeutically effective blood levels of *praziquantel* may not be achieved. In patients receiving *rifampin* who need immediate treatment for schistosomiasis, alternative agents for schistosomiasis should be considered. However, if treatment with *praziquantel* is necessary, *rifampin* should be discontinued 4 weeks before administration of *praziquantel*. Treatment with *rifampin* can then be restarted 1 day after completion of *praziquantel* treatment. Concomitant administration of other P450 inducers (e.g., antiepileptic drugs such as *phenytoin, phenobarbital, carbamazepine*) and *dexamethasone* may also reduce plasma levels of *praziquantel*. Concomitant administration of P450 inhibitors (e.g., *cimetidine, ketoconazole, itraconazole, erythromycin*) may increase plasma levels of *praziquantel*. Patients should be warned not to drive a car or operate machinery on the day of **Biltricide** treatment and the following day. There are no adequate or well-controlled studies in pregnant females. This drug should be used during pregnancy only if clearly needed. *Praziquantel* appears in the milk of nursing women at a concentration of about 1/4 that of maternal serum. It is not known whether a pharmacologic effect is likely to occur in children. Women should not nurse on the day of **Biltricide** treatment and during the subsequent 72 hours.

SCHIZOPHRENIA, SCHIZOPHRENIA WITH COMORBID PERSONALITY DISORDER

Other Antipsychosis Drugs *see* Antipsychosis Drugs
See Tardive Dyskinesia

Comment: A team of researchers examined the effects of antipsychotics on mortality risk in schizophrenia patients. They studied data on 29,823 patients with schizophrenia in Sweden aged 16-64 years and found mortality among patients with schizophrenia was 40% lower when they used antipsychotics as compared to when they did not. Long-acting injection (LAI) use was associated with an approximately 33% lower risk of death compared with the oral use of the same medication. The lowest mortality was observed with use of once-monthly *paliperidone* LAI, oral *aripiprazole*, and *risperidone* LAI.

ATYPICAL ANTIPSYCHOTICS
▷ *aripiprazole*
    Oral Forms
    Adult: initially 15 mg once daily; may increase to max 30 mg/day
    Pediatric: <10 years: safety and efficacy not established; ≥10-17 years: initially 2 mg/day in a single dose for 2 days; then increase to 5 mg/day in a single dose for 2 days; then increase to the target dose of 10 mg/day in a single dose; may increase by 5 mg/day at weekly intervals as needed to max 30 mg/day
    Abilify (G) *Tab:* 2, 5, 10, 15, 20, 30 mg
    Abilify Discmelt (G) *Tab:* 15 mg orally-disint (vanilla) (phenylalanine)
    Parenteral Forms
    Comment: Parenteral forms require administration by a qualified healthcare provider. Parenteral forms must be administered IM in the gluteal muscle. Parenteral forms are approved for patients ≥18-59 years only. Patients <18 years and ≥60 years: safety and efficacy not established. Dose adjustment is required for missed doses. See mfr pkg insert for full preparation and administration procedures. See mfr pkg insert for dosing adjustments for patients who are CYP2D6 poor metabolizers and for patients taking CYP2D6 inhibitors, CYP3A4 inhibitors, or CYP3A4 inducers for greater than 14 days. To report suspected adverse reactions, contact Otsuka America Pharmaceutical at 800-438-9927 or FDA at 800-FDA-1088 or www.fda.gov/medwatch.
    Abilify Asimtufii administration is once every 2 months
    Prefilled syringe: 720 mg (2.4 ml), 960 mg (3.2 ml), single-dose, ext-rel susp
    Comment: For patients naïve to *aripiprazole*, establish tolerability with oral *aripiprazole* prior to initiating treatment with **Abilify Asimtufii**. Recommended starting and maintenance dose is 960 mg administered once every 2 months as a single injection. Some patients may benefit from a reduction to a 720 mg dose.
    Abilify Maintena administration is once monthly
    Vial: 300, 400 mg, single-dose, ext-rel pwdr for IM injection after reconstitution (to a suspension)
    Comment: For patients naïve to *aripiprazole*, establish tolerability with oral *aripiprazole* prior to initiating treatment with **Abilify Maintena**. Recommended starting and maintenance dose is 400 mg administered once monthly as a single injection. In conjunction with the first dose, take 14 consecutive days of concurrent once-daily oral *aripiprazole* (10-20 mg) or current oral antipsychotic. Some patients may benefit from a reduction to a 300 mg dose.
▷ *aripiprazole lauroxil*
    ALERT: Aripiprazole lauroxil is available in two parenteral delivery forms, **Aristada** and **Aristada Initio**, with differing doses and frequency of administration. Therefore, **Aristada Initio** is not interchangeable with **Aristada**. **Aristada Initio** is a smaller particle-size version of extended-release injectable *aripiprazole*. It is the first and only long-acting atypical antipsychotic that can be initiated on day 1. Combining **Aristada Initio** with a single 30 mg dose of oral *aripiprazole* provides an alternative regimen to initiate patients onto any dose of **Aristada** on day 1. Previously, the initiation process for the older *aripiprazole* product was to give the first dose and to then give oral *aripiprazole* for 21 consecutive days. **Aristada Initio** releases

(continued)

relevant levels of *aripiprazole* within 4 days of initiation. **Aristada Initio** carries a warning that it is not approved for use by older patients with dementia-related psychosis as this patient population is at risk for increased mortality when treated with antipsychotics. For patients naïve to *aripiprazole*, establish tolerability with oral *aripiprazole* prior to initiating treatment with **Aristada Initio**.

Pediatric: <18 years: not recommended; ≥18 years: same as adult

    Aristada administer by IM injection in the deltoid (441 mg dose only) or gluteal (441, 662, 882, or 1,064 mg) muscle by a qualified healthcare professional; initiate at a dose of 441, 662, or 882 mg administered monthly, or 882 mg every 6 weeks, or 1064 mg, every 2 months

      Prefilled syringe: 441, 662, 882, 1,064 mg, single-use, ext-rel susp, single-use

    Aristada Initio administer a single 675 mg **Aristada Initio** injection (plus a single 30 mg dose of oral *aripiprazole* in conjunction with the first **Aristada Initio** injection); administer the IM injection into the deltoid or gluteal muscle; must be administered only by a qualified healthcare professional; **Aristada Initio** is only to be used as a single dose and is not for repeated dosing

      Prefilled pen: 675 mg/2.4 ml, single-dose, ext-rel susp

Comment: Aristada and Aristada Initio are atypical antipsychotics. **Aristada** is available in 4 doses with 3 dosing duration options for flexible dosing. **Aristada initio** is a single-dose *longer-acting* form of *aripiprazole lauroxil*. For patients naïve to *aripiprazole*, establish tolerability with oral *aripiprazole* prior to initiating treatment with **Aristada**. **Aristada** can be initiated at any of the 4 doses at the appropriate dosing duration option. In conjunction with the first injection, administer treatment with oral *aripiprazole* for 21 consecutive days for all 4 dose sizes. The most common adverse event associated with **Aristada/Aristada Initio** is akathisia. Patients are also at increased risk for developing neuroleptic malignant syndrome (NMS), tardive dyskinesia (TD), pathologic gambling or other compulsive behaviors, orthostatic hypotension, hyperglycemic, dyslipidemia, and weight gain. Hypersensitive reactions can occur and range from pruritus or urticaria to anaphylaxis. Stroke, transient ischemic attacks (TIAs), and falls have been reported in elderly patients with dementia-related psychosis who were treated with *aripiprazole*. **Aristada/Aristada Initio** are not for treatment of people who have lost touch with reality (psychosis) *due to* confusion and memory loss dementia. Avoid use in known CYP2D6 poor metabolizers. Avoid use with strong CYP2D6 or CYP 3A4 inhibitors and strong CYP3A4 inducers. *Aripiprazole* may cause extrapyramidal and/or withdrawal symptoms in neonates exposed *in utero* in the third trimester of pregnancy. *Aripiprazole* is present in human breast milk; however, there are insufficient data to assess the amount in human milk or the effects on the breastfed infant. The development and health benefits of breastfeeding should be considered along with the mother's clinical need for *aripiprazole* and any potential adverse effects on the breastfed infant from **Aristada/Aristada Initio** or from the underlying maternal condition. For more information or to report suspected adverse side effects (ASEs), contact the National Pregnancy Registry for Atypical Antipsychotics at 1-866-961-2388 or http://womensmentalhealth. org/clinical-and-research programs/pregnancy registry. Limited published data on *aripiprazole* use in pregnant females are not sufficient to inform any drug-associated risks of birth defects or miscarriage.

▷ **asenapine** apply 1 transdermal system q 24 hours to the upper back, upper arm, abdomen, or hip; rotate sites; recommended starting dose is 3.8 mg/24 hours; may increase to 5.7 mg/24 hours or 7.6 mg/24 hours after 1 week

Pediatric: safety and efficacy not established

    Secuado *Transdermal system:* 3.8 mg/24 hours, 5.7 mg/24 hours, 7.6 mg/24 hours

Comment: Secuado *(asenapine)* is an atypical antipsychotic indicated for the treatment schizophrenia in a transdermal drug delivery system (TDDS) that provides sustained concentrations during wear time (24 hours). Commonly observed adverse reactions to **Secuado** (incidence ≥5%) have included extrapyramidal disorder, application site reaction, and weight gain. **Secuado** is contraindicated in patients with severe hepatic impairment (Child-Pugh C). **Secuado** is not approved for treatment of patients with dementia-related psychosis. Elderly patients with dementia-related psychosis treated with antipsychotic drugs are at an increased risk of death and increased incidence of cerebrovascular adverse reactions (e.g., stroke, TIA). Manage neuroleptic malignant syndrome (NMS) with immediate discontinuation and close monitoring. Manage tardive dyskinesia (TD) with discontinuation. Monitor for hyperglycemia/diabetes mellitus, dyslipidemia, and weight gain. Monitor for orthostatic hypotension. Monitor HR and BP and warn patients with known cardiovascular or cerebrovascular disease of risk of dehydration or syncope. Monitor for leukopenia, neutropenia, and agranulocytosis; monitor complete blood count (CBC) in patients with preexisting low white blood cells (WBC) or history of leukopenia or neutropenia and consider discontinuation if a clinically significant decline in WBC occurs in the absence of other causative factors. Monitor for increases in QT interval; avoid use with drugs that also increase the QT interval and in patients with risk factors for prolonged QT interval. Use cautiously in patients with a history of seizures or with conditions that lower the seizure threshold. Use caution when operating machinery; there is potential for cognitive and motor impairment. Avoid exposing **Secuado** to external heat sources during wear because both the rate and extent of absorption are increased. During wear time or immediately after removal of **Secuado**, local skin reactions may occur; advise patient to be sure to remove the expiring transdermal patch when applying the new patch. **Secuado** may enhance the antihypertensive effects of the patient's antihypertensive medications; monitor BP and adjust antihypertensive drug dosage accordingly. Based on clinical response, consider **Secuado** dose reduction when co-administered with strong CYP1A2 inhibitors. *Paroxetine* is a CYP2D6 substrate and inhibitor; therefore, reduce *paroxetine* dose by half. **Secuado** may cause extrapyramidal and/or withdrawal symptoms in neonates with 3rd-trimester exposure. In animal studies, *asenapine* increased postimplantation loss and decreased pup weight and survival at doses similar to or less than recommended clinical doses. In these studies, there was no increase in the incidence of structural abnormalities caused by *asenapine*. Lactation studies have not been conducted to assess the presence of *asenapine* in human milk or effects on the breastfed infant. *Asenapine* is excreted in rat milk. The development and health benefits of breastfeeding should be considered along with the mother's clinical need for **Secuado** and any potential adverse effects on the breastfed infant from **Secuado** or from the underlying maternal condition. There is a pregnancy exposure registry that monitors pregnancy outcomes in women exposed to atypical antipsychotics, including **Secuado**, during pregnancy. For more information, contact the National Pregnancy Registry for Atypical Antipsychotics at 1-866-961-2388 or http://womensmentalhealth.org/clinical-andresearch-programs/pregnancyregistry/.

▷ *lumateperone* 42 mg once daily; no titration required; take with or without food
Pediatric: safety and efficacy not established
    Caplyta *Cap:* 42 mg
    Comment: **Caplyta** *(lumateperone)* is the first-in-class atypical antipsychotic for the treatment of schizophrenia in adults. **Caplyta** is also indicated for the treatment of adult patients with depressive episodes associated with bipolar disorder (i.e., bipolar depression), as monotherapy and as adjunctive therapy with a mood stabilizer (such as *lithium* or *valproate)*. **Caplyta** is not approved for the treatment of patients with dementia-related psychosis due to increased incidence of cerebrovascular adverse reactions (e.g., stroke, TIA) and death in these patients. Avoid **Caplyta** use with moderate-to-severe hepatic impairment. Avoid use with concomitant CYP3A4 inducers and moderate or strong CYP3A4 inhibitors. Discontinue **Caplyta** immediately and monitor the patient closely if signs of neuroleptic malignant syndrome (NMS) develop. Manage signs of tardive dyskinesia (TD) with discontinuation if clinically appropriate. Monitor for hyperglycemia/diabetes mellitus, dyslipidemia, and weight gain. Leukopenia, neutropenia, and agranulocytosis may develop; therefore, monitor CBC—especially in patients with preexisting low WBC or history of leukopenia or neutropenia. Consider discontinuing **Caplyta** if clinically significant decline in WBC occurs in the absence of other causative factors. Orthostatic hypotension and syncope may occur; therefore, monitor HR and BP and warn patients with known cardiovascular or cerebrovascular disease, and caution to avoid dehydration. Use caution in patients with a history of seizure or with conditions that lower seizure threshold. There is potential for cognitive and motor impairment; therefore, advise caution when operating hazardous equipment or machinery and monitor as appropriate. The most common adverse reactions reported in clinical trials (incidence >5% and >2 x placebo) have been somnolence/sedation and dry mouth. Based on findings from animal studies, *lumateperone* may impair male and female fertility. There is risk to the mother from untreated schizophrenia or untreated bipolar depression, including increased risk of relapse, hospitalization, and suicide, and schizophrenia is associated with increased adverse perinatal outcomes, including preterm birth. It is not known if this is a direct result of the illness or other comorbid factors. Extrapyramidal and/or withdrawal symptoms, including agitation, hypertonia, hypotonia, tremor, somnolence, respiratory distress, and feeding disorder, have been reported in neonates who were exposed to antipsychotic drugs during the third trimester of pregnancy. These symptoms have varied in severity. Developmental and health benefits of breastfeeding should be considered along with the mother's clinical need for **Caplyta** and any potential adverse effects on the breastfed infant from **Caplyta** or from the underlying maternal condition. Use of effective contraception during treatment with **Caplyta** is advisable. There is a pregnancy exposure registry that monitors pregnancy outcomes in women exposed to atypical antipsychotics, including **Caplyta**, during pregnancy. Healthcare providers are encouraged to register patients by contacting the National Pregnancy Registry for Atypical Antipsychotics at 1-866-961-2388 or online at http://womensmentalhealth.org/clinical-and-research-programs/pregnancyregistry/. There are published reports of sedation, failure to thrive, jitteriness, and extrapyramidal symptoms (tremors and abnormal muscle movements) in breastfed infants exposed to antipsychotics. Based on findings of toxicity in animal studies and the potential for serious adverse reactions in the breastfed infant, breastfeeding is not recommended during treatment with **Caplyta**.

▷ *brexpiprazole* administer once daily with or without food; *Starting dose:* 1 mg once daily on days 1-4; titrate to 2 mg once daily on Day 5 through day 7, then to 4 mg on day 8 based on the patient's clinical response and tolerability; For patients with moderate, severe, or end-stage renal impairment (CrCl <60 ml/min), the max recommended dose is 3 mg once daily; for patients with moderate-to-severe hepatic impairment (Child-Pugh score ≥7/Class B), the max recommended dose is 3 mg once daily
Pediatric: <13 years: safety and efficacy not been established; 13-17 years: 0.5 mg once daily on Days 1 to 4, with or without food; titrate to 1 mg once daily on Day 5 through day 7, then to 2 mg on Day 8 based on the patient's clinical response and tolerability; Weekly dose increases can be made in 1 mg increments; Recommended target dose: 2-4 mg once daily; max 4 mg once daily; ≥18 years: same as adult
    Rexulti *Tab:* 0.25, 0.5, 1, 2, 3, 4 mg
    Comment: **Rexulti** is an atypical antipsychotic indicated for the treatment of major depressive disorder (MDD), schizophrenia, and agitation associated with dementia due to Alzheimer's disease. The most common adverse reaction (incidence ≥4% and at least twice the rate for placebo) was weight gain. Closely monitor patients for signs and symptoms of neuroleptic malignant syndrome (NMS); if this occurs, immediately discontinue **Rexulti** and treat as appropriate. The **Rexulti** drug label (mfr pkg insert) contains a boxed warning that elderly patients with dementia-related psychosis treated with antipsychotic drugs

(continued)

are at an increased risk of death. Therefore, use of **Rexulti** in these patients is contraindicated. Closely monitor patients for signs and symptoms of tardive dyskinesia (TD). If this occurs, discontinue **Rexulti** if clinically appropriate. Monitor patients for metabolic changes such as hyperglycemia/diabetes mellitus, dyslipidemia, and weight gain. Leukopenia, neutropenia, and agranulocytosis may develop. Obtain complete blood counts (CBCs) in patients with preexisting low white blood cell (WBC) count or history of leukopenia or neutropenia. Consider discontinuing **Rexulti** if a clinically significant decline in WBC occurs in the absence of other causative factor. Advise patients and caregivers that orthostatic hypotension and/or syncope may occur; Monitor HR and BP, especially patients with known cardiovascular or cerebrovascular disease, and avoid dehydration. Use **Rexulti** cautiously in patients with a history of seizures or with conditions that lower the seizure threshold. Adequate and well-controlled studies have not been conducted with **Rexulti** in human pregnancy to inform drug-associated risks. In animal reproduction studies, no teratogenicity was observed with oral administration of *brexpiprazole* during organogenesis at doses up to 73 and 146 times, respectively, of maximum recommended human dose (MRHD) of 4 mg/day on a mg/m² basis. However, when administered *brexpiprazole* during the period of organogenesis through lactation, the number of perinatal deaths of pups was increased at 73 times the MRHD. Extrapyramidal and/or withdrawal symptoms, including agitation, hypertonia, hypotonia, tremor, somnolence, respiratory distress, and feeding disorder, have been reported in neonates whose mothers were exposed to antipsychotic drugs during the third trimester of pregnancy. These symptoms have varied in severity. Some neonates recovered within hours or days without specific treatment; others required prolonged hospitalization. Monitor neonates for extrapyramidal and/or withdrawal symptoms and manage symptoms appropriately. There is a pregnancy exposure registry that monitors pregnancy outcomes in women exposed to **Rexulti** during pregnancy. For more information, contact the National Pregnancy Registry for Atypical Antipsychotics at 1-866-961-2388 or http://womensmentalhealth.org/clinical-and-research-programs/pregnancyregistry/. Lactation studies have not been conducted to assess the presence of *brexpiprazole* in human milk or effects of *brexpiprazole* on the breastfed infant. However, *brexpiprazole* is present in animal milk. Developmental and health benefits of breastfeeding should be considered along with the mother's clinical need for **Rexulti** and any potential adverse effects on the breastfed infant from **Rexulti** or from the underlying maternal condition. To report suspected adverse reactions, contact Otsuka America Pharmaceutical at 800-438-9927 or FDA at 800-FDA-1088 or www.fda.gov/medwatch.

▷ *lurasidone* (G) initially 40 mg once daily; usual range 40 to max 160 mg/day; take with food; *CrCl <50 ml/ min, moderate hepatic impairment (Child-Pugh 7-9)*: max 80 mg/day; *Child-Pugh 10-15*: max 40 mg/day
Pediatric: <13 years: not established; 13-17 years: initially 40 mg once daily; may titrate up to max 80 mg/day
   Latuda *Tab*: 20, 40, 60, 80, 120 mg
   Comment: Latuda is contraindicated with concomitant strong CYP3A4 inhibitors (e.g., *ketoconazole, voriconazole, clarithromycin, ritonavir*) and inducers (e.g., *phenytoin, carbamazepine, rifampin*, St. John's wort); see mfr pkg insert if the patient is taking moderate CYP3A4 inhibitors (e.g., *diltiazem, atazanavir, erythromycin, fluconazole, verapamil*).

▷ *paliperidone palmitate* administration by a healthcare professional via gluteal IM injection once every 6 months; do not administer by any other route; do not mix with any other product or diluent; store at room temperature; the switch to **Invega Hafyera** is based on when the last once-a-month (**Invega Sustenna**) or every-3-month (**Invega Trinza**) product was administered; initiate **Invega Hafyera** when the next once-a-month (**Invega Sustenna**) or every-3-month (**Invega Trinza**) dose is scheduled; see mfr pkg insert for *paliperidone palmitate* full prescribing information; see **Invega Sustenna** and **Invega Trinza** dose forms and dosing information which alpha follow **Invega Hafyera** below and refer to **Invega Hafyera** for essential *paliperidone palmitate* information; to report suspected adverse reactions, contact Janssen Pharmaceuticals at 1-800-JANSSEN (1-800-526-7736) or FDA at 1-800-FDA-1088 or www.fda.gov/medwatch

Switching to Every-6-Month **Invega Hafyera** From Once-a-Month **Invega Sustenna**	
Last Dose of **Invega Sustenna**	Initial Dose of **Invega Hafyera**
156 mg	1,092 mg
234 mg	1,560 mg
Switching To Every-6-Month **Invega Hafyera** From Every-3-Month **Invega Trinza**	
Last Dose of **Invega Trinza**	Initial Dose of **Invega Hafyera**
546 mg	1,092 mg
819 mg	1,560 mg

Pediatric: <18 years: safety and efficacy not established; ≥18 years: same as adult
   Invega Hafyera (*6-month paliperidone palmitate*) *Prefilled syringe*: 1,092 mg/3.5 ml, 1,560 mg/5 ml, single-dose, suspension w. 20 gauge 1½ inch safety needle
   Comment: Invega Hafyera is a long-acting extended-release injectable atypical antipsychotic for the twice-yearly treatment of adults with schizophrenia. Before switching to **Invega Hafyera**, patients must have been adequately treated with **Invega Sustenna** (*1-month paliperidone palmitate*) for at least 4 months or have been

adequately treated with **Invega Trinza** *(3-month paliperidone palmitate)* for at least one 3-month injection cycle. *Boxed Warning:* Elderly patients with dementia-related psychosis treated with antipsychotic drugs are at an increased risk of cerebrovascular adverse reactions (e.g., stroke, TIA, and death). **Invega Hafyera** is not indicated for use in patients with dementia-related psychosis The safety profile of **Invega Hafyera** is consistent with previous studies relating to **Invega Sustenna** and **Invega Trinza**. Known hypersensitivity to *paliperidone, risperidone,* or to any excipients in **Invega Hafyera** is the only contraindication. The most common adverse reactions have been upper respiratory tract infection (URI), injection site reaction, weight gain, headache, and parkinsonism. Monitor patients for neuroleptic malignant syndrome (NMS) and manage with immediate discontinuation of **Invega Hafyera** and close monitoring. Avoid use with drugs that also increase QT interval and in patients with risk factors for prolonged QT interval. Monitor patients for tardive dyskinesia (TD) and discontinue treatment if clinically appropriate. Monitor for metabolic changes, including hyperglycemia/diabetes mellitus, dyslipidemia, and weight gain. Monitor for orthostatic hypotension and syncope; use with caution in patients with known cardiovascular or cerebrovascular disease and patients predisposed to hypotension. Monitor lab tests for leukopenia, neutropenia, and agranulocytosis, especially those with pre-existing low white blood cell (WBC) count or a history of leukopenia or neutropenia. Consider discontinuing **Invega Hafyera** if a clinically significant decline in WBC occurs in the absence of other causative factors. Hyperprolactinemia occurs and persists during chronic administration. Monitor for development of cognitive and/or motor impairment. Advise patients to use caution when operating machinery. Use **Invega Hafyera** cautiously in patients with a history of seizures or with conditions that lower the seizure threshold. Avoid using strong CYP3A4 and/or P-gp inducers during an **Invega Hafyera** dosing interval. If administering a strong inducer is necessary, consider managing the patient using *paliperidone* extended-release tablets. Use of **Invega Hafyera** is not recommended in pediatric patients because of the potential longer duration of an adverse event. In clinical trials of oral *paliperidone,* there were notably higher incidences of dystonia, hyperkinesia, tremor, and parkinsonism in the adolescent population as compared to the adults. Based on the pharmacologic action of *paliperidone* (D2 receptor antagonism), treatment with **Invega Hafyera** may result in an increase in serum prolactin levels, which may lead to a reversible reduction in fertility in females of reproductive potential. *Paliperidone* has been detected in plasma in adult subjects up to 18 months after a single-dose administration of 3-month *paliperidone palmitate* extended-release injectable suspension. Extrapyramidal and/or withdrawal symptoms (including agitation, hypertonia, hypotonia, tremor, somnolence, respiratory distress, and feeding disorder) have been reported in neonates who were exposed to antipsychotic drugs during the third trimester of pregnancy. These symptoms varied in severity. Monitor neonates for extrapyramidal and/or withdrawal symptoms and manage symptoms appropriately. Some neonates recovered within hours or days without specific treatment; others required prolonged hospitalization. Limited data from published literature report the presence of *risperidone* and its metabolite, 9-hydroxyrisperidone, in human breast milk. Infants exposed to **Invega Hafyera** through breast milk should be monitored for excess sedation, failure to thrive, jitteriness, and extrapyramidal symptoms (EPS) (tremors and abnormal muscle movements). Developmental and health benefits of breastfeeding should be considered along with the mother's clinical need for **Invega Hafyera** and any potential adverse effects on the breastfed infant from **Invega Hafyera** or from the mother's underlying condition.

Invega Sustenna (*1-month paliperidone palmitate*) is an extended-release injectable atypical antipsychotic for the once-monthly treatment of adults with schizophrenia. Each injection must be administered by a qualified healthcare professional. Initiate **Invega Sustenna** with a dose of 234 mg on treatment day 1 and 156 mg 1 week later, with both doses administered in the deltoid muscle. The recommended once monthly maintenance dose is 117 mg. Some patients may benefit from a lower or higher maintenance dose within the recommended range of 39-234 mg, based on individual patient tolerability and/or efficacy. Following the second dose, monthly maintenance doses can be administered in either the deltoid or gluteal muscle. Administer doses via IM injection only, using appropriate needle size. For deltoid injection, use a 1½ inch 22 gauge needle for patients ≥90 kg (≥200 lb) or 1 inch 23 gauge needle for patients <90 kg (<200 lb). For gluteal injection, use a 1½ inch 22 gauge needle regardless of patient weight. Refer to *paliperidone palmitate* and the **Invega Hafyera** comment above for warnings, precautions, interactions, and other prescribing information.

Pediatric: <18 years: safety and efficacy not established; ≥18 years: same as adult

Invega Sustenna (*1-month paliperidone palmitate*) *Prefilled syringe:* 39 mg/0.25 ml, 78 mg/0,5 ml, 117 mg/0.75 ml, 156 mg/ml, 234 mg/1.5 ml, single-dose, ext-rel suspension for IM injection

Invega Trinza (*3-month paliperidone palmitate*) is a long-acting injectable atypical antipsychotic for the once every 3 months treatment of adults with schizophrenia who have been adequately treated with **Invega Sustenna** (1-month *paliperidone palmitate* extended-release injectable suspension) for at least 4 months. Each injection must be administered only by a qualified healthcare professional. *For deltoid injection:* For patients weighing <90 kg, use the 1 inch 22 gauge thin-wall needle. For patients weighing ≥90 kg use the 1½ inch 22 gauge thin-wall needle. *For gluteal injection:* Regardless of patient weight, use the1½ inch 22 gauge thin-wall needle. Prior to administration, shake the prefilled syringe vigorously for at least 15 seconds within 5 minutes prior to administration to ensure a homogeneous suspension. Initiate **Invega Trinza** when the next 1-month *paliperidone palmitate* dose is scheduled with the **Invega Trinza** dose based on the previous 1-month injection dose (**Invega Sustenna**) as shown in the

(continued)

table below. Refer to *paliperidone palmitate* and the **Invega Hafyera** comment above for warnings, precautions, interactions, and other prescribing information.

Switching to **Invega Trinza** for Adult Patients Adequately Treated **With Invega Sustenna**	
Last Dose of **Invega Sustenna**	Initial Dose of **Invega Trinza**
78 mg	273 mg
117 mg	410 mg
156 mg	546 mg
234 mg	819 mg

Pediatric: <18 years: safety and efficacy not established; ≥18 years: same as adult
Invega Trinza *Prefilled syringe:* 273 mg/0.88 ml, 410 mg/1.32 ml, 546 mg/1.75 ml, 819 mg/2.63 ml, single-dose, suspension for IM injection

SEIZURE, CLUSTER

▷ *diazepam nasal spray* (IV) *Initial dose:* 5 mg and 10 mg doses are administered as a single spray intranasally into one nostril (administration of 15 mg and 20 mg doses requires two nasal spray devices, one spray into each nostril); *Second dose:* when required, may be administered at least 4 hours after the initial dose; if administered, use a new blister pack; *Max dose and treatment frequency:* do not use more than 2 doses to treat a single episode; it is recommended that **Valtoco** be used to treat no more than one episode every 5 days and no more than 5 episodes per month
Pediatric: <6 years: safety and efficacy not established; ≥6 years: dosage is dependent on the patient's age and weight (see mfr pkg insert)
Valtoco *Nasal spray:* 5, 7.5, 10 mg in 0.1 ml, single-dose
Comment: Valtoco is a benzodiazepine indicated for the acute treatment of intermittent, stereotypic episodes of frequent seizure activity (i.e., seizure clusters, acute repetitive seizures) that are distinct from the patient's usual seizure pattern in patients with epilepsy 6 years of age and older. Benzodiazepines may cause an increased central nervous system (CNS)-depressant effect when used with alcohol or other CNS depressants. Antiepileptic drugs increase the risk of suicidal ideation and behavior. **Valtoco** is contraindicated in patients with acute narrow-angle glaucoma. The most common adverse reactions (incidence 4%) have been somnolence, headache, and nasal discomfort. Concomitant CYP2C19 and CYP3A4 inhibitors may increase adverse reactions to **Valtoco**. Concomitant CYP2C19 and CYP3A4 inducers may decrease *diazepam* exposure. Advise pregnant females and women of childbearing age of potentially serious embryo/fetal risk. *Diazepam* is excreted in human milk. There are no data to assess the effects of **Valtoco** and/or its active metabolite(s) on the breastfed infant. Postmarketing experience suggests that breastfed infants of mothers taking benzodiazepines, such as **Valtoco**, may have effects of lethargy, somnolence, and poor sucking. There is a pregnancy exposure registry that monitors pregnancy outcomes in women exposed to antiepileptic drugs (AEDs), such as **Valtoco**, during pregnancy. Encourage women who are taking **Valtoco** during pregnancy to enroll in the North American Antiepileptic Drug (NAAED) Pregnancy Registry by calling 1-888-233-2334 or http://www.aedpregnancyregistry.org.

SEIZURE DISORDER

Cluster Seizures *see* **Seizure, Cluster**
Status Epilepticus *see* **Status Epilepticus**
See **Anticonvulsant Drugs**

SEXUAL ASSAULT (STD/STI/VD EXPOSURE)

Comment: The following treatment regimens for victims of sexual assault are published in the **2021 CDC** Sexually Transmitted Diseases Treatment Guidelines.

RECOMMENDED PROPHYLAXIS REGIMEN
▷ *ceftriaxone* 250 mg IM in a single dose plus *metronidazole* 2 gm in a single dose plus *azithromycin* 1 gm in a single dose

ALTERNATE PROPHYLAXIS REGIMENS
Regimen 1
▷ *ceftriaxone* 250 mg IM in a single dose plus *metronidazole* 2 gm in a single dose plus *doxycycline* 100 mg bid x 7 days

Regimen 2

▷ *cefixime* 400 mg in a single dose plus *metronidazole* 2 gm in a single dose plus *azithromycin* 1 gm in a single dose

Regimen 3

▷ *cefixime* 400 mg in a single dose plus *metronidazole* 2 gm in a single dose plus *doxycycline* 100 mg bid x 7 days

Regimen 4

▷ *azithromycin* 1 gm as a single dose plus *metronidazole* 2 gm in a single dose

DRUG BRANDS AND DOSE FORMS

▷ *azithromycin* (G)

Zithromax *Tab:* 250, 500, 600 mg; *Oral susp:* 100 mg/5 ml (15 ml); 200 mg/5 ml (15, 22.5, 30 ml) (cherry); *Pkt:* 1 gm for reconstitution (cherry-banana)
Zithromax Tri-Pak *Tab:* 3 x 500 mg tabs/pck
Zithromax Z-Pak *Tab:* 6 x 250 mg tabs/pck
Zmax *Oral susp:* 2 gm ext-rel for reconstitution (cherry-banana) (148 mg Na$^+$)

▷ *cefixime* (G)

Suprax *Tab:* 400 mg; *Cap:* 400 mg; *Oral susp:* 100, 200, 500 mg/5 ml (50, 75, 100 ml) (strawberry)

▷ *ceftriaxone* (G)

Rocephin *Vial:* 250, 500 mg; 1, 2 gm

▷ *doxycycline* (G)

Acticlate *Tab:* 75, 150**mg
Adoxa *Tab:* 50, 75, 100, 150 mg ent-coat
Doryx *Tab:* 50, 75, 100, 150, 200 mg del-rel
Doxteric *Tab:* 50 mg del-rel
Monodox *Cap:* 50, 75, 100 mg
Oracea *Cap:* 40 mg del-rel
Vibramycin *Tab:* 100 mg; *Cap:* 50, 100 mg; *Syr:* 50 mg/5 ml (raspberry-apple) (sulfites); *Oral susp:* 25 mg/5 ml (raspberry)
Vibra-Tab *Tab:* 100 mg film-coat

▷ *metronidazole*

Flagyl *Tab:* 250*, 500*mg
Flagyl 375 *Cap:* 375 mg
Flagyl ER *Tab:* 750 mg ext-rel

SHIGELLOSIS (GENUS *SHIGELLA*)

ANTI-INFECTIVES

▷ *azithromycin* (G) 500 mg x 1 dose on day 1, then 250 mg once daily on days 2-5 or 500 mg once daily x 3 days or Zmax 2 gm in a single dose
Pediatric: <6 months: not recommended; ≥6 months: 10 mg/kg x 1 dose on day 1; then 5 mg/kg/day on days 2-5; max 500 mg/day; see Appendix BB.7. *azithromycin* (G) (Zithromax Suspension, Zmax Suspension) *for dose by weight*
Zithromax *Tab:* 250, 500, 600 mg; *Oral susp:* 100 mg/5 ml (15 ml); 200 mg/5 ml (15, 22.5, 30 ml) (cherry); *Pkt:* 1 gm for reconstitution (cherry-banana)
Zithromax Tri-Pak *Tab:* 3 x 500 mg tabs/pck
Zithromax Z-Pak *Tab:* 6 x 250 mg tabs/pck
Zmax *Oral susp:* 2 gm ext-rel for reconstitution (cherry-banana) (148 mg Na$^+$)

▷ *ciprofloxacin* 500 mg bid x 3 days
Pediatric: <18 years: not recommended; ≥18 years: same as adult
Cipro (G) *Tab:* 250, 500, 750 mg; *Oral susp:* 250, 500 mg/5 ml (100 ml) (strawberry)
Cipro XR *Tab:* 500, 1,000 mg ext-rel
ProQuin XR *Tab:* 500 mg ext-rel

▷ *ofloxacin* (G) 400 mg bid x 3 days
Pediatric: <18 years: not recommended; ≥18 years: same as adult
Floxin *Tab:* 200, 300, 400 mg

▷ *tetracycline* (G) 250-500 mg qid x 5 days
Pediatric: <8 years: not recommended; ≥8 years, <100 lb: 25-50 mg/kg/day in 4 divided doses x 5 days; ≥8 years, ≥100 lb: same as adult; see Appendix BB.31. *tetracycline* (G) (Sumycin Suspension) *for dose by weight*
Achromycin V *Cap:* 250, 500 mg
Sumycin *Tab:* 250, 500 mg; *Cap:* 250, 500 mg; *Oral susp:* 125 mg/5 ml (100, 200 ml) (fruit) (sulfites)

▷ *trimethoprim+sulfamethoxazole* (TMP-SMX) (G)
Bactrim, Septra 2 tabs bid x 10 days
Tab: trim 80 mg+sulfa 400 mg*

(continued)

Bactrim DS, Septra DS 1 tab bid x 10 days
Tab: trim 160 mg+sulfa 800 mg*
Bactrim Pediatric Suspension, Septra Pediatric Suspension 20 ml bid x 10 days
Oral susp: trim 40 mg+sulfa 200 mg per 5 ml (100 ml) (cherry) (alcohol 0.3%)

SHOCK: SEPTIC, DISTRIBUTIVE

Comment: Septic shock is the most common form of distributive shock and is characterized by considerable mortality (treated, around 30%; untreated, probably >80%). In the United States, septic shock is the leading cause of non-cardiac death in intensive care units. **Giapreza (angiotensin II)** is indicated to increase blood pressure, when added to conventional interventions used to raise blood pressure, to prevent/treat dangerously low hypotension resulting from septic and other distributive shock states. There is a potential for venous and arterial thrombotic and thromboembolic events in patients who receive **Giapreza**. Therefore, use concurrent venous thromboembolism (VTE) prophylaxis.

ANGIOTENSIN II

▷ *angiotensin II* dilute in 0.9% NaCl; must be administered as an IV infusion; initial infusion rate 20 ng/kg/min; titrate as frequently as q 5 minutes by increments of up to 15 ng/kg/min as needed; during the first 3 hours, max 80 ng/kg/min; max maintenance dose 40 ng/kg/min; diluted solution may be stored at room temperature or refrigerated; discard after 24 hours
Dilution/Concentration:
Giapreza 1 ml (2.5 mg/ml) in 500 ml 0.9% NaCl = 5,000 ng/ml
       1 ml (2.5.mg/ml in 250 ml 0.9% NaCl = 10,000 ng/ml
       2 ml (5 mg/ml) in 500 ml 0.9% NaCl = 10,000 ng/ml
    Giapreza *Vial:* 2.5 mg in ml, 5 mg/2 ml (2.5 mg/ml)
Comment: The safety and efficacy of **Giapreza** in pediatric patients have not been established. It is not known whether **Giapreza** is present in human milk and no data are available on the effects of angiotensin II on the breastfed infant. The published data on angiotensin II use in pregnant females are not sufficient to determine a drug-associated risk of adverse developmental outcomes. However, delaying treatment in pregnant females with hypotension associated with septic or other distributive shock is likely to increase the risk of shock-associated maternal and fetal morbidity and mortality.

SICKLE CELL DISEASE (SCD)

▷ *hydroxyurea*
Comment: *Hydroxyurea* has an FDA-approved "orphan drug" designation for the treatment of sickle cell disease (SCD). It is an antimetabolite indicated to reduce the frequency of painful crises and to reduce the need for blood transfusions in patients with sickle cell anemia (SCA) with recurrent moderate-to-severe painful crises. *Boxed Warning: Hydroxyurea* may cause severe myelosuppression. Do not administer if bone marrow function is markedly depressed. Monitor blood counts at baseline and every 2 weeks throughout treatment. Blood counts within an acceptable range are defined as *neutrophils* ≥ 2,500 cells/mm³, *platelets* ≥95,000 cells/mm³, Hgb ≥5.3 gm/dL, *reticulocytes* ≥95,000 cells/mm³ if the Hgb <9 gm/dL. Discontinue *hydroxyurea* until hematologic recovery if blood counts are considered toxic. Treatment may be resumed after reducing the *hydroxyurea* dose by 2.5 mg/kg/day from the dose associated with hematologic toxicity. *CrCl <60 ml/min:* reduce dose by 50%. *Hydroxyurea* is carcinogenic. Advise sun protection and monitor patients for malignancies. Avoid live vaccines when using *hydroxyurea*. Discontinue *hydroxyurea* if vasculitic toxicity occurs. Risks with concomitant use of antiretroviral drugs include pancreatitis, hepatotoxicity, and neuropathy. Monitor for signs and symptoms in patients with HIV infection using antiretroviral drugs. If patients with HIV infection are treated with *hydroxyurea*, and in particular in combination with *didanosine* and/or *stavudine*, close monitoring for signs and symptoms of pancreatitis is recommended. Permanently discontinue *hydroxyurea* in patients who develop signs and symptoms of pancreatitis. *Hydroxyurea* can cause fetal harm (embryotoxic and teratogenic effects in animal studies). Advise patients regarding potential risk to the fetus and use of effective contraception during and after treatment with **hydroxyurea** for at least 6 months after therapy is ended. Advise females to immediately report pregnancy. *Hydroxyurea* may damage spermatozoa and testicular tissue, resulting in possible genetic abnormalities. Azoospermia or oligospermia, sometimes reversible, has been observed in men. Inform male patients about the possibility of sperm conservation before the initiation of *hydroxyurea* therapy. Males with female sexual partners of reproductive potential should use effective contraception during and after treatment for at least 1 year. *Hydroxyurea* is excreted in human milk. Discontinue breastfeeding during treatment.
Droxia use actual or ideal body weight (whichever is less) for dosing; initially 15 mg/kg once daily; if the blood counts are within an acceptable range, increase the dose by 5 mg/kg/day every 12 weeks to the highest dose that does not produce toxic blood counts over 24 consecutive weeks (dosage should not exceed 35 mg/kg/day)
Pediatric: <18 years: not established: ≥18 years: same as adult
    Cap: 200, 300, 400 mg

Hydrea (see **Droxia** for prescribing information)
Tab: 500 mg
Siklos use actual or ideal body weight (whichever is less) for dosing; *initially* 20 mg/kg once daily; may be increased by 5 mg/kg/day every 8 weeks, or sooner if a severe painful crisis occurs, until a maximum tolerated dose or 35 mg/kg/day is reached; reduce the dose of **Siklos** by 50% (10 mg) in patients with CrCl <60 ml/min or with end-stage renal disease (ESRD)
Pediatric: <2 years: not recommended; ≥2 years: same as adult
Tab: 100 mg; 1,000***mg
Comment: Safety and effectiveness of **Siklos** have been established in pediatric patients aged 2-18 years with sickle cell disease (SSD) and recurrent moderate-to-severe painful crises and is the only *hydroxyurea* approved for use in children. Use of **Siklos** in these age groups is supported by evidence from a non-interventional cohort study, the European Sickle Cell Disease prospective Cohort study, ESCORT-HU, in which 405 pediatric patients ages 2 to <18 were treated with **Siklos**: n = 274 children (2-11 years) and n = 108 adolescents (12-16 years). Pediatric patients aged 2-16 years had a higher risk of neutropenia than patients >16 years. Continuous follow-up of the growth of treated children is recommended.

AMINO ACID

▶ *L-glutamine powder* take 5-15 gm orally, bid, based on body weight; <30 kg, <66 lb (1 pkt bid), 30-65 kg, 66-143 lb (2 pkts bid), >65 kg, >143 lb (3 pkts bid); mix each dose in 8 oz (240 ml) of cold or room temperature beverage or 4-6 oz of food before ingestion
Pediatric: <5 years: not established; ≥5 years: same as adult
Endari *Oral powder:* 5 gm/paper-foil-plastic laminate pkt (60 pkts/carton)
Comment: Endari is an amino acid indicated to reduce the acute complications of sickle cell disease (SSD). Common adverse reactions include constipation, nausea, abdominal pain, headache, cough, pain in extremity, back pain, and chest pain. There are no available data on **Endari** use in pregnancy to inform a drug-associated risk of major birth defects and miscarriage. There are no data on the presence of **Endari** in human milk or effects on the breastfed infant. The developmental and health benefits from breastfeeding should be considered along with the mother's clinical need for **Endari** and any potential adverse effects on the breastfed infant from **Endari** or from the underlying maternal condition.

CHIMERIC (MURINE/HUMAN) MONOCLONAL ANTIBODY

▶ *basiliximab*
Pediatric: <6 months: not recommended; 6 months-12 years: 14 mg/kg/day in a single or 2 divided doses x 10 days; 12 years: same as adult
Simulect *Vial:* 10, 20 mg (6 ml) for reconstitution and IV infusion (preservative-free); 10 mg vial: contains 10 mg *basiliximab*, 3.61 mg monobasic potassium phosphate, 0.50 mg disodium hydrogen phosphate (anhydrous), 0.80 mg sodium chloride, 10 mg sucrose, and 40 mg mannitol, 20 mg glycine, to be reconstituted in 2.5 ml of Sterile Water for Injection, USP; 20 mg *vial; contains* 20 mg *basiliximab*, 7.21 mg monobasic potassium phosphate, 0.99 mg disodium hydrogen phosphate (anhydrous), 1.61 mg sodium chloride, 20 mg sucrose, 80 mg mannitol, and 40 mg glycine, to be reconstituted with 5 ml of Sterile Water for Injection, USP
Comment: Simulect is indicated for the prophylaxis of acute organ rejection in patients receiving renal transplantation when used as part of an immunosuppressive regimen that includes *cyclosporine* (modified) and corticosteroids. The efficacy of **Simulect** for the prophylaxis of acute rejection in recipients of other solid organ allografts has not been demonstrated. No dose adjustment is necessary when **Simulect** is added to triple immunosuppression regimens including *cyclosporine*, corticosteroids, and either *azathioprine* or *mycophenolate mofetil*. It is not known whether **Simulect** is excreted in human milk. A decision should be made to discontinue nursing or to discontinue the drug, taking into account the importance of the drug to the mother.

P-SELECTIN INHIBITOR

▶ *crizanlizumab-tmca* administer 5 mg/kg by intravenous infusion (IVF) over a period of 30 minutes on Week 0, Week 2, and every 4 weeks thereafter; see mfr pkg insert for preparation and administration instructions
Pediatric: <16 years: not established; ≥16 years: same as adult
Adakveo *Vial:* 100 mg/10 ml (10 mg/ml,10 ml), single-dose
Comment: Adakveo (*crizanlizumab-tmca*) is a P-selectin inhibitor for the prevention of vaso-occlusive crises (VOCs) in patients ≥16 years of age with sickle cell disease (SCD). Monitor the patient for signs and symptoms of an infusion-related reaction; discontinue **Adakveo** infusion for severe reaction and manage medically. **Adakveo** may interfere with automated platelet counts (platelet clumping); run test as soon as possible (within 4 hours of collection or use tubes containing citrate tubes; do not use tubes containing EDTA). The most common adverse reactions (incidence >10%) have been nausea, arthralgia, back pain, and pyrexia. There are insufficient human data on **Adakveo** use in pregnant females to evaluate for a drug-associated risk of major birth defects, miscarriage, or adverse maternal

(continued)

or fetal outcomes; however, animal studies have demonstrated potential of **Adakveo** to cause fetal harm. Advise pregnant females of the potential risk to the fetus. **Adakveo** should only be used during pregnancy if the expected benefit to the patient justifies the potential risk to the fetus. Advise women of potential embryo/risk. **Adakveo** should only be used during pregnancy if the expected benefit to the patient justifies potential embryo/fetal risk. There are no data on the presence of *crizanlizumab-tmca* in human or animal milk or effects on the breastfed infant. Maternal immunoglobulin G (IgG) is known to be present in human milk. The effects of local gastrointestinal exposure and limited systemic exposure in the breastfed infant to *crizanlizumab-tmca* are unknown. The developmental and health benefits of breastfeeding should be considered along with the mother's clinical need for **Adakveo** and any potential adverse effects on the breastfed infant from **Adakveo** or from the underlying maternal condition.

HEMOGLOBIN S (sHgb) POLYMERIZATION INHIBITOR

▶ **voxelotor** administer 1,500 mg once daily (3 x 500 mg or 5 x 300 mg); *Child-Pugh C:* 1,000 mg once daily (2 x 500 mg); take with or without food
Pediatric: <4 years: safety and efficacy not established; 4-<12 years: refer to weight-based dosing table below; *Child-Pugh C:* reduce dose according to weight-based dosing table below; take with or without food; ≥12 years: same as adult

Daily Dose: 4 to <12 Years of age	
Weight	Dose
≥40 kg	1,500 mg
20-<40 kg	900 mg
10-<20 kg	600 mg

Daily Dose: 4 to <12 Years of age, Child-Pugh Class C	
Weight	Dose
≥40 kg	1,000 mg (2 x 500 mg) or 900 mg (3 x 300 mg)
20 to <40 kg	600 mg
10 to <20 kg	300 mg

Oxbryta *Tab:* 500 mg, film-coat; *Tab for oral susp:* 300 mg
Comment: Oxbryta is an HbS (sickle hemoglobin) polymerization inhibitor for the treatment of patients ≥4 years of age with sickle cell disease (SCD). This indication is approved under accelerated approval based on increase in hemoglobin (Hb). Continued approval for this indication may be contingent upon verification and description of clinical benefit in confirmatory trial(s). **Oxbryta** is contraindicated in patients with prior drug hypersensitivity to *voxelotor* or excipients. Observe for signs and symptoms of a hypersensitivity reaction and manage appropriately and promptly. Obtain quantification of hemoglobin species when the patient is not receiving **Oxbryta**. Avoid co-administration of sensitive CYP3A4 substrates with a narrow therapeutic index. Avoid co-administration with strong or moderate CYP3A4 inducers; if unavoidable, increase the dose of **Oxbryta**. The most common adverse reactions in subjects (incidence ≥10% with a difference of >3% compared to placebo) have been headache, diarrhea, abdominal pain, nausea, rash, and pyrexia. The most common adverse reactions (incidence >10%) reported in pediatric patients 4 to <12 years have been pyrexia, vomiting, rash, abdominal pain, diarrhea, and headache. Females with SCD have an increased risk of adverse pregnancy outcomes for the mother and the fetus. Pregnant patients are at greater risk for vaso-occlusive crises (VOC), preeclampsia, eclampsia, and maternal mortality. For the fetus, there is an increased risk for intrauterine growth restriction, preterm delivery, low birth weight (LBW), and perinatal mortality. In animal embryo/fetal development studies, *voxelotor* was administered orally at 15, 50, and 250 mg/kg/day (gestation days 7 through 17) and at 25, 75, and 150 mg/kg/day (gestation days 7 through 19) through organogenesis. Maternal toxicity was observed at the highest dose levels in these studies, equivalent to 2.8-times and 0.3-times the exposures in patients receiving **Oxbryta** at the recommended daily dose, and there were no evidence of adverse developmental outcomes. In a pre- and postnatal animal development study, *voxelotor* was administered orally at 15, 50, and 250 mg/kg/day (gestation day 6 through lactation day 20). Maternal gestational body weights were decreased at 250 mg/kg/day, which continued to the end of lactation. Findings in offspring included reduced survival and reduced body weights throughout lactation, weaning, and maturation. The observed effects in offspring were seen at the maternal dose of 250 mg/kg/day with exposure approximately 2.8-times the exposure in patients at the recommended dose. There are adverse effects on maternal and fetal outcomes associated with SCD in pregnancy. However, there are no available data on use in human pregnancy to evaluate for a drug-associated risk of major birth defects, miscarriage, or adverse maternal or fetal outcomes. Oxbryta should only be used during pregnancy if the benefit of the drug outweighs the potential risk. Because of the potential

for serious adverse reactions in the breastfed infant, including changes in the hematopoietic system, advise mothers that breastfeeding is not recommended during treatment with **Oxbryta** and for at least 2 weeks after the last dose. To report suspected adverse reactions, contact Global Blood Therapeutics at 1-833-GBT-4YOU (1-833-428-4968) or FDA at 1-800-FDA-1088 or www.fda.gov/medwatch.

SINUSITIS, RHINOSINUSITIS: ACUTE BACTERIAL (ABRS)

ANTI-INFECTIVES
➤ *amoxicillin* (G) 500-875 mg bid or 250-500 mg tid x 10 days
   Pediatric: <40 kg (88 lb): 20-40 mg/kg/day in 3 divided doses x 10 days or 25-45 mg/kg/day in 2 divided doses x 10 days; *see* Appendix BB.3. *amoxicillin* (G) (Amoxil Suspension, Trimox Suspension) *for dose by weight*
   Amoxil *Cap:* 250, 500 mg; *Tab:* 875*mg; *Chew tab:* 125, 200, 250, 400 mg (cherry-banana-peppermint) (phenylalanine); *Oral susp:* 125, 250 mg/5 ml (80, 100, 150 ml) (strawberry); 200, 400 mg/5 ml (50, 75, 100 ml) (bubble gum); *Oral drops:* 50 mg/ml (30 ml) (bubble gum)
   Moxatag *Tab:* 775 mg ext-rel
   Trimox *Tab:* 125, 250 mg; *Cap:* 250, 500 mg; *Oral susp:* 125, 250 mg/5 ml (80, 100, 150 ml) (raspberry-strawberry)
➤ *amoxicillin+clavulanate* (G)
   Augmentin 500 mg tid or 875 mg bid x 10 days
   Pediatric: 40-45 mg/kg/day divided tid x 10 days or 90 mg/kg/day divided bid x 10 days; *see* Appendix BB.4. *amoxicillin+clavulanate* (G) (Augmentin Suspension) *for dose by weight*
      Tab: 250, 500, 875 mg; *Chew tab:* 125, 250 mg (lemon-lime); 200, 400 mg (cherry-banana) (phenylalanine); *Oral susp:* 125 mg/5 ml (banana), 250 mg/5 ml (75, 100, 150 ml) (orange); 200, 400 mg/5 ml (50, 75, 100 ml) (orange) (phenylalanine)
   Augmentin ES-600 not recommended for adults
   Pediatric: <3 months: not recommended; ≥3 months, <40 kg: 90 mg/kg/day in 2 divided doses x 10 days; ≥40 kg: not recommended
      Oral susp: 42.9 mg/5 ml (50, 75, 100, 125, 150, 200 ml) (strawberry cream) (phenylalanine)
   Augmentin XR 2 tabs q 12 hours x 10 days
   Pediatric: <16 years: use other forms; ≥16 years: same as adult
      Tab: 1,000*mg ext-rel
➤ *cefaclor* (G)
   Ceclor 250 mg tid or 375 mg bid 3-10 days
   Pediatric: <1 month: not recommended; 1 month-12 years: 20-40 mg/kg divided bid or q 12 hours x 3-10 days; max 1 gm/day; *see* Appendix BB.8. *cefaclor* (G) (Ceclor Suspension) *for dose by weight;* >12 years: same as adult
      Tab: 500 mg; *Cap:* 250, 500 mg; *Susp:* 125 mg/5 ml (75, 150 ml) (strawberry), 187 mg/5 ml (50, 100 ml) (strawberry), 250 mg/5 ml (75, 150 ml) (strawberry), 375 mg/5 ml (50, 100 ml) (strawberry)
   Cefaclor Extended Release 375-500 mg bid x 3-10 days
   Pediatric: <16 years: ext-rel not recommended; ≥16 years: same as adult
      Tab: 375, 500 mg ext-rel
➤ *cefdinir* 300 mg bid or 600 mg once daily x 10 days
   Pediatric: <6 months: not recommended; 6 months-12 years: 14 mg/kg/day in a single or 2 divided doses x 10 days; 12 years: same as adult; *see* Appendix BB.10. *cefdinir* (G) (Omnicef Suspension) *for dose by weight*
      Omnicef *Cap:* 300 mg; *Oral susp:* 125 mg/5 ml (60, 100 ml) (strawberry)
➤ *cefixime* (G) 400 mg once daily x 10 days
   Pediatric: <6 months: not recommended; 6 months-12 years, <50 kg: 8 mg/kg/day in 1-2 divided doses x 10 days; *see* Appendix BB.11. *cefixime* (G) (Suprax Oral Suspension) *for dose by weight;* >12 years, >50 kg: same as adult
      Suprax *Tab:* 400 mg; *Cap:* 400 mg; *Oral susp:* 100, 200, 500 mg/5 ml (50, 75, 100 ml) (strawberry)
➤ *cefpodoxime proxetil* 200 mg bid x 10 days
   Pediatric: <2 months: not recommended; 2 months-12 years: 10 mg/kg/day (max 400 mg/dose) or 5 mg/kg/day bid (max 200 mg/dose) x 10 days; *see* Appendix BB.12. *cefpodoxime proxetil* (G) (Vantin Suspension) *for dose by weight*
      Vantin *Tab:* 100, 200 mg; *Oral susp:* 50, 100 mg/5 ml (50, 75, 100 mg) (lemon creme)
➤ *cefprozil* 250-500 mg bid x 10 days
   Pediatric: <6 months: not recommended; 6 months-12 years: *Mild:* 7.5 mg/kg bid x 10 days; *Moderate/ Severe:* 15 mg/kg q 12 hours x 10 days; *see* Appendix BB.13. *cefprozil* (G) (Cefzil Suspension) *for dose by weight;* >12 years: same as adult
      Cefzil *Tab:* 250, 500 mg; *Oral susp:* 125, 250 mg/5 ml (50, 75, 100 ml) (bubble gum) (phenylalanine)
➤ *ceftibuten* 400 mg once daily x 10 days
   Pediatric: <12 years: 9 mg/kg once daily x 10 days; max 400 mg/day; *see* Appendix BB.14. *ceftibuten* (G) (Cedax Suspension) *for dose by weight;* ≥12 years: 400 mg once daily x 10 days
      Cedax *Cap:* 400 mg; *Oral susp:* 90 mg/5 ml (30, 60, 90, 120 ml); 180 mg/5 ml (30, 60, 120 ml) (cherry)

(continued)

▷ *ciprofloxacin* 500 mg bid x 10 days
Pediatric: <18 years: <u>not</u> recommended; ≥18 years: same as adult
    Cipro (G) *Tab:* 250, 500, 750 mg; *Oral susp:* 250, 500 mg/5 ml (100 ml) (strawberry)
    Cipro XR *Tab:* 500, 1,000 mg ext-rel
    ProQuin XR *Tab:* 500 mg ext-rel
▷ *clarithromycin* **(G)** 500 mg bid <u>or</u> 1,000 mg ext-rel once daily x 10 days
Pediatric: <6 months: <u>not</u> recommended; ≥6 months: 7.5 mg/kg bid x 10 days; *see* Appendix BB.16.
clarithromycin (Biaxin Suspension) *for dose by weight*
    Biaxin *Tab:* 250, 500 mg
    Biaxin Oral Suspension *Oral susp:* 125, 250 mg/5 ml (50, 100 ml) (fruit punch)
    Biaxin XL *Tab:* 500 mg ext-rel
▷ *levofloxacin* *Uncomplicated:* 500 mg once daily x 10-14 days; *Complicated:* 750 mg once daily x 10-14 days
Pediatric: <18 years: <u>not</u> recommended; ≥18 years: same as adult
    Levaquin *Tab:* 250, 500, 750 mg; *Oral soln:* 25 mg/ml (480 ml) (benzyl alcohol); *Inj conc:* 25 mg/ml for IV infusion after dilution (20, 30 ml single-use vial) (preservative-free); *Premix soln:* 5 mg/ml for IV infusion (50, 100, 150 ml) (preservative-free)
▷ *loracarbef* 400 mg bid x 10 days
Pediatric: 15 mg/kg/day in 2 divided doses x 10 days; *see* Appendix BB.27. *loracarbef* (Lorabid Suspension) *for dose by weight*
    Lorabid *Pulvule:* 200, 400 mg; *Oral susp:* 100 mg/5 ml (50, 100 ml), 200 mg/5 ml (50, 75, 100 ml) (strawberry bubble gum)
▷ *moxifloxacin* **(G)** 400 mg once daily x 10 days
Pediatric: <18 years: <u>not</u> recommended; ≥18 years: same as adult
    Avelox *Tab:* 400 mg
▷ *trimethoprim+sulfamethoxazole (TMP-SMX)* **(G)**
Pediatric: <2 months: <u>not</u> recommended; ≥2 months: 40 mg/kg/day of *sulfamethoxazole* in 2 divided doses bid x 10 days; *see* Appendix BB.33. *trimethoprim+sulfamethoxazole* (Bactrim Suspension, Septra Suspension) *for dose by weight*
    Bactrim, Septra 2 tabs bid x 10 days
      Tab: trim 80 mg+sulfa 400 mg*
    Bactrim DS, Septra DS 1 tab bid x 10 days
      Tab: trim 160 mg+sulfa 800 mg*
    Bactrim Pediatric Suspension, Septra Pediatric Suspension
      Oral susp: trim 40 mg+sulfa 200 mg per 5 ml (100 ml) (cherry) (alcohol 0.3%)

SJÖGREN-LARSSON SYNDROME (SLS)

Comment: Sjögren-Larsson syndrome (SLS) is a chronic autoimmune disorder that causes the white blood cells to attack the moisture-producing glands. Sjögren's syndrome can occur in association with other autoimmune diseases, including systemic lupus erythematosus, rheumatoid arthritis, scleroderma, systemic sclerosis, cryoglobulinemia, or polyarteritis nodosa. The disease can affect the eyes, mouth, parotid gland, pancreas, gastrointestinal system, blood vessels, lungs, kidneys, skin, and nervous system. Erythrocyte sedimentation rate (ESR) is elevated in 80% of patients. Rheumatoid factor is present in 52% of primary cases and 98% of secondary-type cases. A mild normochromic normocytic anemia is present in 50% of patients and leukopenia occurs in up to 42% of patients. Creatinine clearance is diminished in up to 50% of patients. Antinuclear antibody (ANA) is positive in 70% of patients. SS-A and SS-B are marker antibodies for Sjögren's syndrome; 70% of patients are positive for SS-A and 40% are positive for SS-B.

CHOLINERGIC (MUSCARINIC) AGONIST COMBINATION
▷ *cevimeline* **(G)** 30 mg tid
    Evoxac *Cap:* 30 mg
  Comment: *Cevimeline* is contraindicated in acute iritis, narrow-angle glaucoma, and uncontrolled asthma.
▷ *pilocarpine* **(G)** 5 mg qid <u>or</u> 7.5 mg tid
    Salagen *Tab:* 5, 7.5 mg

ORAL ENZYME RINSE
▷ *xylitol+solazyme+selectobac* swish 5 ml for 30 seconds bid-tid
    Orazyme Dry Mouth Relief Rinse *Oral soln:* 1.5, 16 oz

SKIN: CALLUSED

KERATOLYTICS
▷ *salicylic acid* (OTC) apply lotion, cream, <u>or</u> gel to affected area once daily-bid; apply patch to affected area and leave on x 48 hours with max 5 applications/14 days
Pediatric: <12 years: <u>not</u> recommended; ≥12 years: same as adult

▷ *urea*
Pediatric: <12 years: not recommended; ≥12 years: same as adult
Carmol 40 apply to affected area with applicator stick provided once daily-tid; smooth over until cream is absorbed; protect surrounding tissue; may cover with adhesive bandage or gauze secured with adhesive tape
Crm/Gel: 40% (30 gm)
Keratol 40 apply to affected area with applicator stick provided once daily-tid; smooth over until cream is absorbed; protect surrounding tissue; may cover with adhesive bandage or gauze secured with adhesive tape
Crm: 40% (1, 3, 7 oz); *Gel:* 40% (15 ml); *Lotn:* 40% (8 oz)
Comment: The moisturizing effect of **Carmol 40** and **Keratol 40** is enhanced by applying while the skin is still moist (after washing or bathing).

SKIN INFECTION: BACTERIAL (CARBUNCLE, FOLLICULITIS, FURUNCLE)

Comment: Abscesses usually require surgical incision and drainage.

ANTIBACTERIAL SKIN CLEANSERS

▷ *hexachlorophene* dispense 5 ml into wet hand, work up into lather; then apply to area to be cleansed; rinse thoroughly
pHisoHex *Liq clnsr:* 5, 16 oz

TOPICAL ANTI-INFECTIVES

▷ *mupirocin* (G) apply to lesions bid
Pediatric: same as adult
Bactroban *Oint:* 2% (22 gm); *Crm:* 2% (15, 30 gm)
Centany *Oint:* 2% (15, 30 gm)
▷ *polymyxin b+neomycin* oint apply once daily-tid
Neosporin (OTC) *Oint:* 15 gm

ORAL ANTI-INFECTIVES

▷ *amoxicillin* (G) 500-875 mg bid or 250-500 mg tid x 10 days
Pediatric: <40 kg (88 lb): 20-40 mg/kg/day in 3 divided doses x 10 days or 25-45 mg/kg/day in 2 divided doses x 10 days; *see* Appendix BB.3. *amoxicillin* (G) (Amoxil Suspension, Trimox Suspension) *for dose by weight*
Amoxil *Cap:* 250, 500 mg; *Tab:* 875*mg; *Chew tab:* 125, 200, 250, 400 mg (cherry-banana-peppermint) (phenylalanine); *Oral susp:* 125, 250 mg/5 ml (80, 100, 150 ml) (strawberry); 200, 400 mg/5 ml (50, 75, 100 ml) (bubble gum); *Oral drops:* 50 mg/ml (30 ml) (bubble gum)
Moxatag *Tab:* 775 mg ext-rel
Trimox *Tab:* 125, 250 mg; *Cap:* 250, 500 mg; *Oral susp:* 125, 250 mg/5 ml (80, 100, 150 ml) (raspberry-strawberry)
▷ *azithromycin* (G) 500 mg x 1 dose on day 1, then 250 mg once daily on days 2-5 or 500 mg once daily x 3 days or **Zmax** 2 gm in a single dose
Pediatric: 12 mg/kg/day x 5 days; max 500 mg/day; *see* Appendix BB.7. *azithromycin* (G) (Zithromax Suspension, Zmax Suspension) *for dose by weight*
Zithromax *Tab:* 250, 500, 600 mg; *Oral susp:* 100 mg/5 ml (15 ml); 200 mg/5 ml (15, 22.5, 30 ml) (cherry); *Pkt:* 1 gm for reconstitution (cherry-banana)
Zithromax Tri-Pak *Tab:* 3 x 500 mg tabs/pck
Zithromax Z-Pak *Tab:* 6 x 250 mg tabs/pck
Zmax *Oral susp:* 2 gm ext-rel for reconstitution (cherry-banana) (148 mg Na$^+$)
▷ *cefaclor* (G)
Ceclor 250 mg tid or 375 mg bid 3-10 days
Pediatric: <1 month: not recommended; 1 month-12 years: 20-40 mg/kg divided bid or q 12 hours x 3-10 days; max 1 gm/day; *see* Appendix BB.8. *cefaclor* (G) (Ceclor Suspension) *for dose by weight;* >12 years: same as adult
Tab: 500 mg; *Cap:* 250, 500 mg; *Susp:* 125 mg/5 ml (75, 150 ml) (strawberry); 187 mg/5 ml (50, 100 ml) (strawberry); 250 mg/5 ml (75, 150 ml) (strawberry); 375 mg/5 ml (50, 100 ml) (strawberry)
Cefaclor Extended Release 375-500 mg bid x 3-10 days
Pediatric: <16 years: ext-rel not recommended; ≥16 years: same as adult
Tab: 375, 500 mg ext-rel
▷ *cefadroxil* 1-2 gm in a single or 2 divided doses x 10 days
Pediatric: 15-30 mg/kg/day in 2 divided doses x 10 days; *see* Appendix BB.9. *cefadroxil* (G) (Duricef Suspension) *for dose by weight*
Duricef *Cap:* 500 mg; *Tab:* 1 gm; *Oral susp:* 250 mg/5 ml (100 ml); 500 mg/5 ml (75, 100 ml) (orange-pineapple)

(continued)

▷ *cefdinir* 300 mg bid x 10 days
  Pediatric: <6 months: <u>not</u> recommended; 6 months-12 years: 14 mg/kg/day in 1-2 divided doses x 10 days; *see* Appendix BB.10. *cefdinir* (G) (Omnicef Suspension) *for dose by weight*
    Omnicef *Cap:* 300 mg; *Oral susp:* 125 mg/5 ml (60, 100 ml) (strawberry)
▷ *cefditoren pivoxil* 200 mg bid x 10 days
  Pediatric: <12 years: <u>not</u> recommended; ≥12 years: same as adult
    Spectracef *Tab:* 200 mg
  Comment: Contraindicated with milk protein allergy <u>or</u> carnitine deficiency.
▷ *cefpodoxime proxetil* 400 mg bid x 7-14 days
  Pediatric: <2 months: <u>not</u> recommended; 2 months-12 years: 10 mg/kg/day (max 400 mg/dose) <u>or</u> 5 mg/kg/day bid (max 200 mg/dose) x 7-14 days; *see* Appendix BB.12. *cefpodoxime proxetil* (G) (Vantin Suspension) *for dose by weight*
    Vantin *Tab:* 100, 200 mg; *Oral susp:* 50, 100 mg/5 ml (50, 75, 100 mg) (lemon creme)
▷ *cefprozil* 250-500 mg bid <u>or</u> 500 mg once daily x 10 days
  Pediatric: 2-12 years: 7.5 mg/kg bid x 10 days; >12 years: same as adult; *see* Appendix BB.13. *cefprozil* (G) (Cefzil Suspension) *for dose by weight*
    Cefzil *Tab:* 250, 500 mg; *Oral susp:* 125, 250 mg/5 ml (50, 75, 100 ml) (bubble gum) (phenylalanine)
▷ *ceftriaxone* (G) 1-2 gm IM once daily; max 4 gm/day
  Pediatric: 50-75 mg/kg IM in 1-2 divided doses; max 2 gm/day
    Rocephin *Vial:* 250, 500 mg; 1, 2 gm
▷ *cephalexin* (G) 500 mg bid x 10 days
  Pediatric: 25-50 mg/kg/day in 4 divided doses x 10 days; *see* Appendix BB.15. *cephalexin* (G) (Keflex Suspension) *for dose by weight*
    Keflex *Cap:* 250, 333, 500, 750 mg; *Oral susp:* 125, 250 mg/5 ml (100, 200 ml) (strawberry)
▷ *clarithromycin* (G) 250-500 mg bid <u>or</u> 500-1,000 mg ext-rel once daily x 7-14 days
  Pediatric: <6 months: <u>not</u> recommended; ≥6 months: 7.5 mg/kg bid x 7-14 days; *see* Appendix BB.16. *Clarithromycin* (G) (Biaxin Suspension) *for dose by weight*
    Biaxin *Tab:* 250, 500 mg
    Biaxin Oral Suspension *Oral susp:* 125, 250 mg/5 ml (50, 100 ml) (fruit punch)
    Biaxin XL *Tab:* 500 mg ext-rel
▷ *dicloxacillin* 500 mg qid x 10 days
  Pediatric: 12.5-25 mg/kg/day in 4 divided doses x 10 days; *see* Appendix BB.18. *dicloxacillin* (G) (Dynapen Suspension) *for dose by weight*
    Dynapen *Cap:* 125, 250, 500 mg; *Oral susp:* 62.5 mg/5 ml (80, 100, 200 ml)
▷ *dirithromycin* (G) 500 mg once daily x 5-7 days
  Pediatric: <12 years: <u>not</u> recommended; ≥12 years: same as adult
    Dynabac *Tab:* 250 mg
▷ *doxycycline* (G) 100 mg bid x 9 days
  Pediatric: <8 years: <u>not</u> recommended; ≥8 years, <100 lb: 1 mg/lb in a single dose once daily x 9 days; *see* Appendix BB.19. *doxycycline* (G) (Vibramycin Syrup/Suspension) *for dose by weight;* >8 years, ≥100 lb: same as adult
    Acticlate *Tab:* 75, 150**mg
    Adoxa *Tab:* 50, 75, 100, 150 mg ent-coat
    Doryx *Tab:* 50, 75, 100, 150, 200 mg del-rel
    Doxteric *Tab:* 50 mg del-rel
    Monodox *Cap:* 50, 75, 100 mg
    Oracea *Cap:* 40 mg del-rel
    Vibramycin *Tab:* 100 mg; *Cap:* 50, 100 mg; *Syr:* 50 mg/5 ml (raspberry-apple) (sulfites); *Oral susp:* 25 mg/5 ml (raspberry)
    Vibra-Tab *Tab:* 100 mg film-coat
▷ *erythromycin base* (G) 250-500 mg tid x 10 days
  Pediatric: 30-50 mg/kg/day in 2-4 divided doses x 10 days
    Ery-Tab *Tab:* 250, 333, 500 mg ent-coat
    PCE *Tab:* 333, 500 mg
▷ *erythromycin estolate* (G) 250-500 mg q 6 hours x 10 days
  Pediatric: 20-50 mg/kg q 6 hours x 10 days; *see* Appendix BB.20. *erythromycin estolate* (G) (Ilosone Suspension) *for dose by weight*
    Ilosone *Pulvule:* 250 mg; *Tab:* 500 mg; *Liq:* 125, 250 mg/5 ml (100 ml)
▷ *erythromycin ethylsuccinate* (G) 400 mg qid x 10 days
  Pediatric: 30-50 mg/kg/day in 4 divided doses x 10 days; may double dose with severe infection; max 100 mg/kg/day; *see* Appendix BB.21. *erythromycin ethylsuccinate* (G) (E.E.S. Suspension, EryPed Drops/ Suspension) *for dose by weight*
    EryPed *Oral susp:* 200 mg/5 ml (100, 200 ml) (fruit); 400 mg/5 ml (60, 100, 200 ml) (banana); *Oral drops:* 200, 400 mg/5 ml (50 ml) (fruit); *Chew tab:* 200 mg wafer (fruit)
    E.E.S. *Oral susp:* 200, 400 mg/5 ml (100 ml) (fruit)
    E.E.S. Granules *Oral susp:* 200 mg/5 ml (100, 200 ml) (cherry)
    E.E.S. 400 Tablets *Tab:* 400 mg

▷ **gemifloxacin** (G) 320 mg once daily x 5-7 days
  Pediatric: <18 years: <u>not</u> recommended; ≥18 years: same as adult
    Factive *Tab:* 320*mg
▷ **levofloxacin** *Uncomplicated:* 500 mg once daily x 7-10 days; *Complicated:* 750 mg once daily x 7-10 days
  Pediatric: <18 years: <u>not</u> recommended; ≥18 years: same as adult
    Levaquin *Tab:* 250, 500, 750 mg; *Oral soln:* 25 mg/ml (480 ml) (benzyl alcohol); *Inj conc:* 25 mg/ml
    for IV infusion after dilution (20, 30 ml single-use vial) (preservative-free); *Premix soln:* 5 mg/ml for
    IV infusion (50, 100, 150 ml) (preservative-free)
▷ **linezolid** (G) 400-600 mg q 12 hours x 10-14 days
  Pediatric: <5 years: 10 mg/kg q 8 hours x 10-14 days; 5-11 years: 10 mg/kg q 12 hours x 10-14 days; >11
  years: same as adult
    Zyvox *Tab:* 400, 600 mg; *Oral susp:* 100 mg/5 ml (150 ml) (orange) (phenylalanine)
  Comment: *Linezolid* is indicated to treat susceptible **vancomycin**-resistant *Enterococcus faecium* infections.
▷ **loracarbef** 200 mg bid x 7 days
  Pediatric: 15 mg/kg/day in 2 divided doses x 7 days; *see* Appendix BB.27. *loracarbef* (G) (Lorabid
  Suspension) *for dose by weight*
    Lorabid *Pulvule:* 200, 400 mg; *Oral susp:* 100 mg/5 ml (50, 100 ml); 200 mg/5 ml (50, 75, 100 ml)
    (strawberry bubble gum)
▷ **minocycline** (G) 200 mg on first day; then 100 mg q 12 hours x 9 more days
  Pediatric: <8 years: <u>not</u> recommended; ≥8 years, <100 lb: 2 mg/lb on first day in 2 divided doses, followed by
  1 mg/lb q 12 hours x 9 more days; ≥8 years, ≥100 lb: same as adult
    Dynacin *Cap:* 50, 100 mg
    Minocin *Cap:* 50, 75, 100 mg; *Oral susp:* 50 mg/5 ml (60 ml) (custard) (sulfites, alcohol 5%)
▷ **moxifloxacin** (G) 400 mg once daily x 10 days
  Pediatric: <18 years: <u>not</u> recommended; ≥18 years: same as adult
    Avelox *Tab:* 400 mg
▷ **ofloxacin** (G) 400 mg bid x 10 days
  Pediatric: <18 years: <u>not</u> recommended; ≥18 years: same as adult
    Floxin *Tab:* 200, 300, 400 mg
▷ **tetracycline** (G) 500 mg qid x 10 days
  Pediatric: <8 years: <u>not</u> recommended; ≥8 years, <100 lb: 25-50 mg/kg/day in 4 divided doses x 10 days; ≥8
  years, ≥100 lb: same as adult; *see* Appendix BB.31. *tetracycline* (G) (Sumycin Suspension) *for dose by weight*
    Achromycin V *Cap:* 250, 500 mg
    Sumycin *Tab:* 250, 500 mg; *Cap:* 250, 500 mg; *Oral susp:* 125 mg/5 ml (100, 200 ml) (fruit) (sulfites)

SLEEP APNEA: OBSTRUCTIVE (HYPOPNEA SYNDROME)

ANTI-NARCOLEPTIC AGENTS

▷ **armodafinil** (IV)(G) *Obstructive sleep apnea/hypopnea syndrome (OSAHS):* 150-250 mg once daily in the
  AM; *Shift-work sleep disorder (SWSD):* 150 mg 1 hour before starting shift; reduce dose with severe hepatic
  impairment
  Pediatric: <17 years: <u>not</u> recommended; ≥17 years: same as adult
    Nuvigil *Tab:* 50, 150, 200, 250 mg
▷ **modafinil** (IV) 100-200 mg q AM; max 400 mg/day
  Pediatric: <16 years: <u>not</u> recommended; ≥16 years: same as adult
    Provigil *Tab:* 100, 200*mg
  Comment: *Modafinil* promotes wakefulness in patients with excessive sleepiness due to OSAHS.

SELECTIVE DOPAMINE AND NOREPINEPHRINE REUPTAKE INHIBITOR (DNRI)

▷ **solriamfetol** administer once daily upon awakening; avoid administration within 9 hours of planned bedtime
  because of the potential to interfere with sleep; *Starting dose for patients with narcolepsy:* 75 mg once daily;
  Starting dose for patients with obstructive sleep apnea (OSA): 37.5 mg once daily; dose may be increased at
  intervals of at least 3 days; max 150 mg once daily; *Moderate renal impairment:* starting dose is 37.5 mg once
  daily; may increase to 75 mg once daily after at least 7 days; *Severe renal impairment:* starting dose and max
  dose is 37.5 mg once daily; *End-stage renal disease (ESRD):* <u>not</u> recommended
  Pediatric: safety and efficacy <u>not</u> established
    Sunosi *Tab:* 75*, 150 mg film-coat
  Comment: **Sunosi** (*solriamfetol*) is a dopamine and norepinephrine reuptake inhibitor (DNRI) indicated
    to improve wakefulness in adult patients with excessive daytime sleepiness associated with narcolepsy
    <u>or</u> obstructive sleep apnea (OSA). **Sunosi** is <u>not</u> indicated to treat the underlying airway obstruction in
    OSA. Ensure that the underlying airway obstruction is treated (e.g., with continuous positive airway
    pressure [CPAP]) for at least 1 month prior to initiating **Sunosi** for excessive daytime sleepiness.
    Modalities to treat the underlying airway obstruction should be continued during treatment with
    Sunosi. **Sunosi** is <u>not</u> a substitute for these modalities. Use caution when co-administering **Sunosi** with
    drugs that increase BP <u>and/or</u> HR and dopaminergic drugs. Measure HR and BP prior to initiating,

(continued)

and periodically throughout, treatment. Control hypertension before and during therapy. Avoid use in patients with unstable cardiovascular disease, serious heart arrhythmias, or other serious heart problems. Use caution in treating patients with a history of psychosis or bipolar disorder. Consider **Sunosi** dose reduction or discontinuation if psychiatric symptoms develop. **Sunosi** is contraindicated in patients receiving treatment with a MAOI and within 14 days following discontinuation of an MAOI. Available data from case reports are not sufficient to determine drug-associated risks of major birth defects, miscarriage, or adverse maternal or fetal outcomes. There are no data available on the presence of *solriamfetol* or its metabolites in human milk or effects on the breastfed infant. The developmental and health benefits of breastfeeding should be considered along with the mother's clinical need for **Sunosi** and any potential adverse effects on the breastfed infant from **Sunosi** or from the underlying maternal condition. Healthcare providers are encouraged to register pregnant patients, or pregnant females may enroll themselves in the **Sunosi** Pregnancy Exposure Registry by calling 1-877-283-6220 or www.SunosiPregnancyRegistry.com

SLEEPINESS: EXCESSIVE, SHIFT-WORK SLEEP DISORDER (SWSD)

ANTINARCOLEPTIC AGENT
➤ *armodafinil* (IV) (G) *OSAHS:* 150-250 mg once daily in the AM; *Shift-work sleep disorder (SWSD):* 150 mg 1 hour before starting shift; reduce dose with severe hepatic impairment
Pediatric: <17 years: not recommended; ≥17 years: same as adult
  Nuvigil *Tab:* 50, 150, 200, 250 mg
➤ *modafinil* (IV) 100-200 mg q AM; max 400 mg/day
Pediatric: <16 years: not recommended; ≥16 years: same as adult
  Provigil *Tab:* 100, 200*mg
  Comment: Provigil promotes wakefulness in patients with narcolepsy, shift work sleep disorder, and excessive sleepiness due to obstructive sleep apnea/hypopnea syndrome.

SMALLPOX (*VARIOLA MAJOR*), MONKEYPOX

PROPHYLAXIS
➤ *smallpox and monkeypox vaccine, live, non-replicating* administer 2 SC doses (0.5 ml each) 4 weeks apart
Pediatric: <18 years: not established; ≥18 years: same as above if determined to be at high risk for smallpox or monkeypox infection
  Jynneos *Vial:* 0.5 ml, single-dose
  Comment: In smallpox vaccine-naïve healthy adults, the most common (incidence >10%) solicited injection site reactions have been pain (84.9%), redness (60.8%), swelling (51.6%), induration (45.4%), and itching (43.1%). The most common solicited systemic adverse reactions have been muscle pain (42.8%), headache (34.8%), fatigue (30.4%), nausea (17.3%), and chills (10.4%). In healthy adults previously vaccinated with a smallpox vaccine, the most common (incidence >10%) solicited injection site reactions were redness (80.9%), pain (79.5%), induration (70.4%), swelling (67.2%), and itching (32.0%). The most common solicited systemic adverse reactions have been fatigue (33.5%), headache (27.6%), and muscle pain (21.5%). Frequencies of solicited local and systemic adverse reactions among adults with HIV infection and adults with atopic dermatitis have generally been similar to those observed in healthy adults.
➤ *vaccina virus* vaccine *(dried, calf lymph type)*
Pediatric: <12 months: not recommended; 12 months-18 years, non-emergency: not recommended
  Dryvax
    Kit: vial dried smallpox vaccine (1), 0.25 ml diluent in syringe (1), vented needle (1), 100 individually wrapped bifurcated needles (5 needles/strip, 20 strips) (polymyxin b sulfate+dihydrostreptomycin+sulfate, chlortetracycline hcl+neomycin sulfate+glycerin+phenol)
  Comment: Dryvax is a dried live vaccine with approximately 100 million *Infectious vaccina* viruses (pock-forming units [pfu] per ml). Contact with immunosuppressed individuals should be avoided until the scab has separated from the skin (2-3 weeks) and/or a protective occlusive dressing covers the inoculation site. Scarification only. Do not inject IV, IM, or SC. Revaccination is recommended every 10 years.

TREATMENT
Comment: On July 11, 2018, the U.S. FDA approved **Tpoxx** *(tecovirimat)*, the first drug with an indication for treatment of smallpox. Although the World Health Organization (WHO) declared smallpox, a contagious and sometimes fatal infectious disease, eradicated in 1980, there have been longstanding concerns that smallpox could be used as a bioweapon. To address the risk of bioterrorism, Congress has taken steps to enable the development and approval of countermeasures to thwart pathogens that could be employed as weapons. **Tpoxx** is the first product to be awarded a Material Threat Medical Countermeasure priority review voucher.

➤ *tecovirimat* 600 mg bid x 14 days; take within 30 minutes after a full meal of moderate or high fat
Pediatric: <13 kg: not recommended; 13 to <25 kg: 200 mg bid x 14 days; 25 kg to <40 kg: 400 mg bid x 14 days; ≥40 kg: 600 mg bid x 14 days
  Tpoxx *Cap:* 200 mg

Comment: Tpoxx is an inhibitor of the orthopoxvirus VP37 envelope wrapping protein and is indicated for the treatment of human smallpox disease in adults and pediatric patients weighing ≥13 kg. The effectiveness of Tpoxx for treatment of smallpox disease has not been determined in humans because adequate and well-controlled field trials have not been feasible, and inducing smallpox disease in humans to study the drug's efficacy is not ethical. Tpoxx efficacy may be reduced in immunocompromised patients based on studies demonstrating reduced efficacy in immunocompromised animal models. Co-administration of Tpoxx with *repaglinide* may cause hypoglycemia. Monitor blood glucose and monitor for hypoglycemic symptoms during co-administration. No adequate and well-controlled studies in pregnancy have been conducted; therefore, there are no human data to establish the presence or absence of Tpoxx associated risk. In animal reproduction studies, no embryo fetal developmental toxicity has been observed. There are no data to assess the presence of *tecovirimat* in human milk or effects on the breastfed infant; however, *tecovirimat* has been found in animal milk. Developmental and health benefits of breastfeeding should be considered along with the mother's clinical need for Tpoxx and any potential adverse effects on the breastfed infant from Tpoxx or from the underlying maternal condition. Common adverse reactions in healthy adult subjects (incidence ≥2%) were headache, nausea, abdominal pain, and vomiting.

SPASTICITY OF CEREBRAL OR SPINAL ORIGIN

GAMMA AMINOBUTYRIC ACID (GABA-ERGIC) AGONIST
▷ *baclofen*
 Pediatric: **Fleqsuvy** *Oral susp:* 25 mg/5 ml (grape)
 Comment: Fleqsuvy is a gamma-aminobutyric acid (GABA-ergic) agonist for the treatment of spasticity resulting from multiple sclerosis (MS), particularly from the relief of flexor spasms and concomitant pain, pain clonus, and muscular rigidity. Fleqsuvy may also be used in patients with spinal cord injuries and other spinal cord diseases. Fleqsuvy is not indicated in the treatment of skeletal muscle spasms resulting from rheumatic disorders.

INTRATHECAL BACLOFEN THERAPY
▷ *Prometra II Programmable Pump*
 Comment: In February 2020, the FDA granted market approval to Flowonix Medical's implantable **Prometra II Programmable Pump System** for use with intrathecal *baclofen* for patients with severe spasticity of cerebral or spinal origin. The device offers a pressure-driven, valve-gated delivery mechanism that allows for novel programming modes of intermittent flow followed by periods of no flow. This indication expanded **Flowonix's** previous market entry in November 2019, when the **Prometra II** 40 ml pump was introduced.

REFERENCES

Flowonix Receives FDA Approval to Market Prometra® II Pump for use with Intrathecal Baclofen [press release]. Mount Olive, NJ: Flowonix Medical; Published February 19, 2020. prnewswire.com/news-releases/flowonix-receives-fda-approval-to-market-prometra-ii-pump-for-use-with-intrathecal-baclofen-301007586.html. Accessed February 19, 2023.

Neurological Surgeons website. Updated 2020. aans.org/Patients/Neurosurgical-Conditions-and-Treatments/Spasticity. Accessed February 18, 2023.

SPINAL MUSCULAR ATROPHY (SMA)

Comment: Spinal muscular atrophy (SMA) is a group of inherited disorders characterized by motor neuron loss in the spinal cord and lower brainstem, muscle weakness, and atrophy. Survival motor neuron (SMN) protein is essential for the maintenance of motor neurons. Because of a defect in, or loss of, the SMN1 gene, patients with SMA do not produce enough SMN protein. It is the most common genetic cause of death in infants, but can affect people at any age. **Spinraza** (*nusinersen*) is the first FDA-approved drug to treat SMA.

SURVIVAL MOTOR NEURON-2 (SMN2)-DIRECTED ANTISENSE OLIGONUCLEOTIDE
▷ *nusinersen* 12 mg per intrathecal administration; initially 4 loading doses: the first 3 loading doses administered at 14-day intervals; the 4th loading dose administered 30 days after the 3rd loading dose; the maintenance dose is administered every 4 months after the 4th loading dose; prior to administration, 5 ml cerebral spinal fluid (CSF) should be removed; the intrathecal bolus injection should be administered over 1-3 minutes using a spinal anesthetic needle
 Pediatric: same as adult
  Spinraza *Vial:* 12 mg/5 ml (2.4 mg/ml), single-dose, solution for intrathecal administration (preservative-free)
  Comment: At baseline and prior to each dose, obtain a platelet count and coagulation laboratory testing (there is increased risk for thrombocytopenia and coagulation abnormalities) and quantitative spot urine protein testing (to monitor for renal toxicity). Store **Spinraza** in a refrigerator between 2°C to 8°C (36°F to 46°F) in the original carton to protect from light. Do not freeze. Prior to administration, unopened vials of **Spinraza** can be removed from and returned to the refrigerator, if necessary. If removed from the original carton, the total combined time out of refrigeration should

(continued)

not exceed 30 hours at a temperature that does not exceed 25°C (77°F). **Spinraza** has no labeled contraindications. **Spinraza** has not been studied in pregnant or lactating females, or in patients with renal or hepatic impairment.

SURVIVAL OF MOTOR NEURON 2 (SMN2) SPLICING MODIFIER

▶ *risdiplam* administer orally once daily, after a meal, using the provided oral syringe

Pediatric: <2 months: not established; 2 months to <2 years: 0.2 mg/kg once daily; ≥2 years, <20 kg: 0.25 mg/kg once daily; ≥2 years, ≥20 kg: 5 mg once daily

Evrysdi *Oral soln:* 60 mg, pwdr for constitution to provide 0.75 mg/ml solution

Comment: **Evrysdi** *(risdiplam)* is a survival of motor neuron 2 (SMN2) splicing modifier indicated for treatment of SMA in patients ≥2 months of age. **Evrysdi** must be constituted by a pharmacist prior to dispensing (see mfr pkg insert for full prescribing information for important preparation and administration instructions). The most common adverse reactions in infantile-onset SMA have been similar to those observed in later-onset SMA. Additionally, adverse reactions (incidence ≥10%) have been upper respiratory infection (URI), pneumonia, constipation, and vomiting. The most common adverse reactions in later-onset SMA (incidence ≥10%) have been fever, diarrhea, and rash. Avoid co-administration with drugs that are substrates of multidrug and toxin extrusion (MATE) transporters. Avoid in patients with hepatic impairment. Based on animal data, *risdiplam* may cause embryo/fetal harm. There are no data on presence of *risdiplam* in human milk or effects on breastfed infant. *Risdiplam* was excreted in milk of lactating rats after orally administered *risdiplam*. Developmental and health benefits of breastfeeding should be considered along with mother's clinical need for **Evrysdi** and any potential adverse effects on breastfed infant from **Evrysdi** or underlying maternal condition.

ADENO-ASSOCIATED VIRUS VECTOR-BASED GENE THERAPY

▶ *onasemnogene abeparvovec-xioi* initially, assess baseline liver function, check platelet (PLT) count and troponin 1, and test for the presence of anti-AAV9 antibodies; recommended dose is 1.1×10 vector genomes (vg) per kg of body weight; administered as a one-time single IV infusion over 60 minutes via peripheral venous access, using an infusion pump primed with normal saline; dose volume of **Zolgensma** is calculated using the upper limit of the patient weight range for pediatric patients <2 years of age between 2.6 kg and 13.5 kg; dose volume for pediatric patients <2 years of age weighing ≥13.6 kg requires a combination of **Zolgensma** kits; refer to the **Zolgensma** dosing table (dose volume in ml for weight range in kg) in the mfr pkg insert; starting 1 day prior to the infusion, administer systemic corticosteroids equivalent to oral *prednisolone* at 1 mg/kg of body weight per day and continue for a total of 30 days; then assess liver function by clinical examination and by laboratory testing; for patients with unremarkable findings, taper the corticosteroid dose over the next 28 days; if liver function abnormalities persist, continue systemic corticosteroids (equivalent to oral *prednisolone* at 1 mg/kg/day) until findings become unremarkable, and then taper the corticosteroid dose over the next 28 days; consult medical expert(s) if the patient does not respond adequately to the equivalent of 1 mg/kg/day oral *prednisolone*

Zolgensma *Vial:* 5.5, 8.3 ml/vial (2-9 vials/kit); keep the kit frozen until infusion day; contents of the **Zolgensma** kit will thaw in approximately 12 hours in a refrigerator, or approximately 4 hours at room temperature; if thawed in a refrigerator, remove from refrigerator on the day of dosing; do not shake

Comment: **Zolgensma** *(onasemnogene abeparvovec-xioi)* is an adeno-associated virus vector-based gene therapy indicated for the treatment of pediatric patients <2 years of age with spinal muscular atrophy (SMA) with biallelic mutations in the survival motor neuron 1 (SMN1) gene. **Zolgensma** is designed to address the genetic root cause of SMA type 1. Safety and effectiveness of repeat administration of **Zolgensma** have not been evaluated. Use of **Zolgensma** in patients with advanced SMA (e.g., complete paralysis of limbs, permanent ventilator dependence) has not been evaluated.

SPRAIN

Comment: RICE: Rest, Ice, Compression, Elevation.

Injectable Acetaminophen *see Pain*

NSAIDs *see* Appendix I. NSAIDs online at https://connect.springerpub.com/content/reference-book/978-0-8261-7935-7/back-matter/part02/back-matter/bmatter10

Opioid Analgesics *see Pain*

Topical and Transdermal Analgesics *see Pain*

Parenteral Corticosteroids *see* Appendix L. Parenteral Corticosteroids

Oral Corticosteroids *see* Appendix K. Oral Corticosteroids

Topical Analgesic and Anesthetic Agents *see* Appendix H. Anesthetic Agents for Local Infiltration and Dermal/Mucosal Membrane Application online at https://connect.springerpub.com/content/reference-book/978-0-8261-7935-7/back-matter/part02/back-matter/bmatter9

STATUS ASTHMATICUS

Inhaled Beta-2 Agonists (Bronchodilators) *see Asthma*

Oral Beta-2 Agonists (Bronchodilators) *see Asthma*

Inhaled Anticholinergics *see Asthma*

Inhaled Anticholinergic+Beta-2 Agonist Combination *see Asthma*

Methylxanthines *see* Asthma
Parenteral Corticosteroids *see* Appendix L. Parenteral Corticosteroids
Oral Corticosteroids *see* Appendix K. Oral Corticosteroids

EPINEPHRINE

▷ *epinephrine* (G) 0.3-0.5 mg (0.3-0.5 ml of a 1:1,000 soln) SC q 20-30 minutes as needed up to 3 doses
  Pediatric: <2 years: 0.05-0.1 ml; 2-6 years: 0.1 ml; 6-12 years: 0.2 ml; all: q 20-30 minutes as needed up to 3 doses; >12 years: same as adult

ANAPHYLAXIS EMERGENCY TREATMENT KITS

▷ *epinephrine* 0.3 ml IM <u>or</u> SC in thigh; may repeat if needed
  Pediatric: 0.01 mg/kg SC <u>or</u> IM in thigh; may repeat if needed; <15 kg: <u>not</u> recommended; 15-30 kg: 0.15 mg; >30 kg: same as adult
    AdrenaClick *Autoinjector:* 0.15, 0.3 mg (1 mg/ml; 2/carton) (sulfites)
    Auvi-Q *Autoinjector:* 0.15, 0.3 mg (1 mg/ml; 2/carton w. 1 non-active training device) (sulfites)
    EpiPen *Autoinjector* 0.3 mg (epi 1:1,000, 0.3 ml (2/carton) (sulfites)
    EpiPen Jr *Autoinjector* 0.15 mg (epi 1:2,000, 0.3 ml (2/carton) (sulfites)
    Twinject *Autoinjector:* 0.15, 0.3 mg (epi 1:1,000, 2/carton) (sulfites)
▷ *epinephrine+chlorpheniramine* epinephrine 0.3 ml SC <u>or</u> IM <u>plus</u> 4 tabs chlorpheniramine by mouth
  Pediatric: infants-2 years: 0.05-0.1 ml SC <u>or</u> IM; 2-6 years: 0.15 ml SC <u>or</u> IM <u>plus</u> 1 tab chlor; 6-12 years: 0.2 ml SC <u>or</u> IM <u>plus</u> 2 tabs chlor; >12 years: same as adult
    Ana-Kit: 0.3 ml syringes of epi 1:1,000 (2/carton) for self-injection <u>plus</u> chlor 2 mg chewable tabs x 4

STATUS EPILEPTICUS

Anticonvulsant Drugs *see* Appendix Q. Anticonvulsant Drugs
▷ *diazepam* (IV) initially 5-10 mg IV in large vein; may repeat q 10-15 minutes; max 30 mg; may repeat in 2-4 hours if needed; do <u>not</u> dilute; may give IM if IV <u>not</u> accessible
  Pediatric: 1 month-5 years: 0.2-0.5 mg IV q 2-5 minutes; max 5 mg; >5 years: 1 mg IV q 2-5 minutes; max 10 mg; may repeat in 2-4 hours if needed
    Diastat *Rectal gel delivery system:* 2.5 mg
    Diastat AcuDial *Rectal gel delivery system:* 10, 20 mg
    Valium Injectable *Vial:* 5 mg/ml (10 ml); *Amp:* 5 mg/ml (2 ml); *Prefilled syringe:* 5 mg/ml (5 ml)
    Valium Intensol Oral Solution *Conc oral soln:* 5 mg/ml (30 ml w. dropper) (alcohol 19%)
    Valium Oral Solution *Oral soln:* 5 mg/5 ml (500 ml) (wintergreen-spice)
▷ *diazepam nasal spray* (IV) *Initial dose:* 5 mg and 10 mg doses are administered as a single spray intranasally into one nostril (administration of 15 mg and 20 mg doses requires two nasal spray devices, one spray into each nostril); *Second dose:* when required, may be administered at least 4 hours after the initial dose; if administered, use a new blister pack; *Max dose and treatment frequency:* do <u>not</u> use more than 2 doses to treat a single episode; it is recommended that **Valtoco** be used to treat <u>no more</u> than one episode every 5 days and <u>no more</u> than five episodes per month
  Pediatric: <6 years: <u>not</u> established; ≥6 years: dosage is dependent on the patient's age and weight (see mfr pkg insert)
    Valtoco *Nasal spray:* 5, 7.5, 10 mg in 0.1 ml, single-dose
    Comment: Valtoco is a benzodiazepine indicated for the acute treatment of intermittent, stereotypic episodes of frequent seizure activity (i.e., seizure clusters, acute repetitive seizures) that are distinct from the patient's usual seizure pattern in patients with epilepsy 6 years of age and older. Benzodiazepines may cause an increased central nervous system (CNS) depressant effect when used with alcohol <u>or</u> other CNS depressants. Antiepileptic drugs (AEDs) increase the risk of suicidal ideation and behavior. **Valtoco** is contraindicated in patients with acute narrow-angle glaucoma. The most common adverse reactions (incidence 4%) have been somnolence, headache, and nasal discomfort. Concomitant CYP2C19 and CYP3A4 inhibitors may increase adverse reactions to **Valtoco**. Concomitant CYP2C19 and CYP3A4 inducers may decrease *diazepam* exposure. Advise pregnant females and women of childbearing age of potentially serious embryo/fetal risk. *Diazepam* is excreted in human milk. There are <u>no</u> data to assess the effects of **Valtoco** and/<u>or</u> its active metabolite(s) on the breastfed infant. Postmarketing experience suggests that breastfed infants of mothers taking benzodiazepines, such as **Valtoco**, may have effects of lethargy, somnolence, and poor sucking. There is a pregnancy exposure registry that monitors pregnancy outcomes in women exposed to antiepileptic drugs (AEDs), such as **Valtoco**, during pregnancy. Encourage women who are taking **Valtoco** during pregnancy to enroll in the North American Antiepileptic Drug (NAAED) Pregnancy Registry by calling 1-888-233-2334 <u>or</u> http://www.aedpregnancyregistry.org.
▷ *lorazepam* injectable (IV) 4 mg IV over 2 minutes (dilute first); may repeat in 10-15 minutes; may give IM if needed (undiluted)
  Pediatric: <18 years: <u>not</u> recommended; ≥18 years: same as adult
    Ativan Injectable *Vial:* 2 mg/ml (1, 10 ml); *Tubex:* 2 mg/ml (0.5 ml); *Cartridge:* 2, 4 mg/ml (1 ml)

(continued)

▷ *midazolam* (IV) *Initial dose:* 1 spray (5 mg) into one nostril; *Second dose:* 1 additional spray (5 mg) into the opposite nostril may be administered after 10 minutes if the patient has not responded to the initial dose; *Maximum dose and treatment frequency:* do not use more than 2 doses to treat a seizure cluster; it is recommended that **Nayzilam** be used to treat no more than one episode every 3 days and treat no more than five episodes per month
  Pediatric: <12 years: not established; ≥12 years: same as adult
    Nayzilam *Nasal spray:* 5 mg/0.1 ml, single dose, nasal spray unit
    Comment: Nayzilam (*midazolam*) is a nasally administered benzodiazepine indicated for the acute treatment of intermittent, stereotypic episodes of frequent seizure activity (i.e., seizure clusters, acute repetitive seizures) that are distinct from the patient's usual seizure pattern in patients with epilepsy 12 years of age and older. **Nayzilam** is contraindicated in patients with narrow-angle glaucoma. **Nayzilam** may cause an increased CNS depressant effect when used with alcohol or other CNS depressants. Concomitant use with moderate or strong CYP3A4 inhibitors may result in prolonged sedation because of a decrease in plasma clearance of *midazolam*. AEDs increase the risk of suicidal ideation and behavior. *Midazolam* is associated with a high incidence of partial or complete impairment of recall for the next several hours. Based on animal data, *midazolam* may cause fetal harm. *Midazolam* is excreted in human milk and effects on the breastfed infant are unknown. Patients with renal impairment may have a longer elimination half-life for *midazolam* and its metabolites which may result in prolonged exposure.
▷ *phenytoin (injectable)* (G) 10-15 mg/kg IV, not to exceed 50 mg/minute; follow with 100 mg orally or IV q 6-8 hours; do not dilute in IV fluid
  Pediatric: 15-20 mg/kg IV, not to exceed 1-2 mg/kg/min
    Dilantin *Vial:* 50 mg/ml (2, 5 ml); *Amp:* 50 mg/ml (2 ml)
    Comment: Monitor *phenytoin* serum levels. Therapeutic serum level is 10-20 gm/ml. Side effects include gingival hyperplasia.

STYE (HORDEOLUM)

OPHTHALMIC ANTI-INFECTIVES
▷ *erythromycin* ophthalmic ointment 1 cm up to 6 x/day
  Pediatric: same as adult
    Ilotycin Ophthalmic Ointment *Ophth oint:* 5 mg/gm (1/8 oz)
▷ *erythromycin* ophthalmic solution initially 1-2 drops q 1-2 hours; may then increase dose interval
  Pediatric: same as adult
    Isopto Cetamide Ophthalmic Solution *Ophth soln:* 15% (15 ml)
▷ *gentamicin* ophthalmic ointment 1 cm bid-tid
  Pediatric: same as adult
    Garamycin Ophthalmic Ointment *Ophth oint:* 3 mg/gm (3.5 gm)
    Genoptic Ophthalmic Ointment *Ophth oint:* 3 mg/gm (3.5 gm)
    Gentacidin Ophthalmic Ointment *Ophth oint:* 3 mg/gm (3.5 gm)
▷ *polymyxin b+bacitracin* ophthalmic ointment apply 1/2 inch q 3-4 hours
  Pediatric: same as adult
    Polysporin *Ophth oint:* poly b 10,000 U+bac 500 units per gm (3.75 gm)
▷ *polymyxin b+bacitracin+neomycin* ophthalmic ointment (G) apply 1/2 inch q 3-4 hours
  Pediatric: same as adult
    Neosporin Ophthalmic Ointment *Ophth oint:* poly b 10,000 U+bac 400 U+neo 3.5 mg/gm (3.75 gm)
▷ *polymyxin b+neomycin+gramicidin* ophthalmic solution 1-2 drops 2-3 times q 1 hour; then 1-2 drops bid-qid x 7-10 days
  Pediatric: same as adult
    Neosporin Ophthalmic Solution
    Ophth soln: poly b 10,000 U+neo 1.75 mg/gm 0.025 mg/ml (10 ml)
▷ *sodium sulfacetamide* ophthalmic solution and ointment
    Bleph-10 Ophthalmic Solution 2 drops q 4 hour x 7-14 days
    Pediatric: <2 years: not recommended; ≥2 years: 1-2 drops q 2-3 hours during the day
      Ophth soln: 10% (2.5, 5, 15 ml; benzalkonium chloride)
    Bleph-10 Ophthalmic Ointment apply 1/2 inch qid and HS
    Pediatric: <2 years: not recommended; ≥2 years: apply 1/4-1/3 inch qid and HS
      Ophth oint: 10% (3.5 gm) (phenylmercuric acetate)

SUNBURN

▷ *prednisone* (G) 10 mg qid x 4-6 days if severe and extensive
▷ *silver sulfadiazine* (G) apply topically to burn once daily-bid
  Pediatric: <12 years: not recommended; ≥12 years: same as adult

Silvadene Crm: 1% (20, 50, 85, 400, 1,000 gm jar; 20 gm tube)

Comment: *Silver sulfadiazine* is contradicted in sulfa allergy, late pregnancy, within the first 2 months after birth, and premature infants.

SYPHILIS (*TREPONEMA PALLIDUM*)

Comment: The following treatment regimens for *Treponema pallidum* are published in the **2021 CDC Sexually Transmitted Diseases Treatment Guidelines.** Treat all sexual contacts. Consider testing for other sexually transmitted infections (STIs). *Penicillin g,* administered parenterally, is the preferred drug for treating all stages of syphilis. The preparation used (i.e., benzathine, aqueous procaine, or aqueous crystalline), the dosage, and the length of treatment depend on the stage and clinical manifestations of the disease. Combinations of *benzathine penicillin, procaine penicillin,* and oral *penicillin* preparations are not appropriate (e.g., **Bicillin C-R**). All women should be screened serologically for syphilis early in pregnancy. There are no proven alternatives to *penicillin* for the treatment of syphilis during pregnancy. Pregnant patients who are allergic to penicillin should be desensitized and treated with *penicillin.* Sexual transmission of *T. pallidum* is thought to occur only when mucocutaneous syphilitic lesions are present. Such manifestations are uncommon after the first year of infection. Persons exposed through sexual contact with a person who has primary, secondary, or early latent syphilis at any stage should be evaluated clinically and serologically and treated with a recommended regimen according to CDC guidelines.

PRIMARY, SECONDARY, AND EARLY LATENT (<1 YEAR) SYPHILIS
Regimen 1
➤ *penicillin g (benzathine)* 2.4 million units IM in a single dose

LATE LATENT, LATENT SYPHILIS OF UNKNOWN DURATION, AND TERTIARY SYPHILIS
Regimen 1
➤ *penicillin g (benzathine)* 7.2 million units total administered in 3 divided doses of 2.4 million units each IM at 1-week intervals

REGIMEN: ADULT, NEUROSYPHILIS
Regimen 1
➤ *aqueous crystalline penicillin g* 18-24 million units per day, administered as 3-4 million units IV q 4 hours or continuous IV infusion, for 10-14 days

ALTERNATIVE REGIMEN: ADULT, NEUROSYPHILIS
Regimen 1
➤ *penicillin g (procaine)* 2.4 million units IM once daily x 10-14 days plus *probenecid* 500 mg qid x 10-14 days

PRIMARY AND SECONDARY SYPHILIS IN HIV-INFECTED PERSONS
Regimen 1
➤ *penicillin g (benzathine)* 2.4 million units IM in a single dose

LATENT SYPHILIS AMONG HIV-INFECTED PERSONS
Comment: Treatment is the same as for HIV-negative persons.

CONGENITAL SYPHILIS
Regimen 1
➤ *aqueous crystalline penicillin g* 100,000-150,000 units/kg/day, administered as 50,000 units IV q 12 hours during the first 7 days of life and q 8 hours thereafter for a total of 10 days

ALTERNATE REGIMEN
Regimen 1
➤ *penicillin g (benzathine)* 50,000 units/kg IM in a single dose

Regimen 2
➤ *penicillin g (procaine)* 50,000 units/kg/dose IM, administered in a single daily dose x 10 days

OLDER INFANTS AND CHILDREN
Regimen 1
➤ *aqueous crystalline penicillin g* 200,000-300,000 units/kg/day, administered as 50,000 units IV q 12 hours during the first 7 days of life and every 4-6 hours thereafter for a total of 10 days

DRUG BRANDS AND DOSE FORMS
➤ *aqueous crystalline penicillin g* (G)

(continued)

▷ *penicillin g (benzathine)* (G)
  Bicillin L-A *Cartridge-needle unit:* 600,000 million units (1 ml); 1.2 million units (2 ml); 2.4 million units (4 ml)
▷ *penicillin g (procaine)* (G)
  Bicillin C-R *Cartridge-needle unit:* 600,000 units (1 ml); 1.2 million units (2 ml); 2.4 million units (4 ml)
▷ *probenecid* (G)
  Benemid *Tab:* 500*mg; *Cap:* 500 mg

SYSTEMIC LUPUS ERYTHEMATOSUS (SLE)

NSAIDs *see* Appendix I. NSAIDs online at https://connect.springerpub.com/content/reference-book/978-0-8261-7935-7/back-matter/part02/back-matter/bmatter10
Oral Corticosteroids *see* Appendix K. Oral Corticosteroids

Comment: All systemic lupus erythematosus (SLE) patients should routinely be given *hydroxychloroquine* (HCQ) and supplemental vitamin D as low levels of vitamin D are associated with higher rates of end-stage renal disease (ESRD); supplemental vitamin D reduces urine protein (the best predictor of future renal failure). Vitamin D insufficiency and deficiency are more common in patients with SLE than in the general population. Vitamin D supplementation may decrease disease activity and improve fatigue. In addition, supplementation may improve endothelial function, which may reduce cardiovascular disease. A disease-modifying antirheumatic drug (DMARD) should be added when the patient's prednisone dose cannot be tapered and also when hemolysis is present and hemoglobin is abnormally low in the setting of mild-to-moderate hematologic involvement. Other DMARDs, such as *methotrexate* (MTX), *azathioprine, mycophenolate mofetil* (MMF), *cyclosporine* (CYC), and other calcineurin inhibitors should be considered in cases of arthritis, cutaneous disease, serositis, vasculitis, or cytopenia if HCQ is insufficient. For refractory cases, *belimumab* (Benlysta) or *rituximab* (Rituxan) may be considered. The recommended dose of *rituximab*, if required, is either 750 mg/m^2 (to a maximum of 1 gm/day) at day 1 and day 15, or 375 mg/m^2 once a week for 4 doses. In patients with SLE without major organ manifestations, glucocorticoids and antimalarial agents may be beneficial. Non-steroidal anti-inflammatory drugs (NSAIDs) may be used for short periods in patients at low risk for complications from these drugs. Consider immunosuppressive agents (e.g., *azathioprine*, MMF, MTX), in refractory cases or when steroid doses cannot be reduced to levels for long-term use.

CD20 ANTIBODY

▷ *rituximab* administer corticosteroid 30 minutes prior to each infusion; concomitant *methotrexate* (MTX) therapy, administer a 1,000 mg IV infusion at 0 and 2 weeks; then q 24 weeks or based on response, but not sooner than q 16 weeks
  Pediatric: <6 years: not recommended; >6 years: same as adult
    Rituxan *Vial:* 100 mg/10 ml (10 mg/ml), 500 mg/50 ml (10 mg/ml), single-use (preservative-free)

B-LYMPHOCYTE STIMULATOR (BLyS)-SPECIFIC INHIBITOR

Comment: Benlysta was initially approved as an IV formulation administered in a hospital or clinic setting as a weight-dosed IV infusion every 4 weeks. Patients can now self-administer **Benlysta** as a once-weekly SC injection after being trained by a healthcare provider.
▷ *belimumab SC administration:* 200 mg SC once weekly; may be self-administered by the patient in the home setting; *IV infusion:* 10 mg/kg at 2-week intervals for the first 3 doses and at 4-week intervals thereafter; reconstitute, dilute, and administer as an IV infusion over a period of 1 hour; consider administering premedication for prophylaxis against infusion reactions and hypersensitivity reactions; must be administered in a hospital or clinic setting by a qualified healthcare provider
  Pediatric: <5 years: not established; ≥5 years: same as adult
    Benlysta *Prefilled syringe:* 200 mg/ml (1 ml), single-dose (4/carton); *Autoinjector:* 200 mg (1 ml), single-dose (4/carton); *Vial:* 120 mg/5 ml, 400 mg/ 20 ml, single-dose, pwdr for reconstitution and IV infusion (4/carton)
    Comment: Benlysta is indicated for the treatment of patients with active, autoantibody-positive, SLE who are receiving standard therapy. Common adverse reactions include nausea, diarrhea, pyrexia, nasopharyngitis, bronchitis, insomnia, pain in extremity, depression, migraine, and pharyngitis. The efficacy of **Benlysta** has not been evaluated in patients with severe active lupus nephritis or severe active central nervous system lupus. **Benlysta** has not been studied in combination with other biologics or IV *cyclophosphamide*. Therefore, use of **Benlysta** is not recommended in these situations. Limited data on use of **Benlysta** in pregnancy women, from observational studies, published case reports, and postmarketing surveillance, are insufficient to determine whether there is a drug-associated risk of major birth defects or miscarriage. Monoclonal antibodies, such as *belimumab,* are actively transported across the placenta during the third trimester of pregnancy and may affect immune response in the *in utero*-exposed infant. Monoclonal antibodies are increasingly transported across the placenta as pregnancy progresses, with the largest amount transferred during the third

trimester. No information is available on the presence of *belimumab* in human milk or the effects of the drug on the breastfed infant. As there are risks to the mother and the fetus associated with SLE, risks and benefits should be considered prior to administering live or live attenuated vaccines to infants exposed to **Benlysta** *in utero*. Monitor the infant of a treated mother for B-cell reduction and other immune dysfunction. There is a pregnancy exposure registry that monitors pregnancy outcomes in females exposed to **Benlysta** during pregnancy. Healthcare professionals are encouraged to register patients by calling 1-877-681-6296.

TYPE I INTERFERON (IFN) RECEPTOR ANTAGONIST

▶ *anifrolumab Recommended dose:* 300 mg via IV infusion 30 minutes q 4 weeks; see mfr pkg insert for complete dilution and IV administration instructions
  Pediatric: <18 years: safety and efficacy not established; ≥18 years: same as adult
    Saphnelo *Vial:* 300 mg/2 ml (150 mg/ml), single-dose, soln for dilution and IV infusion
    Comment: Saphnelo is a type I interferon (IFN) receptor antagonist indicated for the treatment of adult patients with moderate-to-severe SLE who are receiving standard therapy. Efficacy of **Saphnelo** has not been evaluated in patients with severe active lupus nephritis or severe active central nervous system lupus; **Saphnelo** is not recommended in these situations. **Saphnelo** is contraindicated in patients with a history of anaphylaxis with *anifrolumab-fnia*. The most common adverse drug reactions (incidence ≥5%) have been nasopharyngitis, upper respiratory tract infections (URIs), bronchitis, infusion-related reactions, herpes zoster, and cough. Serious and sometimes fatal infections have occurred in patients receiving **Saphnelo**. **Saphnelo** increases the risk of respiratory infections and herpes zoster. Avoid initiating treatment during an active infection. Consider the individual benefit/risk if using in patients with severe or chronic infections. Consider interrupting therapy with **Saphnelo** if patients develop a new infection during treatment. Serious hypersensitivity reactions, including anaphylaxis and angioedema, have been reported. Consider the individual benefit/risk in patients with known risk factors for malignancy prior to prescribing **Saphnelo**. Avoid use of live or live attenuated vaccines in patients receiving **Saphnelo**. **Saphnelo** is not recommended for use with other biologic therapies. Pregnant women with SLE are at increased risk of adverse pregnancy outcomes, including worsening of the underlying disease, premature birth, miscarriage, and intrauterine growth restriction. Maternal lupus nephritis increases the risk of hypertension and preeclampsia/eclampsia. Passage of maternal autoantibodies across the placenta may result in adverse neonatal outcomes, including neonatal lupus and congenital heart block. In animal studies, there was no evidence of *anifrolumab-fnia*-related maternal toxicity, embryo/fetal toxicity, or postnatal developmental effects. No *anifrolumab-fnia*-related effect on T-cell-dependent antibody response in the infants was noted up to Day 180. *Anifrolumab-fnia* was detected in the milk of female cynomolgus monkeys. Due to species-species differences in lactation physiology, animal data may not reliably predict drug levels in humans. Maternal immunoglobulin G (IgG) is known to be present in human milk. If *anifrolumab-fnia* is transferred into human milk, the effects of local gastrointestinal exposure and limited systemic exposure in the breastfed infant are unknown. The developmental and health benefits of breastfeeding should be considered along with the mother's clinical need for *anifrolumab-fnia* and any potential adverse effects on the breastfed child from *anifrolumab-fnia* or from the underlying maternal condition.

DISEASE MODIFYING ANTIRHEUMATIC DRUGS (DMARDS)

Comment: DMARDs include *penicillamine*, gold salts (*auranofin, aurothioglucose*), immunosuppressants, and *hydroxychloroquine* (HCQ). The DMARDs reduce erythrocyte sedimentation rate (ESR), reduce rheumatoid factor (RF), and favorably affect SLE symptoms. Immunosuppressants may require 6 weeks to see some improvement and 6 months for full improvement.

▶ *auranofin (gold salt)* 3 mg bid or 6 mg once daily; if inadequate response after 6 months, increase to 3 mg tid
  Pediatric: <12 years: not recommended; ≥12 years: same as adult
    Ridaura *Vial:* 100 mg/20 ml
▶ *azathioprine* 1 mg/kg/day in a single or divided doses; may increase by 0.5 mg/kg/day q 4 weeks; max 2.5 mg/kg/day; minimum trial to ascertain effectiveness is 12 weeks
  Pediatric: <12 years: not recommended; ≥12 years: same as adult
    Azasan *Tab* 75*, 100*mg
    Imuran *Tab* 50*mg
▶ *cyclosporine (immunosuppressant)* 1.25 mg/kg bid; may increase after 4 weeks by 0.5 mg/kg/day; then adjust at 2-week intervals; max 4 mg/kg/day; administer with meals
  Pediatric: <12 years: not recommended; ≥12 years: same as adult
    Neoral *Cap:* 25, 100 mg (alcohol)
    Neoral Oral Solution *Oral soln:* 100 mg/ml (50 ml), may dilute in room temperature apple juice or orange juice (alcohol)
    Comment: Neoral is indicated for rheumatoid arthritis (RA) unresponsive to *methotrexate (MTX)*.
▶ *leflunomide* (G) initially 100 mg once daily x 3 days; maintenance dose 20 mg once daily; max 20 mg daily
  Pediatric: <18 years: not recommended; ≥18 years: same as adult
    Arava *Tab:* 10, 20, 100 mg
    Comment: Arava is contraindicated with breastfeeding.

(continued)

▶ *methotrexate (MTX)* 7.5 mg x 1 dose per week <u>or</u> 2.5 mg x 3 at 12-hour intervals once a week; max 20 mg/ week; therapeutic response begins in 3-6 weeks; administer *methotrexate (MTX)* injection SC <u>only</u> into the abdomen <u>or</u> thigh

Pediatric: <2 years: <u>not</u> recommended; ≥2 years: 10 mg/m² once weekly; max 20 mg/m²

    Rasuvo *Autoinjector:* 7.5 mg/0.15 ml, 10 mg/0.20 ml, 12.5 mg/0.25 ml, 15 mg/0.30 ml, 17.5 mg/0.35 ml, 20 mg/0.40 ml, 22.5 mg/0.45 ml, 25 mg/0.50 ml, 27.5 mg/0.55 ml, 30 mg/0.60 ml (solution concentration for SC injection is 50 mg/ml)

    Rheumatrex *Tab:* 2.5*mg (5, 7.5, 10, 12.5, 15 mg/week, 4/card unit-of-use dose pack)

    Trexall *Tab:* 5*, 7.5*, 10*, 15*mg (5, 7.5, 10, 12.5, 15 mg/week, 4/card unit-of-use dose pack)

Comment: *Methotrexate (MTX)* is contraindicated with immunodeficiency, blood dyscrasias, alcoholism, and chronic liver disease.

▶ *penicillamine* administer on an empty stomach, at least 1 hour before meals <u>or</u> 2 hours after meals, <u>and</u> at least 1 hour apart from any other drug, food, milk, antacid, and zinc- <u>or</u> iron-containing preparation; maintenance dosage must be individualized and may require adjustment during the course of treatment; *initially* a single daily dose of 125-250 mg; then increase at 1 to 3-month intervals by 125-250 mg/day, as patient response and tolerance indicate; if a satisfactory remission of symptoms is achieved, the dose associated with the remission should be continued as the patient's maintenance therapy; if there is <u>no</u> improvement and there are <u>no</u> signs of potentially serious toxicity after 2-3 months of treatment with doses of 500-750 mg/day, increase by 250 mg/day at 2 to 3-month intervals until a satisfactory remission occurs <u>or</u> signs of toxicity develop; if there is <u>no</u> discernible improvement after 3-4 months of treatment with 1,000-1,500 mg/day, discontinue **Cuprimine**; changes in maintenance dosage levels may <u>not</u> be reflected clinically <u>or</u> in the ESR for 2-3 months after each dosage adjustment

    Cuprimine *Cap:* 125, 250 mg

    Depen: 250 mg

Comment: The use of *penicillamine* has been associated with fatalities due to certain diseases such as aplastic anemia, agranulocytosis, thrombocytopenia, Goodpasture's syndrome, and myasthenia gravis. Because of the potential for serious hematologic and renal adverse reactions to occur at any time, routine urinalysis, white and differential blood cell count, hemoglobin, and direct platelet count must be checked twice weekly, together with monitoring of the patient's skin, lymph nodes and body temperature, during the first month of therapy, every 2 weeks for the next 5 months, and monthly thereafter. Patients should be instructed to report promptly the development of signs and symptoms of granulocytopenia <u>and/or</u> thrombocytopenia such as fever, sore throat, chills, bruising <u>or</u> bleeding; the above laboratory studies should then be promptly repeated.

▶ *sulfasalazine* (G) initially 0.5 gm once daily bid; gradually increase every 4 days; usual maintenance 2-3 gm/ day in equally divided doses at regular intervals; max 4 gm/day

Pediatric: <6 years: <u>not</u> recommended; 6-16 years: initially 1/4 to 1/3 of maintenance dose; increase weekly; maintenance 30-50 mg/kg/day in 2 divided doses at regular intervals; max 2 gm/day

    Azulfidine *Tab:* 500 mg

    Azulfidine EN *Tab:* 500 mg ent-coat

ANTIMALARIALS

▶ *atovaquone* (G) take as a single dose with food <u>or</u> a milky drink at the same time each day; repeat dose if vomited within 1 hour; *Prophylaxis:* 1,500 mg once daily; *Treatment:* 750 mg bid x 21 days

Pediatric: <13 years: <u>not</u> established; ≥13 years: same as adult

    Mepron *Susp:* 750 mg/5 ml

▶ *atovaquone+proguanil* (G) >40 kg: take as a single dose with food <u>or</u> a milky drink at the same time each day; repeat dose if vomited within 1 hour; *Prophylaxis:* 1 tab daily starting 1-2 days before entering endemic area, during stay, and for 7 days after return; *Treatment (acute, uncomplicated):* 4 tabs daily x 3 days

Pediatric: <5 kg: <u>not</u> recommended; 5-40 kg: *Prophylaxis:* daily dose starting 1-2 days before entering endemic area, during stay, and for 7 days after return; 5-20 kg: 1 ped tab; 21-30 kg: 2 ped tabs; 31-40 kg: 3 ped tabs; ≥40 kg: same as adult; *Treatment (acute, uncomplicated):* daily dose x 3 days; 5-8 kg: 2 ped tabs; 9-10 kg: 3 ped tabs; 11-20 kg: 1 adult tab; 21-30 kg: 2 adult tabs; 31-40 kg: 3 adult tabs; >40 kg: same as adult

    Malarone *Tab:* atov 250 mg+prog 100 mg

    Malarone Pediatric *Tab:* atov 62.5 mg+prog 25 mg

Comment: *Atovaquone* is antagonized by *tetracycline* and *metoclopramide*. Concomitant *rifampin* is <u>not</u> recommended (may elevate liver function tests [LFTs]).

▶ *chloroquine* (G) *Prophylaxis:* 500 mg once weekly (on the same day of each week); start 2 weeks prior to exposure, continue while in the endemic area, and continue 4 weeks after departure; *Treatment:* initially 1 gm; then 500 mg 6 hours, 24 hours, and 48 hours after initial dose <u>or</u> initially 200-250 mg IM; may repeat in 6 hours; max 1 gm in the first 24 hours; continue to 1.875 gm in 3 days

Pediatric: *Suppression:* 8.35 mg/kg (max 500 mg) weekly (on the same day of each week); *Treatment:* initially 16.7 mg/kg (max 1 gm); then 8.35 mg/kg (max 500 mg) 6 hours, 24 hours, and 48 hours after initial dose, <u>or</u> initially 6.25 mg/kg IM; may repeat in 6 hours; max 12.5 mg/kg/day

    Aralen *Tab:* 500 mg; *Amp:* 50 mg/ml (5 ml)

Comment: There are no adequate and well-controlled studies evaluating the safety and efficacy of *chloroquine* in pregnant females. Usage of *chloroquine* during pregnancy should be avoided except in the suppression or treatment of malaria when the benefit outweighs the potential risk to the fetus. Because of the potential for serious adverse reactions in nursing infants from *chloroquine*, a decision should be made whether to discontinue nursing or to discontinue the drug, taking into account the potential clinical benefit of the drug to the mother. Since this drug is known to concentrate in the liver, it should be used with caution in patients with hepatic disease or alcoholism or in conjunction with known hepatotoxic drugs.

▶ *hydroxychloroquine* (G) 400-600 mg/day
Pediatric: <12 years: not recommended; ≥12 years: same as adult
   Plaquenil *Tab:* 200 mg
Comment: May require several weeks to achieve beneficial effects. If no improvement in 6 months, discontinue.

▶ *mefloquine Prophylaxis:* 250 mg once weekly (on the same day of each week); start 1 week prior to exposure, continue while in the endemic area and continue for 4 weeks after departure; *Treatment:* 1,250 mg as a single dose
Pediatric: <6 months: not recommended; *Prophylaxis:* ≥6 months: 3-5 mg/kg (max 250 mg) weekly (on the same day of each week); start 1 week prior to exposure, continue while in the endemic area and continue for 4 weeks after departure; *Treatment:* ≥6 months: 25-50 mg/kg as a single dose; max 250 mg
   Lariam *Tab:* 250*mg
Comment: *Mefloquine* is contraindicated with active or recent history of depression, generalized anxiety disorder, psychosis, schizophrenia or any other psychiatric disorder, or history of convulsions.

▶ *quinine sulfate* (G) 1 tab or cap q 8 hours x 7 days
Pediatric: <16 years: not recommended; ≥16 years: same as adult
   quinine sulfate Tab: 260 mg; *Cap:* 260, 300, 325 mg
   Qualaquin *Cap:* 324 mg
Comment: *Qualaquin* is indicated in the treatment of uncomplicated *Plasmodium falciparum* malaria (including *chloroquine*-resistant strains).

TAKAYASU ARTERITIS (TA)

Comment: Takayasu arteritis is a rare yet well-described large-vessel vasculitis with a predilection for the aorta and its primary branches. Treatment options focus on preventing disease progression. There is no consensus on regimen, but high-dose pulse corticosteroid therapy is favored for induction, and long-term therapy includes immunosuppressants and biologics such as *cyclophosphamide, mycophenolate mofetil, methotrexate (MTX), infliximab,* or *tocilizumab,* as well as revascularization surgery. Disease recurrence is common, and mortality rates can range from 16% to 40%. Therefore, prompt identification and treatment is imperative to prevent further morbidity and mortality.

TAPEWORM (CESTODE)

ANTHELMINTICS
Comment: Oral bioavailability of anthelmintics is enhanced when administered with a fatty meal (estimated fat content 40 gm).

▶ *albendazole* (G) take with a meal; may crush and mix with food; 400 mg bid x 7 days; may repeat in 3 weeks if needed
Pediatric: <2 years: 200 mg once daily x 3 days; may repeat in 3 weeks; ≥2-12 years: 400 mg once daily x 3 days; may repeat in 3 weeks; ≥12 years: same as adult
   Albenza *Tab:* 200 mg
Comment: *Albendazole* is a broad-spectrum benzimidazole carbamate anthelmintic.

▶ *nitazoxanide* (G) take with a meal; may crush and mix with food; 500 mg q 12 hours x 3 days
Pediatric: <12 months: not recommended; ≥12 months: treat q 12 hours x 3 days; <11 years: (susp) 12-47 months: 5 ml; 4-11 years: 10 ml; ≥11 years: (tab/susp) 500 mg
   Alinia *Tab:* 500 mg; *Oral susp:* 100 mg/5 ml (60 ml)

▶ *praziquantel* (G) take with a meal; may crush and mix with food; 5-10 mg/kg as a single dose
Pediatric: <4 years: not established; ≥4 years: same as adult
   Biltricide *Tab:* 600 mg film-coat (scored for half or quarter dose)
Comment: Therapeutically effective levels of **Biltricide** may not be achieved when administered concomitantly with strong P450 inducers, such as *rifampin*. Females should not breastfeed on the day of Biltricide treatment and during the subsequent 72 hours. Use caution with hepatosplenic patients who have moderate-to-severe liver impairment (Child-Pugh Class B and C).

TARDIVE DYSKINESIA (TD)

Comment: Tardive dyskinesia is a treatable, albeit irreversible, neurologic disorder characterized by repetitive involuntary movements, usually of the jaw, lips, and tongue, such as grimacing, sticking out the tongue, and smacking the lips. Some affected people also experience involuntary movement of the extremities or difficulty breathing. This condition is most often an adverse side effect associated with the older "typical" antipsychotic drugs. Risk is decreased with the newer "atypical" antipsychotic drugs. The first and only FDA-approved treatment for this disorder is *valbenazine* (Ingrezza), a vesicular monoamine transporter 2 (VMAT2) inhibitor.

VESICULAR MONOAMINE TRANSPORTER 2 (VMAT2) INHIBITOR

▷ *valbenazine* initially 40 mg once daily; after 1 week, increase to the recommended 80 mg once daily; take with or without food; recommended dose for patients with moderate or severe hepatic impairment is 40 mg once daily; consider dose reduction based on tolerability in known CYP2D6 poor metabolizers; concomitant use of strong CYP3A4 inducers is not recommended; avoid concomitant use of monoamine oxidase inhibitors (MAOIs)

Pediatric: <18 years: not established; ≥18 years: same as adult

    Ingrezza *Cap:* 40 mg

    Comment: Safety and effectiveness of **Ingrezza** have not been established in pediatric patients. No dose adjustment is required for elderly patients. The limited available data on **Ingrezza** use in pregnant females are insufficient to inform a drug-associated risk. There is no information regarding the presence of **Ingrezza** or its metabolites in human milk, the effects on the breastfed infant, or the effects on milk production. However, women are advised not to breastfeed during treatment and for 5 days after the final dose.

TEMPOROMANDIBULAR JOINT (TMJ) DISORDER

Injectable Acetaminophen *see Pain*
NSAIDs *see* Appendix I. NSAIDs online at https://connect.springerpub.com/content/reference-book/978-0-8261-7935-7/back-matter/part02/back-matter/bmatter10
Opioid Analgesics *see Pain*
Topical and Transdermal Analgesics *see Pain*
Parenteral Corticosteroids *see* Appendix L. Parenteral Corticosteroids
Oral Corticosteroids *see* Appendix K. Oral Corticosteroids
Topical Analgesic and Anesthetic Agents *see* Appendix H. Anesthetic Agents for Local Infiltration and Dermal/Mucosal Membrane Application online at https://connect.springerpub.com/content/reference-book/978-0-8261-7935-7/back-matter/part02/back-matter/bmatter9

SKELETAL MUSCLE RELAXANTS

▷ *baclofen* (G) 5 mg tid; titrate up by 5 mg every 3 days to 20 mg tid; max 80 mg/day

    Pediatric: <12 years: not recommended; ≥12 years: same as adult

        Lioresal *Tab:* 10*, 20*mg

    Comment: *Baclofen* is indicated for muscle spasm pain and chronic spasticity associated with multiple sclerosis and spinal cord injury or disease. Potential for seizures or hallucinations on abrupt withdrawal.

▷ *carisoprodol* (G) 1 tab tid or qid

    Pediatric: <12 years: not recommended; ≥12 years: same as adult

        Soma *Tab:* 350 mg

▷ *chlorzoxazone* (G) 1 caplet qid; max 750 mg qid

    Pediatric: <12 years: not recommended; ≥12 years: same as adult

        Parafon Forte DSC *Cplt:* 500*mg

▷ *cyclobenzaprine* (G) 10 mg tid; usual range 20-40 mg/day in divided doses; max 60 mg/day x 2-3 weeks or 15 mg ext-rel once daily; max 30 mg ext-rel/day x 2-3 weeks

    Pediatric: <15 years: not recommended; ≥15 years: same as adult

        Amrix *Cap:* 15, 30 mg ext-rel

        Fexmid *Tab:* 7.5 mg

        Flexeril *Tab:* 5, 10 mg

▷ *dantrolene* 25 mg daily x 7 days; then 25 mg tid x 7 days; then 50 mg tid x 7 days; max 100 mg qid

    Pediatric: 0.5 mg/kg daily x 7 days; then 0.5 mg/kg tid x 7 days; then 1 mg/kg tid x 7 days; then 2 mg/kg tid; max 100 mg qid

        Dantrium *Tab:* 25, 50, 100 mg

    Comment: *Dantrolene* is indicated for chronic spasticity associated with multiple sclerosis and spinal cord injury or disease.

▷ *diazepam* (IV) 2-10 mg bid-qid; may increase gradually

    Pediatric: <6 months: not recommended; ≥6 months: initially 1-2.5 mg bid-qid; may increase gradually

        Diastat *Rectal gel delivery system:* 2.5 mg

        Diastat AcuDial *Rectal gel delivery system:* 10, 20 mg

Valium *Tab:* 2, 5, 10 mg
Valium Intensol Oral Solution *Conc oral soln:* 5 mg/ml (30 ml w. dropper) (alcohol 19%)
Valium Oral Solution *Oral soln:* 5 mg/5 ml (500 ml) (wintergreen spice)
➤ *metaxalone* 1 tab tid-qid
Pediatric: <12 years: not recommended; ≥12 years: same as adult
Skelaxin *Tab:* 800*mg
➤ *methocarbamol* (G) initially 1.5 gm qid x 2-3 days; maintenance, 750 mg qid or 1.5 gm tid; max 8 gm/day
Pediatric: <16 years: not recommended; ≥16 years: same as adult
Robaxin *Tab:* 500 mg
Robaxin 750 *Tab:* 750 mg
Robaxin Injection 10 ml IM or IV; max 30 ml/day; max 3 days; max 5 ml/gluteal injection q 8 hours;
max IV rate 3 ml/min
Vial: 100 mg/ml (10 ml)
➤ *nabumetone*
Pediatric: <12 years: not recommended; ≥12 years: same as adult
Relafen *Tab:* 500, 750 mg
Relafen 500 *Tab:* 500 mg
➤ *orphenadrine citrate* (G) 1 tab bid
Pediatric: <12 years: not recommended; ≥12 years: same as adult
Norflex *Tab:* 100 mg sust-rel
➤ *tizanidine* 1-4 mg q 6-8 hours; max 36 mg/day
Pediatric: <12 years: not recommended; ≥12 years: same as adult
Zanaflex *Tab:* 2*, 4**mg; *Cap:* 2, 4, 6 mg

SKELETAL MUSCLE RELAXANT+NON-STEROIDAL ANTI-INFLAMMATORY DRUG (NSAID) COMBINATIONS

Comment: *Aspirin*-containing medications are contraindicated with history of allergic-type reaction to *aspirin*, children and adolescents with *varicella* or other viral illness, and 3rd trimester of pregnancy.
➤ *carisoprodol+aspirin* (III)(G) 1-2 tabs qid
Pediatric: <12 years: not recommended; ≥12 years: same as adult
Soma Compound *Tab:* caris 200 mg+asp 325 mg (sulfites)
➤ *meprobamate+aspirin* (IV) 1-2 tabs tid or qid
Pediatric: <12 years: not recommended; ≥12 years: same as adult
Equagesic *Tab:* mepro 200 mg+asp 325*mg

SKELETAL MUSCLE RELAXANT+NSAID+CAFFEINE COMBINATIONS

Comment: *Aspirin*-containing medications are contraindicated with history of allergic-type reaction to *aspirin*, children and adolescents with *varicella* or other viral illness, and 3rd trimester of pregnancy.
➤ *orphenadrine+aspirin+caffeine* (G)
Pediatric: <12 years: not recommended; ≥12 years: same as adult
Norgesic 1-2 tabs tid-qid
Tab: orphen 25 mg+asp 385 mg+caf 30 mg
Norgesic Forte 1 tab tid or qid; max 4 tabs/day
Tab: orphen 50 mg+asp 770 mg+caf 60*mg

SKELETAL MUSCLE RELAXANT+NSAID+CODEINE COMBINATIONS

➤ *carisoprodol+aspirin+codeine* (III)(G) 1-2 tabs qid prn
Pediatric: <18 years: not recommended; ≥18 years: not recommended
Soma Compound w. Codeine *Tab:* caris 200 mg+asp 325 mg+cod 16 mg (sulfites)
Comment: *Codeine* is known to be excreted in breast milk. <12 years: not recommended; 12 to <18 years: use extreme caution; not recommended for children and adolescents with asthma or other chronic breathing problem. The FDA and the European Medicines Agency (EMA) are investigating the safety of using *codeine* containing medications to treat pain, cough, and colds in children 12-<18 years because of the potential for serious side effects, including slowed or difficult breathing. *Aspirin*-containing medications are contraindicated with history of allergic-type reaction to *aspirin*, children and adolescents with *varicella* or other viral illness, and 3rd trimester of pregnancy.

TENOSYNOVIAL GIANT CELL TUMOR (TGCT)

KINASE INHIBITOR

➤ *pexidartinib* 400 mg (2 x 200 mg) bid until disease progression or unacceptable toxicity; swallow whole, do not open or chew; take on an empty stomach, at least 1 hour before or 2 hours after a meal/snack
Pediatric: safety and efficacy not established
Turalio *Cap:* 200 mg

(continued)

Comment: Turalio *(pexidartinib)* is a kinase inhibitor indicated for treatment of adults with symptomatic tenosynovial giant cell tumor (TGCT) associated with severe morbidity or functional limitations not amenable to improvement with surgery. *CrCl 15-89 ml/min:* 200 mg in the AM and 400 mg in the PM. Turalio can cause serious and potential fatal liver injury. Monitor liver function tests (LFTs) prior to initiation and at intervals during treatment as appropriate. If hepatotoxicity develops, withhold doses, reduce doses, or permanently discontinue **Turalio** based on severity. Reduce the dose as appropriate for patients with mild-to-severe renal impairment. Avoid co-administration of **Turalio** with other products known to cause hepatotoxicity. Reduce the dose of **Turalio** if concomitant use of strong CYP3A inhibitors cannot be avoided. Avoid co-ncomitant use of strong CYP3A inducers. Reduce the dose of **Turalio** if concomitant use of UGT inhibitors cannot be avoided. Avoid concomitant use of proton pump inhibitors (PPIs); use H2 receptor antagonists or antacids if needed. The most common adverse reactions (incidence >20%) have been increased lactate dehydrogenase, increased aspartate aminotransferase, hair color changes, fatigue, increased alanine aminotransferase, decreased neutrophils, increased cholesterol, increased alkaline phosphatase, decreased lymphocytes, eye edema, decreased hemoglobin, rash, dysgeusia, and decreased phosphate. **Turalio** may cause embryo/fetal harm; advise pregnant females of the embryo/fetal risk. Advise women not to breastfeed during treatment and for at least 1 week after the last dose. **Turalio** is available only through the **Turalio** Risk Evaluation and Mitigation Strategy (REMS) program. Prescribers must be certified with the program by enrolling and completing training. Patients must complete and sign an enrollment for inclusion in the patient registry. Pharmacies must be certified with the program and must only dispense to patients who are authorized to receive **Turalio**. For further information, contact the Turalio REMS Program at 1-833-887-2546 or www.turalioREMS.com

TESTOSTERONE DEFICIENCY, HYPOTESTOSTERONEMIA, HYPOGONADISM

Comment: *Testosterone* is contraindicated in male breast cancer and prostate cancer. *Testosterone* replacement therapy is indicated in males with primary hypogonadism (congenital or acquired due to cryptorchidism, bilateral torsion, orchitis, vanishing testis syndrome, or orchidectomy), or hypogonadotropic hypogonadism (congenital or acquired), and delayed puberty not secondary to a pathologic disorder (x-ray of the hand and wrist to determine bone age should be obtained every 6 months to assess the effect of treatment on the epiphyseal centers).

ORAL ANDROGENS

▷ *fluoxymesterone* (III) *Hypogonadism:* <12 years: use by specialist only; *Puberty:* 5-20 mg once daily; *Delayed puberty:* use low dose and limit duration to 4-6 months

    Halotestin *Tab:* 2*, 5*, 10*mg (tartrazine)

▷ *methyltestosterone* (III) usually 10-50 mg once daily; for delayed puberty, use low dose and limit duration to 4-6 months

    Android *Cap:* 10 mg

    Methitest *Tab:* 10*mg

    Testred *Cap:* 10 mg

▷ *testosterone* (III) 30 mg q 12 hours to gum region, just above the incisor tooth on either side of the mouth; hold system in place for 30 seconds; rotate sites with each application

    Striant *Buccal tab:* 30 mg (6 blister pks; 10 buccal systems/blister pck)

Comment: Serum total *testosterone* concentrations may be checked 4-12 weeks after initiating treatment with Striant. To capture the maximum serum concentration, an early morning sample (just prior to applying the AM dose) is recommended.

▷ *testosterone Recommended dose:* 225 mg bid (2 x 112.5 mg caps), once in the morning and once in the evening with food; *Prior to initiating treatment:* confirm the diagnosis of hypogonadism by ensuring that serum testosterone concentrations have been measured in the morning, on at least two separate days, and that these serum testosterone concentrations are below the normal range; *After initiating treatment:* monitor serum testosterone to determine if treatment should be continued or discontinued; *Monitor serum testosterone:* 8-9 hours after the morning dose, 3 to 4 weeks after initiating Tlando, and periodically thereafter; *300-1,080 ng/dL:* continue treatment; *<300 ng/dL or >1,080 ng/dL:* discontinue treatment

Pediatric: <18 years: safety and efficacy not established; ≥18 years: same as adult

    Tlando *Cap:* 112.5 mg

    Comment: Tlando is an androgen indicated for testosterone replacement therapy in adult males for conditions associated with a deficiency or absence of endogenous testosterone. *Contraindications:* (1) Carcinoma of the breast or known or suspected carcinoma of the prostate; (2) women who are pregnant; testosterone may cause fetal harm; (3) hypersensitivity to Tlando or any of its ingredients; and (4) hypogonadal conditions not associated with structural or genetic etiologies. Geriatric patients (≥65 years) treated with androgens may also be at risk for worsening of signs and symptoms of benign prostatic hyperplasia (BPH) and hypertension. **Boxed Warning:** Tlando can cause blood pressure (BP) increases that can increase the risk of major adverse cardiovascular events (MACE), including non-fatal myocardial infarction, non-fatal stroke, and cardiovascular death. Before initiating Tlando, consider the patient's baseline cardiovascular risk and ensure BP is adequately controlled. Periodically monitor for and treat new-onset hypertension or exacerbations of preexisting hypertension and re-evaluate whether the benefits of **Tlando** outweigh its risks in patients who develop cardiovascular risk factors or cardiovascular disease on treatment. Use **Tlando** <u>only</u> for the treatment of men with hypogonadal conditions associated with structural or genetic etiologies. The most common adverse reactions (incidence ≥2%): increased blood prolactin, hypertension, increased hematocrit, upper respiratory tract infection (URI), weight gain, headache, and musculoskeletal pain. Monitor hematocrit approximately every 3 months during the first year after beginning **Tlando** and then every 6 months thereafter during treatment. Monitor patients with benign prostatic hyperplasia (BPH) for worsening of signs and symptoms of BPH. Evaluate patients for prostate cancer, including monitoring prostate-specific antigen (PSA) prior to initiating and during treatment with androgens. Venous thromboembolism (VTE), including deep vein thrombosis (DVT) and pulmonary embolism (PE), has been reported in patients using testosterone products. Discontinue **Tlando** if VTE is suspected and initiate appropriate workup and management. *Abuse of Testosterone:* If testosterone use at doses higher than recommended for the approved indication or in combination with other anabolic androgenic steroids is suspected, check serum testosterone concentration. **Tlando** may cause azoospermia. Edema with or without congestive heart failure (CHF) may occur in patients with preexisting cardiac, renal, or hepatic disease; discontinue **Tlando** and initiate appropriate workup. **Tlando** may potentiate sleep apnea in those with risk factors. Testosterone may affect serum lipid profile; monitor patient lipid concentrations and, if necessary, adjust dosage of lipid-lowering drug(s) or discontinue **Tlando**. Monitor serum prolactin levels prior to initiation of treatment and 3 to 4 months after starting treatment; discontinue **Tlando** if serum prolactin levels remain elevated. In patients with diabetes, concomitant use of **Tlando** may decrease blood glucose and insulin requirements. Concomitant use of **Tlando** with oral coagulants may cause changes in anticoagulant activity; monitor international normalized ratio (INR) and prothrombin time (PT) frequently. Concomitant use of corticosteroids with **Tlando** may result in increased fluid retention; use with caution, particularly in patients with cardiac, renal, or hepatic disease. Concomitant use of antihypertensive agents with **Tlando** may lead to additional increases in BP.

▶ *testosterone undecanoate* Prior to initiating *Jatenzo:* confirm the diagnosis of hypogonadism by ensuring that serum testosterone concentrations have been measured in the morning on at least 2 separate days and that these concentrations are below the normal range; take with food; *starting dose:* 237 mg orally once in the morning and once in the evening; *Dose adjustment:* to a minimum of 158 mg bid, and maximum of 396 mg bid, based on serum testosterone drawn 6 hours after the morning dose at least 7 days after starting treatment or following dose adjustment and periodically thereafter

Pediatric: <18 years: <u>not</u> established; ≥18 years: same as adult

Jatenzo *Cap:* 158, 198, 237 mg

Comment: Jatenzo *(testosterone undecanoate)* is an oral testosterone replacement therapy for the treatment of low testosterone in hypogonadal men. Monitor patients with benign prostatic hyperplasia (BPH) for worsening of signs and symptoms of BPH. Monitor prostate specific antigen (PSA) and lipid concentrations periodically. Edema with or without (CHF), may occur in patients with preexisting cardiac, renal, <u>or</u> hepatic disease. Venous thromboembolism (VTE), including deep vein thrombosis (DVT) and pulmonary embolism (PE), has been reported in patients using testosterone. Evaluate patients with signs or symptoms consistent with DVT or PE. Monitor hematocrit approximately every 3 months to detect increased red blood cell (RBC) mass and polycythemia. Testosterone has been subject to abuse, typically at doses higher than recommended for the approved indication and in combination with other anabolic androgenic steroids. Exogenous administration of androgens may lead to azoospermia. Depression and suicidal ideation have occurred during clinical trials in patients treated with **Jatenzo**. *Contraindications:* men with breast cancer or known or suspected prostate cancer and women who are pregnant.

TOPICAL ANDROGENS

Comment: Wash hands after application. Allow solution to dry before it touches clothing. Do <u>not</u> wash site for at least 2 hours after application. Pregnant and nursing women and children must avoid skin contact with application sites on men. If there is contact, wash the area as soon as possible with soap and water.

▶ *testosterone* (III)(G)
Pediatric: <18 years: <u>not</u> recommended; ≥18 years: same as adult

AndroGel 1% (G) initially apply 25 mg once daily in the AM to clean, dry, intact skin of the shoulders, upper arms, <u>and/or</u> abdomen; do <u>not</u> apply to scrotum; may increase to 75 mg/day and then to 100 mg/day if needed

Gel: 25 mg/2.5 gm pkt (30 pkts/carton); 50 mg/5 gm pkt (30 pkts/carton)

AndroGel 1.62% (G) initially apply 25 mg once daily in the AM to clean, dry, intact skin of the shoulders and upper arms; do <u>not</u> apply to abdomen <u>or</u> genitals; may adjust dose between 1 and 4 pump actuations based on the pre-dose morning serum testosterone concentration at approximately 14 and 28 days after starting treatment <u>or</u> adjusting dose

Gel: 20.25 mg/1.25 gm pkt; 40.5 mg/2.5 gm pkt; 20.25 mg/1.25 gm pump actuation (60 metered dose actuations)

Axiron apply to clean, dry, intact skin of the axillae; do <u>not</u> apply to the scrotum, penis, abdomen, shoulders, <u>or</u> upper arms; initially apply 60 mg (30 mg/axilla) once daily in the AM; adjust dose based on serum testosterone concentration 2-8 hours after applying and at least 14 days after starting therapy

(continued)

or following dose adjustment; may increase dose in 30 mg increments if serum testosterone <300 ng/dL up to 120 mg; reduce dose to 30 mg if levels >1,050 ng/dL; discontinue if serum testosterone remains at >1,050 ng/dL; to apply a 120 mg dose, apply 30 mg to each axilla and allow to dry, then repeat

Soln: 30 mg/1.5 ml pump actuation (60 metered dose actuations) (alcohol, latex-free)

Fortesta (G) initially 40 mg of testosterone (4 pump actuations) applied to the thighs once daily in the AM; may adjust between 10 mg minimum and 70 mg maximum

Gel: 10 mg/0.5 gm pump actuation (120 metered dose actuations) (ethanol)

Comment: The Fortesta dose should be based on the serum *testosterone* concentration 2 hours after applying **Fortesta** and at approximately 14 days and 35 days after starting treatment or following dose adjustment. Dose adjustment criteria: ≤500 ng/dL, increase daily dose by 10 mg; 500-≤1,250 ng/dL, no change; 1,250 to 2,500 ng/dL, decrease daily dose by 10 mg; ≥2,500 ng/dL, decrease daily dose by 20 mg.

Testim (G) initially apply 5 gm once daily in the AM to clean, dry, intact skin of the shoulders and/or upper arms; do not apply to the genitals or abdomen; may increase to 10 gm after 2 weeks

Gel: 1%, clear, hydroalcoholic (5 mg/5 gm pkt, 30 pkts/carton)

Vogelxo Gel (G) 1% initially apply 5 gm once daily in the AM to clean, dry, intact skin of the shoulders, upper arms, and/or abdomen; do not apply to scrotum; may increase to 7.5 gm/day and then to 10 gm/day if needed

Gel: 50 mg/5 gm pkt (30 pkts/carton); 50 mg/5 gm tube (30 tubes/carton); *Pump:* 12.5 mg/1.25 gm pump actuation, 60 metered dose actuations)

INTRANASAL ANDROGENS

▷ *testosterone (nasal gel)* (III) initially 1 pump actuation each nostril (33 mg) 3 tid, at least 6-8 hours apart, at the same time each day max: 6 pump actuation/day

Pediatric: <18 years: not established; ≥18 years: same as adult

Natesto *Gel:* 5.5 mg/0.122 gm pump actuation (60 metered dose actuations)

TRANSDERMAL ANDROGEN PATCH

▷ *testosterone* (III)

Androderm initially apply 4 mg nightly at approximately 10 PM to clean, dry area of the arm, back, or upper buttocks; leave on x 24 hours; may increase to 7.5 mg or decrease to 2.5 mg based on confirmed AM serum testosterone concentrations

Pediatric: <15 years: not recommended; ≥15 years: same as adult

Transdermal patch: 2, 4 mg/24 Hr

PARENTERAL ANDROGENS

Comment: Contraindications include males with carcinoma of the breast or known or suspected carcinoma of the prostate and women who are pregnant (exogenous testosterone may cause fetal harm). *Prior to initiation of treatment:* confirm the diagnosis of hypogonadism by ensuring that serum testosterone has been measured in the morning on at least 2 separate days and that these concentrations are below the normal range. *Starting dose:* administer 75 mg SC in the abdominal region once weekly. Avoid intramuscular and intravascular administration. *Dose Adjustment:* Based upon total testosterone trough concentrations (measured 7 days after most recent dose) obtained following 6 weeks of dosing and periodically thereafter. *Testosterone enanthate* and *testosterone cypionate* are long-acting testosterone esters suspended in oil to prolong absorption. Peak levels occur about 72 hours after intramuscular injection and are followed by a slow decline during the subsequent 1-2 weeks. For complete androgen replacement, the regimen should be between 50 and 100 mg of *testosterone enanthate* administered every 7-10 days, which will achieve relatively normal levels of testosterone throughout the time interval between injections. Longer time intervals are more convenient but are associated with greater fluctuations in testosterone levels. Higher doses of testosterone produce longer-term effects but also higher peak levels and wider swings between peak and nadir circulating testosterone levels; the result is fluctuating symptoms in many patients. The use of 100-150 mg of testosterone every 2 weeks is a reasonable compromise. Use of 300 mg injections every 3 weeks is associated with wider fluctuations of testosterone levels and is generally inadequate to ensure a consistent clinical response. With use of these longer-interval regimens, many men will have pronounced symptoms during the week preceding the next injection. In such instances, a smaller dose at closer intervals should be tried. When full androgen replacement is not required, patients should receive lower doses of testosterone. One such category includes male patients with prepubertal onset of hypogonadism who are going through puberty for the first time during therapy and who often may require psychologic counseling, especially when a spouse is involved as well. In these patients, testosterone therapy should be initiated at 50 mg every 3-4 weeks and then gradually increased during subsequent months, as tolerated, up to full replacement within 1 year. Men with appreciable benign prostatic hypertrophy who have hypogonadism and symptoms may be given 50-100 mg of testosterone every 2 weeks as an initial regimen and maintained on this dosage with careful monitoring of urinary symptoms and prostate examinations; therapy can be withdrawn if necessary. Attaining full virilization in the patient with hypogonadism may take as long as 3-4 years. Follow-up intervals should be between 4 and 6 months to monitor progress, review compliance, and determine whether any complications or psychological adjustment problems are present. As a guide, testosterone levels should be above the lower limit of normal, in the range of 250-300 ng/dL, just before the next injection. Excessive peak levels and side effects should also be monitored and used to adjust the dosing regimens. During exogenous administration of androgens, endogenous testosterone release is inhibited through feedback inhibition of pituitary luteinizing hormone (LH). At large doses of exogenous androgens, spermatogenesis may also be suppressed through feedback inhibition of pituitary follicle-stimulating hormone (FSH). Androgen therapy should be used very cautiously in pediatric patients and <u>only</u> by specialists who are aware of the adverse effects on bone maturation. Skeletal maturation must be monitored every 6 months by an x-ray of the hand and wrist. There is a lack of substantial evidence that androgens are effective in fractures, surgery, convalescence, and functional uterine bleeding.

▷ **testosterone cypionate** (III)
   Comment: *Testosterone cypionate* is the oil-soluble 17 (beta)-cyclopentyl propionate ester of the androgenic hormone testosterone. The half-life of **testosterone cypionate** when injected intramuscularly is approximately 8 days.
   Depot-Testosterone Injection (G) *Usual starting dose:* 75-100 mg deep IM in the gluteal muscle; *Dose/ frequency adjustment:* dose and frequency based upon morning total testosterone trough concentrations (measured 7 days after most recent dose) periodically thereafter; *Maintenance:* usually 100-400 mg deep IM in the gluteal muscle q 4 weeks; total doses above 400 mg per month are <u>not</u> required because of the prolonged action of the preparation; injections more frequently than q 2 weeks are rarely indicated
   Pediatric: <12 years: <u>not</u> established; ≥12 years: same as adult
   Vial: 100, 200 mg/ml (5 ml) (benzyl alcohol)
▷ **testosterone enanthate** (III)
   Comment: The half-life of **testosterone enanthate** when injected intramuscularly is approximately 4.5 days.
   Delatestryl (G) *Usual starting dose:* 75-100 mg deep IM in the gluteal muscle; *Dose/frequency adjustment:* is based upon morning total testosterone trough concentrations (measured 7 days after most recent dose) periodically thereafter; *Maintenance:* usually 100-400 mg deep IM in the gluteal muscle every 4 weeks; total doses above 400 mg per month are <u>not</u> required because of the prolonged action of the preparation; injections more frequently than every 2 weeks are rarely indicated
   Pediatric: <12 years: <u>not</u> established; ≥12 years: same as adult
   Vial: 100, 200 mg/ml (5 ml) (chlorobutanol [chloral derivative] as preservative)
   Xyosted *Initially:* 75 mg SC in the abdominal region once weekly; *Dose adjustment:* based upon morning total testosterone trough concentrations (measured 7 days after most recent dose) obtained following 6 weeks of dosing and periodically thereafter
   Pediatric: <18 years: <u>not</u> established; ≥18 years: same as adult
   Autoinjector: 50, 75, 100 mg/0.5 ml, single-dose (4/carton) (preservative-free)
   Comment: Use **Xyosted** <u>only</u> for the treatment of hypogonadal conditions associated with structural or genetic etiologies. Safety and efficacy of **Xyosted** in males with "age-related hypogonadism" (also referred to as "late-onset hypogonadism") have <u>not</u> been established.

TETANUS (*CLOSTRIDIUM TETANI*)

Comment: For individuals who have received 3 <u>or</u> more doses of tetanus toxoid-containing vaccine, for clean and minor wounds, **Tdap** <u>or</u> **Td** should be administered if more than 10 years have passed since the last dose. For all other wounds, **Tdap** <u>or</u> **Td** should be administered if more than 5 years have passed since the last dose of tetanus toxoid-containing vaccine. For those who have <u>not</u> previously received **Tdap** <u>or</u> whose Tdap history is unknown, **Tdap** is the preferred vaccine. Additionally, **Tdap** should be used to vaccinate pregnant women if a tetanus toxoid-containing vaccine is indicated (ACIP, 2021).

COMBINATION VACCINES

▷ **Pentacel** (DTaP-IPV/Hib) is commercially available as a kit containing single-dose vial of fixed-combination vaccine containing diphtheria, tetanus, pertussis, and poliovirus antigens (DTaP-IPV vaccine) and single-dose vial of lyophilized Hib vaccine (PRP-T; ActHIB). Prior to administration, reconstitute vial of lyophilized PRP-T (ActHIB) vaccine by adding the entire content of a vial of DTaP-IPV vaccine in the kit according to manufacturer's instructions to provide a combination vaccine containing diphtheria, tetanus, pertussis, IPV, and Hib antigens. Gently swirl until cloudy, uniform, white to off-white (yellow tinge) suspension is obtained. Administer IM immediately after reconstitution. **Pentacel** is approved for use as a four-dose series in children 6 weeks through 4 years of age (prior to the 5th birthday). **Pentacel** is to be administered as a 4-dose series at 2, 4, 6, and 15-18 months of age. The first dose may be given as early as 6 weeks of age. Four doses of **Pentacel** constitute a primary immunization course against pertussis. Three doses of **Pentacel** constitute an immunization course against diphtheria, tetanus, *Haemophilus influenzae* type b invasive disease, and poliomyelitis; the fourth dose is a booster for diphtheria, tetanus, *H. influenzae* type b invasive disease, and poliomyelitis immunizations. See mfr pkg insert for full prescribing information, including product storage, preparation, administration, contraindications, warnings, and precautions.
▷ **Vaxelis** *Vial:* 0.5 ml susp, single-dose; *Prefilled syringe:* 0.5 ml susp, single-dose (preservative-free)
   Comment: Vaxelis is a single fixed-dose combination of six vaccines: diphtheria, tetanus toxoid, acellular pertussis, inactivated poliovirus, *Haemophilus* b conjugate, and hepatitis B. The 3-dose immunization series consists of a 0.5 ml IM injection, administered at 2, 4, and 6 months of age. See mfr pkg insert for full prescribing information, including product storage, preparation, administration, contraindications, warnings, and precautions.

POST-EXPOSURE PROPHYLAXIS IN PREVIOUSLY NON-IMMUNIZED PERSONS

▷ *tetanus immune globulin, human* 250 mg deep IM in a single dose
Pediatric: >7 years: same as adult
　　BayTET, Hyper-TET
　　　Vial: 250 units, single-dose; *Prefilled syringe:* 250 units
▷ *tetanus toxoid* vaccine 0.5 ml IM x 3 dose series
　　　Vial: 5 Lf units/0.5 ml (0.5, 5 ml); *Prefilled syringe:* 5 Lf units/0.5 ml (0.5 ml)
Comment: Dose of **BayTET/HyperTET** S/D is calculated as 4 units/kg. However, it may be advisable to administer the entire contents of the syringe of **BayTET/HyperTET** S/D (250 units) regardless of the child's size, since theoretically the same amount of toxin will be produced in the child's body by the infecting tetanus organism as it will in an adult's body. At the same time but in a different extremity and with a different syringe, administer Diphtheria and Tetanus Toxoids and Pertussis Vaccine Adsorbed (DTP) or Diphtheria and Tetanus Toxoids Adsorbed (For Pediatric Use) (DT), if pertussis vaccine is contraindicated, should be administered per mfr pkg insert. Tetanus immune globulin may interact with live viral vaccines such as measles, mumps, rubella, and polio. It is also unknown if **BayTET/HyperTET** can cause fetal harm when administered to a pregnant woman or can affect reproduction capacity. The single injection of tetanus toxoid only initiates the series for producing active immunity in the recipient. Impress upon the patient the need for further toxoid injections in 1 month and 1 year, otherwise the active immunization series is incomplete. If a contraindication to using tetanus toxoid-containing preparations exists for a person who has not completed a primary series of tetanus toxoid immunization and that person has a wound that is neither clean nor minor, only passive immunization should be given using tetanus immune globulin.

PARENTERAL MUSCLE RELAXANT

▷ *methocarbamol for injection* for IM or intravenous push (IVP) or IV infusion; IVP 1-2 vials directly into the tubing of the previously inserted indwelling needle; an additional 10 ml or 20 ml may be added to the infusion bottle (i.e., total up to 30 ml [3 vials]) as the initial dose; repeat q 6 hours until conditions allow for the insertion of a nasogastric (NG) tube; then administer crushed *methocarbamol* tablets suspended in water or saline via the NG tube; total daily oral doses up to 24 gm may be required as judged by patient response
Pediatric: Minimum initial dose: 15 mg/kg or 500 mg/m²; may repeat q 6 hours, if required; *Total dose:* should not exceed 1.8 gm/m² for 3 consecutive days; *maintenance dose:* may be administered via IVP into tubing or by IV infusion with an appropriate quantity of fluid
　　Robaxin Injectable *Vial:* 100 mg/ml (10 ml), single-dose (no natural rubber latex)
　　Comment: **Robaxin Injectable** is a parenteral carbamate derivative of guaifenesin, a central nervous system (CNS) depressant with sedative and musculoskeletal relaxant properties, indicated for the treatment of tetanus (in adults and pediatric patients) and acute, painful musculoskeletal conditions only in adults. The mode of action of *methocarbamol* has not been clearly identified, but its effectiveness may be explained by its sedative properties. *Methocarbamol* does not directly relax tense skeletal muscles. There is clinical evidence which suggests that *methocarbamol* may have a beneficial effect in the control of the neuromuscular manifestations of tetanus. It does not, however, replace the usual procedure of debridement, tetanus antitoxin, penicillin, tracheotomy, attention to fluid balance, and supportive care. **Robaxin Injectable** should be added to the regimen as soon as possible. **Robaxin Injectable** should not be administered to patients with known or suspected renal pathology. This caution is necessary because of the presence of polyethylene glycol 300 in the vehicle. A much larger amount of polyethylene glycol 300 than is present in recommended doses of **Robaxin Injectable** is known to have increased preexisting acidosis and urea retention in patients with renal impairment. Although the amount present in **Robaxin Injectable** is well within the limits of safety, caution dictates this contraindication. Caution should be observed using the **Robaxin Injectable** in patients with suspected or known seizure disorder. Patients should be cautioned that *methocarbamol* may cause drowsiness or dizziness, which may impair ability to operate a motor vehicle or hazardous machinery. Because *methocarbamol* may possess a general CNS depressant effect, patients should be cautioned about combined effects with alcohol and other CNS depressants. *Adverse Reactions/Side Effects: General*—anaphylaxis, angioneurotic edema, fever, and headache; *Cardiovascular*—thrombophlebitis, bradycardia, flushing, hypotension, and syncope (in most cases of syncope, there has been spontaneous recovery, and in other cases epinephrine, injectable steroid, and/or injectable antihistamine have been employed to hasten recovery); *Gastrointestinal*—dyspepsia, jaundice (including cholestatic jaundice), nausea and vomiting; *Hemic/Lymphatic*—leukopenia; *Immune System*—hypersensitivity reactions; *Neurologic*—amnesia, confusion, diplopia, dizziness or lightheadedness, drowsiness, insomnia, mild muscular incoordination, nystagmus, sedation, vertigo, and seizures (including grand mal; (NOTE: Onset of convulsive seizures during IVP or IV infusion of *methocarbamol* has been reported in patients with seizure disorder. The psychic/emotional response to the procedure may be a contributing factor. Although several observers have reported success in terminating epileptiform seizures with **Robaxin Injectable**, administration to patients with epilepsy is not recommended.); *Skin/Special Senses*—blurred vision, conjunctivitis, nasal congestion, metallic taste, pruritus, rash, urticaria, and pain and sloughing at the injection site. If the reaction or side effects persist, a like course may be repeated after a drug-free interval of 48 hours. Dosage and frequency of administration should be based on the severity of the condition being treated and therapeutic response noted. For the relief of symptoms of moderate degree, 1 dose of 100 mg (10 ml) may be adequate. Ordinarily, a single dose does not need to be repeated,

as switching to the oral form will usually sustain the relief initiated by the injection or infusion. For the severest cases or in postoperative conditions in which oral administration is not feasible, additional doses of 100 mg may be repeated every 8 hours up to a maximum of 300 mg/day for a maximum of 3 consecutive days. When satisfactory relief of symptoms is achieved and the patient is able, it can usually be maintained with the tablet form of **methocarbamol**. There have been reports of fetal congenital abnormalities following *in utero* exposure to **methocarbamol**. Therefore, **Robaxin Injectable** should not be used in females who are, or may become, pregnant and particularly during early pregnancy, unless clearly needed. **Methocarbamol** and/or its metabolites are excreted in breast milk as demonstrated in animal lactation studies; however, it is not known whether **methocarbamol** or its metabolites are excreted in human milk or effects on the breastfed infant. No human data are available to indicate the presence or absence of drug-associated risk to the breastfed infant. Developmental and health benefits of breastfeeding should be considered along with the mother's clinical need for **Robaxin Injectable** and any potential adverse effects on the breastfed infant from **Robaxin Injectable** or from the underlying maternal condition.

THREADWORM (*STRONGYLOIDES STERCORALIS*)

ANTHELMINTICS
Comment: Oral bioavailability of anthelmintics is enhanced when administered with a fatty meal (estimated fat content 40 gm).
➤ *albendazole* take with a meal; may crush and mix with food; may repeat in 3 weeks if needed; 400 mg bid x 7 days
　Pediatric: <2 years: 200 mg bid x 7 days; 2-12 years: 400 mg once daily x 7 days; >12 years: same as adult
　　Albenza *Tab:* 200 mg
　Comment: *Albendazole* is a broad-spectrum benzimidazole carbamate anthelmintic.
➤ *ivermectin* take with water; chew or crush and mix with food; may repeat in 3 months if needed; 200 mcg/kg as a single dose
　Pediatric: <15 kg: not recommended; ≥15 kg: same as adult
　　Stromectol *Tab:* 3, 6*mg
➤ *mebendazole* (G) take with a meal; chew or crush and mix with food; may repeat in 3 weeks if needed; 100 mg bid x 3 days
　Pediatric: <2 years: not recommended; ≥2 years: same as adult
　　Emverm *Chew tab:* 100 mg
　　Vermox *Chew tab:* 100 mg
➤ *praziquantel* (G) take with a meal; may crush and mix with food; 5-10 mg/kg as a single dose
　Pediatric: <4 years: not established; ≥4 years: same as adult
　　Biltricide *Tab:* 600**mg film-coat (cross-scored for half or quarter dose)
　　Comment: Therapeutically effective levels of **Biltricide** may not be achieved when administered concomitantly with strong P450 inducers, such as rifampin. Females should not breastfeed on the day of **Biltricide** treatment and during the subsequent 72 hours. Use caution with hepatosplenic patients who have moderate-to-severe liver impairment (Child-Pugh Class B and C).
➤ *pyrantel pamoate* take with a meal; may open capsule and sprinkle or mix with food; treat x 3 days; may repeat in 2-3 weeks if needed; treat x 3 days; 11 mg/kg/dose; max 1 gm/dose; <25 lb: not recommended; 25-37 lb: ½ tsp/dose; 38-62 lb: 1 tsp/dose; 63-87 lb: 1 tsp/dose; 88-112 lb: 2 tsp/dose; 113-137 lb: 2 tsp/dose; 138-162 lb: 3 tsp/dose; 163-187 lb: 3 tsp/dose; >187 lb: 4 tsp/dose
　　Antiminth *Cap:* 180 mg; *Liq:* 50 mg/ml (30 ml); 144 mg/ml (30 ml); *Oral susp:* 50 mg/ml (60 ml)
　　Pin-X *Cap:* 180 mg; *Liq:* 50 mg/ml (30 ml); 144 mg/ml (30 ml); *Oral susp:* 50 mg/ml (30 ml)
➤ *nitazoxanide* (G) take with a meal; may crush and mix with food; <12 months: not recommended; ≥12 months: treat q 12 hours x 3 days; <11 years: (use suspension); 1-3 years: 5 ml; 4-11 years: 10 ml; >11 years: (use tab or suspension) 500 mg
　　Alinia *Tab:* 500 mg; *Oral susp:* 100 mg/5 ml (60 ml)
➤ *thiabendazole* take with a meal; may crush and mix with food; treat x 7 days; <30 lb: consult mfr pkg insert; ≥30 lb: 25 mg/kg/dose bid with meals; 30-50 lb: 250 mg bid with meals; >50 lb: 10 mg/lb/dose bid with meals; max 1.5 gm/dose; max 3 gm/day
　　Mintezol *Chew tab:* 500*mg (orange); *Oral susp:* 500 mg/5 ml (120 ml) (orange)
　Comment: *Thiabendazole* is not for prophylaxis. May impair mental alertness. May not be available in the United States.

THROMBOCYTOPENIA PURPURA, IDIOPATHIC (IMMUNE) (ITP)

THROMBOPOIETIN (TPO) RECEPTOR AGONIST
Comment: Doptelet *(avatrombopag)* is the first oral thrombopoietin (TPO) receptor agonist approved by the FDA for the treatment of adults with chronic liver disease who are scheduled to undergo a procedure. Doptelet is a second-generation, once-daily, orally administered TPO receptor agonist that works by increasing platelet counts to the target level of greater or equal to 50,000 per microliter.

(continued)

➤ *avatrombopag* <18 years: not recommended; ≥18 years: begin dosing 10-13 days prior to a scheduled procedure; the patient should undergo the procedure within 5-8 days after the last dose; take with food, as a single dose x 5 consecutive days; *PLT count <40 x 10⁹/L:* 60 mg (3 tabs) once daily x 5 days; *PLT count 40-50 x 10⁹/L:* 40 mg (2 tabs) once daily x 5 days

Doptelet *Tab:* 20 mg film-coat

Comment: TPO receptor agonists have been associated with thrombotic and thromboembolic complications in patients with chronic liver disease. Monitor platelet counts and for thromboembolic events and institute treatment promptly. Potential adverse reactions include pyrexia, abdominal pain, nausea, headache, fatigue, and peripheral edema. Based on animal studies, *avatrombopag* may cause fetal harm when administered to a pregnant female. There is no information regarding the presence of *avatrombopag* in human milk or effects on the breastfed infant. However, breastfeeding is not recommended during treatment with **Doptelet** and for at least 2 weeks after the last dose. Safety and effectiveness in patients (<18 years of age) have not been established.

➤ *lusutrombopag* 3 mg orally once daily with or without food x 7 days; administer first dose 8-14 days prior to the scheduled procedure; the procedure should occur 2-8 days after the last dose

Pediatric: <18 years: not established; ≥18 years: same as adult

Mulpleta *Tab:* 3 mg

Comment: Mulpleta *(lusutrombopag)* is a thrombopoietin (TPO) receptor agonist indicated for the treatment of thrombocytopenia in adult patients with chronic liver disease who are scheduled to undergo a procedure. TPO receptor agonists have been associated with thrombotic and thromboembolic complications in patients with chronic liver disease. Monitor platelet counts and for thromboembolic events and institute treatment promptly. The most common adverse reaction (incidence 3%) is headache. There are no available data on **Mulpleta** in pregnant females to inform drug-associated fetal risk. However, in animal reproduction studies, oral administration of *lusutrombopag* during organogenesis and the lactation period resulted in adverse developmental fetal outcomes. Advise pregnant females of the potential risk to a fetus. Breastfeeding is not recommended during treatment.

SPLEEN TYROSINE KINASE (SYK) INHIBITOR

➤ *fostamatinib disodium hexahydrate* <18 years: not recommended; ≥18 years: initially 100 mg bid; increase to 150 mg bid if platelet count not at ≥50 x 10⁹/L after 4 weeks; discontinue if insufficient increase in platelet count after 12 weeks; *Dose modifications:* see full labeling

Tavalisse *Tab:* 100, 150 mg

Comment: Tavalisse *(fostamatinib)* is an oral spleen tyrosine kinase (SYK) inhibitor for the treatment of patients with chronic idiopathic (immune) thrombocytopenia purpura (ITP). Monitor complete blood counts (CBCs), including platelets, monthly until stable count (≥50 x 10⁹/l) achieved, then periodically thereafter. Monitor liver function tests (LFTs) monthly. Discontinue if aspartate aminotransferase/alanine aminotransferase (AST/ALT) is >5 x the upper limit of normal (ULN) for ≥2 weeks or ≥3 x ULN and total bilirubin >2 x ULN. Monitor blood pressure every 2 weeks until stable dose established, then monthly thereafter. Interrupt or discontinue dose if hypertensive crisis (>180/120 mm Hg) occurs; discontinue if repeat BP >160/100 mm Hg for >4 weeks. Temporarily interrupt if severe diarrhea (grade ≥3) occurs; resume at next lower daily dose if improved to grade 1. Monitor absolute neutrophil count (ANC) monthly and for infection. Temporarily interrupt if ANC <1 x 10⁹/L occurs and remains low after 72 hours until resolved; resume at next lower daily dose. Use lowest effective dose. Due to potential for embryo/fetal toxicity, use effective contraception during and for ≥1 months after last dose. Confirm negative pregnancy status prior to initiation. Breastfeeding not recommended (during and for ≥1 month after last dose). Concomitant strong CYP3A4 inducers: not recommended. Concomitant strong CYP3A4 inhibitors or substrates; monitor for toxicity. May potentiate concomitant breast cancer resistance protein (BCRP) (e.g., *rosuvastatin*) or P-glycoprotein (P-gp) (e.g., *digoxin*) substrates; monitor for toxicity. Adverse reactions include diarrhea, hypertension, nausea, respiratory infection, dizziness, ALT/AST increase, rash, abdominal pain, fatigue, chest pain, and neutropenia.

THROMBOCYTOPENIA PURPURA, THROMBOTIC, ACQUIRED AUTOIMMUNE (ATTP)

VON WILLEBRAND FACTOR (vWF)-DIRECTED ANTIBODY FRAGMENT

➤ *caplacizumab-yhdp* initial administration should be upon the initiation of plasma exchange therapy, by a qualified healthcare provider

First day of treatment: 11 mg via IV bolus at least 15 minutes *prior to* plasma exchange; followed by 11 mg SC *after completion* of plasma exchange

Subsequent treatment: during daily plasma exchange: 11 mg SC once daily once daily following plasma exchange

Treatment after the plasma exchange period: 11 mg SC once daily x 30 days beyond the last plasma exchange

After initial treatment course: if signs of persistent underlying disease, such as suppressed ADAMTS13 activity levels, remain present, treatment may be extended for a maximum of 28 days

Discontinue treatment with Cablivi: if the patient experiences more than 2 recurrences of acquired autoimmune thrombotic thrombocytopenic purpura (aTTP)

Pediatric: safety and efficacy not established

Cablivi *Vial:* 11 mg powder, single-dose, for reconstitution and IV or SC administration

Comment: Cablivi *(caplacizumab-yhdp)* is indicated for the treatment of adult patients with aTTP, in combination with plasma exchange and immunosuppressive therapy. The ADAMTS13 gene provides instructions for making an enzyme that is involved in blood clotting. The most common adverse reactions to Cablivi (incidence >15%) are epistaxis, headache, and gingival bleeding. Severe bleeding can occur; risk is increased in patients with underlying coagulopathies and patients taking an anticoagulant. If clinically significant bleeding occurs, interrupt treatment. Withhold Cablivi for 7 days prior to elective surgery, dental procedures, or any other invasive intervention. Monitor pregnant patients/fetus and neonates closely for signs of bleeding. There is no information regarding the presence of *caplacizumab-yhdp* in human milk or effects on the breastfed infant. Developmental and health benefits of breastfeeding should be considered along with the mother's clinical need for Cablivi, potential adverse effects on the breastfed infant, and the underlying maternal condition.

CD20-TARGETING MONOCLONAL ANTIBODY

▶ *rituximab* initially (Month 0) 1,000 mg x 2 IV infusions separated by 2 weeks in combination with a tapering course of glucocorticoids; then a 500 mg IV infusion at Month 12 and every 6 months thereafter or based on clinical evaluation; *Relapse:* 1,000 mg IV infusion with considerations to resume or increase the glucocorticoid dose based on clinical evaluation; subsequent infusions may be no sooner than 16 weeks after the previous infusion; methylprednisolone 100 mg IV or equivalent glucocorticoid recommended 30 minutes prior to each infusion

Pediatric: <6 years: not recommended; ≥6 years: same as adult

Rituxan *Vial:* 100 mg/10 ml (10 mg/ml), 500 mg/50 ml (10 mg/ml), single-use (preservative-free)

Comment: Rituxan *(rituximab)* is a CD20-targeting cytolytic monoclonal antibody that received FDA Breakthrough Therapy Designation for treatment of pemphigus vulgaris (PV) in 2017. Safety and efficacy in recalcitrant PV have been demonstrated in approximately 500 patients across several small trials and case studies, with clinical remission occurring within 8 weeks in up to 95% of cases. In a recent phase 2 trial comparing *rituximab* plus *prednisone* with *prednisone* alone in patients with newly diagnosed PV, a 55% increase in 2-year remission rate (89% vs 34%) was observed in those receiving *rituximab* plus *prednisone*. Consider intravenous immunoglobulin (IVIG).

THYROID CANCER

KINASE INHIBITOR

▶ *selpercatinib* <*50 kg:* 120 mg bid; >*50 kg:* 160 mg bid; reduce dose in patients with severe hepatic impairment

Pediatric: <12 years: not established; ≥12 years: same as adult

Retevmo *Cap:* 40, 80 mg

Comment: Retevmo *(selpercatinib)* is a kinase inhibitor indicated for adult patients with metastatic RET (rearranged during transfection) fusion-positive non-small cell lung cancer; adult and pediatric patients ≥12 years of age with advanced or metastatic RET-mutant medullary thyroid cancer (MTC) who require systemic therapy; and adult and pediatric patients ≥12 years of age with advanced or metastatic RET fusion-positive thyroid cancer who require systemic therapy and who are radioactive iodine-refractory (if radioactive iodine is appropriate). The most common adverse reactions (incidence ≥25%), including laboratory abnormalities, have been increased aspartate aminotransferase (AST), increased alanine aminotransferase (ALT), increased glucose, decreased leukocytes, decreased albumin, decreased calcium, dry mouth, diarrhea, increased creatinine, increased alkaline phosphatase, hypertension, fatigue, edema, decreased platelets, increased total cholesterol, rash, decreased sodium, and constipation. Monitor ALT and AST prior to initiating Retevmo, every 2 weeks during the first 3 months, then monthly thereafter and as clinically indicated. Do not initiate Retevmo in patients with uncontrolled hypertension; optimize BP prior to initiating Retevmo and monitor BP after 1 week, at least monthly thereafter and as clinically indicated. Monitor patients who are at significant risk of developing QTc prolongation. Assess QT interval, electrolytes, and thyroid-stimulating hormone (TSH) at baseline and periodically during treatment. Monitor QT interval more frequently when Retevmo is concomitantly administered with strong and moderate CYP3A inhibitors or drugs known to prolong QTc interval. Permanently discontinue Retevmo in patients with severe or life-threatening hemorrhage. Withhold Retevmo and initiate corticosteroids in the occurrence of any hypersensitivity reaction and, upon resolution, resume at a reduced dose and increase dose by 1 dose level each week until reaching the dose taken prior to onset of hypersensitivity. Continue steroids until the patient reaches target dose of Retevmo and then taper. Withhold Retevmo for at least 7 days prior to elective surgery. Do not administer for at least 2 weeks following major surgery and until adequate wound healing. The safety of resumption of Retevmo after resolution of wound healing complications has not been established. Avoid co-administration with proton pump inhibitors (PPIs); if co-administration cannot be avoided, take Retevmo with food (with PPI) or modify its administration time (with H2 receptor antagonist or locally acting antacid). Avoid co-administration of strong and moderate CYP3A inhibitors; if

(continued)

co-administration cannot be avoided, reduce the **Retevmo** dose. Avoid co-administration with strong and moderate CYP3A inducers. Avoid co-administration with CYP2C8 and CYP3A substrates; if co-administration cannot be avoided, modify the substrate dosage as recommended in its product labeling. Based on findings from animal studies, and its mechanism of action, **Retevmo** can cause fetal harm. There are no available data on **Retevmo** use in pregnant females to inform drug-associated risk. Therefore, verify pregnancy status in females of reproductive potential prior to initiating **Retevmo** and advise of the possible risk to the fetus and to use effective contraception. There are no data on the presence of *selpercatinib* or its metabolites in human milk or effects on the breastfed infant. Because of the potential for serious adverse embryo/fetal effects, advise women not to breastfeed during treatment with **Retevmo** and for 1 week after the final dose.

THYROID EYE DISEASE/GRAVE'S EYE DISEASE

MONOCLONAL ANTIBODY AND INSULIN-LIKE GROWTH FACTOR-1 RECEPTOR INHIBITOR

▷ *teprotumumab-trbw* 10 mg/kg for the first IV infusion, followed by 20 mg/kg once every 3 weeks x 7 additional IV infusions; administer the IV infusions over 60-90 minutes

Tepezza *Vial:* 500 mg pwdr, single-dose, for reconstitution, dilution, and IV infusion

Comment: Tepezza *(teprotumumab-trbw)* is a fully human monoclonal antibody (mAb) and a targeted inhibitor of the insulin-like growth factor 1 receptor (IGF-1R) for the treatment of active thyroid eye disease (TED). The most common adverse reactions (incidence >5%) have been muscle spasm, nausea, alopecia, diarrhea, fatigue, hyperglycemia, hearing impairment, dry skin, dysgeusia, and headache. If an infusion reaction occurs, interrupt or slow the rate of infusion and use appropriate medical management. Monitor patients with preexisting inflammatory bowel disease (IBD) for disease flare; discontinue **Tepezza** if IBD worsens. Monitor glucose levels in all patients; treat hyperglycemia with glycemic control medications. Appropriate forms of contraception should be implemented prior to initiation of **Tepezza**, during treatment, and for 6 months following the last dose. There is no information regarding the presence of **Tepezza** in human milk or effects on the breastfed infant.

TICKBORNE ENCEPHALITIS PROPHYLAXIS

▷ *tickborne encephalitis vaccine* each dose 0.5 ml SC; Dose 1: Day 0; Dose 2: 14 days to 3 months after the first dose; Dose 3: 5 to 12 months after the second dose

Pediatric: <1 year: safety and efficacy not established; 1-15 years: each dose 0.25 ml SC; Dose 1: day 0; Dose 2: 1-3 months after the first dose; Dose 3: 5 to 12 months after the second dose; ≥16 years: same as adult

TicoVac *Prefilled syringe:* 0.25, 0.5 ml susp, single-dose

Comment: TicoVac is a 3-dose inactivated whole virus vaccine indicated for active immunization to prevent tickborne encephalitis (TBE) in individuals ≥1 year of age. The only contraindication is severe allergic reaction (e.g., anaphylaxis) to any component of the **TicoVac** vaccine. **TicoVac** contains albumin, a derivative of human blood. Based on effective donor screening and product manufacturing processes, it carries an extremely remote risk for transmission of viral diseases and variant Creutzfeldt-Jakob disease (vCJD). There is a theoretical risk for transmission of Creutzfeldt-Jakob disease (CJD), but if that risk actually exists, the risk of transmission would also be considered extremely remote. No cases of transmission of viral diseases, CJD or vCJD, have ever been identified for licensed albumin or albumin contained in other licensed products. In clinical studies, the most common adverse reactions in subjects 1 through 15 years of age who received **TicoVac** were local tenderness (18.1%), local pain (11.2%), headache (11.1%), fever (9.6%), and restlessness (9.1%). In clinical trials (n = 3,240), the following additional adverse reactions to the vaccine in <1% of subjects 1 through 15 years of age were vertigo, dizziness, sensory abnormalities, abdominal pain, diarrhea, dyspepsia, injection site pruritus, and urticaria. The most common adverse reactions in subjects 16 through 65 years of age who received **TicoVac** were local tenderness (29.9%), local pain (13.2%), fatigue (6.6%), headache (6.3%), and muscle pain (5.1%). In clinical trials (n = 4,427), the following additional adverse reactions to the vaccine in <1% of subjects 16 through <65 years of age were hypersensitivity, somnolence, vertigo, diarrhea, abdominal pain, injection site pruritus, and injection site warmth. There are no adequate and well-controlled studies of **TicoVac** in pregnant females. Available human data are insufficient to establish the presence or absence of vaccine-associated fetal risk during pregnancy. Developmental and reproductive toxicity studies in animals have not been conducted with **TicoVac**. Human data are not available to assess for presence of **TicoVac** in breast milk or potential effects on the breastfed infant. Developmental and health benefits of breastfeeding should be considered along with the mother's clinical need for **TicoVac** and any adverse effects on the breastfed infant from **TicoVac** or from the underlying maternal condition.

REFERENCES

Heinz FX, Holzmann H, Essl A, et al. Field effectiveness of vaccination against tick-borne encephalitis. *Vaccine* 2007, 25(43), 7559–7567.

Heinz FX, Stiasny K, Holzmann H, et al. Vaccination and tick-borne encephalitis, central Europe. *Emerg Infect Dis* 2013, 19(1), 69–76.

TINEA CAPITIS

Comment: Tinea capitis must be treated with a systemic antifungal.

FOR SEVERE KERION PRURITUS

➤ *prednisone* 1 mg/kg/day for 7-14 days
   See **Oral Corticosteroids** Appendix K. Oral Corticosteroids

SYSTEMIC ANTIFUNGALS

➤ *griseofulvin, microsize* (G) 500 mg once daily x 4-6 weeks <u>or</u> longer; max 1 gm/day
   Pediatric: <30 lb: 5 mg/lb/day; 30-50 lb: 125-250 mg/day; >50 lb: 250-500 mg/day; 5 mg/lb/day x 4-6 weeks <u>or</u> longer; *see* Appendix BB.25. *griseofulvin, microsize* (G) (Grifulvin V Suspension) *for dose by weight*
   Grifulvin V *Tab:* 250, 500 mg; *Oral susp:* 125 mg/5 ml (120 ml) (alcohol 0.02%)
➤ *griseofulvin, ultramicrosize* (G) 375 mg/day in a single <u>or</u> divided doses x 4-6 weeks <u>or</u> longer
   Pediatric: <2 years: <u>not</u> recommended; ≥2 years: 3.3 mg/lb/day in a single <u>or</u> divided doses x 4-6 weeks <u>or</u> longer
   Gris-PEG *Tab:* 125, 250 mg
   Comment: *Griseofulvin* should be taken with fatty foods (e.g., milk, ice cream). Liver enzymes should be monitored.
➤ *ketoconazole* (G) initially 200 mg once daily; max 400 mg/day x 4 weeks
   Pediatric: <2 years: <u>not</u> recommended; ≥2 years: 3.3-6.6 mg/kg once daily x 4 weeks
   Nizoral *Tab:* 200 mg
   Comment: Caution with *ketoconazole* due to concerns about potential for hepatotoxicity.

TINEA CORPORIS

TOPICAL ANTIFUNGALS

➤ *butenafine* (G) apply bid x 1 week <u>or</u> once daily x 4 weeks
   Pediatric: <12 years: <u>not</u> recommended; ≥12 years: same as adult
   Lotrimin Ultra (OTC) *Crm:* 1% (12, 24 gm)
   Mentax *Crm:* 1% (15, 30 gm)
   Comment: *Butenafine* is a benzylamine, <u>not</u> an azole. Fungicidal activity continues for at least 5 weeks after last application.
➤ *ciclopirox*
   Loprox Cream apply bid; max 4 weeks
   Pediatric: <10 years: <u>not</u> recommended; ≥10 years: same as adult
   Crm: 0.77% (15, 30, 90 gm)
   Loprox Lotion apply bid; max 4 weeks
   Pediatric: <10 years: <u>not</u> recommended; ≥10 years: same as adult
   Lotn: 0.77% (30, 60 ml)
   Loprox Gel apply bid; max 4 weeks
   Pediatric: <16 years: <u>not</u> recommended; ≥16 years: same as adult
   Gel: 0.77% (30, 45 gm)
➤ *clotrimazole* (G) apply to affected area bid x 7 days
   Pediatric: same as adult
   Lotrimin *Crm:* 1% (15, 30, 45 gm)
   Lotrimin AF (OTC) *Crm:* 1% (12 gm); *Lotn:* 1% (10 ml); *Soln:* 1% (10 ml)
➤ *econazole* apply once daily x 14 days
   Pediatric: same as adult
   Spectazole *Crm:* 1% (15, 30, 85 gm)
➤ *ketoconazole* apply once daily x 14 days
   Pediatric: <12 years: <u>not</u> recommended; ≥12 years: same as adult
   Nizoral Cream *Crm:* 2% (15, 30, 60 gm)
➤ *luliconazole* apply to affected area and 1 inch into the immediate surrounding area(s) once daily
   Pediatric: <18 years: <u>not</u> recommended; ≥18 years: same as adult
   Luzu Cream 1% *Crm:* 1% (30, 60 gm)
➤ *miconazole* 2% apply once daily-bid x 2 weeks
   Pediatric: same as adult
   Lotrimin AF Spray Liquid (OTC) *Spray liq:* 2% (113 gm) (alcohol 17%)
   Lotrimin AF Spray Powder (OTC) *Spray pwdr:* 2% (90 gm) (alcohol 10%)
   Monistat-Derm *Crm:* 2% (1, 3 oz); *Spray liq:* 2% (3.5 oz); *Spray pwdr:* 2% (3 oz)
➤ *naftifine* (G)
   Pediatric: <12 years: <u>not</u> recommended; ≥12 years: same as adult
   Naftin Cream apply once daily x 14 days
   Crm: 1% (15, 30, 60 gm)
   Naftin Gel apply bid x 14 days
   Gel: 1% (20, 40, 60 gm)

(continued)

▷ *oxiconazole nitrate* (G) apply once daily-bid x 2 weeks
  Pediatric: same as adult
    Oxistat *Crm:* 1% (15, 30, 60 gm); *Lotn:* 1% (30 ml)
▷ *sulconazole* apply once daily-bid x 3 weeks
  Pediatric: <12 years: <u>not</u> recommended; ≥12 years: same as adult
    Exelderm *Crm:* 1% (15, 30, 60 gm); *Lotn:* 1% (30 mg)
▷ *terbinafine* (G)
  Pediatric: <12 years: <u>not</u> recommended; ≥12 years: same as adult
    Lamisil Cream (OTC) apply to affected and surrounding area once daily-bid x 1-4 weeks until significantly improved
      Crm: 1% (15, 30 gm)
    Lamisil AT Cream (OTC) apply to affected and surrounding area once daily-bid x 1-4 weeks until significantly improved
      Crm: 1% (15, 30 gm)
    Lamisil Solution (OTC) apply to affected and surrounding area once daily x 1 week
      Soln: 1% (30 ml spray bottle)

TOPICAL ANTIFUNGAL+STEROID COMBINATION
▷ *clotrimazole+betamethasone* (G) apply bid x 2 weeks; max 4 weeks
  Pediatric: <12 years: <u>not</u> recommended; ≥12 years: same as adult
    Lotrisone *Crm:* clotrim 1 mg+beta 0.5 mg (15, 45 gm); *Lotn:* clotrim 1 mg+beta 0.5 mg (30 ml)

SYSTEMIC ANTIFUNGALS
▷ *griseofulvin, microsize* (G) 500 mg/day x 2-4 weeks; max 1 gm/day
  Pediatric: <30 lb: 5 mg/lb/day; 30-50 lb: 125-250 mg/day; >50 lb: 250-500 mg/day; *see* Appendix BB.25.
  griseofulvin, microsize (G) (Grifulvin V Suspension) *for dose by weight*
    Grifulvin V *Tab:* 250, 500 mg; *Oral susp:* 125 mg/5 ml (120 ml) (alcohol 0.02%)
▷ *griseofulvin, ultramicrosize* (G) 375 mg/day in a single <u>or</u> divided doses x 2-4 weeks
  Pediatric: <2 years: <u>not</u> recommended; ≥2 years: 3.3 mg/lb/day in a single <u>or</u> divided doses
    Gris-PEG *Tab:* 125, 250 mg
  Comment: *Griseofulvin* should be taken with fatty foods (e.g., milk, ice cream). Liver enzymes should be monitored.
▷ *ketoconazole* initially 200 mg once daily; max 400 mg/day x 4 weeks
  Pediatric: <2 years: <u>not</u> recommended; ≥2 years: 3.3-6.6 mg/kg/day x 4 weeks
    Nizoral *Tab:* 200 mg
  Comment: Caution with *ketoconazole* due to concerns about potential for hepatotoxicity.

TINEA CRURIS (JOCK ITCH)

TOPICAL ANTIFUNGALS
▷ *butenafine* (G) apply bid x 1 week <u>or</u> once daily x 4 weeks
  Pediatric: <12 years: <u>not</u> recommended; ≥12 years: same as adult
    Lotrimin Ultra (OTC) *Crm:* 1% (12, 24 gm)
    Mentax *Crm:* 1% (15, 30 gm)
  Comment: *Butenafine* is a benzylamine, <u>not</u> an azole. Fungicidal activity continues for at least 5 weeks after last application.
▷ *ciclopirox*
    Loprox Cream apply bid; max 4 weeks
      Pediatric: <10 years: <u>not</u> recommended; ≥10 years: same as adult
      Crm: 0.77% (15, 30, 90 gm)
    Loprox Lotion apply bid; max 4 weeks
      Pediatric: <10 years: <u>not</u> recommended; ≥10 years: same as adult
      Lotn: 0.77% (30, 60 ml)
    Loprox Gel apply bid; max 4 weeks
      Pediatric: <16 years: <u>not</u> recommended; ≥16 years: same as adult
      Gel: 0.77% (30, 45 gm)
▷ *clotrimazole* (G) apply to affected area bid x 7 days
  Pediatric: same as adult
    Lotrimin *Crm:* 1% (15, 30, 45 gm)
    Lotrimin AF (OTC) *Crm:* 1% (12 gm); *Lotn:* 1% (10 ml); *Soln:* 1% (10 ml)
▷ *econazole* apply once daily x 2 weeks
  Pediatric: same as adult
    Spectazole *Crm:* 1% (15, 30, 85 gm)
▷ *ketoconazole* (G) apply bid x 4 weeks
  Pediatric: <12 years: <u>not</u> recommended; ≥12 years: same as adult
    Nizoral Cream *Crm:* 2% (15, 30, 60 gm)

▷ *luliconazole* apply to affected area and 1 inch into the immediate surrounding area(s) once daily
   Pediatric: <18 years: not recommended; ≥18 years: same as adult
     Luzu Cream 1% *Crm:* 1% (30, 60 gm)
▷ *miconazole* **2% (G)** apply once daily-bid x 2 weeks
   Pediatric: same as adult
     Lotrimin AF Spray Liquid (OTC) *Spray liq:* 2% (113 gm) (alcohol 17%)
     Lotrimin AF Spray Powder (OTC) *Spray pwdr:* 2% (90 gm) (alcohol 10%)
     Monistat-Derm *Crm:* 2% (1, 3 oz); *Spray liq:* 2% (3.5 oz); *Spray pwdr:* 2% (3 oz)
▷ *naftifine* **(G)**
   Pediatric: <12 years: not recommended; ≥12 years: same as adult
     Naftin Cream apply once daily x 2 weeks
       Crm: 1% (15, 30, 60 gm)
     Naftin Gel apply bid x 2 weeks
       Gel: 1% (20, 40, 60 gm)
▷ *oxiconazole nitrate* **(G)** apply once daily-bid x 2 weeks
   Pediatric: same as adult
     Oxistat *Crm:* 1% (15, 30, 60 gm); *Lotn:* 1% (30 ml)
▷ *sulconazole* apply once daily-bid x 3 weeks
   Pediatric: <12 years: not recommended; ≥12 years: same as adult
     Exelderm *Crm:* 1% (15, 30, 60 gm); *Lotn:* 1% (30 mg)
▷ *terbinafine* **(G)**
   Pediatric: <12 years: not recommended; ≥12 years: same as adult
     Lamisil Cream (OTC) apply bid x 1-4 weeks
       Crm: 1% (15, 30 gm)
     Lamisil AT Cream (OTC) apply to affected and surrounding area once daily-bid x 1-4 weeks until
     significantly improved
       Crm: 1% (15, 30 gm)
     Lamisil Solution (OTC) apply to affected and surrounding area once daily x 1 week
       Soln: 1% (30 ml spray bottle)
▷ *tolnaftate* **(OTC)(G)** apply sparingly bid x 2-4 weeks
   Pediatric: <2 years: not recommended; ≥2 years: same as adult
     Tinactin *Crm:* 1% (15, 30 gm); *Pwdr:* 1% (45, 90 gm); *Soln:* 1% (10 ml); *Aerosol liq:* 1% (4 oz); *Aerosol*
     pwdr: 1% (3.5, 5 oz)
▷ *undecylenic acid* apply bid x 4 weeks
   Pediatric: same as adult
     Desenex (OTC) *Pwdr:* 25% (1.5, 3 oz); *Spray pwdr:* 25% (2.7 oz); *Oint:* 25% (0.5, 1 oz)

TOPICAL ANTIFUNGAL+ANTI-INFLAMMATORY AGENTS
▷ *clotrimazole+betamethasone* **(G)** apply bid x 4 weeks; max 4 weeks
   Pediatric: <12 years: not recommended; ≥12 years: same as adult
   Crm: clotrim 10 mg+beta 0.5 mg (15, 45 gm); *Lotn:* clotrim 10 mg+beta 0.5 mg (30 ml)

SYSTEMIC ANTIFUNGALS
▷ *griseofulvin, microsize* **(G)** 1 gm once daily x 2 weeks
   Pediatric: <30 lb: 5 mg/lb/day; 30-50 lb: 125-250 mg/day; >50 lb: 250-500 mg/day; 5 mg/lb/day x 4-6 weeks
   or longer; see Appendix BB.25. *griseofulvin, microsize* **(G)** (Grifulvin V Suspension) *for dose by weight*
     Grifulvin V *Tab:* 250, 500 mg; *Oral susp:* 125 mg/5 ml (120 ml) (alcohol 0.02%)
▷ *griseofulvin, ultramicrosize* 375 mg/day in a single or divided doses x 2 weeks
   Pediatric: <2 years: not recommended; ≥2 years: 3.3 mg/lb/day in a single or divided doses
     Gris-PEG *Tab:* 125, 250 mg
Comment: *Griseofulvin* should be taken with fatty foods (e.g., milk, ice cream). Liver enzymes should be
monitored.
▷ *ketoconazole* initially 200 mg once daily; max 400 mg once daily x 4 weeks
   Pediatric: <2 years: not recommended; ≥2 years: 3.3-6.6 mg/kg/day
     Nizoral *Tab:* 200 mg
Comment: Caution with *ketoconazole* due to concerns about potential for hepatotoxicity.

TINEA PEDIS (ATHLETE'S FOOT)

TOPICAL ANTIFUNGALS
▷ *butenafine* **(G)** apply bid x 1 week or once daily x 4 weeks
   Pediatric: <12 years: not recommended; ≥12 years: same as adult
     Lotrimin Ultra (OTC) *Crm:* 1% (12, 24 gm)
     Mentax *Crm:* 1% (15, 30 gm)
Comment: *Butenafine* is a benzylamine, not an azole. Fungicidal activity continues for at least 5 weeks after
last application.

(continued)

▷ *Burow's solution* wet dressings
▷ *ciclopirox*
    Loprox Cream apply bid; max 4 weeks
      Pediatric: <10 years: <u>not</u> recommended; ≥10 years: same as adult
      Crm: 0.77% (15, 30, 90 gm)
    Loprox Lotion apply bid; max 4 weeks
      Pediatric: <10 years: <u>not</u> recommended; ≥10 years: same as adult
      Lotn: 0.77% (30, 60 ml)
    Loprox Gel apply bid; max 4 weeks
      Pediatric: <16 years: <u>not</u> recommended; ≥16 years: same as adult
      Gel: 0.77% (30, 45 gm)
▷ *clotrimazole* (G) apply bid to affected area x 4 weeks
  Pediatric: same as adult
    Desenex *Crm:* 1% (0.5 oz)
    Lotrimin *Crm:* 1% (15, 30, 45, 90 gm); *Lotn:* 1% (30 ml); *Soln:* 1% (10, 30 ml)
    Lotrimin AF (OTC) *Crm:* 1% (15, 30, 45, 90 gm); *Lotn:* 1% (20 ml); *Soln:* 1% (20 ml)
▷ *econazole* apply once daily x 4 weeks
  Pediatric: same as adult
    Spectazole *Crm:* 1% (15, 30, 85 gm)
▷ *ketoconazole* apply once daily x 6 weeks
  Pediatric: <12 years: <u>not</u> recommended; ≥12 years: same as adult
    Nizoral Cream *Crm:* 2% (15, 30, 60 gm)
▷ *luliconazole* apply to affected area and 1 inch into the immediate surrounding area(s) once daily
  Pediatric: <18 years: <u>not</u> recommended; ≥18 years: same as adult
    Luzu Cream 1% *Crm:* 1% (30, 60 gm)
▷ *miconazole 2%* (G) apply bid x 4 weeks
  Pediatric: same as adult
    Lotrimin AF Spray Liquid (OTC) *Spray liq:* 2% (113 gm) (alcohol 17%)
    Lotrimin AF Spray Powder (OTC) *Spray pwdr:* 2% (90 gm) (alcohol 10%)
    Monistat-Derm *Crm:* 2% (1, 3 oz); *Spray liq:* 2% (3.5 oz); *Spray pwdr:* 2% (3 oz)
▷ *naftifine* (G)
  Pediatric: <12 years: <u>not</u> recommended; ≥12 years: same as adult
    Naftin Cream apply once daily x 4 weeks
      Crm: 1% (15, 30, 60 gm)
    Naftin Gel apply bid x 4 weeks
      Gel: 1% (20, 40, 60 gm)
▷ *oxiconazole nitrate* (G) apply once daily-bid x 4 weeks
  Pediatric: same as adult
    Oxistat *Crm:* 1% (15, 30, 60 gm); *Lotn:* 1% (30 ml)
▷ *sertaconazole* apply once daily-bid x 4 weeks
  Pediatric: <12 years: <u>not</u> recommended; ≥12 years: same as adult
    Ertaczo *Crm:* 2% (15, 30 gm)
▷ *sulconazole* apply once daily-bid x 4 weeks
  Pediatric: <12 years: <u>not</u> recommended; ≥12 years: same as adult
    Exelderm *Crm:* 1% (15, 30, 60 gm); *Lotn:* 1% (30 mg)
▷ *terbinafine* (G)
  Pediatric: <12 years: <u>not</u> recommended; ≥12 years: same as adult
    Lamisil Cream (OTC) apply bid x 1-4 weeks
      Crm: 1% (15, 30 gm)
    Lamisil AT Cream (OTC) apply to affected and surrounding area once daily-bid x 1-4 weeks until significantly improved
      Crm: 1% (15, 30 gm)
    Lamisil Solution (OTC) apply to affected and surrounding area bid x 1 week
      Soln: 1% (30 ml spray bottle)
▷ *tolnaftate* (OTC)(G) apply sparingly bid x 2-4 weeks
  Pediatric: <2 years: <u>not</u> recommended; ≥2 years: same as adult
    Tinactin *Crm:* 1% (15, 30 gm); *Pwdr:* 1% (45, 90 gm); *Soln:* 1% (10 ml); *Aerosol liq:* 1% (4 oz); *Aerosol pwdr:* 1% (3.5, 5 oz)

TOPICAL ANTIFUNGAL+ANTI-INFLAMMATORY COMBINATION
  ▷ *clotrimazole+betamethasone* (G) apply bid x 4 weeks; max 4 weeks
    Pediatric: <12 years: <u>not</u> recommended; ≥12 years: same as adult
      Lotrisone *Crm:* clotrim 1 mg+beta 0.5 mg (15, 45 gm); *Lotn:* clotrim 1 mg+beta 0.5 mg (30 ml)

SYSTEMIC ANTIFUNGALS
  ▷ *griseofulvin, microsize* (G) 1 gm once daily x 4-8 weeks

Pediatric: <30 lb: 5 mg/lb/day; 30-50 lb: 125-250 mg/day; >50 lb: 250-500 mg/day; 5 mg/lb/day x 4-6 weeks or longer; *see* Appendix BB.25. *griseofulvin, microsize* (G) (Grifulvin V Suspension) *for dose by weight*
    Grifulvin V *Tab:* 250, 500 mg; *Oral susp:* 125 mg/5 ml (120 ml) (alcohol 0.02%)
▷ *griseofulvin, ultramicrosize* 750 mg/day in a single or divided doses x 4-6 weeks
    Pediatric: <2 years: <u>not</u> recommended; ≥2 years: 3.3 mg/lb/day in a single or divided doses
        Gris-PEG *Tab:* 125, 250 mg
Comment: *Griseofulvin* should be taken with fatty foods (e.g., milk, ice cream). Liver enzymes should be monitored.
▷ *ketoconazole* initially 200 mg once daily; max 400 mg/day x 4 weeks
    Pediatric: <2 years: <u>not</u> recommended; ≥2 years: 3.3-6.6 mg/kg once daily x 4 weeks
        Nizoral *Tab:* 200 mg
Comment: Caution with *ketoconazole* due to concerns about potential for hepatotoxicity.

TINEA VERSICOLOR

Comment: Resolution may take 3-6 months.

TOPICAL ANTIFUNGALS
▷ *butenafine* (G) apply once daily x 2 weeks
    Pediatric: <12 years: <u>not</u> recommended; ≥12 years: same as adult
        Lotrimin Ultra (OTC) *Crm:* 1% (12, 24 gm)
        Mentax *Crm:* 1% (15, 30 gm)
Comment: *Butenafine* is a benzylamine, <u>not</u> an azole. Fungicidal activity continues for at least 5 weeks after last application.
▷ *ciclopirox*
    Loprox Cream apply bid; max 4 weeks
    Pediatric: <10 years: <u>not</u> recommended; ≥10 years: same as adult
      Crm: 0.77% (15, 30, 90 gm)
    Loprox Lotion apply bid; max 4 weeks
    Pediatric: <10 years: <u>not</u> recommended; ≥10 years: same as adult
      Lotn: 0.77% (30, 60 ml)
    Loprox Gel apply bid; max 4 weeks
    Pediatric: <16 years: <u>not</u> recommended; ≥16 years: same as adult
      Gel: 0.77% (30, 45 gm)
▷ *clotrimazole* (G) apply bid x 7 days
    Pediatric: same as adult
        Lotrimin *Crm:* 1% (15, 30, 45 gm)
        Lotrimin AF (OTC) *Crm:* 1% (12 gm); *Lotn:* 1% (10 ml); *Soln:* 1% (10 ml)
▷ *econazole* apply once daily x 2 weeks
    Pediatric: same as adult
        Spectazole *Crm:* 1% (15, 30, 85 gm)
▷ *miconazole* **2%** (G) apply once daily x 2 weeks
    Pediatric: same as adult
        Lotrimin AF Spray Liquid (OTC) *Spray liq:* 2% (113 gm) (alcohol 17%)
        Lotrimin AF Spray Powder (OTC) *Spray pwdr:* 2% (90 gm) (alcohol 10%)
        Monistat-Derm *Crm:* 2% (1, 3 oz); *Spray liq:* 2% (3.5 oz); *Spray pwdr:* 2% (3 oz)
▷ *ketoconazole* (G)
    Pediatric: <12 years: <u>not</u> recommended; ≥12 years: same as adult
        Nizoral Cream apply once daily x 2 weeks
      Crm: 2% (15, 30, 60 gm)
        Nizoral Shampoo lather into area and leave on 5 minutes x 1 application
      Shampoo: 2% (4 oz)
▷ *oxiconazole nitrate* (G) apply once daily x 2 weeks
    Pediatric: same as adult
        Oxistat *Crm:* 1% (15, 30, 60 gm); *Lotn:* 1% (30 ml)
▷ *selenium sulfide* shampoo (G) apply after shower, allow to dry, leave on overnight; then scrub off vigorously in the AM; repeat in 1 week and again q 3 months until resolution occurs
    Pediatric: same as adult
        Selsun Blue *Shampoo:* 1% (120, 210, 240, 330 ml); 2.5% (120 ml)
▷ *sulconazole* apply once daily-bid x 3 weeks
    Pediatric: <12 years: <u>not</u> recommended; ≥12 years: same as adult
        Exelderm *Crm:* 1% (15, 30, 60 gm); *Lotn:* 1% (30 mg)
▷ *terbinafine* apply bid to affected and surrounding area x 1 week
    Pediatric: <12 years: <u>not</u> recommended; ≥12 years: same as adult
        Lamisil Solution (OTC) *Soln:* 1% (30 ml spray bottle)

ORAL ANTIFUNGALS

▷ *ketoconazole* initially 200 mg once daily; max 400 mg/day x 4 weeks
  Pediatric: <2 years: not recommended; ≥2 years: 3.3-6.6 mg/kg once daily x 4 weeks
    Nizoral *Tab:* 200 mg

TOBACCO DEPENDENCE, TOBACCO CESSATION, NICOTINE WITHDRAWAL SYNDROME

Comment: According to findings from the Population Assessment of Tobacco and Health (PATH) Study (respondents = 10, 384, mean age = 14.3), any use of e-cigarettes, hookah, non-cigarette combustible tobacco, or smokeless tobacco was independently associated with traditional cigarette smoking 1 year later and use of more than 1 of these products increases the odds of progressing to traditional cigarette use.

NON-NICOTINE PRODUCTS
Alpha4-Beta4 Nicotinic Acetylcholine Receptor Partial Agonist

▷ *varenicline* (G) set target quit date; begin therapy 1 week prior to target quit date; take after eating with a full glass of water; initially 0.5 mg once daily for 3 days; then 0.5 mg bid x 4 days; then 1 mg bid; treat x 12 weeks; may continue treatment for 12 more weeks
  Pediatric: <16 years: not studied; ≥16 years: same as adult
    Chantix *Tab:* 0.5, 1 mg; *Starting Month Pak:* 0.5 mg x 11 tabs + 1 mg x 42 tabs; *Continuing Month Pak:* 1 mg x 56 tabs
    Comment: Caution with **Chantix** due to potential risk for anxiety or suicidal ideation.

AMINOKETONES

▷ *bupropion HBr* (G)
  Pediatric: safety and efficacy not established; when considering the use of **Aplenzin** in a child or adolescent, balance the potential risks with the clinical need
    Aplenzin initially 100 mg bid for at least 3 days; may increase to 375 or 400 mg/day after several weeks; then after at least 3 more days, 450 mg in 4 divided doses; max 450 mg/day, 174 mg/single dose
      Tab: 174, 348, 522 mg
▷ *bupropion HCl* (G)
  Pediatric: safety and efficacy not established; when considering the use of **Forfivo XL** in a child or adolescent, balance the potential risks with the clinical need
    Forfivo XL do not use for initial treatment; use immediate-release *bupropion* forms for initial titration; switch to **Forfivo XL** 450 mg once daily when total dose/day reaches 450 mg; may switch to **Forfivo XL** when total dose/day reaches 300 mg for 2 weeks and the patient needs 450 mg/day to reach therapeutic target; swallow whole, do not crush or chew
      Tab: 450 mg ext-rel
    Wellbutrin initially 100 mg bid for at least 3 days; may increase to 375 or 400 mg/day after several weeks; then after at least 3 more days, 450 mg in 4 divided doses; max 450 mg/day, 150 mg/single dose
      Tab: 75, 100 mg
    Wellbutrin SR initially 150 mg in the AM for at least 3 days; may increase to 150 mg bid if well tolerated; usual dose 300 mg/day; max 400 mg/day
      Tab: 100, 150 mg sust-rel
    Wellbutrin XL initially 150 mg in the AM for at least 3 days; increase to 150 mg bid if well tolerated; usual dose 300 mg/day; max 400 mg/day
      Tab: 150, 300 mg sust-rel
    Zyban 150 mg once daily x 3 days; then 150 mg bid x 7-12 weeks; max 300 mg/day
      Tab: 150 mg sust-rel
  Comment: Contraindications to *bupropion* include seizure disorder, eating disorder, concurrent monoamine oxidase inhibitor (MAOI), and alcohol use. Smoking should be discontinued after the 7th day of therapy with *bupropion*. Avoid bedtime dose.

TRANSDERMAL NICOTINE SYSTEMS

Habitrol (OTC) initially one 21 mg/24 hours patch/day x 4-6 weeks; then one 14 mg/24 hours patch/day x 2-4 weeks; then one 7 mg/24 hours patch/day x 2-4 weeks; then discontinue
  Pediatric: <12 years: not recommended; ≥12 years: same as adult
    Transdermal patch: 7, 14, 21 mg/24 hours
Nicoderm CQ (OTC) initially one 21 mg/24 hours patch/day x 6 weeks, then one 14 mg/24 hours patch/day x 2 weeks; then one 7 mg/24 hours patch/day x 2 weeks
  Pediatric: <12 years: not recommended; ≥12 years: same as adult
    Transdermal patch: 7, 14, 21 mg/24 hours
  Comment: Nicoderm CQ is available as a clear patch.
Nicotrol Step-down Patch (OTC) 1 patch/day x 6 weeks
  Pediatric: <12 years: not recommended; ≥12 years: same as adult
    Transdermal patch: 7, 14, 21 mg/24 hours (7/pck)
Nicotrol Transdermal (OTC) 1 patch/day x 6 weeks
  Pediatric: <12 years: not recommended; ≥12 years: same as adult

Transdermal patch: 15 mg/24 hours (7/pck)

Prostep initially one 22 mg/24 hours patch/day x 4-8 weeks; then discontinue <u>or</u> one 11 mg/24 hours patch/day x 2-4 additional weeks

Pediatric: <12 years: <u>not</u> recommended; ≥12 years: same as adult

Transdermal patch: 11, 22 mg/24 hours (7/pck)

NICOTINE GUM

▷ *nicotine polacrilex* chew one piece of gum slowly and intermittently over 30 minutes q 1-2 hours x 6 weeks; then q 2-4 hours x 3 weeks; then q 4-8 hours x 3 weeks; max 24 pieces/day; 2 mg if smoked <25 cigarettes/day; 4 mg if smoked >24 cigarettes/day

Pediatric: <12 years: <u>not</u> recommended; ≥12 years: same as adult

Nicorette (OTC) *Gum squares:* 2, 4 mg (108 piece starter kit and 48 piece refill) (orange, mint, <u>or</u> original, sugar-free)

NICOTINE LOZENGE

▷ *nicotine polacrilex* (OTC)(G) dissolve over 20-30 minutes; minimize swallowing; do <u>not</u> eat <u>or</u> drink for 15 minutes before and during use; use 2 mg lozenge if first cigarette smoked >30 minutes after waking; use 4 mg lozenge if first cigarette smoked within 30 minutes of waking; 1 lozenge q 1-2 hours (at least 9/day) x 6 weeks; then q 2-4 hours x 3 weeks; then q 4-8 hours x 3 weeks; then stop; max 5 lozenges/6 hours and 20 lozenges/day

Pediatric: <18 years: <u>not</u> recommended; ≥18 years: same as adult

Commit Lozenge *Loz:* 2, 4 mg (72/pck) (phenylalanine)

Nicorette Mini Lozenge (G) *Loz:* 2, 4 mg (72/pck) (mint; phenylalanine)

NICOTINE INHALATION PRODUCTS

▷ *nicotine* 0.5 mg aqueous nasal spray

Pediatric: <12 years: <u>not</u> recommended; ≥12 years: same as adult

Nicotrol NS 1-2 doses/hour nasally; max 5 doses/hour <u>or</u> 40 doses/day; usual max 3 months

Nasal spray: 0.5 mg/spray; 10 mg/ml (10 ml, 200 doses)

▷ *nicotine* 10 mg inhalation system

Pediatric: <12 years: <u>not</u> recommended; ≥12 years: same as adult

Nicotrol Inhaler individualize therapy; at least 6 cartridges/day x 3-6 weeks; max 16 cartridges/day x first 12 weeks; then reduce gradually over 12 more weeks

Inhaler: 10 mg/cartridge, 4 mg delivered (42 cartridge/pck) (menthol)

Comment: Nicotrol Inhaler is a smoking replacement; to be used with decreasing frequency. Smoking should be discontinued before starting therapy. Side effects include cough, nausea, mouth, <u>or</u> throat irritation. This system delivers nicotine, but no tars <u>or</u> carcinogens. Each cartridge lasts about 20 minutes with frequent continuous puffing and provides nicotine equivalent to 2 cigarettes.

TONSILLITIS: ACUTE

ANTI-INFECTIVES

▷ *amoxicillin* (G) 500-875 mg bid <u>or</u> 250-500 mg tid x 10 days

Pediatric: <40 kg (88 lb): 20-40 mg/kg/day in 3 divided doses x 10 days <u>or</u> 25-45 mg/kg/day in 2 divided doses x 10 days; *see* Appendix BB.3. *amoxicillin* (G) (Amoxil Suspension, Trimox Suspension) *for dose by weight*

Amoxil *Cap:* 250, 500 mg; *Tab:* 875*mg; *Chew tab:* 125, 200, 250, 400 mg (cherry-banana-peppermint) (phenylalanine); *Oral susp:* 125, 250 mg/5 ml (80, 100, 150 ml) (strawberry); 200, 400 mg/5 ml (50, 75, 100 ml) (bubble gum); *Oral drops:* 50 mg/ml (30 ml) (bubble gum)

Moxatag *Tab:* 775 mg ext-rel

Trimox *Tab:* 125, 250 mg; *Cap:* 250, 500 mg; *Oral susp:* 125, 250 mg/5 ml (80, 100, 150 ml) (raspberry-strawberry)

▷ *azithromycin* (G) 500 mg x 1 dose on day 1, then 250 mg once daily on days 2-5 <u>or</u> 500 mg once daily x 3 days <u>or</u> Zmax 2 gm in a single dose

Pediatric: 12 mg/kg/day x 5 days; max 500 mg/day; *see* Appendix BB.7. *azithromycin* (G) (Zithromax Suspension, Zmax Suspension) *for dose by weight*

Zithromax *Tab:* 250, 500, 600 mg; *Oral susp:* 100 mg/5 ml (15 ml); 200 mg/5 ml (15, 22.5, 30 ml) (cherry); *Pkt:* 1 gm for reconstitution (cherry-banana)

Zithromax Tri-Pak *Tab:* 3 x 500 mg tabs/pck

Zithromax Z-Pak *Tab:* 6 x 250 mg tabs/pck

Zmax *Oral susp:* 2 gm ext-rel for reconstitution (cherry-banana) (148 mg Na+)

▷ *cefaclor* (G)

Ceclor 250 mg tid <u>or</u> 375 mg bid 3-10 days

Pediatric: <1 month: <u>not</u> recommended; 1 month-12 years: 20-40 mg/kg divided bid <u>or</u> q 12 hours x 3-10 days; max 1 gm/day; *see* Appendix BB.8. *cefaclor* (G) (Ceclor Suspension) *for dose by weight;* >12 years: same as adult

(continued)

Tab: 500 mg; *Cap:* 250, 500 mg; *Susp:* 125 mg/5 ml (75, 150 ml) (strawberry); 187 mg/5 ml (50, 100 ml) (strawberry), 250 mg/5 ml (75, 150 ml) (strawberry), 375 mg/5 ml (50, 100 ml) (strawberry)

Cefaclor Extended Release 375-500 mg bid x 3-10 days
Pediatric: <16 years: ext-rel <u>not</u> recommended; ≥16 years; same as adult
    Tab: 375, 500 mg ext-rel

▷ *cefadroxil* 1 gm once daily <u>or</u> divided bid x 10 days
Pediatric: 30 mg/kg/day in 2 divided doses x 10 days; *see Appendix BB.9. cefadroxil* (G) (Duricef Suspension) *for dose by weight*
    Duricef *Cap:* 500 mg; *Tab:* 1 gm; *Oral susp:* 250 mg/5 ml (100 ml), 500 mg/5 ml (75, 100 ml) (orange-pineapple)

▷ *cefdinir* 300 mg bid x 5-10 days <u>or</u> 600 mg once daily x 10 days
Pediatric: <6 months: <u>not</u> recommended; 6 months-12 years: 14 mg/kg/day in a single <u>or</u> 2 divided doses x 10 days; >12 years: same as adult; *see Appendix BB.10. cefdinir* (G) (Omnicef Suspension) *for dose by weight*
    Omnicef *Cap:* 300 mg; *Oral susp:* 125 mg/5 ml (60, 100 ml) (strawberry)

▷ *cefditoren pivoxil* 200 mg bid x 10 days
Pediatric: <12 years: <u>not</u> recommended; ≥12 years: same as adult
    Spectracef *Tab:* 200 mg
    Comment: Contraindicated with milk protein allergy <u>or</u> carnitine deficiency.

▷ *ceftibuten* 200 mg once daily x 10 days
Pediatric: 9 mg/kg once daily x 10 days; max 400 mg/day; *see Appendix BB.14. ceftibuten* (G) (Cedax Suspension) *for dose by weight*
    Cedax *Cap:* 400 mg; *Oral susp:* 90 mg/5 ml (30, 60, 90, 120 ml); 180 mg/5 ml (30, 60, 120 ml) (cherry)

▷ *cefixime* (G) 400 mg once daily x 10 days
Pediatric: <6 months: <u>not</u> recommended; 6 months-12 years, <50 kg: 8 mg/kg/day in a single <u>or</u> 2 divided doses x 10 days; *see Appendix BB.11. cefixime* (G) (Suprax Oral Suspension) *for dose by weight*; >12 years, >50 kg: same as adult
    Suprax *Tab:* 400 mg; *Cap:* 400 mg; *Oral susp:* 100, 200, 500 mg/5 ml (50, 75, 100 ml) (strawberry)

▷ *cefpodoxime proxetil* 200 mg bid x 5-7 days
Pediatric: <2 months: <u>not</u> recommended; 2 months-12 years: 10 mg/kg/day (max 400 mg/dose) <u>or</u> 5 mg/kg/day bid (max 200 mg/dose) x 5-7 days; *see Appendix BB.12. cefpodoxime proxetil* (G) (Vantin Suspension) *for dose by weight*
    Vantin *Tab:* 100, 200 mg; *Oral susp:* 50, 100 mg/5 ml (50, 75, 100 mg) (lemon creme)

▷ *cefprozil* 500 mg once daily x 10 days
Pediatric: 2-12 years: 7.5 mg/kg bid x 10 days; >12 years: same as adult; *see Appendix BB.13. cefprozil* (G) (Cefzil Suspension) *for dose by weight*
    Cefzil *Tab:* 250, 500 mg; *Oral susp:* 125, 250 mg/5 ml (50, 75, 100 ml) (bubble gum) (phenylalanine)

▷ *cephalexin* (G) 250 mg tid x 10 days
Pediatric: 25-50 mg/kg/day in 4 divided doses x 10 days; *see Appendix BB.15. cephalexin* (G) (Keflex Suspension) *for dose by weight*
    Keflex *Cap:* 250, 333, 500, 750 mg; *Oral susp:* 125, 250 mg/5 ml (100, 200 ml) (strawberry)

▷ *clarithromycin* (G) 250 mg bid <u>or</u> 500 mg ext-rel once daily x 10 days
Pediatric: <6 months: <u>not</u> recommended; ≥6 months: 7.5 mg/kg bid x 10 days; *see Appendix BB.16. clarithromycin* (G) (Biaxin Suspension) *for dose by weight*
    Biaxin *Tab:* 250, 500 mg
    Biaxin Oral Suspension *Oral susp:* 125, 250 mg/5 ml (50, 100 ml) (fruit punch)
    Biaxin XL *Tab:* 500 mg ext-rel

▷ *dirithromycin* (G) 500 mg once daily x 10 days
Pediatric: <12 years: <u>not</u> recommended; ≥12 years: same as adult
    Dynabac *Tab:* 250 mg

▷ *erythromycin base* (G) 300-400 mg tid x 10 days
Pediatric: 30-50 mg/kg/day in 2-4 divided doses x 10 days
    Ery-Tab *Tab:* 250, 333, 500 mg ent-coat
    PCE *Tab:* 333, 500 mg

▷ *erythromycin ethylsuccinate* (G) 400 mg qid x 7 days
Pediatric: 30-50 mg/kg/day in 4 divided doses x 7 days; may double dose with severe infection; max 100 mg/kg/day; *see Appendix BB.21. erythromycin ethylsuccinate* (G) (E.E.S. Suspension, EryPed Drops/Suspension) *for dose by weight*
    EryPed *Oral susp:* 200 mg/5 ml (100, 200 ml) (fruit); 400 mg/5 ml (60, 100, 200 ml) (banana); *Oral drops:* 200, 400 mg/5 ml (50 ml) (fruit); *Chew tab:* 200 mg wafer (fruit)
    E.E.S. *Oral susp:* 200, 400 mg/5 ml (100 ml) (fruit)
    E.E.S. Granules *Oral susp:* 200 mg/5 ml (100, 200 ml) (cherry)
    E.E.S. 400 Tablets *Tab:* 400 mg

▷ *loracarbef* 200 mg bid x 10 days
Pediatric: 15 mg/kg/day in 2 divided doses x 10 days; *see Appendix BB.27. loracarbef* (G) (Lorabid Suspension) *for dose by weight*

Lorabid *Pulvule:* 200, 400 mg; *Oral susp:* 100 mg/5 ml (50, 100 ml); 200 mg/5 ml (50, 75, 100 ml) (strawberry bubble gum)

➤ *penicillin v potassium* (G) 250 mg tid x 10 days
Pediatric: 25-50 mg/kg day in 4 divided doses x 10 days; ≥12 years: same as adult; *see* Appendix BB.29.
penicillin v potassium (Pen-Vee K Solution, Veetids Solution) *for dose by weight*
Pen-Vee K *Tab:* 250, 500 mg; *Oral soln:* 125 mg/5 ml (100, 200 ml); 250 mg/5 ml (100, 150, 200 ml)

TOXOPLASMOSIS

➤ *pyrimethamine* (G) 50-75 mg daily (together with 1-4 gm daily of a sulfonamide of the sulfapyrimidine type, e.g., *sulfadoxine*) x 1-3 weeks, depending on patient response and tolerance; then reduce dose of each drug to about one-half and continue for an additional 4-5 weeks; tolerated best with food
Pediatric: 1 mg/kg/day divided into 2 equal daily doses (together with the usual pediatric sulfonamide dose) x 2-4 days; then reduce dose of each drug to about one-half and continue for approximately 1 month; tolerated best with food

Daraprim *Tab:* 25*mg
Comment: Daraprim is indicated for the treatment of toxoplasmosis when used conjointly with a sulfonamide, since synergism exists with this combination. *Pyrimethamine* is a folic acid antagonist. The rationale for its therapeutic action is based on the differential requirement between the host and the parasite for nucleic acid precursors involved in growth. This activity is highly selective against *Toxoplasma gondii.* Daraprim is contraindicated in patients with documented megaloblastic anemia due to folate deficiency. Doses used in toxoplasmosis may produce megaloblastic anemia, leukopenia, thrombocytopenia, pancytopenia, neutropenia, atrophic glossitis, hematuria, and disorders of cardiac rhythm. *Pyrimethamine* has a narrow therapeutic index. If signs of folate deficiency develop, reduce the dosage or discontinue according to the response of the patient. Folinic acid *(leucovorin)* should be administered in a dosage of 5-15 mg daily (orally, IV, or IM) until normal hematopoiesis is restored. A small starting dose is recommended for patients with a convulsive disorder to avoid potential central nervous system (CNS) toxicity. Daraprim should be used with caution in patients with impaired renal or hepatic function and patients with possible folate deficiency, such as individuals with malabsorption syndrome, alcoholism, or pregnancy, and those receiving therapy, such as *phenytoin,* affecting folate levels. Patients should be warned that at the first appearance of a skin rash they should stop use of Daraprim and seek medical attention immediately. Patients should also be warned that the appearance of sore throat, pallor, purpura, or glossitis may be early indications of serious disorders which require the discontinuation of Daraprim and immediate medical attention. *Pyrimethamine* may be used with sulfonamides, quinine and other antimalarials, and with other antibiotics. However, the concomitant use of other antifolic drugs or agents associated with myelosuppression, including sulfonamides or *trimethoprim-sulfamethoxazole* combinations, *proguanil, zidovudine,* or cytostatic agents (e.g., *methotrexate [MTX]*), while the patient is receiving *pyrimethamine,* may increase the risk of bone marrow suppression. If signs of folate deficiency develop, *pyrimethamine* should be discontinued and folinic acid *(leucovorin)* should be administered until normal hematopoiesis is restored. There are no adequate and well-controlled studies of *pyrimethamine* use in pregnant females. However, in animal studies, *pyrimethamine* has been shown to be teratogenic in oral doses 2.5 times the human dose for treatment of toxoplasmosis; a significant increase in abnormalities such as cleft palate, brachygnathia, oligodactyly, and microphthalmia have been reported. *Pyrimethamine* has also been shown to produce terata (significantly malformed fetus) such as meningocele cleft palate with oral doses 5 times the human dose for the treatment of toxoplasmosis. Daraprim should be used during pregnancy only if the potential benefit justifies the potential risk to the fetus. Females of childbearing potential who are taking Daraprim should be warned against becoming pregnant. Concurrent administration of folinic acid is strongly recommended when Daraprim is used during pregnancy. *Pyrimethamine* is excreted in human milk. Because of the potential for serious adverse reactions in nursing infants from *pyrimethamine* and from concurrent use of a sulfonamide with Daraprim for treatment of patients with toxoplasmosis, a decision should be made whether to discontinue nursing or to discontinue the drug, taking into account the importance of the drug to the mother.

TRICHINOSIS (*TRICHINELLA SPIRALIS*)

Comment: Trichinosis is caused by eating raw or undercooked pork or wild game infected with the larvae of a parasitic worm, *Trichinella spiralis.* The initial symptoms are abdominal discomfort, nausea, vomiting, diarrhea, fatigue, and fever beginning 1-2 days following ingestion. These parasites then invade other organs (e.g., muscles) causing muscle aches, itching, fever, chills, and joint pains that begin about 2-8 weeks after ingestion. The treatment is oral anthelmintics, which may cause abdominal pain, diarrhea, and (rarely) hypersensitivity reactions, convulsions, neutropenia, agranulocytosis, and hepatitis.

ANTHELMINTICS
Comment: Oral bioavailability of anthelmintics is enhanced when administered with a fatty meal (estimated fat content 40 gm).

(continued)

▷ *albendazole* take with a meal; may crush and mix with food; may repeat in 3 weeks if needed; 400 mg as once daily x 7 days
Pediatric: <2 years: 200 mg once daily x 3 days; may repeat in 3 weeks; 2-12 years: 400 mg once daily x 3 days; may repeat in 3 weeks; >12 years: same as adult
    Albenza *Tab:* 200 mg
    Comment: *Albendazole* is a broad-spectrum benzimidazole carbamate anthelmintic.
▷ *ivermectin* take with water; chew or crush and mix with food; may repeat in 3 months if needed; 200 mcg/kg as a single dose
Pediatric: <15 kg: not recommended; ≥15 kg: same as adult
    Stromectol *Tab:* 3, 6*mg
▷ *mebendazole* (G) take with a meal; chew or crush and mix with food; may repeat in 3 weeks if needed; <2 years: not recommended; ≥2 years: 100 mg bid x 3 days
Pediatric: <2 years: not recommended; ≥2 years: same as adult
    Emverm *Chew tab:* 100 mg
    Vermox (G) *Chew tab:* 100 mg
▷ *pyrantel pamoate* take with a meal; may open capsule and sprinkle or mix with food; treat x 3 days; may repeat in 2-3 weeks if needed; treat x 3 days; 11 mg/kg/dose; max 1 gm/dose; <25 lb: not recommended; 25-37 lb: 1/2 tsp/dose; 38-62 lb: 1 tsp/dose; 63-87 lb: 1 tsp/dose; 88-112 lb: 2 tsp/dose; 113-137 lb: 2 tsp/dose; 138-162 lb: 3 tsp/dose; 163-187 lb: 3 tsp/dose; >187 lb: 4 tsp/dose
    Antiminth *Cap:* 180 mg; *Liq:* 50 mg/ml (30 ml); 144 mg/ml (30 ml); *Oral susp:* 50 mg/ml (60 ml)
    Pin-X (OTC) *Cap:* 180 mg; *Liq:* 50 mg/ml (30 ml); 144 mg/ml (30 ml); *Oral susp:* 50 mg/ml (30 ml)
▷ *thiabendazole* take with a meal; may crush and mix with food; treat x 7 days; 25 mg/kg bid x 7 days; max 1.5 gm/dose; take with a meal
Pediatric: same as adult; <30 lb: consult mfr pkg insert; ≥30 lb: 25 mg/kg in 2 divided doses/day with meals; 30-50 lb: 250 mg bid with meals; >50 lb: 10 mg/lb/dose bid with meals; max 3 gm/day
    Mintezol *Chew tab:* 500*mg (orange); *Oral susp:* 500 mg/5 ml (120 ml) (orange)
    Comment: *Thiabendazole* is not for prophylaxis. May impair mental alertness. May not be available in the United States.

TRICHOMONIASIS (*TRICHOMONAS VAGINALIS*)

Comment: The following treatment regimens for *trichomoniasis* are published in the **2021 CDC Sexually Transmitted Diseases Treatment Guidelines**. Treat all sexual contacts. A multidose treatment regimen should be considered in HIV-positive women.

REGIMEN 2
▷ *secnidazole*
    Solosec *Oral granules:* 2 gm/pkt
    Comment: Solosec is a nitroimidazole antimicrobial. Do not dissolve **Solosec** in liquid. Sprinkle contents onto applesauce, yogurt, or pudding. Consume within 30 minutes without chewing or crunching. May follow with a glass of water. Potential adverse side effects are vulvovaginal pruritus, vulvovaginal candidiasis, headache, nausea, dysgeusia, vomiting, diarrhea, and abdominal pain. Whereas *metronidazole* and *tinidazole* are contraindicated during the 1st trimester of pregnancy, no adverse developmental outcomes have been found in animal reproductive studies and the labeling for *secnidazole* does not include a restriction for use in pregnancy. Breastfeeding is not recommended during and for 96 hours after a dose; may pump and discard milk during this time period.

RECOMMENDED REGIMENS (NON-PREGNANT)
Regimen 1
▷ *metronidazole* 2 gm once in a single dose

Regimen 2
▷ *tinidazole* 2 gm once in a single dose

RECOMMENDED ALTERNATE REGIMEN
Regimen 1
▷ *metronidazole* 500 mg bid x 7 days

DRUG BRANDS AND DOSE FORMS
▷ *metronidazole*
    Flagyl *Tab:* 250*, 500*mg
    Flagyl 375 *Cap:* 375 mg
    Flagyl ER *Tab:* 750 mg ext-rel

▷ *tinidazole*
    Tindamax *Tab:* 250*, 500*mg

RECOMMENDED REGIMENS: PREGNANCY/LACTATION
Comment: All pregnant females should be considered for treatment. Women can be treated with 2 gm *metronidazole* in a single dose at any stage of pregnancy. Lactating women who are administered *metronidazole* should be instructed to interrupt breastfeeding for 12-24 hours after receiving the 2 gm dose of *metronidazole*.

OTHER NITROIMIDAZOLE ANTIMICROBIAL
▷ *secnidazole*
    Solosec *Oral granules:* 2 gm/pkt
    Comment: **Solosec** is a nitroimidazole antimicrobial. Do not dissolve **Solosec** in liquid. Sprinkle contents onto applesauce, yogurt, or pudding. Consume within 30 minutes without chewing or crunching. May follow with a glass of water. Potential adverse side effects are vulvovaginal pruritus, vulvovaginal candidiasis, headache, nausea, dysgeusia, vomiting, diarrhea, and abdominal pain. Whereas *metronidazole* and *tinidazole* are contraindicated during the first trimester of pregnancy, no adverse developmental outcomes have been found in animal reproductive studies and the labeling for *secnidazole* does not include a restriction for use in pregnancy. Breastfeeding is not recommended during and for 96 hours after dose; may pump and discard milk during this time period.

TRICHOTILLOMANIA

Comment: Trichotillomania is on the obsessive-compulsive spectrum within the larger DSM-5 category, anxiety disorders, and depression is frequently a comorbid disorder. Hence, medications used to treat obsessive-compulsive disorder (OCD) can be helpful in treating trichotillomania. Recommended psychotropic agents include *clomipramine* (Anafranil) and *fluvoxamine* (Luvox). Other medications that research suggests may have some benefit include the selective serotonin reuptake inhibitors (SSRIs) *fluoxetine* (Prozac), *sertraline* (Zoloft), and *paroxetine* (Paxil), the mood stabilizer *lithium carbonate* (Lithobid, Eskalith), the OTC supplement N-acetylcysteine, an amino acid that influences neurotransmitters related to mood, *olanzapine* (Zyprexa), an atypical antipsychotic, and *valproate* (Depakote), an anticonvulsant.

TRICYCLIC ANTIDEPRESSANT (TCA) COMBINATIONS
▷ *clomipramine* (G) initially 25 mg daily in divided doses; gradually increase to 100 mg during the first 2 weeks; max 250 mg/day; total maintenance dose may be given at HS
    Pediatric: <10 years: not recommended; ≥10 years: initially 25 mg daily in divided doses; gradually increase; max 3 mg/kg or 100 mg, whichever is smaller
    Anafranil *Cap:* 25, 50, 75 mg

SELECTIVE SEROTONIN REUPTAKE INHIBITORS (SSRIs)
▷ *fluoxetine* (G)
    Prozac initially 20 mg daily; may increase after 1 week; doses >20 mg/day should be divided into AM and noon doses; max 80 mg/day
    Pediatric: <8 years: not recommended; 8-17 years: initially 10 mg/day; may increase after 1 week to 20 mg/day; range 20-60 mg/day; range for lower weight children, 20-30 mg/day
      Cap: 10, 20, 40 mg; *Tab:* 30*, 60*mg; *Oral soln:* 20 mg/5 ml (4 oz) (mint)
    Prozac Weekly following daily fluoxetine therapy at 20 mg/day for 13 weeks, may initiate Prozac Weekly 7 days after the last 20 mg fluoxetine dose
    Pediatric: <12 years: not recommended; ≥12 years: same as adult
      Cap: 90 mg ent-coat del-rel pellets
▷ *fluvoxamine* (G)
    Comment: *Fluvoxamine* has a specific FDA indication for OCD.
    Luvox initially 50 mg q HS; adjust in 50 mg increments at 4 to 7-day intervals; range 100-300 mg/day; over 100 mg/day, divide into 2 doses giving the larger dose at HS
    Pediatric: <8 years: not recommended; 8-17 years: initially 25 mg q HS; adjust in 25 mg increments q 4-7 days; usual range 50-200 mg/day; over 50 mg/day, divide into 2 doses giving the larger dose at HS; >17 years: same as adult
      Tab: 25, 50*, 100*mg
    Luvox CR initially 100 mg once daily at HS; may increase by 50 mg increments at 1-week intervals; max 300 mg/day; swallow whole
    Pediatric: <18 years: not recommended; ≥18 years: same as adult
      Cap: 100, 150 mg ext-rel

(continued)

▷ **paroxetine maleate (G)**
  Pediatric: <12 years: <u>not</u> recommended; ≥12 years: same as adult
    Paxil initially 20 mg daily in the AM; may increase by 10 mg/day at weekly intervals as needed; max 60 mg/day
      Tab: 10*, 20*, 30, 40 mg
    Paxil CR initially 25 mg daily in the AM; may increase by 12.5 mg at weekly intervals as needed; max 62.5 mg/day
      Tab: 12.5, 25, 37.5 mg cont-rel ent-coat
    Paxil Oral Suspension initially 20 mg daily in the AM; may increase by 10 mg/day at weekly intervals as needed; max 60 mg/day
      Oral susp: 10 mg/5 ml (250 ml) (orange)
▷ **paroxetine mesylate (G)** <12 years: <u>not</u> recommended; ≥12 years: initially 7.5 mg daily in the AM; may increase by 10 mg/day at weekly intervals as needed; max 60 mg/day
    Brisdelle *Cap:* 7.5 mg
▷ **sertraline (G)** initially 50 mg daily; increase at 1-week intervals if needed; max 200 mg daily; dilute oral concentrate immediately prior to administration in 4 oz water, ginger ale, lemon-lime soda, lemonade, <u>or</u> orange juice
  Pediatric: <6 years: <u>not</u> recommended; 6-12 years: initially 25 mg daily; max 200 mg/day; 13-17 years: initially 50 mg daily; max 200 mg/day; >17 years: same as adult
    Zoloft *Tab:* 25*, 50*, 100*mg; *Oral conc:* 20 mg per ml (60 ml) (alcohol 12%)

Lithium Salts Mood Stabilizer

▷ **lithium carbonate (G)** swallow whole; *Usual maintenance:* 900-1,200 mg/day in 2-3 divided doses
  Pediatric: <12 years: <u>not</u> recommended; ≥12 years: same as adult
    Lithobid *Tab:* 300 mg slow-rel
  Comment: Signs and symptoms of *lithium* toxicity can occur below 2 mEq/L and include blurred vision, tinnitus, weakness, dizziness, nausea, abdominal pains, vomiting, diarrhea to (severe) hand tremors, ataxia, muscle twitches, nystagmus, seizures, slurred speech, decreased level of consciousness, coma, and death.

Valproate Mood Stabilizer

▷ **divalproex sodium (G)** take once daily; swallow ext-rel form whole; initially 25 mg/kg/day in divided doses; max 60 mg/kg/day; *Elderly:* reduce initial dose and titrate slowly
  Pediatric: <12 years: <u>not</u> recommended; ≥12 years: same as adult
    Depakene *Cap:* 250 mg; *Syr:* 250 mg/5 ml (16 oz)
    Depakote *Tab:* 125, 250 mg
    Depakote ER *Tab:* 250, 500 mg ext-rel
    Depakote Sprinkle *Cap:* 125 mg

ANTIPSYCHOTIC

▷ **olanzapine** initially 2.5-10 mg daily; increase to 10 mg/day within a few days; then by 5 mg/day at weekly intervals; max 20 mg/day
    Zyprexa *Tab:* 2.5, 5, 7.5, 10 mg
    Zyprexa Zydis *ODT:* 5, 10, 15, 20 mg (phenylalanine)

TRIGEMINAL NEURALGIA (TIC DOULOUREUX)

ANTICONVULSANTS

▷ **baclofen (G)** initially 5-10 mg tid with food; usual dose 10-80 mg/day
  Pediatric: <12 years: <u>not</u> recommended; ≥12 years: same as adult
    Lioresal *Tab:* 10*, 20*mg
  Comment: Potential for seizures <u>or</u> hallucinations on abrupt withdrawal of *baclofen*.
▷ **carbamazepine**
    Carbatrol initially 200 mg bid; may increase weekly as needed by 200 mg/day; usual maintenance 800 mg-1.2 gm/day
  Pediatric: <12 years: max <35 mg/kg/day; use ext-rel form above 400 mg/day; 12-15 years: max 1 gm/day in 2 divided doses; >15 years: usual maintenance 1.2 gm/day in 2 divided doses
      Cap: 200, 300 mg ext-rel
    Tegretol (G) initially 100 mg bid <u>or</u> 1/2 tsp susp qid; may increase dose by 100 mg q 12 hours <u>or</u> by 1/2 tsp susp q 6 hours; usual maintenance 400-800 mg/day; max 1200 mg/day
  Pediatric: <6 years: initially 10-20 mg/kg/day in 2 divided doses; increase weekly as needed in 3-4 divided doses; max 35 mg/kg/day in 3-4 divided doses; ≥6 years: initially 100 mg bid; increase weekly as needed by 100 mg/day in 3-4 divided doses; max 1 gm/day in 3-4 divided doses
      Tab: 200*mg; *Chew tab:* 100*mg; *Oral susp:* 100 mg/5 ml (450 ml) (citrus-vanilla)
    Tegretol XR (G) initially 200 mg bid; may increase weekly by 200 mg/day in 2 divided doses

Pediatric: <6 years: use other forms; ≥6 years: initially 100 mg bid; may increase weekly by 100 mg/day in 2 divided doses; max 1 gm/day
Tab: 100, 200, 400 mg ext-rel

➤ *clonazepam* (IV)(G) initially 0.25 mg bid; increase to 1 mg/day after 3 days
Pediatric: <10 years, <30 kg: initially 0.1-0.3 mg/kg/day; may increase up to 0.05 mg/kg/day bid-tid; usual maintenance 0.1-0.2 mg/kg/day tid
    Klonopin *Tab:* 0.5*, 1, 2 mg
    Klonopin Wafers dissolve in mouth with or without water
    Wafer: 0.125, 0.25, 0.5, 1, 2 mg orally-disint

➤ *divalproex sodium* initially 250 mg bid; gradually increase to max of 1,000 mg/day if needed
Pediatric: <10 years: not recommended; ≥10 years: same as adult
    Depakene *Cap:* 250 mg; *Syr:* 250 mg/5 ml
    Depakote *Tab:* 125, 250 mg
    Depakote ER *Tab:* 250, 500 mg ext-rel
    Depakote Sprinkle *Cap:* 125 mg

➤ *phenytoin* 400 mg/day in divided doses
    Dilantin *Cap:* 30, 100 mg; *Oral susp:* 125 mg/5 ml (8 oz); *Infatab:* 50 mg
    Comment: Monitor *phenytoin* serum levels. Therapeutic serum level is 10-20 gm/ml. Side effects include gingival hyperplasia.

➤ *valproic acid* initially 15 mg/kg/day; may increase weekly by 5-10 mg/kg/day; max 60 mg/kg/day or 250 mg/day
    Depakene *Cap:* 250 mg; *Syr:* 250 mg/5 ml

TRICYCLIC ANTIDEPRESSANTS (TCAs)
Comment: Co-administration of tricyclic antidepressants (TCAs) with selective serotonin reuptake inhibitors (SSRIs) requires extreme caution.

➤ *amitriptyline* (G) titrate to achieve pain relief; max 300 mg/day
Pediatric: <12 years: not recommended; ≥12 years: same as adult
    Tab: 10, 25, 50, 75, 100, 150 mg

➤ *amoxapine* titrate to achieve pain relief; if total dose exceeds 300 mg/day, give in divided doses; max 400 mg/day
Pediatric: <12 years: not recommended; ≥12 years: same as adult
    Tab: 25, 50, 100, 150 mg

➤ *desipramine* (G) titrate to achieve pain relief; max 300 mg/day
Pediatric: <12 years: not recommended; ≥12 years: same as adult
    Norpramin *Tab:* 10, 25, 50, 75, 100, 150 mg

➤ *doxepin* (G) titrate to achieve pain relief; max 150 mg/day
Pediatric: <12 years: not recommended; ≥12 years: same as adult
    Cap: 10, 25, 50, 75, 100, 150 mg; *Oral conc:* 10 mg/ml (4 oz w. dropper)

➤ *imipramine* (G)
Pediatric: <12 years: not recommended; ≥12 years: same as adult
    Tofranil titrate to achieve pain relief; max 200 mg/day; adolescents max 100 mg/day; if maintenance dose exceeds 75 mg/day, may switch to **Tofranil PM** at bedtime
    Tab: 10, 25, 50 mg
    Tofranil PM titrate to achieve pain relief; initially 75 mg at HS; max 200 mg at HS
    Cap: 75, 100, 125, 150 mg
    Tofranil Injection 50 mg IM; lower dose for adolescents; switch to oral form as soon as possible
    Amp: 25 mg/2 ml (2 ml)

➤ *nortriptyline* (G) titrate to achieve pain relief; initially 10-25 mg tid-qid; max 150 mg/day; lower doses for elderly and adolescents
Pediatric: <12 years: not recommended; ≥12 years: same as adult
    Pamelor titrate to achieve pain relief; max 150 mg/day
    Cap: 10, 25, 50, 75 mg; *Oral soln:* 10 mg/5 ml (16 oz)

➤ *protriptyline* titrate to achieve pain relief; initially 5 mg tid; max 60 mg/day
Pediatric: <12 years: not recommended; ≥12 years: same as adult
    Vivactil *Tab:* 5, 10 mg

➤ *trimipramine* titrate to achieve pain relief; max 200 mg/day
Pediatric: <12 years: not recommended; ≥12 years: same as adult
    Surmontil *Cap:* 25, 50, 100 mg

TUBERCULOSIS (TB): PULMONARY (*MYCOBACTERIUM TUBERCULOSIS*)

SCREENING
➤ *purified protein derivative* (PPD) 0.1 ml intradermally; examine inoculation site for induration at 48-72 hours
Pediatric: same as adult
    Aplisol, Tubersol *Soln:* 5 US units/0.1 ml (1, 5 ml)

PROPHYLAXIS VACCINE

The <u>only</u> tuberculosis (TB) vaccine uses attenuation of the related organism *Mycobacterium bovis* by culture in bile-containing media to create the *Bacillus Calmette-Guerin* (BCG) vaccination strain. It was first used experimentally in 1921 by Albert Calmette and Camille Guerin and is currently in widespread use outside of the United States. It is <u>not</u> available in the United States. The BCG vaccine protects newborns against TB-related meningitis and other systemic TB infections, but it has limited protection against active pulmonary disease. Once vaccinated, the patient will be purified protein derivative (PPD)-positive.

Comment: Active TB in pregnancy is associated with adverse maternal and neonatal outcomes, including maternal anemia, Cesarean delivery, preterm birth, low birth weight, birth asphyxia, and perinatal infant death.

ANTITUBERCULAR AGENTS

Comment: Avoid *streptomycin* in pregnancy. *Pyridoxine* (*vitamin B6*) 25 mg once daily x 6 months should be administered concomitantly with *isoniazid* (*INH*) for prevention of side effects. *Rifapentine* produces red-orange discoloration of body tissues and body fluids and may stain contact lenses.

▷ *bedaquiline* (G)
  Sirturo *Tab:* 100 mg
  Comment: *Bedaquiline* is a diarylquinoline antimycobacterial ATP synthase for the treatment of pulmonary multidrug resistant tuberculosis (MDR-TB).
▷ *ethambutol* (*EMB*) (G)
  Myambutol *Tab:* 100, 400*mg
▷ *isoniazid* (*INH*) *Tab:* 300*mg
▷ *pyrazinamide* (*PZA*) *Tab:* 500*mg
▷ *rifampin* (*RIF*) (G)
  Rifadin, Rimactane *Cap:* 150, 300 mg
▷ *rifapentine*
  Priftin *Tab:* 150 mg (24, 32 pck)
  Comment: The 32-count packs of **Priftin** are intended for patients with active TB infection. The 24-count packs are intended for patients with latent tuberculosis infection (LTBI) who are at high risk for progression to TB disease. **Priftin** for active TB is indicated for patients ≥12 years of age. **Priftin** for LTBI is indicated for patients ≥2 years of age.
▷ *rilpivirine Tab:* 25 mg
  Rifabutin *Cap:* 150 mg
▷ *streptomycin* (*SM*) (G) *Amp:* 1 gm/2.5 ml <u>or</u> 400 mg/ml (2.5 ml)

COMBINATION AGENTS

▷ *rifampin+isoniazid*
  Rifamate *Cap:* rif 300 mg+iso 150 mg
▷ *rifampin+isoniazid+pyrazinamide*
  Rifater *Tab:* rif 120 mg+iso 50 mg+pyr 300 mg

PROPHYLAXIS AFTER EXPOSURE TO TUBERCULOSIS, WITH NEGATIVE PURIFIED PROTEIN DERIVATIVE (PPD)

▷ *isoniazid* 300 mg once daily in a single dose x at least 6 months
  Pediatric: 10-20 mg/kg/day x 9 months

PROPHYLAXIS AFTER EXPOSURE, WITH NEW PPD CONVERSION

▷ *isoniazid* 300 mg once daily in a single dose x 12 months
  Pediatric: 10-20 mg/kg/day x 9 months
  Tab: 100, 300*mg; *Syr:* 50 mg/5 ml; *Inj:* 100 mg/ml
▷ *rifampin* 600 mg once daily + *isoniazid* 300 mg once daily x 4 months
  Pediatric: rifampin 10-20 mg/kg + *isoniazid* 10-20 mg/kg once daily x 4 months
▷ *rifapentine* 600 mg once weekly + *isoniazid* 300 mg once weekly x 12 weeks
  Pediatric: ≤12 years: treat x 12 weeks; 10-14 kg: *rifapentine* 300 mg once weekly + *isoniazid* 25 mg/kg (max 900 mg) once weekly; 14.1-25 kg: *rifapentine* 450 mg once weekly + *isoniazid* 25 mg/kg (max 900 mg) once weekly; 25.1-32 kg: *rifapentine* 600 mg once weekly + *isoniazid* 25 mg/kg (max 900 mg) once weekly; 32.1-50 kg: *rifapentine* 750 mg once weekly + *isoniazid* 25 mg/kg (max 900 mg) once weekly; >50 kg: *rifapentine* 900 mg once weekly + *isoniazid* 25 mg/kg (max 900 mg) once weekly; >12 years: same as adult

TREATMENT REGIMENS (≥12 YEARS)

Regimen 1

▷ *rifampin* 600 mg + *isoniazid* 300 mg + *pyrazinamide* 2 gm + *ethambutol* 15-25 mg/kg <u>or</u> *streptomycin* 1 gm once daily x 8 weeks; then *isoniazid* 300 mg + *rifampin* 600 mg once daily x 16 weeks <u>or</u> *isoniazid* 900 mg + *rifampin* 600 mg 2-3 x/week x 16 weeks

Regimen 2

▷ *rifampin* 600 mg + *isoniazid* 300 mg + *pyrazinamide* 2 gm + *ethambutol* 15-25 mg/kg <u>or</u> *streptomycin* 1 gm once daily x 2 weeks; then *rifampin* 600 mg + *isoniazid* 900 mg + *pyrazinamide* 4 gm + *ethambutol* 50 mg/kg <u>or</u> *streptomycin* 1.5 gm 2 x/week x 6 weeks; then *isoniazid* 300 mg + *rifampin* 600 mg once daily x 16 weeks <u>or</u> 2 x/week x 16 weeks *rifampin* 600 mg once daily x 16 weeks <u>or</u> 2 x/week x 16 weeks

Regimen 3

▷ *rifampin* 600 mg + *isoniazid* 900 mg + *pyrazinamide* 3 gm + *ethambutol* 25-30 mg/kg or *streptomycin* 1.5 gm 3 x/week x 6 months

Regimen 4 (for smear and culture negative for pulmonary TB in adult)

▷ Options 1, 2, or 3 x 8 weeks; then *isoniazid* 300 mg + *rifampin* 600 mg once daily x 16 weeks; then *rifampin* 600 mg + *isoniazid* 300 mg + *pyrazinamide* 2 gm + *ethambutol* 15-25 mg/kg or *streptomycin* 1 gm once daily x 8 weeks or 2-3 x/week x 8 weeks

Regimen 5 (for smear and culture negative for pulmonary TB in adult)

▷ *rifapentine* 600 mg twice weekly x 2 months (at least 72 hours between doses) + once-daily *isoniazid* 300 mg, *ethambutol* 15-25 mg/kg + *pyrazinamide* 2 gm; then *rifapentine* 600 mg once weekly x 4 months + once daily *isoniazid* 300 mg + another appropriate antituberculosis agent for susceptible organisms

Regimen 6 (when pyrazinamide is contraindicated)

▷ *rifampin* 600 mg + *isoniazid* 300 mg + *ethambutol* 15-25 mg/kg + *streptomycin* 1 gm once daily x 4-8 weeks; then *isoniazid* 300 mg + *rifampin* 600 mg once daily x 24 weeks or 2 x/week x 24 weeks

PEDIATRIC TREATMENT REGIMENS (<12 YEARS)
Regimen 1

▷ *rifampin* 10-20 mg/kg + *isoniazid* 10-20 mg/kg + *pyrazinamide* 15-20 mg/kg + *ethambutol* 15-25 mg/kg or *streptomycin* 20-40 mg/kg once daily x 8 weeks; then *isoniazid* 10-20 mg/kg + *rifampin* 10-20 mg/kg once daily x 16 weeks or *isoniazid* 20-40 mg/kg + *rifampin* 10-20 mg/kg 2-3 x/week x 16 weeks

Regimen 2

▷ *rifampin* 10-20 mg/kg + *isoniazid* 10-20 mg/kg + *pyrazinamide* 15-30 mg/kg + *ethambutol* 15-25 mg/kg or *streptomycin* 20-40 mg/kg once daily x 2 weeks; then *rifampin* 10-20 mg/kg + *isoniazid* 20-40 mg/kg + *pyrazinamide* 50-70 mg/kg + *ethambutol* 50 mg/kg or *streptomycin* 25-30 mg/kg 2 x/week x 6 weeks; then *isoniazid* 10-20 mg/kg + *rifampin* 10-20 mg/kg once daily x 16 weeks or *rifampin* 10-20 mg/kg + *isoniazid* 20-40 mg/kg 2 x/week x 16 weeks

Regimen 3

▷ *rifampin* 10-20 mg/kg + *isoniazid* 20-40 mg/kg + *pyrazinamide* 50-70 mg/kg + *ethambutol* 25-30 mg/kg or *streptomycin* 25-30 mg/kg 3 x/week x 6 months

Regimen 4 (when pyrazinamide is contraindicated)

▷ *rifampin* 10-20 mg/kg + *isoniazid* 10-20 mg/kg + *ethambutol* 15-25 mg/kg + *streptomycin* 20-40 mg/kg once daily x 4-8 weeks; then *isoniazid* 10-20 mg/kg + *rifampin* 10-20 mg/kg once daily x 24 weeks or *rifampin* 10-20 mg/kg + *isoniazid* 20-40 mg/kg 2 x/week x 24 weeks

POLYPEPTIDE ANTIBIOTIC ISOLATED FROM STREPTOMYCES CAPREOLUS

Comment: *Capreomycin sulfate* is a complex of four microbiologically active components which have been characterized in part; however, complete structural determination of all the components has not been established. **Capastat Sulfate**, which is to be used concomitantly with other appropriate antituberculosis agents, is indicated in pulmonary infections caused by *capreomycin*-susceptible strains of *M. tuberculosis* when the primary agents (i.e., *isoniazid, rifampin, ethambutol, aminosalicylic acid,* and *streptomycin*) have been ineffective or cannot be used because of toxicity or the presence of resistant tubercle bacilli.

▷ *capreomycin sulfate* (G) may be administered deep IM in a large muscle mass after reconstitution with 2 ml 0.9%NS or sterile water or via IV infusion over 60 minutes after reconstitution and dilution in 100 ml 0.9%NS; usual dose is 1 gm daily (not to exceed 20 mg/kg/day) via IM or IV infusion for 60-120 days; see mfr pkg insert for dosage table based on kg body weight and route of administration
   Pediatric: <18 years: not recommended; ≥18 years: same as adult
   Capastat *Vial:* 1 gm pwdr for reconstitution with 2 ml 0.9%NS or sterile water
Comment: *Boxed Warning:* The use of *capreomycin sulfate* in patients with renal insufficiency or preexisting auditory impairment must be undertaken with great caution, and the risk of additional cranial nerve VIII impairment or renal injury should be weighed against the benefits to be derived from therapy. Since other parenteral antituberculosis agents (e.g., *streptomycin, viomycin*) also have similar and sometimes irreversible toxic effects, particularly on cranial nerve VIII and renal function, simultaneous administration of these agents with **Capastat Sulfate** is not recommended. Use with non-antituberculosis drugs (e.g., *polymyxin a sulfate, colistin sulfate, amikacin, gentamicin, tobramycin, vancomycin, kanamycin,* and *neomycin*) having ototoxic or nephrotoxic potential should be undertaken only with great caution. Audiometric measurements and assessment of vestibular function should be performed prior to initiation of therapy with **Capastat Sulfate** and at regular intervals during treatment. Renal injury, with tubular necrosis, elevation of the blood urea nitrogen (BUN) or serum creatinine, and abnormal urinary sediment, has been noted. Slight elevation of the BUN and serum creatinine (sCr) has been observed in a significant number of patients receiving prolonged therapy. The appearance of casts, red cells, and white cells in the urine has been

(continued)

noted in a high percentage of these cases. The safety of the use of **Capastat Sulfate** in pregnancy has not been determined. Safety and effectiveness in pediatric patients have not been established. It is not known whether this drug is excreted in human milk.

PULMONARY MULTIDRUG-RESISTANT TUBERCULOSIS (PMRT)

▷ *bedaquiline* 400 mg (4 x 100 mg tablets or 20 x 20 mg tablets) once daily x 2 weeks; then 200 mg (2 x 100 mg tablets or 10 x 20 mg tablets) 3 times per week (at least 48 hours between doses) x 22 weeks; administer doses via directly observed therapy (DOT); must be taken with food; if a dose is missed during the first 2 weeks of treatment, do not administer the missed dose (skip the dose and then continue the daily dosing regimen); from Week 3 onward, if a dose is missed, administer the missed dose as soon as possible, and then resume the 3 x/ week dosing regimen
Pediatric: <5 years, <15 kg: not established; ≥5 years, ≥15 kg: see mfr pkg insert for weight-based chart
    Sirturo *Tab:* 20*, 100 mg
    Comment: Sirturo *(bedaquiline)* is an oral diarylquinoline antimycobacterial drug indicated as part of combination therapy in adult and pediatric patients (≥5 years, ≥15 kg) with pulmonary multi-drug resistant tuberculosis (MDR-TB). Reserve **Sirturo** for use when an effective treatment regimen cannot otherwise be provided. This indication is approved under accelerated approval based on time to sputum culture conversion. Continued approval for this indication may be contingent upon verification and description of clinical benefit in confirmatory trials. Do not use **Sirturo** for the treatment of latent, extrapulmonary, or drug-sensitive TB, or for the treatment of infections caused by non-tuberculous mycobacteria. Safety and efficacy of **Sirturo** in HIV-infected patients with MDR-TB have not been established, as clinical data are limited. Emphasize need for compliance with full course of therapy. Prior to administration, obtain ECG, liver enzymes, and electrolytes. Obtain susceptibility information for the background regimen against *Mycobacterium tuberculosis* isolate if possible. Only use **Sirturo** in combination with at least three other drugs to which the patient's MDR-TB isolate has been shown to be susceptible *in vitro*. If *in vitro* testing results are unavailable, may initiate **Sirturo** in combination with at least 4 other drugs to which the patient's MDR-TB isolate is likely to be susceptible. Monitor ECGs and discontinue **Sirturo** if significant ventricular arrhythmia or QTcF interval >500 msec develops. Monitor liver-related laboratory tests. Discontinue **Sirturo** if evidence of liver injury occurs. The most common adverse reactions reported (incidence ≥10%) of adult patients treated with **Sirturo** have been nausea, arthralgia, headache, hemoptysis, and chest pain. The most common adverse reactions reported (incidence ≥10%) in patients 12 to <18 years have been arthralgia, nausea, and abdominal pain. The most common adverse reaction reported (incidence ≥10%) in patients 5 to <12 years has been elevated liver enzymes. Avoid use of strong and moderate CYP3A4 inducers with **Sirturo**. Avoid use for more than 14 consecutive days of systemic strong CYP3A4 inhibitors with **Sirturo** unless the benefit outweighs the risk. Available data from published literature of **Sirturo** use in pregnant females are insufficient to evaluate a drug-associated risk of major birth defects, miscarriage, or adverse maternal or fetal outcomes. Monitor infants exposed to *bedaquiline* through breast milk for signs of *bedaquiline*-related adverse reactions, such as hepatotoxicity.

TREATMENT-RESISTANT TUBERCULOSIS: 3-PART COMBINATION REGIMEN FOR ADULTS
Nitroimidazooxazine Antimycobacterial+Diarylquinoline Antimycobacterial+Oxazolidinone Antibacterial

Comment: Take each drug in the 3-part regimen daily, with food, for a total of 26 weeks. Doses of the regimen missed for safety reasons can be made up at the end of treatment. Doses of *linezolid* alone missed due to *linezolid* adverse reactions should not be made up. *Pretomanid* and *bedaquiline* are indicated for use in a limited and specific population of patients with TB. *Pretomanid* (a nitroimidazooxazine antimycobacterial) and *bedaquiline* (a diarylquinoline antimycobacterial ATP synthase) are indicated as part of a the 3-part combination regimen with *linezolid* (an oxazolidinone-class antibacterial) for the treatment of adults with pulmonary extensively drug-resistant (XDR) and treatment-intolerant or non-responsive MDR-TB, when an effective treatment regimen cannot otherwise be provided. Approval of this indication is based on limited clinical safety and efficacy data. *Pretomanid* and *bedaquiline* are not indicated for patients with drug-sensitive TB, latent infection due to *Mycobacterium tuberculosis,* extra-pulmonary infection due to *Mycobacterium tuberculosis,* and MDR-TB that is not treatment-intolerant or non-responsive to standard therapy. Safety and effectiveness of *pretomanid* have not been established for use in combination with any drugs other than *bedaquiline* and *linezolid* as part of the recommended dosing regimen. Administration of this medication regimen by directly observed therapy (DOT) is recommended. Emphasize the need for compliance with the full 26-day treatment regimen.

▷ *pretomanid* take 200 mg once daily; swallow whole with water; take with food; x total 26 weeks
    Pretomanid Tablet *Tab:* 200 mg
▷ *bedaquiline* take 400 mg once daily x 2 weeks; followed by 200 mg 3 x/week (separate doses by at least 48 hours) x 22 weeks; swallow whole
    Sirturo *Tab:* 100 mg
▷ *linezolid* take 1,200 mg daily, with dose adjustments for known *linezolid* toxicities, x total 26 weeks
    Zyvox *Tab:* 400, 600 mg; *Oral susp:* 100 mg/5 ml (150 ml) (orange) (phenylalanine)

Comment: Target glycosylated hemoglobin (HbA1c) is <7%. Addition of daily angiotensin-converting enzyme inhibitor (ACEI) and angiotensin II receptor blockers (ARB) therapy is strongly recommended for renal protection. Insulin may be indicated in the management of type 2 diabetes mellitus (T2DM) with or without concomitant oral antidiabetic agents.

TREATMENT FOR ACUTE HYPOGLYCEMIA

▷ *glucagon (recombinant)* administer SC, IM, or IV; if the patient does not respond in 15 minutes, may administer a single dose or 2 divided doses; <20 kg: 0.5 mg or 20-30 mg/kg; ≥20 kg: 1 mg

Comment: Necrolytic migratory erythema (NME), a skin rash, has been reported postmarketing following continuous *glucagon* infusion and resolved with discontinuation of the *glucagon*. Should NME occur, consider whether the benefits of continuous *glucagon* infusion outweigh the risks and consider using an oral or IV glucose preparation instead.

Gvoke 1 mg SC; administer via SC injection only in the upper outer arm, lower abdomen, or outer thigh; call for emergency assistance immediately after administration of the dose; if there has been no response after 15 minutes, an additional weight-appropriate dose may be administered while waiting for emergency assistance; do not reuse an injection device when the patient has responded to treatment; administer oral carbohydrates

Pediatric: <2 years: not established; 2-12 years: <45 kg: 0.5 mg SC; ≥45 kg: same as adult; administer via SC injection only in the upper outer arm, lower abdomen, or outer thigh; call for emergency assistance immediately after administering the dose; if there has been no response after 15 minutes, an additional weight-appropriate dose may be administered while waiting for emergency assistance; do not reuse an injection device; when the patient has responded to treatment, administer oral carbohydrates

HypoPen autoinjector: 0.5 mg/0.1 ml, 1 mg/0.2 ml, single-use; *Prefilled syringe:* 0.5 mg/0.1 ml, 1 mg/0.2 ml, single-use

Comment: Gvoke (*glucagon injection*) is a ready-to-use, room-temperature stable, liquid *glucagon* for the treatment of severe hypoglycemia in adult and pediatric patients ≥2 years of age with diabetes. Patients taking a beta-blocker may have a transient increase in pulse and blood pressure. In patients taking *indomethacin*, Gvoke may lose its ability to raise glucose or may produce hypoglycemia. Gvoke may increase the anticoagulant effect of *warfarin*. Gvoke is contraindicated in patients with pheochromocytoma because Gvoke may stimulate the release of catecholamines from the tumor. In patients with insulinoma, Gvoke administration may produce an initial increase in blood glucose; however, Gvoke may stimulate exaggerated insulin release from an insulinoma and cause hypoglycemia; if the patient develops symptoms of hypoglycemia after a dose of Gvoke, administer glucose orally or intravenously. Allergic reactions have been reported and include generalized rash, anaphylactic shock with breathing difficulties, and hypotension. Gvoke is effective in treating hypoglycemia only if sufficient hepatic glycogen is present; patients in states of starvation, with adrenal insufficiency, or chronic hypoglycemia may not have adequate levels of hepatic glycogen for Gvoke to be effective (use glucose instead). *Glucagon* administered to patients with glucagonoma may cause secondary hypoglycemia. Test patients suspected of having glucagonoma for blood levels of glucagon prior to treatment, and monitor blood glucose levels during treatment; if hypoglycemia develops, administer glucose orally or intravenously.

▷ *glucagon nasal powder* 3 mg administered as one actuation of the intranasal device into one nostril; administer the dose by inserting the tip into one nostril and pressing the device plunger all the way in until the green line is no longer showing; the dose does not need to be inhaled; call for emergency assistance immediately after administering the dose; when the patient responds to treatment, administer oral carbohydrates; do not attempt to reuse the device (each device contains only 1 dose of *glucagon*); if there has been no response after 15 minutes, administer an additional 3 mg using an unused device

Pediatric: <4 years: not approved: ≥4 years: same as adult

Baqsimi *Intranasal device:* 3 mg pwdr, single-dose

Comment: Baqsimi is a nasally administered antihypoglycemic agent indicated for the treatment of severe hypoglycemia in diabetes patients ≥4 years of age. Pheochromocytoma (Baqsimi may stimulate the release of catecholamines from the tumor) and insulinoma (Baqsimi may stimulate exaggerated insulin release from an insulinoma) are contraindications to Baqsimi use. Patients taking a beta-blocker may experience a transient increase in HR and BP. For patients taking *indomethacin*, Baqsimi may lose its ability to raise glucose or may produce hypoglycemia. Baqsimi may increase the anticoagulant effect of *warfarin*. Baqsimi is effective in treating hypoglycemia only if sufficient hepatic glycogen is present. Patients in states of starvation, with adrenal insufficiency, or chronic hypoglycemia may not have adequate levels of hepatic glycogen for Baqsimi to be effective; therefore, patients with any of these conditions should be treated with glucose. The most common (incidence ≥10%) adverse reactions associated with Baqsimi are nausea, vomiting, headache, upper respiratory tract irritation (i.e., rhinorrhea, nasal discomfort, nasal congestion, cough, and epistaxis), watery eyes, redness of eyes, and itchy nose, throat, and eyes.

(continued)

▷ *dasiglucagon* 0.6 mg SC into the outer upper arm, lower abdomen, thigh, or buttocks; if there has been no response after 15 minutes, an additional dose from a new device may be administered while waiting for emergency assistance; when the patient has responded to treatment, give oral carbohydrates
Pediatric: <6 years: safety and efficacy not established; ≥6 years: same as adult
    Zegalogue *Prefilled syringe:* 0.6 mg/0.6 ml, single-dose; *Autoinjector:* 0.6 mg/0.6 ml, single-dose
    Comment: Zegalogue is a glucagon analog for the treatment of severe hypoglycemia in patients with diabetes. Contraindications to Zegalogue include pheochromocytoma and insulinoma. In patients with pheochromocytoma, Zegalogue may stimulate the release of catecholamines from the tumor. In patients with insulinoma, Zegalogue may produce an initial increase in blood glucose, but then stimulate exaggerated insulin release from an insulinoma, causing subsequent hypoglycemia. If the patient develops symptoms of hypoglycemia after a dose of Zegalogue, administer glucose orally or intravenously. Zegalogue is effective in treating hypoglycemia only if sufficient hepatic glycogen is present. Patients in states of starvation, with adrenal insufficiency, or chronic hypoglycemia may not have adequate levels of hepatic glycogen for Zegalogue to be effective and patients with these conditions should be treated with glucose. Drug interactions with Zegalogue include beta-blockers, *indomethacin*, and *warfarin*. Patients taking a beta-blocker may have a transient increase in HR and BP. With patients taking *indomethacin*, Zegalogue may lose its ability to raise serum glucose or may produce hypoglycemia. Co-administration of Zegalogue with *warfarin* may increase *warfarin's* anticoagulant effect. The most common adverse reactions (incidence ≥2%) associated with Zegalogue have been nausea, vomiting, headache, diarrhea, and injection site pain; *Pediatric:* nausea, vomiting, headache, and injection site pain in pediatrics. Allergic reactions have been reported with glucagon products. These reactions may include generalized rash, and in some cases anaphylactic shock with breathing difficulties and hypotension.

NON-DIURETIC BENZOTHIADIAZINE DERIVATIVE

▷ *diazoxide* (G)
    Proglycem *Cap:* 50 mg; *Oral susp:* 50 mg/ml (chocolate mint) (sodium benzoate) (alcohol 7.25%)
    Comment: Proglycem is useful in the management of hypoglycemia due to hyperinsulinism associated with the following conditions: *adults:* inoperable islet cell adenoma or carcinoma, or extrapancreatic malignancy; *infants and children:* leucine sensitivity, islet cell hyperplasia, nesidioblastosis, extrapancreatic malignancy, islet cell adenoma, or adenomatosis. Proglycem may be used preoperatively as a temporary measure, and postoperatively if hypoglycemia persists. Treatment with Proglycem should be initiated under close clinical supervision, with careful monitoring of blood glucose and clinical response until the patient's condition has stabilized. This usually requires several days. If not effective in 2-3 weeks, Proglycem should be discontinued. Proglycem-induced hyperglycemia is reversed by the administration of insulin or *tolbutamide*. The inhibition of insulin release by Proglycem is antagonized by alpha-adrenergic blocking agents. The antidiuretic property of *diazoxide* may lead to significant fluid retention, which in patients with compromised cardiac reserve may precipitate congestive heart failure (CHF). The fluid retention will respond to conventional therapy with diuretics. There have been postmarketing reports of pulmonary hypertension occurring in infants and neonates treated with *diazoxide*. The cases were reversible upon discontinuation of the drug. Monitor patients, especially those with risk factors for pulmonary hypertension, for respiratory distress and discontinue *diazoxide* if pulmonary hypertension is suspected. Development of abnormal facial features in four children treated chronically (>4 years) with Proglycem for hypoglycemia hyperinsulinism has been reported. *Diazoxide* is highly bound to serum proteins (>90%) and therefore may displace other substances which are also protein-bound, such as bilirubin or *coumarin* and its derivatives, resulting in higher blood levels of these substances. Concomitant administration of oral *diazoxide* and *diphenylhydantoin* may result in a loss of seizure control. IV administration of Proglycem during labor may cause cessation of uterine contractions, and administration of oxytocic agents may be required to reinstate labor; caution is advised in administering Proglycem at that time. *Diazoxide* crosses the placental barrier and appears in cord blood. When given to the mother prior to delivery of the infant, the drug may produce fetal or neonatal hyperbilirubinemia, thrombocytopenia, altered carbohydrate metabolism, and possibly other side effects that have occurred in adults. Alopecia and hypertrichosis lanuginosa have occurred in infants whose mothers received oral *diazoxide* during the last 19-60 days of pregnancy. Reproduction animal studies using the oral preparation have revealed increased fetal resorptions and delayed parturition, as well as fetal skeletal anomalies; evidence of skeletal and cardiac teratogenic effects has also been noted with IV administration. Proglycem has also been demonstrated to cross the placental barrier in animals and to cause degeneration of the fetal pancreatic beta cells. When use of Proglycem is considered, potential benefits to the mother must be weighed against possible harmful effects to the fetus. Information is not available concerning the passage of *diazoxide* in breast milk. Because many drugs are excreted in human milk and because of the potential for adverse reactions from *diazoxide* in nursing infants, a decision should be made whether to discontinue nursing or to discontinue the drug, taking into account the importance of the drug to the mother.

INHALED INSULIN
Rapid-Acting Inhalation Powder Insulin

▷ *insulin human (inhaled)* 1 inhaler may be used for up to 15 days, then discard; dose at meal times as follows: *Insulin-naïve:* initially 4 units at each meal; adjust according to blood glucose monitoring
Conversion from SC to inhaled mealtime insulin:
SC 1-4 units: inhal 4 units
SC 5-8 units: inhal 8 units
SC 9-12 units: inhal 12 units
SC 13-16 units: inhal 16 units
SC 17-20 units: inhal 20 units
SC 21-24 units: inhal 24 units
Pediatric: <18 years: <u>not</u> established; ≥18 years: same as adult
   Afrezza Inhalation Powder administer at the beginning of the meal; *Mealtime insulin-naïve:* initially 4 units at each meal; *Using SC prandial insulin:* convert dose to **Afrezza** using a conversion table (see mfr pkg insert); *Using SC premixed:* divide 1/2 of total daily injected premixed insulin equally among 3 meals of the day; administer 1/2 total injected premixed dose as once-daily injected basal insulin dose
   Inhal: 4, 8, 12 unit single-inhalation color-coded cartridges (30, 60, 90/pkg w. 2 disposable inhalers)
   Comment: **Afrezza** is <u>not</u> a substitute for long-acting insulin. **Afrezza** must be used in combination with long-acting insulin in patients with type 1 diabetes mellitus (T1DM). **Afrezza** is <u>not</u> recommended for the treatment of diabetic ketoacidosis. **Afrezza** is contraindicated with chronic lung disease because of the risk of acute bronchospasm. The use of **Afrezza** is <u>not</u> recommended in patients who smoke <u>or</u> who have recently stopped smoking. Each card contains 5 blister strips with 3 cartridges each (total 15 cartridges). The doses are color-coded. **Afrezza** is contraindicated with chronic respiratory disease (e.g., asthma, chronic obstructive pulmonary disease [COPD]) and patients prone to episodes of hypoglycemia.

INJECTABLE INSULINS
Rapid-Acting Insulins

▷ *insulin aspart (recombinant)* onset <15 minutes; peak 1-3 hours; duration 3-5 hours; administer 5-10 minutes prior to a meal; SC <u>or</u> infusion pump <u>or</u> IV infusion
Pediatric: <3 years: <u>not</u> recommended; ≥3 years: same as adult
   Fiasp *Vial:* 1,000 units/10 ml (100 units/ml, 10 ml), multi-dose; *FlexTouch pen:* 300 units/3 ml (100 units/ml, 3 ml), single-use; *PenFill:* 300 units/3 ml (100 units/ml, 3 ml), single-use
   Comment: **Fiasp** is a newer formulation of **NovoLog**, in which the addition of *niacinamide* (vitamin B3) helps to increase the speed of initial insulin absorption.
   NovoLog *Vial:* 100 U/ml (10 ml); *PenFill cartridge:* 100 U/ml (3 ml, 5/pck) (zinc, m-cresol)
▷ *insulin glulisine (rDNA origin)* onset <15 minutes; peak 1 hour; duration 2-4 hours; administer up to 15 minutes before <u>or</u> within 20 minutes after starting a meal; use with an intermediate- <u>or</u> long-acting insulin; SC <u>only</u>; may administer via insulin pump; do <u>not</u> dilute <u>or</u> mix with other insulin in pump
Pediatric: <4 years: <u>not</u> recommended; ≥4 years: same as adult
   Apidra *Vial:* 100 U/ml (10 ml); *Cartridge:* 100 U/ml (3 ml, 5/pck; m-cresol)
▷ *insulin lispro (recombinant)* onset <15 minutes; peak 1 hour; duration 3.5-4.5 hours; administer up to 15 minutes before <u>or</u> immediately after a meal; SC <u>or</u> IV infusion pump <u>only</u>
Pediatric: <3 years: <u>not</u> recommended; ≥3 years: same as adult
   Admelog *Vial:* 100 U/ml (10 ml) (zinc, m-cresol); *Prefilled disposable SoloStar pen (disposable):* 100 U/ml (3 ml) (5/carton) (zinc, m-cresol)
   Humalog *Vial:* 100 U/ml (10 ml); *Prefilled disposable KwikPen:* 100 U/ml (3 ml, 5/pck) (zinc, m-cresol); *HumaPen Memoir* and *HumaPen Luxura* HD inj device for *Humalog cartridges* (100 U/ml, 3 ml 5/pck) (zinc, m-cresol)
▷ *insulin regular*
   Humulin R U-100 *(human, recombinant)* (OTC) onset 30 minutes; peak 2-4 hours; duration up to 6-8 hours; SC <u>or</u> IV <u>or</u> IM
     Vial: 100 U/ml (10 ml)
   Humulin R U-500 *(human, recombinant)* onset 30 minutes; peak 1.75-4 hours; duration up to 24 hours; SC <u>only</u>; for in-hospital use <u>only</u>
     Vial: 500 U/ml (20 ml); *KwikPen:* 3 ml (2, 5/carton)
   Comment: **Humulin R U-500** formulation is 5 times more concentrated than standard U-100 concentration, indicated for adults and children who require ≥200 units of insulin/day, allowing patients to inject 80% less liquid to receive the desired dose. Recommend using U-500 syringe (BD, Eli Lilly). The U-500 syringe (0.5 ml, 6 mm x 31 gauge) is marked in 5-unit increments and allows for dosing up to 250 units.
   Iletin II Regular *(pork)* (OTC) onset 30 minutes; peak 2-4 hours; duration 6-8 hours; SC, IV, <u>or</u> IM
     Vial: 100 U/ml (10 ml)

(continued)

Novolin R *(human)* (OTC) onset 30 minutes; peak 2.5-5 hours; duration 8 hours; SC, IV, or IM
Vial: 100 U/ml (10 ml); *PenFill cartridge:* 100 U/ml (1.5 ml, 5/pck); *Prefilled syringe:* 100 U/ml (1.5 ml, 5/pck)

▶ *pramlintide (amylin analog/amylinomimetic)* administer immediately before major meals (≥250 kcal or ≥30 gm carbohydrates); initially 15 mcg; titrate in 15 mcg increments for 3 days if no significant nausea occurs; if nausea occurs at 45 or 60 mcg, reduce to 30 mcg; if not tolerated, consider discontinuing therapy; *Maintenance:* 60 mcg (30 mcg *only* if 60 mcg not tolerated)

Symlin *Vial:* 0.6 mg/ml (5 ml) (m-cresol, mannitol)

Comment: Symlin is indicated as adjunct to mealtime insulin with or without a sulfonylurea and/or *metformin* when blood glucose control is suboptimal despite optimal insulin therapy. Do not mix with insulin. When initiating **Symlin**, reduce preprandial short/rapid-acting insulin dose by 50% and monitor pre- and postprandial and bedtime blood glucose. Do not use in patients with poor compliance, HgbA1c is >9%, recurrent hypoglycemia requiring assistance in the previous 6 months, or if taking a prokinetic drug. With T2DM, initial therapy is 60 mcg/dose and max is 120 mcg/dose.

RAPID-ACTING+INTERMEDIATE-ACTING INSULIN
Insulin Aspart Protamine Suspension+Insulin Aspart Combinations

▶ *insulin aspart protamine suspension 70%/insulin aspart 30% (recombinant)* **(G)** onset 15 min; peak 2.4 hours; duration up to 24 hours; SC only
Pediatric: not recommended

NovoLog Mix 70/30 (OTC) *Vial:* 100 U/ml (10 ml)
NovoLog Mix 70/30 FlexPen (OTC) *Prefilled disposable pen:* 100 U/ml (3 ml, 5/pck); *PenFill cartridge:* 100 U/ml (3 ml, 5/pck)

LONG-ACTING INSULINS

▶ *insulin detemir (human)* administer SC once daily with evening meal or at HS as a basal insulin; may administer bid (AM/PM); administer in the deltoid, abdomen, or thigh; onset 1-2 hours; peak 6-8 hours; duration 24 hours; switching from another basal insulin, dose should be the same on a unit-to-unit basis; may need more *insulin detemir* when switching from NPH; *Type 1:* starting dose ⅓ of total daily insulin requirements; rapid-acting or short-acting, pre-meal insulin should be used to satisfy the remainder of daily insulin requirements; *Type 2 (inadequately controlled on oral antidiabetic agents):* initially 10 units or 0.1-0.2 units/kg, once daily in the evening or divided bid (AM/PM); do not add-mix or dilute *insulin detemir* with other insulins
Pediatric: <2 years: not recommended; ≥2 years: same as adult

Levemir *Vial:* 100 U/ml (10 ml); *FlexPen:* 100 U/ml (3 ml, 5/pck; (zinc, m-cresol)

▶ *insulin glargine (recombinant)*

Basaglar administer SC once daily, at the same time each day, as a basal insulin in the deltoid, abdomen, or thigh; onset 1-1.5 hours, no pronounced peak, duration 20-24 hours; *T1DM (adults and children >6 years of age):* initially ⅓ of total daily insulin dose; administer the remainder of the total dose as short- or rapid-acting preprandial insulin; *T2DM (adults only):* initially 2 units/kg or up to 10 units once daily; *Switching from once daily insulin glargine 300 units/ml (i.e., Toujeo) to 100 units/ml:* initially 80% of the insulin glargine 300 units/ml; *Switching from twice daily NPH:* initially 80% of the total daily NPH dose; do not add-mix or dilute *insulin glargine* with other insulins.
Pediatric: <6 years: not established; ≥6 years: individualize and adjust as needed

Prefilled KwikPen (disposable): 100 U/ml (3 ml) (5/carton) (m-cresol)

Lantus administer SC once daily at the same time each day as a basal insulin; onset 1-1.5 hours, no pronounced peak, duration 20-24 hours; initial average starting dose 10 units for insulin-naïve patients; *Switching from once daily NPH or Ultralente insulin:* initial dose of *insulin glargine* should be on a unit-for-unit basis; *Switching from twice daily NPH insulin:* start at 20% lower than the total daily NPH dose
Pediatric: <6 years: not recommended; ≥6 years: same as adult

Vial: 100 U/ml (10 ml); *Cartridge:* 100 U/ml (3 ml, for use in the *OptiPen One Insulin Delivery Device*) (5/carton) (m-cresol); *SoloStar pen (disposable):* 100 U/ml (3 ml) (5/carton)

▶ *insulin glargine-yfgn* individualize dosage based on metabolic needs, blood glucose monitoring, glycemic control, type of diabetes, prior insulin use; administer SC into the abdominal area, thigh, buttocks, or upper arms once daily at any time of day, but at the same time every day; do not dilute or mix with any other insulin or solution; rotate injection sites to reduce the risk of lipodystrophy and localized cutaneous amyloidosis
Pediatric: T2DM: not approved; *T1DM:* same as adult

Semglee *Vial:* 100 units/ml (10 ml), multidose; *Prefilled pen:* 100 units/ml (3 ml), single-patient

Comment: Semglee is the first interchangeable long-acting human insulin analog biosimilar to **Lantus** *(insulin glargine)* indicated to improve glycemic control in adults and pediatric patients with T1DM and adults with T2DM.

Toujeo administer SC once daily at the same time each day as a basal insulin; in the upper arm, abdomen, or thigh; onset of action 6 hours; duration 20-24 hours; *T2DM, insulin-naïve:* initially 0.2 units/kg; titrate every 3-4 days; *T1DM, insulin-naïve:* initially ⅓-½ total daily insulin dose; remainder as short-acting insulin divided between each meal; *Switch from once daily long- or intermediate-acting insulin:* on a unit-for-unit basis; *Switching from Lantus:* a higher daily dose is expected; *Switching from twice daily NPH:* reduce initial dose by 20% of total daily NPH dose

Pediatric: <18 years: <u>not</u> established; ≥18 years: same as adult
> *Soln for SC injection:* 450 units/1.5 ml prefilled disposable SoloStar pen (1.5 ml, 3/pck); 300 units/ml prefilled Max SoloStar pen (3 ml, 2/pck)
> **Comment:** The Toujeo Max SoloStar pen contains 900 units of *insulin glargine* for administration of up to 160 units in a single injection and need for fewer prescribed pens and fewer refills.

▶ *insulin isophane suspension (NPH)*
Pediatric: <18 years: <u>not</u> recommended; ≥18 years: same as adult
> **Humulin N** *(human, recombinant)* (OTC) onset 1-2 hours; peak 6-12 hours; duration 18-24 hours; SC <u>only</u>
> *Vial:* 100 U/ml (10 ml); *Prefilled disposable pen:* 100 U/ml (3 ml, 5/pck)
> **Novolin N** *(recombinant)* (OTC) onset 1.5 hours; peak 4-12 hours; duration 24 hours; SC <u>only</u>
> *Vial:* 100 U/ml (10 ml); *PenFill cartridge:* 1.5 ml (5/pck); *KwikPens:* 1.5 ml (5/pck)
> **Iletin II NPH** *(pork)* (OTC) onset 1-2 hours; peak 6-12 hours; duration 18-26 hours; SC <u>only</u>
> *Vial:* 100 U/ml (10 ml)

▶ *insulin zinc suspension (lente)*
Pediatric: <18 years: <u>not</u> recommended; ≥18 years: same as adult
> **Humulin L** *(human)* (OTC) onset 1-3 hours; peak 6-12 hours; duration 18-24 hours; SC <u>only</u>
> *Vial:* 100 U/ml (10 ml)
> **Iletin II Lente** *(pork)* (OTC) onset 1-3 hours; peak 6-12 hours; duration 18-26 hours; SC <u>only</u>
> *Vial:* 100 U/ml (10 ml)
> **Novolin L** *(human)* (OTC) onset 2.5 hours; peak 7-15 hours; duration 22 hours; SC <u>only</u>
> *Vial:* 100 U/ml (10 ml)

Ultra Long-Acting Insulin

▶ *insulin degludec (insulin analog)* administer by SC injection once daily at any time of day, with <u>or</u> without food, into the upper arm, abdomen, <u>or</u> thigh; titrate every 3-4 days; *Insulin-naïve with T1DM:* initially 1/3-1/2 of total daily insulin dose, usually 0.2-0.4 units/kg; administer the remainder of the total dose as short-acting insulin divided between each daily meal; *Insulin-naive with T2DM:* initially 10 units once daily; adjust dose of concomitant oral antidiabetic agent; *Already on insulin (type 1 <u>or</u> type 2):* initiate at same unit dose as total daily long- <u>or</u> intermediate-acting insulin unit dose
Pediatric: <1 year: <u>not</u> established; ≥1 year: same as adult
> **Tresiba FlexTouch Pen:** 100 U/ml (3 ml, 5 pens/carton), 200 U/ml (3 ml, 3 pens/carton) (zinc, m-cresol)
> **Comment:** Tresiba U-200 FlexTouch is the <u>only</u> long-acting insulin in a 160-unit pen allowing up to 160 units in a single injection. The U-200 dose counter always shows the desired dose (i.e., no conversion from U/100 to U-200 is required)

▶ *insulin extended zinc suspension (Ultralente) (human)* onset 4-6 hours; peak 8-20 hours; duration 24-48 hours; SC <u>only</u>
Pediatric: <18 years: <u>not</u> recommended; ≥18 years: same as adult
> **Humulin U** (OTC) *Vial:* 100 U/ml (10 ml)

Insulin Lispro Protamine+Insulin Lispro Combinations
▶ *insulin lispro protamine75%+insulin lispro 25%*
Pediatric: <18 years: <u>not</u> recommended; ≥18 years: same as adult
> **Humalog Mix 75/25** *(human)* onset 15 minutes; peak 30 minutes to 1 hour; duration 24 hours; SC <u>only</u>
> *Vial:* 100 U/ml (10 ml); *Prefilled disposable KwikPen:* 100 U/ml (3 ml, 5/pck) (zinc, m-cresol); *HumaPen Memoir* and *HumaPen Luxura HD* inj device for *Humalog cartridges* (100 U/ml, 3 ml, 5/pck) (zinc, m-cresol)

▶ *insulin lispro protamine 50%+insulin lispro 50%*
Pediatric: <18 years: <u>not</u> recommended; ≥18 years: same as adult
> **Humalog Mix 50/50** *(recombinant)* onset 15 minutes; peak 2.3 hours; range 1-5 hours; SC <u>only</u>
> *Vial:* 100 U/ml (10 ml); *Prefilled disposable KwikPen:* 100 U/ml (3 ml, 5/pck) (zinc, m-cresol); *HumaPen Memoir* and *HumaPen LUXURA HD* inj device for *Humalog cartridges* (100 U/ml, 3 ml, 5/pck) (zinc, m-cresol)

Insulin Isophane Suspension (NPH)+Insulin Regular Combinations
▶ *NPH 70%+regular 30%*
Pediatric: <18 years: <u>not</u> recommended; ≥18 years
> **Humulin 70/30** *(human, recombinant)* (OTC) onset 30 minutes; peak 2-12 hours; duration up to 24 hours; SC <u>only</u>
> *Vial:* 100 U/ml (10 ml)
> **Novolin 70/30** *(recombinant)* (OTC) onset 30 minutes; peak 2-12 hours; duration up to 24 hours; SC <u>only</u>
> *Vial:* 100 U/ml (10 ml)

▶ *NPH 50%+regular 50%*
Pediatric: <18 years: <u>not</u> recommended; ≥18 years: same as adult
> **Humulin 50/50** *(human)* (OTC) onset 30 minutes; peak 3-5 hours; duration up to 24 hours; SC <u>only</u>
> *Vial:* 100 U/ml (10 ml)

Insulin Lispro Protamine+Insulin Lispro Combinations

▷ **insulin lispro protamine 75%+insulin lispro 25%**
  Pediatric: <18 years: <u>not</u> recommended; ≥18 years: same as adult
    Humalog Mix 75/25 *(recombinant)* onset 15 minutes; peak 30-90 minutes; duration 24 hours; SC <u>only</u>
    Vial: 100 U/ml (10 ml); *Prefilled disposable KwikPen:* 100 U/ml (3 ml, 5/pck) (zinc, m-cresol); *Huma-Pen Memoir* and *HumaPen LUXURA* HD inj device for *Humalog cartridges* (100 U/ml, 3 ml 5/pck) (zinc, m-cresol)

▷ **insulin lispro protamine 50%+insulin lispro 50%**
  Pediatric: <18 years: <u>not</u> recommended; ≥18 years: same as adult
    Humalog Mix 50/50 *(recombinant)* onset 15 minutes; peak 1 hour; duration up to 16 hours; SC <u>only</u>
    Vial: 100 U/ml (10 ml); *Prefilled disposable KwikPen:* 100 U/ml (3 ml, 5/pck) (zinc, m-cresol); *HumaPen Memoir* and *HumaPen LUXURA* HD inj device for *Humalog cartridges* (100 U/ml, 3 ml 5/pck) (zinc, m-cresol); U/ml (3 ml, 5/pck) (zinc, m-cresol); *HumaPen Memoir* and *HumaPen LUXURA* HD inj device for *Humalog cartridges* (100 U/ml, 3 ml 5/pck) (zinc, m-cresol) (100 U/ml, 3 ml 5/pck) (zinc, m-cresol)

Basal Insulin+Glucagon-Like Peptide-1 Receptor Agonists (GLP-1 RA) Combinations

▷ **insulin degludec (insulin analog)+liraglutide** for treatment of T2DM <u>only</u> in adults inadequately controlled on <50 units of basal insulin daily <u>or</u> ≤1.8 mg of *liraglutide* daily; administer by SC injection once daily, with <u>or</u> without food, into the upper arm, abdomen, <u>or</u> thigh; titrate every 3-4 days
  Pediatric: <18 years: <u>not</u> recommended; ≥18 years: same as adult
    Xultophy *Prefilled pen:* 100/3.6 U/ml (3 ml, 5 pens/carton)

▷ **insulin glargine (insulin analog)+lixisenatide** for treatment of T2DM <u>only</u> in adults inadequately controlled on <60 units of basal insulin daily <u>or</u> *lixisenatide*; administer by SC injection once daily, with <u>or</u> without food, into the upper arm, abdomen, <u>or</u> thigh; titrate every 3-4 days
  Pediatric: <18 years: <u>not</u> recommended; ≥18 years: same as adult
    Soliqua *Prefilled pen:* 100/33 U/ml (3 ml, 5 pens/carton) covering 15-60 mg **insulin glargine** 100 units/ml and 15-20 mcg of *lixisenatide* (*m-cresol*)

▷ **teplizumab-mzwv** dosing is once daily x 14 days, based on the patient's body surface area (BSA)

Dose Escalation and Body Surface Area	
Day 1	65 mcg/m^2
Day 2	125 mcg/m^2
Day 3	250 mcg/m^2
Day 4	500 mcg/m^2
Days 5-14	1,030 mcg/m^2

Do <u>not</u> administer 2 doses on the same day; if a planned **Tzield** infusion is missed, resume dosing by administering all remaining doses on consecutive days to complete the 14-day treatment course Confirm Stage 2 T1D by documenting at least two positive pancreatic islet autoantibodies in those who have dysglycemia without overt hyperglycemia using an oral glucose tolerance test (OGTT) <u>or</u> alternative method if appropriate and OGTT is <u>not</u> available. In patients who meet criteria for a diagnosis of stage 2 T1DM, ensure the clinical history of the patient does <u>not</u> suggest T2DM. Review the patient's prior age-appropriate immunizations; if any immunizations are needed, administer vaccinations prior to starting **Tzield**. Administer live attenuated (live) vaccines at least 8 weeks prior to treatment. Administer inactivated (killed) vaccines <u>or</u> mRNA vaccines at least 2 weeks prior to treatment. Prior to initiating **Tzield**, obtain a complete blood count (CBC) and liver enzyme tests (LFTs). Use of **Tzield** is <u>not</u> recommended in patients with the following laboratory abnormalities: lymphocytes <1,000/mcL; hemoglobin <10 g/dL; platelets <150,000/mcL; absolute neutrophils <1,500/mcL; elevated alanine aminotransferase (ALT) <u>or</u> aspartate aminotransferase (AST) >2 x the upper limit of normal (ULN); bilirubin >1.5 x ULN; laboratory <u>or</u> clinical evidence of acute infection with Epstein-Barr virus (EBV) <u>or</u> cytomegalovirus (CMV). Dilute **Tzield** in 0.9% NaCl Injection, USP; see full prescribing information for detailed preparation and administration instructions. Premedicate with (1) a non-steroidal anti-inflammatory drug (NSAID) <u>or</u> *acetaminophen*, (2) an antihistamine, <u>and/or</u> (3) an antiemetic before each **Tzield** dose for the first 5 days of the 14-day treatment course. Administer **Tzield** via IV infusion, over a minimum of 30 minutes, once daily x 14 days; see mfr pkg insert for dosing schedule. Refrigerate **Tzield** vials at 2°C to 8°C (36°F to 46°F) in the original carton to protect from light; store upright; do <u>not</u> freeze <u>or</u> shake the vials.
  Pediatric: <8 years: safety and efficacy <u>not</u> established; >8 years: same as adult
    Tzield *Vial:* 2 mg/2 ml (1 mg/ml), single-dose (1, 10, 14/carton)
    Comment: **Tzield** is a CD3-directed antibody indicated to delay the onset of stage 3 T1DM in adults and pediatric patients ≥8 years of age with stage T1DM. The most common adverse reactions (incidence >10%) have been lymphopenia, rash, leukopenia, and headache. Discontinue **Tzield** in patients who develop elevated ALT <u>or</u> AST more than five times the ULN, and if severe cytokine release syndrome

(CRS) develops consider temporarily pausing dosing. Use of **Tzield** is not recommended in patients with active serious infection or chronic infection; monitor for signs and symptoms of infection during and after **Tzield** treatment. If a serious infection develops, discontinue **Tzield**. Monitor white blood cell counts (WBCs) during the treatment period. If prolonged severe lymphopenia develops (<500 cells/mcL lasting 1 week or longer), discontinue **Tzield**. If a severe hypersensitivity reaction occurs, discontinue **Tzield** and treat promptly. Available case reports from clinical trials with **Tzield** are insufficient to identify a drug-associated risk of major birth defects, miscarriage, or other adverse maternal or fetal outcomes. Although there are no data on *teplizumab-mzwv*, monoclonal antibodies can be actively transported across the placenta, and **Tzield** may cause immunosuppression in the utero-exposed infant. To minimize exposure to the fetus, avoid use of **Tzield** during pregnancy and at least 30 days (6 half-lives) prior to a planned pregnancy. Report pregnancies to the Provention Bio Adverse Event reporting line at 844-778-2246. Although the developmental and health benefits of breastfeeding should be considered along with the mother's clinical need for **Tzield** and any potential adverse effects on the breastfed infant from **Tzield** or from the underlying maternal condition, a lactating mother may interrupt breastfeeding and pump and discard breast milk during treatment and for 20 days after **Tzield** administration to minimize drug exposure to the breastfed infant. To report suspected adverse reactions, contact Provention Bio at 844-778-2246 or FDA at 800-FDA-1088 or www.fda.gov/medwatch. The most common adverse reactions (>10%) were lymphopenia, rash, leukopenia, and headache. To report suspected adverse reactions, contact Provention Bio at 1-844-778-2246 or FDA at 1-800-FDA-1088 or www.fda.gov/medwatch

TYPE 2 DIABETES MELLITUS (T2DM)

Comment: Normal fasting glucose is <100 mg/dL. Impaired glucose tolerance is a risk factor for type 2 diabetes and a marker for cardiovascular disease risk; it occurs early in the natural history of these two diseases. Impaired fasting glucose is >100 mg/dL and <125 mg/dL. Impaired glucose tolerance is OGTT, 2 hour post-load 75 gm glucose >140 mg/dL and <200 mg/dL. Target pre-prandial glucose is 80 mg/dL to 120 mg/dL. Target bedtime glucose is 100 mg/dL to 140 mg/dL. Target glycosylated hemoglobin (HbA1c) is <7.0%. Additional medications to be considered for initiation at onset of T2DM, particularly in the presence of hypertension, include an angiotensin-converting enzyme inhibitor (ACEI), angiotensin II receptor blocker (ARB), thiazide-like diuretic, or a calcium channel blocker (CCB). Consider diabetes screening at age 25 years for persons in high-risk groups (non-Caucasian, positive family history for diabetes mellitus [DM], obesity). Hypertension and hyperlipidemia are common comorbid conditions. Macrovascular complications include cerebral vascular disease, coronary artery disease, and peripheral vascular disease. Microvascular complications include retinopathy, nephropathy, neuropathy, and cardiomyopathy. Oral hypoglycemics are contraindicated in pregnancy.

Insulins *see Type 1 Diabetes Mellitus*

TREATMENT FOR ACUTE HYPOGLYCEMIA

▷ *dasiglucagon* 0.6 mg SC into the outer upper arm, lower abdomen, thigh, or buttocks; if there has been no response after 15 minutes, an additional dose from a new device may be administered while waiting for emergency assistance; when the patient has responded to treatment, give oral carbohydrates
  Pediatric: <6 years: safety and efficacy not established; ≥6 years: same as adult
    Zegalogue *Prefilled syringe:* 0.6 mg/0.6 ml, single-dose; *Autoinjector:* 0.6 mg/0.6 ml, single-dose
    Comment: Zegalogue is a glucagon analog for the treatment of severe hypoglycemia in patients with diabetes.
▷ *glucagon (recombinant)* administer SC, IM, or IV; if the patient does not respond in 15 minutes, may administer a single or 2 divided doses *Adults and children:* <20 kg: 0.5 mg or 20-30 mg/kg; ≥20 kg: 1 mg

SULFONYLUREAS

Comment: Sulfonylureas are secretagogues (i.e., stimulate pancreatic insulin secretion); therefore, the patient taking a sulfonylurea should be alerted to the risk for hypoglycemia. Action is dependent on functioning beta cells in the pancreatic islets.

First-Generation Sulfonylureas

▷ *chlorpropamide* (G) initially 250 mg/day with breakfast; max 750 mg
  Pediatric: <12 years: not recommended; ≥12 years: same as adult
    Diabinese *Tab:* 100*, 250*mg
▷ *tolazamide* (G) initially 100-250 mg/day with breakfast; increase by 100-250 mg/day at weekly intervals; maintenance 100 mg 1 gm/day; max 1 gm/day
  Pediatric: <12 years: not recommended; ≥12 years: same as adult
    Tolinase *Tab:* 100, 250, 500 mg

(continued)

▷ **tolbutamide** initially 1-2 gm in divided doses; max 2 gm/day
Pediatric: <12 years: <u>not</u> recommended; ≥12 years: same as adult
  Tab: 500 mg

Second-Generation Sulfonylureas

▷ **glimepiride** initially 1-2 mg once daily with breakfast; after reaching dose of 2 mg, increase by 2 mg at 1 to 2-week intervals as needed; usual maintenance 1-4 mg once daily; max 8 mg/day
Pediatric: <12 years: <u>not</u> recommended; ≥12 years: same as adult
  Amaryl *Tab:* 1*, 2*, 4*mg
▷ **glipizide** (G)
Pediatric: <12 years: <u>not</u> recommended; ≥12 years: same as adult
  Glucotrol initially 5 mg before breakfast; increase by 2.5-5 mg every few days if needed; max 15 mg/day; max 40 mg/day in divided doses
    Tab: 5*, 10*mg
  Glucotrol XL initially 5 mg with breakfast; usual range 5-10 mg/day; max 20 mg/day
    Tab: 2.5, 5, 10 mg ext-rel
▷ **glyburide** (G) initially 2.5-5 mg/day with breakfast; increase by 2.5 mg at weekly intervals; maintenance 1.25-20 mg/day in a single <u>or</u> 2 divided doses; max 20 mg/day
Pediatric: <12 years: <u>not</u> recommended; ≥12 years: same as adult
  DiaBeta, Micronase *Tab:* 1.25*, 2.5*, 5*mg
▷ **glyburide, micronized**
Pediatric: <12 years: <u>not</u> recommended; ≥12 years: same as adult
  Glynase PresTab initially 1.5-3 mg/day with breakfast; increase by 1.5 mg at weekly intervals if needed; usual maintenance 0.75-12 mg/day in single <u>or</u> divided doses; max 12 mg/day
    Tab: 1.5*, 3*, 6*mg

ALPHA-GLUCOSIDASE INHIBITORS

Comment: Alpha-glucosidase inhibitors block the enzyme that breaks down carbohydrates in the small intestine, delaying digestion and absorption of complex carbohydrates, and lowering peak postprandial glycemic concentrations. Use as monotherapy <u>or</u> in combination with a sulfonylurea. Contraindicated in inflammatory bowel disease, colon ulceration, and intestinal obstruction. Side effects include flatulence, diarrhea, and abdominal pain.

▷ **acarbose** initially 25 mg tid ac, increase at 4 to 8-week intervals; <u>or</u> initially 25 mg once daily, increase gradually to 25 mg tid; usual range 50-100 mg tid; max 100 mg tid
Pediatric: <12 years: <u>not</u> recommended; ≥12 years: same as adult
  Precose *Tab:* 25, 50, 100 mg
▷ **miglitol** initially 25 mg tid at the start of each main meal, titrated to 50 mg tid at the start of each main meal; max 100 mg tid
Pediatric: <12 years: <u>not</u> recommended; ≥12 years: same as adult
  Glyset *Tab:* 25, 50, 100 mg

BIGUANIDE

Comment: The biguanides decrease gluconeogenesis by the liver in the presence of insulin. Action is dependent on the presence of circulating insulin. Lower hepatic glucose production leads to lower overnight, fasting, and preprandial plasma glucose levels. Common side effects include gastrointestinal (GI) distress, nausea, vomiting, bloating, and flatulence which usually eventually resolve. May be used as monotherapy (in adults <u>only</u>) <u>or</u> with a sulfonylurea <u>or</u> insulin. The <u>only</u> biguanide is *metformin*.

▷ **metformin** (G) take with meals
Comment: *Metformin* is contraindicated with renal impairment, metabolic acidosis, and ketoacidosis. *Metformin* is contraindicated in patients with decreased tissue perfusion <u>or</u> hemodynamic instability, alcohol abuse, advanced liver disease, acute unstable acute congestive heart failure, <u>or</u> any condition that may lead to lactic acidosis. Suspend *metformin* prior to and for 48 hours after surgery <u>or</u> receiving IV iodinated contrast agents. *Metformin* is associated with weight loss. Clinicians should consider adding either a sulfonylurea, a thiazolidinedione (TZD), a sodium-glucose co-transporter 2 (SGLT2) inhibitor, <u>or</u> a dipeptidyl peptidase-4 (DPP-4) inhibitor to *metformin* to improve glycemic control when a second oral therapy is considered.
  Fortamet initially 500 mg by mouth every evening; may increase by 500 mg/day at 1-week intervals; max 2 gm/day
  Pediatric: <10 years: <u>not</u> recommended; ≥10-16 years: use immediate-release form; >16 years: same as adult
    Tab: 500, 1,000 mg ext-rel
  Glucophage initially 500 mg bid; may increase by 500 mg/day at 1-week intervals; max 1 gm bid <u>or</u> 2.5 gm in 3 divided doses; <u>or</u> initially 850 mg once daily in the AM; may increase by 850 mg/day in divided doses at 2-week intervals; max 2,000 mg/day; take with meals
  Pediatric: <10 years: <u>not</u> recommended; ≥10-16 years: use <u>only</u> as monotherapy; >16 years: same as adult
    Tab: 500, 850, 1,000*mg

Glucophage XR initially 500 mg by mouth every evening; may increase by 500 mg/day at 1-week intervals; max 2 gm/day
Pediatric: <10 years: not recommended; ≥10-16 years: use immediate-release form; >16 years: same as adult
 Tab: 500, 750 mg ext-rel
Glumetza ER (G) initially 1,000 mg once daily; may increase by 500 mg/day at 1-week intervals; max 2 gm/day
Pediatric: <18 years: not recommended; ≥18 years: same as adult
 Tab: 500, 1,000 mg ext-rel
Riomet XR initially 500 mg once daily; may increase by 500 mg/day at 1-week intervals; max 2 gm/day in divided doses; take with meals
Pediatric: <10 years: not recommended; ≥10 years: monotherapy only
 Oral soln: 500 mg/ml (4 oz; cherry)

MEGLITINIDES
Comment: Meglitinides are secretagogues (i.e., stimulate pancreatic insulin secretion) in response to a meal. Action is dependent on functioning beta cells in the pancreatic islets. Use as monotherapy or in combination with *metformin.*
➤ *nateglinide* 60-120 mg tid ac 1-30 minutes prior to start of the meal
Pediatric: <12 years: not recommended; ≥12 years: same as adult
 Starlix *Tab:* 60, 120 mg
➤ *repaglinide* (G) initially 0.5 mg with 2-4 meals/day; take 30 minutes ac; titrate by doubling dose at intervals of at least 1 week; range 0.5-4 mg with 2-4 meals/day; max 16 mg/day
Pediatric: <12 years: not recommended; ≥12 years: same as adult
 Prandin *Tab:* 0.5, 1, 2 mg

THIAZOLIDINEDIONES (TZDs)
Comment: The TZDs decrease hepatic gluconeogenesis and reduce insulin resistance (i.e., increase glucose uptake and utilization by the muscles). Liver function tests are indicated before initiating these drugs. Do not start if alanine aminotransferase (ALT) more than 3 times greater than normal. Recheck ALT monthly for the first 6 months of therapy; then every 2 months for the remainder of the first year and periodically thereafter. Liver function tests should be obtained at the first symptoms suggestive of hepatic dysfunction (nausea, vomiting, fatigue, dark urine, anorexia, abdominal pain).
➤ *pioglitazone* (G) initially 15-30 mg once daily; max 45 mg/day as a monotherapy; usual max 30 mg/day in combination with *metformin*, insulin, or a sulfonylurea
Pediatric: <18 years: not recommended; ≥18 years: same as adult
 Actos *Tab:* 15, 30, 45 mg
➤ *rosiglitazone* (G) initially 4 mg/day in a single or 2 divided doses; may increase after 8-12 weeks; max 8 mg/day as a monotherapy or combination therapy with *metformin* or a sulfonylurea; not for use with *insulin*
Pediatric: <18 years: not recommended; ≥18 years: same as adult
 Avandia *Tab:* 2, 4, 8 mg

DIPEPTIDYL PEPTIDASE-4 (DPP-4) INHIBITOR+THIAZOLIDINEDIONE COMBINATION
Comment: The FDA has reported that *alogliptin*-containing drugs may increase the risk of heart failure, especially in patients who already have cardiovascular or renal disease. The drug Oseni (*alogliptin+pioglitazone*) is in this risk group.
➤ *alogliptin+pioglitazone* take 1 dose once daily with first meal of the day; max: *rosiglitazone* 8 mg and max *glimepiride* per day; same precautions as *alogliptin* and *pioglitazone*
Pediatric: <18 years: not recommended; ≥18 years: same as adult
 Oseni
 Tab: **Oseni 12.5/15** alo 12.5 mg+pio 15 mg;
   Oseni 12.5/30 alo 12.5 mg+pio 30 mg
   Oseni 12.5/45 alo 12.5 mg+pio 45 mg
   Oseni 25/15 alo 25+pio 15 mg
   Oseni 25/30 alo 25+pio 30 mg
   Oseni 25/45 alo 25 mg+pio 45 mg

SECOND-GENERATION SULFONYLUREA+BIGUANIDE COMBINATIONS
Comment: Metaglip and Glucovance are combination secretagogues (sulfonylureas) and insulin sensitizers (biguanides). *Sulfonylurea:* Action is dependent on functioning beta cells in the pancreatic islets; the patient should be alerted to the risk for hypoglycemia. Common side effects of the biguanide include GI distress, nausea, vomiting, bloating, and flatulence which usually eventually resolve. Take with food. *Metformin* is contraindicated with renal impairment, metabolic acidosis, and ketoacidosis. Suspend *metformin* prior to and for 48 hours after surgery or receiving IV iodinated contrast agents.

(continued)

▷ *glipizide+metformin* take with meals; *Primary therapy:* 2.5/250 once daily or if FBS is 280-320 mg/dl, may start at 2.5/250 bid; may increase by 1 tab/day q 2 weeks; max 10/2,000 per day in 2 divided doses; *Second-line therapy:* 2.5/500 or 5/500 bid; may increase by up to 5/500 q 2 weeks; max: 20/2,000 per day; same precautions as *glipizide* and *metformin*
Pediatric: <12 years: not recommended; ≥12 years: same as adult
 Metaglip
  Tab: Metaglip **2.5/250** glip 2.5 mg+met 250 mg
   Metaglip **2.5/500** glip 2.5 mg+met 500 mg
   Metaglip **5/500** glip 5 mg+met 500 mg

▷ *glyburide+metformin* take with meals; *Primary therapy (initial therapy if HgbA1c <9.0%):* initially 1.25/250 once daily; max *glyburide* 20 mg and *metformin* 2,000 mg per day; *Primary therapy (initial therapy if HbA1c >9.0% or FBS >200):* initially 1.25/250 bid; max *glyburide* 20 mg and *metformin* 2,000 mg per day; *Second-line therapy (initial therapy if HbA1c >7.0%):* initially 2.5/500 or 5/500 bid; max *glyburide* 20 mg and *metformin* 2,000 mg per day; *Previously treated with a sulfonylurea and metformin:* dose to approximate total daily doses of *glyburide* and *metformin* already being taken; max: *glyburide* 20 mg and *metformin* 2,000 mg per day; same precautions as *glyburide* and *metformin*
Pediatric: <12 years: not recommended; ≥12 years: same as adult
 Glucovance
  Tab: Glucovance **1.25/250** glyb 1.25 mg+met 250 mg
   Glucovance **2.5/500** glyb 2.5 mg+met 500 mg
   Glucovance **5/500** glyb 5 mg+met 500 mg
Comment: *Metformin* is contraindicated with renal impairment, metabolic acidosis, and ketoacidosis. Suspend *metformin* prior to and for 48 hours after surgery or receiving IV iodinated contrast agents.

THIAZOLIDINEDIONE+BIGUANIDE COMBINATION

▷ *pioglitazone+metformin* take in divided doses with meals; *Previously on metformin alone:* initially 15 mg/500 mg or 15 mg/850 mg once or twice daily; *Previously on pioglitazone alone:* initially 15 mg/500 mg bid; *Previously on pioglitazone and metformin:* switch on a mg/mg basis; may increase after 8-12 weeks; max: *pioglitazone* 45 mg and *metformin* 2,000 mg per day; same precautions as *pioglitazone* and *metformin*
Pediatric: <12 years: not recommended; ≥12 years: same as adult
 Actoplus Met, Actoplus Met R (G)
  Tab: Actoplus Met **15/500** pio 15 mg+met 500 mg
   Actoplus Met **15/850** pio 15 mg+met 850 mg
   Actoplus Met XR **15/1000** pio 15 mg+met 1,000 mg
   Actoplus Met XR **30/1000** pio 30 mg+met 1,000 mg
Comment: *Metformin* is contraindicated with renal impairment, metabolic acidosis, and ketoacidosis. Suspend *metformin* prior to and for 48 hours after surgery or receiving IV iodinated contrast agents.

▷ *rosiglitazone+metformin* (G) take in divided doses with meals; *Previously on metformin alone:* add *rosiglitazone* 4 mg/day; may increase after 8-12 weeks; *Previously on rosiglitazone alone:* add *metformin* 1,000 mg/day; may increase after 1-2 weeks; *Previously on rosiglitazone and metformin:* switch on a mg/mg basis; may increase *rosiglitazone* by 4 mg and/or *metformin* by 500 mg per day; max: *rosiglitazone* 8 mg and *metformin* 2,000 mg per day; same precautions as *rosiglitazone* and *metformin*
Pediatric: <12 years: not recommended; ≥12 years: same as adult
 Avandamet
  Tab: Avandamet **2/500** rosi 2 mg+met 500 mg
   Avandamet **2/1000** rosi 2 mg+met 1,000 mg
   Avandamet **4/500** rosi 4 mg+met 500 mg
   Avandamet **4/1000** rosi 4 mg+met 1,000 mg
Comment: *Rosiglitazone* has been withdrawn from retail pharmacies. In order to enroll and receive *rosiglitazone*, healthcare providers and patients must enroll in the *Avandia-Rosiglitazone Medicines Access Program.* The program limits the use of *rosiglitazone* to patients already being treated successfully and those whose blood sugar cannot be controlled with other antidiabetic medicines. *Metformin* is contraindicated with renal impairment, metabolic acidosis, and ketoacidosis. Suspend *metformin* prior to and for 48 hours after surgery or receiving IV iodinated contrast agents.

THIAZOLIDINEDIONE (TZD)+SULFONYLUREA COMBINATIONS

▷ *pioglitazone+glimepiride* (G) take 1 dose daily with first meal of the day; *Previously on sulfonylurea alone:* initially 30 mg/2 mg; *Previously on pioglitazone and glimepiride:* switch on a mg/mg basis; max: *pioglitazone* 30 mg and *glimepiride* 4 mg per day; same precautions as *pioglitazone* and *glimepiride*
Pediatric: <18 years: not recommended; ≥18 years: same as adult
 Duetact
  Tab: Duetact **30/2** pio 30 mg+glim 2 mg
   Duetact **304** pio 30 mg+glim 4 mg

▷ *rosiglitazone+glimepiride* take 1 dose daily with first meal of the day; max: *rosiglitazone* 8 mg and *glimepiride* 4 mg per day; same precautions as *rosiglitazone* and *glimepiride*
Pediatric: <18 years: not recommended; ≥18 years: same as adult

Avandaryl
Tab: **Avandaryl 4/1** rosi 4 mg+glim 1 mg
Avandaryl 4/2 rosi 4 mg+glim 2 mg
Avandaryl 4/4 rosi 4 mg+glim 4 mg
Avandaryl 8/2 rosi 8 mg+glim 2 mg
Avandaryl 8/4 rosi 8 mg+glim 4 mg

GLUCAGON-LIKE PEPTIDE-1 (GLP-1) RECEPTOR AGONISTS

Comment: Glucagon-like peptide-1 (GLP-1) receptor agonists act as an agonist at the GLP-1 receptors. They have a longer half-life than the native protein allowing them to be dosed once daily. They increase intracellular cAMP resulting in *insulin* release in the presence of increased serum concentration, decrease *glucagon* secretion, and delay gastric emptying, thus reducing fasting, pre-meal, and postprandial glucose throughout the day. GLP-1 receptor agonists are not a substitute for *insulin*, not for treatment of diabetic ketoacidosis, and not for postprandial administration.

▷ *dulaglutide* administer by SC injection into the upper arm, abdomen, or thigh once weekly on the same day and the same time of day, with or without food; initially 0.75 mg SC once weekly; may increase to 1.5 mg SC once weekly

Pediatric: <18 years: not established; ≥18 years: same as adult

Trulicity *Prefilled pen/syringe:* 0.75, 1.5, 3.0, 4.5 mg/0.5 ml, single-dose disposable autoinjector (4/pck)
Comment: Trulicity is a GLP-1 receptor agonist indicated (1) for the treatment of patients ≥10 years of age with T2DM and (2) to reduce the risk of major adverse cardiovascular events in adults with T2DM who have established cardiovascular disease or multiple cardiovascular risk factors. **Trulicity** is not for treatment of type 1 diabetes mellitus (T1DM). **Trulicity** has not been studied in patients with a history of pancreatitis; consider other antidiabetic therapies in these patients. **Trulicity** is contraindicated in patients with a serious hypersensitivity reaction to *dulaglutide* or any of the product components, in patients with severe GI disease, patients with severe gastroparesis, patients with a personal or family history of medullary thyroid carcinoma (MTC), and patients with multiple endocrine neoplasia syndrome type 2 (MENS-2). *Black Box Warning:* Risk of thyroid C-cell tumors: *Dulaglutide* causes thyroid C-cell tumors in animal studies. It is unknown whether **Trulicity** causes thyroid C-cell tumors, including medullary thyroid carcinoma (MTC), in humans as the human relevance of *dulaglutide*-induced thyroid C-cell tumors in animals has not been determined. Pancreatitis has been reported in **Trulicity** clinical trials; discontinue promptly if pancreatitis is suspected and do not restart if pancreatitis is confirmed. Concomitant use of **Trulicity** with an insulin secretagogue or insulin may increase the risk of hypoglycemia, including severe hypoglycemia. Reducing the dose of insulin secretagogue or insulin may be necessary. Serious hypersensitivity reactions (e.g., anaphylactic reactions and angioedema) have occurred; discontinue **Trulicity** and treat the reaction appropriately. Monitor renal function in patients with renal impairment. **Trulicity** has not been studied in patients with severe GI disease and is not recommended in these patients. Diabetic retinopathy complications have been reported in a cardiovascular outcomes trial; monitor patients with a history of diabetic retinopathy. If cholelithiasis or cholecystitis is suspected, gallbladder studies are indicated. The most common adverse reactions (incidence ≥5%) have been nausea, diarrhea, vomiting, abdominal pain, and decreased appetite. There are clinical considerations regarding the risks of poorly controlled diabetes in pregnancy. Poorly controlled diabetes in pregnancy increases the maternal risk for diabetic ketoacidosis, preeclampsia, spontaneous abortions, preterm delivery, and delivery complications. Poorly controlled diabetes increases the fetal risk for major birth defects, stillbirth, and macrosomia-related morbidity. Limited data with **Trulicity** in pregnant women are not sufficient to determine a drug-associated risk of major birth defects and miscarriage. Based on animal reproduction studies, there may be risks to the fetus from exposure to *dulaglutide* during pregnancy. In studies where animals received *dulaglutide* during organogenesis, early embryonic deaths, fetal growth reductions, and fetal abnormalities occurred at systemic exposures at least six times human exposure at the maximum recommended human dose (MRHD) of 4.5 mg/week. In pregnant animals administered *dulaglutide* during organogenesis, major fetal abnormalities occurred at five times human exposure at the MRHD. Adverse embryo/fetal effects in animals occurred in association with decreased maternal weight and food consumption attributed to the pharmacology of *dulaglutide*. **Trulicity** should be used during pregnancy after consideration of risk/benefit and only if the potential benefit justifies the potential risk to the fetus. There are no data on the presence of *dulaglutide* in human milk or effects on the breastfed infant. The presence of *dulaglutide* in milk of treated lactating animals was not determined. Developmental and health benefits of breastfeeding should be considered along with the mother's clinical need for **Trulicity** and any potential adverse effects on the breastfed infant from **Trulicity** or from the underlying maternal condition.

▷ *exenatide* administer by SC injection into the upper arm, abdomen, or thigh once weekly
Pediatric: <12 years: not recommended; ≥12 years: same as adult

Bydureon inject immediately after mixing; administer 2 mg SC once weekly; administer on the same day, at any time of day; with or without meals; if switching from **Byetta**, discontinue **Byetta** and instead administer **Bydureon** and continue the same once weekly administration schedule with **Bydureon**
Vial: 2 mg w. 0.65 ml diluent, single-dose; *Prefilled pen:* 2 mg w. 0.65 ml diluent, single-dose

(continued)

Bydureon BCise administer 2 mg by SC injection once weekly; at any time of day; with or without meals; if switching from **Byetta** to **Bydureon**, discontinue **Byetta** and start **Bydureon BCise** SC once weekly on the same day of the week
> *Autoinjector:* 2 mg (0.85 ml), single-dose

Byetta inject within 60 minutes before AM and PM meals, or before the two main meals of the day, approximately ≥6 hours apart; initially 5 mcg/dose; may increase to 10 mcg/dose after 1 month
> *Prefilled pen:* 250 mcg/ml (5, 10 mcg/dose; 60 doses, needles not included) (m-cresol, mannitol)

Comment: *Exenatide* is indicated as an adjunctive therapy to basal insulin among patients whose blood sugar remains uncontrolled on one or more antidiabetic medications, along with diet and exercise.

▷ *liraglutide* administer by SC injection into the upper arm, abdomen, or thigh once daily; initially 0.6 mg/day for 1 week; then 1.2 mg/day; may increase to 1.8 mg/day
Pediatric: <10 years: not recommended; ≥10 years: same as adult
> **Victoza** *Prefilled pen:* 6 mg/ml (3 ml; needles not included)

▷ *lixisenatide* administer SC in the upper arm, abdomen, or thigh once daily; initially 10 mcg SC x 14 days;
Maintenance: 20 mcg beginning on day 15; administer within 1 hour of the first meal of the day and the same meal of the day
Pediatric: <18 years: not established; ≥18 years: same as adult
> **Adlyxin** *Soln for SC inj;* *Starter pen:* 50 mcg/ml (14 doses of 10 mcg; 3 ml); *Maintenance pen:* 100 mcg/ml (14 doses of 20 mcg); *Starter pack:* 1 prefilled starter pen and 1 prefilled maintenance pen; *Maintenance pack:* 2 prefilled maintenance pens

Comment: **Adlyxin** is indicated as an adjunct to diet and exercise for T2DM. Not indicated for treatment of T1DM. Do not use with **Victoza, Saxenda**, other GLP-1 receptor agonists, or insulin. Contraindicated with gastroparesis and glomerular filtration rate (GFR) <15 ml/min. Poorly controlled diabetes in pregnancy increases the maternal risk for diabetic ketoacidosis, preeclampsia, spontaneous abortions, preterm delivery, stillbirth, and delivery complications. Poorly controlled diabetes increases the fetal risk for major birth defects, stillbirth, and macrosomia-related morbidity. **Adlyxin** should be used during pregnancy only if the potential benefit justifies the potential risk to the fetus. Estimated background risk of major birth defects and miscarriage in clinically recognized pregnancies is 2%-4% and 15%-20%, respectively.

▷ *semaglutide*
Comment: *Semaglutide* is not recommended as first-line therapy for patients inadequately controlled on diet and exercise and is not indicated for use in patients with T1DM or treatment of diabetic ketoacidosis. *Semaglutide* is contraindicated with a personal or family history of medullary thyroid carcinoma or in patients with multiple endocrine neoplasia syndrome type 2 (MENS-2). Pancreatitis has been reported in *semaglutide* clinical trials; discontinue promptly if pancreatitis is suspected and do not restart if pancreatitis is confirmed. Diabetic retinopathy complications have been reported in a cardiovascular outcomes trial with *semaglutide* injection. Patients with a history of diabetic retinopathy should be monitored. When used with an insulin secretagogue or insulin, consider lowering the dose of the secretagogue or insulin to reduce the risk of hypoglycemia. *Semaglutide* is not recommended as first-line therapy for patients inadequately controlled on diet and exercise. There may be potential risks to the fetus from exposure to *semaglutide* during pregnancy; therefore, *semaglutide* should be used during pregnancy only if the potential benefit justifies the potential risk to the fetus. *Semaglutide* is not recommended in females or males with reproductive potential. Discontinue in women at least 2 months before a planned pregnancy due to the long washout period for *semaglutide*. There are no data on the presence of *semaglutide* in human milk or the effects on the breastfed infant.
> **Ozempic** administer SC in the upper arm, abdomen, or thigh once weekly at any time of day, with or without meals; initially 0.25 mg once weekly; after 4 weeks, increase the dose to 0.5 mg once weekly; if after at least 4 weeks additional glycemic control is needed, increase to 1 mg once weekly (usual maintenance dose); if a dose is missed, administer within 5 days of the missed dose
> *Pediatric:* <18 years: not established: ≥18 years: same as adult
> *Prefilled pen:* 2 mg/1.5 ml (1.34 mg/ml), single-patient-use; 0.25, 0.5, 1 mg/injection

Comment: The most common adverse reactions (incidence ≥5%) have been nausea, vomiting, diarrhea, abdominal pain, and constipation. **Rybelsus** initially 3 mg once daily x 30 days; then increase dose to 7 mg once daily; then dose may be increased to 14 mg once daily if additional glycemic control is needed
Pediatric: <18 years: not established; ≥18 years: same as adult
> *Tab:* 3, 7, 14 mg

Comment: Waiting less than 30 minutes, or taking with food, beverages (other than plain water), or other oral medications will lessen the effect of **Rybelsus**. Waiting more than 30 minutes to eat may increase absorption. The most common adverse reactions (incidence ≥5%) have been nausea, abdominal pain, diarrhea, decreased appetite, vomiting, and constipation.

▷ *semaglutide* **(Oral)** Administer: at least 30 minutes before the first food, beverage, or other oral medications of the day with no more than 4 oz of plain water only; swallow whole, do not break, crush, or chew;
Initial dose: 3 mg once daily x 30 days; then, increase dose to 7 mg once daily x 30 days; then, if additional glycemic control is needed, may increase to max 14 mg once daily; see mfr pkg insert for switching between **Ozempic** and **Rybelsus**

Pediatric: safety and efficacy not established

Rybelsus *Tab:* 3, 7, 14 mg

Comment: Rybelsus is a GLP-1 receptor agonist to improve glycemic control in adults with T2DM. Rybelsus is not for the treatment of T1DM. *Boxed Warning:* In animal studies, *semaglutide* causes thyroid C-cell tumors. It is unknown whether **Rybelsus** causes thyroid C-cell tumors, including MTC, in humans as the human relevance of *semaglutide*-induced thyroid C-cell tumors in animals has not been determined. **Rybelsus** is contraindicated in patients with a personal or family history of MTC or in patients with MENS-2. Counsel patients regarding the potential risk of MTC and symptoms of thyroid tumors. See full prescribing information for complete boxed warning. **Rybelsus** has not been studied in patients with a history of pancreatitis; however, pancreatitis has been reported in clinical trials. Discontinue promptly if pancreatitis is suspected and do not restart if pancreatitis is confirmed. The most common adverse reactions (incidence ≥5%) have been nausea, abdominal pain, diarrhea, decreased appetite, vomiting, and constipation. Because **Rybelsus** delays gastric emptying, instruct patients to adhere to **Rybelsus** administration instructions, especially with the taking of other oral medications. Diabetic retinopathy complications have been reported in a cardiovascular outcomes trial with *semaglutide* injection. Patients with a history of diabetic retinopathy should be monitored. Concomitant use of **Rybelsus** with insulin or an oral insulin secretagogue may increase the risk of hypoglycemia, including severe hypoglycemia. Reducing the dose of insulin or oral insulin secretagogue may be necessary. Monitor renal function in patients with renal impairment reporting severe adverse GI reactions. Serious hypersensitivity reactions (e.g., anaphylaxis, angioedema) have been reported; discontinue **Rybelsus** if suspected and promptly seek medical advice. If cholelithiasis or cholecystitis is suspected, gallbladder studies are indicated. **Rybelsus** can cause fetal harm. Discontinue **Rybelsus** at least 2 months before a planned pregnancy due to the long washout period for *semaglutide*. There are alternative formulations of *semaglutide* that can be used during lactation; advise patients that breastfeeding is not recommended during treatment with **Rybelsus**.

▶ **semaglutide** (parenteral) initially 0.25 mg SC once weekly: *After 4 weeks at 0.25 mg:* may increase dose to 0.5 mg SC once weekly; *After 4 weeks at 0.5 mg:* may increase the dose to 1 mg SC once weekly; *After 4 weeks at 1 mg:* may increase the dose to 2 mg SC once weekly; administer at any time of day, with or without meals, in the upper arm, abdomen, or thigh; rotate sites; *If a dose is missed:* administer within 5 days of the missed dose

Pediatric: <18 years: safety and efficacy not established; ≥18 years: same as adult

Ozempic *Prefilled, disposable, single-patient-use pen:* 2 mg/3 ml (0.68 mg/ml), 2 mg/1.5 ml (1.34 mg/ml), 4 mg/3 ml (1.34 mg/ml), 8 mg/3 ml (2.68 mg/ml)

Comment: Ozempic is a GLP-1 receptor agonist indicated to improve glycemic control in adults with T2DM and to reduce the risk of major adverse cardiovascular events in adults with T2DM and established cardiovascular disease. **Ozempic** has not been studied in patients with a history of pancreatitis; consider another antidiabetic therapy. **Ozempic** is not for treatment of T1DM. *Boxed Warning:* In animal studies, *semaglutide* causes thyroid C-cell tumors. It is unknown whether **Ozempic** causes thyroid C-cell tumors, including medullary thyroid carcinoma (MTC), in humans as the human relevance of *semaglutide*-induced animal thyroid C-cell tumors has not been determined. **Ozempic** is contraindicated in patients with a personal or family history of MTC or in patients with multiple endocrine neoplasia syndrome type 2 (MEN 2, counsel patients regarding the potential risk of MTC and symptoms of thyroid tumors) and in patients who have a serious hypersensitivity reaction to *semaglutide* or any of the excipients in **Ozempic**. The most common adverse reactions reported in ≥5% of patients treated with **Ozempic** have been nausea, vomiting, diarrhea, abdominal pain, and constipation. Pancreatitis has been reported in clinical trials; discontinue **Ozempic** promptly if pancreatitis is suspected and do not restart **Ozempic** if pancreatitis is confirmed. Diabetic retinopathy complications have been reported in a clinical trial; patients with a history of diabetic retinopathy should be monitored. Advise patients to never share an **Ozempic** pen, even if the needle is changed. Concomitant use with an insulin secretagogue or insulin may increase the risk of hypoglycemia, including severe hypoglycemia; reducing the insulin secretagogue dose or insulin dose may be necessary. Monitor for signs of acute kidney injury (AKI); monitor renal function in patients with renal impairment reporting severe adverse GI reaction. Serious hypersensitivity reactions (e.g., anaphylaxis and angioedema) have been reported; discontinue **Ozempic** if suspected and promptly treat as appropriate. If cholelithiasis or cholecystitis is suspected, gallbladder studies are indicated. **Ozempic** delays gastric emptying and therefore may impact absorption of concomitantly administered oral medications. There are well-known clinical considerations regarding the risks of poorly controlled diabetes in pregnancy. Hypoglycemia and hyperglycemia occur more frequently during pregnancy in patients with pregestational diabetes. Poorly controlled diabetes during pregnancy increases the maternal risk for diabetic ketoacidosis, preeclampsia, spontaneous abortion, preterm delivery, and delivery complications. Poorly controlled diabetes increases the fetal risk for major birth defects, stillbirth, and macrosomia-related morbidity. There are limited data with *semaglutide* use in human pregnancy to inform a drug-associated risk of adverse fetal developmental outcomes. In animal studies, *semaglutide* administration during organogenesis has demonstrated embryo/fetal mortality, structural abnormalities, and alterations to growth occurrence at maternal clinical exposure based on the area under the curve (AUC). Also, *semaglutide* administration in animal studies during organogenesis,

(continued)

resulted in early pregnancy loss or structural abnormalities were observed at clinical exposure and ≥2-fold the MRHD. These findings coincided with a marked maternal body weight loss. Based on animal reproduction studies, there may be potential risks to the human fetus from exposure to *semaglutide* during pregnancy. **Ozempic** should not be used during pregnancy unless the potential benefit justifies the potential risk to the fetus. It is advisable to determine pregnancy status in females and males of reproductive potential prior to initiating **Ozempic** therapy and to advise use of effective contraception. Discontinue **Ozempic** in females at least 2 months before a planned pregnancy due to the long washout period for *semaglutide*. During therapy with **Ozempic**, discontinue **Ozempic** if pregnancy is suspected and do not resume **Ozempic** if pregnancy is confirmed. There are no data on the presence of *semaglutide* in human milk or effects on the breastfed infant. *Semaglutide* was detected in the milk of lactating animals at levels 3- to 12-fold lower than in maternal plasma. However, due to species-specific differences in lactation physiology, the clinical relevance of these data is not clear. Developmental and health benefits of breastfeeding should be considered along with the mother's clinical need for **Ozempic** and any potential adverse effects on the breastfed infant from **Ozempic** or from the underlying maternal condition.

BASAL INSULIN+GLUCAGON-LIKE PEPTIDE-1 RECEPTOR AGONISTS (GLP-1 RA) COMBINATIONS

▷ *insulin degludec (insulin analog)+liraglutide* for treatment of T2DM only when inadequately controlled on <50 units of basal *insulin* daily or ≤1.8 mg of *liraglutide* daily; administer by SC injection once daily, with or without food, into the upper arm, abdomen, or thigh; titrate every 3-4 days
Pediatric: <18 years: not recommended: ≥18 years: same as adult
 Xultophy *Prefilled pen:* 100/3.6 U/ml (3 ml, 5 pens/carton)

▷ *insulin glargine (insulin analog)+lixisenatide* for treatment of T2DM only when inadequately controlled on <60 units of basal *insulin* daily or *lixisenatide*; administer by SC injection once daily, with or without food, into the upper arm, abdomen, or thigh; titrate every 3-4 days
Pediatric: <18 years: not recommended: ≥18 years: same as adult
 Soliqua *Prefilled pen:* 100/33 U/ml (3 ml, 5 pens/carton), covering 15-60 mg *insulin glargine* 100 units/ml and 15-20 mcg of *lixisenatide* (*m-cresol*)

SODIUM-GLUCOSE CO-TRANSPORTER 2 (SGLT2) INHIBITORS

Comment: SGLT2 inhibitors block the SGLT2 protein involved in 90% of glucose reabsorption in the proximal renal tubule, resulting in increased renal glucose excretion (typically >2,000 mg/dL), and lower blood glucose levels (low risk of hypoglycemia), modest weight loss, and mild reduction in blood pressure (probably due to sodium loss). These agents probably also increase insulin sensitivity, decrease gluconeogenesis, and improve *insulin* release from pancreatic beta cells. SGLT2 inhibitors are contraindicated in T1DM and are decreased or contraindicated with decreased GFR, increased serum creatinine (sCr), renal failure, renal disease (ESRD), renal dialysis, metabolic acidosis, or diabetic ketoacidosis. The most common adverse side effects (ASEs) are increased urination, urinary tract infection (UTI), and female genital mycotic infection (due to the glycosuria). These effects may be managed with adequate oral hydration and postvoiding genital hygiene. OTC **Vagisil** wet wipes are recommended to completely remove any postvoiding glucose film, and thus reduce potential risk of UTI and vaginal candidiasis, and reverse initial signs/symptoms of candida vaginalis. The SGLT2 inhibitors are not recommended in nursing women. There is potential for a hypersensitivity reaction to include angioedema and anaphylaxis. Caution with SGLT2 use due to reports of increased risk of treatment-emergent bone fractures. Serious, life-threatening cases of necrotizing fasciitis (Fournier's gangrene) have been reported in both females and males taking an SGLT2 inhibitor. Assess patients presenting with pain or tenderness, erythema, or swelling in the genital or perineal area, along with fever or malaise. If suspected, initiate prompt diagnosis and treatment.

▷ *bexagliflozin* 20 mg once daily, in the morning, with or without food; do not break, crush, or chew;
Pediatric: safety and efficacy not established
 Brenzavvy *Tab:* 20 mg
 Comment: Brenzavvy is an SGLT2 inhibitor indicated to improve glycemic control in adults with T2DM. **Brenzavvy** is not recommended for patients with T1DM or for the treatment of diabetic ketoacidosis. **Brenzavvy** is contraindicated in patients who are hypersensitive to *bexagliflozin* or any tablet ingredient and is not indicated for the treatment of T2DM in patients with ESRD or who are on renal dialysis. Correct volume depletion and assess renal function before initiating **Brenzavvy** and as clinically indicated. **Brenzavvy** is not recommended if estimated glomerular filtration rate (eGFR) <30 ml/min/1.73 m². Assess patients who present with signs and symptoms of metabolic acidosis for ketoacidosis, regardless of blood glucose level. If suspected, discontinue **Brenzavvy**, evaluate, and treat promptly. Before initiating, consider risk factors for ketoacidosis. Patients may require monitoring and temporary discontinuation of therapy in clinical situations known to predispose to ketoacidosis. Consider factors that may increase the risk for amputations before initiating **Brenzavvy**. Monitor patients for signs and symptoms of infection or ulcers of the lower limbs, and discontinue **Brenzavvy** if either of these conditions occur. Necrotizing fasciitis of the perineum (Fournier's gangrene) can be serious and life-threatening. Cases have occurred in both females and males treated with SGLT2 inhibitors. Assess patients presenting with pain or tenderness, erythema, or swelling in the genital or

perineal area, along with fever <u>or</u> malaise. If suspected, institute prompt treatment. **Brenzavvy** is <u>not</u> recommended for patients with Child-Pugh Class C hepatic failure.

▷ *canagliflozin* take 1 tab before the first meal of the day; initially 100 mg; may titrate up to max of 300 mg once daily; *GFR <45 ml/min:* do <u>not</u> initiate
Pediatric: <18 years: <u>not</u> established; ≥18 years: same as adult
    Invokana *Tab:* 100, 300 mg
    Comment: Invokana is contraindicated with GFR <45 ml/min; if GFR 45-≤60 ml/min, max 100 mg once daily <u>or</u> consider other antihyperglycemic

▷ *dapagliflozin* (G) take 1 tab before the first meal of the day; initially 5 mg; may increase to max 10 mg once daily
Pediatric: <18 years: <u>not</u> established; ≥18 years: same as adult
    Farxiga *Tab:* 5, 10 mg
    Comment: Farxiga is contraindicated with GFR <60 ml/min. **Farxiga** is also indicated to (1) reduce the risk of hospitalization for heart failure in adults with T2DM and either established cardiovascular disease <u>or</u> multiple cardiovascular risk factors, (2) reduce the risk of cardiovascular death and hospitalization for heart failure in adults with heart failure (New York Heart Association [NYHA] class II-IV) with reduced ejection fraction (EF), and (3) reduce the risk of sustained eGFR decline, ESRD, cardiovascular death, and hospitalization for heart failure in adults with chronic kidney disease at risk of progression.

▷ *ertugliflozin* (G) take 1 tab before the first meal of the day; initially 5 mg; may increase to max 15 mg once daily
Pediatric: <18 years: <u>not</u> established; ≥18 years: same as adult
    Steglatro *Tab:* 5, 15 mg

▷ *lacosamide Recommended dose:* 10 mg once daily, taken in the morning, with <u>or</u> without food; may increase to 25 mg once daily; assess renal function before initiating **Jardiance**; do <u>not</u> initiate **Jardiance** if eGFR <45 ml/min/1.73 m²; discontinue **Jardiance** if eGFR persistently falls <45 ml/min/1.73 m²
Pediatric: <18 years: safety and efficacy <u>not</u> established; >18 years: same as adult
    Jardiance *Tab:* 10, 25 mg film-coat
    Comment: Jardiance is an SGLT2 inhibitor indicated for the treatment of adults with T2DM. **Jardiance** is <u>not</u> for the treatment of T1DM <u>or</u> diabetic ketoacidosis. The most common adverse reactions associated with **Jardiance** (incidence ≥5%) have been urinary tract infections (UTIs) and female genital mycotic infection. **Jardiance** is contraindicated in patients with severe renal impairment, ESRD, <u>or</u> dialysis. Before initiating **Jardiance**, assess and correct volume status in patients with renal impairment, the elderly, in patients with low systolic blood pressure (SBP), and in patients taking diuretics. Monitor for signs and symptoms of dehydration and hypotension as these adverse reactions may be increased in patients who become volume-depleted <u>and/or</u> develop decreased renal function. Consider lowering the dose of insulin secretagogue <u>or</u> insulin to reduce the risk of hypoglycemia. Monitor and treat UTIs and genital mycotic infections as appropriate. Monitor and treat low-density lipoprotein cholesterol (LDL-C) as appropriate. There have been <u>no</u> clinical studies establishing conclusive evidence of macrovascular risk reduction with **Jardiance**. It is advisable to assess the patient's pregnancy status prior to initiating treatment with **Jardiance**. Based on results from animal studies, *empagliflozin* may affect renal development and maturation. In animal studies, *empagliflozin* crosses the placenta and reaches fetal tissues. During pregnancy, consider appropriate alternative therapies, especially during the second and third trimesters. Advise females of reproductive potential to use effective contraception. It is <u>not</u> known if **Jardiance** is excreted in human milk. However, *empagliflozin* is secreted in animal milk reaching levels up to 5 times higher than that in maternal plasma. Since human kidney maturation occurs *in utero* and during the first 2 years of life when lactational exposure may occur, there may be risk to the developing human kidney. Because many drugs are excreted in human milk and because of the potential for serious adverse reactions in nursing infants from **Jardiance**, risk/benefit should be considered and a decision should be made whether to discontinue nursing <u>or</u> to discontinue **Jardiance**, taking into account the importance of the drug to the mother.

SODIUM-GLUCOSE CO-TRANSPORTER 2 (SGLT2) INHIBITOR+BIGUANIDE COMBINATIONS

Comment: Caution with SGLT2 use due to reports of increased risk of treatment-emergent bone fractures. *Metformin* is contraindicated with renal impairment, metabolic acidosis, and ketoacidosis. Suspend *metformin* prior to and for 48 hours after surgery <u>or</u> receiving IV iodinated contrast agents.

▷ *canagliflozin+metformin* take 1 dose bid with meals; max daily dose 300/2,000; *GFR 45-≤60 ml/min:* canagliflozin max 100 mg once daily <u>or</u> consider other antihyperglycemic; *GFR <45 ml/min:* do <u>not</u> initiate
Pediatric: <18 years: <u>not</u> established; ≥18 years: same as adult
    Invokamet
        Tab: Invokamet 50/500 cana 50 mg+met 500 mg
                Invokamet 50/1000 cana 50 mg+met 1,000 mg
                Invokamet 150/500 cana 150 mg+met 500 mg
                Invokamet 150/1000 cana 150 mg+met 1,000 mg

▷ *dapagliflozin+metformin* swallow whole; do <u>not</u> crush <u>or</u> chew; take once daily first meal of the day; max daily dose 10/2,000
Pediatric: <18 years: <u>not</u> established; ≥18 years: same as adult
    Xigduo XR

(continued)

 Tab: **Xigduo XR 5/500** dapa 5 mg+met 500 mg ext-rel
  Xigduo XR 5/1000 dapa 5 mg+met 1,000 mg ext-rel
  Xigduo XR 10/500 dapa 10 mg+met 500 mg ext-rel
  Xigduo XR 10/1000 dapa 10 mg+met 1,000 mg ext-rel
 Comment: Xigduo is contraindicated with GFR <60 ml/min, sCr >1.5 (men) <u>or</u> sCr >1.4 (women)

▷ *empagliflozin+metformin* (G) take 1 dose bid with meals; max daily dose 25/2,000
 Pediatric: <18 years: <u>not</u> established; ≥18 years: same as adult
 Synjardy
 Tab: **Synjardy 5/500** empa 5 mg+met 500 mg
  Synjardy 5/1000 empa 5 mg+met 1,000 mg
  Synjardy 12.5/500 empa 12.5 mg+met 500 mg
  Synjardy 12.5/1000 empa 12.5 mg+met 1,000 mg
 Synjardy XR
 Tab: **Synjardy XR 5/1000** empa 5 mg+met 1,000 mg
  Synjardy XR 12.5/1000 empa 12.5 mg+met 1,000 mg
  Synjardy XR 10/1000 empa 10 mg+met 1,000 mg
  Synjardy XR 25/1000 empa 25 mg+met 1,000 mg
 Comment: Synjardy is contraindicated with GFR <45 ml/min, sCr >1.5 (men), <u>or</u> sCr >1.4 (women).

▷ *ertugliflozin+metformin* take 1 dose bid with meals; max daily dose 15/2,000
 Pediatric: <18 years: <u>not</u> established; ≥18 years: same as adult
 Segluromet
 Tab: **Segluromet 2.5/500** ertu 2.5 mg+met 500 mg
  Segluormet 2.5/1000 ertu 2.5 mg+met 1,000 mg
  Segluromet 7.5/500 ertu 7.5 mg+met 500 mg
  Segluromet 7.5/1000 ertu 7.5 mg+met 1,000 mg
 Comment: Segluormet is contraindicated with GFR <30 ml/min. Do <u>not</u> initiate <u>or</u> continue with eGFR <60 ml/min.

SODIUM-GLUCOSE CO-TRANSPORTER 2 (SGLT2) INHIBITOR+DIPEPTIDYL PEPTIDASE-4 (DPP-4) INHIBITOR COMBINATIONS

Comment: Caution with SGLT2 use due to reports of increased risk of treatment-emergent bone fractures and increased risk for UTI and candida vaginalis secondary to drug-associated glycosuria.

▷ *dapagliflozin+saxagliptin* initially 5/10 once daily, at any time of day, with <u>or</u> without food; if a dose is missed and it is ≥12 hours until the next dose, the dose should be taken; if a dose is missed and it is <12 hours until the next dose, the missed dose should be skipped and the next dose taken at the usual time.
 Pediatric: <18 years: <u>not</u> recommended: ≥18 years: same as adult
 Qtern *Tab:* dapa 10 mg+saxa 5 mg film-coat
 Comment: Qtern should <u>not</u> be used during pregnancy. If pregnancy is detected, treatment with **Qtern** should be discontinued. It is unknown whether **Qtern** and/or its metabolites are excreted in human milk. Do <u>not</u> use with CrCl <60 ml/min <u>or</u> eGFR <60 ml/min/1.73 m² <u>or</u> ESRD <u>or</u> severe hepatic impairment <u>or</u> history of pancreatitis.

▷ *empagliflozin+linagliptin* initially 10/5 once daily with the first meal of the day; max daily dose 25/5
 Pediatric: <18 years: <u>not</u> established; ≥18 years: same as adult
 Glyxambi
 Tab: **Glyxambi 10/5** empa 10 mg+lina 5 mg
  Glyxambi 25/5 empa 25 mg+lina 5 mg
 Comment: Glyxambi is contraindicated with GFR <45 ml/min.

▷ *ertugliflozin+sitagliptin* initially 5/100 once daily with the first meal of the day; max daily dose 15/100
 Pediatric: <18 years: <u>not</u> established; ≥18 years: same as adult
 Steglujan
 Tab: **Steglujan 5/100** ertu 5 mg+sita 100 mg
  Steglujan 15/100 ertu 15 mg+sita 100 mg
 Comment: Steglujan is contraindicated with GFR <45 ml/min.

SODIUM-GLUCOSE CO-TRANSPORTER 2 (SGLT-2) INHIBITOR+DIPEPTIDYL PEPTIDASE-4 (DPP-4) INHIBITOR+BIGUANIDE

▷ *dapagliflozin+saxagliptin+metformin* assess renal function before initiation of therapy and periodically thereafter; individualize the starting total daily dose based on the patient's current regimen, effectiveness, and tolerability; take once daily in the morning with food; for patients <u>not</u> currently taking *dapagliflozin,* the recommended starting dose is **Qternmet XR 5/5/1000** (dapa 5 mg/saxa 5 mg/met 1,000 mg) once daily; max dose is **Qternmet XR 10/5/2000** (dapa 10 mg/saxa 5 mg/met 2,000 mg) once daily; swallow tablet whole, do <u>not</u> crush, cut, <u>or</u> chew
 Pediatric: <18 years: <u>not</u> recommended: ≥18 years: same as adult
 Qternmet XL

Tab: **Qternmet XL 2.5/2.5/1000** dapa 2.5 mg+saxa 2.5 mg+met 1,000 mg film-coat ext-rel
Qternmet XL 5/2.5/1000 dapa 5 mg+saxa 2.5 mg+met 1,000 mg film-coat ext-rel
Qternmet XL 5/5/1000 dapa 5 mg+saxa 5 mg+met 1,000 mg film-coat ext-rel
Qternmet XL 10/5/1000 dapa 10 mg+saxa 5 mg+met 1,000 mg film-coat ext-rel

Comment: **Qternmet XL** is <u>not</u> indicated for the treatment of T1DM <u>or</u> diabetic ketoacidosis. **Qternmet** initiation is intended only for patients currently taking *metformin*. Discontinue **Qternmet XL** at the time of <u>or</u> prior to an iodinated contrast imaging procedure. **Qternmet XL** should <u>not</u> be used during pregnancy. If pregnancy is detected, treatment with **Qternmet** should be discontinued. It is unknown whether **Qtern** <u>and/or</u> its metabolites are excreted in human milk. Do <u>not</u> use with CrCl <60 ml/min <u>or</u> eGFR <60 ml/min/1.73 m² <u>or</u> ESRD <u>or</u> severe hepatic impairment <u>or</u> history of pancreatitis.

▷ *empagliflozin+linagliptin+metformin* 1 tablet once daily with a meal; swallow whole, do <u>not</u> split, crush, dissolve, <u>or</u> chew; individualize the starting dose based on the patient's current regimen; daily max *empagliflozin* 25 mg, *linagliptin* 5 mg, *metformin* 2,000 mg
Trijardy XR

Tab: **Trijardy XR 5/2.5/1000** empa 5 mg+lina 2.5 mg+met 1,000 mg, film-coat, ext-rel
Trijardy XR 10/5/1000 empa 10 mg+lina 5 mg+met 1,000 mg, film-coat, ext-rel
Trijardy XR 12.5/2.5/1000 empa 12.5 mg+lina 2.5 mg+met 1,000 mg film-coat, ext-rel
Trijardy XR 25/5/1000 empa 25 mg+lina 5 mg+met 1,000 mg

Comment Trijardy XR *(empagliflozin+linagliptin+metformin hydrochloride)* is a three-drug fixed-dose combination of the SGLT2 inhibitor *empagliflozin* (Jardiance), the DPP-4 inhibitor *linagliptin* (Tradjenta), and the biguanide *metformin*. Assess renal function prior to initiation of **Trijardy XR** and periodically thereafter. *eGFR <45 ml/min:* Do <u>not</u> initiate <u>or</u> continue. *eGFR <30 ml/min, ESRD, <u>or</u> dialysis:* Contraindicated. **Trijardy XR** may need to be discontinued at time of, <u>or</u> prior to, iodinated contrast imaging procedures. Do <u>not</u> initiate **Trijardy XR** in patients with acute <u>or</u> chronic metabolic acidosis, including diabetic ketoacidosis; discontinue **Trijardy XR** immediately if risk of, <u>or</u> occurrence of, metabolic acidosis occurs. Hypersensitivity reactions to *empagliflozin, linagliptin, metformin*, and any of the excipients in **Trijardy XR** have occurred, including anaphylaxis, angioedema, exfoliative skin conditions, urticaria, and bronchial hyperreactivity. The most common adverse reactions associated with **Trijardy XR** (incidence ≥5%) have been upper respiratory infection (URI), UTI, headache, diarrhea, constipation, and gastroenteritis. *Metformin* may lower serum vitamin B12 level; monitor hematologic parameters annually. Severe and disabling arthralgia has been reported in patients taking DPP-4 inhibitors; therefore, consider **Trijardy XR** as a possible cause of new onset <u>or</u> increased severity of severe joint pain and discontinue drug if appropriate. Advise females of potential embryo/fetal risk, especially during the second and third trimesters. **Trijardy XR** is <u>not</u> recommended when breastfeeding.

DIPEPTIDYL PEPTIDASE-4 (DPP-4) INHIBITOR

Comment: DPP-4 is an enzyme that degrades incretin hormones GLP-1 and glucose-dependent insulinotropic polypeptide (GIP). Thus, DPP-4 inhibitors increase the concentration of active incretin hormones, stimulating the release of *insulin* in a glucose-dependent manner and decreasing the levels of circulating *glucagon*. The FDA has reported that *saxagliptin-* and *alogliptin*-containing drugs may increase the risk of heart failure, especially in patients who already have cardiovascular <u>or</u> renal disease. Drugs in this risk group include **Nesina** *(alogliptin)* and **Onglyza** *(saxagliptin)*

▷ *alogliptin* take bid with meals; max 25 mg day
Pediatric: <18 years: <u>not</u> recommended; ≥18 years: same as adult
Nesina *Tab:* 6.25, 12.5, 25 mg
▷ *linagliptin* (G) 5 mg once daily
Pediatric: <18 years: <u>not</u> recommended; ≥18 years: same as adult
Tradjenta *Tab:* 5 mg
▷ *saxagliptin* (G) 2.5-5 mg once daily
Pediatric: <18 years: <u>not</u> recommended; ≥18 years: same as adult
Onglyza *Tab:* 2.5, 5 mg
▷ *sitagliptin* as monotherapy <u>or</u> as combination therapy with metformin <u>or</u> a TZD
Pediatric: <18 years: <u>not</u> recommended; ≥18 years: same as adult
Januvia 25-100 mg once daily
Tab: 25, 50, 100 mg

DIPEPTIDYL PEPTIDASE-4 (DPP-4) INHIBITOR+BIGUANIDE COMBINATIONS

Comment: DPP-4 inhibitor+*metformin* combinations are contraindicated with renal impairment (men: sCr ≥1.5 mg/dL; women: sCr ≥1.4 mg/dL) <u>or</u> abnormal CrCl, metabolic acidosis, ketoacidosis, <u>or</u> history of angioedema. Suspend *metformin* prior to and for 48 hours after surgery <u>or</u> receiving IV iodinated contrast agents. Avoid in the elderly, malnourished, dehydrated, <u>or</u> with clinical <u>or</u> lab evidence of hepatic disease. For other DPP-4 <u>and/or</u> *metformin* precautions, see mfr pkg insert. The FDA has reported that *saxagliptin-* and *alogliptin*-containing drugs may increase the risk of heart failure, especially in patients who already have cardiovascular <u>or</u> renal disease. These drugs include **Onglyza** *(saxagliptin)*, **Kombiglyze XR** *(saxagliptin+metformin)*, **Nesina** *(alogliptin)*, **Kazano** *(alogliptin+metformin)*, and **Oseni** *(alogliptin+pioglitazone)*.

(continued)

▷ *alogliptin+metformin* take bid with meals; max *alogliptin* 25 mg/day, max *metformin* 2,000 mg/day
Pediatric: <18 years: not recommended; ≥18 years: same as adult
    Kazano
      Tab: Kazano 12.5/500 algo 12.5 mg+met 500 mg
             Kazano 2.5/1,000 algo 12.5 mg+met 1,000 mg
▷ *linagliptin+metformin* (G)
Pediatric: <18 years: not recommended; ≥18 years: same as adult
    Jentadueto take bid with meals; max *linagliptin* 5 mg/day, max *metformin* 2,000 mg/day
      Tab: Jentadueto 2.5/500 lina 2.5 mg+met 500 mg film-coat
             Jentadueto 2.5/850 lina 2.5 mg+met 850 mg film-coat
             Jentadueto 2.5/1000 lina 2.5 mg+met 1,000 mg film-coat
    Jentadueto XR *Currently not treated with metformin:* initiate Jentadueto XR 5/1000 once daily; *Already treated with metformin:* initiate Jentadueto XR 5 mg *linagliptin* total daily dose and a similar total daily dose of *metformin* once daily; *Already treated with linagliptin and metformin or Jentadueto:* switch to Jentadueto XR containing 5 mg of *linagliptin* total daily dose and a similar total daily dose of *metformin* once daily; max *linagliptin* 5 mg and *metformin* 2,000 mg; take as a single dose once daily; take with food; do not crush or chew; *eGFR <30 ml/min:* contraindicated; *eGFR 30-45 ml/min:* not recommended
      Tab: Jentadueto 2.5/1000 lina 2.5 mg+met 1,000 mg film-coat ext-rel
             Jentadueto 5/1000 lina 5 mg+met 1,000 mg film-coat ext-rel
▷ *saxagliptin+metformin* (G) take once daily with meals; max *saxagliptin* 5 mg/day, max *metformin* 2,000 mg/day; do not crush or chew
Pediatric: <18 years: not recommended; ≥18 years: same as adult
    Kombiglyze XR
      Tab: Kombiglyze XR 5/500 saxa 5 mg+met 500 mg
             Kombiglyze XR 2.5/1,000 saxa 2.5 mg+met 1,000 mg
             Kombiglyze XR 5/1,000 saxa 5 mg+met 1,000 mg
Comment: The FDA has reported that *saxagliptin*-containing drugs may increase the risk of heart failure, especially in patients who already have cardiovascular or renal disease. The drug **Kombiglyze XR** (*saxagliptin+metformin*) is in this risk group. *Metformin* is contraindicated with renal impairment, metabolic acidosis and ketoacidosis. Suspend *metformin* prior to and for 48 hours after surgery or receiving IV iodinated contrast agents.
▷ *sitagliptin+metformin* take bid with meals; max *sitagliptin* 100 mg/day, max *metformin* 2,000 mg/day
Pediatric: <18 years: not recommended; ≥18 years: same as adult
    Janumet
      Tab: Janumet 50/500 sita 50 mg+met 500 mg
             Janumet 50/1000 sita 50 mg+met 1,000 mg
    Janumet XR
      Tab: Janumet XR 50/500 sita 50 mg+met 500 mg ext-rel
             Janumet XR 50/1000 sita 50 mg+met 1,000 mg ext-rel
             Janumet XR 100/1000 sita 100 mg+met 1,000 mg ext-rel
Comment: *Metformin* is contraindicated with renal impairment, metabolic acidosis, and ketoacidosis. Suspend *metformin* prior to and for 48 hours after surgery or receiving IV iodinated contrast agents.

SODIUM-GLUCOSE CO-TRANSPORTER 2 (SGLT2) INHIBITOR+DIPEPTIDYL PEPTIDASE-4 (DPP-4) INHIBITOR+BIGUANIDE COMBINATION

▷ *dapagliflozin+saxagliptin+metformin* assess renal function before initiation of therapy and periodically thereafter; individualize the starting total daily dose based on the patient's current regimen, effectiveness, and tolerability; take once daily in the morning with food; for patients not currently taking *dapagliflozin*, the recommended starting dose is Qternmet XR 5/5/1000 (dapa 5 mg/saxa 5 mg/met 1,000 mg) once daily; max dose is Qternmet XR 10/5/2000 (dapa 10 mg/saxa 5 mg/met 2,000 mg) once daily; swallow tablet whole, do not crush, cut, or chew
Pediatric: <18 years: not recommended: ≥18 years: same as adult
    Qternmet XL
      Tab: Qternmet XL 2.5/2.5/1000 dapa 2.5 mg+saxa 2.5 mg+met 1,000 mg film-coat ext-rel
             Qternmet XL 5/2.5/1000 dapa 5 mg+saxa 2.5 mg+met 1,000 mg film-coat ext-rel
             Qternmet XL 5/5/1000 dapa 5 mg+saxa 5 mg+met 1,000 mg film-coat ext-rel
             Qternmet XL 10/5/1000 dapa 10 mg+saxa 5 mg+met 1,000 mg film-coat ext-rel
Comment: Qternmet XR is not indicated for the treatment of T1DM or diabetic ketoacidosis. Qternmet initiation is intended only for patients currently taking *metformin*. Discontinue Qternmet XR at the time of or prior to an iodinated contrast imaging procedure. Qternmet XR should not be used during pregnancy. If pregnancy is detected, treatment with Qternmet should be discontinued. It is unknown whether Qtern and/or its metabolites are excreted in human milk. Do not use with CrCl <60 ml/min or eGFR <60 ml/min/1.73 m² or ESRD or severe hepatic impairment or history of pancreatitis.

MEGLITINIDE+BIGUANIDE COMBINATION

▶ *repaglinide+metformin* (G) take in 2-3 divided doses within 30 minutes before food; max 4/1,000 per meal and 10/2,000 per day

Pediatric: <18 years: not recommended; ≥18 years: same as adult

Prandimet

Tab: Prandimet 1/500 repa 1 mg+met 500 mg

Prandimet 2/500 repa 2 mg+met 500 mg

Comment: *Metformin* is contraindicated with renal impairment, metabolic acidosis, and ketoacidosis. Suspend *metformin* prior to and for 48 hours after surgery or receiving IV iodinated contrast agents.

SODIUM-GLUCOSE CO-TRANSPORTER 2 (SGLT2) INHIBITOR+DIPEPTIDYL PEPTIDASE-4 (DPP-4) INHIBITOR+BIGUANIDE

▶ Qternmet EX individualize the starting total daily dose of Qternmet EX based on the patient's current regimen, effectiveness, and tolerability; take once daily in the morning with food; swallow tablet whole, do not crush, cut, or chew; *Patients not currently taking dapagliflozin:* recommended starting total daily dose of Qternmet EX is 5 mg *dapagliflozin*+5 mg *saxagliptin*+1,000 mg or 2,000 mg *metformin hcl* once daily; max recommended daily dose is 10 mg *dapagliflozin*, 5 mg *saxagliptin*, and 2,000 mg *metformin hcl*

Pediatric: <18 years: not recommended; ≥18 years: same as adult

Tab: Qternmet EX 2.5/2.5/1000 dapa 2.5 mg+saxa 2.5 mg+met hcl 1,000 mg ext-rel

Qternmet EX 5/2.5/1000 dapa 5 mg+saxa 2.5 mg+met hcl 1,000 mg ext-rel

Qternmet EX 5/5/1000 dapa 5 mg+saxa 5 mg+met hcl 1,000 mg ext-rel

Qternmet EX 10/5/1000 dapa 10 mg+saxa 5 mg+met hcl 1,000 mg ext-rel

Comment: Qternmet XR is triple fixed-dose combination indicated for adults with T2DM. Assess renal function before initiating Qternmet EX and periodically thereafter. Discontinue Qternmet EX at the time of, or prior to, an iodinated contrast imaging procedure. Contraindications to Qternmet EX include history of a serious hypersensitivity reaction to *dapagliflozin, saxagliptin,* or *metformin,* including anaphylaxis, angioedema, or exfoliative skin conditions; moderate-to-severe renal impairment (eGFR <45 ml/min/1.73 m^2), ESRD, or patient on dialysis, acute or chronic metabolic acidosis, including diabetic ketoacidosis, with or without coma. Diabetic ketoacidosis should be treated with insulin. Do not co-administer Qternmet XR with strong cytochrome P450 3A4/5 inhibitors. Co-administration with carbonic anhydrase inhibitors may increase the risk of lactic acidosis (consider more frequent monitoring). Drugs that reduce *metformin* clearance (such as *ranolazine, vandetanib, dolutegravir,* and *cimetidine*) may increase the accumulation of *metformin* (consider the benefits and risks of concomitant use). Alcohol can potentiate the effects of *metformin* on lactate metabolism (warn patients against excessive alcohol intake). Advise females of reproductive potential of embryo/fetal risk, especially during the second and third trimesters. Qternmet EX is not recommended when breastfeeding. There is a higher incidence of adverse reactions related to volume depletion and reduced renal function in the geriatric population. Avoid use of Qternmet EX in patients with clinical or laboratory evidence of hepatic impairment.

GLUCOSE-DEPENDENT INSULINOTROPIC POLYPEPTIDE (GIP) RECEPTOR+GLUCAGON-LIKE PEPTIDE-1 (GLP-1) RECEPTOR AGONIST

▶ *tirzepatide* administer SC in the upper arm, abdomen, or thigh once weekly, at any time of day, with or without food; rotate sites; *Recommended starting dose;* 2.5 mg SC once weekly; after 4 weeks, increase to 5 mg SC once weekly; then if additional glycemic control is needed, increase in 2.5 mg increments after at least 4 weeks on the current dose; *Max:* 15 mg SC once weekly

Pediatric: <18 years: safety and efficacy not established; ≥18 years: same as adult

Mounjaro *Single-dose pen:* 2.5, 5, 7.5, 10, 12.5. 15 mg per 0.5 ml, soln per single-dose pen for SC injection (4 pens/carton)

Comment: Mounjaro is a GIP receptor and GLP-1 receptor agonist indicated to improve glycemic control in adults with T2DM. Mounjaro is not indicated for use in patients with T1DM. Mounjaro delays gastric emptying and has the potential to impact the absorption of concomitantly administered oral medications. The most common adverse reactions, reported in ≥5% of patients treated with Mounjaro, have been nausea, diarrhea, decreased appetite, vomiting, constipation, dyspepsia, and abdominal pain. Contraindications include patients with personal family history of MTC, patients with MENS-2, and patients with known serious hypersensitivity to *tirzepatide* or any of the excipients in Mounjaro. Mounjaro has not been studied in patients with a history of pancreatitis. *Boxed Warning: Tirzepatide* causes thyroid C-cell tumors in rats. It is unknown whether Mounjaro causes thyroid C-cell tumors, including MTC, in humans as the human relevance of *tirzepatide*-induced rodent thyroid C-cell tumors has not been determined. Counsel patients regarding the potential risk of MTC and symptoms of thyroid tumors. Pancreatitis has been reported in clinical trials; discontinue Mounjaro promptly if pancreatitis is suspected. Concomitant use of an insulin secretagogue or insulin may increase the risk of hypoglycemia, including severe hypoglycemia; reducing the dose of the insulin secretagogue or insulin may be necessary. Hypersensitivity reactions have been reported; discontinue Mounjaro if suspected. Monitor the patient for an acute kidney injury (AKI); monitor renal function in patients with renal impairment reporting severe adverse gastrointestinal (GI) reactions. Mounjaro may be associated with

(continued)

GI adverse reactions, sometimes severe. **Mounjaro** has not been studied in patients with severe GI disease and is not recommended in these patients. Complications may develop in patients with a history of diabetic retinopathy. **Mounjaro** has not been studied in patients with non-proliferative diabetic retinopathy (NPDR) requiring acute therapy, proliferative diabetic retinopathy, or diabetic macular edema; monitor patients with a history of diabetic retinopathy for progression. Acute gallbladder disease has occurred in clinical trials; if cholelithiasis is suspected, gallbladder studies and clinical follow-up are indicated. Based on animal studies, **Mounjaro** may cause fetal harm; advise females of reproductive potential using oral contraceptives to switch to a non-oral contraceptive method or add a barrier method of contraception for 4 weeks after initiation and for 4 weeks after each dose escalation. There are no data on the presence of *tirzepatide* in animal or human milk or effects on the breastfed infant. Developmental and health benefits of breastfeeding should be considered along with the mother's clinical need for **Mounjaro** and any potential adverse effects on the breastfed infant from **Mounjaro** or from the underlying maternal condition. To report suspected adverse reactions, contact Eli Lilly and Company at 1-800-LillyRx (1-800-545-5979) or FDA at 1-800-FDA-1088 or www.fda.gov/medwatch.

DIPEPTIDYL PEPTIDASE-4 (DPP-4) INHIBITOR+HMG-COA REDUCTASE INHIBITOR COMBINATION
▷ *sitagliptin+simvastatin* take once daily in the PM; swallow whole; adjust dose if needed after 4 weeks; *Concomitant* **verapamil** *or* **diltiazem**: max 100/10 once daily; *Concomitant* **amiodarone, amlodipine,** *or* **ranolazine**: max 100/20 once daily; *Homogenous familial hypercholesterolemia*: max 100/40 once daily; *Chinese patients taking lipid-modifying doses (>1 gm/day niacin) of* **niacin**-*containing products*: caution with 100/40 dose; increase risk of myopathy
Pediatric: <18 years: not recommended; ≥18 years: same as adult
    Juvisync
      Tab: Juvisync 100/10 sita 100 mg+simva 10 mg
           Juvisync 100/20 sita 100 mg+simva 20 mg
           Juvisync 100/40 sita 100 mg+simva 40 mg

DOPAMINE RECEPTOR AGONIST
▷ *bromocriptine mesylate* take with food in the morning within 2 hours of waking; initially 0.8 mg once daily; may increase by 0.8 mg/week; max 4.8 mg/week; *Severe psychotic disorders*: not recommended
Pediatric: <12 years: not recommended; ≥12 years: same as adult
    Cycloset *Tab:* 0.8 mg
    Comment: Cycloset is an adjunct to diet and exercise to improve glycemic control. Contraindicated with syncopal migraines, nursing mothers, and other ergot-related drugs.

Bile Acid Sequestrant
▷ *colesevelam* (G)
    WelChol recommended dose is 6 tablets once daily or 3 tablets bid; take with a meal and liquid
    Pediatric: <10 years: not recommended; ≥10 years: same as adult
      Tab: 625 mg
    WelChol for Oral Suspension recommended dose is one 3.75 gm packet once daily or one 1.875 gm packet bid; empty 1 packet into a glass or cup; add 1/2 to 1 cup (4-8 oz) of water, fruit juice, or diet soft drink; stir well and drink immediately; do not swallow dry form; take with meals
    Pediatric: <12 years: not established; ≥12 years: same as adult
      Pwdr: 3.75 gm/pkt (30 pkt/carton), 1.875 gm/pkt (60 pkt/carton) for oral suspension
    Comment: WelChol is indicated as adjunctive therapy to improve glycemic control in adults with T2DM. It can be added to **metformin**, sulfonylureas, or insulin alone or in combination with other antidiabetic agents.

TYPHOID FEVER (*SALMONELLA TYPHI*)

PRE-EXPOSURE PROPHYLAXIS
▷ *typhoid* vaccine, oral, live, attenuated strain
    Vivotif Berna 1 cap every other day, 1 hour before a meal, with a lukewarm (not > body temperature) or cold drink for a total of 4 doses; do not crush or chew; complete therapy at least 1 week prior to expected exposure; reimmunization recommended q 5 years if repeated exposure
      Pediatric: <6 years: not recommended; ≥6 years: same as adult
      Cap: ent-coat
▷ *typhoid* Vi polysaccharide vaccine
    Pediatric: <2 years: not recommended; ≥2 years: same as adult
    Typhim Vi 0.5 ml IM in deltoid; reimmunization recommended q 2 years if repeated exposure
      Vial: 20, 50 dose; *Prefilled syringe:* 0.5 ml
    Comment: Febrile illness may require delaying administration of the vaccine; have *epinephrine* 1:1,000 readily available.

TREATMENT

➤ *azithromycin* (G) 8-10 mg/kg/day; *Mild illness:* treat x 7 days; *Severe illness:* treat x 14 days
 Pediatric: 8-10 mg/kg/day; max 500 mg/day; *Mild illness:* treat x 7 days; *Severe illness:* treat x 14 days; *see* Appendix BB.7. *azithromycin* (Zithromax Suspension, Zmax Suspension) *for dose by weight*
 Zithromax *Tab:* 250, 500, 600 mg; *Oral susp:* 100 mg/5 ml (15 ml); 200 mg/5 ml (15, 22.5, 30 ml) (cherry); *Pkt:* 1 gm for reconstitution (cherry-banana)
 Zithromax Tri-Pak *Tab:* 3 x 500 mg tabs/pck
 Zithromax Z-Pak *Tab:* 6 x 250 mg tabs/pck
 Zmax *Oral susp:* 2 gm ext-rel for reconstitution (cherry-banana) (148 mg Na⁺)
➤ *cefixime* (G) *Mild illness:* 15-20 mg/kg/day x 7-14 days; *Severe illness:* 20 mg/kg/day x 10-14 days
 Pediatric: <6 months: not recommended; 6 months-12 years, <50 kg: *Mild illness:* 15-20 mg/kg/day x 7-14 days; *Severe illness:* 20 mg/kg/day x 10-14 >50 kg: same as adult; *see* Appendix BB.11. *cefixime* (G) (Suprax Oral Suspension) *for dose by weight*
 Suprax *Tab:* 400 mg; *Cap:* 400 mg; *Oral susp:* 100, 200, 500 mg/5 ml (50, 75, 100 ml) (strawberry)
➤ *ciprofloxacin* 15 mg/kg/day; *Mild illness:* treat x 5-7 days; *Severe illness:* treat x 10-14 days
 Pediatric: <18 years: not recommended; ≥18 years: same as adult
 Cipro (G) *Tab:* 250, 500, 750 mg; *Oral susp:* 250, 500 mg/5 ml (100 ml) (strawberry)
 Cipro XR *Tab:* 500, 1,000 mg ext-rel
 ProQuin XR *Tab:* 500 mg ext-rel
➤ *ofloxacin* 15 mg/kg/day; *Mild illness:* treat x 5-7 days; *Severe illness:* treat x 10-14 days
 Pediatric: <18 years: not recommended; ≥18 years: same as adult
 Floxin *Tab:* 200, 300, 400 mg
➤ *cefotaxime* 80 mg/kg/day IM/IV x 10-14 days; max 2 gm/day
 Pediatrics: 80 mg/kg/day IM/IV x 10-14 days; max 2 gm/day
 Claforan *Vial:* 500 mg; 1, 2 gm
➤ *ceftriaxone* (G) 75 mg/kg/day IM/IV x 10-14 days; max 2 gm/day
 Pediatrics: 75 mg/kg/day IM/IV x 10-14 days; max 2 gm/day
 Rocephin *Vial:* 250, 500 mg; 1, 2 gm
➤ *trimethoprim+sulfamethoxazole (TMP-SMX)* (G) 8-40 mg/kg/day x 14 days
 Pediatric: <2 months: not recommended; ≥2 months: 8-40 mg/kg/day of *sulfamethoxazole* in 2 divided doses bid x 10 days; *see* Appendix BB.33. *trimethoprim+sulfamethoxazole* (G) (Bactrim Suspension, Septra Suspension) *for dose by weight*
 Bactrim, Septra 2 tabs bid x 10 days
 Tab: trim 80 mg+sulfa 400 mg*
 Bactrim DS, Septra DS 1 tab bid x 10 days
 Tab: trim 160 mg+sulfa 800 mg*
 Bactrim Pediatric Suspension, Septra Pediatric Suspension 20 ml bid x 10 days
 Oral susp: trim 40 mg+sulfa 200 mg per 5 ml (100 ml) (cherry) (alcohol 0.3%)

ULCER: DIABETIC, NEUROPATHIC (LOWER EXTREMITY); VENOUS INSUFFICIENCY (LOWER EXTREMITY)

NUTRITIONAL SUPPLEMENT

➤ *L-methylfolate calcium (as* Metafolin)+*pyridoxal 5-phosphate+methylcobalamin* take 1 cap daily
 Pediatric: <12 years: not recommended; ≥12 years: same as adult
 Metanx *Cap:* metafo 3 mg+pyrid 35 mg+methyl 2 mg (gluten-free, yeast-free, lactose-free)
 Comment: Metanx is indicated as adjunct treatment of endothelial dysfunction and/or hyperhomocysteinemia in patients who have lower extremity ulceration.

DEBRIDING+CAPILLARY STIMULANT AGENT

➤ *trypsin+balsam peru+castor oil* apply at least bid; may cover with a wet bandage
 Granulex *Aerosol liq:* tryp 0.12 mg+bal peru 87 mg+cast 788 mg per 0.82 ml

GROWTH FACTOR

➤ *becaplermin* apply once daily with a cotton swab or tongue depressor; then cover with saline-moistened gauze dressing; rinse after 12 hours; then re-cover with a clean saline dressing
 Regranex *Gel:* 0.01% (2, 7.5, 15 gm) (parabens)
 Comment: Store in refrigerator; do not freeze. Not for use in wounds that close by primary intention.

ULCER: PRESSURE, DECUBITUS

DEBRIDING/CAPILLARY STIMULANT AGENT

 Granulex (*trypsin 0.1 mg+balsam peru* 72.5 mg+*castor oil* 650 mg per 0.82 ml) apply at least bid; may cover with a wet bandage
 Aerosol liq: (2, 4 oz)

GROWTH FACTOR

▷ *becaplermin* apply once daily with a cotton swab or tongue depressor; then cover with saline-moistened gauze dressing; rinse after 12 hours; then re-cover with a clean saline dressing
    Regranex *Gel:* 0.01% (2, 7.5, 15 gm) (parabens)
Comment: Store in refrigerator; do not freeze. Not for use in wounds that close by primary intention.

ULCERATIVE COLITIS (UC)

Comment: Standard treatment regimen is anti-infective, antispasmodic, and bowel rest; progressing to clear liquids; then to high fiber.
Parenteral Corticosteroids *see* Appendix L. Parenteral Corticosteroids
Oral Corticosteroids *see* Appendix K. Oral Corticosteroids
▷ *budesonide micronized* (G) 9 mg once daily in the AM for up to 8 weeks; may repeat an 8-week course;
    Maintenance of remission: 6 mg once daily for up to 3 months; taper other systemic steroids when transferring to *budesonide*
    Pediatric: <12 years: not recommended; ≥12 years: same as adult
        Entocort EC *Cap:* 3 mg ent-coat granules
        Uceris *Tab:* 9 mg ext-rel

RECTAL CORTICOSTEROIDS

Comment: Rectally administered corticosteroid is indicated for the induction of remission in patients with active mild-to-moderate distal ulcerative colitis (UC) extending up to 40 cm from the anal verge. Children who are treated with corticosteroids by any route may experience a decrease in their growth velocity. This negative impact of corticosteroids on growth has been in the absence of laboratory evidence of hypothalamic-pituitary-adrenal (HPA) axis suppression. The long-term effects of this reduction in growth velocity associated with corticosteroid treatment, including the impact on final adult height, are unknown. Growth velocity may therefore be a more sensitive indicator of systemic corticosteroid exposure in children than some commonly used tests of HPA axis function. The linear growth of children treated with corticosteroids by any route should be monitored (e.g., via stadiometry), and the potential growth effects of prolonged treatment should be weighed against clinical benefits obtained and the availability of other treatment alternatives. In order to minimize the potential growth effects of corticosteroids, children should be titrated to the lowest effective dose. Monitor patients for indications of impaired adrenal function, especially patients switching from other glucocorticoids: Taper slowly from glucocorticosteroids with high systemic effects; monitor for withdrawal symptoms and unmasking of allergies (rhinitis, eczema). Glucocorticosteroid use increases patient risk for infection, including serious and fatal chickenpox and measles. Monitor patients with active or quiescent tuberculosis infection, untreated fungal, bacterial, systemic viral, or parasitic infections, or ocular herpes simplex. There are no adequate and well-controlled studies with corticosteroid in pregnant women. Hypoadrenalism may occur in neonates with *in utero* exposure to corticosteroids via maternal use of rectally administered corticosteroid. Corticosteroid rectal foam should be used in human pregnancy only if the potential benefit justifies the potential risk to the fetus. Carefully observe these neonates for signs and symptoms of hypoadrenalism. Use of corticosteroid rectal foam is likely to result in presence of the steroid in human milk as corticosteroids delivered by inhalation from a dry powder inhaler is present in human milk at low concentrations. Developmental and health benefits of breastfeeding should be considered along with the mother's clinical need for the corticosteroid rectal foam and any potential adverse effects on the breastfed infant from the exposure to corticosteroid via the mother's use of the locally applied rectal foam or from the underlying maternal condition.

▷ *budesonide rectal foam* (G) *Recommended dose:* 1 metered dose administered bid for 2 weeks, followed by 1 metered dose administered once daily for 4 weeks; warm the canister in the hands while shaking it vigorously for 10-15 seconds prior to use; do not refrigerate
    Pediatric: safety and efficacy not established; however, if used, refer to comment above for warnings and precautions of use
        Uceris *Rectal foam:* 2 mg *budesonide* per metered dose (33.4 gm, 14 metered doses/cannister); 2 aerosol canisters w. 28 applicators per kit
▷ *hydrocortisone* rectal
    Pediatric: <12 years: not recommended; ≥12 years: same as adult
        Anusol-HC Suppositories 1 supp rectally tid or 2 supp rectally bid for 2 weeks; max 8 weeks
          Rectal supp: 25 mg (12, 24/pck)
        Cortenema 1 enema q HS x 21 days or until symptoms controlled
          Enema: 100 mg/60 ml (1, 7/pck)
        Cortifoam 1 applicator full once daily-bid x 2-3 weeks and every 2nd day thereafter until symptoms are controlled
          Aerosol: 80 mg/applicator (14 application/container)
        Proctocort 1 supp rectally in AM and PM x 2 weeks; for more severe cases, may increase to 1 supp rectally 3 times daily or 2 supp rectally bid; max 4-8 weeks
          Rectal supp: 30 mg (12, 24/pck)
    Comment: Use *hydrocortisone* foam as adjunctive therapy in the distal portion of the rectum when *hydrocortisone* enemas cannot be retained.

RECTAL CORTICOSTEROID+ANESTHETIC
Hydrocortisone+Pramoxine

Proctofoam HC apply to anal/rectal area 3-4 times daily; max 4-8 weeks
Rectal foam: hydrocort 1%+pram 1% (10 gm w. applicator)

SALICYLATES

Comment: Symptoms of salicylate toxicity include hematemesis, tachypnea, hyperpnea, tinnitus, deafness, lethargy, seizures, confusion, or dyspnea. Severe intoxication may lead to electrolyte and blood pH imbalance and potentially to other organ (e.g., renal and liver) involvement. There is no specific antidote for mesalamine overdose; however, conventional therapy for salicylate toxicity may be beneficial in the event of acute overdosage. This includes prevention of further gastrointestinal tract absorption by emesis and, if necessary, by gastric lavage. Fluid and electrolyte imbalance should be corrected by the administration of appropriate IV therapy. Adequate renal function should be maintained.

▷ *balsalazide disodium*
Comment: *Balsalazide* 6.75 gm provides 2.4 gm of *mesalazine* to the colon.
Colazal 3 x 750 mg caps/day (6.75 gm/day), with or without food, x 8 weeks; may require treatment for up to 12 weeks; swallow whole or may be opened and sprinkled on applesauce, then chewed or swallowed immediately
Pediatric: <5 years: not recommended; 5-17 years: 1 x 750 mg cap 3 tid (2.25 gm/day), with or without food for up to 8 weeks, or 3 x 750 mg caps/day (6.75 gm/day), with or without food, x 8 weeks; swallow whole or may be opened and sprinkled on applesauce, then chewed or swallowed immediately
Cap: 750 mg
Comment: Colazal is a locally acting aminosalicylate indicated for the treatment of mildly to moderately active UC in patients ≥5 years. Safety and effectiveness of Colazal >8 weeks in children (5-17 years) and >12 weeks in patients ≥18 years have not been established.
Giazo is a locally acting aminosalicylate indicated for the treatment of mildly to moderately active UC only in male patients ≥18 years; take 3 x 1.1 gm tabs bid (6.6 gm/day) for up to 8 weeks
Pediatric: <18 years: not recommended; >18 years: same as adult
Tab: 1.1 gm (sodium 126 mg/tab), film-coat
Comment: Effectiveness of Giazo in female patients has not been demonstrated in clinical trials. Safety and effectiveness of Giazo >8 weeks have not been established.

▷ *mesalamine*
Apriso *Maintenance of remission:* 4 x 0.375 gm caps (1.5 gm/day) once daily in the morning, with or without food; do not co-administer with antacids
Pediatric: <18 years: not recommended; ≥18 years: same as adult
Cap: 0.375 gm ext-rel (phenylalanine 0.56 mg/cap)
Comment: Apriso is a locally acting aminosalicylate indicated for the maintenance of remission of ulcerative colitis in adults.
Asacol HD (G) *Induction of remission:* 2 x 800 mg tab (1,600 mg) tid x 6 weeks; *Maintenance of remission:* 1.6 gm/day in divided doses; take on an empty stomach, at least 1 hour before or 2 hours after a meal; swallow whole, do not crush, break, or chew
Pediatric: <18 years: not recommended; ≥18 years: same as adult
Tab: 800 mg del-rel
Comment: Asacol HD is an aminosalicylate indicated for the treatment of moderately active UC in adults. Do not substitute 1 Asacol HD 800 tablet for 2 *mesalamine* delayed-release 400 mg oral products
Canasa 1 x 1,000 mg suppository administered rectally once daily at bedtime for 3 to 6 weeks
Pediatric: <18 years: not recommended; ≥18 years: same as adult
Rectal supp: 1 gm del-rel (30, 42/pck)
Comment: Canasa is an aminosalicylate indicated in adults for the treatment of mildly to moderately active ulcerative proctitis. Safety and effectiveness of Canasa beyond 6 weeks have not been established.
Delzicol *Treatment:* 2 x 400 mg caps (800 mg/day) tid x 6 weeks; *Maintenance:* 4 x 400 mg caps (1.6 gm/day) in 2-4 divided doses once daily; swallow whole; take with or without food; do not crush or chew
Pediatric: ≥5-17 years: twice-daily dosing for 6 weeks; see mfr pkg insert for weight-based dosing table; ≥18 years: same as adult
Cap: 400 mg del-rel
Comment: 2 x 400 mg Delzicol caps have not been shown to be interchangeable or substitutable with 1 *mesalamine* delayed-release 80 mg tablet. Evaluate renal function prior to initiation of Delzicol.
Lialda (G) *Induction of remission:* 2-4 x 1.2 gm tabs (2.4-4.8 gm) once daily for up to 8 weeks; *Maintenance of remission:* 2 x 1.2 gm tabs (2.4 gm) once daily; swallow whole, do not crush or chew
Pediatric: <18 years: not recommended; ≥18 years: same as adult
Tab: 1.2 gm del-rel
Comment: Lialda is a locally acting 5-aminosalicylic acid (5-ASA) indicated for the induction of remission in adults with active, mild-to-moderate UC and for the maintenance of remission of ulcerative colitis (UC). Safety and effectiveness of Lialda in pediatric patients have not been established.

(continued)

Pentasa *Induction of remission:* 1 gm qid for up to 8 weeks
Pediatric: <18 years: <u>not</u> recommended; ≥18 years: same as adult
    Cap: 250, 500 mg ext-rel
Comment: Pentasa is an aminosalicylate anti-inflammatory agent indicated for the induction of remission and for the treatment of patients with mildly to moderately active ulcerative colitis (UC).
Rowasa Suppository 1 supp rectally bid x 3-6 weeks; retain for 1-3 hours <u>or</u> longer
Pediatric: <18 years: <u>not</u> recommended; ≥18 years: same as adult
    Rectal supp: 500 mg (12, 24/pck)
Rowasa Rectal Suspension 4 gm (60 ml) rectally by enema q HS; retain for 8 hours x 3-6 weeks (sulfite-free)
Pediatric: <18 years: <u>not</u> recommended; ≥18 years: same as adult
    Enema: 4 gm/60 ml (7, 14, 28/pck; kit, 7, 14, 28/pck w. wipes)
Comment: Rowasa Rectal Suspension enema is indicated for the treatment of active mild-to-moderate distal UC, proctosigmoiditis, and proctitis.
▸ *olsalazine* *Maintenance of remission:* 1 gm/day in 2 divided doses; take with food
Pediatric: <18 years: <u>not</u> recommended; ≥18 years: same as adult
    Dipentum *Cap:* 250 mg
Comment: *Olsalazine* is the sodium salt of a salicylate, disodium 3,3'-azobis (6-hydroxybenzoate), a compound that is effectively bioconverted to 5-ASA, which has anti-inflammatory activity in UC. The conversion of *olsalazine* to *mesalamine* (5-ASA) in the colon is similar to that of *sulfasalazine*, which is converted into *sulfapyridine* and *mesalamine*. *Olsalazine* is indicated for the maintenance of remission of UC in patients who are intolerant of *sulfasalazine*.
▸ *sulfasalazine* *Induction of remission:* 3-4 gm/day in evenly divided doses with dosage intervals <u>not</u> exceeding eight hours; in some cases, it is advisable to initiate therapy with a smaller dosage, for example, 1-2 gm/day, to reduce possible gastrointestinal intolerance. If daily doses exceeding 4 gm are required to achieve desired effects, the increased risk of toxicity should be kept in mind; *Maintenance of remission:* 4 gm/day in divided doses
Pediatric: <2 years: <u>not</u> recommended; 2-16 years: initially 40-60 mg/kg/day in 3-6 divided doses; max 30 mg/kg/day in 4 divided doses; max 2 gm/day in divided doses; >16 years: same as adult
    Azulfidine *Tab:* 500*mg
    Azulfidine EN-Tabs *Tab:* 500 mg ent-coat

TUMOR NECROSIS FACTOR (TNF) BLOCKER

▸ *adalimumab* 160 mg on Day 1 (given in 1 day <u>or</u> split over 2 consecutive days), 80 mg on Day 15, and 40 mg every other week starting on Day 29; discontinue in patients without evidence of clinical remission by 8 weeks (Day 57); administer in abdomen <u>or</u> thigh; rotate sites
Pediatric: <5 years, <20 kg: <u>not</u> recommended; 5-18 years, living with moderate-to-severe UC, weight-based: 20 kg (44 lb) to <40 kg (<88 lb): Day 1: 80 mg; Day 8: 40 mg; Day 15: 20 mg; Starting on Day 29: 20 mg every week <u>or</u> 40 mg every other week; >40 kg (>88 lb): Day 1: 160 mg (as a single dose <u>or</u> split over 2 consecutive days); Day 8: 80 mg; Day 15: 80 mg; Starting on Day 29: 40 mg every week <u>or</u> 80 mg every other week; it is recommended to continue the recommended pediatric dosage in patients who turn 18 years of age and who are well-controlled on their **Humira** regimen
    Humira *Prefilled syringe:* 20 mg/0.4 ml; 40 mg/0.8 ml, single-dose (2/pck; 2, 6/starter pck) (preservative-free)
▸ *adalimumab-aacf* administer 160 mg SC on Day 1 (may split dose over 2 consecutive days); then 80 mg SC on Day 15; then 40 mg SC every other week starting on Day 29; discontinue in patients without evidence of clinical remission by eight weeks (Day 57)
    Idacio *Prefilled pen (Idacio Pen):* 40 mg/0.8 ml, single-dose; *Prefilled glass syringe:* 40 mg/0.8 ml, single dose
    Comment: Idacio is biosimilar to Humira (*adalimumab*).
▸ *adalimumab-adbm* *First dose (Day 1):* 160 mg SC (4 x 40 mg injections in one day <u>or</u> 2 x 40 mg injections per day for 2 consecutive days); *Second dose 2 weeks later (day 15):* 80 mg SC; *2 weeks later* (Day 29): begin a maintenance dose of 40 mg SC every other week; <u>only</u> continue in patients who have shown evidence of clinical remission by 8 weeks (Day 57) of therapy
Pediatric: <18 years: <u>not</u> recommended; ≥18 years: same as adult
    Cyltezo *Prefilled syringe:* 40 mg/0.8 ml, single-dose (preservative-free)
    Comment: Cyltezo is biosimilar to Humira (*adalimumab*).
▸ *adalimumab-afzb* 40 mg SC every other week; some patients with rheumatoid arthritis (RA) <u>not</u> receiving *methotrexate (MTX)* may benefit from increasing the frequency to 40 mg SC every week
    Abrilada *Prefilled pen:* 40 mg/0.8 ml, single-dose; *Prefilled syringe:* 40 mg/0.8 ml, 20 mg/0.4 ml, 10 mg/0.2 ml, single-dose (for institutional use only) (preservative-free)
    Comment: Abrilada is biosimilar to Humira (*adalimumab*).
▸ *adalimumab-bwwd* *Initial dose* (Day 1): 160 mg SC; *Second dose, 2 weeks later* (Day 15): 80 mg SC; *2 weeks later* (Day 29): begin maintenance dose of 40 mg every other week
    Hadlima *Prefilled autoinjector:* 40 mg/0.8 ml, single-dose (Hadlima PushTouch); *Prefilled syringe:* 40 mg/0.8 ml, single-dose
    Comment: Hadlima is biosimilar to Humira (*adalimumab*).

▷ *infliximab* must be refrigerated at 2°C-8°C (36°F-46°F); administer dose via IV infusion over a period of not less than 2 hours; do not use beyond the expiration date as this product contains no preservative; 5 mg/kg at 0, 2, and 6 weeks, then q 8 weeks

Pediatric: <6 years: safety and efficacy not established; ≥6-17 years: 5 mg/kg at 0, 2, and 6 weeks, then every 8 weeks; ≥18 years: same as adult

> Remicade *Vial:* 100 mg pwdr for reconstitution to 10 ml administration volume, single-dose (preservative-free)
>
> **Comment:** Remicade is indicated to reduce signs and symptoms, and induce and maintain clinical remission, in adults and children ≥6 years of age with moderately to severely active disease who have had an inadequate response to conventional therapy, and reduce the number of draining enterocutaneous and rectovaginal fistulas, and maintain fistula closure, in adults with fistulizing disease. Common adverse effects associated with **Remicade** included abdominal pain, headache, pharyngitis, sinusitis, and upper respiratory infections. In addition, **Remicade** might increase the risk for serious infections, including tuberculosis, bacterial sepsis, and invasive fungal infections. Available data from published literature on the use of *infliximab* products during pregnancy have not reported a clear association with *infliximab* products and adverse pregnancy outcomes. *Infliximab* products cross the placenta and infants exposed *in utero* should not be administered live vaccines for at least 6 months after birth. Otherwise, the infant may be at increased risk of infection, including disseminated infection, which can become fatal. Available information is insufficient to inform the amount of *infliximab* products present in human milk or the effects on the breastfed infant.

▷ *infliximab-abda*

> Renflexis *Vial:* 100 mg for reconstitution to 10 ml administration volume, single-dose
>
> **Comment:** Renflexis is biosimilar to Remicade (*infliximab*).

▷ *infliximab-dyyb*

> Inflectra *Vial:* 100 mg pwdr for reconstitution to 10 ml administration volume, single-dose
>
> **Comment:** Inflectra is biosimilar to Remicade (*infliximab*).

▷ *infliximab-axxq*

> Avsola *Vial:* 100 mg pwdr in a 20 ml single-dose vial, for reconstitution, dilution, and IV infusion
>
> **Comment:** Avsola is biosimilar to Remicade (*infliximab*).

▷ *infliximab-qbtx*

> Ixifi *Vial:* 100 mg pwdr for reconstitution to 10 ml administration volume, single-dose
>
> **Comment:** Ixifi is biosimilar to Remicade (*infliximab*).

INTERLEUKIN-12+INTERLEUKIN-23 ANTAGONIST

▷ *ustekinumab* rotate sites; ≤100 kg: 45 mg SC once; then 45 mg SC once 4 weeks later; then 45 mg SC once every 12 weeks thereafter; >100 kg: 90 mg SC once; then 90 mg SC once 4 weeks later; then 90 mg SC once every 12 weeks thereafter

Pediatric: <18 years: not recommended; ≥18 years: same as adult

> Stelara *Prefilled syringe:* 45 mg/0.5 ml, single-dose; *Vial:* 45 mg/0.5 ml, 90 mg/ml, single-dose; 130 mg/26 ml, single-dose (preservative-free)

JANUS KINASE (JAK) INHIBITOR (JAKI)

▷ *tofacitinib* Xeljanz *Induction:* 10 mg bid or Xeljanz XR 22 mg once daily for 8 weeks; transition to maintenance therapy depending on therapeutic response; if needed, continue **Xeljanz** 10 mg bid or **Xeljanz XR** 22 mg once daily for a maximum of 16 weeks; discontinue **Xeljanz** 10 mg bid or **Xeljanz XR** 22 mg once daily after 16 weeks if adequate therapeutic response is not achieved; *Maintenance:* Xeljanz 5 mg bid or **Xeljanz XR** 11 mg once daily; if loss of response during maintenance treatment, **Xeljanz** 10 mg bid or **Xeljanz XR** 22 mg once daily may be considered and limited to the shortest duration, with careful consideration of the benefits and risks for the individual patient; use the lowest effective dose needed to maintain response; dose adjustment is needed in patients with moderate and severe renal impairment or moderate hepatic impairment; see mfr pkg insert; FDA has not approved the 10 mg twice-daily dosing regimen for RA; this dosing regimen is only approved for patients with UC.

Pediatric: safety and efficacy of **Xeljanz** tabs and **Xeljanz Oral Solution** in pediatric patients for indications other than pcJIA not established

> Xeljanz *Tab:* 5, 10 mg
>
> Xeljanz Oral Solution *Oral soln:* 1 mg/ml (240 ml) with press-in bottle adapter and oral dosing syringe (no latex)
>
> Xeljanz XR *Tab:* 11, 22 mg ext-rel
>
> **Comment:** Xeljanz is the first oral Janus kinase (JAK) inhibitor approved for chronic treatment of moderately to severely active UC. Other FDA-approved treatments for the treatment of moderately to severely active UC must be administered through an IV infusion or SC injection. Use with caution in patients who may be at increased risk for gastrointestinal perforation. The most common adverse events associated with **Xeljanz** treatment for UC are diarrhea, elevated cholesterol level, headache, herpes zoster (shingles), increased blood creatine phosphokinase, nasopharyngitis, rash, and upper respiratory

(continued)

tract infection (URI). Avoid use of **Xeljanz/Xeljanz XR** during an active serious infection, including localized infection. Patients treated with **Xeljanz** are at increased risk for developing serious infections that may lead to hospitalization or death. **Xeljanz** has a black box warning for serious infections (e.g., opportunistic infections) and malignancy (e.g., lymphoma). Use of **Xeljanz** in combination with biological therapies for UC or with potent immunosuppressants, such as *azathioprine* and *cyclosporine*, is not recommended. Avoid live vaccines administration during treatment with **Xeljanz**. Prior to starting **Xeljanz**, perform a test for latent tuberculosis; if it is positive, start treatment for tuberculosis prior to starting **Xeljanz**. Monitor all patients for active tuberculosis during treatment, even if the initial latent tuberculosis test is negative. Recommend lab monitoring due to potential for changes in lymphocytes, neutrophils, hemoglobin, liver enzymes, and lipids. Do not initiate **Xeljanz** if absolute lymphocyte count <500 cells/mm³, an absolute neutrophil count (ANC) <1,000 cells/mm³, or hemoglobin <9 g/dl. The safety and effectiveness of **Xeljanz/Xeljanz XR** in pediatric patients have not been established. Available data with **Xeljanz** use in pregnancy are insufficient to establish a drug-associated risk of major birth defects, miscarriage, or adverse maternal or fetal outcomes. In animal reproduction studies, fetocidal and teratogenic effects were noted. There is a pregnancy exposure registry that monitors pregnancy outcomes in women exposed to **Xeljanz/Xeljanz XR** during pregnancy. Consider pregnancy planning and prevention for females of reproductive potential. Patients should be encouraged to enroll in the **Xeljanz/Xeljanz XR** pregnancy registry if they become pregnant. To enroll or obtain information from the registry, patients can call the toll free number at 1-877-311-8972. There are no data on the presence of *tofacitinib* in human milk or the effects on the breastfed infant; however, patients should be advised not to breastfeed.

INTEGRIN RECEPTOR ANTAGONIST
▷ *vedolizumab* administer by IV infusion over 30 minutes; 300 mg at weeks 0, 2, and 6; then once q 8 weeks
   Pediatric: <12 years: not established; ≥12 years: same as adult
      Entyvio *Vial:* 300 mg (20 ml), single-dose, pwdr for IV infusion after reconstitution (preservative-free)

ANTIDIARRHEAL AGENTS
▷ *difenoxin+atropine* 2 tabs; then 1 tab after each loose stool or 1 tab q 3-4 hours; max 8 tabs/day x 2 days
      Motofen *Tab:* dif 1 mg+atro 0.025 mg
▷ *diphenoxylate+atropine* (G) 2 tabs or 10 ml qid
      Lomotil *Tab:* diphen 2.5 mg+atro 0.025 mg; *Liq:* diphen 2.5 mg+atro 0.025 mg/5 ml (2 oz w. dropper)
▷ *loperamide* (G)
      Imodium (OTC) 4 mg initially; then 2 mg after each loose stool; max 16 mg/day
         Cap: 2 mg
      Imodium A-D (OTC) 4 mg initially; then 2 mg after each loose stool; usual max 8 mg/day x 2 days
         Cplt: 2 mg; *Liq:* 1 mg/5 ml (2, 4 oz)
▷ *loperamide+simethicone* (G)
      Imodium Advanced (OTC) 2 tabs chewed after first loose stool; then 1 after the next loose stool; max 4 tabs/day
         Chew tab: loper 2 mg+simeth 125 mg

URETHRITIS: NON-GONOCOCCAL (NGU)

Comment: The following treatment regimens for non-gonococcal urethritis (NGU) are published in the **2021 CDC Sexually Transmitted Diseases Treatment Guidelines**. Treatment regimens are for adults only; consult a specialist for treatment of patients less than 18 years of age. Treatment regimens are presented by generic drug name first, followed by information about brands and dose forms. All persons who have confirmed or suspected urethritis should be tested for gonorrhea and chlamydia. Men treated for NGU should be instructed to abstain from sexual intercourse for 7 days after a single-dose regimen or until completion of a 7-day regimen.

RECOMMENDED REGIMEN: UNCOMPLICATED NON-GONOCOCCAL URETHRITIS (NGU)
▷ *azithromycin* 1 gm in a single dose or 100 mg orally bid x 7 days
   plus
▷ *doxycycline* 100 mg bid x 7 days

PERSISTENT-RECURRENT NGU
Men Initially Treated With Azithromycin+Doxycycline
▷ *azithromycin* 1 gm PO in a single dose

Men Who Fail a Regimen of Azithromycin
▷ *moxifloxacin* 400 mg PO once daily x 7 days

Heterosexual Men Who Live in Areas Where *Trichomonas Vaginalis* **Is Highly Prevalent**

▷ *metronidazole* 2 gm PO in a single dose

or

▷ *tinidazole* 2 gm PO in a single dose

ALTERNATIVE REGIMENS

▷ *erythromycin base* 500 mg PO qid x 7 days

or

▷ *erythromycin ethylsuccinate* 800 mg PO qid x 7 days

or

▷ *levofloxacin* 500 mg once daily x 7 days

or

▷ *ofloxacin* 300 mg PO bid x 7 days

DRUG BRANDS AND DOSE FORMS

▷ *azithromycin* (G)
Zithromax *Tab:* 250, 500, 600 mg; *Oral susp:* 100 mg/5 ml (15 ml), 200 mg/5 ml (15, 22.5, 30 ml) (cherry); *Pkt:* 1 gm for reconstitution (cherry-banana)
Zithromax Tri-Pak *Tab:* 3 x 500 mg tabs/pck
Zithromax Z-Pak *Tab:* 6 x 250 mg tabs/pck
Zmax *Oral susp:* 2 gm ext-rel for reconstitution (cherry-banana) (148 mg Na$^+$)
▷ *doxycycline* (G)
Acticlate *Tab:* 75, 150**mg
Adoxa *Tab:* 50, 75, 100, 150 mg ent-coat
Doryx *Tab:* 50, 75, 100, 150, 200 mg del-rel
Doxteric *Tab:* 50 mg del-rel
Monodox *Cap:* 50, 75, 100 mg
Oracea *Cap:* 40 mg del-rel
Vibramycin *Tab:* 100 mg; *Cap:* 50, 100 mg; *Syr:* 50 mg/5 ml (raspberry-apple) (sulfites); *Oral susp:* 25 mg/5 ml (raspberry)
Vibra-Tab *Tab:* 100 mg film-coat
▷ *erythromycin base*
Ery-Tab *Tab:* 250, 333, 500 mg ent-coat
PCE *Tab:* 333, 500 mg
▷ *erythromycin ethylsuccinate* (G)
EryPed *Oral susp:* 200 mg/5 ml (100, 200 ml) (fruit), 400 mg/5 ml (60, 100, 200 ml) (banana); *Oral drops:* 200, 400 mg/5 ml (50 ml) (fruit); *Chew tab:* 200 mg wafer (fruit)
E.E.S. *Oral susp:* 200, 400 mg/5 ml (100 ml) (fruit)
E.E.S. Granules *Oral susp:* 200 mg/5 ml (100, 200 ml) (cherry)
E.E.S. 400 Tablets *Tab:* 400 mg
▷ *levofloxacin*
Levaquin *Tab:* 250, 500, 750 mg; *Oral soln:* 25 mg/ml (480 ml) (benzyl alcohol); *Inj conc:* 25 mg/ml for IV infusion after dilution (20, 30 ml, single-use vial) (preservative-free); *Premix soln:* 5 mg/ml for IV infusion (50, 100, 150 ml) (preservative-free)
▷ *metronidazole* (**not** for use in first; B in second and third) (G)
Flagyl *Tab:* 250*, 500*mg
Flagyl 375 *Cap:* 375 mg
Flagyl ER *Tab:* 750 mg ext-rel
▷ *moxifloxacin* (G)
Avelox *Tab:* 400 mg
▷ *ofloxacin* (G)
Floxin *Tab:* 200, 300, 400 mg
▷ *tinidazole* (**not** for use in first; B in second and third)
Tindamax *Tab:* 250*, 500*mg

URINARY RETENTION: UNOBSTRUCTIVE

▷ *bethanechol* 10-30 mg tid
Urecholine *Tab:* 5, 10, 25, 50 mg
Comment: Contraindicated in presence of urinary obstruction. *Atropine* 0.4 mg administered SC reverses *bethanechol* toxicity.

URINARY TRACT INFECTION, COMPLICATED (cUTI)

SIDEROPHORE CEPHALOSPORIN

▷ *cefiderocol* administer 2 gm via IV infusion q 8 hours; infuse dose over 3 hours in patients with CrCl 60-119 ml/min; see mfr pkg insert for dose adjustments required in patients with CrCl <60 ml/min and CrCl ≥120 ml/min; see mfr pkg insert for dose preparation

  Fetroja *Vial:* 1 gm pwdr for reconstitution and IV infusion, single-dose

  Comment: Fetroja *(cefiderocol)* is a siderophore cephalosporin for the treatment of complicated urinary tract infection (cUTI), including pyelonephritis, caused by susceptible gram-negative microorganisms, in patients ≥18 years of age with limited or no alternative treatment options. Approval of this indication is based on limited clinical safety and efficacy data. An increase in all-cause mortality was observed in Fetroja-treated patients compared to those treated with best available therapy (BAT). Closely monitor the clinical response to therapy in patients with cUTI. Serious and occasionally fatal hypersensitivity (anaphylactic) reactions have been reported in patients receiving beta-lactam antibacterial drugs. Hypersensitivity was observed with Fetroja. Cross-hypersensitivity may occur in patients with a history of penicillin allergy. If an allergic reaction occurs, discontinue Fetroja. *Clostridioides difficile*-associated diarrhea (CDAD) has been reported with nearly all systemic antibacterial agents, including Fetroja. Seizures and other central nervous system (CNS) adverse reactions have been reported with Fetroja. If focal tremors, myoclonus, or seizures occur, evaluate patients to determine whether Fetroja should be discontinued. The most frequently occurring adverse reactions (incidence ≥2%) of patients treated with Fetroja have been diarrhea, infusion site reactions, constipation, rash, candidiasis, cough, elevations in liver tests, headache, hypokalemia, nausea, and vomiting. There are no available data on Fetroja use in pregnant females to evaluate for a drug-associated risk of major birth defects, miscarriage, or adverse maternal or fetal outcomes. Available data from published prospective cohort studies, case series, and case reports over several decades with *cephalosporin* use in pregnant females have not established drug-associated risks of major birth defects, miscarriage, or adverse maternal or fetal outcomes. Developmental toxicity studies with *cefiderocol* administered during organogenesis in animal studies showed no evidence of embryo/fetal toxicity, including drug-induced fetal malformations. It is not known whether *cefiderocol* is excreted into human milk. No information is available on the effects of Fetroja on the breastfed infant. Developmental and health benefits of breastfeeding should be considered along with the mother's clinical need for Fetroja and any potential adverse effects on the breastfed infant or from the underlying maternal condition.

PARENTERAL CEPHALOSPORIN ANTIBACTERIAL+BETA-LACTAMASE INHIBITOR

▷ *ceftazidime+avibactam* infuse dose over 2 hours; recommended duration of treatment is 4-5 days; *CrCl 31-50 ml/min:* 1.25 gm q 8 hours; *CrCl 16-30 ml/min:* 0.94 gm q 12 hours; *CrCl 6-15 ml/min:* 0.94 gm q 24 hours; *CrCl ≤5 ml/min:* 0.94 gm q 48 hours; both *ceftazidime* and *avibactam* are hemodialyzable; thus, administer Avycaz after hemodialysis on hemodialysis days

Pediatric: <18 years: not recommended; ≥18 years: same as adult

  Avycaz *Vial:* 2.5 gm, single-dose, pwdr for reconstitution and IV infusion

  Comment: Avycaz 2.5 gm contains *ceftazidime* (a cephalosporin) 2 gm (equivalent to 2.635 gm of *ceftazidime pentahydrate/sodium carbonate powder*) and *avibactam* (a beta-lactam inhibitor) 0.5 gm (equivalent to 0.551 gm of *avibactam sodium*). As only limited clinical safety and efficacy data for Avycaz are currently available, reserve Avycaz for use in patients who have limited or no alternative treatment options. To reduce the development of drug-resistant bacteria and maintain the effectiveness of Avycaz and other antibacterial drugs, Avycaz should be used only to treat infections that are proven or strongly suspected to be caused by susceptible bacteria. Seizures and other neurologic events may occur, especially in patients with renal impairment. Adjust dose in patients with renal impairment. Decreased efficacy in patients with baseline CrCl 30-≤50 ml/min. Monitor CrCl at least daily in patients with changing renal function and adjust the dose of Avycaz accordingly. Monitor for hypersensitivity reactions, including anaphylaxis and serious skin reactions. Cross-hypersensitivity may occur in patients with a history of penicillin allergy. If an allergic reaction occurs, discontinue Avycaz. CDAD has been reported with nearly all systemic antibacterial agents, including Avycaz. There are no adequate and well-controlled studies of Avycaz, *ceftazidime*, or *avibactam* in pregnant females. *Ceftazidime* is excreted in human milk in low concentrations. It is not known whether *avibactam* is excreted into human milk. There are no studies to inform effects on the breastfed infant.

▷ *ceftolozane+tazobactam* administer 1.5 gm q 8 hours via IV infusion over 1 hour x 4-14 days; *CrCl 30-50 ml/min:* 750 mg via IV infusion q 8 hours; *CrCl 15-29 ml/min:* 375 mg via IV infusion q 8 hours; *End-stage renal disease (ESRD):* a single loading dose of 750 mg via IV infusion, followed by 150 mg via IV infusion q 8 hours for the remainder of the treatment period (on hemodialysis days, administer the dose at the earliest possible time following completion of dialysis)

Pediatric: <18: not established; ≥18 years: same as adult

  Zerbaxa *Vial:* 1.5 gm (*ceftolozane* 1 gm+*tazobactam* 0.5 gm), single-dose, pwdr for reconstitution and IV infusion

Comment: For doses >1.5 gm, reconstitute a second vial in the same manner as the first one, withdraw an appropriate volume (see Table 3 in the mfr pkg insert) and add to the same infusion bag. The most common adverse reactions in patients with complicated intra-abdominal infection (cIAI) (incidence ≥5%) have been nausea, diarrhea, headache, and pyrexia.

PARENTERAL PENEM ANTIBACTERIAL+RENAL DEHYDROPEPTIDASE INHIBITOR+ BETA-LACTAMASE INHIBITOR

➤ *imipenem+cilastatin+relebactam* administer dose via IV infusion over 30 minutes q 6 hours; *CrCl ≥90 ml/min:* 1.25 gm/dose (*imipenem* 500 mg, *cilastatin* 500 mg, *relebactam* 250 mg); *CrCl 60-89 ml/min:* 1 gm/dose (*imipenem* 400 mg, *cilastatin* 400 mg, *relebactam* 200 mg); *CrCl 30-59 ml/min:* 0.75 gm/dose (*imipenem* 300 mg, *cilastatin* 300 mg, *relebactam* 150 mg); *CrCl 15-29 ml/min:* 0.5 gm/dose (*imipenem* 200 mg, *cilastatin* 200 mg, *relebactam* 100 mg); *ESRD/Dialysis:* 0.5 gm/dose (*imipenem* 200 mg, *cilastatin* 200 mg, *relebactam* 100 mg)

Pediatric: <18 years: <u>not</u> established; ≥18 years: same as adult

Recarbrio *Vial:* imipen 500 mg+cilast 500 mg+relebac 250 mg, single-dose, pwdr for reconstitution, dilution, and IV infusion

Comment: Recarbrio *(imipenem+cilastatin+relebactam)* is a fixed-dose triple combination of *imipenem* (a penem antibacterial), *cilastatin* (a renal dehydropeptidase inhibitor), and *relebactam* (a beta-lactamase inhibitor) indicated for the treatment of cUTI, including pyelonephritis, and cIAI caused by susceptible gram-negative bacteria in patients who have limited <u>or</u> no alternative treatment options, hospital-acquired bacterial pneumonia (HABP), and ventilator-associated bacterial pneumonia (VABP) in adults. Avoid concomitant use of **Recarbrio** with *ganciclovir, valproic acid,* <u>or</u> *divalproex sodium.* Based on clinical reports on patients treated with *imipenem/cilastatin* plus *relebactam* 250 mg, the most frequent adverse reactions (incidence ≥2%) have been diarrhea, nausea, headache, vomiting, increased alanine aminotransferase, increased aspartate aminotransferase, phlebitis/infusion site reactions, pyrexia, and hypertension. There are insufficient human data to establish whether there is a drug-associated risk of major birth defects, miscarriage, <u>or</u> adverse maternal <u>or</u> fetal outcomes with *imipenem, cilastatin,* <u>or</u> *relebactam* in pregnancy. However, embryonic loss has been observed in monkeys treated with *imipenem/cilastatin,* and fetal abnormalities have been observed in *relebactam*-treated mice; therefore, advise pregnant females of the potential risks to pregnancy and the fetus. There are insufficient data on the presence of *imipenem/cilastatin* and *relebactam* in human milk, and no data on the effects on the breastfed infant. However, *relebactam* is present in the milk of lactating rats and therefore developmental and health benefits of breastfeeding should be considered along with the mother's clinical need for **Recarbrio** and any potential adverse effects on the breastfed infant from **Recarbrio** <u>or</u> from the underlying maternal condition.

PARENTERAL AMINOGLYCOSIDE ANTIBACTERIAL

➤ *plazomicin* recommended dose is 15 mg/kg once q 24 hours by IV infusion over 30 minutes x 4-7 days in patients with *CrCl ≥90 ml/min; CrCl ≥60-<90 ml/min:* 15 mg/kg q 24 hours; *CrCl ≥30-<60 ml/min:* 10 mg/kg q 24 hours; *CrCl ≥15-<30 ml/min:* 10 mg/kg q 48 hours

Pediatric: <18 years: <u>not</u> recommended; ≥18 years: same as adult

Zemdri *Injection Vial:* 500 mg/10 ml (50 mg/ml), single-dose

Comment: Zemdri *(plazomicin)* is an aminoglycoside antibacterial for the treatment of cUTI, including pyelonephritis. As <u>only</u> limited clinical safety and efficacy data are available, reserve **Zemdri** for use in patients who have limited <u>or</u> no alternative treatment options. Assess creatinine clearance in all patients prior to initiating therapy and daily during therapy. Adjustment of initial dose and therapeutic drug monitoring (TDM) is recommended in patients with renal impairment. There is insufficient information to recommend a dosing regimen in patients with CrCl <15 ml/min <u>or</u> on hemodialysis <u>or</u> continuous renal replacement therapy. For patients with CrCl ≥15 ml/min and <90 ml/min, TDM is recommended in order to avoid *plazomicin*-induced nephrotoxicity. Monitor *plazomicin* trough concentrations and adjust **Zemdri** as described in the mfr pkg insert. *Black Box Warning:* Aminoglycosides are associated with nephrotoxicity, ototoxicity, and neuromuscular blockade; therefore, administer **Zemdri** no faster than 30 minutes, monitor for adverse reactions, and stop the infusion if any of these adverse events occur. Aminoglycosides can cause fetal harm in pregnancy. There are <u>no</u> available data on the use of **Zemdri** in pregnancy to inform a drug-related risk of adverse developmental outcomes. *Streptomycin,* an aminoglycoside, can cause total, irreversible, bilateral congenital deafness in children whose mothers received *streptomycin* in pregnancy. There are <u>no</u> data on the presence of **Zemdri** in human milk <u>or</u> effects on the breastfed infant; therefore, potential risk/benefit should be discussed with the mother. The most common adverse reactions (incidence ≥1%) are decreased renal function, diarrhea, hypertension, headache, nausea, vomiting, and hypotension.

URINARY TRACT INFECTION (UTI, CYSTITIS: ACUTE)

URINARY TRACT ANALGESIA

Comment: Except when contraindicated, *ibuprofen* <u>or</u> other inflammatory agent of choice is a recommended adjunct <u>or</u> monotherapy in the treatment of urinary tract infection (UTI) dysuria, frequency, and urgency which is due to inflammation and associated smooth muscle spasms/colic.

(continued)

OTC AZO Standard
OTC AZO Standard Maximum Strength
OTC Prodium
OTC Uristat

ANTISPASMODIC AGENT

▷ *flavoxate* (G) 100-200 mg tid-qid
  Pediatric: <12 years: not recommended; >12 years: same as adult
    Urispas *Tab:* 100 mg
Comment: *Flavoxate* hydrochloride tablets are indicated for symptomatic relief of dysuria, urgency, nocturia, suprapubic pain, frequency, and incontinence as may occur in cystitis, prostatitis, urethritis, and urethrocystitis/urethrotrigonitis. *Flavoxate* is not indicated for definitive treatment, but is compatible with drugs used for the treatment of UTI. *Flavoxate* is contraindicated in patients who have any of the following obstructive conditions: pyloric or duodenal obstruction, obstructive intestinal lesions, ileus, achalasia, gastrointestinal (GI) hemorrhage, and obstructive uropathies of the lower urinary tract. Used with caution with glaucoma. It is not known whether *flavoxate* is excreted in human milk.

URINARY TRACT ANALGESIC-ANTISPASMODIC AGENTS

▷ hyoscyamine (G)
    Anaspaz 1-2 tabs q 4 hours prn; max 12 tabs/day
      Tab: 0.125*mg
    Pediatric: <2 years: not recommended; 2-12 years: 0.0625-0.125 mg q 4 hours prn, max 0.75 mg/day; >12 years: same as adult
    Levbid 1-2 tabs q 12 hours prn; max 4 tabs/day
    Pediatric: <12 years: not recommended; ≥12 years: same as adult
      Tab: 0.375*mg ext-rel
    Levsin 1-2 tabs q 4 hours prn; max 12 tabs/day
    Pediatric: <6 years: not recommended; 6-12 years: 1 tab q 4 hours prn; ≥12 years: same as adult
      Tab: 0.125*mg
    Levsin Drops use SL or PO forms
    Pediatric: 3.4 kg: 4 drops q 4 hours prn, max 24 drops/day; 5 kg: 5 drops q 4 hours prn, max 30 drops/day; 7 kg: 6 drops q 4 hours prn, max 36 drops/day; 10 kg: 8 drops q 4 hours prn, max 40 drops/day
      Oral drops: 0.125 mg/ml (15 ml) (orange) (alcohol 5%)
    Levsin Elixir 5 ml q 4 hours prn
    Pediatric: <10 kg: use drops; 10-19 kg: 1.25 ml q 4 hours prn; 20-39 kg: 2.5 ml q 4 hours prn; 40-49 kg: 3.75 ml q 4 hours prn; >50 kg: same as adult
      Elix: 0.125 mg/5 ml (16 oz) (orange) (alcohol 20%)
    Levsinex SL 1-2 tabs q 4 hours; max 12 tabs/day
    Pediatric: <2 years: not recommended; 2-12 years: 1 tab q 4 hours, max 6 tabs/day; >12 years: same as adult
      Tab: 0.125 mg sublingual
    Levsinex Timecaps 1-2 caps q 12 hours; may adjust to 1 cap q 8 hours
    Pediatric: <2 years: not recommended; 2-12 years: 1 cap q 12 hours, max 2 caps/day; >12 years: same as adult
      Cap: 0.375 mg time-rel
    NuLev dissolve 1-2 tabs on tongue, with or without water, q 4 hours prn; max 12 tabs/day
    Pediatric: <2 years: not recommended; 2-12 years: dissolve 1 tab on tongue, with or without water, q 4 hours prn, max 6 tabs/day; >12 years: same as adult
      ODT: 0.125 mg (mint) (phenylalanine)
▷ *methenamine+phenyl salicylate+methylene blue+benzoic acid+atropine sulfate+hyoscyamine* (G) 2 tabs qid prn
  Pediatric: <6 years: not recommended; ≥6 years: same as adult
    Urised *Tab:* meth 40.8 mg+phenyl salic 18.1 mg+meth blue 5.4 mg+benz acid 4.5 mg+atro sulf 0.03 mg+hyoscy 0.03 mg
    Comment: Urised imparts a blue-green color to urine which may stain fabrics.
▷ *methenamine+phenyl salicylate+methylene blue+sod phosphate monobasic+hyoscyamine* 1 cap qid prn
  Pediatric: <6 years: not recommended; ≥6 years: same as adult
    Uribel *Cap:* meth 118 mg+phenyl salic 36 mg+meth blue 10 mg+sod phos mono 40.8 mg+hyoscy 0.12 mg
▷ *methenamine+phenyl salicylate+methylene blue+sod biphosphate+hyoscyamine* 1 tab qid prn
  Pediatric: <6 years: not recommended; ≥6 years: same as adult
    Urelle *Cap:* meth 81 mg+phenyl salic 32.4 mg+meth blue 10.8 mg+sod biphos 40.8 mg+hyoscy 0.12 mg
▷ *phenazopyridine* (G) 100-200 mg q 6 hours prn; max 2 days
  Pediatric: <12 years: not recommended; ≥12 years: same as adult
    AZO Standard, Prodium, Uristat (OTC) *Tab:* 95 mg

AZO Standard Maximum Strength (OTC) *Tab*: 97.5 mg
Pyridium, Urogesic *Tab*: 100, 200 mg
Comment: *Phenazopyridine* imparts an orange-red color to urine which may stain fabrics.

ANTI-INFECTIVES
▷ *acetyl sulfisoxazole* (G)
Gantrisin initially 2-4 gm in a single or divided doses; then 4-8 gm/day in 4-6 divided doses x 3-10 days
Pediatric: <12 years: not recommended; ≥12 years: same as adult
Tab: 500 mg
Gantrisin initially 2-4 gm in a single or divided doses; then 4-8 gm/day in 4-6 divided doses x 3-10 days
Pediatric: <2 months: not recommended; 2 months-12 years: initial dose 75 mg/kg/day; then 150 mg/kg/day in 4-6 divided doses x 3-10 days; max 6 gm/day; >12 years: same as adult
Oral susp: 500 mg/5 ml (4, 16 oz); *Syr:* 500 mg/5 ml (16 oz)
▷ *amoxicillin* (G) 500-875 mg bid or 250-500 mg tid x 3-10 days
Pediatric: <40 kg (88 lb): 20-40 mg/kg/day in 3 divided doses x 10 days or 25-45 mg/kg/day in 2 divided doses 3-10 days; *see Appendix BB.3.* Amoxicillin (G) *(Amoxil Suspension, Trimox Suspension) for dose by weight table;* ≥40 kg: same as adult
Amoxil *Cap:* 250, 500 mg; *Tab:* 875*mg; *Chew tab:* 125, 200, 250, 400 mg (cherry-banana-peppermint) (phenylalanine); *Oral susp:* 125, 250 mg/5 ml (80, 100, 150 ml) (strawberry); 200, 400 mg/5 ml (50, 75, 100 ml) (bubble gum); *Oral drops:* 50 mg/ml (30 ml) (bubble gum)
Moxatag *Tab:* 775 mg ext-rel
Trimox *Tab:* 125, 250 mg; *Cap:* 250, 500 mg; *Oral susp:* 125, 250 mg/5 ml (80, 100, 150 ml) (raspberry-strawberry)
▷ *amoxicillin+clavulanate* (G)
Augmentin 500 mg tid or 875 mg bid x 3-10 days
Pediatric: <40 kg: 40-45 mg/kg/day divided tid x 3-10 days or 90 mg/kg/day divided bid x 10 days; *see Appendix BB.4.* Amoxicillin+Clavulanate (G) *(Augmentin Suspension) for dose by weight table;* ≥40 kg: same as adult
Tab: 250, 500, 875 mg; *Chew tab:* 125, 250 mg (lemon-lime); 200, 400 mg (cherry-banana) (phenylalanine); *Oral susp:* 125 mg/5 ml (banana), 250 mg/5 ml (75, 100, 150 ml) (orange); 200, 400 mg/5 ml (50, 75, 100 ml) (orange) (phenylalanine)
Augmentin ES-600 <3 months: not recommended; ≥3 months, <40 kg: 90 mg/kg/day divided q 12 hours x 3-10 days; *see Appendix BB.5.* Amoxicillin+Clavulanate (G) *(Augmentin ES 600 Suspension) for dose by weight table;* ≥40 kg: not recommended
Oral susp: 600 mg/5 ml (50, 75, 100, 125, 150, 200 ml) (strawberry cream) (phenylalanine)
Augmentin XR <16 years: use other forms; ≥16 years: 2 tabs q 12 hours x 3-10 days
Tab: 1,000*mg ext-rel
▷ *ampicillin* 500 mg qid x 3-10 days
Pediatric: <12 years: 50-100 mg/kg/day in 4 divided doses x 3-10 days; *see Appendix BB.6.* Ampicillin (G) *(Omnipen Suspension, Principen Suspension) for dose by weight table;* ≥12 years: same as adult
Omnipen, Principen *Cap:* 250, 500 mg; *Oral susp:* 125, 250 mg/5 ml (100, 150, 200 ml) (fruit)
▷ *carbenicillin* 1-2 tabs qid x 3-10 days
Pediatric: <12 years: not recommended; ≥12 years: same as adult
Geocillin *Tab:* 382 mg
Tab: 375, 500 mg ext-rel
▷ *cefaclor* (G)
Ceclor 250 mg tid or 375 mg bid 3-10 days
Pediatric: <1 month: not recommended; 1 month-12 years: 20-40 mg/kg divided bid or q 12 hours x 3-10 days; max 1 gm/day; *see Appendix BB.8.* Cefaclor (G) *(Ceclor Suspension) for dose by weight;* >12 years: same as adult
Tab: 500 mg; *Cap:* 250, 500 mg; *Susp:* 125 mg/5 ml (75, 150 ml) (strawberry), 187 mg/5 ml (50, 100 ml) (strawberry), 250 mg/5 ml (75, 150 ml) (strawberry), 375 mg/5 ml (50, 100 ml) (strawberry)
Cefaclor Extended Release 375-500 mg bid x 3-10 days
Pediatric: <16 years: not recommended; ≥16 years: same as adult
Tab: 375, 500 mg ext-rel
▷ *cefadroxil* 1-2 gm in a single or 2 divided doses x 3-10 days
Pediatric: <12 years: 30 mg/kg/day in 2 divided doses x 3-10 days; *see Appendix BB.9.* Cefadroxil (G) *(Duricef Suspension) for dose by weight table;* ≥12 years: same as adult
Duricef *Cap:* 500 mg; *Tab:* 1 gm; *Oral susp:* 250 mg/5 ml (100 ml), 500 mg/5 ml (75, 100 ml) (orange-pineapple)
▷ *cefixime* (G) 400 mg once daily x 5 days
Pediatric: <6 months: not recommended; 6 months-12 years, <50 kg: 8 mg/kg/day in 1-2 divided doses x 5 days; *see Appendix BB.11.* Cefixime (G) *(Suprax Oral Suspension) for dose by weight table;* >12 years, >50 kg: same as adult
Suprax *Tab:* 400 mg; *Cap:* 400 mg; *Oral susp:* 100, 200, 500 mg/5 ml (50, 75, 100 ml) (strawberry)

(continued)

▷ *cefpodoxime proxetil* 100 mg bid x 3-10 days
   Pediatric: <2 months: <u>not</u> recommended; 2 months-12 years: 10 mg/kg/day (max 400 mg/dose) <u>or</u> 5 mg/kg/day bid (max 200 mg/dose) x 3-10 days: *see Appendix BB.12.* Cefpodoxime Proxetil (G) *(Vantin Suspension) for dose by weight table;* ≥12 years: same as adult
      Vantin *Tab:* 100, 200 mg; *Oral susp:* 50, 100 mg/5 ml (50, 75, 100 mg) (lemon creme)
▷ *cephalexin* (G) 500 mg bid x 3-10 days
   Pediatric: <12 years: 25-50 mg/kg/day in 4 divided doses x 3-10 days; *see Appendix BB.15.* Cephalexin (G) *(Keflex Suspension) for dose by weight table;* ≥12 years: same as adult
      Keflex *Cap:* 250, 333, 500, 750 mg; *Oral susp:* 125, 250 mg/5 ml (100, 200 ml) (strawberry)
▷ *ciprofloxacin* 500 mg bid <u>or</u> 1000 mg XR once daily x 3-7 days
   Pediatric: <18 years: <u>not</u> recommended; ≥18 years: same as adult
      Cipro (G) *Tab:* 250, 500, 750 mg; *Oral susp:* 250, 500 mg/5 ml (100 ml) (strawberry)
      Cipro XR *Tab:* 500, 1,000 mg ext-rel
      ProQuin XR *Tab:* 500 mg ext-rel
▷ *doxycycline* (G) 100 mg bid x 3-10 days
   Pediatric: <8 years: <u>not</u> recommended; ≥8 years, <100 lb: 2 mg/lb on first day in 2 divided doses, followed by 1 mg/lb/day in a single <u>or</u> 2 divided doses x 3-10 days; ≥8 years, ≥100 lb: same as adult
      Acticlate *Tab:* 75, 150**mg
      Adoxa *Tab:* 50, 75, 100, 150 mg ent-coat
      Doryx *Tab:* 50, 75, 100, 150, 200 mg del-rel
      Doxteric *Tab:* 50 mg del-rel
      Monodox *Cap:* 50, 75, 100 mg
      Oracea *Cap:* 40 mg del-rel
      Vibramycin *Tab:* 100 mg; *Cap:* 50, 100 mg; *Syr:* 50 mg/5 ml (raspberry-apple) (sulfites); *Oral susp:* 25 mg/5 ml (raspberry)
      Vibra-Tab *Tab:* 100 mg film-coat
▷ *enoxacin* 200 mg q 12 hours x 3-10 days
   Pediatric: <18 years: <u>not</u> recommended; ≥18 years: same as adult
      Penetrex *Tab:* 200, 400 mg
▷ *fosfomycin* (G) take as a single dose on an empty stomach; dissolve 1 sachet pkt in 3-4 oz cold water and drink immediately
   Pediatric: <12 years: <u>not</u> established; ≥12 years: same as adult
      Monurol *Single-dose sachet pkts:* 3 gm (mandarin orange) (saccharin, sucrose)
   Comment: *Fosfomycin tromethamine* is a single-dose, synthetic, broad-spectrum, bactericidal antibiotic for treatment of uncomplicated UTI. Repeat dosing does <u>not</u> improve clinical efficacy. Safety and effectiveness in children ≥12 years have <u>not</u> been established in adequate and well-controlled studies.
▷ *levofloxacin* 250 mg once daily x 3-7 days
   Pediatric: <18 years: <u>not</u> recommended; ≥18 years: same as adult
      Levaquin *Tab:* 250, 500, 750 mg; *Oral soln:* 25 mg/ml (480 ml) (benzyl alcohol); *Inj conc:* 25 mg/ml for IV infusion after dilution (20, 30 ml, single-use vial) (preservative-free); *Premix soln:* 5 mg/ml for IV infusion (50, 100, 150 ml) (preservative-free)
▷ *lomefloxacin* 400 mg once daily x 3-7 days
   Pediatric: <18 years: <u>not</u> recommended; ≥18 years: same as adult
      Maxaquin *Tab:* 400 mg
▷ *minocycline* (G) 100 mg q 12 hours x 3-10 days
   Pediatric: <8 years: <u>not</u> recommended; ≥8 years, <100 lb: 1-2 mg/lb in 2 divided doses x 3-10 days; ≥8 years, ≥100 lb: same as adult
      Dynacin *Cap:* 50, 100 mg
      Minocin *Cap:* 50, 75, 100 mg; *Oral susp:* 50 mg/5 ml (60 ml) (custard) (sulfites, alcohol 5%)
▷ *nalidixic acid* 1 gm qid x 3-10 days
   Pediatric: <3 months: <u>not</u> recommended; ≥3 months-<12 years: 25 mg/lb/day in 4 divided doses x 3-10 days; ≥12 years: same as adult
      NegGram *Tab:* 250, 500 mg; 1 gm; *Cap:* 250, 500 mg; *Oral susp:* 250 mg/5 ml
▷ *nitrofurantoin* (G)
      Furadantin 50-100 mg qid x 3-10 days
      Pediatric: <1 month: <u>not</u> recommended; ≥1 month-12 years: 5-7 mg/kg/ day in 4 divided doses x 3-10 days; *see Appendix BB.28.* Nitrofurantoin (G) *(Furadantin Suspension) for dose by weight table;* >12 years: same as adult
         Oral susp: 25 mg/5 ml (60 ml)
      Macrobid 100 mg q 12 hours x 3-10 days
      Pediatric: <12 years: <u>not</u> recommended; ≥12 years: same as adult
         Cap: 100 mg
      Macrodantin 50-100 mg qid x 3-10 days
      Pediatric: <12 years: <u>not</u> recommended; ≥12 years: same as adult
         Cap: 25, 50, 100 mg

➤ *norfloxacin* 400 mg once daily x 3-7 days
   Pediatric: <18 years: <u>not</u> recommended; ≥18 years: same as adult
     Noroxin *Tab:* 400 mg
➤ *ofloxacin* (G) 200 mg q 12 hours x 3-7 days
   Pediatric: <18 years: <u>not</u> recommended; ≥18 years: same as adult
     Floxin *Tab:* 200, 300, 400 mg
     Floxin UroPak *Tab:* 200 mg (6/pck)
➤ *trimethoprim* (G)
     Primsol 100 mg q 12 hours <u>or</u> 200 mg once daily x 10 days
   Pediatric: <6 months: <u>not</u> recommended; ≥6 months-12 years: 10 mg/kg/ day in 2 divided doses x 10 days; >12 years: same as adult
      Oral soln: 50 mg/5 ml (bubble gum) (dye-free, alcohol-free)
     Proloprim 100 mg q 12 hours <u>or</u> 200 mg once daily x 10 days
   Pediatric: <12 years: <u>not</u> recommended; ≥12 years: same as adult
      Tab: 100, 200 mg
     Trimpex 100 mg q 12 hours <u>or</u> 200 mg once daily x 10 days
   Pediatric: <12 years: <u>not</u> recommended; ≥12 years: same as adult
      Tab: 100 mg
➤ *trimethoprim+sulfamethoxazole (TMP-SMX)* (G)
     Bactrim, Septra 2 tabs bid x 3-10 days
   Pediatric: <12 years: <u>not</u> recommended; ≥12 years: same as adult
      Tab: trim 80 mg+sulfa 400 mg*
     Bactrim DS, Septra DS 1 tab bid x 3-10 days
   Pediatric: <12 years: <u>not</u> recommended; ≥12 years: same as adult
      Tab: trim 160 mg+sulfa 800 mg*
     Bactrim Pediatric Suspension, Septra Pediatric Suspension use tabs
   Pediatric: <2 months: <u>not</u> recommended; ≥2 months-12 years: 40 mg/kg/day of *sulfamethoxazole* in 2 doses bid; >12 years: use tabs
      Oral susp: trim 40 mg+sulfa 200 mg per 5 ml (100 ml) (cherry) (alcohol 0.3%)

PARENTERAL THERAPY FOR COMPLICATED URINARY TRACT INFECTION (cUTI)

➤ *ertapenem* 1 gm once daily; *CrCl <30 ml/min:* 500 mg once daily; treat x 10-14 days; may switch to an oral antibiotic after 3 days if warranted; *IV infusion:* administer over 30 minutes; *IM injection:* reconstitute
   Pediatric: <18 years: <u>not</u> recommended; ≥18 years same as adult
     Invanz *Vial:* 1 gm pwdr for reconstitution
➤ *meropenem+vaborbactam* administer 4 gm (*meropenem* 2 gm and *vaborbactam* 2 gm) q 8 hours by IV infusion; administer over 3 hours; treat for up to 14 days; monitor urine cultures and estimated glomerular filtration rate (eGFR); *eGFR 30-49 ml/min:* 2 gm (*meropenem* 1 gm and *vaborbactam* 1 gm) q 8 hours; *eGFR 15-29 ml/min:* 2 gm (*meropenem* 1 gm and *vaborbactam* 1 gm) q 12 hours; *eGFR <15 ml/min:* 1 gm (*meropenem* 0.5 gm and *vaborbactam* 0.5 gm) q 12 hours; *End-stage renal disease (ESRD):* administer 1 gm (*meropenem* 0.5 gm and *vaborbactam* 0.5 gm) q 12 hours <u>after</u> dialysis
   Pediatric: <18 years: <u>not</u> recommended; ≥18 years same as adult
     Vabomere *Vial:* mero 1 gm+vabor 1 gm pwdr for reconstitution and dilution
     Comment: Vabomere (formerly Carbavance) is a carbapenem (*meropenem*) and beta-lactamase inhibitor (*vaborbactam*) combination indicated for the treatment of complicated urinary tract infection (cUTI), including pyelonephritis caused by *Escherichia coli*, *Klebsiella pneumoniae*, and *Enterobacter cloacae* species complex. Administer Vabomere with caution with history of hypersensitivity to penicillin, cephalosporin, other beta-lactams, <u>or</u> other allergens. Discontinue immediately if allergic reaction occurs. Vabomere is <u>not</u> recommended with concomitant *valproic acid* <u>or</u> *divalproex sodium*. Discontinue Vabomere if *Clostridioides difficile*-associated diarrhea is suspected <u>or</u> confirmed. Monitor and reevaluate risk/benefit if signs of neuromotor impairment (e.g., seizures, focal tremors, myoclonus, delirium, paresthesias), renal impairment, thrombocytopenia, <u>and/or</u> superinfection.

LONG-TERM PROPHYLACTIC SUPPRESSION THERAPY

➤ *methenamine hippurate* 1 gm once daily
   Pediatric: <6 years: 0.25 gm/30 lb once daily; 6-12 years: 25-50 mg/kg/day once daily <u>or</u> 0.5-1 gm once daily; >12 years: same as adult
     Hiprex *Tab:* 1 gm; *Oral susp:* 500 mg/5 ml (480 ml)
     Urex *Tab:* 1 gm; *Oral susp:* 500 mg/5 ml (480 ml)
➤ *nitrofurantoin* (G)
     Furadantin 50-100 mg as a single dose at bedtime
   Pediatric: <1 month: <u>not</u> recommended; ≥1 month-12 years: 1 mg/kg as a single dose at bedtime; >12 years: same as adult
      Oral susp: 25 mg/5 ml (60 ml)
     Macrobid 50-100 mg as a single dose at bedtime

(continued)

Pediatric: <12 years: not recommended; ≥12 years: same as adult
  Cap: 100 mg
Macrodantin 50-100 mg as a single dose at bedtime
Pediatric: <12 years: not recommended; ≥12 years: same as adult
  Cap: 25, 50, 100 mg
Furadantin 50-100 mg as a single dose at bedtime
Pediatric: <12 years: not recommended; ≥12 years: same as adult
  Oral susp: 25 mg/5 ml (60 ml)
Macrobid 100 mg as a single dose at bedtime
Pediatric: <12 years: not recommended; ≥12 years: same as adult
  Cap: 100 mg
Macrodantin 50-100 mg as a single dose at bedtime
Pediatric: <12 years: not recommended; ≥12 years: same as adult
  Cap: 25, 50, 100 mg

UROLITHIASIS (RENAL CALCULI, KIDNEY STONES)

Acetaminophen for IV Infusion *see Pain*
NSAIDs *see* Appendix I. NSAIDs online at https://connect.springerpub.com/content/reference-book/978-0-8261-7935-7/back-matter/part02/back-matter/bmatter10
Opioid Analgesics *see Pain*

PREVENTION OF CALCIUM STONES
▷ *chlorothiazide* (G) 50 mg bid
  Pediatric: <6 months: up to 15 mg/lb/day in 2 divided doses; ≥6 months-12 years: 10 mg/lb/day in 2 divided doses; max 375 mg/day; >12 years: same as adult
    Diuril *Tab:* 250*, 500*mg; *Oral susp:* 250 mg/5 ml (237 ml)
▷ *hydrochlorothiazide* (G) 50 mg bid
  Pediatric: <12 years: not recommended; ≥12 years: same as adult
    Esidrix *Tab:* 25, 50 mg
    Microzide *Cap:* 12.5 mg

PREVENTION OF CYSTINE STONES
▷ *penicillamine* administer on an empty stomach, at least 1 hour before meals or 2 hours after meals, and at least 1 hour apart from any other drug, food, milk, antacid, and zinc- or iron-containing preparation; usual dose is 2,000-4,000 mg/day; maintenance dosage must be individualized and may require adjustment during the course of treatment; initially a single daily dose of 125-250 mg; then increase at 1- to 3-month intervals by 125-250 mg/day, as patient response and tolerance indicate; if a satisfactory remission of symptoms is achieved, the dose associated with the remission should be continued as the patient's maintenance therapy; if there is no improvement and there are no signs of potentially serious toxicity after 2-3 months of treatment with doses of 500-750 mg/day, increase by 250 mg/day at 2- to 3-month intervals until a satisfactory remission occurs or signs of toxicity develop; if there is no discernible improvement after 3-4 months of treatment, discontinue **Cuprimine**. Changes in maintenance dosage levels may not be reflected clinically or in the erythrocyte sedimentation rate (ESR) for 2-3 months after each dosage adjustment
    Cuprimine *Cap:* 125, 250 mg
    Depen: 250 mg
  Comment: The use of *penicillamine* has been associated with fatalities due to certain diseases such as aplastic anemia, agranulocytosis, thrombocytopenia, Goodpasture's syndrome, and myasthenia gravis. Because of the potential for serious hematologic and renal adverse reactions to occur at any time, routine urinalysis, white and differential blood cell count, hemoglobin, and direct platelet count must be checked twice weekly, together with monitoring of the patient's skin, lymph nodes, and body temperature, during the first month of therapy, every 2 weeks for the next 5 months, and monthly thereafter. Patients should be instructed to report promptly the development of signs and symptoms of granulocytopenia and/or thrombocytopenia, such as fever, sore throat, chills, bruising, or bleeding; the above laboratory studies should then be promptly repeated.
▷ *potassium citrate* (G) 30 mEq qid
  Pediatric: <12 years: not recommended; ≥12 years: same as adult
    Urocit-K *Tab:* 5, 10, 15 mEq ext-rel
  Comment: *Potassium citrate* is contraindicated in hyperkalemia. Encourage patients to limit salt intake and maintain liberal hydration (urine volume should be at least 2 liters/day). Target urine pH is 6.0-7.0 and urine citrate at least 320 mg/day and close to the normal mean of 640 mg/day. Take with food.

PREVENTION OF URIC ACID STONES
▷ *allopurinol* (G) 200-300 mg in 1-3 doses; max 800 mg/day; max single dose 300 mg
  Pediatric: <6 years: max 150 mg/day; 6-10 years: max 400 mg/day; max single dose 300 mg; >10 years: same as adult

Zyloprim *Tab:* 100*, 300*mg

▷ *potassium citrate* (G) 30 mEq qid

Urocit-K *Tab:* 5, 10, 15 mEq ext-rel

Comment: *Potassium citrate* is contraindicated in hyperkalemia. Encourage patients to limit salt intake and maintain liberal hydration (urine volume should be at least 2 liters/day). Target urine pH is 6.0-7.0 and urine citrate at least 320 mg/day and close to the normal mean of 640 mg/day. Take with food.

ALPHA-1A BLOCKERS

Comment: Alpha-1A blockers facilitate stone passage.

▷ *alfuzosin* (G) 10 mg once daily taken immediately after the same meal each day

UroXatral *Tab:* 10 mg ext-rel

▷ *tamsulosin* (G) initially 0.4 mg once daily; may increase to 0.8 mg once daily after 2-4 weeks if needed
Pediatric: ≤18 years: with radiopaque lower ureteral stones of 10-12 mm or smaller receive the following doses: *tamsulosin* 0.2 mg PO at bedtime (≤4 years) and 0.4 mg PO at bedtime (>4 years); administer x 28 days or until definite stone passage (i.e., evidence of stone on urine straining); >18 years: same as adult

Flomax *Cap:* 0.4 mg

Comment: *Tamsulosin* 0.4 mg may be taken with **Avodart** 0.5 mg once daily as combination therapy. *Tamsulosin* is taken with standard analgesia (e.g., *ibuprofen*); mild somnolence is common. If pain is controlled with oral analgesia, clear liquids are tolerated, and there is no evidence of infection, monitor closely for spontaneous passage for 3-4 weeks prior to definitive therapy, since most data demonstrate safe lower ureteral stone expulsion in the first 10 days of conservative medical management.

ANTISPASMODIC AGENT

▷ *flavoxate* (G) 100-200 mg tid-qid
Pediatric: <12 years: not recommended; >12 years: same as adult

Urispas *Tab:* 100 mg

Comment: *Flavoxate* hydrochloride tablets are indicated for symptomatic relief of dysuria, urgency, nocturia, suprapubic pain, frequency, and incontinence as may occur in cystitis, prostatitis, urethritis, and urethrocystitis/urethrotrigonitis. *Flavoxate* is not indicated for definitive treatment, but is compatible with drugs used for the treatment of urinary tract infection (UTI). *Flavoxate* is contraindicated in patients who have any of the following obstructive conditions: pyloric or duodenal obstruction, obstructive intestinal lesions, ileus, achalasia, gastrointestinal (GI) hemorrhage, and obstructive uropathies of the lower urinary tract. Used with caution with glaucoma. It is not known whether *flavoxate* is excreted in human milk.

ACETAMINOPHEN FOR IV INFUSION

▷ *acetaminophen* injectable administer by intravenous infusion (IVF) over 15 minutes; 1,000 mg q 6 hours prn or 650 mg q 4 hours prn; max 4,000 mg/day
Pediatric: <2 years: not recommended; 2-13 years <50 kg: 15 mg/kg q 6 hours prn or 2.5 mg/kg q 4 hours prn; max 750 mg/single dose; max 75 mg/kg per day; >13 years: same as adult

Ofirmev *Vial:* 10 mg/ml (100 ml) (preservative-free)

Comment: The **Ofirmev** vial is intended for single-use. If any portion is withdrawn from the vial, use within 6 hours. Discard the unused portion. For pediatric patients, withdraw the intended dose and administer via syringe pump. Do not admix **Ofirmev** with any other drugs. **Ofirmev** is physically incompatible with *diazepam* and *chlorpromazine hydrochloride*.

IBUPROFEN FOR IV INFUSION

▷ *ibuprofen* dilute dose in 0.9% NS, D5W, or lactated Ringer's solution; administer by IVF over at least 10 minutes; do not administer via IV bolus or IM; 400-800 mg q 6 hours prn; maximum 3,200 mg/day
Pediatric: <6 months; not recommended; 6 months-<12 years: 10 mg/kg q 4-6 hours prn; max 400 mg/dose; max 40 mg/kg or 2,400 mg/24 hours, whichever is less; 12-17 years: 400 mg q 4-6 hours prn; max 2,400 mg/24 hours

Caldolor *Vial:* 800 mg/8 ml, single-dose

Comment: Prepare **Caldolor** solution for IV administration as follows: 100 mg dose: dilute 1 ml of **Caldolor** in at least 100 ml of diluent (IVF); 200 mg dose: dilute 2 ml of **Caldolor** in at least 100 ml of diluent; 400 mg dose: dilute 4 ml of **Caldolor** in at least 100 ml of diluent; 800 mg dose: dilute 8 ml of **Caldolor** in at least 200 ml of diluent. **Caldolor** is also indicated for management of fever. For adults with fever, 400 mg via IVF, followed by 400 mg q 4-6 hours or 100-200 mg q 4 hours prn.

MU OPIOID ANALGESICS

▷ *tramadol* (IV) (G)

Rybix ODT initially 100 mg once daily; may increase by 100 mg q 5 days; max 300 mg/day; *CrCl <30 ml/min or severe hepatic impairment:* not recommended; *Cirrhosis:* max 50 mg q 12 hours
Pediatric: <12 years: contraindicated; 12-<18: use extreme caution; not recommended for children and adolescents with obesity, asthma, obstructive sleep apnea, or other chronic breathing problem, or for posttonsillectomy/adenoidectomy pain; ≥18 years: same as adult

ODT: 50 mg (mint) (phenylalanine)

(continued)

Ryzolt initially 100 mg once daily; may increase by 100 mg q 5 days; max 300 mg/day; *CrCl <30 ml/min or severe hepatic impairment:* not recommended
Pediatric: <12 years: contraindicated; 12-<18 years: use extreme caution; not recommended for children and adolescents with obesity, asthma, obstructive sleep apnea, or other chronic breathing problem, or for posttonsillectomy/adenoidectomy pain; ≥18 years: same as adult
  Tab: 100, 200, 300 mg ext-rel
Ultram 50-100 mg q 4-6 hours prn; max 400 mg/day; *CrCl <30 ml/min:* max 100 mg q 12 hours; *Cirrhosis:* max 50 mg q 12 hours
Pediatric: <12 years: contraindicated; 12-<18 years: use extreme caution; not recommended for children and adolescents with obesity, asthma, obstructive sleep apnea, or other chronic breathing problem, or for posttonsillectomy/ adenoidectomy pain; ≥18 years: same as adult
  Tab: 50*mg
Ultram ER initially 100 mg once daily; may increase by 100 mg q 5 days; max 300 mg/day; *CrCl <30 ml/min or severe hepatic impairment:* not recommended
Pediatric: <12 years: contraindicated; 12-<18 years: use extreme caution; not recommended for children and adolescents with obesity, asthma, obstructive sleep apnea, or other chronic breathing problem, or for posttonsillectomy/adenoidectomy pain; ≥18 years: same as adult
  Tab: 100, 200, 300 mg ext-rel

▶ *tramadol+acetaminophen* **(IV) (G)** 2 tabs q 4-6 hours; max 8 tabs/day x 5 days; *CrCl <30 ml/min:* max 2 tabs q 12 hours; max 4 tabs/day x 5 days
Pediatric: <12 years: contraindicated; 12-<18 years: use extreme caution; not recommended for children and adolescents with obesity, asthma, obstructive sleep apnea, or other chronic breathing problem, or for posttonsillectomy/adenoidectomy pain; same as adult
  Ultracet *Tab:* tram 37.5+acet 325 mg

INTRANASAL (TRANSMUCOSAL) OPIOID ANALGESICS

▶ *butorphanol tartrate* nasal spray **(IV)** initially 1 spray (1 mg) in one nostril and may repeat after 60-90 minutes in opposite nostril if needed or 1 spray in each nostril and may repeat q 3-4 hours prn
Pediatric: <18 years: not recommended; ≥18 years: same as adult
  Butorphanol Nasal Spray *Nasal spray:* 1 mg/actuation (10 mg/ml, 2.5 ml)
  Stadol Nasal Spray *Nasal spray:* 1 mg/actuation (10 mg/ml, 2.5 ml)

▶ *fentanyl* nasal spray **(II)** initially 1 spray (100 mcg) in one nostril and may repeat after 2 hours; when adequate analgesia is achieved, use that dose for subsequent breakthrough episodes; *Titration steps:* 100 mcg using 1 x 100 mcg spray; 200 mcg using 2 x 100 mcg spray (1 spray in each nostril); 400 mcg using 1 x 400 mcg spray; 800 mcg using 2 x 400 mcg (1 spray in each nostril); max 800 mcg; limit to ≤4 doses per day
Pediatric: <18 years: not recommended; ≥18 years: same as adult
  Lazanda Nasal Spray *Nasal spray:* 100, 400 mcg/100 mcl (8 sprays/bottle)
  Comment: Lazanda Nasal Spray is available by restricted distribution program.
  Call 855-841-4234 or https://www.fda.gov/downloads/drugs/drugsafety/ postmarketdrugsafetyinformationforpatientsandproviders/ucm261983.pdf to enroll. **Lazanda Nasal Spray** is indicated for the management of breakthrough pain in cancer patients who are already receiving and who are tolerant to opioid therapy for their underlying persistent cancer pain. Patients considered opioid-tolerant are those who are taking at least 60 mg of oral morphine/day, 25 mcg of transdermal *fentanyl*/hour, 30 mg oral *oxycodone*/day, 8 mg oral *hydromorphone*/day, 25 mg oral *oxymorphone*/day, or an equianalgesic dose of another opioid for a week or longer. Patients must remain on around-the-clock opioids when using **Lazanda Nasal Spray**. As such, it is contraindicated in the management of acute or postop pain, including headache/migraine or dental pain.
Comment: The Transmucosal Immediate Release Fentanyl (TIRF) Risk Evaluation and Mitigation Strategy (REMS) Program is an FDA-required program designed to ensure informed risk-benefit decisions before initiating treatment and while patients are treated to ensure appropriate use of TIRF medicines. The purpose of the TIRF REMS Access Program is to mitigate the risk of misuse, abuse, addiction, overdose, and serious complications due to medication errors with the use of TIRF medicines. You must enroll in the TIRF REMS Access Program to prescribe, dispense, or distribute TIRF medicines.

URTICARIA: MILD-TO-ACUTE HIVES AND CHRONIC SPONTANEOUS/IDIOPATHIC URTICARIA (CSU/CIU)

Topical Corticosteroids *see* Appendix J. Topical Corticosteroids by Potency
Oral Corticosteroids *see* Appendix K. Oral Corticosteroids
Parenteral Corticosteroids *see* Appendix L. Parenteral Corticosteroids

MILD-TO-MODERATE URTICARIA (HIVES, ANGIOEDEMA)
Second-Generation Oral Antihistamines

Comment: The following drugs are second-generation antihistamines. As such they are minimally sedating, much less so than the first-generation antihistamines. All antihistamines are excreted into breast milk.

▷ *cetirizine* (OTC) (G) initially 5-10 mg once daily; 5 mg once daily; ≥*65 years:* use with caution
   Pediatric: <6 years: <u>not</u> recommended; ≥6 years: same as adult
   cetirizine Cap: 10 mg
   Children's Zyrtec Chewable *Chew tab:* 5, 10 mg (grape)
   Children's Zyrtec Allergy Syrup *Syr:* 1 mg/ml (4 oz) (grape, bubble gum) (sugar-free, dye-free)
   Zyrtec *Tab:* 10 mg
   Zyrtec Hives Relief *Tab:* 10 mg
   Zyrtec Liquid Gels *Liq gel:* 10 mg
▷ *desloratadine*
   Clarinex ½-1 tab once daily
   Pediatric: <6 years: <u>not</u> recommended; ≥6 years: same as adult
   Tab: 5 mg
   Clarinex RediTabs 5 mg once daily
   Pediatric: <6 years: <u>not</u> recommended; 6-12 years: 2.5 mg once daily; ≥12 years: same as adult
   ODT: 2.5, 5 mg (tutti-frutti) (phenylalanine)
   Clarinex Syrup 5 mg (10 ml) once daily
   Pediatric: <6 months: <u>not</u> recommended; 6-11 months: 1 mg (2 ml) once daily; 1-5 years: 1.25 mg (2.5 ml)
   once daily; 6-11 years: 2.5 mg (5 ml) once daily; ≥12 years: same as adult
   Syr: 0.5 mg per ml (4 oz) (tutti-frutti) (phenylalanine)
   Desloratadine ODT 1 tab once daily
   Pediatric: <6 years: <u>not</u> recommended; 6-11 years: ½ tab once daily; ≥12 years: same as adult
   ODT: 5 mg
▷ *fexofenadine* (OTC) (G) 60 mg once daily-bid <u>or</u> 180 mg once daily; *CrCl <90 ml/min:* 60 mg once daily
   Pediatric: <6 months: <u>not</u> recommended; 6 months-2 years: 15 mg bid; *CrCl ≤90 ml/min:* 15 mg once daily;
   2-11 years: 30 mg bid; *CrCl ≤90 ml/min:* 30 mg once daily; ≥12 years: same as adult
   Allegra *Tab:* 30, 60, 180 mg film-coat
   Allegra Allergy *Tab:* 60, 180 mg film-coat
   Allegra ODT *ODT:* 30 mg (phenylalanine)
   Allegra Oral Suspension *Oral susp:* 30 mg/5 ml (6 mg/ml) (4 oz)
▷ *levocetirizine* (OTC) (G) administer dose in the PM; *Seasonal allergic rhinitis:* <2 years: <u>not</u>
   recommended; may start at ≥2 years; *Chronic idiopathic urticaria (CIU), perennial allergic rhinitis:* <6
   months: <u>not</u> recommended; may start at ≥ 6 months; *Dosing by age:* 6 months-5 years: max 1.25 mg once
   daily; 6-11 years: max 2.5 mg once daily; ≥12 years: 2.5-5 mg once daily; *Renal dysfunction <12 years:*
   contraindicated; *Renal dysfunction ≥12 years:* CrCl 50-80 ml/min: 2.5 mg once daily; CrCl 30-50 ml/min:
   2.5 mg every other day; CrCl 10-30 ml/min: 2.5 mg twice weekly (q 3-4 days); CrCl <10 ml/min, end-
   stage renal disease (ESRD), <u>or</u> hemodialysis: contraindicated
   Children's Xyzal Allergy 24HR *Oral Soln:* 0.5 mg/ml (150 ml)
   Xyzal Allergy 24HR *Tab:* 5*mg
▷ *loratadine* (OTC) (G) 5 mg bid <u>or</u> 10 mg once daily; *Hepatic <u>or</u> renal insufficiency:* see mfr pkg insert
   Pediatric: <2 years: <u>not</u> recommended; 2-5 years: 5 mg once daily; ≥6 years: same as adult
   Children's Claritin Chewables *Chew tab:* 5 mg (grape) (phenylalanine)
   Children's Claritin Syrup 1 mg/ml (4 oz) (fruit) (sugar-free, alcohol-free, dye-free; sodium 6 mg/5 ml)
   Claritin *Tab:* 10 mg
   Claritin Hives Relief *Tab:* 10 mg
   Claritin Liqui-Gels *Liq gel:* 10 mg
   Claritin RediTabs 12 Hours *ODT:* 5 mg (mint)
   Claritin RediTabs 24 Hours *ODT:* 10 mg (mint)

First-Generation Oral Antihistamines

▷ *diphenhydramine* (G) 25-50 mg q 6-8 hours; max 100 mg/day
   Pediatric: <2 years: <u>not</u> recommended; 2-6 years: 6.25 mg q 4-6 hours, max 37.5 mg/day; >6-12 years: 12.5-
   25 mg q 4-6 hours, max 150 mg/day; >12 years: same as adult
   Benadryl (OTC) *Chew tab:* 12.5 mg (grape) (phenylalanine); *Liq:* 12.5 mg/5 ml (4, 8 oz); *Cap:* 25 mg;
   Tab: 25 mg; *Dye-free soft gel:* 25 mg; *Dye-free liq:* 12.5 mg/5 ml (4, 8 oz)
▷ *hydroxyzine* (G) 50 mg/day divided qid prn; 50-100 mg/day divided qid prn
   Pediatric: <6 years: 50 mg/day divided qid prn; ≥6 years: same as adult
   Atarax *Tab:* 10, 25, 50, 100 mg; *Syr:* 10 mg/5 ml (alcohol 0.5%)
   Vistaril *Cap:* 25, 50, 100 mg; *Oral susp:* 25 mg/5 ml (4 oz) (lemon)
Comment: *Hydroxyzine* is contraindicated in early pregnancy and in patients with a prolonged QT interval.
It is <u>not</u> known whether this drug is excreted in human milk; therefore, *hydroxyzine* should <u>not</u> be given to
nursing mothers.

SEVERE URTICARIA
Parenteral Antihistamine

▷ *cetirizine* for IV injection 10 mg IV once q 24 hours prn
  Pediatric: <6 months: not established; 6 months-5 years: 2.5 mg IV; 6-11 years: 5-10 mg IV (depending on severity); ≥12 years: same as adult
  Quzyttir *Vial:* 10 mg/ml (1 ml), single-use
  Comment: Quzyttir *(cetirizine)* is a histamine-1 (H1) receptor antagonist indicated for the treatment of acute urticaria in adults and children ≥6 months of age. Contraindications to **Quzyttir** include known hypersensitivity to *cetirizine hcl* or any of its ingredients, *levocetirizine,* or *hydroxyzine.* Patients should be warned about potential somnolence/sedation and to exercise caution when driving a car or operating potentially dangerous machinery. The most common adverse reactions (incidence <1%) with **Quzyttir** have been dysgeusia, headache, paresthesia, presyncope, dyspepsia, feeling hot, and hyperhidrosis.

▷ *diphenhydramine* injectable (G) 25-50 mg IM immediately; then q 6 hours prn
  Pediatric: <12 years: see mfr pkg insert: 1.25 mg/kg up to 25 mg IM x 1 dose; then q 6 hours prn; ≥12 years: same as adult
  Benadryl Injectable *Vial:* 50 mg/ml (1 ml single-use), 50 mg/ml (10 ml multidose); *Amp:* 10 mg/ml (1 ml); *Prefilled syringe:* 50 mg/ml (1 ml)

Parenteral Epinephrine

▷ *epinephrine* 1:1,000 0.01 ml/kg SC; max 0.3 ml
  Pediatric: 0.01 mg/kg SC

CHRONIC SPONTANEOUS/IDIOPATHIC URTICARIA
Immunoglobulin E (IgE) Blocker (Immunoglobulin G1k [IgG1k] Monoclonal Antibody)

Comment: *Xolair (omalizumab)* is a humanized monoclonal antibody that specifically binds to free immunoglobulin E in the blood and on the surface of selected B-lymphocytes, but not on the surface of mast cells, antigen-presenting dendritic cells, or basophils. In the United States, *omalizumab* is approved for adults at 150 mg or 300 mg subcutaneously administered every 4 weeks for the treatment of chronic spontaneous urticaria (CSU) not responsive to high-dose antihistamines. In three published, pivotal, phase 3 randomized trials, the clinical response rate to **omalizumab** at 300 mg every 4 weeks, as defined by a weekly 7-day Urticaria Activity Score (UAS7) ≤6 at 12 weeks, was 52% in ASTERIA I, 66% in ASTERIA II, and 52% in GLACIAL. Good control of disease activity was defined as a UAS7 score of ≤6 on the 0- to 42-point UAS7, which correlates well with minimal or no patient symptoms

Comment: A multicenter, open-label study of 286 patients with CSU, conducted by the Catalan and Balearic Chronic Urticaria Network (XUrCB) at 15 hospitals, found about two-thirds of patients with CSU treated with the approved dose of *omalizumab* achieved good disease control. Three-quarters of the non-responders achieved good disease control upon up-dosing to 450 or 600 mg (twice the approved dose) every 4 weeks, without increase in adverse events.

▷ *omalizumab* 150-375 mg SC q 2-4 weeks based on body weight and pretreatment serum total IgE level; max 150 mg/injection site; approved for patient self-administration after education by a qualified healthcare provider
  Pediatric: <12 years: not recommended; ≥12 years: 30-90 kg + IgE >30-100 IU/ml: 150 mg q 4 weeks; 90-150 kg + IgE >30-100 IU/ml or 30-90 kg + IgE >100-200 IU/ml or 30-60 kg + IgE >200-300 IU/ml: 300 mg q 4 weeks; >90-150 kg + IgE >100-200 IU/ml or >60-90 kg + IgE >200-300 IU/ml or 30-70 kg + IgE >300-400 IU/ml: 225 mg q 2 weeks; >90-150 kg + IgE >200-300 IU/ml or >70-90 kg + IgE >300-400 IU/ml or 30-70 kg + IgE >400-500 IU/ml or 30-60 kg + IgE >500-600 IU/ml or 30-60 kg + IgE >600-700 IU/ml: 375 mg q 2 weeks
  Xolair *Vial:* 150 mg, single-dose, pwdr for SC injection after reconstitution; *Prefilled syringe:* 75 mg/0.5 ml, 150 mg/1 ml, single-dose (preservative-free)

UTERINE LEIOMYOMATA (FIBROID TUMOR)

See See Appendix G.5. Progesterone-Only Oral Contraceptives ("Mini-Pill")

▷ *medroxyprogesterone acetate* 10 mg daily
  Provera *Tab:* 2.5, 5, 10 mg
▷ *Oral contraceptives* with 35 mcg estrogen equivalent

SELECTIVE PROGESTERONE RECEPTOR MODULATOR

▷ *ulipristal acetate (UPA)* (G) 5-10 mg once daily
  Comment: *Ulipristal acetate (UPA)* is currently approved in the United States as an emergency contraceptive (a single 30 mg dose), but is marketed for treating symptomatic fibroids in Canada and Europe. It is not yet available in a dose form appropriate for treatment of uterine fibroids (i.e., 5, 10 mg). The drug reduced

dysfunctional uterine bleeding in about 90% of patients in the European trials. Women with uterine fibroids taking *UPA* experienced significant improvement of quality of life, compared with those taking placebo, according to researchers' reported outcomes of VENUS II, a phase 3, prospective, randomized, double-blind, double-dummy, placebo-controlled study. Its design incorporated both parallel and crossover elements: Some patients who were on placebo crossed over to one of two doses of *UPA* after a washout period, and some patients on each active arm crossed over to placebo. The women (n = 432) were between 18 and 50 years and premenopausal. At 13 weeks, uterine bleeding was controlled in 91% of the women receiving 5 mg of *UPA*, 92% of those receiving 10 mg of *UPA*, and 19% of those receiving placebo (P<.001). Of women taking 5 mg of *UPA*, 91% achieved control (40.5%-42% became amenorrheic); of those taking 10 mg, 92% achieved control (54.8%-57.3% became amenorrheic) (controlled in 92%). These results compared to amenorrhea rates of 0%-8% (controlled in 19%) for women on placebo (p<.0001 for all values).
Ella *Tab:* 30 mg
Logilia *Tab:* 30 mg

GONADOTROPIN-RELEASING HORMONE (GnRH) RECEPTOR AGONIST+ESTROGEN+PROGESTIN

▶ *elagolix* 300 mg+*estradiol* 1 mg+*norethindrone acetate* 0.5 mg plus *elagolix* 300 mg take one Morning (AM) capsule (*elagolix* 300 mg, *estradiol* 1 mg, *norethindrone acetate* 0.5 mg) in the morning and take one Evening (PM) capsule (*elagolix* 300 mg) in the evening for up to 24 months; exclude pregnancy before starting Oriahnn or start Oriahnn within 7 days from the onset of menses; take doses at approximately the same time each day; take with or without food

  Oriahnn *Morning (AM) Cap:* *elagolix* 300 mg+*estradiol* 1 mg+*norethindrone acetate* 0.5 mg plus *Evening (PM) Cap:* *elagolix* 300 mg (tartrazine)
  Comment: Oriahnn is a gonadotropin-releasing hormone (GnRH) receptor antagonist, estrogen, and progestin coformulation indicated for the management of heavy menstrual bleeding associated with uterine leiomyomas (fibroids) in premenopausal women. The following are contraindications to use of Oriahnn: pregnancy, high risk of arterial, venous thrombotic, or thromboembolic disorder, known osteoporosis, current or history of breast cancer or other hormonally sensitive malignancy, known liver impairment or disease, undiagnosed abnormal uterine bleeding, women over 35 years of age who smoke, women with uncontrolled hypertension, known hypersensitivity to ingredients of Oriahnn, and organic anion transporting polypeptide (OATP)1B1 inhibitors that are known or expected to significantly increase *elagolix* plasma concentrations. Use of Oriahnn should be limited to 24 months due to the risk of continued bone loss, which may not be reversible. The most common adverse reactions (incidence >5%) in clinical trials have been hot flashes, headache, fatigue, and metrorrhagia. Exclude pregnancy before initiating treatment with Oriahnn and discontinue Oriahnn if pregnancy occurs during treatment. There is no information on the presence of *elagolix* in human milk or effects on the breastfed infant.

ORAL GnRH RECEPTOR ANTAGONIST+ESTROGEN+PROGESTIN COMBINATION

▶ *relugolix*+*estradiol*+*norethindrone acetate* exclude pregnancy and discontinue hormonal contraceptives prior to initiation of treatment; take 1 tablet once daily; take a missed dose as soon as possible the same day; then resume regular dosing the next day at the usual time; if concomitant use of oral P-glycoprotein (P-gp) inhibitors is unavoidable, take the Myfembree dose 6 hours before taking the P-gp inhibitor; use of Myfembree should be limited to 24 months due to the risk of continued bone loss, which may not be reversible
Pediatric: safety and efficacy not established

  Myfembree *Tab:* fixed-dose combination of *relugolix* 40 mg+*estradiol* 1 mg+*norethindrone acetate* 0.5 mg, film-coat
  Comment: Myfembree is a fixed-dose combination of *relugolix* (GnRH) receptor antagonist), *estradiol* (estrogen), and *norethindrone acetate* (progesterone) indicated for the management of heavy menstrual bleeding associated with uterine leiomyomas (fibroid tumors) and endometriosis in premenopausal females. In patients with heavy menstrual bleeding associated with uterine fibroids, the most common adverse reactions (incidence ≥3%) have been vasomotor symptoms, uterine bleeding, alopecia, and decreased libido. In patients with moderate-to-severe pain associated with endometriosis, the most common adverse reactions (incidence ≥3%) have been headache, vasomotor symptoms, mood disorders, abnormal uterine bleeding, nausea, toothache, back pain, decreased sexual desire and arousal, arthralgia, fatigue, and dizziness. *Black Box Warning:* Estrogen and progestin combinations, including Myfembree, increase the risk of thrombotic or thromboembolic disorders, especially in females at increased risk for these events. Myfembree is contraindicated in women with current or a history of thrombotic or thromboembolic disorders and in females at increased risk for these events, including females >35 years of age who smoke or females with uncontrolled hypertension. Other contraindications are pregnancy, known osteoporosis, current or history of breast cancer or other hormone-sensitive malignancy, known hepatic impairment or disease, undiagnosed abnormal uterine bleeding, and known hypersensitivity to components of Myfembree. (See mfr pkg insert for complete boxed warning.) Discontinue Myfembree if an arterial or venous thrombotic, cardiovascular, or cerebrovascular event occurs. Discontinue Myfembree if there is sudden unexplained partial or complete loss of vision, proptosis, diplopia, papilledema, or retinal vascular lesion, and evaluate for retinal vein thrombosis immediately. Baseline bone marrow density (BMD) assessment is recommended in all patients receiving

(continued)

treatment with **Myfembree**. In patients with heavy menstrual bleeding associated with uterine fibroids, periodic BMD assessments are recommended. In patients with moderate-to-severe pain associated with endometriosis, annual BMD assessments are recommended. Assess risk-benefit for patients with additional risk factors for bone loss. Advise patients to seek medical attention for new-onset or worsening depression, anxiety, or other mood changes, or suicidal ideation. Monitor transaminase for elevation and other signs and symptoms of liver injury and inform patients regarding the signs and symptoms. Do not use **Myfembree** in patients with uncontrolled hypertension. For patients with well-controlled hypertension, continue to monitor blood pressure and stop **Myfembree** if blood pressure rises significantly. **Myfembree** may cause a change in menstrual bleeding pattern and reduced ability to recognize pregnancy. Inform patients that **Myfembree** can cause early pregnancy loss and advise using an effective form of non-hormonal contraception during treatment and for 1 week after discontinuing **Myfembree**. Perform testing if pregnancy is suspected and discontinue **Myfembree** if pregnancy is confirmed. Advise patients to seek medical attention for severe uterine bleeding which could signal miscarriage or uterine fibroid prolapse or expulsion. Immediately discontinue **Myfembree** if a hypersensitivity reaction occurs. Epidemiologic studies and meta-analyses have not found an increased risk of genital or non-genital birth defects (including cardiac anomalies and limb-reduction defects) following exposure to estrogens and progestins before conception or during early pregnancy. In animal studies of exposure to *relugolix* during organogenesis, no fetal malformations were present at any dose level; however, exposure to *relugolix* resulted in spontaneous abortion and total litter loss at *relugolix* exposures about half those at the maximum recommended human dose (MRHD) of 40 mg. Therefore, **Myfembree** is contraindicated in pregnancy. There is a pregnancy exposure registry that monitors pregnancy outcomes in females exposed to **Myfembree** during pregnancy. Pregnant females exposed to **Myfembree** and healthcare providers are encouraged to call the Myfembree Pregnancy Exposure Registry at 1-855-428-0707. There are no data on the presence of *relugolix* or its metabolites in human milk or effects on the breastfed infant. However, *relugolix* has been detected in lactating animals. When a drug is present in animal milk, it is likely that the drug will be present in human milk. Detectable amounts of estrogen and progestin have been identified in the breast milk of patients receiving estrogen plus progestin therapy and can reduce milk production in breastfeeding patients. This reduction can occur at any time but is less likely to occur once breastfeeding is well established. Developmental and health benefits of breastfeeding should be considered along with the mother's clinical need for **Myfembree** and any potential adverse effects on the breastfed infant from **Myfembree** or from the underlying maternal condition.

UVEITIS: POSTERIOR, CHRONIC, NON-INFECTIOUS

INTRAVITREAL IMPLANT

▷ *fluocinolone acetonide* surgical intravitreal injection is administered by a qualified healthcare provider under sterile conditions in the office/clinic/hospital setting; the implant is a 36-month sustained-release system

   Yutiq 0.18 mg non-bioerodible intravitreal implant, single-dose, preloaded applicator w. 25 g needle , for ophthalmic intravitreal injection
   Comment: Yutiq is indicated for the treatment of macular edema, diabetic macular edema, and chronic non-infectious posterior uveitis. Placement of a **Yutiq** intravitreal implant is contraindicated with active infection (e.g., ocular herpes simplex, acute blepharoconjunctivitis) or glaucoma. Use of **Yutiq** may increase risk of cataract development. Postprocedure blurring of vision should clear within 4 weeks. Avoid driving and hazardous activity until vision returns to baseline. If both eyes require treatment, the implants should be placed on separate dates to decrease risk of infection in both eyes.

VAGINAL IRRITATION: EXTERNAL

OTC Replens Vaginal Moisturizer
OTC Vagisil Intimate Moisturizer
Comment: Vagisil products have no effect on condom integrity.

VARICOSE VEINS

▷ *sodium tetradecyl sulfate* generally, the 1% solution will be found most useful, with the 3% solution preferred for larger varicosities; volume should be kept small, using 0.5-2 ml per site (preferably 1 ml max); max 10 ml per treatment session

   Sotradecol *Vial:* 1% (20 mg/2ml, 10 mg/ml, 2 ml), 3% (60 mg/2 ml, 30 mg/ml, 2 ml), multidose
   Comment: Sotradecol *(sodium tetradecyl sulfate)* is indicated in the treatment of small uncomplicated varicose veins of the lower extremities that show simple dilation with competent valves. Benefit-to-risk ratio should be considered in selected patients who are great surgical risks. It is not known whether **Sotradecol** can cause fetal harm when administered to a pregnant female or whether **Sotradecol** is excreted in human milk.

VERTIGO

▷ **meclizine (G)** 25-100 mg/day in divided doses
 Pediatric: <12 years: not established; ≥12 years: same as adult
  Antivert *Tab:* 12.5, 25, 50*mg
  Bonine (OTC) *Cap:* 15, 25, 30 mg; *Tab:* 12.5, 25, 50 mg; *Chew tab/Film-coat tab:* 25 mg
  Dramamine II (OTC) *Tab:* 25*mg
  Zentrip *Strip:* 25 mg orally-disint
▷ **methscopolamine bromide** 1 tab q 6 hours prn
 Pediatric: <12 years: not recommended; ≥12 years: same as adult
  Pamine *Tab:* 2.5 mg
  Pamine Forte *Tab:* 5 mg
▷ **scopolamine** 0.4-0.8 mg tab (may repeat in 8 hours) or 1 x 1.5 mg transdermal patch behind ear (effective x 3 days; may replace every fourth day)
 Pediatric: <12 years: not recommended; ≥12 years: same as adult
  Scopace *Tab:* 0.4 mg
  Transderm Scop *Transdermal patch:* 1.5 mg (4/carton)

VITILIGO

REPIGMENTATION AGENTS

▷ **methoxsalen** apply to well-defined area of vitiligo; then expose area to source of UVA (ultraviolet A) or sunlight; initial exposure no more than ½ predicted minimal erythemal dose; repeat weekly
 Pediatric: <12 years: not recommended; ≥12 years: same as adult
  Oxsoralen *Lotn:* 1% (30 ml)
 Comment: *Methoxsalen* may only be applied by a healthcare provider. Do not dispense to patient.
▷ **trioxsalen** 10 mg daily, taken 2-4 hours before UV light exposure; max 14 days and 28 tabs
 Pediatric: <12 years: not recommended; ≥12 years: same as adult
  Trisoralen *Tab:* 5 mg

DEPIGMENTING AGENTS

▷ **hydroquinone (G)** apply sparingly to affected area and rub in bid
  Lustra *Crm:* 4% (1, 2 oz) (sulfites)
  Lustra AF *Crm:* 4% (1, 2 oz) (sunscreen, sulfites)
▷ **monobenzone** apply sparingly to affected area and rub in bid-tid; depigmentation occurs in 1-4 months
 Pediatric: same as adult
  Benoquin *Crm:* 20% (1.25 oz)
▷ **tazarotene (G)** apply daily at HS
 Pediatric: <12 years: not recommended; ≥12 years: same as adult
  Avage Cream *Crm:* 0.1% (30 gm)
  Tazorac Cream *Crm:* 0.05, 0.1% (15, 30, 60 gm)
  Tazorac Gel *Gel:* 0.05, 0.1% (30, 100 gm)
▷ **tretinoin (G)** apply daily at HS
 Pediatric: <12 years: not recommended; ≥12 years: same as adult
  Avita *Crm/Gel:* 0.025% (20, 45 gm)
  Renova *Crm:* 0.02% (40 gm), 0.05% (40, 60 gm)
  Retin-A Cream *Crm:* 0.025, 0.05, 0.1% (20, 45 gm)
  Retin-A Gel *Gel:* 0.01, 0.025% (15, 45 gm) (alcohol 90%)
  Retin-A Liquid *Liq:* 0.05% (28 ml) (alcohol 55%)
  Retin-A Micro *Microspheres:* 0.04, 0.1% (20, 45 gm)

COMBINATION AGENTS

▷ **hydroquinone+fluocinolone+tretinoin** apply sparingly to affected area and rub in daily at HS
 Pediatric: <12 years: not recommended; ≥12 years: same as adult
  Tri-Luma *Crm:* hydroquin 4%+fluo 0.01%+tretin 0.05% (30 gm) (parabens, sulfites)
▷ **hydroquinone+padimate o+oxybenzone+octyl methoxycinnamate** apply sparingly to affected area and rub in bid
 Pediatric: <12 years: not recommended; ≥16 years: same as adult
  Glyquin *Crm:* 4% (1 oz jar)
▷ **hydroquinone+ethyl dihydroxypropyl PABA+dioxybenzone+oxybenzone** apply sparingly to affected area and rub in bid; max 2 months
 Pediatric: <12 years: not recommended; ≥12 years: same as adult
  Solaquin *Crm:* hydroquin 2%+PABA 5%+dioxy 3%+oxy 2% (1 oz) (sulfites)
▷ **hydroquinone+padimate+dioxybenzone+oxybenzone** apply sparingly to affected area and rub in bid; max 2 months
 Pediatric: <12 years: not recommended; ≥12 years: same as adult
  Solaquin Forte *Crm:* hydroquin 4%+pad 0.5%+dioxy 3%+oxy 2% (1oz) (sunscreen, sulfites)

(continued)

▶ *hydroquinone+padimate+dioxybenzone* apply sparingly to affected area and rub in bid; max 2 months
Pediatric: <12 years: <u>not</u> recommended; ≥12 years: same as adults
    Solaquin Forte Gel hydroquin 4%+pad 0.5%+dioxy 3% (1 oz) (alcohol, sulfites)

JANUS KINASE (JAK) INHIBITOR

▶ *ruxolitinib* apply a thin layer bid to affected areas of up to 10% body surface area (BSA); do <u>not</u> use more than one 60 gm tube per week <u>or</u> one 100 gm tube per 2 weeks
Pediatric: <12 years: safety and efficacy <u>not</u> established; ≥12 years: same as adult
    Opzelura *Crm:* 1.5% (60, 100 gm tube)
    Comment: **Opzelura** is a Janus kinase (JAK) inhibitor indicated for the topical, short-term, and non-continuous chronic treatment of mild-to-moderate atopic dermatitis in non-immunocompromised adult and pediatric patients ≥12 years of age whose disease is <u>not</u> adequately controlled with topical prescription therapies <u>or</u> when those therapies are <u>not</u> advisable and for the topical treatment of non-segmental vitiligo in adult and pediatric patients ≥12 years of age. Use of **Opzelura** in combination with therapeutic biologics, other JAK inhibitors, <u>or</u> potent immunosuppressants such as **azathioprine** <u>or</u> **cyclosporine** is <u>not</u> recommended. *Black Box Warning:* Serious infections, mortality, malignancy, major adverse cardiovascular events (MACE), and thrombosis. The following are conditions seen in patients treated with JAK inhibitors for inflammatory conditions: (1) serious infections leading to hospitalization <u>or</u> death, including tuberculosis (TB), and bacterial, invasive fungal, viral, and other opportunistic infections; (2) a higher rate of all-cause mortality, including sudden cardiovascular death; (3) lymphoma and other malignancies; (4) a higher rate of MACE, including cardiovascular death, acute myocardial infarction (AMI), and stroke; and (5) thrombosis including deep venous thrombosis (DVT), pulmonary embolism (PE), and arterial thrombosis, with some fatal. Regularly monitor patients for bacterial, mycobacterial, fungal, and viral infections, and initiate treatment promptly. Monitor patients for skin cancers (i.e., melanoma, basal cell carcinoma [BCC] and squamous cell carcinoma [SCC]) periodically during treatment and following treatment as appropriate. Monitor complete blood count (CBC) for thrombocytopenia, anemia, and neutropenia as clinically indicated. When used in the treatment of non-segmental vitiligo, the most common adverse reactions (incidence ≥1%) are application site acne, application site pruritus, nasopharyngitis, headache, urinary tract infection, application site erythema, and pyrexia. Available data from pregnancies reported in clinical trials with **Opzelura** are <u>not</u> sufficient to evaluate a drug-associated risk of major birth defects, miscarriage, <u>or</u> other adverse maternal <u>or</u> fetal outcomes. There is a pregnancy registry that monitors pregnancy outcomes in pregnant persons exposed to **Opzelura** during pregnancy. Pregnant persons exposed to **Opzelura** and healthcare providers should report **Opzelura** exposure by calling 1-855-463-3463. Because of the more serious adverse findings in adults, including risks of serious infections, thrombocytopenia, anemia, and neutropenia, advise females <u>not</u> to breastfeed during treatment with **Opzelura** and for approximately 4 weeks after the last dose.

WALDENSTRÖM'S MACROGLOBULINEMIA

BRUTON'S TYROSINE KINASE (BTK) INHIBITOR

▶ *zanubrutinib* 160 mg (2 x 80 mg) bid <u>or</u> 320 mg (4 x 80 mg) once daily; swallow whole with water, with <u>or</u> without food; do <u>not</u> open, break, <u>or</u> chew capsules; *Child-Pugh Class C:* reduce dose; manage toxicity with dose reduction, treatment interruption, <u>or</u> discontinuation
Pediatric: safety and efficacy <u>not</u> established
    Brukinsa *Cap:* 80 mg
    Comment: **Brukinsa** is a Bruton's tyrosine kinase (BTK) inhibitor indicated for the treatment of patients with mantle cell lymphoma (MCL) who have received at least one prior therapy. This indication is approved under accelerated approval based on overall response rate. Continued approval for this indication may be contingent upon verification and description of clinical benefit in a confirmatory trial. Marginal zone lymphoma (MZL) relapsed <u>or</u> refractory marginal zone lymphoma (MZL) who have received at least one anti–CD20-based regimen, chronic lymphocytic leukemia (CLL) <u>or</u> small lymphocytic lymphoma (SLL), and Waldenström's macroglobulinemia (WM). There are <u>no</u> contraindications to the use of **Brukinsa**. Monitor for bleeding and manage appropriately. Monitor patients for signs and symptoms of infection, including opportunistic infections, and treat as needed. Monitor complete blood counts (CBCs) for cytopenias during treatment. Other malignancies have developed, including skin cancers and non-skin carcinomas; advise patients to use sun protection. Monitor for signs and symptoms of cardiac arrhythmias and manage appropriately. Modify **Brukinsa** dose with moderate <u>or</u> strong CYP3A inhibitors. Avoid co-administration with strong <u>or</u> moderate CYP3A inducers. Dose adjustment may be recommended with moderate CYP3A inducers. The most common adverse reactions (≥30%), including laboratory abnormalities, are decreased neutrophil count, upper respiratory tract infection, decreased platelet count, hemorrhage, and musculoskeletal pain. *Embryo/Fetal Toxicity:* Can cause fetal harm. Advise patients of reproductive potential of potential risk to the fetus and to use effective contraception. Advise <u>not</u> to breastfeed.

WART: COMMON (*VERRUCA VULGARIS*)

▷ *salicylic acid* (G)
  Pediatric: same as adult
    Duo Film (OTC) apply daily-bid; max 12 weeks;
    Liq: 17% (½ oz w. applicator)
    Duo Film Patch for Kids (OTC) apply 1 patch q 48 hours; max 12 weeks
      Patch: 40% (18/pck)
    Occlusal HP (OTC) apply daily-bid; max 12 weeks
      Liq: 17% (10 ml w. applicator)
    Wart-Off (OTC) apply 1 drop at a time to sufficiently cover wart, let dry; repeat 1-2 times daily; max 12 weeks
      Liq: 17% (0.45 oz)
▷ *trichloroacetic acid* apply after wart is pared and repeat weekly
▷ Cryotherapy with liquid nitrogen or cryoprobe or cryospray; repeat applications q 1-2 weeks as needed to destroy lesion
    Histofreezer see pkg insert for application freeze time

ORAL RETINOID
▷ *acitretin* (G) 25-50 mg once daily with main meal
  Pediatric: <18 years: not recommended; ≥18 years: same as adult
    Soriatane *Cap:* 10, 25 mg

WART: PLANTAR (*VERRUCA PLANTARIS*)

▷ *salicylic acid* (G)
    Duo Plant Gel (OTC) apply daily bid; max 12 weeks
      Gel: 17% (½ oz)
    Mediplast cut to size of wart and apply; remove q 1-2 days, peel keratin, and reapply; repeat as long as needed
    Occlusal-HP (OTC) apply once daily-bid; max 12 weeks
      Liq: 17% (10 ml w. applicator)
    Wart-Off (OTC) apply 1 drop at a time to sufficiently cover wart, let dry; repeat 1-2 times daily; max 12 weeks
      Liq: 17% (0.45 oz)
▷ *trichloroacetic acid* apply after wart is pared and repeat weekly

ORAL RETINOID
▷ *acitretin* (G) 25-50 mg once daily with main meal
  Pediatric: <12 years: not recommended; ≥12 years: same as adult
    Soriatane *Cap:* 10, 25 mg

WART: VENEREAL, HUMAN PAPILLOMAVIRUS (HPV), CONDYLOMA ACUMINATA

Comment: Due to the increased risk of cervical cancer with human papillomavirus (HPV), Pap smears should be done q 3 months during active disease and then q 3-6 months for the next 2 years.

PATIENT-APPLIED AGENTS
Regimen 1

▷ *imiquimod* (G)
  Pediatric: <12 years: not recommended; ≥12 years: same as adult
    Aldara (G) rub into lesions before bedtime and remove with soap and water 6-10 hours later; treat 3 times per week; max 16 weeks
      Crm: 5% (12 single-use pkts/carton)
    Zyclara rub into lesions before bedtime and remove with soap and water 8 hours later; treat 3 times per week; max 1 packet per treatment; max 8 weeks
      Crm: 3.75% (28 single-use pkts/carton) (parabens)

Regimen 2

▷ *podofilox 0.5% cream* apply bid (q 12 hours) x 3 days; then discontinue for 4 days; may repeat if needed; max 4 treatment cycles
    Condylox *Soln:* 0.5% (3.5 ml); *Gel:* 0.5% (3.5 gm)

Regimen 3

▷ *sinecatechins 15% ointment* apply to each lesion tid for up to 16 weeks
    Veregen *Oint:* 15% (15, 30 gm)

PROVIDER-ADMINISTERED AGENTS
Regimen 1
▷ Cryotherapy with liquid nitrogen or cryoprobe; repeat applications every 1-2 weeks as needed

Regimen 2
▷ *trichloroacetic acid (TCA) 80-90%* apply to warts; repeat weekly if needed
Comment: TCA is the preferred treatment during pregnancy. Immediate application of sodium bicarbonate paste following treatment decreases pain.

Regimen 3
▷ *podofilox 0.5% cream* apply bid (q 12 hours) x 3 days; then discontinue for 4 days; may repeat if needed; max 4 treatment cycles
    Condylox *Soln:* 0.5% (3.5 ml); *Gel:* 0.5% (3.5 gm)

Regimen 4
▷ *interferon alfa-n3* 0.05 ml injected into base of wart twice weekly for up to 8 weeks; max 0.5 ml/session (20 warts/session)
    Alferon N *Vial:* 5 million units/ml (1 ml)

Regimen 5
▷ *interferon alfa-2b* 0.1 ml injected into base of wart 3 times weekly for up to 3 weeks; max 0.5 ml/session (5 warts/session)
    Intron A *Vial:* 1 million units/0.1 ml (0.5, 1 ml)

Regimen 6
▷ Surgical removal either by tangential scissor excision, tangential shave excision, curettage, or electrosurgery

WEST NILE VIRUS (WNV)

Comment: The principal route of human infection with West Nile virus is through the bite of an infected mosquito. Additional routes of infection have become apparent during the 2002 West Nile epidemic. It is important to note that these other methods of transmission represent a very small proportion of cases. Other methods of transmission include blood transfusion, organ transplantation, mother-to-child (ingestion of breast milk and transplacental), and occupational. Symptoms of mild disease will generally last a few days. Symptoms of severe disease may last several weeks, although neurologic effects may be permanent. There is no specific treatment for West Nile virus infection; treatment is symptomatic and supportive. About 8 in 10 infected with West Nile virus do not develop any symptoms. About 1 in 5 develop a fever with other symptoms such as headache, body aches, joint pains, vomiting, diarrhea, or rash. Most people with this level of disease recover completely, but fatigue and weakness can last for weeks to months. About 1 in 150 people who are infected develop a severe illness affecting the central nervous system (encephalitis meningitis). Symptoms of severe illness include high fever, headache, neck stiffness, stupor, disorientation, coma, tremors, convulsions, muscle weakness, vision loss, numbness, and paralysis. About 1 in 10 who develop severe illness affecting the central nervous system die. There is currently no preventive vaccine. However, the National Institutes of Health has announced that an experimental vaccine to protect against West Nile Virus has entered human trial. The developers say because the vaccine uses inactivated virus it should be suitable for a wide range of people. The trial tested the safety of the vaccine, called **HydroVax-001**, and its ability to produce an immune response in human subjects. The randomized, placebo-controlled, double-blind clinical trial was conducted by researchers at Duke University School of Medicine, Durham, North Carolina, and enrolled 50 healthy volunteers, men and women 18-50 years of age. Participants were randomly assigned to one of the three groups. One group volunteers (n = 20) received a low dose of the vaccine (1 mcg), another group (n = 20) received a higher dose (4 mcg), and a third group (n = 10) received a placebo. All participants received their doses via IM injection on day 1 and day 29 of the trial and are followed for 14 months. Results of the completed trial are pending.

WHIPWORM (TRICHURIASIS)

ANTHELMINTICS
▷ *albendazole* 400 mg as a single dose; may repeat in 3 weeks; take with a meal
    Pediatric: <2 years: 200 mg daily x 3 days; may repeat in 3 weeks; 2-12 years: 400 mg daily x 3 days; may repeat in 3 weeks; >12 years: same as adult
        Albenza *Tab:* 200 mg
▷ *mebendazole* chew, swallow, or mix with food; 100 mg bid x 3 days; may repeat in 3 weeks if needed; take with a meal
    Pediatric: <2 years: not recommended; ≥2 years: same as adult
        Emverm *Chew tab:* 100 mg
        Vermox (G) *Chew tab:* 100 mg

▷ *pyrantel pamoate* 11 mg/kg x 1 dose; max 1 gm/dose; take with a meal
Pediatric: 25-37 lb: ½ tsp x 1 dose; 38-62 lb: 1 tsp x 1 dose; 63-87 lb: 1 tsp x 1 dose; 88-112 lb: 2 tsp x 1 dose; 113-137 lb: 2 tsp x 1 dose; 138-162 lb: 3 tsp x 1 dose; 163-187 lb: 3 tsp x 1 dose; >187 lb: 4 tsp x 1 dose
    Antiminth (OTC) *Cap:* 180 mg; *Liq:* 50 mg/ml (30 ml), 144 mg/ml (30 ml); *Oral susp:* 50 mg/ml (60 ml)
    Pin-X (OTC) *Cap:* 180 mg; *Liq:* 50 mg/ml (30 ml), 144 mg/ml (30 ml); *Oral susp:* 50 mg/ml (30 ml)
▷ *thiabendazole* 25 mg/kg bid x 7 days; max 1.5 gm/dose; take with a meal
Pediatric: same as adult; <30 lb: consult mfr pkg insert; >30 lb: 2 doses/day with meals; 30-50 lb: 250 mg bid with meals; >50 lb: 10 mg/lb/dose bid with meals; max 3 gm/day
    Mintezol *Chew tab:* 500*mg (orange); *Oral susp:* 500 mg/5 ml (120 ml) (orange)
Comment: *Thiabendazole* is not for prophylaxis. May impair mental alertness. May not be available in the United States.

WILSON'S DISEASE

Comment: Wilson's disease (hepatolenticular degeneration) occurs in individuals who have inherited an autosomal recessive defect that leads to an accumulation of copper far in excess of metabolic requirements. The excess copper is deposited in several organs and tissues, and eventually produces pathologic effects primarily in the liver, where damage progresses to postnecrotic cirrhosis, and in the brain, where degeneration is widespread. Copper is also deposited as characteristic, asymptomatic, golden-brown Kayser-Fleischer rings in the corneas of all patients with cerebral symptomatology. Treatment has two objectives: (1) to minimize dietary intake of copper; and (2) to promote excretion and complex formation (i.e., detoxification) of excess tissue copper.

COPPER CHELATING AGENTS

▷ *penicillamine* administer on an empty stomach, at least 1 hour before meals or 2 hours after meals, and at least 1 hour apart from any other drug, food, milk, antacid, and zinc- or iron-containing preparation; dosage must be individualized and may require adjustment during the course of treatment; initially a single daily dose of 125-250 mg; then increase at 1- to 3-month intervals by 125-250 mg/day, as patient response and tolerance indicate; if a satisfactory remission of symptoms is achieved, the dose associated with the remission should be continued as the patient's maintenance therapy; if there is no improvement and there are no signs of potentially serious toxicity after 2-3 months of treatment with doses of 500-750 mg/day, increase by 250 mg/day at 2- to 3-month intervals until a satisfactory remission occurs or signs of toxicity develop; if there is no discernible improvement after 3-4 months of treatment with 1,000-1,500 mg/day, discontinue **Cuprimine**; changes in maintenance dosage levels may not be reflected clinically or in the erythrocyte sedimentation rate (ESR) for 2-3 months after each dosage adjustment
    Cuprimine *Cap:* 125, 250 mg
    Depen: 250 mg
Comment: Taking *penicillamine* on an empty stomach permits maximum absorption and reduces the likelihood of inactivation by metal binding in the gastrointestinal (GI) tract. Optimal dosage can be determined by measurement of urinary copper excretion and the determination of free copper in the serum. The urine must be collected in copper-free glassware and should be quantitatively analyzed for copper before and soon after initiation of therapy with **Cuprimine**. Determination of 24-hour urinary copper excretion is of greatest value in the first week of therapy with *penicillamine*. In the absence of any drug reaction, a dose between 0.75 and 1.5 gm that results in an initial 24-hour cupriuresis of over 2 mg should be continued for about 3 months, by which time the most reliable method of monitoring maintenance treatment is the determination of free copper in the serum. This equals the difference between quantitatively determined total copper and ceruloplasmin-copper. Adequately treated patients will usually have less than 10 mcg free copper/dl of serum. It is seldom necessary to exceed a dosage of 2 gm/day, In patients who cannot tolerate as much as 1 g/day initially, initiating dosage with 250 mg/day and increasing gradually to the requisite amount give closer control of the effects of the drug and may help to reduce the incidence of adverse reactions. If the patient is intolerant to therapy with **Cuprimine**, alternative treatment is *trientine* (**Syprine**).
The use of *penicillamine* has been associated with fatalities due to certain diseases such as aplastic anemia, agranulocytosis, thrombocytopenia, Goodpasture's syndrome, and myasthenia gravis. Because of the potential for serious hematologic and renal adverse reactions to occur at any time, routine urinalysis, white and differential blood cell count, hemoglobin, and direct platelet count must be checked twice weekly, together with monitoring of the patient's skin, lymph nodes, and body temperature, during the first month of therapy, every 2 weeks for the next 5 months, and monthly thereafter. Patients should be instructed to report promptly the development of signs and symptoms of granulocytopenia and/or thrombocytopenia, such as fever, sore throat, chills, bruising, or bleeding; the above laboratory studies should then be promptly repeated.

▷ *trientine* (G) recommended initial dose is 500-750 mg/day for pediatric patients and 750-1,250 mg/day for adults administered in divided doses 2, 3, or 4 x a day; may be increased to max of 2,000 mg/day for adults or 1,500 mg/day for patients ≤12 years of age; the daily dose of **Syprine** should be increased only when the clinical response is not adequate or the concentration of free serum copper is persistently above 20 mcg/dl; optimal long-term maintenance dose should be determined at 6- to 12-month intervals; administer on an

(continued)

empty stomach, at least 1 hour before meals or 2 hours after meals and at least 1 hour apart from any other drug, food, or milk; swallow whole with water; do not open the cap or chew the contents

Syrine *Cap:* 250 mg

Comment: Syrine is a chelating agent indicated in the treatment of patients with Wilson's disease who are intolerant of *penicillamine*. Clinical experience with **Syrine** is limited and alternate dosing regimens have not been well-characterized; all endpoints in determining an individual patient's dose have not been well defined. **Syrine** and *penicillamine* cannot be considered interchangeable. **Syrine** should be used when continued treatment with *penicillamine* is no longer possible because of intolerable or life-endangering side effects. Unlike *penicillamine*, **Syrine** is not recommended in cystinuria or rheumatoid arthritis. The absence of a sulfhydryl moiety renders it incapable of binding cystine and therefore it is of no use in cystinuria. In 15 patients with rheumatoid arthritis, **Syrine** was reported not to be effective in improving any clinical or biochemical parameter after 12 weeks of treatment. The most reliable index for monitoring treatment is the determination of free copper in the serum, which equals the difference between quantitatively determined total copper and ceruloplasmin-copper. Adequately treated patients will usually have less than 10 mcg free copper/dl of serum. Therapy may be monitored with a 24-hour urinary copper analysis periodically (i.e., every 6-12 months). Urine must be collected in copper-free glassware. Since a low copper diet should keep copper absorption down to less than 1 mg a day, the patient probably will be in the desired state of negative copper balance if 0.5-1.0 mg of copper is present in a 24-hour collection of urine. In general, mineral supplements should not be used since they may block the absorption of **Syrine**. However, iron deficiency may develop, especially in children and menstruating or pregnant females, or as a result of the low copper diet recommended for Wilson's disease. If necessary, iron may be given in short courses, but since iron and **Syrine** each inhibits absorption of the other, 2 hours should elapse between administration of **Syrine** and iron. *Trientine* was teratogenic in animals at doses similar to the human dose. The frequencies of both resorptions and fetal abnormalities, including hemorrhage and edema, increased while fetal copper levels decreased when *trientine* was given in the maternal diets. There are no adequate and well-controlled studies in pregnant females. **Syrine** should be used during pregnancy only if the potential benefit justifies the potential risk to the fetus. It is not known whether this drug is excreted in human milk. Caution should be exercised when **Syrine** is administered to a nursing mother. Clinical studies of **Syrine** did not include sufficient numbers of subjects ≥65 years of age to determine whether they respond differently from younger subjects. Other reported clinical experience is insufficient to determine differences in responses between the elderly and younger patients. In general, dose selection should be cautious, usually starting at the low end of the dosing range, reflecting the greater frequency of decreased hepatic, renal, or cardiac function, and of concomitant disease or other drug therapy. Clinical experience with **Syrine** has been limited. The following adverse reactions have been reported in a clinical study in patients with Wilson's disease who were on therapy with *trientine*: iron deficiency and systemic lupus erythematosus. In addition, the following adverse reactions have been reported in marketed use: dystonia, muscular spasm, and myasthenia gravis.

WOUND: INFECTED, NON-SURGICAL, MINOR

TETANUS PROPHYLAXIS VACCINE
Previously Immunized (within previous 5 years)

▷ *tetanus toxoid* vaccine 0.5 ml IM x 1 dose
   Vial: 5 Lf units/0.5 ml (0.5, 5 ml); *Prefilled syringe:* 5 Lf units/0.5 ml (0.5 ml)

Not Previously Immunized

See Tetanus

TOPICAL ANTI-INFECTIVES
▷ *mupirocin* (G) apply to lesions bid
   Pediatric: same as adult
      Bactroban *Oint:* 2% (22 gm); *Crm:* 2% (15, 30 gm)
      Centany *Oint:* 2% (15, 30 gm)

ORAL ANTI-INFECTIVES
▷ *azithromycin* (G) 500 mg x 1 dose on day 1, then 250 mg daily on days 2-5 or 500 mg daily x 3 days or Zmax 2 gm in a single dose
   Pediatric: 10 mg/kg x 1 dose on day 1, then 5 mg/kg/day on days 2-5; max 500 mg/day; *see Appendix BB.7.*
   Azithromycin (G) (*Zithromax Suspension, Zmax Suspension*) for dose by weight
      Zithromax *Tab:* 250, 500, 600 mg; *Oral susp:* 100 mg/5 ml (15 ml), 200 mg/5 ml (15, 22.5, 30 ml) (cherry); *Pkt:* 1 gm for reconstitution (cherry-banana)
      Zithromax Tri-Pak *Tab:* 3 x 500 mg tabs/pck
      Zithromax Z-Pak *Tab:* 6 x 250 mg tabs/pck
      Zmax *Oral susp:* 2 gm ext-rel for reconstitution (cherry-banana) (148 mg Na+)
▷ *amoxicillin+clavulanate* (G)
      Augmentin 500 mg tid or 875 mg bid x 10 days

Pediatric: 40-45 mg/kg/day divided tid x 10 days <u>or</u> 90 mg/kg/day divided bid x 10 days; *see Appendix BB.4. Amoxicillin+Clavulanate (G) (Augmentin Suspension) for dose by weight*
> *Tab:* 250, 500, 875 mg; *Chew tab:* 125, 250 mg (lemon-lime); 200, 400 mg (cherry-banana) (phenylalanine); *Oral susp:* 125 mg/5 ml (banana), 250 mg/5 ml (75, 100, 150 ml) (orange); 200, 400 mg/5 ml (50, 75, 100 ml) (orange) (phenylalanine)

Augmentin ES-600 <u>not</u> recommended for adults
Pediatric: <3 months: <u>not</u> recommended; ≥3 months, <40 kg: 90 mg/kg/day in 2 divided doses x 10 days; ≥40 kg: <u>not</u> recommended
> *Oral susp:* 42.9 mg/5 ml (50, 75, 100, 125, 150, 200 ml) (strawberry cream) (phenylalanine)

Augmentin XR 2 tabs q 12 hours x 10 days
Pediatric: <16 years: use other forms; ≥16 years: same as adult
> *Tab:* 1,000*mg ext-rel

▷ *cefaclor* **(G)**
Ceclor 250 mg tid <u>or</u> 375 mg bid 3-10 days
Pediatric: <1 month: <u>not</u> recommended; 1 month-12 years: 20-40 mg/kg divided bid <u>or</u> q 12 hours x 3-10 days; max 1 gm/day; *see Appendix BB.8. Cefaclor (G) (Ceclor Suspension) for dose by weight;* >12 years: same as adult
> *Tab:* 500 mg; *Cap:* 250, 500 mg; *Susp:* 125 mg/5 ml (75, 150 ml) (strawberry), 187 mg/5 ml (50, 100 ml) (strawberry), 250 mg/5 ml (75, 150 ml) (strawberry), 375 mg/5 ml (50, 100 ml) (strawberry)

Cefaclor Extended Release 375, 500 mg bid x 3-10 days
Pediatric: <16 years: ext-rel <u>not</u> recommended; ≥16 years: same as adult
> *Tab:* 375, 500 mg ext-rel

▷ *cefadroxil* 1 gm/day in 1-2 divided doses x 10 days
Pediatric: 15-30 mg/kg/day in 2 divided doses x 10 days; *see Appendix BB.9. Cefadroxil (G) (Duricef Suspension) for dose by weight*
> **Duricef** *Cap:* 500 mg; *Tab:* 1 gm; *Oral susp:* 250 mg/5 ml (100 ml), 500 mg/5 ml (75, 100 ml) (orange-pineapple)

▷ *cefdinir* 300 mg bid <u>or</u> 600 mg daily x 10 days
Pediatric: <6 months: <u>not</u> recommended; 6 months-12 years: 14 mg/kg/day in 1-2 divided doses x 10 days; *see Appendix BB.10. Cefdinir (G) (Omnicef Suspension) for dose by weight*
> **Omnicef** *Cap:* 300 mg; *Oral susp:* 125 mg/5 ml (60, 100 ml) (strawberry)

▷ *cefpodoxime proxetil* 400 mg bid x 7-14 days
Pediatric: <2 months: <u>not</u> recommended; 2 months-12 years: 10 mg/kg/day (max 400 mg/dose) <u>or</u> 5 mg/kg/day bid (max 200 mg/dose) x 7-14 days; *see Appendix BB.12. Cefpodoxime Proxetil (G) (Vantin Suspension) for dose by weight*
> **Vantin** *Tab:* 100, 200 mg; *Oral susp:* 50, 100 mg/5 ml (50, 75, 100 mg; lemon creme)
> *Pediatric: see Appendix BB.12. Cefpodoxime Proxetil (G) (Vantin Suspension) for dose by weight*

▷ *cefprozil* 250-500 mg q 12 hours <u>or</u> 500 mg daily x 10 days
Pediatric: <2 years: <u>not</u> recommended; 2-12 years: 7.5 mg/kg-15 mg/kg q 12 hours x 10 days; *see Appendix BB.13. Csefprozil (G) (Cefzil Suspension) for dose by weight;* >12 years: same as adult
> **Cefzil** *Tab:* 250, 500 mg; *Oral susp:* 125, 250 mg/5 ml (50, 75, 100 ml) (bubble gum, phenylalanine)

▷ *cephalexin* **(G)** 2 gm 1 hour before procedure
Pediatric: 50 mg/kg/day in 4 divided doses x 10 days; *see Appendix BB.15. Cephalexin (G) (Keflex Suspension) for dose by weight*
> **Keflex** *Cap:* 250, 333, 500, 750 mg; *Oral susp:* 125, 250 mg/5 ml (100, 200 ml) (strawberry)
> *Pediatric: see Appendix BB.15. Cephalexin (G) (Keflex Suspension) for dose by weight*

▷ *clarithromycin* **(G)** 500 mg bid <u>or</u> 500 mg ext-rel once daily x 7-10 days
Pediatric: see Appendix BB.16. Clarithromycin (G) (Biaxin Suspension) for dose by weight
> **Biaxin** *Tab:* 250, 500 mg
> **Biaxin Oral Suspension** *Oral susp:* 125, 250 mg/5 ml (50, 100 ml) (fruit punch)
> **Biaxin XL** *Tab:* 500 mg ext-rel

▷ *dirithromycin* **(G)** 500 mg daily x 7 days
Pediatric: <12 years: <u>not</u> recommended
> **Dynabac** *Tab:* 250 mg

▷ *erythromycin base* **(G)** 500 mg qid x 14 days
Pediatric: 30-50 mg/kg/day in 2-4 divided doses x 10 days
> **Ery-Tab** *Tab:* 250, 333, 500 mg ent-coat
> **PCE** *Tab:* 333, 500 mg

▷ *erythromycin ethylsuccinate* **(G)** 400 mg qid x 7 days
Pediatric: 30-50 mg/kg/day in 4 divided doses x 7 days; may double dose with severe infection; max 100 mg/kg/day; *see Appendix BB.21. Erythromycin Ethylsuccinate (G) (E.E.S. Suspension, EryPed Drops/Suspension) for dose by weight*
> **EryPed** *Oral susp:* 200 mg/5 ml (100, 200 ml) (fruit), 400 mg/5 ml (60, 100, 200 ml) (banana); *Oral drops:* 200, 400 mg/5 ml (50 ml) (fruit); *Chew tab:* 200 mg wafer (fruit)
> **E.E.S.** *Oral susp:* 200, 400 mg/5 ml (100 ml) (fruit)
> **E.E.S. Granules** *Oral susp:* 200 mg/5 ml (100, 200 ml) (cherry)
> **E.E.S. 400 Tablets** *Tab:* 400 mg

(continued)

▷ **gemifloxacin (G)** 320 mg daily x 5-7 days
  Pediatric: <18 years: <u>not</u> recommended; ≥18 years: same as adult
      Factive *Tab:* 320*mg
▷ **levofloxacin** *Uncomplicated:* 500 mg daily x 7 days; *Complicated:* 750 mg daily x 7 days
  Pediatric: <18 years: <u>not</u> recommended; ≥18 years: same as adult
      Levaquin *Tab:* 250, 500, 750 mg
▷ **loracarbef** 200-400 mg bid x 7 days
  Pediatric: 15 mg/kg/day in 2 divided doses x 7 days; *see Appendix BB.27. Loracarbef (G) (Lorabid*
  Suspension) for dose by weight
      Lorabid *Pulvule:* 200, 400 mg; *Oral susp:* 100 mg/5 ml (50, 100 ml), 200 mg/5 ml (50, 75, 100 ml)
      (strawberry bubble gum)
▷ **ofloxacin (G)** 400 mg bid x 10 days
  Pediatric: <18 years: <u>not</u> recommended; ≥18 years: same as adult
      Floxin *Tab:* 200, 300, 400 mg

WRINKLES: FACIAL

TOPICAL RETINOIDS
Comment: Wash the affected area with a soap-free cleanser; pat dry and wait 20-30 minutes; then apply topical retinoid sparingly to affected area; use <u>only</u> once daily in the PM; avoid the eyes, ears, nostrils, and mouth
▷ **adapalene (G)**
  Pediatric: <12 years: <u>not</u> recommended; ≥12 years: same as adult
      Differin *Crm:* 0.1% (15, 45 gm); *Gel:* 0.1% (15, 45 gm); *Pad:* 0.1% (30/pck) (alcohol 30%)
      Differin Solution *Soln:* 0.1% (30 ml; alcohol 30%)
▷ **tazarotene (G)** apply daily at HS
  Pediatric: <12 years: <u>not</u> recommended; ≥12 years: same as adult
      Avage Cream *Crm:* 0.1% (5, 30 gm)
      Tazorac Cream *Crm:* 0.05, 0.1% (15, 30, 60 gm)
      Tazorac Gel *Gel:* 0.05, 0.1% (30, 100 gm)
▷ **tretinoin (G)** apply daily at HS
  Pediatric: <12 years: <u>not</u> recommended; ≥12 years: same as adult
      Atralin Gel *Gel:* 0.05% (45 gm)
      Avita *Crm:* 0.025% (20, 45 gm); *Gel:* 0.025% (20, 45 gm)
      Renova *Crm:* 0.02% (40 gm); 0.05% (40, 60 gm)
      Retin-A Cream *Crm:* 0.025, 0.05, 0.1% (20, 45 gm)
      Retin-A Gel *Gel:* 0.01, 0.025% (15, 45 gm; alcohol 90%)
      Retin-A Liquid *Soln:* 0.05% (alcohol 55%)
      Retin-A Micro Gel *Gel:* 0.04, 0.08, 0.1% (20, 45 gm)
      Tretin-X Cream *Crm:* 0.075% (35 gm) (parabens-free, alcohol-free, propylene glycol-free)
      Retin-A Micro *Microspheres:* 0.04, 0.1% (20, 45 gm)
  Comment: Topical **tretinoin** is effective for mitigation of fine wrinkles, mottled hyperpigmentation, and tactile roughness of skin. No mitigating effect on deep wrinkles, skin yellowing, lentigines, telangiectasia, skin laxity, keratinocytic atypia, melanocytic atypia, <u>or</u> dermal elastosis. Avoid sun exposure. Cautious use of concomitant astringents, alcohol-based products, sulfur-containing products, salicylic acid-containing products, soap, and other topical agents.

BOTULISM TOXIN PRODUCT
▷ **prabotulinumtoxina-xvfs** *Glabellar lines administration:* using a 30-33 gauge needle, 0.1 ml (4 units) by IM injection into each of five sites, for a max total dose of 20 units; consult pkg insert for exact injection sites; must be administered by a qualified healthcare provider with knowledge of the relevant neuromuscular and/ or orbital anatomy of the area involved <u>and</u> any alterations to the anatomy due to prior surgical procedures; avoid injection near the levator palpebrae superioris, particularly in patients with larger brow depressor complexes; lateral corrugator injections should be placed at least 1 cm above the bony supraorbital ridge; ensure the injected volume/dose is accurate and where feasible kept to a minimum; avoid injecting toxin closer than 1 cm above the central eyebrow
      Jeuveau *Vial:* 100 units vacuum-dried pwdr, single-use, for reconstitution with 2.5 ml sterile, preservative-free 0.9% NaCl diluent, to obtain a solution concentration of 4 units/0.1 ml (total 20 units in 0.5 ml)
      Comment: **Jeuveau** is an acetylcholine release inhibitor and a neuromuscular blocking agent indicated for the temporary improvement in the appearance of moderate-to-severe glabellar lines ("worry lines" between the brows) associated with corrugator <u>and/</u>or procerus muscle activity in adult patients. The effects of all botulinum toxin products may spread from the area of injection to produce symptoms consistent with botulinum toxin effects. These symptoms have been reported hours to weeks after injection. Swallowing and breathing difficulties can be life-threatening. Adverse event reports have also involved the cardiovascular system, some with fatal outcomes. Use caution when administering to patients with preexisting cardiovascular disease. **Jeuveau** is <u>not</u> approved for the treatment of spasticity <u>or</u> any conditions other than glabellar lines. Potency units of **Jeuveau** are <u>not</u> interchangeable with other preparations of botulinum toxin products. Animal studies have <u>not</u> demonstrated treatment-related

effects to the developing fetus when administered intramuscularly during organogenesis at doses up to 12 times the maximum recommended human dose (MRHD). There is no information regarding the presence of *prabotulinumtoxina-xvfs* in human <u>or</u> its effects on the breastfed infant.

XEROSIS

MOISTURIZING AGENTS

Aquaphor Healing Ointment (OTC) *Oint:* 1.75, 3.5, 14 oz (alcohol)
Eucerin Daily Sun Defense (OTC) *Lotn:* 6 oz (fragrance-free)
Comment: Eucerin Daily Sun Defense is a moisturizer with SPF-15 sunscreen.
Eucerin Facial Lotion (OTC) *Lotn:* 4 oz
Eucerin Light Lotion (OTC) *Lotn:* 8 oz
Eucerin Lotion (OTC) *Lotn:* 8, 16 oz
Eucerin Original Creme (OTC) *Crm:* 2, 4, 16 oz (alcohol)
Eucerin Plus Creme (OTC) *Crm:* 4 oz
Eucerin Plus Lotion (OTC) *Lotn:* 6, 12 oz
Eucerin Protective Lotion (OTC) *Lotn:* 4 oz (alcohol)
Comment: Eucerin Protective is a moisturizer with SPF-25 sunscreen.
Lac-Hydrin Cream (OTC) *Crm:* 280, 385 gm
Lac-Hydrin Lotion (OTC) *Lotn:* 225, 400 gm
Lubriderm Dry Skin Scented (OTC) *Lotn:* 6, 10, 16, 32 oz
Lubriderm Dry Skin Unscented (OTC) *Lotn:* 3.3, 6, 10, 16 oz (fragrance-free)
Lubriderm Sensitive Skin Lotion (OTC) *Lotn:* 3.3, 6, 10, 16 oz (lanolin-free)
Lubriderm Dry Skin (OTC) *Lotn:* 2.5, 6, 10, 16 oz (scented); 1, 2.5, 6, 10, 16 oz (fragrance-free)
Lubriderm Bath & Shower Oil (OTC) 1-2 capfuls in bath <u>or</u> rub onto wet skin as needed, then rinse; *Oil:* 8 oz
Moisturel *Crm:* 4, 16 oz; *Lotn:* 8, 12 oz; *Clnsr:* 8.75 oz

Topical Oil

➤ *fluocinolone acetonide* 0.01% topical oil
  Pediatric: <6 years: <u>not</u> recommended; ≥6 years: apply sparingly bid for up to 4 weeks
    Derma-Smoothe/FS Topical Oil apply sparingly tid
      Topical oil: 0.01% (4 oz; peanut oil)

YELLOW FEVER

Comment: The yellow fever vaccine is recommended for people ≥9 months of age who are traveling to <u>or</u> living in areas at risk for the yellow fever virus in Africa and South America (www.cdc.gov/yellowfever/maps/africa.html). The vaccine is a live, weakened form of the virus. A single dose provides lifelong protection for most people. Sanofi Pasteur, the manufacturer of the <u>only</u> yellow fever vaccine (YF-Vax) licensed in the United States, announced that **YF-Vax** for civilian use is expected to be available from the manufacturer again by mid-2019. However, **YF-Vax** might be available at some clinics, until remaining supplies at those sites are used up. Sanofi Pasteur applied and received approval from the U.S. FDA to make another yellow fever vaccine available in the United States under an investigational new drug (IND) program. Although the name of the FDA program is "investigational new drug," **Stamaril** is <u>not</u> investigational <u>or</u> experimental. **Stamaril** has been used in European and other countries for decades but is <u>not</u> licensed in the United States. IND is the mechanism through which FDA gives approval for **Stamaril** to be imported. Manufactured by Sanofi Pasteur in France, this vaccine, **Stamaril**, is registered and distributed in more than 70 countries. It is comparable in safety and efficacy to **YF-Vax**. In order to meet the requirements of the IND program, Sanofi Pasteur can provide **Stamaril** to <u>only</u> a limited number of clinics. Sanofi has identified sites throughout the United States to include in the program so patients can have continued access to yellow fever vaccine. Travelers and healthcare providers can find locations that can administer **Stamaril**, and those clinics with remaining doses of **YF-Vax**, by visiting the yellow fever vaccination clinic search page. For information about which countries require yellow fever vaccination for entry and which countries the CDC recommends yellow fever vaccination, visit the CDC Traveler's Health website (www.cdc.gov/travel). For more information, contact Sanofi Pasteur at 1-800-VACCINE (1-800-822-2463) <u>or</u> https://wwwnc.cdc.gov/travel/news-announcements/yellow-fever-vaccine-access.

ZIKA VIRUS

Comment: The Zika virus is transmitted via the bite of an infected mosquito and is associated with severe teratogenicity: a unique and distinct pattern of birth defects, called congenital Zika syndrome, characterized by the following five features: (1) severe microcephaly in which the skull has partially collapsed; (2) decreased brain tissue with a specific pattern of brain damage, including subcortical

(continued)

calcifications; (3) damage to the back of the eye, including macular scarring and focal pigmentary retinal mottling; (4) congenital contractures, such as clubfoot and arthrogryposis; and (5) hypertonia restricting body movement. Congenital Zika virus infection has also been associated with other abnormalities, including but not limited to brain atrophy and asymmetry, abnormally formed or absent brain structures, hydrocephalus, and neuronal migration disorders. Other anomalies include excessive and redundant scalp skin. Reported neurologic findings include hyperreflexia, irritability, tremors, seizures, brainstem dysfunction, and dysphagia. Reported eye abnormalities include, but are not limited to, focal pigmentary mottling and chorioretinal atrophy in the macula, optic nerve hypoplasia, cupping, and atrophy, other retinal lesions, iris colobomas, congenital glaucoma, microphthalmia, lens subluxation, cataracts, and intraocular calcifications. **A synthetic DNA-based preventive vaccine showed promising immune responses with no severe adverse reactions in humans**, an interim analysis of a phase 1 trial found. Following 3 doses of vaccine, 100% of patients produced binding antibodies and 95% of patients produced binding antibodies following 2 doses of the vaccine. Examining immunogenicity, 41% of participants had detectable binding antibody responses 4 weeks after the first dose, the authors said, with a 74% antibody response at week 6 (2 weeks after the second dose). **The vaccine is not yet available to the public.** The FDA formally approved Roche's cobas Zika molecular test for use on whole donor blood and blood products and living organ donors; it is the first such approval granted.

ZOLLINGER-ELLISON SYNDROME

Comment: Zollinger-Ellison syndrome is a condition in which a gastrin-secreting tumor or hyperplasia of the islet cells in the pancreas causes overproduction of gastric acid, resulting in recurrent peptic ulcers.

PROTON PUMP INHIBITORS (PPIs)
Comment: If hepatic impairment, or if the patient is Asian, consider reducing the proton pump inhibitor (PPI) dose.
▷ *dexlansoprazole* (G) 30-60 mg daily for up to 4 weeks
  Pediatric: <18 years: not recommended; ≥18 years: same as adult
    Dexilant *Cap:* 30, 60 mg ent-coat del-rel granules; may open and sprinkle on applesauce; do not crush or chew granules
    Dexilant SoluTab *Tab:* 30 mg del-rel orally-disint
▷ *esomeprazole* (OTC) (G) 20-40 mg daily; max 8 weeks; take 1 hour before food; swallow whole or mix granules with food or juice and take immediately; do not crush or chew granules
  Pediatric: <1 year: not recommended; 1-11 years, <20 kg: 10 mg; ≥20 kg: 10-20 mg once daily; 12-17 years: 20-40 mg once daily; max 8 weeks
    Nexium *Cap:* 20, 40 mg ent-coat del-rel pellets
    Nexium for Oral Suspension *Oral susp:* 10, 20, 40 mg ent-coat del-rel granules/pkt; mix in 2 tbsp water and drink immediately; 30 pkt/carton
▷ *esomeprazole+aspirin* take 1 dose daily; max 8 weeks; take 1 hour before food
    Yosprala
    Tab: Yosprala 40/81 esom 40 mg+asp 81 mg del-rel
      Yosprala 40/325 esom 40 mg+asp 325 mg del-rel
▷ *lansoprazole* (OTC) (G) 15-30 mg daily for up to 8 weeks; may repeat course; take before eating
  Pediatric: <1 year: not recommended; 1-11 years, <30 kg: 15 mg once daily; >11 years: same as adult
    Prevacid *Cap:* 15, 30 mg ent-coat del-rel granules; swallow whole or mix granules with food or juice and take immediately; do not crush or chew granules; follow with water
    Prevacid for Oral Suspension *Oral susp:* 15, 30 mg ent-coat del-rel granules/pkt; mix in 2 tbsp water and drink immediately; 30 pkt/carton (strawberry)
    Prevacid SoluTab *ODT:* 15, 30 mg (strawberry) (phenylalanine)
    Prevacid 24HR *Oral granules:* 15 mg ent-coat del-rel granules; swallow whole or mix granules with food or juice and take immediately; do not crush or chew granules; follow with water
▷ *omeprazole* (OTC) (G) 20-40 mg daily; take before eating; swallow whole or mix granules with applesauce and take immediately; do not crush or chew; follow with water
    Prilosec *Cap:* 10, 20, 40 mg ent-coat del-rel granules
    Pediatric: <18 years: not recommended; ≥18 years: same as adult
    Prilosec *Tab:* 20 mg del-rel (regular, wild berry)
    Pediatric: <1 year: not recommended; 5-<10 kg: 5 mg daily; 10-<20 kg: 10 mg daily; ≥20 kg: same as adult
▷ *pantoprazole* (G) initially 40 mg bid
  Pediatric: <12 years: not recommended; ≥12 years: same as adult
    Protonix *Tab:* 40 mg ent-coat del-rel
    Protonix for Oral Suspension *Oral susp:* 40 mg ent-coat del-rel granules/pkt; mix in 1 tsp apple juice for 5 seconds or sprinkle on 1 tsp apple sauce, and swallow immediately; do not mix in water or any other liquid or food; take approximately 30 minutes prior to a meal; 30 pkt/carton any other liquid or food; take approximately 30 minutes prior to a meal; 30 pkt/carton
▷ *rabeprazole* (OTC) (G) initially 20 mg daily; then titrate; may take 100 mg daily in divided doses or 60 mg bid
  Pediatric: <12 years: not recommended; ≥12 years: 20 mg once daily; max 8 weeks
    AcipHex *Tab:* 20 mg ent-coat del-rel

SECTION II

APPENDICES

Appendix A. U.S. Schedule of Controlled Substances **665**
*Appendix B. Blood Pressure Guidelines
  *Appendix B.1. Blood Pressure Classifications (≥18 Years)
  *Appendix B.2. Blood Pressure Classifications (<18 Years)
  *Appendix B.3. Identifiable Causes of Hypertension (JNC-9)
  *Appendix B.4. Cardiovascular Disease (CVD) Risk Factors (JNC-9)
  *Appendix B.5. Diagnostic Workup of Hypertension (JNC-9)
  *Appendix B.6. Recommendations for Measuring Blood Pressure (JNC-9)
  *Appendix B.7. Patient-Specific Factors to Consider When Selecting Drug Treatment for Hypertension
    (JNC-9 and ASH)
  *Appendix B.8. Blood Pressure Treatment Recommendations (JNC-9)
*Appendix C. Target Lipid Recommendations (ATP-IV)
  *Appendix C.1. Target TC, TRG, HDL-C, Non-HDL-C
  *Appendix C.2. Target LDL-C (ATP-IV)
  *Appendix C.3. Non-HDL-C Classifications (ATP-IV)
*Appendix D. Effects of Selected Drugs on Insulin Activity
*Appendix E. Glycosylated Hemoglobin (HbA1c) and 90-Day Average Blood Glucose Equivalent
*Appendix F. Routine Immunization Recommendations
  *Appendix F.1. Administration of Vaccines
  *Appendix F.2. Contraindications to Vaccines
  *Appendix F.3. Route of Administration and Dose of Vaccines
  *Appendix F.4. Adverse Reactions to Vaccines
  *Appendix F.5. Minimum Interval Between Vaccine Doses
  Appendix F.6. Childhood (Birth-12 Years) Immunization Schedule **665**
  Appendix F.7. Childhood (Birth-12 Years) Immunization Catch-Up Schedule **666**
  Appendix F.8. Recommended Adult Immunization Schedule **666**
Appendix G. Contraceptives **666**
  Appendix G.1. Non-Hormonal Vaginal Contraceptives **666**
  Appendix G.2. Hormonal Contraceptive Contraindications and Recommendations **666**
  Appendix G.3. 28-Day Oral Contraceptives With Estrogen and Progesterone Content **667**
  Appendix G.4. Extended-Cycle Oral Contraceptives **673**
  Appendix G.5. Progesterone-Only Oral Contraceptives ("Mini-Pill") **674**
  *Appendix G.6. Injectable Contraceptives
    *Appendix G.6.1. Injectable Progesterone
  Appendix G.7. Transdermal Contraceptives **674**
  Appendix G.8. Contraceptive Vaginal Rings **674**
  Appendix G.9. Subdermal Contraceptives **675**
  Appendix G.10. Intrauterine Contraceptives **675**
  Appendix G.11. Emergency Contraception **675**
*Appendix H. Anesthetic Agents for Local Infiltration and Dermal/Mucosal Membrane Application
*Appendix I. NSAIDs
Appendix J. Topical Corticosteroids by Potency **676**
Appendix K. Oral Corticosteroids **678**
Appendix L. Parenteral Corticosteroids **679**
Appendix M. Inhalational Corticosteroids **680**
Appendix N. Antiarrhythmia Drugs **681**
Appendix O. Antineoplasia Drugs **682**
Appendix P. Antipsychosis Drugs **692**
Appendix Q. Anticonvulsant Drugs **694**
Appendix R. Anti-HIV Drugs **696**
Appendix S. Anticoagulants **698**
  Appendix S.1. Coumadin Titration and Dose Forms **698**
  Appendix S.2. Coumadin Over-Anticoagulation Reversal **699**
  Appendix S.3. Agents That Inhibit Coumadin's Anticoagulation Effects **699**

---

*Online only; available at connect.springerpub.com/content/reference-book/978-0-8261-7935-7/section/sectionII/appendix.

Appendix T. Low Molecular Weight Heparins   *699*
Appendix U. Factor Xa Inhibitors   *699*
Appendix V. Direct Thrombin Inhibitors   *701*
Appendix W. Platelet Aggregation Inhibitors   *702*
Appendix X. Protease-Activated Receptor-1 (PAR-1) Inhibitors   *703*
*Appendix Y. Prescription Prenatal Vitamins
*Appendix Z. Drugs for the Management of Allergy, Cough, and Cold Symptoms
Appendix AA. Systemic Anti-Infectives   *703*
Appendix BB. Antibiotic Dosing by Weight for Liquid Forms   *710*
  Appendix BB.1. *acyclovir* (G) (Zovirax Suspension)   *710*
  Appendix BB.2. *amantadine* (G) (Symmetrel Syrup)   *711*
  Appendix BB.3. *amoxicillin* (G) (Amoxil Suspension, Trimox Suspension)   *711*
  Appendix BB.4. *amoxicillin+clavulanate* (G) (Augmentin Suspension)   *712*
  Appendix BB.5. *amoxicillin+clavulanate* (G) (Augmentin ES 600 Suspension)   *712*
  Appendix BB.6. *ampicillin* (G) (Omnipen Suspension, Principen Suspension)   *712*
  Appendix BB.7. *azithromycin* (G) (Zithromax Suspension, Zmax Suspension)   *713*
  Appendix BB.8. *cefaclor* (G) (Ceclor Suspension)   *713*
  Appendix BB.9. *cefadroxil* (G) (Duricef Suspension)   *714*
  Appendix BB.10. *cefdinir* (G) (Omnicef Suspension)   *714*
  Appendix BB.11. *cefixime* (G) (Suprax Oral Suspension)   *714*
  Appendix BB.12. *cefpodoxime proxetil* (G) (Vantin Suspension)   *715*
  Appendix BB.13. *cefprozil* (G) (Cefzil Suspension)   *715*
  Appendix BB.14. *ceftibuten* (G) (Cedax Suspension)   *715*
  Appendix BB.15. *cephalexin* (G) (Keflex Suspension)   *716*
  Appendix BB.16. *clarithromycin* (G) (Biaxin Suspension)   *716*
  Appendix BB.17. *clindamycin* (G) (Cleocin Pediatric Granules)   *716*
  Appendix BB.18. *dicloxacillin* (G) (Dynapen Suspension)   *717*
  Appendix BB.19. *doxycycline* (G) (Vibramycin Syrup/Suspension)   *717*
  Appendix BB.20. *erythromycin estolate* (G) (Ilosone Suspension)   *717*
  Appendix BB.21. *erythromycin ethylsuccinate* (G) (E.E.S. Suspension, EryPed Drops/Suspension)   *718*
  Appendix BB.22. *erythromycin+sulfamethoxazole* (G) (Eryzole, Pediazole)   *719*
  Appendix BB.23. *fluconazole* (G) (Diflucan Suspension)   *719*
  Appendix BB.24. *furazolidone* (G) (Furoxone Liquid)   *719*
  Appendix BB.25. *griseofulvin, microsize* (G) (Grifulvin V Suspension)   *719*
  Appendix BB.26. *itraconazole* (G) (Sporanox Solution)   *720*
  Appendix BB.27. *Loracarbef* (G) (Lorabid Suspension)   *720*
  Appendix BB.28. *nitrofurantoin* (G) (Furadantin Suspension)   *720*
  Appendix BB.29. *penicillin v potassium* (G) (Pen-Vee K Solution, Veetids Solution)   *720*
  Appendix BB.30. *rimantadine* (G) (Flumadine Syrup)   *721*
  Appendix BB.31. *tetracycline* (G) (Sumycin Suspension)   *721*
  Appendix BB.32. *trimethoprim* (G) (Primsol Suspension)   *721*
  Appendix BB.33. *trimethoprim+sulfamethoxazole* (G) (Bactrim Suspension, Septra Suspension)   *722*
  Appendix BB.34. *vancomycin* (G) (Vancocin Suspension)   *722*

---

*Online only; available at connect.springerpub.com/content/reference-book/978-0-8261-7935-7/section/sectionII/appendix.

APPENDIX A. U.S. SCHEDULE OF CONTROLLED SUBSTANCES

Schedule	Description
I	High potential for abuse and of no currently accepted medical use. Not obtainable by prescription but may be legally procured for research, study, or instructional use. (e.g., *heroin, LSD, marijuana, mescaline, peyote*).
II	High-abuse potential and high liability for severe psychological or physical dependence potential. Prescription required and cannot be refilled. Prescription must be written in ink or typed and signed. A verbal prescription may be allowed in an emergency by the dispensing pharmacist but must be followed by a written prescription within 72 hours. Includes opium derivatives, other opioids, and short-acting barbiturates.
III	Potential for abuse is less than that for drugs in schedules I and II. Moderate-to-low physical dependence and high psychological dependence potential. Prescription required. May be refilled up to five times in 6 months. Prescription may be verbal (telephone) or written. Includes certain stimulants and depressants not included in the above schedules, and preparations containing limited quantities of certain opioids.
IV	Lower potential for abuse than Schedule III drugs. Prescription required. May be refilled up to five times in 6 months. Prescription may be verbal (telephone) or written.
V	Abuse potential less than that for Schedule IV drugs. Preparations contain limited quantities of certain narcotic drugs. Generally intended for antitussive and antidiarrheal purposes and may be distributed without a prescription provided that • such distribution is made only by a pharmacist; • not more than 240 ml or not more than 48 solid dosage units of any substance containing opium, nor more than 120 ml or not more than 24 solid dosage units of any other controlled substance may be distributed at retail to the same purchaser in any given 48-hour period without a valid prescription order; • the purchaser is at least 18 years old; • the pharmacist knows the purchaser or requests suitable identification;
	• the pharmacist keeps an official written record of name and address of the purchaser, name, and quantity of controlled substance purchased, date of sale, and initials of the dispensing pharmacist; this record is to be made available for inspection and copying by the U.S. officers authorized by the Attorney General; and • other federal, state, or local law does not require a prescription order; under jurisdiction of the Federal Controlled Substances Act; refillable up to five times within 6 months.

APPENDIX F. ROUTINE IMMUNIZATION RECOMMENDATIONS

APPENDIX F.6. CHILDHOOD (BIRTH-12 YEARS) IMMUNIZATION SCHEDULE

Type	Birth	1 Month	2 Months	4 Months	6 Months	6-18 Months	12-15 Months	15-18 Months	4-6 Years	11-12 Years
HBV	✔	✔			✔					
DTaP			✔	✔	✔		✔		✔	
IPV			✔	✔		✔			✔	
Hib			✔	✔	✔		✔			
Rotavirus			✔	✔	✔					
MMR							✔		✔	
Tdap										✔
Varicella							✔		✔	
PVC-13			✔	✔	✔		✔			
HAV							✔	✔		
Meningitis										✔
HPV										✔✔✔

Source: DHHS CDC 2021

✔ = immunization due

✔✔✔ = HPV 3-dose series: months 0, 1, and 6

APPENDIX F.7. CHILDHOOD (BIRTH-12 YEARS) IMMUNIZATION CATCH-UP SCHEDULE

Vaccine	Minimum Interval Between Doses				
	#1 to #2	#2 to #3		#3 to #4	#4 to #5
HBV	4 weeks	8 weeks (16 weeks after #1)			
DTaP	4 weeks	4 weeks		6 months	6 months
IPV	4 weeks	4 weeks		4 weeks	
MMR	4 weeks				
Var	4 weeks				
Rotavirus	4 weeks	4 weeks; do not administer >32 weeks of age			
PCV	2 months	2 months		2 months	6-15 months
HPV	4 weeks	20 weeks (24 weeks after #1)			

Source: DHHS CDC 2021

APPENDIX F.8. RECOMMENDED ADULT IMMUNIZATION SCHEDULE

Type	19-21 Years	22-26 Years	27-49 Years	50-59 Years	60-65 Years	≥65 Years
Influenza	1 dose annually					
HBV	3-dose series: months 0, 1, and 6					
Td/Tdap	Substitute Tdap for Td one time; then continue Td once every 10 years					
MMR*	Born >1957: 2 doses, 4 weeks apart					
Varicella*	Without evidence of immunity: 2 doses, 4 weeks apart					
Herpes zoster*					1 time dose	
PVC-13/PVC-23					1 time dose	
HAV	Single antigen, 2 doses: months 0, 6-12 (**Havrix**); 0, 6-18 (**Vaqta**)					
Meningitis	1 or more doses					
HPV (female)*[β]	3 doses; months 0, 1, 6					
HPV (male)[β]	3 doses; months 0, 1, 6					

Source: ACIP 2021

*Contraindicated in pregnancy

[β] Only if not previously vaccinated between 11 and 12 years of age.

APPENDIX G. CONTRACEPTIVES

APPENDIX G.1. NON-HORMONAL VAGINAL CONTRACEPTIVES

▷ *lactic acid, citric acid, and potassium bitartrate vaginal gel* administer 1 prefilled applicatorful (5 gm) vaginally immediately before or up to 1 hour before each episode of vaginal intercourse; may use during any part of the menstrual cycle

Phexxi *Prefilled vaginal applicator:* single-dose, delivers 5 gm of gel containing lactic acid (1.8%), citric acid (1%), and potassium bitartrate (0.4%)

Comment: **Phexxi** is a combination of lactic acid, citric acid, and potassium bitartrate indicated for the prevention of pregnancy in females of reproductive potential for use as an on-demand method of contraception. **Phexxi** is not effective for the prevention of pregnancy when administered after intercourse. The most common adverse reactions (incidence ≥2%) have been vulvovaginal burning sensation, vulvovaginal pruritus, vulvovaginal mycotic infection, urinary tract infection, vulvovaginal discomfort, bacterial vaginosis, vaginal discharge, genital discomfort, dysuria, and vulvovaginal pain. Avoid use in females with a history of recurrent urinary tract infection (UTI), pyelonephritis, or urinary tract abnormalities. To report suspected adverse reactions, contact Evofem at 1-833-EVFMBIO or FDA at 1-800-FDA-1088 or www.fda.gov/medwatch.

APPENDIX G.2. HORMONAL CONTRACEPTIVE CONTRAINDICATIONS AND RECOMMENDATIONS

- All contraceptives are pregnancy category X
- No non-barrier contraceptives protect against sexually transmitted infections (STIs)

(*continued*)

Appendix G.2 (*continued*)

- **Absolute Contraindication**
  - HTN >35 years of age
  - DM >35 years of age
  - LDL-C >160 or TG >250
  - Known or suspected pregnancy
  - Known or suspected carcinoma of the breast
  - Known or suspected carcinoma of the endometrium
  - Known or suspected estrogen-dependent neoplasia
  - Undiagnosed abnormal genital bleeding
  - Cerebral vascular or coronary artery disease
  - Cholestatic jaundice of pregnancy or jaundice with prior use
  - Hepatic adenoma or carcinoma or benign liver tumor
  - Active or history of thrombophlebitis or thromboembolic disorder
- **Relative Contraindications**
  - Lactation
  - Asthma
  - Ulcerative colitis
  - Migraine or vascular headache
  - Cardiac or renal dysfunction
  - Gestational diabetes, prediabetes, diabetes mellitus
  - Diastolic BP 90 mmHg or greater or hypertension by any other criteria
  - Psychic depression
  - Varicose veins
  - Smoker >35 years of age
  - Sickle-cell or sickle-hemoglobin C disease
  - Cholestatic jaundice during pregnancy, active gallbladder disease
  - Hepatitis or mononucleosis during the preceding year
  - First-order family history of fatal or non-fatal rheumatic CVD or diabetes prior to age 50 years
  - Drug(s) with known interaction(s)
  - Elective surgery or immobilization within 4 weeks
  - Age >50 years
- **Recommendations**
  - Start the first pill on the first Sunday after menses begins. Thereafter, each new pill pack will be started on a Sunday.
  - Take each daily pill in the same 3-hour window (e.g., 9A-12N, 12N-3P; a 4-hour window prior to bedtime is not recommended).
  - If 1 pill is missed, take it as soon as possible and the next pill at the regular time.
  - If 2 pills are missed, take both pills as soon as possible and then two pills the following day. A barrier method should be used for the remainder of the pill pack.
  - If 3 pills are missed before the 10th cycle day, resume taking oral contraceptives (OCs) on a regular schedule and take precautions.
  - If 3 pills are missed after the 10th cycle day, discard the current pill pack and begin a new one 7 days after the last pill was taken.
  - If very low-dose OCs are used or if combination OCs are begun after the 5th day of the menstrual cycle, an additional method of birth control should be used for the first 7 days of OC use.
  - If nausea occurs as a side effect, select an OC with *lower **estrogen*** content.
  - If breakthrough bleeding occurs during the first half of the cycle, select an OC with *higher **progesterone*** content.
  - Symptoms of a serious nature include loss of vision, diplopia, unilateral numbness, weakness, or tingling, severe chest pain, severe pain in the left arm or neck, severe leg pain, slurring of speech, and abdominal tenderness or mass.

APPENDIX G.3. 28-DAY ORAL CONTRACEPTIVES WITH ESTROGEN AND PROGESTERONE CONTENT

Comment: Beyaz, Loryna, Rajani, Syeda, Safyral, Tydemy, Yasmin, and Yaz are contraindicated with renal insufficiency and adrenal insufficiency. Monitor K^+ level during the first cycle if the patient is at risk of hyperkalemia for any reason. If the patient is taking drugs that increase potassium (e.g., angiotensin-converting enzymes [ACEs], angiotensin receptor blockers [ARBs], non-steroidal anti-inflammatory drugs [NSAIDs], K^+ sparing diuretics), the patient is at risk for hyperkalemia.

Combined Oral Contraceptive	Estrogen (mcg)	Progesterone (mg)
Alesse-21, Alesse-28 (G) *ethinyl estradiol+levonorgestrel*	20	0.1
Altavera *ethinyl estradiol+levonorgestrel*	30	0.15

(continued)

Appendix G.3 (*continued*)

Combined Oral Contraceptive	Estrogen (mcg)	Progesterone (mg)
Apri (G) *ethinyl estradiol+desogestrel*	30	0.15
Aranelle (G) *ethinyl estradiol+norethindrone*	35	0.5 1 0.5
Aviane (G) *ethinyl estradiol+levonorgestrel*	20	0.1
Balcoltra *ethinyl estradiol+levonorgestrel* <u>plus</u> *ferrous bisglycinate 36.5 mg*	20	0.1
Balziva (G) *ethinyl estradiol+norethindrone*	35	0.4
Beyaz (G) *ethinyl estradiol+drospirenone* <u>plus</u> levomefolate calcium 0.451 mcg (28 tabs)	20	3
Blisovi 24Fe (G) *ethinyl estradiol+norethindrone* <u>plus</u> *ferrous fumarate 75 mg (4 tabs)*	20	1
Brevicon-21, Brevicon-28 (G) *ethinyl estradiol+norethindrone*	35	0.5
Camrese *ethinyl estradiol+levonorgestrel*	30 10	0.15
Camrese Lo *ethinyl estradiol+levonorgestrel*	20 10	0.1
Cesia (G) *ethinyl estradiol+desogestrel*	25 25 25	0.1 0.125 0.15
Cryselle (G) *ethinyl estradiol+norgestrel*	30	0.3
Cyclessa (G) *ethinyl estradiol+desogestrel*	25 25 25	0.1 0.125 0.15
Demulen 1/35-21, Demulen 1/35-28 (G) *ethinyl estradiol+ethynodiol diacetate*	35	1
Demulen 1/50-21, Demulen 1/50-28 (G) *ethinyl estradiol+ethynodiol diacetate*	50	1
Desogen (G) *ethinyl estradiol+desogestrel diacetate*	30	0.15
Enpresse (G) *ethinyl estradiol+levonorgestrel*	30 40 30	0.05 0.075 0.125
Estarylla *ethinyl estradiol+norgestimate*	35	0.25
Estrostep Fe *ethinyl estradiol+norethindrone* <u>plus</u> *ferrous fumarate 75 mg*	20 30 35	1 1 1
Femcon Fe (G) *ethinyl estradiol+norethindrone* <u>plus</u> *ferrous fumarate 75 mg*	35	0.4

(*continued*)

Appendix G.3 (*continued*)

Combined Oral Contraceptive	Estrogen (mcg)	Progesterone (mg)
Generess Fe Chew tab (G) *ethinyl estradiol+norethindrone* <u>plus</u> *ferrous fumarate* 75 mg	25	0.8
Genora (G) *ethinyl estradiol+norethindrone*	35 35 35	0.5 1 0.5
Gianvi (G) *ethinyl estradiol+drospirenone*	20	3
Gildess 1.5/30 (G) *ethinyl estradiol+norethindrone*	30	1.5
Introvale *ethinyl estradiol+levonorgestrel*	30	0.15
Jenest-28 *ethinyl estradiol+norethindrone*	35 35	0.5 1
Jolessa (G) *ethinyl estradiol+levonorgestrel*	30	0.15
Junel 1/20 (G) *ethinyl estradiol+norethindrone*	20	1
Junel 1.5/30 (G) *ethinyl estradiol+norethindrone*	30	1.5
Junel Fe 1/20 (G) *ethinyl estradiol+norethindrone* <u>plus</u> *ferrous fumarate* 75 mg	20	1
Junel Fe 1.5/30 (G) *ethinyl estradiol+norethindrone* <u>plus</u> *ferrous fumarate* 75 mg	30	1.5
Kaitlib Fe Chew Tab (G) *ethinyl estradiol+norethindrone* <u>plus</u> *ferrous fumarate* 75 mg	25	0.8
Kariva (G) *ethinyl estradiol+desogestrel*	20 10	0.15 0.15
Kelnor 1/35 (G) *ethinyl estradiol+ethynodiol diacetate*	35	1
Kurvelo-28 *ethinyl estradiol/levonorgestrel*	30	0.15
Leena *ethinyl estradiol+norethindrone*	35 35 35	0.5 1 0.5
Lessina 28 (G) *ethinyl estradiol+levonorgestrel*	20	0.1
Levlen 21, Levlen 28 (G) *ethinyl estradiol+levonorgestrel*	30	0.15
Levlite 28 (G) *ethinyl estradiol+levonorgestrel*	20	0.1
Levora-21, Levora-28 (G) *ethinyl estradiol+levonorgestrel*	30	0.15
Loestrin 21 1/20 (G) *ethinyl estradiol+norethindrone*	20	1

(*continued*)

Appendix G.3 (*continued*)

Combined Oral Contraceptive	Estrogen (mcg)	Progesterone (mg)
Loestrin 21 1.5/30 (G) *ethinyl estradiol+norethindrone*	30	1.5
Loestrin Fe 1/20 (G) *ethinyl estradiol+norethindrone* plus *ferrous fumarate* 75 mg	20	1
Loestrin Fe 1.5/30 (G) *ethinyl estradiol+norethindrone* plus *ferrous fumarate* 75 mg (4 tabs)	30	1.5
Loestrin 24 Fe (G) *ethinyl estradiol+norethindrone* plus *ferrous fumarate* 75 mg (4 tabs)	20	1
Lo Loestrin Fe *ethinyl estradiol+norethindrone* plus *ferrous fumarate* 75 mg (2 tabs)	10	1
Lomedia 24 Fe (G) *ethinyl estradiol+norethindrone* plus *ferrous fumarate* 75 mg	20	1
Lo/Ovral-21, Lo/Ovral-28 (G) *ethinyl estradiol+norgestrel*	30	0.3
Loryna *ethinyl estradiol+drospirenone*	20	3
Low-Ogestrel-21, Low-Ogestrel-28 (G) *ethinyl estradiol/norgestrel*	30	0.3
Lutera (G) *ethinyl estradiol+levonorgestrel*	20	0.1
Lybrel *ethinyl estradiol+levonorgestrel*	20	0.09
Mibelas 24 FE (G) *ethinyl estradiol+norethindrone* plus *ferrous fumarate* 75 mg	20	1
Microgestin 1/20 (G) *ethinyl estradiol+norethindrone*	20	1
Microgestin Fe 1/20 (G) *ethinyl estradiol+norethindrone* plus *ferrous fumarate* 75 mg	20	1
Microgestin 1.5/30 (G) *ethinyl estradiol+norethindrone*	30	1.5
Microgestin Fe 1.5/30 (G) *ethinyl estradiol+norethindrone* plus *ferrous fumarate* 75 mg	30	1.5
Mircette (G) *ethinyl estradiol+desogestrel diacetate*	20 10	0.15
Minastrin 24 FE (G) *ethinyl estradiol+norethindrone* plus *ferrous fumarate* 75 mg	20	1
Modicon 0.5/35-28 (G) *ethinyl estradiol+norethindrone*	35	0.5
MonoNessa (G) *ethinyl estradiol+norgestimate*	35	0.25

(*continued*)

Appendix G.3 (*continued*)

Combined Oral Contraceptive	Estrogen (mcg)	Progesterone (mg)
Natazia (G) *estradiol valerate+dienogest*	30 20 20 10	— 2 3 —
Necon 0.5/35-21, Necon 0.5/35-28 (G) *ethinyl estradiol+norethindrone*	35	0.5
Necon 1/35-21, Necon 1/35-28 (G) *ethinyl estradiol+norethindrone*	35	0.5
Necon 10/11-21, Necon 10/11-28 (G) *ethinyl estradiol+norethindrone*	35 35	0.5 1
Necon 1/50-21, Necon 1/50-28 (G) *mestranol+norethindrone*	50	1
Nelova 0.5/35-21, Nelova 0.5/35-28 (G) *ethinyl estradiol+norethindrone*	35	0.5
Nelova 1/35-21, Nelova 1/35-28 (G) *ethinyl estradiol+norethindrone*	35	1
Nelova 10/11-21, Nelova 10/11-28 (G) *ethinyl estradiol/norethindrone*	35 35	0.5 1
Nelova 1/50-21, Nelova 1/50-28 (G) *mestranol+norethindrone*	50	1
Neocon 7/7/7 (G) *ethinyl estradiol+norethindrone*	35 35 35	0.5 0.75 1
Nextstellis *estetrol+drospirenone* (*estetrol* is plant-derived estrogen)	14,200	3
Nordette-21, Nordette-28 (G) *ethinyl estradiol+levonorgestrel*	30	0.15
Norinyl 1/35-21, Norinyl 1/35-28 (G) *ethinyl estradiol+norethindrone*	35	1
Norinyl 1/50-21, Norinyl 1/50-28 (G) *mestranol+norethindrone*	50	1
Nortrel 0.5/35 (G) *ethinyl estradiol/norethindrone*	35	0.5
Nortrel 1/35-21, Nortrel 1/35-28 (G) *ethinyl estradiol+norethindrone*	35	1
Nortrel 7/7/7-28 (G) *ethinyl estradiol+norethindrone*	35 35 35	0.5 0.75 1
Ocella (G) *ethinyl estradiol+drospirenone*	30	3
Ortho-Cept 28 (G) *ethinyl estradiol+desogestrel*	30	0.15
Ortho-Cyclen 28 (G) *ethinyl estradiol+norgestimate*	35	0.25
Ortho-Novum 1/35-21, Ortho-Novum 1/35-28 (G) *ethinyl estradiol+norethindrone*	35	1
Ortho-Novum 1/50-21, Ortho-Novum 1/50-28 (G) *mestranol+norethindrone*	50	1

(*continued*)

Appendix G.3 (*continued*)

Combined Oral Contraceptive	Estrogen (mcg)	Progesterone (mg)
Ortho-Novum 7/7/7-28 (G) *ethinyl estradiol+norethindrone*	35 35 35	0.5 0.75 1
Ortho-Novum 10/11-28 *ethinyl estradiol+norethindrone*	35 35	0.5 1
Ortho Tri-Cyclen 21, Ortho Tri-Cyclen 28 (G) *ethinyl estradiol+norgestimate*	35 35 35	0.18 0.215 0.25
Ortho Tri-Cyclen Lo (G) *ethinyl estradiol+norgestimate*	25 25 25	0.18 0.215 0.25
Ovcon 35 Fe (G) *ethinyl estradiol+norethindrone* <u>plus</u> *ferrous fumarate 75* mg (4 tabs)	35	0.4
Ovcon 50-28, Ovcon 50-28 (G) *ethinyl estradiol+norethindrone*	50	1
Ovral-21, Ovral-28 (G) *ethinyl estradiol+norgestrel*	50	0.5
Portia (G) *ethinyl estradiol+levonorgestrel*	30	0.15
Previfem *ethinyl estradiol+norgestimate*	35	0.25
Quasense *ethinyl estradiol+levonorgestrel*	30	0.15
Rajani *ethinyl estradiol + drospirenone* <u>plus</u> *levomefolate calcium 0.451 mg*	20	3
Reclipsen (G) *ethinyl estradiol+desogestrel* <u>plus</u> *ferrous fumarate 75 mg (4 tabs)*	30	0.15
Safyral (G) *ethinyl estradiol+drospirenone* <u>plus</u> *levomefolate calcium 0.451 mg*	30	3
Sprintec 28 (G) *ethinyl estradiol+norgestimate*	35	0.25
Syeda *ethinyl estradiol+drospirenone*	30	3
Tarina Fe 1/20 (G) *ethinyl estradiol+norethindrone* <u>plus</u> *ferrous fumarate 75 mg (7 tabs)*	20	1
Taytulla Fe 1/20 (G) (softgel caps) *ethinyl estradiol+norethindrone* <u>plus</u> *ferrous fumarate 75* mg (4 softgel caps)	20	1
Tilia Fe (G) *ethinyl estradiol+norethindrone* <u>plus</u> *ferrous fumarate 75 mg (7 tabs)*	20 30 35	1 1 1
Tri-Legest 21 (G) *ethinyl estradiol+norethindrone*	20 30 35	1 1 1

(*continued*)

Appendix G.3 (*continued*)

Combined Oral Contraceptive	Estrogen (mcg)	Progesterone (mg)
Tri-Legest Fe (G) *ethinyl estradiol+norethindrone* plus *ferrous fumarate* 75 mg (7 tabs)	20 30 35	1 1 1
Tri-Levlen 21, Tri-Levlen 28 (G) *ethinyl estradiol+levonorgestrel*	30 40 30	0.05 0.075 0.125
Tri-Lo-Estarylla (G) *ethinyl estradiol+norgestimate*	25 25 25	0.18 0.215 0.25
Tri-Lo-Sprintec (G) *ethinyl estradiol+norgestimate*	25 25 25	0.18 0.215 0.25
TriNessa (G) *ethinyl estradiol+norgestimate*	35 35 35	0.18 0.215 0.25
Tri-Norinyl 21, Tri-Norinyl 28 (G) *ethinyl estradiol+norethindrone*	35 35 35	0.5 1 0.5
Triphasil-21, Triphasil-28 (G) *ethinyl estradiol+levonorgestrel*	30 40 30	0.050 0.075 0.125
Tri-Previfem (G) *ethinyl estradiol+norgestimate*	35 35 35	0.18 0.215 0.25
Tri-Sprintec (G) *ethinyl estradiol+norgestimate*	35 35 35	0.18 0.215 0.25
Trivora (G) *ethinyl estradiol+levonorgestrel*	30 40 30	0.05 0.075 0.125
Tydemy *ethinyl estradiol+drospirenone* plus *levomefolate calcium* 0.451 mg	30	3
Velivet (G) *ethinyl estradiol+desogestrel*	25 25 25	0.1 0.125 0.15
Vienva *ethinyl estradiol+levonorgestrel*	20	0.1
Yasmin (G) *ethinyl estradiol+drospirenone*	30	3
Yaz (G) *ethinyl estradiol+drospirenone*	20	3
Zovia 1/35E-28 (G) *ethinyl estradiol+ethynodiol diacetate*	35	1
Zovia 1/50E-28 (G) *ethinyl estradiol+ethynodiol diacetate*	50	1

APPENDIX G.4. EXTENDED-CYCLE ORAL CONTRACEPTIVES
91-Day

➤ *ethinyl estradiol+levonorgestrel* 1 tab daily x 91 days; repeat (no tablet-free days)
    Ashlyna (G) *Tab:* levonor 15 mcg+eth est 30 mcg (84)+eth est 10 mcg (7) (91 tabs/pck)
    Jolessa (G) *Tab:* levonor 15 mcg+eth est 30 mcg (84)+inert tabs (7) (91 tabs/pck)
    LoSeasonique (G) *Tab:* levonor 0.1 mcg+eth est 20 mcg (84)+eth est 10 mcg (7) (91 tabs/pck)
    Quartette (G) *Tab:* levonor 15 mcg+eth est 30 mcg (84)+eth est 10 mcg (7) (91 tabs/pck)

(*continued*)

Appendix G.4 (*continued*)

    Quasense (G) *Tab:* levonor 15 mcg+eth est 30 mcg (84)+inert tabs (7) (91 tabs/pck)
    Seasonale (G) *Tab:* levonor 15 mcg+eth est 30 mcg (84)+inert tabs (7) (91 tabs/pck)
    Seasonique (G) *Tab:* levonor 15 mcg+eth est 30 mcg (84)+eth est 10 mcg (7) (91 tabs/pck)
365-Day
▷ *ethinyl estradiol+levonorgestrel* 1 tab daily x 28 days; repeat (no tablet-free days)
    Lybrel *Tab:* levonor 0.09 mcg+eth est 20 mcg (28 tabs/pck)

APPENDIX G.5. PROGESTERONE-ONLY ORAL CONTRACEPTIVES ("MINI-PILL")

Brand	Progesterone	mcg
Comment: Take progestin-only pills at the same time each day (within a 3-hour time window). If a pill is missed, another method of contraception should be used for the remainder of the pill pack.		
Camila (G)	*norethindrone*	35
Errin (G)	*norethindrone*	35
Jolivette (G)	*norethindrone*	35
Micronor (G)	*norethindrone*	35
Nora-BE (G)	*norethindrone*	35
Nor-QD (G)	*norethindrone*	35
Ortho Micronor (G)	*norethindrone*	35
Ovrette (G)	*norgestrel*	7.5

APPENDIX G.7. TRANSDERMAL CONTRACEPTIVES

Ethinyl Estradiol+Norelgestromin
Comment: Apply the transdermal patch to the abdomen, buttock, upper-outer arm, <u>or</u> upper torso. *Do* <u>not</u> apply the transdermal patch to the breast. Rotate the site (however, may use the same anatomical area).

▷ *ethinyl estradiol+levonorgestrel* apply 1 patch once weekly x 3 weeks; then 1 patch-free week; then repeat
    sequence
        Twirla *Transdermal patch:* eth est 30 mcg+levo 120 mcg per day (1, 3/pck)

▷ *ethinyl estradiol+norelgestromin* (G) apply 1 patch once weekly x 3 weeks; then 1 patch-free week; then
    repeat sequence
        Ortho Evra *Transdermal patch:* eth est 20 mcg+norel 150 mcg per day (1, 3/pck)

APPENDIX G.8. CONTRACEPTIVE VAGINAL RINGS

Ethinyl Estradiol+Etonogestrel
Comment: The vaginal ring should be inserted prior to, <u>or</u> on the 5th day, of the menstrual cycle. Use of a backup method is recommended during the first week. When switching from oral contraceptives, the vaginal ring should be inserted anytime within 7 days after the last active tablet and no later than the day a new pill pack would have been started (no backup method is needed). If the ring is accidently expelled for less than 3 hours, it should be rinsed with cool-to-lukewarm water and reinserted promptly. If ring removal lasts for more than 3 hours, an additional contraceptive method should be used. If the ring is lost, a new ring should be inserted and the regimen continued without alteration.

▷ *etonogestrel+ethinyl estradiol* insert 1 ring vaginally and leave in place for 3 weeks; then remove for 1 ring-
    free week; then repeat
        EluRyng (G) *Vag ring:* eth est 2.7 mg (0.015 mg/day)+etonor 11.7 mg (0.12 mg/day) (1, 3/pck)
        (polymeric)
        NuvaRing (G) *Vag ring:* eth est 2.7 mg (0.015 mg/day)+etonor 11.7 mg (0.12 mg/day) (1, 3/pck)
        (polymeric)

▷ *segesterone acetate+ethinyl estradiol* insert 1 ring vaginally and leave in place for 3 weeks (21 on-days); then
    remove, clean, and store in the compact storage case suppled; after 7 off-days, clean and reinsert for the next
    21 on-day/7 off-day cycle; discard the ring after 13 cycles
        Annover *Vag ring:* eth est 17.4 mg (0.013 mg/day)+segest 103 mg (0.15 mg/day) (1/pck w. compact
        case) (silicone elastomer)
    Comment: Contraindications to **Annovera/NuvaRing** include co-administration with hepatitis C drug
    combinations containing *ombitasvir+paritaprevir+ritonavir*, with <u>or</u> without *dasabuvir*, age >35 years,

(*continued*)

Appendix G.8 (*continued*)

smoking, risk of arterial or venous thrombotic diseases, breast cancer or other estrogen or progestin-sensitive cancer, liver tumors or liver disease, acute hepatitis or cirrhosis, undiagnosed abnormal uterine bleeding, and pregnancy. Stop **Annovera/NuvaRing** at least 4 weeks before and through 2 weeks after major surgery. **Annovera/NuvaRing** are not recommended with breastfeeding. Start no earlier than 4 weeks after delivery in females who are not breastfeeding. Drugs or herbal products that induce certain enzymes, including CYP3A4, may decrease the effectiveness of **Annovera/NuvaRing** or increase breakthrough bleeding. Counsel patients to use a backup or alternative method of contraception when enzyme inducers are used.
Comment: NuvaRing is a polymeric vaginal ring containing 11.7 mg *etonogestrel* and 2.7 mg *ethinyl estradiol* which releases on average 0.12 mg/day of *etonogestrel* and 0.015 mg/day of *ethinyl estradiol*. Do not reuse **NuvaRing** (discard after 3 weeks in-use and, after 7 days, start the next cycle with a new **NuvaRing**).
Comment: The Annovera vaginal system (ring) is a silicone elastomer vaginal system containing 103 mg *segesterone acetate* and 17.4 mg *ethinyl estradiol* which releases on average 0.15 mg/day of *segesterone acetate* and 0.013 mg/day of *ethinyl estradiol*. Annovera is the first and only vaginal system/ring that provides contraception for 13 cycles. The removed vaginal system should be cleaned with mild soap and warm water, patted dry with a clean cloth towel or paper towel, and stored in the case provided during the 1-week dose-free interval. At the end of the dose-free interval, the vaginal system should be cleaned prior to being placed back in the vagina for the next cycle.

APPENDIX G.9. SUBDERMAL CONTRACEPTIVES
Comment: Implants must be inserted within 7 days of the onset of menses. A complete physical examination is required annually. Remove if pregnancy, thromboembolic disorder including thrombophlebitis, jaundice, and visual disturbances. Not for use by patients with hypertension, diabetes, hyperlipidemia, impaired liver function, epilepsy, asthma, migraine, depression, cardiac or renal insufficiency, thromboembolic disorder including thrombophlebitis, prolonged immobilization, or who are smokers.

➤ *etonogestrel* implant rod subdermally in the upper inner non-dominant arm; remove and replace at the end of 3 years
 Implanon, Nexplanon
  Implantable rod: 68 mg implant for subdermal insertion (w. insertion device; latex-free)
➤ *levonorgestrel* implant rods subdermally in the upper inner non-dominant arm; remove and replace at the end of 5 years
 Norplant
  Implantable rods: 6-36 mg implants (total 216 mg) for subdermal insertion (1 kit w. sterile supplies)

APPENDIX G.10. INTRAUTERINE CONTRACEPTIVES
Comment: Indicated in women who have had at least one child and who are in a stable, mutually monogamous relationship. Reexamine after menses within 3 months (recommend 4-6 weeks) to check placement.

➤ *levonorgestrel*
 Kyleena *IUD:* 19.5 mg (replace at least every 5 years)
 Liletta *IUD:* 52 mg (replace at least every 8 years)
 Mirena *IUD:* 52 mg (replace at least every 6 years)
 Skyla *IUD:* 13.5 mg (replace at least every 3 years)

APPENDIX G.11. EMERGENCY CONTRACEPTION
Comment: Emergency contraception must be started within 72 hours after unprotected intercourse following a negative urine human chorionic gonadotropin (hCG) pregnancy test. If vomiting occurs within 1 hour of taking a dose, repeat the dose.

➤ *ethinyl estradiol+levonorgestrel* 2 tabs as soon as possible after unprotected intercourse or contraceptive failure, then 2 more 12 hours after the first dose
Premenarchal: not applicable
 Preven *Tab:* eth est 50 mcg+levonor 250 mcg (4/pck) plus 1 hCG home pregnancy test
 Yuzpe Regimen *Tab:* eth est 50 mcg+levonor 250 mcg (4/pck)
➤ *levonorgestrel* (OTC)(G) 1 tab as soon as possible, within 72 hours, after unprotected sex or suspected contraceptive failure
Premenarchal: not applicable; <17 years (prescription required); ≥17 years (OTC)
 EContra EZ *Tab:* 1.5 mg single-dose
 My Way *Tab:* 1.5 mg single-dose
 Plan B One Step *Tab:* 1.5 mg single-dose
 EContra EZ *Tab:* 1.5 mg single-dose
 Preventeza *Tab:* 1.5 mg single-dose

(*continued*)

Appendix G.11 (*continued*)

▶ *ulipristal* (G) take 1 tab as soon as possible within 120 hours (5 days) after unprotected intercourse <u>or</u> contraceptive failure; may repeat dose if vomiting occurs within 3 hours
Pediatric: premenarchal: <u>not</u> applicable
   ella *Tab:* 30 mg (1/pck)
   Logilia *Tab:* 30 mg (1/pck)

APPENDIX J. TOPICAL CORTICOSTEROIDS BY POTENCY

Comment: All topical, oral, and parenteral corticosteroids are pregnancy category C. Use with caution in infants and children. Steroids should be applied sparingly and for the shortest time necessary. Do <u>not</u> use in the diaper area. Do <u>not</u> use an occlusive dressing. Systemic absorption of topical corticosteroids can induce reversible hypothalamic–pituitary–adrenal (HPA) axis suppression with the potential for clinical glucocorticoid insufficiency.

Potency guide: Face: low potency
                  Ears/Scalp margin: Intermediate potency
                  Eyelids: hydrocortisone in ophthalmic ointment base 1%
                  Chest/Back: intermediate potency
                  Skin folds: low potency

Generic Name and Pregnancy Category	Brands, Formulation, and Dosing Frequency	Strength and Volume
Low Potency		
alclometasone dipropionate	**Aclovate** Crm bid-tid **Aclovate** Oint bid-tid	0.05% (15, 45, 60 gm) 0.05% (15, 45, 60 gm)
fluocinolone acetonide	**Synalar** Crm bid-qid	0.025% (15, 60 gm)
hydrocortisone base <u>or</u> *acetate* (G)	**Anusol-HC** Crm bid-qid **Hytone** Crm bid-qid **Hytone** Oint bid-qid **Hytone** Lotn bid-qid	2.5% (30 gm) 1% (1, 2 oz) 1% (1 oz) 1% (2 oz)
	Hytone Crm bid-qid **Hytone** Oint bid-qid **Hytone** Lotn bid-qid **U-cort** Crm bid-qid	2.5% (1, 2 oz) 2.5% (1 oz) 2.5% (1 oz) 1% (7, 28, 35 gm)
triamcinolone acetonide (G)	**Kenalog** Crm bid-qid **Kenalog** Lotn bid-qid **Kenalog** Oint bid-qid	0.025% (15, 80 gm) 0.025% (60 ml) 0.025% (15, 60, 80 gm)
Intermediate Potency		
betamethasone valerate (G)	**Luxiq** Foam bid	0.12% (100 gm)
clocortolone pivalate (G)	**Cloderm** Crm bid	0.1% (30, 45, 75, 90 gm)
desonide (G)	**Desonate** Gel/Formulation bid-tid **DesOwen** Crm bid-tid **DesOwen** Lotn bid-tid **DesOwen** Oint bid-tid **Tridesilon** Crm bid-qid **Tridesilon** Oint bid-qid **Verdeso** Foam	0.05% (15, 60 gm) 0.05% (15, 60 gm) 0.05% (2, 4 fl oz) 0.05% (15, 60 gm) 0.05% (15, 60 gm) 0.05% (15, 60 gm)
desoximetasone (G)	**Topicort-LP** Emol Crm bid	0.05% (15, 60 gm; 4 oz)
fluocinolone acetonide (G)	**Capex** Shampoo **Derma-Smoothe/FS** Oil tid **Derma-Smoothe/FS** Shampoo **Synalar** Crm bid-qid **Synalar** Oint bid-qid	0.01% (4 oz) 0.01% (4 oz) 0.01% (4 oz) 0.025% (15, 30, 60 gm) 0.025% (15, 60 gm)

(*continued*)

Appendix J (*continued*)

Generic Name and Pregnancy Category	Brands, Formulation, and Dosing Frequency	Strength and Volume
flurandrenolide (G)	**Cordran SP** Crm bid-tid **Cordran** Oint bid-tid **Cordran SP** Crm bid-tid **Cordran** Lotn bid-tid **Cordran** Oint bid-tid	0.025% (30, 60 gm) 0.025% (30, 60 gm) 0.05% (15, 30, 60 gm) 0.05% (15, 60 ml) 0.05% (15, 30, 60 gm)
fluticasone propionate (G)	**Cutivate** Oint bid **Cutivate** Crm qd-bid **Cutivate** Lotn qd-bid	0.005% (15, 30, 60 gm) 0.05% (15, 30, 60 gm) 0.05%
hydrocortisone probutate	**Pandel** Crm qd-bid	0.1% (15, 45 gm)
hydrocortisone butyrate (G)	**Locoid** Crm bid-tid **Locoid** Oint bid-tid **Locoid** Soln bid-tid	0.1% (15, 45 gm) 0.1% (15, 45 gm) 0.1% (30, 60 ml)
hydrocortisone valerate (G)	**Westcort** Crm bid-tid **Westcort** Oint bid-tid	0.2% (15, 45, 60, 120 gm) 0.2% (15, 45, 60 gm)
mometasone furoate	**Elocon** Crm qd **Elocon** Lotn qd **Elocon** Oint qd	0.1% (15, 45 gm) 0.1% (30, 60 ml) 0.1% (15, 45 gm)
prednicarbate	**Dermatop** Emol Crm bid **Dermatop** Oint bid	0.1% (15, 60 gm)
triamcinolone acetonide (G)	**Kenalog** Crm bid-tid **Kenalog** Lotn bid-tid **Kenalog** Emul Spray bid-tid	0.1% (15, 60, 80 gm) 0.1% (60 ml) 0.2% (63, 100 gm)
High Potency		
amcinonide (G)	Crm bid-tid Lotn bid Oint bid	0.1% (15, 30, 60 gm) 0.1% (20, 60 ml) 0.1% (15, 30, 60 gm)
betamethasone dipropionate	**Sernivo Spray** Emul Spray bid	0.05% (60, 120 ml)
betamethasone dipropionate, augmented	**Diprolene AF** Emol Crm qd-bid **Diprolene** Lotn qd-bid	0.05% (15, 50 gm) 0.05% (30, 60 ml)
clobetasol propionate (G)	**Bryhali** Lotn bid **Impoyz** Crm bid	0.01% (60, 112 gm) 0.025% (60, 112 gm)
desoximetasone (G)	**Topicort** Gel bid **Topicort** Emol Crm bid **Topicort** Oint bid	0.05% (15, 60 gm) 0.25% (15, 60 gm) 0.25% (15, 60 gm)
diflorasone diacetate	**Psorcon E** Emol Crm bid **Psorcon E** Emol Oint qd-tid	0.05% (15, 30, 60 gm) 0.05% (15, 30, 60 gm)
fluocinonide	**Lidex** Crm bid-qid **Lidex** Gel bid-qid **Lidex** Oint bid-qid **Lidex** Soln bid-qid **Lidex-E** Emol Crm bid-qid	0.05% (15, 30, 60, 120 gm) 0.05% (15, 30, 60 gm) 0.05% (15, 30, 60, 120 gm) 0.05% (20, 60 ml) 0.05% (15, 30, 60 gm)
flurandrenolide	**Cordran** Oint bid-tid **Cordran** Crm bid-tid	0.05% (15, 30, 60 gm) 0.025% (30, 60, 120 gm) 0.05% (15, 30, 60, 120 gm)

(*continued*)

Appendix J (*continued*)

Generic Name and Pregnancy Category	Brands, Formulation, and Dosing Frequency	Strength and Volume
halcinonide	Halog Crm bid-tid Halog Oint bid-tid Halog Soln bid-tid Halog-E Emol Crm qd-tid	0.1% (15, 30, 60, 240 gm) 0.1% (15, 30, 60, 120 gm) 0.1% (20, 60 ml) 0.1% (15, 30, 60 gm)
triamcinolone acetonide (G)	Kenalog Crm bid-tid	0.5% (20 gm)
Super High Potency		
betamethasone dipropionate, augmented (G)	Diprolene Oint qd-bid Diprolene Gel qd-bid	0.05% (15, 50 gm) 0.05% (15, 50 gm)
clobetasol propionate (G)	Bryhali Lotn bid Clobex Shampoo daily Clobex Spray bid Cormax Oint bid Cormax Scalp App Olux Foam Olux E Foam Temovate Crm bid Temovate Gel bid Temovate Oint bid	0.01% (60, 112 gm) 0.05% (4 oz) 0.05% (2, 4.5 oz) 0.05% (15, 45 gm) 0.05% (15, 45 gm) 0.05% (50, 100 gm) 0.05% (50, 100 gm) 0.05% (15, 30, 45, 60 gm) 0.05% (15, 30, 60 gm) 0.05% (15, 30, 45, 60 gm)
	Temovate Scalp App bid Temovate-E Emol Crm bid	0.05% (25, 50 ml) 0.05% (15, 30, 60 gm)
fluocinonide (G)	Vanos Oint qd-tid	0.1% (30, 60, 120 gm)
flurandrenolide	Cordran Tape q 12 hours	4 mcg/cm^2 (roll of 3″ x 80″)
halobetasol propionate	Ultravate Crm qd-bid Ultravate Oint qd-bid	0.05% (15, 45 gm) 0.05% (15, 45 gm)

APPENDIX K. ORAL CORTICOSTEROIDS

Comment: Systemic corticosteroids increase glucose intolerance, reduce the action of insulin and oral hypoglycemic agents, reduce adrenal cortex activity, decrease immunity, mask signs of infection, impair wound healing, suppress growth in children, and promote osteoporosis, fluid retention, and weight gain. Use systemic steroids with caution, using the lowest possible dose to affect clinical response, and withdraw (wean) gradually in tapering doses to avoid adrenal insufficiency. The American Academy of Rheumatology (AAR) recommends the following daily doses for anyone on a chronic systemic corticosteroid regimen: calcium 1,200-1,500 mg/day and vitamin D 800-1,000 IU/day.

Oral Corticosteroids

▷ *betamethasone* (G) initially 0.6-7.2 mg daily
   Pediatric: <12 years: <u>not</u> recommended; ≥12 years: same as adult
      Celestone *Tab:* 0.6 mg; *Syr:* 0.6 mg/5 ml (120 ml)

▷ *cortisone* (G) initially 25-300 mg daily <u>or</u> every other day
   Pediatric: <12 years: <u>not</u> recommended; ≥12 years: same as adult
      Cortone Acetate *Tab:* 25 mg

▷ *dexamethasone* (G) initially 0.75-9 mg/day
   Pediatric: <12 years: <u>not</u> recommended; ≥12 years: same as adult
      Decadron *Tab:* 0.5*, 0.75*, 4*mg; *Syr:* 0.5 mg/5 ml (100 ml)
      Decadron 5-12 Pak *Tabs:* 0.75*mg (12/pck)

▷ *hydrocortisone* (G) 20-240 mg daily
   Pediatric: <12 years: 2-8 mg/day; ≥12 years: same as adult
      Cortef *Tab:* 5, 10, 20 mg; *Oral susp:* 10 mg/5 ml
      Hydrocortone *Tab:* 10 mg

(*continued*)

Appendix K (*continued*)

▷ *methylprednisolone* (G) 4-48 mg/day
　　Pediatric: <12 years: not recommended; ≥12 years: same as adult
　　　　Medrol *Tab:* 2*, 4*, 8*, 16*, 24*, 32*mg
　　　　Medrol Dosepak *Dosepak:* 4*mg tabs (21/pck)

▷ *prednisolone* (G) initially 5-60 mg/day in 1-2 doses x 3-5 days
　　Pediatric: 0.14-2 mg/kg/day in 3-4 doses x 3-5 days
　　　　Flo-Pred *Susp:* 5, 15 mg/5 ml
　　　　Orapred *Soln:* 15 mg/5 ml (grape) (dye-free, alcohol 2%)
　　　　Orapred ODT *Tab:* 10, 15, 30 mg orally disintegrating (grape)
　　　　Pediapred *Soln:* 5 mg/5 ml (raspberry) (sugar-, alcohol-, dye-free)
　　　　Prelone *Syr:* 15 mg/5 ml
　　　　Comment: Flo-Pred does not require refrigeration or shaking prior to use.

▷ *prednisone* (G) initially 5-60 mg/day in 1-2 doses x 3-5 days
　　Pediatric: 0.14-2 mg/kg/day in 3-4 doses x 3-5 days
　　　　Deltasone *Tab:* 2.5*, 5*, 10*, 20*, 50*mg

▷ *prednisone (delayed release)* (G) initially 5-60 mg/day in 1-2 doses x 3-5 days
　　Pediatric: 0.14-2 mg/kg/day in 3-4 doses x 3-5 days
　　　　Rayos *Tab:* 1, 2, 5 mg del-rel

▷ *triamcinolone* (G) initially 4-48 mg/day in 1-2 doses x 3-5 days
　　Pediatric: 0.14-2 mg/kg/day in 3-4 doses x 3-5 days
　　　　Aristocort *Tab:* 4*mg
　　　　Aristocort Forte *Susp:* 40 mg/ml (benzoyl alcohol)
　　　　Aristocort Aristopak *Tab:* 4*mg (16/pck)

APPENDIX L. PARENTERAL CORTICOSTEROIDS

Comment: Systemic glucocorticosteroids increase glucose intolerance, reduce the action of insulin and oral hypoglycemic agents, reduce adrenal cortex activity, decrease immunity, mask signs of infection, impair wound healing, suppress growth in children, and promote osteoporosis, fluid retention, and weight gain. Use systemic steroids with caution, using the lowest possible dose to affect clinical response, and withdraw (wean) gradually in tapering doses to avoid adrenal insufficiency. The American Academy of Rheumatology (AAR) recommends the following daily doses for anyone on a chronic systemic corticosteroid regimen: calcium 1,200-1,500 mg/day and vitamin D 800-1,000 IU/day.

▷ *betamethasone* (G)
　　　　Celestone 0.5-9 mg IM/IV x 1 dose
　　　　　Vial: 3 mg/ml (10 ml)
　　　　Celestone Soluspan 0.5-9 mg IM/IV x 1 dose; usual IM dose 6 mg
　　　　　Vial: 6 mg/ml (10 ml)

▷ *cortisone* (G) 20-300 mg IM
　　Pediatric: <12 years: not recommended; ≥12 years: same as adult
　　　　Cortone Acetate *Vial:* 50 mg/ml (10 ml)

▷ *dexamethasone* (G) initially 0.5-9 mg IM/IV daily
　　Pediatric: <12 years: not recommended; ≥12 years: same as adult
　　　　Decadron *Vial:* 4, 24 mg/ml for IM use (5 ml, sulfites)
　　　　Dalalone D.P. *Vial:* 16 mg/ml (1, 5 ml)
　　　　Decadron-LA *Vial:* 8 mg/ml (1, 5 ml)

▷ *hydrocortisone* (G) initially 100-500 mg IM/IV daily
　　Pediatric: 2-8 mg/kg loading dose (max 250 mg); then 8 mg/kg/day
　　　　Hydrocortone *Vial:* 50 mg/ml (5 ml)
　　　　Solu-Cortef *Vial:* 100 mg (2 ml), 250 mg (2 ml), 500 mg (4 ml), 1 gm (8 ml)

▷ *hydrocortisone phosphate* (G) for IM, IV, and SC injection
　　Pediatric: <12 years: not recommended; ≥12 years: same as adult
　　　　Hydrocortone *Vial:* 50 mg/ml (2 ml)

▷ *methylprednisolone* (G) 40-120 mg IM/week for 1-4 weeks
　　Pediatric: <12 years: not recommended; ≥12 years: same as adult
　　　　Depo-Medrol *Vial:* 20 mg/ml (5 ml), 40 mg/ml (5, 10 ml), 80 mg/ml (5 ml)

▷ *methylprednisolone sodium succinate* (G) 10-40 mg IV initially; then IM or IV
　　Pediatric: 1-2 mg/kg loading dose; then 1.6 mg/kg/day in divided doses at least 6 hours apart
　　　　Solu-Medrol *Vial:* 40 mg (1 ml), 125 mg (2 ml), 500 mg (4 ml), 1 g (8 ml), 2 g (8 ml)

(*continued*)

Appendix L (*continued*)

▷ **triamcinolone** (G) 40 mg IM/week
  Pediatric: <12 years: not recommended; ≥12 years: same as adult
    Aristocort *Vial:* 25 mg/ml (5 ml)
    Aristocort Forte *Vial:* 40 mg/ml (1, 5 ml) (*do not administer IV*)
    Aristospan *Vial:* 5 mg/ml (5 ml), 20 mg/ml (1, 5 ml)
    TAC-3 *Vial:* 3 mg/ml (5 ml) for intralesional and intradermal use

Injectable Corticosteroid/Anesthetic

▷ **dexamethasone/lidocaine** 0.1-0.75 ml into painful area
    Decadron Phosphate with Xylocaine *Vial:* dexa 4 mg/lido 10 mg per ml (5 ml)

APPENDIX M. INHALATIONAL CORTICOSTEROIDS

Comment: Inhaled corticosteroids are indicated for the long-term control of asthma. Inhaled corticosteroids are not indicated for exercise-induced asthma or for relief of acute symptoms (i.e., "rescue"). Low doses are indicated for mild persistent asthma, medium doses are indicated for moderate persistent asthma, and high doses are reserved for severe cases. Titrate to lowest effective dose. To reduce the potential for adverse effects with inhalers, the patient should use a spacer or holding chamber and rinse the mouth and spit after every inhalation treatment. Linear growth should be monitored in children. When inhaled doses exceed 1,000 mcg/day, consider supplements of calcium (1-1.5 gm/day) and vitamin D (400 IU/day).

▷ **beclomethasone**
  Beclovent 2 inhalations tid-qid or 4 inhalations bid; max 20 inhalations/day
  Pediatric: <6 years: not recommended; 6-12 years: 1-2 inhalations tid-qid or 4 inhalations bid; max 10 inhalations/day
    Inhaler: 42 mcg/actuation (6.7 g, 80 inh; 16.8 g, 200 inh)
  Qvar *Previously using only bronchodilators:* initiate 40-80 mcg bid, max 320 mcg/day; *previously using an inhaled corticosteroid:* initiate 40-160 mcg bid; max 320 mcg/day; *Previously taking a systemic corticosteroid:* attempt to wean off the systemic drug after approximately 1 week after initiating **Qvar**
  Pediatric: <12 years: not recommended; ≥12 years: same as adult
    Inhaler: 40, 80 mcg/actuation metered-dose aerosol w. dose counter (8.7 g, 120 inh) (chlorofluorocarbon [CFC]-free)
  Vanceril 2 inhalations tid to qid or 4 inhalations bid
  Pediatric: <6 years: not recommended; 6-12 years: 1-2 inhalations tid to qid
    Inhaler: 42 mcg/actuation (16.8 g, 200 inh)
  Vanceril Double Strength 2 inhalations bid
  Pediatric: <6 years: not recommended; 6-12 years: 1-2 inhalations bid; >12 years: same as adult
    Inhaler: 84 mcg/actuation (12.2 g, 120 inh)

▷ **budesonide** (G)
  Pulmicort Respules use turbuhaler
  Pediatric: <12 months: not recommended; ≥12 months to 8 years: *Previously using only bronchodilators:* initiate 0.5 mg/day once daily or in 2 divided doses; may start at 0.25 mg/day; *Previously using inhaled corticosteroids:* initiate 0.5 mg/day daily or in 2 divided doses; max 1 mg/day; *Previously using oral corticosteroids:* initiate 1 mg/day daily or in 2 divided doses
    Inhal susp: 0.25 mg/2 ml (30/box)
  Pulmicort Turbuhaler 1-2 inhalations bid; *Previously on oral corticosteroids:* 2-4 inhalations bid
  Pediatric: <6 years: not recommended; 6-12 years: 1-2 inhalations bid; >12 years: same as adult
    Turbuhaler: 200 mcg/actuation (200 inh)

▷ **flunisolide** (G)
  AeroBid, AeroBid M initially 2 inhalations bid; max 8 inhalations/day
  Pediatric: <6 years: not recommended; 6-15 years: 2 inhalations bid; ≥16 years: same as adult
    Inhaler: 250 mcg/actuation (7 gm, 100 inh)

▷ **fluticasone** (G)
  Flovent HFA initially 88 mcg bid; *If previously using an inhaled corticosteroid:* initially 88-220 mcg bid; *If previously taking an oral corticosteroid:* initially 880 mcg/day
  Pediatric: use **Rotadisk:** initially 50-88 mcg inh bid; <4 years: not recommended; 4-11 years: initially 50-88 mcg bid; >11 years: initially 100 mcg bid; if previously using an inhaled corticosteroid, initially 100-200 mcg bid; *Previously taking an oral corticosteroid,* initially 1,000 mcg bid
    Inhaler: 44 mcg/actuation (7.9 g, 60 inh; 13 g, 120 inh), 110 mcg/actuation (13 g, 120 inh), 220 mcg/actuation (13 g, 120 inh)

(continued)

Appendix M (*continued*)

    Rotadisk 50 mcg/actuation (60 blisters/disk), 100 mcg/actuation (60 blisters/disk), 250 mcg/actuation (60 blisters/disk)
    Pediatric: <12 years: <u>not</u> recommended; ≥12 years: same as adult

▶ **mometasone furoate** *Previously using a bronchodilator <u>or</u> inhaled corticosteroid: 220 mcg q PM <u>or</u> bid, max 440 mcg q PM <u>or</u> 220 mcg bid; Previously using an oral corticosteroid: 440 mcg bid, max 880 mcg/day*
    Pediatric: <12 years: <u>not</u> recommended; ≥12 years: same as adult
    Asmanex Twisthaler *Inhaler:* 220 mcg/actuation (6.7 gm, 80 inh; 16.8 gm, 200 inh)

APPENDIX N. ANTIARRHYTHMIA DRUGS

Antiarrhythmics by Classification With Dose Forms		
Brand/Generic and Pregnancy Category	**Class and Indication(s)**	**Dose Form(s)**
Betapace *sotalol*	*Class:* Class II and III Antiarrhythmic *Indications:* Documented life-threatening ventricular arrhythmias	*Tab:* 80*, 120*, 160*, 240*mg
Betapace AF *sotalol*	*Class:* Class II and III Antiarrhythmic *Indications:* Maintenance of normal sinus rhythm in patients with highly symptomatic atrial fibrillation <u>or</u> atrial flutter who are currently in sinus rhythm	*Tab:* 80*, 120*, 160*mg
Calan *verapamil* **(G)**	*Class:* Calcium Channel Blocker *Indications:* Control (with *digitalis*) of ventricular rate in patients with chronic atrial fibrillation <u>or</u> atrial flutter; prophylaxis of repetitive paroxysmal supraventricular tachycardia	*Tab:* 40, 80*, 120*mg
Cordarone *amiodarone* **(G)**	*Class:* Class III Antiarrhythmic *Indications:* Documented life-threatening recurrent refractory ventricular fibrillation <u>or</u> hemodynamically unstable ventricular tachycardia	*Tab:* 200*mg
Quinidex *quinidine sulfate* **(G)**	*Class:* Class I Antiarrhythmic *Indications:* Atrial and ventricular arrhythmias	*Tab:* 300 mg ext-rel
Inderal *propranolol* **(G)** Inderal XL *propranolol* ext-rel **(G)** InnoPran XL *Propranolol ext-rel*	*Class:* Beta-Blocker *Indications:* Atrial and ventricular arrhythmias; tachyarrhythmias due to *digitalis* intoxication; reduce mortality and risk of reinfarction in stabilized patients after myocardial infarction	*Tab:* 10*, 20*, 40*, 60*, 80* mg *Cap:* 60, 80, 120, 160 mg sust-rel *Cap:* 80, 120 mg ext-rel
Mexitil *mexiletine*	*Class:* Class IB Antiarrhythmic *Indications:* Documented life-threatening ventricular arrhythmias	*Cap:* 150, 200, 250 mg
Multaq *dronedarone*	*Class:* IB Antiarrhythmic *Indications:* Paroxysmal <u>or</u> persistent atrial fibrillation <u>or</u> atrial flutter	*Tab:* 400 mg
Norpace *disopyramide*	*Class:* Class I Antiarrhythmic *Indications:* Documented life-threatening ventricular arrhythmias	*Cap:* 100, 150 mg
Procanbid *procainamide* **(G)**	*Class:* Class IA Antiarrhythmic *Indications:* Life-threatening ventricular arrhythmias	*Tab:* 500, 1,000 mg ext-rel
Quinaglute *quinidine gluconate* **(G)**	*Class:* Class I Antiarrhythmic *Indications:* Atrial and ventricular arrhythmias	*Tab:* 324 mg ext-rel
Rythmol *propafenone* **(G)**	*Class:* Class IC Antiarrhythmic *Indications:* Documented life-threatening ventricular arrhythmias, prolonged recurrence of paroxysmal atrial fibrillation, <u>and/or</u> atrial flutter <u>or</u> paroxysmal supraventricular tachycardia associated with disabling symptoms in patients without structural heart disease	*Tab:* 150*, 225*, 300*mg *Cap:* 225, 325, 425 mg ext-rel

(continued)

Appendix N (*continued*)

Antiarrhythmics by Classification With Dose Forms		
Brand/Generic and Pregnancy Category	**Class and Indication(s)**	**Dose Form(s)**
Sectral *acebutolol* (G)	*Class:* Beta-Blocker *Indications:* Ventricular arrhythmias	*Cap:* 200, 400 mg
Sotylize *sotalol*	*Class:* Class II and III Antiarrhythmic *Indications:* Documented life-threatening ventricular arrhythmias, and highly symptomatic A-flutter/A-fib	*Oral soln:* 5 mg/ml
Tambocor *flecainide acetate* (G)	*Class:* Class IC Antiarrhythmic *Indications:* Documented life-threatening ventricular arrhythmias; paroxysmal atrial fibrillation and/or atrial flutter or paroxysmal supraventricular tachycardia in patients without structural heart disease	*Tab:* 50, 100*, 150* mg
Tenormin *atenolol* (G)	*Class:* Beta-Blocker *Indications:* Reduce mortality and in stabilized patients after myocardial infarction	*Tab:* 25, 50, 100 mg *Inj:* 5 mg/ml (10 ml) for IV administration
timolol maleate (G)	*Class:* Beta-Blocker *Indications:* Reduce mortality and in stabilized patients after myocardial infarction	*Tab:* 5, 10*, 20*mg
dofetilide (G)	*Class:* Class III Antiarrhythmic *Indications:* Maintenance of normal sinus rhythm in patients with atrial fibrillation or atrial flutter of >1 week duration who were converted to normal sinus rhythm (only for highly symptomatic patients); conversion to normal sinus rhythm	*Cap:* 125, 250, 500 mcg
Tonocard *tocainide* (G)	*Class:* Class I Antiarrhythmic *Indications:* Documented life-threatening ventricular arrhythmias	*Tab:* 400*, 600*mg
Toprol XL *metoprolol* (G)	*Class:* Beta-Blocker *Indications:* Ischemic, hypertensive, or cardiomyopathic heart failure	*Tab:* 25*, 50*, 100*, 200*mg

APPENDIX O. ANTINEOPLASIA DRUGS

Comment: A new lab test offers potential for early detection of multiple cancer types with a single blood sample. Researchers studied 1,005 persons with non-metastatic, clinically detected, stage 2 and 3 cancers of the ovary, liver, stomach, pancreas, esophagus, colorectum, lung, or breast. The blood test, CancerSEEK, accurately identified cancer cases 33%-98% (M = 70%) of the time in the study cohort, with accuracy reportedly 69%-98% for the five cancers that currently have no widely used screening test: ovarian, pancreatic, stomach, liver, and esophageal cancers. CancerSEEK combines tests that look for 16 genes and 10 proteins (mutations in cell-free DNA) linked to cancer. The researchers also tested blood samples from 812 healthy people to see how often the test gave false-positive results and were reported to be less than 1%. These findings represent a promising future for screening and early detection of cancer in asymptomatic persons. Optimally, cancers would be detected early enough that they could be cured by surgery alone, but even cancers that are not curable by surgery alone will respond better to systemic therapies when there is less advanced disease.

Anne Marie Lennon, MD, PhD, Johns Hopkins Kimmel Cancer Center, Baltimore, and Len Lichtenfeld, MD, Deputy Chief Medical Officer, American Cancer Society, Atlanta. Online and print announcements, January 2018: PR Newswire, Science, U.S. News & World Report, Los Angeles Times, Forbes, The Guardian, Chicago Tribune

REFERENCE
Cohen, J. D., Li, L., Wang, Y., Thoburn, C., Afsari, B., Danilova, L., et al. (2018). Detection and localization of surgically resectable cancers with a multi-analyte blood test. *Science, 359*(6378), 926–930. doi:10.1126/science.aar3247

Appendix O (*continued*)

Antineoplastics With Classification and Dose Forms		
Brand, Generic, and Pregnancy Category	**Class and Indications**	**Dose Form(s)**
Adstiladrin *nadofaragene firadenovec-vncg*		
Adcetris *brentuximab vedotin*	CD30-Directed Antibody-Drug Conjugate	*Vial:* 50 mg single-use, pwdr for reconstitution
Afinitor *everolimus*	Kinase Inhibitor	*Tab:* 2.5, 5, 7.5, 10 mg
Afinitor Disperz *everolimus*	Kinase Inhibitor	*Tab:* 2, 3, 5 mg for oral suspension
Alecensa *alectinib*	Kinase Inhibitor	*Cap:* 150 mg
Alimta *pemetrexed* (G)	Folate Analog Metabolic Inhibitor	*Vial:* 100, 500 mg, single-dose, pwdr for reconstitution, dilution, and IV infusion
Aliqopa *copanlisib*	Kinase Inhibitor	*Vial:* 60 mg pwdr for injection, single-dose
Alkeran *melphalan* (G)	Alkylating Agent	*Tab:* 2*mg
Alunbrig *brigatinib*	Kinase Inhibitor	*Tab:* 30, 90, 180 mg
Arimidex *anastrozole*	Aromatase Inhibitor	*Tab:* 1 mg
Aromasin *exemestane*	Aromatase Inactivator	*Tab:* 25 mg
Arranon *nelarabine* (G)	Nucleoside Analog	*Vial:* 250 mg/50 ml (5 mg/ml) single-dose, soln for dilution and IV infusion
Arzerra *ofatumumab*	CD20-Directed Cytolytic Monoclonal Antibody	*Vial:* 100 mg/5 ml (20 mg/ml), single-use soln (3, 10 vials/carton with 2 filters)(preservative-free)(latex-free)
Asparlas *calaspargase pegol-mknl*	Asparagine-Specific Enzyme	*Vial:* 3750 units/5 ml (750 units/ml, 5 ml), single-dose' soln for dilution and IV infusion
Avastin *bevacizumab*	Vascular Endothelial Growth Factor (VEGF) Inhibitor	*Vial:* 100 mg/4 ml (25 mg/ml), 400 mg/16 ml (25 mg/ml), single-dose, soln for dilution and IV infusion
Ayvakit *avapritinib*	Kinase Inhibitor	*Tab:* 100, 200, 300 mg
Azedra *iobenguane I[131]*	Radioactive Therapeutic Agent	*Vial:* 555 MBq/ml (15 mCi/ml), single-dose, soln for dilution and IV infusion
Balversa *erdafitinib*	Kinase Inhibitor	*Tab:* 3, 4, 5 mg
Bavencio *avelumab*	Programmed Death Ligand-1 (PD-L1) Blocking Antibody	*Vial:* 200 mg/10 ml (20 mg/ml), single-dose, soln for dilution and IV infusion

(*continued*)

Appendix O (*continued*)

Antineoplastics With Classification and Dose Forms		
Brand, Generic, and Pregnancy Category	Class and Indications	Dose Form(s)
Besponsa *inotuzumab ozogamicin*	CD22-Directed Antibody-Drug Drug Conjugate Mixture of	*Vial:* 0.9 mg, single-dose pwdr for reconstitution, dilution, and IV infusion
Bevyxxa *betrixaban*	Factor Xa (FXa) Inhibitor	*Cap:* 40, 80 mg
Blenrep *belantamab mafodotin-blmf*	B-Cell Maturation Antigen (BCMA)-Directed Antibody and Microtubule Inhibitor Conjugate	*Vial:* 100 mg, single-dose pwdr for reconstitution, dilution, and IV infusion
bleomycin sulfate (G)	Cytotoxic Glycopeptide Antibiotics Isolated from a Strain of *Streptomyces verticillus*	*Vial:* 15, 30 units, pwdr for reconstitution and IV, IM, SC, intrapleural administration
Blincyto *blinatumomab*	Bispecific CD19-directed CD3 T-cell Engager	*Vial:* 35 mcg, pwdr for reconstitution, dilution, and IV infusion, single-dose
bortezomib	Kinase Inhibitor	*Vial:* 3.5 mg, pwdr for reconstitution, dilution, and IV infusion, single-dose
Bosulif *bosutinib*	Kinase Inhibitor	*Tab:* 100, 400, 500 mg
Braftovi *encorafenib*	Kinase Inhibitor	*Cap:* 50, 75 mg
Breyanzi *lisocabtagene maraleucel*	Chimeric Antigen Receptor T-Cell (CAR-T) Therapy	*Vial:* 50 to 110 × 10⁶ CAR-positive viable T-cells/5 ml
Brukinsa *zanubrutinib*	Bruton's Tyrosine Kinase (BTK) Inhibitor	*Cap:* 160, 320 mg
Cabometyx *cabozantinib*	Kinase Inhibitor	*Tab:* 20, 40, 60 mg
Calquence *acalabrutinib*	Kinase Inhibitor	*Cap:* 100 mg
Casodex *bicalutamide*	Antiandrogen	*Tab:* 50 mg
Clolar *clofarabine*	Purine Nucleoside Metabolic Inhibitor	*Vial:* 20 mg/20 ml (1 mg/ml), single-dose, for dilution and IV infusion
Copiktra *duvelisib*	Dual phosphoinositide-3-kinase (PI3K)-delta/PI3K-gamma Inhibitor	*Cap:* 15, 25 mg
Cosela *trilaciclib*	Kinase Inhibitor	*Tab:* 300 mg pwdr, single-dose, for reconstitution, dilution, and IV infusion
Cytoxan *Cyclophosphamide*	Alkylating Agent	*Tab:* 25, 50 mg
Darzalex ***daratumumab***	Human CD38-directed Monoclonal Antibody	*Vial:* 100 mg/5 ml, (20 mg/ml), 400 mg/20 ml (20 mg/ml), soln for dilution and IV infusion, single-dose
Darzalex Faspro *daratumumab+hyaluronidase-fihj*	CD38-Directed Cytolytic Antibody+Hyaluronidase	*Vial:* 1,800 mg *daratumumab*+30,000 units *hyaluronidase-fihi* (15 ml, 120 mg/2,000 units/ml), single-dose, soln for SC administration

(continued)

Appendix O (*continued*)

Antineoplastics With Classification and Dose Forms		
Brand, Generic, and Pregnancy Category	**Class and Indications**	**Dose Form(s)**
Daurismo *glasdegib*	Hedgehog Pathway Inhibitor	*Tab:* 25, 100 mg
Doxil *doxorubicin HCl*	Anthracycline Topoisomerase Inhibitor	*Vial:* 10 mg/10 ml, 50 mg/30 ml (10 mg/ml), single-use
Elahere *mirvetuximab soravtansine-gynx*	Folate Receptor Alpha (FRα)-Directed Antibody and Microtubule Inhibitor Conjugate	*Vial:* 100 mg/20 ml (5 mg/ml), single-dose, for dilution and IV infusion
Eligard *leuprolide acetate*	GnRH Analog	*Inj:* 7.5 mg ext-rel per monthly SC injection
Elzonris *tagraxofusp-erzs*	CD123-directed Cytotoxin	*Vial:* 1,000 mcg/ml (1 ml), single-dose for IV infusion
Endari *l-glutamine*	Amino Acid	*Oral Pwdr:* 5 gm of L-glutamine pwdr per paper-foil-plastic laminate pkt
Enhertu *fam-trastuzumab deruxtecan-nxki*	HER2-directed Antibody and Topoisomerase Conjugate	*Vial:* 100 mg, single-dose, pwdr for reconstitution, dilution, and IV infusion
Eulexin *flutamide*	Antiandrogen	*Cap:* 125 mg
Fareston *toremifene* (G)	Selective Estrogen Receptor Modulator (SERM)	*Tab:* 60 mg
Faslodex *fulvestrant* (G)	Estrogen Receptor Antagonist	*Prefilled syringe for IM inj:* 50 mg/ml (2.5, 5 ml/syringe)
Femara *letrozole*	Aromatase Inhibitor	*Tab:* 2.5 mg
Gavreto *pralsetinib*	RET Kinase Inhibitor	*Cap:* 100 mg
Gleevec *imatinib mesylate*	Signal Transduction Inhibitor	*Cap:* 100 mg
Herceptin *trastuzumab*	HER2/neu Receptor Antagonist	*Vial:* 420 mg, multidose pwdr for reconstitution, dilution, and IV infusion
Herceptin Hylecta *trastuzumab+hyaluronidase*	HER2/neu Receptor Antagonist+Endoglycosidase	*trastuzumab* 600 mg+*hyaluronidase* 10,000 units/5 ml (120 mg/2,000 units per ml), single-dose soln for SC administration
Herzuma *trastuzumab-pkrb*	HER2/neu Receptor Antagonist	*Vial:* 150 mg, single-dose, 420 mg multidose, pwdr for reconstitution, dilution, and IV infusion
Hydrea *hydroxyurea* (G)	Substituted Urea	*Cap:* 500 mg
Ibrance *palbociclib*	Kinase Inhibitor	*Cap:* 75, 100, 150 mg
Idhifa *enasidenib*	Isocitrate Dehydrogenase-2 (IDH2) Inhibitor	*Tab:* 50, 100 mg
Imbruvica *ibrutinib*	Kinase Inhibitor	*Tab:* 140 mg

(*continued*)

Appendix O (*continued*)

Antineoplastics With Classification and Dose Forms		
Brand, Generic, and Pregnancy Category	**Class and Indications**	**Dose Form(s)**
Imfinzi *durvalumab*	Programmed Death Ligand-1 (PD-L1) Blocking Antibody	*Vial:* 120 mg/2.4 ml (50 mg/ml), 500 mg/10 ml (50 mg/ml), soln for dilution and single-dose
Imjudo *tremelimumab*	Cytotoxic T-Lymphocyte-Associated Antigen 4 (CTLA-4) Blocking Antibody	*Vial:* 25 mg/1.25 ml (20 mg/ml), 300 mg/15 ml (20 mg/ml), single-dose, soln for dilution and IV infusion
Inqovi *decitabine+cedazuridine*	Nucleoside Metabolic Inhibitor+Cytidine Deaminase Inhibitor	*Tabs:* 35 mg *decitabine* and 100 mg *cedazuridine*
Iressa *gefitinib* (G)	Epidermal Growth Factor Receptor Tyrosine Kinase Inhibitor	*Tab:* 250 mg
Istodax *romidepsin* (G)	Histone Deacetylase (HDAC) Inhibitor	*Kit: Vial:* romidepsin 10 mg, single-dose, pwdr for reconstitution plus *Vial:* diluent, 2.2 ml, single-use, for dilution and IV infusion
Jakafi *ruxolitinib*	Kinase Inhibitor	*Tab:* 5, 10, 15, 20, 25 mg
Jaypirca *pirtobrutinib*	Non-Covalent (Reversible) Bruton's Tyrosine Kinase (BTK) Inhibitor	*Tab:* 50, 100 mg
Jemperli *dostarlimab-gxly*	Programme Death Receptor-1 (PD-1)–Blocking Antibody	*Vial:* 500 mg/10 ml (50 mg/ml), single-dose, soln for dilution and IV infusion
Jevtana *cabazitaxel* (G)	Microtubule Inhibitor	*Vial:* 60 mg/1.5 ml, single-dose w. diluent (5.7 ml) for further dilution and IV infusion (polysorbate 80)
Kanjinti *trastuzumab-anns*	HER2/neu Receptor Antagonist	*Vial:* 420 mg (21 mg/ml), multidose, pwdr for reconstitution, dilution, and IV infusion
Keytruda *pembrolizumab*	Programmed Death Receptor-1 (PD-1)-Blocking Antibody	*Vial:* 100 mg/4 ml (25 mg/ml), single-dose soln for dilution and IV infusion
Kisqali Femara Co-Pack *ribociclib+letrozole*	Cyclin-dependent Kinase Inhibitor+Aromatase Inhibitor	*Tab:* 600/2.5, 400/2.5, 200/2.5 mg
Krazati *adagrasib* brentuximab vedotin	Inhibitor of the RAS GTPase Family	*Tab:* 200 mg *Vial:* 10 mg, single-dose, pwdr for reconstitution, dilution, and IV infusion
Kymriah *tisagenlecleucel*	CD19-directed Genetically Modified Autologous T cell Immunotherapy	*IV bag:* frozen suspension for IV infusion after thawing
Kyprolis, *carfilzomib*	Protease Inhibitor	*Vial:* 10, 30, 60 mg, single-dose, pwdr for reconstitution, dilution, and IV infusion
Lartruvo *olaratumab*	Platelet-derived Growth Factor Receptor Alpha (PDGFR-α) Blocking Antibody	*Vial:* 500 mg/50 ml (10 mg/ml), single-dose, soln for dilution and IV infusion

(*continued*)

Appendix O (*continued*)

Antineoplastics With Classification and Dose Forms		
Brand, Generic, and Pregnancy Category	**Class and Indications**	**Dose Form(s)**
Lenvima *lenvatinib*	Kinase Inhibitor	*Cap:* 4, 10 mg
Leukeran *chlorambucil* (G)	Alkylating Agent	*Tab:* 2 mg
Libtayo *cemiplimab-rwlc*	Programmed Death Receptor-1 (PD-1) Blocking Antibody	*Vial:* 350 mg/7 ml (50 mg/ml), single-dose, soln for dilution and IV infusion
Lorbrena *lorlatinib*	Kinase Inhibitor	*Tab:* 25, 100 mg
Lumoxiti *moxetumomab pasudotox-tdfk*	Anti-CD22 Recombinant Immunotoxin	*Vial:* 1 mg, single-dose, pwdr for reconstitution, dilution, and IV infusion
Lunsumio *mosunetuzumab-axgb*	Bispecific CD20-Directed CD3 T-Cell Engager	*Vial:* 1 mg/ml (1 ml), 30 mg/30 ml (30 ml), single-dose, soln for dilution and IV infusion
Lupron *leuprolide* (G)	GnRH Analog	*Vial:* 5 mg/ml (2.8 ml), multidose, soln for SC inj: 1 mg (daily); 7.5 mg depot (monthly); 22.5 mg depot (every 3 months); 30 mg depot (every 4 months)
Lynparza *olaparib*	Poly(ADP-ribose) Polymerase (PARP)-Inhibitor	*Tab:* 100, 150 mg
Lytgobi *futibatinib*	Kinase Inhibitor	*Tab:* 4 mg
Margenza *margetuximab-cmkb*	HER2/neu Receptor Antagonist	*Vial:* 250 mg/10 ml (25 mg/ml), single-dose, soln for dilution and IV infusion
Megace, Megace Oral Suspension, Megace ES, *megestrol acetate* (G)	Progestin	*Tab:* 20*, 40*mg; *Susp:* 40 mg/ml; *ES concentrate:* 125 mg/ml, 625 mg/5 ml
Mekinist *trametinib*	Kinase Inhibitor	*Tab:* 0.5, 2 mg
Mektovi *binimetinib*	Kinase Inhibitor	*Tab:* 15 mg
Nerlynx *neratinib*	Tyrosine Kinase Inhibitor (TKI)	*Tab:* 40 mg
Nexavar *sorafenib* (G)	Multikinase Inhibitor	*Tab:* 200 mg
Nilandron *nilutamide*	Nonsteroidal Orally Active Antiandrogen	*Tab:* 150 mg
Nubeqa *darolutamide*	Androgen Receptor Inhibitor (ARi)	*Tab:* 300 mg
Nyvepria *pegfilgrastim-apgf*	Leukocyte Growth Factor (LGF)	*Prefilled syringe:* 6 mg/0.6 ml, single-dose, soln for SC administration
Ogivri *trastuzumab-dkst*	HER2/neu Receptor Antagonist	*Vial:* 420 mg, multidose, pwdr for reconstitution, dilution, and IV infusion

(*continued*)

Appendix O (*continued*)

Antineoplastics With Classification and Dose Forms		
Brand, Generic, and Pregnancy Category	Class and Indications	Dose Form(s)
Ontruzant for Injection *trastuzumab-dttb*	HER2/neu Receptor Antagonist	*Vial:* 150 mg, single-use; 420 mg pwdr, multiuse; pwdr for reconstitution, dilution, and IV infusion
Onureg *azacitidine*	Nucleoside Metabolic Inhibitor (NMI)	*Tab:* 200, 300 mg
Opdivo *nivolumab*	Anti-Programmed Death Receptor-1 (PD-1) Monoclonal Antibody	*Vial:* 40 mg/4 ml, 100 mg/10 ml, 240 mg/24 ml (10 mg/ml), single-use, soln for dilution and IV infusion
Opdualag *nivolumab* and *relatlimab-rmbw*	Programmed Death Receptor-1 (PD-1) Blocking and Lymphocyte Activation Gene-3 (LAG-3) Blocking Antibody	*Vial:* nivolumab 240 mg and relatlimab 80 mg per 20 ml (12 mg and 4 mg per ml, respectively), soln, fixed single-dose
Orgovyx *relugolix*	Gonadotropin-Releasing Hormone (GnRH) Receptor Antagonist	*Tab:* 120 mg
Orserdu	Selective Estrogen Receptor Down Regulator (SERD)	*Tab:* 86, 345 mg
Padcev *enfortumab vedotin-ejfv*	Nectin-4-directed Antibody and Microtubule Inhibitor Conjugate	*Vial:* 20, 30 mg, single-dose, pwdr for reconstitution, dilution, and IV infusion
Pemazyre *pemigatinib*	Kinase Inhibitor	*Tab:* 4.5, 9, 13.5 mg
Pemfexy *pemetrexed*	Folate Analog Metabolic Inhibitor	*Vial:* 100, 500 mg, single-dose, pwdr for reconstitution, dilution, and IV infusion
Pepaxto *melphalan flufenamide*	Anti-Cancer Peptide-Drug Conjugate	*Vial:* 20 mg, single-dose, pwdr for reconstitution, dilution, and IV infusion
Perjeta *pertuzumab*	HER2/neu Receptor Antagonist	*Vial:* 420 mg/14 ml, single-dose
Piqray *alpelisib*	Kinase Inhibitor	*Tab:* 50, 150, 200 mg
Polivy *polatuzumab vedotin-piiq*	CD79b-Directed Antibody-Drug Conjugate	*Vial:* 140 mg, single-dose, pwdr for reconstitution, dilution, and IV infusion
Poteligeo *mogamulizumab*	CC Chemokine Receptor Type 4 (CCR4)-Directed Monoclonal Antibody	*Vial:* 420 mg, multidose, pwdr for reconstitution, dilution, and IV infusion
Qinlock *ripretinib*	Kinase Inhibitor	*Tab:* 50 mg
Retevmo *selpercatinib*	Kinase Inhibitor	*Cap:* 40, 80 mg
Revlimid *lenalidomide* (G)	Thalidomide Analogue	*Cap:* 2.5, 5, 10, 15, 20, 25 mg
Rezlidhia *olutasidenib*	Isocitrate Dehydrogenase-1 (IDH1) Inhibitor	*Cap:* 150 mg

(*continued*)

Appendix O (*continued*)

Antineoplastics With Classification and Dose Forms		
Brand, Generic, and Pregnancy Category	**Class and Indications**	**Dose Form(s)**
Riabni rituximab-arrx	CD20-Directed Cytolytic Antibody	*Vial:* 100 mg/10 ml (10 mg/ml), 500 mg/50 ml (10 mg/ml), single-dose, soln for dilution and IV infusion
Rituxan *rituximab*	CD20-Directed Cytolytic Antibody	*Vial:* 100 mg/10 ml (10 mg/ml), 500 mg/50 ml (10 mg/ml), single-dose, soln for dilution and IV infusion
Rituxan Hycela *rituximab+ hyaluronidase human*	Combination of *rituximab*, a CD20-Directed Cytolytic Antibody and *hyaluronidase human*, an Endoglycosidase	*Vial:* 1400 mg *rituximab* and 23,400 units *hyaluronidase human* per 11.7 ml (120 mg/2,000 units per ml) single-dose; 1,600 mg *rituximab* and 26,800 units *hyaluronidase human* per 13.4 ml (120 mg/2,000 units per ml), single-dose, soln for SC administration
Rozlytrek *entrectinib*	Selective Tyrosine Kinase Inhibitor (TKI)	*Cap:* 100, 200 mg
Rubraca *rucaparib*	Poly ADP-ribose Polymerase (PARP)-Inhibitor	*Tab:* 200, 300 mg
Ruxience *rituximab-pvvr*	CD20-directed Cytolytic Antibody	*Vial:* 100 mg/10 ml (10 mg/ml), 500 mg/50 ml (10 mg/ml), single-dose, soln for dilution and IV infusion
Rybrevant *amivantamab-vmjw*	Bispecific EGF Receptor-Directed and MET Receptor-Directed Antibody	*Vial:* 350 mg/7 ml (50 mg/ml), single-dose, soln for dilution and IV infusion (preservative-free)
Rydapt *midostaurin*	Kinase Inhibitor	*Tab:* 40 mg
Sarclisa *isatuximab-irfc*	CD38-directed Cytolytic Antibody	*Vial:* 100 mg/5 ml (20 mg/ml), 500 mg/20 ml (20/ml), single-dose, soln for dilution and IV infusion
Sprycel *dasatini*	Tyrosine Kinase Inhibitor (TKI)	*Tab:* 20, 50, 70, 80, 100, 140 mg
Stivarga *regorafenib*	Kinase Inhibitor	*Tab:* 40 mg
Sutent *sunitinib malate* (G)	Kinase Inhibitor	*Cap:* 12.5, 25, 37.5, 50 mg
Tabrecta *capmatinib*	Kinase Inhibitor	*Tab:* 150, 200 mg
Tafinlar *dabrafenib*	Kinase Inhibitor	*Cap:* 50, 75 mg *Tab for oral susp:* 10 mg
Tagrisso *osimertinib*	Kinase Inhibitor	*Tab:* 40, 80 mg
Talzenna *talazoparib*	Poly (ADP-ribose) (PARP) Inhibitor	*Tab:* 0.5, 1 mg
tamoxifen citrate (G)	Antiestrogen	*Tab:* 10, 20 mg
Tarceva *erlotinib*	Kinase Inhibitor	*Tab:* 25, 100, 150 mg
Targretin *bexarotene* (G)	Retinoid X Receptor (RXR) Activator	*Gelcap:* 75 mg

(continued)

Appendix O (*continued*)

Antineoplastics With Classification and Dose Forms		
Brand, Generic, and Pregnancy Category	Class and Indications	Dose Form(s)
Targretin 1% Topical Gel *bexarotene* (G)	Topical Retinoid X Receptor (RXR) Activator	*Topical gel:* 1% (60 gm tube)
Tasigna *nilotinib*	Kinase Inhibitor	*Cap:* 50, 150, 200 mg
Taxotere *docetaxel* (G)	Microtubule Inhibitor	*Vial:* 20 mg/2 ml (10 mg/ml), single-dose; 80 mg/8 ml (10 mg/ml), 160 mg/16 ml (10 mg/ml), multidose
Tazverik *tazemetostat*	Methyltransferase Inhibitor	*Tab:* 200 mg, film-coat
Tecentriq *atezolizumab*	Programmed Death Ligand-1 (PD-L1)-Blocking Antibody	*Vial:* 1,200 mg/20 ml (60 mg/ml), single-dose, for dilution and IV infusion
Tecvayli *teclistamab-cqyv*	Bispecific B-Cell Maturation Antigen (BCMA)-Directed CD3 T-Cell Engager	*Vial:* 30 mg/3 ml (10 mg/ml), single-dose; 153 mg/1.7 ml (90 mg/ml), single-dose
Tepmetko *tepotinib*	Kinase Inhibitor	*Tab:* 225 mg
Tibsovo *ivosidenib*	Isocitrate Dehydrogenase-1 (IDH1) Inhibitor	*Tab:* 250 mg
Trazimera *trastuzumab-qyyp*	HER2/neu receptor antagonist	*Vial:* 420 mg, multidose, pwdr for reconstitution, dilution, and IV infusion
Treanda *bendamustine* (G)	Alkylating Agent	*Vial:* 45 mg/0.5 ml, 180 mg/2 ml soln, single-dose; 25, 100 mg pwdr, single-dose, for reconstitution, dilution, and IV infusion
Trisenox *arsenic trioxide*	Arsenical	*Vial:* 12 mg/6 ml (2 mg/ml), single-dose, soln for dilution and IV infusion
Trodelvy *sacituzumab govitecan-hziy*	Trop-2-Directed Antibody and Topoisomerase Inhibitor Conjugate	*Vial:* 180 mg, single-dose, pwdr for reconstitution, dilution, and IV infusion
Truxima *rituximab-abbs*	CD20-Directed Cytolytic Antibody	*Vial:* 100 mg/10 ml, 500 mg/50 ml (10 mg/ml), single-use, for dilution and IV infusion
Tukysa *tucatinib*	Kinase Inhibitor	*Tab:* 50 mg
Turalio *pexidartinib*	Kinase Inhibitor	*Cap:* 200 mg
Uplizna *inebilizumab-cdon*	CD19-Directed Cytolytic Antibody	*Vial:* 100 mg/10 ml (10 mg/ml), single-dose, soln for dilution and IV infusion
Vectibix	Epidermal Growth Factor Receptor (EGFR) Antagonist	*Vial:* 100 mg/5 ml, 200 mg/10 ml, 400 mg/20 ml (20 mg/ml), single-use, soln for dilution and IV infusion
Vegzelma *bevacizumab-adcd*	Vascular Endothelial Growth Factor Inhibitor	*Vial:* 100 mg/4 ml (25 mg/ml), 400 mg/16 ml (25 mg/ml), single-dose, soln for dilution and IV infusion

(continued)

Appendix O (*continued*)

Antineoplastics With Classification and Dose Forms		
Brand, Generic, and Pregnancy Category	**Class and Indications**	**Dose Form(s)**
Velcade *bortezomib*	Proteasome Inhibitor	*Vial:* 3.5 mg, single dose, pwdr for reconstitution, dilution, and IV infusion
Venclexta *venetoclax*	BCL-2 Inhibitor	*Tab:* 10, 50, 100 mg
Verzenio *abemaciclib*	Kinase Inhibitor	*Tab:* 50, 100, 150, 200 mg
Viadur *leuprolide acetate*	GnRH Analog	*SC implant:* 65 mg depot (12 months)
Vitrakvi *larotrectinib*	Selective Tropomyosin Receptor Kinase (TRK) Inhibitor	*Caps:* 25, 100 mg *Oral soln:* 20 mg/ml (100 ml)
Vizimpro *dacomitinib*	Irreversible Pan-Human Epidermal Growth Factor Receptor Tyrosine Kinase Inhibitor (TKI)	*Tab:* 15, 30, 45 mg
Vyxeos *daunorubicin+cytarabine*	Anthracycline Topoisomerase Inhibitor (ATI)+Nucleoside Metabolic Inhibitor (NMI)	*Vial: daunorubicin* 44 mg/*cytarabine* 100 mg, single-dose, pwdr for reconstitution, dilution, and IV infusion
Xalkori *crizotinib*	Kinase Inhibitor	*Cap:* 25, 100 mg
Xeloda *capecitabine*	*fluoropyrimidine* (prodrug of *5-fluorouracil*)	*Tab:* 150, 500 mg
Xermelo *telotristat*	Tryptophan Hydroxylase Inhibitor (THI)	*Tab:* 150 mg
Xospata *gilteritinib*	Kinase Inhibitor	*Tab:* 40 mg
Xpovio *selinexor*	Selective Inhibitor of Nuclear Export (SINE) XPO1 Antagonist	*Tab:* 20 mg
Yervoy *ipilimumab*	CD19-Directed Genetically Human Cytotoxic T-lymphocyte Antigen 4 (CTLA-4)-Blocking Antibody	*Vial:* 100 mg/5 ml (20 mg/ml), 400 mg/20 ml (20 mg/ml), single-dose, soln for dilution and IV infusion
Yescarta *axicabtagene*	CD19-Directed Genetically Modified Autologous T cell	*Infusion bag:* 68 ml, single autologous use immunotherapy
Zynyz *retifanlimab-dlwr*	Programmed Death Receptor-1 (PD-1) Blocking Antibody	*Vial:* 500 mg/20 ml (25 mg/ml), single-dose, soln for dilution and IV infusion
Zejula *niraparib*	Poly ADP-Ribose Polymerase (PARP)-Inhibitor	*Cap:* 100 mg
Zelboraf *vemurafenib*	Kinase Inhibitor	*Tab:* 240 mg
Zepzelca *lurbinectedin*	Selective Oncogenic Transcription Inhibitor	*Vial:* 4 mg, single-dose, pwdr for reconstitution, dilution, and IV infusion
Zirabev *bevacizumab-bvzr*	Vascular Endothelial Growth Factor (VEGF) Inhibitor	*Vial:* 100 mg/4 ml (25 mg/ml), 400 mg/16 ml (25 mg/ml), single-dose, soln for dilution and IV infusion

(*continued*)

Appendix O (*continued*)

Antineoplastics With Classification and Dose Forms		
Brand, Generic, and Pregnancy Category	**Class and Indications**	**Dose Form(s)**
Zoladex *goserelin acetate*	GnRH Analog	*SC implant:* 3.6 mg depot (28 days), 10.8 mg depot (3 months)
Zometa *zoledronic acid*	Bisphosphonate	*Vial:* 4 mg, single-dose, pwdr for reconstitution, dilution, and IV infusion
Zykadia *ceritinib*	Kinase Inhibitor	*Cap:* 150 mg
Zynlonta *loncastuximab tesirine-lpyl*	CD19-Directed Antibody and Alkylating Agent Conjugate	*Vial:* 10 mg, single-dose, pwdr for reconstitution, dilution, and IV infusion

ARi, androgen receptor inhibitor; BCMA, B-cell maturation antigen; BTK, Bruton's tyrosine kinase; CAR, chimeric antigen receptor; CCR4, CC chemokine receptor type 4; CTLA-4, cytotoxic T-lymphocyte antigen 4; EGFR, epidermal growth factor receptor; FRα, folate receptor alpha; GnRH, gonadotropin-releasing hormone; HDAC, histone deacetylase; HER2, human epidermal growth factor receptor 2; IDH2, isocitrate dehydrogenase-2; LAG-3, lymphocyte activation gene-3; PARP, poly(ADP-ribose) polymerase; PD-1, programmed death receptor-1; PDGFR-α, platelet-derived growth factor receptor alpha; PD-L1, programmed death ligand-1; PI3K, phosphoinositide-3-kinase; RET, rearranged during transfection; RXR, retinoid X receptor; SERDs, selective estrogen receptor downregulators; SERM, selective estrogen receptor modulator; SINE, selective inhibitor of nuclear export; THI, tryptophan hydroxylase inhibitor; TKI, tyrosine kinase inhibitor; TRK, tropomyosin receptor kinase; VEGF, vascular endothelial growth factor.

APPENDIX P. ANTIPSYCHOSIS DRUGS

ANTIPSYCHOTICS WITH DOSE FORMS

Comment: Patients receiving an antipsychotic agent should be monitored closely for the following adverse side effects: neuroleptic malignant syndrome, extrapyramidal reactions, tardive dyskinesia, blood dyscrasias, anticholinergic effects, drowsiness, hypotension, photosensitivity, retinopathy, and lowered seizure threshold. Use lower doses for elderly or debilitated patients. Prescriptions should be written for the smallest practical amount. Foods and beverages containing alcohol are contraindicated in patients receiving any psychotropic drug. *Neuroleptic malignant syndrome* (NMS) and *tardive dyskinesia* (TD) are adverse side effects (ASEs), most often associated with the older antipsychotic drugs. Risk is decreased with the newer "atypical" antipsychotic drugs. However, these syndromes can develop, although much less commonly, after relatively brief treatment periods at low doses. Given these considerations, antipsychotic drugs should be prescribed in a manner that is most likely to minimize the occurrence. NMS, a potentially fatal symptom complex, is characterized by hyperpyrexia, muscle rigidity, altered mental status, and evidence of autonomic instability (irregular pulse or blood pressure, tachycardia, diaphoresis, and cardiac dysrhythmia). Additional signs may include elevated creatine phosphor-kinase (CPK), myoglobinuria (rhabdomyolysis), and acute renal failure (ARF). TD is a syndrome consisting of potentially irreversible, involuntary, dyskinetic movements that can develop in patients with antipsychotic drugs. Characteristics include repetitive involuntary movements, usually of the jaw, lips, and tongue, such as grimacing, sticking out the tongue, and smacking the lips. Some affected people also experience involuntary movement of the extremities or difficulty breathing. The syndrome may remit, partially or completely, if antipsychotic treatment is withdrawn. If signs and symptoms of NMS and/or TD appear in a patient, management should include immediate discontinuation of antipsychotic drugs and other drugs not essential to concurrent therapy, intensive symptomatic treatment, medical monitoring, and treatment of any concomitant serious medical problems. The risk of developing NMS and/or TD and the likelihood that either syndrome will become irreversible are believed to increase as the duration of treatment and the total cumulative dose of antipsychotic drugs administered to the patient increase. The first and <u>only</u> FDA-approved treatment for TD is ***valbenazine*** (**Ingrezza**) (*see* Tardive Dyskinesia).

ANTIPSYCHOTICS WITH DOSE FORMS

➤ *aripiprazole* (G)
    Abilify *Tab:* 2, 5, 10, 15, 20, 30 mg; *Oral soln:* 1 mg/ml (150 ml) (orange crèam; parabens)
    Abilify Discmelt *Tab:* 15 mg orally disintegrating (vanilla) (phenylalanine)
    Abilify Maintena *Vial:* 300, 400 mg ext-rel pwdr for IM injection after reconstitution; 300, 400 mg single-dose prefilled dual-chamber syringes w. supplies
    Aristada *Prefilled syringe:* 441, 662, 882, 1,064 mg, ext-rel susp for IM injection, single-dose w. safety needle

(*continued*)

Appendix P (*continued*)

▷ *aripiprazole lauroxil*
    Aristada *Prefilled syringe:* single-use, ext-rel injectable suspension: 441mg (1.6 ml), 662 mg (2.4 ml), 882 mg (3.2 ml), 1,064 mg (3.9 ml)

▷ *asenapine*
    Saphris *SL tab:* 2.5, 5, 10 mg
    Secuado *Transdermal system:* 3.8 mg/24 hours, 5.7 mg/24 hours, 7.6 mg/24 hours

▷ *brexpiprazole* (G)
    Rexulti *Tab:* 0.25, 0.5, 1, 2, 3, 4 mg

▷ *bupropion*
    Forfivo XL *Tab:* 450 mg ext-rel

▷ *cariprazine* (G)
    Vraylar *Cap:* 1.5, 3, 4.5, 6 mg

▷ *chlorpromazine* (G)
    Thorazine *Tab:* 10, 25, 50, 100, 200 mg; *Cap:* 30, 75, 150 mg sust-rel; *Syr:* 10 mg/5 ml (4 oz) (orange-custard); *Vial/Amp:* 25 mg/ml (1, 2 ml) (sulfites)

▷ *clozapine* (G)
    Clozapine ODT *ODT:* 150, 200 mg
    Clozaril *Tab:* 25*, 100*mg; *ODT:* 150, 200 mg
    FazaClo ODT *ODT:* 12.5, 25, 100, 150, 200 mg (phenylalanine)
    Versacloz *Oral susp:* 50 mg/ml (100 ml)

▷ *fluphenazine* (G)
    Prolixin *Tab:* 1, 2.5, 5*, 10 mg (tartrazine); *Conc:* 5 mg/ml (4 oz w. calib dropper) (alcohol 14%); *Elix:* 5 mg/ml (2 oz w. calib dropper) (alcohol 14%); *Vial:* 25 mg/ml (10 ml)

▷ *fluphenazine decanoate* (G)
    Prolixin Decanoate *Vial:* 25 mg/ml (5 ml) (benzyl alcohol)

▷ *fluphenazine* (G)
    Prolixin Enanthate *Vial:* 25 mg (5 ml) (benzyl alcohol)

▷ *fluphenazine decanoate* (G)
    Prolixin Decanoate *Vial:* 25 mg/ml (5 ml) (benzyl alcohol)

▷ *haloperidol* (G)
    Haldol *Tab:* 0.5*, 1*, 2*, 5*, 10*, 20*mg
    Haldol Lactate *Vial:* 5 mg for IM injection, single-dose
    Haldol Decanoate *Vial:* 50, 100 mg for IM injection, single-dose

▷ *iloperidone*
    Fanapt *Tab:* 1, 2, 4, 6, 8, 10, 12 mg

▷ *loxapine*
    Adasuve *Oral inhal pwdr:* 10 mg single-use disposable inhaler (5/box)

▷ *lumateperone*
    Caplyta *Cap:* 42 mg

▷ *lurasidone* (G)
    Latuda *Tab:* 20, 40, 80 mg

▷ *olanzapine fumarate* (G)
    Zyprexa *Tab:* 2.5, 5, 7.5, 10, 15, 20 mg
    Zyprexa Zydis *ODT:* 5, 10, 15, 20 mg (phenylalanine)

▷ *paliperidone* (G)
    Invega *Tab:* 3, 6, 9 mg ext-rel

▷ *paliperidone palmitate* (G)
    Invega Hafyera *Prefilled syringe:* 1,092, 1,560 mg, long-acting suspension
    Invega Sustenna *Prefilled syringe:* 39, 78, 117, 156, 234 mg ext-rel suspension
    Invega Trinza *Prefilled syringe:* 273, 410, 546, 819 mg long-acting suspension

▷ *pimozide* (G)
    Orap *Tab:* 1, 2 mg

(*continued*)

Appendix P (*continued*)

▷ *prochlorperazine* (G)
    Compazine *Tab:* 5, 10 mg; *Cap:* 10, 15 mg sus-rel; *Syr:* 5 mg/5 ml (4 oz) (fruit); *Supp:* 2.5, 5, 25 mg

▷ *quetiapine* (G)
    Seroquel *Tab:* 25, 100, 200, 300 mg
    Seroquel XR *Tab:* 50, 150, 200, 300, 400 mg ext-rel

▷ *risperidone* (G)
    Risperdal *Tab:* 0.25, 0.5, 1, 2, 3, 4 mg; *Soln:* 1 mg/ml (30 ml w. pipette); *Consta Inj:* 25, 37.5, 50 mg
    Risperdal M-Tabs *M-tab:* 0.5, 1, 2, 3, 4 mg orally disint (phenylalanine)

▷ *thioridazine* (G) *Tab:* 10, 25, 50, 100 mg

▷ *trifluoperazine* (G)
    Stelazine *Tab:* 1, 2, 5, 10 mg; *Conc:* 10 mg/ml; 2 oz w. calib dropper (banana-vanilla) (sulfites); *Vial:* 2 mg/ml (10 ml)

▷ *ziprasidone* (G)
    Geodon *Cap:* 20, 40, 60, 80 mg

APPENDIX Q. ANTICONVULSANT DRUGS

ANTICONVULSANTS WITH DOSE FORMS

▷ *brivaracetam* (G)
    Briviact *Tab:* 10, 25, 50, 75, 100 mg; *Oral soln:* 10 mg/ml (300 ml); *Vial:* 50 mg/5 ml single-dose for IV inj

▷ *carbamazepine* (G)
    Carbatrol *Cap:* 200, 300 mg ext-rel
    Carnexiv *Vial:* 200 mg/20 ml (10 mg/ml), single-dose for IV infusion
    Equetro *Cap:* 100, 200, 300 mg ext-rel
    Tegretol *Tab:* 100*, 200*mg; *Chew tab:* 100*mg
    Tegretol Suspension *Oral susp:* 100 mg/5 ml (450 ml) (citrus vanilla) (sorbitol)
    Tegretol-XR *Tab:* 100, 200, 400 mg ext-rel

▷ *cenobamate*
    Xcopri *Tab:* 12.5, 25, 50, 100, 150, 200 mg film-coat

▷ *clobazam* (IV)
    Onfi *Tab:* 10*, 20*mg
    Onfi Oral Suspension *Oral susp:* 2.5 mg/ml (120 ml w. 2 dosing syringes) (berry)

▷ *clonazepam* (IV)(G)
    Clonazepam ODT *ODT:* 0.125, 0.25, 0.5, 1, 2, oral-disint
    Klonopin *Tab:* 0.5*, 1, 2 mg

▷ *diazepam* (IV)(G)
    Diastat *Rectal gel delivery system:* 2.5 mg
    Diastat AcuDial *Rectal gel delivery system:* 10, 20 mg
    Valium *Tab:* 2*, 5*, 10*mg
    Valium Injectable *Vial:* 5 mg/ml (10 ml); *Amp:* 5 mg/ml (2 ml); *Prefilled syringe:* 5 mg/ml (5 ml)
    Valium Intensol *Conc oral soln:* 5 mg/ml (30 ml w. dropper) (alcohol 19%)
    Valium Oral Solution *Oral soln:* 5 mg/5 ml (500 ml) (winter green-spice)
    Valtoco *Nasal spray:* 5, 7.5, 10 mg

▷ *divalproex sodium* (G)
    Depakene *Cap:* 250 mg; *Syr:* 250 mg/5 ml (16 oz)
    Depakote *Tab:* 125, 250, 500 mg
    Depakote ER *Tab:* 250, 500 mg ext-rel
    Depakote Sprinkle *Cap:* 125 mg

▷ *eslicarbazepine* (G)
    Aptiom *Tab:* 200*, 400, 600*, 800*mg

▷ *felbamate* (G)
    Felbatol *Tab:* 400*, 600*mg
    Felbatol Oral Suspension *Oral susp:* 600 mg/5 ml (4, 8, 32 oz)
    Peganone *Tab:* 250, 500 mg

▷ *fosphenytoin sodium*
    Cerebyx *Vial:* 100 mg PE (2 ml), 500 mg PE (10 ml), 50 mg PE/ml, ready-mixed solution in water for injection

(*continued*)

Appendix Q (*continued*)

▷ *gabapentin*
Horizant *Tab:* 300, 600 ext-rel
Neurontin (G) *Cap:* 100, 300, 400 mg; *Tab:* 600*, 800*mg
Neurontin Oral Solution *Oral soln:* 250 mg/5 ml (480 ml) (strawberry-anise)

▷ *lacosamide* (V)(G)
Vimpat *Tab:* 50, 100, 150, 200 mg; *Oral soln:* 10 mg/ml (200, 465 ml); *Vial:* 10 mg/ml soln for IV infusion, single-use (20 ml)

▷ *lamotrigine* (G)
Lamictal *Tab:* 25*, 100*, 150*, 200*mg
Lamictal Chewable Dispersible Tab *Chew tab:* 2, 5, 25, 50 mg (black current)
Lamictal ODT *ODT:* 25, 50, 100, 200 mg oral-disint
Lamictal XR *Tab:* 25, 50, 100, 200, 250, 300 mg ext-rel

▷ *levetiracetam* (G)
Elepsia *Tab:* 1,000, 1,500 mg ext-rel
Keppra *Tab:* 250*, 500*, 750*, 1,000*mg
Keppra Oral Solution *Oral soln:* 100 mg/ml (16 oz) (grape) (dye-free)
Keppra XR *Tab:* 500, 750 mg ext-rel
Levetiracetam IV *Premixed:* 500, 1,000, 1,500 mg for IV infusion (100 ml)
Roweepra *Tab:* 250, 500, 750 mg; 1 gm

▷ *mephobarbital* (II)
Mebaral *Tab:* 32, 50, 100 mg

▷ *methsuximide*
Celontin Kapseals *Cap:* 150, 300 mg

▷ *midazolam* (IV)
Nayzilam Nasal Spray *Nasal spray:* 5 mg/0.1 ml spray, single-dose

▷ *oxcarbazepine* (G)
Trileptal *Tab:* 150, 300, 600 mg; *Oral susp:* 300 mg/5 ml (lemon) (alcohol)
Oxtellar XR *Tab:* 150, 300, 600 mg ext-rel

▷ *perampanel* (III)
Fycompa *Tab:* 2, 4, 6, 8, 10, 12 mg
Fycompa Oral Suspension *Oral susp:* 0.5 mg/ml (340 ml w. dosing syringe)

▷ *phenytoin* (G), *primidone* (G)
Dilantin *Cap:* 30, 100 mg ext-rel
Dilantin Infatabs *Chew tab:* 50 mg
Dilantin Oral Suspension *Oral susp:* 125 mg/5 ml (237 ml) (alcohol 6%)
Phenytek *Cap:* 200, 300 mg ext-rel

▷ *pregabalin* (V)(G)
Lyrica *Cap:* 25, 50, 75, 100, 200, 225, 300 mg
Lyrica CR *Tab:* 82.5, 165, 330 mg ext-rel
Lyrica Oral Solution *Oral soln:* 20 mg/ml

▷ *primidone*
Mysoline *Tab:* 50*, 250*mg
Mysoline Oral Solution *Oral susp:* 250 mg/5 ml (8 oz)

▷ *rufinamide* (G)
Banzel *Tab:* 200*, 400*mg
Banzel Oral Solution *Susp:* 40 mg/ml (orange) (lactose-free, gluten-free, dye-free)

▷ *stiripentol*
Diacomit *Cap:* 250, 500 mg; *Pwdr for oral susp:* 250, 500 mg/pkt (60/carton) (fruit)

▷ *tiagabine* (G)
Gabitril *Tab:* 2, 4, 12, 16 mg

▷ *topiramate* (G)
Eprontia *Oral soln:* 25 mg/ml (473 ml)
Topamax *Tab:* 25, 50, 100, 200 mg
Topamax Sprinkle Caps *Cap:* 15, 25, 50 mg
Trokendi XR *Cap:* 25, 50, 100, 200 mg ext-rel
Qudexy *Tab:* 25, 50, 100, 150, 200 mg ext-rel
Qudexy XR *Cap:* 25, 50, 100, 150, 200 mg ext-rel

(*continued*)

Appendix Q (*continued*)

▷ *vigabatrin* (G)
    Sabril *Tab:* 500 mg
    Sabril for Oral Solution 500 mg/pkt pwdr for reconstitution

▷ *zonisamide*
    Zonegran *Cap:* 25, 50, 100 mg
    Zonisade *Oral liq:* 100 mg/5 ml (strawberry)

APPENDIX R. ANTI-HIV DRUGS

ANTI-HIV DRUGS WITH DOSE FORMS

▷ **Aptivus** *tipranavir*
    Gel cap: 250 mg (alcohol); *Oral soln:* 100 mg/ml (95 ml w. dosing syringe) (vitamin E 116 IU/ml) (buttermint-butter, toffee)

▷ **Atripla** *efavirenz+emtricitabine+tenofovir disoproxil*
    Tab: efa 600 mg+emtri 200 mg+teno diso 300 mg

▷ **Biktarvy** *bictegravir+emtricitabine+tenofovir alafenamide*
    Tab: bict 50 mg+emtri 200 mg+teno alaf 25 mg

▷ **Cabenuva** *cabotegravir+rilpivirine*
    Tab: 600 mg ext-rel

▷ **Cimduo** *lamivudine+tenofovir disoproxil fumarate*
    Tab: lami 300 mg+teno diso 300 mg

▷ **Combivir** (G) *lamivudine+zidovudine*
    Tab: aba+lami 150+zido 300 mg

▷ **Complera** *emtricitabine+tenofovir disoproxil*
    Tab: emtri 200 mg+teno diso 300 mg+rilpiv 25 mg

▷ **Crixivan** *indinavir sulfate*
    Cap: 100, 200, 333, 400 mg

▷ **Cytovene** (G) *ganciclovir*
    Cap: 250, 500 mg; *Vial:* 50 mg/ml single-dose (500 mg, 10 ml)

▷ **Delstrigo** *doravirine+lamivudine+tenofovir disoproxil fumarate*
    Tab: dora 100 mg+lami ala 300 mg+teno dis 300 mg

▷ **Descovy** *emtricitabine+tenofovir alafenamide+rilpivirine*
    Tab: emtri 200 mg+teno ala 25 mg

▷ **Dovato** *dolutegravir+lamivudine*
    Tab: dolu 50 mg+lami 300 mg film-coat

▷ **Edurant** *rilpivirine*
    Tab: 25 mg

▷ **Emtriva** (G) *emtricitabine*
    Cap: 200 mg; *Oral soln:* 10 mg/ml (170 ml) (cotton candy)

▷ **Epivir** (G) *lamivudine*
    Tab: 150*, 300*mg; *Oral soln:* 10 mg/ml (240 ml) (strawberry-banana) (sucrose 3 gm/15 ml)

▷ **Epzicom** *abacavir sulfate+lamivudine*
    Tab: aba 600 mg+lami 300 mg

▷ **Evotaz** *atazanavir+cobicistat*
    Tab: ataz 300+cobi 150 mg

▷ **Fortovase** *aquinavir*
    Soft gelcap: 200 mg

▷ **Fuzeon** *enfuvirtide*
    Vial: 90 mg/ml pwdr for SC inj after reconstitution (1 ml, 60 vials/kit) (preservative-free)

(*continued*)

Appendix R (*continued*)

▷ Genvoya *elvitegravir+cobicistat+emtricitabine+tenofovir alafenamide (TAF)*
Tab: elv 150 mg+cob 150 mg+emtri 200 mg+teno alafen 10 mg

▷ Intelence *etravirine*
Tab: 25*, 100, 200 mg

▷ Invirase *saquinavir mesylate*
Hard gelcap: 200 mg

▷ Isentress *raltegravir (potassium)*
Tab: 400 mg film-coat; *Chew tab:* 25, 100*mg (orange-banana) (phenylalanine); *Oral susp:* 100 mg/pkt pwdr for oral susp (banana)

▷ Juluca *dolutegravir+rilpivirine*
Tab: dolu 50 mg+rilp 25 mg

▷ Kaletra (G) *lopinavir plus ritonavir*
Cap: lopin 100 mg+riton 25 mg, lopin 200 mg+riton 50 mg; *Oral soln:* lopin 80 mg+riton 20 mg per ml (160 ml w. dose cup) (cotton candy) (alcohol 42%)
Hard gelcap: 200 mg

▷ Lexiva (G) *fosamprenavir*
Tab: 700 mg; *Oral soln:* 50 mg/ml (grape, bubble gum) (peppermint)

▷ Norvir *ritonavir*
Soft gelcap: 100 mg (alcohol); *Oral soln:* 80 mg/ml (8 oz) (peppermint-caramel) (alcohol)

▷ Odefsey *emtricitabine+rilpivirine+tenofovir alafenamide*
Tab: emtri 200 mg+rilpiv 25 mg+tenof alafen 25 mg

▷ Pifeltro *doravirine*
Tab: 100 mg

▷ Prezcobix *darunavir+cobicistat*
Tab: daru 800+cobi 150 mg

▷ Prezista (G) *darunavir*
Tab: 75, 150, 600, 800 mg; *Oral susp:* 100 mg/ml (200 ml) (strawberry cream)

▷ Rescriptor *delavirdine mesylate*
Tab: 100, 200 mg

▷ Retrovir (G) *zidovudine*
Tab: 300 mg; *Cap:* 100 mg; *Syr:* 50 mg/5 ml (240 ml) (strawberry); *Vial:* 10 mg/ml (20 ml vial for IV infusion) (preservative-free)

▷ Reyataz *atazanavir*
Cap: 100, 150, 200, 300 mg

▷ Rukobia *fostemsavir*
Tab: 600 mg ext-rel

▷ Selzentry (G) *maraviroc*
Tab: 150, 300 mg

▷ Stribild *elvitegravir+cobicistat+emtricitabine+tenofovir disoproxil fumarate*
Tab: elv 150 mg+cob 150 mg+emtri 200 mg+teno diso fumar 300 mg

▷ Sunlenca *lenacapavir*
Tab: 300 mg; *Vial:* 463.5 mg/1.5 ml (309 mg/ml), single-dose for SC administration

▷ Sustiva *efavirenz*
Tab: 75, 150, 600, 800 mg; *Cap:* 50, 200 mg

▷ Symfi *efavirenz+lamivudine+tenofovir disoproxil fumarate*
Tab: efav 600 mg+lami 300 mg+teno diso fum 300 mg

▷ Symfi Lo *efavirenz+lamivudine+tenofovir disoproxil fumarate*
Tab: efav 400 mg+lami 300 mg+teno diso fum 300 mg

(*continued*)

Appendix R (*continued*)

▷ **Temixys** *lamivudine+tenofovir disoproxil fumarate*
Tab: lami 300 mg+teno diso fum 300 mg

▷ **Tivicay** *dolutegravir*
Tab: 50 mg

▷ **Temixys** *lamivudine+tenofovir disoproxil fumarate*
Tab: lami 300 mg+teno diso fum 300 mg

▷ **Triumeq** *abacavir sulfate+dolutegravir+lamivudine*
Tab: aba 600 mg+dolu 50 mg+lami 300 mg

▷ **Trizivir (G)** *abacavir sulfate+lamivudine+zidovudine*
Tab: aba 300 mg+lami 150 mg+zido 300 mg

▷ **Trogarzo** *ibalizumab-uiyk* administer as an IV injection once every 14 days
Vial: 200 mg/1.33 ml (1.33 ml), single-dose

▷ **Truvada (G)** *emtricitabine+tenofovir disoproxil fumarate*
Tab: emt 100 mg+teno 150 mg, 133 mg+teno 200 mg, emt 167 mg+teno 250 mg, emt 200 mg+teno 300 mg

▷ **Valcyte (G)** *valganciclovir*
Tab: 450 mg
Comment: *valganciclovir* is indicated for the treatment of AIDS-related cytomegalovirus (CMV) retinitis.

▷ **Videx EC (G)** *didanosine*
Cap: 125, 200, 250, 400 mg ent-coat del-rel; *Chew tab:* 25, 50, 100, 150, 200 mg (mandarin orange; buffered with calcium carbonate and magnesium hydroxide) (phenylalanine); *Pwdr for oral soln:* 2, 4 gm (120, 240 ml)

▷ **Videx Pediatric Pwdr for Oral Solution** *didanosine*
Pwdr for oral soln: 2, 4 gm (120, 240 ml)

▷ **Viracept** *nelfinavir mesylate*
Tab: 250, 625 mg; *Pwdr for oral soln:* 50 mg/gm (144 gm) (phenylalanine)

▷ **Viramune (G)** *nevirapine*
Tab: 200*mg; *Oral susp:* 50 mg/5 ml (240 ml)

▷ **Viramune XR** *nevirapine*
Tab: 100, 400 mg ext-rel

▷ **Viread (G)** *tenofovir disoproxil fumarate*
Tab: 150, 200, 250, 300 mg; *Oral pwdr:* 40 mg/1 gm pwdr (60 gm w. dosing scoop)

▷ **Vistide** *cidofovir*
Inj: 75 mg/ml (5 ml vials for IV infusion) (preservative free)
Comment: *Cidofovir* is indicated for the treatment of AIDS-related *Cytomegalovirus* (CMV) retinitis.

▷ **Vitekta** *elvitegravir*
Inj: 75 mg/ml (5 ml vials for IV infusion) (preservative free)

▷ **Vocabria**
Tab: 30 mg film-coat

▷ **Zerit (G)** *stavudine*
Cap: 15, 20, 30, 40 mg; *Oral soln:* 1 mg/ml pwdr for reconstitution (200 ml) (fruit) (dye-free)

▷ **Ziagen (G)** *abacavir sulfate*
Tab: 300*mg; *Oral soln:* 20 mg/ml (240 ml) (strawberry-banana) (parabens, propylene glycol)

APPENDIX S. ANTICOAGULANTS

APPENDIX S.1. COUMADIN TITRATION AND DOSE FORMS

▷ *warfarin* **(G)** dosage initially 2-5 mg/day; usual maintenance 2-10 mg/day; adjust dosage to maintain INR in therapeutic range:
Venous thrombosis: 2.0-3.0
Atrial fibrillation: 2.0-3.0
Post MI: 2.5-3.5
Mechanical and bioprosthetic heart valves: 2.0-3.0 for 12 weeks after valve insertion, then 2.5-3.5 long-term

(*continued*)

Appendix S.1 (*continued*)

Pediatric: <18 years: not recommended
Coumadin *Tab:* 1*, 2*, 2.5*, 3*, 4*, 5*, 6*, 7.5*, 10*mg
Coumadin for Injection *Vial:* 2 mg/ml (2.5 ml)
Comment: Coumadin for Injection is for peripheral IV administration only.

APPENDIX S.2. COUMADIN OVER-ANTICOAGULATION REVERSAL

▷ *phytonadione (vitamin K)* (G) 2.5-10 mg PO or IM; max 25 mg
   AquaMEPHYTON *Vial:* 1 mg/0.5 ml (0.5 ml), 10 mg/ml (1, 2.5, 5 ml)
   Mephyton *Tab:* 5 mg

APPENDIX S.3. AGENTS THAT INHIBIT COUMADIN'S ANTICOAGULATION EFFECTS

Increase Metabolism	Decrease Absorption	Other Mechanism(s)
azathioprine carbamazepine dicloxacillin (G) ethanol griseofulvin nafcillin pentobarbital phenobarbital phenytoin primidone rifabutin rifampin	azathioprine cholestyramine colestipol sucralfate	coenzyme Q10 estrogen griseofulvin oral contraceptives ritonavir spironolactone trazodone vitamin C (high dose) vitamin K

APPENDIX T. LOW MOLECULAR WEIGHT HEPARINS

Comment: Administer by subcutaneous injection *only*, in the abdomen, and rotate sites. Avoid concomitant drugs that affect hemostasis (e.g., oral anticoagulants and platelet aggregation inhibitors, including *aspirin*, NSAIDs, *dipyridamole, sulfinpyrazone, ticlopidine*). <18 years: not recommended

Low Molecular Weight Heparins With Dose Forms

▷ *ardeparin*
   Normiflo *Soln for inj:* 5,000 anti-factor Xa U/0.5 ml; 10,000 anti-Factor Xa U/0.5 ml (sulfites, parabens)

▷ *dalteparin*
   Fragmin *Prefilled syringe:* 2,500 IU/0.2 ml, 5,000 IU/0.2 ml (10/box) (preservative-free); *Multidose vial:* 1,000 IU/ml (95,000 IU, 9.5 ml) (benzyl alcohol)

▷ *danaparoid*
   Orgaran *Amp:* 750 anti-Xa units/0.6 ml (0.6 ml, 10/box); *Prefilled syringe:* 750 anti-Xa units/0.6 ml (0.6 ml, 10/box) (sulfites)

▷ *enoxaparin* (G)
   Lovenox *Prefilled syringe:* 30 mg/0.3 ml, 40 mg/0.4 ml, 60 mg/0.6 ml, 80 mg/0.8 ml (100 mg/ml) (preservative-free); *Vial:* 100 mg/ml (3 ml)

▷ *tinzaparin*
   Innohep *Vial:* 20,000 anti-Factor Xa IU/ml (2 ml) (sulfites, benzyl alcohol)

APPENDIX U. FACTOR XA INHIBITORS

Comment: Factor Xa inhibitors are anticoagulants that reversibly and competitively inhibit free and clot-bound factor Xa. **Andexxa** *(andexanet alfa, coagulation factor Xa [recombinant] inactivated-zhzo)* is only indicated for patients treated with *apixaban* (Eliquis) or *rivaroxaban* (Xarelto) or when reversal of anticoagulation is needed due to life-threatening or uncontrolled bleeding. This indication is approved under accelerated approval based on the change from baseline in anti-factor Xa activity in healthy volunteers. An improvement in hemostasis has not been established. Continued approval for this indication may be contingent upon the results of studies that demonstrate an improvement in hemostasis in patients. As of April 2023, **Andexxa** has not been shown to be effective for, and is not indicated for, treatment of bleeding related to any factor Xa inhibitors *other than* **apixaban** (Eliquis) or *rivaroxaban* (Xarelto).

(*continued*)

Appendix U (*continued*)

Factor Xa Inhibitor Dose Forms and Therapy

▶ *apixaban* 5 mg bid; reduce to 2.5 mg bid if any two of the following: ≥80 years, ≤60 kg, serum creatinine (sCr) >1.5 mg/dL
Pediatric: not recommended
    Eliquis *Tab:* 2.5, 5 mg
Comment: Eliquis is indicated to reduce the risk of stroke and systemic embolism in patients with non-valvular atrial fibrillation (NVAF). Eliquis is not recommended for use in patients with a prosthetic heart valve, in pregnancy, in breastfeeding mothers, or patients with severe hepatic failure (Child-Pugh Class C). Strong dual inhibitors of CYP3A4 and P-glycoprotein (P-gp) increase blood levels of *apixaban*; therefore, reduce Eliquis dose to 2.5 mg or avoid concomitant use. Simultaneous use of strong inducers of CYP3A4 and P-gp reduces blood levels of *apixaban*; therefore, avoid concomitant use. See mfr pkg insert for full prescribing information. The reversal agent for *apixaban* is Andexxa (*andexanet alfa, coagulation factor Xa [recombinant] inactivated-zhzo*).

▶ *betrixaban Recommended dose:* an initial single dose of 160 mg, followed by 80 mg once daily, taken at the same time each day with food; *Recommended duration of treatment:* 35-42 days; reduce dose with severe renal impairment or with P-gp inhibitors
Pediatrics: safety and efficacy not established
    Bevyxxa *Cap:* 40, 80 mg
Comment: Bevyxxa is indicated for the prophylaxis of venous thromboembolism (VTE) in adults who are hospitalized for acute mental illness and at risk for thromboembolic complications due to moderate or severe restricted mobility and other VTE risk factors. There are no data with use of *betrixaban* in pregnancy, but treatment is likely to increase the risk of hemorrhage during pregnancy and delivery. No data are available regarding the presence of *betrixaban* or its metabolites in human milk or the effects of the drug on the breastfed infant.

▶ *edoxaban* Transition to and from Savaysa; assess CrCl prior to initiation:
NVAF CrCl >50 ml/min: 60 mg once daily; *CrCl 15-50 ml/min:* 30 mg once daily
DVT/PE CrCl >50 ml/min: 60 mg once daily following initial parenteral anticoagulant; *CrCl 15-50 ml/min, <60 kg, or concomitant P-gp inhibitors:* 30 mg once daily
Pediatric: safety and efficacy not established
    Savaysa *Tab:* 15, 30, 60 mg
Comment: Savaysa is indicated to reduce the risk of stroke and systemic embolism in patients with nonvalvular atrial fibrillation (NVAF), treatment of DVT and pulmonary embolism (PE), following 5-10 days of initial therapy with parenteral anticoagulant. Renal clearance accounts for approximately 50% of the total clearance of *edoxaban*. Consequently, *edoxaban* blood levels are increased in patients with poor renal function compared with those with higher renal function. Reduce Savaysa dose to 30 mg once daily in patients with CrCL 15-50 ml/min. There are limited clinical data with Savaysa in patients with CrCL <15 ml/min; Savaysa is, therefore, not recommended in these patients. Hemodialysis does not significantly contribute to Savaysa clearance. Savaysa is not for use in persons with NVAF with CrCl >95 ml/min. There are no adequate and well-controlled studies in pregnant women. Savaysa should be used during pregnancy only if the potential benefit justifies the potential risk to the fetus. Safety and effectiveness of Savaysa during labor and delivery have not been evaluated in clinical studies. The risk of bleeding should be balanced with the risk of thrombotic events when considering the use of Savaysa in this setting. A decision should be made to discontinue Savaysa or discontinue breastfeeding, taking into account the importance of the drug to the mother.

▶ *fondaparinux* administer SC; administer first dose no earlier than 6-8 hours after hemostasis is achieved, start warfarin usually within 72 hours of last dose of *fondaparinux*
Postop: 2.5 mg once daily x 5-9 days
Hip/Knee Replacement: once daily x 11 days
Hip Fracture: once daily x 32 days
Abdominal Surgery: once daily x 10 days
Prophylaxis: do not use <50 kg
Treatment: once daily for at least 5 days until INR = 2-3 (usually 5-9 days); max 26 days; <50 kg: 5 mg; 50-100 kg: 7.5 mg; >100 kg: 10 mg
Pediatric: safety and efficacy not established
    Arixtra *Soln for SC inj:* 2.5 mg/0.5 ml, 5 mg/0.4 ml, 7.5 mg/0.6 ml, 10 mg/0.8 ml; *Prefilled syringe* and 27-gauge x ½ inch needle with automatic needle protection system (10/box) (preservative-free)

▶ *prasugrel* (G) *Loading dose:* 60 mg once in a single dose; *Maintenance:* 10 mg once daily; *<60 kg:* consider 5 mg once daily; take with aspirin 75-325 mg once daily
Pediatric: safety and efficacy not recommended
    Effient *Tab:* 5, 10 mg
Comment: Effient is indicated to reduce the risk of thrombotic cardiovascular events in persons with acute coronary syndrome (ACS) who are to be managed with percutaneous coronary intervention (PCI), including unstable angina, non-ST elevation myocardial infarction (NSTEMI), and ST elevation myocardial infarction

(*continued*)

Appendix U (*continued*)

(STEMI). Do not start if there is active pathologic bleeding (e.g., peptic ulcer, intracranial hemorrhage), prior transient ischemic attack (TIA) or stroke, or if the patient is likely to undergo urgent coronary artery bypass graft (CABG). Discontinue 7 days before surgery and if TIA or stroke occurs.

▶ **rivaroxaban** take with food
  Treatment of DVT or PE: 15 mg bid for the first 21 days; then 20 mg once daily
  Reduction in risk of DVT or PE recurrence: 20 mg once daily with the evening meal; *CrCl <30 ml/min:* avoid
  Prophylaxis of DVT: take 6-10 hours after surgery when hemostasis established, then 10-20 mg once daily with the evening meal; *CrCl 30-50 ml/min:* 10 mg; *CrCl <30 ml/min:* avoid; discontinue if acute renal failure develops; monitor closely for blood loss
  Hip: treat for 35 days; *Knee:* treat for 12 days
  Nonvalvular AF: take once daily with the evening meal; *CrCl >50 ml/min:* 20 mg; *CrCl 15-50 ml/min:* 15 mg; *CrCl >15 ml/min:* avoid
  Pediatric: not recommended
    Xarelto *Cap:* 10, 15, 20 mg
Comment: Xarelto is indicated to reduce the risk of stroke and systemic embolism in NVAF, to treat DVT and PE, to reduce the risk of recurrence of DVT and/or PE following 6 months treatment for DVT and/or PE, and prophylaxis of DVT, which may lead to PE in patients undergoing knee or hip replacement surgery. **Xarelto** eliminates the need for bridging with heparin or low molecular heparin; no need for routine monitoring of INR or other coagulation parameters; no need for dose adjustments for age, weight, or gender; no known dietary restrictions. Switching from **warfarin** or other anticoagulant, see mfr pkg insert.

Factor Xa Inhibitor Reversal Agent

Comment: Andexxa (*coagulation factor Xa [recombinant] inactivated-zhzo*) is indicated to reverse the anticoagulation effects of factor Xa inhibitors (i.e., reversal agent specific to **rivaroxaban** [Xarelto] and **apixaban** [Eliquis]) when needed due to life-threatening or uncontrolled bleeding or emergency surgery. **Andexxa** was approved under the FDA's accelerated approval pathway based on effects in healthy volunteers, and continued approval may be contingent on postmarketing studies to demonstrate an improvement in hemostasis in patients. A clinical trial comparing this agent or usual care that was started in 2019 is scheduled to be reported in 2023. As of April 2023, **Andexxa** is not indicated for, the treatment of bleeding related to any factor Xa inhibitors other than **apixaban** (Eliquis) and **rivaroxaban** (Xarelto).

COAGULATION FACTOR A (RECOMBINANT) INACTIVATED-ZHZO

▶ **andexanet alfa** (*coagulation factor Xa [recombinant] inactivated-zhzo*) administer as an IV bolus, with a target rate of 30 mg/min, followed by continuous infusion for up to 120 minutes; select a high-dose or low-dose regimen based on the specific factor Xa inhibitor, dose of factor Xa inhibitor, and time since the patient's last dose of factor Xa inhibitor (see pkg insert); resume anticoagulant therapy as soon as medically appropriate following treatment with **Andexxa**
  High Dose Regimen: initial IV bolus: 800 mg at a target rate of 30 mg/min; follow-on IV infusion: 8 mg/min for up to 120 min
  Low Dose Regimen: initial IV bolus: 400 mg at a target rate of 30 mg/min; follow-on IV infusion: 4 mg/min for up to 120 min
  Pediatric: >18 years: not studied; ≥18 years: same as adult
    Andexxa *Vial:* 100 mg, single-dose, pwdr for reconstitution and IV infusion
Comment: There are no adequate and well-controlled studies of **Andexxa** in pregnant females to inform patients of associated risks. The safety and effectiveness of **Andexxa** during labor and delivery have not been evaluated. There is no information regarding the presence of **Andexxa** in human milk or effects on the breastfed infant. Safety and efficacy of **Andexxa** in the pediatric population have not been studied. *Black Boxed Warning:* Treatment with **Andexxa** has been associated with serious and life-threatening adverse events, including arterial and venous thromboembolic events, ischemic events, including myocardial infarction and ischemic stroke, cardiac arrest, and sudden deaths.

APPENDIX V. DIRECT THROMBIN INHIBITORS

Direct Thrombin Inhibitor Dosing and Dose Forms

▶ **aspirin** single dose once daily
  Pediatric: safety and efficacy not established
    Durlaza *Cap:* 162.5 mg 24-hour ext-rel (30, 90/bottle)
▶ **dabigatran etexilate mesylate** (**G**) *Recommended dose: CrCl >30 ml/min:* 150 mg bid; *CrCl 15-30 ml/min:* 75 mg bid; swallow whole; do not chew, break, or open capsules; see mfr pkg insert recommendations for converting to or from other oral or parenteral anticoagulants; temporarily discontinue **Pradaxa** before invasive or surgical procedures when possible, then restart promptly
  Pediatric: <8 years: safety and efficacy not established; 8-18 years: venous thromboembolic event (VTE): patients who have been treated with a parenteral anticoagulant for at least 5 days may be switched to weight-based dosing of **Pradaxa** bid; >18 years: same as adult; see mfr pkg insert for weight-based dosing table

(*continued*)

Appendix V (*continued*)

Pradaxa *Cap (oral pellets):* 75, 150 mg
Pediatric: Safety and efficacy of **Pradaxa Oral Pellets** for the treatment and the reduction in risk of recurrence of venous thromboembolism (VTE) have been established in pediatric patients <12 years-of-age. Approval for this indication is supported by evidence from adequate and well-controlled studies in pediatric patients. These studies included an open-label, randomized, parallel-group study and an open-label, single-arm safety study and Clinical Studies. Other age-appropriate pediatric formulations of *dabigatran etexilate* are available for pediatric patients aged ≥12 years for these indications. Safety and efficacy of **Pradaxa** have not been established in pediatric patients with non-valvular atrial fibrillation or those who have undergone hip replacement surgery.
Comment: **Pradaxa** is a direct thrombin inhibitor indicated (1) to reduce the risk of stroke and systemic embolism in adult patients with non-valvular atrial fibrillation (AF); (2) for treatment of deep venous thrombosis (DVT) and pulmonary embolism (PE) in adult patients who have been treated with a parenteral anticoagulant for 5-10 days; (3) to reduce the risk of recurrence of DVT and PE in adult patients who have been previously treated; (4) for prophylaxis of DVT and PE in adult patients who have undergone hip replacement surgery.
Pediatric: <18 years: safety and efficacy not established; ≥18 years: same as adult

▷ *desirudin (recombinant hirudin)* 15 mg SC every 12 hours, preferably in the abdomen or thigh, starting up to 5-15 minutes before surgery (after induction of regional block anesthesia, if used); may continue for 9-12 days postop; *CrCl <60 ml/min:* reduce dose (see mfr pkg insert)
Pediatric: not recommended
Iprivask *Pwdr for SC inj after reconstitution:* 15 mg/single-use vial (10/box) (preservative-free, diluent contains mannitol)
Comment: Iprivask is indicated for DVT prophylaxis in patients undergoing hip replacement surgery. It is not interchangeable with other hirudins.

Idarucizumab Reversal Agent: Humanized Monoclonal–Antibody Fragment (FAB)

▷ *idarucizumab* administer 5 gm (2 vials) IV drip or push; administer within 1 hour of removal from vial
Pediatric: safety and efficacy not established
Praxbind *Vial:* 2.5 g/50 ml, single-use (preservative-free)
Comment: Presently, there are inadequate human and animal data to assess risk of *idarucizumab* (Praxbind) use in pregnancy. Risk/benefit should be considered prior to use.

APPENDIX W. PLATELET AGGREGATION INHIBITORS

Platelet Aggregation Inhibitor Dosing and Dose Forms

▷ *cilostazol* (G) *Tab:* 100 mg bid
Pediatric: not recommended
Pletal *Tab:* 50, 100 mg
Comment: Pletal is an antiplatelet/vasodilator phosphodiesterase ([PDE] III) inhibitor.

▷ *clopidogrel* (G) 75 mg once daily
Pediatric: not recommended
Plavix *Tab:* 75, 300 mg
Comment: Plavix is indicated for the reduction of atherosclerotic events in recent myocardial infarction or stroke, established peripheral arterial disease (PAD), non-ST-segment elevation acute coronary syndrome (unstable angina/NSTEMI), or ST elevation myocardial infarction (STEMI).

▷ *dipyridamole* (G) 75-100 mg qid
Pediatric: not recommended
Persantine *Tab:* 25, 50, 75 mg
Comment: *Dipyridamole* is indicated as an adjunct to oral anticoagulants after cardiac valve replacement surgery to prevent thromboembolism.

▷ *dipyridamole+aspirin* (G) swallow whole; one cap bid
Pediatric: not recommended
Aggrenox *Cap:* dipyr 200 mg+asa 25 mg

▷ *pentoxifylline* (hemorrheologic [xanthine])
Pediatric: not recommended
Trental *Tab:* 400 mg sust-rel

▷ *prasugrel* (G)
Pediatric: not recommended
Effient *Tab:* 5, 10 mg
Comment: Effient is indicated to reduce the risk of cardiovascular events in patients with acute coronary syndrome (ACS), who are to be managed with percutaneous coronary intervention (PCI) (unstable angina or non-STEMI), and STEMI when managed with either primary or delayed PCI.

(*continued*)

Appendix W (*continued*)

➤ *ticagrelor* initiate 180 mg loading dose once in a single dose with *aspirin* 325 mg loading dose in a single dose; maintenance 90 mg bid with *aspirin* 75-100 mg once daily; ACS patients may start *ticagrelor* after a loading dose of *clopidogrel*
  Brilinta *Tab:* 90 mg
Comment: Brilinta is indicated to reduce the risk of cardiovascular events in patients with acute coronary syndrome (ACS) (unstable angina, Non-ST elevation [NSTEMI], myocardial infarction, or STEMI).

➤ *ticlopidine* 250 mg bid
  Pediatric: not recommended
  Ticlid *Tab:* 250 mg
Comment: Ticlid is indicated to reduce the risk of thrombotic stroke in selected patients intolerant of *aspirin*.

APPENDIX X. PROTEASE-ACTIVATED RECEPTOR-1 (PAR-1) INHIBITORS

Protease-Activated Receptor-1 (PAR-1) Inhibitor Dosing And Dose Form

➤ *vorapaxar* administer 2.08 mg once daily; use with *aspirin* or *clopidogrel*
  Pediatric: <12 years: not established; ≥12 years: same as adult
  Zontivity *Tab:* 2.08 mg (equivalent to 2.5 mg vorapaxar sulfate)
Comment: Zontivity is indicated to reduce thrombotic cardiovascular events in patients with a history of myocardial infarction or with peripheral arterial disease (PAD). Contraindicated with active pathologic bleeding (e.g., peptic ulcer, intracranial hemorrhage); prior TIA or stroke. Not recommended with severe hepatic impairment.

APPENDIX AA. SYSTEMIC ANTI-INFECTIVES

Comment:
- Adverse effects of aminoglycosides include nephrotoxicity and ototoxicity.
- Use cephalosporins with caution in persons with penicillin allergy due to potential cross allergy.
- Sulfonamides are contraindicated with sulfa allergy and glucose-6-phosphate dehydrogenase (G6PD) deficiency. A high fluid intake is indicated during sulfonamide therapy.
- Tetracyclines should be taken on an empty stomach to facilitate absorption. Tetracyclines should not be taken with milk.
- Tetracyclines are contraindicated during pregnancy and breastfeeding and in children <8 years of age, due to the risk of developing tooth enamel discoloration.
- Systemic quinolones and fluoroquinolones are contraindicated in pregnancy and children <18 years of age due to the risk of joint dysplasia.

Anti-Infectives by Class With Dose Forms		
Generic Name	Brand Name	Dose Form/Volume
Amebicides		
chloroquine phosphate (**G**)	Aralen	*Tab:* 500 mg
chloroquine phosphate+ primaquine phosphate (**G**)	Aralen Phosphate+ Primaquine Phosphate	*Tab:* chlor 300 mg+prim 45 mg
iodoquinol	Yodoxin	*Tab:* 210, 650 mg
metronidazole (**G**)	Flagyl	*Tab:* 250*, 500*mg
	Flagyl 375	*Cap:* 375 mg
	Flagyl ER	*Tab:* 750 mg ext-rel
tinidazole	Tindamax	*Tab:* 250*, 500*mg
Aminoglycosides		
amikacin (**G**)	Amikin	*Vial:* 500 mg, 1 gm (2 ml)
gentamicin (**G**)	Garamycin	*Vial:* 20, 80 mg/2 ml
streptomycin (**G**)	Streptomycin	*Amp:* 1 gm/2.5 ml or 400 mg/ml (2.5 ml)
Antifungals		
atovaquone	Mepron	*Susp:* 750 mg/5ml (210 ml)
clotrimazole (**G**)	Mycelex Troche	10 mg (70, 40/bottle)

(*continued*)

Appendix AA (*continued*)

Anti-Infectives by Class With Dose Forms		
Generic Name	Brand Name	Dose Form/Volume
fluconazole (G)	Diflucan	*Tab:* 50, 100, 150, 200 mg; *Oral susp:* 10, 40 mg/ml (35 ml) (orange)
griseofulvin, microsize (G)	Grifulvin V	*Tab:* 250, 500 mg; *Oral susp:* 125 mg/ 5 ml (120 ml) (alcohol 0.02%)
griseofulvin, ultramicrosize (G)	Gris-PEG	*Tab:* 125, 250 mg
itraconazole (G)	Sporanox	*Cap:* 100 mg; *Soln:* 10 mg/ml (150 ml); *Pulse pack:* 100 mg caps (7/pck)
ketoconazole (G)	Nizoral	*Tab:* 200 mg
nystatin (G)	Mycostatin	*Pastille:* 200,000 units/pastille (30 pastilles/pck); *Oral susp:* 100,000 units/ml (60 ml w. dropper)
posaconazole (G)	Noxafil	*Tab:* 100 mg ext-rel; *Oral susp:* 40 mg/ml (105 ml); *Vial:* 300 mg/16.7 ml (18 mg/ml), soln for IV infusion
terbinafine (G)	Lamisil	*Tab:* 250 mg
voriconazole (G)	Vfend	*Tab:* 50, 200 mg
Antihelmintics		
albendazole (G)	Albenza	*Tab:* 200 mg
ivermectin (G)	Stromectol	*Tab:* 3 mg
mebendazole (G)	Emverm, Vermox	*Chew tab:* 100 mg
pyrantel pamoate (G)	Antiminth Pin-X	*Cap:* 180 mg; *Liq:* 50 mg/ml (30 ml), 144 mg/ml (30 ml); *Oral susp:* 50 mg/ml (30 ml) (caramel) (sodium benzoate, tartrazine-free)
thiabendazole (G)	Mintezol (currently <u>not</u> available in the United States)	*Chew tab:* 500*mg (orange); *Oral susp:* 500 mg/5 ml (120 ml) (orange)
Antimalarials		
atovaquone	Mepron	*Susp:* 750 mg/5 ml
atovaquone+ proguanil	Malarone	*Tab:* atov 250 mg+proq 100 mg
	Malarone Pediatric	*Tab:* atov 62.5 mg+proq 25 mg
chloroquine (G)	Aralen	*Tab:* 500 mg; *Amp:* 50 mg/ml (5 ml)
doxycycline (G)	Acticlate	*Tab:* 75, 150**mg
	Adoxa	*Tab:* 50, 75, 100, 150 mg ent-coat
	Doryx	*Cap:* 100 mg; *Tab:* 50, 75, 100, 150, 200 mg
	Doxsteric	*Tab:* 50 mg del-rel
	Monodox	*Cap:* 50, 75, 100 mg
	Oracea	*Cap:* 40 mg del-rel
	Vibramycin	*Cap:* 50, 100 mg; *Syr:* 50 mg/5 ml (raspberry-apple) (sulfites); *Oral susp:* 25 mg/5 ml (raspberry)
	Vibra-Tab	*Tab:* 100 mg film-coat
	Xerava	*Vial:* 50 mg, pwdr for dilution and IV infusion
hydroxychloroquine (G)	Plaquenil	*Tab:* 200 mg
mefloquine	Lariam	*Tab:* 250 mg
minocycline (G)	Dynacin	*Cap:* 50, 100 mg

(continued)

Appendix AA (*continued*)

Anti-Infectives by Class With Dose Forms		
Generic Name	**Brand Name**	**Dose Form/Volume**
	Minocin	*Cap:* 50, 75, 100 mg; *Oral susp:* 50 mg/5 ml (60 ml) (custard) (sulfites, alcohol 5%)
	Minolira	*Tab:* 105, 135 mg ext-rel
	Solodyn	*Tab:* 55, 65, 80, 105, 115 mg ext-rel
Antiprotozoal/Antibacterials		
quinine sulfate **(G)**	Qualaquin	*Cap:* 324 mg
metronidazole **(G)**	Flagyl, Protostat	*Tab:* 250*, 500*mg
	Flagyl 375	*Cap:* 375 mg
	Flagyl ER	*Tab:* 750 mg ext-rel
nitazoxanide **(G)**	Alinia	*Tab:* 500 mg; *Oral susp:* 100 mg/5 ml (60 ml) (strawberry)
tinidazole	Tindamax	*Tab:* 250*, 500*mg
Antituberculars		
ethambutol (EMB) **(G)**	Myambutol	*Tab:* 100, 400*mg
isoniazid (INH) **(G)**	*generic only*	*Tab:* 100, 300*mg; *Syr:* 50 mg/5 ml; *Inj:* 100 mg/ml
pyrazinamide (PZA)	*generic only*	*Tab:* 500*mg
rifampin **(G)**	Priftin	*Tab:* 150 mg
	Rifadin	*Cap:* 150, 300 mg
rifampin+isoniazid	Rifamate	*Cap:* rif 300 mg+iso 150 mg
rifampin+isoniazid+ pyrazinamide	Rifater	*Tab:* rif 120 mg+iso 50 mg+pyr 300 mg
Antivirals (for HIV-antiretroviral drugs, see page 592)		
acyclovir **(G)**	Zovirax	*Cap:* 200 mg; *Tab:* 400, 800 mg; *Oral susp:* 200 mg/5 ml (banana)
amantadine **(G)**	Symmetrel	*Tab:* 100 mg; *Syr:* 50 mg/5ml (16 oz) (raspberry)
famciclovir	Famvir	*Tab:* 125, 250, 500 mg
lamivudine	Epivir-HBV	*Tab:* 100 mg; *Oral soln:* 5 mg/ml (240 ml) (strawberry-banana)
oseltamivir	Tamiflu	*Cap:* 75 mg
rimantadine **(G)**	Flumadine	*Tab:* 100 mg
valacyclovir	Valtrex	*Tab:* 500 mg; 1 gm
zanamivir	Relenza	*Tab:* lami 150+zido 300 mg
Cephalosporins		
First-generation cephalosporins		
cefadroxil **(G)**	Duricef	*Cap:* 500 mg; *Tab:* 1 gm; *Oral susp:* 250 mg/5 ml (100 ml), 500 mg/5 ml (75, 100 ml) (orange-pineapple)
cefazolin	Ancef, Zolicef	*Vial:* 500 mg; 1, 10 gm
cephalexin **(G)**	Keflex	*Cap:* 250, 333, 500, 750 mg; *Oral susp:*125, 250 mg/5 ml (100, 200 ml)

(*continued*)

Appendix AA (*continued*)

Anti-Infectives by Class With Dose Forms		
Generic Name	**Brand Name**	**Dose Form/Volume**
Second-generation cephalosporins		
cefaclor (G)	*generic <u>only</u>*	*Tab:* 500 mg; *Cap:* 250, 500 mg; *Susp:* 125 mg/5 ml (75, 150 ml) (strawberry), 187 mg/5 ml (50, 100 ml) (strawberry), 250 mg/5 ml (75, 150 ml) (strawberry), 375 mg/5 ml (50, 100 ml) (strawberry)
cefaclor ext-rel (G)	Cefaclor Extended Release	*Tab:* 375, 500 mg ext-rel
cefamandole	Mandol	*Vial:* 1, 2 gm
cefotetan	Cefotan	*Vial:* 1, 2 gm
cefoxitin	Mefoxin	*Vial:* 1, 2 gm
cefprozil (G)	Cefzil	*Tab:* 250, 500 mg; *Oral susp:* 125, 250 mg/5 ml (50, 75, 100 ml) (bubble gum) (phenylalanine)
ceftaroline	Teflaro	*Vial:* 400, 600 mg
cefuroxime sodium (G)	Zinacef	*Vial:* 750 mg; 1.5 gm
loracarbef (G)	Lorabid	*Pulvule:* 200, 400 mg; *Oral susp:* 100 mg/5 ml (50, 100 ml), 200 mg/5 ml (50, 75, 100 ml; strawberry bubble gum)
Third-generation cephalosporins		
cefoperazone	Cefobid	*Vial:* 1, 2 gm pwdr for reconstitution
cefotaxime	Claforan	*Vial:* 500 mg; 1, 2 gm pwdr for reconstitution
cefpodoxime	Vantin	*Tab:* 100, 200 mg; *Oral susp:* 50, 100 mg/5 ml (50, 75, 100 ml) (lemon creme)
ceftazidime	Ceptaz	*Vial:* 1, 2 gm pwdr for reconstitution
	Fortaz	*Vial:* 500 mg; 1, 2 gm pwdr for reconstitution
	Tazicef	*Vial:* 1, 2 gm pwdr for reconstitution
	Tazidime	*Vial:* 1, 2 gm pwdr for reconstitution
ceftazidime/avibactam	Avycaz	*Vial:* 2.5 gm pwdr for reconstitution
ceftibuten (G)	Cedax	*Cap:* 400 mg; *Oral susp:* 90 mg/5 ml (30, 60, 90, 120 ml), 180 mg/5 ml (30, 60, 120 ml) (cherry)
Third-/fourth-generation cephalosporins		
cefdinir (G)	Omnicef	*Cap:* 300 mg; *Oral susp:* 125 mg/5 ml (60, 100 ml) (strawberry)
cefditoren pivoxil	Spectracef	*Tab:* 200 mg
cefepime	Maxipime	*Vial:* 1 gm pwdr for reconstitution
cefixime (G)	Suprax	*Tab/Cap:* 400 mg; *Oral Susp:* 100 mg/5 ml (50, 75, 100 ml) (strawberry)
ceftaroline	Teflaro	*Vial:* 400, 600 mg
ceftriaxone (G)	Rocephin	*Vial:* 250, 500 mg; 1, 2 gm
ceftolozane+tazobactam	Zerbaxa	*Vial:* 1.5 gm pwdr for reconstitution

(*continued*)

Appendix AA (*continued*)

Anti-Infectives by Class With Dose Forms		
Generic Name	Brand Name	Dose Form/Volume
Lipoglycopeptide Antibacterials		
oritavancin	Kimyrsa	*Vial:* 1,200 mg single-dose, pwdr for reconstitution, dilution, and IV infusion
	Orbactiv	*Vial:* 400 mg single-dose, pwdr for reconstitution, dilution, and IV infusion
Penicillins		
amoxicillin (G)	Amoxil	*Cap:* 250, 500 mg; *Tab:* 500, 875* mg; *Chew tab:* 125, 200, 250, 400 mg (cherry-banana-peppermint) (phenylalanine); *Oral susp:*125, 250 mg/ml (80, 100, 150 ml) (bubble gum); 200, 400 mg/5 ml (50, 75, 100 ml) (bubble gum); *Oral drops:* 50 mg/ml (30 ml) (bubble gum)
	Moxatag	*Tab:* 775 mg ext-rel
	Trimox	*Cap:* 250, 500 mg; *Oral susp:* 125, 250 mg/5ml (80, 100, 150 ml) (raspberry-strawberry)
amoxicillin+ clavulanate (G)	Augmentin	*Tab:* 250, 500, 875 mg; *Chew tab:* 125, 250 mg (lemon lime); 200, 400 mg (cherry-banana; phenylalanine); *Oral susp:* 125 mg/5 ml (banana), 250 mg/5 ml (orange) (75, 100, 150 ml); 200, 400 mg/5 ml (50, 75, 100 ml) (orange)
	Augmentin ES-600	*Oral susp:* 600 mg/5 ml (50, 75, 100, 125, 150, 200 ml) (strawberry cream) (phenylalanine)
	Augmentin XR	*Tab:* 1,000*mg ext-rel
ampicillin (G)	Omnipen	*Cap:* 250, 500 mg; *Oral susp:* 125, 250 mg/ml (100, 150, 200 ml)
	Principen	*Cap:* 250, 500 mg; *Syr:* 125, 250 mg/5 ml
ampicillin+ sulbactam (G)	Unasyn	*Vial:* 1.5, 3 gm
carbenicillin	Geocillin	*Tab:* 382 mg film-coat
dicloxacillin (G)	Dynapen	*Cap:* 125, 250, 500 mg; *Oral susp:* 62.5 mg/5 ml (80, 100, 200 ml)
ertapenem	Invanz	*Vial:* 1 gm pwdr for reconstitution
meropenem (G)	Merrem	*Vial:* 500 mg; 1 gm pwdr for reconstitution (sodium 3.92 mEq/gm)
penicillin g benzathine (G)	Bicillin LA, Bicillin C-R	*Cartridge-needle unit:* 600,000 million units (1 ml), 1.2 million units (2 ml), 2.4 million units (4 ml)
	Permapen	*Prefilled syringe:* 1.2 million units
penicillin g potassium (G)	Generic <u>only</u>	*Vial:* 5, 20 MU pwdr for reconstitution; *Premixed bag:* 1, 2, 3 MU (50 ml)
penicillin g procaine (G)	Generic <u>only</u>	*Prefilled syringe:* 1.2 million units
penicillin v potassium (G)	Pen-Vee K	*Tab:* 250, 500 mg; *Oral soln:* 125 mg/5 ml (100, 200 ml), 250 mg/5 ml (100, 150, 200 ml)
piperacillin+ tazobactam (G)	Zosyn	*Vial:* 2, 3, 4 gm pwdr for reconstitution

(*continued*)

Appendix AA (*continued*)

Anti-Infectives by Class With Dose Forms		
Generic Name	**Brand Name**	**Dose Form/Volume**
Quinolone and Fluoroquinolones		
First-generation quinolone		
enoxacin	Penetrex	*Tab:* 200, 400 mg
First-generation fluoroquinolones		
ciprofloxacin (G)	Cipro	*Tab:* 250, 500, 750 mg; *Oral susp:* 250, 500 mg/5 ml (100 ml) (strawberry); *IV conc:* 10 mg/ml after dilution (20, 40 ml); *Premixed bag:* 2 mg/ml (100, 200 ml)
	Cipro XR	*Tab:* 500, 1,000 mg ext-rel
	ProQuin XR	*Tab:* 500 mg ext-rel
lomefloxacin	Maxaquin	*Tab:* 400 mg
norfloxacin (G)	Noroxin	*Tab:* 400 mg
ofloxacin (G)	Floxin	*Tab:* 200, 300, 400 mg
lomefloxacin	Floxin	*Tab:* 200, 300, 400 mg
Third-generation fluoroquinolone		
levofloxacin (G)	Levaquin	*Tab:* 250, 500, 750 mg
Fourth-generation fluoroquinolones		
delafloxacin	Baxdela	*Tab:* 400 mg; *Vial:* 300 mg pwdr for reconstitution
gemifloxacin (G)	Factive	*Tab:* 320*mg
moxifloxacin (G)	Avelox	*Tab:* 400 mg
Ketolide		
telithromycin	Ketek	*Tab:* 300, 400 mg
Macrolides		
azithromycin (G)	Zithromax	*Tab:* 250, 500, 600 mg; *Granules:* 1 gm/pck for reconstitution (cherry-banana); Pwdr for oral susp
	Zithromax Tri-Pak	*Tab:* 3 x 500 mg tabs/pck
	Zithromax Z-Pak	*Tab:* 6 x 250 mg tabs/pck
	Zmax	*Granules:* 2 gm/pkt for reconstitution (cherry-banana)
clarithromycin (G)	Biaxin	*Tab:* 250, 500 mg; *Oral susp:* 125, 250 mg/5 ml (50, 100 ml) (fruit punch)
	Biaxin XL	*Tab:* 500 mg ext-rel
dirithromycin (G)	generic <u>only</u>	*Tab:* 250 mg
erythromycin base (G)	Ery-Tab	*Tab:* 250, 333, 500 mg ent-coat
	PCE	*Tab:* 333, 500 mg
erythromycin estolate (G)	Ilosone	*Pulvule:* 250 mg; *Tab:* 500 mg; *Liq:* 125, 250 mg/5 ml (100 ml)
erythromycin ethylsuccinate (G)	E.E.S.	*Tab:* 400 mg; *Oral susp:* 200 mg/5 ml (100, 200 ml) (cherry); 200, 400 mg/5 ml (100 ml) (fruit)

(*continued*)

Appendix AA *(continued)*

Anti-Infectives by Class With Dose Forms		
Generic Name	**Brand Name**	**Dose Form/Volume**
erythromycin ethylsuccinate **(G)**	EryPed	*Oral susp:* 200 mg/5 ml (100, 200 ml) (fruit), 400 mg/5 ml (60, 100, 200 ml) (banana); *Oral drops:* 200, 400 mg/5 ml (50 ml) (fruit); *Chew tab:* 200 mg (fruit)
erythromycin stearate **(G)**	Erythrocin	*Film tab:* 250, 500 mg
Macrolide+Sulfonamide		
erythromycin ethylsuccinate+ sulfisoxazole **(G)**	Pediazole	*Oral susp:* eryth 200 mg+sulf 600 mg per 5 ml (100, 150, 200 ml) (strawberry-banana)
Sulfonamides		
sulfamethoxazole **(G)**	Gantrisin Pediatric	*Oral susp:* 500 mg/5 ml; *Syr:* 500 mg/5 ml
trimethoprim **(G)**	Primsol	*Oral soln:* 50 mg/5 ml (bubble gum) (dye-free, alcohol-free)
	Trimpex	*Tab:* 100 mg
	Proloprim	*Tab:* 100, 200 mg
trimethoprim+ sulfamethoxazole **(G)**	Bactrim, Septra	*Tab:* trim 80 mg+sulfa 400 mg*
	Bactrim DS, Septra DS	*Tab:* trim 160 mg+sulfa 800 mg*; *Oral susp:* trim 40 mg+sulfa 200 mg per 5 ml (100 ml) (cherry) (alcohol 0.3%)
Tetracyclines		
demeclocycline	Declomycin	*Tab:* 300 mg
doxycycline **(G)**	Adoxa	*Tab:* 50, 100 mg ent-coat
	Doryx	*Cap:* 100 mg
	Monodox	*Cap:* 50, 100 mg
doxycycline **(G)**	Vibramycin	*Cap:* 50, 100 mg; *Syr:* 50 mg/5 ml (raspberry) (sulfites); *Oral susp:* 25 mg/5 ml (raspberry-apple); *IV conc:* doxy 100 mg+asc acid 480 mg after dilution, doxy 200 mg+asc acid 960 mg after dilution
	Vibra-Tab	*Tab:* 100 mg film-coat
	Xerava	*Vial:* 50 mg pwdr for IV infusion
minocycline **(G)**	Dynacin	*Cap:* 50, 100 mg
	Minocin	*Cap:* 50, 100 mg; *Oral susp:* 50 mg/5 ml (60 ml) (custard) (sulfites, alcohol 5%); *Vial:* 100 mg soln for inj
	Minolira	*Tab:* 105, 135 mg ext-rel
tetracycline **(G)**	Achromycin V	*Cap:* 250, 500 mg
	Sumycin	*Tab:* 250, 500 mg; *Oral susp:* 125 mg/5 ml (fruit) (sulfites)
Unclassified/Miscellaneous		
aztreonam	Cayston	*Vial:* 75 mg pwdr for reconstitution (preservative-free)
chloramphenicol **(G)**	Chloromycetin	*Vial:* 1 gm

(continued)

Appendix AA (*continued*)

Anti-Infectives by Class With Dose Forms		
Generic Name	**Brand Name**	**Dose Form/Volume**
clindamycin (G)	Cleocin	*Cap:* 75 (tartrazine), 150 (tartrazine), 300 mg; *Oral susp:* 75 mg/5 ml (100 ml) (cherry); *Vial:* 150 mg/ml (2, 4 ml) (benzyl alcohol)
dalbavancin	Dalvance	*Vial:* 500 mg pwdr for reconstitution (preservative-free)
daptomycin (G)	Cubicin	*Vial:* 500 mg pwdr for reconstitution
doripenem	Doribax	*Vial:* 500 mg pwdr for reconstitution
fosfomycin (G)	Monurol	*Sachet:* 3 gm single-dose (mandarin orange; sucrose)
imipenem+ cilastatin (G)	Primaxin	*Vial:* imip 500 mg+cila 500 mg, imip 750 mg+cila 750 mg pwdr for reconstitution
lincomycin (G)	Lincocin	*Vial:* 300 mg/ml (10 ml)
linezolid (G)	Zyvox	*Tab:* 400, 600 mg; *Oral susp:* 100 mg/5 ml (orange) (phenylalanine); *IV:* 2 mg ml (100, 200, 300 ml)
meropenem	Merrem	*Vial:* 500 mg; 1 gm (sodium 3.92 mEq/gm)
meropenem+ vaborbactam	Vabomere	*Vial:* mero 1 gm+vabor 1 gm pwdr for reconstitution, single-dose
nitrofurantoin (G)	Furadantin	*Oral susp:* 25 mg/5 ml (60 ml)
	Macrobid	*Cap:* 100 mg
	Macrodantin	*Cap:* 25, 50, 100 mg
quinupristin+ dalfopristin	Synercid	*Vial:* quin 150 mg+dalfo 350 mg, quin 180 mg+dalfo 420 mg single-dose
rifaximin	Xifaxan	*Tab:* 200, 550 mg
telavancin	Vibativ	*Vial:* 250, 750 mg pwdr for reconstitution (preservative-free)
tigecycline (G)	Tygacil	*Vial:* 50 mg pwdr for reconstitution
vancomycin (G)	Vancocin	*Cap:* 125, 250 mg; *Vial:* 500 mg, 1 gm pwdr for reconstitution
vancomycin oral solution	Firvanq	*Oral soln:* 25, 55 mg (base)/ml

APPENDIX BB. ANTIBIOTIC DOSING BY WEIGHT FOR LIQUID FORMS

APPENDIX BB.1. *ACYCLOVIR* (G) (ZOVIRAX SUSPENSION)

Weight												
Pounds	15	20	25	30	35	40	45	50	55	60	65	70
Kilograms	6.8	9	11.4	13.6	15.9	18.2	20.5	22.7	25	27.3	29.5	31.8
Single Dose (ml)/Frequency/Strength/5-Day Volume (ml)												
20 mg/kg/day ml/dose qid	3.5	4.5	5.5	6.5	8	9	10	11.5	12.5	13.5	14.5	16
mg/5 ml	200	200	200	200	200	200	200	200	200	200	200	200
Volume (ml)	70	90	110	130	160	180	200	230	250	270	290	320

Zovirax Oral Suspension <2 years: not recommended; >2 years, <40 kg: 20 mg/kg dosed qid x 5 days; ≥2 years, >40 kg: 800 mg dosed qid x 5 days; *Oral susp:* 200 mg/5 ml (banana).

APPENDIX BB.2. *AMANTADINE* (G) (SYMMETREL SYRUP)

Weight												
Pounds	15	20	25	30	35	40	45	50	55	60	65	70
Kilograms	6.8	9	11.4	13.6	15.9	18.2	20.5	22.7	25	27.3	29.5	31.8
Single Dose (ml)/Frequency/Strength/10-Day Volume (ml)												
4 mg/kg/day ml/dose bid	3	4	5	6	7	8	9	10	11	12	13	14
mg/5 ml	50	50	50	50	50	50	50	50	50	50	50	50
Volume (ml)	30	40	50	60	70	80	90	100	110	120	130	140
8 mg/lb/day ml/dose bid	6	8	10	12								
mg/5 ml	50	50	50	50								
Volume (ml)	60	80	100	60								

Symmetrel Suspension (G) Symmetrel <1 year: not recommended; 1-8 years: max 150 mg/day; 9-12 years: 2 tsp bid; >12 years: 100 mg bid or 200 mg once daily; *Syr*: 50 mg/5 ml (raspberry).

APPENDIX BB.3. *AMOXICILLIN* (G) (AMOXIL SUSPENSION, TRIMOX SUSPENSION)

Weight												
Pounds	15	20	25	30	35	40	45	50	55	60	65	70
Kilograms	6.8	9	11.4	13.6	15.9	18.2	20.5	22.7	25	27.3	29.5	31.8
Single Dose (ml)/Frequency/Strength/10-Day Volume (ml)												
20 mg/kg/day ml/dose tid	2	2.5	3	3.5	4	5	5.5	6	7	7.5	8	9
mg/5 ml	125	125	125	125	125	125	125	125	125	125	125	125
Volume (ml)	60	75	90	105	120	150	165	180	210	225	240	270
30 mg/kg/day ml/dose tid	3	3.5	2.5	3	3	3.5	4	4.5	5	5.5	6	6.5
mg/5 ml	125	125	250	250	250	250	250	250	250	250	250	250
Volume (ml)	90	105	75	90	90	105	120	135	150	165	180	195
40 mg/kg/day ml/dose bid	5	7	4.5	5	6	7	8	9	10	11	12	13
mg/5 ml	125	125	250	250	250	250	250	250	250	250	250	250
Volume (ml)	100	140	90	100	120	140	160	180	200	220	240	250
45 mg/kg/day ml/dose bid	4	2.5	3	4	4.5	5	6	6.5	7	7.5	8.5	9
mg/5 ml	200	400	400	400	400	400	400	400	400	400	400	400
Volume (ml)	80	50	60	80	90	100	120	130	140	150	170	180
90 mg/kg/day ml/dose bid	8	5	6	7	9	10	12	13	14	15	17	18
mg/5 ml	200	400	400	400	400	400	400	400	400	400	400	400
Volume (ml)	160	100	120	140	180	200	240	260	280	300	340	360

<40 kg (88 lb): 20-30 mg/kg/day in 3 divided doses or 40-90 mg/kg/day in 2 divided doses; >40 kg: same as adult.

Amoxil Suspension (G) 125, 250 mg/5 ml (80, 100, 150 ml) (strawberry); 200, 400 mg/5 ml (50, 75, 100 ml) (bubble gum).

Trimox Suspension (G) 125, 250 mg/5 ml (80, 100, 150 ml) (raspberry-strawberry).

APPENDIX BB.4. *AMOXICILLIN+CLAVULANATE* (G) (AUGMENTIN SUSPENSION)

Weight												
Pounds	15	20	25	30	35	40	45	50	55	60	65	70
Kilograms	6.8	9	11.4	13.6	15.9	18.2	20.5	22.7	25	27.3	29.5	31.8
Single Dose (ml)/Frequency/Strength/10-Day Volume (ml)												
40 mg/kg/day ml/dose bid	5.5	7	4.5	5.5	6.5	7	8	9	10	11	12	13
mg/5 ml	125	125	250	250	250	250	250	250	250	250	250	250
Volume (ml)	110	140	90	110	130	140	160	180	200	220	240	260
45 mg/kg/day ml/dose bid	3	4	5	6	7	8	9	10	11.5	12.5	13.5	14.5
mg/5 ml	250	250	250	250	250	250	250	250	250	250	250	250
Volume (ml)	60	80	100	120	140	160	180	200	230	250	270	290
45 mg/kg/day ml/dose bid	4	2.5	3	4	4.5	5	6	6.5	7	7.5	8.5	9
mg/5 ml	200	400	400	400	400	400	400	400	400	400	400	400
Volume (ml)	80	50	60	80	90	100	120	130	140	150	170	180
90 mg/kg/day ml/dose bid	4	5	6.5	8	9	10	11.5	13	14	15.5	16.5	18
mg/5 ml	400	400	400	400	400	400	400	400	400	400	400	400
Volume (ml)	80	100	130	160	180	200	240	260	280	300	340	360

Augmentin Suspension (G) 40-45 mg/kg/day divided tid or 90 mg/kg/day divided bid; 125 mg/5 ml (75, 100, 150 ml) (banana), 250 mg/5 ml (75, 100, 150 ml) (orange); 200, 400 mg/5 ml (50, 75, 100 ml) (orange-raspberry) (phenylalanine).

APPENDIX BB.5. *AMOXICILLIN+CLAVULANATE* (G) (AUGMENTIN ES 600 SUSPENSION)

Weight												
Pounds	15	20	25	30	35	40	45	50	55	60	65	70
Kilograms	6.8	9	11.4	13.6	15.9	18.2	20.5	22.7	25	27.3	29.5	31.8
Single Dose (ml)/Frequency/Strength/10-Day Volume (ml)												
40 mg/kg/day ml/dose bid	1	1.5	2	2	2.5	3	3.5	4	4	4.5	5	5
mg/5 ml	600	600	600	600	600	600	600	600	600	600	600	600
Volume (ml)	30	40	40	40	50	60	70	80	80	90	100	100
45 mg/kg/day ml/dose bid	1.25	1.5	2	2.5	3	3.5	4	4.5	5	5	5.5	6
mg/5 ml	600	600	600	600	600	600	600	600	600	600	600	600
Volume (ml)	25	30	40	50	60	70	80	90	100	100	110	120
90 mg/kg/day ml/dose bid	2.5	3.5	4	5	6	7	8	8.5	9.5	10	11	12
mg/5 ml	600	600	600	600	600	600	600	600	600	600	600	600
Volume (ml)	50	70	80	100	120	140	160	170	190	200	220	240

Augmentin ES 600 Suspension <3 months: not recommended; ≥3 months, <40 kg: 90 mg/kg/day in 2 divided doses; ≥40 kg: not recommended; 600 mg/5 ml (50, 75, 100, 125, 150, 200 ml) (strawberry cream) (phenylalanine).

APPENDIX BB.6. *AMPICILLIN* (G) (OMNIPEN SUSPENSION, PRINCIPEN SUSPENSION)

Weight												
Pounds	15	20	25	30	35	40	45	50	55	60	65	70
Kilograms	6.8	9	11.4	13.6	15.9	18.2	20.5	22.7	25	27.3	29.5	31.8

(continued)

Appendix BB.6 (*continued*)

Single Dose (ml)/Frequency/Strength/10-Day Volume (ml)						
50 mg/kg/day ml/dose q 6 hours	3.5	4.5	3	3.5	4	4.5
mg/5 ml	125	125	250	250	250	250
Volume (ml)	140	180	120	140	160	180
100 mg/kg/d ml/dose q 6 hours	3.5	4.5	6	7	8	9
mg/5 ml	250	250	250	250	250	250
Volume (ml)	140	180	240	280	320	360

Omnipen Suspension, Principen Suspension (G) >20 kg: 250-500 mg q 6 hours, 125, 250 mg/5 ml (100, 150, 200 ml) (fruit).

APPENDIX BB.7. *AZITHROMYCIN* (G) (ZITHROMAX SUSPENSION, ZMAX SUSPENSION)

Weight								
Pounds	11	22	33	44	55	66	77	88
Kilograms	5	10	15	20	25	30	35	40
Single Dose (ml)/Frequency/Strength/Volume (ml)								
3-Day Regimen								
10 mg/kg qd	2.5	5	7.5	5	6	7.5	9	10
mg/5 ml	100	100	100	200	200	200	200	200
Volume (ml)	7.5	15	22.5	15	18	22.5	27	30
5-Day Regimen								
10 mg/kg qd								
Day 1	2.5	5	7.5	5	6	7.5	7.5	10
Days 2–5	1.25	2.5	4	2.5	3	4	4	5
Volume (ml)	10	15	23.5	15	18	23.5	23.5	30

Zithromax ES 600 Suspension (G) 100 mg/5 ml (15 ml), 200 mg/5 ml (15, 22.5, 30 ml) (cherry-vanilla-banana).

APPENDIX BB.8. *CEFACLOR* (G) (CECLOR SUSPENSION)

Weight											
Pounds	15	20	25	30	35	40	45	50	55	60	65	70
Kilograms	6.8	9	11.4	13.6	15.9	18.2	20.5	22.7	25	27.3	29.5	31.8
Single Dose (ml)/Frequency/Strength/10-Day Volume (ml)											
20 mg/kg/day ml/dose tid	2	2.5	3	3.5	4	5	5.5	6	7	7.5	8	8.5
mg/5 ml	125	125	125	125	125	125	125	125	125	125	125	125
Volume (ml)	60	75	90	105	120	150	165	180	210	225	240	255
20 mg/kg/day ml/dose tid	1.5	1.5	2	2.5	3	3	4	4	4.5	5	5.5	6
mg/5 ml	187	187	187	187	187	187	187	187	187	187	187	187
Volume (ml)	45	45	60	75	90	90	105	120	135	150	165	180
40 mg/kg/day ml/dose tid	2	2.5	3	3.5	4	5	5.5	6	6.5	7	8	8.5
mg/5 ml	250	250	250	250	250	250	250	250	250	250	250	250
Volume (ml)	60	75	90	105	120	150	165	180	195	210	240	255
40 mg/kg/day ml/dose tid	1.5	1.5	2	2.5	3	3	3.5	4	4.5	5	5	5.5

(*continued*)

Appendix BB.8 (*continued*)

mg/5 ml	375	375	375	375	375	375	375	375	375	375	375	375
Volume (ml)	45	45	60	75	90	90	105	120	135	150	150	165

Ceclor Suspension <6 months: not recommended; 125, 250 mg/5 ml (75, 150 ml) (strawberry); 187, 375 mg/5 ml (50, 100 ml) (strawberry).

APPENDIX BB.9. *CEFADROXIL* (G) (DURICEF SUSPENSION)

Weight												
Pounds	15	20	25	30	35	40	45	50	55	60	65	70
Kilograms	6.8	9	11.4	13.6	15.9	18.2	20.5	22.7	25	27.3	29.5	31.8
Single Dose (ml)/Frequency/Strength/10-Day Volume (ml)												
30 mg/kg/day ml/dose bid	2	3	3.5	4	5	5.5	6	7	7.5	8	9	9.5
mg/5 ml	250	250	250	250	250	250	250	250	250	250	250	250
Volume (ml)	40	60	75	80	100	110	120	140	150	160	180	190
30 mg/kg/day ml/dose qd	2	3	3.5	4	5	5.5	6	7	7.5	8	9	9.5
mg/5 ml	500	500	500	500	500	500	500	500	500	500	500	500
Volume (ml)	20	30	35	40	50	55	60	70	75	80	90	95

Duricef Suspension 250 mg/5 ml (100 ml) (orange-pineapple), 500 mg/5 ml (75, 100 ml) (orange-pineapple).

APPENDIX BB.10. *CEFDINIR* (G) (OMNICEF SUSPENSION)

Weight												
Pounds	15	20	25	30	35	40	45	50	55	60	65	70
Kilograms	6.8	9	11.4	13.6	15.9	18.2	20.5	22.7	25	27.3	29.5	31.8
Single Dose (ml)/Frequency/Strength/10-Day Volume (ml)												
7 mg/kg/day ml/dose bid	2	2.5	3	4	4.5	5	6	6.5	7	7.5	8	9
mg/5 ml	125	125	125	125	125	125	125	125	125	125	125	125
Volume (ml)	40	50	60	80	90	100	120	130	140	150	160	180
14 mg/kg ml/dose bid	4	5	6	8	9	10	12	13	14	15	16	18
mg/5 ml	125	125	125	125	125	125	125	125	125	125	125	125
Volume (ml)	40	50	60	80	90	100	120	130	140	150	160	180

Omnicef Suspension <6 months: not recommended; 125 mg/5 ml (60, 100 ml) (strawberry).

APPENDIX BB.11. *CEFIXIME* (G) (SUPRAX ORAL SUSPENSION)

Weight												
Pounds	15	20	25	30	35	40	45	50	55	60	65	70
Kilograms	6.8	9	11.4	13.6	15.9	18.2	20.5	22.7	25	27.3	29.5	31.8
Single Dose (ml)/Frequency/Strength/10-Day Volume (ml)												
8 mg/kg/day ml/dose bid	1.3	1.8	2.2	2.5	3.1	3.5	4	4.5	5	5.5	6	6.5
mg/5 ml	100	100	100	100	100	100	100	100	100	100	100	100
8 mg/kg/day ml/dose qd	2.7	3.6	4.5	5.5	6.3	7.2	8.2	9	10	11	12	13
mg/5 ml	100	100	100	100	100	100	100	100	100	100	100	100
Volume (ml)	27	36	45	55	65	70	80	90	100	110	120	130

Supra Oral Suspension (G) <6 months: not recommended; 100 mg/5 ml (50, 75, 100 ml) (strawberry).

APPENDIX BB.12. *CEFPODOXIME PROXETIL* (G) (VANTIN SUSPENSION)

Weight												
Pounds	15	20	25	30	35	40	45	50	55	60	65	70
Kilograms	6.8	9	11.4	13.6	15.9	18.2	20.5	22.7	25	27.3	29.5	31.8
Single Dose (ml)/Frequency/Strength/10-Day Volume (ml)												
5 mg/kg/day ml/dose bid	3.5	4.5	5.5	7	8	9	10	11	12.5	13.5	15	16
mg/5 ml	50	50	50	50	50	50	50	50	50	50	50	50
Volume (ml)	70	90	110	140	160	180	200	220	250	270	300	320
5 mg/kg/day ml/dose bid	2	2	3	3.5	4	4.5	5	5.5	6	7	7.5	8
mg/5 ml	100	100	100	100	100	100	100	100	100	100	100	100
Volume (ml)	40	40	60	70	80	90	100	110	120	140	150	160

Vantin Suspension <2 months: not recommended; 50, 100 mg/5 ml (50, 75, 100 ml) (lemon-crème).

APPENDIX BB.13. *CEFPROZIL* (G) (CEFZIL SUSPENSION)

Weight												
Pounds	15	20	25	30	35	40	45	50	55	60	65	70
Kilograms	6.8	9	11.4	13.6	15.9	18.2	20.5	22.7	25	27.3	29.5	31.8
Single Dose (ml)/Frequency/Strength/10-Day Volume (ml)												
7.5 mg/kg/day ml/dose bid	2	3	3.5	4	5	5.5	6	7	7.5	4	4.5	5
mg/5 ml	125	125	125	125	125	125	125	125	125	250	250	250
Volume (ml)	40	60	70	80	100	110	120	140	150	80	90	100
15 mg/kg/day ml/dose bid	2	3	3.5	4	5	5	6	7	7.5	8	9	9.5
mg/5 ml	250	250	250	250	250	250	250	250	250	250	250	250
Volume (ml)	40	60	70	80	100	100	120	140	150	160	180	190
20 mg/kg/day ml/dose qd	3	3.5	4.5	5.5	6.5	7	8	9	10	11	12	13
mg/5 ml	250	250	250	250	250	250	250	250	250	250	250	250
Volume (ml)	60	70	90	110	130	140	160	180	200	220	240	260

Cefzil Suspension ≤6 months: not recommended; 2-12 years: 7.5-20 mg/kg bid; >12 years: same as adult, 250-500 mg bid or 500 mg once daily; 125, 250 mg/5 ml (50, 75, 100 ml) (bubble gum) (phenylalanine).

APPENDIX BB.14. *CEFTIBUTEN* (G) (CEDAX SUSPENSION)

Weight												
Pounds	15	20	25	30	35	40	45	50	55	60	65	70
Kilograms	6.8	9	11.4	13.6	15.9	18.2	20.5	22.7	25	27.3	29.5	31.8
Single Dose (ml)/Frequency/Strength/10-Day Volume (ml)												
9 mg/kg/day ml/dose qd	3.5	4.5	6	7	8	9	10	11.5	12.5	13.5	15	16
mg/5 ml	90	90	90	90	90	90	90	90	90	90	90	90
Volume (ml)	35	45	60	70	80	90	100	115	125	135	150	160
9 mg/kg/day ml/dose qd	1.75	2.3	3	3.5	4	4.5	5	5.4	6.2	6.6	7.5	8

(continued)

Appendix BB.14 (*continued*)

mg/5 ml	180	180	180	180	180	180	180	180	180	180	180	180
Volume (ml)	20	25	30	35	40	45	50	55	60	65	70	80

Cedax Suspension 90 mg/5 ml (30, 60, 90, 120 ml) (cherry), 180 mg/5 ml (30, 60, 120 ml) (cherry).

APPENDIX BB.15. *CEPHALEXIN* (G) (KEFLEX SUSPENSION)

Weight												
Pounds	15	20	25	30	35	40	45	50	55	60	65	70
Kilograms	6.8	9	11.4	13.6	15.9	18.2	20.5	22.7	25	27.3	29.5	31.8
Single Dose (ml)/Frequency/Strength/10-Day Volume (ml)												
25 mg/kg/day ml/dose tid	1	1.5	2	2	3	3	3.5	4	4	4.5	5	5
mg/5 ml	125	125	125	125	125	125	125	125	125	125	125	125
Volume (ml)	30	45	60	60	90	90	105	120	120	135	150	150
25 mg/kg/day ml/dose qid	1	1	1.5	2	2	2.5	2.5	3	3	3.5	4	4
mg/5 ml	250	250	250	250	250	250	250	250	250	250	250	250
Volume (ml)	40	40	60	80	80	100	100	120	120	140	160	160
50 mg/kg/day ml/dose tid	2	3	4	4.5	5	6	7	7.5	8	9	10	10.5
mg/5 ml	250	250	250	250	250	250	250	250	250	250	250	250
Volume (ml)	60	90	120	135	150	180	210	225	240	270	300	315
50 mg/kg/day ml/dose qid	2	2	3	3.5	4	4.5	5	6	6	7	7.5	8
mg/5 ml	250	250	250	250	250	250	250	250	250	250	250	250
Volume (ml)	80	80	120	140	160	180	200	240	240	280	300	320

Keflex Suspension (G) <2 months: not recommended; 125, 250 mg/5 ml (100, 200 ml) (strawberry).

APPENDIX BB.16. *CLARITHROMYCIN* (G) (BIAXIN SUSPENSION)

Weight												
Pounds	15	20	25	30	35	40	45	50	55	60	65	70
Kilograms	6.8	9	11.4	13.6	15.9	18.2	20.5	22.7	25	27.3	29.5	31.8
Single Dose (ml)/Frequency/Strength/10-Day Volume (ml)												
7.5 mg/kg/day ml/dose bid	2	3	3.5	4	5	5.5	6	7	7.5	8	9	10
mg/5 ml	125	125	125	125	125	125	125	125	125	125	125	125
Volume (ml)	40	60	70	80	100	110	120	140	150	160	180	200
7.5 mg/kg/day ml/dose bid	1	1.5	2	2	2.5	3	3	3.5	4	4	4.5	5
mg/5 ml	250	250	250	250	250	250	250	250	250	250	250	250
Volume (ml)	20	30	40	40	50	60	60	70	80	80	90	100

Biaxin Suspension <6 months: not recommended; 125, 250 mg/5 ml (50, 100 ml) (fruit punch).

APPENDIX BB.17. *CLINDAMYCIN* (G) (CLEOCIN PEDIATRIC GRANULES)

Weight												
Pounds	15	20	25	30	35	40	45	50	55	60	65	70
Kilograms	6.8	9	11.4	13.6	15.9	18.2	20.5	22.7	25	27.3	29.5	31.8

(*continued*)

Appendix BB.17 (*continued*)

Single Dose (ml)/Frequency/Strength/10-Day Volume (ml)												
8 mg/kg/day ml/dose tid	1	1.5	2	2.5	3	3	3.5	4	4.5	5	5	5.5
mg/5 ml	75	75	75	75	75	75	75	75	75	75	75	75
Volume (ml)	30	45	60	75	90	90	105	120	135	150	150	165
16 mg/kg/day ml/dose tid	2.5	3	4	5	5.5	6.5	7	8	9	9.5	10.5	11
mg/5 ml	75	75	75	75	75	75	75	75	75	75	75	75
Volume (ml)	75	90	120	150	165	105	210	240	270	285	315	330

Cleocin Pediatric Granules (G) 75 mg/5 ml (100 ml) (cherry).

APPENDIX BB.18. *DICLOXACILLIN* (G) (DYNAPEN SUSPENSION)

Weight												
Pounds	15	20	25	30	35	40	45	50	55	60	65	70
Kilograms	6.8	9	11.4	13.6	15.9	18.2	20.5	22.7	25	27.3	29.5	31.8
Single Dose (ml)/Frequency/Strength/10-Day Volume (ml)												
12.5 mg/kg/day ml/dose qid	2	2.5	3	3.5	4	4.5	5	6	6	7	7.5	8
mg/5 ml	62.5	62.5	62.5	62.5	62.5	62.5	62.5	62.5	62.5	62.5	62.5	62.5
Volume (ml)	80	100	120	140	160	180	200	240	240	280	300	320
25 mg/kg/day ml/dose qid	3.5	4.5	6	7	8	9	10	11.5	12.5	13.5	15	16
mg/5 ml	62.5	62.5	62.5	62.5	62.5	62.5	62.5	62.5	62.5	62.5	62.5	62.5
Volume (ml)	140	180	240	280	320	360	400	460	500	540	600	640

Dynapen Suspension (G) 6.25 mg/5 ml (80, 100 ml) (raspberry-strawberry).

APPENDIX BB.19. *DOXYCYCLINE* (G) (VIBRAMYCIN SYRUP/SUSPENSION)

Weight												
Pounds	15	20	25	30	35	40	45	50	55	60	65	70
Kilograms	6.8	9	11.4	13.6	15.9	18.2	20.5	22.7	25	27.3	29.5	31.8
Single Dose (ml)/Frequency/Strength/10-Day Volume (ml)												
1 mg/lb/day ml/dose qd	1.5	2	2.5	3	3.5	4	4.5	5	5.5	6	6.5	7
50 mg/5 ml	50	50	50	50	50	50	50	50	50	50	50	50
Volume (ml)	15	20	25	30	35	40	45	50	55	60	65	70
1 mg/lb/day ml/dose qd	3	4	5	6	7	8	9	10	11	12	13	14
25 mg/5 ml	25	25	25	25	25	25	25	25	25	25	25	25
Volume (ml)	30	40	50	60	70	80	90	100	110	120	130	140

Vibramycin Syrup (G) <8 years: not recommended; double dose first day; 50 mg/5 ml (80, 100, ml) (raspberry-apple) (sulfites).
Vibramycin Suspension (G) <8 years: not recommended; double dose first day; 25 mg/5 ml (80, 100, ml) (raspberry).

APPENDIX BB.20. *ERYTHROMYCIN ESTOLATE* (G) (ILOSONE SUSPENSION)

Weight												
Pounds	15	20	25	30	35	40	45	50	55	60	65	70
Kilograms	6.8	9	11.4	13.6	15.9	18.2	20.5	22.7	25	27.3	29.5	31.8

(*continued*)

Appendix BB.20 (*continued*)

Dose/Volume (10 days) in ml												
10 mg/kg/day ml/dose bid	3	3.5	4.5	5.5	6	7	8	9	10	5.5	6	6.5
mg/5 ml	125	125	125	125	125	125	125	125	125	250	250	250
Volume (ml)	60	70	90	110	120	140	160	180	200	110	120	130
15 mg/kg/day ml/dose bid	4	5.5	7	8	9.5	5.5	6	7	7.5	8	9	9.5
mg/5 ml	125	125	125	125	125	250	250	250	250	250	250	250
Volume (ml)	80	110	140	160	190	110	120	140	150	160	180	190
20 mg/kg/day ml/dose bid	3	3.5	4.5	5.5	6.5	7	8	9	10	11	12	13
mg/5 ml	250	250	250	250	250	250	250	250	250	250	250	250
Volume (ml)	60	70	90	110	120	140	160	180	200	220	240	260
25 mg/kg/day ml/dose bid	3.5	4.5	5.5	7	8	9	10	11.5	12.5	13.5	15	16
mg/5 ml	250	250	250	250	250	250	250	250	250	250	250	250
Volume (ml)	70	90	110	140	160	180	200	230	250	280	300	320

Ilosone Suspension (G) 125, 250 mg/5 ml (100 ml).

APPENDIX BB.21. *ERYTHROMYCIN ETHYLSUCCINATE* (G) (E.E.S. SUSPENSION, ERYPED DROPS/ SUSPENSION)

Weight												
Pounds	15	20	25	30	35	40	45	50	55	60	65	70
Kilograms	6.8	9	11.4	13.6	15.9	18.2	20.5	22.7	25	27.3	29.5	31.8
Single Dose (ml)/Frequency/Strength/10-Day Volume (ml)												
30 mg/kg/day ml/dose qid	1.5	2	2	2.5	3	3.5	4	4	4.5	5	5.5	6
mg/5 ml	200	200	200	200	200	200	200	200	200	200	200	200
Volume (ml)	60	80	80	100	120	140	160	160	180	200	220	240
30 mg/kg/day ml/dose qid			1	1.5	1.5	2	2	2	2.5	2.5	3	3
mg/5 ml			400	400	400	400	400	400	400	400	400	
Volume (ml)			60	60	80	80	80	100	100	120	120	
50 mg/kg/day ml/dose qid	2	3	3.5	4.5	5	5.5	6.5	7	8	8.5	9	10
mg/5 ml	200	200	200	200	200	200	200	200	200	200	200	200
Volume (ml)	80	120	140	180	200	220	260	280	320	340	360	400
50 mg/kg/day ml/dose qid	1	1.5	2	2	2.5	3	3	3.5	4	4.5	4.5	5
mg/5 ml	400	400	400	400	400	400	400	400	400	400	400	400
Volume (ml)	40	60	80	80	100	120	140	140	160	180	180	200

Ery-Ped Drops/Suspension (G) 200 mg/5 ml (100, 200 ml) (fruit), 400 mg/5 ml (60, 100, 200 ml) (banana); Oral drops: 200, 400 mg/5 ml (50 ml) (fruit).

E.E.S. Suspension (G) 200 mg/5 ml, 400 mg/5 ml (100 ml) (fruit).

E.E.S. Granules (G) 200 mg/5 ml (100, 200 ml) (cherry).

APPENDIX BB.22. *ERYTHROMYCIN+SULFAMETHOXAZOLE* (G) (ERYZOLE, PEDIAZOLE)

Weight												
Pounds	15	20	25	30	35	40	45	50	55	60	65	70
Kilograms	6.8	9	11.4	13.6	15.9	18.2	20.5	22.7	25	27.3	29.5	31.8
Single Dose (ml)/Frequency/Strength/10-Day Volume (ml)												
10 mg/kg/day ml/dose bid	3	4	5	6	6.5	7.5	8.5	9.5	10	11	12	13.5
mg/5 ml	200	200	200	200	200	200	200	200	200	200	200	200
Volume (ml)	90	120	150	180	200	225	255	285	300	330	360	400

Eryzole (G) <2 months: not recommended; *eryth* 200 mg/*sulf* 600 mg/5 ml (100, 150, 200, 250 ml).

Pediazole (G) <2 months: not recommended; *eryth* 200 mg/*sulf* 600 mg/5 ml (100, 150, 200 ml) (strawberry-banana).

APPENDIX BB.23. *FLUCONAZOLE* (G) (DIFLUCAN SUSPENSION)

Weight												
Pounds	15	20	25	30	35	40	45	50	55	60	65	70
Kilograms	6.8	9	11.4	13.6	15.9	18.2	20.5	22.7	25	27.3	29.5	31.8
Single Dose (ml)/Frequency/Strength/21-Day Volume (ml)												
3 mg/kg/day ml/dose qd	2	3	3.5	4	5	5.5	6	7	7.5	8	9	9.5
mg/ml	10	10	10	10	10	10	10	10	10	10	10	10
Volume (ml)	44	66	77	88	110	121	132	154	165	176	198	209
6 mg/kg/day ml/dose qd	4	5.5	2	2	2.5	3	3	3.5	4	4	4.5	5
mg/ml	10	10	40	40	40	40	40	40	40	40	40	40
Volume (ml)	88	121	44	44	55	66	66	77	88	88	99	110

Diflucan Suspension (G) double-dose first day; 10, 40 mg/5 ml (35 ml) (orange).

APPENDIX BB.24. *FURAZOLIDONE* (G) (FUROXONE LIQUID)

Weight												
Pounds	15	20	25	30	35	40	45	50	55	60	65	70
Kilograms	6.8	9	11.4	13.6	15.9	18.2	20.5	22.7	25	27.3	29.5	31.8
Single Dose (ml)/Frequency/Strength/7-Day Volume (ml)												
5 mg/kg/day ml/dose qid	2.5	3.5	4	5	6	7	8	8.5	9.5	10	11	12
mg/15 ml	50	50	50	50	50	50	50	50	50	50	50	50
Volume (ml)	100	140	160	200	240	280	320	340	380	400	440	480

Furoxone Liquid (G) double-dose first day; 50 mg/15 ml (35 ml).

APPENDIX BB.25. *GRISEOFULVIN, MICROSIZE* (G) (GRIFULVIN V SUSPENSION)

Weight												
Pounds	15	20	25	30	35	40	45	50	55	60	65	70
Kilograms	6.8	9	11.4	13.6	15.9	18.2	20.5	22.7	25	27.3	29.5	31.8
Single Dose (ml)/Frequency/Strength/30-Day Volume (ml)												
5 mg/lb/day ml/dose day	3	4	5	6	7	8	9	10	11	12	13	14
mg/5 ml	125	125	125	125	125	125	125	125	125	125	125	125
Volume (ml)	90	120	150	180	210	240	270	300	330	360	390	420

Grifulvin V Suspension (G) double-dose first day; 125 mg/5 ml (120 ml) (orange) (alcohol 0.02%).

APPENDIX BB.26. *ITRACONAZOLE* (G) (SPORANOX SOLUTION)

Weight												
Pounds	15	20	25	30	35	40	45	50	55	60	65	70
Kilograms	6.8	9	11.4	13.6	15.9	18.2	20.5	22.7	25	27.3	29.5	31.8
Single Dose (ml)/Frequency/Strength/7-Day Volume (ml)												
5 mg/kg/day ml/dose qd	3.5	4.5	6	7	8	9	10	11.5	12.5	14	15	16
mg/ml	10	10	10	10	10	10	10	10	10	10	10	10
Volume (ml)	25	32	42	49	56	63	70	71	88	98	105	112

Sporanox V Solution (G) double-dose first day; 10 mg/ml (150 ml) (cherry-caramel).

APPENDIX BB.27. *LORACARBEF* (G) (LORABID SUSPENSION)

Weight												
Pounds	15	20	25	30	35	40	45	50	55	60	65	70
Kilograms	6.8	9	11.4	13.6	15.9	18.2	20.5	22.7	25	27.3	29.5	31.8
Single Dose (ml)/Frequency/Strength/10-Day Volume (ml)												
15 mg/kg/day ml/dose bid	2.5	3.5	4	5	3	3.5	4	4	5	5	5.5	6
mg/5 ml	100	100	100	100	200	200	200	200	200	200	200	200
Volume (ml)	50	70	80	100	60	70	80	80	100	100	110	120
30 mg/kg/day ml/dose bid	2.5	3.5	4	5	6	7	8	8.5	9.5	10	11	12
mg/5 ml	200	200	200	200	200	200	200	200	200	200	200	200
Volume (ml)	50	70	80	100	120	140	160	170	190	200	220	240

Lorabid Suspension 100 mg/5 ml (50, 100 ml) (strawberry bubble gum), 200 mg/5 ml (50, 75, 100 ml) (strawberry bubble gum).

APPENDIX BB.28. *NITROFURANTOIN* (G) (FURADANTIN SUSPENSION)

Weight												
Pounds	15	20	25	30	35	40	45	50	55	60	65	70
Kilograms	6.8	9	11.4	13.6	15.9	18.2	20.5	22.7	25	27.3	29.5	31.8
Single Dose (ml)/Frequency/Strength/10-Day Volume (ml)												
5 mg/kg ml/dose qid	1.5	2.5	3	3.5	4	4.5	5	5.5	6	7	7.5	8
mg/5 ml	25	25	25	25	25	25	25	25	25	25	25	25
Volume (ml)	60	100	120	140	160	190	200	220	240	280	300	320

Furadantin Suspension (G) 25 mg/5 ml (60 ml).

APPENDIX BB.29. *PENICILLIN V POTASSIUM* (G) (PEN-VEE K SOLUTION, VEETIDS SOLUTION)

Weight												
Pounds	15	20	25	30	35	40	45	50	55	60	65	70
Kilograms	6.8	9	11.4	13.6	15.9	18.2	20.5	22.7	25	27.3	29.5	31.8
Single Dose (ml)/Frequency/Strength/10-Day Volume (ml)												
25 mg/kg/day ml/dose qid	2	2.5	3	3.5	4	4.5	5	5.5	6	7	7.5	8
mg/5 ml	125	125	125	125	125	125	125	125	125	125	125	125
Volume (ml)	80	90	120	140	160	180	200	220	240	280	300	320

(continued)

Appendix BB.29 *(continued)*

25 mg/kg/day ml/dose qid	1	1	1.5	2	2	2.5	2.5	3	3	3.5	4	4
mg/5 ml	250	250	250	250	250	250	250	250	250	250	250	250
Volume (ml)	40	40	60	80	80	100	100	120	120	140	160	160
50 mg/kg/day ml/dose qid	2	2.5	3	3.5	4	4.5	5	6	6.5	7	7.5	8
mg/5 ml	250	250	250	250	250	250	250	250	250	250	250	250
Volume (ml)	80	100	120	140	160	180	200	240	260	280	300	320

Pen-Vee K Solution (G) 125 mg/5 ml (100, 200 ml), 250 mg/5 ml (100, 150, 200 ml).

Veetids Solution (G) 125, 250 mg/5 ml (100, 200 ml).

APPENDIX BB.30. *RIMANTADINE* (G) (FLUMADINE SYRUP)

Weight												
Pounds	15	20	25	30	35	40	45	50	55	60	65	70
Kilograms	6.8	9	11.4	13.6	15.9	18.2	20.5	22.7	25	27.3	29.5	31.8
Single Dose (ml)/Frequency/Strength/10-Day Volume (ml)												
5 mg/kg/day ml/dose qd	3.5	4.5	6	7	8	9	10	11.5	12.5	13.5	15	16
mg/5 ml	50	50	50	50	50	50	50	50	50	50	50	50
Volume (ml)	35	45	60	70	80	90	100	115	125	135	150	160

Flumadine Syrup >10 years: same as adult; 50 mg/5 ml (2, 8, 16 oz) (raspberry).

APPENDIX BB.31. *TETRACYCLINE* (G) (SUMYCIN SUSPENSION)

Weight												
Pounds	15	20	25	30	35	40	45	50	55	60	65	70
Kilograms	6.8	9	11.4	13.6	15.9	18.2	20.5	22.7	25	27.3	29.5	31.8
Single Dose (ml)/Frequency/Strength/10-Day Volume (ml)												
25 mg/kg/day ml/dose qid	1.5	2.5	3	3.5	4	4.5	5	6	6.5	7	7.5	8
mg/5 ml	125	125	125	125	125	125	125	125	125	125	125	125
Volume (ml)	60	100	120	140	160	180	200	240	260	280	300	320
50 mg/kg/day ml/dose qid	3.5	4.5	6	7	8	9	10	11.5	12.5	13.5	15	16
mg/5 ml	125	125	125	125	125	125	125	125	125	125	125	125
Volume (ml)	140	180	240	280	320	360	400	460	500	540	600	640

Sumycin Suspension (G) <8 years: not recommended; 125 mg/5 ml (100, 200 ml) (fruit) (sulfites).

APPENDIX BB.32. *TRIMETHOPRIM* (G) (PRIMSOL SUSPENSION)

Weight												
Pounds	15	20	25	30	35	40	45	50	55	60	65	70
Kilograms	6.8	9	11.4	13.6	15.9	18.2	20.5	22.7	25	27.3	29.5	31.8
Single Dose (ml)/Frequency/Strength/10-Day Volume (ml)												
5 mg/kg/day ml/dose bid	3.5	4.5	6	7	8	9	10	11.5	12.5	13.5	15	16
mg/5 ml	50	50	50	50	50	50	50	50	50	50	50	50
Volume (ml)	70	90	120	140	160	180	200	230	250	270	300	320

Primsol Suspension (G) 50 mg/5 ml (50 mg/5 ml) (bubble gum) (dye-free, alcohol-free).

APPENDIX BB.33. *TRIMETHOPRIM+SULFAMETHOXAZOLE* (G) (BACTRIM SUSPENSION, SEPTRA SUSPENSION)

Weight											
Pounds	15	20	25	30	35	40	45	50	55	60	65	70
Kilograms	6.8	9	11.4	13.6	15.9	18.2	20.5	22.7	25	27.3	29.5	31.8
Single Dose (ml)/Frequency/Strength/10-Day Volume (ml)											
10 mg/kg/day ml/dose bid	2	2	3	3.5	4	4.5	5	5.5	6	7	7.5	8
mg/5 ml	200	200	200	200	200	200	200	200	200	200	200	200
Volume (ml)	40	40	60	70	80	90	100	110	120	140	150	160
20 mg/kg/day ml/dose bid	4	4	6	7	8	9	10	11	12	14	15	16
mg/5 ml	200	200	200	200	200	200	200	200	200	200	200	200
Volume (ml)	80	80	120	140	160	180	200	220	240	280	300	320

Bactrim Pediatric Suspension, Septra Pediatric Suspension (G) trim 40 mg/sulfa 200 mg/5 ml (100 ml) (cherry) (alcohol 0.3%).

APPENDIX BB.34. *VANCOMYCIN* (G) (VANCOCIN SUSPENSION)

Weight											
Pounds	15	20	25	30	35	40	45	50	55	60	65	70
Kilograms	6.8	9	11.4	13.6	15.9	18.2	20.5	22.7	25	27.3	29.5	31.8
Single Dose (ml)/Frequency/Strength/10-Day Volume (ml)											
40 mg/kg/day ml/dose tid	2	2.5	3	3.5	4.5	5	5.5	6	7	7.5	8	8.5
mg/5 ml	250	250	250	250	250	250	250	250	250	250	250	250
Volume (ml)	60	75	90	105	135	150	165	180	210	225	240	255
40 mg/kg/day ml/dose qid	1.5	2	2.5	3	3	3.5	4	4.5	5	5.5	6	6.5
mg/5 ml	250	250	250	250	250	250	250	250	250	250	250	250
Volume (ml)	60	80	100	120	120	140	160	180	200	220	240	260
40 mg/kg/day ml/dose tid	1	1	1.5	2	2	2.5	3	3	3.5	3.5	4	4
mg/6 ml	500	500	500	500	500	500	500	500	500	500	500	500
Volume (ml)	30	30	45	60	60	75	90	90	105	105	120	120
40 mg/kg/day ml/dose qid	1	1	1.5	1.5	1.5	2	2	2.5	2.5	3	3	3.5
mg/6 ml	500	500	500	500	500	500	500	500	500	500	500	500
Volume (ml)	40	40	60	60	60	80	80	100	100	120	120	140

Vancomycin Suspension (G).

ACC/AHA/AAPA/ABC/ACPM/AGS/APhA/ASH/ASPC/NMA/PCNA. (2017). *2017 Guideline for the prevention, detection, evaluation, and management of high blood pressure in adults: A report of the American College of Cardiology/American Heart Association Task Force on clinical practice guidelines.*
http://hyper.ahajournals.org/content/hypertensionaha/early/2017/11/10/HYP.0000000000000065.full.pdf

ACR guidelines on prevention & treatment of glucocorticoid-induced osteoporosis [press release, June 7, 2017]. Atlanta, GA: American College of Rheumatology.
https://www.rheumatology.org/About-Us/Newsroom/Press-Releases/ID/812/ACR-Releases-Guideline-on-Prevention-Treatment-of-Glucocorticoid-Induced-Osteoporosis

Advance for Nurse Practitioners.
http://nurse-practitioners.advanceweb.com

American Academy of Dermatology.
https://www.aad.org/home

American Academy of Pediatrics (AAP).
http://aapexperience.org

American Association of Nurse Practitioners.
www.aanp.org

American College of Cardiology. *Then and now: ATP III vs. IV: Comparison of ATP III and ACC/AHA guidelines.*
http://www.acc.org/latest-in-cardiology/articles/2014/07/18/16/03/then-and-now-atp-iii-vs-iv

American College of Obstetricians and Gynecologists (ACOG).
http://www.acog.org

American Diabetes Association (ADA), Professional Diabetes Resources Online.
http://professional.diabetes.org/content/clinical-practice-recommendations/?loc=rp-slabnav

American Diabetes Association. (2018). Children and adolescents: Standards of medical care in diabetes—2018. *Diabetes Care, 41*(Suppl 1), S126–S136. doi:10.2337/dc18-S012

American Diabetes Association. (2018). Management of diabetes in pregnancy: Standards of medical care in diabetes—2018. *Diabetes Care, 41*(Suppl 1), S137–S143. doi:10.2337/dc18-S013

American Diabetes Association. (2018). Microvascular complications and foot care: Standards of medical care in diabetes—2018. *Diabetes Care, 41*(Suppl 1), S105–S118. doi:10.2337/dc18-S010

American Diabetes Association. (2018). Older adults: Standards of medical care in diabetes—2018. *Diabetes Care, 41*(Suppl 1), S119–S125. doi:10.2337/dc18-S011

American Diabetes Association. (2018). Pharmacologic approaches to glycemic treatment: Standards of medical care in diabetes—2018. *Diabetes Care, 41*(Suppl 1), S73–S85. doi:10.2337/dc18-S008

American Diabetes Association. (2018). Summary of revisions: Standards of medical care in diabetes—2018. *Diabetes Care, 41*(Suppl 1), S4–S6. doi:10.2337/dc18-Srev01

American Family Physician.
http://www.aafp.org/online/en/home.html

American Geriatrics Society.
http://www.americangeriatrics.org

American Geriatrics Society. (2015). Updated Beers Criteria for potentially inappropriate medication use in older adults. *Journal of the American Geriatrics Society, 63*(11), 2227–2246.

American Headache Society.
www.americanheadachesociety.org

American Pain Society.
http://americanpainsociety.org

American Pharmacists Association. (2018). *Pediatric and neonatal dosage handbook: A universal resource for clinicians treating pediatric and neonatal patients* (25th ed.). Hudson, OH: Lexicomp.

Anderson, E., Fantus, R. J., & Haddadin, R. I. (2017). Diagnosis and management of herpes zoster ophthalmicus. *Disease-a-Month, 63*(2), 38–44.

Andorf, S., Purington, N., Block, W. M., Long, A. J., Tupa, D., Brittain, E., . . . Chinthrajah, R. S. (2018). Anti-IgE treatment with oral immunotherapy in multi-food allergic participants: A double-blind, randomised, controlled trial. *Lancet Gastroenterology Hepatology, 3*(2), 85–94. doi:10.1016/S2468-1253(17)30392-8

Antiretroviral Pregnancy Registry. Address: Research Park, 1011 Ashes Drive, Wilmington, NC 28405; telephone: 800-258-4263; fax: 800-800-1052; email: registies@kendle.com.
http://www.apregistry.com/index.htm

Aronow, W. S. *Initiation of antihypertensive therapy.* Presented at the American Heart Association (AHA) Scientific Sessions 2017; November 11–15, 2017; Anaheim, CA.
http://www.abstractsonline.com/pp8/-!/4412/presentation/55060

Auron, M., & Raissouni, N. (2015). Adrenal insufficiency. *Pediatric Review, 36*(3), 92–102.

Bosworth, T. (2017). *Testosterone deficiency treatment recommendation.*
https://www.medpagetoday.com/resource-center/hypogonadism/treatment- recommendations/a/64511

Bradley, J. S., & Nelson, J. D. (2021). *Nelson's pediatric antimicrobial therapy* (27th ed.). Itasca, IL: American Academy of Pediatrics.

Brunk, D. (2018). Learn 'four Ds' approach to heart failure in diabetes. *Clinician Reviews* [Online]. https://www.mdedge.com/clinicalendocrinologynews/article/157198/diabetes/learn-four-ds-approach-heart-failure-diabetes

Canestaro, W. J., Forrester, S. H., Raghu, G., Ho, L., & Devine, B. E. (2016). Drug treatment of idiopathic pulmonary fibrosis: Systematic review and network meta-analysis. *Chest, 149,* 756–766.

CDC 2015 sexually transmitted diseases treatment guidelines. http://www.cdc.gov/std/tg2015/default.htm

CDC Cases of Public Health Importance (COPHI) Coordinator (for reporting HIV infections in HCP and failures of PEP); telephone: 404-639-2050.

CDC guidelines for conception in HIV positive women stress the use of PrEP in sexual partners. https://www.medpagetoday.com/resource-centers/contemporary-hiv-prevention/cdc-guide-lines-conception-hiv-positive-women-stress-use-prep-sexual- partners/775?xid=NL_MPT_MPT_HIV_2017-09-26&eun=g766320d0r

CDC Morbidity and Mortality Weekly Report (MMWR). http://www.cdc.gov/mmwr/mmwr_wk.html

CDC provider information sheet - PrEP during conception, pregnancy, and breastfeeding information for clinicians counseling patients about PrEP use during conception, pregnancy, and breastfeeding. https://www.cdc.gov/hiv/pdf/prep_gl_clinician_factsheet_pregnancy_english.pdf

CDC Travelers' Health. https://wwwnc.cdc.gov/travel/destinations/list

Centers for Disease Control and Prevention. *Parasites—American trypanosomiasis (also known as Chagas disease).* Resources for health professionals.

Centers for Disease Control and Prevention. (2016). *Diphtheria, tetanus, and pertussis vaccine recommendations.* http://www.cdc.gov/vaccines/vpd/dtap-tdap-td/hcp/recommendations.htm

Centers for Disease Control and Prevention. (2016). *Facts about ADHD.* www.cdc.gov/ncbddd/adhd/facts.html

Centers for Disease Control and Prevention. (2020). *Update to CDC's treatment guidelines for gonococcal infection, 2020.* https://www.cdc.gov/mmwr/volumes/69/wr/mm6950a6.htm?s_cid=mm6950a6_w

Chang, A., Martins, K. A. O., Encinales, L., Reid, S. P., Acuña, M., & Encinales, C., . . . Firestein, G. S. (2017). A cross-sectional analysis of chikungunya arthritis patients 22 months post-infection demonstrates no detectable viral persistence in synovial fluid. *Arthritis Rheumatology.* doi:10.1002/art.40383

Chang, A., Encinales, L., Porras, A., Pachecho, N., Reid, S. P., Martins, K. A. O., . . . Simon, G. L. (2017). Frequency of chronic joint pain following chikungunya infection: A Colombian cohort study. *Arthritis Rheumatology.* doi:10.1002/art.40384

Chow, A. W., Benninger, M. S., Brook, I., Brozek, J. L., Goldstein, E. J., Hicks, L. A., . . . Infectious Disease Society of America. (2012). IDSA clinical practice guideline for acute and bacterial rhinosinusitis in children and adults. *Clinical Infectious Diseases, 54*(8), e72–e112.

Chutka, D. S., Takahashi, P. Y., & Hoel, R. W. (2004). Inappropriate medications for elderly patients. *Mayo Clinic Proceedings, 79*(1), 122–139.

Clinician Reviews. http://www.clinicianreviews.com

Cohen, J. D., Li, L., Wang, Y., Th oburn, C., Afsari, B., Danilova, L. et al. (2018). Detection and localization of surgically resectable cancers with a multi-analyte blood test. *Science, 359*(6378), 926–930. doi:10.1126/science.aar3247

Coker, T. J., & Dierfeldt, D. M. (2016). Acute bacterial prostatitis: Diagnosis and management. *American Family Physician, 93*(2), 114–120.

Consultant360. http://www.consultant360.com/home

DailyMed: NIH. U.S. Library of Medicine. https://dailymed.nlm.nih.gov/dailymed/index.cfm

Davis, M. C., Miller, B. J., Kalsi, J. K., Birkner, T., & Mathis, M. V. (2017). Efficient trial design—FDA approval of valbenazine for tardive dyskinesia. *New England Journal of Medicine, 376,* 2503–2506.

Dietrich, E. A., & Davis, K. (2017). Antibiotics for acute bacterial prostatitis: Which agent, and for how long? *Consultant, 57*(9), 564–565.

Domino, F. J., Baldor, R. A., Golding, J., & Stephens, M. B. (2021). *The 5-minute clinical consult.* Philadelphia, PA: Wolters Kluwer.

Dowell, D., Haegerich, T. M., & Chou, R. (2016). CDC guidelines for prescribing opioids for chronic pain. *Journal of the American Medical Association, 315*(15), 1624–1645. doi:10.1001/jama.2016.1464

Drugs.com. www.drugs.com

Drugs.com: Drugs Interaction Checker. https://www.drugs.com/drug_interactions.php

Drugs@FDA: FDA-Approved Drugs. http://www.accessdata.fda.gov/scripts/cder/drugsatfda/index.cfm

Durkin, M. J., Jafarzadeh, S. R., Hsueh, K., Sallah, Y. H., Munshi, K. D., Henderson, R. R., & Fraser, V. J. (2018). Outpatient antibiotic prescription trends in the United States: A national cohort study. *Infection Control & Hospital Epidemiology, 39*(05), 584–589. doi:10.1017/ice.2018.26

eMPR: Monthly Prescribing Reference (new FDA-approved products, new generics, new drug withdrawals, safety alerts). http://www.empr.com

Engorn, B., & Flerlage, J. (Eds.). (2021). *The Harriet Lane handbook: A handbook for pediatric house officers* (20th ed.). Philadelphia, PA: Elsevier.

epocrates. https://online.epocrates.com/drugs

FDA Drug Safety Communication. (2018). *FDA review finds additional data supports the potential for increased long-term risks with antibiotic clarithromycin (Biaxin) in patients with heart disease* [Online]. https://www.fda.gov/downloads/Drugs/DrugSafety/ucm597723.pdf

FDA. (2017). *FDA approves drug to treat Duchenne muscular dystrophy* [news release]. https://www.fda.gov/NewsEvents/Newsroom/PressAnnouncements/ucm540945.htm

FDA: Recalls, Market Withdrawals, and Safety Alerts. http://www.fda.gov/Safety/Recalls/default.htm

FDA: Reporting Unusual or Severe Toxicity to Antiretroviral Agents). Address: MedWatch, The FDA Safety Information and Adverse Event Reporting Program, Food and Drug Administration, 5600 Fishers Lane, Rockville, MD 20852; telephone: 800-332-1088. http://www.fda.gov/medwatch/

Fleming, J. E., & Lockwood, S. (2017). Cannabinoid hyperemesis syndrome. *Federal Practitioner, 34*(10), 33–36.

Freedberg, D. E., Kim, L. S., & Yang, Y.-X. (2017). The risks and benefits of long-term use of proton pump inhibitors: Expert review and best practice advice from the American Gastroenterological Association. *Gastroenterology, 152*(4), 706–715. doi:10.1053/j.gastro.2017.01.031

Freedman, M. S., Ault, K., & Bernstein, H. Advisory Committee on Immunization Practices recommended immunization schedule for adults aged 19 years or older—United States, 2021. *MMWR Morbidity and Mortality Weekly Report, 70,* 193–196. doi:10.15585/mmwr.mm7006a2

Garber, A. J., Abrahamson, M. J., Barzilay, J. I., Blonde, L., Bloomgarden, Z. T., Bush, M. A., . . . Umpierrez, G. E. (2017). Consensus statement by the American Association of Clinical Endocrinologists and American College of Endocrinology on the comprehensive type 2 diabetes management algorithm—2017 executive summary. *Endocrine Practice, 23*(2), 207–238. doi:10.4158/ep161682.cs

Gilbert, D. N., Chambers, H. F., Eliopoulos, G. M., Saag, M. S., & Pavia, A. T. (Eds.). (2020). *The Sanford guide to antimicrobial therapy, 2020* (50th ed.). Sperryville, VA: Antimicrobial Therapy.

Global Initiative for Chronic Obstructive Lung Disease. *GOLD guidelines, 2017.* http://goldcopd.org

Gordon, C., Amissah-Arthur, M. B., Gayed, M., Brown, S., Bruce, I. N., D'Cruz D., . . . British Society for Rheumatology Standards, Audit and Guidelines Working Group. (2017). The British Society for Rheumatology guideline for the management of systemic lupus erythematosus in adults: Executive summary. *Rheumatology (Oxford).* doi:10.1093/rheumatology/kex291 [Epub ahead of print]

Gordon, C., Amissah-Arthur, M. B., Gayed, M., Brown, S., Bruce, I. N., D'Cruz D., . . . British Society for Rheumatology Standards, Audit and Guidelines Working Group. (2017). The British Society for Rheumatology guideline for the management of systemic lupus erythematosus in adults. *Rheumatology (Oxford).* doi:10.1093/rheumatology/kex286

Greenhawt, M., Turner, P. J., & Kelso, J. M. (2018). Allergy experts set the record straight on flu shots for patients with egg sensitivity. *Annals of Allergy, Asthma & Immunology, 120*(1), 49–52. doi:10.1016/j.anai.2017.10.020

Groot, N., de Graaff, N., Avcin, T., Bader-Meunier, B., Brogan, P., Dolezalova, P., . . . Beresford, M. W. (2017). European evidence-based recommendations for diagnosis and treatment of childhood-onset systemic lupus erythematosus (cSLE): The (Single Hub and Access point for paediatric Rheumatology in Europe) SHARE initiative. *Annals of the Rheumatic Diseases, 76*(11), 1788–1796. doi:10.1136/annrheumdis-2016-210960

Groot, N., de Graeff, N., Marks, S. D., Brogan, P., Avcin, T., Bader-Meunier, B., . . . Kamphuis, S. (2017). European evidence-based recommendations for the diagnosis and treatment of childhood-onset lupus nephritis (cLN): The SHARE initiative. *Recommendation.* doi:10.1136/annrheumdis-2017-211898

Guidelines updated for thyroid disease in pregnancy and postpartum. (2017). *American Journal of Nursing, 4*(117), 16.

Handbook of antimicrobial therapy (20th ed.). (2015). New Rochelle, NY: The Medical Letter.

Harrison's infectious diseases (3rd ed.). (2016). New York, NY: McGraw Hill Education.

Huang, A. R., Mallet, L., & Rochefort, C. M. (2012). Medication-related falls in the elderly: Causative factors and preventive strategies. *Drugs & Aging, 29*(5), 359–376.

Hughes, H. K., & Kahl, K. (Eds.). (2018). *The Johns Hopkins Hospital: The Harriet Lane handbook for pediatric house officers* (21st ed.). Philadelphia, PA: Elsevier.

International Diabetes Federation (IDF) Clinical Practice Guidelines. http://www.idf.org/guidelines

JAMA Network. www.jamanetwork.com

Jarrett, J. B., & Moss, D. (2017, July). Oral agent offers relief from generalized hyperhidrosis—An inexpensive and well-tolerated anticholinergic reduces sweating in patients with localized—and generalized—hyperhidrosis. *Clinician Reviews* [Online]. https://www.mdedge.com/sites/default/files/Document/June-2017/CR02707024.PDF

JNC 8 Guideline Summary. *Pharmacist's Letter/Prescriber's Letter.*
    https://www.scribd.com/doc/290772273/JNC-8-guideline-summary

Journal of the American Academy of Nurse Practitioners.
    https://www.aanp.org/publications/jaanp

Journal of the American Geriatrics Society.
    http://onlinelibrary.wiley.com/journal/10.1111/(ISSN)1532-5415

Journal of the American Medical Association (JAMA) Internal Medicine.
    http://archinte.jamanetwork.com/journal.aspx

Justesen, K., & Prasad, S. (2016). On-demand pill protocol protects against HIV. *Clinician Reviews, 26*(9), 18–19, 22.
    https://www.mdedge.com/authors/kathryn-justesen-md
    https://www.mdedge.com/authors/shaliendra-prasad-mbbs-mph

Kasper, D. L., & Fauci, A. S. (2017). Listeria monocytogenes infections. In: *Harrison's infectious diseases* (3rd ed.). New York, NY: McGraw Hill Education.

Khera, M., Adaikan, G., Buvat, J, Carrier, S., El-Meliegy, A., Hatzimouratidis, K., . . . Salonia, A. (2016). Diagnosis and treatment of testosterone deficiency: Recommendations from the Fourth International Consultation for Sexual Medicine (ICSM 2015). *The Journal of Sexual Medicine, 13*, 1787–1804.

Kuhar, D. T., Henderson, D. K., Struble, K. A., Heneine, W., Thomas, V., . . . Cheever, L. W. (2013). Updated US Public Health Service guidelines for the management of occupational exposures to human immunodeficiency virus and recommendations for postexposure prophylaxis. *Infection Control & Hospital Epidemiology, 34*(09), 875–892. doi:10.1086/672271

Kumar, S., Yegneswaran, B., & Pitchumoni, C. S. (2017). Preventing the adverse effects of glucocorticoids: A reminder. *Consultant, 57*(12), 726–728.

Langer, R., Simon, J. A., Pines, A., Lobo, R. A., Hodis, H. N., Pickar, J. H., . . . Utian, W. H. (2017). Menopausal hormone therapy for primary prevention: Why the USPSTF is wrong. *The North American Menopause Society, 24*(10), 1101–1112. doi:10.1097/GME.0000000000000983

Leach, M. Z. (2017, November 7). First UK guidelines for adults with lupus. *Rheumatology Network.*
    http://www.rheumatologynetwork.com/article/first-uk-guidelines-adults-lupus

Lexicomp. (2021). *Pediatric and neonatal dosage handbook: An extensive resource for clinicians treating pediatric and neonatal patients* (25th ed.). Lexicomp.

Lortscher, D., Admani, S., Satur, N., & Eichenfield, L. F. (2016). Hormonal contraceptives and acne: A retrospective analysis of 2147 patients. *Journal of Drugs in Dermatology, 15*(6), 670–674.
    http://jddonline.com/articles/dermatology/S1545961616P0670X

Manchikanti, L., Kaye, A. M., Knezevic, N. N., McAnally, H., Slavin, K., Trescot, A. M., . . . Hirsch, J. A. (2017). Responsible, safe, and effective prescription of opioids for chronic non-cancer pain: American Society of Interventional Pain Physicians (ASIPP) guidelines. *Pain Physician, 20*(2S), S3–S92.

McDonald, J., & Mattingly, J. (2016). Chagas disease: Creeping into family practice in the United States. *Clinician Reviews, 26*(11), 38–45.

McNeill, C., Sisson, W., & Jarrett, A. (2017). Listeriosis: A resurfacing menace. *International Journal of Nursing Practice, 13*(10), 647–654.

MDedge: Family Practice News.
    https://www.mdedge.com/familypracticenews/

MedlinePlus.
    https://www.nlm.nih.gov/medlineplus/ency/article/000165.htm

MedPage Today.
    http://www.medpagetoday.com

Medscape.
    http://www.medscape.com

Medscape: Drug Interaction Checker.
    http://reference.medscape.com/drug-interactionchecker?src=wnl_drugguide
    _170410_mscpref &uac=123859AY&impID=1324737&faf=1

Merel, S. E., & Paauw, D. S. (2017). Common drug side effects and drug-drug interactions in elderly adults in primary care. *Journal of the American Geriatrics Society, 65*(7), 1578–1585.

Miller, G. E., Sarpong, E. M., Davidoff, A. J., Yang, E. Y., Brandt, N. J., & Fick, D. M. (2016). Determinants of potentially inappropriate medication use among community-dwelling older adults. *Health Services Research, 52*(4), 1534–1549.

Molina, J. M., Capitant, C., Spire, B., Pialoux, G., Cotte, L., Charreau, I., . . . ANRS IPERGAY Study Group. (2015). On-demand preexposure prophylaxis in men at high risk for HIV-1 infection. *The New England Journal of Medicine, 373*, 2237–2246.

Monaco, K. (2017). *HRT benefits outweigh risks for certain menopausal women—Menopause Society statement aims to clear up confusion.*
    https://www.medpagetoday.com/Endocrinology/Menopause/66158?xid=NL_MPT_IRXHealthWomen_2017-12-27&eun=g766320d0r

Morales, A., Bebb, R. A., Manoo, P., Assimakopoulos, P., Axler, J., Collier, C., . . . Lee, J. (2015). *Appendix 1 (as supplied by the authors): Full-text guidelines. Multidisciplinary Canadian Clinical Practice Guideline on the diagnosis and management of testosterone deficiency syndrome in adult males.*
    http://www.cmaj.ca/content/suppl/2015/10/26/cmaj.150033.DC1/15-0033-1-at.pdf

National Academy of Medicine.
http://nam.edu

National Center for Emerging and Zoonotic Infectious Diseases (NCEZID).
https://www.cdc.gov/ncezid/index.html

National Heart Lung, and Blood Institute (NHLBI).
http://www.nhlbi.nih.gov

National Institute of Diabetes and Digestive and Kidney Diseases. *Adrenal insufficiency and Addison's disease.*
http://www.nidk.nih.gov/health-infromation/health-topics/endocrine/adren [Accessed May 31, 2016]

New England Journal of Medicine (NEJM) Journal Watch General Medicine.
http://www.jwatch.org/general-medicine

Ní Chróinín, D., Neto, H. M., Xiao, D., Sandhu, A., Brazel, C., Farnham, N., . . . Beveridge, A. (2016). Potentially inappropriate medications (PIMs) in older hospital in-patients: Prevalence, contribution to hospital admission and documentation of rationale for continuation. *Australasian Journal on Ageing, 35*(4), 262–265.

NIH, HIV/AIDS Treatment Information Service.
http://aidsinfo.nih.gov/

Oliver, S. E., Gargano, J. W., Marin, M., Wallace, M., Curran, K. G., Chamberland, M., . . . Dooling, K. (2020). The Advisory Committee on Immunization Practices' interim recommendation for use of Pfizer-BioNTech COVID-19 vaccine—United States, December 2020. *MMWR Morbidity and Mortality Weekly Report, 69,*1922–1924. doi:10.15585/mmwr.mm6950e2

Oliver, S. E., Gargano, J. W., Marin, M., Wallace, M., Curran, K. G., Chamberland, M., . . . Dooling, K. (2021). The Advisory Committee on Immunization Practices' interim recommendation for use of Moderna COVID-19 vaccine—United States, December 2020. *MMWR Morbidity and Mortality Weekly Report, 69*:1653-1656. doi:10.15585/mmwr.mm695152e1

Ostergaard, L., Vesikari, T., Absalon, J., Beeslaar, J., Ward, B. J., Senders, S., . . . B1971009 and B1971016 Trial Investigators. (2017). A bivalent meningococcal b vaccine in adolescents and young adults. *The New England Journal of Medicine, 35*(4), 262–265. doi:10.1111/ ajag.12312

PEPline. Telephone: 888-448-4911.
http://www.nccc.ucsf.edu/about_nccc/pepline/

Pharmacist's Letter.
www.pharmacistsletter.com

Physician's Desk Reference (PDR).
http://www.pdr.net

Pregnancy and Lactation Labeling Final Rule (PLLR).
https://www.drugs.com/pregnancy-categories.html

Prescriber's Letter.
http://prescribersletter.therapeuticresearch.com/pl/sample.aspx?cs=&s=PRL&AspxAutoDetectCookieSupport=1

Psychopharmacology.
http://link.springer.com/journal/213

Reference for Interpretation of Hepatitis C Virus (HCV) Test Results.
www.cdc.gov/hepatitis

Rosenberg, E. S., Doyle, K., Munoz-Jordan, J. L., Klein, L., Adams, L., Lozier, M., Weiss, K., & Sharp, T. M. (2017, November 5–9). *Prevalence and incidence of Zika virus infection among household contacts of Zika patients, Puerto Rico, 2016–2017. ASTMH 2017* . Paper presented at the 66th Annual Meeting of the American Society of Tropical Medicine and Hygiene, Baltimore, MD.

RxList.
http://www.rxlist.com/script/main/hp.asp

RxList: Drugs A-Z.
http://www.rxlist.com/drugs/alpha_a.htm

Sáez-Llorens, X., Tricou, V., Yu, D., Rivera, L., Jimeno, J., Villarreal, A. C., ... Wallace, D. (2018). Immunogenicity and safety of one versus two doses of tetravalent dengue vaccine in healthy children aged 2–17 years in Asia and Latin America: 18-month interim data from a phase 2, randomised, placebo-controlled study. *The Lancet Infectious Diseases, 18*(2), 162–170. doi:10.1016/s1473-3099(17)30632-1

Sanford Guide Web Edition.
https://webedition.sanfordguide.com

Saunders, K. H., Shukla, A. P., Igel, L. I., & Aronne, L. J. (2017). Obesity: When to consider medication. *The Journal of Family Practice, 66*(10), 608–616.
http://www.mdedge.com/sites/default/files/Document/September-2017/JFP06610608.PDF

Schaeffer, A. J., & Nicolle, L. E. (2016). Urinary tract infections in older men. *The New England Journal of Medicine, 374*(6), 562–571.

Schwartz, S. R., Magit, A. E., Rosenfeld, R. M., Ballachanda, B. B., Hackell, J. M., Krouse, H. J., . . . Cunningham, E. R. (2017). Clinical practice guideline (update): Earwax (cerumen impaction). *Otolaryngology Head Neck Surgery, 156*(1S), S1–S29.

Solutions for safer ER/LA opioid prescribing in a new era of health care. *American Nurses Credentialing Center, Post Graduate Institute of Medicine.*
www.cmeuniversity.com

Sterling, T. R., Villarino, M. E., Borisov, A. S., Shang, N., Gordin, F., Bliven-Sizemore, E., . . . TB Trials Consortium PREVENT TB Study Team. (2011). Three months of rifapentine and isoniazid for latent tuberculosis infection. *The New England Journal of Medicine, 365,* 2155–2166. doi:10.1056/NEJMoa1104875

Taipale, H., Mittendorfer-Rutz, E., Alexanderson, K., Majak, M., Mehtälä, J., Hoti, F., . . . Tiihonen, J. (2017, December 20). Antipsychotics and mortality in a nationwide cohort of 29,823 patients with schizophrenia. *Schizophrenia Research,* pii: S0920-9964(17), 30762–30764. doi:10.1016/j.schres.2017.12.010

Tebas, P., Roberts, C. C., Muthumani, K., Reuschel, E. L., Kudchodkar, S. B., Zaidi, F. I., . . . Maslow, J. N. (2017). Safety and immunogenicity of an anti-zika virus DNA vaccine—Preliminary report. *New England Journal of Medicine.* doi:10.1056/nejmoa1708120

The 2017 Hormone Therapy Position Statement of the North American Menopause Society. (2017). *Menopause: The North American Menopause Society.* doi:10.1097/GME.0000000000000921

The Journal for Nurse Practitioners.
www.elsevier.com/locate/tjnp

The Medical Letter on Drugs and Therapeutics.
http://secure.medicalletter.org

The Nurse Practitioner Journal.
www.tnpj.com

Third Report of the National Cholesterol Education Program (NCEP) expert panel on detection, evaluation, and treatment of high blood cholesterol in adults (Adult Treatment Panel III) final report.
http://www.ncbi.nlm.nih.gov/pubmed/12485966

Tomaselli, G. F., Mahaffey, K. W., Cuker, A., Dobesh, P. P., Doherty, J. U., Eikelboom, J. W., . . . Wiggins, B. S. (2017). 2017 ACC expert consensus decision pathway on management of bleeding in patients on oral anticoagulants. *Journal of the American College of Cardiology, 70*(24), 3042–3067. doi:10.1016/j.jacc.2017.09.1085

Turner, P. J., Southern, J., Andrews, N. J., Miller, E., Erlewyn-Lajeunesse, M., & Doyle, C. (2015). Safety of live attenuated influenza vaccine in atopic children with egg allergy. *Journal of Allergy and Clinical Immunology, 136*(2), 376–381. doi:10.1016/j.jaci.2014.12.1925

Updated CDC guidance: Superbugs threaten hospital patients. *Medscape Education Clinical Briefs.* (2016, March 31). http://www.medscape.org/viewarticle/859361?nlid=105320_2713&src=wnl_cmemp_160523_mscpedu_nurs&impID=1106718&faf=1

UpToDate.com.
http://www.uptodate.com

U.S. Pharmacist Weekly Newsletter.
http://www.uspharmacist.com

Vogt, C. (2017, November 14). New AHA/ACC guidelines lower high BP threshold. *Consultant360.* https://www.consultant360.com/exclusives/new-ahaacc-guidelines-lower- high-bp-threshold

Vrcek, I., Choudhury, E., & Durairaj, V. (2017). Herpes zoster ophthalmicus: A review for the internist. *The American Journal of Medicine, 130*(1), 21–26.

Wald, E. R., Applegate, K. E., Bordley, C., Darrow, D. H., Glode, M. P., Marcy, S. M., . . . American Academy of Pediatrics. (2013). Clinical practice guidelines for the diagnosis and management of acute bacterial sinusitis in children 1 to 18 years. *Pediatrics, 132*(1), e262–e280.

Wallace, D. V., Dykewicz, M. S., Oppenheimer, J., Portnoy, J. M., & Lang, D. M. (2017). Pharmacologic treatment of seasonal allergic rhinitis: Synopsis of guidance from the 2017 joint task force on practice parameters. *Annals of Internal Medicine, 167*(12), 876. doi:10.7326/m17-2203

Watkins, S. L., Glantz, S. A., & Chaffee, B. W. (2018). Association of noncigarette tobacco product use with future cigarette smoking among youth in the Population Assessment of Tobacco and Health (PATH) study, 2013–2015. *JAMA Pediatrics, 172*(2), 181. doi:10.1001/jamapediatrics.2017.4173

WebMD: Drugs and Medications A to Z. Latest Drug News.
http://www.webmd.com/drugs

Wimmer, B. C., Cross, A. J., Jokanovic, N., Wiese, M. D., George, J., Johnell, K., . . . Bell, J. S. (2016). Clinical outcomes associated with medication regimen complexity in older people: A systematic review. *Journal of the American Geriatrics Society, 65*(4), 747–753. doi:10.1111/jgs.14682

Winkel, P., Hilden, J., Hansen, J. F., Kastrup, J., Kolmos, H. J., Kjøller, E., . . . Gluud, C. (2015). Clarithromycin for stable coronary heart disease increases all-cause and cardiovascular mortality and cerebrovascular morbidity over 10 years in the CLARICOR randomised, blinded clinical trial. *International Journal of Cardiology, 182,* 459–465. doi:10.1016/j.ijcard.2015.01.020

Wodi, A. P., Ault, K., Hunter, P., McNally, V., Szilagyi, P. G., & Bernstein, H. (2021). Advisory Committee on Immunization Practices—Recommended immunization schedule for children and adolescents aged 18 years or younger—United States, 2021. *MMWR Morbidity and Mortality Weekly Report, 70,* 189–192. doi:10.15585/mmwr.mm7006a1

Wong, J., Marr, P., Kwan, D., Meiyappan, S., & Adcock, L. (2014). Identification of inappropriate medication use in elderly patients with frequent emergency department visits. *Canadian Pharmacists Journal/Revue Des Pharmaciens Du Canada, 147*(4), 248–256. doi:10.1177/1715163514536522

World Health Organization. (2016, August 30.). *Growing antibiotic resistance forces updates to recommended treatments for sexually transmitted infections.*
http://www.who.int/mediacentre/news/releases/2016/antibiotics-sexual-infections/en

World Health Organization. (2016). *WHO guidelines for the treatment of Chlamydia trachomatis.*
http://www.who.int/reproductivehealth/publications/rtis/chlamydia-treatment-guidelines/en

World Health Organization. (2016). *WHO guidelines for the treatment of Neisseria gonorrhoeae.*
http://www.who.int/reproductivehealth/publications/rtis/gonorrhoea-treatment-guidelines/en

World Health Organization. (2016). *WHO guidelines for the treatment of Treponema pallidum (syphilis).*
http://www.who.int/reproductivehealth/publications/rtis/syphilis-treatment-guidelines/en

World Health Organization. (2017, March). *WHO model list of essential medicines* (20th list). Geneva, Switzerland: Author.
http://www.who.int/medicines/publications/essentialmedicines/20th_EML2017.pdf?ua=1

World Health Organization. (2017, March). *WHO model list of essential medicines for children* (6th list). Geneva, Switzerland: Author.
http://www.who.int/medicines/publications/essentialmedicines/6th_EMLc2017.pdf?ua=1

World Health Organization. (2017, June 6). *WHO updates essential medicines list with new advice on use of antibiotics, and adds medicines for hepatitis C, HIV, tuberculosis and cancer.* Geneva, Switzerland: Author.
http://www.who.int/mediacentre/news/releases/2017/essential-medicines-list/en

Xie, Y., Bowe, B., Li, T., Xian, H., Yan, Y., & Al-Aly, Z. (2017, February 22). Long-term kidney outcomes among users of proton pump inhibitors without intervening acute kidney injury. *Kidney International, 91*(6), 1482–1494. doi:10.1016/j.kint.2016.12.021

Yılmaz, D., Heper, Y., & Gözler, L. (2017). Effect of the use of buzzy during phlebotomy on pain and individual satisfaction in blood donors. *Pain Management Nursing, 18*(4), 260–267.

Yoon, I.-K., & Thomas, S. J. (2017). Encouraging results but questions remain for dengue vaccine. *The Lancet Infectious Diseases, 18*(2), 125–126. doi:10.1016/S1473-3099(17)30634-5

Zarrabi, H., Khalkhali, M., Hamidi, A., Ahmadi, R., & Zavarmousavi, P. (2016). Clinical features, course and treatment of methamphetamine-induced psychosis in psychiatric inpatients. *BMC, 44.* doi:10.1186/s12888-016-0745-5

NOTE: Generic names are in italics; FDA pregnancy categories and controlled drug categories appear in parentheses.

A-200, *pyrethrins with piperonyl butoxide* (G)
  pediculosis humanus capitis, 475
A/B Otic, *antipyrine+benzocaine+ glycerine* (G)
  otitis externa, 445
  otitis media: acute, 447
abacavir sulfate, Ziagen (G), 698
  human immunodeficiency virus (HIV) infection, 308
abaloparatide, Tymlos (G)
  hypoparathyroidism, 344–345
  osteoporosis, 442
abametapir, Xeglyze Lotion
  pediculosis humanus capitis, 475
abatacept, Orencia (G)
  graft versus host disease (GVHD), 264–265
  juvenile idiopathic arthritis, 373–374
  polyarticular juvenile idiopathic arthritis (PJIA), 370–371
  psoriatic arthritis, 531
  rheumatoid arthritis, 549
abdominal cramps
  chlordiazepoxide+clidinium, Librax (IV), 175
  dicyclomine, Bentyl, 174
  hyoscyamine, Anaspaz, Levbid, Levsin, Levsinex, NuLev (G), 174–175
  methscopolamine bromide, Pamine, Pamine Forte, 174
  phenobarbital+hyoscyamine+ atropine+scopolamine, Donnatal (G), 175
  simethicone, Mylicon Drop (G), 175
abemaciclib, Verzenio
  breast cancer, 78–79
Abilify, *aripiprazole* (G), 692
  bipolar disorder, 62
  major depressive disorder, 194
  methamphetamine-induced psychosis, 394
  schizophrenia, 561
abiraterone acetate, Yonsa, Zytiga
  prostate cancer, 128–129
Abreva, *docosanol*
  herpes labialis/herpes facialis, 301
Abrilada, *adalimumab-afzb*
  Crohn's disease, 177
  osteoarthritis (OA), 438
  psoriasis, 525
  psoriatic arthritis, 530
  rheumatoid arthritis (RA), 547
  ulcerative colitis (UC), 636
abrocitinib, Cibinqo
  asthma, 45
  atopic dermatitis, 200
Abrysvo, respiratory syncytial virus vaccine
  respiratory syncytial virus (RSV), 539
Absorica/Absorica LD, *isotretinoin*
  acne vulgaris, 7
Abstral, *fentanyl*
  pain, 461
acamprosate, Campral (G)
  alcohol withdrawal syndrome, 11
Acanya, *clindamycin+benzoyl peroxide*
  acne vulgaris, 4
  folliculitis barbae, 246
acarbose, Precose
  type 2 diabetes mellitus, 620
Accolate, *zafirlukast*
  allergic rhinitis/sinusitis, 551

asthma, 41
AccuNeb Inhalation Solution, *albuterol sulfate* (G)
  asthma, 39
Accupril, *quinapril* (G)
  heart failure, 280
  hypertension, 329
Accuretic, *quinapril+hydrochlorothiazide*
  hypertension, 333
Accutane, *isotretinoin*
  acne vulgaris, 7
acebutolol, Sectral
  hypertension, 326
Aceon, *perindopril*
  hypertension, 330
Acetadote, *acetylcysteine*
  acetaminophen overdose, 1
acetaminophen, Ofirmev, Children's Tylenol, Extra Strength Tylenol, FeverAll Extra Strength Tylenol, Maximum Strength Tylenol Sore Throat, Tylenols
  fever (pyrexia), 241–242
  pain, 450–451
  postherpetic neuralgia (PHN), 509
  urolithiasis, 647
acetaminophen overdose
  acetylcysteine, Acetadote, 1
acetazolamide, Diamox (G)
  glaucoma, 257
acetic acid 2% in aluminum sulfate, Domeboro Otic (G)
  otitis externa, 444
acetyl sulfisoxazole, Gantrisin (G)
  urinary tract infection, 643
acetylcysteine, Acetadote, Mucomyst
  acetaminophen overdose, 1
  cystic fibrosis (CF), 182
achondroplasia
  vosoritide, Voxzogo, 1–2
Achromycin V, *tetracycline*, 709
  acne vulgaris, 6
  acute exacerbation of chronic bronchitis, 71
  aphthous stomatitis, 37
  bacterial skin infection, 575
  blepharitis, 67
  hidradenitis suppurativa, 304
  Lyme disease, 383
  malaria, 385
  mycoplasma pneumonia, 497
  psittacosis, 519
  rocky mountain spotted fever, 557
  shigellosis, 567
AcipHex, *rabeprazole*
  gastroesophageal reflux (GER), 251
  peptic ulcer disease (PUD), 479
  Zollinger-Ellison syndrome, 662
acitretin, Soriatane
  common wart, 655
  plantar wart, 655
  psoriasis, 521
aclidinium bromide, Tudorza Pressair (G)
  chronic obstructive pulmonary disease, 72
  emphysema, 230
Aclovate, *alclometasone dipropionate* (G), 676
acne rosacea
  azelaic acid, Azelex, Finacea, 2
  brimonidine, Mirvaso, 2
  Clenia Emollient Cream, Clenia Foaming Wash, *sodium sulfacetamide+sulfur* (G), 3

doxycycline, Acticlate, Adoxa, Doryx, Doxteric, Monodox, Oracea, Vibramycin, Vibra-Tab, 3
ivermectin, Soolantra (G), 2
metronidazole, MetroCream, MetroGel, MetroLotion, 2
minocycline, Amzeeq, Dynacin, Minocin, 2, 3
oxymetazoline hcl, Rhofade, 2
sodium sulfacetamide, Klaron (G), 3
acne vulgaris
  adapalene, Differin (G), 6
  adapalene+benzoyl peroxide, Epiduo Gel, Epiduo Forte Gel (G), 6
  azelaic acid, Azelex, Finacea, 4
  benzaClin, *clindamycin+benzoyl peroxide*, 5
  Benzamycin Topical Gel, *erythromycin+ benzoyl peroxide* (G), 4
  benzoyl peroxide, Benzac-W, Benzac-W Wash, Benzagel, Benzagel Wash, Desquam X, Triaz, ZoDerm (G), 4
  clindamycin, Cleocin T, Clindagel, Evoclin Foam, 4
  clindamycin+benzoyl peroxide, Acanya, BenzaClin, Duac, Onexton Gel, 4
  clascoterone, Winlevi, 4
  dapsone, Aczone (G), 4
  doxycycline, Acticlate, Adoxa, Doryx, Doxteric, Monodox, Oracea, Vibramycin, Vibra-Tab (G), 5
  erythromycin base, Ery-Tab, PCE, 5
  erythromycin ethylsuccinate, EryPed, E.E.S. Granules, E.E.S. 400 Tablets, 5
  isotretinoin, Absorica/Absorica LD, Accutane, Amnesteem, 7
  minocycline, Amzeeq, Dynacin, Minocin, Minolira, Solodyn, 5
  sarecycline, Seysara, 5–6
  sodium sulfacetamide, Klaron (G), 5
  tazarotene, Avage, Tazorac, 6
  tetracycline, Achromycin V, Sumycin, 6
  tretinoin, Altreno, Atralin, Avita, Retin-A, Tretin-X (G), 6
  tretinoin 0.1% cream+benzoyl peroxide 3%, Twyneo, 6–7
  trifarotene 0.005% cream, Aklief, 6
  Ziana, *tretinoin+clindamycin* (G), 7
acquired autoimmune thrombotic thrombocytopenia purpura (aTTP)
  caplacizumab-yhdp, Cablivi, 594–595
  rituximab, Rituxan, 595
acromegaly
  octreotide acetate Bynfezia Pen, Mycapssa, Sandostatin, Sandostatin LAR Depot, 8
  pasireotide, Signifor LAR (G), 7
  pegvisomant, Somavert, 7
Actemra, *tocilizumab*
  COVID-19 (coronavirus), 174
  giant cell arteritis (GCA), 254
  idiopathic pulmonary fibrosis (IPF), 535
  juvenile idiopathic arthritis, 370
  juvenile rheumatoid arthritis (JRA), 373
  pemphigus vulgaris, 477
  rheumatoid arthritis, 548–549

Acticin, *permethrin*
  scabies, 559
Acticlate, *doxycycline*
  acne rosacea, 3
  acne vulgaris, 5
  acute exacerbation of chronic
    bronchitis, 70
  anthrax (bacillus anthracis), 32
  bacterial skin infection, 574
  cat bite, 65
  cat scratch fever, 141
  Chlamydia trachomatis, 151
  cholera *(Vibrio cholerae)*, 155, 156
  community-acquired pneumonia, 494
  dog bite, 66
  dose forms, 639, 644, 704
  epididymitis, 237
  gonorrhea, 256
  granuloma inguinale, 266
  hidradenitis suppurativa, 303
  lyme disease, 383
  lymphogranuloma venereum, 384
  malaria, 384
  nongonococcal urethritis, 639
  pelvic inflammatory disease, 476
  proctitis: acute, 516
  rocky mountain spotted fever, 556
  sexual assault, 567
Actigall, *ursodiol*
  bile acid deficiency, 60
  cholelithiasis, 153
actinic keratosis
  aminolevulinic acid, Ameluz, 8
  diclofenac sodium, Solaraze Gel,
    Voltaren Gel (G), 9
  fluorouracil, Carac, Efudex,
    Fluoroplex, 9
  imiquimod, Aldara, Zyclara, 9
  ingenol mebutate, Picato (G), 9
  tirbanibulin, Klisyri, 9
Activella, FemHRT, Fyavolv (G), Mimvey
  LO, *estradiol+norethindrone*
  menopause, 391
  osteoporosis, 440
Actonel, *risedronate (as sodium)* (G)
  osteoporosis, 442
  Paget's disease, 442
Actonel with Calcium,
    risedronate+calcium (G), 343
  osteoporosis, 442
  Paget's disease, 450
Actoplus Met, Actoplis Met R,
    pioglitazone+metformin (G)
  type 2 diabetes mellitus, 622
Acular, Acular LS, Acular PF, *ketorolac*
    tromethamine (G)
  allergic (vernal) conjunctivitis, 168
  eye pain, 241
acute bacterial sinusitis, rhinosinusitis
    (ABSR)
  amoxicillin, Amoxil, Moxatag, Trimox,
    571
  Augmentin, Augmentin
    ES-600, Augmentin XR,
    amoxicillin+clavulanate, 571
  cefaclor, Cefaclor Extended Release, 571
  cefixime, Suprax, 571
  cefpodoxime proxetil, Vantin, 571
  ceftibuten, Cedax, 571
  ciprofloxacin, Cipro (G), Cipro XR,
    ProQuin XR (G), 572
  clarithromycin, Biaxin (G), 572
  levofloxacin, Levaquin (G), 572
  loracarbef, Lorabid, 572
  moxifloxacin, Avelox (G), 572
  trimethoprim+sulfamethoxazole
    (TMP-SMX), Bactrim, Septra
    (G), 572
acute bacterial skin and skin structure
    infection (ABSSSI). *See cellulitis*

acute diarrhea
  attapulgite, Donnagel, Kaopectate
    (G), 211
  bismuth subsalicylate, Pepto-Bismol
    (G), 211
  calcium polycarbophil, Fibercon (G),
    211
  crofelemer, Mytesi (G), 212
  difenoxin+atropine, Motofen (G), 212
  diphenoxylate+atropine, Lomotil
    (G)(V), 212
  loperamide, Imodium, Imodium
    A-D, 212
  loperamide+simethicone, Imodium
    Advanced, 212
  oral electrolyte replacement, CeraLyte,
    KaoLectrolyte, Pedialyte (OTC),
    212
acute exacerbation of chronic bronchitis
    (AECB)
  amoxicillin, Amoxil, Moxatag, Trimox,
    68–69
  amoxicillin+clavulanate, Augmentin,
    Augmentin ES-600, Augmentin
    XR, 69
  ampicillin, Omnipen, Principen, 69
  azithromycin, Zithromax, Zmax, 69
  cefaclor, Cefaclor Extended Release, 69
  cefadroxil, Duricef, 69
  cefdinir, Omnicef, 69
  cefditoren pivoxil, Spectracef, 69
  cefixime, Suprax, 69
  cefpodoxime proxetil, Vantin, 69
  cefprozil, Cefzil, 70
  ceftibuten, Cedax, 70
  ceftriaxone, Rocephin, 70
  cephalexin, Keflex, 70
  clarithromycin, Biaxin, Biaxin Oral
    Suspension, Biaxin XL (G), 70
  dirithromycin, Dynabac (G), 70
  doxycycline, Acticlate, Adoxa, Doryx,
    Doxteric, Monodox, Oracea,
    Vibramycin, Vibra-Tab, 70
  erythromycin ethylsuccinate, EryPed,
    E.E.S., 70
  gemifloxacin, Factive (G), 70
  levofloxacin, Levaquin (G), 70
  loracarbef, Lorabid, 70
  moxifloxacin, Avelox (G), 70
  ofloxacin, Floxin (G), 70
  telithromycin, Ketek (G), 70–71
  tetracycline, Achromycin V, Sumycin,
    71
  trimethoprim/sulfamethoxazole
    (TMP-SMX), Bactrim, Septra, 71
acute prostatitis
  ciprofloxacin, Cipro (G), Cipro XR,
    ProQuin XR (G), 516
  norfloxacin, Noroxin (G), 516
  ofloxacin, Floxin (G), 516
  trimethoprim+sulfamethoxazole
    (TMP-SMX), Bactrim, Septra
    (G), 516
acute tonsillitis
  amoxicillin, Amoxil, Moxatag, Trimox,
    603
  azithromycin, Zithromax, Zmax, 603
  cefaclor, Cefaclor Extended Release,
    603–604
  cefadroxil, Duricef, 604
  cefdinir, Omnicef, 604
  cefditoren pivoxil, Spectracef, 604
  cefixime, Suprax, 604
  cefpodoxime proxetil, Vantin, 604
  cefprozil, Cefzil, 604
  ceftibuten, Cedax, 604
  cephalexin, Keflex, 604
  clarithromycin, Biaxin, 604
  dirithromycin, Dynabac (G), 604
  erythromycin base, Ery-Tab, PCE, 604

  erythromycin ethylsuccinate, EryPed,
    E.E.S., 604
  loracarbef, Lorabid, 604–605
  penicillin v potassium, Pen-Vee K, 605
acyclovir, Avaclyr, Zovirax, Sitavig (G),
  616
  chickenpox (Varicella), 150
  dose forms, 610
  herpes genitalis (HSV TYPE II), 300
  herpes labialis/herpes facialis, 300, 301
  herpes simplex, keratitis/
    keratoconjunctivitis, 374
  herpes zoster, 301
  herpes zoster ophthmicus, 303
Aczone, *dapsone* (G)
  acne vulgaris, 4
  folliculitis barbae, 247
  Hansen's disease, 296
  pemphigus vulgaris, 177
A&D Ointment, *vitamin a and e* (G)
  diaper rash, 211
A&D Ointment with Zinc Oxide, *zinc*
    oxide (G)
  diaper rash, 211
adagrasib, Krazati
  lung cancer, 108
Adakveo, *crizanlizumab-tmca*
  sickle cell disease (SCD), 569–570
Adalat, Adalat CC, *nifedipine* (G)
  angina pectoris: stable, 28
  headache, 276
  hypertension: primary, 331
adalimumab, Humira
  Crohn's disease, 176–177
  hidradenitis suppurativa, 304
  juvenile idiopathic arthritis, 371
  osteoarthritis, ankylosing spondylitis,
    437
  psoriasis, 525
  psoriatic arthritis, 529
  rheumatoid arthritis, 546–547
  ulcerative colitis, 636
adalimumab-aacf, Idacio
  Crohn's disease, 177
  juvenile idiopathic arthritis (JIA), 371
  osteoarthritis (OA), 438
  psoriasis, 525
  psoriatic arthritis, 529
  rheumatoid arthritis (RA), 547
  ulcerative colitis (UC), 636
adalimumab-adaz, Hyrimoz
  Crohn's disease, 177
  juvenile idiopathic arthritis, 371
  osteoarthritis, 438
  psoriasis, 525
  psoriatic arthritis, 529
adalimumab-adbm, Cyltezo
  Crohn's disease, 177
  juvenile idiopathic arthritis, 371
  osteoarthritis, 438
  psoriasis, 525
  psoriatic arthritis, 529
  rheumatoid arthritis, 547
  ulcerative colitis, 636
adalimumab-afzb, Abrilada
  Crohn's disease, 177
  osteoarthritis (OA), 438
  psoriasis, 525
  psoriatic arthritis, 530
  rheumatoid arthritis (RA), 547
  ulcerative colitis (UC), 636
adalimumab-bwwd, Hadlim
  juvenile idiopathic arthritis (JIA), 371
  osteoarthritis (OA), 438
adapalene, Differin (G)
  acne vulgaris, 6
  facial wrinkles, 660
Adcetris, *brentuximab vedotin*, 583
  dose forms, 683
  lymphoma, 114

Adderall, Adderall XR,
  *dextroamphetamine saccharate+
  dextroamphetamine sulfate+
  amphetamine aspartate+
  amphetamine sulfate* (G)(II)
  attention deficit hyperactivity disorder
    (ADHD), 50–52
  narcolepsy, 411–412
Addyi, *flibanserin*
  low libido, hypoactive sexual desire
    disorder (HSDD), 380
adefovir dipivoxil, Hepsera (G)
  hepatitis B, 293
Adempas, *riociguat*
  pulmonary arterial hypertension
    (PAH), 533
Adhansia XR, *methylphenidate
  (long-acting)* (II)
  narcolepsy, 412
Adlarity, *donepezil transdermal system*
  Alzheimer's disease, 14–15
adrenocortical insufficiency
  hydrocortisone granules, Alkindi
    Sprinkle, 9–10
Adoxa, *doxycycline*
  acne rosacea, 3
  acne vulgaris, 5
  acute exacerbation of chronic
    bronchitis, 70
  anthrax (bacillus anthracis), 32
  bacterial skin infection, 574
  cat bite, 65
  cat scratch fever, 141
  Chlamydia trachomatis, 151
  cholera (Vibrio cholerae), 155, 156
  community-acquired pneumonia, 494
  dog bite, 66
  dose forms, 639, 644, 704
  epididymitis, 237
  gonorrhea, 256
  granuloma inguinale, 266
  hidradenitis suppurativa, 303
  lyme disease, 383
  lymphogranuloma venereum, 384
  malaria, 384
  nongonococcal urethritis, 639
  pelvic inflammatory disease, 476
  proctitis: acute, 516
  rocky mountain spotted fever, 556
  sexual assault, 567
aducanumab-avwa, Aduhelm
  Alzheimer's disease, 14
Aduhelm, *Aducanumab-avwa*
  Alzheimer's disease, 14
Adrenaclick, *epinephrine* (G)
  anaphylaxis, 21
  status asthmaticus, 579
Advair HFA, Advair Diskus, *fluticasone
  propionate+salmeterol* (G)
  asthma, 43
Advanced Relief Visine,
  *tetrahydrozoline+polyethylene
  glycol 400+povidone+dextran
  70* (G)
  allergic (vernal) conjunctivitis, 167
Advicor, *niacin+lovastatin*
  dyslipidemia, 224
  hypertriglyceridemia, 339
Advil, *ibuprofen*
  fever (pyrexia), 242
Advil *Dual* Action with Acetaminophen,
  ibuprofen+acetaminophen (G)
  pain, 451
Adzenys ER, *amphetamine, mixed salts of
  single entity amphetamine* (G)(II)
  attention deficit hyperactivity disorder
    (ADHD), 50–51
Adzenys XR-ODT, *amphetamine, mixed
  salts of single entity amphetamine*
  (G)(II)

attention deficit hyperactivity disorder
    (ADHD), 50–51
Aemcolo, *rifamycin* (G)
  Traveler's diarrhea, 213–214
AeroBid, AeroBid-M, *flunisolide* (G), 680
  asthma, 41
Aerospan HFA, *flunisolide* (G)
  asthma, 41
Afinitor, *everolimus,* 683
aflibercept, Eylea (G)
  diabetic retinopathy, 206
African sleeping sickness
  fexinidazole, Fexinidazole Tablets,
    10–11
Afrin Allergy Nasal Spray, Afrin Nasal
  Decongestant Childrens Pump
  Mist, *phenylephrine*
  common cold, 160–161
Afrin Moisturizing Saline Mist (OTC),
  saline nasal spray (G)
  common cold, 160–161
Afrin, *oxymetazoline* (G)
  common cold, 161
Afrin Saline Mist w. Eucalyptol and
  Menthol (OTC), *saline nasal
  spray* (G)
  common cold, 160–161
AirDuo RespiClick, *fluticasone
  propionate+salmeterol* (G)
  asthma, 43–44
Akineton, *biperiden hydrochloride* (G)
  Parkinson's disease, 471
Akynzeo, *fosnetupitant+palonosetron*
  chemotherapy-induced nausea/
    vomiting, 148, 413
Alamast, *pemirolast potassium* (G)
  allergic (vernal) conjunctivitis, 166
Alaway, *ketotifen fumarate* (G)
  allergic (vernal) conjunctivitis, 167
albendazole, Albenza (G)
  hookworm, 304
  pinworm, 488
  roundworm, 557
  tapeworm, 585
  threadworm, 593
  trichinosis, 606
  whipworm, 656
Albenza, *albendazole* (G)
  hookworm, 304
  pinworm, 488
  roundworm, 557
  tapeworm, 585
  threadworm, 593
  trichinosis, 606
  whipworm, 656
albuterol, Albuterol Syrup, Proventil,
  Ventolin, VoSpire ER (G)
  asthma, 39
Albuterol Inhalation Solution, Albuterol
  Nebules, *albuterol sulfate* (G)
  asthma, 39
albuterol sulfate, AccuNeb Inhalation
  Solution, Albuterol Inhalation
  Solution, Albuterol Nebules,
  Proair HFA Inhaler, Proair
  RespiClick, Proventil HFA
  Inhaler, Proventil Inhalation
  Solution, Ventolin (G)
  asthma, 39
Albuterol Syrup, *albuterol* (G)
  asthma, 44
alcaftadine, Lastacaft
  allergic (vernal) conjunctivitis, 166
alclometasone dipropionate, Aclovate
  (G), 676
alcohol withdrawal syndrome
  acamprosate, Campral (G), 11
  chlordiazepoxide (IV)(G), 11
  clorazepate, Tranxene, Librium (G)
    (IV), 11

diazepam, Diastat, Valium (IV), 11
  disulfiram, Antabuse, 11
  oxazepam (G), 11
Aldactazide, *spironolactone+
  hydrochlorothiazide*
  edema, 230
  heart failure, 282
  hypertension, primary, 329
Aldactone, *spironolactone*
  edema, 228
  fibrocystic breast disease, 243
  heart failure, 281
  hypertension, primary, 327
  premenstrual dysphoric disorder,
    514
Aldara, *imiquimod*
  actinic keratosis, 9
  venereal wart, 655
Aldoril, *methyldopa+hydrochlorothiazide*
  (G)
  hypertension, 334
Alecensa, *alectinib,* 683
alefacept, Amevive
  psoriasis, 521
alemtuzumab, Lemtrada (G)
  multiple sclerosis (MS), 398
alendronate (as sodium), Binosto,
  Fosamax (G)
  osteoporosis, 441
  Paget's disease, 450
Alesse-21, Alesse-28, *ethinyl estradiol/
  levonorgestrel*
  estrogen and progesterone, 667
Aleve, *naproxen*
  fever (pyrexia), 243
Alferon N, *interferon alfa-n3* (G)
  venereal wart, 656
alfuzosin, UroXatral
  benign prostatic hyperplasia, 58
  urolithiasis, 647
Alinia, *nitazoxanide*
  criptosporidiosis, 179
  dose forms, 705
  giardiasis, 254
  nitazoxanide, Alinia, 585
  threadworm, 593
Aliqopa, *copanlisib,* 683
alirocumab, Praluent (G)
  dyslipidemia, 221
aliskiren, Tekturna
  hypertension, 332
Alkeran, *melphalan,* 683
Allegra, *fexofenadine* (G)
  allergic rhinitis/sinusitis, 550
  atopic dermatitis, 198
  contact dermatitis, 202
  genus rhus dermatitis, 204
  rhinitis medicamentosa, 555
  urticaria, 649
allergic reaction
  diphenhydramine, Benadryl, 12
  hydroxyzine, Atarax, Vistaril (G), 12
allergic rhinitis/sinusitis
  azelastine, Astelin Ready Spray, Astepro
    0.15% Nasal Spray, 552
  azelastine+fluticasone, Dymista (G),
    552
  budesonide, Rhinocort (G), 552
  cetirizine, Children's Zyrtec Chewable,
    Children's Zyrtec Allergy Syrup,
    Zyrtec (G), 549
  ciclesonide, Alvesco (G), 552
  cromolyn sodium, Children's
    NasalCrom, NasalCrom, 552
  desloratadine, Clarinex, Desloratadine
    ODT (G), 550
  dexamethasone, Dexacort Turbinaire,
    552
  diphenhydramine, Benadryl, 550
  dupilumab, Dupixent, 553

allergic rhinitis/sinusitis (cont.)
  fexofenadine, Allegra (G), 550
  flunisolide, Nasalide, Nasarel (G), 552
  fluticasone furoate, Veramyst, 552
  fluticasone propionate, Flonase (OTC) (G), 552
  hydroxyzine, Atarax, Vistaril (G), 550
  ipratropium bromide, Atroven, 553
  levocetirizine, Children's Xyzal Allergy 24HR, Xyzal Allergy 24HR, 550
  loratadine, Claritin (G), 550
  mepolizumab, Nucala, 554
  mometasone furoate, Nasonex (G), 552
  montelukast, Singulair, 551
  olopatadine, Patanase (G), 552
  olopatadine hydrochloride+mometasone furoate, Ryaltris, 553
  short ragweed pollen allergen extract, Ragwitek (G), 551
  sweet vernal, orchard, perennial rye, timothy, Kentucky blue grass mixed pollen allergen extract, Oralair (G), 551
  tetrahydrozoline, Tyzine, Tyzine Pediatric Nasal Drops (G), 551
  Timothy grass pollen allergen extract, Grastek (G), 551
  triamcinolone acetonide, Nasacort Allergy 24HR, Tri-Nasal, Zilretta (G), 552
  zafirlukast, Accolate, 551
  zileuton, Zyflo, Zyflo-CR (G), 551
allergic (vernal) conjunctivitis
  alcaftadine, Lastacaft, 166
  azelastine, Optivar, 167
  bepotastine besilate, Bepreve, 167
  bromfenac, Bromday Ophthalmic Solution, Xibrom Ophthalmic Solution (G), 167
  cetirizine, Zerviate (G), 166
  cromolyn sodium, Crolom, 166
  cyclosporine, Verkazia, 168
  dexamethasone, Maxidex (G), 165
  dexamethasone phosphate, Decadron (G), 165
  diclofenac, Voltaren Ophthalmic Solution, 167
  emedastine, Emadine (G), 166
  epinastine, Elestat (G), 167
  fluorometholone acetate, Flarex (G), 165
  fluorometholone, FML, FML Forte, FML S.O.P. Ointment (G), 165
  ketorolac tromethamine, Acular, Acular LS, Acular PF (G), 168
  ketotifen fumarate, Alaway, Claritin Eye, Refresh Eye Itch Relief, Zaditor, Zyrtec Itchy Eye (G), 167
  levocabastine, Livostin (G), 166
  lodoxamide tromethamine, Alomide, 166
  loteprednol etabonate, Alrex, Lotemax (G), 166
  medrysone, HMS (G), 166
  naphazoline, Vasocon-A (G), 167
  naphazoline+pheniramine, Naphcon-A (G), 167
  nedocromil, Alocril, 166
  nepafenac, Nevanac Ophthalmic Suspension (G), 168
  olopatadine, Pataday, Patanol, Pazeo (G), 167
  oxymetazoline, Visine L-R (G), 167
  pemirolast potassium, Alamast (G), 166
  prednisolone acetate, Econopred, Econopred Plus, Pred Forte, Pred Mild (G), 166

  prednisolone sodium phosphate, Inflamase Forte, Inflamase Mild (G), 166
  rimexolone, Vexol (G), 166
  tetrahydrozoline, Visine (G), 167
  tetrahydrozoline+polyethylene glycol 400+povidone+dextran 70, Advanced Relief Visine (G), 167
  tetrahydrozoline+zinc sulfate, Visine AC (G), 167
allergies: multi-food
  omalizumab, Xolair, 12
Alli, orlistat (G)
  obesity, 418
allopurinol, Zyloprim (G)
  gout (hyperuricemia), 206
  urolithiasis, 646–647
almotriptan, Axert (G)
  migraine and cluster headache, 270
Alocril, nedocromil
  allergic (vernal) conjunctivitis, 166
alogliptin, Nesina
  type 2 diabetes mellitus, 629
Alomide, lodoxamide tromethamine
  allergic (vernal) conjunctivitis, 166, 375
alopecia areata
  baricitinib, Olumiant, 12–13
alosetron, Lotronex
  irritable bowel syndrome with diarrhea, 279
Aloxi, palonosetron
  cannabinoid hyperemesis syndrome, 140
  chemotherapy-induced nausea/vomiting, 149
  opioid-induced nausea/vomiting (OINV), 429
  post-anesthesia nausea/vomiting, 414
alpelisib, Piqray
  breast cancer, 79
alpha-1 antitrypsin (AAT) deficiency
  alpha-1 proteinase inhibitor (human), Aralast (G), 13
alpha-1 proteinase inhibitor (human), Aralast (G)
  alpha-1 antitrypsin (AAT) deficiency, 13
alprazolam, Niravam, Xanax, Xanax XR (IV)
  anxiety disorder, 33
  panic disorder, 465
alprostadil, Caverject, Edex, Muse
  erectile dysfunction (ED), 237
Alrex, loteprednol etabonate (G)
  allergic (vernal) conjunctivitis, 166
Alrex Ophthalmic Solution, etabonate (G)
  eye pain, 166
Altace, ramipril (G)
  heart failure, 200
  hypertension, primary, 330
Altavera, ethinyl estradiol/levonorgestrel
  estrogen and progesterone, 667
Altoprev, lovastatin
  dyslipidemia, 222
Altreno, tretinoin (G)
  acne vulgaris, 6
Altuviiio, antihemophilic factor (recombinant), Fc-VWF-XTEN fusion protein-ehtl
  hemophilia A, 286–287
aluminum chloride, Drysol
  hyperhidrosis, 320
aluminum hydroxide, ALTernaGEL, Amphojel (G)
  gastroesophageal reflux disease, 248
Alunbrig, brigatinib
  dose forms, 683
  lung cancer, 103

Alupent, metaproterenol (G)
  asthma, 40
Alvesco, ciclesonide (G)
  allergic rhinitis/sinusitis, 552
  asthma, 41
  polyps, nasal, 505
alvimopan, Entereg
  bowel resection with primary anastomosis, 68
Alzheimer's disease
  aducanumab-avwa, Aduhelm, 14
  brexpiprazole, Rexulti, 15–17
  donepezil, Aricept, Aricept ODT (G), 14
  donepezil transdermal system, Adlarity, 14–15
  ergoloid mesylate, Hydergine (G), 15
  galantamine, Razadyne, 15
  lecanemab-irmb, Leqembi, 14
  L-methylfolate calcium (as metafolin)+methylcobalamin+n-acetylcysteine, Cerefolin, 13
  memantine, Namenda, 15
  memantine+donepezil, Namzaric (G), 15
  rivastigmine, Exelon, 15
  tacrine, Cognex (G), 15
amantadine, Gocovri, Osmolex ER, Symadine (G), Symmetrel (G), 711
  benign essential tremor, 58
  dose forms, 705
  extrapyramidal side effects (EPS), 240
  Parkinson's disease, 468
Ambien, Ambien CR, zolpidem
  aphasia, 26
  fibromyalgia, 245
  insomnia, 359
ambrisentan, Letairis (G)
  pulmonary arterial hypertension (PAH), 533
amebiasis
  extra-intestinal
    chloroquine phosphate, Aralen (G), 17
  intestinal
    diiodohydroxyquin (iodoquinol) (G), 17
    metronidazole, Flagyl, Flagyl 375, Flagyl ER (G), 17
    paromomycin, Humatin, 17
    tinidazole, Tindamax (G), 17
amebic liver abscess
  metronidazole, Flagyl, Flagyl 375, Flagyl ER (G), 17
  tinidazole, Tindamax (G), 17
Ameluz, aminolevulinic acid
  actinic keratosis, 8
Amen, medroxyprogesterone
  amenorrhea, secondary, 18
amenorrhea, secondary
  estrogen+progesterone, Premarin, Provera, 17
  human chorionic gonadotropin, Pregnyl, 17
  medroxyprogesterone, Amen, Provera, 18
  norethindrone, Aygestin, 18
  progesterone, micronized, Prometrium, 18
Americaine Otic, benzocaine (G)
  otitis externa, 445
  otitis media: acute, 448
American trypanosomiasis, 146
amiloride, Midamor
  edema, 228
  heart failure, 281
  hypertension, 327
aminolevulinic acid, Ameluz
  actinic keratosis, 8–9

Amitiza, *lubiprostone* (G)
chronic idiopathic constipation, 169
irritable bowel syndrome with
constipation, 365
opioid-induced constipation, 428
amitriptyline (G)
anxiety disorder, 34
diabetic peripheral neuropathy
(DPN), 210
fibromyalgia, 244
interstitial cystitis, 362
irritable bowel syndrome with
diarrhea, 368
major depressive disorder, 193
migraine and cluster headache, 276
nocturnal enuresis, 235
post-herpetic neuralgia, 507, 509
post-traumatic stress disorder, 512
tension headache, 278
trigeminal neuralgia, 609
amivantamab-vmjw, Rybrevant
lung cancer, 107–108
amlodipine, Norvasc (G)
angina pectoris: stable, 28
hypertension, primary, 331
amlodipine benzoate, Katerzia
angina pectoris: stable, 28
hypertension, 331
Amnesteem, *isotretinoin*
acne vulgaris, 7
Amondys, *casimersen*
duchenne muscular dystrophy
(DMD), 218–219
amoxapine (G)
anxiety disorder, 34
diabetic peripheral neuropathy
(DPN), 210
major depressive disorder, 193
nocturnal enuresis, 235
post-herpetic neuralgia, 507, 509
trigeminal neuralgia, 609
amoxicillin, Amoxil, Moxatag, Trimox,
707, 711
acute bacterial sinusitis, rhinosinusitis,
571
acute exacerbation of chronic
bronchitis, 68–69
acute tonsillitis, 603
bacterial endocarditis prophylaxis, 55
bacterial skin infection, 573
cellulitis, 142
community acquired pneumonia,
493
diverticulitis, 215
dose form/volume, 707
impetigo contagiosa, 351
Lyme disease, 382
otitis media: acute, 445
streptococcal pharyngitis, 484
urinary tract infection, 643
Amoxil, *amoxicillin*, 711
acute bacterial sinusitis, rhinosinusitis,
571
acute exacerbation of chronic
bronchitis, 68–69
acute tonsillitis, 603
bacterial endocarditis prophylaxis, 55
bacterial skin infection, 573
cellulitis, 142
community acquired pneumonia, 493
diverticulitis, 215
dose form/volume, 707
impetigo contagiosa, 351
Lyme disease, 382
otitis media: acute, 445
streptococcal pharyngitis, 484
urinary tract infection, 643
*amphetamine, mixed salts of single entity
amphetamine*, Adzenys ER,
Adzenys XR-ODT, Dyanavel

XR Oral Suspension, Evekeo,
Mydayis (G)(II)
attention deficit hyperactivity disorder
(ADHD), 50–51
amphetamine sulfate, Evekeo (G)(II)
narcolepsy, 409
obesity, 418
amphotericin b, Fungizone
skin candidiasis, 136
ampicillin, Omnipen, Principen, Unasyn,
712–717
acute exacerbation of chronic
bronchitis, 69
bacterial endocarditis prophylaxis, 55
dose form/volume, 707
listeriosis, 379
otitis media: acute, 446
urinary tract infection, 643
dalfampridine, Ampyra (G)
multiple sclerosis, 397
Amrix, *cyclobenzaprine*
fibromyalgia, 244
muscle strain, 403
temporomandibular joint disorder,
586
Amturnide, *aliskiren+amlodipine+
hydrochlorothiazide*
hypertension, 252–253
amyotrophic lateral sclerosis (ALS)
edaravone, Radicava, 18–19
riluzole, Exservan, 19
sodium phenylbutyrate+taurursodiol,
Relyvrio, 18
tofersen, Qalsody, 19–20
Amzeeq, *minocycline*
acne rosacea, 2, 3
acne vulgaris, 5
anacaulase-bcdb, NexoBrid
burn, major, 75
Anacin, *aspirin+caffeine*
fever (pyrexia), 242
Anafranil, *clomipramine* (G)
anxiety disorder, 34
nocturnal enuresis, 235
obsessive-compulsive disorder, 422
trichotillomania, 607
*anakinra (interleukin-1 receptor
antagonist)*, Kineret
rheumatoid arthritis, 548
ana-Kit, *epinephrine+chlorpheniramine*
(G)
anaphylaxis, 21
status asthmaticus, 579
AnaMantle HC, *hydrocortisone+lidocaine*
hemorrhoids, 289
anaphylaxis
ana-Kit,
epinephrine+chlorpheniramine
(G), 21
epinephrine, Adrenaclick, Auvi-Q,
EpiPen, EpiPen Jr, Symjepi,
Twinject (G), 21
Anaprox, *naproxen*
fever (pyrexia), 165243
Anaspaz, *hyoscyamine* (G)
abdominal cramps, 174
interstitial cystitis, 361
irritable bowel syndrome with
diarrhea, 367
urinary overactive bladder, 354
urinary tract infection (UTI), 642
Ancef, *cefazolin*
bacterial endocarditis prophylaxis, 55
Androderm, *testosterone* (III)
testosterone deficiency, 590
AndroGel, *testosterone* (III)
testosterone deficiency, 589
anemia
beta thalassemia-associated, 21–22
chronic kidney disease, 22–24

folic acid deficiency, 24
hemolytic/anemia, 24–25
anemia of chronic kidney disease
daprodustat, Jesduvroq, 24
darbepoetin alpha, Aranesp (G), 23
epoetin alfa-epbx, Retacrit, 23
epoetin alpha, Epogen, Procrit (G), 23
ferric citrate, Aurexia, 22
finerenone, Kerendia, 22
peginesatide, Omontys (G), 23
Angeliq, *estradiol+drospirenone*, 303
angina pectoris, stable
amlodipine benzoate, Katerzia, 28
amlodipine besylate, Norliqva, 28
amlodipine, Norvasc (G), 28
atenolol, Tenormin, 29
Bidil, *isosorbide+hydralazine HCl*
(G), 30
*diltiazem, Cardizem, Cartia XT,
Dilacor XR, Tiazac* (G), 28
hydralazine (G), 30
*isosorbide dinitrate, Dilatrate-SR,
Isordil Titradose* (G), 29
isosorbide mononitrate, Imdur, Ismo
(G), 29
metoprolol succinate, Toprol-XL
(G), 29
metoprolol tartrate, Lopressor (G), 29
nadolol, Corgard (G), 29
nicardipine, Cardene (G), 28
*nifedipine, Adalat, Adalat CC,
Procardia, Procardia XL* (G), 28
*nitroglycerin, Nitro-Bid Ointment,
Nitrodisc, Nitrolingual Pump
Spray, Nitromist, Nitrostat,
Transderm-Nitro* (G), 29–30
*propranolol, Inderal, Inderal LA,
InnoPran XL* (G), 29
ranolazine, Ranexa (G), 30
*verapamil, Calan, Calan SR, Isoptin
SR* (G), 29
angiotensin II, Giapreza
shock, septic, distributive, 458
angular stomatitis, 482
anifrolumab, Saphnelo
systemic lupus erythematosis (SLE),
583
Anjeso, *meloxicam*
pain, 451
Annovera, *segesterone acetate+ethinyl
estradiol*, 674
anorexia/cachexia
cyproheptadine, Periactin (G), 30
dronabinol, Marinol, Syndros (III), 30
megestrol (progestin), Megace, Megace
ES, Megace Oral Suspension,
Megestrol Acetate Oral
Suspension (G), 31
Anoro Ellipta, *umeclidinium+vilanterol*
(G)
chronic obstructive pulmonary
disease (COPD), 73
emphysema, 232
ansuvimab-zykl, Ebanga
ebola zaire disease (zaire ebolavirus),
227–228
Antabuse, *disulfiram* (G)
alcohol withdrawal syndrome, 11
Antara, *fenofibrate* (G)
dyslipidemia, 223
hypertriglyceridemia, 338
anthralin, Zithranol-RR (G)
psoriasis, 521
Anthrasil, *bacillus anthracis immune
globulin intravenous (human)*
anthrax (bacillus anthracis), 31
anthrax (bacillus anthracis)
*bacillus anthracis immune globulin
intravenous (human)*, Anthrasil,
31

anthrax (bacillus anthracis) (cont.)
  ciprofloxacin, Cipro (G), Cipro XR, ProQuin XR (G), 31, 32
  doxycycline, Acticlate, Adoxa, Doryx, Doxteric, Monodox, Oracea, Vibramycin, Vibra-Tab, 32
  minocycline, Dynacin, Minocin, 32
  obiltoxaximab, Anthim, 31
  raxibacumab, 31
antihemophilic factor (recombinant), Fc-VWF-XTEN fusion protein-ehtl, Altuviiio, 286–287
  hemophilia A
Antiminth, pyrantel pamoate (G)
  dose forms, 704
  hookworm, 305
  pinworm, 557
  threadworm, 593
  trichinosis, 606
  whipworm, 657
Antivert, meclizine
  labyrinthitis, 375
  Meniere's disease, 388
  motion sickness, 396
  vertigo, 653
Anusol-HC, hydrocortisone (G)
  hemorrhoids, 289
  ulcerative colitis (UC), 634
anxiety disorder
  alprazolam, Niravam, Xanax, Xanax XR (IV), 33
  amitriptyline (G), 34
  amoxapine (G), 34
  buspirone, BuSpar, 33
  chlordiazepoxide, Librium (IV), 33
  citalopram, Celexa (G), 35
  clomipramine, Anafranil (G), 34
  clonazepam, Klonopin (IV), 34
  clorazepate, Tranxene (IV), 34
  desipramine, Norpramin (G), 34
  desvenlafaxine, Pristiq (G), 36
  diazepam, Diastat, Valium (IV), 34
  diphenhydramine, Benadryl, 32
  doxepin, Sinequan (G), 34
  duloxetine, Cymbalta (G), 36
  escitalopram, Lexapro (G), 35
  Etrafon, perphenazine+amitriptyline (G)(G), 36
  fluoxetine, Prozac, Prozac Weekly (G), 35
  generalized, 32–36
  hydroxyzine, Atarax, Vistaril (G), 33
  imipramine, Tofranil PM (G), 34
  Librax, chlordiazepoxide+clidinium (IV), 33
  Limbitrol, chlordiazepoxide+amitriptyline (G), 36
  lorazepam, Ativan, Lorazepam Intensol (IV), 33
  nortriptyline, Pamelor, 34
  oxazepam (G), 33
  paroxetine maleate, Paxil, Paxil CR, Paxil Suspension, 35
  paroxetine mesylate, Brisdelle, 35
  prochlorperazine, Compazine (G), 35
  protriptyline, Vivactil (G), 34
  sertraline, Zoloft (G), 35
  social, 32–36
  trifluoperazine, Stelazine (G), 35
  trimipramine, Surmontil (G), 34
  venlafaxine, Effexor, Effexor XR (G), 36
Anzemet, dolasetron
  cannabinoid hyperemesis syndrome, 139
  chemotherapy-induced nausea/vomiting, 148
  opioid-induced nausea/vomiting, 429

Apadaz, benzhydrocodone+acetaminophen (II)
  pain, 454
apalutamide, Erleada
  prostate cancer, 129
aphasia
  zolpidem, Ambien (IV), 36
  zolpidem, Edluar, Intermezzo, ZolpiMist (G)(IV), 36–37
aphthous stomatitis
  benzocaine, Cepacol Spray, Chloraseptic Spray (G), 37
  carbamide peroxide, Gly-Oxide (A), 37
  dexamethasone elixir, 37
  lidocaine, Xylocaine Viscous Solution, 37
  minocycline, Dynacin, Minocin, 37
  tetracycline, Achromycin V, Sumycin, 37
  triamcinolone acetonide, Oralone (G), 37
  triamcinolone, Kenalog, 37
Aplenzin, bupropion HBr (G)
  attention deficit hyperactivity disorder (ADHD), 54
  major depressive disorder, 193
  tobacco dependence, 602
Aplisol, purified protein derivative (PPD), (G)
  tuberculosis, 609
Apokyn, apomorphine hcl (G)
  Parkinson's disease, 467–468
apomorphine hcl, Apokyn (G)
  Parkinson's disease, 467–468
apomorphine sublingual film, Kynmobi
  Parkinson's disease, 468
Aponvie, omidenepag isopropyl
  nephropathy:primary, immunoglobulin A (IGAN), 415
aqueous crystalline penicillin g (G)
  syphilis, 581
apraclonidine, Iopidine (G)
  glaucoma, 255
apremilast, Otezla (G)
  psoriatic arthritis, 528
aprepitant, Emend
  cannabinoid hyperemesis syndrome, 139
  chemotherapy-induced nausea/vomiting, 148
  opioid-induced nausea/vomiting, 430
Apri, ethinyl estradiol+desogestrel
  estrogen and progesterone, 668
Aptivus, tipranavir (G)
  dose forms, 696
  human immunodeficiency virus infection, 312
Aquaphor Healing Ointment
  atopic dermatitis, 197
arachis hypogaea allergen powder-dnfp, Palforzia
  peanut (arachis hypogaea) allergy, 474–475
Arakoda, tafenoquine (G)
  malaria, 386
Aralast, alpha-1 proteinase inhibitor (human) (G)
  alpha-1 antitrypsin (AAT) deficiency, 13
Aralen, chloroquine phosphate (G)
  amebiasis, 17
  dose form/volume, 703, 704
  malaria, 386
  systemic lupus erythematosis, 584
Aranelle, ethinyl estradiol+norethindrone
  estrogen and progesterone, 668
Aranesp, darbepoetin alpha (G)

anemia of chronic kidney disease, 23
Arava, leflunomide
  rheumatoid arthritis, 546
  systemic lupus erythematosis, 583
Arcapta Neohaler, indacaterol (G)
  chronic obstructive pulmonary disease (COPD), 71
  emphysema, 230
ardeparin, Normiflo (G), 399
arformoterol, Brovana (G)
  asthma, 42
Aricept, Aricept ODT, donepezil (G)
  Alzheimer's disease, 14
Arimidex, anastrozole, 683
aripiprazole, Abilify (G)
  dose forms, 692
  bipolar disorder, 62
  major depressive disorder, 194
  methamphetamine-induced psychosis, 394
  schizophrenia, 561
aripiprazole lauroxil, Aristada (G)
  dose forms, 693
  methamphetamine-induced psychosis, 394–395
  schizophrenia, 561–562
Aristada, aripiprazole lauroxil (G)
  dose forms, 693
  methamphetamine-induced psychosis, 394–395
  schizophrenia, 561–562
Aristada Initio
  methamphetamine-induced psychosis, 394–395
armodafinil, Nuvigil (G)(IV), 464
  narcolepsy, 410
  obstructive sleep apnea, 575
  sleepiness, 576
Armour Thyroid, liothyronine+levothyroxine (A)
  hypothyroidism, 346
Arnuity Ellipta, fluticasone furoate (G)
  asthma, 41
Aromasin, exemestane, 683
Arranon, nelarabine (G)
  leukemia, 96–97
Artane, trihexyphenidyl (G)
  Parkinson's disease, 471
artesunate, Artesunate for Injection
  malaria, 385
Artesunate for Injection, artesunate
  malaria, 385
Asacol, Asacol HD, mesalamine (B)
  Crohn's disease, 175
  ulcerative colitis, 635
asenapine, Saphris, Secuado (G)
  dose forms, 693
  schizophrenia, 562–563
asfotase alfa, Strensiq
  hypophosphatasia, 345
Ashlyna, ethinyl estradiol+levonorgestrel (G), 673
Asmanex HFA, Asmanex Twisthaler, mometasone furoate (G)
  asthma, 41
asparaginase erwinia chrysanthemi (recombinant)-rywn, Rylaze
  leukemia, 96–97
Asparlas, calaspargase pegol-mknl, 683
aspergillosis
  isavuconazonium, Cresemba (G), 38
  itraconazole, Tolsura, 38
  posaconazole, Noxafil, 38
  voriconazole, Vfend, 38
aspirin, Bayer, Ecotrin
  fever (pyrexia), 242
  peripheral vascular disease, 482
  post-herpetic neuralgia, 509
Astepro, azelastine
  allergic rhinitis/sinusitis, 552

asthma
abrocitinib, Cibinqo, 45
albuterol, Albuterol Syrup, Proventil, Ventolin, VoSpire ER (G), 44
albuterol+budesonide, Airsupra, 40
albuterol sulfate, AccuNeb Inhalation Solution, Albuterol Inhalation Solution, Albuterol Nebules, Proair HFA Inhaler, Proair RespiClick, Proventil HFA Inhaler, Proventil Inhalation Solution, Ventolin (G), 39
arformoterol, Brovana (G), 42
beclomethasone dipropionate, Qvar (G), 40
benralizumab, Fasenra, 49
bevespi Aerosphere, glycopyrrolate+formoterol fumarate (G), 44
budesonide, Entocort EC, Pulmicort Flexhaler, Pulmicort Respules, Rhinocort, Rhinocort Aqua Nasal Spray, Uceris
budesonide, Pulmicort Flexhaler, Pulmicort Respules, 40
budesonide+formoterol, Symbicort (G), 43
ciclesonide, Alvesco (G), 41
cromolyn sodium, Intal, Intal Inhalation Solution, 42
dupilumab, Dupixent (G), 46, 47
dyphylline+guaifenesin, Lufyllin GG (G), 45
epinephrine inhalation aerosol, Primatene MIST Pump inhal (G), 38
flunisolide, AeroBid, AeroBid-M, Aerospan HFA (G), 41
fluticasone furoate, Arnuity Ellipta (G), 41
fluticasone furoate+vilanterol, Breo Ellipta (G), 44
fluticasone propionate, ArmorAir, Flovent, Flovent HFA, Flovent Diskus (G), 41
fluticasone propionate+salmeterol, Advair HFA, Advair Diskus, AirDuo RespiClick (G), 43–44
formoterol fumarate, Foradil Aerolizer, Perforomist (G), 43
glycopyrrolate+formoterol fumarate, Bevespi Aerosphere (G), 44
ipratropium bromide, Atrovent (G), 40
ipratropium bromide+albuterol sulfate, Combivent, Duoneb (G), 42
isoproterenol, Medihaler-ISO, 40
levalbuterol tartrate, Xopenex (G), 40
mepolizumab, Nucala (G), 48
metaproterenol, Alupent (G), 44
mometasone furoate, Asmanex HFA, Asmanex Twisthaler (G), 41
mometasone furoate+formoterol fumarate, Dulera (G), 44
montelukast, Singulair, Singulair Chewable, Singulair Oral Granules (G), 41
nedocromil sodium, Tilade, Tilade Nebulizer Solution, 42
olodaterol, Striverdi Respimat (G), 43
omalizumab, Xolair, 42, 49
pirbuterol, Maxair (G), 40
racepinephrine, Asthmanefrin (G), 39
reslizumab, Cinqair, 48
ruxolitinib, Opzelura, 45
salmeterol, Serevent Diskus (G), 43
terbutaline, 40
theophylline, Theo-24, Theo-Dur, Theolair-SR, Uniphyl (G), 45
tiotropium (as bromide monohydrate), Spiriva HandiHaler, Spiriva Respimat (G), 42
triamcinolone, Azmacort (G), 41
zafirlukast, Accolate, 41
zileuton, Zyflo, Zyflo-CR (G), 41
asthma-COPD overlap syndrome (ACOS)
fluticasone furoate+umeclidinium bromide+vilanterol trifenatate, Trelegy Ellipta, 47
omalizumab, Xolair, 47
Asthmanefrin, racepinephrine (G)
asthma, 39
Atacand, candesartan (G)
hypertension, 330
Atacand HCT, candesartan+hydrochlorothiazide
hypertension, 333
Atarax, 603
Atarax, hydroxyzine (G)
allergic reaction, 12
allergic rhinitis/sinusitis550
anxiety disorder, 33
atopic dermatitis, 199
chickenpox (Varicella), 150
contact dermatitis, 203
genus rhus dermatitis, 204
panic disorder, 465
rhinitis medicamentosa, 555
urticaria, 649
atazanavir, Reyataz (G)
human immunodeficiency virus infection, 310
Atelvia, risedronate (as sodium) (G)
osteoporosis, 442
Paget's disease, 450
atenolol, Tenormin
angina pectoris: stable, 29
dose forms, 682
headache, 275
hypertension, 326
Ativan, lorazepam (IV)
anxiety disorder, 33
delirium, 188
panic disorder, 466
status epilepticus, 579
atomoxetine, Strattera (G)
attention deficit hyperactivity disorder (ADHD), 50
atopic dermatitis
abrocitinib, Cibinqo, 200
Aveeno (OTC), 197–198
capsaicin 8% patch, Qutenza, 199
capsaicin, Axsain, Capsin, Capzasin-HP, Capzasin-P, Dolorac, Double Cap (OTC), R-Gel, Zostrix, Zostrix HP (G), 199
cetirizine, Children's Zyrtec Chewable, Children's Zyrtec Allergy Syrup, Zyrtec (G), 198
crisaborole, Eucrisa (G), 197
desloratadine, Clarinex, Desloratadine ODT (G), 198
desonide, Desonate (G), 198
diclofenac sodium, Pennsaid, Solaraze Gel, Voltaren Gel (G), 199
diphenhydramine, Benadryl, 199, 124
doxepin, Prudoxin, Zonalon, 199
dupilumab, Dupixent, 201
fexofenadine, Allegra (G), 198
fluocinolone acetonide, Derma-Smoothe/FS Topical Oil (G), 198
hydroxyzine, Atarax, Vistaril (G), 199
levocetirizine, Children's Xyzal Allergy 24HR, Xyzal Allergy 24HR, 198
lidocaine 2.5%+prilocaine 2.5%, Emla Cream, 200
lidocaine, LidaMantle, Lidoderm, ZTlido lidocaine, 200
lidocaine+dexamethasone, Decadron Phosphate with Xylocaine, 200
lidocaine+hydrocortisone, LidaMantle HC, 200
loratadine, Claritin (G), 198
moisturizing agents, 197
pimecrolimus, Elidel (G), 199
ruxolitinib, Opzelura, 200–201
trolamine salicylate, Mobisyl Creme, 200
atorvastatin, Lipitor
dyslipidemia, 222
hypertriglyceridemia, 339
atovaquone, Mepron (G)
malaria, 385
dose form/volume, 704
Pneumocystis jiroveci pneumonia, 498
systemic lupus erythematosis, 584
Atralin, tretinoin (G)
acne vulgaris, 6
facial wrinkles, 247
folliculitis barbae, 1660
Atripla, efavirenz+emtricitabine+tenofovir disoproxil fumarate
human immunodeficiency virus infection, 314, 696
AtroPen, atropine sulfate (G)
nerve agent poisoning, 415
atrophic vaginitis
estradiol, Estrace Vaginal Cream, 49
estradiol, Vagifem Vaginal Tablet, Yuvafem Vaginal Tablet, 49
estrogens, conjugated, Premarin Cream, 49
estropipate, Ogen Cream, 49
atropine sulfate, AtroPen (G)
nerve agent poisoning, 415
Atrovent, ipratropium
emphysema, 230
Atrovent, ipratropium bromide
allergic rhinitis/sinusitis, 553
asthma, 40
chronic obstructive pulmonary disease, 72
rhinitis medicamentosa, 554
vasomotor rhinitis, 554
attapulgite, Donnagel, Kaopectate (G)
chronic diarrhea, 213
diarrhea: acute, 211
attention deficit hyperactivity disorder (ADHD)
amphetamine, mixed salts of single entity amphetamine, Adzenys ER, Adzenys XR-ODT, Dyanavel XR Oral Suspension, Evekeo, Mydayis (G)(II), 50–51
atomoxetine, Strattera (G), 50
bupropion HBr, Aplenzin (G), 54
bupropion HCl, Forfivo XL, Wellbutrin (G), 54
clonidine, Catapres, Kapvay, Nexiclon XR (G), 54
dextroamphetamine, Xelstrym (II), 51
dexmethylphenidate, Focalin (G)(II), 51
dextroamphetamine saccharate+dextroamphetamine sulfate+amphetamine aspartate+amphetamine sulfate, Adderall, Adderall XR (G)(II), 52
dextroamphetamine sulfate, Dexedrine, Dextrostat (G)(II), 52
guanfacine, Intuniv, 54
lisdexamfetamine dimesylate, Vyvanse (G)(II), 52

attention deficit hyperactivity disorder
(ADHD)(*cont.*)
methylphenidate (long-acting),
Concerta, Cotempla XR-ODT,
Metadate CD, Metadate ER,
QuilliChew ER, Quillivant XR,
Ritalin (G)(II), 52–53
methylphenidate (transdermal patch),
Daytrana (G)(II), 53
methylphenidate (regular-acting),
Methylin, Ritalin (G)(II), 52
serdexmethylphenidate+
dexmethylphenidate, Azstarys,
53
viloxazine, Qelbree, 50
atypical hemolytic uremic syndrome
(aHUS)
eculizumab, Soliris (G), 284–285
Augmentin, Augmentin
ES-600, Augmentin XR,
amoxicillin+clavulanate (G)
acute bacterial sinusitis, rhinosinusitis,
571
acute exacerbation of chronic
bronchitis, 69
cat bite, 65
cellulitis, 142
community acquired pneumonia,
493
dental abscess, 190
diverticulitis, 215
dog bite, 66
dose form/volume, 707, 717–718
human bite, 66
impetigo contagiosa, 351
lymphadenitis, 382
mastitis (breast abscess), 387
otitis externa, 445
otitis media: acute, 446
streptococcal pharyngitis, 484
urinary tract infection, 643
wound, 658–659
auranofin (gold salt), Ridaura (G)
rheumatoid arthritis, 546
systemic lupus erythematosis, 583
Auryxia, *ferric citrate*
anemia of chronic kidney disease, 22
hyperphosphatemia, 324
Austedo, *deutetrabenazine*
Huntington disease-associated chorea,
318
autosomal dominant polycystic kidney
disease (ADPKD)
tolvaptan, Jynarque, Samsca, 500
Auvi-Q, *epinephrine* (G)
anaphylaxis, 21
status asthmaticus, 579
Avage, *tazarotene*
acne vulgaris, 6
facial wrinkles, 660
folliculitis barbae, 247
hyperpigmentation, 325
lentigines, 379
plaque psoriasis, 521
vitiligo, 653
Avalide, *irbesartan+hydrochlorothiazide*
hypertension, 334
avanafil, Stendra
erectile dysfunction (ED), 237
Avandamet, *rosiglitazone+metformin* (G)
type 2 diabetes mellitus, 622
Avandaryl, *rosiglitazone+glimepiride* (G)
type 2 diabetes mellitus, 622–623
avapritinib, Ayvakit
gastrointestinal stromal tumor (GIST),
91
Avapro, *irbesartan* (G)
hypertension, 330
avatrombopag, Doptelet

idiopathic thrombocytopenia
purpura, 594
Aveeno (OTC)
atopic dermatitis, 197
contact dermatitis, 202
genus rhus dermatitis, 203
Avelox, *moxifloxacin* (G)
acute bacterial sinusitis, rhinosinusitis,
572
acute exacerbation of chronic
bronchitis, 70
bacterial skin infection, 575
cellulitis, 144
community-acquired pneumonia,
494
dose forms, 708
nongonococcal urethritis, 639
plague, 489
avelumab, Bavencio
renal cell carcinoma (RCC), 95
Aviane, *ethinyl estradiol/levonorgestrel*
estrogen and progesterone, 668
Avita, *tretinoin* (G)
acne vulgaris, 6
facial wrinkles, 660
folliculitis barbae, 247
hyperpigmentation, 325
lentigines, 379
vitiligo, 653
Avodart, *dutasteride*
benign prostatic hyperplasia, 58
Avsola, *infliximab-axxq*
osteoarthritis (OA), 439
psoriasis, 526
psoriatic arthritis, 530
rheumatoid arthritis (RA), 548
ulcerative colitis (UC), 637
Avycaz, *ceftazidime+avibactam*
acute, complicated pyelonephritis,
536–537
complicated intra-abdominal
infection, 363
complicated urinary tract infection,
640
hospital-acquired bacterial
pneumonia (HABP), 489
ventilator associated bacterial
pneumonia (VABP), 490
Axid, *nizatidine*
gastroesophageal reflux, 250
peptic ulcer disease (PUD), 478
Axiron, *testosterone* (III)
testosterone deficiency, 589
Axsain, *capsaicin*
atopic dermatitis, 199
diabetic peripheral neuropathy
(DPN), 208
gouty arthritis, 261
juvenile idiopathic arthritis, 369
juvenile rheumatoid arthritis, 372
muscle strain, 404
osteoarthritis, 434
pain, 453
peripheral neuritis, 480
pruritus, 517
psoriatic arthritis, 527
rheumatoid arthritis, 541
Aygestin, *norethindrone*
amenorrhea, secondary, 18
endometriosis, 233
menopause, 392
Ayvakit, *avapritinib*
gastrointestinal stromal tumor (GIST),
91
Azasan, *azathioprine*
idiopathic pulmonary fibrosis, 534
pemphigus vulgaris, 477
rheumatoid arthritis, 546
systemic lupus erythematosis, 583

AzaSite Ophthalmic Solution,
azithromycin
bacterial conjunctivitis, 161
azathioprine, Azasan, Imuran
Crohn's disease, 176
idiopathic pulmonary fibrosis (IPF),
534
pemphigus vulgaris, 477
rheumatoid arthritis, 546
systemic lupus erythematosis, 583
Azedra, *iobenguane*
dose forms, 683
pheochromocytoma, 487
azelaic acid, Azelex, Finacea
acne rosacea, 2
acne vulgaris, 4
azelastine, Astelin, Astepro, Optivar
allergic (vernal) conjunctivitis, 167
allergic rhinitis/sinusitis, 552
rhinitis medicamentosa, 555
Azilect, *rasagiline* (G)
Parkinson's disease, 470
Azelex, *azelaic acid*
acne rosacea, 2
acne vulgaris, 4
azilsartan medoxomil, Edarbi (G)
hypertension, 330
azithromycin, AzaSite Ophthalmic
Solution
bacterial conjunctivitis, 161
azithromycin, Zithromax, Zmax (G),
713
acute exacerbation of chronic
bronchitis, 69
acute tonsillitis, 603
bacterial endocarditis prophylaxis, 55
bacterial skin infection, 573
cat scratch fever, 141
cellulitis, 142
chancroid, 146–147
Chlamydia trachomatis, 151
chlamydial conjunctivitis, 164
chlamydial pneumonia, 492
cholera (*Vibrio cholerae*), 155, 156
community acquired pneumonia, 493
dose form/volume, 708
gonococcal conjunctivitis, 165
gonococcal pharyngitis, 483
gonorrhea, 258, 259
granuloma inguinale, 266
impetigo contagiosa, 365
lymphogranuloma venereum, 384
mycoplasma pneumonia, 496
nongonococcal urethritis, 639
otitis media: acute, 446
pertussis, 483
scarlet fever, 560
sexual assault, 567
shigellosis, 567
streptococcal pharyngitis, 484
typhoid fever, 633
wound, 658
Azmacort, *triamcinolone* (G)
asthma, 411
AZO Standard, *phenazopyridine*
interstitial cystitis, 361, 362
pyelonephritis: acute, 536
urinary tract infection, 642
Azor, *amlodipine+olmesartan medoxomil*
hypertension, 336
Azstarys, *serdexmethylphenidate+*
dexmethylphenidate
attention deficit hyperactivity disorder
(ADHD), 53
aztreonam, Cayston
cystic fibrosis (CF), 184
Azulfidine, Azulfidine EN, *sulfasalazine*
Crohn's disease, 176
rheumatoid arthritis, 546

systemic lupus erythematosis, 584
ulcerative colitis, 636

bacillus anthracis immune globulin intravenous (human), Anthrasil
anthrax (bacillus anthracis), 31
bacitracin, Bacitracin Ophthalmic Ointment (G)
   bacterial conjunctivitis, 162
Bacitracin Ophthalmic Ointment, *bacitracin* (G)
   bacterial conjunctivitis, 162
baclofen, Lioresal, Fleqsuvy (G)
   muscle strain, 403
   temporomandibular joint disorder, 586
   trigeminal neuralgia, 608
   spasticity of cerebral/spinal origin, 577
bacterial conjunctivitis
   azithromycin, AzaSite Ophthalmic Solution, 161–162
   bacitracin, Bacitracin Ophthalmic Ointment (G), 12
   besifloxacin, Besivance Ophthalmic Solution (G), 162
   ciprofloxacin, Ciloxan Ophthalmic Ointment (G), 162
   erythromycin, Ilotycin Ophthalmic Ointment, 162
   gatifloxacin, Zymar Ophthalmic Solution, Zymaxid Ophthalmic Solution (G), 162
   gentamicin sulfate, Garamycin Ophthalmic Ointment, Genoptic Ophthalmic Ointment, Gentacidin Ophthalmic Ointment (G), 9162
   gentamicin sulfate+prednisolone acetate, Pred-G Ophthalmic Suspension, Pred-G Ophthalmic Ointment (G), 163
   levofloxacin, Quixin Ophthalmic Solution (G), 162
   moxifloxacin, Moxeza Ophthalmic Solution, Vigamox Ophthalmic Solution (G), 162
   neomycin sulfate+polymyxin b sulfate+dexamethasone, Maxitrol Ophthalmic Suspension, Maxitrol Ophthalmic Ointment (G), 163
   neomycin sulfate+polymyxin b sulfate+prednisolone acetate ophthalmic suspension, Poly-Pred Ophthalmic Suspension (G), 163
   ofloxacin, Ocuflox Ophthalmic Solution (G), 162
   polymyxin b sulfate+bacitracin, Polysporin Ophthalmic Ointment (G), 163
   polymyxin b sulfate+bacitracin zinc+ neomycin sulfate, Neosporin Ophthalmic Ointment (G), 163
   polymyxin b sulfate+gramicidin+neomycin, Neosporin Ophthalmic Solution (G), 163
   polymyxin b sulfate+neomycin sulfate+bacitracin zinc+hydrocortisone, Cortisporin Ophthalmic Ointment (G), 162
   polymyxin b sulfate+neomycin sulfate+hydrocortisone, Cortisporin Ophthalmic Suspension (G), 163
   sulfacetamide, Bleph-10, Cetamide Ophthalmic Solution, Isopto Cetamide Ophthalmic Ointment (G), 164

sulfacetamide sodium+fluorometholone suspension, FML-S (G), 164
sulfacetamide sodium+prednisolone acetate, Blephamide Liquifilm, Blephamide S.O.P. Ophthalmic Ointment (G), 164
sulfacetamide sodium+prednisolone sodium phosphate, Vasocidin Ophthalmic Solution (G), 164
tobramycin, Tobrex Ophthalmic Solution, Tobrex Ophthalmic Ointment, 164
tobramycin+dexamethasone, TobraDex, TobraDex ST (G), 164
tobramycin+loteprednol etabonate, Zylet (G), 164
trimethoprim+polymyxin b sulfate, Polytrim (G), 163
bacterial endocarditis prophylaxis
   amoxicillin, Amoxil, Trimox, 55
   ampicillin, Omnipen, Principen, Unasyn, 55
   azithromycin, Zithromax, 55
   cefazolin, Ancef, Kefzol, 55
   ceftriaxone, Rocephin, 55
   clarithromycin, Biaxin, 55
   clarithromycin, Biaxin, Biaxin Oral Suspension, Biaxin XL (G), 55
   clindamycin, Cleocin, Cleocin Pediatric Granules, 55
   erythromycin estolate, Ilosone, 55
   penicillin v potassium, Pen-Vee K, 56
bacterial skin infection
   amoxicillin, Amoxil, Moxatag, Trimox, 573
   azithromycin, Zithromax (G), 573
   cefaclor, Cefaclor Extended Release, 573
   cefadroxil, Duricef, 573
   cefdinir, Omnicef, 574
   cefditoren pivoxil, Spectracef, 574
   cefpodoxime proxetil, Vantin, 574
   cefprozil, Cefzil, 574
   ceftriaxone, Rocephin, 574
   cephalexin, Keflex, 574
   clarithromycin, Biaxin, 574
   dicloxacillin, Dynapen, 574
   doxycycline, Acticlate, Adoxa, Doryx, Doxteric, Monodox, Oracea, Vibramycin, Vibra-Tab, 574
   erythromycin base, Ery-Tab, PCE, 574
   erythromycin estolate, Ilosone, 574
   erythromycin ethylsuccinate, EryPed, E.E.S, 574
   gemifloxacin, Factive (G), 575
   hexachlorophene, pHisoHex (G), 573
   levofloxacin, Levaquin (G), 575
   linezolid, Zyvox (G), 575
   loracarbef, Lorabid, 575
   minocycline, Dynacin, Minocin, 575
   moxifloxacin, Avelox (G), 575
   mupirocin, Bactroban, Centany, 573
   Neosporin, *polymyxin b+neomycin* (G), 573
   ofloxacin, Floxin (G), 575
   tetracycline, Achromycin V, Sumycin, 575
bacterial vaginosis
   clindamycin, Cleocin (G), Cleocin Pediatric Granules, Cleocin Vaginal Cream, Cleocin Vaginal Ovules, 57
   clindamycin phosphate, Xaciato, 57
   metronidazole, Flagyl, MetroGel-Vaginal, Vandazole, 46
   secnidazole, Solosec, 57
   tinidazole, Tindamax (G), 57
Bactrim, *trimethoprim+sulfamethoxazole (TMP-SMX)*, 722

acute bacterial sinusitis, rhinosinusitis, 572
acute exacerbation of chronic bronchitis, 71
cat scratch fever, 141
chronic prostatitis, 517
community acquired pneumonia, 495
cyclosporiasis, 182
diverticulitis, 216
dose forms, 709
granuloma inguinale, 266
human bite, 67
legionella pneumonia, 496
otitis externa, 445
otitis media: acute, 447
pertussis, 483
Pneumocystis jiroveci pneumonia, 498
pyelonephritis: acute, 516
salmonellosis, 559
shigellosis, 567
Traveler's diarrhea, 214
typhoid fever, 633
urinary tract infection (UTI), 645
Bactroban, *mupirocin*
   bacterial skin infection, 573
   impetigo contagiosa, 351
   wound, 658
Bafiertam, *monomethyl fumarate*
   multiple sclerosis (MS), 401–402
Balcoltra, *ethinyl estradiol+levonorgestrel plus ferrous bisglycinate 36.5 mg*
   estrogen and progesterone, 668
Baldness: male pattern
   finasteride, Propecia, 57
   minoxidil, Rogaine, 57
Balmex, *aloe+vitamin e+zinc oxide*
   diaper rash, 210
baloxavir marboxil, Xofluza
   influenza, seasonal (FLU), 358
balsalazide disodium, Colazal, Giazo
   ulcerative colitis, 635
Balversa, *erdafitinib*
   urothelial carcinoma, 133–134
Balziva, *ethinyl estradiol+norethindrone*
   estrogen and progesterone, 668
Baqsimi, *glucagon nasal powder*
   type 1 diabetes mellitus (T1DM), 613
Baraclude, *entecavir* (G)
   hepatitis B, 293
baricitinib, Olumiant
   alopecia areata, 12
   COVID-19 (coronavirus), 174
   rheumatoid arthritis, 544
basiliximab, Simulect
   organ transplant rejection prophylaxis, 432
   sickle cell disease, 569
Bavencio, *avelumab*
   dose form, 683
   renal cell carcinoma, 95
Baxdela, *delafloxacin*
   cellulitis, 143–144
Bayer, *aspirin*
   fever (pyrexia), 242
BayRab, *rabies immune globulin, human (HRIG)* (G)
   rabies, 538
BayTET, *tetanus immune globulin, human* (G), 592
becaplermin, Regranex (G)
   diabetic ulcer, 633
   pressure ulcer, 634
beclomethasone dipropionate, Beconase, Qvar, Vancenase, QNASL Nasal Aerosol (G), 580
   allergic rhinitis/sinusitis, 551
   asthma, 40
   polyps, nasal (G), 505

Beconase, *beclomethasone dipropionate* (G)
    allergic rhinitis/sinusitis, 551
bedaquiline, Sirturo
    tuberculosis, 610, 612
belantamab mafodotin-blmf, Blenrep
    multiple myeloma, 121
belimumab, Benlysta
    pemphigus vulgaris, 477
    systemic lupus erythematosis, 582
Bell's palsy
    prednisone, Deltasone (G), 57
Belsomra, *suvorexant* (G)(IV)
    insomnia, 359
    non-24 sleep-wake disorder, 418
bempedoic acid, Nexletol
    dyslipidemia, 221–222
Benadryl, *diphenhydramine*
    allergic reaction, 12
    allergic rhinitis/sinusitis, 550
    anxiety disorder, 32
    atopic dermatitis, 199
    chickenpox (Varicella), 150
    contact dermatitis, 202, 203
    genus rhus dermatitis, 204
    Meniere's disease, 388
    rhinitis medicamentosa, 555
    urticaria, 649
benazepril (G)
    hypertension, 329
Benemid, *probenecid*
    gonorrhea, 259
    pelvic inflammatory disease, 476
    syphilis, 582
Benicar HCT, *olmesartan medoxomil+hydrochlorothiazide*
    hypertension, 334
benign essential tremor
    amantadine, Symmetrel (G), 58
    propranolol, Inderal, Inderal LA, InnoPran XL (G), 58
benign prostatic hyperplasia (BPH)
    alfuzosin, UroXatral, 58
    doxazosin, Cardura, Cardura XL (G), 58
    dutasteride, Avodart, 58
    dutasteride+tamsulosin, Jalyn, 58
    finasteride, Proscar, 58
    finasteride+tadalafil, Entadfi, 59
    silodosin, Rapaflo, 58
    tadalafil, Cialis, 59
    tamsulosin, Flomax, 58
    terazosin, Hytrin (G), 58
Benlysta, *belimumab*
    pemphigus vulgaris, 477
    systemic lupus erythematosis, 582
Benoquin, *monobenzone* (G)
    hyperpigmentation, 325
    vitiligo, 653
benralizumab, Fasenra
    asthma, 49
    eosinophilia, 49
bentoquatam, IvyBlock (OTC)
    contact dermatitis, 201
    genus rhus dermatitis, 203
Bentyl, *dicyclomine*
    abdominal cramps, 174
    irritable bowel syndrome with diarrhea, 367
    urinary overactive bladder, 354
BenzaClin, *clindamycin+benzoyl peroxide*
    acne vulgaris, 4
Benzac-W, Benzac-W Wash, *benzoyl peroxide* (G)
    acne vulgaris, 4
    folliculitis barbae, 246
Benzagel, Benzagel Wash, *benzoyl peroxide* (G)
    acne vulgaris, 4

Benzamycin Topical Gel, *erythromycin+ benzoyl peroxide* (G)
    acne vulgaris, 4
benznidazole (G)
    Chagas disease, 146
benzocaine, Americaine Otic, Benzotic, Cepacol Spray, Chloraseptic Spray (G)
    aphthous stomatitis, 37
    otitis externa, 445
    otitis media: acute, 448
Benzotic, *benzocaine* (G)
    otitis externa, 445
    otitis media: acute, 448
benzoyl peroxide, Benzac-W, Benzac-W Wash, Benzagel, Benzagel Wash, Desquam X, Triaz, ZoDerm (G)
    acne vulgaris, 4
    folliculitis barbae, 246
benzphetamine, Didrex (III)
    obesity, 418
benztropine mesylate, Cogentin (G)
    Parkinson's disease, 471
bepotastine besilate, Bepreve
    allergic (vernal) conjunctivitis, 167
Bepreve, *bepotastine besilate*
    allergic (vernal) conjunctivitis, 167
Berinert, *C1 esterase inhibitor (human)*
    hereditary angioedema, 298
besifloxacin, Besivance Ophthalmic Solution (G)
    bacterial conjunctivitis, 162
Besivance Ophthalmic Solution, *besifloxacin* (G)
    bacterial conjunctivitis, 162
Besponsa, *inotuzumab ozogamicin*, 684
Besremi, *ropeginterferon-alfa-2b-njft*
    polycythemia vera, 500–501
betamethasone, Celestone (G), 678, 679
betamethasone valerate, Luxiq, Diprolene (G)
    seborrheic dermatitis, 205
    strength and volume, 676
Betapace, *sotalol*, 681
beta thalassemia
    betibeglogene autotemcel, Zynteglo, 59–60
betaxolol, Betoptic, Betoptic S, Kerlone (G)
    glaucoma, 256
    hypertension, 326
bethanechol, Urecholine (G)
    unobstructive urinary retention, 639
    urinary overactive bladder, 355
Betoptic, Betoptic S, *betaxolol*
    glaucoma, 256
betibeglogene autotemcel, Zynteglo
    beta thalassemia, 59–60
bevacizumab-adcd, Vegzelma
    cervical cancer, 86
    colorectal cancer, 87
    fallopian tube cancer, 90
    glioblastoma multiforme, 92–93
    lung cancer, 102
    ovarian cancer, 122
    peritoneal cancer, 127
    renal cell carcinoma (RCC), 94
bevacizumab-bvzr, Zirabev
    colorectal cancer, 87
    glioblastoma multiforme, 93
    lung cancer, 103
Bevespi Aerosphere, *glycopyrrolate+ formoterol fumarate* (G)
    asthma, 44
Bevyxxa, *betrixiban*, 684
bexaglifl, Brenzavvy
    type 2 diabetes mellitus (T2DM), 626–627
bexarotene, Targretin
    lymphoma, 114–115

Bexsero, *Meningococcal group b vaccine [recombinant, absorbed]*
    meningitis, 388
Beyaz, *ethinyl estradiol+drospirenone plus levomefolate calcium*
    estrogen and progesterone, 668
    premenstrual dysphoric disorder, 514
bezlotoxumab, Zinplava (G)
    Clostridioides difficile infection, 167
Biaxin, Biaxin Oral Suspension, Biaxin XL, *clarithromycin* (G), 708, 716
    acute exacerbation of chronic bronchitis, 70
    acute tonsillitis, 604
    bacterial endocarditis prophylaxis, 55
    cellulitis, 143
    community acquired pneumonia, 494
    Hansen's disease, 270
    impetigo contagiosa, 352
    legionella pneumonia, 496
    Lyme disease, 383
    mycoplasma pneumonia, 496
    otitis media: acute, 447
    pertussis, 483
    scarlet fever, 560
    streptococcal pharyngitis, 485
    wound, 659
Bicillin L-A, Bicillin C-R, *penicillin g (benzathine)*
    impetigo contagiosa, 353
    scarlet fever, 560
    streptococcal pharyngitis, 485
    syphilis, 581
Bidil, *isosorbide+hydralazine HCl* (G)
    angina pectoris: stable, 30
    heart failure, 282
Bijuva, estradiol+progesterone
    menopause, 392
Biktarvy, *bictegravir+emtricitabine+ tenofovir alafenamide*, 594
    human immunodeficiency virus infection, 314
bile acid deficiency
    ursodiol, Actigall, 60
Biltricide, *praziquantel*
    liver flukes, 380
    schistosomiasis, 560
    tapeworm, 585
    threadworm, 593
bimatoprost, Latisse, Lumigan (G)
    glaucoma, 256
    hypotrichosis, 347
binge eating disorder
    lisdexamfetamine dimesylate, Vyvanse (G)(II), 60
Binosto, *alendronate (as sodium)* (G)
    Osteoporosis, 441
    Paget's disease, 450
bioengineered replica of human parathyroid hormone, Natpara (G)
    hypocalcemia, 341
    hypoparathyroidism, 345
    osteoporosis, 443
Bion Tears, *dextran 70+hypromellose*
    dry eye syndrome, 217
biperiden hydrochloride, Akineton (G)
    Parkinson's disease, 471
bipolar disorder
    aripiprazole, Abilify, Abilify Discmelt, Abilify Maintena (G), 62
    asenapine, Saphris (G), 52
    carbamazepine, Carbatrol, Carnexiv, Equetro, Tegretol, Tegretol XR (G), 61
    cariprazine, Vraylar (G), 62
    divalproex sodium, Depakene, Depakote (G), 61
    lamotrigine, Lamictal (G), 61
    lithium carbonate, Lithobid (G), 61

lumateperone, *Caplyta*, 63
lurasidone, *Latuda* (G), 63
olanzapine+fluoxetine, *Symbyax* (G), 65
quetiapine fumarate, *SeroQUEL, SeroQUEL XR* (G), 63
risperidone, *Risperdal, Risperdal Consta, Risperdal M-Tab, Rykindo*, 63
ziprasidone, *Geodon* (G), 64–65
bisacodyl, Dulcolax, Gentlax, Senokot
encopresis, 232
occasional constipation, 170
bismuth subgallate powder, Devron
fecal odor, 241
bismuth subsalicylate, Pepto-Bismol (G)
acute diarrhea, 211
bisoprolol, Zebeta (G)
hypertension, 326
bleomycin sulfate (G), 684
Blenrep, belantamab mafodotin-blmf
multiple myeloma, 121
Bleph-10, sulfacetamide (G)
bacterial conjunctivitis, 162
blepharitis, 67
stye (hordeolum), 580
Blephamide Liquifilm, Blephamide S.O.P. Ophthalmic Ointment, *sulfacetamide sodium+prednisolone acetate* (G)
bacterial conjunctivitis, 164
blepharitis
erythromycin, Ilotycin, 67
polymyxin b+bacitracin, Polysporin (G), 67
polymyxin b+bacitracin+neomycin, Neosporin (G), 67
sodium sulfacetamide, Bleph-10 (G), 67
tetracycline, Achromycin V, Sumycin, 67
blepharoptosis, acquired (droopy eyelid)
oxymetazoline hydrochloride ophthalmic solution, 0.1%, Upneeq, 67–68
Blincyto, blinatumomab, 584
Blisovi 24Fe, ethinyl estradiol+norethindrone plus ferrous fumarate
estrogen and progesterone, 668
Blocadren, timolol (G)
hypertension, 327
blood pressure guidelines, 684
Bonine (OTC), *meclizine*
labyrinthitis, 375
Meniere's disease, 388
motion sickness, 396
vertigo, 653
Boniva, ibandronate (as monosodium monohydrate) (G)
osteoporosis, 441
Paget's disease, 450
Bonjesta, doxylamine
hyperemesis gravidarum, 320
bosentan, Tracleer (G)
pulmonary arterial hypertension (PAH), 532
Bosulif, bosutinib, 684
bowel resection with primary anastomosis
alvimopan, Entereg, 68
Braftovi, encorafenib, 684
breast cancer
abemaciclib, Verzenio, 78–79
alpelisib, Piqray, 79
elacestrant, Orserdu, 85
fam-trastuzumab deruxtecan-nxki, Enhertu, 83
fulvestrant, Faslodex, 78
lapatinib ditosylate, Tykerb, 79–80
letrozole, Femara, 78

margetuximab-cmkb, Margenza, 81–82
Olaparib, Lynparza, 81
pembrolizumab, Keytruda, 78
sacituzumab govitecan-hziy, Trodelvy, 84
sodium neratinib, Nerlynx, 80
talazoparib, Talzenna, 81
tamoxifen citrate, 84
toremifene, Fareston, 85
trastuzumab, Herceptin for Injection, 82
trastuzumab-anns, Kanjinti, 82
trastuzumab-dkst, Ogivri for Injection, 82
trastuzumab-dttb, Ontruzant for Injection, 82
trastuzumab+hyaluronidase, Herceptin Hylecta, 93
trastuzumab-pkrb, Herzuma, 83
trastuzumab-qyyp, Trazimera, 83
tucatinib, Tukysa, 80
bremelanotide, Vyleesi
low libido, hypoactive sexual desire disorder (HSDD), 381
brentuximab vedotin, Adcetris
lymphoma, 114
Brenzavvy, bexaglifl
type 2 diabetes mellitus (T2DM), 626–627
Breo Ellipta, *fluticasone furoate+vilanterol* (G)
asthma, 44
chronic obstructive pulmonary disease (COPD), 73
emphysema, 230
Brevicon-21, Brevicon-28, *ethinyl estradiol+norethindrone*
estrogen and progesterone, 668
brexpiprazole, Rexulti (G), 693
Alzheimer's disease, 15–16
major depressive disorder, 195
schizophrenia, 563
Brexafemme, ibrexafungerp
vulvovaginal (moniliasis) candidiasis, 136–137
brexpiprazole, Rexulti
Alzheimer's disease, 15–17
brigatinib, Alunbrig
lung cancer, 103
brimonidine, Mirvaso
acne rosacea, 2
brimonidine tartrate, Alphagan P
glaucoma, 255
brinzolamide, Azopt (G)
glaucoma, 255
Brisdelle, paroxetine mesylate
anxiety disorder, 35
major depressive disorder, 192
obsessive-compulsive disorder, 422
panic disorder, 465
post-traumatic stress disorder, 510
premenstrual dysphoric disorder, 515
trichotillomania, 608
Briumvi, ublituximab-xiiy
multiple sclerosis (MS), 400
Brixadi, *buprenorphine extended-release for subcutaneous injection*
opioid dependence, 424–425
brodalumab, Siliq
psoriasis, 522
Bromday Ophthalmic Solution, *bromfenac* (G)
allergic (vernal) conjunctivitis, 167
bromfenac, Bromday Ophthalmic Solution, Xibrom Ophthalmic Solution (G)
allergic (vernal) conjunctivitis, 167
bromocriptine mesylate, Cycloset
type 2 diabetes mellitus, 632
bromocriptine, Parlodel

Parkinson's disease, 469
bronchiolitis. *See* asthma
bronchitis
acute (*see* acute exacerbation of chronic bronchitis)
chronic (*see* chronic obstructive pulmonary disease)
Brovana, arformoterol (G)
asthma, 42
Brukinsa, *zanubrutinib*
Waldenström's macroglobulinemia, 654
budesonide micronized, Entocort EC (G)
Crohn's disease, 176
ulcerative colitis, 634
budesonide, Pulmicort Flexhaler, Pulmicort Respules, Rhincort, Tarpeyo, 580
allergic rhinitis/sinusitis, 552
asthma, 40
immunoglobulin A nephropathy, 414
nephropathy:primary, immunoglobulin A (IGAN), 414
polyps, nasal, 505
budesonide rectal foam, Uceris (G)
ulcerative colitis (UC), 634
Bufferin, *aspirin+antacid*
fever (pyrexia), 242
bulimia nervosa
fluoxetine, Prozac, Prozac Weekly (G), 75
bumetanide, Bumex (G)
edema, 228
heart failure, 281
hypertension, primary, 327–328
Bumex, *bumetanide* (G)
edema, 228
heart failure, 281
hypertension, primary, 327–328
Bunavail, Suboxone, Sucartonone, Zubsolv, *buprenorphine+naloxone* (G)(III)
opioid dependence, 427
Buprenex, *buprenorphine hcl*
opioid dependence, 426
pain, 462
buprenorphine, Belbuca, Butrans Transdermal System, Probuphine, Subutex, Sublocade (G)(III)
opioid dependence, 426
pain, 461
buprenorphine extended-release for subcutaneous injection, Brixadi
opioid dependence, 424–425
bupropion HBr, Aplenzin (G)
attention deficit hyperactivity disorder (ADHD), 54
major depressive disorder, 193
tobacco dependence, 602
bupropion HCl, Buprenex, Forfivo XL, Wellbutrin (G)
attention deficit hyperactivity disorder (ADHD), 54
dose forms, 693
major depressive disorder, 193
opioid dependence, 426
pain, 462
tobacco dependence, 602
burn, major
anacaulase-bcdb, NexoBrid, 75
burn, minor
lidocaine 2.5%+prilocaine 2.5%, Emla Cream, 76
lidocaine, LidaMantle, Lidoderm, ZTlido lidocaine, 76
lidocaine+dexamethasone, Decadron Phosphate with Xylocaine, 76
lidocaine+hydrocortisone, LidaMantle HC, 76

burosumab-twza, Crysvita (G)
  X-linked hypophosphatemia, 345
bursitis, 76
BuSpar, *buspirone*
  anxiety disorder, 33
  panic disorder, 465
buspirone, BuSpar
  anxiety disorder, 33
  panic disorder, 465
butenafine, Lotrimin Ultra, Mentax
  diaper rash, 211
  skin candidiasis, 135
  tinea corporis, 597
  tinea cruris, 598
  tinea pedis, 599
  tinea versicolor, 601
butoconazole cream 2%, Gynazole-12%
  Vaginal Cream, Femstat-3
  Vaginal Cream (OTC) (G)
  vulvovaginal (moniliasis) candidiasis,
  138
Butorphanol Nasal Spray, *butorphanol
  tartrate* (G)(IV)
  pain, 462
  tension headache, 277
  ulcerative colitis, 462
  urolithiasis, 648
butorphanol tartrate, Butorphanol Nasal
  Spray, Stadol Nasal Spray (G)(IV)
  pain, 462
  tension headache, 277
  ulcerative colitis, 462
  urolithiasis, 648
Bylvay, odevixibat
  cholestasis, 154
Bynfezia Pen, *octreotide acetate*
  acromegaly, 8
Byvalson, *nebivolol+valsartan*
  hypertension, 335
Bystolic, *nebivolol* (G)
  hypertension, 326

C1 esterase inhibitor deficiency See
  Hereditary angioedema
C1 esterase inhibitor (human), Berinert,
  Haegarda
  hereditary angioedema, 297, 298
C1 esterase inhibitor [recombinant],
  Ruconest
  hereditary angioedema, 298
cabazitaxel, Jevtana (G)
  prostate cancer, 130
Cabergoline, dostinex
  hyperprolactinemia, 326
cabenuva, cabotegravir and rilpivirine
  human immunodeficiency virus
  (HIV) infection, 314
Cabenuva, cabotegravir+rilpivirine
  human immunodeficiency virus
  (HIV) infection, 314, 317
Cablivi, *caplacizumab-yhdp*
  acquired autoimmune thrombotic
  thrombocytopenia purpura,
  594–595
Cabometyx, *cabozantinib,* 684
cabotegravir, Vocabria
  human immunodeficiency virus
  (HIV) infection, 308
Caduet, *amlodipine+atorvastatin*
  dyslipidemia, 224–225
  hypertension, 337
Calan, Calan SR, *verapamil* (G)
  angina pectoris: stable, 29
  dose form(s), 681
  headache, migraine, 276
  hypertension, primary, 331
calcifediol, Rayaldee (G)
  hyperparathyroidism (HPT), 323
calcipotriene, Dovonex (G)

psoriasis, 519
calcitonin-salmon, Fortical, Miacalcin (G)
  hypocalcemia, 340
  osteoporosis, 440
calcitriol, Rocaltrol, Vectical (G)
  hypocalcemia, 340
  hypoparathyroidism, 344
  osteoporosis, 441
  psoriasis, 520
calcium acetate, PhosLo (G)
  hyperphosphatemia, 325
calcium carbonate, Rolaids, Tums,
  Os-Cal 500 (G)
  gastroesophageal reflux disease, 249
  hypocalcemia, 340
  osteoporosis, 340
calcium citrate, Citracal (G)
  hypocalcemia, 340
  osteoporosis, 441
Calcium Disodium Versenate, *edetate
  calcium disodium (EDTA)*
  lead poisoning, 376
*calcium, magnesium, potassium, and
  sodium oxybate oral solution
  (CIII),* Xywav
  narcolepsy, 413
calcium polycarbophil, FiberCon, Konsyl
  Fiber Tablets (G)
  acute diarrhea, 211
  occasional constipation, 169
Caldolor, *ibuprofen*
  pain, 451
  urolithiasis, 647
callused skin
  salicylic acid (G), 572
  urea, Carmol 40, Keratol 40 (G), 473
Calquence, *acalabrutinib,* 684
Camcevi, *leuprolide mesylate*
  prostate cancer, 128
Campral, *acamprosate* (G)
  alcohol withdrawal syndrome, 11
Camrese, *ethinyl estradiol+levonorgestrel*
  estrogen and progesterone, 668
Camrese Lo, *ethinyl
  estradiol+levonorgestrel*
  estrogen and progesterone, 668
canagliflozin, Invokana (G)
  type 2 diabetes mellitus, 627
Canasa, *mesalamine*
  Crohn's disease, 175
  ulcerative colitis, 635
cancer
  cervical, 86
  colorectal, 86–87
  endometrial, 87–88
  epithelioid sarcoma, 88
  fallopian tube, 88–90
  gastric/gastroesophageal/esophageal,
  90–91
  gastrointestinal stromal tumor (GIST),
  91–92
  glioblastoma multiforme, 92–93
  hepatocellular carcinoma (HCC),
  99–101
  leukemia, 96–99
  lung, 102–108
  lymphoma, 108–115
  melanoma, 116–119
  merkel cell carcinoma, 119–120
  multiple myeloma, 120–122
  ovarian, 122–124
  pancreatic, 124–125
  peritoneal, 125–127
  prostate, 127–130
  renal cell carcinoma (RCC), 93–96
  solid tumor, 132–133
  squamous cell carcinoma (SCC),
  130–131
  thyroid carcinoma, 131–132

  urothelial, 133–134
candesartan, Atacand (G)
  hypertension, 330
candidiasis
  abdomen, bladder, esophagus, kidney,
  134
  oral (*see* oral (thrush) candidiasis)
  skin (*see* skin candidiasis)
  vulvovaginal (*see* vulvovaginal
  (moniliasis) candidiasis)
canker sore. *See* aphthous stomatitis
cannabinoid hyperemesis syndrome
  (CHS)
  aprepitant, Emend, 139
  chlorpromazine, Thorazine (G), 139
  dolasetron, Anzemet, 139
  granisetron, Kytril, Sancuso, Sustol,
  139
  granisetron extended-release injection,
  Sustol, 139
  ondansetron, Zofran, Zuplenz Oral
  Soluble Film (G), 140
  palonosetron, Aloxi, 140
  perphenazine, Trilafon (G), 139
  prochlorperazine, Compazine (G),
  139
  promethazine, Phenergan (G), 139
cannabidiol, Epidiolex
  Lennox-Gastaut syndrome (LGS),
  377
Cantil, *mepenzolate*
  peptic ulcer disease (PUD), 480
Capastat, *capreomycin sulfate* (G)
  tuberculosis, 611
Capitrol Shampoo, *chloroxine* (G)
  seborrheic dermatitis, 204
caplacizumab-yhdp, Cablivi
  acquired autoimmune thrombotic
  thrombocytopenia purpura,
  594–595
Caplyta, *lumateperone*
  bipolar disorder, 63
  schizophrenia, 563
capmatinib, Tabrecta
  lung cancer, 103
  mesothelioma, 393
Capoten, *captopril* (G)
  heart failure, 279
  hypertension, 329
Capozide, *captopril+hydrochlorothiazide*
  hypertension, 333
capreomycin sulfate, Capastat (G)
  tuberculosis, 611
capsaicin 8% patch, Qutenza
  atopic dermatitis, 199
  diabetic peripheral neuropathy, 208
  gouty arthritis, 262
  hemorrhoids, 289
  juvenile idiopathic arthritis, 369
  juvenile rheumatoid arthritis, 372
  muscle strain, 404
  osteoarthritis, 434
  pain, 453
  peripheral neuritis, 480
  post-herpetic neuralgia, 508
  pruritus, 517
  psoriatic arthritis, 527
  rheumatoid arthritis, 542
capsaicin, Axsain, Capsin, Capzasin-HP,
  Capzasin-P, Dolorac, Double
  Cap (OTC), R-Gel, Zostrix,
  Zostrix HP
  atopic dermatitis, 199
  diabetic peripheral neuropathy
  (DPN), 208
  gouty arthritis, 261–262
  juvenile idiopathic arthritis, 369
  juvenile rheumatoid arthritis, 372
  muscle strain, 404

osteoarthritis, 434
pain, 453
peripheral neuritis, 480
pruritus, 517
psoriatic arthritis, 527
rheumatoid arthritis, 541
Capsin, *capsaicin*
atopic dermatitis, 199
diabetic peripheral neuropathy
(DPN), 208
gouty arthritis, 261–262
juvenile idiopathic arthritis, 369
juvenile rheumatoid arthritis, 372
muscle strain, 404
osteoarthritis, 434
pain, 453
peripheral neuritis, 480
pruritus, 517
psoriatic arthritis, 527
rheumatoid arthritis, 541
captopril, Capoten (G)
heart failure, 279
hypertension, 329
Capzasin-HP, Capzasin-P, *capsaicin*
atopic dermatitis, 199
diabetic peripheral neuropathy
(DPN), 208
gouty arthritis, 261–262
juvenile idiopathic arthritis, 369
juvenile rheumatoid arthritis, 372
muscle strain, 404
osteoarthritis, 434
pain, 453
peripheral neuritis, 480
pruritus, 517
psoriatic arthritis, 527
rheumatoid arthritis, 541
Carac, *fluorouracil*
actinic keratosis, 9
Carafate, *sucralfate*
eophagitis, erosive, 238
peptic ulcer disease (PUD), 480
carbamazepine, Carbatrol, Carnexiv,
Equetro, Tegretol, Tegretol XR
bipolar disorder, 61
dose forms, 694
trigeminal neuralgia, 608–609
carbamide peroxide, Gly-Oxide (A)
aphthous stomatitis, 37
cerumen impaction, 145
denture irritation, 191
Carbatrol, *carbamazepine* (G)
bipolar disorder, 61
dose forms, 694
carbenicillin, Geocillin
chronic prostatitis, 516
dose forms, 707
urinary tract infection, 643
carbidopa, Lodosyn (G)
Parkinson's disease, 466
carcinoid syndrome diarrhea (CSD)
telotristat, Xermelo, 75, 140
Cardene, *nicardipine* (G)
angina pectoris: stable, 28
hypertension, primary, 331
cardiomyopathy of transthyretin-
mediated amyloidosis
tafamidis, Vyndamax, 140
tafamidis meglumine, Vyndaqel, 140
Cardizem, *diltiazem* (G)
angina pectoris: stable, 28
headache, migraine, 275–276
hypertension, primary, 330
Cardura, Cardura XL, *doxazosin* (G)
benign prostatic hyperplasia, 58
hypertension: primary, 332
urinary overactive bladder, 356
carfilzomib, Kyprolis
multiple myeloma, 120

cariprazine, Vraylar (NE)
bipolar disorder, 62
dose forms, 693
major depressive disorder, 195
carisoprodol, Soma (G)
muscle strain, 403
temporomandibular joint disorder,
586
Carmol 40, *urea* (G)
callused skin, 573
Carnexiv, *carbamazepine* (G)
bipolar disorder, 61
dose forms, 694
CaroSpir, *spironolactone*
edema, 228
fibrocystic breast disease, 243
heart failure, 281
hypertension, primary, 327
carpal tunnel syndrome (CTS), 140–141
carteolol, Cartrol, Ocupress (G)
glaucoma, 256
hypertension, 326
Cartrol, *carteolol*
hypertension, 326
Cartia XT, *diltiazem* (G)
angina pectoris: stable, 28
hypertension, primary, 330
carvedilol, Coreg, Coreg CR (G)
heart failure, 280
hypertension, 327
Casodex, *bicalutamide*, 684
casimersen, Amondys
duchenne muscular dystrophy
(DMD), 218–219
cat bite
amoxicillin+clavulanate, Augmentin,
Augmentin ES-600, Augmentin
XR, 65
doxycycline, Acticlate, Adoxa, Doryx,
Doxteric, Monodox, Oracea,
Vibramycin, Vibra-Tab, 65
penicillin v potassium, Pen-Vee K, 65
tetanus toxoid vaccine (G), 65
cat scratch fever
azithromycin, Zithromax, Zmax, 141
doxycycline, Acticlate, Adoxa, Doryx,
Doxteric, Monodox, Oracea,
Vibramycin, Vibra-Tab, 141
erythromycin base, Ery-Tab, PCE,
141
erythromycin ethylsuccinate, EryPed,
E.E.S, 141
*trimethoprim/sulfamethoxazole (TMP-
SMX)*, Bactrim, Septra, 141
cataplexy, 409–413. *See also* narcolepsy
Catapres, Catapres-TTS, *clonidine* (G)
attention deficit hyperactivity disorder
(ADHD), 54
hypertension: primary, 322
post-traumatic stress disorder, 511
Caverject, *alprostadil*
erectile dysfunction (ED), 237
Cayston, *aztreonam*
cystic fibrosis (CF), 184
Cedax, *ceftibuten*, 706, 715, 716
acute bacterial sinusitis, rhinosinusitis,
571
acute exacerbation of chronic
bronchitis, 70
acute tonsillitis, 604
otitis media: acute, 446
streptococcal pharyngitis, 485
cefaclor, Cefaclor Extended Release (G),
703, 706
acute bacterial sinusitis, rhinosinusitis,
571
acute exacerbation of chronic
bronchitis, 69
acute tonsillitis, 603–604

bacterial skin infection, 573
cellulitis, 142
community acquired pneumonia, 493
dose form/volume, 706
impetigo contagiosa, 352
mastitis (breast abscess), 387
otitis externa, 445
otitis media: acute, 446
streptococcal pharyngitis, 484
urinary tract infection, 643
wound, 659
Cefaclor Extended Release, *cefaclor* (G)
acute bacterial sinusitis, rhinosinusitis,
571
acute exacerbation of chronic
bronchitis, 69
acute tonsillitis, 603–604
bacterial skin infection, 573
cellulitis, 142
community acquired pneumonia, 493
dose form/volume, 706
impetigo contagiosa, 352
mastitis (breast abscess), 387
otitis externa, 445
otitis media: acute, 446
streptococcal pharyngitis, 484
urinary tract infection, 643
wound, 659
cefadroxil, Duricef (G), 714
acute exacerbation of chronic
bronchitis, 69
acute tonsillitis, 604
dose form/volume, 705
impetigo contagiosa, 352
scarlet fever, 560
streptococcal pharyngitis, 484
urinary tract infection, 643
wound, 659
cefazolin, Ancef, Kefzol (G)
bacterial endocarditis prophylaxis, 55
dose forms, 705
cefdinir, Omnicef (G), 714
acute bacterial sinusitis, rhinosinusitis,
571
acute exacerbation of chronic
bronchitis, 69
acute tonsillitis, 604
bacterial skin infection, 574
community acquired pneumonia, 493
dose form/volume, 706
otitis media: acute, 446
streptococcal pharyngitis, 484
wound, 659
cefditoren pivoxil, Spectracef (G)
acute exacerbation of chronic
bronchitis, 69
acute tonsillitis, 604
bacterial skin infection, 574
dose form/volume, 704
streptococcal pharyngitis, 484
cefiderocol, Fetroja
complicated urinary tract infection
(CUTI), 640
hospital-acquired bacterial
pneumonia (HABP), 490
ventilator-associated bacterial
pneumonia (VABP), 491–492
cefixime, Suprax (G), 714
acute bacterial sinusitis, rhinosinusitis,
571
acute exacerbation of chronic
bronchitis, 69
acute tonsillitis, 604
dose form/volume, 706
otitis media: acute, 446
sexual assault, 567
streptococcal pharyngitis, 484
typhoid fever, 633
urinary tract infection, 643

cefotaxime, Claforan
  dose form/volume, 706
  gonorrhea, 259
  typhoid fever, 633
cefoxitin, Mefoxin
  dose form/volume, 706
  gonorrhea, 259
  human bite, 66
  pelvic inflammatory disease, 476
cefpodoxime proxetil, Vantin, 715
  acute bacterial sinusitis, rhinosinusitis,
    571
  acute exacerbation of chronic
    bronchitis, 69
  acute tonsillitis, 604
  bacterial skin infection, 574
  cellulitis, 142
  community acquired pneumonia, 493
  gonorrhea, 259
  impetigo contagiosa, 352
  otitis media: acute, 446
  streptococcal pharyngitis, 485
  urinary tract infection, 644
  wound, 659
cefprozil, Cefzil (G), 715
  acute bacterial sinusitis, rhinosinusitis,
    571
  acute exacerbation of chronic
    bronchitis, 70
  acute tonsillitis, 604
  bacterial skin infection, 574
  cellulitis, 143
  dose form/volume, 706
  impetigo contagiosa, 352
  otitis media: acute, 446
  streptococcal pharyngitis, 485
  wound, 659
ceftaroline fosamil, Teflaro
  cellulitis, 143
  community acquired pneumonia,
    493
  dose form/volume, 706
  impetigo contagiosa, 352
ceftibuten, Cedax (G), 715–716
  acute bacterial sinusitis, rhinosinusitis,
    571
  acute exacerbation of chronic
    bronchitis, 70
  acute tonsillitis, 604
  dose forms, 706
  otitis media: acute, 446
  streptococcal pharyngitis, 485
ceftriaxone, Rocephin
  acute exacerbation of chronic
    bronchitis, 70
  bacterial endocarditis prophylaxis, 55
  bacterial skin infection, 574
  cellulitis, 143
  chancroid, 147
  community acquired pneumonia,
    493
  dose forms, 706
  epididymitis, 237
  gonococcal conjunctivitis, 165
  gonococcal ophthalmia neonatorum,
    423
  gonococcal pharyngitis, 483
  gonorrhea, 259
  mastitis (breast abscess), 387
  otitis media: acute, 446
  pelvic inflammatory disease, 476
  proctitis: acute, 516
  sexual assault, 567
  typhoid fever, 633
Cefzil, *cefprozil*, 715
  acute bacterial sinusitis, rhinosinusitis,
    571
  acute exacerbation of chronic
    bronchitis, 70

acute tonsillitis, 604
bacterial skin infection, 574
cellulitis, 143
  dose form/volume, 706
  impetigo contagiosa, 352
  otitis media: acute, 446
  streptococcal pharyngitis, 485
  wound, 659
Celebrex, *celecoxib* (G)
  dysmenorrhea: primary, 225
  gouty arthritis, 263
  muscle strain, 406
  osteoarthritis, 436
  psoriatic arthritis, 528
  rheumatoid arthritis, 544
celecoxib, Celebrex (G), 571
  dysmenorrhea: primary, 225
  gouty arthritis, 263
  muscle strain, 406
  osteoarthritis, 436
  psoriatic arthritis, 528
  rheumatoid arthritis, 544
Celexa, *citalopram* (G)
  anxiety disorder, 35
  major depressive disorder, 191
CellCept, *mycophenolate mofetil (MMF)*
  organ transplant rejection prophylaxis,
    432
cellulitis
  amoxicillin, Amoxil, Moxatag, Trimox,
    142
  amoxicillin+clavulanate, Augmentin,
    Augmentin ES-600, Augmentin
    XR, 142
  azithromycin, Zithromax, Zmax, 142
  cefaclor, Cefaclor Extended Release,
    142
  cefpodoxime proxetil, Vantin, 142
  cefprozil, Cefzil, 143
  ceftaroline fosamil, Teflaro, 143
  ceftriaxone, Rocephin, 143
  cephalexin, Keflex, 143
  clarithromycin, Biaxin, Biaxin Oral
    Suspension, Biaxin XL (G), 143
  dalbavancin, Dalvance (G), 143
  delafloxacin, Baxdela, 143–144
  dicloxacillin, Dynapen, 144
  dirithromycin, Dynabac (G), 144
  erythromycin base, Ery-Tab, PCE, 144
  erythromycin ethylsuccinate, EryPed,
    E.E.S, 144
  linezolid, Zyvox (G), 144
  loracarbef, Lorabid, 144
  moxifloxacin, Avelox (G), 144
  omadacycline, Nuzyra, 144
  oritavancin, Orbactiv (G), 145
  penicillin v potassium, Pen-Vee K, 145
  tedizolid phosphate, Sivextro (G), 145
  tigecycline, Tygacil, 145
cenegermin-bkbj, Oxervat
  neurotrophic keratitis, 374–375
Centany, *mupirocin*
  bacterial skin infection, 573
  impetigo contagiosa, 351
  wound, 658
central precocious puberty (CPP)
  leuprolide acetate, Fensolvi, 512–513
  triptorelin, Triptodur, 513
Cepacol Spray, *benzocaine* (G)
  aphthous stomatitis, 37
cephalexin, Keflex, 716
  acute exacerbation of chronic
    bronchitis, 70
  acute tonsillitis, 604
  bacterial endocarditis prophylaxis, 55
  bacterial skin infection, 574
  cellulitis, 143
  dose forms, 705
  impetigo contagiosa, 352

lymphadenitis, 383
mastitis (breast abscess), 387
otitis media: acute, 447
paronychia, 472
pyelonephritis: acute, 536
scarlet fever, 560
streptococcal pharyngitis, 485
urinary tract infection, 644
wound, 659
Cequa, *cyclosporine* (G)
  dry eye syndrome, 214, 374
CeraLyte, *oral electrolyte replacement*
  (OTC)
  acute diarrhea, 212
Cerefolin, *L-methylfolate calcium (as*
  metafolin)+methylcobalamin+
  n-acetylcysteine
  Alzheimer's disease, 13
  hyperhomocysteinemia, 321
certolizumab, Cimzia
  Crohn's disease, 177
  rheumatoid arthritis, 547
cerumen impaction
  antipyrine+benzocaine+zinc acetate
    dihydrate otic, Otozin (G), 145
  carbamide peroxide, Debrox (G), 145
  triethanolamine, Cerumenex (G), 145
Cerumenex, *triethanolamine* (G)
  cerumen impaction, 145
Cesamet, *nabilone* (G)(II)
  chemotherapy-induced nausea/
    vomiting, 149
Cesia, *ethinyl estradiol+desogestrel*
  estrogen and progesterone, 668
Cetamide Ophthalmic Solution,
  sulfacetamide (G)
  bacterial conjunctivitis, 162
cetirizine, Children's Zyrtec Chewable,
  Children's Zyrtec Allergy Syrup,
  Zerviate, Zyrtec (G)
  allergic (vernal) conjunctivitis, 166
  allergic rhinitis/sinusitis, 549
  atopic dermatitis, 198
  contact dermatitis, 203
  genus rhus dermatitis, 128
  rhinitis medicamentosa, 555
  urticaria, 649
cevimeline, Evoxac (G)
  Sjögren-Larsson-syndrome (SLS),
    572
Chagas disease
  benznidazole (G), 146
  nifurtimox (G), 146
chancroid
  azithromycin, Zithromax, Zmax,
    146–147
  ceftriaxone, Rocephin, 147
  ciprofloxacin, Cipro, Cipro XR,
    ProQuin XR (G), 147
  erythromycin base, Ery-Tab, PCE, 147
  erythromycin ethylsuccinate, EryPed,
    E.E.S, 147
Chantix, *varenicline* (G)
  tobacco dependence, 602
Chemet, *succimer* (G)
  iron overload, 278
  lead poisoning, 376
chemotherapy-induced nausea/vomiting
  (CINV)
  aprepitant, Emend, 148
  chlorpromazine, Thorazine (G), 147
  dolasetron, Anzemet, 148
  dronabinol, Marinol (G)(III), 149
  fosnetupitant+palonosetron, Akynzeo,
    148, 413
  granisetron, Kytril, Sancuso, 148
  granisetron, Kytril, Sancuso, Sustol S,
    148
  nabilone, Cesamet (G)(II), 149

ondansetron, Zofran, Zuplenz (G), 148–149
palonosetron, Aloxi, 149
perphenazine, Trilafon (G), 147
prochlorperazine, Compazine (G), 147
promethazine, Phenergan (G), 147
chest wall syndrome, 171
chickenpox (Varicella)
　acyclovir, Zovirax, 150
　diphenhydramine, Benadryl, 150
　hydroxyzine, AtaraxR, Vistaril (G), 150
　immune globulin (human), GamaSTAN S/D, 149
　Varicella virus vaccine, Varivax, 149
Chikungunya-related arthritis, 150
Children's Advil, *ibuprofen*
　fever (pyrexia), 242
Children's Tylenol, Extra Strength Tylenol, FeverAll Extra Strength Tylenol, *acetaminophen*
　fever (pyrexia), 198
Children's Xyzal Allergy 24HR, Xyzal Allergy 24HR, *levocetirizine*
　atopic dermatitis, 198
　contact dermatitis, 202
　genus rhus dermatitis, 204
　rhinitis medicamentosa, 555
　rhinitis/sinusitis, allergic, 550
　urticaria, 649
Children's Zyrtec Chewable, Children's Zyrtec Allergy Syrup, *cetirizine* (G)
　atopic dermatitis, 198
　contact dermatitis, 202
　genus rhus dermatitis, 203
　rhinitis medicamentosa, 555
　rhinitis/sinusitis, allergic, 549
　urticaria, 649
Chlamydia trachomatis
　azithromycin, Zithromax, Zmax, 151
　doxycycline, Acticlate, Adoxa, Doryx, Doxteric, Monodox, Oracea, Vibramycin, Vibra-Tab, 151
　erythromycin base, Ery-Tab, PCE, 152
　erythromycin ethylsuccinate, EryPed, E.E.S, 152
　levofloxacin, Levaquin (G), 152
　ofloxacin, Floxin (G), 152
chlamydial conjunctivitis
　azithromycin, Zithromax, Zmax, 164
　erythromycin base, Ery-Tab, PCE, 164
　erythromycin ethylsuccinate, EryPed, E.E.S, 164
chlamydial ophthalmia neonatorum
　erythromycin base, Ery-Tab, PCE, 423
　erythromycin ethylsuccinate, EryPed, E.E.S, 423
　erythromycin, Ilotycin, 423
chlamydial pneumonia
　azithromycin, Zithromax, Zmax, 492
　erythromycin base, Ery-Tab, PCE, 492
　erythromycin ethylsuccinate, EryPed, E.E.S, 492
　levofloxacin, Levaquin (G), 492
Chloraseptic Spray, *benzocaine* (G)
　aphthous stomatitis, 37
chlordiazepoxide, Librium (IV)
　alcohol withdrawal syndrome, 11
　anxiety disorder, 33
　panic disorder, 466
chlorhexidine gluconate, Peridex, PerioGard
　gingivitis/periodontitis, 254
chloroquine phosphate, Aralen (G)
　amebiasis, 17
　dose form/volume, 703, 704
　malaria, 386
　systemic lupus erythematosis, 584

chlorothiazide, Diuril
　edema, 228
　heart failure, 280
　hypertension, 327
　urolithiasis, 646
chloroxine, Capitrol Shampoo (G)
　seborrheic dermatitis, 204
chlorpromazine, Thorazine (G)
　cannabinoid hyperemesis syndrome, 139
　chemotherapy-induced nausea/vomiting, 147
　dose forms, 63
　hiccups: intractable, 303
chlorpropamide, Diabinese (G)
　type 2 diabetes mellitus, 619
chlorthalidone, Thalitone
　edema, 228
　hypertension, primary, 327
chlorzoxazone, Parafon Forte DSC (G)
　muscle strain, 403
　temporomandibular joint disorder, 586
cholelithiasis
　cholestyramine, Prevalite (G), 153
　colesevelam, WelChol, 154
　colestipol, Colestid (G), 153
　ursodeoxycholic acid (UDCA), Ursofalk (G), 153
　ursodiol, Actigall, 153
cholera (*Vibrio cholerae*)
　azithromycin, Zithromax, Zmax, 155, 156
　ciprofloxacin, Cipro (G), Cipro XR, ProQuin XR (G), 155, 156
　doxycycline, Acticlate, Adoxa, Doryx, Doxteric, Monodox, Oracea, Vibramycin, Vibra-Tab, 155, 156
　erythromycin base, Ery-Tab, PCE, 155–156
　erythromycin ethylsuccinate, EryPed, E.E.S, 91–92
　Vibrio cholerae vaccine, Vaxchora, 155
cholestyramine, Prevalite, Questran (G)
　cholelithiasis, 153
　diarrhea, chronic, 213
　dyslipidemia, 223–224
　primary biliary cholangitis, 152–153
chronic diarrhea
　attapulgite, Donnagel, Kaopectate (G), 213
　cholestyramine, Questran (G), 213
　crofelemer, Mytesi (G), 213
　difenoxin+atropine, Motofen (G), 213
　diphenoxylate+atropine, Lomotil (G)(V), 213
　loperamide, Imodium, Imodium A-D, 213
　loperamide+simethicone, Imodium Advanced, 213
chronic idiopathic constipation (CIC)
　linaclotide, Linzess (G), 168
　lubiprostone, Amitiza (G), 169
　plecanatide, Trulance (G), 168
　prucalopride, Motegrity (G), 169
chronic inflammatory demyelinating polyneuropathy (CIDP)
　immune globulin subcutaneous [human] 20% liquid, Hizentra, 503–504
chronic obstructive pulmonary disease (COPD)
　aclidinium bromide, Tudorza Pressair (G), 72
　aclidinium bromide+formoterol fumarate, Duaklir Pressair, 73
　budesonide+glycopyrrolate +formoterol fumarate, Breztri Aerosphere

　dyphylline+guaifenesin, Lufyllin GG (G), 74
　fluticasone furoate+vilanterol, Breo Ellipta (G), 73
　glycopyrrolate inhalation solution, Lonhala Magnair, Seebri Neohaler (G), 71, 72, 67–68
　indacaterol, Arcapta Neohaler (G), 71
　indacaterol+glycopyrrolate, Utibron Neohaler (G), 71
　ipratropium bromide, Atroven, 72
　ipratropium/albuterol, Combivent Respimat (G), 73
　olodaterol, Striverdi Respimat (G), 71
　revefenacin inhalation solution, Yupelri (G), 72
　roflumilast, Daliresp (G), 74
　salmeterol, Serevent Diskus (G), 71
　theophylline, Theo-24, Theo-Dur, Theolair-SR, Uniphyl (G), 74
　tiotropium (as bromide monohydrate), Spiriva HandiHaler (G), 66
　tiotropium+olodaterol, Stiolto Respimat (G), 73
　umeclidinium, Incruse Ellipta (G), 72
　umeclidinium+vilanterol, Anoro Ellipta (G), 73
chronic prostatitis
　carbenicillin, Geocillin, 516
　ciprofloxacin, Cipro (G), Cipro XR, ProQuin XR (G), 516
　norfloxacin, Noroxin (G), 517
　ofloxacin, Floxin (G), 517
　trimethoprim+sulfamethoxazole (TMP-SMX), Bactrim, Septra (G), 517
Churg-Strauss syndrome, 235–236
Cialis, *tadalafil*
　benign prostatic hyperplasia, 58
　erectile dysfunction (ED), 237
ciclesonide, Alvesco (G)
　allergic rhinitis/sinusitis, 552
　asthma, 41
　polyps, nasal, 505
ciclopirox, Loprox, Penlac Nail Lacquer
　onychomycosis (fungal nail), 422
　seborrheic dermatitis, 204
　skin candidiasis, 135
　tinea corporis, 597
　tinea cruris, 598
　tinea pedis, 600
　tinea versicolor, 601
cidofovir, Vistide V (G)
　COVID-19 (coronavirus), 173
　cytomegalovirus (CMV) retinitis, 186–187
　posttransplant cytomegalovirus, 185, 186
cilostazol (G)
　dose forms, 702
　peripheral vascular disease, 482
Ciloxan Ophthalmic Ointment, *ciprofloxacin* (G)
　bacterial conjunctivitis, 162
Cimduo, *lamivudine+tenofovir disoproxil fumarate*
　dose forms, 696
　human immunodeficiency virus infection, 314
cimetidine, Tagamet
　gastroesophageal reflux disease, 249
　peptic ulcer disease (PUD), 477–478
Cimzia, *certolizumab*
　Crohn's disease, 177
　rheumatoid arthritis, 547
cinacalcet, Sensipar (G)
　hypercalcemia, 319
　hyperparathyroidism (HPT), 323–324
Cinqair, *reslizumab*
　eosinophilia, 48

Cipro (G), Cipro XR, *ciprofloxacin* (G)
  acute bacterial sinusitis, rhinosinusitis, 572
  acute prostatitis, 516
  anthrax (bacillus anthracis), 31, 32
  chancroid, 147
  cholera *(Vibrio cholerae)*, 155, 156
  chronic prostatitis, 516–517
  cystic fibrosis (CF), 184
  diverticulitis, 215
  dose forms, 708
  granuloma inguinale (donovanosis), 266
  human bite, 66–67
  legionella pneumonia, 496
  pyelonephritis: acute, 536
  salmonellosis, 559
  shigellosis, 567
  Traveler's diarrhea, 213
  typhoid fever, 633
  urinary tract infection, 644
Cipro HC Otic, *ciprofloxacin+ hydrocortisone* (G)
  otitis externa, 444
  otitis media: acute, 447
Ciprodex, *ciprofloxacin+dexamethasone* (G)
  otitis media, acute, 447
  otitis externa, 444
ciprofloxacin, Cipro (G), Cipro XR, Ciloxan Ophthalmic Ointment, ProQuin XR (G)
  acute bacterial sinusitis, rhinosinusitis, 572
  acute prostatitis, 516
  anthrax (bacillus anthracis), 31, 32
  chancroid, 147
  cholera *(Vibrio cholerae)*, 155, 156
  chronic prostatitis, 516–517
  cystic fibrosis (CF), 184
  diverticulitis, 215
  dose forms, 708
  granuloma inguinale (donovanosis), 266
  human bite, 66–67
  legionella pneumonia, 496
  pyelonephritis: acute, 536
  salmonellosis, 559
  shigellosis, 567
  Traveler's diarrhea, 213
  typhoid fever, 633
  urinary tract infection, 644
ciprofloxacin otic suspension, Otiprio
  serous otitis media (SOM), 448
citalopram, Celexa (G)
  anxiety disorder, 35
  major depressive disorder, 191
Citracal, *calcium citrate* (OTC)
  hypocalcemia, 340
Citracal+D, Citracal 250+D, *calcium citrate+vitamin D* (G)
  hypocalcemia, 340
  osteoporosis, 441
Citrate of Magnesia (OTC), *magnesium citrate*
  occasional constipation, 170
Claforan, *cefotaxime*
  dose form/volume, 706
  gonorrhea, 259
  typhoid fever, 633
Clarinex, *desloratadine* (G)
  allergic rhinitis/sinusitis, 550
  atopic dermatitis, 198
  contact dermatitis, 202
  genus rhus dermatitis, 203
  rhinitis medicamentosa, 555
  urticaria, 649
clarithromycin, Biaxin, Biaxin Oral Suspension, Biaxin XL (G), 708, 716

acute exacerbation of chronic bronchitis, 70
acute tonsillitis, 604
bacterial endocarditis prophylaxis, 55
cellulitis, 143
community acquired pneumonia, 494
Hansen's disease, 270
impetigo contagiosa, 352
legionella pneumonia, 496
Lyme disease, 383
mycoplasma pneumonia, 496
otitis media: acute, 447
pertussis, 483
scarlet fever, 560
streptococcal pharyngitis, 485
wound, 659
Claritin Eye, *ketotifen fumarate* (G)
  allergic (vernal) conjunctivitis, 167
Claritin, *loratadine* (OTC)(G)
  allergic rhinitis/sinusitis, 550
  atopic dermatitis, 198
  contact dermatitis, 202
  genus rhus dermatitis, 204
  rhinitis medicamentosa, 555
  urticaria, 649
Clenia, *sodium sulfacetamide+sulfur* (G)
  acne rosacea, 3–4
  seborrheic dermatitis, 130
Cleocin (G), Cleocin Pediatric Granules, Cleocin Vaginal Cream, Cleocin Vaginal Ovules, *clindamycin*, 624
  bacterial endocarditis prophylaxis, 55
  bacterial vaginosis, 56
  dog bite, 66
  mastitis (breast abscess), 387
  scarlet fever, 560
Cleocin T, *clindamycin*
  acne vulgaris, 4
  hidradenitis suppurativa, 304
clevidipine butyrate, Cleviprex (G)
  hypertension, 246
Climara Pro, *estradiol+levonorgestrel*
  menopause, 391
  osteoporosis, 440
Clindagel, *clindamycin*
  acne vulgaris, 4
  folliculitis barbae, 246
clindamycin, Cleocin, Cleocin T, Clindagel, Clindets, Evoclin, 624
  acne vulgaris, 4
  bacterial endocarditis prophylaxis, 55
  bacterial vaginosis, 56
  dental abscess, 191
  dog bite, 66
  dose form/volume, 710, 716–717
  folliculitis barbae, 246
  hidradenitis suppurativa, 304
  mastitis (breast abscess), 387
  paronychia, 472
  scarlet fever, 560
clobazam, Onfi, Sympaza Oral Film (G)(IV)
  dose forms, 694
  Lennox-Gastaut syndrome (LGS), 377
clobetasol propionate, Impoyz (G)
  psoriasis, 520
  strength and volume, 667
clofazimine (G)
  Hansen's disease, 269
Clolar, *clofarabine*, 684
clomipramine, Anafranil (G)
  anxiety disorder, 34
  nocturnal enuresis, 235
  obsessive-compulsive disorder, 422
  trichotillomania, 607
clonazepam, Klonopin (IV)
  anxiety disorder, 34
  dose forms, 694
  panic disorder, 466
  trigeminal neuralgia, 609

clonidine, Catapres, Catapres-TTS, Kapvay, Nexiclon XR (G)
  attention deficit hyperactivity disorder (ADHD), 54
  hypertension, 332
  post-traumatic stress disorder, 511
clopidogrel, Plavix, 702
  peripheral vascular disease, 482
clorazepate, Tranxene (IV)
  alcohol withdrawal syndrome, 11
  anxiety disorder, 34
  panic disorder, 466
Clorpres, *clonidine+chlorthalidone* (G)
  hypertension, 337
Clostridioides difficile infection (CDI)
  bezlotoxumab, Zinplava (G), 157
  fecal microbiota, live-jslm, Rebyota, 157–158
  fecal microbiota, spores, live-brpk, Vowst, 158
  fidaxomicin, Dificid, 156
  vancomycin hcl capsule, Vancocin, 157
  vancomycin hcl oral solution, Firvanq, 157
clotrimazole, Gyne-Lotrimin, Mycelex-G, Mycelex Twin Pack, Mycelex-7
  vulvovaginal (moniliasis) candidiasis, 138
clotrimazole, Lotrimin, Lotrimin AF, Mycelex Troches, Gyne-Lotrimin Vaginal Cream, Mycelex-G Vaginal Cream
  diaper rash, 211
  dose forms, 703
  oral candidiasis, 134
  skin candidiasis, 135
  tinea corporis, 597
  tinea cruris, 598
  tinea pedis, 600
  tinea versicolor, 601
  vulvovaginal candidiasis, 138
clozapine, Clozapine ODT, Clozaril (G), FazaClo ODT, Versacloz
  dose forms, 693
coal tar, Scytera, T/Gel (G)
  pityriasis alba, 488
  psoriasis, 521
  seborrheic dermatitis, 205
codeine sulfate (G)(III)
  pain, 455
Cogentin, *benztropine mesylate* (G)
  Parkinson's disease, 471
Cognex, *tacrine* (G)
  Alzheimer's disease, 15
Colazal, *balsalazide disodium*
  ulcerative colitis, 635
colchicine, Colcrys, Gloperba, Mitigare (G)
  gout (hyperuricemia), 260
colesevelam, WelChol
  cholelithiasis, 154
  dyslipidemia, 224
  primary biliary cholangitis, 153
  type 2 diabetes mellitus, 632
Colestid, *colestipol* (G)
  cholelithiasis, 153
  dyslipidemia, 224
  primary biliary cholangitis, 153
colestipol, Colestid (G)
  cholelithiasis, 153
  dyslipidemia, 224
  primary biliary cholangitis, 153
colonoscopy prep/colon cleanse
  polyethylene glycol 3350 with electrolytes, Plenvu, 160
  sodium picosulfate+magnesium oxide+citric acid, Prepopik, 160
Coly-Mycin S, *colistin+neomycin+ hydrocortisone+thonzonium* (G)

otitis externa, 444
otitis media: acute, 447
Combigan, *brimonidine tartrate+timolol*
glaucoma, 256
CombiPatch, *estradiol+norethindrone*
menopause, 391
Combipres, *clonidine+chlorthalidone* (G)
hypertension, 334
Combivent, *ipratropium
bromide+albuterol sulfate* (G)
asthma, 42
Combivent MDI, *ipratropium/albuterol*
(G)
emphysema, 231
Combivent Respimat, *ipratropium+
albuterol* (G)
chronic obstructive pulmonary
disease, 73
emphysema, 231
Combivir, *lamivudine+zidovudine* (G),
594
dose forms, 696
human immunodeficiency virus
infection, 314
Combunox, *oxycodone+ibuprofen* (G)(II)
pain, 459
Commit Lozenge, *nicotine polacrilex* (G)
tobacco dependence, 603
common cold
oxymetazoline, Afrin, Neo-Synephrine
(G), 161
phenylephrine, Afrin Allergy Nasal
Spray, Afrin Nasal Decongestant
Childrens Pump Mist,
Neo-Synephrine, 161
saline nasal spray, Afrin Saline Mist w.
Eucalyptol and Menthol (OTC),
Afrin Moisturizing Saline Mist
(OTC), Ocean Mist (OTC),
Pediamist (OTC)(G), 160–161
tetrahydrozoline, Tyzine, Tyzine
Pediatric Nasal Drops (G), 161
common wart
acitretin, Soriatane, 655
salicylic acid, Duo Film, Occlusal HP,
Wart-Off (G), 655
trichloroacetic acid, 655
community acquired pneumonia
amoxicillin, Amoxil, Moxatag, Trimox,
493
Augmentin, Augmentin
ES-600, Augmentin XR,
amoxicillin+clavulanate, 493
azithromycin, Zithromax, Zmax, 493
Bactrim,
*trimethoprim+sulfamethoxazole
(TMP-SMX)* (G), 495
cefaclor, Cefaclor Extended Release,
493
cefdinir, Omnicef, 493
cefpodoxime proxetil, Vantin, 493
ceftaroline fosamil, Teflaro, 493
ceftriaxone, Rocephin, 493
clarithromycin, Biaxin, 494
dirithromycin, Dynabac (G), 494
doxycycline, Acticlate, Adoxa, Doryx,
Doxteric, Monodox, Oracea,
Vibramycin, Vibra-Tab, 494
ertapenem, Invanz, 494
erythromycin base, Ery-Tab, PCE, 494
erythromycin estolate, Ilosone, 494
gemifloxacin, Factive (G), 494
levofloxacin, Levaquin (G), 494
linezolid, Zyvox (G), 494
loracarbef, Lorabid, 494
moxifloxacin, Avelox (G), 494
ofloxacin, Floxin (G), 494
omadacycline Loading Dose, Nuzyra,
494
penicillin v potassium, Pen-Vee K, 494

*pneumococcal 15-valent conjugate
vaccine,* 493
tedizolid phosphate, Sivextro, 494
telithromycin, Ketek (G), 494
tigecycline, Tygacil, 495
Compazine, *prochlorperazine* (G)
anxiety disorder, 35
cannabinoid hyperemesis syndrome,
139
chemotherapy-induced nausea/
vomiting, 147
motion sickness, 396
opioid-induced nausea/vomiting, 430
panic disorder, 466
Complera, *emtricitabine+tenofovir
disoproxil fumarate+rilpivirine,*
594
dose forms, 696
human immunodeficiency virus
infection, 314
complicated intra-abdominal infection
(cIAI)
ceftazidime+avibactam, Avycaz, 363
ceftolozane+tazobactam, Zerbaxa, 363
eravacycline, Xerava, 364
imipenem+cilastatin+relebactam,
Recarbrio, 363
complicated urinary tract infection
(CUTI)
cefiderocol, Fetroja, 640
ceftazidime +avibactam, Avycaz, 640
ceft olozane+tazobactam, Zerbaxa,
640–641
imipenem+cilastatin+relebactam,
Recarbrio, 641
plazomicin, Zemdri, 96
Comtan, *entacapone* (G)
Parkinson's disease, 471
Concerta, *methylphenidate (long-acting)*
(G)(II)
attention deficit hyperactivity disorder
(ADHD), 52
narcolepsy, 412
Condylox, *podofilox 0.5% cream* (G)
venereal wart, 655, 656
conjunctivitis
allergic (*see* allergic (vernal)
conjunctivitis)
bacterial (*see* bacterial conjunctivitis)
fungal, 165
gonococcal (*see* gonococcal
conjunctivitis)
viral, 168
constipation
chronic (*see* chronic idiopathic
constipation)
occasional (*see* occasional
constipation)
contact dermatitis
Aveeno (OTC), 202
bentoquatam, IvyBlock (OTC), 201
cetirizine, Children's Zyrtec Chewable,
Children's Zyrtec Allergy Syrup,
Zyrtec (G), 202
desloratadine, Clarinex, Desloratadine
ODT (G), 202
diphenhydramine, Benadryl, 202, 203
fexofenadine, Allegra (G), 202
hydroxyzine (G), Atarax, Vistaril
(G), 203
levocetirizine, Children's Xyzal Allergy
24HR, Xyzal Allergy 24HR, 202
loratadine, Claritin (G), 202
Contrave, *naltrexone+bupropion*
obesity, 419
Copegus, *ribavirin*
hepatitis C (HCV), 294
Copiktra, *duvelisib,* 684
Coreg, Coreg CR, *carvedilol* (G)
heart failure, 327

Corgard, *nadolol* (G)
angina pectoris: stable, 29
headache, migraine, 275
hypertension, primary, 326
Corlanor, *ivabradine*
heart failure, 283
corneal edema
sodium chloride (G), 171
corneal ulceration, 171
Cortane B, Cortane B Aqueous, Cortane
Ear Drops, *chloroxylenol+
pramoxine+hydrocortisone* (G)
otitis externa, 444
otitis media: acute, 447
Cortef, *hydrocortisone* (G), 678
cortisone, Cortone Acetate, 678, 679
Cortisporin Ophthalmic Ointment,
*polymyxin b sulfate+neomycin
sulfate+bacitracin
zinc+hydrocortisone* (G)
bacterial conjunctivitis, 163
Cortisporin Ophthalmic Suspension,
*polymyxin b sulfate+neomycin
sulfate+hydrocortisone* (G)
bacterial conjunctivitis, 163
Cortisporin, *polymyxin b+neomycin+
hydrocortisone* (G)
otitis externa, 444
otitis media: acute, 447
Cortisporin-TC Otic, *colistin+neomycin+
hydrocortisone+thonzonium* (G)
otitis externa, 444
Corzide, *nadolol+bendroflumethiazide*
(G)
hypertension, 335
Cosopt, Cosopt PF, *dorzolamide+
timolol* (G)
glaucoma, 257
costochondritis, 171
Cotazym, *pancreatic enzymes* (G)
pancreatic enzyme deficiency, 239
pancreatic enzyme insufficiency, 463
Cotempla XR-ODT, *methylphenidate
(long-acting)* (G)(II)
attention deficit hyperactivity disorder
(ADHD), 52
Coumadin, *warfarin* (G)
dose forms, 698–699
peripheral vascular disease, 482
COVID-19 (coronavirus)
Baricitinib, Olumiant, 174
cidofovir, Vistide, 173
nirmatrelvir+ritonavir, Paxlovid, 173
remdesivir, Veklury, 172
tocilizumab, Actemra, 174
valganciclovir, Valcyte (G), 173
Coxsackievirus infection, 268–269
Creon, *pancreatic enzymes* (G)
pancreatic enzyme deficiency, 239
pancreatic enzyme insufficiency, 463
Cresemba, *isavuconazonium* (G)
aspergillosis, 38
Crestor, *rosuvastatin*
dyslipidemia, 222
hypertriglyceridemia, 339
crisaborole, Eucrisa (G)
atopic dermatitis, 197
crofelemer, Mytesi (G)
acute diarrhea, 212
chronic diarrhea, 213
Crohn's disease
adalimumab, Humira, 176–177
adalimumab-aacf, Idacio, 177
adalimumab-adaz, Hyrimoz, 117
adalimumab-adbm, Cyltezo, 117
adalimumab-afzb, Abrilada, 117
azathioprine, Imuran, 176
budesonide micronized, Entocort EC
(G), 176
certolizumab, Cimzia, 117.

Crohn's disease (*cont.*)
  infliximab, Remicade, 117
  infliximab-abda, Renflexis, 117
  infl iximab-axxq, Avsola, 178
  infliximab-qbtx, Ifixi, 178
  mesalamine, Asacol, Asacol HD,
    Canasa, Delzicol, Lialda,
    Pentasa, Rowasa Enema,
    Rowasa Suppository, Sulfite-Free
    Rowasa Rectal Suspension,
    175–176
  metronidazole, Flagyl, Flagyl 375,
    Flagyl ER (G), 175
  natalizumab, Tysabri (G), 179
  olsalazine, Dipentum (G), 176
  risankizumab-rzaa, Skyrizi, 178
  sulfasalazine, Azulfidine, Azulfidine
    EN, 176
  upadacitinib, Rinvoq Extended-Release
    Tablets, 179
  ustekinumab, Stelara, 178
  vedolizumab, Entyvio, 179
Crolom, *cromolyn sodium*
  allergic (vernal) conjunctivitis, 166
  vernal keratitis, 375
cromolyn sodium, Crolom, Children's
  NasalCrom, Intal, Intal
  Inhalation Solution, NasalCrom,
  Opticrom
  allergic (vernal) conjunctivitis, 166
  allergic rhinitis/sinusitis, 552
  asthma, 42
  vernal keratitis, 375
crotamiton, Eurax (G)
  scabies, 559
cryptosporidiosis
  nitazoxanide, Alinia, 179
Cryselle, *ethinyl estradiol+norgestrel*, 668
Crysvita, *burosumab-twza* (G)
  X-linked hypophosphatemia, 345
Cuprimine, *penicillamine* (G)
  Gaucher disease, type 1 (GD1), 252
  rheumatoid arthritis, 546
  systemic lupus erythematosis, 584
  urolithiasis, 646
  Wilson's disease, 657
Cushing's syndrome
  levoketoconazole, Recorlev, 180–181
  mifepristone, Korlym, 179–180
  osilodrostat, Isturisa, 181
  pasireotide, Signifor, 180
cutaneous larva migrans
  thiabendazole, Mintezol (G), 376
cutaneous leishmaniasis
  miltefosine (G), Impavido, 377
Cyclessa, *ethinyl estradiol+desogestrel*
  estrogen and progesterone, 668
cyclobenzaprine, Amrix, Fexmid, Flexeril
  fibromyalgia, 244
  muscle strain, 403
  temporomandibular joint disorder,
    586
cyclosporiasis
  trimethoprim+sulfamethoxazole
    (TMP-SMX), Bactrim, Septra
    (G), 182
cyclosporine (immunosuppressant),
  Cequa, Neoral (G)
  dry eye syndrome, 217, 374
  psoriasis, 521
  rheumatoid arthritis, 546
  systemic lupus erythematosis, 583
Cyltezo, *adalimumab-adbm*
  Crohn's disease, 177
  juvenile idiopathic arthritis, 371
  osteoarthritis, 438
  psoriasis, 525
  psoriatic arthritis, 529
  rheumatoid arthritis, 547

ulcerative colitis, 636
Cymbalta, *duloxetine* (G)
  anxiety disorder, 36
  fibromyalgia, 244
  major depressive disorder, 192
  peripheral neuritis, 480
  post-traumatic stress disorder, 511
cyproheptadine, Periactin
  anorexia/cachexia, 30
cystic fibrosis (CF)
  acetylcysteine, Mucomyst, 182
  aztreonam, Cayston, 184
  ciprofloxacin, Cipro, Cipro XR,
    ProQuin XR (G), 184
  elexacaftor+ivacaftor+tezacaftor,
    Trikaft, 183
  ivacaftor, Kalydeco, 182
  lumacaftor+ivacaftor, Orkambi, 183
  tezacaftor+ivacaftor plus ivacaftor,
    Symdeko, 183
  ursodeoxycholic acid (UDCA),
    Ursofalk (G), 183–184
cystinuria
  tiopronin, Thiola, Thiola EC (G),
    184–185
cytomegalovirus (CMV) retinitis
  cidofovir, Vistide V (G), 186–187
  letermovir, Prevymis, 187
Cytomel, *liothyronine* (A)
  hypothyroidism, 346
Cytotec, *misoprostol*
  peptic ulcer disease (PUD), 480
Cytoxan, *Cyclophosphamide*, 477
  dose forms, 684
  pemphigus vulgaris/pemphigus
    foliaceus, 477

dabrafenib, Tafinlar
  melanoma, 117
daclatasvir, Daklinza
  hepatitis C (HCV), 294
Daklinza, *daclatasvir*
  hepatitis C (HCV), 294
dalbavancin, Dalvance (G)
  cellulitis, 143
dalfampridine, Ampyra (G)
  multiple sclerosis (MS), 397
Daliresp, *roflumilast* (G)
  chronic obstructive pulmonary
    disease, 74
Dalmane, *flurazepam* (IV)
  fibromyalgia, 245
  insomnia, 359
Dalvance, *dalbavancin* (G)
  cellulitis, 143
danazol, Danocrine
  endometriosis, 233
  fibrocystic breast disease, 243
  hereditary angioedema, 296
Danocrine, *danazol*
  endometriosis, 233
  fibrocystic breast disease, 243
  hereditary angioedema, 296
dantrolene, Dantrium (G)
  muscle strain, 403
  temporomandibular joint disorder,
    586
dapagliflozin, Farxiga (G)
  heart failure, 279
  type 2 diabetes mellitus, 279
daprodustat, Jesduvroq
  anemia of chronic kidney disease, 24
dapsone, Aczone (G)
  acne vulgaris, 4
  folliculitis barbae, 247
  Hansen's disease, 299
  pemphigus vulgaris, 177
Daraprim, *pyrimethamine* (G)
  toxoplasmosis, 605

darbepoetin alpha, Aranesp (G)
  anemia of chronic kidney disease, 23
daridorexant, Quviviq, 360
  insomnia, 360
darifenacin, Enablex (G)
  urinary overactive bladder, 354
darolutamide, Nubeqa
  prostate cancer, 129
darunavir, Prezista (G)
  human immunodeficiency virus
    infection, 311
Darzalex, *daratumumab*, 684
Darzalex Faspro, *daratumumab+
  hyaluronidase*, 684
  melanoma, 118
  multiple myeloma, 120–121
dasiglucagon, Zegalogue
  hypoglycemia: acute, 342
  type 1 diabetes mellitus (T1DM), 614
  type 2 diabetes mellitus (T2DM), 619
Daurismo, *glasdegib*, 685
Daybue, *Trofinetide*
  rett syndrome, 541
Daytrana, *methylphenidate* (transdermal
    patch) (G)(II)
  attention deficit hyperactivity disorder
    (ADHD), 53
Dayvigo, *lemborexant*
  insomnia, 360
DDAVP, DDAVP Rhinal Tube,
    desmopressin acetate (DDAVP)
  nocturnal enuresis, 235
  urinary overactive bladder, 353
Debrox, *carbamide peroxide* (G)
  cerumen impaction, 145
Decadron, *dexamethasone phosphate* (G)
  allergic (vernal) conjunctivitis, 165
Decadron Phosphate with Xylocaine,
    lidocaine+dexamethasone, 680
  atopic dermatitis, 200
  burn: minor, 76
  diabetic peripheral neuropathy
    (DPN), 209
  gouty arthritis, 262
  hemorrhoids, 290
  herpangina, 299
  herpes zoster, 302
  indications, 358
  insect bite/sting, 358
  juvenile idiopathic arthritis, 369
  juvenile rheumatoid arthritis, 373
  muscle strain, 405
  pain, 454
  peripheral neuritis, 481
  post-herpetic neuralgia, 509
Declomycin, *demeclocycline*
  gonorrhea, 259
deep vein thrombosis (DVT)
  prophylaxis, 187
deferasirox (tridentate ligand), Exjade,
    Jadenu (G)
  iron overload, 365
deferoxamine mesylate, Desferal (G)
  lead poisoning, 376
deflazacort, Emflaza
  duchenne muscular dystrophy
    (DMD), 218
degarelix acetate, Firmagon (G)
  prostate cancer, 127
dehydration
  oral electrolyte replacement (OTC),
    KaoLectrolyte, Pedialyte,
    Pedialyte Freezer Pops (G), 187
delafloxacin, Baxdela
  cellulitis, 143–144
delavirdine mesylate, Rescriptor (G)
  human immunodeficiency virus
    infection, 309
delirium

haloperidol, Haldol, Haldol Lactate (G), 188
lorazepam, Ativan, Lorazepam Intensol (IV), 188
mesoridazine, Serentil (G), 188
olanzapine, Zyprexa, Zyprexa Zydis (G), 188
quetiapine fumarate, SeroQUEL, SeroQUEL XR (G), 188
risperidone, Risperdal, Risperdal M-Tab (G), 188
thioridazine, Mellaril (G), 188
Delstrigo, *doravirine+lamivudine+tenofovir disoproxil fumarate*
  human immunodeficiency virus infection, 314
Deltasone, *prednisone* (G)
  Bell's palsy, 57
Delzicol, *mesalamine*
  Crohn's disease, 175–176
  ulcerative colitis, 635
Demadex, *torsemide*
  edema, 229
  heart failure, 281
  hypertension, primary, 328
demecarium bromide, Humorsol Ocumeter
  glaucoma, 255
demeclocycline, Declomycin
  gonorrhea, 259
dementia
  haloperidol, Haldol, Haldol Lactate (G), 188
  mesoridazine, Serentil (G), 188
  olanzapine, Zyprexa, Zyprexa Zydis (G), 188
  quetiapine fumarate, SeroQUEL, SeroQUEL XR (G), 188
  risperidone, Risperdal, Risperdal M-Tab (G), 189
  thioridazine, Mellaril (G), 189
Demulen 1/35-21, Demulen 1/35-28, Demulen 1/50-21, Demulen 1/50-28, *ethinyl estradiol+ethynodiol diacetate*
  estrogen and progesterone, 668
Demser, *metyrosine* (G)
  pheochromocytoma, 486–487
Denavir, *penciclovir*
  herpes labialis/herpes facialis, 301
dengue fever
  Dengue virus vaccine, Dengvaxia, 190
denosumab, Prolia, Xgeva
  osteoporosis, 344–345
dental abscess
  Augmentin, Augmentin ES-600, Augmentin XR, *amoxicillin+clavulanate,* 190
  clindamycin, Cleocin (G), Cleocin Pediatric Granules, 191
  erythromycin base, Ery-Tab, PCE, 191
  erythromycin ethylsuccinate, EryPed, E.E.S, 191
  penicillin v potassium, Pen-Vee K, 191
denture irritation
  carbamide peroxide 10% (OTC), Gly-Oxide, 191
Depakene, *divalproex sodium, valproic acid,* 694
  bipolar disorder, 61
  headache, migraine, 274
  trichotillomania, 608
  trigeminal neuralgia, 609
Depakote, *divalproex sodium,* 694
  bipolar disorder, 61
  headache, migraine, 274
  trichotillomania, 608
  trigeminal neuralgia, 609

Depen, *penicillamine* (G)
  Gaucher disease, type 1 (GD1), 252
  rheumatoid arthritis, 546
  systemic lupus erythematosis, 584
  urolithiasis, 646
  Wilson's disease, 657
Depo-Provera, Depo-SubQ, *medroxyprogesterone*
  endometriosis, 232
  menometrorrhagia, 389
Derma-Smoothe/FS Shampoo, Derma-Smoothe/FS Topical Oil *fluocinolone acetonide, fluocinolone acetonide* (G), 676
  atopic dermatitis, 198
  pruritus, 517
  seborrheic dermatitis, 205
  xerosis, 661
dermatitis
  atopic (see atopic dermatitis)
  contact (see contact dermatitis)
  genus rhus (see genus rhus dermatitis)
dermatomyositis
  immune globulin intravenous (human), 502–503
Descovy, *emtricitabine+tenofovir alafenamide*
  human immunodeficiency virus infection, 305
Desenex, *undecylenic acid*
  tinea cruris, 599
  tinea pedis, 600
Desferal, *deferoxamine mesylate* (G)
  lead poisoning, 376
desipramine, Norpramin (G)
  anxiety disorder, 34
  diabetic peripheral neuropathy (DPN), 210
  major depressive disorder, 193
  nocturnal enuresis, 235
  post-herpetic neuralgia, 508, 509
  tension headache, 278
  trigeminal neuralgia, 609
Desitin, *zinc oxide* (G)
  diaper rash, 211
desloratadine, Clarinex, Desloratadine ODT (G)
  allergic rhinitis/sinusitis, 550
  atopic dermatitis, 198
  contact dermatitis, 202
  genus rhus dermatitis, 203
  rhinitis medicamentosa, 555
  urticaria, 649
Desloratadine ODT, *desloratadine* (G)
  allergic rhinitis/sinusitis, 550
  atopic dermatitis, 198
  contact dermatitis, 202
  genus rhus dermatitis, 203
  rhinitis medicamentosa, 555
  urticaria, 649
desmopressin acetate (DDAVP), DDAVP, DDAVP Rhinal Tube
  nocturnal enuresis, 235
  urinary overactive bladder, 353
desmopressin acetate, Nocdurna
  nocturnal polyuria, 506–507
Desogen, *ethinyl estradiol+desogestrel diacetate*
  estrogen and progesterone, 668
Desonate, *desonide* (G)
  atopic dermatitis, 198
  strength and volume, 676
desonide, Desonate, DesOwen, Tridesilon, Verdeso (G)
  atopic dermatitis, 198
  strength and volume, 676
DesOwen, *desonide* (G)
  atopic dermatitis, 198
Desoxyn, *methamphetamine* (G)(II)

obesity, 419
Desquam X, *benzoyl peroxide* (G)
  acne vulgaris, 4
  folliculitis barbae, 246
desvenlafaxine, Pristiq (G)
  anxiety disorder, 36
  major depressive disorder, 192
  panic disorder, 465
  post-traumatic stress disorder, 511
Desyrel, *trazodone* (G)
  fibromyalgia, 245
Detrol, *tolterodine tartrate* (G)
  interstitial cystitis, 360
  urinary overactive bladder, 354
deutetrabenazine, Austedo
  Huntington disease-associated chorea, 318
Devrom, *bismuth subgallate powder*
  fecal odor, 241
Dexacort Turbinaire, *dexamethasone*
  allergic rhinitis/sinusitis, 552
  polyps, nasal, 506
dexamethasone elixir
  aphthous stomatitis, 37
dexamethasone, Dexacort Turbinaire, Maxidex, Decadron (G), 679
  allergic rhinitis/sinusitis, 552
  allergic (vernal) conjunctivitis, 165
  polyps, nasal, 506
dexamethasone ophthalmic insert, Dextenza
  pain, 453
dexamethasone phosphate, Decadron (G)
  allergic (vernal) conjunctivitis, 65
Dexedrine, *dextroamphetamine sulfate* (G)(II)
  attention deficit hyperactivity disorder (ADHD), 52
  narcolepsy, 411
Dexilant, *dexlansoprazole*
  gastroesophageal reflux disease, 250
  peptic ulcer disease (PUD), 478
  Zollinger-Ellison syndrome, 662
dexlansoprazole, Dexilant
  gastroesophageal reflux disease, 250
  peptic ulcer disease (PUD), 478
  Zollinger-Ellison syndrome, 662
dexmethylphenidate, Focalin (G)(II)
  attention deficit hyperactivity disorder (ADHD), 51
  narcolepsy, 412
Dextenza, *dexamethasone ophthalmic insert*
  pain, 453
dextroamphetamine sulfate, Dexedrine, Dextrostat (G)(II)
  attention deficit hyperactivity disorder (ADHD), 52
  narcolepsy, 411
dextroamphetamine, Xelstrym (II)
  attention deficit hyperactivity disorder (ADHD), 51
Dextrostat, *dextroamphetamine sulfate* (G)(II)
  attention deficit hyperactivity disorder (ADHD), 52
  narcolepsy, 411
diabetic neuropathic pain
  pregabalin (GABA analog), Lyrica, Lyrica CR (G), 480
  capsaicin, Axsain, Capsin, Capzasin-HP, Capzasin-P, Dolorac, Double Cap (OTC), R-Gel, Zostrix, Zostrix HP, 480
  capsaicin 8%, Qutenza, 480
  diclofenac sodium, Pennsaid, Solaraze Gel, Voltaren Gel (G), 480
  doxepin, Prudoxin, Zonalon, 132
  duloxetine, Cymbalta, 480

diabetic neuropathic pain (*cont.*)
  pimecrolimus, Elidel (G), 481
  lidocaine, LidaMantle, Lidoderm, ZTlido lidocaine, 481
  lidocaine+hydrocortisone, LidaMantle HC, 481
  lidocaine 2.5%+prilocaine 2.5%, Emla Cream, 481
  tapentadol, Nucynta, Nucynta ER, 481–482
  tramadol, Rybix ODT, Ryzolt, Ultram (G)(IV), 481
  tramadol+acetaminophen, Ultracet (G)(IV), 481
diabetic peripheral neuropathy (DPN)
  amitriptyline (G), 210
  amoxapine (G), 210
  capsaicin, Axsain, Capsin, Capzasin-HP, Capzasin-P, Dolorac, Double Cap (OTC), R-Gel, Zostrix, Zostrix HP, 208
  capsaicin 8%, Qutenza, 208
  Decadron Phosphate with Xylocaine, *lidocaine+dexamethasone*, 209
  desipramine, Norpramin (G), 210
  diclofenac sodium, Pennsaid, Solaraze Gel, Voltaren Gel (G), 208–209
  doxepin (G), 209
  doxepin, Prudoxin, Zonalon, 209
  gabapentin enacarbil, Horizant (G), 210
  gabapentin, Gralise, Neurontin (G), 209–210
  imipramine, Tofranil (G), 210
  lidocaine 2.5%+prilocaine 2.5%, Emla Cream, 209
  lidocaine, LidaMantle, Lidoderm, ZTlido lidocaine, 209
  lidocaine+hydrocortisone, LidaMantle HC, 209
  L-methylfolate calcium (as metafolin)+ pyridoxyl 5-phosphate+ methylcobalami, Metanx, 208
  nortriptyline, Pamelor, 210
  pimecrolimus, Elidel (G), 209
  pregabalin (GABA analog), Lyrica, Lyrica CR (G), 210
  protriptyline, Vivactil, 210
  tramadol, Rybix ODT, Ryzolt, Ultram (G)(IV), 208
  tramadol+acetaminophen, Ultracet (G)(IV), 208
  trimipramine, Surmontil (G), 210
  trolamine salicylate, Mobisyl Creme, 208
diabetic retinopathy
  aflibercept, Eylea (G), 206
  brolucizumab-dbll, Beovu, 206
  ranibizumab, Lucentis (G), 206–207
  ranibizumab-nuna, Byooviz, 207
diabetic ulcer
  becaplermin, Regranex (G), 633
  L-methylfolate calcium (as metafolin)+ pyridoxyl 5-phosphate+ methylcobalamin, Metanx, 633
  trypsin+balsam peru+castor oil, Granulex, 633
Diacomit, *stiripentol*
  Lennox-Gastaut syndrome (LGS), 378
Diamox, *acetazolamide*, (G)
  glaucoma, 257
diaper rash
  aloe+vitamin e+zinc oxide, Balmex, 210
  butenafine, Lotrimin Ultra, Mentax, 211
  clotrimazole, Lotrimin, Lotrimin AF, 211
  clotrimazole+betamethasone, Lotrisone (G), 211
  econazole, Spectazole (G), 211
  ketoconazole, Nizoral Cream (G), 211

  miconazole, Lotrimin AF, Monistat-Derm (G), 211
  vitamin a and e, A&D Ointment (G), 211
  zinc oxide, A&D Ointment with Zinc Oxide, Desitin (G), 211
diarrhea
  acute (*see* acute diarrhea)
  carcinoid syndrome, 140
  chronic (*see* chronic diarrhea)
  Traveler's diarrhea (*see* Traveler's diarrhea)
Diastat, *diazepam* (IV)
  alcohol withdrawal syndrome, 11
  anxiety disorder, 34
  dose forms, 694
  Meniere's disease, 388
  muscle strain, 403
  panic disorder, 466
  status epilepticus, 579
  temporomandibular joint disorder, 586
diazepam, Diastat, Valium (IV)
  alcohol withdrawal syndrome, 11
  anxiety disorder, 34
  dose forms, 694
  Meniere's disease, 388
  muscle strain, 403
  panic disorder, 466
  status epilepticus, 579
  temporomandibular joint disorder, 586
diazepam nasal spray, Valtoco (IV)
  seizure, cluster, 566
  status epilepticus, 579
diazoxide, Proglycem (G)
  hypoglycemia: acute, 343
  type 1 diabetes mellitus (T1DM), 614
Dibenzyline, *phenoxybenzamine* (G)
  pheochromocytoma, 487
dibucaine, Nupercainal (OTC)(G)
  hemorrhoids, 289
Diclegis, *doxyalamine succinate+ pyridoxine* (A)
  pregnancy, 514
Diclegis, *doxylamine*
  hyperemesis gravidarum, 320
diclofenac potassium powder for oral solution, Cambia (G)
  migraine and cluster headache, 272
diclofenac sodium, Pennsaid, Solaraze Gel, Voltaren Gel, Zorvolex (G), 571–572
  actinic keratosis, 9
  atopic dermatitis, 199
  diabetic peripheral neuropathy (DPN), 208–209
  dysmenorrhea: primary, 225
  gouty arthritis, 262
  hemorrhoids, 289–290
  juvenile idiopathic arthritis, 369
  juvenile rheumatoid arthritis, 372
  muscle strain, 404–405
  osteoarthritis, 434, 435
  pain, 453
  peripheral neuritis, 480
  post-herpetic neuralgia, 508
  pruritus, 518
  psoriatic arthritis, 527
  rheumatoid arthritis, 542
diclofenac, Voltaren Ophthalmic Solution
  allergic (vernal) conjunctivitis, 168
  eye pain, 241
dicloxacillin, Dynapen, 707, 717
  bacterial skin infection, 574
  cellulitis, 144
  impetigo contagiosa, 352
  lymphadenitis, 383
  otitis externa, 445

  paronychia, 472
dicyclomine, Bentyl
  abdominal cramps, 174
  irritable bowel syndrome with diarrhea, 367
  urinary overactive bladder, 354
didanosine, Videx EC, Videx Pediatric Pwdr for Solution (G)
  human immunodeficiency virus infection, 308
Didrex, *benzphetamine* (III)
  obesity, 418
Differin, *adapalene* (G)
  acne vulgaris, 6
  facial wrinkles, 660
Dificid, *fidaxomicin*
  Clostridioides difficile infection, 156–157
Diflucan, *fluconazole* (G), 627
  oral (thrush) candidiasis, 135
  vulvovaginal (moniliasis) candidiasis, 138
difluprednate, Durezol Ophthalmic Solution (G)
  eye pain, 241
  pain, 453
Digibind, *digoxin (immune fab [ovine])*
  digitalis toxicity, 214
digitalis toxicity
  digoxin (immune fab [ovine]), Digibind, 214
digoxin (immune fab [ovine]), Digibind
  digitalis toxicity, 214
dihydroergotamine mesylate, DHE 45, Migranal
  migraine and cluster headache, 270
dihydroxyaluminum, Rolaids (OTC)
  gastroesophageal reflux disease, 249
diiodohydroxyquin (iodoquinol) (G)
  intestinal amebiasis, 17
Dilacor XR, *diltiazem* (G)
  angina pectoris: stable, 28
  hypertension, primary, 330
Dilantin, *phenytoin (injectable)* (G), 695
  status epilepticus, 580
  trigeminal neuralgia, 609
Dilatrate-SR, *isosorbide dinitrate* (G)
  angina pectoris: stable, 29
diltiazem, Cardizem, Cartia XT, Dilacor XR, Tiazac (G)
  angina pectoris: stable, 28
  headache, migraine, 275–276
  hypertension, primary, 330
diltiazem maleate, Tiamate (G)
  hypertension, 331
dimenhydrinate, Dramamine (OTC)
  Meniere's disease, 388
  motion sickness, 396
dimethyl fumarate, Tecfidera (G)
  multiple sclerosis (MS), 397
Diovan HCT, *valsartan+ hydrochlorothiazide*
  hypertension, 334
Diovan, *valsartan*
  heart failure, 280
  hypertension, primary, 330
Dipentum, *olsalazine* (G)
  Crohn's disease, 176
  ulcerative colitis, 636
diphenhydramine, Benadryl
  allergic reaction, 12
  allergic rhinitis/sinusitis, 550
  anxiety disorder, 32
  atopic dermatitis, 199
  chickenpox (Varicella), 150
  contact dermatitis, 202, 203
  genus rhus dermatitis, 204
  Meniere's disease, 388
  rhinitis medicamentosa, 555
  urticaria, 649

diphtheria
  erythromycin base, Ery-Tab, PCE, 214
  erythromycin ethylsuccinate, EryPed,
    E.E.S, 215
  Pentacel, 215
  Vaxelis, 215
diphtheria, tetanus toxoid, acellular
  pertussis, inactivated poliovirus,
  haemophilus b conjugate, and
  hepatitis b, Vaxeli
  haemophilus influenzae B (HIB), 290
dipivefrin, Cosopt, Cosopt PF, 257
  glaucoma, 257
dipyridamole, Persantine
  dose forms, 702
  peripheral vascular disease, 482
dirithromycin, Dynabac (G)
  acute exacerbation of chronic
    bronchitis, 70
  acute tonsillitis, 604
  bacterial skin infection, 574
  cellulitis, 144
  community acquired pneumonia, 494
  dose form/volume, 708
  legionella pneumonia, 496
  streptococcal pharyngitis, 485
  wound, 659
diroximel fumarate, Vumerity
  multiple sclerosis (MS), 402
disulfiram, Antabuse
  alcohol withdrawal syndrome, 11
Ditropan, *oxybutynin chloride*
  hyperhidrosis, 320
  interstitial cystitis, 362
  urinary overactive bladder, 355
Diuril, *chlorothiazide*
  edema, 228
  heart failure, 280
  hypertension, 327
  urolithiasis, 646
divalproex sodium, Depakene, Depakote
  bipolar disorder, 61
  dose forms, 694
  migraine and cluster headache, 274
  trichotillomania, 608
  trigeminal neuralgia, 609
diverticulitis
  amoxicillin, Amoxil, Moxatag, Trimox,
    215
  Augmentin, Augmentin
    ES-600, Augmentin XR,
    amoxicillin+clavulanate, 215
  ciprofloxacin, Cipro (G), Cipro XR,
    ProQuin XR (G), 215
  metronidazole, Flagyl, Flagyl 375,
    Flagyl ER (G), 216
  trimethoprim/sulfamethoxazole (TMP-
    SMX), Bactrim, Septra, 216
diverticulosis, 216
docosanol, Abreva
  herpes labialis/herpes facialis, 301
docusate enema, DocuSol Kids
  occasional constipation, 170
docusate sodium, Dialose, Surfak (OTC)
  occasional constipation, 169
DocuSol Kids, docusate enema
  occasional constipation, 170
dofetilide (G), 682
dog bite
  amoxicillin+clavulanate, Augmentin,
    Augmentin ES-600, Augmentin
    XR, 66
  clindamycin, Cleocin, Cleocin
    Pediatric Granules, 66
  doxycycline, Acticlate, Adoxa, Doryx,
    Doxteric, Monodox, Oracea,
    Vibramycin, Vibra-Tab, 66
  penicillin v potassium, Pen-Vee K, 66
  tetanus *toxoid* vaccine, 65
dolasetron, Anzemet

cannabinoid hyperemesis syndrome,
  139
chemotherapy-induced nausea/
  vomiting, 148
opioid-induced nausea/vomiting, 429
Dolorac, *capsaicin* (G)
  atopic dermatitis, 199
  diabetic peripheral neuropathy
    (DPN), 208
  gouty arthritis, 261–262
  juvenile idiopathic arthritis, 369
  juvenile rheumatoid arthritis, 372
  muscle strain, 404
  osteoarthritis, 434
  pain, 453
  peripheral neuritis, 480
  pruritus, 517
  psoriatic arthritis, 527
  rheumatoid arthritis, 541
dolutegravir, Tivicay (G)
  human immunodeficiency virus
    infection, 308
Domeboro Otic, *acetic acid 2% in*
  aluminum sulfate (G)
  otitis externa, 444
donepezil, Aricept, Aricept ODT (G)
  Alzheimer's disease, 14
donepezil transdermal system, Adlarity
  Alzheimer's disease, 14–15
Donnagel, *attapulgite* (G)
  acute diarrhea, 211
  chronic diarrhea, 213
Donnatal, *phenobarbital+hyoscyamine+*
  atropine+scopolamine (G)
  abdominal cramps, 175
  irritable bowel syndrome with
    diarrhea, 367
Donnazyme, *pancreatic enzymes* (G)
  pancreatic enzyme deficiency, 239
  pancreatic enzyme insufficiency, 463
Doptelet, *avatrombopag*
  idiopathic thrombocytopenia
    purpura, 594
doravirine, Pifeltro
  human immunodeficiency virus
    infection, 309
Doryx, *doxycycline*
  acne rosacea, 3
  acne vulgaris, 5
  acute exacerbation of chronic
    bronchitis, 70
  anthrax (bacillus anthracis), 32
  bacterial skin infection, 574
  cat bite, 65
  cat scratch fever, 141
  Chlamydia trachomatis, 151
  cholera *(Vibrio cholerae),* 155, 156
  community-acquired pneumonia, 494
  dog bite, 66
  dose forms, 639, 644, 704
  epididymitis, 237
  gonorrhea, 256
  granuloma inguinale, 266
  hidradenitis suppurativa, 303
  lyme disease, 383
  lymphogranuloma venereum, 384
  malaria, 384
  nongonococcal urethritis, 639
  pelvic inflammatory disease, 476
  proctitis: acute, 516
  rocky mountain spotted fever, 556
  sexual assault, 567
dorzolamide, Trusopt (G)
  glaucoma, 255
dostinex, Cabergoline
  hyperprolactinemia, 326
Double Cap (OTC), *capsaicin*
  atopic dermatitis, 199
  diabetic peripheral neuropathy
    (DPN), 208

gouty arthritis, 261–262
juvenile idiopathic arthritis, 369
juvenile rheumatoid arthritis, 372
muscle strain, 404
osteoarthritis, 434
pain, 453
peripheral neuritis, 480
pruritus, 517
psoriatic arthritis, 527
rheumatoid arthritis, 541
Dovato, *dolutegravir+lamivudine*
  human immunodeficiency virus
    (HIV) infection, 315
doxazosin, Cardura, Cardura XL (G)
  benign prostatic hyperplasia, 58
  hypertension: primary, 332
  urinary overactive bladder, 356
doxercalciferol, Hectorol (G)
  hypocalcemia, 340–341
  hypoparathyroidism, 344
  osteoporosis, 441
doxepin (G)
  anxiety disorder, 34
  diabetic peripheral neuropathy
    (DPN), 210
  headache: migraine, 276
  major depressive disorder, 193
  nocturnal enuresis, 235
  panic disorder, 465
  post-herpetic neuralgia, 508, 510
  post-traumatic stress disorder, 512
  trigeminal neuralgia, 609
doxepin, Prudoxin, Zonalon, Silenor
  atopic dermatitis, 199
  diabetic peripheral neuropathy
    (DPN), 209
  gouty arthritis, 262
  hemorrhoids, 290
  insomnia, 360
  juvenile idiopathic arthritis, 369
  juvenile rheumatoid arthritis, 372
  muscle strain, 405
  osteoarthritis, 434
  pain, 453
  peripheral neuritis, 480–481
  post-herpetic neuralgia, 508
  pruritus, 518
  psoriatic arthritis, 527
  rheumatoid arthritis, 542
doxercalciferol, Hectorol (G)
  osteoporosis, 441
Doxidan, *docusate+casanthranol* (G)
  occasional constipation, 170
Doxil, *doxorubicin HCl,* 685
Doxteric, *doxycycline*
  acne rosacea, 3
  acne vulgaris, 5
  acute exacerbation of chronic
    bronchitis, 70
  anthrax (bacillus anthracis), 32
  bacterial skin infection, 574
  cat bite, 65
  cat scratch fever, 141
  Chlamydia trachomatis, 151
  cholera *(Vibrio cholerae),* 155, 156
  community-acquired pneumonia, 494
  dog bite, 66
  dose forms, 639, 644, 704
  epididymitis, 237
  gonorrhea, 256
  granuloma inguinale, 266
  hidradenitis suppurativa, 303
  lyme disease, 383
  lymphogranuloma venereum, 384
  malaria, 384
  nongonococcal urethritis, 639
  pelvic inflammatory disease, 476
  proctitis: acute, 516
  rocky mountain spotted fever, 556
  sexual assault, 567

doxycycline, Acticlate, Adoxa, Doryx,
   Doxteric, Monodox, Oracea,
   Vibramycin, Vibra-Tab
   acne rosacea, 3
   acne vulgaris, 5
   acute exacerbation of chronic
      bronchitis, 70
   anthrax (bacillus anthracis), 32
   bacterial skin infection, 574
   cat bite, 65
   cat scratch fever, 141
   Chlamydia trachomatis, 151
   cholera (Vibrio cholerae), 155, 156
   community-acquired pneumonia, 494
   dog bite, 66
   dose forms, 639, 644, 704
   epididymitis, 237
   gonorrhea, 256
   granuloma inguinale, 266
   hidradenitis suppurativa, 303
   lyme disease, 383
   lymphogranuloma venereum, 384
   malaria, 384
   nongonococcal urethritis, 639
   pelvic inflammatory disease, 476
   proctitis: acute, 516
   rocky mountain spotted fever, 556
   sexual assault, 567
doxylamine, Bonjesta, Diclegis
   hyperemesis gravidarum, 320
Dramamine (OTC), dimenhydrinate
   Meniere's disease, 388
   motion sickness, 396
Dramamine II (OTC), meclizine
   labyrinthitis, 375
   Meniere's disease, 388
   motion sickness, 396
   vertigo, 653
dronabinol, Marinol, Syndros (III)
   anorexia/cachexia, 30
   chemotherapy-induced nausea/
      vomiting, 149
droxidopa, Northera (G)
   neurogenic hypotension, 316
dry eye syndrome, 287
   cyclosporine, Cequa (G), 217
   dextran 70+hypromellose, Bion Tears,
      217
   hydroxypropyl cellulose, Lacrisert,
      Hypotears Ophthalmic
      Ointment, 217
   hydroxypropyl methylcellulose, GenTeal
      Mild, GenTeal Moderate,
      GenTeal Severe, 217
   lifitegrast, Xiidra, 216
   loteprednol etabonate, Eysuvis, 218
   perfluorohexyloctane, Miebo, 218
   petrolatum+lanolin+mineral oil,
      Duratears Naturale, 217
   petrolatum+mineral oil, Hypotears,
      Lacri-Lube, 217
   polyethylene glycol, Systane, Systane
      Balance, Systane Ultra, 217
   polyethylene glycol+glycerin+
      hydroxypropyl methylcellulose,
      Visine Tears, 217
   polyvinyl alcohol, Hypotears,
      Hypotears PF, 142
   varenicline, Tyrvaya, 216
Drysol, aluminum chloride
   hyperhidrosis, 320
DRYvax, vaccina virus vaccine (dried, calf
   lymph type) (G)
   smallpox, 576
Duac, clindamycin+benzoyl peroxide
   acne vulgaris, 54
   folliculitis barbae, 246
Duavee, estrogen, conjugated+
   bazedoxifene

menopause, 392
   osteoporosis, 341
Duavee, estrogen, conjugated+
   bazedoxifene
   menopause, 392
   osteoporosis, 440
duchenne muscular dystrophy (DMD)
   casimersen, Amondys, 218–219
   deflazacort, Emflaza, 218
   eteplirsen, Exondys, 219
   golodirsen, Vyondys, 219
   viltolarsen, Viltepso, 219
Duetact, pioglitazone+glimepiride (G)
   type 2 diabetes mellitus, 622
Duexis, ibuprofen+famotidine
   osteoarthritis (OA), 436
   pain, 451–452
   rheumatoid arthritis (RA), 543–544
dulaglutide, Trulicity (G)
   type 2 diabetes mellitus, 623
Dulcolax, bisacodyl
   encopresis, 232
   occasional constipation, 170
Dulera, mometasone furoate+formoterol
   fumarate (G)
   asthma, 44
duloxetine, Cymbalta (G)
   anxiety disorder, 36
   fibromyalgia, 244
   major depressive disorder, 192
   peripheral neuritis, 480
   post-traumatic stress disorder, 511
Duobrii, halobetasol propionate+
   tazarotene
   psoriasis, 521
Duo Film, salicylic acid
   common wart, 655
Duoneb, ipratropium bromide+albuterol
   sulfate (G)
   asthma, 42
Duopa, carbidopa+levodopa (G)
   Parkinson's disease, 469
dupilumab, Dupixent
   allergic rhinitis/sinusitis, 553
   asthma, 46
   atopic dermatitis, 201
   eosinophilia, 47
Dupixent, dupilumab
   allergic rhinitis/sinusitis, 553
   asthma, 46
   atopic dermatitis, 201
   eosinophilia, 47
Duo Plant Gel, salicylic acid
   plantar wart, 655
Duratears Naturale, petrolatum+lanolin+
   mineral oil
   dry eye syndrome, 217
Durezol Ophthalmic Solution,
   difluprednate (G)
   eye pain, 241
   pain, 453
Duricef, cefadroxil, 714
   acute exacerbation of chronic
      bronchitis, 69
   acute tonsillitis, 604
   dose form/volume, 705
   impetigo contagiosa, 352
   scarlet fever, 560
   streptococcal pharyngitis, 484
   urinary tract infection, 643
   wound, 659
Durolane, sodium hyaluronate
   osteoarthritis, 437
dust mite allergy
   dermatophagoides farinae+
      dermatophagoides pteronyssinus
      allergen extract, Odactra, 219
dutasteride, Avodart
   benign prostatic hyperplasia, 58

Dutoprol, metoprolol succinate+ext-rel
   hydrochlorothiazide (G)
   hypertension, 334–335
Duzallo, allopurinol+lesinurad
   gout (hyperuricemia), 261
Dyanavel XR Oral Suspension,
   amphetamine, mixed salts of
   single entity amphetamine (G)(II)
   attention deficit hyperactivity disorder
      (ADHD), 50–51
Dyazide, triamterene+
   hydrochlorothiazide (G)
   edema, 230
   heart failure, 282
   hypertension, 329
Dymista, azelastine+fluticasone (G)
   allergic rhinitis/sinusitis, 552
Dynabac, dirithromycin (G)
   acute exacerbation of chronic
      bronchitis, 70
   acute tonsillitis, 604
   bacterial skin infection, 574
   cellulitis, 144
   community acquired pneumonia, 494
   dose form/volume, 708
   legionella pneumonia, 496
   streptococcal pharyngitis, 485
   wound, 659
Dynacin, minocycline, 704, 709
   acne rosacea, 3
   acne vulgaris, 5
   anthrax, 32
   aphthous stomatitis, 37
   bacterial skin infection, 575
   Hansen's disease, 270
   hidradenitis suppurativa, 304
   Lyme disease, 383
   malaria, 384–385
   urinary tract infection, 644
Dynapen, dicloxacillin, 707, 717
   bacterial skin infection, 574
   cellulitis, 144
   impetigo contagiosa, 352
   lymphadenitis, 383
   otitis externa, 445
   paronychia, 472
Dyrenium, triamterene
   edema, 228
   hypertension, primary, 327
dysfunctional uterine bleeding (DUB)
   medroxyprogesterone acetate, Provera,
      220
dyshidrosis, 220
dyshidrotic eczema, 220
dyslipidemia
   alirocumab, Praluent (G), 221
   amlodipine+atorvastatin, Caduet,
      224–225
   atorvastatin, Lipitor, 222
   bempedoic acid, Nexletol, 221–222
   cholestyramine, Questran (G),
      223–224
   colesevelam, WelChol, 224
   colestipol, Colestid (G), 224
   evolocumab, Repatha, 221
   evinacumab-dgnb, Evkeeza, 220–221
   ezetimibe, Zetia (G), 220
   ezetimibe+atorvastatin, Liptruzet, 222
   ezetimibe+rosuvastatin, Roszet,
      222–223
   ezetimibe+simvastatin, Vytorin, 223
   fenofibrate, Antara, Fenoglide,
      FibriCor, TriCor, TriLipix,
      Lipofen, Lofibra (G), 223
   fluvastatin, Lescol, Lescol XL, 222
   gemfibrozil, Lopid, 223
   icosapent ethyl (omega 3-fatty acid
      ethyl ester of EPA), Vascepa sgc
      (G), 220

inclisiran, Leqvio, 221
lomitapide mesylate, Juxtapid, 220
lovastatin, Mevacor, Altoprev, 222
mipomersen, Kynamro, 220
niacin, Niaspan, Slo-Niacin (G), 223
niacin+lovastatin, Advicor, 224
niacin+simvastatin, Simcor, 224
omega 3-acid ethyl esters, Lovaza, Epanova (G), 220
pitavastatin, Livalo, Nikita, Zypitamag, 222
pravastatin, Pravachol, 222
rosuvastatin, Crestor, 222
simvastatin, Zocor, 222
dysmenorrhea: primary
  celecoxib, Celebrex (G), 225
  diclofenac, Cataflam, Voltaren, Voltaren-XR (G), 225
  mefenamic acid, Ponstel (G), 225
  meloxicam, Mobic, Vivlodex (G), 225
dyspareunia
  estradiol, Invexxy, 226
  ospemifene, Osphena, 226
  prasterone (dehydroepiandrosterone [DHEA]), Intrarosa, 226

Ebanga, *ansuvimab-zykl*
  ebola zaire disease (zaire ebolavirus), 227–228
ebola zaire disease (zaire ebolavirus)
  ansuvimab-zykl, Ebanga, 227–228
  atoltivimab+maft ivimab+odesivimab, Inmazeb, 227
  ebola zaire vaccine, live, Ervebo, 226–227
ebola zaire vaccine, live, Ervebo
  ebola zaire disease (zaire ebolavirus), 226–227
ecallantide, Kalbitor (G)
  hereditary angioedema, 298
echothiophate iodide, Phospholine Iodide
  glaucoma, 255
EC-Naprosyn, *naproxen*
  fever (pyrexia), 243
econazole, Spectazole (G)
  diaper rash, 211
  skin candidiasis, 135
  tinea corporis, 597
  tinea cruris, 598
  tinea pedis, 600
  tinea versicolor, 601
Econopred, Econopred Plus, *prednisolone acetate* (G)
  allergic (vernal) conjunctivitis, 166
EContra EZ, *levonorgestrel*, 675
Ecotrin, *aspirin*
  peripheral vascular disease, 482
eculizumab, Soliris (G)
  atypical hemolytic uremic syndrome (aHUS), 284–285
  neuromyelitis optica spectrum disorder, 416
  myesthenia gravis, 406–407
  paroxysmal nocturnal hemoglobinuria, 472–473
edaravone, Radicava
  amyotrophic lateral sclerosis (ALS), 18–19
Edarbi, *azilsartan medoxomil* (G)
  hypertension, 330
Edarbyclor, *azilsartan+chlorthalidone*
  hypertension, 333
Edecrin, *ethacrynic acid*
  edema, 228
  heart failure, 281
  hypertension, primary, 328
edema
  amiloride, 228

amiloride+hydrochlorothiazide, Moduretic, 229
bumetanide (G), 228
chlorothiazide, Diuril, 228
chlorthalidone, Thalitone, 228
ethacrynate sodium, Sodium Edecrin, 228–229
ethacrynic acid, Edecrin, 228
furosemide, Lasix (G), 229
hydrochlorothiazide, Esidrix, Microzide, 228
hydroflumethiazide, Saluron, 228
indapamide, Lozol, 229
methyclothiazide+deserpidine, Enduronyl, Enduronyl Forte, 228
metolazone, Mykrox, Zaroxolyn, 229
polythiazide, Renese (G), 228
spironolactone, Aldactone, CaroSpir, 228
spironolactone+hydrochlorothiazide, Aldactazide, 229–230
torsemide, Demadex, Soaanz, 229
triamterene, Dyrenium, 228
triamterene+hydrochlorothiazide, Dyazide, Maxzide (G), 230
edetate calcium disodium (EDTA), Calcium Disodium Versenate
  lead poisoning, 376
Edex, *alprostadil*
  erectile dysfunction (ED), 238
Edluar, *zolpidem* (G)(IV)
  aphasia, 36–37
  fibromyalgia, 245
  insomnia, 359
E.E.S., E.E.S. Granules, E.E.S. 400 Tablets, *erythromycin ethylsuccinate*, 708, 709, 718
  acne vulgaris, 5
  acute exacerbation of chronic bronchitis, 70
  acute tonsillitis, 604
  bacterial skin infection, 574
  cat scratch fever, 141
  cellulitis, 144
  chancroid, 147
  Chlamydia trachomatis, 152
  chlamydial conjunctivitis, 164
  chlamydial ophthalmia neonatorum, 423
  chlamydial pneumonia, 492
  cholera (*Vibrio cholerae*), 156
  dental abscess, 191
  diphtheria, 215
  erysipelas, 238
  gonococcal conjunctivitis, 165
  granuloma inguinale, 266
  hidradenitis suppurativa, 303–304
  human bite, 67
  impetigo contagiosa, 352
  lymphogranuloma venereum, 384
  mycoplasma pneumonia, 496
  nongonococcal urethritis, 639
  paronychia, 472
  pertussis, 483
  scarlet fever, 560
  streptococcal pharyngitis, 485
  wound, 659
efavirenz, Sustiva
  human immunodeficiency virus infection, 309–310
Effexor, Effexor XR, *venlafaxine* (G)
  anxiety disorder, 36
  major depressive disorder, 192
  panic disorder, 465
  post-traumatic stress disorder, 511–512
efinaconazole, Jublia (G)
  onychomycosis (fungal nail), 422
eflornithine, Vaniqa (G)

facial hair: excessive/unwanted, 241
Efudex, *fluorouracil*
  actinic keratosis, 9
elacestrant, Orserdu
  breast cancer, 85
elagolix, Orlissa, Oriahnn
  endometriosis, 233
  uterine leiomyomata, 651
Elahere, *mirvetuximab soravtansine-gynx*
  fallopian tube cancer, 89–90
  ovarian cancer, 123–124
  peritoneal cancer, 126
Elestat, *epinastine* (G)
  allergic (vernal) conjunctivitis, 167
eletriptan, Relpax (G)
  migraine and cluster headache, 270
Elidel, *pimecrolimus* (G)
  atopic dermatitis, 190
  diabetic peripheral neuropathy (DPN), 209
  gouty arthritis, 262
  hemorrhoids, 290
  juvenile idiopathic arthritis, 369
  juvenile rheumatoid arthritis, 372
  muscle strain, 405
  osteoarthritis, 434
  pain, 454
  peripheral neuritis, 481
  post-herpetic neuralgia, 508
  pruritus, 518
  psoriatic arthritis, 527
  rheumatoid arthritis, 542
Eligard, *leuprolide acetate*, 685
Elimite, *permethrin*
  scabies, 559
ElixSure IB, *ibuprofen*
  fever (pyrexia), 242
Ella, *ulipristal acetate (UPA)* (G), 676
  uterine fibroids, 650–651
Elmiron, *pentosan*
  interstitial cystitis, 362
EluRyng, *etonogestrel+ethinyl estradiol* (G), 674
eluxadoline, Viberzi (NA)(IV)
  irritable bowel syndrome with diarrhea, 366
Elzonris, *tagraxofusp-erzs*, 685
Emadine, *emedastine* (G)
  allergic (vernal) conjunctivitis, 166
Embeda, *morphine sulfate+naltrexone* (G)(II)
  pain, 458
emedastine, Emadine (G)
  allergic (vernal) conjunctivitis, 166
Emend, *aprepitant*
  cannabinoid hyperemesis syndrome, 139
  chemotherapy-induced nausea/vomiting, 148
  opioid-induced nausea/vomiting, 430
Emflaza, *deflazacort*
  duchenne muscular dystrophy (DMD), 218
emicizumab-kxwh, Hemlibra
  hemophilia A, 285–286
Emla Cream, *lidocaine 2.5%+prilocaine 2.5%*
  atopic dermatitis, 200
  burn: minor, 76
  diabetic peripheral neuropathy (DPN), 209
  gouty arthritis, 262
  hemorrhoids, 290
  herpangina, 299
  herpes zoster, 302
  indication(s), 570
  insect bite/sting, 358
  juvenile idiopathic arthritis, 370
  juvenile rheumatoid arthritis, 373

Emla Cream, *lidocaine 2.5%+prilocaine 2.5% (cont.)*
  muscle strain, 405
  pain, 454
  peripheral neuritis, 481
  post-herpetic neuralgia, 509
Empaveli, *pegcetacoplan*
  paroxysmal nocturnal hemoglobinuria (PNH), 473
emphysema
  aclidinium bromide, Tudorza Pressair (G), 230
  dyphylline+guaifenesin, Lufyllin GG (G), 232
  fluticasone furoate+umeclidinium+ vilanterol, Trelegy Ellipta, 232
  fluticasone furoate/vilanterol, Breo Ellipta (G), 230
  glycopyrrolate inhalation solution, Lonhala Magnair (G), 230–231
  glycopyrrolate inhalation solution, Seebri Neohaler (G), 230
  indacaterol, Arcapta Neohaler (G), 230
  indacaterol+glycopyrrolate, Utibron Neohaler (G), 231
  ipratropium, Atrovent, 230
  ipratropium/albuterol, Combivent MDI (G), 231
  ipratropium+albuterol, Combivent Respimat (G), 231
  olodaterol, Striverdi Respimat (G), 152
  revefenacin inhalation solution, Yupelri, 231
  theophylline+potassium iodide+ ephedrine+phenobarbital, Quadrinal (II), 232
  tiotropium (as bromide monohydrate), Spiriva HandiHaler, Spiriva Respimat (G), 231
  tiotropium+olodaterol, Stiolto Respimat (G), 232
  umeclidinium, Incruse Ellipta (G), 231
  umeclidinium+vilanterol, Anoro Ellipta (G), 232
Emsam, *selegiline* (G)
  major depressive disorder, 194
  post-traumatic stress disorder, 512
emtricitabine, Emtriva
  human immunodeficiency virus infection, 309
Emverm, *mebendazole* (G), 704
  hookworm, 305
  pinworm, 488
  roundworm, 557
  threadworm, 593
  trichinosis, 606
  whipworm, 656
Enablex, *darifenacin* (G)
  urinary overactive bladder, 354
enalapril, Epaned Oral Solution, Vasotec
  heart failure, 279
  hypertension, 329
Enbrel, *etanercept*
  juvenile idiopathic arthritis, 371
  osteoarthritis, 438
  plaque psoriasis, 525
  psoriatic arthritis, 530
  rheumatoid arthritis, 547
encopresis
  bisacodyl, Dulcolax, 232
  glycerin suppository (A), 232
  mineral oil (G), 232
Endari, *L-glutamine powder*, 685
  sickle cell disease, 569
endometrial carcinoma
  dostarlimab-gxly, Jemperli, 87
  pembrolizumab, Keytruda, 88
endometriosis

danazol, Danocrine, 233
elagolix, Orlissa, 233
goserelin (GnRH analog), Zoladex, 233
leuprolide acetate (GnRH analog), Lupron Depot, 233
medroxyprogesterone acetate, Depo-Provera, 232
medroxyprogesterone, Provera, 232
nafarelin acetate, Synarel, 233
norethindrone acetate, Aygestin, 233
relugolix+estradiol+norethindrone acetate, Myfembree, 234
Enduronyl, Enduronyl Forte, *methylclothiazide+deserpidine*
  edema, 228
  heart failure, 281
  hypertension, 327
enfortumab vedotin-ejfv, Padcev
  urothelial carcinoma, 134
enfuvirtide, Fuzeon
  human immunodeficiency virus infection, 312, 696
Engerix-B, *hepatitis B recombinant vaccine* (G)
  hepatitis B, 292
Enhertu, *fam-trastuzumab deruxtecan-nxki*
  breast cancer, 83
enoxacin, Penetrex, 708
  gonorrhea, 259
  urinary tract infection, 644
Enpresse, *ethinyl estradiol/levonorgestrel*
  estrogen and progesterone, 668
Enstilar, *calcipotriene+betamethasone dipropionate* (G)
  psoriasis, 520
entacapone, Comtan (G)
  Parkinson's disease, 471
Entadfi, *finasteride+tadalafil*
  benign prostatic hyperplasia (BPH), 59
entecavir, Baraclude (G)
  hepatitis B, 293
Entereg, *alvimopan*
  bowel resection with primary anastomosis, 68
Entocort EC, *budesonide micronized* (G)
  Crohn's disease, 176
  ulcerative colitis (UC), 634
Entresto, *sacubitril+valsartan*
  heart failure, 280
Entyvio, *vedolizumab*
  Crohn's disease, 179
  ulcerative colitis, 638
Envarsus XR, *tacrolimus*
  organ transplant rejection prophylaxis, 433
eosinophilia
  benralizumab, Fasenra, 49
  dupilumab, Dupixent, 47
  mepolizumab, Nucala, 48
  omalizumab, Xolair, 49
  reslizumab, Cinqair, 48
eosinophilic granulomatosis with polyangitis
  mepolizumab, Nucala, 235–236
leoteprednol etabonate, Inveltys (G)
  eye pain, 241
Epaned Oral Solution, *enalapril*
  heart failure, 279
  hypertension, primary, 329
Epanova, *omega 3-fatty acid ethyl esters* (G)
  dyslipidemia, 220
  hypertriglyceridemia, 338
Epclusa, *sofosbuvir+velpatasvir*
  hepatitis C (HCV), 295
epcoritamab-bysp, Epkinly

lymphoma, 109–110
epicondylitis, 236
epididymitis
  ceftriaxone, Rocephin, 237
  doxycycline, Acticlate, Adoxa, Doryx, Doxteric, Monodox, Oracea, Vibramycin, Vibra-Tab, 327
  levofloxacin, Levaquin (G), 237
  ofloxacin, Floxin (G), 237
Epidiolex, *cannabidiol*
  Lennox-Gastaut syndrome (LGS), 377
epiduo Gel, Epiduo Forte Gel, *adapalene+benzoyl peroxide* (G)
  acne vulgaris, 6
epinastine, Elestat (G)
  allergic (vernal) conjunctivitis, 167
epinephrine (G)
  anaphylaxis, 21
  insect bite/sting, 358
  status asthmaticus, 579
  urticaria, 650
epinephrine, Adrenaclick, Auvi-Q, EpiPen, EpiPen Jr, Symjepi, Twinject (G)
  anaphylaxis, 21
  status asthmaticus, 579
epinephrine inhalation aerosol, Primatene MIST Pump inhal (G)
  asthma, 38
EpiPen, EpiPen Jr, *epinephrine* (G)
  anaphylaxis, 21
  status asthmaticus, 579
epithelioid sarcoma
  tazemetostat, Tazverik, 88
Epivir-HBV, *lamivudine* (G)
  dose forms, 705
  hepatitis B, 293
eplerenone, Inspra
  heart failure, 280
  hypertension, 332
epoetin alfa-epbx, Retacrit
  anemia of chronic kidney disease, 23
epoetin alpha, Epogen, Procrit (G)
  anemia of chronic kidney disease, 23
Epogen, *epoetin alpha*
  anemia of chronic kidney disease, 23
eprosartan, Teveten (G)
  hypertension, 330
Epzicom, *abacavir sulfate+lamivudine*
  dose forms, 696
  human immunodeficiency virus infection, 315
Equagesic, *meprobamate+aspirin* (IV)
  muscle strain, 404
  temporomandibular joint disorder, 587
Equetro, *carbamazepine* (G)
  bipolar disorder, 61
  dose forms, 694
eravacycline, Xerava
  complicated intra-abdominal infection, 364
erdafitinib, Balversa
  urothelial carcinoma, 133–134
erectile dysfunction (ED)
  alprostadil, Caverject, Edex, Muse, 237–238
  avanafil, Stendra, 237
  sildenafil citrate, Viagra, 237
  tadalafil, Cialis, 237
  vardenafil (as HCl), Staxyn, 237
  vardenafil, Levitra, 237
erenumab-aooe, Aimovig
  migraine and cluster headache, 273
ergoloid mesylate, Hydergine (G)
  Alzheimer's disease, 15
ergotamine
  migraine and cluster headache, 270
Erleada, *apalutamide*

prostate cancer, 129
ertapenem, Invanz
  pneumonia, 494
  urinary tract infection, 645
Ertaczo, *sertaconazole*
  tinea pedis, 600
ertugliflozin, Steglatro *(G)*
  type 2 diabetes mellitus, 627
EryPed, *erythromycin ethylsuccinate,* 408,
  709, 718
  acne vulgaris, 5
  acute exacerbation of chronic
    bronchitis, 70
  acute tonsillitis, 604
  bacterial skin infection, 574
  cat scratch fever, 141
  cellulitis, 144
  chancroid, 147
  Chlamydia trachomatis, 152
  chlamydial conjunctivitis, 164
  chlamydial ophthalmia neonatorum,
    423
  chlamydial pneumonia, 492
  cholera *(Vibrio cholerae),* 156
  dental abscess, 191
  diphtheria, 215
  erysipelas, 238
  gonococcal conjunctivitis, 165
  granuloma inguinale, 266
  hidradenitis suppurativa, 303–304
  human bite, 67
  impetigo contagiosa, 352
  lymphogranuloma venereum, 384
  mycoplasma pneumonia, 496
  nongonococcal urethritis, 639
  paronychia, 472
  pertussis, 483
  scarlet fever, 560
  streptococcal pharyngitis, 485
  wound, 659
erysipelas
  erythromycin base, Ery-Tab, PCE,
    238
  erythromycin ethylsuccinate, EryPed,
    E.E.S, 238
  penicillin v potassium, Pen-Vee K, 238
Ery-Tab, *erythromycin base*
  acne vulgaris, 5
  acute exacerbation of chronic
    bronchitis, 70
  acute tonsillitis, 604
  bacterial skin infection, 574
  cat scratch fever, 141
  cellulitis, 144
  chancroid, 147
  Chlamydia trachomatis, 152
  chlamydial conjunctivitis, 164
  chlamydial ophthalmia neonatorum,
    423
  chlamydial pneumonia, 492
  cholera *(Vibrio cholerae),* 156
  dental abscess, 191
  diphtheria, 215
  erysipelas, 238
  gonococcal conjunctivitis, 165
  granuloma inguinale, 266
  hidradenitis suppurativa, 303–304
  human bite, 67
  impetigo contagiosa, 352
  lymphogranuloma venereum, 384
  mycoplasma pneumonia, 496
  nongonococcal urethritis, 639
  paronychia, 472
  pertussis, 483
  scarlet fever, 560
  streptococcal pharyngitis, 485
  wound, 659
erythromycin base, Ery-Tab, PCE
  acne vulgaris, 5

acute exacerbation of chronic
  bronchitis, 70
acute tonsillitis, 604
bacterial skin infection, 574
cat scratch fever, 141
cellulitis, 144
chancroid, 147
Chlamydia trachomatis, 152
chlamydial conjunctivitis, 164
chlamydial ophthalmia neonatorum,
  423
chlamydial pneumonia, 492
cholera *(Vibrio cholerae),* 156
dental abscess, 191
diphtheria, 215
erysipelas, 238
gonococcal conjunctivitis, 165
granuloma inguinale, 266
hidradenitis suppurativa, 303
human bite, 67
impetigo contagiosa, 352
lymphogranuloma venereum, 384
mycoplasma pneumonia, 496
nongonococcal urethritis, 639
paronychia, 472
pertussis, 483
scarlet fever, 560
streptococcal pharyngitis, 485
wound, 659
erythromycin estolate, Ilosone, 717–718
  bacterial endocarditis prophylaxis, 55
  bacterial skin infection, 574
  community-acquired pneumonia, 494
  dose form/volume, 708
  legionella pneumonia, 496
  scarlet fever, 560
  streptococcal pharyngitis, 485
erythromycin ethylsuccinate, EryPed,
  E.E.S
  acne vulgaris, 5
  acute exacerbation of chronic
    bronchitis, 70
  acute tonsillitis, 604
  bacterial skin infection, 574
  cat scratch fever, 141
  cellulitis, 144
  chancroid, 147
  Chlamydia trachomatis, 152
  chlamydial conjunctivitis, 164
  chlamydial ophthalmia neonatorum,
    423
  chlamydial pneumonia, 492
  cholera *(Vibrio cholerae),* 156
  dental abscess, 191
  diphtheria, 215
  erysipelas, 238
  gonococcal conjunctivitis, 165
  granuloma inguinale, 266
  hidradenitis suppurativa, 303–304
  human bite, 67
  impetigo contagiosa, 352
  lymphogranuloma venereum, 384
  mycoplasma pneumonia, 496
  nongonococcal urethritis, 639
  paronychia, 472
  pertussis, 483
  scarlet fever, 560
  streptococcal pharyngitis, 485
  wound, 659
erythromycin, Ilotycin
  bacterial conjunctivitis, 162
  blepharitis, 67
  chlamydial ophthalmia neonatorum,
    423
  gonococcal ophthalmia neonatorum,
    423
  stye (hordeolum), 580
erythromycin, Isopto Cetamide
  Ophthalmic Solution

stye (hordeolum), 580
Eryzole, *erythromycin+sulfisoxazole* (G),
  719
  otitis media: acute, 447
Esbriet, *pirfenidone* (G)
  idiopathic pulmonary fibrosis, 535
escitalopram, Lexapro, Lexapro Oral
  Solution (G)
  anxiety disorder, 35
  major depressive disorder, 192
  panic disorder, 464
  posttraumatic stress disorder, 510
Esidrix, *hydrochlorothiazide*
  edema, 228
  heart failure, 281
  hypertension, primary, 327
  urolithiasis, 646
Esimil, *guanethidine+hydrochlorothiazide*
  hypertension, 335
Eskata, hydrogen peroxide 40% (G)
  seborrheic dermatitis, 205
esomeprazole, Nexium
  gastroesophageal reflux disease, 250
  peptic ulcer disease (PUD), 478
  Zollinger-Ellison syndrome, 662
Esperoct, *turoctocog alfa pegol, N8-GP*
  hemophilia A, 287
estazolam, ProSom (IV)
  insomnia, 359
Estrace Vaginal Cream, *estradiol*
  atrophic vaginitis, 49
estradiol, acetate, Femring Vaginal Ring
  menopause, 390
estradiol, Alora, Climara, Esclim,
  Estrace, Estrasorb, EstroGel,
  Estraderm, Imvexxy Menostar,
  Minivelle, Vivelle, Vivelle-Dot,
  Vagifem Tabs, Yuvafem Vaginal
  Tablet (G)
  atrophic vaginitis, 49
  dyspareunia, 226
  menopause, 391–393
  osteoporosis, 341
estradiol, micronized, Estrace Vaginal
  Cream (G)
  menopause, 390
estrogen, conjugated (synthetic), Cenestin,
  Enjuvia
  menopause, 392
estrogen, conjugated, Premarin
  atrophic vaginitis, 49
  menopause, 390, 392
  osteoporosis, 440
estrogen, esterified (plant derived),
  Estratab, Menest
  menopause, 391, 392
estropipate, Ogen Cream
  atrophic vaginitis, 49
estropipate, piperazine estrone sulfate,
  Ogen, Ortho-Est
  atrophic vaginitis, 49
  menopause, 391–392
  osteoporosis, 440
Estrostep Fe, *ethinyl estradiol+*
  norethindrone plus ferrous
  fumarate
  estrogen and progesterone, 668
eszopiclone, Lunesta (G)(IV)
  fibromyalgia, 244
  insomnia, 359
etabonate, Alrex Ophthalmic Solution
  (G)
  eye pain, 241
etanercept, Enbrel, Eticovo
  juvenile idiopathic arthritis, 371
  osteoarthritis, 438
  plaque psoriasis, 525
  psoriatic arthritis, 530
  rheumatoid arthritis, 547

etanercept-ykro, Eticovo
  osteoarthritis (OA), 438
  psoriatic arthritis, 530
  rheumatoid arthritis (RA), 547
etelcalcetide, Parsabiv
  hyperhidrosis, 321
eteplirsen, Exondys
  duchenne muscular dystrophy
    (DMD), 219
ethacrynate sodium, Sodium Edecrin
  edema, 228–229
  heart failure, 281
  hypertension, 328
ethacrynic acid, Edecrin
  edema, 228
  heart failure, 281
  hypertension, primary, 328
ethambutol (EMB), Myambutol
  tuberculosis, 610
ethinyl estradiol, Estinyl
  menopause, 391, 392
Eticovo, etanercept
  juvenile idiopathic arthritis (JIA), 371
  osteoarthritis (OA), 438
  psoriatic arthritis, 530
  rheumatoid arthritis (RA), 547
etonogestrel, Implanon, Nexplanon, 675
Etrafon, perphenazine+amitriptyline (G)
  anxiety disorder, 36
etravirine, Intelence, 594
  dose forms, 697
  human immunodeficiency virus
    infection, 310
Eucerin Facial Lotion
  atopic dermatitis, 197
  psoriasis, 526
  xerosis, 661
Eucerin Original Creme (OTC)
  atopic dermatitis, 197
  psoriasis, 526
  xerosis, 661
Eucerin Protective Lotion (OTC)
  atopic dermatitis, 197
  psoriasis, 526
  xerosis, 661
Eucrisa, *crisaborole* (G)
  atopic dermatitis, 197
Euflexx, *sodium hyaluronate*
  osteoarthritis, 437
Eulexin, *flutamide,* 685
Eurax, *crotamiton* (G)
  scabies, 559
Evekeo, *amphetamine, mixed salts of
    single entity amphetamine* (G)(II)
  attention deficit hyperactivity disorder
    (ADHD), 51
  narcolepsy, 409
  obesity, 418
Evenity, *romosozumab-aqqg*
  osteoporosis, 443–444
everolimus, Zortress (G)
  organ transplant rejection prophylaxis,
    432
Evoclin Foam, *clindamycin*
  acne vulgaris, 4
  folliculitis barbae, 246
evinacumab-dgnb, Evkeeza
  dyslipidemia, 220–221
Evkeeza, evinacumab-dgnb
  dyslipidemia, 220–221
evolocumab, Repatha
  dyslipidemia, 221
Evotaz, *atazanavir+cobicistat*
  dose form, 696
  human immunodeficiency virus
    infection, 315
Evoxac, *cevimeline* (G)
  Sjögren-Larsson-syndrome (SLS),
    572

Evrysdi, *risdiplam*
  spinal muscular atrophy (SMA), 578
Evzio, *naloxone*
  opioid overdose, 431
exanthem subitum, 557
Excedrin Migraine (OTC),
    acetaminophen+aspirin+caffeine
  migraine and cluster headache, 272
Excedrin PM, *acetaminophen+
    diphenhydramine*
  insomnia, 360
excessive daytime sleepiness (EDS),
    409–413. See also narcolepsy
exocrine pancreas insufficiency (EPI).
    See pancreatic enzyme deficiency
Exelderm, *sulconazole* (G)
  tinea corporis, 598
  tinea cruris, 599
  tinea pedis, 600
  tinea versicolor, 601
Exelon, *rivastigmine*
  Alzheimer's disease, 15
exenatide, Bydureon, Byetta (G)
  type 2 diabetes mellitus, 623–624
Exforge 5/160, *amlodipine+valsartan
    medoxomil*
  hypertension, 336
Exforge HCT, *amlodipine+valsartan
    medoxomil+hydrochlorothiazide*
  hypertension, 337
Exjade, *deferasirox (tridentate ligand)* (G)
  iron overload, 365
Exondys, *eteplirsen*
  duchenne muscular dystrophy
    (DMD), 219
expressive aphasia
  zolpidem, Ambien (IV), 36
  zolpidem, Edluar, Intermezzo,
    ZolpiMist (G)(IV), 36–37
Exsel Shampoo, *selenium sulfide* (G)
  seborrheic dermatitis, 205
Exservan, *riluzole*
  amyotrophic lateral sclerosis (ALS), 19
Extra Strength Bayer Plus,
    aspirin+antacid
  fever (pyrexia), 242
extrapyramidal side effects (EPS)
  amantadine, Osmolex ER, 240
eye pain
  diclofenac, Voltaren Ophthalmic
    Solution, 241
  difluprednate, Durezol Ophthalmic
    Solution (G), 241
  eoteprednol etabonate, Inveltys (G),
    241
  etabonate, Alrex Ophthalmic Solution
    (G), 241
  ketorolac tromethamine, Acular,
    Acular LS, Acular PF (G), 241
  nepafenac, Nevanac Ophthalmic
    Suspension (G), 241
Eylea, *aflibercept* (G)
  diabetic retinopathy, 206
Eysuvis, *loteprednol etabonate*
  dry eye syndrome, 218
ezetimibe, Zetia (G)
  dyslipidemia, 220

facial hair: excessive/unwanted
  eflornithine, Vaniqa (G), 241
facial wrinkles
  adapalene, Differin (G), 660
  prabotulinumtoxinA-xvfs, Jeuveau, 660
  tazarotene, Avage, Tazorac, 660
  tretinoin, Altreno, Atralin, Avita,
    Retin-A, Tretin-X (G), 660
Factive, *gemifloxacin* (G)
  acute exacerbation of chronic
    bronchitis, 70

fallopian tube cancer
  bevacizumab-adcd, Vegzelma, 90
  mirvetuximab soravtansine-gynx,
    Elahere, 89–90
  niraparib tosylate, Zejula, 88
  olaparib, Lynparza, 89
famciclovir, Famvir, 705
  herpes genitalis (HSV TYPE II), 300
  herpes zoster, 301
  herpes zoster ophthmicus, 303
famotidine, Pepcid
  gastroesophageal reflux disease,
    249–250
  peptic ulcer disease (PUD), 478
fam-trastuzumab deruxtecan-nxki,
    Enhertu
  breast cancer, 83
Famvir, *famciclovir*
  herpes genitalis (HSV TYPE II), 300
  herpes zoster, 301
  herpes zoster ophthmicus, 303
Fareston, *toremifene,* 585
  dose forms, 685
  breast cancer, 85
Farxiga, *dapagliflozin* (G)
  heart failure, 279
Fasenra, *benralizumab*
  asthma, 49
  eosinophilia, 49
Faslodex, *fulvestrant,* 585
  dose forms, 685
  breast cancer, 78
febuxostat, Uloric (G)
  gout (hyperuricemia), 260
fecal incontinence
  *dextranomer microspheres+sodium
    hyaluronate,* Solesta, 353
fecal microbiota, live-jslm, Rebyota
  clostridioides difficile infection (CDI),
    157–158
fecal odor
  bismuth subgallate powder, Devron,
    241
fedratinib, Inrebic
  myelofibrosis, 408
felodipine, Plendil (G)
  hypertension, 331
Femara, *letrozole,* 585
  dose forms, 685
  breast cancer, 78
Femcon Fe, *ethinyl estradiol+
    norethindrone plus ferrous
    fumarate*
  estrogen and progesterone, 668
Femstat-3 Vaginal Cream (OTC),
    butoconazole cream 2% (G)
  vulvovaginal (moniliasis) candidiasis,
    138
fenofibrate, Antara, Fenoglide, FibriCor,
    TriCor, TriLipix, Lipofen,
    Lofibra (G)
  dyslipidemia, 223
  hypertriglyceridemia, 338
Fenoglide, *fenofibrate* (G)
  dyslipidemia, 223
fentanyl citrate, Actiq, Fentora (G)(II)
  pain, 641
fentanyl, Abstral, Onsolis, Duragesic,
    Lazanda Nasal Spray, Onsolis
    (G)(II)
  pain, 461
  urolithiasis, 648
*fentanyl iontophoretic transdermal
    system,* Ionsys
  pain, 461
fentanyl sublingual spray, Subsys (G)(II)
  pain, 461
fentanyl sublingual tab, Abstral (G)(II)
  pain, 461

Feosol, *ferrous sulfate* (A)
  iron deficiency anemia, 25
Fergon, *ferrous gluconate* (A)
  iron deficiency anemia, 25
Fer-In-Sol, *ferrous sulfate* (A)
  iron deficiency anemia, 25
ferric citrate, Aurexia
  anemia of chronic kidney disease, 22
  hyperphosphatemia, 324
ferrous gluconate, Fergon (A), 25
  iron deficiency anemia, 25
ferrous sulfate, Feosol, Fer-In-Sol (A)
  iron deficiency anemia, 25
fesoterodine, Toviaz (G)
  urinary overactive bladder, 354
Fetroja, *cefiderocol*
  complicated urinary tract infection
    (CUTI), 640
  hospital-acquired bacterial
    pneumonia (HABP), 490
  ventilator-associated bacterial
    pneumonia (VABP), 491–492
Fetzima, *levomilnacipran* (G)
  major depressive disorder, 192
fever (pyrexia)
  acetaminophen, Ofirmev, Children's
    Tylenol, Extra Strength Tylenol,
    FeverAll Extra Strength Tylenol,
    Maximum Strength Tylenol Sore
    Throat, Tylenol, 241, 242
  aspirin, Bayer, 242
  aspirin+antacid, Extra Strength Bayer
    Plus, Bufferin, 242
  aspirin+caffeine, Anacin, 242
  ibuprofen, Advil, Children's Advil,
    ElixSure IB, Motrin, Nuprin,
    PediaCare, PediaProfen, 242–243
  naproxen, Aleve, Anaprox,
    EC-Naprosyn, Naprelan,
    Naprosyn, 243
Fexmid, *cyclobenzaprine*
  fibromyalgia, 244
  muscle strain, 403
  temporomandibular joint disorder,
    586
fexofenadine, Allegra (G)
  allergic rhinitis/sinusitis, 550
  atopic dermatitis, 198
  contact dermatitis, 202
  genus rhus dermatitis, 204
  rhinitis medicamentosa, 555
  urticaria, 649
FiberCon, *calcium polycarbophil* (G)
  acute diarrhea, 169
  occasional constipation, 211
FibriCor, *fenofibrate* (G)
  dyslipidemia, 223
  hypertriglyceridemia, 338
fibrocystic breast disease
  danazol, Danocrine, 243
  spironolactone, Aldactone, CaroSpir,
    243
  vitamin B6 (A), 243
  vitamin E (A), 243
fibromyalgia
  amitriptyline (G), 244
  cyclobenzaprine, Amrix, Fexmid,
    Flexeril, 245
  duloxetine, Cymbalta (G), 244
  eszopiclone, Lunesta (G)(IV), 244–245
  flurazepam, Dalmane (IV), 245
  gabapentin enacarbil, Horizant (G),
    244
  gabapentin, Gralise, Neurontin (G),
    244
  milnacipran, Savella (G), 244
  pregabalin (GABA analog), Lyrica,
    Lyrica CR (G)(V), 244
  trazodone, Desyrel (G), 245

triazolam, Halcion (IV)(G), 245
zaleplon, Sonata (IV), 245
zolpidem, Ambien, Ambien CR, 245
zolpidem, Edluar, Intermezzo,
  ZolpiMist (G)(IV), 245
fidaxomicin, Dificid
  Clostridioides difficile infection, 156
fifth disease, 245
filgrastim
  neutropenia, 417
filgrastim-aafi
  neutropenia, 417
filgrastim-cbqv (G)
  neutropenia, 417
filgrastim-sndz (G)
  neutropenia, 418
Finacea, *azelaic acid*
  acne rosacea, 3
  acne vulgaris, 4
finafloxacin, Xtoro (G)
  otitis externa, 444
finasteride, Proscar, Propecia
  baldness: male pattern, 57
  benign prostatic hyperplasia, 58
  urinary overactive bladder, 356
fingolimod, Gilenya (G)
  multiple sclerosis (MS), 398
Fioricet, *butalbital+acetaminophen+*
  caffeine (G)
  tension headache, 277
Fioricet with Codeine, *butalbital+*
  acetaminophen+codeine+caffeine
  (G)(III)
  tension headache, 277
Fioricet, Zebutal, *butalbital+*
  acetaminophen+caffeine (G)
  pain, 455
  tension headache, 277
Fiorinal, *butalbital+aspirin+caffeine*
  (G)(III)
  pain, 455
  tension headache, 277
Fiorinal with Codeine, *butalbital+*
  aspirin+codeine+caffeine (G)(III)
  pain, 455
  tension headache, 277
Firazyr, *icatibant* (G)
  hereditary angioedema, 298
Firvanq, *vancomycin hcl oral solution*, 770
  Clostridioides difficile infection, 157
  pseudomembranous colitis, 519
Flagyl, Flagyl 375, Flagyl ER,
  metronidazole (G), 703, 705
  amebiasis, 17
  amebic liver abscess, 17
  bacterial vaginosis, 56
  Crohn's disease, 175
  diverticulitis, 216
  giardiasis, 254
  nongonococcal urethritis, 639
  pelvic inflammatory disease, 476
  pseudomembranous colitis, 519
  sexual assault, 567
  trichomoniasis, 606
Flarex, *fluorometholone acetate* (G)
  allergic (vernal) conjunctivitis, 166
flatulence
  simethicone, Gas-X, Mylicon,
    Phazyme-95 (G), 245
flavoxate, Urispas
  urinary tract infection, 642
  urolithiasis, 647
Fleets Adult, Fleets Pediatric, *sodium*
  biphosphate+sodium phosphate
  enema (G)
  occasional constipation, 171
Flexeril, *cyclobenzaprine*
  fibromyalgia, 244
  muscle strain, 403

temporomandibular joint disorder,
  586
flibanserin, Addyi
  low libido, hypoactive sexual desire
    disorder (HSDD), 380
Flomax, *tamsulosin*
  benign prostatic hyperplasia, 58
  urinary overactive bladder, 356
  urolithiasis, 647
Floxin, *ofloxacin* (G), 708
  acute exacerbation of chronic
    bronchitis, 70
  acute prostatitis, 516
  bacterial skin infection, 575
  Chlamydia trachomatis, 152
  chronic prostatitis, 517
  community-acquired pneumonia, 494
  epididymitis, 237
  Hansen's disease, 270
  nongonococcal urethritis, 639
  otitis externa, 444
  otitis media: acute, 447
  shigellosis, 567
  typhoid fever, 633
  urinary tract infection, 645
  wound, 660
Fluarix, *trivalent inactivated influenza*
  subvirion vaccine, types a
  and b (G)
  influenza, seasonal (FLU), 356–357
Flublok, *trivalent inactivated influenza*
  subvirion vaccine, types a
  and b (G)
  influenza, seasonal (FLU), 356–357
fluconazole, Diflucan (G), 719
  oral (thrush) candidiasis, 135
  vulvovaginal (moniliasis) candidiasis,
    138
FluLaval, *trivalent inactivated influenza*
  subvirion vaccine, types a
  and b (G)
  influenza, seasonal (FLU), 356–357
FluMist Nasal Spray, *trivalent, live*
  attenuated influenza vaccine,
    types A and B (G)
  influenza, seasonal (FLU), 356
flunisolide, AeroBid, AeroBid-M,
  Aerospan HFA, Nasalide, Nasarel
  (G), 680
  allergic rhinitis/sinusitis, 552
  asthma, 41
  polyps, nasal, 506
fluocinolone acetonide, Derma-Smoothe/
  FS Shampoo, Derma-Smoothe/
  FS Topical Oil fluocinolone
  acetonide, Synalar (G), 575
  atopic dermatitis, 198
  pruritus, 517
  seborrheic dermatitis, 205
  xerosis, 661
fluoridation, water
  fluoride, Luride (G), 246
  fluoride+vitamin a+vitamin d+
    vitamin c, Tri-Vi-Flor Drops (G),
    246
  fluoride+vitamin a+vitamin d+
    vitamin c+iron, Tri-Vi-Flor w.
    Iron Drops, 246
fluoride, Luride (G)
  fluoridation, water, 246
fluorometholone acetate, Flarex (G)
  allergic (vernal) conjunctivitis, 166
fluorometholone, FML, FML Forte, FML
  S.O.P. Ointment (G)
  allergic (vernal) conjunctivitis, 165
Fluoroplex, *fluorouracil*
  actinic keratosis, 9
fluorouracil, Carac, Efudex, Fluoroplex
  actinic keratosis, 9

fluoxetine, Prozac, Prozac Weekly (G)
  anxiety disorder, 35
  bulimia nervosa, 75
  major depressive disorder, 192
  migraine and cluster headache, 276
  obsessive-compulsive disorder, 421
  panic disorder, 464
  premenstrual dysphoric disorder, 514
  trichotillomania, 607
fluoxymesterone, Halotestin (III)
  testosterone deficiency, 588
fluphenazine decanoate [Prolixin Decanoate] (G), 693
  methamphetamine-induced psychosis, 395
fluphenazine hcl [Prolixin] (G)
  methamphetamine-induced psychosis, 395
flurazepam, Dalmane (IV)
  fibromyalgia, 245
  insomnia, 359
FluShield, *trivalent inactivated influenza subvirion vaccine, types a and b* (G)
  influenza, seasonal (FLU), 356–357
fluticasone furoate, Arnuity Ellipta, Veramyst (G)
  allergic rhinitis/sinusitis, 552
  asthma, 41
  polyps, nasal, 506
fluticasone propionate, ArmorAir, Flonase, Flovent, Flovent HFA, Flovent Diskus (G), 580
  allergic rhinitis/sinusitis, 552
  asthma, 41
  polyps, nasal, 506
  strength and volume, 677
fluvastatin, Lescol, Lescol XL
  dyslipidemia, 222
  hypertriglyceridemia, 339
fluvoxamine, Luvox (G)
  obsessive-compulsive disorder, 421
  trichotillomania, 607
Fluzone, *trivalent inactivated influenza subvirion vaccine, types a and b* (G)
  influenza, seasonal (FLU), 357
FML, FML Forte, FML S.O.P. Ointment, *fluorometholone* (G)
  allergic (vernal) conjunctivitis, 165
FML-S, *sulfacetamide sodium+ fluorometholone suspension* (G)
  bacterial conjunctivitis, 164
Focalin, *dexmethylphenidate* (G)(II)
  attention deficit hyperactivity disorder (ADHD), 51
  narcolepsy, 412
folic acid (A)(OTC)
  folic acid deficiency, 24
folic acid deficiency
  folic acid (A)(OTC), 24
folliculitis barbae
  benzoyl peroxide, Benzac-W, Benzac-W Wash, Benzagel, Benzagel Wash, Desquam X, Triaz, ZoDerm (G), 246
  clindamycin, Cleocin T, Clindagel, Clindets, Evoclin, 246
  clindamycin+benzoyl peroxide, Acanya, BenzaClin, Duac, Onexton Gel, 246
  dapsone, Aczone (G), 247
  tazarotene, Avage, Tazorac, 247
  tretinoin, Altreno, Atralin, Avita, Retin-A, Tretin-X (G), 247
Foradil Aerolizer, *formoterol fumarate* (G)
  asthma, 43

foreign body: esophagus
  glucagon, Glucagon, 247
foreign body: eye
  proparacaine, Ophthaine, 247
Forfivo XL, *bupropion HCl* (G)
  attention deficit hyperactivity disorder (ADHD), 54
  dose forms, 693
  major depressive disorder, 193
  tobacco dependence, 602
formoterol fumarate, Foradil Aerolizer, Perforomist (G)
  asthma, 43
Forteo, *teriparatide* (G)
  hypoparathyroidism, 344
Fortesta, *testosterone* (III)
  testosterone deficiency, 590
Fosamax, *alendronate (as sodium)* (G)
  osteoporosis, 441
  Paget's disease, 450
Fosamax Plus D, *alendronate+ cholecalciferol (vit d3)* (G)
  osteoporosis, 441
  Paget's disease, 450
fosamprenavir, Lexiva (G), 697
  human immunodeficiency virus infection, 311
fosfomycin, Monurol
  dose forms, 710
  urinary tract infection, 644
fosinopril, Monopril (G)
  heart failure, 279
  hypertension, 329
fosnetupitant and palonosetron, Akynzeo
  chemotherapy-induced nausea/ vomiting, 148, 413
Fosrenol, *lanthanum carbonate* (G)
  hyperphosphatemia, 325
fostamatinib disodium hexahydrate, Tavalisse
  idiopathic thrombocytopenia purpura, 348, 594
fostemsavir, Rukobia
  human immunodeficiency virus (HIV) infection, 312
fremanezumab-vfrm, Ajovy
  migraine and cluster headache, 273
frovatriptan, Frova (G)
  migraine and cluster headache, 270
Fulphila, *pegfilgrastim-jmd*
  neutropenia, 416
fulvestrant, Faslodex
  breast cancer, 78
  dose forms, 685
fungal conjunctivitis
  natamycin, Natacyn Ophthalmic Suspension (G), 165
Fungizone, *amphotericin b*
  skin candidiasis, 136
furazolidone, Furoxone liquid, 719
furosemide, Lasix (G)
  edema, 229
  heart failure, 281
  hypertension, 328
futibatinib, Lytgobi
  hepatocellular carcinoma (HCC), 101

gabapentin enacarbil, Horizant (G)
  diabetic peripheral neuropathy (DPN), 210
  fibromyalgia, 244
  post-herpetic neuralgia, 507
  restless legs syndrome, 540
gabapentin, Gralise, Neurontin (G)
  diabetic peripheral neuropathy (DPN), 209–210
  fibromyalgia, 244
  post-herpetic neuralgia, 507
  restless legs syndrome, 540

galantamine, Razadyne
  Alzheimer's disease, 15
galcanezumab-gnlm, Emgality
  migraine and cluster headache, 273
GamaSTAN S/D, *immune globulin (human)* (G)
  chickenpox (Varicella), 149
  hepatitis A, 291
  rubella, 558
  rubeola, 558–559
ganciclovir, Zirga (G)
  herpes simplex keratitis, 374
Garamycin Ophthalmic Ointment, *gentamicin sulfate* (G)
  bacterial conjunctivitis, 162
  stye, 580
Gardasil 9, *human papillomavirus 9-valent (types 6, 11, 16, 18, 31, 33, 45, 52, and 58) vaccine, recombinant, aluminum adsorbed*
  human papillomavirus (HPV), 318
gastritis/dyspepsia, 247
gastritis-related nausea/vomiting
  ondansetron, Zofran, Zuplenz (G), 247
  phosphorylated carbohydrate solution, Emetrol (G), 247
  promethazine, Phenergan (G), 248
gastroesophageal reflux disease (GERD)
  aluminum hydroxide, ALTernaGEL, Amphojel (G), 248
  aluminum hydroxide+magnesium carbonate, Maalox HRF (G), 248
  aluminum hydroxide+magnesium hydroxide+simethicone, Maalox Plus, Extra Strength Maalox Plus, Mylanta (G), 249
  aluminum hydroxide+magnesium trisilicate, Gaviscon (G), 248–249
  calcium carbonate, Rolaids, Tums, Os-Cal 500 (G), 249
  calcium carbonate+magnesium carbonate, Mylanta Gel (G), 249
  calcium carbonate+magnesium hydroxide, Mylanta, Rolaids Sodium (G), 249
  cimetidine, Tagamet, 249
  dexlansoprazole, Dexilant, 250
  dihydroxyaluminum, Rolaids (OTC), 249
  esomeprazole, Nexium, 250
  famotidine, Pepcid, 249–250
  lansoprazole, Prevacid, 250
  Maalox, *aluminum hydroxide+ magnesium hydroxide* (G), 249
  metoclopramide, Metozolv ODT, Reglan, 251
  nizatidine, Axid, 250
  omeprazole, Prilosec (G), 250–251
  pantoprazole, Protonix, 251
  rabeprazole, AcipHex, 251
  ranitidine bismuth citrate, Tritec (G), 250
  ranitidine, Zantac, 250
gastrointestinal stromal tumor (GIST)
  avapritinib, Ayvakit, 91
  ripretinib, Qinlock, 91
  sunitinib malate, Sutent, 91–92
Gas-X, *simethicone* (G)
  flatulence, 245
gatifloxacin, Zymar Ophthalmic Solution, Zymaxid Ophthalmic Solution (G)
  bacterial conjunctivitis, 162
Gaucher disease, type 1 (GD1)
  eliglustat tartrate, Cerdelga (G), 251
  miglustat, Zavesca (G), 252
  penicillamine, Cuprimine, Depen (G), 252
  trientine, Syprine (G), 253

Gaviscon, *aluminum hydroxide+ magnesium trisilicate* (G)
gastroesophageal reflux disease, 248–249
gefitinib, Iressa (G)
lung cancer, 105
GelnIQUE, *oxybutynin chloride*
hyperhidrosis, 320
urinary overactive bladder, 355
Gel-One, *sodium hyaluronate*
osteoarthritis, 437
GelSyn-3, *sodium hyaluronate*
osteoarthritis, 437
gemfibrozil, Lopid
dyslipidemia, 233
hypertriglyceridemia, 338
gemifloxacin, Factive (G), 708
acute exacerbation of chronic bronchitis, 70
bacterial skin infection, 575
community-acquired pneumonia, 494
wound, 660
Generess Fe Chew tab, *ethinyl estradiol+norethindrone plus ferrous fumarate*
estrogen and progesterone, 669
Genoptic Ophthalmic Ointment, *gentamicin sulfate* (G)
bacterial conjunctivitis, 182
stye, 580
Genora, *ethinyl estradiol+norethindrone*
estrogen and progesterone, 669
Genotropin, *somatropin*
growth failure, 266–267
Genotropin Miniquick, *somatropin*
growth failure, 267
Gentacidin Ophthalmic Ointment, *gentamicin sulfate* (G)
bacterial conjunctivitis, 162
gentamicin sulfate, Garamycin Ophthalmic Ointment, Genoptic Ophthalmic Ointment, Gentacidin Ophthalmic Ointment (G)
bacterial conjunctivitis, 162
stye (hordeolum), 580
GenTeal Mild, GenTeal Moderate, GenTeal Severe, *hydroxypropyl methylcellulose*
dry eye syndrome, 217
gentian violet (G)
oral (thrush) candidiasis, 135
Gentlax, *bisacodyl*
occasional constipation, 170
genus rhus dermatitis
Aveeno (OTC), 127
bentoquatam, IvyBlock (OTC), 203
cetirizine, Children's Zyrtec Chewable, Children's Zyrtec Allergy Syrup, Zyrtec (G), 203
desloratadine, Clarinex, Desloratadine ODT (G), 203
diphenhydramine, Benadryl, 204
fexofenadine, Allegra (G), 204
hydroxyzine, Atarax, Vistaril (G), 204
levocetirizine, Children's Xyzal Allergy 24HR, Xyzal Allergy 24HR, 204
loratadine, Claritin (G), 204
GenVisc 850, *sodium hyaluronate*
osteoarthritis, 437
Genvoya, *elvitegravir+cobicistat+ emtricitabine+tenofovir alafenamide,* 697
human immunodeficiency virus infection, 315
Geocillin, *carbenicillin*
chronic prostatitis, 516
dose forms, 707
urinary tract infection, 643

Geodon, *ziprasidone* (G)
bipolar disorder, 64–65
giant cell arteritis (GCA)
tocilizumab, Actemra, 253–254
Gianvi, *ethinyl estradiol+drospirenone,* 669
Giapreza, *angiotensin II*
shock: septic, distributive, 586
giardiasis
metronidazole, Flagyl, Flagyl 375, Flagyl ER (G), 254
nitazoxanide, Alinia, 254
tinidazole, Tindamax (G), 254
Giazo, *balsalazide disodium*
ulcerative colitis, 635
gingivitis/periodontitis
chlorhexidine gluconate, Peridex, PerioGard, 254
Givlaari, *givosiran*
hepatic porphyria, acute (AHP), 291
givosiran, Givlaari
hepatic porphyria, acute (AHP), 291
glatiramer acetate, Copaxone, Glatopa
multiple sclerosis (MS), 398
glaucoma
acetazolamide, Diamox (G), 257
apraclonidine, Iopidine (G), 255
betaxolol, Betoptic, Betoptic S (G), 256
bimatoprost, Lumigan (G), 256
brimonidine tartrate, Alphagan P, 255
brimonidine tartrate+timolol, Combigan, 256
brimonidine+brinzolamide, Simbrinza (G), 255
brinzolamide, Azopt (G), 255
carbachol+hydroxypropyl methylcellulose, Isopto Carbachol (G), 255
carteolol, Ocupress (G), 256
demecarium bromide, Humorsol Ocumeter, 255
dipivefrin, Cosopt, Cosopt PF, 257
dorzolamide, Trusopt (G), 255
dorzolamide+timolol, Cosopt, Cosopt PF (G), 257
echothiophate iodide, Phospholine Iodide, 255
latanoprost, Xalatan, Xelpros (G), 256
latanoprostene bunod, Vyzulta, 257
levobunolol, Betagan (G), 256
methazolamide, Neptazane (G), 257
metipranolol, OptiPranolol (G), 256
netarsudil, Rhopressa (G), 257
netarsudil+latanoprost, Rocklatan, 257
pilocarpine, Isopto Carpine, Ocusert Pilo, Pilocar Ophthalmic Sol, Pilopine HS (G), 255
tafluprost, Zioptan (G), 256
timolol, Betimol, Istalol, Timoptic (G), 256
travoprost, Travatan, Travatan Z (G), 256
unoprostone isopropyl, Rescula (G), 257
Gleevec, *imatinib mesylate,* 685
glimepiride, Amaryl (G)
type 2 diabetes mellitus, 620
glioblastoma multiforme
bevacizumab-adcd, Vegzelma, 92–93
bevacizumab-bvzr, Zirabev, 93
glipizide, Glucotrol, Glucotrol XL (G)
type 2 diabetes mellitus, 620
Gloperba, *colchicine*
gout (hyperuricemia), 260
glucagon, Glucagon
foreign body: esophagus, 247
type 1 diabetes mellitus, 613
type 2 diabetes mellitus, 619
glucagon injection, Gvoke

hypoglycemia: acute, 341–342
glucagon nasal powder, Baqsimi
hypoglycemia: acute, 342
type 1 diabetes mellitus (T1DM), 613
Glucovance, *glyburide+metformin*
type 2 diabetes mellitus, 622
glyburide, DiaBeta, Micronase (G)
type 2 diabetes mellitus, 620
glycerin suppository (A)
encopresis, 232
GlycoLax Powder for Oral Solution, *polyethylene glycol (PEG)* (G)
occasional constipation, 170
glycopyrrolate inhalation solution, Lonhala Magnair, Seebri Neohaler (G)
chronic obstructive pulmonary disease (COPD), 71–72
emphysema, 230
glycopyrrolate, Robinul
peptic ulcer disease (PUD), 479
glycopyrronium, Qbrexza
hyperhidrosis, 320
Gly-Oxide, *carbamide peroxide* (A)
aphthous stomatitis, 37
denture irritation, 191
Glyquin, *hydroquinone+padimate o+oxybenzone+octyl methoxycinnamate* (G)
hyperpigmentation, 325
vitiligo, 653
Glyxambi, *empagliflozin+linagliptin* (G)
type 2 diabetes mellitus, 628
Gocovri, *amantadine* (G)
benign essential tremor, 58
extrapyramidal side effects (EPS), 240
Parkinson's disease, 468
golimumab, Simponi
juvenile idiopathic arthritis, 371
psoriasis, 525
psoriatic arthritis, 530
rheumatoid arthritis, 547
golodirsen, Vyondys
duchenne muscular dystrophy (DMD), 219
duchenne muscular dystrophy (DMD), 219
gonococcal conjunctivitis
azithromycin, Zithromax, Zmax, 165
ceftriaxone, Rocephin, 165
erythromycin base, Ery-Tab, PCE, 165
erythromycin ethylsuccinate, EryPed, E.E.S, 165
gonococcal ophthalmia neonatorum
ceftriaxone, Rocephin, 423
erythromycin, Ilotycin, 423
gonococcal pharyngitis
azithromycin, Zithromax, Zmax, 483
ceftriaxone, Rocephin, 483
gonorrhea
azithromycin, Zithromax, Zmax, 258
cefotaxime, Claforan, 259
cefoxitin, Mefoxin Injectable, 259
cefpodoxime proxetil, Vantin, 259
ceftibuten, Cedax, 259
ceftriaxone, Rocephin, 259
demeclocycline, Declomycin, 259
doxycycline, Acticlate, Adoxa, Doryx, Doxteric, Monodox, Oracea, Vibramycin, Vibra-Tab, 256
enoxacin, Penetrex, 259
imipramine, Maxaquin (G), 259
norfloxacin, Noroxin (G), 259
probenecid, Benemid, 259
spectinomycin, Trobicin, 259
goserelin (GnRH analog), Zoladex, 692
endometriosis, 233
gout (hyperuricemia)
allopurinol, Zyloprim (G), 260
allopurinol+lesinurad, Duzallo, 261

gout (hyperuricemia)(cont.)
  colchicine, Colcrys, Mitigare (G), 260
  febuxostat, Uloric (G), 260
  lesinurad, Zurampic (G), 261
  pegloticase, Krystexxa (G), 260
  probenecid (G), 260
  probenecid+colchicine (G), 260
  sulfinpyrazone, Anturane (G), 260
gouty arthritis
  capsaicin 8% patch, Qutenza, 262
  capsaicin, Axsain, Capsin, Capzasin-HP,
    Capzasin-P, Dolorac, Double Cap
    (OTC), R-Gel, Zostrix, Zostrix
    HP, 261–262
  celecoxib, Celebrex (G), 263
  Decadron Phosphate with Xylocaine,
    lidocaine+dexamethasone, 262
  diclofenac sodium, Pennsaid, Solaraze
    Gel, Voltaren Gel (G), 262
  doxepin, Prudoxin, Zonalon, 262
  Emla Cream, *lidocaine 2.5%+*
    prilocaine 2.5%, 262
  esomeprazole+naproxen, Vimovo
    (G), 263
  indomethacin (G), 263
  LidaMantle HC, *lidocaine+*
    hydrocortisone, 262
  lidocaine, LidaMantle, Lidoderm,
    ZTlido lidocaine, 262
  meloxicam, Mobic, Vivlodex (G), 263
  pimecrolimus, Elidel (G), 262
  trolamine salicylate, Mobisyl Creme,
    262
Gralise, *gabapentin* (G), 166
  diabetic peripheral neuropathy
    (DPN), 209–210
  fibromyalgia, 244
  post-herpetic neuralgia, 507
  restless legs syndrome, 540
granisetron, Kytril, Sancuso, Sustol
  cannabinoid hyperemesis syndrome,
    139
  chemotherapy-induced nausea/
    vomiting, 148
  opioid-induced nausea/vomiting, 429
Granix, *tbo-filgrastim*
  neutropenia, 418
Granulex, *trypsin+balsam peru+castor oil*
  diabetic ulcer, 633
  pressure ulcer, 633
granuloma inguinale
  azithromycin, Zithromax, Zmax, 266
  ciprofloxacin, Cipro (G), Cipro XR,
    ProQuin XR (G), 266
  doxycycline, Acticlate, Adoxa, Doryx,
    Doxteric, Monodox, Oracea,
    Vibramycin, Vibra-Tab, 266
  erythromycin base, Ery-Tab, PCE, 266
  erythromycin ethylsuccinate, EryPed,
    E.E.S, 266
  trimethoprim+sulfamethoxazole
    (TMP-SMX), Bactrim, Septra,
    (G), 266
granulomatosis
  rituximab, Rituxan, 265
  rituximab-arrx, Riabni
Grastek, *Timothy grass pollen allergen*
  extract (G)
  allergic rhinitis/sinusitis, 551
Grifulvin V, *griseofulvin, microsize* (G),
    704, 719
  onychomycosis (fungal nail), 422
  tinea capitis, 597
  tinea corporis, 598
  tinea cruris, 599
  tinea pedis, 600–601
griseofulvin, microsize, Grifulvin V (G),
    628
  onychomycosis (fungal nail), 422

tinea capitis, 597
tinea corporis, 598
tinea cruris, 599
tinea pedis, 600–601
griseofulvin, ultramicrosize, Gris-PEG
  (G)
  onychomycosis (fungal nail), 422
  tinea capitis, 597
  tinea corporis, 598
  tinea cruris, 599
  tinea pedis, 601
Gris-PEG, *griseofulvin, ultramicrosize* (G)
  tinea capitis, 597
  tinea corporis, 598
  tinea cruris, 599
  tinea pedis, 601
growth failure
  mecasermin, Increlex, 266
  somatropin, Genotropin, Genotropin
    Miniquick, Humatrope (G),
    Norditropin (G), Nutropin (G),
    Nutropin AQ (G), Nutropin
    Depot (G), Omnitrope, Saizen,
    Serostim, 266–267
guanabenz (G)
  hypertension, 332
guanethidine, Ismelin (G)
  hypertension, 332
guanfacine, Intuniv, Tenex
  attention deficit hyperactivity disorder
    (ADHD), 54
  hypertension, 332
guselkumab, Tremfya
  psoriasis, 523
  psoriatic arthritis, 528
Gynazole-12% Vaginal Cream,
  butoconazole cream 2% (G)
  vulvovaginal (moniliasis) candidiasis,
    138
Gyne-Lotrimin, *clotrimazole*
  vulvovaginal (moniliasis) candidiasis,
    138

Habitrol, *transdermal nicotine system*
  tobacco dependence, 602
Hadlima, *adalimumab-bwwd*
  juvenile idiopathic arthritis (JIA),
    371
  osteoarthritis (OA), 438
  psoriasis, 525
  psoriatic arthritis, 530
  rheumatoid arthritis (RA), 547
Haegarda,
  C1 esterase inhibitor (human)
  hereditary angioedema, 297
Haemophilus influenzae B (HIB)
  diphtheria, tetanus toxoid, acellular
    pertussis, inactivated poliovirus,
    haemophilus b conjugate, and
    hepatitis b, Vaxelis, 290
Halcion, *triazolam* (IV)
  fibromyalgia, 245
  insomnia, 360
Haldol, Haldol Lactate, *haloperidol* (G),
    693
  delirium, 188
  dementia, 188
  methamphetamine-induced
    psychosis, 395
halobetasol propionate, Bryhali, Ultravate
  (G)
  psoriasis, 521
haloperidol, Haldol, Haldol Lactate (G)
  delirium, 188
  dementia, 188
  dose forms, 693
  methamphetamine-induced
    psychosis, 395
  hand, foot, & mouth disease, 268

Hansen's disease
  clarithromycin, Biaxin, Biaxin Oral
    Suspension, Biaxin XL (G), 270
  clofazimine (G), 295
  dapsone, Aczone (G), 296
  minocycline, Dynacin, Minocin, 296
  ofloxacin, Floxin (G), 296
  rifampin, Rifadin, Rimactane (G), 295
Harvoni, *ledipasvir+sofosbuvir*
  hepatitis C (HCV), 295
Havrix, *hepatitis A vaccine, inactivated*
  (G)
  hepatitis A, 291
heart failure
  amiloride, Midamor, 281
  amiloride+hydrochlorothiazide,
    Moduretic, 202
  bumetanide, Bumex (G), 201
  captopril, Capoten (G), 279
  carvedilol, Coreg, Coreg CR (G), 200
  chlorothiazide, Diuril (G), 280
  enalapril, Epaned Oral Solution,
    Vasotec, 279
  eplerenone, Inspra, 280
  ethacrynic acid, Edecrin, 201
  dapagliflozin, Farxiga (G), 279
  fosinopril, Monopril (G), 279
  furosemide, Lasix (G), 201
  hydrochlorothiazide, Esidri,
    Hydrochlorothiazide, Microzide,
    281
  indapamide, Lozol, 201
  ivabradine, Corlanor, 203
  lisinopril, Prinivil, Qbrelis Oral
    Solution, Zestril, 279–280
  methyclothiazide+deserpidine,
    Enduronyl, 281
  metoprolol succinate, Toprol-XL (G),
    280
  metoprolol tartrate Lopressor (G), 280
  polythiazide, Renese (G), 281
  quinapril, Accupril (G), 280
  ramipril, Altace (G), 280
  sacubitril+valsartan, Entresto, 280
  sotaglifl ozin, Inpefa, 279
  spironolactone, Aldactone, CaroSpir
    (G), 281
  trandolapril, Mavik (G), 200
  valsartan, Diovan, Prexxartan Oral
    Solution, 280
Hectorol, *doxecalciferol* (G)
  hypocalcemia, 340–341
  hypoparathyroidism, 344
  osteoporosis, 441
Helicobacter pylori (*H.pylori*) infection
  Helidac Therapy, 284
  Omeclamox-Pak (G), 284
  PrevPac, 284
  Pylera, 284
Helidac Therapy
  Helicobacter pylori (*H.pylori*)
    infection, 84
Hemlibra, *emicizumab-kxwh*
  hemophilia A, 284
hemophilia A
  antihemophilic factor (recombinant),
    Fc-VWF-XTEN fusion protein-
    ehtl, Altuviiio, 286–287
  coagulation factor VIIa (recombinant)-
    jncw, Sevenfact, 286
  emicizumab-kxwh, Hemlibra, 284
  Stimate Nasal Spray, 287–288
  turoctocog alfa pegol, N8-GP, Esperoct
  von Willebrand factor (recombinant)
    (rVWF), Vonvendi, 288–289
hemorrhoids
  capsaicin 8% patch, Qutenza, 289
  dibucaine, Nupercainal (OTC)(G),
    289

diclofenac sodium, Pennsaid, Solaraze Gel, Voltaren Gel (G), 289–290
doxepin, Prudoxin, Zonalon, 290
Emla Cream, *lidocaine 2.5%+ prilocaine 2.5%,* 290
hydrocortisone, Anusol-HC, Nupercainal, Proctocort, Proctocream (G), 289
hydrocortisone+lidocaine, AnaMantle HC, LidaMantle HC, 289
hydrocortisone+pramoxine, Procort (G), 290
lidocaine, LidaMantle, Lidoderm, ZTlido lidocaine, 290
petrolatum+mineral oil+shark liver oil+phenylephrine, Preparation H Ointment (G), 289
phenylephrine+cocoa butter+shark liver oil, Preparation H Suppositories (G), 289
pimecrolimus, Elidel (G), 290
trolamine salicylate, Mobisyl Crème, 290
witch hazel, Tucks, 290
hepatic porphyria, acute (AHP)
givosiran, Givlaari, 291
hepatitis A
hepatitis A inactivated+hepatitis b surface antigen (recombinant vaccine), Twinrix (G), 291
hepatitis A vaccine, inactivated, Havrix, Vaqta (G), 291
immune globulin (human), GamaSTAN S/D, 291–292
hepatitis A vaccine, inactivated, Havrix, Vaqta (G)
hepatitis A, 291
hepatitis B
adefovir dipivoxil, Hepsera *(G),* 293
entecavir, Baraclude (G), 293
hepatitis A inactivated+hepatitis b surface antigen (recombinant) vaccine, Twinrix (G), 293
hepatitis B recombinant vaccine, Engerix-B, Recombivax HB (G), 292
interferon alfa-2b, Intron A (G), 293
lamivudine, Epivir-HBV (G), 293
telbivudine, Tyzeka (G), 293
tenofovir alafenamide (TAF), Vemlidy (G), 293
tenofovir disoproxil fumarate, Viread (G), 293
Twinrix, 292
Vaxelis, 292–293
hepatitis B recombinant vaccine, Engerix-B, Recombivax HB (G)
hepatitis B, 292
hepatitis C (HCV)
daclatasvir, Daklinza, 294
elbasvir+grazoprevir, Zepatier, 294
glecaprevir+pibrentasvir, Mavyret, 294–295
interferon alfa-2b, Intron A (G), 294
interferon alfacon-1, Infergen (G), 294
ledipasvir+sofosbuvir, Harvoni, 295
ombitasvir+paritaprevir+ritonavir plus dasabuvir, Viekira Pak, 295–296
ombitasvir+paritaprevir+ritonavir, Technivie, 295
peginterferon alfa-2a, PEGasys, PEG-Intron, 294
ribavirin, Copegus, Rebetol, Ribasphere RibaPak, Virazole, 294
simeprevir, Olysio (G), 295
sofosbuvir+velpatasvir, Epclusa, Viekira XR, 295

sofosbuvir+velpatasvir+voxilaprevir, Vosevi, 296
hepatocellular carcinoma (HCC)
futibatinib, Lytgobi, 101
olutasidenib, Imjudo, Treanda, 101
pembrolizumab, Keytruda, 86
sorafenib, Nexavar (G), 99
Hepsera, *adefovir dipivoxil (G)*
hepatitis B, 293
Herceptin, *trastuzumab,* 685
breast cancer, 82
Herceptin Hylecta, *trastuzumab+ hyaluronidase*
breast cancer, 93
hereditary angioedema (HAE)
berotralstat, Orladeyo, 297
C1 esterase inhibitor (human), Berinert, Cinryze, Haegarda, 297, 298
C1 esterase inhibitor [recombinant], Ruconest, 298
danazol, Danocrine, 296
ecallantide, Kalbitor (G), 298
icatibant, Firazyr (G), 298
lanadelumab-flyo, Takhzyro, 297
herpangina
Decadron Phosphate with Xylocaine, *lidocaine+dexamethasone,* 299
Emla Cream, *lidocaine 2.5%+ prilocaine 2.5%,* 299
LidaMantle HC, *hydrocortisone+ lidocaine,* 299
lidocaine, LidaMantle, Lidoderm, ZTlido lidocaine, 299
tramadol, Rybix ODT, Ryzolt, Ultram (G)(IV), 299
Ultracet, *tramadol+acetaminophen* (G)(IV), 299
herpes genitalis (HSV TYPE II)
acyclovir, Zovirax, (G), 300
famciclovir, Famvir, 300
valacyclovir, Valtrex, 301
herpes labialis/herpes facialis
acyclovir, Sitavig, Zovirax, 300, 301
acyclovir+hydrocortisone, 301
docosanol, Abreva, 301
penciclovir, Denavir, 301
valacyclovir, Valtrex, 301
herpes zoster
acyclovir, Zovirax, Sitavig, 301
famciclovir, Famvir, 301
lidocaine, LidaMantle, Lidoderm, ZTlido lidocaine, 299
silver sulfadiazine, Silvadene, 301, 302
tramadol, Rybix ODT, Ryzolt, Ultram (G)(IV), 302
valacyclovir, Valtrex, 301
Ultracet, *tramadol+acetaminophen* (G)(IV), 299
zoster vaccine recombinant, adjuvanted, Shingrix, 301
herpes zoster ophthmicus (HZO)
acyclovir, Zovirax, Sitavig, 303
famciclovir, Famvir, 303
valacyclovir, Valtrex, 303
herpes simplex keratitis
acyclovir, Avaclyr, 374
ganciclovir, Zirga (G), 374
idoxuridine, Herplex (G), 374
trifluridine, Viroptic (G), 374
vidarabine, Vira-A (G), 374
Herplex, *idoxuridine (G)*
herpes simplex keratitis, 374
Herzuma, *trastuzumab-pkrb,* 585
breast cancer, 83
Hetlioz, *tasimelteon (G)*
non-24 sleep-wake disorder, 418
hexachlorophene, pHisoHex (G)
bacterial skin infection, 573

hiccups: intractable
chlorpromazine, Thorazine (G), 303
hidradenitis suppurativa
adalimumab, Humira, 304
clindamycin, Cleocin T, Clindagel, Clindets, Evoclin, 304
doxycycline, Acticlate, Adoxa, Doryx, Doxteric, Monodox, Oracea, Vibramycin, Vibra-Tab, 303
erythromycin base, Ery-Tab, PCE, 303
erythromycin ethylsuccinate, EryPed, E.E.S., 304
minocycline, Dynacin, Minocin, 304
tetracycline, Achromycin V, Sumycin, 304
Hizentra, *immune globulin subcutaneous [human] 20% liquid*
chronic inflammatory demyelinating polyneuropathy, 503–504
immunodeficiency, 349–350
HMS, *medrysone (G)*
allergic (vernal) conjunctivitis, 166
hookworm
albendazole, Albenza (G), 304
ivermectin, Stromectol (G), 305
mebendazole, Emverm, Vermox (G), 305
pyrantel pamoate, Antiminth, Pin-X (G), 305
thiabendazole, Mintezol (G), 305
Horizant, *gabapentin enacarbil (G)*
diabetic peripheral neuropathy (DPN), 210
fibromyalgia, 244
post-herpetic neuralgia, 507
restless legs syndrome, 540
hospital-acquired bacterial pneumonia (HABP)
ceftazidime+avibactam, Avycaz, 489
ceftolozane+tazobactam, Zerbaxa, 489
cefiderocol, Fetroja, 490
imipenem+cilastatin+relebactam, Recarbrio, 489–490
Humalog Mix 50/50, *insulin lispro protamine 50%+insulin lispro 50%*
type 1 diabetes mellitus, 617
Humalog Mix 75/25, *insulin lispro protamine75%+insulin lispro 25%*
type 1 diabetes mellitus, 617
human bite
amoxicillin+clavulanate, Augmentin, Augmentin ES-600, Augmentin XR, 66
cefoxitin, Mefoxin Injectable, 66
ciprofloxacin, Cipro (G), Cipro XR, ProQuin XR (G), 66
erythromycin base, Ery-Tab, PCE, 67
erythromycin ethylsuccinate, EryPed, E.E.S., 67
trimethoprim+sulfamethoxazole (TMP-SMX), Bactrim, Septra, 67
human chorionic gonadotropin, Pregnyl
amenorrhea, secondary, 18
human immunodeficiency virus (HIV) infection
abacavir sulfate, Ziagen (G), 308
atazanavir, Reyataz, 310
atazanavir+cobicistat, Evotaz, 315
Biktarvy *bictegravir+emtricitabine+ tenofovir alafenamide,* 314
Cabenuva *cabotegravir and rilpivirine,* 314
cabotegravir, Vocabria, 308
cabotegravir+rilpivirine, Cabenuva, 317
Cimduo, *lamivudine+tenofovir disoproxil fumarate,* 314

human immunodeficiency virus (HIV) infection (*cont.*)
cobicistat, Tybost, 313
Combivir, *lamivudine+zidovudine* (G), 314
Complera, *emtricitabine+tenofovir disoproxil fumarate+rilpivirine*, 314, 696
darunavir, Prezista (G), 311
delavirdine mesylate, Rescriptor (G), 309
didanosine, Videx EC, Videx Pediatric Pwdr for Solution (G), 308
dolutegravir, Tivicay (G), 308
doravirine, Pifeltro, 309
doravirine+lamivudine+tenofovir disoproxil fumarate, Delstrigo, 314–315
Dovato, *dolutegravir+lamivudine*, 315
efavirenz, Sustiva, 309–310
efavirenz+emtricitabine+tenofovir disoproxil fumarate, Atripla, 314
emtricitabine, Emtriva, 309
emtricitabine+tenofovir alafenamide, Descovy, 314
emtricitabine+tenofovir disoproxil fumarate, Truvada, 316
emtricitabine+tenofovir disoproxil fumarate+rilpivirine, Complera, 314, 696
enfuvirtide, Fuzeon, 312
Epzicom, *abacavir sulfate+lamivudine*, 315
etravirine, Intelence, 310
Evotaz, *atazanavir+cobicistat*, 315, 696
fosamprenavir, Lexiva (G), 311
fostemsavir, Rukobia, 312
Genvoya, *elvitegravir+cobicistat+ emtricitabine+tenofovir alafenamide*, 315
ibalizumab-uiyk, Trogarzo, 312
indinavir sulfate, Crixivan (G), 311
Juluca, *dolutegravir+rilpivirine*, 315
Kaletra, Kaletra Oral Solution, *lopinavir+ritonavir* (G), 315
lamivudine, Epivir (G), 309
lenacapavir, Sunlenca, 313–314
maraviroc, Selzentry, 312
nelfinavir mesylate, Viracept, 311
nevirapine, Viramune, 310
Odefsey, *emtricitabine+rilpivirine+ tenofovir alafenamide*, 315
Prezcobix, *darunavir+cobicistat*, 316
raltegravir (as potassium), Isentress (G), 308
rilpivirine, Edurant, 310
ritonavir, Norvir (G), 312
saquinavir mesylate, Fortovase, Invirase, 312
stavudine, Zerit (G), 309
Stribild, *elvitegravir+cobicistat+ emtricitabine+tenofovir disoproxil fumarate*, 316, 697
Symfi, *efavirenz+lamivudine+tenofovir disoproxil fumarate*, 316
Symtuza, *darunavir+cobicistat+ emtricitabine+tenofovir alafenamide*, 316
Temixys, *lamivudine+tenofovir disoproxil fumarate*, 316
tenofovir disoproxil fumarate, Virea (G), 309
tipranavir, Aptivus (G), 312
Triumeq, *abacavir sulfate+ dolutegravir+lamivudine* (G), 316

Trizivir, *abacavir sulfate+ lamivudine+zidovudine* (G), 316
zidovudine, Retrovir (G), 309
human papillomavirus (HPV)
human papillomavirus 9-valent (types 6, 11, 16, 18, 31, 33, 45, 52, and 58) vaccine, recombinant, aluminum adsorbed, Gardasil 9, 318
human papillomavirus 9-valent (types 6, 11, 16, 18, 31, 33, 45, 52, and 58) vaccine, recombinant, aluminum adsorbed, Gardasil 9
human papillomavirus (HPV), 318
Humatin, *paromomycin*
intestinal amebiasis, 17
Humatrope, *somatropin*
growth failure, 267
Humira, *adalimumab*
Crohn's disease, 176–177
hidradenitis suppurativa, 304
juvenile idiopathic arthritis, 371
osteoarthritis, ankylosing spondylitis, 437
psoriasis, 525
psoriatic arthritis, 529
rheumatoid arthritis, 546–547
ulcerative colitis, 636
Humulin 50/50, *NPH 50%+regular 50%*
type 1 diabetes mellitus, 617
Humulin 70/30, Novolin 70/30, *NPH 70%+regular 30%*
type 1 diabetes mellitus,617
Huntington disease-associated chorea
deutetrabenazine, Austedo, 318
trabenazine, Xenazine, 318
valbenazine, Ingrezza, 318
Hyalgan, *sodium hyaluronate*
osteoarthritis, 437
rheumatoid arthritis, 549
Hycet, *hydrocodone bitartrate+ acetaminophen* (G)(II)
pain, 455–456
Hydergine, *ergoloid mesylate* (G)
Alzheimer's disease, 15
hydralazine (G)
angina pectoris: stable, 30
hypertension, 333
Hydrea, *hydroxyurea*
dose forms, 685
sickle cell disease (SCD), 568–569
hydrochlorothiazide, Esidri, Hydrochlorothiazide, Microzide
edema, 228
heart failure, 281
hypertension, 327
urolithiasis, 646
hydrocodone bitartrate, Hysingla ER, Vantrela ER, Zohydro ER (G)(II)
pain, 455
hydrocortisone, Anusol-HC, Cortef, Hydrocortone, Hytone, Nupercainal, Proctocort, Proctocream (G), 579
hemorrhoids, 289
strength and volume, 678, 679
ulcerative colitis, 634
hydrocortisone butyrate, Locoid (G), 677
hydrocortisone probutate, Pandel (G), 677
hydrocortisone valerate, Westcort (G), 677
Hydrocortone, *hydrocortisone* (G), 678, 679
hydroflumethiazide, Saluron
edema, 228
hydrogen peroxide 40%, Eskata (G)
seborrheic dermatitis, 205
hydromorphone (II)(G), Dilaudid
pain, 456

hydroquinone, Lustra, Lustra AF (G)
hyperpigmentation, 325
melasma/chloasma, 387
vitiligo, 653
hydroxychloroquine, Plaquenil (G)
malaria, 386
rheumatoid arthritis, 546
systemic lupus erythematosis, 858
hydroxypropyl methylcellulose, GenTeal Mild, GenTeal Moderate, GenTeal Severe
dry eye syndrome, 217
hydroxyurea, Hydrea, Siklos
sickle cell disease (SCD), 568–589
hydroxyzine, Atarax, Vistaril (G)
allergic reaction, 12
allergic rhinitis/sinusitis, 550
anxiety disorder, 33
atopic dermatitis, 199
chickenpox (Varicella), 150
contact dermatitis, 203
genus rhus dermatitis, 204
panic disorder, 465
rhinitis medicamentosa, 555
urticaria, 649
hyoscyamine, Anaspaz, Levbid, Levsin, Levsinex, NuLev (G)
abdominal cramps, 174
interstitial cystitis, 361
irritable bowel syndrome with diarrhea, 367
urinary overactive bladder, 354
urinary tract infection (UTI), 642
hypercalcemia
cinacalcet, Sensipar (G), 319
hypercholesterolemia. See dyslipidemia
hyperemesis gravidarum
doxylamine, Bonjesta, Diclegis, 320
hyperhidrosis
aluminum chloride, Drysol, 320
etelcalcetide, Parsabiv, 321
glycopyrronium, Qbrexza, 320
oxybutynin chloride, Ditropan, GelniQUE, Oxytrol Transdermal Patch, 320
hyperhomocysteinemia
betaine anhydrous for oral solution, Cystadane (G)
L-methylfolate calcium (as metafolin)+ methylcobalamin+n-acetylcysteine, Cerefolin, 236
L-methylfolate calcium (as metafolin)+ pyridoxyl 5-phosphate+ methylcobalamin, Metanx, 236
hyperkalemia
patiromer sorbitex calcium, Veltassa, 322
sodium polystyrene sulfonate, Kayexalate (G), 322
sodium zirconium cyclosilicate, Lokelma, 322–323
hyperlipidemia. See dyslipidemia
hyperparathyroidism (HPT)
calcifediol, Rayaldee (G), 323
cinacalcet, Sensipar (G), 323–324
etelcalcetide, Parsabiv, 324
paricalcitol, Zemplar (G), 323
hyperphosphatemia
calcium acetate, PhosLo (G), 325
ferric citrate, Aurexia, 324
lanthanum carbonate, Fosrenol (G), 325
sevelamer, Renagel, Renvela (G), 325
hyperpigmentation
hydroquinone, Lustra, Lustra AF (G), 325
hydroquinone+ethyl dihydroxypropyl PABA+dioxybenzone+ oxybenzone, Solaquin (G), 325

hydroquinone+fluocinolone+tretinoin, Tri-Luma (G), 325
hydroquinone+padimate o+ oxybenzone+octyl methoxycinnamate, Glyquin (G), 325
hydroquinone+padimate+ dioxybenzone+oxybenzone, Solaquin Forte (G), 325
monobenzone, Benoquin (G), 325
tazarotene, Avage, Tazorac, 325
tretinoin, Avita, Renova, Retin-A (G), 325
hyperprolactinemia
dostinex, Cabergoline, 326
HyperRAB S/D, *rabies immune globulin, human (HRIG)* (G)
rabies, 538
hypertension
Accuretic, *quinapril+ hydrochlorothiazide,* 333
acebutolol, Sectral, 326
Aldactazide, *spironolactone+ hydrochlorothiazide,* 329
Aldoril, *methyldopa+ hydrochlorothiazide* (G), 334
aliskiren, Tekturna, 332
amiloride, Midamor, 327
amlodipine, Norvasc (G), 331
amlodipine benzoate, Katerzia (G), 331
Amturnide, *aliskiren+amlodipine+ hydrochlorothiazide,* 336
Atacand HCT, *candesartan+ hydrochlorothiazide,* 333
atenolol, Tenormin, 326
Avalide, *irbesartan+ hydrochlorothiazide,* 334
azilsartan medoxomil, Edarbi (G), 330
Azor, *amlodipine+olmesartan medoxomil,* 336–337
benazepril (G), 329
Benicar HCT, *olmesartan medoxomil+ hydrochlorothiazide,* 334
betaxolol, Kerlone (G), 326
bisoprolol, Zebeta (G), 326
bumetanide (G), 327–328
Byvalson, *nebivolol+valsartan,* 335
Caduet, *amlodipine+atorvastatin,* 337
candesartan, Atacand (G), 330
Capoten, captopril (G), 329
Capozide, *captopril+ hydrochlorothiazide,* 333
carteolol, Cartrol, 327
carvedilol, Coreg, Coreg CR (G), 327
chlorothiazide, Chlorthalidone, Diuril, Thalitone (G), 327
clevidipine butyrate, Cleviprex (G), 331
clonidine, Catapres, Catapres-TTS, Kapvay, Nexiclon XR (G), 332
Clorpres, *clonidine+chlorthalidone* (G), 337
Combipres, *clonidine+chlorthalidone* (G), 334
Corzide, *nadolol+bendroflumethiazide* (G), 335
Cosensi, *amlodipine+celecoxib,* 254
diagnostic workup, 549
diltiazem, Cardizem, Cartia XT, Dilacor XR, Tiazac (G), 330
diltiazem maleate, Tiamate (G), 331
Diovan HCT, *valsartan+ hydrochlorothiazide,* 334
doxazosin, Cardura, Cardura XL (G), 332
Dutoprol, *metoprolol succinate+ext-rel hydrochlorothiazide* (G), 335
Dyazide, Maxzide, *triamterene+ hydrochlorothiazide* (G), 329

Edarbyclor, *azilsartan+chlorthalidone,* 333
enalapril, Epaned Oral Solution, Vasotec, 329
Enduronyl, Enduronyl Forte, *methyclothiazide+deserpidine,* 327
Enduronyl, *methyclothiazide+ deserpidine* (G), 327
eplerenone, Inspra, 332
eprosartan, Teveten (G), 330
Esimil, *guanethidine+ hydrochlorothiazide,* 335
ethacrynate sodium, Sodium Edecrin, 328
ethacrynic acid, Edecrin, 328
Exforge 5/160, *amlodipine+valsartan medoxomil,* 336
Exforge HCT, *amlodipine+valsartan medoxomil+hydrochlorothiazide,* 337
felodipine, Plendil (G), 331
fosinopril, Monopril (G), 329
furosemide, Lasix (G), 348
guanabenz (G), 332
guanethidine, Ismelin (G), 332
guanfacine, Tenex, 332
hydralazine (G), 333
hydrochlorothiazide, Esidri, Hydrochlorothiazide, Microzide, 327
Hyzaar, *losartan+hydrochlorothiazide,* 334
identifiable causes, 549
indapamide, Lozol, 328
Inderide, *propranolol+ hydrochlorothiazide* (G), 335
irbesartan, Avapro (G), 330
isradipine, DynaCirc (G), 331
labetalol, Normodyne, Trandate (G), 327
levamlodipine maleate, Conjupri, 331
Lexxel, *enalapril+felodipine,* 336
lisinopril, Prinivil, Qbrelis Oral Solution, Zestril, 329–330
Lopressor HCT, *metoprolol succinate+ hydrochlorothiazide* (G), 334–335
losartan, Cozaar (G), 330
Lotensin HCT, *benazepril+ hydrochlorothiazide,* 333
Lotrel, *amlodipine+benazepril,* 335
methyldopa, Aldomet, 248
metolazone, Zaroxolyn, 328
metoprolol succinate, Toprol-XL (G), 346
metoprolol tartrate, Lopressor (G), 346
Micardis HCT, *telmisartan+ hydrochlorothiazide,* 334
Minizide, *prazosin+polythiazide* (G), 335
minoxidil, Loniten (G), 333
Moduretic, *amiloride+ hydrochlorothiazide* (G), 328
moexipril, Univasc, 330
nadolol, Corgard (G), 326
nebivolol, Bystolic (G), 326
nifedipine, Adalat, Adalat CC, Cardene, Procardia, Procardia XL (G), 331
nisoldipine, 331
olmesartan medoxomil, Benicar, 334
penbutolol, Levatol, 326
perindopril, Aceon, 330
polythiazide, Renese (G), 327
prazosin, Minipres, 332
Prestalia, *perindopril+amlodipin,* 335
Prinzide, Zestoretic, *lisinopril+ hydrochlorothiazide* (D), 333

Prestalia, *amlodipine+perindopril,* 335
propranolol, Inderal (G), 346
quinapril, Accupril (G), 330
ramipril, Altace (G), 330
Salutensin, *reserpine+ hydroflumethiazide* (G), 337
spironolactone, Aldactone, CaroSpir (G), 327
Tarka, *trandolapril+verapamil,* 336
Teczem, *enalapril+diltiazem,* 336
Tekamlo, *aliskiren+amlodipine,* 336
Tekturna HCT, *aliskiren+ hydrochlorothiazide,* 336
Tenoretic, *atenolol+chlorthalidone,* 334
terazosin, Hytrin (G), 332
Teveten HCT, *eprosartan+ hydrochlorothiazide,* 334
Timolide, *timolol+hydrochlorothiazide* (G), 335
timolol, Blocadren (G), 327
torsemide, Demadex, Soaanz, 328
trandolapril, Mavik (G), 330
triamterene, Dyrenium, 327
triamterene+hydrochlorothiazide, Dyazide (G)
Tribenzor, *olmesartan medoxomil+ amlodipine+hydrochlorothiazide,* 337
Twynsta, *telmisartan+amlodipine,* 337
Uniretic, *moexipril+ hydrochlorothiazide,* 333
valsartan, Diovan, Prexxartan Oral Solution, 330
Valturna, *aliskiren+valsartan,* 336
Vaseretic, *enalapril+ hydrochlorothiazide,* 333
verapamil, Calan, Calan SR, Isoptin SR (G), 331
Ziac, *bisoprolol+hydrochlorothiazide,* 334
Hyper-TET, *tetanus immune globulin, human* (G), 478
hyperthyroidism
methimazole, Tapazole, 254
propranolol, Inderal (G), 254
propylthiouracil (ptu), Propyl-Thyracil, 254
hypertriglyceridemia
atorvastatin, Lipitor (G), 339
fenofibrate, Antara, Fenoglide, FibriCor, TriCor, TriLipix, Lipofen, Lofibra (G), 338
fluvastatin, Lescol, Lescol XL (G), 339
gemfibrozil, Lopid (G), 338
icosapent ethyl (omega 3-fatty acid ethyl ester of EPA), Vascepa sgc (G), 338
lovastatin, Mevacor, Altoprev, 339
niacin, Niaspan, Slo-Niacin (G), 338–339
niacin+lovastatin, Advicor, 339
omega 3-fatty acid ethyl esters, Lovaza, Epanova (G), 338
pravastatin, Pravachol, 256
rosuvastatin, Crestor, 256
simvastatin, Zocor, 339
hypocalcemia
bioengineered replica of human parathyroid hormone, Natpara (G), 341
calcitonin-salmon, Miacalcin (G), 340
calcitriol, Rocaltrol (G), 340
calcium carbonate, Rolaids, Tums, Os-Cal 500 (G), 340
calcium carbonate+vitamin D, Os-Cal 250+D, Os-Cal 500+D, Viactiv (OTC)(G), 340
calcium citrate, Citracal (OTC), 340

hypocalcemia (cont.)
  calcium citrate+vitamin D, Citracal+D, Citracal 250+D (G), 340
  doxecalciferol, Hectorol (G), 340–341
  paricalcitol, Zemplar (G), 341
hypoglycemia, acute
  dasiglucagon, Zegalogue, 342
  diazoxide, Proglycem (G), 343
  glucagon injection, Gvoke, 341–342
  glucagon nasal powder, Baqsimi, 342
hypokalemia
  potassium, KCL Solution Oral soln, K-Dur, K-Lor for Oral Solution, Klor-Con, Klorvess, Klotrix, K-Lyte, K-Tab, Micro-K, Potassium Chloride (G), 343–344
hypomagnesemia
  magnesium oxide, Mag-Ox 400, 344
  magnesium, Slow-Mag, 344
hypoparathyroidism
  abaloparatide, Tymlos (G), 344–345
  bioengineered replica of human parathyroid hormone, Natpara (G), 345
  calcitriol, Rocaltrol (G), 344
  doxecalciferol, Hectorol (G), 344
  teriparatide, Forteo (G), 344
hypophosphatasia
  asfotase alfa, Strensiq, 345
hypopnea syndrome, 575–576
Hypotears, Hypotears PF, *polyvinyl alcohol*
  dry eye syndrome, 217
Hypotears Ophthalmic Ointment, *hydroxypropyl cellulose*
  dry eye syndrome, 217
Hypotears, *petrolatum+mineral oil*
  dry eye syndrome, 217
hypothyroidism
  levothyroxine, Levoxyl, Synthroid, Unithroid (A), 346
  levothyroxine sodium, T4 (A), 347
  liothyronine, Cytomel (A), 346
  liothyronine+levothyroxine, Armour Thyroid, Thyrolar (A), 346
hypotrichosis
  bimatoprost, Latisse (G), 347
Hyrimoz, *adalimumab-adaz*
  Crohn's disease, 177
  juvenile idiopathic arthritis, 371
  osteoarthritis, 438
  psoriasis, 525
  psoriatic arthritis, 529
Hytone, *hydrocortisone* (G)
  strength and volume, 676
Hytrin, *terazosin* (G)
  benign prostatic hyperplasia, 58
  hypertension, primary, 332
  urinary overactive bladder, 356
Hyzaar, *losartan+hydrochlorothiazide*
  hypertension, 334

ibalizumab-uiyk, Trogarzo
  human immunodeficiency virus infection, 312, 698
ibandronate (as monosodium monohydrate), Boniva (G)
  osteoporosis, 441
  Paget's disease, 450
Ibrance, *palbociclib*, 685
ibrexafungerp, Brexafemme
  vulvovaginal (moniliasis) candidiasis, 136–137
Ibudone, *hydrocodone+ibuprofen* (G)(II)
  pain, 456
ibuprofen, Advil, Caldolor, Children's Advil, ElixSure IB, Motrin, Nuprin, PediaCare, PediaProfen
  fever (pyrexia), 242–243

  pain, 451
  urolithiasis, 647
Ibsrela, *tenapanor*
  irritable bowel syndrome with constipation (IBS-C), 365–366
icatibant, Firazyr (G)
  hereditary angioedema, 298
icosapent ethyl (omega 3-fatty acid ethyl ester of EPA), Vascepa sgc (G)
  dyslipidemia, 220
  hypertriglyceridemia, 338
Idacio, *adalimumab-aacf*
  Crohn's disease, 177
  juvenile idiopathic arthritis (JIA), 371
  osteoarthritis (OA), 438
  psoriasis, 525
  psoriatic arthritis, 529
  rheumatoid arthritis (RA), 547
  ulcerative colitis (UC), 636
Idhifa, *enasidenib*, 685
idiopathic pulmonary fibrosis (IPF)
  azathioprine, Azasan, Imuran, 534
  nintedanib, Ofev, 535
  pirfenidone, Esbriet (G), 535
idiopathic thrombocytopenia purpura (ITP)
  avatrombopag, Doptelet, 593–594
  fostamatinib disodium hexahydrate, Tavalisse, 594
  lusutrombopag, Mulpleta, 594
idoxuridine, Herplex (G)
  herpes simplex keratitis, 374
Ilosone, *erythromycin estolate*, 708, 717–718
  bacterial endocarditis prophylaxis, 55
  legionella pneumonia, 496
  scarlet fever, 560
  streptococcal pharyngitis, 485
Ilotycin, *erythromycin*
  bacterial conjunctivitis, 162
  blepharitis, 67
  chlamydial ophthalmia neonatorum, 423
  gonococcal ophthalmia neonatorum, 423
  stye (hordeolum), 580
Ilumya, *tildrakizumab-asmn*
  psoriasis, 524
Imbruvica, *imbrutinib*, 686
Imdur, *isosorbide mononitrate* (G)
  angina pectoris: stable, 29
Imfinzi, *durvalumab*, 686
imipramine, Tofranil (G)
  anxiety disorder, 34
  diabetic peripheral neuropathy (DPN), 210
  gonorrhea, 259
  interstitial cystitis, 362
  irritable bowel syndrome with diarrhea, 386
  major depressive disorder, 193
  migraine and cluster headache, 276
  nocturnal enuresis, 235
  obsessive-compulsive disorder, 422
  panic disorder, 465
  post-herpetic neuralgia, 508, 510s
  post-traumatic stress disorder, 512
  tension headache, 278
  trigeminal neuralgia, 609
imiquimod, Aldara, Zyclara
  actinic keratosis, 9
  venereal wart, 655
Imjudo, *olutasidenib, tremelimumab-actl*
  hepatocellular carcinoma (HCC), 99–101
immune globulin (human), GamaSTAN S/D (G)
  chickenpox (Varicella), 149
  dermatomyositis, 502–503

  hepatitis A, 291
  polymyositis, 502–503
  rubella, 558
  rubeola, 558–559
immune globulin subcutaneous [human] 20% liquid, Hizentra
  chronic inflammatory demyelinating polyneuropathy, 503
  primary humoral immunodeficiency (PHI), 349–350
immunization recommendations, 665–666
Imodium Advanced, *loperamide+ simethicone*
  acute diarrhea, 212
  chronic diarrhea, 213
  irritable bowel syndrome with diarrhea, 366
  ulcerative colitis, 638
Imodium, Imodium A-D, *loperamide*
  acute diarrhea, 212
  chronic diarrhea, 213
  irritable bowel syndrome with diarrhea, 366
  ulcerative colitis, 638
Imogam Rabies HT, *rabies immune globulin, human (HRIG)* (G)
  rabies, 538
Imovax, *rabies vaccine, human diploid cell [HDVC]* (G)
  rabies, 538
Impavido, *miltefosine*
  leishmaniasis, 376–377
impetigo contagiosa
  amoxicillin, Amoxil, Moxatag, Trimox, 351
  Augmentin, Augmentin ES-600, Augmentin XR, *amoxicillin+clavulanate*, 351–352
  azithromycin, Zithromax, Zmax, 352
  cefaclor, Cefaclor Extended Release, 352
  cefadroxil, Duricef, 352
  cefpodoxime proxetil, Vantin, 352
  cefprozil, Cefzil, 352
  ceftaroline fosamil, Teflaro, 352
  cephalexin, Keflex, 352
  clarithromycin, Biaxin, 352
  dicloxacillin, Dynapen, 353
  erythromycin base, Ery-Tab, PCE, 352
  erythromycin ethylsuccinate, EryPed, E.E.S, 352
  loracarbef, Lorabid, 353
  mupirocin, Bactroban, Centany, 351
  ozenoxacin, Xepi, 353
  penicillin g (benzathine), Bicillin L-A, Bicillin C-R, 353
  penicillin v potassium, Pen-Vee K, 353
Implanon, *etonogestrel*, 675
Imuran, *azathioprine*
  Crohn's disease, 176
  idiopathic pulmonary fibrosis (IPF), 534
  pemphigus vulgaris, 477
  rheumatoid arthritis, 546
  systemic lupus erythematosis, 583
Imvexxy, *estradiol*
  dyspareunia, 226
Inbrija, *levodopa inhalation powder*
  Parkinson's disease, 467
inclisiran, Leqvio
  dyslipidemia, 221
Increlex, *mecasermin*
  growth failure, 266
Incruse Ellipta, *umeclidinium* (G)
  chronic obstructive pulmonary disease (COPD), 72
  emphysema, 231

indacaterol, Arcapta Neohaler (G)
  chronic obstructive pulmonary
    disease (COPD), 71
  emphysema, 230
indapamide, Lozol
  edema, 229
  heart failure, 282
  hypertension, 328
Inderal, Inderal LA, *propranolol* (G), 681
  angina pectoris: stable, 29
  benign essential tremor, 58
  headache, migraine, 275
  hypertension: primary, 326
  hyperthyroidism, 338
  mitral valve prolapse (MVP), 396
  post-traumatic stress disorder, 511
Inderide, propranolol+
    hydrochlorothiazide (G)
  hypertension, 335
indinavir sulfate, Crixivan (G), 696
  human immunodeficiency virus
    infection, 311
indomethacin (G)
  gouty arthritis, 263
  juvenile idiopathic arthritis, 370
  juvenile rheumatoid arthritis, 373
  osteoarthritis, 434–435
  psoriatic arthritis, 527
  rheumatoid arthritis, 542
infantile colic
  hyoscyamine, Levsin Drops (G), 159
  simethicone, Mylicon Drops (G), 159
Infergen, *interferon alfacon-1* (G)
  hepatitis C (HCV), 294
Inflamase Forte, Inflamase Mild,
    prednisolone sodium phosphate
    (G)
  allergic (vernal) conjunctivitis, 166
Inflectra, *infliximab-dyyb*
  osteoarthritis, 438
  psoriasis, 526
  psoriatic arthritis, 530
  rheumatoid arthritis, 538
  ulcerative colitis, 637
infliximab, Remicade
  Crohn's disease, 117
  osteoarthritis, 438
  psoriasis, 526
  psoriatic arthritis, 530
  rheumatoid arthritis, 547
  ulcerative colitis, 637
infliximab-abda, Renflexis
  Crohn's disease, 177
  osteoarthritis, 439
  psoriasis, 526
  psoriatic arthritis, 530
  rheumatoid arthritis, 548
  ulcerative colitis, 637
infliximab-axxq, Avsola
  osteoarthritis (OA), 439
  psoriasis, 526
  psoriatic arthritis, 530
  rheumatoid arthritis (RA), 548
  ulcerative colitis (UC), 637
infliximab-dyyb, Inflectra
  osteoarthritis, 438
  psoriasis, 526
  psoriatic arthritis, 530
  rheumatoid arthritis, 548
  ulcerative colitis, 637
infliximab-qbtx, Ixifi
  osteoarthritis, 439
  psoriasis, 526
  psoriatic arthritis, 530
  rheumatoid arthritis, 548
  ulcerative colitis, 637
infliximab, Remicade
  rheumatoid arthritis (RA), 547–548
influenza, seasonal (FLU)

baloxavir marboxil, Xofluza, 358
oseltamivir phosphate, Tamiflu (G),
  357
peramivir, Rapivab, 357
*quadrivalent inactivated infl uenza
    subvirion vaccine, types a and b,
    Fluad, Fluarix Quadrivalent*, 356
*trivalent inactivated influenza
    subvirion vaccine, types a and
    b, Fluarix, Flublok, FluLaval,
    FluShield, Fluzone* (G), 356–357
*trivalent, live attenuated influenza
    vaccine, types A and B, FluMist
    Nasal Spray* (G), 356
zanamivir, Relenza Inhaler (G), 357
ingenol mebutate, Picato (G)
  actinic keratosis, 9
Ingrezza, *valbenazine*
  Huntington disease-associated chorea,
    318
  tardive dyskinesia, 586
InnoPran XL, *propranolol* (G), 681
  angina pectoris: stable, 29
  benign essential tremor, 58
  headache: migraine, 275
  hypertension: primary, 326
  hyperthyroidism, 338
  mitral valve prolapse (mvp), 396
Inmazeb, *atoltivimab+maft ivimab+
    odesivimab*
  ebola zaire disease (zaire ebolavirus),
    227
Inpefa, *sotagliflozin*
  heart failure, 279
Inrebic, *fedratinib*
  myelofibrosis, 408
insect bite/sting
  Decadron Phosphate with Xylocaine,
    lidocaine+dexamethasone, 358
  Emla Cream, *lidocaine
    2.5%+prilocaine 2.5%*, 358
  epinephrine (G), 358
  LidaMantle HC,
    hydrocortisone+lidocaine, 358
  lidocaine, LidaMantle, Lidoderm,
    ZTlido lidocaine, 358
  tetanus toxoid vaccine (G), 359
insomnia
  *acetaminophen+diphenhydramine,
    Excedrin PM, Tylenol PM*, 360
  daridorexant, Quviviq, 360
  doxepin, Silenor (G), 360
  estazolam, ProSom (IV), 3
  eszopiclone, Lunesta (G)(IV), 359
  flurazepam, Dalmane (IV), 359
  lemborexant, Dayvigo, 360
  pentobarbital, Nembutal (II), 360
  ramelteon, Rozerem (G), 359
  suvorexant, Belsomra (G)(IV), 359
  temazepam, Restoril (IV)(G), 359
  triazolam, Halcion (IV), 360
  zaleplon, Sonata (IV), 359
  zolpidem, Ambien, Edluar,
    Intermezzo, ZolpiMist (G)
    (IV), 359
Inspra, *eplerenone*
  heart failure, 280
  hypertension: primary, 332
insulin aspart (recombinant), NovoLog
  type 1 diabetes mellitus, 615
*insulin aspart protamine suspension
    70%/insulin aspart 30%
    (recombinant)*, NovoLog Mix
    70/30, NovoLog Mix 70/30
    FlexPen
  type 1 diabetes mellitus, 626
insulin degludec (insulin analog), Tresiba
    FlexTouch (G)
  type 1 diabetes mellitus, 617

*insulin degludec (insulin analog)+
    liraglutide*, Xultophy (G)
  type 1 diabetes mellitus, 618
  type 2 diabetes mellitus, 626
insulin detemir (human), Levemir
  type 1 diabetes mellitus, 616
*insulin extended zinc suspension
    (Ultralente) (human)*,
    Humulin U
  type 1 diabetes mellitus, 617
insulin glargine (recombinant), Basaglar,
    Lantus, Toujeo, NPH, Soliqua
    (G)
  type 1 diabetes mellitus, 616
  type 2 diabetes mellitus, 626
insulin glulisine (rDNA origin),
    Apidra (G)
  type 1 diabetes mellitus, 615
insulin human (inhaled), Afrezza
    Inhalation Powder (G)
  type 1 diabetes mellitus, 615
insulin isophane suspension (NPH),
    Humulin N, Novolin N,
    Iletin II NPH
  type 1 diabetes mellitus, 617
insulin lispro (recombinant), Admelog,
    Humalog
  type 1 diabetes mellitus, 615
insulin regular, Humulin R U-100,
    Humulin R U-500, Iletin II
    Regular, Novolin R
  type 1 diabetes mellitus, 615–616
insulin zinc suspension, Humulin L, Iletin
    II Lente, Novolin L
  type 1 diabetes mellitus, 617
Intal, Intal Inhalation Solution, *cromolyn
    sodium*
  asthma, 42
interferon alfa-2b, Intron A (G)
  hepatitis B, 293
  hepatitis C (HCV), 294
  venereal wart, 656
interferon alfacon-1, Infergen (G)
  hepatitis C (HCV), 294
interferon alfa-n3, Alferon N (G)
  venereal wart, 656
interferon beta-1a, Avonex, Rebif, Rebif
    Rebidose (G)
  multiple sclerosis (MS), 398, 399
interferon beta-1b, Actimmune,
    Betaseron, Extavia (G)
  multiple sclerosis (MS), 399
Intermezzo, *zolpidem* (G)(IV)
  aphasia, 36–37
  fibromyalgia, 245
  insomnia, 359
interstitial cystitis
  amitriptyline (G), 362
  chlordiazepoxide+clidinium, Librax
    (IV), 362
  hyoscyamine, Anaspaz, Levbid, Levsin,
    Levsinex, NuLev (G), 361
  imipramine, Tofranil (G), 362
  *methenamine+phenyl salicylate+
    methylene blue+benzoic
    acid+atropine sulfate+-
    hyoscyamine sulfate*, Urised (G),
    362
  *methenamine+sod phosphate
    monobasic+phenyl
    salicylate+methylene
    blue+hyoscyamine sulfate*,
    Uribel (G), 362
  oxybutynin chloride, Ditropan, 362
  pentosan, Elmiron, 362
  phenazopyridine, AZO Standard,
    Prodium, Uristat, 361, 362
  propantheline, Pro-Banthine (G), 362
  tolterodine tartrate, Detrol (G), 362

intertrigo, 362–363
intestinal cramps. *See* abdominal cramps
Intrarosa, *prasterone
(dehydroepiandrosterone
[DHEA])*
  dyspareunia, 226
Intron A, *interferon alfa-2b* (G)
  hepatitis B, 293
  hepatitis C (HCV), 294
  venereal wart, 656
Introvale, *ethinyl estradiol/levonorgestrel*
  estrogen and progesterone, 669
Intuniv, *guanfacine*
  attention deficit hyperactivity disorder
    (ADHD), 54
Invega Hafyera, Invega Sustenna,
    paliperidone palmitate
  schizophrenia, 564–566
Inveltys, *eoteprednol etabonate* (G)
  eye pain, 241
Invokamet, *canagliflozin+metformin* (G)
  type 2 diabetes mellitus, 627
iobenguane, Azedra
  pheochromocytoma, 487
Ipol, *trivalent poliovirus vaccine,
    inactivated (type 1, 2, and 3)* (G)
  poliomyelitis, 498
ipratropium bromide, Atrovent
  allergic rhinitis/sinusitis, 553
  asthma, 40
  chronic obstructive pulmonary
    disease, 72
  rhinitis medicamentosa, 554
  vasomotor rhinitis, 447
Iressa, *gefitinib*, 686
  lung cancer, 105
iritis: acute
  loteprednol etabonate, Lotemax
    Ophthalmic Solution (G), 364
  prednisone acetate, Pred Forte (G), 364
iron deficiency anemia
  ferric carboxymaltose, Injectafer, 25–26
  ferric maltol, Accrufer, 25
  ferrous gluconate, Fergon (A), 25
  ferrous sulfate, Feosol, Fer-In-Sol (A),
    25
  ferumoxytol, Feraheme, 26
iron overload
  deferasirox (tridentate ligand), Exjade,
    Jadenu (G), 365
  Succimer, Chemet (G), 365
irritable bowel syndrome with
    constipation (IBS-C)
  linaclotide, Linzess (G), 365
  lubiprostone, Amitiza (G), 365
  plecanatide, Trulance, 366
  tenapanor, Ibsrela, 365–366
irritable bowel syndrome with diarrhea
    (IBS-D)
  alosetron, Lotronex, 367
  amitriptyline (G), 368
  dicyclomine, Bentyl, 367
  diphenoxylate+atropine, Lomotil (G),
    366
  Donnatal,
    *phenobarbital+hyoscyamine+
    atropine+scopolamine* (G), 367
  eluxadoline, Viberzi (NA)(IV), 366
  hyoscyamine, Anaspaz, Levbid, Levsin,
    Levsinex, NuLev (G), 367
  imipramine, Tofranil (G), 368
  Imodium Advanced, *loperamide+
    simethicone*, 366
  Librax, *chlordiazepoxide+
    clidinium* (IV), 367
  loperamide, Imodium, Imodium
    A-D, 366
  methscopolamine bromide, Pamine,
    367
  Motofen, *difenoxin+atropine* (G), 366

nortriptyline, Pamelor, 368
  protriptyline, Vivactil (G), 368
  simethicone, Mylicon (G), 367
  trimipramine, Surmontil (G), 368
isavuconazonium, Cresemba (G)
  aspergillosis, 38
Ismo, *isosorbide mononitrate* (G)
  angina pectoris: stable, 29
isocarboxazid, Marplan (G)
  major depressive disorder, 194
isoniazid (INH) (G)
  dose forms, 705
  tuberculosis, 610
isoproterenol, Medihaler-ISO
  asthma, 40
Isoptin SR, *verapamil* (G)
  angina pectoris: stable, 29
  headache, migraine, 276
  hypertension, primary, 331–332
Isopto Carbachol, *carbachol+
    hydroxypropyl methylcellulose* (G)
  glaucoma, 255
Isopto Cetamide Ophthalmic Ointment,
    sulfacetamide (G)
  bacterial conjunctivitis, 162
Isopto Cetamide Ophthalmic Solution,
    erythromycin
  stye (hordeolum), 580
Isordil Titradose, *isosorbide dinitrate* (G)
  angina pectoris: stable, 29
isosorbide dinitrate, Dilatrate-SR, Isordil
    Titradose (G)
  angina pectoris: stable, 29
isosorbide mononitrate, Imdur, Ismo (G)
  angina pectoris: stable, 29
istradefylline, Nourianz
  parkinson's disease, 470
isotretinoin, Accutane, Amnesteem
  acne vulgaris, 7
isradipine, DynaCirc (G)
  hypertension, 331
Isturisa, *osilodrostat*
  cushing's syndrome, 181
itraconazole, Sporanox, Pulse Pack,
    Tolsura (G), 628
  aspergillosis, 38
  onychomycosis (fungal nail), 422
  oral (thrush) candidiasis, 135
ivabradine, Corlanor
  heart failure, 283
ivacaftor, Kalydeco
  cystic fibrosis (CF), 182
ivermectin, Sklice, Soolantra, Stromectol
    (G), 704
  acne rosacea, 2
  hookworm, 305
  pediculosis humanus capitis, 475
  threadworm, 593
  trichinosis, 606
IvyBlock (OTC), *bentoquatam*
  contact dermatitis, 201
  genus rhus dermatitis, 203
ixekizumab, Taltz
  psoriasis, 522
Ixiaro, *Japanese encephalitis vaccine*
  Japanese encephalitis virus (JEV), 368
Ixifi, *infliximab-qbtx*
  Crohn's disease, 178
  osteoarthritis, 439
  psoriatic arthritis, 526, 530
  rheumatoid arthritis, 548
  ulcerative colitis, 637

Jadenu, *deferasirox (tridentate ligand)* (G)
  iron overload, 365
Jakafi, *ruxolitinib*, 686
  graft versus host disease, 263
  myelofibrosis, 409
  polycythemia vera, 501
Jalyn, *dutasteride+tamsulosin*

benign prostatic hyperplasia, 58
Janumet, *sitagliptin+metformin*
  type 2 diabetes mellitus, 630
Japanese encephalitis vaccine, Ixiaro
  Japanese encephalitis virus (JEV),
    368
Japanese encephalitis virus (JEV)
  Japanese encephalitis vaccine, Ixiaro,
    368
Jardiance, *lacosamide*
  type 2 diabetes mellitus (T2DM), 627
Jatenzo, *testosterone undecanoate*
  testosterone deficiency, 589
Jenest-28, *ethinyl estradiol+norethindrone*
  estrogen and progesterone, 669
Jentadueto, *linagliptin+metformin*
  type 2 diabetes mellitus, 630
Jeuveau, *prabotulinumtoxinA-xvfs*
  facial wrinkles, 660
Jevtana, *cabazitaxel* (G)
  prostate cancer, 130
Jesduvroq, *daprodustat*
  anemia of chronic kidney disease, 24
Jolessa, *ethinyl estradiol/levonorgestrel*
    (G), 673
  estrogen and progesterone, 669
Jublia, *efinaconazole* (G)
  onychomycosis (fungal nail), 442
Juluca, *dolutegravir+rilpivirine*, 697
  human immunodeficiency virus
    infection, 315
Junel 1.5/30, *ethinyl estradiol+
    norethindrone*
  estrogen and progesterone, 669
Junel 1/20, *ethinyl estradiol+
    norethindrone*
  estrogen and progesterone, 669
Junel Fe 1.5/30, *ethinyl estradiol+
    norethindrone plus ferrous
    fumarate*
  estrogen and progesterone, 669
Junel Fe 1/20, *ethinyl estradiol+
    norethindrone plus ferrous
    fumarate*
  estrogen and progesterone, 669
juvenile idiopathic arthritis (JIA)
  abatacept, Orencia (G), 370–371
  adalimumab, Humira, 371
  adalimumab-aacf, Idacio, 371
  adalimumab-adaz, Hyrimoz, 371
  adalimumab-adbm, Cyltezo, 371
  adalimumab-bwwd, Hadlim, 371
  capsaicin 8% patch, Qutenza, 369
  capsaicin, Axsain, Capsin,
    Capzasin-HP, Capzasin-P,
    Dolorac, Double Cap (OTC),
    R-Gel, Zostrix, Zostrix HP, 369
  Decadron Phosphate with Xylocaine,
    lidocaine+dexamethasone, 282
  diclofenac sodium, Pennsaid, Solaraze
    Gel, Voltaren Gel (G), 369
  doxepin, Prudoxin, Zonalon, 369
  Emla Cream, *lidocaine 2.5%+
    prilocaine 2.5%*, 370
  etanercept, Eticovo, 371
  golimumab, Simponi, 371
  indomethacin (G), 370
  LidaMantle HC, *hydrocortisone+
    lidocaine*, 369
  lidocaine, LidaMantle, Lidoderm,
    ZTlido lidocaine, 369
  methotrexate, Rasuvo, Rheumatrex,
    Trexall, 370
  pimecrolimus, Elidel (G), 369
  tocilizumab, Actemra, 370
  trolamine salicylate, Mobisyl Creme,
    369
juvenile rheumatoid arthritis (JRA)
  abatacept, Orencia (G), 373–374
  capsaicin 8% patch, Qutenza, 372

capsaicin, Axsain, Capsin, Capzasin-HP, Capzasin-P, Dolorac, Double Cap (OTC), R-Gel, Zostrix, Zostrix HP, 372
Decadron Phosphate with Xylocaine, *lidocaine+dexamethasone,* 373
diclofenac sodium, Pennsaid, Solaraze Gel, Voltaren Gel (G), 372
doxepin, Prudoxin, Zonalon, 372
Emla Cream, *lidocaine 2.5%+ prilocaine 2.5%,* 373
indomethacin (G), 373
LidaMantle HC, *hydrocortisone+ lidocaine,* 285
lidocaine, LidaMantle, Lidoderm, ZTlido lidocaine, 372
methotrexate, Rasuvo, Rheumatrex, Trexall, 373
pimecrolimus, Elidel (G), 372
tocilizumab, Actemra, 373
trolamine salicylate, Mobisyl Creme, 285
Juvisync, sitagliptin+simvastatin
type 2 diabetes mellitus, 632
Juxtapid, *lomitapide mesylate*
dyslipidemia, 220
Jynarque, *tolvaptan*
autosomal dominant polycystic kidney disease, 500
Jynneos, *smallpox and monkeypox vaccine, live, non-replicating,* smallpox, 576

Kaitlib Fe Chew Tab, *ethinyl estradiol+ norethindrone plus ferrous fumarate*
estrogen and progesterone, 669
Kalbitor, *ecallantide* (G)
hereditary angioedema, 298
Kaletra, Kaletra Oral Solution, *lopinavir+ritonavir* (G), 697
human immunodeficiency virus infection, 315
Kalydeco, *ivacaftor*
cystic fibrosis (CF), 182
KamRAB, *rabies immune globulin, human (HRIG)* (G)
rabies, 538
Kanjinti, *trastuzumab-anns*
breast cancer, 82
Kao Lectrolyte, *oral electrolyte replacement* (OTC)
acute diarrhea, 212
dehydration, 187
Kaopectate, *attapulgite* (G)
diarrhea: acute, 211
Kapvay, *clonidine* (G)
attention deficit hyperactivity disorder (ADHD), 54
hypertension: primary, 332
post-traumatic stress disorder, 511
Kariva, *ethinyl estradiol+desogestrel*
estrogen and progesterone, 669
Katerzia, *amlodipine benzoate* (G)
angina pectoris: stable, 28
hypertension, 331
Kayexalate, *sodium polystyrene sulfonate* (G)
hyperkalemia, 322
Kazano, *alogliptin+metformin*
type 2 diabetes mellitus, 630
KCL Solution Oral soln, *potassium* (G)
hypokalemia, 344
K-Dur, *potassium* (G)
hypokalemia, 344
Keflex, *cephalexin,* 716
acute exacerbation of chronic bronchitis, 70
acute tonsillitis, 604
bacterial endocarditis prophylaxis, 55

bacterial skin infection, 574
cellulitis, 143
dose forms, 705
impetigo contagiosa, 352
lymphadenitis, 383
mastitis (breast abscess), 387
otitis media: acute, 447
paronychia, 472
pyelonephritis: acute, 536
scarlet fever, 560
streptococcal pharyngitis, 485
urinary tract infection, 644
wound, 659
Kefzol, *cefazolin*
bacterial endocarditis prophylaxis, 55
Kelnor 1/35, *ethinyl estradiol+ethynodiol diacetate*
estrogen and progesterone, 669
Kemadrin, *procyclidine* (G)
Parkinson's disease, 471
Kenalog, *triamcinolone*
aphthous stomatitis, 37
keratitis/keratoconjunctivitis
allergic. (*see* allergic (vernal) conjunctivitis)
dry eye syndrome, 2374
herpes simplex, 374
neurotrophic, 374–375
vernal, 375
Keratol 40, *urea* (G)
callused skin, 573
Kerendia, *finerenone*
anemia of chronic kidney disease, 22
Kerydin, *tavaborole* (G)
onychomycosis (fungal nail), 423
Kesimpta, *ofatumumab*
multiple sclerosis (MS), 400
Ketek, *telithromycin* (G), 708
acute exacerbation of chronic bronchitis, 70–71
pneumonia, 494
ketoconazole, Nizoral Cream, Xolegel, Xolex (G)
diaper rash, 211
seborrheic dermatitis, 205
skin candidiasis, 135, 136
tinea capitis, 597
tinea corporis, 597, 598
tinea cruris, 598, 599
tinea pedis, 600
tinea versicolor, 601
ketorolac tromethamine, Acular, Acular LS, Acular PF, Sprix, Toradol (G), 572–573
allergic (vernal) conjunctivitis, 168
eye pain, 241
ketotifen fumarate, Alaway, Claritin Eye, Refresh Eye Itch Relief, Zaditor, Zyrtec Itchy Eye (G)
allergic (vernal) conjunctivitis, 167
Kevzara, *sarilumab*
polymyalgia rheumatica, 502
rheumatoid arthritis, 548
Keytruda, *pembrolizumab,* 686
bladder cancer, 77–78
breast cancer78
cervical cancer, 86
colorectal cancer, 86
endometrial carcinoma, 88
gastric/gastroesophageal/esophageal cancer, 90, 95
kidney, 95
liver, 99
lung, 106
lymphoma, 108
melanoma, 116
merkel cell carcinoma, 119
squamous cell carcinoma, 131
tumor, solid, 133
urothelial carcinoma, 134

Kineret, *anakinra (interleukin-1 receptor antagonist)*
rheumatoid arthritis, 548
Kisqali Femara Co-Pack, *ribociclib+ letrozole,* 686
Klaron, *sodium sulfacetamide* (G)
acne rosacea, 3
acne vulgaris, 5
Klisyri, *tirbanibulin*
actinic keratosis, 9
Klonopin, *clonazepam* (IV)
anxiety disorder, 34
dose forms, 694
panic disorder, 466
trigeminal neuralgia, 609
K-Lor for Oral Solution, *potassium* (G)
hypokalemia, 344
Klor-Con, *potassium* (G)
hypokalemia, 344
Klorvess, *potassium* (G)
hypokalemia, 344
Klotrix, *potassium* (G)
hypokalemia, 344
Kloxxado, *naloxone* (G)
opioid overdose/opioid reversal, 431
K-Lyte, *potassium* (G)
hypokalemia, 344
Kombiglyze XR, *saxagliptin+metformin*
type 2 diabetes mellitus, 630
Konsyl Fiber Tablets, *calcium polycarbophil* (G)
occasional constipation, 169
Konsyl, *psyllium*
occasional constipation, 169
Korlym, *mifepristone*
Cushing's syndrome, 179–180
Koselugo, *selumetinib*
neurofibromatosis type 1, 415–416
Krintafe, *tafenoquine*
malaria, 386
Kristalose (OTC), *lactulose*
occasional constipation, 170
K-Tab, *potassium* (G)
hypokalemia, 344
Kutrase, *pancreatic enzymes* (G)
pancreatic enzyme deficiency, 239
pancreatic enzyme insufficiency, 463
Kuvan, *sapropterin*
phenylketonuria, 486
Ku-Zyme, *pancreatic enzymes* (G)
pancreatic enzyme deficiency, 463
pancreatic enzyme insufficiency, 239
Kwell, *lindane*
scabies, 559
Kwell Shampoo, *lindane* (G)
pediculosis humanus capitis, 475
Kyleena, *levonorgestrel,* 575
Kymriah, *tisagenlecleucel,* 686
Kynamro, *mipomersen*
dyslipidemia, 220
Kynmobi, *apomorphine sublingual film*
Parkinson's disease, 468
Kyprolis, *carfilzomib,* 686
multiple myeloma, 120
Kytril, *granisetron*
cannabinoid hyperemesis syndrome, 139
chemotherapy-induced nausea/vomiting, 148
opioid-induced nausea/vomiting, 429

labetalol, Normodyne, Trandate (G)
hypertension, 327
labyrinthitis
meclizine, Antivert, Bonine (OTC), Dramamine II (OTC), Zentrip, 375
promethazine, Phenergan (G), 375
scopolamine, Transderm Scop (G), 375

Lac-Hydrin Cream
  atopic dermatitis, 197
  psoriasis, 526
lacosamide, Jardiance
  type 2 diabetes mellitus (T2DM), 627
Lacri-Lube, *petrolatum+mineral oil*
  dry eye syndrome, 217
Lacrisert, *hydroxypropyl cellulose*
  dry eye syndrome, 217
Lactaid, *lactase*
  lactose intolerance, 375
lactase, Lactaid
  lactose intolerance, 375
lactose intolerance
  lactase, Lactaid, 375
lactulose, Kristalose (OTC)
  occasional constipation, 170
Lamictal, *lamotrigine* (G), 695
  bipolar disorder, 61
Lamisil, *terbinafine,* 704
  onychomycosis (fungal nail), 422
  tinea corporis, 598
  tinea cruris, 599
  tinea pedis, 600
  tinea versicolor, 601
lamivudine, Epivir, Epivir-HBV (G)
  dose forms, 696, 707
  hepatitis B, 293
  human immunodeficiency virus
    infection, 309
lamotrigine, Lamictal (G), 695
  bipolar disorder, 61
lanadelumab-flyo, Takhzyro
  hereditary angioedema, 297
lansoprazole, Prevacid
  gastroesophageal reflux disease, 250
  peptic ulcer disease (PUD), 478
  Zollinger-Ellison syndrome, 662
lanthanum carbonate, Fosrenol (G)
  hyperphosphatemia, 325
lapatinib ditosylate, Tykerb
  breast cancer, 79–80
Lariam, *mefloquine* (G), 704
  malaria, 386
  systemic lupus erythematosis, 585
Lartruvo, *olaratumab,* 686
Lasix, *furosemide* (G)
  edema, 229
  heart failure, 281
  hypertension, 328
Lastacaft, *alcaftadine*
  allergic (vernal) conjunctivitis, 166
latanoprost, Xalatan, Xelpros (G)
  glaucoma, 256
latanoprostene bunod, Vyzulta
  glaucoma, 256
Latisse, *bimatoprost* (G)
  hypotrichosis, 347
Latuda, *lurasidone*
  bipolar disorder, 63
  schizophrenia, 564
Lazanda Nasal Spray, *fentanyl* (G)(II)
  pain, 462
  urolithiasis, 648
lead poisoning
  deferoxamine mesylate, Desferal (G),
    376
  edetate calcium disodium (EDTA),
    Calcium Disodium Versenate,
    376
  succimer, Chemet (G), 376
lecanemab-irmb, Leqembi
  Alzheimer's disease, 14
Leena, *ethinyl estradiol+norethindrone*
  estrogen and progesterone, 669
leflunomide, Arava
  rheumatoid arthritis, 546
  systemic lupus erythematosis, 583
leg cramps
  quinine sulfate, Qualaquin (G), 376

legionella pneumonia
  ciprofloxacin, Cipro (G), Cipro XR,
    ProQuin XR (G), 496
  clarithromycin, Biaxin, 496
  dirithromycin, Dynabac (G), 496
  erythromycin base, Ery-Tab, PCE, 496
  erythromycin estolate, Ilosone, 496
  trimethoprim+sulfamethoxazole,
    Bactrim (TMP-SMX) (G), 496
leishmaniasis
  miltefosine, Impavido, 376–377
lemborexant, Dayvigo
  insomnia, 360
Lemvima, *lenvatinib,* 687
lenacapavir, Sunlenca
  human immunodeficiency virus
    (HIV) infection, 313–314
lenalidomide, Revlimid
  multiple myeloma, 121–122
Lennox-Gastaut syndrome (LGS)
  cannabidiol, Epidiolex, 377
  clobazam, Onfi, Sympaza Oral Film
    (G)(IV), 377
  stiripentol, Diacomit, 378
  topiramate, Eprontia, 378
lentigines
  tazarotene, Avage, Tazorac, 379
  tretinoin, Altreno, Atralin, Avita,
    Retin-A, Tretin-X (G), 379
Leqembi, *lecanemab-irmb*
  Alzheimer's disease, 14
Leqvio, *inclisiran*
  dyslipidemia, 221
Lescol, Lescol XL, *fluvastatin*
  dyslipidemia, 222
  hypertriglyceridemia, 339
lesinurad, Zurampic (G)
  gout (hyperuricemia), 261
Lessina 28, *ethinyl estradiol/levonorgestrel*
  estrogen and progesterone, 669
Letairis, *ambrisentan*
  pulmonary arterial hypertension
    (PAH), 533
letermovir, Prevymis
  cytomegalovirus (CMV) retinitis, 187
letrozole, Femara
  breast cancer, 78
  dose forms, 685
leukemia
  *asparaginase erwinia chrysanthemi
    (recombinant)-rywn,* Rylaze,
    96–97
  azacytidine, Onureg, 96
  ofatumumab, Arzerra, 97
  rituximab-arrx, Riabni, 98
  rituximab+hyaluronidase, Rituxan
    Hycela, 98–99
  rituximab, Rituxan, 98
  zanubrutinib, Brukinsa, 96
Leukeran, *chlorambucil,* 687
leuprolide acetate, Eligard, Fensolvi,
    Lupron Depot, 685
  endometriosis, 233
  precocious puberty, central, 512–513
leuprolide mesylate, Camcevi
  prostate cancer, 128
levalbuterol tartrate, Xopenex (G)
  asthma, 40
levamlodipine maleate, Conjupri
  hypertension, 331
Levaquin, *levofloxacin* (G), 708
  acute bacterial sinusitis, rhinosinusitis,
    572
  acute exacerbation of chronic
    bronchitis, 70
  bacterial skin infection, 575
  Chlamydia trachomatis, 152
  chlamydial pneumonia, 492
  community-acquired pneumonia, 494
  epididymitis, 237

  nongonococcal urethritis, 639
  pyelonephritis: acute, 536
  urinary tract infection, 644
  wound, 660
Levatol, penbutolol
  hypertension, 326
Levbid, *hyoscyamine* (G)
  abdominal cramps, 174
  interstitial cystitis, 361
  irritable bowel syndrome with
    diarrhea, 367
  urinary overactive bladder, 354
  urinary tract infection (UTI), 642
Levitra, *vardenafil*
  erectile dysfunction (ED), 237
Levlen 21, Levlen 28, *ethinyl estradiol/
    levonorgestrel*
  estrogen and progesterone, 669
Levlite 28, *ethinyl estradiol/levonorgestrel*
  estrogen and progesterone, 669
levobunolol, Betagan (G)
  glaucoma, 256
levocabastine, Livostin (G)
  allergic (vernal) conjunctivitis, 166
levocetirizine, Children's Xyzal Allergy
    24HR, Xyzal Allergy 24HR
  atopic dermatitis, 198
  contact dermatitis, 202
  genus rhus dermatitis, 204
  rhinitis medicamentosa, 555
  rhinitis/sinusitis, allergic, 550
  urticaria, 649
levodopa inhalation powder, Inbrija
  Parkinson's disease, 467
levofloxacin, Levaquin, Quixin
    Ophthalmic Solution (G)
  acute bacterial sinusitis, rhinosinusitis,
    572
  acute exacerbation of chronic
    bronchitis, 70
  bacterial skin infection, 575
  Chlamydia trachomatis, 152
  chlamydial pneumonia, 492
  community-acquired pneumonia,
    494
  epididymitis, 237
  nongonococcal urethritis, 639
  pyelonephritis: acute, 536
  urinary tract infection, 644
  wound, 660
levoketoconazole, Recorlev
  Cushing's syndrome, 180–181
levomilnacipran, Fetzima (G)
  major depressive disorder, 192
levonorgestrel, EContra EZ, My Way,
    Plan B One Step, EContra EZ,
    Preventeza, Kyleena, Liletta,
    Mirena, Norplant, Skyla, 675
Levora-21, Levora-28, *ethinyl estradiol/
    levonorgestrel*
  estrogen and progesterone, 669
levothyroxine, Levoxyl, Synthroid,
    Unithroid (A)
  hypothyroidism, 346
levothyroxine sodium, T4 (A)
  hypothyroidism, 347
Levoxyl, *levothyroxine* (A)
  hypothyroidism, 346
Levsin, *hyoscyamine* (G), 93
  abdominal cramps, 174
  infantile colic, 159
  interstitial cystitis, 361
  irritable bowel syndrome with
    diarrhea, 367
  urinary overactive bladder, 354
  urinary tract infection (UTI), 642
Levsinex, *hyoscyamine*
  abdominal cramps, 174
  infantile colic, 159
  interstitial cystitis, 361

irritable bowel syndrome with
diarrhea, 367
urinary overactive bladder, 354
urinary tract infection (UTI), 642
Lexapro, Lexapro Oral Solution,
escitalopram (G)
anxiety disorder, 35
major depressive disorder, 192
panic disorder, 464
posttraumatic stress disorder, 510
Lexxel, *enalapril+felodipine*
hypertension, 336
L-glutamine powder, Endari
sickle cell disease, 569
Lialda, *mesalamine*
Crohn's disease, 176
ulcerative colitis, 635
Librax, *chlordiazepoxide+clidinium* (IV)
abdominal cramps, 175
anxiety disorder, 33
interstitial cystitis, 362
irritable bowel syndrome with
diarrhea, 367
panic disorder, 466
Librium, *chlordiazepoxide* (IV)
alcohol withdrawal syndrome, 11
anxiety disorder, 33
panic disorder, 466
Libtayo, *cemiplimab-rwlc*, 687
basal cell carcinoma, 76–77
lung cancer, 105–106
squamous cell carcinoma, 130–131
LidaMantle HC, *lidocaine+hydrocortisone*
atopic dermatitis, 200
burn: minor, 76
diabetic peripheral neuropathy
(DPN), 209
gouty arthritis, 262
hemorrhoids, 290
herpangina, 299
herpes zoster, 302
insect bite/sting, 2358
juvenile idiopathic arthritis, 369
juvenile rheumatoid arthritis, 373
muscle strain, 405
pain, 454
peripheral neuritis, 481
postherpetic neuralgia, 509
LidaMantle, *lidocaine*, 509
atopic dermatitis, 200
burn: minor, 76
diabetic peripheral neuropathy, 209
gouty arthritis, 262
hemorrhoids, 292
herpangina, 299
herpes zoster, 302
insect bite/sting, 358
juvenile idiopathic arthritis, 369
juvenile rheumatoid arthritis, 372
muscle strain, 405, 406
pain, 454
peripheral neuritis, 481
post-herpetic neuralgia, 509
lidocaine, LidaMantle, Lidoderm, ZTlido
lidocaine, 509
atopic dermatitis, 200
burn: minor, 76
diabetic peripheral neuropathy, 209
gouty arthritis, 262
hemorrhoids, 292
herpangina, 299
herpes zoster, 302
insect bite/sting, 358
juvenile idiopathic arthritis, 369
juvenile rheumatoid arthritis, 372
muscle strain, 405, 406
pain, 454
peripheral neuritis, 481
post-herpetic neuralgia, 509
lidocaine, Xylocaine Viscous Solution

aphthous stomatitis, 37
Lidoderm, *lidocaine*
atopic dermatitis, 200
burn: minor, 76
diabetic peripheral neuropathy, 209
gouty arthritis, 262
hemorrhoids, 292
herpangina, 299
herpes zoster, 302
insect bite/sting, 358
juvenile idiopathic arthritis, 369
juvenile rheumatoid arthritis, 372
muscle strain, 405, 406
pain, 454
peripheral neuritis, 481
post-herpetic neuralgia, 509
lifitegrast, Xiidra (G)
dry eye syndrome, 216
Liletta, *levonorgestrel*, 675
Limbitrol, *chlordiazepoxide+amitriptyline*
anxiety disorder, 36
major depressive disorder, 194
linaclotide, Linzess (G)
chronic idiopathic constipation, 168
irritable bowel syndrome with
constipation, 365
linagliptin, Tradjenta
type 2 diabetes mellitus, 629
lindane, Kwell (G)
pediculosis humanus capitis, 475
scabies, 559
linezolid, Zyvox (G), 710
cellulitis, 144
community-acquired pneumonia,
494
Linzess, *linaclotide* (G)
chronic idiopathic constipation, 168
irritable bowel syndrome with
constipation, 365
Lioresal, *baclofen* (G)
muscle strain, 403
temporomandibular joint disorder,
586
trigeminal neuralgia, 608
liothyronine, Cytomel (A)
hypothyroidism, 346
Lipitor, *atorvastatin*
dyslipidemia, 222
hypertriglyceridemia, 339
Lipofen, *fenofibrate* (G)
dyslipidemia, 223
hypertriglyceridemia, 338
Liptruzet, *ezetimibe+atorvastatin*
dyslipidemia, 222
liraglutide, Saxenda, Victoza (G)
obesity, 420
type 2 diabetes mellitus, 624
lisdexamfetamine dimesylate, Vyvanse
(G)(II)
attention deficit hyperactivity disorder
(ADHD), 52
binge eating disorder, 60
lisinopril, Prinivil, Qbrelis Oral Solution,
Zestril
heart failure, 279
hypertension, 329–330
lisocabtagene maraleucel, Breyanzi
lymphoma, 110–111
listeriosis
ampicillin, Unasyn, 379
penicillin g potassium, 379
*trimethoprim-sulfamethoxazole
(TMP-SMX)* (G), 379
lithium carbonate, Lithobid
bipolar disorder, 61
trichotillomania, 608
Lithobid, *lithium carbonate*
bipolar disorder, 61
trichotillomania, 608
Livalo, *pitavastatin*

dyslipidemia, 222
liver flukes
praziquantel, Biltricide, 380
triclabendazole, Egaten, 379
Livostin, *levocabastine* (G)
allergic (vernal) conjunctivitis, 166
Livtencity, *maribavir*
posttransplant cytomegalovirus
(CMV), 185
lixisenatide, Adlyxin (G)
type 2 diabetes mellitus, 624
Lodosyn, *carbidopa* (G)
Parkinson's disease, 466
lodoxamide tromethamine, Alomide
allergic (vernal) conjunctivitis, 166
vernal keratitis, 375
Loestrin 21, *ethinyl estradiol+
norethindrone plus ferrous
fumarate*
estrogen and progesterone, 570
Loestrin 21 1.5/30, *ethinyl estradiol+
norethindrone*
estrogen and progesterone, 670
Loestrin 21 1/20, *ethinyl estradiol+
norethindrone*
estrogen and progesterone, 670
Loestrin 24 Fe, *ethinyl estradiol+
norethindrone plus ferrous
fumarate*
estrogen and progesterone, 670
Loestrin Fe 1.5/30, *ethinyl estradiol+
norethindrone plus ferrous
fumarate*
estrogen and progesterone, 670
Loestrin Fe 1/20, *ethinyl estradiol+
norethindrone plus ferrous
fumarate*
estrogen and progesterone, 670
lofexidine, Lucemyra (G)
opioid dependence, 424
Lofibra, *fenofibrate* (G)
dyslipidemia, 223
hypertriglyceridemia, 338
Logilia, *ulipristal acetate* (UPA), 676
uterine fibroids, 651
Lokelma, *sodium zirconium cyclosilicate*
hyperkalemia, 322–323
Lomedia 24 Fe, *ethinyl estradiol+
norethindrone plus ferrous
fumarate*
estrogen and progesterone, 670
lomefloxacin, Maxaquin (G)
urinary tract infection, 644
lomitapide mesylate, Juxtapid
dyslipidemia, 220s
Lomotil, *diphenoxylate+atropine* (G)(V)
acute diarrhea, 212
chronic diarrhea, 213
irritable bowel syndrome with
diarrhea, 366
ulcerative colitis, 638
loncastuximab tesirine-lpyl, Zynlonta
lymphoma, 109
Lonhala Magnair, *glycopyrrolate
inhalation solution* (G)
chronic obstructive pulmonary
disease (COPD), 71, 72
emphysema, 230–231
Lo/Ovral-21, Lo/Ovral-28, *ethinyl
estradiol+norgestrel*
estrogen and progesterone, 670
loperamide, Imodium, Imodium A-D
acute diarrhea, 212
chronic diarrhea, 213
irritable bowel syndrome with
diarrhea, 366
ulcerative colitis, 638
Lopid, *gemfibrozil*
dyslipidemia, 223
hypertriglyceridemia, 338

Lopressor HCT, *metoprolol succinate+ hydrochlorothiazide* (G)
  hypertension, 334–335
Lopressor, *metoprolol tartrate* (G)
  angina pectoris: stable, 29
  headache: migraine, 275
  heart failure, 280
  hypertension: primary, 326
Loprox, *ciclopirox*
  onychomycosis (fungal nail), 422
  seborrheic dermatitis, 204
  skin candidiasis, 135
  tinea corporis, 597
  tinea cruris, 598
  tinea pedis, 600
  tinea versicolor, 601
Lorabid, *loracarbef*, 706, 720
  acute bacterial sinusitis, rhinosinusitis, 572
  acute exacerbation of chronic bronchitis, 70
  acute tonsillitis, 604–605
  bacterial skin infection, 575
  cellulitis, 144
  community-acquired pneumonia, 494
  impetigo contagiosa, 353
  otitis media: acute, 447
  pyelonephritis: acute, 536
  streptococcal pharyngitis, 485
  wound, 660
loracarbef, Lorabid, 706, 720
  acute bacterial sinusitis, rhinosinusitis, 572
  acute exacerbation of chronic bronchitis, 70
  acute tonsillitis, 604–605
  bacterial skin infection, 575
  cellulitis, 144
  community-acquired pneumonia, 494
  impetigo contagiosa, 353
  otitis media: acute, 447
  pyelonephritis: acute, 536
  streptococcal pharyngitis, 485
  wound, 660
loratadine, Claritin (OTC)(G)
  allergic rhinitis/sinusitis, 550
  atopic dermatitis, 198
  contact dermatitis, 202
  genus rhus dermatitis, 204
  rhinitis medicamentosa, 555
  urticaria, 649
lorazepam, Ativan, Lorazepam Intensol (IV)
  anxiety disorder, 33
  delirium, 188
  panic disorder, 466
  status epilepticus, 579
Lorazepam Intensol, *lorazepam* (IV)
  anxiety disorder, 33
  delirium, 188
  panic disorder, 466
Lorbrena, *lorlatinib*, 687
lorcaserin, Belviq
  obesity, 420
Lorcet, *hydrocodone bitartrate+ acetaminophen* (G)(II)
  pain, 455–456
Loryna, *ethinyl estradiol+drospirenone*
  estrogen and progesterone, 670
losartan, Cozaar (G)
  hypertension, 330
LoSeasonique, *ethinyl estradiol+levonorgestrel* (G), 673
Lotemax, *loteprednol etabonate* (G)
  allergic (vernal) conjunctivitis, 166
  iritis: acute, 364
Lotensin HCT, *benazepril+ hydrochlorothiazide*
  hypertension, 333

loteprednol etabonate, Alrex, Eysuvis, Lotemax (G)
  allergic (vernal) conjunctivitis, 166
  dry eye disease, 218
  eye pain, 241
  iritis: acute, 364
Lotrel, *amlodipine+benazepril*
  hypertension, 335
Lotrimin AF, *miconazole* (G)
  diaper rash, 211
  skin candidiasis, 136
  tinea corporis, 597
  tinea cruris, 509
  tinea pedis, 600
  tinea versicolor, 601
Lotrimin, Lotrimin AF, *clotrimazole*
  diaper rash, 211
  skin candidiasis, 135
  tinea corporis, 597
  tinea cruris, 508
  tinea pedis, 600
  tinea versicolor, 601
Lotrimin Ultra, *butenafine*
  diaper rash, 211
  skin candidiasis, 135
  tinea corporis, 597
  tinea cruris, 598
  tinea pedis, 599
  tinea versicolor, 601
Lotrisone, *clotrimazole+betamethasone* (G)
  diaper rash, 211
  tinea corporis, 598
  tinea pedis, 600
Lou Gehrig's disease. *See* amyotrophic lateral sclerosis
lovastatin, Mevacor, Altoprev
  dyslipidemia, 222
  hypertriglyceridemia, 339
Lovaza, *omega 3-fatty acid ethyl esters* (G)
  dyslipidemia, 222
  hypertriglyceridemia, 339
low back strain (LBS), 380
low libido, hypoactive sexual desire disorder (HSDD)
  bremelanotide, Vyleesi, 381
  flibanserin, Addyi, 293
  selpercatinib, Retevmo, 381
Low-Ogestrel-21, Low-Ogestrel-28, *ethinyl estradiol+norgestrel*
  estrogen and progesterone, 670
Lozol, *indapamide*
  edema, 229
  heart failure, 282
  hypertension, 328
lubiprostone, Amitiza (G)
  chronic idiopathic constipation, 169
  irritable bowel syndrome with constipation, 365
  opioid-induced constipation, 428
Lubriderm Dry Skin Lotion
  atopic dermatitis, 197
  psoriasis, 526
  xerosis, 661
Lubriderm Sensitive Skin Lotion
  atopic dermatitis, 197
  psoriasis, 526
  xerosis, 661
Lucentis, *ranibizumab* (G)
  diabetic macular edema, 206
Ludiomil, *maprotiline*
  major depressive disorder, 194
Lufyllin GG, *dyphylline+guaifenesin* (G)
  asthma, 45
  chronic obstructive pulmonary disease, 74
  emphysema, 232
luliconazole, Luzu Cream (G)

tinea corporis, 597
tinea cruris, 599
tinea pedis, 600
lumateperone, Caplyta
  bipolar disorder, 63
  schizophrenia, 563
Lumoxiti, *moxetumomab pasudotox-tdfk*, 687
Lumryz, *sodium oxybate, extended-release* (III)
  narcolepsy, 410–411
lung cancer
  adagrasib, Krazati, 108
  amivantamab-vmjw, Rybrevant, 107–108
  bevacizumab-adcd, Vegzelma, 102
  bevacizumab-bvzr, Zirabev, 103
  brigatinib, Alunbrig, 103
  capmatinib, Tabrecta, 103
  cemiplimab-rwlc, Libtayo, 105–106
  gefitinib, Iressa (G), 105
  pembrolizumab, Keytruda, 106
  pemetrexed, Pemfexy (G), 105
  pralsetinib, Gavreto, 103
  selpercatinib, Retevmo, 103–104
  sodium thiosulfate, Pedmark, 102
  tepotinib, Tepmetko, 104
  tremelimumab-actl, Imjudo, 106–107
  trilaciclib, Cosela, 104
Lunesta, *eszopiclone* (G)(IV)
  fibromyalgia, 244
  insomnia, 359
Lupron Depot, *leuprolide acetate (GnRH analog)*
  endometriosis, 233
Lupron, *leuprolide*, 687
lurasidone, Latuda
  bipolar disorder, 63
  schizophrenia, 564
luspatercept-aamt, Reblozyl
  beta thalassemia-associated anemia, 21–22
Lustra, Lustra AF, *hydroquinone* (G)
  hyperpigmentation, 325
  melasma/chloasma, 387
  vitiligo, 653
lusutrombopag, Mulpleta
  idiopathic thrombocytopenia purpura, 594
Lutera, *ethinyl estradiol/levonorgestrel*
  estrogen and progesterone, 670
Luvox, *fluvoxamine* (G)
  obsessive-compulsive disorder, 421
  trichotillomania, 607
Luxiq, *betamethasone valerate* (G)
  seborrheic dermatitis, 205
Luzu Cream, *luliconazole* (G)
  tinea corporis, 597
  tinea cruris, 599
  tinea pedis, 600
Lybrel, *ethinyl estradiol/levonorgestrel*, 670
  estrogen and progesterone, 670, 674
Lyme disease
  amoxicillin, Amoxil, Moxatag, Trimox, 382
  clarithromycin, Biaxin, 383
  doxycycline, Acticlate, Adoxa, Doryx, Doxteric, Monodox, Oracea, Vibramycin, Vibra-Tab, 383
  minocycline, Dynacin, Minocin, 383
  tetracycline, Achromycin V, Sumycin, 383
lymphadenitis
  augmentin, Augmentin ES-600, Augmentin XR, *amoxicillin+clavulanate*, 383
  cephalexin, Keflex, 383
  dicloxacillin, Dynapen, 383

lymphogranuloma venereum
  azithromycin, Zithromax, Zmax, 384
  doxycycline, Acticlate, Adoxa, Doryx,
    Doxteric, Monodox, Oracea,
    Vibramycin, Vibra-Tab, 384
  erythromycin base, Ery-Tab, PCE, 384
  erythromycin ethylsuccinate, EryPed,
    E.E.S, 384
lymphoma
  bexarotene, Targretin, 114–115
  brentuximab vedotin, Adcetris, 114
  epcoritamab-bysp, Epkinly, 109–110
  lisocabtagene maraleucel, Breyanzi,
    110–111
  loncastuximab tesirine-lpyl, Zynlonta,
    109
  mosunetuzumab-axgb, Lunsumio,
    113–114
  pembrolizumab, Keytruda, 108–109
  pemetrexed, Pemfexy (G), 111
  rituximab-arrx, Riabni, 113
  rituximab+hyaluronidase human,
    Rituxan Hycela, 112–113
  rituximab, Rituxan, 111–112
  zanubrutinib, Brukinsa, 109
Lynparza, *olaparib,* 687
  breast cancer, 81
  fallopian tube cancer, 59
  pancreatic cancer, 124
  peritoneal cancer, 125
Lyrica, Lyrica CR, *pregabalin (GABA
    analog)* (G)(V), 695
  diabetic peripheral neuropathy
    (DPN), 210
  fibromyalgia, 244
  peripheral neuritis, 480
  postherpetic neuralgia, 507, 508
  restless legs syndrome, 540
Lysteda, *tranexamic acid*
  menometrorrhagia, 389
Lytgobi, *futibatinib*
  hepatocellular carcinoma (HCC), 101

Maalox, *aluminum hydroxide+
    magnesium hydroxide* (G)
  gastroesophageal reflux disease, 248
Maalox HRF, *aluminum hydroxide+
    magnesium carbonate* (G)
  gastroesophageal reflux disease, 248
Maalox Plus, Extra Strength Maalox
    Plus, Mylanta, *aluminum
    hydroxide+magnesium
    hydroxide+simethicone,* (G)
  gastroesophageal reflux disease, 248
magnesium citrate, Citrate of Magnesia
    (OTC)
  occasional constipation, 170
magnesium hydroxide, Milk of Magnesia
  occasional constipation, 170
magnesium oxide, Mag-Ox 400
  hypomagnesemia, 344
  migraine and cluster headache, 277
  tension headache, 278
magnesium, Slow-Mag
  hypomagnesemia, 344
  migraine and cluster headache, 277
  tension headache, 278
Mag-Ox 400, *magnesium oxide*
  hypomagnesemia, 344
  migraine and cluster headache, 277
  tension headache, 278
major depressive disorder (MDD)
  amitriptyline (G), 193
  amoxapine (G), 193
  aripiprazole, Abilify (G), 194
  brexpiprazole, Rexulti (G), 194–195
  bupropion HBr, Aplenzin (G), 193
  bupropion HCl, Forfivo XL, Wellbutrin
    (G), 193–194

cariprazine, Vraylar, 195
chlordiazepoxide+amitriptyline,
    Limbitrol (G)(IV), 194
citalopram, Celexa (G), 191
desipramine, Norpramin (G), 193
desvenlafaxine, Pristiq (G), 192
doxepin, 193
duloxetine, Cymbalta (G), 192
escitalopram, Lexapro, Lexapro Oral
    Solution (G), 192
fluoxetine, Prozac, Prozac Weekly (G),
    192
imipramine, Tofranil (G), 193
isocarboxazid, Marplan (G), 194
levomilnacipran, Fetzima (G), 192
maprotiline, Ludiomil, 194
mirtazapine, Remeron (G), 194
nortriptyline, Pamelor, 193
olanzapine+fluoxetine, Symbyax (G),
    193
paroxetine maleate, Paxil, 192
paroxetine mesylate, Brisdelle, 192
phenelzine, Nardil (G), 194
protriptyline, Vivactil, 193
selegiline, Emsam (G), 194
sertraline, Zoloft (G), 192
tranylcypromine, Parnate (G), 194
trazodone, Oleptro (G), 194
trimipramine, Surmontil, 193
venlafaxine, Effexor, Effexor XR (G),
    192
vilazodone, Viibryd (G), 193
vortioxetine, Trintellix (G), 192
malaria
  artesunate, Artesunate for Injection, 385
  atovaquone, Mepron (G), 385
  atovaquone+proguanil, Malarone (G),
    385
  chloroquine, Aralen (G), 385–386
  doxycycline, Acticlate, Adoxa, Doryx,
    Doxteric, Monodox, Oracea,
    Vibramycin, Vibra-Tab, 384
  hydroxychloroquine, Plaquenil (G), 386
  mefloquine, Lariam (G), 386
  minocycline, Dynacin, Minocin,
    384–385
  quinine sulfate, Qualaquin (G), 386
  tafenoquine, Arakoda (G), 386
  tafenoquine, Krintafe, 386
  tetracycline, Achromycin V, Sumycin,
    385
Malarone, *atovaquone+proguanil* (G),
    704
  malaria, 385
  systemic lupus erythematosis, 584
malathion, Ovide (OTC)
  pediculosis humanus capitis, 475
maprotiline, Ludiomil, 697
  major depressive disorder, 194
maraviroc, Selzentry
  human immunodeficiency virus
    infection, 312
Margenza, *margetuximab-cmkb*
  breast cancer, 81–82
margetuximab-cmkb, Margenza,
  breast cancer, 81–82
maribavir, Livtencity
  posttransplant cytomegalovirus
    (CMV), 185
Marinol, *dronabinol* (G)(III)
  anorexia/cachexia, 30
  chemotherapy-induced nausea/
    vomiting, 149
Marplan, *isocarboxazid* (G)
  major depressive disorder, 194
mastitis (breast abscess)
  augmentin, Augmentin
    ES-600, Augmentin XR,
    amoxicillin+clavulanate, 387

cefaclor, Cefaclor Extended Release, 387
ceftriaxone, Rocephin, 387
cephalexin, Keflex, 387
clindamycin, Cleocin, Cleocin
    Pediatric Granules, 387
erythromycin base, Ery-Tab, PCE, 387
Mavenclad, *cladribine*
  multiple sclerosis (MS), 397
Mavik, *trandolapril* (G)
  heart failure, 280
  hypertension: primary, 330
Mavyret, *glecaprevir+pibrentasvir*
  hepatitis C (HCV), 294–295
Maxair, *pirbuterol* (G)
  asthma, 40
Maxaquin, *imipramine* (G), 708
  gonorrhea, 259
  urinary tract infection, 644
Maxidex, *dexamethasone* (G)
  allergic (vernal) conjunctivitis, 165
Maxidone, *hydrocodone bitartrate+
    acetaminophen* (G)(II)
  pain, 455–456
Maximum Strength Tylenol Sore Throat,
    acetaminophen
  fever (pyrexia), 242
Maxitrol Ophthalmic Suspension,
    Maxitrol Ophthalmic Ointment,
    *neomycin sulfate+polymyxin b
    sulfate+dexamethasone* (G)
  bacterial conjunctivitis, 163
Maxzide, *triamterene+
    hydrochlorothiazide* (G)
  edema, 230
  heart failure, 282
  hypertension: primary, 329
Mayzent, *siponimod*
  multiple sclerosis (MS), 401
*measles, mumps, rubella, live, attenuated,
    neomycin vaccine,* MMR II (G)
  mumps, 403
  rubella, 558
  rubeola, 558
mebendazole, Emverm, Vermox (G)
  hookworm, 305
  pinworm, 488
  roundworm, 557
  threadworm, 593
  trichinosis, 606
  whipworm, 656
mecasermin, Increlex
  growth failure, 266
meclizine, Antivert, Bonine (OTC),
    Dramamine II (OTC), Zentrip
  labyrinthitis, 375
  Meniere's disease, 388
  motion sickness, 396
  vertigo, 653
Medihaler-1SO, *isoproterenol*
  asthma, 40
medroxyprogesterone, Amen, Depo-
    Provera, Depo-SubQ, Provera
  amenorrhea, secondary, 18
  endometriosis, 232
  menometrorrhagia, 389
  menopause, 392
medroxyprogesterone acetate, Provera
  dysfunctional uterine bleeding, 220
  endometriosis, 232
  uterine leiomyomata, 650
medrysone, HMS (G)
  allergic (vernal) conjunctivitis, 166
mefenamic acid, Ponstel (G)
  dysmenorrhea: primary, 225
mefloquine, Lariam (G)
  malaria, 386
  systemic lupus erythematosis, 585
Mefoxin, *cefoxitin*
  dose form/volume, 706

Mefoxin, *cefoxitin (cont.)*
  gonorrhea, 259
  human bite, 66
  pelvic inflammatory disease, 476
Megace, Megace ES, Megace Oral
    Suspension, *megestrol*
    (progestin) (G), 587
  anorexia/cachexia, 31
megestrol (progestin), Megace, Megace
    ES, Megace Oral Suspension,
    Megestrol Acetate Oral
    Suspension (G)
  anorexia/cachexia, 31
Megestrol Acetate Oral Suspension,
    megestrol (progestin) (G)
  anorexia/cachexia, 31
Mekinist, *trametinib*, 687
  melanoma, 117
Mektovi, *binimetinib*, 687
melanoma, 116–119
  dabrafenib, Tafinlar, 117
  *daratumumb+hyaluronidase, Darzalex
    Faspro*, 118
  nivolumab, Opdivo, 118
  *nivolumab+relatlimab-rmbw,
    Opdualag*, 116
  pembrolizumab, Keytruda, 116
  trametinib, Mekinist, 117–118
melasma/chloasma
  hydroquinone, Lustra, Lustra AF (G),
    387
  tri-Luma, *hydroquinone+fluocinolone+
    tretinoin* (G), 387
Mellaril, *thioridazine* (G)
  delirium, 188
  dementia, 189
  methamphetamine-induced
    psychosis, 396
meloxicam, Anjeso, Mobic, Vivlodex (G),
    573
  dysmenorrhea: primary, 225
  gouty arthritis, 263
  muscle strain, 406
  osteoarthritis, 436
  pain, 451
  psoriatic arthritis, 528
  rheumatoid arthritis, 544
melphalan flufenamide, Pepaxto
  multiple myeloma, 121
memantine, Namenda
  Alzheimer's disease, 15
Menactra, *Neisseria meningitidis
    polysaccharides* (G)
  meningitis, 389
Meniere's disease
  diazepam, Diastat, Valium (IV), 388
  dimenhydrinate, Dramamine (OTC),
    388
  diphenhydramine, Benadryl, 388
  meclizine, Antivert, Bonine (OTC),
    Dramamine II (OTC), Zentrip,
    388
  promethazine, Phenergan (G), 388
  scopolamine, Transderm Scop (G),
    388
meningitis
  *Meningococcal group b vaccine
    [recombinant, absorbed]*,
    Bexsero, Trumenba, 388
  *Neisseria meningitides oligosaccharide
    conjugate*, Menveo, 389
  Neisseria meningitides polysaccharides,
    Menactra, Menomune-A/C/
    Y/W-135 (G), 389
  *Meningococcal group b vaccine
    [recombinant, absorbed]*,
    Bexsero, Trumenba
  meningitis, 388
menometrorrhagia

medroxyprogesterone, Depo-Provera,
    Depo-SubQ, 389
tranexamic acid, Lysteda, 389
Menomune-A/C/Y/W-135, *Neisseria
    meningitidis polysaccharides* (G)
  meningitis, 389
menopause
  Bijuvia, estradiol+projesterone, 392
  Duavee, *estrogen,
    conjugated+bazedoxifene*, 392
  estradiol, acetate, Femring Vaginal
    Ring, 390
  estradiol, Alora, Climara, Divigel,
    Esclim, Estraderm, Estrace,
    Estrasorb, EstroGel, Evamist,
    Menostar, Vivelle, Vivelle-Dot
    (G), 391–393
  estradiol, micronized, Estrace Vaginal
    Cream (G), 390
  estradiol, Vagifem Tabs, Yuvafem
    Vaginal Tablet, 390, 392
  estradiol+drospirenone, Angeliq, 391
  estradiol+levonorgestrel, Climara
    Pro, 391
  estradiol+norethindrone, Activella,
    FemHRT, Fyavolv (G), Mimvey
    LO, 391
  estradiol+norethindrone, CombiPatch,
    391
  estradiol+norgestimate, Ortho-Prefest,
    391
  estradiol+progesterone, Bijuva (G),
    391, 392
  estrogen, conjugated+bazedoxifene,
    Duavee, 392
  estrogen, conjugated (synthetic),
    Cenestin, Enjuvia, 392
  estrogen, conjugated equine, Premarin
    Vaginal Cream, 390, 392
  *estrogen, conjugated+
    medroxyprogesterone*, Prempro,
    Premphase, 391
  estrogen, esterified (plant derived),
    Estratab, Menest, 391, 392
  estropipate, piperazine estrone sulfate,
    Ogen, Ortho-Est, 391–392
  ethinyl estradiol, Estinyl, 391, 392
  medroxyprogesterone, Provera, 392
  norethindrone acetate, Aygestin, 392
  progesterone, micronized, Prometrium,
    392
Mentax, *butenafine*
  diaper rash, 211
  skin candidiasis, 135
  tinea corporis, 597
  tinea cruris, 598
  tinea pedis, 599
  tinea versicolor, 601
Menveo, *Neisseria meningitides
    oligosaccharide conjugate*
  meningitis, 388–389
mepenzolate, Cantil
  peptic ulcer disease (PUD), 480
Mepergan, *meperidine+promethazine* (G)
  pain, 457
meperidine, Demerol (G)
  pain, 457
mepolizumab, Nucala
  allergic rhinitis/sinusitis, 554
  eosinophilia, 48
  eosinophilic granulomatosis with
    polyangitis, 235–236
Mepron, *atovaquone* (G)
  malaria, 385
  dose form/volume, 704
  Pneumocystis jiroveci pneumonia,
    498
  systemic lupus erythematosis, 584
merkel cell carcinoma, 119–120

pembrolizumab, Keytruda, 119
retifanlimab-dlwr, Zynyz, 119
Meruvax II, *rubella virus, live, attenuated+
    neomycin vaccine* (G)
  rubella, 558
mesalamine, Asacol, Asacol HD, Canasa,
    Delzicol, Lialda, Pentasa, Rowasa
    Enema, Rowasa Suppository,
    Sulfite-Free Rowasa Rectal
    Suspension
  Crohn's disease, 175
  ulcerative colitis, 635
mesoridazine, Serentil (G)
  delirium, 188
  dementia, 188
  methamphetamine-induced
    psychosis, 395
mesothelioma
  capmatinib, Tabrecta, 393
  pemetrexed, Pemfexy (G), 393–394
Metadate CD, Metadate ER,
    methylphenidate (long-acting)
    (G)(II)
  attention deficit hyperactivity disorder
    (ADHD), 53
  narcolepsy, 412
Metaglip, *glipizide+metformin* (G)
  type 2 diabetes mellitus, 622
Metamucil (OTC), *psyllium husk*
  occasional constipation, 169
Metanx, *L-methylfolate calcium
    (as metafolin)+pyridoxyl
    5-phosphate+methylcobalamin*
  diabetic peripheral neuropathy, 208
  diabetic ulcer, 633
  hyperhomocysteinemia, 321
metaproterenol, Alupent (G)
  asthma, 40, 44
metaxalone, Skelaxin
  muscle strain, 404
  temporomandibular joint disorder,
    587
metformin, Fortamet, Glucophage,
    Glumetza ER, Riomet XR
  type 2 diabetes mellitus, 620
methadone, Dolophine (G)(II)
  opioid dependence, 424
  pain, 457
methamphetamine, Desoxyn (G)(II)
  obesity, 419
methamphetamine-induced psychosis
  aripiprazole, Abilify (G), 394
  aripiprazole lauroxil, Aristada,
    Aristada Initio (G), 394–395
  fluphenazine decanoate [Prolixin
    Decanoate] (G), 395
  fluphenazine hcl [Prolixin] (G), 395
  haloperidol, Haldol (G), 395
  mesoridazine, Serentil, 395
  olanzapine, Zyprexa, Zyprexa Zydis,
    395
  quetiapine fumarate, SeroQUEL,
    SeroQUEL XR (G), 395
  risperidone, Risperdal, Risperdal
    M-Tab, 396
  thioridazine, Mellaril (G), 396
methazolamide, Neptazane (G)
  glaucoma, 257
methenamine hippurate, Hiprex, Urex (G)
  urinary tract infection, 257
methimazole, Tapazole
  hyperthyroidism, 337
methocarbamol, Robaxin (G)
  muscle strain, 404
  temporomandibular joint disorder, 587
  tetanus, 592–593
methotrexate, Abrilada, Rasuvo,
    Rheumatrex, Trexall
  Crohn's disease, 177

juvenile idiopathic arthritis, 370
juvenile rheumatoid arthritis, 373
polymyalgia rheumatica, 502
psoriasis, 525
rheumatoid arthritis, 546
systemic lupus erythematosis, 584
methoxsalen, Oxsoralen (G)
vitiligo, 653
methscopolamine bromide, Pamine,
Pamine Forte
abdominal cramps, 174
irritable bowel syndrome with
diarrhea, 367
vertigo, 653
methylcellulose, Citrucel, Citrucel
Sugar-Free
occasional constipation, 169
methyldopa, Aldomet
hypertension, 332
Methylin, *methylphenidate (regular-
acting)* (G)(II)
attention deficit hyperactivity disorder
(ADHD), 52
narcolepsy, 412
methylnaltrexone bromide, Relistor (G)
opioid-induced constipation (OIC),
428
methylphenidate (long-acting), Concerta,
Cotempla XR-ODT, Metadate
CD, Metadate ER, QuilliChew
ER, Quillivant XR, Ritalin (G)(II)
attention deficit hyperactivity disorder
(ADHD), 52
narcolepsy, 412
methylphenidate (transdermal patch),
Daytrana (G)(II)
attention deficit hyperactivity disorder
(ADHD), 53
narcolepsy, 412
methylphenidate (regular-acting),
Methylin, Ritalin (G)(II)
attention deficit hyperactivity disorder
(ADHD), 52
narcolepsy, 412
methyltestosterone, Android, Methitest,
Testred (III)
testosterone deficiency, 588
methysergide, Sansert (G)
migraine and cluster headache, 277
metipranolol, OptiPranolol (G)
glaucoma, 256
metoclopramide, Metozolv ODT, Reglan
gastroesophageal reflux disease, 251
metolazone, Mykrox, Zaroxolyn
edema, 229
heart failure, 282
hypertension, primary, 328
metoprolol succinate, Toprol-XL (G)
angina pectoris: stable, 29
heart failure, 280
hypertension, 326
migraine and cluster headache, 275
metoprolol tartrate, Lopressor (G)
angina pectoris: stable, 29
headache: migraine, 275
heart failure, 280
hypertension: primary, 326
MetroCream, MetroGel, MetroLotion,
metronidazole
acne rosacea, 2
bacterial vaginosis, 56
metronidazole, Flagyl, Flagyl 375, Flagyl
ER, MetroGel, Vandazole (G)
amebiasis, 17
amebic liver abscess, 17
bacterial vaginosis, 56
Crohn's disease, 175
diverticulitis, 216
giardiasis, 254

nongonococcal urethritis, 639
pelvic inflammatory disease, 476
pseudomembranous colitis, 519
sexual assault, 567
trichomoniasis, 606
metyrosine, Demser (G)
pheochromocytoma, 486–487
Mevacor, *lovastatin*
dyslipidemia, 222
hypertriglyceridemia, 339
Mexitil, *mexiletine* (G), 681
Miacalcin, *calcitonin-salmon* (G)
hypocalcemia, 340
Mibelas 24 FE, *ethinyl estradiol+
norethindrone plus ferrous
fumarate*
estrogen and progesterone, 670
Micardis HCT,
telmisartan+hydrochlorothiazide
hypertension, 334
miconazole, Lotrimin AF, Monistat,
Oravig (G)
diaper rash, 211s
oral (thrush) candidiasis, 135
skin candidiasis, 136
vulvovaginal (moniliasis) candidiasis,
138
Microgestin 1.5/30, *ethinyl estradiol+
norethindrone*
estrogen and progesterone, 670
Microgestin 1/20, *ethinyl estradiol+
norethindrone*
estrogen and progesterone, 670
Microgestin Fe 1.5/30, *ethinyl estradiol+
norethindrone*
estrogen and progesterone, 670
Microgestin Fe 1/20, *ethinyl estradiol+
norethindrone*
estrogen and progesterone, 670
Micro-K, *potassium* (G)
hypokalemia, 344
Microzide, *hydrochlorothiazide*
edema, 228
heart failure, 281
hypertension, 327
urolithiasis, 646
Midamor, *amiloride*
heart failure, 281
hypertension, primary, 327
midazolam, Nayzilam (IV)
status epilepticus, 580
midodrine, ProAmatine (G)
neurogenic hypotension, 345
Midrin, *isometheptene mucate+
dichloralphenazone+
acetaminophen* (G)(IV)
migraine and cluster headache, 272
Miebo, *perfluorohexyloctane*
dry eye syndrome, 218
mifepristone, Korlym
Cushing's syndrome, 179–180
miglitol, Glyset
type 2 diabetes mellitus, 620
miglustat, Zavesca (G)
Gaucher disease, type 1 (GD1), 252
migraine and cluster headache
acetaminophen+aspirin+caffeine,
Excedrin Migraine (OTC), 272
Advil Dual Action,
ibuprofen+acetaminophen, 272
almotriptan, Axert (G), 270
amitriptyline (G), 276
atenolol, Tenormin (G), 275
atogepant, Qulipta, 272–273
celecoxib, Elyxyb, 271–272
*diclofenac potassium powder for oral
solution,* Cambia (G), 272
dihydroergotamine mesylate, DHE 45,
Migranal, 270

diltiazem, Cardizem (G), 275
divalproex sodium, Depakene, 274
eletriptan, Relpax (G), 270
erenumab-aooe, Aimovig, 273
ergotamine, 270
ergotamine+caffeine, Cafergot (G), 270
fluoxetine, Prozac, Prozac Weekly (G),
276–277
fremanezumab-vfrm, Ajovy, 273
frovatriptan, Frova (G), 270
galcanezumab-gnlm, Emgality, 273
imipramine, Tofranil (G), 276
*isometheptene mucate+
dichloralphenazone+
acetaminophen,* Midrin (G)(IV),
272
lasmiditan, Reyvow, 271
magnesium oxide, Mag-Ox 400, 277
methysergide, Sansert (G), 277
metoprolol succinate, Toprol-XL (G),
275
metoprolol tartrate, Lopressor (G), 275
nadolol, Corgard (G), 275
naratriptan, Amerge (G), 270
nifedipine, Adalat, Procardia,
Procardia XL (G), 276
propranolol, Inderal, Inderal LA,
InnoPran XL (G), 275
rimegepant, Nurtec ODT, 273
rizatriptan, Maxalt, Maxalt-MLT (G),
270
sumatriptan, Alsuma, Imitrex,
Onzetra Xsail, Sumavel DosePro,
Zembrace SymTouch (G),
192–271
sumatriptan+naproxen, Treximet (G),
272
timolol, Blocadren (G), 275
topiramate, Topamax, Topamax
Sprinkle Caps, Trokendi XR,
Qudexy XR, 274
ubrogepant, Ubrelvy, 273
verapamil, Calan, Covera HS, Isoptin,
Isoptin SR (G), 276
zavegepant, Zavzpret, 274
zolmitriptan, Zomig (G), 270
Milk of Magnesia, *magnesium hydroxide*
occasional constipation, 170
milnacipran, Savella (G)
fibromyalgia, 244
miltefosine, Impavido
leishmaniasis, 376–377
Minastrin 24 FE, *ethinyl estradiol+
norethindrone plus ferrous
fumarate*
estrogen and progesterone, 670
mineral oil (G)
encopresis, 232
Minipres, *prazosin*
hypertension: primary, 332
post-traumatic stress disorder, 511
urinary overactive bladder, 356
Minizide, *prazosin+polythiazide* (G)
hypertension, 335
Minocin, *minocycline,* 705, 709
acne rosacea, 3
acne vulgaris, 5
anthrax, 32
aphthous stomatitis, 37
bacterial skin infection, 575
Hansen's disease, 270
hidradenitis suppurativa, 304
Lyme disease, 383
malaria, 384–385
urinary tract infection, 644
minocycline, Amzeeq, Dynacin, Minocin,
Minocin, Minolira, Solodyn,
704–705, 709
acne rosacea, 2, 3

minocycline, Amzeeq, Dynacin, Minocin,
   Minocin, Minolira, Solodyn
   (cont.)
   acne vulgaris, 5
   anthrax, 32
   aphthous stomatitis, 37
   bacterial skin infection, 575
   Hansen's disease, 270
   hidradenitis suppurativa, 304
   Lyme disease, 383
   malaria, 384–385
   urinary tract infection, 644
Minolira, minocycline
   acne vulgaris, 5
minoxidil, Loniten, Rogaine (G)
   baldness: male pattern, 57
   hypertension, 333
Mintezol, thiabendazole (G), 704
   cutaneous larva migrans, 376
   hookworm, 305
   pinworm, 488
   roundworm, 558
   threadworm, 593
   trichinosis, 606
   whipworm, 657
mipomersen, Kynamro
   dyslipidemia, 220s
mirabegron, Myrbetriq, VESIcare (G)
   urinary overactive bladder, 354s
MiraLAX Powder for Oral Solution,
   polyethylene glycol (PEG) (G)
   occasional constipation, 170
Mirapex, pramipexole, pramipexole
   dihydrochloride (G)
   Parkinson's disease, 469
   restless legs syndrome, 540
Mircette, ethinyl estradiol+desogestrel
   diacetate
   estrogen and progesterone, 670
Mirena, levonorgestrel, 675
mirtazapine, Remeron (G)
   major depressive disorder, 194
   post-traumatic stress disorder, 512
Mirvaso, brimonidine
   acne rosacea, 2
mirvetuximab soravtansine-gynx, Elahere
   fallopian tube cancer, 89–90
   ovarian cancer, 123–124
   peritoneal cancer, 126
misoprostol, Cytotec
   peptic ulcer disease (PUD), 480
mitapivat, Pyrukynd
   hemolytic/anemia, 24–25
mitral valve prolapse (MVP)
   propranolol, Inderal (G), 396
MMR II, measles, mumps, rubella, live,
   attenuated, neomycin vaccine (G)
   mumps, 403
   rubella, 558
   rubeola, 558
Mobic, meloxicam (G), 573
   dysmenorrhea: primary, 225
   gouty arthritis, 263
   muscle strain, 406
   osteoarthritis, 436
   psoriatic arthritis, 528
   rheumatoid arthritis, 544
Mobisyl Creme, trolamine salicylate
   atopic dermatitis, 200
   diabetic peripheral neuropathy
      (DPN), 209
   gouty arthritis, 262
   hemorrhoids, 290
   juvenile idiopathic arthritis, 369
   juvenile rheumatoid arthritis, 372
   muscle strain, 405
   osteoarthritis, 434
   pain, 454
   peripheral neuritis, 481

post-herpetic neuralgia, 508
   pruritus, 518
   psoriatic arthritis, 527
   rheumatoid arthritis, 542
modafinil, Provigil (G)(IV)
   narcolepsy, 410
   obstructive sleep apnea, 575
   sleepiness, 576
Modicon 0.5/35-28, ethinyl estradiol+
   norethindrone
   estrogen and progesterone, 670
Moduretic, amiloride+
   hydrochlorothiazide
   edema, 229
   heart failure, 282
   hypertension, 282
moexipril, Univasc
   hypertension, 330
mometasone furoate, Asmanex HFA,
   Asmanex Twisthaler, Nasonex,
   Sinuva Sinus Implant (G)
   allergic rhinitis/sinusitis, 552
   asthma, 41
   polyps, nasal, 506
Monistat 1 Vaginal Ointment,
   tioconazole (G)
   vulvovaginal (moniliasis) candidiasis,
      138
Monistat-Derm, miconazole (G)
   diaper rash, 211
   skin candidiasis, 136
   tinea corporis, 597
   tinea cruris, 599
   tinea pedis, 600
   tinea versicolor, 601
   vulvovaginal (moniliasis) candidiasis,
      138
Monkeypox, 576–577
monobenzone, Benoquin (G)
   hyperpigmentation, 325
   vitiligo, 653
Monodox, doxycycline
   acne rosacea, 3
   acne vulgaris, 5
   acute exacerbation of chronic
      bronchitis, 70
   anthrax (bacillus anthracis), 32
   bacterial skin infection, 574
   cat bite, 65
   cat scratch fever, 141
   Chlamydia trachomatis, 151
   cholera (Vibrio cholerae), 155, 156
   community-acquired pneumonia, 494
   dog bite, 66
   dose forms, 639, 644, 704
   epididymitis, 237
   gonorrhea, 256
   granuloma inguinale, 266
   hidradenitis suppurativa, 303
   lyme disease, 383
   lymphogranuloma venereum, 384
   malaria, 384
   nongonococcal urethritis, 639
   pelvic inflammatory disease, 476
   proctitis: acute, 516
   rocky mountain spotted fever, 556
   sexual assault, 567
monomethyl fumarate, Bafiertam
   multiple sclerosis (MS), 401–402
MonoNessa, ethinyl estradiol+
   norgestimate
   estrogen and progesterone, 670
mononucleosis (MONO)
   prednisone (G), 396
Monopril, fosinopril (G)
   heart failure, 279
   hypertension, primary, 329
Monovisc, sodium hyaluronate
   osteoarthritis, 437

montelukast, Singulair, Singulair
   Chewable, Singulair Oral
   Granules (G)
   allergic rhinitis/sinusitis, 551
   asthma, 41
morphine sulfate (immed- and sust-
   rel), Arymo ER, Duramorph,
   Infumorph, Kadian (G), MS
   Contin (G), MSIR, Oramorph
   SR, Roxanol (G)(II)
   pain, 457
morphine sulfate (ext-rel), MorphaBond
   ER (G)(II)
   pain, 457
Mounjaro, tirzepatide
   type 2 diabetes mellitus (T2DM),
      631–632
Motegrity, prucalopride (G)
   chronic idiopathic constipation, 169
motion sickness
   dimenhydrinate, Dramamine (OTC),
      396
   meclizine, Antivert, Bonine (OTC),
      Dramamine II (OTC), Zentrip,
      396
   prochlorperazine, Compazine (G),
      396
   promethazine, Phenergan (G), 396
   scopolamine, Scopace, Transderm
      Scop, 396
Motofen, difenoxin+atropine (G)
   acute diarrhea, 212
   chronic diarrhea, 213
   irritable bowel syndrome with
      diarrhea, 366
   ulcerative colitis, 638
Motrin, ibuprofen
   fever (pyrexia), 242–243
mouth ulcer. See aphthous stomatitis
Movantik, naloxegol (G)
   opioid-induced constipation (OIC),
      429
Moxatag, amoxicillin (G)
   acute bacterial sinusitis, rhinosinusitis,
      571
   acute exacerbation of chronic
      bronchitis, 69
   acute tonsillitis, 603
   bacterial skin infection, 573
   cellulitis, 142
   community acquired pneumonia, 493
   diverticulitis, 215
   dose forms, 707
   impetigo contagiosa, 351
   Lyme disease, 382
   otitis media: acute, 446
   streptococcal pharyngitis, 484
   urinary tract infection (UTI), 643
Moxeza Ophthalmic Solution,
   moxifloxacin (G)
   bacterial conjunctivitis, 162
moxidectin (G)
   river blindness, 556
moxifloxacin, Avelox, Moxeza
   Ophthalmic Solution, Vigamox
   Ophthalmic Solution (G)
   acute bacterial sinusitis, rhinosinusitis,
      572
   acute exacerbation of chronic
      bronchitis, 70
   bacterial conjunctivitis, 162
   bacterial skin infection, 575
   cellulitis, 144
   community-acquired pneumonia, 494
   dose forms, 508
   nongonococcal urethritis, 638, 639
   plague, 489
Mucomyst, acetylcysteine
   cystic fibrosis (CF), 182

miltefosine, Impavido, 376–377
mucosal leishmaniasis
  miltefosine, Impavido, 376–377
Mulpleta, *lusutrombopag*
  idiopathic thrombocytopenia
    purpura, 594
Multaq, *dronedarone* (G), 681
multiple sclerosis (MS)
  alemtuzumab, Lemtrada (G), 398
  cladribine, Mavenclad, 397
  dalfampridine, Ampyra (G), 397
  dextromethorphan+quinidine,
    Nuedexta (G), 402
  dimethyl fumarate, Tecfidera (G),
    397
  diroximel fumarate, Vumerity, 402
  fingolimod, Gilenya (G), 398
  glatiramer acetate, Copaxone, Glatopa,
    398
  interferon beta-1a, Avonex, Rebif,
    Rebif Rebidose (G), 398, 399
  interferon beta-1b, Actimmune,
    Betaseron, Extavia (G), 399
  monomethyl fumarate, Bafiertam,
    401–402
  natalizumab, Tysabri (G), 399
  ocrelizumab, Ocrevus, 399–400
  ofatumumab, Kesimpta, 400
  ozanimod, Zeposia, 401
  peginterferon beta-1a, Plegridy,
    398–399
  siponimod, Mayzent, 401
  teriflunomide, Aubagio, 398
  ublituximab-xiiy, Briumvi, 400
mumps
  measles, mumps, rubella, live,
    attenuated, neomycin vaccine,
    MMR II (G), 403
mupirocin, Bactroban, Centany
  bacterial skin infection, 573
  impetigo contagiosa, 351
  wound, 658
muscle strain
  baclofen, Lioresal (G), 403
  capsaicin 8% patch, Qutenza, 404
  capsaicin, Axsain, Capsin,
    Capzasin-HP, Capzasin-P,
    Dolorac, Double Cap (OTC),
    R-Gel, Zostrix, Zostrix HP, 404
  carisoprodol, Soma (G), 403
  celecoxib, Celebrex (G), 406
  chlorzoxazone, Parafon Forte DSC (G),
    403
  cyclobenzaprine, Amrix, Fexmid,
    Flexeril, 403
  dantrolene, Dantrium (G), 403
  Decadron Phosphate with Xylocaine,
    lidocaine+dexamethasone, 405
  diazepam, Diastat, Valium (IV), 403
  diclofenac, Zorvolex, 405
  diclofenac sodium, Pennsaid, Solaraze
    Gel, Voltaren Gel (G), 404–405
  doxepin, Prudoxin, Zonalon, 405
  Emla Cream, *lidocaine 2.5%+*
    prilocaine 2.5%, 405
  Equagesic, *meprobamate+aspirin*
    (IV), 404
  LidaMante HC, *lidocaine+*
    hydrocortisone, 405
  lidocaine, LidaMante, Lidoderm,
    ZTlido lidocaine, 405, 406
  meloxicam, Anjeso, Mobic, Vivlodex
    (G), 406
  metaxalone, Skelaxin, 405
  methocarbamol, Robaxin (G), 404
  nabumetone, Relafen (G), 404
  Norgesic, *orphenadrine+*
    aspirin+caffeine (G), 404
  orphenadrine citrate, Norflex (G), 404

pimecrolimus 1% cream (G), Elidel,
  405
Soma Compound, *carisoprodol+*
  aspirin (G)(III), 404
Soma Compound w. *Codeine,*
  carisoprodol+aspirin+codeine
  (G)(III), 404
  tizanidine, Zanaflex (G), 404
  trolamine salicylate, Mobisyl Creme,
    405
  Vimovo, *esomeprazole+naproxen* (G),
    406
Muse, *alprostadil*
  erectile dysfunction (ED), 237
Mycapssa, *octreotide acetate*
  acromegaly, 8
My Way, *levonorgestrel,* 675
Myambutol, *ethambutol (EMB)*
  dose forms, 610
  tuberculosis, 610
myasthenia gravis (MG)
  eculizumab, Soliris, 406–407
  efgartigimod alfa-fcab, Vyvgart, 407
Mycelex Troches, *clotrimazole* (G)
  oral (thrush) candidiasis, 134
Mycelex-G, Mycelex Twin Pack,
  Mycelex-7, *clotrimazole*
  vulvovaginal (moniliasis) candidiasis,
    138
mycophenolate mofetil (MMF), CellCept
  organ transplant rejection prophylaxis,
    432
mycoplasma pneumonia
  azithromycin, Zithromax, Zmax, 496
  clarithromycin, Biaxin, 496
  erythromycin base, Ery-Tab, PCE, 496
  erythromycin ethylsuccinate, EryPed,
    E.E.S, 496
  tetracycline, Achromycin V, Sumycin,
    496–497
Mycostatin, Mycostatin Suspension,
  nystatin (G)
  diaper rash, 211
  dose forms, 704
  oral (thrush) candidiasis, 135
  vulvovaginal (moniliasis) candidiasis,
    138
Mydayis, *amphetamine, mixed salts of*
  single entity amphetamine (G)(II)
  attention deficit hyperactivity disorder
    (ADHD), 51
Mykrox, *metolazone*
  edema, 229
Mylanta Gel, *calcium carbonate+*
  magnesium carbonate (G)
  gastroesophageal reflux disease, 249
Mylanta, Rolaids Sodium, *calcium*
  carbonate+magnesium
  hydroxide (G)
  gastroesophageal reflux disease, 248,
    249
Mylicon, *simethicone* (G)
  abdominal cramps, 175
  flatulence, 245
  infantile colic, 159
  irritable bowel syndrome with
    diarrhea, 367
myelodysplastic syndromes (MDS)
  decitabine+cedazuridine, Inqovi, 407
myelofibrosis
  fedratinib, Inrebic, 408
  pacritinib, Vonjo, 408–408
  ruxolitinib, Jakafi, 409
Myfembree, *relugolix+estradiol+*
  norethindrone acetate
  uterine leiomyomata (fibroid tumor)
  uterine fibroids, 651–652
Myrbetriq, *mirabegron* (G)
  urinary overactive bladder, 354

Mytesi, *crofelemer* (G)
  acute diarrhea, 212
  chronic diarrhea, 213

nabilone, Cesamet (II)
  chemotherapy-induced nausea/
    vomiting, 149
nabumetone, Relafen
  muscle strain, 404
  temporomandibular joint disorder,
    587
nadolol, Corgard
  angina pectoris: stable, 29
  hypertension, 326
  migraine and cluster headache, 275
nafarelin acetate, Synarel
  endometriosis, 233
naftifine, Naftin (G)
  tinea corporis, 597
  tinea cruris, 599
  tinea pedis, 600
Naftin, *naftifine* (G)
  tinea corporis, 597
  tinea cruris, 599
  tinea pedis, 600
nalbuphine, Nubain (G)
  pain, 462
naldemedine, Symproic
  opioid-induced constipation (OIC),
    429
nalidixic acid, NegGram
  urinary tract infection, 644
nalmefene
  opioid overdose/opioid reversal,
    430–431
naloxegol, Movantik
  opioid-induced constipation (OIC),
    429
naloxone, Evzio, Kloxxado, Narcan (G)
  opioid overdose, 431
naltrexone, ReVia, Vivitrol
  opioid dependence, 424
Namzaric, *memantine+donepezil*
  Alzheimer's disease, 15
naphazoline, Vasocon-A
  allergic (vernal) conjunctivitis, 167
Naphcon-A, *naphazoline+pheniramine*
  allergic (vernal) conjunctivitis, 167
Naprelan, *naproxen*
  fever (pyrexia), 243
Naprosyn, *naproxen*
  fever (pyrexia), 243
naproxen, Aleve, Anaprox, EC-Naprosyn,
  Naprelan, Naprosyn (G)
  fever (pyrexia), 243
naratriptan, Amerge
  migraine and cluster headache, 270
Narcan, *naloxone,* (G)
  opioid overdose/opioid reversal, 431
narcolepsy
  Adderall, Adderall XR,
    dextroamphetamine
    saccharate+dextroamphetamine
    sulfate+amphetamine
    aspartate+amphetamine sulfate
    (II)(G), 411–412
  amphetamine sulfate, Evekeo (II), 409
  armodafinil, Nuvigil (IV)(G), 410
  calcium, magnesium, potassium, and
    sodium oxybate oral solution
    (CIII), Xywav, 413
  dexmethylphenidate, Focalin (II)
    (G), 412
  dextroamphetamine sulfate, Dexedrine,
    Dextrostat (II)(G), 411
  methylphenidate (long-acting) (II),
    Adhansia XR, Concerta (G),
    Metadate CD (G), Metadate ER,
    Ritalin LA, Ritalin SR, 412

narcolepsy (cont.)
  methylphenidate (regular-acting),
    Methylin, Methylin Chewable,
    Methylin Oral Solution (II)(G),
    412
  methylphenidate (transdermal patch),
    Daytrana (II)(G), 412
  modafinil, Provigil (IV)(G), 410
  pitolisant, Wakix, 412–413
  sodium oxybate, extended-release,
    Lumryz (III), 410–411
  sodium oxybate, Xyrem (III)(G), 410
  solriamfetol, Sunosi, 411
Nardil, phenelzine
  major depressive disorder, 194
  post-traumatic stress disorder, 512
Nasacort Allergy 24HR, triamcinolone
    acetonide
  allergic rhinitis/sinusitis, 552
Nasalide, flunisolide
  allergic rhinitis/sinusitis, 552
Nascobal Nasal Spray, vitamin B12
    (cyanocobalamin) (A)
  pernicious/megaloblastic anemia, 26
Nasonex, mometasone furoate
  allergic rhinitis/sinusitis, 552
Nasonex 24HR Allergy, mometasone
    furoate monohydrate (OTC)(G)
  polyps, nasal, 506
Natacyn Ophthalmic Suspension,
    natamycin
  fungal conjunctivitis, 165
natalizumab, Tysabri
  Crohn's disease, 179
  multiple sclerosis (MS), 399
natamycin, Natacyn Ophthalmic
    Suspension
  fungal conjunctivitis, 165
Natazia, estradiol valerate+dienogest (G)
  estrogen and progesterone, 671
nateglinide, Starlix
  type 2 diabetes mellitus, 621
Natesto, testosterone (III)
  testosterone deficiency, 590
Natpara, bioengineered replica of human
    parathyroid hormone
  hypocalcemia, 341
  hypoparathyroidism, 345
Natroba, spinosad
  scabies, 559
nausea and vomiting
  chemotherapy-induced. see
    chemotherapy-induced nausea/
    vomitingstanesthesia
  of pregnancy, 235
Nayzilam, midazolam (IV)
  status epilepticus, 580
nebivolol, Bystolic (G)
  hypertension, 326
Necon 0.5/35-21, Necon 0.5/35-28,
    ethinyl estradiol+norethindrone
  estrogen and progesterone, 671
Necon 1/35-21, Necon 1/35-28, ethinyl
    estradiol+norethindrone
  estrogen and progesterone, 671
Necon 1/50-21, Necon 1/50-28,
    mestranol+norethindrone
  estrogen and progesterone, 671
Necon 10/11-21, Necon 10/11-28, ethinyl
    estradiol+norethindrone
  estrogen and progesterone, 671
nedocromil, Alocril
  allergic (vernal) conjunctivitis, 166
nedocromil sodium, Tilade, Tilade
    Nebulizer Solution
  asthma, 42
Neisseria meningitides oligosaccharide
    conjugate, Menveo
  meningitis, 388–389

Neisseria meningitidis
    polysaccharides, Menactra,
    Menomune-A/C/Y/W-135
  meningitis, 389
nelfinavir mesylate, Viracept
  human immunodeficiency virus
    infection, 311
Nelova 0.5/35-21, Nelova 0.5/35-28,
    ethinyl estradiol+norethindrone
  estrogen and progesterone, 671
Nelova 1/35-21, Nelova 1/35-28, ethinyl
    estradiol+norethindrone
  estrogen and progesterone, 671
Nelova 1/50-21, Nelova 1/50-28,
    mestranol+norethindrone
  estrogen and progesterone, 671
Nelova 10/11-21, Nelova 10/11-28,
    ethinyl estradiol+norethindrone
  estrogen and progesterone, 671
Nembutal, pentobarbital (II)
  insomnia, 360
Neocon 7/7/7, ethinyl estradiol+
    norethindrone
  estrogen and progesterone, 671
Neoral, cyclosporine
    (immunosuppressant)
  rheumatoid arthritis, 546
  systemic lupus erythematosis, 583
Neosporin Ophthalmic Ointment,
    polymyxin b sulfate+bacitracin
    zinc+neomycin sulfate
  bacterial conjunctivitis, 163
Neosporin Ophthalmic Solution,
    polymyxin b sulfate+
    gramicidin+neomycin
  bacterial conjunctivitis, 163
  stye (hordeolum), 580
Neosporin, polymyxin b+bacitracin+
    neomycin
  blepharitis, 67
  stye (hordeolum), 580
Neosporin, polymyxin b+neomycin
  bacterial skin infection, 573
Neo-Synephrine, oxymetazoline,
    phenylephrine
  common cold, 161
nepafenac, Nevanac Ophthalmic
    Suspension
  allergic (vernal) conjunctivitis, 168
  eye pain, 241
  pain, 453
nephropathy:primary, immunoglobulin
    A (IGAN)
  budesonide, Tarpeyo, 414
  omidenepag isopropyl, Aponvie, 415
Nerlynx, neratinib, sodium neratinib, 687
  breast cancer, 80
nerve agent poisoning
  atropine sulfate, AtroPen (G), 415
netarsudil, Rhopressa
  glaucoma, 257
Neulasta, pegfilgrastim
  neutropenia, 416
Neupro, rotigotine, rotigotine transdermal
    patch
  Parkinson's disease, 469
  restless legs syndrome, 540
neurofibromatosis type 1
  selumetinib, Koselugo, 415–416
neurogenic detrusor overactivity (NDO)
  solifenacin, 415
  solifenacin succinate, VESIcare LS, 415
neurogenic hypotension
  droxidopa, Northera, 346
  midodrine, ProAmatine, 345
neuromyelitis optica spectrum disorder
    (NMOSD)
  eculizumab, Soliris, 416
Neurontin, gabapentin

diabetic peripheral neuropathy (DPN),
    209–210
  fibromyalgia, 244
  post-herpetic neuralgia, 507
  restless legs syndrome, 540
neurotrophic keratitis
  cenegermin-bkbj, Oxervat, 374–375
neutropenia
  filgrastim, 417
  filgrastim-aa, 417
  filgrastim-ayow, 417
  filgrastim-cbqv, 417
  filgrastim-sndz, 418
  pegfilgrastim, Neulasta, 416
  pegfilgrastim-jmd, Fulphila, 416
  tbo-filgrastim, Granix, 418
Nevanac Ophthalmic Suspension,
    nepafenac
  allergic (vernal) conjunctivitis, 168
  eye pain, 241
nevirapine, Viramune
  human immunodeficiency virus
    infection, 310
Nexavar, sorafenib (G), 687
  hepatocellular carcinoma (HCC), 99
  renal cell carcinoma (RCC), 93
  thyroid carcinoma, 132
Nexiclon XR, clonidine
  attention deficit hyperactivity disorder
    (ADHD), 54
  post-traumatic stress disorder, 511
Nexium, esomeprazole
  peptic ulcer disease (PUD), 478
  Zollinger-Ellison syndrome, 662
Nexletol, bempedoic acid
  dyslipidemia, 221–222
NexoBrid, anacaulase-bcdb
  burn, major, 75
Nexplanon, etonogestrel, 675
niacin, Niaspan, Slo-Niacin
  dyslipidemia, 146
  hypertriglyceridemia, 255
Niaspan, niacin
  dyslipidemia, 223
  hypertriglyceridemia, 338–339
nicardipine, Cardene
  angina pectoris: stable, 28
  hypertension, primary, 331
Nicoderm CQ, transdermal nicotine
    system
  tobacco dependence, 602
Nicorette Mini Lozenge, nicotine
    polacrilex (G)
  tobacco dependence, 603
nicotin, Nicotrol NS, Nicotrol Inhaler
  tobacco dependence, 603
nicotine polacrilex, Commit Lozenge,
    Nicorette Mini Lozenge (G)
  tobacco dependence, 603
Nicotrol NS, Nicotrol Inhaler, nicotin
  tobacco dependence, 603
Nicotrol Step-down Patch, transdermal
    nicotine system
  tobacco dependence, 602
Nicotrol Transdermal, Prostep,
    transdermal nicotine system
  tobacco dependence, 602–603
nifedipine, Adalat, Adalat CC, Procardia,
    Procardia XL
  angina pectoris: stable, 28
  hypertension: primary, 331
  migraine and cluster headache, 276
nifurtimox (NR)(G)
  Chagas disease, 146
Nikita, pitavastatin
  dyslipidemia, 222
Nilandron, nilutamide, 687
nintedanib, Ofev
  idiopathic pulmonary fibrosis, 535

niraparib tosylate, Zejula
  fallopian tube cancer, 88
  ovarian cancer, 122–123
  peritoneal cancer, 125
  prostate cancer, 129
Niravam, *alprazolam* (IV)
  anxiety disorder, 33
  panic disorder, 465
nisoldipine
  hypertension, 331
nitazoxanide, Alinia
  criptosporidiosis, 179
  dose forms, 705
  giardiasis, 254
  threadworm, 593
Nitro-Bid Ointment, *nitroglycerin*
  angina pectoris: stable, 29
Nitrodisc, *nitroglycerin*
  angina pectoris: stable, 29
nitrofurantoin, Furadantin, Macrobid,
    Macrodantin, 710, 720
  urinary tract infection, 644–646
nitroglycerin, Nitro-Bid Ointment,
    Nitrodisc, Nitrolingual Pump
    Spray, Nitromist, Nitrostat,
    Transderm-Nitro
  angina pectoris: stable, 29–30
Nitrolingual Pump Spray, *nitroglycerin*
  angina pectoris: stable, 29
Nitromist, *nitroglycerin*
  angina pectoris: stable, 30
Nitrostat, *nitroglycerin*
  angina pectoris: stable, 30
nivolumab, Opdivo
  melanoma, 118
Nix (OTC), *permethrin*
  pediculosis humanus capitis, 475
nizatidine, Axid
  gastroesophageal reflux disease, 250
  peptic ulcer disease (PUD), 478
Nizoral Cream, *ketoconazole*
  diaper rash, 211
  seborrheic dermatitis, 205
  skin candidiasis, 135
  tinea capitis, 597
  tinea corporis, 597, 598
  tinea cruris, 598, 599
  tinea pedis, 600
  tinea versicolor, 601
Nocdurna, *desmopressin acetate*
  nocturnal polyuria, 506–507
nocturnal enuresis
  amitriptyline (G), 235
  amoxapine (G), 235
  clomipramine, Anafranil (G), 235
  desipramine, Norpramin (G), 235
  desmopressin acetate, DDAVP, DDAVP
    Rhinal Tube, 235
  doxepin (G), 235
  imipramine, Tofranil (G), 235
  nortriptyline, Pamelor (G), 235
  protriptyline, Vivactil, 235
  trimipramine, Surmontil, 235
nocturnal polyuria
  desmopressin acetate, Nocdurna,
    506–507
non-24 sleep-wake disorder
  suvorexant, Belsomra (IV), 418
  tasimelteon, Hetlioz, 418
nongonococcal urethritis (NGU)
  azithromycin, Zithromax, Zmax (G),
    639
  doxycycline, Acticlate, Adoxa, Doryx,
    Doxteric, Monodox, Oracea,
    Vibramycin, Vibra-Tab (G), 639
  erythromycin base, Ery-Tab, PCE, 639
  erythromycin ethylsuccinate, EryPed,
    E.E.S (G), 639
  levofloxacin, Levaquin, 639

metronidazole, Flagyl, Flagyl 375,
    Flagyl ER (G), 639
ofloxacin, Floxin (G), 639
tinidazole, Tindamax, 639
Norco, *hydrocodone bitartrate+*
    acetaminophen (II)
  pain, 456
Nordette-21, Nordette-28, *ethinyl*
    estradiol/levonorgestrel
  estrogen and progesterone, 671
Norditropin, *somatropin*
  growth failure, 267
norethindrone acetate, Aygestin
  endometriosis, 233
  menopause, 392
norethindrone, Aygestin
  amenorrhea, secondary, 18
norfloxacin, Noroxin
  acute prostatitis, 516
  chronic prostatitis, 517
  dose form/volume, 708
  urinary tract infection, 645
Norgesic, *orphenadrine+aspirin+*
    caffeine
  muscle strain, 404
  temporomandibular joint disorder,
    587
Norinyl 1/35-21, Norinyl 1/35-28, *ethinyl*
    estradiol+norethindrone
  estrogen and progesterone, 671
Norinyl 1/50-21, Norinyl 1/50-28, *ethinyl*
    estradiol+norethindrone
  estrogen and progesterone, 671
Noroxin, *norfloxacin*
  acute prostatitis, 516
  chronic prostatitis, 517
Norpace, *disopyramide,* 681
Norplant, *levonorgestrel,* 675
Norpramin, *desipramine* (G)
  anxiety disorder, 34
  diabetic peripheral neuropathy
    (DPN), 210
  major depressive disorder, 193
  nocturnal enuresis, 235
  post-herpetic neuralgia, 508, 509
  tension headache, 278
  trigeminal neuralgia, 609
Northera, *droxidopa*
  neurogenic hypotension, 346
Nortrel 0.5/35, *ethinyl estradiol+*
    norethindrone
  estrogen and progesterone, 671
Nortrel 1/35-21, Nortrel 1/35-28, *ethinyl*
    estradiol+norethindrone
  estrogen and progesterone, 671
Nortrel 7/7/7-28, *ethinyl estradiol+*
    norethindrone
  estrogen and progesterone, 671
nortriptyline, Pamelor
  anxiety disorder, 34
  diabetic peripheral neuropathy
    (DPN), 210
  irritable bowel syndrome with
    diarrhea, 368
  major depressive disorder (MDD),
    193
  nocturnal enuresis, 235
  post-herpetic neuralgia, 508, 510
  post-traumatic stress disorder, 512
  premenstrual dysphoric disorder, 515
  trigeminal neuralgia, 609
Norvasc, *amlodipine*
  angina pectoris: stable, 28
  hypertension, primary, 331
Norvir, *ritonavir* (G)
  human immunodeficiency virus
    (HIV) infection, 312
Nourianz, *istradefylline*
  parkinson's disease, 470

Noxafil, *posaconazole* (G)
  aspergillosis, 38
  oral (thrush) candidiasis, 135
  skin candidiasis, 136
  vulvovaginal (moniliasis) candidiasis,
    138
Nubain, *nalbuphine* (G)
  pain, 462
Nubeqa, *darolutamide*
  prostate cancer, 129
Nucala, *mepolizumab*
  asthma, 48
  allergic rhinitis/sinusitis, 553
  eosinophilia, 48
  eosinophilic granulomatosis with
    polyangitis, 235–236
Nucynta, *tapentadol*
  peripheral neuritis, 481–482
Nuedexta, *dextromethorphan+quinidine*
  multiple sclerosis (MS), 402
  Parkinson's disease, 471
  pseudobulbar affect (PBA) disorder,
    518
NuLev, *hyoscyamine*
  abdominal cramps, 175
  interstitial cystitis, 361
  irritable bowel syndrome with
    diarrhea, 367
  urinary overactive bladder, 355
Nupercainal, *dibucaine* (OTC)
  hemorrhoids, 289
Nupercainal, *hydrocortisone*
  hemorrhoids, 289
Nuplazid, *pimavanserin*
  Parkinson's disease, 471
Nuprin, *ibuprofen* (G)
  fever (pyrexia), 243
nusinersen, Spinraza
  spinal muscular atrophy (SMA),
    577–578
Nutropin, Nutropin AQ, Nutropin
    Depot, *somatropin*
  growth failure, 267
NuvaRing, *etonogestrel+ethinyl estradiol*
    (G), 674
Nuvigil, *armodafinil* (G)(IV)
  narcolepsy, 410
  obstructive sleep apnea, 575
  sleepiness, 576
Nuzyra, *omadacycline*
  cellulitis, 144
nystatin, Mycostatin, Mycostatin
    Suspension, Nystop Powder (G)
  oral (thrush) candidiasis, 135
  skin candidiasis, 136
  vulvovaginal (moniliasis) candidiasis,
    138
Nystop Powder, *nystatin*
  skin candidiasis, 136

obesity
  amphetamine sulfate, Evekeo (II),
    418
  benzphetamine, Didrex (III), 418
  liraglutide, Saxenda, 420
  lorcaserin, Belviq (G), 420
  methamphetamine, Desoxyn (II), 419
  naltrexone+bupropion, Contrave (G),
    419
  orlistat, Alli, Xenical (G), 418
  phendimetrazine, Bontril (III), 419
  phentermine, Adipex-P, Fastin,
    Ionamin, Suprenza ODT (G)(IV),
    419
  phentermine+topiramate ext-rel,
    Qsymia (G)(IV), 419–420
  semaglutide, Wegovy, 420–421
obeticholic acid, Ocaliva
  primary biliary cholangitis, 152

obiltoxaximab, Anthim
  anthrax (*bacillus anthracis*), 31
obsessive-compulsive disorder (OCD)
  clomipramine, Anafranil (G), 422
  fluoxetine, Prozac, Prozac Weekly (G),
    421
  fluvoxamine, Luvox (G), 421
  imipramine, Tofranil (G), 422
  paroxetine maleate, Paxil (G), 422
  paroxetine mesylate, Brisdelle (G), 422
  sertraline, Zoloft, 422
obstructive sleep apnea
  armodafinil, Nuvigil (G)(IV), 575
  modafinil, Provigil (G)(IV), 575
  solriamfetol, Sunosi, 575–576
Ocaliva, *obeticholic acid*
  primary biliary cholangitis, 152
occasional constipation
  bisacodyl, Dulcolax, Gentlax, Senokot,
    170
  calcium polycarbophil, FiberCon,
    Konsyl Fiber Tablets, 169
  docusate enema, DocuSol Kids, 170
  docusate sodium, Dialose, Surfak
    (OTC), 169–170
  docusate+casanthranol, Doxidan,
    Peri-Colace (OTC), 170–171
  docusate+senna, Senokot S (OTC),
    171
  lactulose, Kristalose (G), 170
  magnesium citrate, Citrate of
    Magnesia (OTC)(G), 170
  magnesium hydroxide, Milk of
    Magnesia, 170
  methylcellulose, Citrucel, Citrucel
    Sugar-Free, 169
  polyethylene glycol (PEG), GlycoLax
    Powder for Oral Solution,
    MiraLAX Powder for Oral
    Solution, Polyethylene Glycol
    3350 Powder for Oral Solution
    (G), 170
  psyllium husk, Metamucil (OTC), 169
  psyllium, Konsyl, 169
  psyllium+senna, Perdiem,
    SennaPrompt (OTC), 170
  sodium biphosphate+sodium phosphate
    enema, Fleets Adult, Fleets
    Pediatric (OTC), 171
Occlusal HP, *salicylic acid*
  common wart, 655
  plantar wart, 655
Ocean Mist (OTC), *saline nasal spray* (G)
  common cold, 160–161
Ocella, *ethinyl estradiol+drospirenone*
  estrogen and progesterone, 671
ocrelizumab, Ocrevus
  multiple sclerosis (MS), 399–400
octreotide acetate Bynfezia Pen,
  Mycapssa, Sandostatin,
  Sandostatin LAR Depot
  acromegaly, 8
Ocuflox Ophthalmic Solution, *ofloxacin*
  bacterial conjunctivitis, 162
Odactra, *dermatophagoides*
  farinae+dermatophagoides
  pteronyssinus allergen extract
  dust mite allergy, 219
Odefsey, *emtricitabine+rilpivirine+*
  tenofovir alafenamide
  human immunodeficiency virus
    infection, 315
odevixibat, Bylvay
  cholestasis, 154
ofatumumab, Arzerra, Kesimpta
  leukemia, 97
  multiple sclerosis (MS), 400
Ofev, *nintedanib*
  idiopathic pulmonary fibrosis, 535

Ofirmev, *acetaminophen* (G)
  fever (pyrexia), 241
  urolithiasis, 647
ofloxacin, Floxin, 708
  acute exacerbation of chronic
    bronchitis, 70
  acute prostatitis, 516
  bacterial skin infection, 575
  Chlamydia trachomatis, 152
  chronic prostatitis, 517
  community-acquired pneumonia,
    494
  epididymitis, 237
  Hansen's disease, 270
  nongonococcal urethritis, 639
  otitis externa, 444
  otitis media: acute, 447
  shigellosis, 567
  typhoid fever, 633
  urinary tract infection, 645
  wound, 660
ofloxacin, Ocuflox Ophthalmic Solution
  bacterial conjunctivitis, 162
Ogen Cream, *estropipate*
  atrophic vaginitis, 49
Ogivri for Injection, *trastuzumab-dkst*
  breast cancer, 82
Ogivri, *trastuzumab-dkst,* 687
olanzapine, Zyprexa, Zyprexa Zydis (G)
  delirium, 188
  dementia, 188
  methamphetamine-induced
    psychosis, 395
  post-traumatic stress disorder, 511
  trichotillomania, 608
Olaparib, Lynparza
  breast cancer, 81
  fallopian tube cancer, 89
  pancreatic cancer, 124–125
  peritoneal cancer, 125
olmesartan medoxomil, Benicar (G)
  hypertension, 330
olodaterol, Striverdi Respimat
  asthma, 43
  chronic obstructive pulmonary
    disease, 71
  emphysema, 230
olopatadine, Pataday, Patanol, Patanase,
  Pazeo
  allergic (vernal) conjunctivitis, 167
  allergic rhinitis/sinusitis, 553
  polyps, nasal, 506
olsalazine, Dipentum
  Crohn's disease, 176
  ulcerative colitis, 636
Olumiant, *baricitinib*
  alopecia areata, 12–13
  COVID-19 (coronavirus), 174
  rheumatoid arthritis, 544
olutasidenib, Imjudo, Treanda
  hepatocellular carcinoma (HCC), 101
Olysio, *simeprevir*
  hepatitis C (HCV), 295
omadacycline, Nuzyra
  cellulitis, 144
omalizumab, Xolair
  allergies: multi-food, 12
  asthma, 42
  asthma-COPD overlap syndrome, 47
  eosinophilia, 49
  urticaria, 650
Omeclamox-Pak
  Helicobacter pylori (H. pylori)
    infection, 284
omega 3-fatty acid ethyl esters, Lovaza,
  Epanova
  dyslipidemia, 220
  hypertriglyceridemia, 338
omeprazole, Prilosec (OTC)(G)

gastroesophageal reflux disease,
  250–251
  peptic ulcer disease (PUD), 478–479
  Zollinger-Ellison syndrome, 662
omidenepag isopropyl, Aponvie
  nephropathy:primary,
    immunoglobulin A (IGAN),
    415
Omnaris, *ciclesonide*
  polyps, nasal, 505
Omnicef, *cefdinir* (G), 714
  acute bacterial sinusitis, rhinosinusitis,
    571
  acute exacerbation of chronic
    bronchitis, 69
  acute tonsillitis, 604
  bacterial skin infection, 574
  community acquired pneumonia, 493
  dose form/volume, 706
  otitis media: acute, 446
  streptococcal pharyngitis, 484
  wound, 659
Omnipen, *ampicillin,* 712–717
  acute exacerbation of chronic
    bronchitis, 69
  bacterial endocarditis prophylaxis, 55
  otitis media: acute, 446
Omnitrope, *somatropin*
  growth failure, 267
Omontys, *peginesatide*
  anemia of chronic kidney disease, 23
onasemnogene abeparvovec-xioi,
  Zolgensma
  spinal muscular atrophy (SMA), 578
onchocerciasis, 556
ondansetron, Zofran, Zuplenz (G)
  cannabinoid hyperemesis syndrome,
    140
  chemotherapy-induced nausea/
    vomiting, 148–149
  gastritis-related nausea/vomiting, 247
  post-anesthesia nausea/vomiting, 414
1-Day, *tioconazole*
  vulvovaginal (moniliasis) candidiasis,
    138
Onexton Gel, *clindamycin+benzoyl*
  peroxide
  acne vulgaris, 4
Onfi, *clobazam* (IV)(G)
  dose forms, 694
  Lennox-Gastaut syndrome (LGS), 377
Ongentys, *opicapone*
  parkinson's disease, 471
Onsolis, *fentanyl*
  pain, 461
Ontruzant for Injection,
  trastuzumab-dttb
  breast cancer, 82
onychomycosis (fungal nail)
  ciclopirox, Penlac Nail Lacquer, 422
  efinaconazole, Jublia (G), 422
  griseofulvin, microsize, Grifulvin V (G),
    422
  griseofulvin, ultramicrosize, Gris-PEG
    (G), 422
  itraconazole, Sporanox, Pulse Pack (G),
    422
  tavaborole, Kerydin (G), 423
  terbinafine, Lamisil, 422
Opdivo, *nivolumab,* 688
  melanoma, 118
Opdualag, *nivolumab+relatlimab-rmbw*
  melanoma, 116
opicapone, Ongentys
  parkinson's disease, 471
opioid dependence
  Bunavail, Suboxone, Sucartonone,
    Zubsolv, *buprenorphine+*
    naloxone (G)(III), 427

buprenorphine, Belbuca, Butrans
  Transdermal System,
  Probuphine, Subutex, Sublocade
  (III), 426
*buprenorphine extended-release for
  subcutaneous injection*, Brixadi,
  424–425
buprenorphine hcl, Buprenex, 426
lofexidine, Lucemyra, 424
methadone, Dolophine (G)(II), 424
naltrexone, ReVia, Vivitrol (G), 424
Troxyca ER, *oxycodone+naloxone* (II),
  427–428
opioid overdose/opioid reversal
nalmefene, 430–431
naloxone, Evzio, Kloxxado, Narcan (G),
  431
RiVive Nasal Spray (OTC), 431
opioid-induced constipation (OIC)
lubiprostone, Amitiza (G), 428
methylnaltrexone bromide, Relistor,
  428–429
naldemedine, Symproic, 429
naloxegol, Movantik, 429
opioid-induced nausea/vomiting
  (OINV)
aprepitant, Emend (G), 430
dolasetron, Anzemet, 429
granisetron, Kytril, Sancuso, 429
ondansetron, Zofran, Zuplenz (G), 429
palonosetron, Aloxi (G), 430
prochlorperazine, Compazine (G), 429
Opticrom, *cromolyn sodium*
  vernal keratitis, 375
Optivar, *azelastine*
  allergic (vernal) conjunctivitis, 167
Opzelura, *ruxolitinib*
  asthma, 45
  atopic dermatitis, 200–201
  vitiligo, 654
Oracea, *doxycycline*
  acne rosacea, 3
  acne vulgaris, 5
  acute exacerbation of chronic
    bronchitis, 70
  anthrax (bacillus anthracis), 32
  bacterial skin infection, 574
  cat bite, 65
  cat scratch fever, 141
  Chlamydia trachomatis, 151
  cholera (*Vibrio cholerae*), 155, 156
  community-acquired pneumonia, 494
  dog bite, 66
  dose forms, 639, 644, 704
  epididymitis, 237
  gonorrhea, 256
  granuloma inguinale, 266
  hidradenitis suppurativa, 303
  lyme disease, 383
  lymphogranuloma venereum, 384
  malaria, 384
  nongonococcal urethritis, 639
  pelvic inflammatory disease, 476
  proctitis: acute, 516
  rocky mountain spotted fever, 556
  sexual assault, 567
oral (thrush) candidiasis
  clotrimazole, Mycelex Troches, 134
  fluconazole, Diflucan, 135
  gentian violet (G), 135
  itraconazole, Sporanox (G), 135
  miconazole, Oravig, 135
  nystatin, Mycostatin, Mycostatin
    Suspension (G), 135
  posaconazole, Noxafil (G), 135
oral electrolyte replacement (OTC),
    KaoLectrolyte, Pedialyte,
    Pedialyte Freezer Pops (G)
  acute diarrhea, 212

dehydration, 187
Oralair, *sweet vernal, orchard, perennial
    rye, timothy, Kentucky blue grass
    mixed pollen allergen extract*
  allergic rhinitis/sinusitis, 551
Oralone, *triamcinolone acetonide*
  aphthous stomatitis, 37
Oravig, *miconazole*
  oral (thrush) candidiasis, 135
Orazyme Dry Mouth Rinse, *xylitol+
    solazyme+selectobac*
  Sjögren-Larsson-syndrome, 572
Orbactiv, *oritavancin*
  cellulitis, 145
Orencia, *abatacept*
  graft versus host disease (GVHD),
    264–265
  juvenile idiopathic arthritis, 373–374
  polyarticular juvenile idiopathic
    arthritis (PJIA), 370–371
  psoriatic arthritis, 531
  rheumatoid arthritis, 549
Orenitram, *treprostinil*
  pulmonary arterial hypertension
    (PAH), 534
organ transplant rejection prophylaxis
  basiliximab, Simulect, 432
  everolimus, Zortress (G), 432
  mycophenolate mofetil (MMF),
    CellCept, 432
  sirolimus, Rapamune (G), 432–433
  tacrolimus, Envarsus XR, 433
Orgovyx, *relugolix*
  prostate cancer, 128
Oriahnn, *elagolix*
  uterine leiomyomata, 651
  uterine leiomyomata (fibroid tumor)
    uterine fibroids, 651
orilissa, *elagolix*
  endometriosis, 233
oritavancin, Orbactiv
  cellulitis, 145
Orkambi, *lumacaftor+ivacaftor*
  cystic fibrosis (CF), 183
orlistat, Alli, Xenical (G)
  obesity, 418
orphenadrine citrate, Norflex
  muscle strain, 404
  temporomandibular joint disorder,
    587
Orserdu, *elacestrant*
  breast cancer, 85
Ortho-Cept 28, *ethinyl estradiol+
    desogestrel* (G)
  estrogen and progesterone, 671
Ortho-Cyclen 28, *ethinyl estradiol+
    norgestimate* (G)
  estrogen and progesterone, 671
ortho evra, *ethinyl estradiol+
    norelgestromin* (G), 674
Ortho-Novum 1/35-21, Ortho-
    Novum 1/35-2, *ethinyl
    estradiol+norethindrone*
  estrogen and progesterone, 671
Ortho-Novum 1/50-21, Ortho-
    Novum 1/50-28,
    mestranol+norethindrone
  estrogen and progesterone, 671
Ortho-Novum 7/7/7-28, *ethinyl
    estradiol+norethindrone*, 672
Ortho-Novum 10/11-28, *ethinyl
    estradiol+norethindrone* (G)
  estrogen and progesterone, 672
Ortho-Prefest, *estradiol+norgestimate* (G)
  menopause, 391
  osteoporosis, 440
Ortho Tri-Cyclen 21, Ortho Tri-Cyclen
    28, *ethinyl estradiol+norgestimate*
  estrogen and progesterone, 672

Ortho Tri-Cyclen Lo, *ethinyl
    estradiol+norgestimate*
  estrogen and progesterone, 672
Orthovisc, *sodium hyaluronate*
  osteoarthritis, 437
Os-Cal 250+D, Os-Cal 500+D, *calcium
    carbonate+vitamin D*
  hypocalcemia, 340
Os-Cal 250+D, Viactiv, *calcium
    carbonate+vitamin D*
  osteoporosis, 441
Os-Cal 500, *calcium carbonate*
  hypocalcemia, 340
oseltamivir phosphate, Tamiflu
  influenza, seasonal (FLU), 357
Oseni, *alogliptin+pioglitazone*
  type 2 diabetes mellitus, 621
Osgood-Schlatter disease, 433–434
osilodrostat, Isturisa
  cushing's syndrome, 181
Osmolex ER, *amantadine*
  extrapyramidal side effects (EPS), 240
  Parkinson's disease, 469
ospemifene, Osphena
  dyspareunia, 226
Osphena, *ospemifene*
  dyspareunia, 226
osteoarthritis (OA)
  adalimumab, Humira, 437–438
  adalimumab-aacf, Idacio, 438
  adalimumab-adaz, Hyrimoz, 438
  adalimumab-adbm, Cyltezo, 438
  adalimumab-afzb, Abrilada, 438
  adalimumab-bwwd, Hadlima, 438
  capsaicin 8% patch, Qutenza, 438
  capsaicin, Axsain, Capsin,
    Capzasin-HP, Capzasin-P,
    Dolorac, Double Cap (OTC),
    R-Gel, Zostrix, Zostrix HP (G),
    434
  celecoxib, Celebrex (G), 436
  diclofenac sodium, Pennsaid, Solaraze
    Gel, Voltaren Gel, 434
  diclofenac sodium, Voltaren, 435
  diclofenac, Zorvolex, 435
  doxepin, Prudoxin, Zonalon (G), 434
  Duexis, *ibuprofen+famotidine*, 436
  etanercept, Enbrel, 438
  etanercept-ykro, Eticovo, 438
  indomethacin, 434–435
  infliximab, Remicade, 438
  infliximab-abda, Renflexis, 438
  infliximab-axxq, Avsola, 439
  infliximab-dyyb, Inflectra, 438
  infliximab-qbtx, Ixifi, 439
  meloxicam, Mobic, Vivlodex (D), 436
  pimecrolimus, Elidel, 434
  secukinumab, Cosentyx, 439
  sodium hyaluronate, Durolane,
    Euflexx, Gel-One, GelSyn-3,
    GenVisc 850, Hyalgan,
    Monovisc, Orthovisc, Supartz,
    Supartz FX, Synvisc, Synvisc-
    One, Triluron, *TriVisc*, Visco-3,
    437
  triamcinolone acetonide, Zilretta, 436
  trolamine salicylate, Mobisyl Creme,
    434
  Vimovo, *naproxen+esomeprazole
    magnesium* (G), 435
osteomalacia, 345
osteoporosis
  abaloparatide, Tymlos, 442
  Activella (G), FemHRT,
    estradiol+norethindrone, 440
  Actonel with Calcium, *risedronate+
    calcium*, 442
  alendronate (as sodium), Binosto,
    Fosamax (G), 441

osteoporosis (cont.)
  bioengineered replica of human
    parathyroid hormone, Natpara,
    443
  calcitonin-salmon, Fortical, Miacalcin,
    440
  calcitriol, Rocaltrol, 441
  calcium carbonate, Rolaids, Tums,
    Os-Cal 500 (G), 440
  calcium citrate, Citracal (G), 441
  calcium citrate+vitamin D, Citracal+D,
    Citracal 250+D, 441
  Climara Pro, estradiol+levonorgestrel,
    440
  denosumab, Prolia, Xgeva, 443
  doxercalciferol, Hectorol, 441
  estradiol, Alora, Climara, Estrace,
    Estraderm, Menostar, Minivelle,
    Vivelle, Vivelle-Dot, 440
  estrogen, conjugated (equine),
    Premarin, 440
  estrogen, conjugated+bazedoxifene,
    Duavee, 440
  estropipate, piperazine estrone sulfate,
    Ogen, Ortho-Est (G), 440
  Fosamax Plus D,
    alendronate+cholecalciferol
    (vit d3) (G), 441
  ibandronate (as monosodium
    monohydrate), Boniva, 441–442
  Ortho-Prefest, estradiol+norgestimate,
    440
  Os-Cal 250+D, Os-Cal 500+D, Viactiv,
    calcium carbonate+vitamin D (G),
    441
  raloxifene, Evista (G), 442
  risedronate (as sodium), Actonel,
    Atelvia (G), 442
  romosozumab-aqqg, Evenity, 443–444
  teriparatide, Forteo Multidose Pen,
    442–443
  zoledronic acid, Reclast, Zometa (G),
    442
Otezla, apremilast
  psoriatic arthritis, 528
Otiprio, ciprofloxacin otic suspension
  serous otitis media (SOM), 448
otitis externa
  acetic acid 2% in aluminum sulfate,
    Domeboro Otic, 444
  acetic acid+propylene glycol+
    benzethonium chloride+sodium
    acetate, VoSol (G), 444
  acetic acid+propylene glycol+
    hydrocortisone+benzethonium
    chloride+sodium acetate, VoSol
    HC (G), 444
  antipyrine+benzocaine+glycerine, A/B
    Otic, 445
  antipyrine+benzocaine+zinc acetate
    dihydrate, Otozin, 444
  augmentin, Augmentin
    ES-600, Augmentin XR,
    amoxicillin+clavulanate (G), 445
  benzocaine, Americaine Otic, Benzotic
    (G), 445
  cefaclor, Cefaclor Extended Release
    (G), 445
  chloroxylenol+pramoxine, PramOtic,
    444
  chloroxylenol+pramoxine+
    hydrocortisone, Cortane B,
    Cortane B Aqueous (G), 444
  ciprofloxacin+dexamethasone,
    Ciprodex, 444
  ciprofloxacin+hydrocortisone, Cipro
    HC Otic, 444
  colistin+neomycin+hydrocortisone+
    thonzonium, Coly-Mycin S,
    Cortisporin-TC Otic (G), 444

dicloxacillin, Dynapen, 445
finafloxacin, Xtoro, 445
ofloxacin, Floxin Otic (G), 444
polymyxin b+neomycin+
  hydrocortisone, Cortisporin (G),
  444
trimethoprim+sulfamethoxazole
  (TMP-SMX), Bactrium, septra
  (G), 445
otitis media: acute
  A/B Otic, antipyrine+benzocaine+
    glycerine, 447
  amoxicillin, Amoxil, Moxatag, Trimox,
    445–446
  ampicillin, Omnipen, Principen,
    Unasyn, 446
  Augmentin, Augmentin
    ES-600, Augmentin XR,
    amoxicillin+clavulanate (G), 446
  azithromycin, Zithromax, Zmax (G),
    446
  benzocaine, Americaine Otic, Benzotic
    (OTC), 448
  cefaclor, Cefaclor Extended Release
    (G), 446
  cefdinir, Omnicef, 446
  cefixime, Suprax (G), 446
  cefpodoxime proxetil, Vantin, 446
  cefprozil, Cefzil, 446
  ceftibuten, Cedax, 446
  ceftriaxone, Rocephin (G), 446
  cephalexin, Keflex (G), 447
  chloroxylenol+pramoxine+
    hydrocortisone, Cortane Ear
    Drops, 447
  Ciprodex, ciprofloxacin+
    dexamethasone (G), 447
  Cipro HC Otic, ciprofloxacin+
    hydrocortisone, 447
  clarithromycin, Biaxin (G), 447
  coly-Mycin S, colistin+neomycin+
    hydrocortisone+thonzonium, 447
  cortisporin, PediOtic, polymyxin b+
    neomycin+hydrocortisone (G),
    447
  Cortisporin-TC, polymyxin
    b+neomycin+hydrocortisone+
    surfactant, 447
  erythromycin+sulfisoxazole, Eryzole,
    Pediazole (G), 447
  loracarbef, Lorabid, 447
  ofloxacin, Floxin, 447
  Otozin, antipyrine+benzocaine+zinc
    acetate dihydrate, 445
  trimethoprim+sulfamethoxazole
    (TMP-SMX]), Bactrim, Septra
    (G), 447
Otozin, antipyrine+benzocaine+zinc
    acetate dihydrate
  cerumen impaction, 145
  otitis externa, 444
  otitis media: acute, 445
ovarian cancer
  bevacizumab-adcd, Vegzelma, 122
  mirvetuximab soravtansine-gynx,
    Elahere, 123–124
  niraparib tosylate, Zejula, 122–123
  rucaparib, Rubraca, 123
Ovcon 35 Fe, ethinyl estradiol+
    norethindrone plus ferrous
    fumarate (G)
  estrogen and progesterone, 672
Ovcon 50-28, Ovcon 50-28, ethinyl
    estradiol+norethindrone (G)
  estrogen and progesterone, 672
Ovide (OTC), malathion
  pediculosis humanus capitis, 475
Ovral-21, Ovral-28, ethinyl estradiol+
    norgestrel (G)
  estrogen and progesterone, 672

oxazepam
  alcohol withdrawal syndrome, 11
  anxiety disorder, 33
  panic disorder, 465
Oxbryta, voxelotor
  sickle cell disease (SCD), 570–571
Oxervat, cenegermin-bkbj
  neurotrophic keratitis, 374–375
oxiconazole nitrate, Oxistat
  tinea corporis, 598
  tinea cruris, 599
  tinea pedis, 600
  tinea versicolor, 601
Oxistat, oxiconazole nitrate
  tinea corporis, 598
  tinea cruris, 599
  tinea pedis, 600
  tinea versicolor, 601
Oxsoralen, methoxsalen
  vitiligo, 653
oxybutynin chloride, Ditropan,
    GelniQUE, Oxytrol Transdermal
    Patch
  hyperhidrosis, 320
  interstitial cystitis, 362
  urinary overactive bladder, 355
oxycodone, Oxaydo, OxyContin, OxyFast
    Xtampza ER (II)
  pain, 458
oxymetazoline, Afrin, Neo-Synephrine,
    Rhofade, Visine L-R
  acne rosacea, 2
  allergic (vernal) conjunctivitis, 167
  common cold, 161
oxymetazoline hydrochloride ophthalmic
    solution, 0.1%, Upneeq
  blepharoptosis, acquired (droopy
    eyelid), 67–68
oxymorphone, Numorphan, Opana
    (G)(II)
  pain, 459
Oxytrol Transdermal Patch, oxybutynin
    chloride
  hyperhidrosis, 320
  urinary overactive bladder, 355
ozanimod, Zeposia
  multiple sclerosis (MS), 401
ozenoxacin, Xepi
  impetigo contagiosa, 353

pacritinib, Vonjo
  myelofibrosis, 408–409
Padcev, enfortumab vedotin-ejfv
  urothelial carcinoma, 134
Paget's disease
  alendronate (as sodium), Binosto,
    Fosamax (G), 450
  alendronate+cholecalciferol (vit d3),
    Fosamax Plus D (G), 450
  ibandronate (as monosodium
    monohydrate), Boniva (G), 450
  risedronate (as sodium), Actonel,
    Atelvia (G), 450
  risedronate+calcium, Actonel with
    Calcium (G), 450
  zoledronic acid, Reclast, Zometa (G),
    450
pain
  acetaminophen, Ofirmev, 450–451
  Advil Dual Action with
    Acetaminophen, ibuprofen+
    acetaminophen (G), 451
  Apadaz, benzhydrocodone+
    acetaminophen (II), 454
  buprenorphine, Butrans Transdermal
    System (III), 461
  buprenorphine hcl, Buprenex, 462
  buprenorphine, Subutex, 461
  butorphanol tartrate, Butorphanol Nasal
    Spray, Stadol Nasal Spray, 462

capsaicin 8% patch, Qutenza, 453
capsaicin, Axsain, Capsin, Capzasin-HP, Capzasin-P, Dolorac, Double Cap (OTC), R-Gel, Zostrix, Zostrix HP (G), 453
codeine sulfate (G)(III), 455
Decadron Phosphate with Xylocaine, *lidocaine+dexamethasone,* 454
dexamethasone ophthalmic insert, Dextenza, 453
diclofenac sodium, Pennsaid, Solaraze Gel, Voltaren Gel, 453
difluprednate, Durezol Ophthalmic Solution *(G),* 453
doxepin, Prudoxin, Zonalon (G), 453
Duexis, *ibuprofen+famotidine,* 451–452
Emla Cream, *lidocaine 2.5%+prilocaine 2.5%,* 454
fentanyl citrate, Actiq, Fentora (G)(II), 461
fentanyl, Abstral, 461
fentanyl, Duragesic (II), 461
fentanyl iontophoretic transdermal system, Ionsys, 461
fentanyl, Lazanda Nasal Spray (II), 462
fentanyl, Onsolis, 461
fentanyl sublingual spray, Subsys (II), 461
fentanyl sublingual tab, Abstral (II), 461
Fioricet, Zebutal, *butalbital+ acetaminophen+caffeine* (G), 455
Fiorinal, *butalbital+aspirin+caffeine* (G)(III), 455
Fiorinal with Codeine, *butalbital+ aspirin+codeine+caffeine* (G)(III), 455
hydrocodone bitartrate, Hysingla ER, Vantrela ER, Zohydro ER (G)(II), 455
hydrocodone bitartrate+ acetaminophen, Hycet, Lorcet, Maxidone, Norco, Vicodin, Xodol, Zamicet Oral Solution, Zydone (II), 455–456
hydrocodone+ibuprofen, Ibudone, Reprexain, Vicoprofen (G)(II), 456
hydromorphone (II)(G), Dilaudid, 456
ibuprofen, Caldolor, 451
LidaMantle HC, *lidocaine+ hydrocortisone* (G), 454
lidocaine, LidaMantle, Lidoderm, ZTlido lidocaine, 454
meloxicam, Anjeso, 451
meperidine, Demerol, 457
meperidine+promethazine, Mepergan (G)(II), 457
methadone, Dolophine (G)(II), 457
morphine sulfate (immed-release) (G)(II), 457
morphine sulfate (immed- and sust-rel), Arymo ER, Duramorph, Infumorph, Kadian (G), MS Contin (G), MSIR, Oramorph SR, Roxanol (II), 457–458
morphine sulfate (ext-rel), MorphaBond ER (II), 458
morphine sulfate+naltrexone, Embeda (II), 458
nalbuphine (G), Nubain, 462
nepafenac, Nevanac Ophthalmic Suspension, 453
oxycodone cont-rel, OxyContin, OxyFast Xtampza ER (G)(II), 458–459
oxycodone, Oxaydo (II), 458

oxycodone+acetaminophen, Magnacet, Percocet, Roxicet, Tylox, Xartemis XR (G)(II), 459
oxycodone+aspirin, Percodan (G)(II), 459
oxycodone+ibuprofen, Combunox (G)(II), 459
oxycodone+naloxone, Targiniq (II), 459
oxymorphone, Numorphan, Opana (G)(II), 459
Panlor DC, Panlor SS, *dihydrocodeine+acetaminophen+ caffeine* (III), 455
pentazocine+aspirin, Talwin Compound (IV), 460
pentazocine lactate (IV), Talwin, 460
pentazocine+naloxone, Talwin NX (IV), 460, 462
Phrenilin, Phrenilin Forte, *butalbital+ acetaminophen* (G), 455
pimecrolimus, Elidel, 454
propoxyphene napsylate+ acetaminophen, Balacet (G) (IV), 460
sufentanil, Dsuvia, 461–462
Synalgos-DC, *dihydrocodeine+ aspirin+caffeine (G)(III),* 455
tramadol, Conzip, Rybix ODT, Ryzolt, Ultram (G)(IV), 460
trolamine salicylate, Mobisyl Creme, 454
Tylenol, codeine+acetaminophen (G)(III), 455
Ultracet, *tramadol+acetaminophen* (G)(IV), 461
Vimovo, *naproxen+esomeprazole magnesium* (G), 452–453
ziconotide, Prial, 462
Palforzia, *arachis hypogaea allergen powder-dnfp*
peanut (arachis hypogaea) allergy, 474–475
paliperidone palmitate, Invega Hafyera, Invega Sustenna
schizophrenia, 564–566
palivizumab, Synagis
respiratory syncytial virus (RSV), 539
palonosetron, Aloxi
cannabinoid hyperemesis syndrome, 140
chemotherapy-induced nausea/ vomiting, 149
opioid-induced nausea/vomiting (OINV), 429
post-anesthesia nausea/vomiting, 414
Palynziq, *pegvaliase-pqpz*
phenylketonuria (PKU), 486
Pamelor, *nortriptyline* (G), 193
anxiety disorder, 34
diabetic peripheral neuropathy (DPN), 210
irritable bowel syndrome with diarrhea, 368
major depressive disorder (MDD), 193
nocturnal enuresis, 235
post-herpetic neuralgia, 508, 510
post-traumatic stress disorder, 512
premenstrual dysphoric disorder, 515
trigeminal neuralgia, 609
Pamine, Pamine Forte, *methscopolamine bromide*
abdominal cramps, 174
irritable bowel syndrome with diarrhea, 367
vertigo, 653
pancreatic cancer
olaparib, Lynparza, 124–125
sodium thiosulfate, Pedmark, 124

pancreatic enzyme insufficiency
pancreatic enzymes, Creon, Cotazym, Donnazyme, Ku-Zyme, Kutrase, Pancreaze, Pertyze, Ultrase, Viokace, Zenpep, 463–464
pancreatic enzyme deficiency
pancreatic enzymes, Creon, Cotazym, Donnazyme, Ku-Zyme, Kutrase, Pancreaze, Pertyze, Ultrase, Viokace, Zenpep, 239–240
pancreatic enzymes, Creon, Cotazym, Donnazyme, Ku-Zyme, Kutrase, Pancreaze, Pertyze, Ultrase, Viokace, Zenpep
pancreatic enzyme deficiency, 239–240
pancreatic enzyme insufficiency, 463–464
Pancreaze, *pancreatic enzymes*
pancreatic enzyme deficiency, 463
pancreatic enzyme insufficiency, 463
panic disorder
alprazolam, Niravam, Xanax, Xanax XR (G)(IV), 465
buspirone, BuSpar, 465
chlordiazepoxide, Librium (G)(IV), 466
clonazepam, Klonopin (G)(IV), 466
clorazepate, Tranxene (G)(IV), 466
desvenlafaxine, Pristiq (G), 465
diazepam, Diastat, Valium (G)(IV), 466
doxepin (G), 465
escitalopram, Lexapro (G), 464
fluoxetine, Prozac, Prozac Weekly, 464
hydroxyzine, Atarax, Vistaril (G), 465
imipramine, Tofranil (G), 465
Librax, *chlordiazepoxide+clidinium* (IV), 466
lorazepam, Ativan, Lorazepam Intensol (G)(IV), 466
oxazepam (IV)(G), 465
paroxetine maleate, Paxil (G), 464
paroxetine mesylate, Brisdelle (G), 465
prochlorperazine, Compazine (G), 466
sertraline, Zoloft, 465
trifluoperazine, Stelazine (G), 466
venlafaxine, Effexor, Effexor XR (G), 465
Panlor DC, Panlor SS, *dihydrocodeine+ acetaminophen+caffeine* (III)(G)
pain, 455
pantoprazole, Protonix
gastroesophageal reflux disease, 251
peptic ulcer disease (PUD), 479
Zollinger-Ellison syndrome, 662
paricalcitol, Zemplar (G)
hyperparathyroidism, 323
hypocalcemia, 341
Parkinson's disease
amantadine, Gocovri, Osmolex ER, Symadine (G), Symmetrel (G), 468–469
apomorphine hcl, Apokyn (G), 467–468
apomorphine sublingual film, Kynmobi, 468
benztropine mesylate, Cogentin, 471
biperiden hydrochloride, Akineton, 471
bromocriptine, Parlodel (G), 469
carbidopa, Lodosyn (G), 466
carbidopa+levodopa, Duopa, Sinemet (G), 469
carbidopa+levodopa+entacapone, Stalevo (G), 470
dextromethorphan+quinidine, Nuedexta (G), 471
entacapone, Comtan, 471
istradefylline, Nourianz, 470

Parkinson's disease (*cont.*)
  levodopa (G), 466
  levodopa inhalation powder, Inbrija, 467
  opicapone, Ongentys, 471
  pimavanserin, Nuplazid, 471
  pramipexole, Mirapex (G), 469
  procyclidine, Kemadrin, 471
  rasagiline, Azilect (G), 470
  ropinirole, Requip, 469
  rotigotine, Neupro, 469
  safinamide, Xadago (G), 470
  selegiline (G), 470
  selegiline, Zelapar (G), 470
  tolcapone, Tasmar (G), 471
  trihexyphenidyl, Artane (G), 471
Parlodel, *bromocriptine*
  Parkinson's disease, 469
Parnate, *tranylcypromine*
  major depressive disorder, 194
paromomycin, Humatin
  intestinal amebiasis, 17
paronychia (periungual abscess)
  cephalexin, Keflex (G), 472
  clindamycin, Cleocin (G), 472
  dicloxacillin, Dynapen (G), 472
  erythromycin base, Ery-Tab, PCE (G), 472
  erythromycin ethylsuccinate, EryPed, E.E.S. (G), 472
paroxetine maleate, Paxil, Paxil CR, Paxil Suspension (G)
  anxiety disorder, 35
  major depressive disorder, 192
  obsessive-compulsive disorder, 422
  panic disorder, 464
  post-traumatic stress disorder, 510
  premenstrual dysphoric disorder, 515
  trichotillomania, 608
paroxetine mesylate, Brisdelle (G)
  anxiety disorder, 35
  major depressive disorder, 192
  obsessive-compulsive disorder, 422
  panic disorder, 465
  post-traumatic stress disorder, 510
  premenstrual dysphoric disorder, 515
  trichotillomania, 608
paroxysmal nocturnal hemoglobinuria (PNH)
  eculizumab, Soliris, 472–473
  pegcetacoplan, Empaveli, 473
  ravulizumab-cwvz, Ultomiris, 474
Parsabiv, *etelcalcetide*
  hyperhidrosis, 321
pasireotide, Signifor
  cushing's syndrome, 180
pasireotide, Signifor LAR
  acromegaly, 7
Pataday, *olopatadine*
  allergic (vernal) conjunctivitis, 167
Patanase, *olopatadine*
  allergic rhinitis/sinusitis, 553
Patanol, *olopatadine*
  allergic (vernal) conjunctivitis, 167
patiromer sorbitex calcium, Veltassa
  hyperkalemia, 322
Paxil, Paxil CR, Paxil Suspension, *paroxetine maleate*
  anxiety disorder, 35
  major depressive disorder, 192
  obsessive-compulsive disorder, 422
  panic disorder, 464
  post-traumatic stress disorder, 510
  premenstrual dysphoric disorder, 515
  trichotillomania, 608
Paxlovid, *nirmatrelvir+ritonavir*
  COVID-19 (coronavirus), 173
Pazeo, *olopatadine*
  allergic (vernal) conjunctivitis, 167

PCE, *erythromycin base*
  acne vulgaris, 5
  acute exacerbation of chronic bronchitis, 70
  acute tonsillitis, 604
  bacterial skin infection, 574
  cat scratch fever, 141
  cellulitis, 144
  chancroid, 147
  Chlamydia trachomatis, 152
  chlamydial conjunctivitis, 164
  chlamydial ophthalmia neonatorum, 423
  chlamydial pneumonia, 492
  cholera *(Vibrio cholerae)*, 156
  dental abscess, 191
  diphtheria, 215
  erysipelas, 238
  gonococcal conjunctivitis, 165
  granuloma inguinale, 266
  hidradenitis suppurativa, 303
  human bite, 67
  impetigo contagiosa, 352
  lymphogranuloma venereum, 384
  mycoplasma pneumonia, 496
  nongonococcal urethritis, 639
  paronychia, 472
  pertussis, 483
  scarlet fever, 560
  streptococcal pharyngitis, 485
  wound, 659
peanut (arachis hypogaea) allergy
  arachis hypogaea allergen powder-dnfp, Palforzia, 474–475
PediaCare, *ibuprofen* (G)
  fever (pyrexia), 242–243
Pedialyte, Pedialyte Freezer Pops, *oral electrolyte replacement* (OTC)(G)
  acute diarrhea, 212
  dehydration, 187
Pediamist (OTC), *saline nasal spray* (G)
  common cold, 160–161
PediaProfen, *ibuprofen* (G)
  fever (pyrexia), 242–243
Pediazole, *erythromycin+sulfisoxazole*, 709
  otitis media: acute, 447
pediculosis humanus capitis
  abametapir, Xeglyze Lotion, 475
  ivermectin, Sklice (G), 475
  lindane, Kwell Shampoo (G), 475
  malathion, Ovide (OTC)(G), 475
  permethrin, Nix (OTC)(G), 475
  pyrethrins with piperonyl butoxide, A-200, Rid (G), 475
Pedmark, *sodium thiosulfate*
  pancreatic cancer, 124
  solid tumor, 132–133
PEGasys, *peginterferon alfa-2a*
  hepatitis C (HCV), 294
pegcetacoplan, Empaveli
  paroxysmal nocturnal hemoglobinuria (PNH), 473
pegfilgrastim, Neulasta
  neutropenia, 416
pegfilgrastim-jmdb, Fulphila
  neutropenia, 418
peginesatide, Omontys
  anemia of chronic kidney disease, 23
peginterferon alfa-2a, PEGasys
  hepatitis C (HCV), 294
peginterferon alfa-2b, PEG-Intron
  hepatitis C (HCV), 294
peginterferon beta-1a, Plegridy
  multiple sclerosis (MS), 398–399
PEG-Intron, *peginterferon alfa-2b*
  hepatitis C (HCV), 294
pegloticase, Krystexxa
  gout (hyperuricemia), 260

pegvaliase-pqpz, Palynziq
  phenylketonuria (PKU), 486
pegvisomant, Somavert
  acromegaly, 7
pelvic inflammatory disease (PID)
  cefoxitin, Mefoxin (G), 476
  ceftriaxone, Rocephin (G), 476
  doxycycline, Acticlate, Adoxa, Doryx, Doxteric, Monodox, Oracea, Vibramycin, Vibra-Tab (G), 476
  metronidazole, Flagyl, Flagyl 375, Flagyl ER (G), 476
  probenecid, Benemid (G), 476
pembrolizumab, Keytruda
  breast cancer, 78
  cervical cancer, 86
  colorectal cancer, 86
  hepatocellular carcinoma (HCC), 86
  lung cancer, 106
  lymphoma, 108–109
  renal cell carcinoma (RCC), 95
  solid tumor, 133
  urothelial carcinoma, 134
pemetrexed, Pemfexy (G)
  lung cancer, 105
  lymphoma, 111
  mesothelioma, 393–394
Pemfexy, *pemetrexed* (G)
  lung cancer, 105
  lymphoma, 111
  mesothelioma, 393–394
pemirolast potassium, Alamast
  allergic (vernal) conjunctivitis, 166
pemoline, Cylert (B)(IV)
pemphigus foliaceus (PF), 476–477
pemphigus vulgaris
  azathioprine, Azasan, Imuran, 476–477
  belimumab, Benlysta, 477
  cyclophosphamide, Cytoxan (G), 477
  dapsone, Aczone (G), 477
  prednisone, 476
  rituximab, Rituxan, 477
  tocilizumab, Actemra, 477
penbutolol, Levatol
  hypertension, 326
penciclovir, Denavir
  herpes labialis/herpes facialis, 301
Penetrex, *enoxacin*
  gonorrhea, 259
penicillamine, Cuprimine, Depen
  Gaucher disease, type 1 (GD1), 252
  rheumatoid arthritis, 546
  systemic lupus erythematosis, 584
  urolithiasis, 646
  Wilson's disease, 657
penicillin g (benzathine), Bicillin L-A, Bicillin C-R (G)
  dose form/volume, 707
  impetigo contagiosa, 353
  scarlet fever, 560
  streptococcal pharyngitis, 485
  syphilis, 582
penicillin g potassium (G)
  listeriosis, 379
penicillin v potassium, Pen-Vee K (G), 720–721
  acute tonsillitis, 605
  bacterial endocarditis prophylaxis, 56
  cat bite, 65
  cellulitis, 145
  community acquired pneumonia, 494
  dental abscess, 191
  dog bite, 66
  dose form/volume, 707
  erysipelas, 238
  impetigo contagiosa, 353
  scarlet fever, 560

streptococcal pharyngitis, 485
Penlac Nail Lacquer, *ciclopirox*
  onychomycosis (fungal nail), 422
Pennsaid, *diclofenac sodium*
  atopic dermatitis, 199
  diabetic peripheral neuropathy
    (DPN), 208–209
  gouty arthritis, 262
  hemorrhoids, 289–290
  juvenile idiopathic arthritis, 369
  muscle strain, 404–405
  osteoarthritis, 434
  pain, 453
  peripheral neuritis, 480
  post-herpetic neuralgia, 508
  pruritus, 518
  psoriatic arthritis, 527
  rheumatoid arthritis, 542
Pentacel
  poliomyelitis/poliovirus, 498–499
Pentasa, *mesalamine*
pentazocine lactate (IV), Talwin
  pain, 460
  Crohn's disease, 176
pentobarbital, Nembutal (II)
  insomnia, 360
PentoPak, *pentoxifylline*
  peripheral vascular disease, 482
pentosan, Elmiron
  interstitial cystitis, 362
pentoxifylline, PentoPak, Trental
  peripheral vascular disease, 482
Pen-Vee K, *penicillin v potassium* (G)
  acute tonsillitis, 605
  bacterial endocarditis prophylaxis, 56
  cat bite, 65
  cellulitis, 145
  community acquired pneumonia, 494
  dental abscess, 191
  dog bite, 66
  dose form/volume, 707
  erysipelas, 238
  impetigo contagiosa, 353
  scarlet fever, 560
  streptococcal pharyngitis, 485
Pepaxto, *melphalan flufenamide*
  multiple myeloma, 121
Pepcid, *famotidine* (G)
  peptic ulcer disease (PUD), 478
peptic ulcer disease (PUD)
  cimetidine, Tagamet (G), 477–478
  dexlansoprazole, Dexilant (G), 478
  esomeprazole, Nexium (G), 478
  famotidine, Pepcid (G), 478
  glycopyrrolate, Dartisla, 479
  lansoprazole, Prevacid (G), 478
  mepenzolate, Cantil (G), 480
  misoprostol, Cytotec (G), 480
  nizatidine, Axid (G), 478
  omeprazole, Prilosec (G), 478–479
  pantoprazole, Protonix (G), 479
  rabeprazole, AcipHex (G), 479
  ranitidine bismuth citrate, Tritec, 478
  ranitidine, Zantac (G), 478
  Robinul (G), 479
  Robinul Forte (G), 479
  sucralfate, Carafate (G), 480
Pepto-Bismol, *bismuth subsalicylate*
  acute diarrhea, 211
peramivir, Rapivab
  influenza, seasonal (FLU), 357
Percodan, *oxycodone+aspirin* (G)(II)
  pain, 459
Perdiem, *psyllium+senna*
  occasional constipation, 170
perfluorohexyloctane, Miebo
  dry eye syndrome, 218
Perforomist, *formoterol fumarate*
  asthma, 43

Periactin, *cyproheptadine* (G)
  anorexia/cachexia, 30
Peri-Colace, *docusate+casanthranol*
  occasional constipation, 170
Peridex, *chlorhexidine gluconate*
  gingivitis/periodontitis, 254
perindopril, Aceon
  hypertension, 330
PerioGard, *chlorhexidine gluconate*
  gingivitis/periodontitis, 254
peripheral neuritis
  capsaicin, Axsain, Capsin,
    Capzasin-HP, Capzasin-P,
    Dolorac, Double Cap (OTC),
    R-Gel, Zostrix, Zostrix HP (G),
    480
  Decadron Phosphate with Xylocaine,
    lidocaine+dexamethasone, 481
  diclofenac sodium, Pennsaid, Solaraze
    Gel, Voltaren Gel, 480
  doxepin, Prudoxin, Zonalon (G),
    480–481
  duloxetine, Cymbalta, 480
  Emla Cream, *lidocaine*
    2.5%+prilocaine 2.5%, 481
  LidaMantle HC, *lidocaine+*
    hydrocortisone, 481
  lidocaine, LidaMantle, Lidoderm,
    ZTlido lidocaine, 481
  pimecrolimus, Elidel, 481
  pregabalin (GABA analog), Lyrica,
    Lyrica CR (G), 480
  tapentadol, Nucynta (II), 481–482
  tramadol, Rybix ODT, Ryzolt, Ultram
    (G)(IV), 481
  trolamine salicylate, Mobisyl Creme,
    481
  Ultracet, *tramadol+*
    acetaminophen (IV), 481
peripheral neuropathic pain, 480–482
peripheral vascular disease (PVD)
  aspirin, Ecotrin, 482
  cilostazol, 482
  clopidogrel, Plavix, 482
  dipyridamole, Persantine (G), 482
  pentoxifylline, PentoPak, Trental, 482
  ticlopidine, Ticlid, 482
  warfarin, Coumadin, 482
peritoneal cancer
  bevacizumab-adcd, Vegzelma, 127
  mirvetuximab soravtansine-gynx,
    Elahere, 125
  niraparib tosylate, Zejula, 125
  olaparib, Lynparza, 125
  rucaparib, Rubraca, 126
Perjeta, *pertuzumab*, 688
perleche, 482
permethrin, Acticin, Elimite, Nix
  pediculosis humanus capitis, 475
  scabies, 559
pernicious/megaloblastic anemia
  vitamin B12 (cyanocobalamin),
    Nascobal Nasal Spray (A), 17
perphenazine, Trilafon
  cannabinoid hyperemesis syndrome,
    139
  chemotherapy-induced nausea/
    vomiting, 147
Persantine, *dipyridamole*
  dose forms, 702
  peripheral vascular disease, 482
pertussis
  azithromycin, Zithromax, Zmax (G),
    483
  clarithromycin, Biaxin (G), 483
  erythromycin base, Ery-Tab, PCE (G),
    483
  erythromycin ethylsuccinate, EryPed,
    E.E.S, 483

Pentacel, 482
  Vaxelis, 483
  trimethoprim+sulfamethoxazole
    (TMP-SMX), Bactrim, Septra
    (G), 483
Pertyze, *pancreatic enzymes*
  pancreatic enzyme deficiency, 239
  pancreatic enzyme insufficiency, 463
Phazyme-95, *simethicone*
  flatulence, 245
phenazopyridine, AZO Standard,
    Prodium, Uristat
  interstitial cystitis, 361, 362
  pyelonephritis: acute, 536
  urinary tract infection, 642
phendimetrazine, Bontril (III)
  obesity, 419
phenelzine, Nardil
  major depressive disorder, 194
  post-traumatic stress disorder, 512
Phenergan, *promethazine* (G)
  cannabinoid hyperemesis syndrome
    (CHS), 139
  chemotherapy-induced nausea/
    vomiting, 147
  gastritis-related nausea/vomiting, 248
  labyrinthitis, 375
  Meniere's disease, 388
  motion sickness, 396
  post-anesthesia nausea/vomiting, 414
  pregnancy, 514
phenoxybenzamine, Dibenzyline
  pheochromocytoma, 487
phentermine, Adipex-P, Fastin, Ionamin,
    Suprenza ODT (IV)
  obesity, 419
phenylephrine, Afrin Allergy Nasal
    Spray, Afrin Nasal Decongestant
    Childrens Pump Mist,
    Neo-Synephrine
  common cold, 160–161
phenylketonuria (PKU)
  pegvaliase-pqpz, Palynziq, 486
  sapropterin, Kuvan (G), 486
phenytoin (injectable), Dilantin (G)
  dose forms, 695
  status epilepticus, 580
  trigeminal neuralgia, 609
pheochromocytoma
  iobenguane I 131, Azedra, 487–488
  metyrosine, Demser (G), 486–487
  phenoxybenzamine, Dibenzyline, 487
pHisoHex, *hexachlorophene*
  bacterial skin infection, 573
Phrenilin, Phrenilin Forte, *butalbital+*
    acetaminophen (G)
  pain, 455
  tension headache, 277
Picato, *ingenol mebutate*
  actinic keratosis, 9
pilocarpine, Isopto Carpine, Ocusert Pilo,
    Pilocar Ophthalmic Sol, Pilopine
    HS, Salagen
  glaucoma, 255
  Sjögren-Larsson-syndrome (SLS), 572
pimavanserin, Nuplazid
  Parkinson's disease, 471
pimecrolimus, Elidel
  atopic dermatitis, 190
  diabetic peripheral neuropathy
    (DPN), 209
  gouty arthritis, 262
  hemorrhoids, 290
  juvenile idiopathic arthritis, 369
  juvenile rheumatoid arthritis, 372
  muscle strain, 405
  osteoarthritis, 434
  pain, 454
  peripheral neuritis, 481

pimecrolimus, Elidel (*cont.*)
  post-herpetic neuralgia, 508
  pruritus, 518
  psoriatic arthritis, 527
  rheumatoid arthritis, 542
pinworm
  albendazole, Albenza, 488
  mebendazole, Emverm, Vermox, 488
  pyrantel pamoate, Antiminth, Pin-X, 488
  thiabendazole, Mintezol, 488
Pin-X, *pyrantel pamoate*
  hookworm, 304
  pinworm, 488
  roundworm, 557
  threadworm, 593
  trichinosis, 606
  whipworm, 656
pioglitazone, Actos
  type 2 diabetes mellitus, 621
pirbuterol, Maxair
  asthma, 40
pirfenidone, Esbriet
  idiopathic pulmonary fibrosis, 535
pitavastatin, Livalo, Nikita, Zypitamag
  dyslipidemia, 222
pitolisant, Wakix
  narcolepsy, 412–413
pityriasis alba, 488
  coal tar, Scytera, T/Gel (OTC), 488
pityriasis rosea, 488
plague
  moxifloxacin, Avelox (G), 489
  streptomycin (G), 489
  tetracycline (G), 489
Plan B One Step, *levonorgestrel,* 675
plantar wart
  acitretin, Soriatane, 655
  salicylic acid, Duo Film, Occlusal HP, Wart-Off (G), 655
  trichloroacetic acid, 655
Plaquenil, *hydroxychloroquine*
  malaria, 386
  rheumatoid arthritis, 546
  systemic lupus erythematosis, 585
Plavix, *clopidogrel*
  peripheral vascular disease, 482
plazomicin, Zemdri
  acute, complicated pyelonephritis (ACP), 537–538
  complicated urinary tract infection (cUTI), 641
plecanatide, Trulance
  chronic idiopathic constipation, 168
  irritable bowel syndrome with constipation (IBS-C), 366
Plegridy, *peginterferon beta-1a*
  multiple sclerosis (MS), 398–399
Plenvu, *polyethylene glycol 3350 with electrolytes*
  colonoscopy prep/colon cleanse, 160
pneumococcal 15-valent conjugate vaccine
  community acquired pneumonia, 493
pneumococcal pneumonia
  pneumococcal vaccine, Pneumovax, Pnu-Imune 23, Prevnar 13, 497
pneumococcal vaccine, Pneumovax, Pnu-Imune 23, Prevnar 13
  pneumococcal pneumonia, 497
Pneumocystis jiroveci pneumonia
  atovaquone, Mepron (G), 498
  trimethoprim+sulfamethoxazole (TMP-SMX), Bactrim, Septra, 498
pneumonia
  chlamydial pneumonia, 492
  community-acquired bacterial pneumonia (CABP), 492–495

community-acquired pneumonia (CAP), 492–495
hospital-acquired bacterial pneumonia (HABP), 489–490
legionella pneumonia, 496
mycoplasma, 496–497
pneumococcal, 497–498
Pneumocystis jirovecii, 498
ventilator associated bacterial pneumonia, 490–492
Pneumovax, *pneumococcal vaccine*
  pneumococcal pneumonia, 497
Pnu-Imune 23, *pneumococcal vaccine*
  pneumococcal pneumonia, 497
podofilox 0.5% cream, Condylox
  venereal wart, 655, 656
poliomyelitis/poliovirus, 498–499
  Pentacel, 498–499
  trivalent poliovirus vaccine, inactivated (type 1, 2, and 3), Ipol, 498
  Vaxelis, 499
polyangiitis
  rituximab, Rituxan, 499
  rituximab-arrx, Riabni, 499–500
polyarticular juvenile idiopathic arthritis (PJIA), 368–371
polycystic ovarian syndrome (PCOS), 500
polycythemia vera
  ropeginterferon-alfa-2b-njft, Besremi, 500–501
  ruxolitinib, Jakafi, 501
polyethylene glycol (PEG), GlycoLax Powder for Oral Solution, MiraLAX Powder for Oral Solution, Polyethylene Glycol 3350 Powder for Oral Solution, 160
  occasional constipation, 170
Polyethylene Glycol 3350 Powder for Oral Solution, *polyethylene glycol (PEG)*
  occasional constipation, 170
polyethylene glycol, Systane, Systane Balance, Systane Ultra
  dry eye syndrome, 217
polymyalgia rheumatica
  methotrexate (MTX), Rasuvo, Rheumatrex, Trexall, 502
  sarilumab, Kevzara, 502
polymyositis
  immune globulin intravenous (human), 502–503
Poly-Pred Ophthalmic Suspension, *neomycin sulfate+polymyxin b sulfate+prednisolone acetate ophthalmic suspension*
  bacterial conjunctivitis, 163
polymyositis
  immune globulin intravenous (human), 502–503
polyps, nasal
  beclomethasone dipropionate, Beconase, Qvar, Vancenase, QNASL Nasal Aerosol, 505
  budesonide, Rhinocort, 505
  ciclesonide, Omnaris, Zetonna, 505
  dexamethasone, Dexacort Turbinaire, 506
  flunisolide, Nasalide, Nasarel, 506
  fluticasone furoate, Veramyst, 506
  fluticasone propionate, Flonase (OTC)(G), Xhance 1, 506
  mometasone furoate monohydrate, Nasonex 24HR Allergy (OTC)(G), 506
  mometasone furoate, Nasonex (G), 506
  mometasone furoate, Sinuva Sinus Implant, 505

olopatadine, Patanase, 506
  triamcinolone acetonide, Nasacort Allergy 24HR (OTC), 506
Polysporin Ophthalmic Ointment, *polymyxin b sulfate+bacitracin*
  bacterial conjunctivitis, 163
Polysporin, *polymyxin b+bacitracin*
  blepharitis, 67
  stye (hordeolum), 580
polythiazide, Renese
  edema, 228
  heart failure, 281
  hypertension, 327
Polytrim, *trimethoprim+polymyxin b sulfate*
  bacterial conjunctivitis, 163
polyvinyl alcohol, Hypotears, Hypotears PF
  dry eye syndrome, 217
Ponstel, *mefenamic acid*
  dysmenorrhea: primary, 225
Portia, *ethinyl estradiol/levonorgestrel*
  estrogen and progesterone, 672
posaconazole, Noxafil (G)
  aspergillosis, 38
  oral (thrush) candidiasis, 135
  skin candidiasis, 136
  vulvovaginal (moniliasis) candidiasis, 138
post-anesthesia nausea/vomiting
  amisulpride, Barhemsys, 414
  ondansetron, Zofran, Zuplenz (G), 414
  palonosetron, Aloxi (G), 414
  promethazine, Phenergan (G), 414
postherpetic neuralgia (PHN)
  acetaminophen (G), 509
  amitriptyline (G), 507, 509
  amoxapine (G), 507, 509
  aspirin, Bayer (G), 509
  capsaicin 8% patch, Qutenza, 508
  decadron Phosphate with Xylocaine, *lidocaine+dexamethasone,* 509
  desipramine, Norpramin (G), 508, 509
  diclofenac sodium, Pennsaid, Solaraze Gel, Voltaren Gel, 508
  doxepin (G), 508, 510
  doxepin, Prudoxin, Zonalon (G), 508
  emla Cream, *lidocaine 2.5%+ prilocaine 2.5%,* 509
  gabapentin enacarbil, Horizant, 507
  gabapentin, Gralise, Neurontin (G), 507
  imipramine, Tofranil (G), 508, 510
  lidocaine, LidaMantle, Lidoderm, ZTlido lidocaine, 509
  nortriptyline, Pamelor, 508, 510
  pregabalin (GABA analog), Lyrica (V), 507, 508
  pimecrolimus, Elidel (G), 508
  protriptyline, Vivactil, 508, 510
  tramadol, Rybix ODT, Ryzolt, Ultram (IV), 509
  trimipramine, Surmontil, 508, 510
  trolamine salicylate, Mobisyl Creme, 508
  ultracet, *tramadol+acetaminophen* (G)(IV), 509
postmenopausal painful intercourse. *See dyspareunia*
posttransplant cytomegalovirus (CMV)
  cidofovir, Vistide, 185, 186
  maribavir, Livtencity, 185
  valganciclovir, Valcyte, 186
posttraumatic stress disorder (PTSD)
  amitriptyline (G), 512
  clonidine, Catapres, Kapvay, Nexiclon XR, 511
  desvenlafaxine, Pristiq (G), 511

doxepin (G), 512
imipramine, Tofranil (G), 512
mirtazapine, Remeron, Remeron SolTab (G), 512
nortriptyline, Pamelor (G), 512
olanzapine, Zyprexa, Zyprexa Zydis (G), 511
paroxetine maleate, Paxil (G), 510
paroxetine mesylate, Brisdelle (G), 510
phenelzine, Nardil (G), 512
prazosin, Minipress (G), 511
propranolol, Inderal, Inderal LA (G), 511
quetiapine fumarate, SeroQUEL, SeroQUEL XR, 511
risperidone, Risperdal, Risperdal Consta, Risperdal M-Tab (G), 511
selegiline, Emsamrdil, 512
sertraline, Zoloft, 511
trazodone, Oleptro (G), 512
venlafaxine, Effexor (G), 511–512
Potassium Chloride, *potassium*
hypokalemia, 344
potassium citrate, Urocit-K
urolithiasis, 646, 647
potassium, KCL Solution Oral soln, K-Dur, K-Lor for Oral Solution, Klor-Con, Klorvess, Klotrix, K-Lyte, K-Tab, Micro-K, Potassium Chloride
hypokalemia, 344
Poteligeo, *mogamulizumab*, 688
prabotulinumtoxinA-xvfs, Jeuveau
facial wrinkles, 660
pralsetinib, Gavreto
lung cancer, 103
Praluent, *alirocumab*
dyslipidemia, 221
pramipexole, Mirapex
Parkinson's disease, 469
pramipexole dihydrochloride, Mirapex (G)
restless legs syndrome, 540
pramlintide, Symlin
type 1 diabetes mellitus, 616
PramOtic, *chloroxylenol+pramoxine*
otitis externa, 444
Prandimet, *repaglinide+metformin* (G)
type 2 diabetes mellitus, 619
prasterone (dehydroepiandrosterone [DHEA]), Intrarosa
dyspareunia, 226
Pravachol, *pravastatin*
dyslipidemia, 222
hypertriglyceridemia, 339
pravastatin, Pravachol
dyslipidemia, 222
hypertriglyceridemia, 339
praziquantel, Biltricide
liver flukes, 380
schistosomiasis, 560–561
tapeworm, 585
threadworm, 593
prazosin, Minipres
hypertension, 335
post-traumatic stress disorder, 511
urinary overactive bladder, 356
Pred Forte, Pred Mild, *prednisolone acetate* (G)
allergic (vernal) conjunctivitis, 166
iritis: acute, 364
Pred-G Ophthalmic Ointment, Pred-G Ophthalmic Suspension, *gentamicin sulfate+prednisolone acetate*
bacterial conjunctivitis, 163
prednicarbate, Dermatop, 677
prednisolone acetate, Econopred, Econopred Plus, Pred Forte, Pred Mild

allergic (vernal) conjunctivitis, 166
prednisolone sodium phosphate, Inflamase Forte, Inflamase Mild
allergic (vernal) conjunctivitis, 166
prednisone (G), 679
Bell's palsy, 51
mononucleosis (MONO), 396
pemphigus vulgaris, 476
sunburn, 580
tinea capitis, 597
prednisone acetate, Pred Forte
iritis: acute, 364
pregabalin (GABA analog), Lyrica, Lyrica CR (G)(V)
diabetic peripheral neuropathy (DPN), 210
fibromyalgia, 244
peripheral neuritis, 480
postherpetic neuralgia (PHN), 507, 508
pregnancy
doxyalamine succinate+pyridoxine, Diclegis (G), 514
promethazine, Phenergan (G), 514
Pregnyl, *human chorionic gonadotropin*
amenorrhea, secondary, 18
Premarin, *estrogen+progesterone*
amenorrhea, secondary, 17
atrophic vaginitis, 49
premenstrual dysphoric disorder (PMDD)
ethinyl estradiol+drospirenone plus levomefolate calcium, Beyaz, Rajani (G), 514
fluoxetine, Prozac, Prozac Weekly, Sarafem (G), 514–515
nortriptyline, Pamelor (G), 515
paroxetine maleate, Paxil, Paxil CR, Paxil Suspension (G), 515
paroxetine mesylate, Brisdelle (G), 515
sertraline, Zoloft, 515
spironolactone, Aldactone (G), 514
Yaz, *ethinyl estradiol+drospirenone*, 514
Premphase, *estrogen, conjugated+medroxyprogesterone*
menopause, 391
Prempro, *estrogen, conjugated+medroxyprogesterone*
menopause, 391
Preparation H Ointment, *petrolatum+mineral oil+shark liver oil+phenylephrine* (OTC)(G)
hemorrhoids, 289
Preparation H Suppositories, *phenylephrine+cocoa butter+shark liver oil* (OTC)(G)
hemorrhoids, 289
Prepopik, *sodium picosulfate+magnesium oxide+citric acid*
colonoscopy prep/colon cleanse, 160
presbyopia
pilocarpine hydrochloride, Vuity, 515–516
pressure ulcer
becaplermin, Regranex, 634
Granulex, *trypsin+balsam peru+castor oil*, 633
Prestalia, *amlodipine+perindopril*
hypertension, 335
Prevacid, *lansoprazole* (G)
peptic ulcer disease (PUD), 478
Zollinger-Ellison syndrome, 662
Prevalite, *cholestyramine*
cholelithiasis, 153
primary biliary cholangitis (PBC), 152–153
Preven, *ethinyl estradiol+levonorgestrel*, 675
Preventeza, *levonorgestrel*, 675

Previfem, *ethinyl estradiol+norgestimate*
estrogen and progesterone, 672
Prevnar 13, *pneumococcal vaccine*
pneumococcal pneumonia, 497
PrevPac (G)
Helicobacter pylori (H. pylori) infection, 284
Prevymis, *letermovir*
cytomegalovirus (CMV) retinitis, 187
Prezcobix, *darunavir+cobicistat*
human immunodeficiency virus infection, 316
Priftin, *rifapentine*
tuberculosis, 610
Prilosec, *omeprazole* (OTC)(G)
gastroesophageal reflux disease, 250–251
peptic ulcer disease (PUD), 478–479
Zollinger-Ellison syndrome, 662
primary biliary cholangitis (PBC)
cholestyramine, Prevalite, 152–153
colesevelam, WelChol (G), 153
colestipol, Colestid, Flavored Colestid (G), 153
obeticholic acid, Ocaliva, 152
ursodeoxycholic acid (UDCA), Ursofalk (G), 152
primary humoral immunodeficiency (PHI)
immune globulin subcutaneous [human] 20% liquid, Hizentra, 349–350
Primatene MIST Pump inhal, *epinephrine inhalation aerosol*
asthma, 38
Primsol, *trimethoprim*
urinary tract infection, 645
Principen, *ampicillin*, 619
acute exacerbation of chronic bronchitis, 69
bacterial endocarditis prophylaxis, 55
otitis media: acute, 446
Prinivil, *lisinopril*
heart failure, 279
Prinzide, Zestoretic, *lisinopril+hydrochlorothiazide*
hypertension, 333
Pristiq, *desvenlafaxine* (G)
anxiety disorder, 36
major depressive disorder, 192
panic disorder, 465
post-traumatic stress disorder, 511
Proair HFA Inhaler, Proair RespiClick, *albuterol sulfate*
asthma, 39
ProAmatine, *midodrine*
neurogenic hypotension, 345
Pro-Banthine, *propantheline*
interstitial cystitis, 362
urinary overactive bladder, 355
probenecid, Benemid (G)
gonorrhea, 259
gout (hyperuricemia), 260
pelvic inflammatory disease, 476
syphilis, 582
Procanbid, *procainamide*, 681
Procardia, Procardia XL, *nifedipine*
angina pectoris: stable, 28
prochlorperazine, Compazine
anxiety disorder, 35
cannabinoid hyperemesis syndrome, 139
chemotherapy-induced nausea/vomiting, 147
motion sickness, 396
opioid-induced nausea/vomiting, 430
panic disorder, 466
Procort, *hydrocortisone+pramoxine*
hemorrhoids, 289

Procrit, *epoetin alpha*
anemia of chronic kidney disease, 23
proctitis: acute
  ceftriaxone, Rocephin (G), 516
  doxycycline, Acticlate, Adoxa, Doryx, Doxteric, Monodox, Oracea, Vibramycin, Vibra-Tab, 516
Proctocort, *hydrocortisone*
  hemorrhoids, 289
  ulcerative colitis (UC), 634
Proctocream, *hydrocortisone*
  hemorrhoids, 289
procyclidine, Kemadrin
  Parkinson's disease, 471
Prodium, *phenazopyridine*
  interstitial cystitis, 361, 362
  pyelonephritis: acute, 536
  urinary tract infection, 642
progesterone, micronized,
  Prometrium (G)
  amenorrhea, secondary, 18
  menopause, 392
Proglycem, *diazoxide* (G)
  type 1 diabetes mellitus (T1DM), 614
Proloprim, *trimethoprim*
  urinary tract infection, 645
promethazine, Phenergan (G)
  cannabinoid hyperemesis syndrome (CHS), 139
  chemotherapy-induced nausea/vomiting, 147
  gastritis-related nausea/vomiting, 248
  labyrinthitis, 375
  Meniere's disease, 388
  motion sickness, 396
  post-anesthesia nausea/vomiting, 414
  pregnancy, 514
Prometra II Programmable Pump
  spasticity of cerebral or spinal origin, 577
Prometrium, *progesterone, micronized*
  amenorrhea, secondary, 18
  menopause, 392
propantheline, Pro-Banthine
  interstitial cystitis, 362
  urinary overactive bladder, 355
Propecia, *finasteride*
  baldness: male pattern, 57
propoxyphene napsylate+acetaminophen,
  Balacet (IV)
  pain, 460
propranolol, Inderal, Inderal LA, InnoPran XL
  angina pectoris: stable, 29
  benign essential tremor, 58
  dose form(s), 681
  hypertension, 326
  hyperthyroidism, 338
  migraine and cluster headache, 275
  mitral valve prolapse (MVP), 396
  post-traumatic stress disorder, 511
propylthiouracil (ptu), Propyl-Thyracil
  hyperthyroidism, 338
Propyl-Thyracil, *propylthiouracil (ptu)*
  hyperthyroidism, 338
ProQuin XR, *ciprofloxacin*
  acute prostatitis, 516
  anthrax (bacillus anthracis), 31, 32
  chancroid, 147
  cholera (*Vibrio cholerae)*, 155, 156
  chronic prostatitis, 517
  cystic fibrosis (CF), 184
  dose forms, 708
  granuloma inguinale (donovanosis), 266
  human bite, 66–67
  diverticulitis, 215
  pyelonephritis: acute, 536
  salmonellosis, 559

Traveler's diarrhea, 213
typhoid fever, 633
Proscar, *finasteride*
  benign prostatic hyperplasia , 58
  urinary overactive bladder, 356
ProSom, *estazolam* (IV)
  insomnia, 359
prostate cancer
  abiraterone acetate, Yonsa, Zytiga, 128–129
  apalutamide, Erleada, 129
  cabazitaxel, Jevtana (G), 130
  darolutamide, Nubeqa, 129
  degarelix acetate, Firmagon (G), 127
  leuprolide mesylate, Camcevi, 128
  niraparib tosylate, Zejula, 129
  relugolix, Orgovyx, 128
  rucaparib, Rubraca, 130
Protonix, *pantoprazole*
  peptic ulcer disease (PUD), 479
protriptyline, Vivactil
  anxiety disorder, 34
  diabetic peripheral neuropathy (DPN), 210
  irritable bowel syndrome with diarrhea, 368
  major depressive disorder, 193
  nocturnal enuresis, 235
  post-herpetic neuralgia, 508, 510
  trigeminal neuralgia, 609
Proventil HFA Inhaler, Proventil Inhalation Solution, *albuterol sulfate*
  asthma, 39
Provera, *estrogen+progesterone*
  amenorrhea, secondary, 17
Provera, *medroxyprogesterone*
  amenorrhea, secondary, 18
  dysfunctional uterine bleeding, 220
  endometriosis, 232
  uterine leiomyomata, 650
Provigil, *modafinil* (IV)
  narcolepsy, 410
  obstructive sleep apnea, 575
  sleepiness, 575
Prozac, Prozac Weekly, *fluoxetine* (G)
  anxiety disorder, 35
  bulimia nervosa, 75
  major depressive disorder, 192
  migraine and cluster headache, 276
  obsessive-compulsive disorder, 421
  panic disorder, 464
  premenstrual dysphoric disorder, 514
  trichotillomania, 607
prucalopride, Motegrity
  chronic idiopathic constipation, 169
Prudoxin, *doxepin* (G)
  atopic dermatitis, 199
  diabetic peripheral neuropathy (DPN), 209
  gouty arthritis, 262
  hemorrhoids, 290
  juvenile idiopathic arthritis, 369
  osteoarthritis, 434
  peripheral neuritis, 480–481
  post-herpetic neuralgia, 508
  pruritus, 518
  psoriatic arthritis, 527
  rheumatoid arthritis, 542
pruritus
  capsaicin 8% patch, Qutenza, 517
  capsaicin, Axsain, Capsin, Capzasin-HP, Capzasin-P, Dolorac, Double Cap (OTC), R-Gel, Zostrix, Zostrix HP (G), 517
  diclofenac sodium, Pennsaid, Solaraze Gel, Voltaren Gel, 518
  doxepin, Prudoxin, Zonalon, 518

fluocinolone acetonide, Derma-Smoothe/FS Topical Oil, 517
pimecrolimus, Elidel, 518
trolamine salicylate, Mobisyl Creme, 518
pseudobulbar affect (PBA) disorder
  dextromethorphan+quinidine, Nuedexta (G), 518
pseudogout, 518
pseudomembranous colitis
  metronidazole, Flagyl, Flagyl 375, Flagyl ER (G), 519
  vancomycin hcl capsule, Vancocin (G), 519
  vancomycin hcl oral solution, Firvanq, 519
psittacosis
  tetracycline, Achromycin V, Sumycin, 519
psoriasis
  acitretin, Soriatane (G), 521
  adalimumab-aacf, Idacio, 525
  adalimumab, Humira, 525
  adalimumab-adaz, Hyrimoz, 525
  adalimumab-adbm, Cyltezo, 525
  adalimumab-afzb, Abrilada, 525
  adalimumab-bwwd, Hadlima, 525
  alefacept, Amevive, 521
  anhydrous calcipotriene+betamethasone dipropionate, Wynzora, 519–520
  anthralin, Zithranol-RR, 521
  brodalumab, Siliq, 522
  calcipotriene, Dovonex, Sorilux Foam, 519
  calcipotriene+betamethasone dipropionate, Enstilar, Taclonex (G), 520
  calcitriol, Vectical, 520
  clobetasol propionate, Impoyz, 520–521
  coal tar, Scytera, T/Gel, 521
  cyclosporine (immunosuppressant), Neoral, 521
  etanercept, Enbrel, 525
  golimumab, Simponi, 525
  guselkumab, Tremfya, 525
  halobetasol propionate, Bryhali (G), 521
  halobetasol propionate+tazarotene, Duobrii, 521
  ildrakizumab-asmn, Ilumya, 524
  infliximab, Remicade, 526
  infliximab-abda, Renflexis, 526
  infliximab-axxq, Avsola, 526
  infliximab-dyyb, Inflectra, 526
  infliximab-qbtx, Ifixi, 526
  ixekizumab, Taltz, 522
  risankizumab-rzaa, Skyrizi, 523–524
  roflumilast, Zoryve, 522
  secukinumab, Cosentyx, 522–523
  spesolimab-sbzo, Spevigo (G), 524–525
  tazarotene, Avage, Tazorac (G), 521
  tildrakizumab-asmn, Ilumya, 524
  ustekinumab, Stelara, 524
psoriatic arthritis
  abatacept, Orencia, 531
  adalimumab-aacf, Idacio, 529
  adalimumab-adaz, Hyrimoz, 529
  adalimumab-adbm, Cyltezo, 529
  adalimumab-afzb, Abrilada, 530
  adalimumab-bwwd, Hadlima, 530
  adalimumab, Humira, 529
  apremilast, Otezla (G), 528
  capsaicin 8% patch, Qutenza, 527
  capsaicin, Axsain, Capsin, Capzasin-HP, Capzasin-P, Dolorac, Double Cap (OTC), R-Gel, Zostrix, Zostrix HP (G), 527

celecoxib, Celebrex (G), 528
diclofenac, Zorvolex, 527
diclofenac sodium, Pennsaid, Solaraze
  Gel, Voltaren, Voltaren Gel,
  Voltaren XR, 527
doxepin, Prudoxin, Zonalon, 527
esomeprazole+naproxen (G), Vimovo,
  528
etanercept, Enbrel, 530
etanercept-ykro, Eticovo, 530
golimumab, Simponi, 530
guselkumab, Tremfya, 528
indomethacin, 527
infliximab, Remicade, 530
infliximab-abda, Renflexis, 530
infliximab-axxq, Avsola, 530
infliximab-dyyb, Inflectra, 530
infliximab-qbtx, Ifixi, 530
meloxicam, Mobic, Vivlodex (G), 528
pimecrolimus, Elidel, 527
risankizumab-rzaa, Skyrizi, 528–529
rituximab, Rituxan, 531
trolamine salicylate, Mobisyl Creme,
  527
ustekinumab, Stelara, 529
vimovo, esomeprazole+naproxen (G),
  528
psyllium, Konsyl, Metamucil (OTC)
  occasional constipation, 169
Pulmicort Flexhaler, Pulmicort Respules,
  budesonide
  asthma, 40
pulmonary arterial hypertension (PAH)
  ambrisentan, Letairis (G), 533
  bosentan, Tracleer (G), 532
  macitentan, Opsumit (G), 532–533
  riociguat, Adempas, 533–534
  selexipag, Uptravi (G), 533
  sildenafil citrate, Revatio (G), 534
  tadalafil, Adcirca (G), 534
  treprostinil, Orenitram, 534
Pulse Pack, *itraconazole*
  onychomycosis (fungal nail), 422
pupillary dilation (mydriasis): short-term
  tropicamide+phenylephrine
    hydrochloride, Mydcombi, 531,
    536
purified protein derivative (PPD), Aplisol,
  Tubersol
  tuberculosis, 609
pyelonephritis: acute
  cephalexin, Keflex (G), 536
  ciprofloxacin, Cipro (G), Cipro XR,
    ProQuin XR, 536
  levofloxacin, Levaquin, 536
  loracarbef, Lorabid, 536
  phenazopyridine, AZO Standard,
    Prodium, Uristat, 536
  trimethoprim+sulfamethoxazole
    (TMP-SMX), Bactrim, Septra,
    536
Pylera
  Helicobacter pylori (H. pylori)
    infection, 284
pyrantel pamoate, Antiminth, Pin-X
  dose forms, 704
  hookworm, 305
  pinworm, 557
  roundworm, 557
  threadworm, 593
  trichinosis, 606
  whipworm, 657
pyrazinamide (PZA)
  dose forms, 705
  tuberculosis, 610
pyelonephritis: acute, complicated
  (ACP), 536–538
pyrethrins with piperonyl butoxide,
  A-200, Rid

pediculosis humanus capitis, 475
pyrimethamine (G), Daraprim
  toxoplasmosis, 605
Pyrukynd, *mitapivat*
  hemolytic/anemia, 24–25

Qalsody, *tofersen*
  amyotrophic lateral sclerosis (ALS),
    19–20
Qbrelis Oral Solution, lisinopril
  heart failure, 329
Qbrexza, *glycopyrronium*
  hyperhidrosis, 320
Qelbree, *viloxazine*
  attention deficit hyperactivity disorder
    (ADHD), 50
Qinlock, *ripretinib*
  gastrointestinal stromal tumor (GIST),
    91
QNASL Nasal Aerosol, *beclomethasone*
  dipropionate
  allergic rhinitis/sinusitis, 551
Qsymia, *phentermine+topiramate ext-rel*
  (IV)
  obesity, 419–420
Qtern, *dapagliflozin+saxagliptin*
  type 2 diabetes mellitus, 628
Qternmet XL, *dapagliflozin+*
  saxagliptin+metformin
  type 2 diabetes mellitus (T2DM),
    628–630
Quadrinal, *theophylline+potassium*
  iodide+ephedrine+phenobarbital
  (II)
  emphysema, 232
quadrivalent inactivated infl uenza
  subvirion vaccine, types a and b,
  Fluad, Fluarix Quadrivalent
  influenza, seasonal (FLU), 356
Qualaquin, *quinine sulfate*
  leg cramps, 376
  malaria, 386
  systemic lupus erythematosis, 585
Quartette, *ethinyl estradiol+levonorgestrel*
  (G), 673
Quasense, *ethinyl estradiol+levonorgestrel*
  (G), 674
Questran, *cholestyramine*
  dyslipidemia, 223–224
quetiapine fumarate, SeroQUEL,
  SeroQUEL XR
  bipolar disorder, 63–64
  delirium, 188
  dementia, 188–189
  methamphetamine-induced
    psychosis, 395
  post-traumatic stress disorder, 511
QuilliChew ER, *methylphenidate*
  (long-acting)(II)
  attention deficit hyperactivity disorder
    (ADHD), 53
Quillivant XR, *methylphenidate*
  (long-acting)(II)
  attention deficit hyperactivity disorder
    (ADHD), 53
Quinaglute, *quinidine gluconate,* 681
quinapril, Accupril
  heart failure, 280
  hypertension, 330
Quinidex, *quinidine sulfate,* 681
quinine sulfate, Qualaquin
  leg cramps, 376
  malaria, 386
  systemic lupus erythematosis, 585
Quixin Ophthalmic Solution,
  levofloxacin
  bacterial conjunctivitis, 162
Qutenza, *capsaicin 8% patch*
  atopic dermatitis, 199

diabetic peripheral neuropathy, 208
  gouty arthritis, 262
  hemorrhoids, 289
  juvenile idiopathic arthritis, 369
  juvenile rheumatoid arthritis, 372
  muscle strain, 404
  osteoarthritis, 434
  pain, 453
  peripheral neuritis, 480
  post-herpetic neuralgia, 508
  pruritus, 517
  psoriatic arthritis, 527
  rheumatoid arthritis, 542
Quviviq, *daridorexant*
  insomnia, 360
Quzyttir, *cetirizine*
  urticaria, 650
Qvar, *beclomethasone dipropionate*
  asthma, 40
QWO, *collagenase clostridium*
  histolyticum-aaes
  cellulite, 141–142

RabAvert, *rabies vaccine, human diploid*
  cell [HDVC]
  rabies, 538
rabeprazole, AcipHex (OTC)(G)
  gastroesophageal reflux (GER), 251
  peptic ulcer disease (PUD), 479
  Zollinger-Ellison syndrome, 662
rabies
  rabies immune globulin, human
    (HRIG), BayRab, KamRAB,
    Imogam Rabies HT, HyperRAB
    S/D, 538–539
  rabies vaccine, human diploid cell
    [HDVC], Imovax, RabAvert, 538
rabies immune globulin, human (HRIG),
  BayRab, KamRAB, Imogam
  Rabies HT, HyperRAB S/D
  rabies, 538–539
rabies vaccine, human diploid cell
  [HDVC], Imovax, RabAvert
  rabies, 538
racepinephrine, Asthmanefrin
  asthma, 39
Radicava, *edaravone*
  amyotrophic lateral sclerosis (ALS),
    18–19
Ragwitek, *short ragweed pollen allergen*
  extract
  allergic rhinitis/sinusitis, 551
Rajani, *ethinyl estradiol+drospirenone*
  plus levomefolate calcium
  estrogen and progesterone, 672
  premenstrual dysphoric disorder,
    514
raloxifene, Evista
  osteoporosis, 442
raltegravir (as potassium), Isentress, 697
  human immunodeficiency virus
    infection, 308, 311–312
ramelteon, Rozerem (IV)
  insomnia, 359
ramipril, Altace
  heart failure, 280
  hypertension, 330
Ranexa, *ranolazine*
  angina pectoris: stable, 30
ranibizumab, Lucentis
  diabetic retinopathy, 206
ranitidine bismuth citrate, Tritec
  gastroesophageal reflux disease, 250
  peptic ulcer disease (PUD), 478
ranitidine, Zantac
  gastroesophageal reflux disease, 250
  peptic ulcer disease (PUD), 478
ranolazine, Ranexa
  angina pectoris: stable, 30

Rapaflo, *silodosin*
  benign prostatic hyperplasia, 58
  urinary overactive bladder, 356
Rapamune, *serolimus*
  organ transplant rejection prophylaxis,
    432–433
Rapivab, *peramivir*
  influenza, seasonal (FLU), 357
rasagiline, Azilect
  Parkinson's disease, 470
Rasuvo, *methotrexate*
  juvenile idiopathic arthritis, 370
  polymyalgia rheumatica, 502
  rheumatoid arthritis, 546
  systemic lupus erythematosis, 584
ravulizumab-cwvz, Ultomiris
  paroxysmal nocturnal
    hemoglobinuria, 474
raxibacumab
  anthrax (bacillus anthracis), 31
Rayaldee, *calcifediol*
  hyperparathyroidism (HPT), 323
Razadyne, *galantamine*
  Alzheimer's disease, 15
Rebetol, *ribavirin*
  hepatitis C (HCV), 294
Reblozyl, *luspatercept-aamt*
  beta thalassemia-associated anemia,
    21–22
Rebyota, *fecal microbiota, live-jslm*
  clostridioides difficile infection (CDI),
    157–158
Recarbrio, *imipenem+cilastatin+*
    relebactam
  complicated intra-abdominal
    infection (cIAI), 363
  hospital-acquired bacterial
    pneumonia (HABP), 489–490
  ventilator-associated bacterial
    pneumonia (VABP), 491
Reclast, *zoledronic acid*
  Paget's disease, 450
Reclipsen, *ethinyl estradiol+*
    norethindrone plus ferrous
    fumarate
  estrogen and progesterone, 672
Recombivax HB, *hepatitis B recombinant*
    vaccine
  hepatitis B, 292
Recorlev, *levoketoconazole*
  cushing's syndrome, 180–181
Refresh Eye Itch Relief, *ketotifen*
    fumarate
  allergic (vernal) conjunctivitis, 167
Regranex, *becaplermin*
  diabetic ulcer, 633
  pressure ulcer, 633
Relagard, *acetic acid+oxyquinolone*
  vulvovaginal (moniliasis) candidiasis,
    136
Relenza Inhaler, *zanamivir*
  influenza, seasonal (FLU), 357
Relistor, *methylnaltrexone bromide*
  opioid-induced constipation (OIC),
    428–429
relugolix, Orgovyx
  prostate cancer, 128
Relyvrio, *sodium phenylbutyrate+*
    taurursodiol
  amyotrophic lateral sclerosis (ALS), 18
remdesivir, Veklury
  COVID-19 (coronavirus), 172
Remeron, *mirtazapine*
  major depressive disorder, 194
  post-traumatic stress disorder, 512
Remicade, *infliximab*
  Crohn's disease, 117
  osteoarthritis, 438
  psoriasis, 526

psoriatic arthritis, 530
rheumatoid arthritis, 547–548
ulcerative colitis, 637
Renagel, *sevelamer*
  hyperphosphatemia, 325
renal cell carcinoma (RCC)
  avelumab, Bavencio, 95
  bevacizumab-adcd, Vegzelma, 94
  pembrolizumab, Keytruda, 95
  selpercatinib, Retevmo, 95
  sorafenib, Nexavar (G), 93
  sunitinib malate, Sutent, 93–94
Renese, *polythiazide*
  edema, 228
  heart failure, 281
  hypertension, 327
Renflexis, *infliximab-abda*
  Crohn's disease, 177
  osteoarthritis, 439
  psoriasis, 526
  psoriatic arthritis, 530
  rheumatoid arthritis, 548
  ulcerative colitis, 637
Renova, *tretinoin* (G)
  facial wrinkles, 660
  folliculitis barbae, 247
  hyperpigmentation, 325
  lentigines, 379
  vitiligo, 653
Renvela, *sevelamer*
  hyperphosphatemia, 325
repaglinide, Prandin
  type 2 diabetes mellitus, 621
Repatha, *evolocumab*
  dyslipidemia, 221
Reprexain, *hydrocodone+ibuprofen* (II)
  pain, 456
Requip, *ropinirole*
  Parkinson's disease, 469
  restless legs syndrome, 540
reslizumab, Cinqair
  asthma, 48
  eosinophilia, 48
respiratory syncytial virus (RSV)
  MVA-BN RSV vaccine, 539
  palivizumab, Synagis, 539
  respiratory syncytial virus vaccine,
    Abrysvo, 539
  respiratory syncytial virus vaccine,
    adjuvanted, Arexvy, 539–540
  respiratory syncytial virus vaccine,
    Abrysvo
  respiratory syncytial virus (RSV),
    539
restless legs syndrome (RLS)
  gabapentin enacarbil, Horizant, 540
  gabapentin, Gralise, Neurontin, 540
  pramipexole dihydrochloride,
    Mirapex, 540
  pregabalin (GABA analog), Lyrica (V),
    540
  ropinirole, Requip, 540
  rotigotine transdermal patch, Neupro,
    540
Restoril, *temazepam* (IV)(G)
  insomnia, 359
Retacrit, *epoetin alfa-epbx*
  anemia of chronic kidney disease, 23
Retevmo, *selpercatinib*
  renal cell carcinoma (RCC), 95
  thyroid cancer, 595–596
  thyroid carcinoma, 131–132
retifanlimab-dlwr, Zynyz
  merkel cell carcinoma, 119
Retin-A, *tretinoin*
  acne vulgaris, 6
  facial wrinkles, 660
  folliculitis barbae, 247
  hyperpigmentation, 325

lentigines, 379
vitiligo, 653
Rett syndrome
  trofinetide, Daybue, 541
Revatio, *sildenafil citrate*
  pulmonary arterial hypertension
    (PAH), 534
revefenacin inhalation solution, Yupelri
  chronic obstructive pulmonary
    disease, 72
  emphysema, 231
Revex, *nalmefene*
  opioid overdose, 430–431
Revlimid, *lenalidomide* (G), 688
  multiple myeloma, 121–122
Rexulti, *brexpiprazole*
  alzheimer's disease, 15–17
  major depressive disorder, 194–195
  schizophrenia, 563–564
R-Gel, *capsaicin* (G)
  atopic dermatitis, 199
  diabetic peripheral neuropathy
    (DPN), 208
  gouty arthritis, 261–262
  juvenile idiopathic arthritis, 369
  juvenile rheumatoid arthritis, 372
  muscle strain, 404
  osteoarthritis, 434
  pain, 453
  peripheral neuritis, 480
  pruritus, 517
  psoriatic arthritis, 527
  rheumatoid arthritis, 541
rheumatoid arthritis (RA)
  abatacept, Orencia, 549
  adalimumab, Humira, 546–547
  adalimumab-aacf, Idacio, 547
  adalimumab-adbm, Cyltezo, 547
  adalimumab-afzb, Abrilada, 547
  adalimumab-bwwd, Hadlima, 547
  anakinra (interleukin-1 receptor
    antagonist), Kineret, 548
  auranofin (gold salt), Ridaura, 546
  azathioprine, Azasan, Imuran, 546
  baricitinib, Olumiant, 544
  capsaicin, Axsain, Capsin,
    Capzasin-HP, Capzasin-P,
    Dolorac, Double Cap (OTC),
    R-Gel, Zostrix, Zostrix HP (G),
    541
  capsaicin 8%, Qutenza, 542
  celecoxib, Celebrex (G), 544
  certolizumab pegol, Cimzia, 547
  cyclosporine (immunosuppressant),
    Neoral, 546
  diclofenac sodium, Pennsaid, Solaraze
    Gel, Voltaren Gel (G), 542
  doxepin, Prudoxin, Zonalon, 542
  Duexis, *ibuprofen+famotidine*,
    543–544
  etanercept, Enbrel, 547
  etanercept-ykro, Eticovo, 547
  golimumab, Simponi, 547
  hydroxychloroquine, Plaquenil, 546
  infliximab, Remicade, 547–548
  infliximab-abda, Renflexis, 548
  infliximab-axxq, Avsola, 548
  infliximab-dyyb, Inflectra, 548
  infliximab-qbtx, Ixifi, 548
  indomethacin, 542
  leflunomide, Arava (G), 546
  meloxicam, Mobic, Vivlodex (G), 544
  methotrexate, Rasuvo, Rheumatrex,
    Trexall, 546
  penicillamine, Cuprimine, Depen, 546
  pimecrolimus, Elidel, 542
  rituximab, Rituxan, 549
  sarilumab, Kevzara, 548
  sodium hyaluronate, Hyalgan, 549

sulfasalazine, Azulfidine, Azulfidine
EN, 546
tocilizumab, Actemra, 548–549
tofacitinib, Xeljanz, 544–545
trolamine salicylate, Mobisyl Creme,
542
upadacitinib, Rinvoq, 545
Vimovo, *naproxen+esomeprazole
magnesium* (G), 542–543
Rheumatrex, *methotrexate*
juvenile idiopathic arthritis, 370
juvenile rheumatoid arthritis, 373
polymyalgia rheumatica, 502
rheumatoid arthritis, 546
systemic lupus erythematosis, 584
rhinitis medicamentosa
azelastine, Astelin, 555
cetirizine, Children's Zyrtec Chewable,
Children's Zyrtec Allergy Syrup,
Zyrtec (OTC)(G), 555
desloratadine, Clarinex, Desloratadine
ODT, 555
diphenhydramine, Benadryl (G), 555
fexofenadine, Allegra (OTC)(G), 555
hydroxyzine, Atarax, Vistaril, 555
ipratropium bromide, Atrovent Nasal
Spray (G), 554
levocetirizine, Children's Xyzal Allergy
24HR, Xyzal Allergy 24HR
(OTC)(G), 555
loratadine, Claritin (OTC)(G), 555
rhinitis: vasomotor
ipratropium bromide, Atrovent Nasal
Spray (G), 556
Rhinocort, *budesonide*
allergic rhinitis/sinusitis, 552
Rhofade, *oxymetazoline hcl*
acne rosacea, 2
Riabni, *rituximab-arrx*
granulomatosis, 265
polyangiitis, 499–500
Ribasphere RibaPak, *ribavirin*
hepatitis C (HCV), 294
ribavirin, Copegus, Rebetol, Ribasphere
RibaPak, Virazole
hepatitis C (HCV), 294
rickets, 345
Rid, *pyrethrins with piperonyl butoxide*
pediculosis humanus capitis, 475
Ridaura, *auranofin (gold salt)*
rheumatoid arthritis, 546
systemic lupus erythematosis, 583
Rifabutin, *rilpivirine*
tuberculosis, 495
Rifadin, *rifampin (RIF)*
tuberculosis, 610
Rifamate, *rifampin+isoniazid*
tuberculosis, 610
rifampin (RIF), Rifadin, Rimactane
Hansen's disease, 296
tuberculosis, 610
rifamycin, Aemcolo
Traveler's diarrhea, 213–214
rifapentine, Priftin, 610
tuberculosis, 610
Rifater, *rifampin+isoniazid+
pyrazinamide*
tuberculosis, 610
rifaximin, Xifaxan
Traveler's diarrhea, 214
rilpivirine, Edurant, Rifabutin, 697
human immunodeficiency virus
infection, 310
tuberculosis, 610
riluzole, Exservan
amyotrophic lateral sclerosis (ALS),
19
Rimactane, *rifampin (RIF)*
tuberculosis, 610

rimantadine, Flumadine, 705
rimexolone, Vexol
allergic (vernal) conjunctivitis, 166
Rinvoq Extended-Release Tablets,
upadacitinib
Crohn's disease, 179
Rinvoq, *upadacitinib*
rheumatoid arthritis (RA), 545
riociguat, Adempas
pulmonary arterial hypertension
(PAH), 533–534
ripretinib, Qinlock
gastrointestinal stromal tumor (GIST),
91
risankizumab-rzaa, Skyrizi
crohn's disease, 178
psoriasis, 523–524
risankizumab-rzaa, Skyrizi
psoriatic arthritis, 528–529
risdiplam, Evrysdi
spinal muscular atrophy (SMA), 578
risedronate (as sodium), Actonel, Atelvia
osteoporosis, 442
Paget's disease, 450
Risperdal, Risperdal Consta, Risperdal
M-Tab, *risperidone*
bipolar disorder, 63
delirium, 188
dementia, 189
methamphetamine-induced
psychosis, 396
post-traumatic stress disorder, 511
risperidone, Risperdal, Risperdal Consta,
Risperdal M-Tab
bipolar disorder, 63
delirium, 188
dementia, 189
dose forms, 694
methamphetamine-induced
psychosis, 396
post-traumatic stress disorder, 511
Ritalin LA, Ritalin SR *methylphenidate
(long-acting)* (II)
narcolepsy, 412
Ritalin, *methylphenidate (long-acting)*(II)
attention deficit hyperactivity disorder
(ADHD), 52
narcolepsy, 412
Ritalin, *methylphenidate (regular-acting)*
(II)
attention deficit hyperactivity disorder
(ADHD), 52
narcolepsy, 412
ritonavir, Norvir (G)
human immunodeficiency virus
(HIV) infection, 312
Rituxan, *rituximab*
acquired autoimmune thrombotic
thrombocytopenia purpura, 595
granulomatosis, 265
pemphigus vulgaris, 477
polyangiitis, 499
psoriatic arthritis, 531
rheumatoid arthritis, 549
systemic lupus erythematosis, 582
rituximab-arrx, Riabni
leukemia, 98
lymphoma, 113
polyangiitis, 499–500
rituximab, Rituxan
acquired autoimmune thrombotic
thrombocytopenia purpura, 595
granulomatosis, 265
leukemia, 98
lymphoma, 111–112
pemphigus vulgaris, 477
polyangiitis, 499
psoriatic arthritis, 531
rheumatoid arthritis, 549

systemic lupus erythematosis, 582
rivastigmine, Exelon
Alzheimer's disease, 15
river blindness
moxidectin (G), 556
RiVive Nasal Spray (OTC)
opioid overdose/opioid reversal, 431
rizatriptan, Maxalt, Maxalt-MLT
migraine and cluster headache, 270
Robaxin, *methocarbamol*
tetanus, 592–593
Robinul, *glycopyrrolate*
peptic ulcer disease (PUD), 479
Robinul, Robinul Forte (G)
peptic ulcer disease (PUD), 479
Rocaltrol, *calcitriol*
hypocalcemia, 340
hypoparathyroidism, 344
Rocephin, *ceftriaxone* (G)
acute exacerbation of chronic
bronchitis, 70
bacterial endocarditis prophylaxis, 55
bacterial skin infection, 574
cellulitis, 143
chancroid, 147
community acquired pneumonia, 493
dose forms, 706
epididymitis, 237
gonococcal conjunctivitis, 165
gonococcal ophthalmia neonatorum,
423
gonococcal pharyngitis, 483
gonorrhea, 259
mastitis (breast abscess), 387
otitis media: acute, 446
pelvic inflammatory disease, 476
proctitis: acute, 516
sexual assault, 567
typhoid fever, 633
Rocklatan, *netarsudil+latanoprost*
glaucoma, 257
rocky mountain spotted fever
doxycycline, Acticlate, Adoxa, Doryx,
Doxteric, Monodox, Oracea,
Vibramycin, Vibra-Tab (G),
556–557
tetracycline, Achromycin V, Sumycin
(G), 557
roflumilast, Daliresp
chronic obstructive pulmonary
disease, 74
roflumilast, Zoryve
psoriasis, 522
Rogaine, *minoxidil*
baldness: male pattern, 57
Rolaids, *calcium carbonate*
hypocalcemia, 340
romosozumab-aqqg, Evenity
osteoporosis, 443–444
ropeginterferon-alfa-2b-njft, Besremi
polycythemia vera, 500–501
ropinirole, Requip
Parkinson's disease, 469
restless legs syndrome, 540
roseola infantum, 557
rosiglitazone, Avandia (G)
type 2 diabetes mellitus, 621
Rosula, *sodium sulfacetamide+sulfur*
acne rosacea, 3
seborrheic dermatitis, 205
rosuvastatin, Crestor
dyslipidemia, 222
hypertriglyceridemia, 339
Roszet, *ezetimibe+rosuvastatin*
dyslipidemia, 222–223
RotaTeq, *rotavirus vaccine*
rotavirus gastroenteritis, 557
rotavirus gastroenteritis
rotavirus vaccine, RotaTeq, 557

rotavirus vaccine, RotaTeq
  rotavirus gastroenteritis, 457
rotigotine, Neupro
  Parkinson's disease, 469
rotigotine transdermal patch, Neupro
  restless legs syndrome, 540
roundworm
  albendazole, Albenza, 557
  mebendazole, Emverm, Vermox (G), 557
  pyrantel pamoate, Antiminth, Pin-X (OTC), 557
  thiabendazole, Mintezol, 558
Rowasa Enema, Rowasa Suppository, *mesalamine*
  Crohn's disease, 175–176
  ulcerative colitis, 636
Rozerem, *ramelteon* (IV)
  insomnia, 359
rubella
  immune globulin (human), GamaSTAN S/D, 558
  measles, mumps, rubella, live, attenuated, neomycin vaccine, MMR II, 558
  rubella virus, live, attenuated+ neomycin vaccine, Meruvax II, 558
rubella virus, live, attenuated+neomycin vaccine, Meruvax II
  rubella, 558
rubeola
  immune globulin (human), GamaSTAN S/D, 558–559
  measles, mumps, rubella, live, attenuated, neomycin vaccine, MMR II, 558
Rubraca, *rucaparib*, 689
  ovarian cancer, 123
  peritoneal cancer, 126
  prostate cancer, 130
rucaparib, Rubraca
  ovarian cancer, 123
  peritoneal cancer, 126
  prostate cancer, 130
Ruconest, *C1 esterase inhibitor [recombinant]*
  hereditary angioedema, 298
Rukobia, *fostemsavir*
  human immunodeficiency virus (HIV) infection, 312
ruxolitinib, Jakafi
  myelofibrosis, 409
  polycythemia vera, 501
ruxolitinib, Opzelura
  asthma, 45
  atopic dermatitis, 200–201
  vitiligo, 654
Ryaltris, *olopatadine hydrochloride+mometasone furoate*
  allergic rhinitis/sinusitis, 553
Rybix ODT, *tramadol* (G)(IV)
  diabetic peripheral neuropathy (DPN), 208
  herpangina, 299
  herpes zoster, 302
  pain, 460
  peripheral neuritis, 481
  post-herpetic neuralgia, 509
  tension headache, 278
  urolithiasis, 647
Rydapt, *midostaurin*, 689
Rythmol, *propafenone*, 681
Ryzolt, *tramadol* (G)(IV)
  diabetic peripheral neuropathy (DPN), 208
  herpangina, 299
  herpes zoster, 302

pain, 460
peripheral neuritis, 481
post-herpetic neuralgia, 509
tension headache, 278
urolithiasis, 648

sacituzumab govitecan-hziy, Trodelvy
  breast cancer, 84
safinamide, Xadago (G)
  Parkinson's disease, 470
Safyral, *ethinyl estradiol+drospirenone plus levomefolate calcium*
  estrogen and progesterone, 672
Saizen, *somatropin*
  growth failure, 266–267
Salagen, *pilocarpine*
  Sjögren-Larsson-syndrome (SLS), 572
salicylic acid, Duo Film, Occlusal HP, Wart-Off (G)
  callused skin, 572
  common wart, 655
  plantar wart, 533
saline nasal spray, Afrin Saline Mist w. Eucalyptol and Menthol (OTC), Afrin Moisturizing Saline Mist (OTC), Ocean Mist (OTC), Pediamist (OTC)(G)
  common cold, 160–161
salmeterol, Serevent Diskus
  asthma, 43
  chronic obstructive pulmonary disease, 71
salmonellosis
  Bactrim, Septra, *trimethoprim+ sulfamethoxazole (TMP-SMX)* (G), 559
  ciprofloxacin, Cipro (G), Cipro XR, ProQuin XR, 559
Saluron, *hydroflumethiazide*
  edema, 228
Salutensin, *reserpine+hydroflumethiazide*
  hypertension, 337
Samsca, *tolvaptan*
  autosomal dominant polycystic kidney disease, 500
Sanctura, *trospium chloride* (G)
  urinary overactive bladder, 355
Sancuso, *granisetron*
  cannabinoid hyperemesis syndrome, 139
  chemotherapy-induced nausea/ vomiting, 148
  opioid-induced nausea/vomiting, 429
Sandostatin, Sandostatin LAR Depot, *octreotide acetate*
  acromegaly, 8
Saphnelo, *anifrolumab*
  systemic lupus erythematosis (SLE), 583
Saphris, *asenapine* (G)
  bipolar disorder, 62
sapropterin, Kuvan
  phenylketonuria, 486
saquinavir mesylate, Fortovase, Invirase, 697
  human immunodeficiency virus infection, 312
sarecycline, Seysara
  acne vulgaris, 5–6
sarilumab, Kevzara
  polymyalgia rheumatica, 502
  rheumatoid arthritis, 548
Savella, *milnacipran*
  fibromyalgia, 244
saxagliptin, Onglyza
  type 2 diabetes mellitus, 628
scabies
  crotamiton, Eurax, 559

  lindane, Kwell (G), 559
  permethrin, Acticin, Elimite (G), 559
  spinosad, Natroba, 559
scarlet fever
  azithromycin, Zithromax, Zmax (G), 560
  cefadroxil, Duricef, 560
  cephalexin, Keflex (G), 560
  clarithromycin, Biaxin (G), 560
  clindamycin (G), Cleocin, 560
  erythromycin estolate, Ilosone (G), 560
  erythromycin ethylsuccinate, EryPed, E.E.S. (G), 560
  penicillin g (benzathine and procaine), Bicillin C-R (G), 560
  penicillin v potassium, Pen-Vee K, 560
schizophrenia
  aripiprazole, Abilify, 561
  aripiprazole lauroxil, Aristada, 561–562
  asenapine, Secuado, 562–563
  brexpiprazole, Rexulti, 563–564
  lumateperone, Caplyta, 563
  lurasidone, Latuda (G), 564
  paliperidone palmitate, Invega Hafyera, Invega Sustenna, 564–566
Scopace, *scopolamine*
  motion sickness, 396
  vertigo, 653
scopolamine, Scopace, Transderm Scop
  labyrinthitis, 375
  Meniere's disease, 388
  motion sickness, 396
  vertigo, 653
Scytera, *coal tar*
  pityriasis alba, 488
  seborrheic dermatitis, 205
Seasonale, *ethinyl estradiol+levonorgestrel* (G), 674
Seasonique, *ethinyl estradiol+levonorgestrel* (G), 674
seborrheic dermatitis
  betamethasone valerate, Luxiq, 205
  chloroxine, Capitrol Shampoo, 204
  ciclopirox, Loprox, 204
  coal tar, Scytera, T/Gel (G), 205
  fluocinolone acetonide, Derma-Smoothe/FS Shampoo, Derma-Smoothe/FS Topical Oil fluocinolone acetonide, 205
  hydrogen peroxide 40%, Eskata, 205
  ketoconazole, Nizoral Cream, Xolegel, 205
  selenium sulfide, Exsel Shampoo, Selsun Rx, Selsun Shampoo, 205
  sodium sulfacetamide+sulfur, Clenia, Rosula, 205
secnidazole, Solosec
  bacterial vaginosis, 57
  vulvovaginal (moniliasis) candidiasis, 137
Sectral, *acebutolol*, 682
  hypertension, 326
Secuado, *asenapine*
  schizophrenia, 562–563
secukinumab, Cosentyx
  psoriasis, 522–523
  osteoarthritis (OA), 439
Seebri Neohaler, *glycopyrrolate inhalation solution*
  chronic obstructive pulmonary disease (COPD), 72, 75
  emphysema, 230
Segluromet, *ertugliflozin+metformin*
  type 2 diabetes mellitus, 628
seizure, cluster

diazepam nasal spray, Valtoco (IV),
  566
seizure disorder, 566
selegiline, Emsam, Zelapar
  major depressive disorder, 194
  Parkinson's disease, 470
  post-traumatic stress disorder, 512
selenium sulfide, Exsel Shampoo, Selsun
  Rx, Selsun Shampoo
  seborrheic dermatitis, 205
  tinea versicolor, 601
selexipag, Uptravi
  pulmonary arterial hypertension
    (PAH), 533
selpercatinib, Retevmo
  low libido, hypoactive sexual desire
    disorder (HSDD), 381
  lung cancer, 103–104
  renal cell carcinoma (RCC), 95
  thyroid cancer, 595–596
  thyroid carcinoma, 131–132
Selsun Blue, *selenium sulfide shampoo*
  tinea versicolor, 601
Selsun Rx, Selsun Shampoo, *selenium
  sulfide*
  seborrheic dermatitis, 205
selumetinib, Koselugo
  neurofibromatosis type 1, 415–416
semaglutide, Ozempic
  type 2 diabetes mellitus, 624–626
semaglutide, Wegovy
  obesity, 420–421
SennaPrompt, *psyllium+senna*
  occasional constipation, 170
Senokot, *bisacodyl*
  occasional constipation, 170
Senokot S, *docusate+senna*
  occasional constipation, 170
Sensipar, *cinacalcet*
  hypercalcemia, 319
  hyperparathyroidism (HPT), 323–324
Septra, *trimethoprim/sulfamethoxazole
  (TMP-SMX)* (G), 722
  acute bacterial sinusitis, rhinosinusitis,
    572
  acute exacerbation of chronic
    bronchitis, 71
  cat scratch fever, 141
  chronic prostatitis, 517
  community acquired pneumonia, 495
  cyclosporiasis, 182
  diverticulitis, 216
  granuloma inguinale, 266
  human bite, 67
  legionella pneumonia, 496
  otitis externa, 445
  otitis media: acute, 447
  pertussis, 483
  Pneumocystis jiroveci pneumonia, 498
  pyelonephritis: acute, 536
  salmonellosis, 559
  shigellosis, 567–568
  Traveler's diarrhea, 214
  typhoid fever, 633
  urinary tract infection, 645
Serentil, *mesoridazine*
  delirium, 188
  dementia, 188
  methamphetamine-induced
    psychosis, 395
Serevent Diskus, *salmeterol*
  asthma, 43
  chronic obstructive pulmonary
    disease, 71
serolimus, Rapamune
  organ transplant rejection prophylaxis,
    432–433
SeroQUEL, SeroQUEL XR, *quetiapine
  fumarate*

bipolar disorder, 63–64
  delirium, 188
  dementia, 188–189
  methamphetamine-induced
    psychosis, 395
  post-traumatic stress disorder, 511
Serostim, *somatropin*
  growth failure, 266–267
serous otitis media (SOM)
  ciprofloxacin otic suspension, Otiprio,
    448
sertaconazole, Ertaczo
  tinea pedis, 600
sertraline, Zoloft
  anxiety disorder, 35
  major depressive disorder, 192
  obsessive-compulsive disorder, 422
  panic disorder, 465
  post-traumatic stress disorder, 511
  premenstrual dysphoric disorder,
    515
  trichotillomania, 608
sevelamer, Renagel, Renvela
  hyperphosphatemia, 325
Sevenfact, *coagulation factor VIIa
  (recombinant)-jncw*
  hemophilia A, 286
sexual assault
  azithromycin, Zithromax, Zmax (G),
    567
  cefixime, Suprax (G), 567
  ceftriaxone, Rocephin (G), 567
  doxycycline, Acticlate, Adoxa, Doryx,
    Doxteric, Monodox, Oracea,
    Vibramycin, Vibra-Tab (G), 567
  metronidazole, Flagyl, Flagyl 375,
    Flagyl ER (G), 567
shift work sleep disorder (SWSD), 576
shigellosis
  azithromycin, Zithromax, Zmax (G),
    567
  Bactrim, Septra,
    *trimethoprim+sulfamethoxazole
    (TMP-SMX)* (G), 567–568
  ciprofloxacin, Cipro (G), Cipro XR,
    ProQuin XR, 567
  ofloxacin, Floxin (G), 567
  tetracycline, Achromycin V, Zmax
    (G), 567
shock: septic, distributive
  angiotensin II, Giapreza, 568
short ragweed pollen allergen extract,
  Ragwitek
  allergic rhinitis/sinusitis, 551
sickle cell disease (SCD)
  basiliximab, Simulect, 569
  crizanlizumab-tmca, Adakveo,
    569–570
  hydroxyurea, Hydrea, Siklos, 568–569
  L-glutamine powder, Endari, 569
  voxelotor, Oxbryta, 570–571
Signifo, *pasireotide*
  Cushing's syndrome, 180
Signifor LAR, *pasireotide*
  acromegaly, 7
Siklos, *hydroxyurea*
  sickle cell disease (SCD), 568–569
sildenafil citrate, Revatio, Viagra
  erectile dysfunction (ED), 237
  pulmonary arterial hypertension
    (PAH), 534
Silenor, *doxepin*
  insomnia, 360
silodosin, Rapaflo
  benign prostatic hyperplasia, 58
  urinary overactive bladder, 356
Silvadene, *silver sulfadiazine* (G)
  herpes zoster, 301, 302
  sunburn, 580–581

silver sulfadiazine, Silvadene
  herpes zoster, 301, 302
  sunburn, 580–581
Simbrinza, *brimonidine+brinzolamide*
  glaucoma, 255
Simcor, *niacin+simvastatin*
  dyslipidemia, 224
simeprevir, Olysio
  hepatitis C (HCV), 295
simethicone, Gas-X, Mylicon,
  Phazyme-95
  flatulence, 245
  irritable bowel syndrome with
    diarrhea, 367
simethicone, Mylicon Drops
  abdominal cramps, 175
  infantile colic, 159
Simponi, *golimumab*
  juvenile idiopathic arthritis, 371
  psoriasis, 525
  psoriatic arthritis, 530
  rheumatoid arthritis, 547
Simulect, *basiliximab*
  organ transplant rejection prophylaxis,
    432
  sickle cell disease, 569
simvastatin, Zocor
  dyslipidemia, 222
  hypertriglyceridemia, 339
sinecatechins 15% ointment, Veregen
  venereal wart, 655
Sinemet, *carbidopa+levodopa*
  Parkinson's disease, 469
Sinequan, *doxepin*
  anxiety disorder, 34
Singulair, Singulair Chewable, Singulair
  Oral Granules, *montelukast*
  allergic rhinitis/sinusitis, 551
  asthma, 41
siponimod, Mayzent
  multiple sclerosis (MS), 401
sitagliptin, Januvia
  type 2 diabetes mellitus, 629
Sitavig, *acyclovir*
  herpes labialis/herpes facialis, 300
Sivextro, *tedizolid phosphate*
  cellulitis, 145
Sjögren-Larsson-syndrome (SLS)
  cevimeline, Evoxac (G), 572
  pilocarpine, Salagen (G), 572
  xylitol+solazyme+selectobac, Orazyme
    Dry Mouth Rinse, 572
skin candidiasis
  amphotericin b, Fungizone, 136
  butenafine, Lotrimin Ultra, Mentax
    (G), 135
  ciclopirox, Loprox, 135
  clotrimazole, Lotrimin, Lotrimin
    AF, 135
  econazole, Spectazole, 135
  ketoconazole, Nizoral, Nizoral Cream,
    135, 136
  miconazole, Lotrimin AF Spray,
    Monistat-Derm, 136
  nystatin, Nystop Powder, 136
  posaconazole, Noxafil (G), 136
Sklice, *ivermectin* (G)
  pediculosis humanus capitis, 475
Skyla, *levonorgestrel*, 675
Skyrizi, *risankizumab-rzaa*
  crohn's disease, 178
  psoriasis, 523–524
  psoriatic arthritis, 528–529
sleepiness
  armodafinil, Nuvigil (G)(IV), 576
  modafinil, Provigil (IV), 576
Slo-Niacin, *niacin*
  dyslipidemia, 223
  hypertriglyceridemia, 338–339

Slow-Mag, *magnesium*
  hypomagnesemia, 344
smallpox
  smallpox and monkeypox vaccine, live,
    non-replicating, Jynneos, 576
  tecovirimat, Tpoxx, 576–577
  vaccina virus vaccine (dried, calf lymph
    type), DRYvax, 576
  smallpox and monkeypox vaccine, live,
    non-replicating, Jynneos
    smallpox, 576
Soaanz, *torsemide*
  hypertension, 328
sodium chloride (G)
  corneal edema, 171
Sodium Edecrin, *ethacrynate sodium*
  edema, 228–229
sodium hyaluronate, Durolane, Euflexx,
  Gel-One, GelSyn-3, GenVisc
  850, Hyalgan, Monovisc,
  Orthovisc, Spartz, Supartz FX,
  Synvisc, Synvisc-One, Visco-3
  osteoarthritis, 437
  rheumatoid arthritis, 549
sodium neratinib, Nerlynx
  breast cancer, 80
sodium oxybate, extended-release,
  Lumryz (III)
  narcolepsy, 410–411
sodium oxybate, Xyrem
  narcolepsy, 410
sodium polystyrene sulfonate, Kayexalate
  hyperkalemia, 322
sodium sulfacetamide, Bleph-10,
  Klaron (G)
  acne rosacea, 3
  acne vulgaris, 5
  blepharitis, 67
  stye (hordeolum), 580
sodium tetradecyl sulfate, Sotradecol
  varicose veins, 652
sodium thiosulfate, Pedmark
  lung cancer, 102
  pancreatic cancer, 124
  solid tumor, 132–133
sodium zirconium cyclosilicate, Lokelma
  hyperkalemia, 322–323
Solaquin Forte, *hydroquinone+*
  padimate+dioxybenzone+
  oxybenzone
  hyperpigmentation, 325
Solaquin, *hydroquinone+ethyl*
  dihydroxypropyl PABA+
  dioxybenzone+oxybenzone, 532
  hyperpigmentation, 325
  vitiligo, 653
Solaraze Gel, *diclofenac sodium*
  actinic keratosis, 9
  atopic dermatitis, 199
  diabetic peripheral neuropathy
    (DPN), 208–209
  dysmenorrhea: primary, 225
  gouty arthritis, 262
  hemorrhoids, 289–290
  juvenile idiopathic arthritis, 369
  juvenile rheumatoid arthritis, 372
  muscle strain, 404–405
  osteoarthritis, 434, 435
  pain, 453
  peripheral neuritis, 480
  post-herpetic neuralgia, 508
  pruritus, 518
  psoriatic arthritis, 527
  rheumatoid arthritis, 542
Solesta, *dextranomer microspheres+*
  sodium hyaluronate
  fecal incontinence, 353
solid tumor
  pembrolizumab, Keytruda, 133

sodium thiosulfate, Pedmark, 132–133
solifenacin succinate, VESIcare LS
  neurogenic detrusor overactivity
    (NDO), 415
solifenacin, VESIcar (G)
  neurogenic detrusor overactivity
    (NDO), 415
  urinary overactive bladder, 355
Soliqua, *insulin glargine (insulin*
  analog)+lixisenatide
  type 2 diabetes mellitus, 626
Soliqua Prefilled pen, *insulin glargine*
  (insulin analog)+lixisenatide
  type 1 diabetes mellitus, 618
Soliris, *eculizumab*
  atypical hemolytic uremic syndrome
    (aHUS), 284–285
  neuromyelitis optica spectrum
    disorder, 416
  myasthenia gravis, 406–407
  paroxysmal nocturnal
    hemoglobinuria, 472–473
Solodyn, *minocycline*
  acne vulgaris, 5
Solosec, *secnidazole*
  bacterial vaginosis, 57
  vulvovaginal (moniliasis) candidiasis,
    137
solriamfetol, Sunosi
  narcolepsy, 411
  obstructive sleep apnea, 575–576
Soma Compound, *carisoprodol+*
  aspirin (III)
  muscle strain, 404
  temporomandibular joint disorder,
    587
Soma Compound w. *Codeine,*
  carisoprodol+aspirin+codeine (III)
  muscle strain, 404
  temporomandibular joint disorder,
    587
somatropin, Genotropin, Genotropin
  Miniquick, Humatrope,
  Norditropin, Nutropin,
  Nutropin AQ, Nutropin Depot,
  Omnitrope, Saizen, Serostim
  growth failure, 266–267
Somavert, *pegvEisomant*
  acromegaly, 8
Sonata, *zaleplon* (IV)
  fibromyalgia, 245
  insomnia, 359
Soolantra, *ivermectin*
  acne rosacea, 3
sorafenib, Nexavar (G)
  hepatocellular carcinoma (HCC), 99
  renal cell carcinoma (RCC), 93
  thyroid carcinoma, 132
Soriatane, *acitretin*
  common wart, 655
  plantar wart, 655
sotagliflozin, Inpefa
  heart failure, 279
Sotradecol, *sodium tetradecyl sulfate*
  varicose veins, 652
Sotylize, *sotalol,* 682
Spartz, *sodium hyaluronate*
  osteoarthritis, 437
Spasticity of cerebral or spinal origin
  baclofen, Fleqsuvy, 577
  Prometra II Programmable Pump, 577
Spectazole, *econazole*
  diaper rash, 211
  skin candidiasis, 135
  tinea corporis, 597
  tinea cruris, 598
  tinea pedis, 600
  tinea versicolor, 601
spectinomycin, Trobicin

  gonorrhea, 259
Spectracef, *cefditoren pivoxil* (G)
  acute exacerbation of chronic
    bronchitis, 69
  acute tonsillitis, 604
  bacterial skin infection, 574
  dose form/volume, 704
  streptococcal pharyngitis, 484
spesolimab-sbzo, Spevigo (G)
  psoriasis, 524–525
Spevigo, *spesolimab-sbzo* (G)
  psoriasis, 524–525
spinal muscular atrophy (SMA)
  nusinersen, Spinraza, 577–578
  onasemnogene abeparvovec-xioi,
    Zolgensma, 578
  risdiplam, Evrysdi, 578
spinosad, Natroba
  scabies, 559
Spinraza, *nusinersen*
  spinal muscular atrophy (SMA),
    577–578
Spiriva HandiHaler, Spiriva Respimat,
  tiotropium (as bromide
  monohydrate)
  asthma, 42
  chronic obstructive pulmonary
    disease, 73
  emphysema, 231
spironolactone, Aldactone, CaroSpir
  edema, 228
  fibrocystic breast disease, 243
  heart failure, 281
  hypertension, 327
  premenstrual dysphoric disorder, 514
Sporanox, *itraconazole* (G), 704, 720
  onychomycosis (fungal nail), 422
  oral (thrush) candidiasis, 135
sprain, 578
Sprintec 28, *ethinyl estradiol+*
  norgestimate
  estrogen and progesterone, 672
Stadol Nasal Spray, *butorphanol tartrate*
  (IV)
  pain, 462
  tension headache, 277
  urolithiasis, 648
  ulcerative colitis, 528
Stalevo, *carbidopa+levodopa+entacapone*
  Parkinson's disease, 470
status asthmaticus
  ana-Kit, epinephrine+
    chlorpheniramine, 579
  epinephrine (G), 579
  epinephrine, Adrenaclick, Auvi-Q,
    EpiPen, EpiPen Jr, Symjepi,
    Twinject, 579
status epilepticus
  diazepam, Diastat, Valium (IV), 579
  diazepam nasal spray, Valtoco (IV),
    579
  lorazepam, Ativan (IV), 579
  midazolam, Nayzilam (IV), 580
  phenytoin (injectable), Dilantin, 580
stavudine, Zerit
  human immunodeficiency virus
    infection, 309
Staxyn, *vardenafil (as HCl)*
  erectile dysfunction (ED), 237
Steglatro, *ertugliflozin* (G)
  type 2 diabetes mellitus (T2DM), 627
Steglujan, *ertugliflozin+sitagliptin*
  type 2 diabetes mellitus, 628
Stein-Leventhal disease, 500
Stelara, *ustekinumab*
  psoriatic arthritis, 529
  ulcerative colitis (UC), 637
Stelazine, *trifluoperazine* (G)
  anxiety disorder, 35

panic disorder, 466
Stendra, *avanafil*
  erectile dysfunction (ED), 237
Stimate Nasal Spray
  hemophilia A, 287–288
Stiolto Respimat, *tiotropium+olodaterol*
  chronic obstructive pulmonary
    disease, 73
  emphysema, 232
stiripentol, Diacomit
  Lennox-Gastaut syndrome (LGS),
    378
Stivarga, *regorafenib*, 689
Strensiq, *asfotase alfa*
  hypophosphatasia, 345
streptococcal pharyngitis
  amoxicillin, Amoxil, Moxatag,
    Trimox (G), 484
  Augmentin, *amoxicillin+clavulanate*
    (G), 484
  azithromycin, Zithromax, Zmax (G),
    484
  cefaclor, Cefaclor Extended Release
    (G), 484
  cefadroxil, Duricef, 484
  cefdinir, Omnicef, 484
  cefditoren pivoxil, Spectracef, 484
  cefixime, Suprax (G), 484
  cefpodoxime proxetil, Vantin, 485
  cefprozil, Cefzil, 485
  ceftibuten, Cedax, 485
  cephalexin, Keflex, 485
  clarithromycin, Biaxin (G), 485
  dirithromycin, Dynabac (G), 485
  erythromycin base, Ery-Tab, PCE (G),
    485
  erythromycin estolate, Ilosone (G), 485
  erythromycin ethylsuccinate, EryPed,
    E.E.S (G), 485
  loracarbef, Lorabid, 485
  penicillin g (benzathine and procaine),
    Bicillin C-R (G), 485
  penicillin v potassium, Pen-Vee K (G),
    485
streptomycin (SM) (G)
  dose forms, 703
  plague, 489
  tuberculosis, 610
Striant, *testosterone* (III)
  testosterone deficiency, 588
Stribild, *elvitegravir+cobicistat+*
    emtricitabine+tenofovir
    disoproxil fumarate
  human immunodeficiency virus
    infection, 316
Striverdi Respimat, *olodaterol*
  asthma, 43
  chronic obstructive pulmonary
    disease, 71
  emphysema, 230
stroke-induced aphasia
  zolpidem, Ambien (IV), 36
  zolpidem, Edluar, Intermezzo,
    ZolpiMist (IV), 36–37
Stromectol, *ivermectin*
  hookworm, 305
  threadworm, 593
  trichinosis, 606
stye (hordeolum)
  erythromycin, Ilotycin, 580
  erythromycin, Isopto Cetamide
    Ophthalmic Solution, 580
  gentamicin, Garamycin Ophthalmic
    Ointment, Genoptic Ophthalmic
    Ointment, Gentacidin
    Ophthalmic Ointment, 580
  Neosporin Ophthalmic Solution,
    polymyxin b+neomycin+
    gramicidin, 580

Neosporin Ophthalmic Ointment,
    polymyxin b+bacitracin+
    neomycin (G), 580
  Polysporin, *polymyxin b+bacitracin*,
    580
  sodium sulfacetamide, Bleph-10, 580
succimer, Chemet
  iron overload, 365
  lead poisoning, 376
sucralfate, Carafate
  peptic ulcer disease (PUD), 480
sufentanil, Dsuvia
  pain, 461–462
sulconazole, Exelderm
  tinea corporis, 598
  tinea cruris, 599
  tinea pedis, 600
  tinea versicolor, 601
sulfacetamide, Bleph-10, Cetamide
    Ophthalmic Solution, Isopto
    Cetamide Ophthalmic Ointment
  bacterial conjunctivitis, 164
sulfasalazine, Azulfidine, Azulfidine EN
  Crohn's disease, 176
  rheumatoid arthritis, 546
  systemic lupus erythematosis, 584
  ulcerative colitis, 636
sulfinpyrazone, Anturane
  gout (hyperuricemia), 260
Sulfite-Free Rowasa Rectal Suspension,
    mesalamine
  Crohn's disease, 175–176
sumatriptan, Alsuma, Imitrex, Onzetra
    Xsail, Sumavel DosePro,
    Zembrace SymTouch (G)
  migraine and cluster headache, 271
Sumycin, *tetracycline*, 709, 721
  acne vulgaris, 6
  acute exacerbation of chronic
    bronchitis, 71
  aphthous stomatitis, 37
  bacterial skin infection, 575
  blepharitis, 67
  hidradenitis suppurativa, 304
  Lyme disease, 383
  malaria, 385
  mycoplasma pneumonia, 497
  psittacosis, 519
  rocky mountain spotted fever, 557
  shigellosis, 567
sunburn
  prednisone (G), 580
  silver sulfadiazine, Silvadene (G),
    580–581
sunitinib malate, Sutent
  gastrointestinal stromal tumor (GIST),
    91–92
  renal cell carcinoma (RCC), 93–94
Sunlenca, *lenacapavir*
  human immunodeficiency virus
    (HIV) infection, 313–314
Sunosi, *solriamfetol*
  narcolepsy, 411
  obstructive sleep apnea, 575–576
Supartz FX, *sodium hyaluronate*
  osteoarthritis, 437
Suprax, *cefixime* (G), 714
  acute bacterial sinusitis, rhinosinusitis,
    571
  acute exacerbation of chronic
    bronchitis, 69
  acute tonsillitis, 604
  dose form/volume, 706
  otitis media: acute, 446
  sexual assault, 567
  streptococcal pharyngitis, 484
  typhoid fever, 633
  urinary tract infection, 643
Surmontil, *trimipramine*

  anxiety disorder, 34
  diabetic peripheral neuropathy
    (DPN), 210
  irritable bowel syndrome with
    diarrhea, 368
  major depressive disorder, 193
  nocturnal enuresis, 235
  post-herpetic neuralgia, 508, 510
  trigeminal neuralgia, 609
Sustol, *granisetron*
  cannabinoid hyperemesis syndrome,
    139
  chemotherapy-induced nausea/
    vomiting, 148
Sustol, *granisetron extended-release*
    injection
  cannabinoid hyperemesis syndrome
    (CHS), 139
Sutent, *sunitinib malate*, 689
  gastrointestinal stromal tumor (GIST),
    91–92
  renal cell carcinoma (RCC), 93–94
suvorexant, Belsomra (IV)
  insomnia, 359
  non-24 sleep-wake disorder, 418
sweet vernal, orchard, perennial rye,
    timothy, Kentucky blue grass
    mixed pollen allergen extract,
    Oralair
  allergic rhinitis/sinusitis, 551
Syeda, *ethinyl estradiol+drospirenone*
  estrogen and progesterone, 672
Symadine (G), *amantadine*
  Parkinson's disease, 468–469
Symbicort, *budesonide+formoterol*
  asthma, 43
Symbyax, *olanzapine+fluoxetine*
  bipolar disorder, 65
  major depressive disorder, 193
Symdeko, *tezacaftor+ivacaftor plus*
    ivacaftor
  cystic fibrosis (CF), 183
Symfi, *efavirenz+lamivudine+tenofovir*
    disoproxil fumarate
  human immunodeficiency virus
    infection, 316
Symjepi, *epinephrine*
  anaphylaxis, 21
Symmetrel (G), *amantadine*, 705, 711
  Parkinson's disease, 469
Sympaza Oral Film, *clobazam* (G)(IV)
  Lennox-Gastaut syndrome (LGS),
    377–378
Symproic, *naldemedine*
  opioid-induced constipation (OIC),
    429
Symtuza, *darunavir+cobicistat+*
    emtricitabine+tenofovir
    alafenamide
  human immunodeficiency virus
    infection, 316
Synagis, *palivizumab*
  respiratory syncytial virus (RSV), 539
Synalar, *fluocinolone acetonide*, 676
Synalgos-DC, *dihydrocodeine+*
    aspirin+caffeine (III)
  pain, 455
Synarel, *nafarelin acetate*
  endometriosis, 233
Syndros, *dronabinol* (III)
  anorexia/cachexia, 30
Synjardy, Synjardy XR,
    empagliflozin+metformin
  type 2 diabetes mellitus, 628
Synthroid, *levothyroxine* (A)
  hypothyroidism, 346
Synvisc, Synvisc-One, *sodium*
    hyaluronate
  osteoarthritis, 437

syphilis
  aqueous crystalline penicillin g (G), 581
  penicillin g (benzathine), Bicillin L-A (G), 582
  penicillin g (procaine) (G), Bicillin C-R, 582
  probenecid, Benemid (G), 582
Syprine, *trientine* (G)
  Gaucher disease, type 1 (GD1), 253
  Wilson's disease, 657–658
Systane, Systane Balance, Systane Ultra, *polyethylene glycol*
  dry eye syndrome, 217
systemic juvenile idiopathic arthritis (SJIA), 368–371
systemic lupus erythematosis (SLE)
  anifrolumab, Saphnelo, 583
  atovaquone, Mepron (G), 584
  auranofin (gold salt), Ridaura, 583
  azathioprine, Azasan, Imuran, 583
  belimumab, Benlysta, 582–583
  chloroquine, Aralen (G), 584–585
  cyclosporine (immunosuppressant), Neoral, 583
  hydroxychloroquine, Plaquenil (G), 585
  leflunomide, Arava (G), 583
  Malarone, *atovaquone+proguanil* (G), 584
  mefloquine, Lariam, 585
  methotrexate (MTX), Rasuvo, 584
  penicillamine, Cuprimine, Depen, 584
  quinine sulfate, Qualaquin (G), 585
  rituximab, Rituxan, 582
  sulfasalazine, Azulfidine, Azulfidine EN (G), 584

T4, *levothyroxine sodium* (A)
  hypothyroidism, 347
Tabrecta, *capmatinib*
  mesothelioma, 393
Taclonex, *calcipotriene+betamethasone dipropionate* (G)
  psoriasis, 520
tacrine, Cognex
  Alzheimer's disease, 15
tacrolimus, Envarsus XR
  organ transplant rejection prophylaxis, 433
tadalafil, Cialis
  benign prostatic hyperplasia, 58
  erectile dysfunction (ED), 237
tafamidis meglumine, Vyndaqel
  cardiomyopathy of transthyretin-mediated amyloidosis, 140
tafamidis, Vyndamax
  cardiomyopathy of transthyretin-mediated amyloidosis, 140
tafenoquine, Arakoda, Krintafe
  malaria, 386
Tafinlar, *dabrafenib*
  melanoma, 117
tafluprost, Zioptan
  glaucoma, 256
Tagamet, *cimetidine* (G)
  peptic ulcer disease (PUD), 477–478
Tagrisso, *osimertinib*, 689
Takhzyro, *lanadelumab-flyo*
  hereditary angioedema, 297
talazoparib, Talzenna
  breast cancer, 81
Talwin Compound, *pentazocine+aspirin* (IV)
  pain, 460
Talwin NX, *pentazocine+naloxone* (IV)
  pain, 460, 462
Talwin, *pentazocine lactate* (IV)
  pain, 460

Talzenna, *talazoparib*, 689
  breast cancer, 81
Tambocor, *flecainide acetate*, 682
Tamiflu, *oseltamivir phosphate*
  influenza, seasonal (FLU), 357
tamoxifen citrate (G), 689
  breast cancer, 84–85
tamsulosin, Flomax
  benign prostatic hyperplasia, 58
  urinary overactive bladder, 356
  urolithiasis, 647
Tapazole, *methimazole*
  hyperthyroidism, 337
tapentadol, Nucynta
  peripheral neuritis, 481–482
tapeworm, 585
  albendazole, Albenza (G), 585
  nitazoxanide, Alinia (G), 585
  praziquantel, Biltricide (G), 585
Tarceva, *erlotinib*, 689
tardive dyskinesia (TD)
  valbenazine, Ingrezza, 586
Targiniq, *oxycodone+naloxone* (II)
  pain, 459
Tarina Fe 1/20, *ethinyl estradiol+norethindrone plus ferrous fumarate*
  estrogen and progesterone, 672
Tarka, *trandolapril+verapamil*
  hypertension, 336
Tarpeyo, *budesonide*
  nephropathy:primary, immunoglobulin A (IGAN), 414
  immunoglobulin A nephropathy, 4
Tasigna, *nilotinib*, 690
tasimelteon, Hetlioz (G)
  non-24 sleep-wake disorder, 418
Tasmar, *tolcapone* (G)
  Parkinson's disease, 471
tavaborole, Kerydin (G)
  onychomycosis (fungal nail), 423
Tavalisse, *fostamatinib disodium hexahydrate*
  idiopathic (immune) thrombocytopenia purpura, 594
Taxotere, *docetaxel* (G), 690
Taytulla Fe 1/20, *ethinyl estradiol+norethindrone plus ferrous fumarate*
  estrogen and progesterone, 672
tazarotene, Avage, Tazorac
  acne vulgaris, 6
  facial wrinkles, 660
  folliculitis barbae, 247
  hyperpigmentation, 325
  lentigines, 379
  plaque psoriasis, 521
  vitiligo, 653
Tazorac, *tazarotene* (G)
  acne vulgaris, 6
  facial wrinkles, 660
  folliculitis barbae, 247
  hyperpigmentation, 325
  lentigines, 379
  plaque psoriasis, 521
  vitiligo, 653
tbo-filgrastim, Granix
  neutropenia, 418
Tecentriq, *atezolizumab*, 690
Technivie, *ombitasvir+paritaprevir+ritonavir*
  hepatitis C (HCV), 295
tecovirimat, Tpoxx
  smallpox, 576–577
Teczem, *enalapril+diltiazem*
  hypertension, 336
tedizolid phosphate, Sivextro
  cellulitis, 145
Teflaro, *ceftaroline fosamil*
  cellulitis, 143

community acquired pneumonia, 493
  dose form/volume, 706
  impetigo contagiosa, 352
Tegretol, *carbamazepine*
  trigeminal neuralgia, 608–609
Tegretol, Tegretol XR, *carbamazepine*
  bipolar disorder, 61
Tekamlo, *aliskiren+amlodipine*
  hypertension, 336
Tekturna HCT, *aliskiren+hydrochlorothiazide*
  hypertension, 336
telbivudine, Tyzeka
  hepatitis B, 293
telithromycin, Ketek
  acute exacerbation of chronic bronchitis, 70–71
telotristat, Xermelo, 691
  carcinoid syndrome diarrhea (CSD), 140, 212
temazepam, Restoril (IV)(G)
  insomnia, 359
Temixys, *lamivudine+tenofovir disoproxil fumarate*
  human immunodeficiency virus infection, 316
temporal arteritis, 253–254
temporomandibular joint (TMJ) disorder
  baclofen, Lioresal (G), 586
  carisoprodol, Soma, 586
  chlorzoxazone, Parafon Forte DSC (G), 586
  cyclobenzaprine, Amrix, Fexmid, Flexeril (G), 586
  dantrolene, Dantrium, 586
  diazepam, Diastat, Valium (IV), 586–587
  Equagesic, *meprobamate+aspirin* (IV), 587
  metaxalone, Skelaxin, 587
  methocarbamol, Robaxin (G), 587
  nabumetone, Relafen, 587
  Norgesic, *orphenadrine+aspirin+caffeine* (G), 587
  orphenadrine citrate, Norflex (G), 587
  Soma Compound, *carisoprodol+aspirin* (G)(III), 587
  Soma Compound w. *Codeine*, *carisoprodol+aspirin+codeine* (G)(III), 587
  tizanidine, Zanaflex, 587
tenapanor, Ibsrela
  irritable bowel syndrome with constipation (IBS-C), 365–366
tenofovir alafenamide (TAF), Vemlidy
  hepatitis B, 293
tenofovir disoproxil fumarate, Viread (G)
  hepatitis B, 293
  human immunodeficiency virus infection, 309
Tenoretic, *atenolol+chlorthalidone*
  hypertension, 334
Tenormin, *atenolol* (G), 682
  angina pectoris: stable, 29
  hypertension, 326
  migraine and cluster headache, 275
Tenosynovial giant cell tumor (TGCT)
  pexidartinib, Turalio, 587–588
tension headache
  amitriptyline (G), 278
  butalbital+acetaminophen, Phrenilin (G), 277
  butalbital+acetaminophen+caffeine, Fioricet, Zebutal (G), 277
  butalbital+acetaminophen+codeine+caffeine, Fioricet with Codeine (G)(III), 277

butalbital+aspirin+caffeine, Fiorinal (G)(III), 277
butalbital+aspirin+codeine+caffeine, Fiorinal with Codeine (G)(III), 277
butorphanol tartrate, Butorphanol Nasal Spray, Stadol Nasal Spray (G)(IV), 277
desipramine, Norpramin (G), 278
imipramine, Tofranil (G), 278
magnesium, Slow-Mag, 278
magnesium oxide, Mag-Ox 400, 278
nortriptyline, Pamelor (G), 278
tramadol, Rybix ODT, Ryzolt, Ultram (G)(IV), 278
tramadol+acetaminophen, Ultracet (G)(IV), 278
teplizumab-mzwv, Tzield
  type 1 diabetes mellitus (T1DM), 618–619
tepotinib, Tepmetko
  lung cancer, 104
teprotumumab-trbw
  thyroid eye disease/Grave's eye disease, 596
Terazol, *terconazole*
  vulvovaginal (moniliasis) candidiasis, 138
terazosin, Hytrin
  benign prostatic hyperplasia, 58
  hypertension, primary, 332
  urinary overactive bladder, 356
terbinafine, Lamisil
  onychomycosis (fungal nail), 422
  tinea corporis, 598
  tinea cruris, 599
  tinea pedis, 600
  tinea versicolor, 601
terbutaline
  asthma, 40
terconazole, Terazol
  vulvovaginal (moniliasis) candidiasis, 138
teriflunomide, Aubagio
  multiple sclerosis (MS), 398
teriparatide, Forteo Multidose Pen
  hypoparathyroidism, 344
  osteoporosis, 442–443
testosterone, Androderm, AndroGel, Axiron, Fortesta, Natesto, Vogelxo Gel, Striant (III)
  testosterone deficiency, 590
testosterone cypionate (III)
  testosterone deficiency, 591
testosterone deficiency
  fluoxymesterone, Halotestin (III), 588
  methyltestosterone, Android, Methitest, Testred (III), 588
  testosterone, Androderm, AndroGel, Axiron, Fortesta, Natesto, Vogelxo Gel, Striant, Tlando (G) (III), 588–591
  testosterone cypionate (III), 591
  testosterone enanthate, Delatestryl, Xyosted (III), 591
  testosterone undecanoate, Jatenzo, 589
testosterone enanthate, Delatestryl, Xyosted (III)
  testosterone deficiency, 591
testosterone undecanoate, Jatenzo
  testosterone deficiency, 589
tetanus
  methocarbamol, Robaxin, 592–593
  tetanus immune globulin, human, BayTET, Hyper-TET, 592
  tetanus toxoid vaccine, BayTET/ HyperTET, 592
tetanus immune globulin, human, BayTET, Hyper-TET, 592

tetanus toxoid vaccine
  cat bite, 65
  insect bite/sting, 359
  tetanus, 592
  wound, 658
tetracycline, Achromycin V, Sumycin, 709
  acne vulgaris, 6
  acute exacerbation of chronic bronchitis, 71
  aphthous stomatitis, 37
  bacterial skin infection, 575
  blepharitis, 67
  hidradenitis suppurativa, 304
  Lyme disease, 383
  malaria, 385
  mycoplasma pneumonia, 497
  psittacosis, 519
  rocky mountain spotted fever, 557
  shigellosis, 567
tetrahydrozoline, Tyzine, Tyzine Pediatric Nasal Drops, Visine
  allergic (vernal) conjunctivitis, 167
  allergic rhinitis/sinusitis, 551
  common cold, 161
Teveten, *eprosartan* (G)
  hypertension, 330
Teveten HCT, *eprosartan+ hydrochlorothiazide*
  hypertension, 334
T/Gel, *coal tar*
  pityriasis alba, 488
  seborrheic dermatitis, 205
Thalitone, *chlorthalidone*
  edema, 228
Theo-24, *theophylline* (G)
  asthma, 45
  chronic obstructive pulmonary disease, 74
Theo-Dur, *theophylline* (G)
  asthma, 45
  chronic obstructive pulmonary disease, 74
Theolair-SR, *theophylline* (G)
  asthma, 45
  chronic obstructive pulmonary disease, 74
theophylline, Theo-24, Theo-Dur, Theolair-SR, Uniphyl (G)
  asthma, 45
thiabendazole, Mintezol
  cutaneous larva migrans, 376
  hookworm, 305
  pinworm, 488
  roundworm, 558
  threadworm, 593
  trichinosis, 606
  whipworm, 657
thin/sparse eyelashes, 347
Thiola, Thiola EC, *tiopronin* (G)
  cystinuria, 184–185
thioridazine, Mellaril
  delirium, 188
  dementia, 189
  methamphetamine-induced psychosis, 396
Thorazine, *chlorpromazine*
  cannabinoid hyperemesis syndrome, 139
  chemotherapy-induced nausea/ vomiting, 147
  dose forms, 63
  hiccups: intractable, 303
threadworm
  albendazole, Albenza, 593
  ivermectin, Stromectol, 593
  mebendazole, Emverm, Vermox (G), 593
  nitazoxanide, Alinia (G), 593
  praziquantel, Biltricide (G), 593

  pyrantel pamoate, Antiminth, Pin-X, 593
  thiabendazole, Mintezol, 593
thyroid carcinoma
  selpercatinib, Retevmo, 131–132, 595–596
  sorafenib, Nexavar, 132
thyroid eye disease/Grave's eye disease
  teprotumumab-trbw, 596
Thyrolar, *liothyronine+levothyroxine* (A)
  hypothyroidism, 346
Tiazac, *diltiazem*
  angina pectoris: stable, 28
Tibsovo, *ivosidenib,* 690
tickborne encephalitis prophylaxis, 596
Ticlid, *ticlopidine*
  peripheral vascular disease, 482
  platelet aggregation inhibitors, 703
ticlopidine, Ticlid
  peripheral vascular disease, 482
  platelet aggregation inhibitors, 703
tigecycline, Tygacil
  cellulitis, 145
Tilade, Tilade Nebulizer Solution, *nedocromil sodium*
  asthma, 42
tildrakizumab-asmn, Ilumya
  psoriasis, 524
Tilia Fe, *ethinyl estradiol+norethindrone plus ferrous fumarate*
  estrogen and progesterone, 672
Timolide, *timolol+hydrochlorothiazide*
  hypertension, 335
timolol, Betimol, Blocadren, Istalol, Timoptic (G)
  glaucoma, 256
  hypertension, 327
timolol maleate, 682
Timothy grass pollen allergen extract, Grastek
  allergic rhinitis/sinusitis, 551
Tinactin, *tolnaftate* (OTC)(G)
  tinea cruris, 599
  tinea pedis, 600
Tindamax, *tinidazole*
  amebic liver abscess, 17
  bacterial vaginosis, 57
  dose forms, 703, 705
  giardiasis, 254
  intestinal amebiasis, 17
  nongonococcal urethritis, 639
  trichomoniasis, 607
tinea capitis
  griseofulvin, microsize, Grifulvin V (G), 597
  griseofulvin, ultramicrosize, Gris-PEG (G), 597
  ketoconazole, Nizoral Cream (G), 597
tinea corporis
  butenafine, Lotrimin Ultra, Mentax (G), 597
  ciclopirox, Loprox, 597
  clotrimazole, Lotrimin, Lotrimin AF (G), 597
  clotrimazole+betamethasone, Lotrisone (G), 598
  econazole, Spectazole, 597
  griseofulvin, microsize, Grifulvin V (G), 598
  griseofulvin, ultramicrosize, Gris-PEG (G), 598
  ketoconazole, Nizoral Cream, 597
  luliconazole, Luzu Cream, 597
  miconazole, Lotrimin AF, Monistat-Derm, 597
  naftifine, Naftin, 597
  oxiconazole nitrate, Oxistat (G), 598
  sulconazole, Exelderm, 598
  terbinafine, Lamisil (G), 598

tinea cruris
  butenafine, Lotrimin Ultra, Mentax (G), 598
  ciclopirox, Loprox, 598
  clotrimazole, Lotrimin, Lotrimin AF (G), 598
  clotrimazole+betamethasone (G), 599
  econazole, Spectazole, 598
  griseofulvin, microsize, Grifulvin V (G), 599
  griseofulvin, ultramicrosize, Gris-PEG, 599
  ketoconazole, Nizoral, Nizoral Cream, 598, 599
  luliconazole, Luzu Cream, 599
  miconazole, Lotrimin AF, Monistat-Derm (G), 599
  naftifine, Naftin (G), 599
  oxiconazole nitrate, Oxistat (G), 599
  sulconazole, Exelderm, 599
  terbinafine, Lamisil (G), 599
  tolnaftate, Tinactin (OTC)(G), 599
  undecylenic acid, Desenex, 599
tinea pedis
  butenafine, Lotrimin Ultra, Mentax (G), 599
  ciclopirox, Loprox, 600
  clotrimazole, Desenex, Lotrimin, Lotrimin AF, 600
  clotrimazole+betamethasone, Lotrisone (G), 600
  econazole, Spectazole, 600
  griseofulvin, microsize, Grifulvin V (G), 600–601
  griseofulvin, ultramicrosize, Gris-PEG, 601
  ketoconazole, Nizoral, Nizoral Cream, 600, 601
  luliconazole, Luzu Cream, 600
  miconazole, Lotrimin AF, Monistat-Derm, 600
  naftifine, Naftin (G), 600
  oxiconazole nitrate, Oxistat (G), 600
  sertaconazole, Ertaczo, 600
  sulconazole, Exelderm, 600
  terbinafine, Lamisil (G), 600
  tolnaft ate, Tinactin (OTC)(G), 600
tinea versicolor
  butenafine, Lotrimin Ultra, Mentax (G), 601
  ciclopirox, Loprox, 601
  clotrimazole, Lotrimin, Lotrimin AF (G), 601
  econazole, Spectazole, 601
  ketoconazole, Nizoral, Nizoral Cream (G), 601, 602
  miconazole, Lotrimin AF, Monistat-Derm (G), 601
  oxiconazole nitrate, Oxistat (G), 601
  selenium sulfide shampoo, Selsun Blue, 601
  sulconazole, Exelderm, 601
  terbinafine, Lamisil, 601
tinidazole, Tindamax
  amebic liver abscess, 17
  bacterial vaginosis, 57
  dose forms, 703, 705
  giardiasis, 254
  intestinal amebiasis, 17
  nongonococcal urethritis, 639
  trichomoniasis, 607
tioconazole, 1-Day, Monistat 1 Vaginal Ointment, Vagistat-1 Vaginal Ointment
  vulvovaginal (moniliasis) candidiasis, 138
tiopronin, Thiola, Thiola EC (G)
  cystinuria, 184–185

tiotropium (as bromide monohydrate), Spiriva HandiHaler, Spiriva Respimat
  asthma, 42
  chronic obstructive pulmonary disease, 73
  emphysema, 231
tipranavir, Aptivus
  dose forms, 696
  human immunodeficiency virus infection, 312
tirbanibulin, Klisyri
  actinic keratosis, 9
tizanidine, Zanaflex
  muscle strain, 404
  temporomandibular joint disorder, 587
tirzepatide, Mounjaro
  type 2 diabetes mellitus (T2DM), 631–632
tobacco dependence
  bupropion HBr, Aplenzin (G), 602
  bupropion HCl, Forfivo XL, Wellbutrin, Zyban (G), 602
  nicotin, Nicotrol NS, Nicotrol Inhaler, 603
  nicotine polacrilex, Commit Lozenge, Nicorette Mini Lozenge, 603
  transdermal nicotine system, Habitrol, Nicoderm CQ, Nicotrol Step-down Patch, Nicotrol Transdermal, Prostep, 602–603
  varenicline, Chantix (G), 602
TobraDex, TobraDex ST, *tobramycin+dexamethasone*
  bacterial conjunctivitis, 164
tobramycin, Tobrex Ophthalmic Solution, Tobrex Ophthalmic Ointment
  bacterial conjunctivitis, 164
Tobrex Ophthalmic Solution, Tobrex Ophthalmic Ointment, *tobramycin*
  bacterial conjunctivitis, 164
tocilizumab, Actemra
  COVID-19 (coronavirus), 174
  giant cell arteritis (GCA), 254
  idiopathic pulmonary fibrosis (IPF), 535
  juvenile idiopathic arthritis, 370
  juvenile rheumatoid arthritis (JRA), 373
  pemphigus vulgaris, 477
  rheumatoid arthritis, 548–549
tofacitinib, Xeljanz
  rheumatoid arthritis, 544–545
  ulcerative colitis, 637–638
tofersen, Qalsody
  amyotrophic lateral sclerosis (ALS), 19–20
Tofranil, *imipramine*
  anxiety disorder, 34
  diabetic peripheral neuropathy (DPN), 210
  gonorrhea, 259
  interstitial cystitis, 362
  irritable bowel syndrome with diarrhea, 386
  major depressive disorder, 193
  migraine and cluster headache, 276
  nocturnal enuresis, 235
  obsessive-compulsive disorder, 422
  panic disorder, 465
  post-herpetic neuralgia, 508, 510s
  post-traumatic stress disorder, 512
  tension headache, 278
  trigeminal neuralgia, 609
tolazamide, Tolinase
  type 2 diabetes mellitus, 619
tolcapone, Tasmar

Parkinson's disease, 471
tolnaftate, Tinactin (OTC)(G)
  tinea cruris, 599
  tinea pedis, 600
Tolsura, *itraconazole*
  aspergillosis, 38
tolterodine tartrate, Detrol
  interstitial cystitis, 362
  urinary overactive bladder, 354
tolvaptan, Jynarque, Samsca
  autosomal dominant polycystic kidney disease, 500
Tonocard, *tocainide,* 682
topiramate, Topamax, Topamax Sprinkle Caps, Trokendi XR, Qudexy XR
  dose forms, 695
  migraine and cluster headache, 274
Toprol-XL, *metoprolol succinate*
  angina pectoris: stable, 29
  heart failure, 280
  hypertension, 326
  migraine and cluster headache, 275
toremifene, Fareston
  breast cancer, 85
torsemide, Demadex, Soaanz
  edema, 229
  heart failure, 281
  hypertension, 328
Toviaz, *fesoterodine*
  urinary overactive bladder, 354
toxoplasmosis
  pyrimethamine (G), Daraprim, 605
Tpoxx, *tecovirimat*
  smallpox, 576–577
trabenazine, Xenazine
  Huntington disease-associated chorea, 318
Tracleer, *bosentan* (G)
  pulmonary arterial hypertension (PAH), 532
tramadol, Rybix ODT, Ryzolt, Ultram (IV)
  diabetic peripheral neuropathy (DPN), 208
  herpangina, 299
  herpes zoster, 302
  pain, 460
  peripheral neuritis, 481
  post-herpetic neuralgia, 509
  tension headache, 278
  urolithiasis, 648
trandolapril, Mavik
  heart failure, 280
  hypertension, 330
tranexamic acid, Lysteda
  menometrorrhagia, 389
Transderm Scop, *scopolamine*
  labyrinthitis, 375
  Meniere's disease, 388
  motion sickness, 396
  vertigo, 653
transdermal nicotine system, Habitrol, Nicoderm CQ, Nicotrol Step-down Patch, Nicotrol Transdermal, Prostep
  tobacco dependence, 602–603
Transderm-Nitro, *nitroglycerin*
  angina pectoris: stable, 29–30
Tranxene, *clorazepate* (G)(IV)
  alcohol withdrawal syndrome, 11
  anxiety disorder, 34
  panic disorder, 466
tranylcypromine, Parnate
  major depressive disorder, 194
trastuzumab, Herceptin for Injection
  breast cancer, 82
trastuzumab-anns, Kanjinti
  breast cancer, 82
trastuzumab-dkst, Ogivri for Injection

breast cancer, 82
trastuzumab-dttb, Ontruzant for Injection
breast cancer, 82
trastuzumab-pkrb, Herzuma
breast cancer, 83
trastuzumab-qyyp, Trazimera
breast cancer, 83
Traveler's diarrhea
ciprofloxacin, Cipro (G), Cipro XR, ProQuin XR, 213
rifamycin, Aemcolo, 213–214
rifaximin, Xifaxan, 214
trimethoprim+sulfamethoxazole (TMP-SMX), Bactrim, Septra, 214
travoprost, Travatan, Travatan Z
glaucoma, 256
Trazimera, *trastuzumab-qyyp*
breast cancer, 83
trazodone, Desyrel, Oleptro
fibromyalgia, 245
major depressive disorder, 194
Treanda, *bendamustine* (G), 690
Treanda, *olutasidenib*
hepatocellular carcinoma (HCC), 101
Treanda, *tremelimumab-actl*
hepatocellular carcinoma (HCC), 99–100
Trelegy Ellipta, *fluticasone furoate+umeclidinium bromide+vilanterol trifenatate*
asthma, 44
asthma-COPD overlap syndrome, 47
chronic obstructive pulmonary disease (COPD), 74
emphysema, 232
tremelimumab-actl, Imjudo, Treanda
hepatocellular carcinoma (HCC), 99–100
lung cancer, 106–107
Tremfya, *guselkumab*
psoriatic arthritis, 528
Trental, *pentoxifylline*
peripheral vascular disease, 482
treprostinil, Orenitram
pulmonary arterial hypertension (PAH), 534
tretinoin, Altreno, Atralin, Avita, Renova, Retin-A, Tretin-X (G)
acne vulgaris, 6
facial wrinkles, 660
folliculitis barbae, 247
hyperpigmentation, 325
lentigines, 379
vitiligo, 653
tretinoin 0.1% cream+benzoyl peroxide 3%, Twyneo
acne vulgaris, 6–7
Tretin-X, *tretinoin*
acne vulgaris, 7
facial wrinkles, 660
folliculitis barbae, 247
Trexall, *methotrexate*
juvenile idiopathic arthritis, 370
polymyalgia rheumatica, 502
rheumatoid arthritis, 546
systemic lupus erythematosis, 584
triamcinolone acetonide, Kenalog, Nasacort Allergy 24HR, Oralone, Tri-Nasal, Zilretta
allergic rhinitis/sinusitis, 552
aphthous stomatitis, 37
osteoarthritis, 436
polyps, nasal, 506
strength and volume, 676–678
triamcinolone, Azmacort, Aristocort, Aristospan, Kenalog (G), 679, 680
aphthous stomatitis, 37

asthma, 41
triamterene, Dyrenium
edema, 228
hypertension, 327
Triaz, *benzoyl peroxide*
acne vulgaris, 4
triazolam, Halcion (IV)(G)
fibromyalgia, 245
insomnia, 360
Tribenzor, *olmesartan medoxomil+amlodipine+hydrochlorothiazide*
hypertension, 337
trichinosis
albendazole, Albenza, 606
ivermectin, Stromectol, 606
mebendazole, Emverm, Vermox (G), 606
pyrantel pamoate, Antiminth, Pin-X, 606
thiabendazole, Mintezol, 606
trichloroacetic acid
common wart, 655
plantar wart, 655
trichomoniasis
metronidazole, Flagyl, Flagyl 375, Flagyl ER (G), 606
secnidazole, Solosec, 607
tinidazole, Tindamax, 607
trichotillomania
clomipramine, Anafranil (G), 607
divalproex sodium, Depakene, Depakote (G), 608
fluoxetine, Prozac, Prozac Weekly, 607
fluvoxamine, Luvox, 607
lithium carbonate, Lithobid (G), 608
olanzapine, Zyprexa, Zyprexa Zydis, 608
paroxetine maleate, Paxil, Paxil CR, PaxilOral Suspension (G), 608
paroxetine mesylate, Brisdelle (G), 608
sertraline, Zoloft, 608
trichuriasis. *See* whipworm
TriCor, *fenofibrate*
dyslipidemia, 223
hypertriglyceridemia, 338
Tridesilon, *desonide*
atopic dermatitis, 198
trientine, Syprine (G)
Gaucher disease, type 1 (GD1), 253
Wilson's disease, 657–658
triethanolamine, Cerumenex (G)
cerumen impaction, 145
trifarotene 0.005% cream, Aklief
acne vulgaris, 6
trifluoperazine, Stelazine (G)
anxiety disorder, 35
panic disorder, 466
trifluridine, Viroptic
herpes simplex keratitis, 374
viral conjunctivitis, 168
trigeminal neuralgia
amitriptyline (G), 609
amoxapine, 609
baclofen, Lioresal, 608
carbamazepine, Carbatrol, Tegretol, 608–609
clonazepam, Klonopin (G)(IV), 609
desipramine, Norpramin (G), 609
divalproex sodium, Depakene, 609
doxepin (G), 609
imipramine, Tofranil (G), 609
nortriptyline, Pamelor (G), 609
phenytoin, Dilantin, 609
protriptyline, Vivactil, 609
trimipramine, Surmontil, 609
valproic acid, Depakene, 609
trihexyphenidyl, Artane
Parkinson's disease, 471

Trijardy XR, *empagliflozin+linagliptin+metformin*
type 2 diabetes mellitus (T2DM), 629
Trikaft, *elexacaftor+ivacaftor+tezacaftor*
cystic fibrosis (CF), 183
trilaciclib, Cosela
lung cancer, 104
Trilafon, *perphenazine*
cannabinoid hyperemesis syndrome, 139
chemotherapy-induced nausea/vomiting, 147
Tri-Legest 21, *ethinyl estradiol+norethindrone*
estrogen and progesterone, 672
Tri-Legest Fe, *ethinyl estradiol+norethindrone plus ferrous fumarate*
estrogen and progesterone, 673
Tri-Levlen 21, Tri-Levlen 28, *ethinyl estradiol/levonorgestrel*
estrogen and progesterone, 673
TriLipix, *fenofibrate*
dyslipidemia, 223
hypertriglyceridemia, 338
Tri-Lo-Estarylla, *ethinyl estradiol+norgestimate*
estrogen and progesterone, 673
Tri-Lo-Sprintec, *ethinyl estradiol+norgestimate*
estrogen and progesterone, 673
Tri-Luma, *hydroquinone+fluocinolone+tretinoin*
hyperpigmentation, 325
melasma/chloasma, 387
vitiligo, 653
trimethoprim, Primsol, Proloprim, Trimpex
dose form/volume, 709
urinary tract infection, 645
trimipramine, Surmontil
anxiety disorder, 34
diabetic peripheral neuropathy (DPN), 210
irritable bowel syndrome with diarrhea, 368
major depressive disorder, 193
nocturnal enuresis, 235
post-herpetic neuralgia, 508, 510
trigeminal neuralgia, 609
Trimox, *amoxicillin*, 711
acute bacterial sinusitis, rhinosinusitis, 571
acute exacerbation of chronic bronchitis, 68–69
acute tonsillitis, 603
bacterial endocarditis prophylaxis, 55
cellulitis, 142
community acquired pneumonia, 493
dose form, 707
impetigo contagiosa, 351
Lyme disease, 382
otitis media: acute, 445
streptococcal pharyngitis, 484
Trimpex, *trimethoprim*
urinary tract infection, 645
Tri-Nasal, *triamcinolone acetonide*
allergic rhinitis/sinusitis, 552
TriNessa, *ethinyl estradiol+norgestimate*
estrogen and progesterone, 673
Tri-Norinyl 21, Tri-Norinyl 28, *ethinyl estradiol+norethindrone*
estrogen and progesterone, 673
trioxsalen, Trisoralen
vitiligo, 653
Triphasil-21, Triphasil-28, *ethinyl estradiol/levonorgestrel*
estrogen and progesterone, 673

Tri-Previfem, *ethinyl estradiol+ norgestimate*
  estrogen and progesterone, 673
Triptodur, *triptorelin*
  central precocious puberty, 513
triptorelin, Triptodur
  central precocious puberty, 513
Trisenox, *arsenic trioxide,* 690
Trisoralen, *trioxsalen*
  vitiligo, 653
Tri-Sprintec, *ethinyl estradiol+ norgestimate*
  estrogen and progesterone, 673
Tritec, *ranitidine bismuth citrate*
  gastroesophageal reflux disease, 250
  peptic ulcer disease (PUD), 478
Triumeq, *abacavir sulfate+dolutegravir+ lamivudine*
  human immunodeficiency virus infection, 316
trivalent inactivated influenza subvirion vaccine, types a and b, Fluarix, Flublok, FluLaval, FluShield, Fluzone
  influenza, seasonal (FLU), 356–357
trivalent, live attenuated influenza vaccine, types A and B, FluMist Nasal Spray
  influenza, seasonal (FLU), 356
trivalent poliovirus vaccine, inactivated (type 1, 2, and 3), Ipol
  poliomyelitis, 498
Tri-Vi-Flor Drops, *fluoride+vitamin a+ vitamin d+vitamin c* (G)
  fluoridation, water, 246
Tri-Vi-Flor w. Iron Drops, *fluoride+ vitamin a+vitamin d+vitamin c+ iron* (G)
  fluoridation, water, 246
Trivora, *ethinyl estradiol/levonorgestrel*
  estrogen and progesterone, 673
Trizivir, *abacavir sulfate+lamivudine+ zidovudine*
  human immunodeficiency virus infection, 316
Trodelvy, *sacituzumab govitecan-hziy*
  breast cancer, 84
Trofinetide, Daybue
  rett syndrome, 541
trolamine salicylate, Mobisyl Creme
  atopic dermatitis, 200
  diabetic peripheral neuropathy (DPN), 209
  gouty arthritis, 262
  hemorrhoids, 290
  juvenile idiopathic arthritis, 369
  juvenile rheumatoid arthritis, 372
  muscle strain, 405
  osteoarthritis, 434
  pain, 454
  peripheral neuritis, 481
  post-herpetic neuralgia, 508
  pruritus, 518
  psoriatic arthritis, 527
  rheumatoid arthritis, 542
trospium chloride, Sanctura
  urinary overactive bladder, 355
Troxyca ER, *oxycodone+naloxone* (II)
  opioid dependence, 427–428
Trulance, *plecanatide*
  chronic idiopathic constipation, 168
  irritable bowel syndrome with constipation (IBS-C), 366
Trumenba, *Meningococcal group b vaccine [recombinant, absorbed]*
  meningitis, 388
Truvada, *emtricitabine+tenofovir disoproxil fumarate*
  human immunodeficiency virus infection, 316

Truxima, *rituximab-abbs,* 690
tuberculosis (TB)
  bedaquiline, Sirturo (G), 610, 612
  capreomycin sulfate, Capastat (G), 611–612
  ethambutol (EMB), Myambutol (G), 610
  isoniazid, 610
  isoniazid (INH), 610
  linezolid, Zyvox, 610
  pretomanid, Pretomanid Tablet, 612
  purified protein derivative (PPD), Aplisol, Tubersol, 609
  pyrazinamide (PZA), 610
  rifampin, 610
  rifampin (RIF), Rifadin, Rimactane (G), 610
  rifampin+isoniazid, Rifamate, 610
  rifampin+isoniazid+pyrazinamide, Rifater, 610
  rifapentine, 610
  rifapentine, Priftin, 610
  rilpivirine, Rifabutin, 610
  streptomycin (SM) (G), 610
Tubersol, *purified protein derivative (PPD)*
  tuberculosis, 609
tucatinib, Tukysa
  breast cancer, 80
Tudorza Pressair, *aclidinium bromide*
  chronic obstructive pulmonary disease, 72
  emphysema, 230
Tukysa, *tucatinib*
  breast cancer, 80
Tums, *calcium carbonate*
  hypocalcemia, 340
turoctocog alfa pegol, N8-GP, Esperoct
  hemophilia A, 287
Twinject, *epinephrine*
  anaphylaxis, 21
  status asthmaticus, 579
Twinrix, *hepatitis A inactivated+hepatitis b surface antigen (recombinant vaccine)*
  hepatitis A, 291
  hepatitis B, 292
Twirla, *ethinyl estradiol+levonorgestrel,* 674
Twynsta, *telmisartan+amlodipine*
  hypertension, 337
Tybost, *cobicistat*
  human immunodeficiency virus (HIV) infection, 313
Tygacil, *tigecycline*
  cellulitis, 145
Tykerb, *lapatinib ditosylate*
  breast cancer, 79–80
Tylenol, *acetaminophen*
  fever (pyrexia), 242
Tylenol, codeine+acetaminophen (III)
  pain, 455
Tylox, *oxycodone+acetaminophen* (II)
  pain, 459
Tymlos, *abaloparatide*
  hypoparathyroidism, 344–345
  osteoporosis, 442
Tylenol PM, *acetaminophen+ diphenhydramine*
  insomnia, 360
type 1 diabetes mellitus (T1DM)
  glucagon (recombinant), Gvoke, 613
  glucagon nasal powder, Baqsimi, 613
  dasiglucagon, Zegalogue, 614
  diazoxide (G), Proglycem, 614
  Humalog Mix 50/50 (recombinant), *insulin lispro protamine 50%+insulin lispro 50%,* 617
  Humalog Mix 50/50, *insulin lispro protamine 50%+insulin lispro 50%,* 618

Humalog Mix 75/25, *insulin lispro protamine 75%+insulin lispro 25%,* 618
Humalog Mix 75/25, *insulin lispro protamine75%+insulin lispro 25%,* 618
Humulin 50/50, *NPH 50%+regular 50%,* 617
Humulin 70/30, Novolin 70/30, *NPH 70%+regular 30%,* 617
insulin aspart (recombinant), Fiasp, NovoLog, 615
insulin aspart protamine suspension 70%/insulin aspart 30% (recombinant), NovoLog Mix 70/30, NovoLog Mix 70/30 FlexPen, 616
insulin degludec (insulin analog), Tresiba FlexTouch, 617
insulin detemir (human), Levemir, 616
insulin extended zinc suspension (Ultralente) (human), Humulin U, 617
insulin glargine (recombinant), Basaglar, Lantus, 616
insulin glargine-yfgn, Semglee, 616–617
insulin glulisine (rDNA origin), Apidra, 615
insulin human (inhaled), Afrezza Inhalation Powder, 615
insulin isophane suspension (NPH), Humulin N, Novolin N, Iletin II NPH, 617
insulin lispro (recombinant), Admelog, Humalog, 615
insulin regular, Humulin R U-100, Humulin R U-500, Iletin II Regular, Novolin R, 615–616
insulin zinc suspension, Humulin L, Iletin II Lente, Novolin L, 617
pramlintide, Symlin, 616
Soliqua Prefilled pen, *insulin glargine (insulin analog)+lixisenatide,* 618
teplizumab-mzwv, Tzield, 618–619
Xultophy Prefilled pen, *insulin degludec (insulin analog)+liraglutide,* 618
type 2 diabetes mellitus (T2DM)
  acarbose, Precose, 620
  Actoplus Met, Actoplis Met R, *pioglitazone+metformin,* 622
  alogliptin, Nesina, 629
  Avandamet, *rosiglitazone+metformin* (G), 622
  Avandaryl, *rosiglitazone+glimepiride,* 622–623
  bexaglifl, Brenzavvy, 626–627
  bromocriptine mesylate, Cycloset, 632
  canagliflozin, Invokana, 627
  chlorpropamide, Diabinese, 619
  colesevelam, WelChol (G), 632
  dapagliflozin, Farxiga, (G) 627
  dasiglucagon, Zegalogue, 619
  Duetact, *pioglitazone+glimepiride* (G), 622
  dulaglutide, Trulicity, 623
  ertugliflozin, Steglatro (G), 627
  exenatide, Bydureon, Bydureon BCise, Byetta, 623–624
  glimepiride, Amaryl, 620
  glipizide, Glucotrol, Glucotrol XL (G), 620
  glucagon (recombinant), 619
  Glucovance, *glyburide+metformin,* 622
  glyburide, DiaBeta, Micronase (G), 620
  glyburide, micronized, Glynase PresTab, 620

Glyxambi, *empagliflozin+linagliptin*, 628
insulin degludec (insulin analog)+ liraglutide, Xultophy, 626
insulin glargine (insulin analog)+ lixisenatide, Soliqua, 626
Invokamet, *canagliflozin+metformin* 627
Janumet, *sitagliptin+metformin*, 630
Jentadueto, *linagliptin+metformin* (G), 630
Juvisync, sitagliptin+simvastatin, 632
Kazano, *alogliptin+metformin*, 630
Kombiglyze XR, *saxagliptin+metformin* (G), 630
lacosamide, Jardiance, 627
linagliptin, Tradjenta, 629
liraglutide, Victoza, 624
lixisenatide, Adlyxin, 624
Metaglip, *glipizide+metformin*, 622
metformin, Fortamet, Glucophage, Glumetza ER, Riomet XR (G), 620–621
miglitol, Glyset, 620
nateglinide, Starlix, 621
Oseni, *alogliptin+pioglitazone*, 621
pioglitazone, Actos (G), 621
Prandimet, *repaglinide+metformin* (G), 631
Qtern, *dapagliflozin+saxagliptin*, 628
Qternmet XL, *dapagliflozin+ saxagliptin+metformin*, 628–630
repaglinide, Prandin, 621
rosiglitazone, Avandia (G), 621
saxagliptin, Onglyza (G), 629
Segluormet, *ertugliflozin+metformin*, 628
semaglutide, Ozempic, Rybelsus, 624–626
sitagliptin, Januvia, 629
Steglujan, *ertugliflozin+sitagliptin*, 628
Synjardy, Synjardy XR, *empagliflozin+ metformin* (G), 628
tolazamide, Tolinase (G), 619
tolbutamide, 620
Trijardy XR, *empagliflozin+ linagliptin+metformin*, 629
tirzepatide, Mounjaro, 631–632
Xigduo XR, *dapagliflozin+metformin*, 627–628
Typhim Vi, *typhoid Vi polysaccharide vaccine*, 632
typhoid fever
  azithromycin, Zithromax, Zmax (G), 633
  Bactrim, *trimethoprim+ sulfamethoxazole (TMP-SMX)* (G), 633
  cefixime, Suprax (G), 633
  cefotaxime, Claforan, 633
  ceftriaxone, Rocephin (G), 633
  ciprofloxacin, Cipro (G), Cipro XR, ProQuin XR, 633
  ofloxacin, Floxin, 633
  typhoid vaccine, oral, live, attenuated strain, Vivotif Berna, 632
  typhoid Vi polysaccharide vaccine, Typhim Vi, 632
typhoid vaccine, oral, live, attenuated strain, Vivotif Berna
  typhoid fever, 633
typhoid Vi polysaccharide vaccine, Typhim Vi
  typhoid fever, 633
Tyrvaya, *varenicline*
  dry eye syndrome, 216
Tysabri, *natalizumab*
  Crohn's disease, 179

Tyzeka, *telbivudine*
  hepatitis B, 293
Tyzine, Tyzine Pediatric Nasal Drops, *tetrahydrozoline*
  allergic rhinitis/sinusitis, 551
  common cold, 161
Tzield, *teplizumab-mzwv*
  type 1 diabetes mellitus (T1DM), 618–619

ublituximab-xiiy, Briumvi
  multiple sclerosis (MS), 400
Uceris, *budesonide rectal foam* (G)
  ulcerative colitis (UC), 634
ulcerative colitis (UC)
  adalimumab-aacf, Idacio, 636
  adalimumab-afzb, Abrilada, 636
  adalimumab-bwwd, Hadlima, 636
  adalimumab, Humira, 636
  balsalazide disodium, Colazal, Giazo, 635
  budesonide micronized, Entocort EC (G), 634
  budesonide rectal foam, Uceris (G), 634
  butorphanol tartrate, Butorphanol Nasal Spray, Stadol Nasal Spray (IV), 648
  diphenoxylate+atropine, Lomotil (G), 638
  hydrocortisone, Anusol-HC, Cortenema, Cortifoam, Proctocort, 634
  Imodium Advanced, *loperamide+ simethicone*, 638
  infliximab-abda, Renflexis, 637
  infliximab-axxq, Avsola, 637
  infliximab-dyyb, inflectra, 637
  infliximab, Remicade, 637
  infliximab-qbtx, Ifixi, 637
  loperamide, Imodium, Imodium A–D (G), 638
  mesalamine, Apriso, Asacol HD, Canasa, Delzicol, Lialda, Pentasa, Rowasa Suppository, Rowasa Rectal Suspension, 635–636
  Motofen, *difenoxin+atropine*, 638
  olsalazine, Dipentum, 636
  sulfasalazine, Azulfidine, Azulfidine EN, 636
  tofacitinib, Xeljanz, 637–638
  ustekinumab, Stelara, 637
  vedolizumab, Entyvio, 638
ulipristal acetate (UPA)(G)
  uterine leiomyomata, 650–651
ulipristal, ella, Logilia, 676
Ultomiris, *ravulizumab-cwvz*
  paroxysmal nocturnal hemoglobinuria, 474
Ultracet, *tramadol+acetaminophen* (G)(IV)
  diabetic neuropathic pain, 481
  diabetic peripheral neuropathy (DPN), 208
  herpangina, 299
  pain, 461
  herpes zoster, 301
  peripheral neuritis, 481
  post-herpetic neuralgia, 509
  tension headache, 278
  urolithiasis, 648
Ultram, *tramadol* (G)(IV)
  diabetic peripheral neuropathy (DPN), 208
  herpangina, 299
  herpes zoster, 302
  pain, 460
  peripheral neuritis, 481
  post-herpetic neuralgia, 509
  tension headache, 278

urolithiasis, 648
Ultrase, *pancreatic enzymes*
  pancreatic enzyme deficiency, 239
  pancreatic enzyme insufficiency, 463
umeclidinium, Incruse Ellipta
  chronic obstructive pulmonary disease (COPD), 72
  emphysema, 231
Unasyn, *ampicillin*
  bacterial endocarditis prophylaxis, 55
  listeriosis, 379
undecylenic acid, Desenex
  tinea cruris, 599
Uniphyl, *theophylline*
  asthma, 45
  chronic obstructive pulmonary disease, 74
Uniretic, *moexipril+hydrochlorothiazide*
  hypertension, 333
Unithroid, *levothyroxine* (A)
  hypothyroidism, 346
Univasc, *moexipril*
  hypertension, 330
unobstructive urinary retention
  bethanechol, Urecholine, 639
unoprostone isopropyl, Rescula
  glaucoma, 257
upadacitinib, Rinvoq, Rinvoq Extended-Release Tablets
  crohn's disease, 179
  rheumatoid arthritis (RA), 545
Upneeq, *oxymetazoline hydrochloride ophthalmic solution, 0.1%*
  blepharoptosis, acquired (droopy eyelid), 67–68
Uptravi, *selexipag*
  pulmonary arterial hypertension (PAH), 533
urea, Carmol 40, Keratol 40
  callused skin, 473
Urecholine, *bethanechol*
  unobstructive urinary retention, 639
  urinary overactive bladder, 355
Urelle, *methenamine+phenyl salicylate+ methylene blue+sod biphosphate+hyoscyamine*
  urinary tract infection, 642
Uribel, *methenamine+sod phosphate monobasic+phenyl salicylate+methylene blue+hyoscyamine sulfate*
  interstitial cystitis, 362
  urinary tract infection, 642
urinary overactive bladder
  bethanechol, Urecholine, 355
  darifenacin, Enablex, 354
  desmopressin acetate (DDAVP), DDAVP, DDAVP Rhinal Tube (G), 353
  dicyclomine, Bentyl, 354
  doxazosin, Cardura, 356
  fesoterodine, Toviaz, 354
  finasteride, Proscar, 356
  flavoxate, Urispas, 354
  hyoscyamine, Anaspaz, Levbid, Levsin, Levsinex, NuLev (G), 354–355
  mirabegron, Myrbetriq, VESIcare, 354
  oxybutynin chloride, Ditropan, GelniQUE, Oxytrol Transdermal Patch (OTC), 355
  prazosin, Minipres (G), 356
  propantheline, Pro-Banthin, 355
  silodosin, Rapaflo, 356
  solifenacin, VESIcar (G), 355
  tamsulosin, Flomax, 356
  terazosin, Hytrin, 356
  tolterodine tartrate, Detrol, 354
  trospium chloride, Sanctura (G), 355
  vibegron, Gemtesa, 354

urinary tract infection (UTI)
  acetyl sulfisoxazole, Gantrisin (G), 643
  amoxicillin, Amoxil, Moxatag, Trimox (G), 643
  ampicillin, Omnipen, Principen, 643
  Augmentin, Augmentin ES-600, Augmentin XR, *amoxicillin+ clavulanate* (G), 643
  carbenicillin, Geocillin, 643
  cefaclor, Cefaclor Extended Release (G), 643
  cefadroxil, Duricef, 643
  cefixime (G), Suprax, 643
  cefpodoxime proxetil, Vantin, 644
  cephalexin, Keflex (G), 644
  ciprofloxacin, Cipro (G), Cipro XR, ProQuin XR, 644
  doxycycline, Acticlate, Adoxa, Doryx, Doxteric, Monodox, Oracea, Vibramycin, Vibra-Tab (G), 644
  enoxacin, Penetrex (G), 644
  ertapenem, Invanz, 645
  flavoxate, Urispas, 642
  fosfomycin, Monurol (G), 644
  hyoscyamine, Anaspaz, Levbid, Levsin, Levsinex, NuLev (G), 642
  levofloxacin, Levaquin, 644
  lomefloxacin, Maxaquin, 644
  methenamine hippurate, Hiprex, Urex, 645
  minocycline, Dynacin, Minocin (G), 644
  nalidixic acid, NegGram, 644
  nitrofurantoin, Furadantin, Macrobid, Macrodantin (G), 644–646
  norfloxacin, Noroxin, 645
  ofloxacin, Floxin (G), 645
  phenazopyridine, AZO Standard, Prodium, Uristat, 642–643
  trimethoprim, Primsol, Proloprim, Trimpex (G), 645
  trimethoprim-sulfamethoxazole (TMP-SMX), Bactrim, Septra (G), 645
  Urelle, *methenamine+phenyl salicylate+methylene blue+sod biphosphate+hyoscyamine,* 642
  Uribel, *methenamine+phenyl salicylate+methylene blue+ sod phosphate monobasic+ hyoscyamine,* 642
  Urised, *methenamine+phenyl salicylate+methylene blue+ benzoic acid+atropine sulfate+- hyoscyamine sulfate* (G), 642
  Vabomere, *meropenem+vaborbactam,* 645
  Urised, *methenamine+phenyl salicylate+ methylene blue+benzoic acid+ atropine sulfate+- hyoscyamine sulfate*
    interstitial cystitis, 362
    urinary tract infection, 642
  Urispas, *flavoxate*
    urinary overactive bladder, 354
    urinary tract infection, 642
    urolithiasis, 647
  Uristat, *phenazopyridine*
    interstitial cystitis, 361, 362
    pyelonephritis: acute, 536
    urinary tract infection, 642
  Urocit-K, *potassium citrate*
    urolithiasis, 646, 647
  Urogesic, *phenazopyridine* (G)
    pyelonephritis: acute, 536
  urolithiasis
    acetaminophen, Ofirmev, 647
    alfuzosin, UroXatral (G), 647

  allopurinol, Zyloprim (G), 646–647
  butorphanol tartrate, Butorphanol Nasal Spray, Stadol Nasal Spray, 648
  chlorothiazide, Diuril (G), 646
  fentanyl, Lazanda Nasal Spray (II), 648
  flavoxate, Urispas, 647
  hydrochlorothiazide, Esidri, Microzide (G), 646
  ibuprofen, Caldolor, 647
  penicillamine, Cuprimine, Depen, 646
  potassium citrate, Urocit-K (G), 646, 647
  tamsulosin, Flomax (G), 647
  tramadol, Rybix ODT, Ryzolt, Ultram (IV)(G), 647–648
  Ultracet, *tramadol+ acetaminophen* (IV)(G), 648
urothelial carcinoma
  enfortumab vedotin-ejfv, Padcev, 134
  erdafitinib, Balversa, 133–134
  pembrolizumab, Keytruda, 134
UroXatral, *alfuzosin*
  benign prostatic hyperplasia, 58
  urolithiasis, 647
ursodeoxycholic acid (UDCA), Ursofalk (G)
  cholelithiasis, 153
  cystic fibrosis (CF), 184
  primary biliary cholangitis, 152
ursodiol, Actigall
  bile acid deficiency, 60
  cholelithiasis, 153
Ursofalk, *ursodeoxycholic acid* (UDCA) (G)
  cholelithiasis, 153
  cystic fibrosis (CF), 184
  primary biliary cholangitis, 152
urticaria
  cetirizine, Children's Zyrtec Chewable, Children's Zyrtec Allergy Syrup, Zyrtec, Quzyttir (OTC)(G),649, 650
  desloratadine, Clarinex, Desloratadine ODT, 649
  diphenhydramine, Benadryl (G), 649
  epinephrine, 650
  fexofenadine, Allegra (OTC)(G), 649
  hydroxyzine, Atarax, Vistaril (G), 649
  levocetirizine, Children's Xyzal Allergy 24HR, Xyzal Allergy 24HR (OTC)(G), 649
  loratadine, Claritin (OTC)(G), 649
  omalizumab, Xolair, 650
ustekinumab, Stelara
  psoriasis, 524
  psoriatic arthritis, 529
  ulcerative colitis (UC), 637
uterine leiomyomata
  elagolix, Oriahnn, 651
  medroxyprogesterone, Provera, 650
  Myfembree, *relugolix+estradiol+ norethindrone acetate,* 651–652
  Oral contraceptives, 650
  ulipristal acetate (UPA) (G), 650–651
Utibron Neohaler, *indacaterol+ glycopyrrolate*
  chronic obstructive pulmonary disease, 71
  emphysema, 231
uveitis
  fluocinolone acetonide, Yutiq, 652

Vabomere, *meropenem+vaborbactam*
  urinary tract infection, 645
vaccina virus vaccine (dried, calf lymph type), DRYvax
  smallpox, 576
Vagifem Vaginal Tablet, *estradiol*

  atrophic vaginitis, 49
  vaginal irritation, 652
Vagistat-1 Vaginal Ointment, *tioconazole*
  vulvovaginal (moniliasis) candidiasis, 138
valacyclovir, Valtrex
  herpes genitalis (HSV TYPE II), 301
  herpes labialis/herpes facialis, 301
  herpes zoster, 301
  herpes zoster ophthmicus, 303
valbenazine, Ingrezza
  Huntington disease-associated chorea, 318
  tardive dyskinesia, 586
Valcyte, *valganciclovir* (G), 698
  COVID-19 (coronavirus), 173
  cytomegalovirus (CMV) retinitis, 185
  posttransplant cytomegalovirus (CMV), 186
valganciclovir, Valcyte (G)
  COVID-19 (coronavirus), 173
  cytomegalovirus (CMV) retinitis, 185
  posttransplant cytomegalovirus (CMV), 186
Valium, *diazepam* (IV)
  alcohol withdrawal syndrome, 11
  anxiety disorder, 34
  dose forms, 694
  Meniere's disease, 388
  muscle strain, 403
  panic disorder, 466
  status epilepticus, 579
  temporomandibular joint disorder, 586–587
valproic acid, Depakene
  trigeminal neuralgia, 609
valsartan, Diovan, Prexxartan Oral Solution (G)
  heart failure, 280
  hypertension, 330
Valtoco, *diazepam nasal spray* (IV)
  seizure, cluster, 566
  status epilepticus, 579
Valtrex, *valacyclovir*
  herpes genitalis (HSV TYPE II), 301
  herpes labialis/herpes facialis, 301
  herpes zoster, 301
  herpes zoster ophthmicus, 303
Valturna, *aliskiren+valsartan*
  hypertension, 336
Vancenase, *beclomethasone dipropionate*
  allergic rhinitis/sinusitis, 551
Vancocin, *vancomycin hcl capsule* (G)
  Clostridioides difficile infection, 157
  pseudomembranous colitis, 519
vancomycin hcl capsule, Vancocin (G), 722
  Clostridioides difficile infection, 157
  dose forms, 710
  pseudomembranous colitis, 519
vancomycin hcl oral solution, Firvanq
  Clostridioides difficile infection, 157
  pseudomembranous colitis, 519
Vandazole, *metronidazole*
  bacterial vaginosis, 46
Vaniqa, *eflornithine*
  facial hair: excessive/unwanted, 241
Vantin, *cefpodoxime proxetil,* 715
  acute bacterial sinusitis, rhinosinusitis, 571
  acute exacerbation of chronic bronchitis, 69
  acute tonsillitis, 604
  bacterial skin infection, 574
  cellulitis, 142
  community acquired pneumonia, 493
  gonorrhea, 259
  impetigo contagiosa, 352
  otitis media: acute, 446

streptococcal pharyngitis, 485
urinary tract infection, 644
wound, 659
Vaqta, *hepatitis A vaccine, inactivated*
hepatitis A, 291
vardenafil (as HCl), Levitra, Staxyn
erectile dysfunction (ED), 237
varenicline, Chantix, Tyrvaya
dry eye syndrome, 216
tobacco dependence, 602
Varicella virus vaccine, Varivax
chickenpox (Varicella), 149
sodium tetradecyl sulfate, Sotradecol,
652
Varivax, *Varicella virus* vaccine
chickenpox (Varicella), 149
Vascepa sgc, *icosapent ethyl (omega
3-fatty acid ethyl ester of EPA)*
dyslipidemia, 220
hypertriglyceridemia, 338
Vaseretic, *enalapril+hydrochlorothiazide*
hypertension, 333
Vasocidin Ophthalmic Solution,
*sulfacetamide sodium+
prednisolone sodium phosphate*
bacterial conjunctivitis, 164
Vasocon-A, *naphazoline*
allergic (vernal) conjunctivitis, 167
Vasotec, *enalapril*
heart failure, 279
Vaxchora, *Vibrio cholerae* vaccine
cholera (*Vibrio cholerae*), 155
Vaxeli, *diphtheria, tetanus toxoid,
acellular pertussis, inactivated
poliovirus, haemophilus b
conjugate, and hepatitis b
haemophilus influenzae B (HIB)*, 290
Vaxelis
hepatitis B, 292–293
poliomyelitis/poliovirus, 499
Vectibix, *panitumumab*, 690
vedolizumab, Entyvio
Crohn's disease, 179
ulcerative colitis, 638
Vegzelma, *bevacizumab-adcd*
cervical cancer, 86
colorectal cancer, 87
fallopian tube cancer, 90
glioblastoma multiforme, 92–93
ovarian cancer, 122
peritoneal cancer, 127
renal cell carcinoma (RCC), 94
Vegzelma, *bevacizumab-bvzr*
cervical cancer, 86
Veklury, *remdesivir*
COVID-19 (coronavirus), 172
Velcade, *bortezomib*, 691
Velivet, *ethinyl estradiol+desogestrel*,
673
Veltassa, *patiromer sorbitex calcium*
hyperkalemia, 322
Vemlidy, *tenofovir alafenamide (TAF)*
hepatitis B, 293
Venclexta, *venetoclax*, 691
venereal wart
imiquimod, Aldara, Zyclara (G), 655
interferon alfa-2b, intron A, 656
interferon alfa-n3, Alferon N, 656
podofilox 0.5% cream, Condylox,
655, 656
sinecatechins 15% ointment, Veregen,
655
trichloroacetic acid (TCA), 656
venlafaxine, Effexor, Effexor XR
anxiety disorder, 36
major depressive disorder, 192
panic disorder, 465
post-traumatic stress disorder,
511–512

ventilator associated bacterial
pneumonia (VABP)
ceftazidime+avibactam, Avycaz,
490–491
ceftolozane+tazobactam, Zerbaxa, 491
imipenem+cilastatin+relebactam,
Recarbrio, 491
cefiderocol, Fetroja, 491
Ventolin, *albuterol, albuterol sulfate*
asthma, 39
Veramyst, *fluticasone furoate*
allergic rhinitis/sinusitis, 552
verapamil, Calan, Covera HS, Isoptin,
Isoptin SR (G)
angina pectoris: stable, 29
dose form(s), 681
hypertension, primary, 331
migraine and cluster headache, 276
Verdeso, *desonide*
atopic dermatitis, 198
Veregen, *sinecatechins 15% ointment*
venereal wart, 655
Verkazia, *cyclosporine*
allergic (vernal) conjunctivitis, 168
Vermox, *mebendazole*
hookworm, 305
pinworm, 488
roundworm, 557
threadworm, 593
trichinosis, 606
whipworm, 656
vernal keratitis
cromolyn sodium, Crolom, Opticrom,
375
lodoxamide tromethamine, Alomide,
375
vertigo
meclizine, Antivert, Bonine (OTC),
Dramamine II (OTC), Zentrip
(G), 653
methscopolamine bromide, Pamine,
653
scopolamine, Scopace, Transderm
Scop, 653
Verzenio, *abemaciclib*
breast cancer, 78–79
VESIcare, *mirabegron, solifenacin* (G)
urinary overactive bladder, 354, 355
VESIcare LS, *solifenacin succinate*
neurogenic detrusor overactivity
(NDO), 415
Vexol, *rimexolone*
allergic (vernal) conjunctivitis, 166
Vfend, *voriconazole*, 704
aspergillosis, 38
candidiasis: abdomen, bladder,
esophagus, kidney, 134
Viactiv (OTC), *calcium carbonate+
vitamin D*
hypocalcemia, 340
Viadur, *leuprolide acetate*, 691
Viagra, *sildenafil citrate*
erectile dysfunction (ED), 237
Viberzi, *eluxadoline (IV)*
irritable bowel syndrome with
diarrhea, 366
Vibramycin, *doxycycline* (G)
acne rosacea, 3
acne vulgaris, 5
acute exacerbation of chronic
bronchitis, 70
anthrax (bacillus anthracis), 32
bacterial skin infection, 574
cat bite, 65
cat scratch fever, 141
Chlamydia trachomatis, 151
cholera (*Vibrio cholerae*), 155, 156
community-acquired pneumonia, 494
dog bite, 66

dose forms, 704
epididymitis, 237
gonorrhea, 256
granuloma inguinale, 266
hidradenitis suppurativa, 303
lyme disease, 383
lymphogranuloma venereum, 384
malaria, 384
nongonococcal urethritis, 639
pelvic inflammatory disease, 476
proctitis: acute, 516
rocky mountain spotted fever, 556
sexual assault, 567
urinary tract infection, 644
Vibra-Tab, *doxycycline* (G)
acne rosacea, 3
acne vulgaris, 5
acute exacerbation of chronic
bronchitis, 70
anthrax (bacillus anthracis), 32
bacterial skin infection, 574
cat bite, 65
cat scratch fever, 141
Chlamydia trachomatis, 151
cholera (*Vibrio cholerae*), 155, 156
community-acquired pneumonia, 494
dog bite, 66
dose forms, 704, 709
epididymitis, 237
gonorrhea, 256
granuloma inguinale, 266
hidradenitis suppurativa, 303
lyme disease, 383
lymphogranuloma venereum, 384
malaria, 384
nongonococcal urethritis, 639
pelvic inflammatory disease, 476
proctitis: acute, 516
rocky mountain spotted fever, 556
sexual assault, 567
urinary tract infection, 644
Vibrio cholerae vaccine, Vaxchora
cholera (*Vibrio cholerae*), 155
Vicodin, *hydrocodone
bitartrate+acetaminophen* (II)
pain, 455–456
Vicoprofen, *hydrocodone+ibuprofen* (II)
pain, 456
vidarabine, Vira-A
herpes simplex keratitis, 374
Viekira Pak, *ombitasvir+paritaprevir+
ritonavir, ombitasvir+
paritaprevir+ritonavir plus
dasabuvir*
hepatitis C (HCV), 296
Viekira XR, *sofosbuvir+velpatasvir*
hepatitis C (HCV), 295
Vigamox Ophthalmic Solution,
moxifloxacin
bacterial conjunctivitis, 162
Viibryd, *vilazodone*
major depressive disorder, 193
vilazodone, Viibryd
major depressive disorder, 193
viloxazine, Qelbree
attention deficit hyperactivity disorder
(ADHD), 50
Viltepso, *viltolarsen*
duchenne muscular dystrophy
(DMD), 219
viltolarsen, Viltepso
duchenne muscular dystrophy
(DMD), 219
Vimovo, *esomeprazole+naproxen* (G), 573
gouty arthritis, 263
muscle strain, 406
osteoarthritis, 435
psoriatic arthritis, 528
rheumatoid arthritis, 542–543

Vimovo, *naproxen+esomeprazole magnesium* (G)
  osteoarthritis (OA), 435
  pain, 452–453
  rheumatoid arthritis (RA), 542–543
Viokace, *pancreatic enzymes*
  pancreatic enzyme deficiency, 239
  pancreatic enzyme insufficiency, 463
Vira-A, *vidarabine*
  herpes simplex keratitis, 374
viral conjunctivitis
  trifluridine, Viroptic Ophthalmic Solution, 168
viral upper respiratory infection. *See* common cold
Virazole, *ribavirin*
  hepatitis C (HCV), 294
Viread, *tenofovir disoproxil fumarate*
  hepatitis B, 293
Viroptic, *trifluridine*
  herpes simplex keratitis, 374
  viral conjunctivitis, 168
visceral leishmaniasis, 376–377
Visco-3, *sodium hyaluronate*
  osteoarthritis, 437
Visine AC, *tetrahydrozoline+zinc sulfate*
  allergic (vernal) conjunctivitis, 167
Visine L-R, *oxymetazoline*
  allergic (vernal) conjunctivitis, 167
Visine Tears, *polyethylene glycol+ glycerin+hydroxypropyl methylcellulose*
  dry eye syndrome, 217
Visine, *tetrahydrozoline*
  allergic (vernal) conjunctivitis, 167
Vistaril, *hydroxyzine*
  allergic reaction, 12
  allergic rhinitis/sinusitis, 550
  anxiety disorder, 33
  atopic dermatitis, 199
  chickenpox (Varicella), 150
  contact dermatitis, 203
  genus rhus dermatitis, 204
  panic disorder, 465
  rhinitis medicamentosa, 555
  urticaria, 649
Vistide, *cidofovir*
  COVID-19 (coronavirus), 173
  posttransplant cytomegalovirus (CMV), 185, 186
Vistide V, *cidofovir*
  cytomegalovirus (CMV) retinitis, 186–187
vitamin a and e, A&D Ointment (G)
  diaper rash, 211
vitamin B6 (A)
  fibrocystic breast disease, 243
vitamin B12 (cyanocobalamin), Nascobal Nasal Spray (A)
  pernicious/megaloblastic anemia, 26
vitamin E (A)
  fibrocystic breast disease, 243
vitiligo
  hydroquinone, Lustra, Lustra AF (G), 653
  hydroquinone+ethyl dihydroxypropyl PABA+dioxybenzone+ oxybenzone, Solaquin, 653
  hydroquinone+fluocinolone+tretinoin, Tri-Luma, 653
  hydroquinone+padimate o+oxybenzone+octyl methoxycinnamate, Glyquin, 653
  methoxsalen, Oxsoralen, 653
  monobenzone, Benoquin, 653
  ruxolitinib, Opzelura, 654
  tazarotene, Avage, Tazorac (G), 653
  tretinoin, Avita, Renova, Retin-A (G), 653

trioxsalen, Trisoralen, 653
Vitrakvi, *larotrectinib*, 691
Vivactil, *protriptyline*
  anxiety disorder, 34
  diabetic peripheral neuropathy (DPN), 210
  irritable bowel syndrome with diarrhea, 368
  major depressive disorder, 193
  nocturnal enuresis, 235
  post-herpetic neuralgia, 508, 510
  trigeminal neuralgia, 609
Vivlodex, *meloxicam*
  dysmenorrhea: primary, 225
  gouty arthritis, 263
  muscle strain, 406
  osteoarthritis, 436
  psoriatic arthritis, 528
  rheumatoid arthritis, 544
Vivotif Berna, *typhoid vaccine, oral, live, attenuated strain*
  typhoid fever, 632
Vizimpro, *dacomitinib*, 691
Vocabria, *cabotegravir*
  human immunodeficiency virus (HIV) infection, 308
Vogelxo Gel, *testosterone* (G)(III)
  testosterone deficiency, 590
Voltaren Gel, *diclofenac sodium*
  actinic keratosis, 9
  atopic dermatitis, 199
  diabetic peripheral neuropathy (DPN), 208–209
  dysmenorrhea: primary, 225
  gouty arthritis, 262
  juvenile idiopathic arthritis, 369
  hemorrhoids, 289–290
  juvenile rheumatoid *arthritis*, 372
  muscle strain, 404–405
  osteoarthritis, 434, 435
  pain, 453
  peripheral neuritis, 480
  pruritus, 518
  psoriatic arthritis, 527
  rheumatoid arthritis, 542
  post-herpetic neuralgia, 508
Vonjo, *pacritinib*
  myelofibrosis, 408–409
von Willebrand factor (recombinant) (rVWF), Vonvendi
  hemophilia A, 288–289
vorapaxar, Zontivity, 703
voriconazole, Vfend, 704
  aspergillosis, 38
  candidiasis: abdomen, bladder, esophagus, kidney, 134
vortioxetine, Brintellix
  major depressive disorder, 192
Vosevi, *sofosbuvir+velpatasvir+ voxilaprevir*
  hepatitis C (HCV), 296
VoSol, *acetic acid+propylene glycol+ benzethonium chloride+sodium acetate*
  otitis externa, 444
VoSol HC, *acetic acid+propylene glycol+ hydrocortisone+benzethonium chloride+sodium acetate*
  otitis externa, 444
vosoritide, Voxzogo
  achondroplasia, 1–2
VoSpire ER, *albuterol*
  asthma, 39
Vowst, *fecal microbiota, spores, live-brpk*
  clostridioides *difficile* infection (CDI), 158
voxelotor, Oxbryta
  sickle cell disease (SCD), 570–571
Voxzogo, *vosoritide*

achondroplasia, 1–2
Vraylar, *cariprazine*
  bipolar disorder, 62
  major depressive disorder (MDD), 195
vulvovaginal (moniliasis) candidiasis
  acetic acid+oxyquinolone, Relagard, 136
  butoconazole cream 2%, Gynazole-12% Vaginal Cream, Femstat-3 Vaginal Cream (OTC), 138
  clotrimazole, Gyne-Lotrimin, Mycelex-G, Mycelex Twin Pack, Mycelex-7, 138
  fluconazole, 136
  ibrexafungerp, Brexafemme, 136–137
  miconazole, Monistat, 138
  nystatin, Mycostatin, 138
  posaconazole, Noxafil, 138
  secnidazole, Solosec, 137
  terconazole, Terazol, 138
  tioconazole, 1-Day, Monistat 1 Vaginal Ointment, Vagistat-1 Vaginal Ointment, 138
Vumerity, *diroximel fumarate*
  multiple sclerosis (MS), 402
Vyndamax, *tafamidis*
  cardiomyopathy of transthyretin-mediated amyloidosis, 140
Vyndaqel, *tafamidis meglumine*
  cardiomyopathy of transthyretin-mediated amyloidosis, 140
Vyondys, *golodirsen*
  duchenne muscular dystrophy (DMD), 219
Vytorin, *ezetimibe+simvastatin*
  dyslipidemia, 223
Vyvanse, *lisdexamfetamine dimesylate* (II)
  attention deficit hyperactivity disorder (ADHD), 52
  binge eating disorder, 60
Vyxeos, *daunorubicin+cytarabine*, 691
Vyzulta, *latanoprostene bunod*
  glaucoma, 257

Wakix, *pitolisant*
  narcolepsy, 412–413
Waldenström's macroglobulinemia
  zanubrutinib, Brukinsa, 654
warfarin, Coumadin (G)
  dose forms, 698–699
  peripheral vascular disease, 482
Wart-Off, *salicylic acid*
  common wart, 655
  plantar wart, 655
Wegovy, *semaglutide*
  obesity, 420–421
WelChol, *colesevelam*
  cholelithiasis, 154
  dyslipidemia, 224
  primary biliary cholangitis, 153
  type 2 diabetes mellitus, 632
Wellbutrin, *bupropion HCl*
  attention deficit hyperactivity disorder (ADHD), 54
  major depressive disorder, 193
  tobacco dependence, 602
West nile virus (WNV), 656
whipworm
  albendazole, Albenza, 656
  mebendazole, Emverm, Vermox, 656
  pyrantel pamoate, Antiminth, Pin-X, 657
  thiabendazole, Mintezol, 657
whooping cough, 482–483
Wilson's disease
  penicillamine, Cuprimine, Depen, 657
  trientine, Syprine (G), 657–658

wound
  Augmentin, Augmentin
    ES-600, Augmentin XR,
    amoxicillin+clavulanate (G),
    658–659
  azithromycin, Zithromax, Zmax (G),
    658
  cefaclor, Cefaclor Extended Release
    (G), 659
  cefadroxil, Duricef, 659
  cefdinir, Omnicef, 659
  cefpodoxime proxetil, Vantin, 659
  cefprozil, Cefzil, 659
  cephalexin, Keflex (G), 659
  clarithromycin, Biaxin (G), 659
  dirithromycin, Dynabac (G), 659
  erythromycin base, Ery-Tab, PCE (G),
    659
  erythromycin ethylsuccinate, EryPed,
    E.E.S (G), 659
  gemifloxacin, Factive (G), 660
  levofloxacin, Levaquin, 660
  loracarbef, Lorabid, 660
  mupirocin, Bactroban, Centany (G), 658
  ofloxacin, Floxin (G), 660
  tetanus toxoid vaccine, 658
Wynzora, *anhydrous calcipotriene+
    betamethasone dipropionate*
  psoriasis, 519–520

Xaciato, *clindamycin phosphate*
  bacterial vaginosis, 57
Xadago, *safinamide*
  Parkinson's disease, 470
Xalkori, *crizotinib,* 691
Xanax, Xanax XR, *alprazolam* (IV)
  anxiety disorder, 33
  panic disorder, 465
Xartemis XR, *oxycodone+acetaminophen*
    (II)
  pain, 459
Xeglyze Lotion, *abametapir*
  pediculosis humanus capitis, 475
Xeljanz, *tofacitinib*
  rheumatoid arthritis, 544–545
  ulcerative colitis, 637–638
Xeloda, *capecitabine,* 691
Xelstrym, *dextroamphetamine* (II)
  attention deficit hyperactivity disorder
    (ADHD), 51
Xenazine, *trabenazine*
  Huntington disease-associated chorea,
    318
Xenical, *orlistat*
  obesity, 418
Xepi, *ozenoxacin*
  impetigo contagiosa, 353
Xerava, *eravacycline*
  complicated intra-abdominal
    infection, 364
Xermelo, *telotristat,* 691
  carcinoid syndrome diarrhea (CSD),
    140, 212
  xerosis, 661
Xibrom Ophthalmic Solution,
    bromfenac
  allergic (vernal) conjunctivitis, 167
Xifaxan, *rifaximin*
  Travelers' diarrhea, 214
Xigduo XR, *dapagliflozin+metformin*
  type 2 diabetes mellitus, 627–628
Xiidra, *lifitegrast*
  dry eye syndrome, 216
X-linked hypophosphatemia (XLH)
  burosumab-twza, Crysvita, 345
Xodol, *hydrocodone
    bitartrate+acetaminophen* (II)
  pain, 455–456
Xofluza, *baloxavir marboxil*

influenza, seasonal (FLU), 358
Xolair, *omalizumab*
  allergies: multi-food, 12
  asthma, 42
  asthma-COPD overlap syndrome, 47
  eosinophilia, 49
  urticaria, 650
Xolegel, *ketoconazole*
  seborrheic dermatitis, 205
Xopenex, *levalbuterol tartrate*
  asthma, 40
Xospata, *gilteritinib,* 691
Xtoro, *finafloxacin*
  otitis externa, 444
Xultophy Prefilled pen, *insulin degludec
    (insulin analog)+liraglutide*
  type 1 diabetes mellitus, 618
Xylocaine Viscous Solution, *lidocaine*
  aphthous stomatitis, 37
Xywav, *calcium, magnesium, potassium,
    and sodium oxybate oral solution
    (CIII)*
  narcolepsy, 413
Xyzal Allergy 24HR, *levocetirizine*
  allergic rhinitis/sinusitis, 550

Yasmin, *ethinyl estradiol+drospirenone*
  estrogen and progesterone, 673
Yaz, *ethinyl estradiol+drospirenone*
  estrogen and progesterone, 673
  premenstrual dysphoric disorder,
    514
yellow fever, 661
Yervoy, *ipilimumab,* 691
Yescarta, *axicabtagene,* 691
Yonsa, *abiraterone acetate*
  prostate cancer, 128–129
Yosprala, *esomeprazole+aspirin*
  Zollinger-Ellison syndrome, 662
Yupelri, *revefenacin inhalation solution*
  chronic obstructive pulmonary
    disease, 72–73
  emphysema, 231
Yutiq, *fluocinolone acetonide*
  uveitis, 652
Yuvafem Vaginal Tablet, *estradiol*
  atrophic vaginitis, 49
Yuzpe Regimen, *ethinyl
    estradiol+levonorgestrel,* 675

Zaditor, *ketotifen fumarate*
  allergic (vernal) conjunctivitis, 167
zafirlukast, Accolate
  allergic rhinitis/sinusitis, 551
  asthma, 41
zaleplon, Sonata (IV)
  fibromyalgia, 245
  insomnia, 359
Zamicet Oral Solution, *hydrocodone
    bitartrate+acetaminophen* (II)
  pain, 455–456
zanamivir, Relenza Inhaler
  influenza, seasonal (FLU), 357
Zantac, *ranitidine*
  gastroesophageal reflux disease, 250
  peptic ulcer disease (PUD), 478
zanubrutinib, Brukinsa
  leukemia, 96
  lymphoma, 109
  Waldenström's macroglobulinemia,
    654
Zaroxolyn, *metolazone*
  edema, 229
  hypertension, 328
Zavesca, *miglustat*
  Gaucher disease, type 1 (GD1), 252
Zebutal, *butalbital+acetaminophen+
    caffeine*
  tension headache, 277

Zegalogue, *dasiglucagon*
  hypoglycemia: acute, 342
  type 1 diabetes mellitus (T1DM), 614
  type 2 diabetes mellitus (T2DM),
    619
Zejula, *niraparib, niraparib tosylate,*
    691
  fallopian tube cancer, 88
  ovarian cancer, 122–123
  peritoneal cancer, 125
  prostate cancer, 129
Zelapar, *selegiline*
  Parkinson's disease, 470
Zelboraf, *vemurafenib,* 691
Zemdri, *plazomicin*
  acute complicated pyelonephritis
    (ACP), 537–538
  complicated urinary tract infection
    (cUTI), 641
Zemplar, *paricalcitol*
  hyperparathyroidism, 323
  hypocalcemia, 341
Zenpep, *pancreatic enzymes*
  pancreatic enzyme deficiency,
    239–240
  pancreatic enzyme insufficiency,
    463–464
Zentrip, *meclizine*
  labyrinthitis, 375
  Meniere's disease, 388
  motion sickness, 396
  vertigo, 653
Zepatier, *elbasvir+grazoprevir*
  hepatitis C (HCV), 294
Zeposia, *ozanimod*
  multiple sclerosis (MS), 401
Zerbaxa, *ceftolozane+tazobactam,* 706
  complicated intra-abdominal
    infection (cIAI), 363
  complicated urinary tract infection
    (CUTI), 640–641
  ventilator-associated bacterial
    pneumonia (VABP), 491
Zerviate, *cetirizine*
  allergic (vernal) conjunctivitis, 166
Zestril, *lisinopril*
  heart failure, 279–280
Zetia, *ezetimibe*
  dyslipidemia, 220
Zetonna, *ciclesonide*
  polyps, nasal, 505
Ziac, *bisoprolol+hydrochlorothiazide*
  hypertension, 334
Ziana, *tretinoin+clindamycin*
  acne vulgaris, 7
ziconotide, Prial
  pain, 462
zidovudine, Retrovir
  human immunodeficiency virus
    infection, 309
Zika virus, 661–662
zileuton, Zyflo, Zyflo-CR
  allergic rhinitis/sinusitis, 551
  asthma, 41
Zilretta, *triamcinolone acetonide*
  osteoarthritis, 436
zinc oxide, A&D Ointment with Zinc
    Oxide, Desitin (G)
  diaper rash, 211
Zinplava, *bezlotoxumab*
  Clostridioides difficile infection, 157
ziprasidone, Geodon (G)
  bipolar disorder, 64–65
  dose forms, 694
Zirabev, *bevacizumab-bvzr*
  colorectal cancer, 87
  glioblastoma multiforme, 93
Zirga, *ganciclovir*
  herpes simplex keratitis, 374

Zithromax, *azithromycin*, 708, 713
  acute exacerbation of chronic
    bronchitis, 69
  acute tonsillitis, 603
  bacterial endocarditis prophylaxis, 55
  bacterial skin infection, 573
  cat scratch fever, 141
  cellulitis, 142
  chancroid, 146–147
  Chlamydia trachomatis, 151
  chlamydial conjunctivitis, 164
  chlamydial pneumonia, 492
  cholera (*Vibrio cholerae*), 155, 156
  community acquired pneumonia, 493
  dose form/volume, 708
  gonococcal conjunctivitis, 165
  gonococcal pharyngitis, 483
  gonorrhea, 258, 259
  granuloma inguinale, 266
  impetigo contagiosa, 365
  lymphogranuloma venereum, 384
  mycoplasma pneumonia, 496
  nongonococcal urethritis, 639
  otitis media: acute, 446
  pertussis, 483
  scarlet fever, 560
  sexual assault, 567
  shigellosis, 567
  streptococcal pharyngitis, 484
  typhoid fever, 633
  wound, 658
Zmax, *azithromycin*, 708, 713
  acute exacerbation of chronic
    bronchitis, 69
  acute tonsillitis, 603
  bacterial endocarditis prophylaxis, 55
  bacterial skin infection, 573
  cat scratch fever, 141
  cellulitis, 142
  chancroid, 146–147
  Chlamydia trachomatis, 151
  chlamydial conjunctivitis, 164
  chlamydial pneumonia, 492
  cholera (*Vibrio cholerae*), 155, 156
  community acquired pneumonia, 493
  dose form/volume, 708
  gonococcal conjunctivitis, 165
  gonococcal pharyngitis, 483
  gonorrhea, 258, 259
  granuloma inguinale, 266
  impetigo contagiosa, 365
  lymphogranuloma venereum, 384
  mycoplasma pneumonia, 496
  nongonococcal urethritis, 639
  otitis media: acute, 446
  pertussis, 483
  scarlet fever, 560
  sexual assault, 567
  shigellosis, 567
  streptococcal pharyngitis, 484
  typhoid fever, 633
  wound, 658
Zocor, *simvastatin*
  dyslipidemia, 222
  hypertriglyceridemia, 339
ZoDerm, *benzoyl peroxide*
  acne vulgaris, 4
Zofran, Zuplenz Oral Soluble Film,
  ondansetron
  cannabinoid hyperemesis syndrome,
    140
  chemotherapy-induced nausea/
    vomiting, 148–149
  gastritis-related nausea/vomiting, 247
  post-anesthesia nausea/vomiting,
    414
Zoladex, *goserelin (GnRH analog)*, 692
  endometriosis, 233

zoledronic acid, Reclast, Zometa
  osteoporosis, 442
  Paget's disease, 450
Zolgensma, *onasemnogene*
  abeparvovec-xioi
  spinal muscular atrophy (SMA), 578
Zollinger-Ellison syndrome
  dexlansoprazole, Dexilant (G), 662
  esomeprazole, Nexium (OTC)(G), 662
  esomeprazole+aspirin, Yosprala, 662
  lansoprazole, Prevacid (OTC)(G), 662
  omeprazole, Prilosec (OTC)(G), 662
  pantoprazole, Protonix (G), 662
  rabeprazole, AcipHex (OTC)(G), 662
zolmitriptan, Zomig
  migraine and cluster headache, 270
Zoloft, *sertraline*
  anxiety disorder, 35
  major depressive disorder, 192
  obsessive-compulsive disorder, 422
  panic disorder, 465
  post-traumatic stress disorder, 511
  premenstrual dysphoric disorder, 515
  trichotillomania, 608
zolpidem, Ambien, Ambien CR, Edluar,
  Intermezzo, ZolpiMist (IV)
  aphasia, 36–37
  fibromyalgia, 245
  insomnia, 359
ZolpiMist, *zolpidem* (IV)
  aphasia, 36–37
  fibromyalgia, 245
  insomnia, 359
Zometa, *zoledronic acid* (G), 442, 450,
  692
Zonalon, *doxepin*
  atopic dermatitis, 199
  diabetic peripheral neuropathy
    (DPN), 209
  gouty arthritis, 262
  hemorrhoids, 290
  insomnia, 360
  juvenile idiopathic arthritis, 369
  juvenile rheumatoid arthritis, 372
  muscle strain, 405
  osteoarthritis, 434
  pain, 453
  peripheral neuritis, 480–481
  post-herpetic neuralgia, 508
  pruritus, 518
  psoriatic arthritis, 527
  rheumatoid arthritis, 542
Zortress, *everolimus*
  organ transplant rejection prophylaxis,
    432
Zorvolex, *diclofenac*
  muscle strain, 405
  osteoarthritis, 435
  psoriatic arthritis, 527
Zoryve, *roflumilast*
  psoriasis, 522
Zostrix, Zostrix HP, *capsaicin*
  atopic dermatitis, 199
  diabetic peripheral neuropathy
    (DPN), 208
  gouty arthritis, 261–262
  juvenile idiopathic arthritis, 369
  juvenile rheumatoid arthritis, 372
  osteoarthritis, 434
  muscle strain, 404
  peripheral neuritis, 480
  pain, 453
  pruritus, 517
  rheumatoid arthritis, 541
  psoriatic arthritis, 527
Zovia 1/35E-28, Zovia 1/50E-28, *ethinyl*
  estradiol+ethynodiol diacetate
  estrogen and progesterone, 673

Zovirax, *acyclovir* (G), 705
  chickenpox (Varicella), 150
  herpes genitalis (HSV TYPE II), 300
  herpes labialis/herpes facialis, 300,
    301
  herpes zoster, 301
  herpes zoster ophthmicus, 303
ZTlido lidocaine, *lidocaine*
  atopic dermatitis, 200
  burn: minor, 76
  diabetic peripheral neuropathy
    (DPN), 209
  gouty arthritis, 262
  hemorrhoids, 292
  herpangina, 299
  herpes zoster, 302
  insect bite/sting, 358
  juvenile idiopathic arthritis, 369
  juvenile rheumatoid arthritis, 372
  muscle strain, 405
  pain, 454
  peripheral neuritis, 481
  post-herpetic neuralgia, 509
Zuplenz, *ondansetron* (G)
  cannabinoid hyperemesis syndrome,
    140
  chemotherapy-induced nausea/
    vomiting, 148–149
  gastritis-related nausea/vomiting, 247
  opioid-induced nausea/vomiting, 429
  post-anesthesia nausea/vomiting,
    414
Zyclara, *imiquimod*
  actinic keratosis, 9
  venereal wart, 655
Zydone, *hydrocodone bitartrate+*
  acetaminophen (II)
  pain, 455–456
Zyflo, Zyflo-CR, *zileuton*
  allergic rhinitis/sinusitis, 551
  asthma, 41
Zykadia, *ceritinib*, 692
Zylet, *tobramycin+loteprednol etabonate*
  bacterial conjunctivitis, 164
Zyloprim, *allopurinol*
  urolithiasis, 646–647
Zymar Ophthalmic Solution, *gatifloxacin*
  bacterial conjunctivitis, 162
Zymase, *pancreatic enzymes*
  pancreatic enzyme insufficiency, 464
Zymaxid Ophthalmic Solution,
  gatifloxacin
  bacterial conjunctivitis, 162
Zynteglo, *betibeglogene autotemcel*
  beta thalassemia, 59–60
Zynyz, *retifanlimab-dlwr*
  merkel cell carcinoma, 119
Zypitamag, *pitavastatin*
  dyslipidemia, 222
Zyprexa, Zyprexa Zydis, *olanzapine*
  delirium, 188
  dementia, 188
  methamphetamine-induced
    psychosis, 395
  post-traumatic stress disorder, 511
  trichotillomania, 608
Zyrtec, *cetirizine*
  allergic rhinitis/sinusitis, 549
  contact dermatitis, 202
  genus rhus dermatitis, 203rhinitis
    medicamentosa, 555
  urticaria, 649
Zyrtec Itchy Eye, *ketotifen fumarate*
  allergic (vernal) conjunctivitis, 167
Zytiga, *abiraterone acetate*
  prostate cancer, 128–129
Zyvox, *linezolid*
  cellulitis, 144